Drug	Adult	Pediatric (Pediatric dose should not generally exceed adult dose)
Dopamine (40, 80, 160 mg/mL)	5–20 μg/kg/min i.v. drip	5–20 μg/kg/min i.v. drip
Enalapril (enalaprilat)	1.25 mg i.v. over 5 min then 1.25–5 mg i.v. q6h	N/A
Enoxaparin (Lovenox)	1 mg/kg	N/A
Epinephrine	*Asystole:* 1 mg i.v. q3–5min *Anaphylaxis/allergy:* 0.3 mL (1:1000) SC q15–20min PRN	*Asystole:* 0.1 mL (1:10,000) (0.01 mg)/kg/dose i.v. q3–5min PRN. ET, IO and subsequent i.v. doses, 0.1 mL (1:1000) (0.1 mg)/kg/dose q3–5min PRN *Anaphylaxis/allergy:* 0.01 mg/kg (0.1 mL of 1:1000) SC, q15–20min PRN
Epinephrine, racemic (Vaponefrin) (2.25% soln)	0.5–0.75 mL/dose by inhalation; may repeat	0.25–0.75 mL/dose by inhalation; may repeat
Eptifibatide (Integrilin)	180 μg/kg i.v., then 2 μg/kg/min infusion	N/A
Esmolol	*Load:* 500 μg/kg over 1 min *Infusion:* 50–200 μg/kg/min to max 0.3 mg/kg/min (max 300 mg total dose)	*Load:* 100–500 μg/kg i.v. over 1 min *Infusion:* 25–100 μg/kg/min
Fentanyl (Sublimaze) (50 μg/mL)	0.5–1 μg/kg/dose slow i.v. up to 50–100 μg/dose	1–2 μg/kg/dose slow i.v. up to 4 mg/kg/dose
Flumazenil	0.2 mg i.v., then 0.3 mg followed by 0.5 mg q min up to 3 mg	0.01 mg/kg i.v. to max of 0.2 mg
Fosphenytoin	15–20 mg phenytoin equivalents/kg i.v./i.m.	15–20 mg phenytoin equivalents/kg i.v./i.m.
Furosemide (Lasix) (10 mg/mL)	20–40 mg i.v.	1 mg/kg i.v.
Glucagon	1 mg q5 min, max 5 mg	0.03–0.1 mg/kg i.v./i.m./SC q5–20 min, max 1 mg
Heparin	80 IU/kg i.v., then 15–18 IU/kg/h	50–75 IU/kg then 15–25 IU/kg/h
Hydralazine (Apresoline) (20 mg/mL)	10–20 mg i.m./i.v.	0.1–0.2 mg/kg/dose i.v./i.m.; max 20 mg
Insulin, regular	DKA: 2–10 units/h i.v.	DKA: 0.05–0.2 units/kg/h i.v. drip
Isoproterenol (200 μg/mL)	2–10 μg/min	0.05–2 μg/kg/min i.v. drip
Labetalol (Normodyne) (5 mg/mL)	*Load:* 20 mg/dose i.v. q10 min up to 300 mg *Maintenance:* 0.5–2 mg/min	*Load:* 0.25–1.0 mg/kg/dose i.v. slow push; may repeat i 0.4–1 mg/kg/h, max 3 mg/kg/h
Lidocaine (Xylocaine) (10, 20 mg/mL)	*Load:* 1–1.5 mg/kg/dose i.v. (or ET) q5–10 min PRN up to 3–5 mg/kg max 3 mg/kg *Maintenance:* 1–4 mg/min i.v. drip	*Load:* 1 mg/kg/dose i.v. (or ET) q5–10 min PRN up to 3–5 mg/kg *Maintenance:* 20 μg/kg/min i.v. drip
Lorazepam (Ativan) (2, 4 mg/mL)	0.5–2 mg i.v./i.m./PO up to 5 mg	0.05–0.15 mg/kg/dose i.v./i.m.
Magnesium sulfate	1–2 g i.v. Pre eclampsia: 4 mg	25–50 mg/kg over 10 min
Mannitol (200, 250 mg/mL)	*Load:* 0.5–1 g/kg *Maintenance:* 0.25–0.5 g/kg	*Load:* 0.5–1 g/kg *Maintenance:* 0.25–0.5 g/kg
Metoprolol	5 mg i.v. q5min to 15 mg total	N/A

Drug	Adult	Pediatric (Pediatric dose should not generally exceed adult dose)
Midazolam (Versed) (1 mg/mL)	1–2.5 mg, max 2.5–5 mg	0.05–0.1 mg/kg/dose i.v.
Morphine (8, 10, 15 mg/mL)	0.1–0.2 mg/kg/dose i.v./i.m. up to 15 mg	0.1–0.2 mg/kg/dose i.v./i.m.
Naloxone (Narcan) (0.4, 1 mg/mL)	1–2 mg i.v., i.m., ET	0.1 mg/kg/dose i.v.
Nitroglycerin (Tridil) (0.5 mg, 0.8 mg, 5 mg, 10 mg/mL)	5 μg/min i.v. drip, titrate up as needed	0.25–0.5 μg/kg/min i.v. drip, titrate up as needed
Nitroprusside	0.10 μg/kg/min up to 5.0 μg/kg/min	0.10 μg/kg/min up to 5.0 μg/kg/min i.v.
Norepinephrine	0.5 μg/min i.v. up to 30 μg/min	0.05–0.1 μg/kg/min i.v. and titrate max 1–2 μg/kg/min
Pancuronium (Pavulon) (1,2 mg/mL)	0.1–0.15 mg/kg/dose i.v. q30–60min	0.04–0.1 mg/kg/dose i.v. q30–60 min
Phenobarbital (65, 130 mg/mL)	*Load:* 15–20 mg/kg/dose i.v. (< 25–50 mg/min)	*Load:* 15–20 mg/kg/dose i.v. (< 1 mg/kg/min)
Phenytoin (Dilantin) (50 mg/mL)	*Seizure load:* 10–20 mg/kg/dose i.v. (<40 mg/min) up to 1000 mg; fosphenytoin (Cerebyx) permits more rapid administration, also	*Seizure load:* 10–20 mg/kg/dose i.v. (<0.5 mg/kg/min); fosphenytoin alternative
Procainamide	*Load:* 20 mg/min i.v. to max dose 17 mg/kg *Infusion:* 1–4 mg/min	*Load:* 2–6 mg/kg/dose over 5 min (max dose: 100 mg/dose); repeat dose q5–10 min PRN up to a total max of 15 mg/kg; do not exceed 500 mg in 30 min *Maintenance:* 20–80 μg/kg/min by continuous infusion
Propranolol (Inderal) (1 mg/mL)	1 mg i.v. over 10 min q5 min to total dose 5 mg	0.01–0.1 mg/kg/dose slow i.v. over 10 min; max 1 mg
Reteplase (Retavase)	10 IU i.v. over 2 min, repeat in 30 min	N/A
Streptokinase	1.5 million IU over 1 h infusion	N/A
Succinylcholine (Anectine) (20 mg/mL)	1–1.5 mg/kg/dose i.v. up to 150 mg	1–1.5 mg/kg/dose i.v.
Tenecteplase (TNKase)	30–50 mg i.v. bolus	N/A
Terbutaline	0.25 mg SC	0.01 mL/kg/dose SC *Nebulized:* 0.01–0.03 mg/kg/dose in 2 mL saline
Thiopental	3–5 mg/kg i.v.	2–5 mg/kg i.v.
Tirofiban (Aggrastat)	0.4 μg/kg/min for 30 min then 0.1 μg/kg/min	N/A
Vasopressin	40 U i.v.	N/A
Vecuronium (Norcuron) (10 mg/mL)	0.1 mg/kg/dose i.v.	0.1 mg/kg/dose i.v.
Verapamil	2.5–5.0 mg i.v.; then 5–10 mg i.v.	N/A

Rosen and Barkin's 5-Minute Emergency Medicine Consult

Second Edition

JEFFREY SCHAIDER, MD

ASSOCIATE CHAIRMAN
DEPARTMENT OF EMERGENCY MEDICINE
COOK COUNTY HOSPITAL
ASSOCIATE PROFESSOR OF EMERGENCY MEDICINE
RUSH MEDICAL COLLEGE
CHICAGO, ILLINOIS

STEPHEN R. HAYDEN, MD

ASSOCIATE PROFESSOR
DIRECTOR, RESIDENCY PROGRAM
DEPARTMENT OF EMERGENCY MEDICINE
UNIVERSITY OF CALIFORNIA SAN DIEGO MEDICAL CENTER
SAN DIEGO, CALIFORNIA

RICHARD WOLFE, MD

CHIEF OF EMERGENCY MEDICINE
BETH ISRAEL DEACONESS MEDICAL CENTER
ASSISTANT PROFESSOR
DIVISION OF EMERGENCY MEDICINE
HARVARD MEDICAL SCHOOL
BOSTON, MASSACHUSETTS

ROGER M. BARKIN, MD

VICE PRESIDENT FOR PEDIATRIC AND NEWBORN PROGRAMS AND
VICE PRESIDENT OF MEDICAL SERVICES
HEALTHONE
PROFESSOR OF SURGERY
DIVISION OF EMERGENCY MEDICINE
UNIVERSITY OF COLORADO HEALTH SCIENCES CENTER
DENVER, COLORADO

PETER ROSEN, MD

ASSOCIATE PROFESSOR
HARVARD UNIVERSITY;
ATTENDING PHYSICIAN
BETH ISRAEL HOSPITAL
BOSTON, MASSACHUSETTS;
ATTENDING PHYSICIAN
ST. JOHN'S HOSPITAL
JACKSON HOLE, WYOMING;
VISITING PROFESSOR
UNIVERSITY OF ARIZONA
TUCSON, ARIZONA

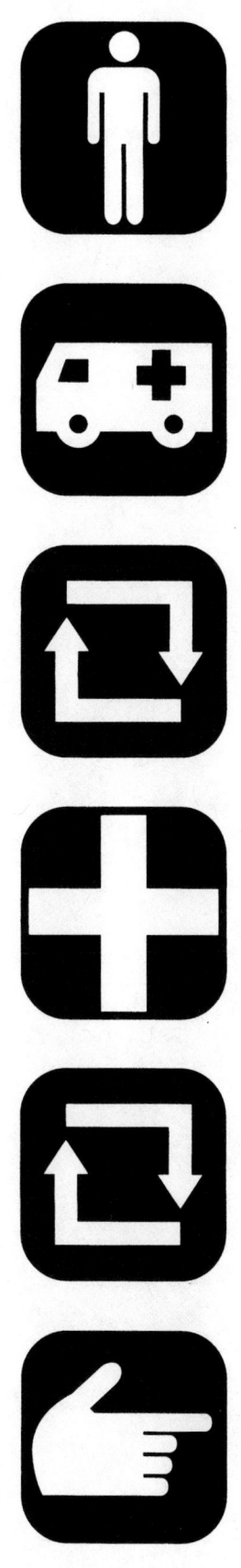

Rosen and Barkin's 5-Minute Emergency Medicine Consult

Second Edition

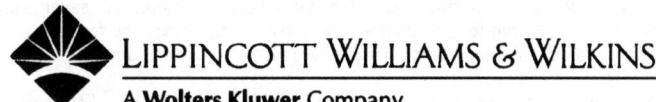

LIPPINCOTT WILLIAMS & WILKINS
A **Wolters Kluwer** Company
Philadelphia • Baltimore • New York • London
Buenos Aires • Hong Kong • Sydney • Tokyo

Acquisitions Editor: Anne M. Sydor
Developmental Editor: Julia Seto
Production Manager: Toni Ann Scaramuzzo
Production Editor: Michael Mallard
Manufacturing Manager: Colin Warnock
Cover Designer: Christine Jenny
Compositor: TechBooks
Printer: Quebecor World Taunton

530 Walnut Street
Philadelphia, PA 19106 USA
LWW.com

Printed in the USA

Library of Congress Cataloging-in-Publication Data

Rosen and Barkin's 5 minute emergency medicince consult/[edited by] Jeffrey J. Schaider...
[et al.].—2nd ed.
p. ; cm.
Rev. ed. of: 5 minute emergency medicine consult. 1999.
Includes bibliographical references and index.
ISBN 0-7817-3917-9
1. Emergency medicine—Handbooks, manuals, etc. 2. Medical emergencies—Handbooks, manuals, etc. I. Title: Rosen and Barkin's five minute emergency medicine consult. II. Title: 5 minute emergency medicine consult. III. Rosen, Peter, 1935– IV. Barkin, Roger M. V. Schaider, Jeffrey.
[DNLM: 1. Emergency Medicine—Handbooks. 2. Emergency Medical Services—Handbooks. 3. Emergency Treatment—Handbooks. WB 39 R813 2003]
RC86.8.A14 2003
616.02′5—dc21 2003047530

Care has been taken to confirm the accuracy of the information presented and to describe generally accepted practices. However, the authors, editors, and publisher are not responsible for errors or omissions or for any consequences from application of the information in this book and make no warranty, expressed or implied, with respect to the currency, completeness, or accuracy of the contents of the publication. Application of this information in a particular situation remains the professional responsibility of the practitioner.

The authors, editors, and publisher have exerted every effort to ensure that drug selection and dosage set forth in this text are in accordance with current recommendations and practice at the time of publication. However, in view of ongoing research, changes in government regulations, and the constant flow of information relating to drug therapy and drug reactions, the reader is urged to check the package insert for each drug for any change in indications and dosage and for added warnings and precautions. This is particularly important when the recommended agent is a new or infrequently employed drug.

Some drugs and medical devices presented in this publication have Food and Drug Administration (FDA) clearance for limited use in restricted research settings. It is the responsibility of the health care provider to ascertain the FDA status of each drug or device planned for use in their clinical practice.

10 9 8 7 6 5 4 3 2 1

Preface

Rosen and Barkin's 5-Minute Emergency Medicine Consult uniquely reflects our clinical practices and specialty of emergency medicine. The focus is to provide concise, formatted information that will allow the busy clinician to respond to challenges in a timely fashion. The book is meant to be readily available and to be frequently used in the midst of the clinical environment rather than be read at one's leisure. It is written and edited by practicing clinicians for practicing clinicians.

All emergency physicians need references to remind us of clinical presentations, differential diagnoses, drugs and dosages and management principles that facilitate our clinical judgment in synthesizing the vast array of data to which we are exposed. We have attempted to supplement the data bank we have acquired through many years of practice. The book is not meant to be a diagnostic engine, but rather a place to turn to confirm a diagnosis that is supported by the clinical presentation.

Our talented authors discuss each topic as if they were in the middle of a busy ED, trying to give a precise and clinically relevant summary to a resident who had queried them on a topic, or with whom they might be seeing a patient with a particular problem. We are indebted to them for their commitment to this task.

The book is intended to be accurate, pointed, and readily integrated into practice, rather than definitive. This new edition incorporates new information and approaches to management, while allowing us to incorporate new topics that reflect some of the new challenges we face.

Rosen and Barkin's 5-Minute Emergency Medicine Consult will be useful to both novices in emergency medicine and experienced clinicians. The information and organization of the book is designed to be optimal in the middle of the "chaos" that surrounds our clinical settings. Each topic focuses on what you need to know about a subject as opposed to what it might be nice to know.

Clinical acumen, judgment and experience remain as the foundation for our clinical practices. It is our hope that this book will serve as a useful and readily used resource and enhance the fulfillment of practicing emergency medicine.

Jeffrey Schaider
Stephen R. Hayden
Richard Wolfe
Roger M. Barkin
Peter Rosen

Acknowledgments

We are tremendously appreciative to the innumerable contributors who have done a superb job in conceptualizing and focusing this reference to be an essential guide to emergency medicine practice. Special thanks are also due to Anne Sydor, Julia Seto and the rest of the editorial and production staff of Lippincott Williams & Wilkins who facilitated the creation of what we hope will be a remarkably user friendly book.

Special thanks to the outstanding Cook County Hospital emergency medicine residents who provide a fertile ground for teaching and training that made this book easy to write and edit since each resident-attending interaction is a shortened 5-Minute Emergency Medicine Consult chapter. Nothing would be possible with the love and support of my wife Anna and children Jacob and Isaac.

J.S.

I would to acknowledge all the wonderful emergency medicine residents, and faculty at UCSD for their contributions to the text, and daily use of it. I am told that for some, they would never be able to do sufficient reading in the ED if it were not for the 5-Minute Emergency Medicine Consult. Lastly, to Marina, without you this project would never have happened. Thank you for keeping me on track, as well as the myriad of contributors.

S.R.H.

To my wife and children who have always supported and inspired me.

R.W.

To the many clinicians who have contributed to the creation of this second edition through suggestions, insights, and their practice. I am indebted to Kathi Thompson who made the process move smoothly through its many steps and coordinated the communication, editing and timetables.

R.M.B.

Contributors

JAMES ADAMS, MD
Division of Emergency Medicine
Northwestern University School of Medicine
Chicago, Illinois

MITCHELL ADELSTEIN, MD
Department of Emergency Medicine
Beth Israel Deaconess Medical Center
Boston, Massachusetts

STEVEN AKS, DO
The Toxikon Consortium
Department of Emergency Medicine
Cook County Hospital
Chicago, Illinois

MARILYN ALTHOFF, MD
Department of Emergency Medicine
Morristown Memorial Hospital
Morristown, New Jersey

PHILIP ANDERSON, MD
Department of Emergency Medicine
Beth Israel Deaconess Medical Center
Boston, Massachusetts

STEPHEN ANDERSON, MD
Resident in Emergency Medicine
University of California, Irvine
Orange, California

ANGELA ANDERSON, MD
Department of Pediatric Emergency Medicine
Hasbro Children's Hospital
Providence, Rhode Island

PAUL A. ANDRULONIS, MD
Department of Emergency Medicine
Pennsylvania Hospital
Philadelphia, Pennsylvania

PAUL ARNOLD, MD
Department of Emergency Medicine
University Health Network
Toronto, Ontario, Canada

L. KRISTIAN ARNOLD, MD
Emergency Medicine
Boston University School of Medicine
Boston, Massachusetts

ANDREW A. ARONSON, MD
Brigham and Women's Hospital
Boston, Massachusetts

VERONIQUE AU, MD
Stanford-Kaiser Emergency Medicine Program
Palo Alto, California

JENNIFER AUDI, MD
Department of Emergency Medicine
Beth Israel Deaconess Medical Center
Boston, Massachusetts

ELISA AUMONT, MD
Department of Emergency Medicine
University of Mississippi Medical Center
Jackson, Mississippi

BRANDON BACKLUND, MD
Department of Emergency Medicine
University of California San Diego Medical Center
San Diego, California

JOHN BAILITZ, MD, PHD
Department of Emergency Medicine
Cook County Hospital
Chicago, Illinois

ADAM Z. BARKIN, MD
Harvard Affilliated Emergency Medicine Residency
Beth Israel Deaconess Medical Center
Boston, Massachussetts

ROGER M. BARKIN, MD
Division of Emergency Medicine
University of Colorado Health Sciences Center
Denver, Colorado

SUZANNE Z. BARKIN, MD
University of Colorado Health Sciences Center
Denver Health Medical Center
Denver, Colorado

DAVID BARLAS, MD
Department of Emergency Medicine
North Shore University Hospital
Manhasset, New York

ERIK D. BARTON, MD, MS
Division of Emergency Medicine
University of Utah Health Science Center
Salt Lake City, Utah

KATHLENE BASSETT, MD
Assistant Professor of Pediatrics
University of Utah School of Medicine
Salt Lake City, Utah

H. PETER BEAUPARLANT JR., MD
Emergency Medicine
Brown University School of Medicine
Rhode Island Hospital
Providence, Rhode Island

B. J. BECK, MD
Harvard Medical School
Massachusetts General Hospital
Boston, Massachusetts;
East Boston Neighborhood Health Center
East Boston, Massachusetts

WALTER G. BELLEZA, MD
Department of Emergency Medicine
University of Maryland School of Medicine
Baltimore, Maryland

DANIEL BELMONT, MD
Department of Emergency Medicine
Cook County Hospital
Chicago, Illinois

KYAN J. BERGER, MD
Beverly Hospital
Beverly, Massachusetts;
Addison Gilbert Hospital
Gloucester, Massachusetts

LAURIE A. BERNARD, MD
Division of Pediatrics
Children's Hospital and Health Center, San Diego
San Diego, California

KRITI BHATIA, MD
Massachusetts General Hospital
Brigham and Women's Hospital
Boston, Massachusetts

HERBERT G. BIVINS, MD
Department of Emergency Medicine
UCSF-Fresno
Fresno, California

ADAM J. BLACK, MD
Department of Emergency Medicine
Resurrection-St. Elizabeth's Hospital
Chicago, Illinois

PAUL BLACKBURN, DO
Department of Emergency Medicine
Maricopa Medical Center
Phoenix, Arizona

KEITH BONIFACE, MD
Department of Emergency Medicne
George Washington University Medical Center
Washington, D.C.

MICHAEL J. BONO, MD
Eastern Virginia Medical School
Norfolk, Virginia

STEVEN H. BOWMAN, MD
Department of Emergency Medicine
Cook County Hospital
Chicago, Illinois

JEFFERSON D. BRACEY, DO
University of Nevada School of Medicine
Las Vegas, Nevada

ANDREA BRACIKOWSKI, MD
Department of Emergency Medicine
Vanderbilt University Medical Center
Nashville, Tennessee

KENNETH BRAMWELL, MD
Pediatric Emergency Medicine
University of Arizona
Tuscon, Arizona

JUDITH BRILLMAN, MD
Department of Emergency Medicine
University of New Mexico School of Medicine
Albuquerque, New Mexico

KATHRYN BRINSFIELD, MD
Department of Emergency Medicine
Boston City Hospital
Boston, Massachusetts

JOSHUA S. BRODER, MD
Department of Emergency Medicine
University of North Carolina at Chapel Hill
Chapel Hill, North Carolina

KERRY B. BRODERICK, MD
University of Colorado Health Sciences
Denver Health Medical Center
Denver, Colorado

DAVID F. M. BROWN, MD
Department of Emergency Medicine
Massachusetts General Hospital
Boston, Massachusetts

CALVIN BROWN III, MD
Department of Emergency Medicine
Brigham and Women's Hospital
Boston, Massachusetts

BRIAN J. BROWNE, MD
Department of Surgery, Division of Emergency Medicine
University of Maryland
Baltimore, Maryland

G. RICHARD BRUNO, MD
University Hospital of Brooklyn/SUNY Downstate
Brooklyn, New York

SEAN BRYANT, MD
Toxikon Consortium
Cook County Hospital
Chicago, Illinois

GARY BUBLY, MD
Department of Emergency Medicine
Miriam Hospital
Providence, Rhode Island

ROBERT BUCKLEY, MD, MPH
Department of Emergency Medicine
Naval Medical Center San Diego
San Diego, California

COLLEEN BUONO-KRASKA, MD
Department of Emergency Medicine
University of California, San Diego Medical Center
San Diego, California

PAUL BYSKOSH, MD
Department of Emergency Medicine
Cook County Hospital
Chicago, Illinois

COLLEEN J. CAMPBELL, MD
Department of Emergency Medicine
University of California San Diego Medical Center
San Diego, California

TAYLOR Y. CARDALL, MD
Department of Emergency Medicine
University of California, San Diego Medical Center
San Diego, California

MARTIN J. CAREY, MD
Department of Emergency Medicine
University of Arkansas for Medical Sciences
Little Rock, Arkansas

WALLACE A. CARTER, MD
Emergency Medicine
New York-Presbyterian
Weill Medical College of Cornell University;
College of Physicians and Surgeons
Columbia University
New York, New York

AUSTEN CHAI, MD
Cook County Hospital
Department of Emergency Medicine
Chicago, Illinois

HARITHA CHALLAPALLI, MD
Emergency Medicine
Brigham and Women's Hospital
Harvard Medical School
Boston, Massachusetts

MICHAEL CHAMALES, MD
Department of Surgery
Texas Tech University Health Sciences Center
Lubbock, Texas

THEODORE C. CHAN, MD
Department of Emergency Medicine
University of California, San Diego Medical Center
San Diego, California

ROBERT S. CHANG, MD
Department of Emergency Medicine
Boston University Medical Center
Boston, Massachusetts

ANDREW CHANG, MD
University of California Irvine
Orange; California

MICHELE CHETHAM, MD
Pediatric Emergency
CarePoint, PC
Denver, Colorado

GORDON CHEW, MD
Emergency Department
Kaiser Permanente Medical Center
Vallejo, California

KARLENE M. CHIN
Section of Emergency Medicine
Mount Vernon Hospital
Mount Vernon, New York

YI-MEI CHNG, MD
Emergency Medicine
Brigham and Women's Hospital
Harvard Medical School
Boston, Massachusetts

THOMAS H. CHUN, MD
Department of Pediatric Emergency Medicine
Hasbro Children's Hospital
Providence, Rhode Island

TERIGGI J. CICCONE, MD
Department of Emergency Medicine
Beth Israel Deaconess Medical Center
Boston, Massachusetts

GREGORY CIOTTONE, MD
Department of Emergency Medicine
Beth Israel Deaconess Medical Center
Boston, Massachusetts

TODD CLARK, MD
Department of Emergency Medicine
Cook County Hospital
Chicago, Illinois

RICHARD F. CLARK, MD
Department of Emergency Medicine
University of California, San Diego, School of Medicine;
Division of Medical Toxicology
University of California, San Diego Medical Center
San Diego, California

G. CAROLYN CLAYTON, MD
Department of Emergency Medicine
Rush Presbyterian St Lukes Medical Center
Chicago, Illinois

KATHLEEN J. CLEM, MD
Emergency Medicine
Duke University School of Medicine
Durham, North Carolina

BRIAN CLYNE, MD
Brown University School of Medicine
Providence, Rhode Island

STEWART R. COFFMAN, MD, FACEP
Emergency Services
Medical Center of Lewisville
Lewisville, Texas;
Division of Emergency Medicine
University of Texas Southwestern School of Medicine
Dallas, Texas

JAMES COLLETTI, MD
Department of Surgery
Division of Emergency Medicine
University of Maryland School of Medicine
Baltimore, Maryland

JAMIE COLLINGS, MD
Division of Emergency Medicine
Northwestern Memorial Hospital
Chicago, Illinois

JAMES A. COMES, MD
Emergency Medicine Program
UCSF-Fresno
Fresno, California

MARCO COPPOLA, DO
Emergency Medicine
Scott and White Memorial Hospital
Texas A&M University
Temple, Texas

STEPHEN C. COPPS, MD
Department of Emergency Medicine
Mayo Clinic
Rochester, Minnesota

MARCO CORDERO, MD
Palos Hospital
Palos Heights, Illinois

KELLY J. CORRIGAN, MD
Emergency Medicine
Beth Israel Deaconess Medical Center
Boston, Massachusetts

BRIAN N. CORWELL
Emergency Medicine
Beth Israel Deaconess Medical Center
Boston, Massachusetts

KAREN S. COSBY, MD
Department of Emergency Medicine
Cook County Hospital
Chicago, Illinois

FRANCIS L. COUNSELMAN, MD
Department of Emergency Medicine
Eastern Virginia Medical School
Emergency Physicians of Tidewater
Norfolk, Virginia

CHRISTO COURBAN, MD
Department of Emergency Medicine
Massachusetts General Hospital
Brigham and Women's Hospital
Boston, Massachusetts

LINDA C. COWELL, MD
Newton Wellesley Hospital
Norfolk, Massachusetts

RICHARD A. CRAVEN, MD
Department of Family and Community Medicine
Eastern Virginia Medical School
Norfolk, Virginia

STEVEN CRESPO, MD
Boston Medical Center
Boston, Massachusetts

KIRK CUMPSTON, MD
Toxikon Consortium
Cook County Hospital
Chicago, Illinois

LIESL CURTIS, MD
Department of Emergency Medicine
Georgetown University Hospital
Medstar Health
Washington, D.C.

KEVIN CURTIS, MD
Department of Emergency Medicine
Hospital of the University of Pennsylvania
Philadelphia, Pennsylvania

RITA CYDULKA, MD
Department of Emergency Medicine
MetroHealth Medical Center
Case Western Reserve University School of Medicine
Cleveland, Ohio

R. DART, MD
Department of Emergency Medicine
Boston Medical Center
Boston, Massachusetts

DANIEL DAVIS, MD
Department of Emergency Medicine
University of California, San Diego
San Diego, California

PETER M.C. DEBLIEUX, MD
Division of Emergency Medicine
Louisiana State University Health Science Center
New Orleans, Louisiana

BETH ANNE DEGENNARO, MD
Department of Emergency Medicine and Traumatology
University of Connecticut Medical School
Farmington, Connecticut

SEAN DEITCH, MD
Department of Emergency Medicine
Pioneers Memorial Hospital
Brawley, California

DAVID DELLA-GIUSTINA, MD
Department of Emergency Medicine
Madigan Army Medical Center
Madigan-University of Washington
Fort Lewis, Washington

PAUL H. DESAN, MD
Department of Psychiatry
Yale University School of Medicine
New Haven, Connecticut

PAUL L. DESANDRE, MD
Department of Emergency Medicine
Beth Israel Medical Center
New York, New York

DIANE DEVITA, MD
Department of Emergency Medicine
Madigan-University of Washington
Tacoma/Seattle, Washington

COLIN B. DEVONSHIRE, MD
Beth Israel Deaconess Medical Center
Harvard Affiliated Emergency Medicine Residency
Boston, Massachusetts

JNO DISCH, MD
Department of Emergency Medicine
Metro Health Medical Center
Cleveland, Ohio

MICHAEL K. DONEY, MD
Department of Emergency Medicine
University of California San Diego Medical Center
San Diego, California

MARK DOUCETTE, MD
Department of Emergency Medicine
Cook County Hospital
Chicago Illinois

SUSAN DUFEL, MD
Department of Emergency Medicine/Traumatology
Hartford Hospital
Hartford, Connecticut

SUSAN J. DUFFY, MD
Pediatric Emergency Medicine
Hasbro Children's Hospital/Rhode Island Hospital
Brown University
Providence, Rhode Island

JONATHAN EDLOW, MD
Department of Emergency Medicine
Beth Israel Deaconess Medical Center
Boston, Massachusetts

NORBERT ELSNER, MD
Jacobi Medical Center
Bronx, New York

JANET ENG, DO
Department of Emergency Medicine
Ingham Regional Medical Center
Lansing, Michigan

STEPHEN EPSTEIN, MD
Department of Emergency Medicine
Beth Israel Deaconess Medical Center
Harvard Medical School
Boston, Massachusetts

TIMOTHY ERICKSON, MD
Division of Clinical Toxicology
University of Illinois Chicago College of Medicine
Chicago, Illinois

MICHELLE GRANT ERVIN, MD, MHPE
Department of Emergency Medicine
Howard University Hospital
Washington, D.C.

CHRISTOPHER ERVIN, MD, FACEP
INPHYNET
Washington, D.C.

BARNET ESKIN, MD, PHD
Department of Emergency Medicine
Morristown Memorial Hospital
Morristown, New Jersey

BRIAN EUERLE, MD
University of Maryland School of Medicine
Baltimore, Maryland

TANYA M. FATOVICH, MD
Emergency Medicine
Massachusetts General Hospital
Brigham and Women's Hospital
Boston, Massachusetts

DAVID P. FELDMAN, MD, MBA
Emergency Medicine
Boston, Massachusetts

JAMES FELDMAN, MD
Department of Emergency Medicine
Boston Medical Center
Boston University School of Medicine
Boston, Massachusetts

STUART FELDMAN, DO
Infinity Healthcare
United Health Systems
Kenosha, Wisconsin

IAN GLEN FERGUSON, DO
Department of Emergency Medicine
Stanford University Medical Center
Palo Alto, California

MICHELLE A. FINKEL, MD
Department of Emergency Medicine
Massachusetts General Hospital
Boston, Massachusetts

STEVEN F. FISHER, MD
Department of Emergency Medicine
Lahey Clinic
Burlington, Massachusetts

KELLY ANNE FOLEY, MD
Emergency Medicine
Eastern Virginia Medical School
Norfolk, Virginia

JESSICA FREEDMAN, MD
Department of Emergency Medicine
Mount Sinai School of Medicine
New York, New York

RYAN FRIEDBERG, MD
Emergency Medicine
Beth Israel Deaconess Medical Center
Boston, Massachusetts

STEVEN FRIEDMAN, MD, MPH
Department of Emergency Medicine
University Health Network, Toronto
Toronto, Ontario, Canada

MARY ANNE FUCHS, MD
Department of Emergency Medicine
University of California San Diego Medical Center
San Diego, California

STEVEN FURER, MD
The Medical Center of Aurora
Aurora, Colorado

TAMI GASH-KIM, MD
Emergency Department
Scripps-Mercy;
Department of Emergency Medicine
University of California San Diego Medical Center
San Diego, California

MARC GELMAN, MD
Department of Emergency Medicine
Mercy Hospital of Buffalo
Buffalo, New York

PAUL GENNIS, MD
Jacobi Medical Center
Albert Einstein College of Medicine
Bronx, New York

DELARAM GHADISHAH, MD
Department of Emergency Medicine
Kaiser Panorama City
Panorama City, California

MICHELLE GILL, MD
Department of Emergency Medicine
Loma Linda University Medical Center
Loma Linda, California

BRET E. GINTHER, MD
California Emergency Physicians Medical Group
Laguna Hills, California

DAREN D. GIRARD, MD
Department of Emergency Medicine
Brown University/The Miriam Hospital
Providence, Rhode Island

JUDD GLASSER, MD
Department of Emergency Medicine
University of California, San Diego Medical Center
San Diego, California

ERIC GLASSER, MD
Department of Emergency Medicine
Georgetown University Hospital
Washington, D.C.

DONALD C. GOFF, MD
Harvard Medical School;
Psychotic Disorders Program
Massachusetts General Hospital
Boston Massachusetts

WILLIAM L. GOLDBERG, MD
Clinical Surgery/Emergency Medicine
Bellevue Hospital Center
New York University School of Medicine
New York, New York

DOLORES GONTHIER
MD2 Healthcare Consulting
Wexford, Pennsylvania

JEFFREY GORDON, MD
Department of Emergency Medicine
Holy Family Medical Center
Des Plaines, Illinois;
Department of Emergency Medicine
University of Illinois
Chicago, Illinois

DEEPI G. GOYAL, MD
Emergency Medicine
Mayo Clinic
Rochester, Minnesota

KIMBERLIE A. GRAEME, MD
Department of EU
Mayo Clinic Scottsdale
Scottsdale, Arizona

CHARLES S. GRAFFEO, MD
Department of Emergency Medicine
Eastern Virginia Medical School
Norfolk, Virginia

MYLES GREENBERG, MD
Department of Emergency Medicine
University of North Carolina
Chapel Hill, North Carolina

CONSTANCE S. GREENE, MD
Rush Medical College
Department of Emergency Medicine
Cook County Hospital
Chicago, Illinois

JILL GRIFFIN, MD
Department of Emergency Medicine
Bayustate Medical Center
Springfield, Massachusetts;
Tufts University School of Medicine
Boston, Massachusetts

LAUREN GROSSMAN, MD
Department of Emergency Medicine
Cook County Hospital
Chicago, Illinois

SHAMAI A. GROSSMAN, MD, MS
Department of Emergency Medicine
Beth Israel Deaconess Medical Center
Harvard Medical School
Boston, Massachusetts

KAMA Z. GULUMA, MD
Department of Emergency Medicine
University of California San Diego Medical Center
San Diego, California

ATUL GUPTA, MD
Stanford/Kaiser Emergency Medicine
Palo Alto, California

DAVID A. GUSS, MD
Department of Emergency Medicine
University of California San Diego Medical Center
San Diego, California

LEON GUSSOW, MD
Department of Emergency Medicine
Cook County Hospital
Chicago, Illinois

ROBERT S. HAMILTON, MD
Palo Cedro, California

ROY HANAKI, MD
Department of Emergency Medicine
Cook County Hospital
Chicago, Illinois

MARY HANCOCK, MD
Emergency Medicine
MetroHealth Medical Center
Case Western Reserve University School of Medicine
Cleveland, Ohio

MATTHEW R. HARMODY, MD, MBA
Sandhills Emergency Physicians
Pinehurst, North Carolina

DAVID A. HARTER, MD
Department of Emergency Medicine
Cook County Hospital
Chicago, Illinois

STEPHEN R. HAYDEN, MD
Department of Emergency Medicine
University of California San Diego Medical Center
San Diego, California

LAWRENCE E. HEISKELL, MD, FACEP, FAAFP
El Centro Regional Medical Center
El Centro, California

ROBYN R. HEISTER, MD
Department of Emergency Medicine
University of California at San Diego Medical Center
San Diego, California

ROBIN R. HEMPHILL, MD
Department of Emergency Medicine
Vanderbilt University
Nashville, Tennessee

SEAN O. HENDERSON, MD
Keck School of Medicine
University of Southern California
Los Angeles, California

GREGORY W. HENDEY, MD
Emergency Medicine
UCSF-Fresno Medical Education Program
Fresno, California

DAVID HERZOG, MD
Psychiatry and Pediatrics
Harvard Medical School;
Eating Disorders Unit
Massachusetts General Hospital
Boston, Massachusetts

RA'ED HIJAZI, MD
Department of Emergency Medicine
King Fahad National Guard Hospital
Riyadh, Saudi Arabia

STEPHEN HOCHEDER, MD
Department of Emergency Medicine
University of Arizona Health Sciences Center
Tuscon; Arizona

FORREST D. HOLDEN, MD
Emergency Residency Program
Maricopa Medical Center
Phoenix, Arizona

JEFFREY HORTON, MD
Department of Emergency Medicine
Memorial Hospital
Martinsville, Virginia

MARK A. HOSTETLER, MD, MPH
Pediatric Emergency Department
University of Chicago
Chicago, Illinois

JEFF C. HUFFMAN, MD
Psychiatric Consultation Service
Massachusetts General Hospital;
Department of Psychiatry
McLean Hospital and Harvard Medical School
Boston, Massachusetts

DANIEL E. HUHN, MD
Naval Medical Center San Diego
San Diego, California

TIMOTHY R. HURTADO, DO
Emergency Medicine
Madigan-University of Washington
Tacoma/Seattle, Washington

CRAIG HUSTON, MD
Department of Emergency Medicine
Cook County Hospital
Chicago, Illinois

ANTHONY HUYNH, MD
University of California San Diego Medical Center
San Diego, California

JASON IMPERATO, MD, MBA
Emergency Medicine
Beth Israel Deaconess Medical Center
Boston, Massachusetts

LISANDRO IRIZARRY, MD
Department of Emergency Medicine
The Brooklyn Hospital Center
Brooklyn, New York;
Cornell/Weill College of Medicine
New York, New York

HAGOP ISNAR, MD
Emergency Medicine
Auburn Memorial Hospital
Auburn, New York

KENNETH JACKIMCZYK, MD
Department of Emergency Medicine
Maricopa Medical Center
Phoenix, Arizona

IRVING "JAKE" JACOBY, MD
Department of Emergency Medicine
University of California San Diego Medical Center
University of California, San Diego School of Medicine
La Jolla, California

LIUDVIKAS JAGMINAS, MD
Department of Emergency Medicine
Rhode Island Hospital
Miriam Hospital
Hasbro Children's Hospital
Brown Medical School
Providence, Rhode Island

THEA JAMES, MD
Emergency Medicine
Boston University School of Medicine
Boston, Massachusetts

JOHN F. JARDINE, MD
Department of Emergency Medicine
Rhode Island Hospital
Brown University School of Medicine
Providence, Rhode Island

GREGORY D. JAY, MD, PHD
Department of Emergency Medicine
Brown University
Providence, Rhode Island

DAVID JERRARD, MD
Department of Emergency Medicine
University of Maryland Medicine
Baltimore, Maryland

ALBERT S. JIN, MD
Emergency Medicine
Orange County, California

DEAN E. JOHNSON, MD
University of Maryland School of Medicine
Baltimore, Maryland

GARY A. JOHNSON, MD
Department of Emergency Medicine
Upstate Medical University
Syracuse, New York

MICHAEL P. JONES, MD
Department of Emergency Medicine
Cook County Hospital
Chicago, Illinois

NICHOLAS J. JOURILLES, MD
Department of Emergency Medicine
Metro Health Medical Center
Cleveland, Ohio

PASCAL S. C. JUANG, MD
Hoag Hospital
Newport Beach, California

JOSEPH H. KAHN, MD
Department of Emergency Medicine
Boston Medical Center
Boston University School of Medicine
Boston, Massachusetts

CHRISTOPHER S. KANG, MD
Department of Emergency Medicine
Madigan Army Medical Center
Tacoma, Washington

ZIAD N. KAZZI, MD
Department of Emergency Medicine
Emory University
Atlanta, Georgia

A. ANTOINE KAZZI, MD
Department of Emergency Medicine
University of California, Irvine
South Orange, California

SAMUEL M. KEIM, MD
Department of Emergency Medicine
University of Arizona Health Science Center
Tuscon, Arizona

SEAN P. KELLY, MD
Department of Emergency Medicine
Beth Israel Deaconess Medical Center
Boston, Massachusetts

AILEEN KENNEDY, MD
Medical Center of Ocean County
Brick, New Jersey

ELICIA SINOR KENNEDY, MD
Emergency Medicine
University of Arkansas for Medical Sciences
Baptist Medical Center-Little Rock
Little Rock, Arkansas

KEVIN KERN, DO
Department of Emergency Medicine
Cook County Hospital
Chicago, Illinois

JAMES KILLEEN, MD
Department of Emergency Medicine
University of California San Diego Medical Center
San Diego, California

TAMAKI KIMBRO, MD
Department of Emergency Medicine
Mendocino Coast District Hospital
Fort Bragg, California

JEFFREY KING, MD
Wayne State University
Detroit, Michigan

BARRY KNAPP, MD
Department of Emergency Medicine
Eastern Virginia Medical School
Norfolk, Virginia

PAUL KOLECKI, MD
Department of Emergency Medicine
Thomas Jefferson University
Philadelphia, Pennsylvania

ANNE KRANTZ, MD, MPH
Division of Occupational Medicine
Cook County Hospital
Chicago, Illinois

RICHARD S. KRAUSE, MD
Department of Emergency Medicine
SUNY Buffalo School of Medicine
Buffalo, New York

JOEL KRAVITZ, MD
Department of Emergency Medicine
Albert Einstein Medical Center
Philadelphia, Pennsylvania

RICK G. KULKARNI, MD
Department of Emergency Medicine
Beth Israel Deaconess Medical Center
Harvard Medical School
Boston, Massachusetts

ANITA KULKARNI, MD
Department of Emergency Medicine
Herman Memorial Northwest
Houston, Texas

ALAN M. KUMAR, MD
Emergency Medicine
Brigham and Women's Hospital
Boston, Massachusetts

DICK KUO, MD
Department of Surgery
University of Maryland School of Medicine
Baltimore, Maryland

NANCY KWON, MD
Clinical Surgery/Emergency Medicine
New York University School of Medicine
Bellevue Hospital Center
New York, New York

TORREY LAACK, MD
Department of Emergency Medicine
Loma Linda University Medical Center
Loma Linda, California

JENNIFER M. LAFAYETTE, MD
Acute Psychiatry Service
Massachusetts General Hospital
Boston, Massachusetts

GREGORY W. LAMPE, MD
Emergency Department Information Systems
Mission Hospital Regional Medical Center
Mission Viejo, California

OWEN M. LANDER, MD
Department of Emergency Medicine
Beth Israel Deaconess Medical Center
Boston, Massachusetts

MARK I. LANGDORF, MD, MHPE
Department of Emergency Medicine
University of California Irvine Medical Center
Orange, California

MINH V. LE, MD
Department of Emergency Medicine
University of California San Diego Medical Center
San Diego, California

JAMES M. LEAMING, MD
Emergency Medicine
University of Alabama at Birmingham
Birmingham, Alabama

THOMAS C. LEE, MD
University of California Davis Medical School
Davis, California

MOSES LEE, MD
Department of Emergency Medicine
Cook County Hospital
Chicago, Illinois

SHIRLEY LEE, MD
Schwartz/Reisman Emergency Centre
Mount Sinai Hospital
University of Toronto
Toronto, Ontario, Canada

ERIC LEGOME, MD
Emergency Medicine
Bellevue Hospital Center/NYU Medical Center
New York, New York

STEVEN LELYVELD, MD
Pediatrics and Medicine
University of Chicago
Chicago, Illinois

THOMAS LEMKE, MD
Brown University School of Medicine
Providence, Rhode Island

RONEET LEV, MD
Scripps Mercy Emergency Department
San Diego, California

DAVID LEVINE, MD
Department of Emergency Medicine
Cook County Hospital
Chicago, Illinois

TREVOR LEWIS, MD
Department of Emergency Medicine
Cook County Hospital
Chicago, Illinois

LAZARO LEZCANO, MD
Division of Neonatalogy
St. Barnabas Hospital
Bronx, New York;
Weill Medical College of Cornell University
New York, New York

RICHARD LICHENSTEIN, MD
Pediatric Emergency Department
University of Maryland Hospital
Baltimore, Maryland

J. BRIAN LIDDY, MD
Department of Emergency Medicine
Baystate Medical Center
Springfield, Massachusetts;
Tufts University School of Medicine
Boston, Massachusetts

HARTWEL LIN, MD
University of Pittsburgh
Pittsburgh, Pennsylvania

CHRISTOPHER A. LIPINSKI, MD
University of Arizona College of Medicine, Phoenix Programs
Maricopa Medical Center
Phoenix, Arizona

SHAN LIU, MD
Emergency Medicine
Brigham and Women's Hospital
Boston, Massachusetts

ANGELA LOH, MD
Department of Emergency Medicine
University of California San Diego Medical Center
San Diego, California

FRANK LOVECCHIO, DO
Department of Medical Toxicology
Good Samaritan Regional Poison Center
Phoenix, Arizona

BORIS LUBAVIN, MD
Department of Emergency Medicine
University of California, Irvine
Orange, California

JON LUDWIG, MD
Department of Emergency Medicine
University of California, San Diego
San Diego, California

THOMAS W. LUKENS, MD, PHD
Department of Emergency Medicine
MetroHealth Medical Center
Cleveland, Ohio

BINH T. LY, MD
Division of Medical Toxicology
Department of Emergency Medicine
University of California San Diego Medical Center
San Diego, California

ELIZABETH L. LYNCH, MD
Department of Emergency Medicine
Loma Linda University Medical Center
Loma Linda, California

GENE MA, MD
Department of Emergency Medicine
Tri City Medical Center
Oceanside, California

JOHN MACKAY, MD
Department of Emergency Medicine
Texas Tech University
El Paso, Texas

LAURA MACNOW, MD
Department of Emergency Medicine
Beth Israel Deaconess Medical Center
Boston, Massachusetts

TIMOTHY J. MADER, MD
Department of Emergency Medicine
Baystate Medical Center, Springfield, Massachusetts
Tufts University School of Medicine
Boston, Massachusetts

JOHN F. MAHONEY, MD
Department of Emergency Medicine
University of Pittsburgh School of Medicine
Pittsburgh, Pennsylvania

MARK MANDELL, MD
Department of Emergency Medicine
Morristown Memorial Hospital
Morristown, New Jersey

JEFFREY MANKO, MD
Emergency Medicine
NYU/Bellevue Medical Center
New York, New York

JON D. MASON, MD
Emergency Medicine
Eastern Virginia Medical School
Norfolk, Virginia

JOHN MATHESON, MD
Emergency Medicine
Maricopa Medical Center
Phoenix, Arizona

CHRISTINA MATTS, MD
University of California Irvine College of Medicine
South Orange, California

SEJAL G. MATTU, MD
Department of Internal Medicine
Anne Arundel Medical Center
Annapolis, Maryland

AMAL MATTU, MD
Emergency Medicine
University of Maryland School of Medicine
Baltimore, Maryland

SUZAN MAZOR, MD
Toxikon Consortium
Cook County Hospital
Chicago Illinois

ANDREW T. MCAFEE, MD, MSC
Department of Emergency Medicine
Brigham and Women's Hospital
Boston, Massachusetts

ROBERT F. MCCORMACK, MD
Buffalo General Hospital
Buffalo, New York

JOHN MCCOURT, MD
Department of Emergency Medicine
University Medical Center of Southern Nevada
Las Vegas, Nevada

MARY PATRICIA MCKAY, MD
Emergency Medicine
MCP/Hahnemann School of Medicine
Allegheny General Hospital
Pittsburgh, Pennsylvania

CATHERINE MCLAREN, MD
Stanford/Kaiser Emergency Medicine
Program
Palo Alto, California

BONNIE MCMANUS, MD
Department of Emergency Medicine
Elmhurst Memorial Hospital
Elmhurst, Illinois

ABHISHEK MEHROTRA, MD
Department of Emergency Medicine
University of North Carolina
Durham, North Carolina

MOSS MENDELSON, MD
Department of Emergency Medicine
Eastern Virginia Medical School
Norfolk, Virginia

NATHAN MICK, MD
Department of Emergency Medicine
Massachusetts General Hospital
Boston, Massachusetts

TREVOR J. MILLS, MD
Division of Emergency Medicine
Louisiana State University Health Science Center
New Orleans, Louisiana

LESLIE MILNE, MD
Department of Emergency Medicine
Massachusetts General Hospital;
Sports Medicine Department
Children's Hospital
Boston, Massachusetts

ANDREW MILSTEN, MD
Emergency Medicine
University of Maryland
Glen Burnie, Maryland

ELIZABETH L. MITCHELL, MD
Department of Emergency Medicine
Boston Medical Center
Boston, Massachusetts

CHRISTY ROSA MOHLER, MD
Alvarado Hospital
San Diego, California

CHRIS MOORE, MD
Department of Emergency Medicine
Virginia Mason Medical Center
Seattle, Washington

LINDA MUELLER, MD
Department of Emergency Medicine
Munster Community Hospital
Munster, Indiana

DAVID W. MUNTER, MD, MBA
TRICARE Mid-Atlantic Region 2
Norfolk, Virginia;
Department of Military and Emergency Medicine
Uniformed Services University of the Health Sciences
Bethesda, Maryland

MICHAEL S. MURPHY, MD
Department of Emergency Medicine
South Shore Hospital
Weymouth, Massachusetts

MARK B. MYCYK, MD
Toxikon Consortium
Cook County Hospital
Northwestern University Medical School
Chicago, Illinois

ERIC S. NADEL, MD
Department of Emergency Medicine
Brigham and Women's Hospital
Boston, Massachusetts

KATHLEEN NASCI, MD
Emergency Department
University of Pennsylvania School of Medicine
Pennsylvania Hospital
Philadelphia, Pennsylvania

ISAM NASR, MD
Department of Emergency Medicine
Cook County Hospital
Chicago, Illinois

SEAN-XAVIER NEATH, MD
University of California, San Diego
San Diego, California

MEIKA NEBLETT, MD
Mount Sinai Hospital-Queens
Long Island City, New York

BRET P. NELSON, MD
Department of Emergency Medicine
Brigham and Women's Hospital
Boston, Massachusetts

EDWARD NEWTON, MD
Department of Emergency Medicine
Keck School of Medicine, University of Southern California
Los Angeles, California

ANN NGUYEN, MD
Department of Emergency Medicine
Cook County Hospital
Chicago, Illinois

SEAN PATRICK NORDT, PHARMD
University College Dublin School of Medicine
Dublin, Ireland

JONATHAN S. OLSHAKER, MD
Department of Emergency Medicine
Boston University School of Medicine
Boston Medical Center
Boston, Massachusetts

CHARLES ORSAY, MD
Division of Colorectal Surgery
Cook County Hospital
Chicago, Illinois

FRANK PALOUCEK, PHARMD
Department of Pharmacy Practice
University of Illinois College of Pharmacy
Chicago, Illinois

PETER S. PANG, MD
Emergency Medicine
Brigham and Women's Hospital/Massachusetts General Hospital
Boston, Massachusetts

LAWRENCE PARK, MD
Acute Psychiatry Service
Massachusetts General Hospital
Boston, Massachusetts

ROBERT PARTRIDGE, MD
Emergency Medicine
Brown University School of Medicine
Rhode Island Hospital
Providence, Rhode Island

CHIRAG PATEL, MD
Department of Emergency Medicine
Hospital of the University of Pennsylvania
Philadelphia, Pennsylvania

RAJ J. PATEL, MD
Department of Emergency Medicine
University of California, San Diego Medical Center
San Diego, California

STEVE C. PATTERSON, MD
Loma Linda University Medical Center
Loma Linda, California

RAHUL PATWARI
Rush St. Lukes-Presbyterian Hospital
Chicago, Illinois

TIMOTHY PAVEK, MD
St. Vincent Hospital Medical Center
Green Bay, Wisconsin

DAVID A. PEAK, MD
Department of Emergency Medicine
Massachusetts General Hospital
Boston, Massachusetts

DAVID A. PERLSTEIN, MD
Division of Ambulatory Pediatrics
St. Barnabas Hospital, Bronx, New York
Weill Medical College of Cornell University

ARYEH J. PESSAH, MD
Boca Raton Hospital
Boca Raton, Florida

KELLY PETTIT, MD
Department of Emergency Medicine
University of California San Diego Medical Center
San Diego, California

MICHAEL POLICASTRO, MD
Department of Emergency Medicine
MetroHealth Medical Center;
Case Western Reserve University School of Medicine
Cleveland, Ohio

CHARLES V. POLLACK, JR., MA, MD
Department of Emergency Medicine
Pennsylvania Hospital
University of Pennsylvania School of Medicine
Philadelphia, Pennsylvania

JANET POPONICK, MD
Department of Emergency Medicine
MetroHealth Medical Center
Case Western Reserve University
Cleveland, Ohio

ROBERT POWERS, MD, MPH
Department of Emergency Medicine
Hartford Hospital
Hartford, Connecticut

JEFFREY PROUDFOOT, DO
Department of Pediatrics
Division of Pediatric Emergency Medicine
Maricopa Medical Center
Phoenix, Arizona

NIELS K. RATHLEV, MD
Department of Emergency Medicine,
Boston Medical Center
Boston, Massachusetts

ERIC F. REICHMAN, MD
Department of Emergency Medicine
Cook County Hospital
Rush Medical College
Chicago, Illinois

KRISTINE M. REID, MD
Department of Emergency Medicine
York Hospital
York, Maine

IAN REILLY, MD
University of California San Diego Medical Center
San Diego, California

CHRISTOPHER F. RICHARDS, MD
Department of Emergency Medicine
Oregon Health Sciences University
Portland, Oregon

MARK G. RICHMOND, MD
Emergency Medicine
Loma Linda University Medical Center;
Santa Barbara Cottage Hospital
Santa Barbara, California

STEVEN RILEY, MD
Emergency Medicine and Pediatrics
Vanderbilt University Medical Center
Nashville, Tennessee

JAIME B. RIVAS, MD
Palomar Medical Center
Escondido, California

COLLEEN N. ROCHE, MD
Department of Emergency Medicine
George Washington University Medical Center
Washington, D.C.

E. JEDD ROE, MD
Department of Emergency Medicine
Legacy Emanuel Hospital
Portland Oregon

ROBERT L. ROGERS, MD
Departments of Medicine and Surgery
Division of Emergency Medicine
University of Maryland School of Medicine
Baltimore, Maryland

CARLO L. ROSEN, MD
Emergency Medicine
Beth Israel Deaconess Medical Center
Boston, Massachusetts

CHRISTOPHER ROSS, MD
Department of Emergency Medicine
Cook County Hospital
Chicago, Illinois

TODD C. ROTHENHAUS, MD
Department of Emergency Medicine
Boston University Medical Center
Boston Massachusetts

DAVID H. RUBIN, MD
Department of Pediatrics
St. Barnabas Hospital
Bronx, New York;
Weill Medical College of Cornell University
New York, New York

NATE RUDMAN, MD
Cape Cod Hospital
Hyannis, Massachusetts

DINO P. RUMORO, DO
Department of Emergency Medicine
Rush-Presbyterian-St. Luke's Medical Center
Chicago, Illinois

GARY S. SACHS, MD
Department of Psychiatry
Harvard Medical School
Boston, Massachusetts

MARK SAGARIN, MD
Mt. Auburn Hospital
Cambridge, Massachusetts

JOHN SAKLES, MD
Department of Emergency Medicine
University of Arizona College of Medicine
Tucson, Arizona

ERICH SALVACION, MD
Department of Emergency Medicine
University of California San Diego Medical Center
San Diego, California

LEON D. SANCHEZ, MD, MPH
Department of Emergency Medicine
Beth Israel Deaconess Medical Center
Boston, Massachusetts

KATHY SANDERS, MD
Department of Psychiatry
Harvard Medical School
Boston, Massachusetts

ARTHUR B. SANDERS, MD
Department of Emergency Medicine
University of Arizona College of Medicine
Tucson, Arizona

MARCELO SANDOVAL, MD
Emergency/Disaster Management
Beth Israel Medical Center
New York, New York

JOHN P. SANTAMARIA, MD
Department of Pediatrics,
University of South Florida School of Medicine
Tampa, Florida

SALLY SANTEN, MD
Department of Emergency Medicine
Vanderbilt University Medical Center
Nashville, Tennessee

ELAINE M. SAPIRO, MD, MPH
Department of Emergency Medicine
University of California San Diego Medical Center
San Diego, California

JOHN E. SATHER, MD
University of Connecticut School of Medicine
Farmington, Connecticut

DANIEL L. SAVITT, MD
Department of Emergency Medicine
The Miriam Hospital
Brown University
Providence, Rhode Island

ASSAAD J. SAYAH, MD
Department of Emergency Medicine
Caritas Good Samaritan Medical Center
Brockton, Massachussetts

SHARI SCHABOWSKI, MD
Department of Emergency Medicine
Cook County Hospital
Chicago, Illinois

JEFFREY J. SCHAIDER, MD
Department of Emergency Medicine
Cook County Hospital
Rush Medical College
Chicago, Illinois

HUGH SCHUCKMAN, MD
Department of Emergency Medicine
Northeast Ohio Universities College of Medicine
Summa Health System
Akron, Ohio

SUZANNE SCHUH, MD
Division of Paediatric Emergency Medicine
Research Institute, The Hospital for Sick Children
University of Toronto
Toronto, Ontario, Canada

THERESA SCHWAB, MD
Christ Medical Center
Oak Lawn, Illinois

GARY SCHWARTZ, MD
Emergency Medicine and Pediatrics
Vanderbilt University Medical Center
Nashville, Tennessee

JAMES SCOTT, MD
Department of Emergency Medicine
George Washington University Medical Center
Washington, D.C.

HANAN SEDIK, MD
Department of Pediatrics
Division of Pediatric Emergency Medicine
Boston Medical Center
Boston, Massachusetts

KAUSHAL SHAH, MD
Emergency Medicine
Beth Israel Deaconess Medical Center
Boston, Massachusetts

NATHAN I. SHAPIRO, MD
Department of Emergency Medicine
Beth Israel Deaconess Medical Center
Boston, Massachusetts

PHILIP SHAYNE, MD
Department of Emergency Medicine
Emory University School of Medicine
Atlanta, Georgia

SAM SHEN, MD
Emergency Medicine
Beth Israel Deaconess Medical Center
Boston, Massachusetts

LORNE SHERMAN, MD
North Shore University Hospital
Manhasset, New York

SCOTT SHERMAN, MD
Department of Emergency Medicine
Cook County Hospital
Chicago, Illinois

CHET SHERMER, MD
Emergency Medicine
University of Mississippi
Jackson, Mississippi

PATRICIA SHIPLEY, MD
Rush-Presbyterian St. Luke's Medical Center
Chicago, Illinois

LEE SHOCKLEY, MD
Department of Emergency Medicine
Denver Health Medical Center
Denver, Colorado

ROBERT SIDMAN, MD
Department of Emergency Medicine
Rhode Island Hospital
Providence, Rhode Island

JULIO SILVA, MD
Department of Emergency Medicine
Rush-Presbyterian-St. Luke's Medical Center
Chicago, Illinois

ALISON SISITSKY, MD
Department of Emergency Medicine
Beth Israel Deaconess Medical Center
Boston, Massachusetts

CHRISTIAN SLOANE, MD
Department of Emergency Medicine
University of California San Diego Medical Center
San Diego, California

REBECCA SMITH-COGGINS, MD
Emergency Medicine
Stanford University
Palo Alto, California

BRIAN SNYDER, MD
Department of Emergency Medicine
University of California San Diego Medical Center
San Diego, California

JULIA SONE, MD, FACS
Section of Surgical Endoscopy
Cook County Hospital;
Department of Surgery
Rush-Presbyterian-St. Luke's Medical Center;
University of Illinois at Chicago
Chicago, Illinois

MATTHEW T. SPENCER, MD
Department of Emergency Medicine
University of Rochester Medical Center
Rochester, New York

LINDA SPILLANE, MD
Department of Emergency Medicine
University of Rochester Medical Center
Rochester, New York

BLAKE SPIRKO, MD
Pediatric Emergency Department
Baystate Medical Center
Springfield, Massachusetts

TIMOTHY STALLARD, MD
Emergency Medicine
Scott and White Memorial Hospital
Texas A&M University
Temple, Texas

DALE W. STEELE, MD
Department of Pediatrics and Section of Emergency Medicine
Brown Medical School
Hasbro Children's Hospital
Providence, Rhode Island

THEODORE A. STERN, MD
Psychiatric Consultation Service
Massachusetts General Hospital;
Harvard Medical School
Boston, Massachusetts

HELEN STRAUS, MD, MS
Department of Emergency Medicine
Cook County Hospital
Rush University
Chicago, Illinois

STACEY A. SUECOFF, MD
Pediatric Emergency Medicine
Weill Medical College of Cornell University
St. Barnabas Hospital
Bronx, New York

HARSH SULÉ, MD
Department of Emergency Medicine
Cook County Hospital
Chicago, Illinois

JOHN E. SULLIVAN, MD
Emergency Medicine
Brigham and Women's Hospital
Boston, Massachusetts

BENJAMIN SUN, MD
Emergency Medicine
Massachusetts General Hospital
Brigham and Women's Hospital
Boston, Massachusetts

PAUL A. SZUCS, MD
Department of Emergency Medicine
Morristown Memorial Hospital
Morristown, New Jersey

DAVID TANEN, MD
Department of Emergency Medicine
Naval Medical Center San Diego
San Deigo, California

ROSS TANNENBAUM, MD
Section of Emergency Medicine
Provean St. Joseph Medical Center
Joliet, Illinois

GUY TARLETON, MD
Emergency Department
St. Francis Medical Center
Santa Barbara, California

ELIZABETH TEMIN, MD
Department of Emergency Medicine
Boston Medical Center
Boston, Massachussets

ADAM THOMAS, MD
Department of Emergency Medicine/Traumatology
Hartford Hospital
Hartford, Connecticut

KRISTINE M. THOMPSON, MD
Department of Emergency Medicine
Mayo Clinic
Rochester, Minnesota

CARRIE TIBBLES, MD
Department of Emergency Medicine
Beth Israel Deaconess Hospital
Boston, Massachusetts

FRED TILDEN, MD
Emergency Services
Midstate Medical Center
Meriden, Connecticut

SUSAN P. TORREY, MD
Department of Emergency Medicine
Baystate Medical Center
Springfield, Massachusetts;
Tufts University School of Medicine
Boston, Massachusetts

SHIRIN H. TRACHIOTIS, MD
Department of Emergency Medicine
Sibley Memorial Hospital
Washington, D.C.

JASON A. TRACY, MD
Emergency Medicine
Beth Israel Deaconess Medical Center
Boston, Massachusetts

OWEN T. TRAYNOR, MD
Department of Emergency Medicine
University of Pittsburgh School of Medicine
Pittsburgh, Pennsylvania

NEIL TROOST, MD
Department of Emergency Medicine
Cook County Hospital
Chicago, Illinois

CHRISTINE L. TSIEN, MD, PHD
Emergency Medicine
Brigham and Women's Hospital,
Massachusetts General Hospital
Boston Massachusetts

CLYDE TURNER, DO
Darnall Army Community Hospital
Fort Hood, Texas

ANDREW S. ULRICH, MD
Department of Emergency Medicine
Boston University Medical Center
Boston, Massachusetts

THOMAS A. UTECHT, MD
Emergency Department
UCSF-Fresno Medical Education Program
Fresno, California

FEDERICO VACA, MD, MPH
Department of Emergency Medicine
University of California Irvine College of Medicine
Orange, California

TYLER VADEBONCOEUR, MD
Department of Emergency Medicine
University of California, San Diego Medical Center
San Diego, California

CARLA VALENTINE, MD
Department of Emergency Medicine
University of California, San Diego Medical Center
San Diego, California

VERENA VALLEY, MD
Department of Emergency Medicine
University of Mississippi Medical Center
Jackson, Mississippi

KAREN B. VAN HOESEN, MD
Department of Emergency Medicine
University of California San Diego
San Diego, California

JAMES T. VANDENBERG, MD
Great River Medical Center
West Burlington, Iowa

BENJAMIN D. VANLANDINGHAM, MD
Department of Emergency Medicine
University of Arizona Health Sciences Center
Tuscon, Arizona

GARY M. VILKE, MD
Department of Emergency Medicine
University of California San Diego Medical Center
San Diego, California

ROBERT J. VISSERS, MD
Department of Emergency Medicine
University of North Carolina
Chapel Hill, North Carolina

MICHELE B. WAGNER, MD
Department of Emergency Medicine
Beth Israel Deaconess Medical Center
Boston, Massachusetts

JAMES S. WALKER, DO
Department of Surgery
University of Oklahoma Health Sciences Center
Oklahoma City, Oklahoma

MATTHEW J. WALSH, MD
Department of Emergency Medicine
Texas Tech University
El Paso, Texas

DAVID WANG, MD
Department of Emergency Medicine
Maricopa Medical Center
Phoenix, Arizona

JAY WEAVER, EMT-P
Boston Medical Center
Boston, Massachusetts

BRUCE WEBSTER, MD
Department of Emergency Medicine
Swedish Medical Center
Seattle, Washington

SCOTT G. WEINER, MD
Emergency Medicine
Beth Israel Deaconess Medical Center
Boston, Massachusetts

REBECAH M. WILKS, MD
Department of Emergency Medicine
University of California San Diego
San Diego, California

SETH K. WILLIAMS, MD
Department of Orthopaedics
University of California, San Diego
San Diego, California

TRACY WIMBUSH, MD
Department of Emergency Medicine
Brigham and Women's Hospital
Boston, Massachusetts

MICHAEL D. WITTING, MD
Department of Emergency Medicine
University of Maryland
Baltimore, Maryland

RUTH M. WOLD, MD
Department of Emergency Medicine
University of California, San Diego Medical Center
San Diego, California

JEANNETTE WOLFE, MD, FACEP
Emergency Medicine
Baystate Medical Center
Springfield Massachusetts;
Tufts University School of Medicine
Boston, Massachusetts

RICHARD E. WOLFE, MD
Emergency Medicine
Beth Israel Deaconess Medical Center
Harvard Medical School
Boston, Massachusetts

ADAM WOS, MD
Department of Emergency Medicine
University of California, San Diego Medical Center
San Diego, California

DANIEL WU, MD
Department of Emergency Medicine
Cook County Hospital
Chicago, Illinois

CHRISTINE YANG-KAUH, MD
Department of Emergency Medicine
Brigham and Women's Hospital
Boston, Massachusetts

RICHARD D. ZANE, MD
Department of Emergency Medicine
Brigham and Women's Hospital
Harvard Medical School
Boston, Massachusetts

SUSAN C. ZAPALAC, MD
Emergency Medicine
Santa Barbara Cottage Hospital
Santa Barbara, California

MICHELE ZELL-KANTER, PHARMD
Division of Occupational Medicine
Section of Clinical Toxicology
Cook County Hospital
Chicago, Illinois

AVIVA JACOBY ZIGMAN, MD
Legacy Good Samaritan Hospital
Portland, Oregon

GARY D. ZIMMER, MD
Department of Emergency Medicine
The Johns Hopkins Hospital
Baltimore, Maryland

KAREN P. ZIMMER, MD
Department of Pediatrics
The Johns Hopkins Hospital
Baltimore, Maryland

STEPHANIE ZIMMERMAN, MD
Division of Emergency Medicine
Phoenix Children's Hospital Phoenix, Arizona

Contents

TOPICAL TABLE OF CONTENTS

PRESENTING SIGNS/SYMPTOMS

CARDIAC EMERGENCIES

DERMATOLOGIC/SOFT TISSUE EMERGENCIES

ENDOCRINE EMERGENCIES

ENVIRONMENTAL EMERGENCIES

GASTROINTESTINAL EMERGENCIES

GENITOURINARY EMERGENCIES

GYNECOLOGIC EMERGENCIES

HEAD AND NECK EMERGENCIES

HEMATOLOGIC EMERGENCIES

IMMUNE SYSTEM EMERGENCIES

INFECTIOUS DISEASE EMERGENCIES

METABOLIC EMERGENCIES

NERVOUS SYSTEM EMERGENCIES

NONTRAUMATIC MUSCULOSKELETAL EMERGENCIES

OBSTETRICAL EMERGENCIES

ONCOLOGIC EMERGENCIES

OPHTHALMOLOGIC EMERGENCIES

ORTHOPEDIC INJURIES

PEDIATRIC EMERGENCIES

PULMONARY-THORACIC EMERGENCIES

PSYCHOBEHAVIORAL EMERGENCIES

RENAL EMERGENCIES

TOXICOLOGIC EMERGENCIES

TRAUMATIC INJURIES

VASCULAR EMERGENCIES

APPENDIX

Rosen and Barkin's 5-Minute Emergency Medicine Consult

Second Edition

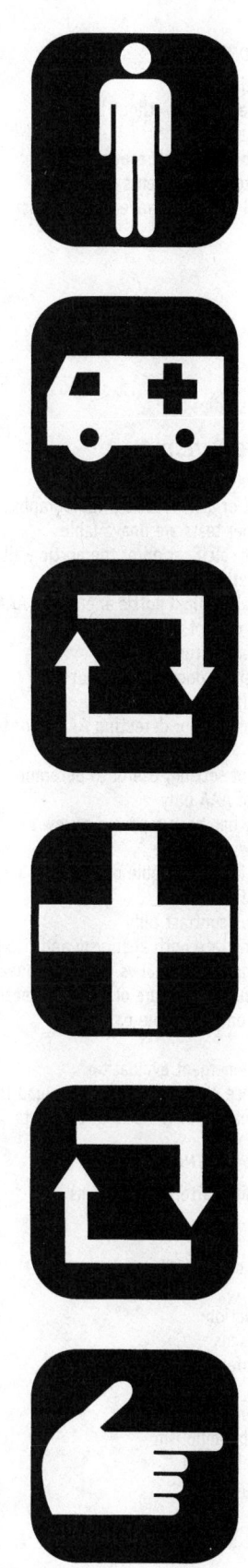

Abdominal Aortic Aneurysm

Clinical Presentation

SIGNS AND SYMPTOMS

- Unruptured
  - —Most often asymptomatic
  - —Abdominal, back, or flank pain
    - -Vague, dull quality
    - -Constant, throbbing, or colicky
  - —Abdominal mass or fullness
  - —Palpable, nontender, pulsatile mass
  - —Intact femoral pulses
- Ruptured
  - —Classic triad
    - -Pain
    - -Hypotension
    - -Pulsatile abdominal mass
    - -Present in 50% of patients
  - —Systemic
    - -Syncope
    - -Hypotension
    - -Tachycardia
    - -Evidence of systemic embolization
  - —Abdomen
    - -Abdominal, back, or flank pain
    - -Acute, severe, and constant
    - -Radiates to chest, thigh, inguinal area, or scrotum
    - -Flank pain radiating to the groin in 10% of cases
    - -Pulsatile, tender abdominal mass
    - -Abdominal tenderness
    - -Abdominal bruit
    - -Gastrointestinal hemorrhage
  - —Extremities
    - -Lower extremity pain
    - -Diminished or asymmetric pulses in the lower extremities
- Complications
  - —Large emboli: acute painful lower extremity
  - —Microemboli: cool, painful, cyanotic toes (blue toe syndrome)
  - —Aneurysmal thrombosis: acutely ischemic lower extremities
  - —Aortoenteric fistula: gastrointestinal hemorrhage

MECHANISM/DESCRIPTION

- Focal dilation of the aortic wall with an increase in diameter by at least 50% (>3 cm)
- 95% are infrarenal
- Gradual expansion and rupture
  - —Intraperitoneally
  - —Retroperitoneally
- Present in 2% of the elderly population
- Peak incidence
  - —Men 5.9% at the age of 80
  - —Women 4.5% at the age of 90
- Average growth rate of 0.2 to 0.5 cm per year
- 5-year risk of rupture
  - —Aneurysms <4.0 cm: 2%
  - —Aneurysms 4.0–5.0 cm: 5%
  - —Aneurysms >5.0–6.0 cm: 25%
  - —Aneurysms >6.0–7.0 cm: 35%
  - —Aneurysms >7.0 cm: 75%
- Intraperitoneal rupture is usually immediately fatal
- 50% of patients who reach the hospital alive survive
- Five-year survival after repair is 67%

ETIOLOGY

- Risk factors
  - —Male gender
  - —Age >65
  - —Family history
  - —Cigarette smoking
  - —Atherosclerosis
  - —Hypertension
- Uncommon causes
  - —Blunt abdominal trauma
  - —Infections of the aorta
  - —Mycotic aneurysm secondary to endocarditis

Pre-Hospital

- Establish two large-bore intravenous lines
- Rapid transport to the nearest facility with surgical backup
- Alert ED staff as soon as possible to prepare the following
  - —Operating room
  - —Universal donor blood
  - —Surgical consultation

Diagnosis

ESSENTIAL WORKUP

- Unstable patients
  - —Explorative surgery without further ancillary studies
  - —Bedside abdominal ultrasound
- Stable symptomatic patients
  - —Abdominal CT with intravenous contrast only

LABORATORY

- CBC
- Type and cross match blood
- Creatinine
- Urinalysis
- Coagulation studies

IMAGING/SPECIAL TESTS

- Plain radiographs
  - —Abdominal or lateral lumbar radiographs
  - —Only if other tests are unavailable
  - —Curvilinear calcification of the aortic wall or a paravertebral soft tissue mass indicates abdominal aortic aneurysm (AAA) in 75% of patients
  - —Cannot identify rupture
  - —Negative study does not rule out AAA
- Abdominal ultrasonography
  - —Highly sensitive for detecting AAA prior to rupture
  - —In emergent setting, useful to determine presence of AAA only
  - —Sensitivity has been reported as low as 10% following rupture
  - —Indicated in the unstable patient
- Abdominal CT scan
  - —Intravenous contrast only
  - —Will demonstrate both aneurysm and site of rupture (intraperitoneal vs. retroperitoneal)
  - —Allows accurate measure of aortic diameter
  - —Indicated only in stable patients
- Aortography
  - —No use in emergent evaluation
  - —The presence of mural thrombi can lead to underestimation of the size of the aorta

DIFFERENTIAL DIAGNOSIS

- Other abdominal arterial aneurysms
- Renal colic
- Biliary colic
- Lumbosacral disc disease
- Pancreatitis
- Bowel obstruction
- Perforated viscus
- Mesenteric infarction
- Diverticulitis
- Gastrointestinal hemorrhage
- Aortic thromboembolism
- Myocardial infarction
- Addisonian crisis
- Sepsis

Treatment

INITIAL STABILIZATION

- Two large-bore intravenous lines
- Crystalloid infusion
- Cardiac monitor
- Early blood transfusion

ED TREATMENT

- For patients suspected of symptomatic AAA:
  —Avoid overaggressive fluid resuscitation: leads to increased bleeding
  —Emergent surgical consult and operative intervention
  —Diagnostic tests should not delay definitive treatment

MEDICATIONS

N/A

Disposition

ADMISSION CRITERIA

- All patients with symptomatic AAA require emergent surgical intervention

DISCHARGE CRITERIA

- Asymptomatic patients only
- Close surgical follow-up
- Instructions to return immediately
  —With any pain in the back, abdomen, or lower extremities
  —With dizziness or syncope

Miscellaneous

ICD9: 441.3

ICD10: I71.4

SUGGESTED READINGS

Bessen HA. Abdominal aortic aneurysms. In: Marx JA, et al, eds. Rosen's emergency medicine: concepts and clinical practice, 5th ed. St. Louis: Mosby, 2002:1176–1186.

Ernst CB. Abdominal aortic aneurysm. N Engl J Med 1993;328:1167–1172.

Hallet JW. Management of abdominal aortic aneurysms. Mayo Clin Proc 2000;75: 395–399.

Walker JS, Dire DJ. Vascular abdominal emergencies. Emerg Med Clin North Am 1996;14:571–591.

Authors: Jason Imperato; Carlo L. Rosen

Abdominal Pain

Clinical Presentation

SIGNS AND SYMPTOMS

General

- Anorexia
- Malaise
- Tachycardia
- Hypotension
- Fever
- Nausea
- Vomiting
  - —Etiology requiring surgical intervention is less likely when vomiting precedes the onset of pain

Abdominal

- Diarrhea
- Constipation
- Distended abdomen
- Abnormal bowel sounds
  - —High-pitched rushes with bowel obstruction
  - —Absence of sound with ileus or peritonitis
  - —Often unreliable
- Pulsatile abdominal mass
- Rovsing's sign
  - —Palpation of LLQ causes pain in RLQ
  - —Suggestive of appendicitis
- McBurney's point tenderness associated with appendicitis
  - —Palpation in RLQ two-thirds distance between umbilicus and right anterior superior iliac crest causes pain
- Murphy's sign
  - —Pause in inspiration while examiner is palpating under liver
  - —Suggestive of cholecystitis
- Psoas sign
  - —Pain on extension of the thigh
  - —Suggests inflammation around psoas muscle
- Obturator sign
  - —Pain on rotation of the flexed thigh, especially internal rotation
  - —Inflammation around internal obturator muscle
- Tender or discolored hernia site
- Rectal and pelvic examination
  - —Tenderness with pelvic peritoneal irritation
  - —Cervical motion tenderness
  - —Adnexal masses
  - —Rectal mass or tenderness

Genitourinary

- Flank pain
- Dysuria
- Hematuria
- Vaginal bleeding
- Tender adnexal mass on pelvis
- Testicular pain
  - —May be referred from renal or appendiceal pathology
- Testicular swelling
- High-riding testes
- Transverse lie of testis

Extremities

- Shoulder pain
  - —Referred pain from diaphragmatic involvement
- Pulse deficit or unequal femoral pulses

Skin

- Jaundice
- Herpes zoster
- Cellulitis

MECHANISM/DESCRIPTION

- Parietal pain
  - —Irritating material applied to the peritoneum
  - —Inflammation of the parietal peritoneum
  - —Pain transmitted by somatic nerves
  - —Exacerbated by changes in tension of the peritoneum
  - —Pain characteristics
    - -Sharp
    - -Well localized
    - -Abdominal tenderness
    - -Involuntary guarding
    - -Rebound tenderness
    - -Guarding
    - -Exacerbated by movement and coughing
- Visceral
  - —Distention of a viscous or organ capsule or spasm of intestinal muscularis fibers
    - -Pain is generally poorly localized
    - -Pain with intestinal distention is colicky
    - -Pain with a distended gallbladder or kidney is steady
  - —Inflammation
    - -Initially the pain is poorly localized
    - -Focal tenderness develops as the inflammation extends to the peritoneum or localizers
  - —Ischemia from vascular disturbances
    - -Pain is severe and diffuse with catastrophic vascular emergencies
    - -The pain is disproportional to the abdominal examination
- Referred
  - —Felt at distant location from diseased organ
  - —Due to an overlapping supply by the affected neurosegment to the perceived location of pain
- Abdominal wall pain
  - —Constant
  - —Aching
  - —Muscle spasm
  - —Involvement of other muscle groups

ETIOLOGY

- Peritoneal irritants
  - —Gastric juice
  - —Fecal material
  - —Pus
  - —Blood
  - —Bile
  - —Pancreatic enzymes
- Visceral obstruction
  - —Small intestines
  - —Large intestines
  - —Gallbladder
  - —Ureters and kidneys
  - —Visceral ischemia
  - —Intestinal
  - —Renal
  - —Splenic
- Visceral inflammation
  - —Appendicitis
  - —Inflammatory bowel disorders
    - -Gastroenteritis
    - -Lymphadenitis
    - -Crohn's disease
    - -Ulcerative colitis
  - —Cholecystitis
  - —Hepatitis
  - —Peptic ulcer disease
  - —Pancreatitis
  - —Pelvic inflammatory disease
  - —Pyelonephritis
- Abdominal wall pain
- Referred pain
  - —The possibility of intrathoracic disease must be considered in every patient with abdominal pain

Pre-Hospital

- Intravenous access and resuscitation if signs of hemodynamic instability
- In patients with epigastric pain who are at risk for coronary artery disease
  —Supplemental oxygen
  —Monitor

Diagnosis

ESSENTIAL WORKUP

- Historical characteristics define the type of pain and suggest underlying causes
  —Nature of onset of pain
  —Time of onset and duration of pain
  —Location of pain initially and at presentation
  —Extraabdominal radiations
  —Quality of pain (sharp, dull, crampy)
  —Palliative or provocative factors
  —Relation of associated finding to onset of pain
  —Changes in bowel habits
  —History of trauma
  —Gynecologic history
  —Visceral obstruction

LABORATORY

- CBC
  —WBC is unreliable in distinguishing surgical and nonsurgical disease
- Urinalysis
  —Pyuria
  —Hematuria
  —Glucosuria
  —Ketones
- Serum lipase
  —More accurate than a serum amylase in diagnosing pancreatic disorders
- Serum hCG
- Serum electrolytes and glucose
- Gonorrhea and chlamydia cultures should be obtained if a pelvic examination is performed

IMAGING/SPECIAL TESTS

EKG

- Indicated in patients with epigastric pain over the age of 40 or with risk factors for coronary artery disease

KUB and Upright

- Indicated primarily if bowel obstruction is suspected
- Of little help in the evaluation of renal colic or gallbladder disease
- Air fluid levels and intestinal distention
  —Bowel obstruction
  —Ileus
  —Volvulus
  —Intussusception
- Intraabdominal mass
- Aortic aneurysm

Upright chest radiograph

- Pneumoperitoneum
  —Perforated stomach, duodenum, or colon
- Extraabdominal causes
  —Pneumonia
  —Pleural effusion

Ultrasound

- Biliary abnormalities
  —Cholelithiasis
  —Evidence of cholecystitis
  —Sonographic Murphy's sign
  —Wall thickening
  —Pericholecystic fluid
  —Ductal dilation
- Hydronephrosis
- Intraperitoneal fluid
  —Aneurysmal rupture
  —Splenic rupture
  —Ruptured ectopic pregnancy
  —Ascites
  —Ruptured ovarian cyst
- Aortic aneurysm
- Pelvic ultrasound
  —Intrauterine pregnancy
  —Adnexal mass
    -Ectopic pregnancy
    -Ovarian cyst
    -Ovarian torsion
    -Ovarian tumor
    -Tuboovarian abscess

Abdominal CT

- Spiral CT without contrast
  —Determines location and size of stone in patients with renal colic
- CT with intravenous contrast only
  —Vascular rupture suspected in a stable patient
- CT with intravenous and oral contrast
  —Indicated when there is a suspicion of a surgical etiology involving bowel or intraperitoneal hemorrhage
    -Ruptured spleen
    -Enlarged pancreas
    -Thickened colonic wall and streaking of the mesocolon is characteristic of diverticulitis
- CT with rectal contrast only
  —High accuracy reported in detecting appendicitis

IVP

- Indicated in patients with suspected ureteral calculi
- More time-consuming than spiral CT

Barium Enema

- Intussusception
- Volvulus

DIFFERENTIAL DIAGNOSIS

- Abdominal aortic aneurysm
- Abdominal epilepsy
- Abdominal migraine
- Abdominal wall hematoma or infection
- Adrenal crisis
- Appendicitis
- Black widow spider bite
- Bowel obstruction
- Cholecystitis
- Constipation
- Depression
- Diabetic ketoacidosis

Abdominal Pain

- Diverticulitis
- Dysmenorrhea
- Ectopic pregnancy
- Esophagitis
- Fecal impaction
- Fitz-Hugh–Curtis syndrome
- Gastroenteritis
- Hepatitis
- Herpes zoster
- Hirschsprung's disease
- Incarcerated hernia
- Inflammatory bowel disease
- Intussusception
- Irritable bowel syndrome
- Ischemic bowel
- Lactose intolerance
- Lead poisoning
- Meckel's diverticulitis
- Myocardial infarction
- Neoplasm
- Ovarian cyst
- Ovarian torsion
- Pancreatitis
- Pelvic inflammatory disease
- Peptic ulcer disease
- Perforated viscus
- Pneumonia
- Renal/ureteral calculi
- Sickle cell crisis
- Splenic infarction
- Splenic rupture
- Spontaneous abortion
- Testicular torsion
- Urinary tract infection
- Volvulus

PEDIATRIC CONSIDERATIONS

- Under 2 years
  —Hirschsprung's disease
  —Incarcerated hernia
  —Intussusception
  —Neoplasm
  —Sickle cell crisis
  —Volvulus
- 2–5 years
  —Appendicitis
  —Incarcerated hernia
  —Meckel's diverticulitis
  —Neoplasm
  —Sickle cell crisis
- Over 5 years
  —Appendicitis
  —Ectopic pregnancy
  —Inflammatory bowel disease
  —PID

Treatment

INITIAL STABILIZATION

- Emergent laparotomy
  —Patients who are hemodynamically unstable with suspected vascular rupture
- IV fluids
- Nasogastric suction

ED TREATMENT

- Antiemetics are important for comfort
- Narcotics or analgesics should not be withheld as they do not impair decision-making
- Antibiotics are needed in potential perforation and in peritonitis
- Surgical consultation
  —Parietal pain
  —Suspicion of appendicitis
  —Hemodynamic instability
  —Bowel obstruction
  —Suspicion of bowel ischemia
  —Cholecystitis

MEDICATIONS

- Cefoxitin: 1 g i.v. (peds 40 mg/kg i.v.)
- Fentanyl: 1–2 μg/kg i.v. q hr
- Gentamicin: 2.5 mg/kg i.v.
- Prochlorperazine: 0.13 mg/kg i.v./PO/IM q 6 PRN nausea; 25 mg PR q 6 in adults
- Promethazine: 1 mg/kg IM/PO/PR

Disposition

ADMISSION CRITERIA

- Surgical intervention
- Peritoneal signs
- Patient unable to keep down fluids
- Lack of pain control
- Medical cause necessitating in-house treatment (MI, DKA)
- IV antibiotics needed

DISCHARGE CRITERIA

- No surgical or severe medical etiology found in patient who is able to keep fluid down, has good pain control, and is able to follow detailed discharge instructions

Miscellaneous

ICD9: 789.0

ICD10: R10.4

SUGGESTED READINGS

Graff LG 4th, Robinson D. Abdominal pain and emergency department evaluation. Emerg Med Clin North Am 2001;19(1):123–136.

Kizer KW, Vassar MJ. Emergency department diagnosis of abdominal disorders in the elderly. Am J Emerg Med 1998;16(4):357–362.

Mason JD. The evaluation of acute abdominal pain in children. Emerg Med Clin North Am 1996;14(3):629–643.

Sanson TG, O'Keefe KP. Evaluation of abdominal pain in the elderly. Emerg Med Clin North Am 1996;14(3):615–627.

Stone R. Acute abdominal pain. Lippincotts Prim Care Pract 1998;2(4):341–357.

Author: Michelle A. Finkel

Abdominal Trauma, Blunt

Clinical Presentation

SIGNS AND SYMPTOMS

- Spectrum of presentation from abdominal pain with or without signs of peritoneal irritation to hypovolemic shock without physical exam findings
- Nausea or vomiting
- Labored respirations due to diaphragm irritation or upper abdominal injury
- Left shoulder pain with inspiration (Kehr's sign) from diaphragmatic irritation due to bleeding
- Delayed presentation possible with small bowel injury

MECHANISM/DESCRIPTION

- Injury results from a sudden increase of pressure to abdomen
- Solid organ injury usually manifests itself as hemorrhage
- Hollow viscous injuries result in bleeding and peritonitis from contamination with bowel contents

ETIOLOGY

- 60% of cases result from motor vehicle accidents
- Solid organs are injured more frequently than hollow viscous organs
- The spleen is the most frequently injured organ (25%), followed by the liver (15%), intestines (15%), retroperitoneal structures (13%), and kidney (12%)
- Less frequently injured are the mesentery, pancreas, diaphragm, urinary bladder, urethra, and vascular structures

PEDIATRIC CONSIDERATIONS

- Children tend to tolerate trauma better due to the more elastic nature of their tissues
- Due to the decreased size of the intrathoracic abdomen, the spleen and liver are more exposed to injury as they lie partially outside the bony rib cage

Pre-Hospital

CONTROVERSIES

- Aggressive fluid resuscitation is still considered standard of care
- Normal vital signs do not preclude significant intraabdominal pathology

Diagnosis

ESSENTIAL WORKUP

- Evaluate and stabilize airway, breathing, and circulation
- Primary objective is to determine the need for operative intervention
- Examine the abdomen to determine presence of intraabdominal bleeding or peritoneal irritation
- Injury in the retroperitoneal space or intrathoracic abdomen is difficult to assess by palpation
- Remember that the limits of the abdomen include the diaphragm superiorly (nipples anteriorly, inferior scapular tip posteriorly) and the intragluteal fold inferiorly and encompasses the entire circumference
- Abrasions or ecchymoses may be indicators of intraabdominal injury; roll the patient to assess the back
- Bowel sounds may be absent secondary to peritoneal irritation, but this is usually a late finding
- Foley catheter (if no blood at the meatus, no perineal hematoma, and normal prostate exam) to obtain urine for urinalysis and record urinary output
- Plain film of the pelvis
  - —Fracture of the pelvis and gross hematuria may indicate genitourinary injury and necessitate further evaluation of these structures with retrograde urethrogram, cystogram, or IVP
- Microscopic hematuria in the presence of shock is an indication for genitourinary evaluation
  - —CT is useful in suspected renal injury
- Objective imaging of the abdomen (see Abdominal Trauma, Imaging)
  - —Ultrasonography (FAST exam) for detection of fluid (as useful as diagnostic peritoneal lavage (DPL) in unstable patients in determining need for laparotomy); ultrasonography is rapid, requires no contrast agents, and is noninvasive; it is, however, operator-dependent
  - —DPL (useful for picking up injuries in the intrathoracic abdomen, pelvic abdomen, and the true abdomen) is primarily indicated for unstable patients; it is positive in the context of blunt abdominal trauma with gross blood, a RBC count of $>100{,}000/mm^3$, WBC count of $500/mm^3$, or the presence of bile, feces, or food particles
  - —CT is most useful in assessing need for operative intervention and for evaluating the retroperitoneal space and solid organs; patient must be stable enough to make trip to scanner

LABORATORY

- Hgb/hematocrit, which may be initially normal due to isovolemic blood loss
- Type and cross is essential
- Urinalysis for blood
- ABG: the base deficit may aid in the diagnosis of hypovolemic shock and help guide the resuscitation

IMAGING

See Essential Workup, above

DIFFERENTIAL DIAGNOSIS

- Lower thoracic injury may cause abdominal pain

Treatment

INITIAL STABILIZATION

- ABCs
- Ensure adequate airway; intubate if needed; O_2 100% by non-rebreather face mask
- Two large-bore IVs with crystalloid infusion
- Begin infusion of PRBCs if no response to 2 L of crystalloid
- If in profound shock, consider transfusion of O-negative or type-specific blood on the way to the operating room

ED TREATMENT

- Continue stabilization begun in field
- NGT to evacuate stomach, decrease distention, and decrease risk of aspiration; this may relieve respiratory distress if caused by a herniated stomach through the diaphragm
- Placement of Foley catheter

MEDICATIONS

- Tetanus toxoid booster: 0.5 cc IM for patients with open wounds
- Tetanus immune globulin: 250 units IM for patients who have not had complete series
- IV antibiotics: Unasyn 1 g IVPB or 2nd-generation cephalosporin

PEDIATRIC CONSIDERATIONS

- Crystalloid infusion for pediatrics is 20 cc/kg if patient is in shock
- Packed RBC dose is 1 cc/kg

Disposition

ADMISSION CRITERIA

- Postoperative cases
- Equivocal findings on DPL or CT

DISCHARGE CRITERIA

- No patient in whom you suspect intraabdominal injury should be discharged home without an appropriate period of observation despite negative exam or imaging studies

Miscellaneous

ICD9: 868.00

ICD10: S39.9

SUGGESTED READINGS

Amoroso TA. Evaluation of the patient with blunt abdominal trauma: an evidence based approach. Emerg Med Clin North Am 1999;17(1):63–75.

Davis JJ, et al. Diagnosis and management of blunt abdominal trauma. Ann Surg 1976;183:672.

McGahan JP, Wang L, Richards JR. Focused abdominal ultrasound for trauma. Radiographics 2001;21:91–99.

Stengel D, Bauwens K, Sehouli J, et al. Systematic review and meta-analysis of emergency ultrasonography for blunt abdominal trauma. Br J Surg 2001;88(7):901–912.

Author: Stewart Coffman

Abdominal Trauma, Imaging

Clinical Presentation

SIGNS AND SYMPTOMS

- Abdominal trauma may present as an unstable patient with multiple associated injuries or as an isolated injury in a stable patient with no physical findings.
- In unstable patients, the management of the ABCs, treatment of hypovolemic shock, and control of major hemorrhage must take precedence
- Assessment of the abdomen focuses on the need for early surgical management; the diagnosis of specific organ injuries should come later

Pre-Hospital

CAUTIONS

- All patients with a significant mechanism of injury or suspicion of major trauma should be triaged to a facility equipped to manage trauma

PEDIATRIC CONSIDERATIONS

- Pediatric patients should be triaged to a pediatric trauma center or to an adult trauma center equipped to manage children

Diagnosis

ESSENTIAL WORKUP

- See Abdominal Trauma, Blunt; and Abdominal Trauma, Penetrating
- History including mechanism of injury, restraint use, airbag or helmet use, pre-hospital vital signs, initial mental status and change in mental status, and any pre-hospital treatments performed and their effect on patient status
- AMPLE history (*a*llergies, especially to radiographic contrast agents, *m*edications, *p*ast medical history, *l*ast meal, *e*vents leading up to the injury)
- Comprehensive physical exam including complete exposure and both a perineal and digital rectal exam
- Abdominal stab wounds should be locally explored after local anesthesia; penetration of the abdominal wall fascia is considered a positive exploration and requires further evaluation
- Gunshot wounds to the abdomen require evaluation by a surgeon; selective laparotomy is still in its infancy for gunshot wounds.
- Caution
  - —Physical exam is accurate in determining serious abdominal injury in only 45–50% of cases

IMAGING/SPECIAL TESTS

General Approach to Imaging in Blunt Abdominal Trauma

- The ideal abdominal imaging study is rapid, cheap, sensitive for operative injury, identifies nonoperative injuries requiring close observation and follow-up, requires minimal training to perform and interpret, and currently does not exist
- Ultrasound has become the initial screening test of choice for hemodynamically stable patients; it has replaced diagnostic peritoneal lavage (DPL) (see below) in many settings
- CT scan is ideal for many patients, especially children, but requires intravenous contrast material
  - —Unstable patients should not be transported to CT scan
  - —Most patients require serial physical examinations and a period of observation after negative imaging studies

Ultrasound

- Advantages
  - —Rapid
  - —Noninvasive
  - —Sensitive for intraperitoneal fluid
  - —Can be performed at the bedside
  - —Does not require contrast agents or ionizing radiation

- Disadvantages
  - —Does not reliably identify specific organ injury
  - —Not well suited for penetrating injuries as may miss significant bowel injuries not accompanied by hemoperitoneum
- Indications
  - —Blunt trauma, stable or unstable patients
- Contraindications
  - —Absolute: preexisting indication for exploratory laparotomy
  - —Relative: obesity, subcutaneous emphysema
- Positive test
  - —Demonstration of free fluid or obvious solid organ injury (approximately 250 cc free fluid required in adults)
- Adequate exam includes visualization of Morrison pouch, pericardium, both paracolic gutters, and the pelvis (pouch of Douglas), and exam of the liver and spleen for parenchymal injuries
- Considerations
  - —Positive test should be followed by CT in a stable patient or laparotomy in an unstable patient
  - —Institutional factors determine who performs the study

CT Scan

- Advantages
  - —Sensitive (85–98%)
  - —Provides specific organ injury information
  - —Fosters nonoperative approach to certain liver and spleen injuries
  - —Detects retroperitoneal injuries
- Disadvantages
  - —Requires IV contrast (acute contrast reactions and renal failure)
  - —Isolated diaphragmatic, pancreatic, bowel injuries may be missed, especially if performed immediately after injury
- Indications
  - —Hemodynamically stable patients
- Contraindications
  - —Absolute: preexisting indication for exploratory laparotomy, hemodynamic instability, previous contrast reaction
  - —Relative: multiple allergies
- Considerations
  - —Modality of choice in children
  - —Many multiple-injury patients require CT imaging of the head, spine, chest, or pelvis; modern equipment provides for rapid scanning of multiple anatomic regions in one session
  - —Monitoring must be continued in the CT suite; patients should be accompanied by appropriate medical personnel
  - —Water may be substituted for oral contrast, but optimal detection of intestinal injury requires oral contrast and a 2- to 4-hour delay for intestinal opacification

Diagnostic Peritoneal Lavage

- Advantages
  - —Rapid
  - —Easy to perform
  - —97.8% accurate in diagnosing injury
- Disadvantages
  - —Invasive
  - —Does not identify specific organ injury
  - —1–2% complication rate
  - —May miss retroperitoneal injuries and intraperitoneal bladder rupture
- Indications
  - —Hemodynamically unstable patients
  - —Patients requiring emergent surgery for other conditions (e.g., craniotomy for epidural hematoma)
  - —Stab wounds that penetrate the abdominal fascia
- Contraindications
  - —Absolute: preexisting indication for exploratory laparotomy
  - —Relative: previous abdominal surgery, severe abdominal distention, pregnancy, pediatric patients
  - —Nasogastric tube and Foley catheter placement mandatory prior to procedure
  - —Positive test
    - -Aspiration of >10 cc of blood, bile, bowel contents, or urine
    - -DPL fluid in the urine or chest tube
    - -Blunt trauma >100,000 RBC/mm^3
    - -Penetrating trauma >1,000 RBC/mm^3
  - —Considerations
    - -Favored in stab wound patients when local wound exploration is positive
    - -Favored in unstable blunt trauma patients as may be performed simultaneously with other emergent surgical interventions (e.g., craniotomy for epidural hematoma)
    - -Must always be accompanied by serial abdominal exams after procedure
    - -In the presence of pelvic fractures, use supraumbilical location
    - -In pregnancy, consider supraumbilical or open technique
    - -False-positive results may be obtained if performed more than 8 hours following injury

PEDIATRIC CONSIDERATIONS

- Because so many pediatric patients can be managed nonoperatively, CT scan, which provides the best anatomic information, is the study of choice in all but the most unstable pediatric patient

DIFFERENTIAL DIAGNOSIS

See Abdominal Trauma, Blunt; and Abdominal Trauma, Penetrating

Treatment

INITIAL STABILIZATION

See Abdominal Trauma, Blunt; and Abdominal Trauma, Penetrating

ED MANAGEMENT

See Abdominal Trauma, Blunt; and Abdominal Trauma, Penetrating

MEDICATIONS

See Abdominal Trauma, Blunt; and Abdominal Trauma, Penetrating

Disposition

ADMISSION CRITERIA

See Abdominal Trauma, Blunt; and Abdominal Trauma, Penetrating

DISCHARGE CRITERIA

See Abdominal Trauma, Blunt; and Abdominal Trauma, Penetrating

Miscellaneous

ICD9: N/A

ICD10: N/A

SEE ALSO: ABDOMINAL TRAUMA, BLUNT; AND ABDOMINAL TRAUMA, PENETRATING

SUGGESTED READINGS

Amoroso TA. Evaluation of the patient with blunt abdominal trauma: an evidence based approach. Emerg Med Clin North Am 1999;17(1):63–75.

Boulanger BR, McLellan BA. Blunt abdominal trauma. Emerg Med Clin North Am 1996;14(1):151–171.

Chiquito PE. Blunt abdominal injuries. Diagnostic peritoneal lavage, ultrasonography and computed tomography scanning. Injury 1996;27(2):117–124.

Demetriades D, Charalambides D, Lakhoo M, et al. Gunshot wound of the abdomen: role of selective conservative management. Br J Surg 1991;78(2):220–222.

McGahan JP, Richards JR. Blunt abdominal trauma: the role of emergent sonography and review of the literature. AJR 1999;172(4):897–903.

Salim A, Velmahos GC. When to operate on abdominal gunshot wounds. Scand J Surg 2002;91(1):62–66.

Author: Chris Richards

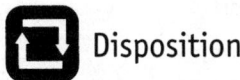

Abdominal Trauma, Penetrating

Clinical Presentation

SIGNS AND SYMPTOMS

- Penetrating wound from knife, gun, or other foreign object
- Spectrum of presentation from localized pain to peritoneal signs
  —High-velocity projectile can cause shock wave in tissues and extensive tissue damage
  —Exit wound may cause greater damage than entrance wound
- Remember the borders of the abdomen: superior from the nipples (anteriorly) or inferior tip of scapula (posteriorly) to the inferior gluteal folds

MECHANISM/DESCRIPTION

- Solid organ injury usually results in hemorrhage
- Hollow viscous injury can lead to bowel content spillage and peritonitis

ETIOLOGY

- 80% of gunshot wounds and 20–30% of stab wounds to the abdomen result in significant intraabdominal injury
- The most commonly injured structures are the liver (37%), small bowel (26%), stomach (19%), colon (17%), major vessel (13%), retroperitoneum (10%), mesentery/omentum (10%), and less often the spleen (7%), diaphragm (5%), kidney (5%), pancreas (4%), duodenum (2%), and biliary tract (1%)
- Injury to both thoracic structures and abdominal structures occurs 25% of the time

Pre-Hospital

CONTROVERSIES

- MAST trousers should not be used in the treatment of penetrating abdominal wounds
- The current standard of care in the treatment of hypovolemic shock is volume resuscitation with crystalloid solutions

CAUTIONS

- Apply sterile dressings to open wounds and eviscerated bowel
- Secure in place impaled foreign objects; do not remove them

Diagnosis

ESSENTIAL WORKUP

- Diagnosis of intraabdominal injury from gunshot wounds to the abdomen are made by laparotomy in the OR
- Locally explore stab wounds to the abdomen
- If the wound penetrates the anterior fascial layer, the patient should receive a diagnostic peritoneal lavage or bedside ultrasound by a skilled sonographer
- Diagnostic laparoscopy is useful in diagnosing diaphragmatic injury, spleen, and liver lacerations; it may help avoid unnecessary laparotomies in equivocal penetrating wounds
- CT is useful in evaluation of patients with a suspected retroperitoneal injury but is not reliable for detection of hollow viscus or diaphragmatic injuries
- If $\geq$1,000 RBC/mm^3 are found in the diagnostic peritoneal lavage (DPL) fluid, the patient should undergo laparotomy
- If $<$1,000 RBC/mm^3 are present, the patient should be observed for 8–24 hours for the development of peritoneal signs

LABORATORY

- Hematocrit should be drawn initially and may be obtained serially to assess for ongoing hemorrhage
- Urinalysis for blood should be performed to assess for possible genitourinary injuries
- ABGs: The base deficit may be helpful in assessing degree of hypovolemia and guide volume resuscitation
- Type and cross should be performed in all patients with significant intraabdominal injuries

IMAGING

- Plain films should be taken after placement of markers for localization of foreign bodies, missiles, and associated fractures, and free air
- Bedside abdominal US may help in identifying intraperitoneal fluid or blood
- CT scan or IVP may be used if there is a suspicion of retroperitoneal injury

DIFFERENTIAL DIAGNOSIS

- Consider the possibility of accompanying intrathoracic injury with upper abdominal wounds
- Likewise, consider the possibility of intraabdominal injury after penetrating wounds to the lower thoracic area

Treatment

INITIAL STABILIZATION

- ABCs
- Two large-bore IVs with crystalloid infusion
- 100% oxygen by non-rebreather face mask
- Packed RBC infusion if no response to 2 L of crystalloid
  - —May use 0-negative blood initially
  - —Type specific and crossmatched blood as it becomes available

ED TREATMENT

- A nasogastric tube (NGT) should be placed to decrease the chance of aspiration; it should be placed prior to DPL to decompress the stomach and decrease chances of iatrogenic injury
  - —An NGT may also relieve respiratory distress if there is a diaphragmatic injury with herniated abdominal contents in the thorax
- A Foley catheter should be placed once urethral injuries have been ruled out to facilitate rapid assessment for genitourinary injury, as well as to assist the monitoring of urinary output
- Tetanus toxoid if appropriate; tetanus immune globulin if primary tetanus vaccination series not administered

MEDICATIONS

- Tetanus toxoid 0.5 cc IM
- Tetanus immunoglobulin 250 units IM for patients who have not had complete series

PEDIATRIC CONSIDERATIONS

- Children in hypovolemic shock should receive 20 cc/kg boluses of crystalloid
- Children in severe hypovolemic shock should receive 1 cc/kg of packed RBCs
- Age less than 8 years is a relative contraindication for DPL

Disposition

ADMISSION CRITERIA

- Patients requiring abdominal surgery
- Observe all patients for at least 8 hours who had negative DPL, US, or CT
  - —These patients should receive frequent abdominal exams
  - —Repeat hematocrits should be performed on these patients at regular intervals

DISCHARGE CRITERIA

- Patients with stab wounds who had no evidence of fascial involvement may be discharged after observation in the emergency department

Miscellaneous

ICD9: 868.00

ICD10: S31.8

SUGGESTED READINGS

Feliciano DV, Rozycki GS. The management of penetrating abdominal trauma. Adv Surg 1995;28:1–39.

Ferrada R, Birolini D. New concepts in the management of patients with penetrating abdominal wounds. Surg Clin North Am 1999;79(6):1331–1356.

Thal ER. Evaluation of peritoneal lavage and local exploration in lower chest and abdominal stab wounds. J Trauma 1979;17:642.

Thompson JS, Moore EE, Van Duzer-Moore S, et al. The evolution of abdominal stab wound management. J Trauma 1980;20:478.

Author: Stewart Coffman

Abortion, Spontaneous

Clinical Presentation

SIGNS AND SYMPTOMS

- Lower abdominal pain, cramping
- Vaginal bleeding with or without the passage of clots or products of conception
- Dizziness or syncope
- Known positive pregnancy test or sexually active with a period of amenorrhea

DEFINITIONS

- *Threatened abortion:* vaginal bleeding, cervical os is closed, viable intrauterine pregnancy confirmed
- *Inevitable abortion:* vaginal bleeding, cervical os is open
- *Incomplete abortion:* vaginal bleeding, cervical os is open with partial passage of products of conception (POC) and some retained POC
- *Complete abortion:* vaginal bleeding, cervical os closed, complete passage of POC
- *Missed abortion:* nonviable intrauterine pregnancy, os closed, +/− vaginal bleeding

MECHANISM/DESCRIPTION

- Spontaneous termination of a <20-week intrauterine pregnancy
- Vaginal bleeding in the first trimester of pregnancy is seen in 20–25% of pregnant patients; approximately 50% of these women will eventually miscarry

ETIOLOGY

- Risk factors include increased age of both the mother and father, increased parity
- Most early miscarriages are from abnormalities of the fetus

Pre-Hospital

CAUTIONS

- Patients with SAB/vaginal bleeding can have severe hemorrhage and present in shock, especially >12 weeks
- Blood pressure drops during the second trimester of pregnancy with an average of 110/70
- These patients need to be fully resuscitated with IV fluids, oxygen, and cardiac monitor

Diagnosis

ESSENTIAL WORKUP

- *History* including last menstrual period (LMP), duration and amount of bleeding (quantify by number of pads used, compare to normal menstrual period for patient), passage of clots, presence of abdominal pain, fevers, dizziness, or light-headedness
- *Physical examination*
  - —Determine hemodynamic status of patient; pregnant patients beginning in the late first trimester have an increased blood volume and can lose substantial amount of blood before having abnormal vital signs
  - —Pelvic exam to *determine whether the internal cervical os is opened or closed,* amount of bleeding, and the presence of any POC; the presence of adnexal tenderness or peritoneal irritation can be consistent with an ectopic pregnancy
  - —Bimanual exam to determine the size of the uterus
    - -Size of an orange: 6–8 weeks
    - -Fundus at the symphysis pubis: 12 weeks
    - -Fundus at the umbilicus: 16–20 weeks
  - —Confirm pregnancy with urine or serum testing
  - —Rapid hemoglobin determination; type and Rh

LABORATORY

- Confirm pregnancy with a urine or serum test
  - —Urine pregnancy test: most are positive at β-hCG levels of 50 mIU/mL approximately 1 week gestational age and remain positive 2–3 weeks after induced or spontaneous abortions
- CBC, type and Rh
- Type and crossmatch for woman with low Hct or signs of active blood loss
- Quantitative β-hCG if indicated (see below)
- Any POC passed should be sent to pathology for confirmation

IMAGING/SPECIAL TESTS

- Vaginal ultrasound: gestational sac seen at 5 weeks; cardiac activity seen at 6.5 weeks
- Abdominal ultrasound: gestational sac at 6 weeks; cardiac activity seen at 8 weeks
- Diagnostic of intrauterine pregnancy (IUP): "double" gestational sac sign, intrauterine fetal pole or yolk sac, intrauterine fetal heart activity

DIFFERENTIAL DIAGNOSIS

- Positive pregnancy test with vaginal bleeding
  - —Cervicitis
  - —Ectopic pregnancy
  - —Trauma
  - —Septic abortions
  - —Molar pregnancy
- Second- and third-trimester vaginal bleeding
  - —Placenta previa
  - —Placental abruption

Treatment

INITIAL STABILIZATION

- Stable patients
  - —IV
  - —Pelvic exam
- Unstable patients
  - —Oxygen, IV fluids via two large-bore IVs, cardiac monitor
  - —Transfuse PRBC if patient does not stabilize after 2–3 L of crystalloid
  - —Gynecologic consultation immediately
  - —Oxytocin or methylergonovine may be necessary to control hemorrhage
  - —These patients are at high risk for having ruptured ectopic pregnancies and may need emergent operative intervention

ED TREATMENT

- Threatened abortion
  - —Pelvic rest, close follow-up with obstetrics
  - —Patients less than 6.5 weeks pregnant with no documented cardiac activity by vaginal ultrasound, need to be followed with serial β-hCG to assess the viability of the fetus and to rule out ectopic pregnancy
- Inevitable and incomplete abortions
  - —Dilation and curettage or evacuation, removal of POC at the cervical os to help decrease bleeding and cramping
  - —The confirmation of POC by pathology rules out ectopic pregnancy
- Complete abortion
  - —May treat with methylergonovine or oxytocin if bleeding is heavy
  - —If quantitative β-hCG is <1,000 and the ultrasound is negative, may follow-up with obstetrics for serial β-hCG to confirm the levels are decreasing
- Missed abortion
  - —These patients are at risk for disseminated intravascular coagulation (DIC) especially if fetus is retained >4–6 weeks
  - —Obtain CBC, PT/PTT, FSP (fibrin split products), and fibrinogen levels
  - —These patients may be followed closely as outpatients if stable with an early, confirmed IUP and no evidence of DIC; these patients may choose to have a dilation and curettage at a later date or miscarry at home with no intervention; this decision should be done with consultation of OB/Gyn

MEDICATIONS

- Oxytocin: 20 IU in 1,000 mL of NS at a rate of 20 mIU/min titrated to decrease bleeding; may repeat for a max dose of 40 mIU/min
- Methylergonovine: 0.2 mg IM/PO qid PRN bleeding
- RHO immune globulin in Rh-negative women: 50 μg for women with threatened or complete abortion <12 weeks; 300 μg for women with threatened or complete abortion $\geq$12 weeks
- Patients need RhoGAM administration within 72 hours to prevent future isoimmunization

Disposition

ADMISSION CRITERIA

- Suspected unstable ectopic pregnancy (see Ectopic Pregnancy)
- Any hemodynamically unstable patients with hypovolemia or anemia
- DIC
- Septic abortions
- Suspected gestational trophoblastic disease

DISCHARGE CRITERIA

- Many dilation and curettages are done in the emergency department for incomplete and inevitable abortions and may be discharged home if stable after 2–3 hours
- Patients with threatened abortions should be told to avoid strenuous activity
- Pelvic rest, i.e., "nothing in the vagina" during active bleeding, as this may increase the risk of infection
- Patients should be instructed to return to the emergency department for any increase in bleeding, dizziness, or temperature >100.4°F
- Patients and their partners should be told that early miscarriages are common and that they are not anyone's fault

Miscellaneous

ICD9: 634.90

ICD10: 003

SUGGESTED READINGS

Hansen WF, Hansen AR. Problems in pregnancy. In: Tintinalli JE, ed. Emergency medicine: a comprehensive study guide, 4th ed. New York: McGraw-Hill, 1996.

Houry D, Abbott J. Acute complications of pregnancy. In: Rosen P, et al., eds. Emergency medicine: concepts and clinical practice, 5th ed. St. Louis: CV Mosby, 2002:2413–2433.

Turner LM. Vaginal bleeding during pregnancy. Emerg Med Clin North Am 1994;12:45.

Author: Aviva Jacoby Zigman

Abruptio Placenta

Clinical Presentation

SIGNS AND SYMPTOMS

- Typically occur in second half of pregnancy
  - —*Painful vaginal bleeding*
  - —*Abdominal pain*
  - —Signs of *hypotensive shock* may be present
  - —*Uterine cramps,* tenderness, frequent contractions, or tetany
  - —Back pain
  - —Nausea, vomiting
  - —Decreased fetal heart tones and movement
  - —Petechiae, bleeding and other signs of disseminated intravascular coagulation (DIC)
  - —Nontender uterus may occur with complete abruption
  - —Bleeding may be concealed in 20–25%

MECHANISM/DESCRIPTION

- Separation of the placenta from the uterine wall; may occur from trauma or spontaneously
- Dissection of blood into the decidua basalis or mechanical shearing between the placenta and uterus results in clot formation, bleeding, development of DIC, and maternal-fetal compromise

INCIDENCE/PREVALENCE

- Approximately 1% of all pregnancies
- 30% of bleeding episodes in the second half of pregnancy
- Accounts for 15% of all fetal deaths
- Accounts for 6% of all maternal mortality
- Risk of recurrence 10–20%

ETIOLOGY

- Primary etiology is unknown
- Blunt abdominal trauma
- Spontaneous dissection of blood into the decidua basalis
- Drugs, especially sympathomimetics

RISK FACTORS

- Maternal hypertension (>140/90)
- Increased maternal age
- Increased parity
- Previous abruption
- Tobacco use
- Premature rupture of membranes with sudden decompression of uterus
- Precipitous first twin delivery endangers second twin
- Fibroids

Pre-Hospital

CAUTIONS

- Patients with abruption may be in shock and need full resuscitative measures
- Hypotension frequently occurs late in the course of hypovolemic shock in pregnancy
- In advanced pregnancy, transport in the left lateral recumbent position

Diagnosis

ESSENTIAL WORKUP

- Blood type, Rh, and crossmatch
- Rapid hemoglobin determination
- Ultrasound
  - —Ultrasound demonstrates evidence of abruption in only 50% of cases
  - —False-negative with posterior abruptions (concealed hemorrhage)
- Determine fetal heart tones by Doppler (10 weeks' gestation or later)
- Fetal monitoring sensitive for detecting early fetal distress
- Uterine tocographic monitoring may demonstrate frequent contractions, rarely tetany
- Sterile vaginal examination
  - —Performed with great caution to avoid further tissue injury, especially if placenta previa suspected
  - —Assess for presence of amniotic fluid (Nitrazine paper turns blue or ferning of fluid on glass slide)
  - —Evaluate for vaginal or cervical lacerations

LABORATORY

- CBC, platelets
- PT/PTT (anticipate consumptive coagulopathy)
- Fibrinogen levels (normally 450 in latter half of pregnancy), fibrin-split products
- Betke-Kleihauer

IMAGING/SPECIAL TESTS

- MRI is most sensitive in detecting small or posterior abruption

DIFFERENTIAL DIAGNOSIS

- Placenta previa
- Vasa previa
- Bleeding during labor
- Vaginal or cervical lacerations
- Uterine rupture
- Preterm labor
- Ovarian torsion
- Pyelonephritis
- Cholelithiasis/cholecystitis
- Preeclampsia complications
- Other blunt intraabdominal injuries

Treatment

INITIAL STABILIZATION

- ABCs, oxygen
- Cardiac monitor
- IV crystalloid resuscitation

ED TREATMENT

- Maternal cardiac and tocographic monitoring
- Fetal monitoring
- PRBCs, FFP, platelets as indicated
- Immediate OB-Gyn consultation
- If abruption is suspected in the setting of trauma, maternal stabilization is of primary importance
  - —All indicated x-rays should be performed as needed

MEDICATIONS

- RhoGAM in Rh-negative women: 50 μg IM in women <12 weeks pregnant; 300 μg IM in women $\geq$12 weeks pregnant

Disposition

ADMISSION CRITERIA

- Patients with abruptio placenta must be admitted for maternal and fetal monitoring
- Admit to ICU setting if DIC, amniotic fluid embolism, or significant hemorrhage occurs
- Victims of multiple trauma with abruption should be admitted and managed in accordance with trauma protocols
- Transportation to higher trauma or obstetric level of care is appropriate if the patient is stable for transfer

DISCHARGE CRITERIA

- Patients with no evidence of abruption or other significant injury may be discharged after 4–6 hours of normal maternal and fetal monitoring
- Discharge instructions include pelvic rest, no intercourse, no heavy lifting, no prolonged standing

Miscellaneous

SYNONYMS

- Placental abruption
- Ablatio placentae
- Premature separation of the placenta

ICD9: 641.20

ICD10: 045.9

SUGGESTED READINGS

Baron F, Hill WC. Placenta previa, placenta abruptio. Clin Obstet Gynecol 1998;41(3):527–532.

Cunningham FG, MacDonald PC, Gant NF, eds. Williams' obstetrics, 20th ed. Stamford, CT: Appleton & Lange, 1997.

Gabbe SG, Niebyl JR, Simpson JL, eds. Obstetrics: normal and problem pregnancies, 4th ed. New York: Churchill Livingstone, 2002.

Marx J, ed. Rosen's emergency medicine, 5th ed. St. Louis: Mosby, 2002.

Author: Rebecah M. Wilks

Abscess, Skin/Soft Tissue

Clinical Presentation

SIGNS AND SYMPTOMS

- Local: erythema, tenderness, pain, heat, swelling, fluctuantes
- Systemic: absent to fever, rigors, malaise, hypotension, and altered mentation
- Regional lymphadenopathy and lymphangitis may occur

MECHANISM/DESCRIPTION

- A localized collection of pus surrounded and walled off by inflamed tissue
  —Bacterial: most abscesses are bacterial, with the microbiology reflective of the microflora of the body part involved
  —Sterile: tend to be associated with IV drug abuse and injection of chemical irritants

ETIOLOGY

Conditions associated with soft tissue abscess formation include

- Soft tissue trauma
- Dog or cat bites
- Bacteremia with hematogenous seeding
- Obstruction of normal drainage (sweat glands)
- Tissue ischemia
- Intravenous drug abuse
- Endocarditis
- Lactation disease
- Crohn's disease

Specific Abscesses and Typical Microbiology

- Dog/cat bites: *Pasteurella* species/anaerobes often involved; usually polymicrobial
- Orbital abscess: associated with paranasal sinusitis, hematogenous spread, or local skin trauma; staphylococci, streptococci, *H. flu*, *E. coli*, polymicrobial
- Breast abscess: microbiology is dependent on type of abscess
  —Puerperal: classically occurs during lactation, location is peripheral wedge and caused by staphylococci
  —Duct ectasia: typically caused by ectatic ducts, location is periareolar, and is polymicrobial with a mix of staphylococci, anaerobic streptococci, bacteroides, and enterococci
- Hidradenitis suppurativa: chronic abscesses of apocrine sweat glands, especially in the groin and axilla; *S. aureus* and *S. viridans* are common pathogens; *E. coli* and *Proteus* may be present in chronic disease
- Pilonidal abscess: caused by epithelial disruption in gluteal fold over coccyx; staphylococcal species most common; also polymicrobial with bacteroides and *E. coli*
- Bartholin's abscess: obstruction of Bartholin duct; composed of mixed vaginal flora and may include *N. gonorrhea, C. trachomatis,* and *E. coli*
- Perirectal abscess: originates in anal crypts and extends through ischiorectal space; inflammatory bowel disease and diabetes are major predisposing factors; *B. fragilis* and *E. coli* are the most common pathogens; requires treatment in the OR
- Pyomyositis: abscess in muscle, typically occurs in tropics; increasingly common with HIV and diabetes; *S. aureus* most common
- Abscesses in association with IVDA: staphylococci species, *S. milleri*, and anaerobes; often isolates of oral origin; may be sterile
- Furuncle: arises from infected hair follicle; most common on back, axilla, and lower extremities; staphylococci species are most common
- Carbuncle: larger and more extensive than furuncle; often multiple in a honeycomb pattern on back of neck; more common in diabetics; invariably caused by staphylococci
- Paronychia: infection surrounding the nail fold; *S. aureus*
- Felon: closed space abscess in distal pulp of finger; *S. aureus*

Pre-Hospital

CAUTIONS

- Septic patients may require rapid transport with intravenous access and volume resuscitation

Diagnosis

ESSENTIAL WORKUP

- History and physical examination
  - —Identify subcutaneous air and involvement of deeper structures
- Gram stain is unnecessary for simple abscesses in healthy individuals
- Wound cultures are not indicated in simple abscesses in healthy patients
  - —May help differentiate aerobic from anaerobic infections and help guide specific therapy in a compromised host, abscesses of the central face or hand, and in treatment failures

LABORATORY

- A glucose determination may be a useful screening test for diabetes
- Blood cultures are indicated only if either endocarditis is suspected or patient is systemically ill

IMAGING/SPECIAL TESTS

- Plain films may demonstrate the presence of gas in the tissue planes
- Ultrasound, CT, or MRI may be helpful when diagnosis is in question

DIFFERENTIAL DIAGNOSIS

- Cellulitis
- Aneurysm (especially with IV drug abusers)
- Cysts
- Hematoma

Treatment

INITIAL STABILIZATION

- Immediate IV access, oxygen, crystalloid volume resuscitation, blood cultures, and antibiotic therapy are indicated for the septic patient with soft tissue abscesses

ED TREATMENT

- Incision and drainage is the mainstay of treatment
- Antibiotics are indicated for the following conditions:
  - —Sepsis
  - —Systemic illness
  - —Endocarditis
  - —Facial abscesses drained into the cavernous sinus
  - —Concurrent cellulitis (see medications below)
  - —Dog and cat bite infections
  - —Immunocompromised hosts

SPECIAL PEDIATRIC CONSIDERATIONS

- Incision and drainage is a painful procedure and often requires sedation and analgesia

MEDICATIONS

- Augmentin 250–500 mg po q8h (peds: 40–80 mg/kg/day divided into 3 doses)
- Cephalexin 250–500 mg po q8h; or 500 mg po q12h (peds: 25–50 mg/kg/day po in 4 doses)
- Clindamycin 150–450 mg po q6h (peds: 10–20 mg/kg/day po or i.v. in 3–4 divided doses)
- Dicloxacillin 250–500 mg po q6h (peds: 50–100 mg/kg/day in 4 divided doses)
- Erythromycin 500 mg–1 g po or i.v. q6h (peds: 40 mg/kg/day po divided q6h)
- Gentamicin 5 mg/kg/day i.v. q24h (peds: 7.5 mg/kg/day i.v. divided q8h)
- Levaquin 500 mg i.v. q24h (contraindicated in peds)
- Unasyn 1.5–3.0 g i.v. q6h (peds: $<$40 kg, 300 mg/kg/d divided q6h, $\geq$40 kg, adult dose)
- Vancomycin 500 mg i.v. q6h (peds: 40 mg/kg/day i.v. divided q6h)
- Levaquin 500 mg i.v. q24h (contraindicated in peds)

Disposition

ADMISSION CRITERIA

- Sepsis, endocarditis, systemic illness, perirectal involvement, abscesses extensive enough to require incision and debridement in the OR

DISCHARGE CRITERIA

- The majority of patients with uncomplicated abscesses can be treated with I&D and close follow-up

Miscellaneous

ICD9: 682.9

ICD10: L02.9

SUGGESTED READINGS

Benson EA. Management of breast abscesses. World J Surg 1989;13: 753–756.

Canales FL, Newmeyer WL, Kilgore ES. The treatment of felons and paronychias. Hand Clin 1989;5(4):515–522.

Chiedozi LC. Pyomyositis: review of 205 cases in 112 patients. Am J Surg 1979;137:255–259.

Loyer EM, DuBrow RA, David CL, et al. Imaging of superficial soft-tissue infections: sonographic findings in cases of cellulitis and abscess. AJR 1995;166: 149–152.

Meislin HW. Pathogen identification of abscesses and cellulitis. Ann Emerg Med 1986;15(3):329–332.

Summanen PH, Talan DA, Strong C, et al. Bacteriology of skin and soft-tissue infections in intravenous drug users and individuals with no history of intravenous drug use. Clin Infect Dis 1995;20(suppl 2):S279–282.

Talan DA, Citron DM, Abrahamian FM, et al. Bacteriologic analysis of infected dog and cat bites. N Engl J Med 1999;340(2): 85–92.

Author: Nate Rudman

Abuse, Elder

Clinical Presentation

SIGNS AND SYMPTOMS

- Inconsistent history or physical findings
  - —Patterns or variable age bruises, burns, lacerations/abrasions
  - —Unusual sites of bruising (inner arm, torso, buttocks, scalp)
  - —Poor hygiene (inadequate care of skin, nails, teeth)
- Unexplained injuries
  - —Bruised or bleeding genital or rectal area
- Multiple visits to doctor or hospital
  - —Previously developed reasonable treatment plan unsuccessful
- Vague explanations
- Delay in obtaining medical care/previously untreated medical condition
  - —Dehydration
  - —Weight loss
  - —Decubitus ulcer
- Medication difficulties
  - —Incorrect doses
  - —Lost medications
  - —Unfilled prescriptions
- Altered interpersonal interactions
  - —Withdrawn
  - —Indifferent
  - —Demoralized
  - —Fearful
  - —Substance abuse
- Caregiver with
  - —Financial dependence on patient
  - —Substance abuse, psychiatric, or violence history
  - —Controlling behavior (may refuse to leave elder alone with physician) or poor knowledge of patient's condition
  - —Significant life stressors
    - -Relationship issues
    - -Financial difficulties
    - -Legal problems

ETIOLOGY

- One million known cases annually in U.S.
  - —Only 2% reported by physicians
- Caregiver stress, dependency, or psychopathology
- Victim dependency, or diminishment of ability to perform activities of daily living

MECHANISM/DESCRIPTION

- Emotional abuse
  - —Insults
  - —Humiliation
  - —Threats (to institutionalize or abandon)
- Physical abuse and/or sexual abuse
  - —Hitting
  - —Slapping
  - —Pushing
  - —Burning
  - —Inappropriate restraining
  - —Forced sexual activity
- Material exploitation
  - —Stealing or coercion involving patient monies or properties
- Neglect
  - —Behaviors by a patient or caregiver that compromise the patient's health or safety
  - —Failure to provide adequate food, shelter, hygiene, medical attention

Pre-Hospital

CAUTIONS

- Observe details of the patient's environment that may not be immediately available to the hospital care team
  - —Interpersonal interactions at the scene
    - -Embarrassment
    - -Shame
    - -Fear of reprisal/abandonment/ institutionalization
  - —Conditions of physical environment to determine potential areas of danger

Diagnosis

ESSENTIAL WORKUP

- Perform any examination, laboratory, or x-ray indicated by the patient's condition
- Obtain history without family members/caregivers present
  - —Abused elders may fear institutionalization if they report caregivers
  - —Many may feel embarrassment and responsibility for the abuse
  - —Frequently will not volunteer information to the health care team
    - -Ask patient specifically about abuse or neglect (in private)
- Obtain history from other relatives/friends/ neighbors
- Document a clear and detailed description of the patient's findings including
  - —Statements of the patient as they pertain to the abuse
  - —Psychosocial history
    - -Family and other social relationships
    - -Caregiver burdens/coping mechanisms
    - -Drug/ethanol (EtOH) use
    - -Prior Adult Protective Services reports
  - —Skin and other physical findings
    - -Photographic documentation
- Safety assessment

DIFFERENTIAL DIAGNOSIS

- Patient may present with any chief complaint
  - —Potential differential diagnosis nonspecific
  - —Abuse best identified by asking the patient about it directly in a setting apart from caregivers/family and correlating with risk factors and provider findings
  - —Findings consistent with other disease etiologies must be differentiated from abuse/neglect (examples: dehydration, ill-fitting dentures, burns, ecchymoses, insomnia, medication noncompliance, dementia, depression)

Treatment

INITIAL STABILIZATION

- ABCs
- Treat life-threatening medical/traumatic condition as appropriate

ED TREATMENT

- May require separation of the patient and the caregiver or family member
- Competent elder patients are free to accept or decline any treatments or dispositions they wish despite the risks they may incur
- Many states have mandatory reporting requirements
  —Call Adult Protective Services

Disposition

ADMISSION CRITERIA

- Medical condition calling for admission
- Abuse or neglect renders home conditions unsafe

DISCHARGE CRITERIA

- Medical conditions addressed
- Safe environment available
- Abuse or neglect successfully countered by social services or law enforcement

Miscellaneous

ICD9: V61.3

ICD10: T74.1

SUGGESTED READINGS

Clarke ME, Pierson W. Management of elder abuse in the emergency department. Emerg Med Clin North Am 1999;17(3):631–644.

Kleinschmidt K. Elder abuse: a review. Ann Emerg Med 1997;30(4):463–472.

Kruger RM, Moon CH. Can you spot the signs of elder mistreatment? Postgrad Med 1999;106(2):169–183.

Lynch SH. Elder abuse: what to look for, how to intervene. Am J Nurs 1997;97(1):26–32.

Marshall CE, Benton D, Brazier JM. Elder abuse: using clinical tools to identify clues of mistreatment. Geriatrics 2000;55(2):42–53.

Vernon MJ, Bennett GC. Elder abuse. Br J Hosp Med 1996:56(5):234–237.

Author: Helen Straus

Abuse, Pediatric (Nonaccidental Trauma, NAT)

Clinical Presentation

SIGNS AND SYMPTOMS

- History and mechanism inconsistent with the injury or illness
  - —Unexplained death, apnea, injury
  - —Unexplained ingestion or toxin exposure
  - —Recurrent injury
- Parent/caregiver reluctant to give information or deny knowledge of how injury occurred
  - —Discrepancy among different caregivers
- Developmentally, child unable to experience mechanism
- Inappropriate response to injury or illness; delay in seeking care
- Cutaneous bruising/contusions
  - —Regular pattern, straight line of demarcation, regular angles, slap marks from fingers, dunking burns (stocking or glove burns or doughnut shaped on buttock), bites, strap, buckle
  - —Location: buttocks, hips, face (not forehead), arms, back, thighs, genitalia, pinna
  - —Aging
    - -Often different ages
    - -Yellow bruises are older than 18 hours
    - -Red, blue and purple, or black color may occur from 1 hour after injury to resolution
    - -Red may be present irrespective of age
    - -Bruises of identical age and cause on the same person may appear to be different
- Skeletal trauma
  - —Usually multiple, unexplained, various stages of healing
  - —Metaphyseal or corner (classic metaphyseal lesions) fractures (pathognomonic)
  - —Skull fractures that cross suture lines
  - —Posterior rib fractures (rib fractures almost never occur in infants from CPR)
  - —Spiral fractures of long bones
  - —Subperiosteal new bone formation
  - —Uncommon fractures (vertebrae, sternum, scapula, spinous process) without significant mechanism
- Central nervous system
  - —Altered mental status, seizure
  - —Head trauma is leading cause of death in child abuse
  - —Skull fracture; must consider child abuse in children <1 year
  - —Subdural hematoma, subarachnoid hemorrhage
  - —"Shaken-baby syndrome" with shearing and rotational injury
- Ocular findings
  - —Retinal hemorrhage or detachment
  - —Hyphema
  - —Corneal abrasion/conjunctival hemorrhage
- Oral trauma
- Abdominal injuries
  - —Lacerated liver, spleen, kidney, pancreas
  - —Intramural hematoma (duodenal most common)
  - —Retroperitoneal hematoma
- Anogenital/sexual abuse
  - —Credible history
  - —Contusion, erythema, open wounds, scarring, foreign material (hair, debris, semen)
  - —Presence of STD or pregnancy in child <12 years
- Death
  - —Unexplained death
- Munchausen by proxy
  - —Recurrent illness without medical explanation
  - —Unexplained metabolic disorder suspicious for poisoning
- Failure to thrive
  - —Inadequate caloric intake secondary to poor maternal bonding/neglect

MECHANISM/DESCRIPTION

- Child abuse effects up to 14 million or 2–3% of U.S. children each year
- Up to 2,000 children die of maltreatment each year, 80% <5 years and 40% <1 year
- Mandated reporters of suspected abuse or neglect including all health care workers
- Risk factors
  - —Child: usually <4 years, often handicapped, retarded or special needs ("vulnerable child"), premature birth, multiple birth
  - —Abusive parent: low self-esteem, abused as child, violent temper, mental illness history, rigid and unrealistic expectations of child, young maternal age
  - —Family: monetary problems, isolated and mobile, marital instability
  - —Poor parent-child relationship, unwanted pregnancy
  - —Abuse crosses all religious and socioeconomic groups

Pre-Hospital

- Diagnosis relies on physical evidence in child and inconsistency with the history and mechanism
- Examination of the scene may be useful
  - —Evaluate validity of mechanisms
  - —General appearance of home
  - —Consistency of history by multiple caregivers
  - —Evaluation of parent-child interaction

Diagnosis

ESSENTIAL WORKUP

- Formal oral and written report to appropriate child welfare agency
- Family and environmental evaluation mandatory, usually in cooperation with responsible child welfare agency
- Diagram or photograph of bruises is helpful

LABORATORY

- Bleeding screen if there is a history of recurrent bruising or bruising is the prominent manifestation; may usually be done electively: CBC, platelets, PT/PTT, bleeding time
- If significant blunt trauma, CBC, LFT, amylase, urinalysis
- Toxicology and metabolic screens in children with altered mental status
- Consider other differential considerations

IMAGING/SPECIAL TESTS

- Global assessment
  - —Indicated for children <2 years to exclude unsuspected injuries
  - —In children 2–5 years, in selected cases where physical abuse is strongly suspected
  - —In older children, radiographs of individual sites of injury suspected on clinical grounds
  - —Radiographic skeletal survey
    - -AP and lateral skull
    - -Lateral cervical spine
    - -AP and lateral thoracic and lumbar spine
    - -AP and obliques of chest
    - -AP pelvis
    - -AP of humerus, forearm, and hands (bilateral)
    - -AP femur, tibia, and feet (bilateral)
  - —If fracture identified, get at least two views, 90 degrees to original view
  - —May need coned-down view of joints for visualization of classic metaphyseal lesions
  - —Skeletal scintigraphy provides adjunctive screening if suspicion exists beyond skeletal survey
- Visceral imaging
  - —Suspected thoracoabdominal injury
    - -Abdominal CT scan with IV and oral contrast
    - -Barium upper GI study for gastric and intestinal hematoma
- Neuroimaging
  - —Nonenhanced head CT with brain, subdural and bone windowing
  - —MRI
  - —Adjunctive in evaluation of acute, subacute and chronic intracranial injury; useful for shear injuries, evolving hemorrhage, contusion, secondary hypoxic/ischemic injury

DIFFERENTIAL DIAGNOSIS

- General
  - —Trauma—accidental or birth/obstetrical
- Cutaneous
  - —Burn—accidental
  - —Infection
  - —Impetigo/cellulitis
  - —Staphylococcal scalded skin syndrome
  - —Henoch-Schönlein purpura
  - —Purpura fulminans/meningococcemia
  - —Sepsis
  - —Dermatitis: contact or photo
  - —Hematologic/oncologic disorder (ITP, leukemia)
  - —Bleeding diathesis (hemophilia, von Willebrand)
  - —Nutritional deficiency: scurvy
  - —Cultural healing practices (coining, cupping)
- Skeletal
  - —Osteogenesis imperfecta
  - —Nutritional (rickets, copper deficiency, scurvy)
  - —Menkes' syndrome
  - —Peripheral sensory impairment (indifference to pain)
- Ocular
  - —Conjunctivitis
- Abdomen and GU
  - —GI disease (obstruction, peritonitis, inflammatory bowel disease)
  - —Genitourinary tract infection/anomaly
- CNS
  - —Intoxication, ingestion (CO, lead, mercury)
- Infection
  - —Metabolic: hypoglycemia
  - —Epilepsy
- Death
  - —SIDS, apparent life-threatening event (ALTE)

Treatment

INITIAL STABILIZATION

- Injury-specific intervention

ED TREATMENT

- Medical and trauma management as required
- Mandatory reporting to local child welfare agency to determine appropriate social disposition
  - —Expedited family, environmental, and social evaluation
- Communication with family about report and primary concern is child's welfare
  - —Security may be required to protect child and staff
- Siblings and other household children must be examined in appropriate time frame

MEDICATIONS

N/A

Disposition

ADMISSION CRITERIA

- Observation and intervention for traumatic injury
- Concerns about disposition or lack of availability of child welfare receiving site, if required

DISCHARGE CRITERIA

- Adequate ED evaluation and medical follow-up
- Safe setting for child

Miscellaneous

ICD9: 995.9

ICD10: T74.8

SEE ALSO: TRAUMA, MULTIPLE

SUGGESTED READINGS

Brodeur AE, Monteleone JA. Child maltreatment: a clinical guide and reference. St Louis: CV Mosby, 1994.

Gayle MO, Kissoon N, Hered RW, et al. Retinal hemorrhage in the young child: a review of etiology, predisposed conditions and clinical implications. J Emerg Med 1995;13:233.

Kleinman PK, ed. Diagnostic imaging of child abuse, 2nd ed. St. Louis: Mosby, 1998.

Schreier HA, Libow JA. Munchausen by proxy syndrome: a modern pediatric challenge. J Pediatr 1994;125:S110–115.

Steward GM, Rosenberg NM. Conditions mistaken for child abuse. Parts I and II. Pediatr Emerg Med 1996;12:116.

Author: Suzanne Z. Barkin

Acetaminophen, Poisoning

Clinical Presentation

SIGNS AND SYMPTOMS

Phase 1: 0.5–24 hours postingestion

- Nausea, vomiting, malaise
  - —Occurs with large overdoses
  - —May not be present with smaller toxic doses

Phase 2: 24–72 hours postingestion

- "Quiescent period"
- Decreased GI symptoms
- Hepatic damage is occurring
  - —Right upper quadrant pain and tenderness
  - —Elevation of liver enzymes, PT/INR, bilirubin
  - —Oliguria
  - —Prolonged (>4 hours) acetaminophen (APAP) half-life implies hepatic toxicity

Phase 3: 72–96 hours postingestion

- Critical time period in the prognosis
- Peak liver function abnormalities
- Hepatic encephalopathy develops
- If the PT/INR continues to rise and/or renal insufficiency develops beyond the third day postingestion, there is high likelihood that the patient will require hepatic transplantation

Phase 4: 96 hours to 10 days postingestion

- Resolution of hepatic injury or progression to complete hepatic failure

MECHANISM/DESCRIPTION

- Liver failure caused by NAPQI, the toxic metabolite of APAP
  - —NAPQI produced when APAP metabolized by cytochrome P-450
  - —NAPQI normally detoxified by glutathione
  - —In overdose, glutathione is quickly depleted
  - —*N*-acetylcysteine (NAC) replenishes the liver's glutathione stores
  - —Children are less likely to suffer toxicity from APAP than adults because of increased sulfation activity
- Increased risk of toxicity
  - —Increased activity of cytochrome P-450 system (phenobarbital, rifampin)
  - —Chronic alcoholism
  - —Patients with poor nutrition have decreased glutathione stores

Pharmacokinetics

- APAP half-life
  - —>4 hours in overdose
  - —2.5–4 hours in a non-overdose setting
- Toxic dose >150 mg/kg acutely
- Probable toxic level is 140 μg/mL at 4 hours postingestion (see Fig. 1 nomogram for acute intoxication)
- Therapeutic plasma concentration is 5–20 μg/mL

Pre-Hospital

CAUTIONS

- Transport all pill bottles/pills involved in overdose for identification in ED
- Over-the-counter cold remedies often contain acetaminophen

CONTROVERSIES

- A shortened NAC protocol may be considered with poison center or toxicology consultation

Diagnosis

ESSENTIAL WORKUP

- APAP level
  - —Obtain 4-hour postingestion level or immediately on presentation if >4 hours postingestion
  - —Use Rumack-Matthew nomogram as guide for the single acute overdose
  - —Do not use nomogram in chronic ingestions or very late ingestions

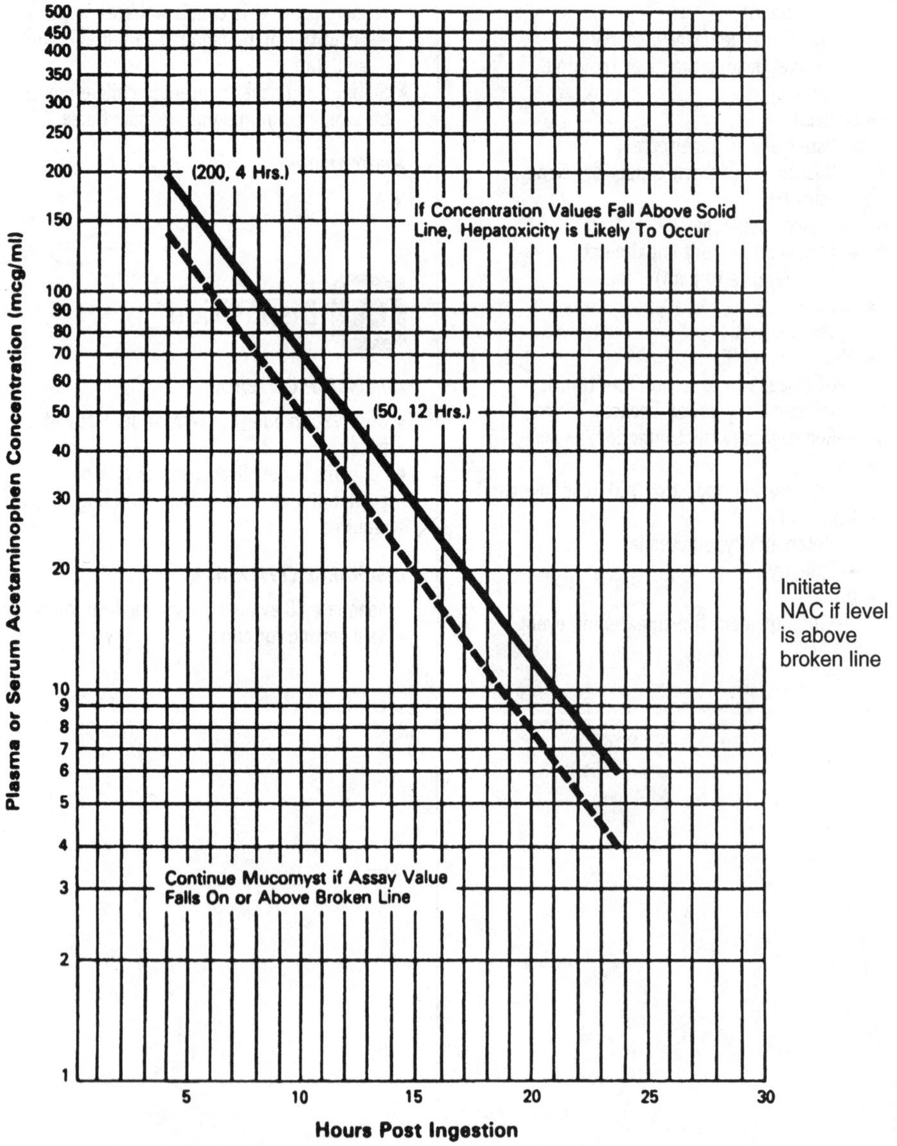

Figure 1.1. Rumack-Matthew nomogram. (Adapted from Rumack BH, Matthew H. Acetaminophen poisoning and toxicity. Pediatrics 1975;55:871–876.)

LABORATORY

- Electrolytes, BUN, Cr, glucose
- Liver enzymes
  - —Baseline value in toxic ingestions
  - —Elevated AST—first abnormality detected
  - —AST/ALT levels may rise >10,000 in stage III of toxicity
- PT/INR
- Bilirubin

DIFFERENTIAL DIAGNOSIS

- Suspect APAP as co-ingestant with other drugs in overdose
- Causes of acute onset hepatotoxicity
  - —Reye's syndrome
  - —Infectious hepatitis
  - —*Amanita* sp. mushrooms toxicity
  - —Other drug ingestions

Treatment

INITIAL STABILIZATION

- ABCs
- Naloxone, thiamine, D50 (or Accucheck) for altered mental status

ED TREATMENT

Gastric Decontamination

- Administer single-dose activated charcoal immediately
  - —Very effective in lowering peak APAP levels
  - —Does not interfere with initial loading dose of NAC
  - —First dose of NAC is so high that some absorption by activated charcoal does not decrease NAC effectiveness
- Avoid syrup of ipecac
  - —Will delay NAC/charcoal administration

NAC Administration

- Administer if toxic level detected as defined by Rumack-Matthew nomogram
- <8 hours postingestion
  - —Check APAP level
  - —Initiate NAC if APAP level will not be available within 8 hours of ingestion and toxic ingestion suspected
  - —NAC virtually 100% hepatoprotective if initiated within 8 hours of overdose
  - —Discontinue NAC if APAP level nontoxic
- ≥8 hours postingestion
  - —Initiate NAC immediately if suspected toxic ingestion
  - —Check APAP level
  - —Discontinue NAC if APAP level is nontoxic
- >24 hours postingestion or chronic repeated APAP ingestion
  - —Initiate NAC if
    - -Ingestion >150 mg/kg APAP
    - -Symptomatic
    - -Abnormal hepatic screening panel
  - —Discontinue NAC if APAP falls to nondetectable level and no AST elevation occurs by 36 hours postingestion
- Pregnancy
  - —No teratogenicity with NAC
  - —NAC may be effective in protecting fetal liver
  - —Fetal liver metabolizes APAP to toxic NAPQI after 14 weeks of gestation
- Oral NAC
  - —Poor taste and odor
  - —Dilute to 5% with fruit juice or soft drink to increase palatability
  - —If the patient vomits NAC within 1 hour of administration, repeat the dose
  - —Use antiemetics (metoclopramide or ondansetron) liberally to facilitate PO administration
  - —Administer NAC as a drip through NG tube if vomiting continues
- IV NAC
  - —Used throughout the world
  - —Not FDA approved, but used commonly in U.S. when vomiting prevents oral administration of NAC
  - —Contact regional poison control center or local toxicologist for assistance with IV NAC administration

Other Measures

- Transplantation for fulminant hepatic failure
- Hemodialysis for renal failure

MEDICATIONS

- Activated charcoal slurry: 1–2 g/kg PO
- Dextrose: D50W 1 amp (50 mL or 25 g) (peds: D25W 2–4 mL/kg) i.v.
- Metoclopramide start with 10 mg (peds: 1 mg/kg) i.v. (1 mg/kg max)
- *N*-acetylcysteine (NAC): 140 mg/kg PO loading (adult and pediatric) followed by 70 mg/kg q4 for 17 additional doses
- Naloxone (Narcan): 0.4–2 mg (peds: 0.1 mg/kg) i.v. or i.m. initial dose
- Ondansetron: >80 kg, 12 mg; 45–80 kg, 8 mg (peds 0.15 mg/kg) i.v.
- Thiamine (vitamin B_1): 100 mg (peds: 50 mg) i.v. or i.m.

Disposition

ADMISSION CRITERIA

- Hepatotoxic level of APAP requiring full course of NAC therapy (see Treatment)
- Nontoxic suicide attempt requiring psychiatric treatment

DISCHARGE CRITERIA

- Asymptomatic patients with nontoxic ingestions not requiring full course of NAC therapy

Miscellaneous

ICD9: 965.4

ICD10: T39.1

SUGGESTED READINGS

Anker AL. Acetaminophen. In: Ford MD, Delaney KA, Ling LJ, et al., eds. Clinical toxicology. Philadelphia: WB Saunders, 2001:265–274.

Jones AL. Mechanism of action and value of N-acetylcysteine in the treatment of early and late acetaminophen poisoning: a critical review. J Toxicol Clin Toxicol 1998;36:277–285.

Smilkstein MJ, Knapp GL, Kulig KW, et al. Efficacy of oral n-acetylcysteine in treatment of acetaminophen overdose. Analysis of the national multicenter study. N Engl J Med 1988;319:1557–1562.

Yip L, Dart RC, Hurlbut KM. Intravenous administration of oral N-acetylcysteine. Crit Care Med 1998;26:40–42.

Author: Mark B. Mycyk

Acidosis

Clinical Presentation

SIGNS AND SYMPTOMS

- Nonspecific
- Vital signs
  - —Tachypnea or Kussmaul respirations with metabolic acidosis
  - —Hypoventilation with respiratory acidosis
- Somnolence
- Confusion
- CO_2 narcosis
- Myocardial conduction and contraction disturbances

MECHANISM/DESCRIPTION

Respiratory Acidosis

- Results from hypoventilation
- Reduced pH due to increased $Paco_2$
- Defined as $Paco_2$ >45 mm Hg
- Classified into three broad categories
  - —Primary failure in CNS drive to ventilate
    - -Sleep apnea
    - -Anesthesia
    - -Sedative overdose
  - —Primary failure in transport of CO_2 from alveolar space
    - -COPD
    - -Myasthenic crisis
    - -Severe hypokalemia
    - -Guillain-Barré
  - —Primary failure in transport of CO_2 from tissue to alveoli
    - -Severe heart failure

Metabolic Acidosis

- Results from reduction in plasma bicarbonate decreasing the pH
- Divided into two groups
  - —Normal anion gap due to abnormally high net bicarbonate losses
    - -Kidneys fail to reabsorb or regenerate bicarbonate
    - -Extrarenal losses of bicarbonate (diarrhea)
    - -Excessive amounts of substances releasing hydrochloric acid have been given
  - —Increased anion gap due to
    - -Kidneys fail to excrete inorganic acids (phosphate, sulfates)
    - -Net accumulation of organic acids
    - -Inborn errors of metabolism in pediatric patients

ETIOLOGY

Nonanion Gap Metabolic Acidosis

- Gastrointestinal losses of bicarbonate
  - —Diarrhea
  - —Small bowel/pancreatic fistula
  - —Ileal loop (obstructed or too long)
  - —Anion exchange resins
  - —Ingestion of $CaCl_2$, $MgCl_2$
- Renal loss of bicarbonate
  - —Renal tubular acidosis
    - -Type I—serum HCO_3^- >15 MEq/L, low K^+, normal BUN, renal stone common
    - -Type II—serum HCO_3^- <15 MEq/L, low K^+, normal BUN, renal stone rare
    - -Type IV—serum HCO_3^- >15 MEq/L, normal/elevated K^+, elevated BUN, renal stone uncommon
  - —Carbonic anhydrase inhibitors
  - —Tubulointerstitial renal disease
  - —Hypoaldosteronism
    - -Deficiency
    - -Drug inhibition
- Addition of hydrochloric acid
  - —Ammonium chloride
  - —Arginine HCL

Anion Gap Acidosis

To remember, use the mnemonic A CAT MUD PILES:

- Alcohol ketoacidosis
- Carbon monoxide/cyanide
- Aspirin
- Toluene
- Methanol
- Uremia
- Diabetic ketoacidosis
- Paraldehyde
- Iron/isoniazid
- Lactic acidosis
- Ethylene glycol
- Starvation

Increased Osmolar Gap

To remember, use the mnemonic ME DIE:

- Methanol
- Ethylene glycol
- Diuretics (mannitol)
- Isopropyl alcohol
- Ethanol

Pre-Hospital

N/A

Diagnosis

ESSENTIAL WORKUP

- Electrolytes, BUN, Cr, glucose
  - —Decreased bicarbonate with metabolic acidosis
  - —Hyperkalemia and hypercalcemia with severe metabolic acidosis
- ABG
  - —pH
  - —CO_2 retention in respiratory acidosis
  - —Carbon monoxide level
  - —Correction factors
    - -Increase/decrease pH by 0.08 for each 10 mm Hg decrease/increase in pco_2
- Calculate anion gap = $Na^+ - (HCO_3^- + Cl^-)$
  - —Normal = 8–15

LABORATORY

- Urinalysis
  - —For glucose/ketones
- Measured serum osmolality
  - —Calculate serum osmolality = 2 Na^+ + glucose/18 + BUN/2.8
  - —Osmolal gap = difference between calculated and measured osmolality ≤10 normal
- Toxicology screen
  - —Methanol/ethylene glycol/ethanol/isopropyl alcohol levels if increase osmol gap
  - —Aspirin/iron levels for suspected ingestion
- Serum ketones
- Serum lactate

Treatment

INITIAL STABILIZATION

- ABCs
  - —Early intubation for severe metabolic acidosis with progressive/potential weakening of respiratory compensation
- Naloxone, D50W (or Accucheck) and thiamine if altered mental status

ED TREATMENT

Respiratory Acidosis

- Treat underlying disorder
- Provide ventilatory support for worsening hypercapnia
- In chronic hypercapnia, identify and correct aggravating factors (e.g., pneumonia)

Metabolic Acidosis

- Identify if concurrent osmolal gap
- Treat underlying disorder
  - —Diabetic ketoacidosis
  - —Lactic acidosis
  - —Alcohol ketoacidosis
  - —Ingestion
- Rehydrate with 0.9% NS if hypovolemic
- Correct electrolyte abnormalities

MEDICATIONS

- Dextrose: D50W 1 amp (50 mL or 25 g) (peds: D25W 2–4 mL/kg) i.v.
- Naloxone (Narcan): 2 mg (peds: 0.1 mg/kg) i.v. or i.m. initial dose
- Thiamine (vitamin B_1): 100 mg (peds: 50 mg) i.v. or i.m.

Disposition

ADMISSION CRITERIA

- Worsening metabolic acidosis
- ICU admission if pH <7.1 or altered mental status
- Respiratory acidosis

DISCHARGE CRITERIA

- Resolving anion gap metabolic acidosis

Miscellaneous

ICD9: 276.2

ICD10: E87.2

SUGGESTED READINGS

Chabli R. Diagnostic use of anion and osmolal gaps in pediatric emergency medicine. Pediatr Emerg Care 1997;3:204.

Levy MM. An evidenced-based evaluation of the use of sodium bicarbonate during cardiopulmonary resuscitation. Crit Care Clin 1998;14:457.

Uribarri J, Oh MS, Carrol HJ. D-lactic acidosis: a review of clinical presentation, biochemical features and pathophysiologic mechanisms. Medicine 1998;77:73.

Author: Michelle Ervin

Acromioclavicular Joint Injury

Clinical Presentation

SIGNS AND SYMPTOMS

- Examine in standing or sitting position
- Acromioclavicular (AC) joint is painful and tender to palpation
- Pain is worsened by any motion of the upper extremity
- Ipsilateral arm is held in adduction supported by the contralateral arm
- Extreme adduction worsens the symptoms
- In more severe injuries the clavicle appears free floating

MECHANISM

- *Most common:* direct force from a fall on the lateral aspect of the shoulder
- *Less common:* indirect force from a fall on the outstretched hand
- Football and hockey are common sports associated with AC joint separation

PEDIATRIC CONSIDERATIONS

- *Seldom* occurs in isolation in the pediatric population
- In children, there is tight approximation of the coracoclavicular and acromioclavicular ligaments to the periosteal tube that protects the AC joint from dislocation
- Distal clavicular fractures are more common than AC joint dislocations in children

Pre-Hospital

- Ice packs
- Sling immobilization
- Cervical spine immobilization if appropriate

Diagnosis

ESSENTIAL WORKUP

- Physical exam
- Radiographic evaluation as outlined below

CLASSIFICATION

Type 1

- Painful and tender but AC joint is stable
- AC ligaments are strained
- All other ligaments are uninjured
- X-rays are normal except for mild swelling

Type 2

- Pain, swelling, and tenderness are greater than in type 1
- Distal clavicle may appear prominent and mildly unstable
- Acromioclavicular ligament *completely torn*
- Coracoclavicular ligaments are either intact or strained
- Slight widening of the AC joint on x-ray (3–5 mm)

Type 3

- Localized symptoms are greater and the distal end of the clavicle is prominent and unstable
- *Disruption of both* the acromioclavicular and coracoclavicular ligament
- Distal end of the clavicle is noted to be displaced above the acromion on x-ray
- Widening of the coracoclavicular interspace by 25–100% (>5 mm)

Type 4

- Rare
- Clavicle is displaced posteriorly into or through the trapezius muscle
- Best visualized on lateral radiograph

Type 5

- Rare
- Severe vertical separation of the clavicle from the scapula

Type 6

- Clavicle is dislocated inferiorly into either a subacromial or subcoracoid position
- Usually associated with severe trauma

RADIOGRAPHY

- Minimum of two views; most commonly the AP and lateral view
- The distal clavicle and acromion may be superimposed on the spine of the scapula so a slight angulation of the beam 15–30 degrees will project the scapular spine out of view
- Additional views: apical oblique and axillary lateral can be used if joint dislocation suspected but not illustrated by routine radiography
- Stress films (holding weights) are not useful in the acute setting as they have low diagnostic yield, require additional patient radiation, and are painful

SPECIAL TESTS

- Ultrasonography may demonstrate instability of the distal clavicle, hematoma formation, or ligament remnant
- Rarely, MRI is used to evaluate tendons and muscles

DIFFERENTIAL DIAGNOSIS

- Clavicular fractures
- Shoulder dislocation
- In the atraumatic patient, consider osteoarthritis, osteomyelitis

PEDIATRIC CONSIDERATIONS

- True acromioclavicular separations are rare
- Most likely there is a clavicle fracture through the distal physis
- Must distinguish between true AC disruption from pseudodislocation and lateral epiphyseal injury

Treatment

INITIAL STABILIZATION

- Sling immobilization
- Ice
- Analgesia (NSAIDs, narcotics)

ED TREATMENT

Types 1 and 2

- Sling immobilization for 10–12 days
- Resume normal range of motion after 14 days
- Long-term prognosis is good

Type 3

- Significant debate in orthopedic literature about management
- Conservative management vs. operative management
- Consider operative repair for athletes, heavy laborers, and severe cosmetic deformities

Types 4, 5, and 6

- Immediate operative repair
- Involves screw or plating

SPECIAL CIRCUMSTANCES

- Operative repair may be considered for those with simultaneous distal clavicle fracture
- Late surgery for those with continuous pain

PEDIATRIC CONSIDERATIONS

Types 1 and 2

- Conservative management
- Should heal without major sequelae

Type 3

- Age $<$15 conservative management
- Age $\geq$15 may require more aggressive treatment

Types 4, 5, and 6

- Operative repair

Disposition

ADMISSION CRITERIA

- Open injury
- Types 4, 5, and 6 require admission for operative repair

DISCHARGE CRITERIA

- Types 1 and 2 can be discharged with orthopedic referral
- Type 3 should have urgent orthopedic referral
- Analgesics (NSAIDs)

Miscellaneous

ICD9: 810.03

ICD10: S43.5

SUGGESTED READINGS

Bossart PJ, Joyce SM, et al. Lack of efficacy of weighted radiographs in diagnosing acute acromioclavicular separation. Ann Emerg Med 1988;17:47–51.

Clarke H, McCann P. Acromioclavicular joint injuries. Orthop Clin North Am 2000;31(2): 177–187.

Gustilo RB, Kyle RF, Templeman DC. Fractures and dislocations. St. Louis: CV Mosby, 1993:303–315.

Kucher MS. Upper extremity injury in the pediatric athlete. Sports Med 2000;30(2): 117–135.

Rockwood CA, Williams GR, Young DC. Rockwood and Green's fractures in adults, 4th ed. Philadelphia: JB Lippincott, 1996:1342–1413.

Authors: Aileen Kennedy; Wallace A. Carter

Acute Coronary Syndrome: Coronary Vasospasm

Clinical Presentation

SIGNS AND SYMPTOMS

- Chest pain
  —Retrosternal
  —Radiates to neck, jaw, left shoulder, or arm
  —Occurs at rest
- Palpitations
- Presyncope or syncope
- Associated with migraine headaches and Raynaud's disease in a minority of patients
- May occur during cold weather or stress
- May be prolonged in duration compared to typical angina
- May be elicited by hyperventilation
- May be relieved with exercise
- Circadian pattern, most commonly in early morning

MECHANISM/DESCRIPTION

- Also called Prinzmetal's angina or variant angina
- Most common in patients age 51 to 57 and males
- Occurs in patients without other cardiac risk factors
- Risk factors
  —Smoking
  —Hyperinsulinemia
  —Insulin resistance
- Associated with minimal coronary artery disease
  —Usually has a normal coronary angiogram

ETIOLOGY

- Abnormal vasodilator function in coronary arteries
- Focal coronary artery vasospasm
- Often adjacent to or at the site of fixed stenoses
- Unopposed alpha sympathetic stimulation
- Sympathetic stimulation by endogenous hormones may cause vasoconstriction
- Hypersensitivity of coronary arteries due to mediators of vasoconstriction
- May or may not be associated with a fixed coronary lesion

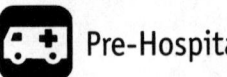

Pre-Hospital

CAUTIONS

- Treat as any other acute coronary syndrome

Diagnosis

ESSENTIAL WORKUP

- EKG
  —Transient ST segment elevation is characteristic
  —May be followed by ST depression or T-wave inversion

LABORATORY

- CK-MB and troponin I or T
- Toxicologic screen
  —Helpful if cocaine is suspected as etiology of chest pain

IMAGING/SPECIAL TESTS

- Chest x-ray
  —May be helpful to rule other etiologies such as pneumonia, pneumothorax, aortic dissection
- Exercise stress testing is controversial
  —Helpful only if there are underlying fixed stenoses
- Thallium scintigraphy may be useful to localize area of spasm
- Coronary angiography
  —Mild atherosclerosis is often the norm
  —Provocative test with ergonovine, acetylcholine, or hyperventilation will induce coronary spasm

DIFFERENTIAL DIAGNOSIS

- Angina pectoris
- Anxiety and panic disorders
- Aortic dissection
- Esophageal rupture
- Esophageal spasm
- Esophagitis
- Gastroesophageal reflux
- Mitral valve prolapse
- Musculoskeletal chest pain
- Myocardial infarction
- Peptic ulcer disease
- Pericarditis
- Pneumothorax
- Pulmonary embolism

Treatment

INITIAL STABILIZATION

- Intravenous access
- Oxygen
- Cardiac monitoring
- Vital signs and oxygen saturation

ED TREATMENT

- All patients with chest pain, in which cardiac ischemia is a consideration, should receive an aspirin on arrival to the emergency department
- Nitroglycerin should then be administered and is appropriate to help relieve both ischemic and vasospastic chest pain
- A trial of calcium channel blockers is indicated if clinical history is consistent with coronary vasospasm
- Heparin and beta-blockers are not helpful

MEDICATIONS

- Aspirin 160–325 mg PO
- Nitroglycerin either 0.4 sublingual or intravenous at 5–10 μg/min titrating to effect, or 1–2 inches of nitropaste
- Diltiazem 30–60 mg PO
- Verapamil 40–80 mg PO

Disposition

ADMISSION CRITERIA

- New-onset chest pain
- Rest chest pain (by definition most patients with coronary vasospasm)
- Accelerated chest pain symptoms

DISCHARGE CRITERIA

- Stable (chronic chest pain)

Miscellaneous

ICD9: 413.1

ICD10: I20.1

SUGGESTED READINGS

Braunwald E. Unstable angina: an etiologic approach to management [editorial]. Circulation 1998;98:2219–2222.

Crea F, Kaski JC, Maseri A. Key references on coronary artery spasm. Circulation 1994;89:2442–2446.

Gersh BJ, Braunwald E, Rutherford JD. Chronic coronary artery disease. In: Braunwald E, ed. Heart disease: a textbook of cardiovascular disease, 5th ed. Philadelphia: WB Saunders, 1997:1340–1343.

Mayer S, Hillis LD. Prinzmetal's variant angina. Clin Cardiol 1998;21:243–246.

Orford JL. Coronary artery vasospasm. Med J 2001;2:1–11.

Prinzmetal M, Kennamer R, Merliss R. A variant form of angina pectoris. Am J Med 1959;27:375–388.

Author: Shamai A. Grossman

Acute Coronary Syndrome: Drug Induced

Clinical Presentation

SIGNS AND SYMPTOMS

- Chest pain
- Substernal pressure
- Heaviness
- Squeezing
- Burning sensation
- Tightness
- Dyspnea
- Sympathomimetic toxidrome symptoms
  - —Agitation
  - —Tremulousness
  - —Tachypnea
  - —Tachycardia
  - —Hypertension
  - —Hyperthermia
  - —Moist skin
  - —No urine retention
- Other agents that may induce coronary syndromes include:
  - —Calcium channel blockers: nifedipine
  - —Beta-blockers: metoprolol and propranolol have rarely been associated with myocardial infarction (MI)
  - —Antimigraine therapy: sumatriptan (commonly used for migraine and cluster headaches), methysergide, ergotamine, isometheptene
  - —Carbon monoxide (found with gas heaters, smoke inhalation, furniture stripping with methylene chloride)
  - —Bromocriptine (particularly in postpartum women and Parkinson's patients)
  - —Other dopaminergic agents (dopamine)
  - —Sildenafil (Viagra)
  - —Oral contraceptives (particularly first and second generation)

MECHANISM/DESCRIPTION

- Imbalance in myocardial blood supply and oxygen requirements
- Sympathomimetics, most notably ephedrine, cocaine, and phenylpropanolamine, may cause hypersensitivity or eosinophilic myocarditis

ETIOLOGY

- Sympathomimetics are associated with myocardial oxygen mismatch due to cocaine-induced vasoconstriction
  - —Cocaine
  - —Amphetamines (Crank)
  - —Ephedrine (dietary supplement)
  - —Ma Huang (herbal diet supplement)
  - —Dipivefrin (glaucoma eye drop)
  - —Phenylpropanolamine (nasal decongestant)
  - —Epinephrine
  - Cocaine-induced chest pain may also be caused by
  - —Increased myocardial workload
  - —Accelerated atherosclerosis
  - —Activation of platelets and promotion of thrombosis
- Sumatriptan, methysergide, ergotamine, and isometheptene are vasoconstrictors and associated with MI and ischemia particularly in patients with cardiac risk factors or known coronary disease
- Nifedipine may induce ischemia by reflex tachycardia and vasoconstriction
- Beta-blockers may cause coronary vasospasm mediated by α-adrenergic receptors
- Carbon monoxide causes myocardial ischemia by
  - —Decreasing oxygen carrying capacity
  - —Shifting the oxyhemoglobin dissociation curve to the left
  - —Binding to myoglobin
- Bromocriptine is a vasoconstrictor and may cause vasospasm
  - —Used for acromegaly, Parkinson's disease, hyperprolactinemia, amenorrhea/galactorrhea, and most commonly for lactation cessation
  - —Predisposing conditions for myocardial ischemia include a history of pregnancy-induced hypertension or other vasospastic conditions, such as Raynaud's disease or migraine headaches
- Other dopaminergic agents also can cause vasoconstriction and vasospasm
- Sildenafil has systemic vasodilatory properties that can cause transient decreases in supine blood pressure and increase the risk of cardiac event during sexual activity in patients with preexisting cardiovascular disease
- Oral contraceptives are prothrombotics and are associated with significantly higher incidence of MI in young women
  - —Oral contraceptives with concomitant smoking increase the risk of MI even in third-generation oral contraceptive formulations

Pre-Hospital

- Remove patient from contaminated environment if carbon monoxide toxicity is a consideration
- Intravenous access
- Oxygen
- Cardiac monitoring
- Sublingual nitroglycerin for symptom relief

CAUTIONS

- All chest pain should be treated and transported as a possible life-threatening emergency

Diagnosis

ESSENTIAL WORKUP

- History is critical in diagnosing and differentiating drug-induced and unusual causes of acute coronary syndromes
- Blood pressure is usually elevated during symptoms
- Physical exam is usually unrevealing
- EKG will be normal approximately 50% of the time
  - —ST segment changes or T-wave inversions most often will be unchanged from previous tracings
  - —Must be compared to prior tracings if available
  - —New ST segment changes or T-wave inversions are suspicious for an acute coronary syndrome regardless of etiology
  - —Serial EKG tracings may be helpful
  - —1-mm depression of the ST segment below the baseline, 80 msec from the J point, is characteristic of ischemia regardless of etiology
- EKG may be helpful in diagnosing other etiologies of chest pain
- EKG in carbon monoxide poisoning:
  - —PVCs
  - —Dysrhythmias
  - —Tachycardia
  - —Nonspecific ST-T wave abnormalities
  - —Acute MI: ST elevation or depression

LABORATORY

- Serial cardiac enzymes may be helpful in diagnosis of acute MI; troponin may be more helpful in cocaine-induced coronary syndromes as cocaine-induced rhabdomyolysis may also elevate CK
- Carboxyhemoglobin level should be obtained in all patients in whom carbon monoxide toxicity is being considered
- Serum toxicology screening specifically for cocaine, amphetamines, and alcohol, which may potentiate the effects of cocaine as cocaethylene

IMAGING/SPECIAL TESTS

- Chest x-ray
  —Usually normal
  —May show cardiomegaly
    -Congestive heart failure (CHF) is suggestive of unstable angina or carbon monoxide–induced CHF
  —May identify other etiologies of chest pain such as pneumonia
- Exercise stress testing may help identify underlying atherosclerosis; however, stress testing cannot differentiate between the primary or secondary etiology
- A technetium Tc-99m perfusion scan may identify myocardial damage and infarction
- Echocardiogram may help identify regional wall motion abnormalities
- Cardiac catheterization is the gold standard and will often be needed to differentiate atherosclerotic versus drug-induced etiologies
- Most patients with drug-induced coronary syndromes will have angiographically normal coronary arteries

DIFFERENTIAL DIAGNOSIS

- Anxiety
- Aortic dissection
- Biliary colic
- Costochondritis
- Esophageal reflux
- Esophageal spasm
- Herpes zoster
- Hiatal hernia
- MI
- Mitral valve prolapse
- Panic disorder
- Peptic ulcer disease
- Pneumonia
- Psychogenic
- Pulmonary embolus
- Unstable angina

Treatment

INITIAL STABILIZATION

- Remove patient from contaminated environment if carbon monoxide toxicity is suspected
- Place patient on a monitor
- Intravenous access should be obtained
- O_2: 100% oxygen should be administered to all patients in whom carbon monoxide toxicity is being considered
- Nitrates

ED TREATMENT

- Aspirin
- β-adrenergic antagonists, such as metoprolol should be avoided in patients who suspected to have used cocaine; these drugs enhance cocaine-induced coronary vasoconstriction, increase blood pressure, fail to control the heart rate, increase the likelihood of seizures, and decrease survival
- Labetalol is both an α- and β-antagonist and may be a safer option in patients suspected of having used cocaine
- Benzodiazepines, besides their anxiolytic effects, reduce blood pressure and heart rate, thereby decreasing myocardial oxygen demand in patients who have used cocaine
- Heparin or enoxaparin
- Thrombolytics should be used with caution in ST elevation acute coronary syndromes of possible vasospastic etiology
- Cardiac catheterization is preferred as both a diagnostic and possibly a therapeutic study if significant atherosclerotic disease is found
- If carbon monoxide toxicity is present
  —Administer 100% O_2
  —Hyperbarics are indicated if
    -Carboxyhemoglobin level is >25–40%
    -Any period of coma
    -Significant persistent neurologic deficits
    -Persistent metabolic acidosis
    -Pregnant and carboxyhemoglobin level is >15%
    -Cardiac instability
    -Acute MI, unless hemodynamically unstable
- Half-life of carboxyhemoglobin
  —Room air 300 minutes
  —100% O_2: 90 minutes
  —Hyperbaric chamber at 3 ATM: 20 minutes

MEDICATIONS

- Aspirin 160–325 mg
- Nitroglycerin 0.4 mg SL, nitropaste 1 to 2 inches to chest wall, or i.v. nitroglycerin starting at 10–20 μg/min and titrating to relief of pain
- Lopressor 5–15 mg i.v. or 25–50 mg PO
- Labetalol 20 mg i.v. or 100 mg PO
- Ativan 1–2 mg i.v.
- Morphine 2–10 mg i.v.
- Heparin 80 units/kg i.v. bolus then 18 unit/kg/hour, or enoxaparin 1 mg/kg s.c.
- Tenecteplase, for 60-kg person, 30 mg; >60–69 kg, 35 mg; 70–79 kg, 40 mg; 80–89 kg, 45 mg, $\geq$90 kg, 50 mg or Reteplase, 10 units over 2 minutes, repeat in 30 minutes

Disposition

ADMISSION CRITERIA

- Similar to patients with acute coronary syndromes of atherosclerotic origin
- New-onset chest pain
- Rest chest pain
- Accelerated chest pain symptoms

DISCHARGE CRITERIA

- Chronic stable chest pain

Miscellaneous

ICD9: 411.1

ICD10: I20.9 T88.7

SUGGESTED READINGS

Lange RA, Hillis LD. Cardiovascular complications of cocaine use. N Engl J Med 2001;345:351–358.

Marius-Nunez AL. Myocardial infarction with normal coronary arteries after acute exposure to carbon monoxide. Chest 1990;97:491–494.

Ottervanger JP, Wilson JH, Stricker BH. Drug-induced chest pain and MI. Reports to a national center and review of the literature. Eur J Clin Pharmacol 1997;53:105–110.

Tanis BC, van den Bosch MA, Kemmeren JM, et al. Oral contraceptives and the risk of myocardial infarction. N Engl J Med 2001;345:1787–1793.

Author: Shamai A. Grossman

Acute Coronary Syndrome: Myocardial Infarction

Clinical Presentation

SIGNS AND SYMPTOMS

- Chest pain
  - —Most common presentation of myocardial infarction
  - —Substernal pressure
  - —Heaviness
  - —Squeezing
  - —Burning sensation
  - —Tightness
- Anginal equivalents (MI without chest pain)
  - —Abdominal pain
  - —Syncope
  - —Diaphoresis
  - —Nausea or vomiting
  - —Weakness
- May localize or radiate to arms, shoulders, back, neck, or jaw
- Associated symptoms
  - —Dyspnea
  - —Syncope
  - —Fatigue
  - —Diaphoresis
  - —Nausea
  - —Vomiting
- Symptoms are usually reproduced by exertion, eating, exposure to cold, or emotional stress
- Symptoms commonly last 30 minutes or more
- Symptoms may occur with rest or during exertion
- Often preceded by crescendo angina
- May be improved or relieved with rest or nitroglycerin
- Symptoms generally unchanged with position or inspiration
- Positive Levine sign or clenched fist over chest is suggestive of angina
- Blood pressure is usually elevated during symptoms
- Physical exam is usually unrevealing
- Occasional physical findings include:
  - —S3 or S4 due to LV systolic or diastolic symptoms
  - —Papillary muscle dysfunction resulting in mitral regurgitation
  - —Diminished peripheral pulses

MECHANISM/DESCRIPTION

- Imbalance in myocardial blood supply and oxygen requirement
- Acute cardiac ischemia (ACI) encompasses a spectrum of disease processes
  - —Unstable angina pectoris (UAP)
  - —Acute myocardial infarction (AMI)
  - —ST elevation MI
  - —Non-ST elevation MI

EPIDEMIOLOGY

- Syndromes of ACI are a leading cause of death in the U.S. and worldwide
- Approximately 10% of ED visits are cardiac related, the majority with chest pain
  - —10% of ED malpractice claims are due to missed diagnosis of AMI
  - —2–8% of patients presenting to the ED with chest pain will be sent home with an AMI
  - —History, physical exam, and EKG miss 1–4% of all AMI
- Chest pain from a cardiac etiology is difficult to categorize along the spectrum of ACI
  - —History is the critical component in diagnosing etiology of cardiac chest pain
  - —All modalities beyond history and EKG are only adjuncts to diagnosing the etiology of chest pain

ETIOLOGY

- Atherosclerotic narrowing of coronary vessels
- Vasospasm, although this is usually at rest and considered unstable if new onset
- Microvascular angina or abnormal relaxation of vessels with diffuse vascular disease
- Plaque disruption
- Thrombosis
- Arteritis
  - —Lupus
  - —Takayasu's disease
  - —Kawasaki's disease
  - —Rheumatoid arthritis
- Anemia: hemoglobin <8 g/dL
- Prolonged hypotension
- Hyperbarism or elevations in carboxyhemoglobin
- Coronary artery gas embolus
- Thyroid storm
- Structural abnormalities of coronary arteries
  - —Radiation fibrosis
  - —Aneurysms
  - —Ectasia
- Cocaine- or amphetamine-induced vasospasm
- Cardiac risk factors include:
  - —Hypercholesterolemia
  - —Diabetes mellitus
  - —Hypertension
  - —Smoking
  - —Family history in a first-degree relative less than age 55
  - —Male, age >55
  - —Postmenopausal women

Pre-Hospital

- Intravenous access
- Aspirin
- Oxygen
- Cardiac monitoring
- Sublingual nitroglycerin for symptom relief
- 12 lead EKG, if possible, with transmission or results relayed to receiving hospital

CAUTIONS

- All chest pain should be treated and transported as a possible life-threatening emergency

CONTROVERSIES

- Do not administer thrombolytics or heparin if aortic dissection is suspected

Diagnosis

ESSENTIAL WORKUP

- History is critical in differentiating myocardial infarction from noncardiac etiologies
- EKG
- See Cardiac Testing

DIFFERENTIAL DIAGNOSIS

- Anxiety
- Aortic dissection
- Biliary colic
- Costochondritis
- Esophageal reflux
- Esophageal spasm
- Herpes zoster
- Hiatal hernia
- Mitral valve prolapse
- Myocardial infarction
- Panic disorder
- Peptic ulcer disease
- Pneumonia
- Psychogenic
- Pulmonary embolus
- Unstable angina

Treatment

INITIAL STABILIZATION

- Intravenous access
- Oxygen
- Cardiac monitoring
- Oxygen saturation
- Continuous blood pressure monitoring and pulse oximetry

ED TREATMENT

- ST elevation MI requires reperfusion therapy as soon as possible
  —Thrombolytics should be used if PCI is not readily available within a 90-minute time frame (see Reperfusion Therapy, Cardiac)
- Patients with non-ST segment elevation M, if started on glycoprotein IIb/IIIa inhibitors and if they subsequently receive a stent, benefit from a PCI within a 48-hour time frame
- Aspirin should be administered first to all patients with suspected myocardial infarction unless the patient has a known allergy
- If blood pressure is >90–100 mm Hg systolic, administer sublingual nitroglycerin, nitropaste, or IV nitroglycerin assuming no EKG criteria of right ventricular infarct
  —Symptoms that persist after three sublingual nitroglycerin tablets are strongly suggestive of AMI or noncardiac etiology
- Beta-blockers should be administered if no contraindications, e.g., bradyarrhythmias, heart rate <60, CHF, hypotension, or obstructive pulmonary disease, are present
- Morphine may be given to relieve pain and increase oxygen carrying capacity
- Enoxaparin or heparin is generally appropriate as the next line of therapy
- Angiotensin-converting enzyme (ACE) inhibitors may effect a small decrease in mortality when given acutely
- If non-ST segment MI is clearly the clinical diagnoses, a glycoprotein IIb/IIIa inhibitor should be started
- If patient is in cardiogenic shock, patient should be transported to a cardiac catheterization laboratory for angioplasty and intraaortic balloon pump as soon as possible (see Congestive Heart Failure)
- Ventricular dysrhythmias
  —See Ventricular Tachycardia
- Bradydysrhythmia associated with hypotension should be treated with atropine or external pacing
- Conduction disturbances
  —First-degree AV block and Mobitz I (Wenckebach) are often self-limited and do not require treatment
  —Mobitz II, complete heart block, new RBBB in anterior MI, RBBB plus LAFB or LPFB, LBBB plus first-degree AV block may require a temporary transvenous pacemaker

MEDICATIONS

- Aspirin 160–325 mg
- Nitroglycerin: 0.4 mg sublingual
- Nitropaste 1–2 inches transdermal
- Nitroglycerin drip at 5–10 μg/min
- Morphine 2 mg i.v., may titrate upward in 2-mg increments for relief of pain assuming no respiratory deterioration and SBP >90 mm Hg
- Metoprolol 5 mg i.v. q5–15 min followed by 25–50 mg PO starting dose as tolerated (Note: beta-blockers contraindicated in cocaine chest pain)
- Enoxaparin (Lovenox) 1 mg/kg s.c. q12h
- Heparin 80 units/kg i.v. bolus, then 18 units/kg/hr
- Glycoprotein IIb/IIIa Inhibitors
  —Eptifibatide (Integrilin) 180 μg/kg i.v. over 1–2 minutes, followed by continuous intravenous infusion of 2 μg/kg/minute up to 72 hours
  —Tirofiban (Aggrastat) 0.4 μg/kg/min for 30 minutes, then 0.1 μg/kg/min for 48–108 hours
  —Abciximab (ReoPro) for use prior to PCI only: 0.25 mg/kg i.v. bolus
- Thrombolytics: see Reperfusion Therapy, Cardiac, for dosing
- Amiodarone: 150 mg i.v. over 5 minutes then 0.5 mg/min
- Lidocaine: 1.5 mg/kg bolus, infusion of 2–4 mg/kg/min
- Magnesium: 2 g bolus i.v.

Disposition

ADMISSION CRITERIA

- Patients with an AMI require hospital admission
- If PCI is unavailable in the treating institution, and particularly if the patient is in cardiogenic shock, patients should be transported to another hospital if PCI can be underway in less than 90 minutes
- If the diagnosis is unclear, admission to the hospital or an ED observation unit may be useful for serial cardiac enzymes, EKGs, and exercise stress testing and/or cardiac catheterization

DISCHARGE CRITERIA

- No patient with an AMI should be discharged from the ED

Miscellaneous

ICD9: 410.0

ICD10: I21.9

SUGGESTED READINGS

Braunwald E, Antman EM, Beasley JW, et al. ACC/AHA guidelines for the management of patients with unstable angina and non-ST-segment elevation myocardial infarction. J Am Coll Cardiol 2000;36:970–1062.

Gibson CM. Primary angioplasty compared with thrombolysis: new issues in the era of glycoprotein IIb/IIIa inhibition and intracoronary stenting. Ann Intern Med 1999;130:841–847.

Lieu TA, Gurley RJ, Lundstrom RJ, et al. Primary angioplasty and thrombolysis for acute myocardial infarction: an evidence based summary. J Am Coll Cardiol 1996;27:737–750.

Ryan TJ, Antman EM, Brooks NH, et al. ACC/AHA practice guidelines for the management of patients with acute myocardial infarction. J Am Coll Cardiol 1996;28:1328–1428. See also 1999 web update at *www.acc.org*.

Schömig A, Kastrati A, Dirschinger J, et al. Coronary stenting plus platelet glycoprotein IIb/IIIa blockade compared with tissue plasminogen activator in acute myocardial infarction. N Engl J Med 2000;343:385–391.

Author: Shamai A. Grossman

Acute Coronary Syndrome: Non–Q-Wave (Non-ST Elevation) MI

Clinical Presentation

SIGNS AND SYMPTOMS

- Pain
  - —Pressure or tightness
  - —Substernal, epigastric
  - —+/− radiation to L arm/jaw, back
- Nausea, vomiting
- Diaphoresis
- Cough
- Dyspnea
- Anxiety
- Light-headedness
- Syncope
- Hypertension
- Hypotension
- Arrhythmias
- S4 heart sound

MECHANISM/DESCRIPTION

- Coronary plaque disruption
  - —Endothelial disruption exposes subendothelial collagen and other platelet-adhering ligands, von Willebrand factor (vWF), and fibronectin
  - —Release of tissue factors activates factor VII and extrinsic pathway
- Thrombus generation
  - —Platelet adhesion via glycoprotein (GP) Ia/IIa to collagen, GP Ib to vWF
    - -Platelet activation: release of ADP, thromboxane A_2, and serotonin alters the platelet GP IIb/IIIa receptor, also causes local vasoconstriction
    - -Platelet aggregation: GP IIb/IIIa receptor binds fibrinogen molecules, cross-links platelets forming local platelet plug
  - —Platelet stabilization: thrombin converts fibrinogen to fibrin, provides fibrin mesh, stabilizes platelet aggregate

ETIOLOGY

- Coronary thrombosis
- Coronary artery spasm, idiopathic or cocaine induced
- *In situ* thrombosis/hypercoagulable states
- Embolic event
- Arteritis

Pre-Hospital

- Intravenous access
- Oxygen administration
- Cardiac monitoring and treatment of arrhythmias
- Aspirin, analgesia, anxiolytics

Diagnosis

ESSENTIAL WORKUP

- EKG, cardiac markers, CXR

LABORATORY

- Cardiac markers
  - —Troponins: specific indicators of myocardial infarction, positive 3–6 hours after MI, peaks at 9–10 days
  - —Creatine kinase (CK): rises following infarction in 4–8 hours, peaks at 18–24 hours, subsiding at 3–4 days; isoenzyme CK-MB more specific for cardiac origin
  - —Myoglobin: rises within 2–6 hours, returns to baseline within 24 hours, highly sensitive but very nonspecific
  - —LDH: rises within 24 hours, peaks at 3–6 days, baseline at 8–12 days
- CBC
- Serum electrolytes
- ESR: nonspecific marker of inflammation, rises within 3 days, elevated for several weeks

IMAGING/SPECIAL TESTS

- EKG
  - —To evaluate for ST segment depression/elevation, T wave inversion, in regional patterns
- CXR
  - —To assess pulmonary edema/congestion or identify other causes of chest pain
- Echocardiography
  - —To identify wall motion abnormalities and assess LV function
- Radionuclide studies
  - —Thallium or sestamibi scanning: identifies viable myocardium
  - —Technetium 99: identifies recently infarcted myocardium

DIFFERENTIAL DIAGNOSIS

- ST-elevation myocardial infarction
- Pulmonary embolus
- Aortic dissection
- Acute pericarditis
- Pancreatitis
- Pneumonia
- Esophageal spasm/gastroesophageal reflux
- Musculoskeletal pain (diagnosis of exclusion)

Treatment

INITIAL STABILIZATION

- Oxygen administration
- Intravenous access
- Cardiac monitoring and treatment of arrhythmias

ED TREATMENT

- Antiischemic therapy to reduce myocardial demand and increase myocardial supply of oxygen: beta-blockers, nitrates, and oxygen
- Calcium channel blockers (non-dihydropyridines, e.g., diltiazem, verapamil) may be used in patients with ongoing ischemia and contraindications to beta-blockade
- Antithrombotic therapy
- Anticoagulation
- Analgesia, anxiolytics to suppress sympathomimetic release
- GP IIb/IIIa inhibitors (eptifibatide, tirofiban)
  —When catheterization and PCI is planned
  —Ongoing ischemia
  —Positive initial cardiac markers

MEDICATIONS

- Aspirin 160–325 mg
- Ativan 1–2 mg i.v.
- Morphine 2–10 mg i.v.
- Heparin 80 units/kg i.v. bolus then 18 unit/kg/hr, or
- Enoxaparin 1 mg/kg sc
- Tenectaplase, for 60-kg person, 30 mg; >60–69 kg, 35 mg; 70–79 kg, 40 mg; 80–89 kg, 45 mg, ≥90 kg, 50 mg
- Reteplase 10 units over 2 minutes, repeat in 30 minutes
- Nitroglycerin: 0.4 mg SL or by spray q 5 min followed by i.v. infusion beginning at 10–20 μg/min if pain persists
- Atenolol: start 5 mg i.v. over 5 minutes, then 5 mg i.v. 10 minutes later, then 50 mg PO q12h
- Metoprolol: start 5 mg i.v. q 2 min × 3, after 15 minutes begin 50 mg PO q6h
- Clopidogrel 300 mg PO × 1, then 75 mg qd
- Eptifibatide: 180 μg/kg i.v. load, then 2 μg/kg/min i.v.
- Tirofiban: 0.4 μg/kg/min i.v. × 30 min, then 0.1 μg/kg/min i.v. infusion

Disposition

ADMISSION CRITERIA

- All patients with positive cardiac markers or significant clinical probability of acute coronary syndrome
- Intensive care unit for monitoring unstable patients

DISCHARGE CRITERIA

- Only those who rule out for acute coronary syndrome/non-Q-wave infarction can be safely sent home

Miscellaneous

ICD9: 410.9

ICD10: I21.4

SUGGESTED READINGS

Braunwald E, et al. ACC/AHA guideline update for the management of patients with unstable angina and non–ST-segment elevation myocardial infarction, 2002, *www.acc.org/clinical/guidelines/unstable/unstable.pdf*.

DeFilippi CR. Evaluating the chest pain patient. Scope of the problem. Cardiol Clin 1999;17(2):307–326.

Storrow AB. Chest pain centers: diagnosis of acute coronary syndromes. Ann Emerg Med 2000;35(5):449–461.

Tatum JL. Comprehensive strategy for the evaluation and triage of the chest pain patient. Ann Emerg Med 1997;29(1):116–125.

Zalenski RJ. National Heart Attack Alert Program position paper: chest pain centers and programs for the evaluation of acute cardiac ischemia. Ann Emerg Med 2000;35(5):462–471.

Zalenski RJ. Evaluation and risk stratification of patients with chest pain in the emergency department. Predictors of life threatening events. Emerg Med Clin North Am 1998;16(3):495–517, vii.

Authors: Tanya M. Fatovich; David F. M. Brown

Acute Coronary Syndrome: Stable Angina

Clinical Presentation

SIGNS AND SYMPTOMS

- Chest pain
  - —Substernal pressure
  - —Heaviness
  - —Squeezing
  - —Burning sensation
  - —Tightness
- May localize or radiate to arms, shoulders, back, neck, or jaw
- May be associated with dyspnea, syncope, fatigue, diaphoresis, nausea, or vomiting
- Usually reproduced by exertion, eating, exposure to cold, or emotional stress
- Symptoms last less than 20 minutes, but more than a few seconds
- Recurrent symptoms of 2 months duration or more
- Usually relieved with rest or nitroglycerin
- Symptoms generally unchanged with position or inspiration
- No changes in pattern or frequency of symptoms
- Occasional anginal equivalents include:
  - —Abdominal pain
  - —Syncope
  - —Diaphoresis
  - —Nausea or vomiting
  - —Weakness
- Positive Levine sign or clenched fist over chest is suggestive of angina
- Blood pressure is usually elevated during symptoms
- Physical exam is usually unrevealing
- Occasional symptoms include:
  - —S3 or S4 due to LV systolic or diastolic symptoms
  - —Mitral regurgitation or pansystolic murmur
  - —Diminished peripheral pulses

MECHANISM/DESCRIPTION

- Imbalance in myocardial blood supply and oxygen requirements
- Canadian Cardiovascular Classification: class I: ordinary physical activity does not cause symptoms
- Canadian Cardiovascular Classification: class II: symptoms that slightly limit normal activity such as:
  - —Walking
  - —Climbing stairs
  - —Emotional stress
  - —Cold

ETIOLOGY

- Cardiac risk factors include:
  - —Hypercholesterolemia
  - —Diabetes mellitus
  - —Hypertension
  - —Smoking
  - —Family history
  - —Male, age >35
  - —Postmenopausal women
- Atherosclerotic narrowing of coronary vessels
- Vasospasm, although this is usually at rest and considered unstable if new onset
- Microvascular angina or abnormal relaxation of vessels with diffuse vascular disease
- Arteritis
  - —Lupus
  - —Takayasu's disease
  - —Kawasaki's disease
  - —Rheumatoid arthritis
- Anemia: hemoglobin <8 g/dL
- Hyperbarism or elevations in carboxyhemoglobin
- Structural abnormalities of coronary arteries
  - —Radiation fibrosis
  - —Aneurysms
  - —Ectasia
- Cocaine- or amphetamine-induced vasospasm

Pre-Hospital

- Intravenous access
- Oxygen
- Cardiac monitoring
- Sublingual nitroglycerin for symptom relief
- Aspirin

CAUTIONS

- All chest pain should be treated and transported as a possible life-threatening emergency

Diagnosis

ESSENTIAL WORKUP

- History is critical in differentiating stable and unstable angina
- EKG
  - —Will be normal approximately 50% of the time
  - —ST segment changes or T-wave inversions most often will be unchanged from previous tracings
  - —Must be compared to prior tracings if available
  - —New ST segment changes or T-wave inversions are suspicious for unstable angina
  - —Serial EKG tracings that remain unchanged may assist in differentiating stable from unstable angina
  - —1-mm depression of the ST segment below the baseline, 80 msec from the J point, is characteristic of angina
- EKG may be helpful in diagnosing other etiologies of chest pain
  - —Pericarditis is suggested by diffuse ST elevations followed by T-wave inversions and PR depression
  - —Pulmonary embolism is suggested by an S1, Q3, T3 pattern and unexplained tachycardia

LABORATORY

- Cardiac enzymes should not be elevated and are not indicated unless the history is suspicious for acute myocardial infarction (AMI)

IMAGING/SPECIAL TESTS

- Chest x-ray
  - —Usually normal
  - —May show cardiomegaly
  - —Congestive heart failure is suggestive of unstable angina
  - —May identify other etiologies of chest pain such as pneumonia
- Exercise stress testing may help establish the diagnosis of stable angina and provide prognostic information
  - —1-mm depression of the ST segment below the baseline, 80 msec from the J point, in three consecutive beats and two consecutive leads is characteristic of cardiac ischemia
  - —Early positive (within 3 minutes) stress tests are worrisome for unstable angina
  - —Six minutes of exercise utilizing a standard Bruce protocol suggests an excellent prognosis
  - —Exercise stress testing with EKG alone has a sensitivity of 68% and specificity of 77%
  - —Exercise stress testing with echocardiography has a sensitivity of 85% and specificity of 77%
  - —Exercise stress testing with thallium-201 or technetium Tc-99m sestamibi has a sensitivity of 87% and specificity of 64%

DIFFERENTIAL DIAGNOSIS

- Anxiety
- Aortic dissection
- Biliary colic
- Costochondritis
- Esophageal reflux
- Esophageal spasm
- Herpes zoster
- Hiatal hernia
- Mitral valve prolapse
- Myocardial infarction
- Panic disorder
- Peptic ulcer disease
- Pneumonia
- Psychogenic
- Pulmonary embolus
- Unstable angina

Treatment

INITIAL STABILIZATION

- Intravenous access
- Oxygen
- Cardiac monitoring
- Oxygen saturation

ED TREATMENT

- Aspirin
- Sublingual nitroglycerin
  - —Symptoms that persist after three sublingual nitroglycerins are strongly suggestive of unstable angina, AMI, or noncardiac etiology
- May require adjustment of patient's outpatient medical regimen including adding or changing the dosage of a beta-blocker

MEDICATIONS

- Aspirin 160–325 mg
- Nitroglycerin 0.4 mg sublingual
- Isosorbide mononitrate 20 mg PO b.i.d. or isosorbide dinitrate 5–40 mg PO t.i.d. or Nitropatch 1–2 inches 10–14 hours daily
- Metoprolol 25–50 mg PO starting dose

Disposition

ADMISSION CRITERIA

- Patients with stable angina generally do not require hospital admission
- If the diagnosis is unclear, admission to the hospital or an ED observation unit may be useful for serial cardiac enzymes, EKGs, and exercise stress testing
- Patients who require additional adjustment of medication or angioplasty to reduce symptoms, and improve quality of life

DISCHARGE CRITERIA

- By definition, patients who meet diagnostic criteria of stable angina are safe to discharge

Miscellaneous

ICD9: 413.9

ICD10: I20.9

SUGGESTED READINGS

Braunwald E, Antman EM, Beasley JW, et al. ACC/AHA guidelines for the management of patients with unstable angina and non-ST-segment elevation myocardial infarction. J Am Coll Cardiol 2000;36:970–1062.

Solomon AJ, Gersh BJ. Management of chronic stable angina: medical therapy, percutaneous transluminal coronary angioplasty, and coronary artery bypass graft surgery. Lessons from the randomized trials. Ann Intern Med 1998;128:216–223.

Thadani U. Management of patients with chronic stable angina at low risk for serious cardiac events. Am J Cardiol 1997;79:24–30.

Author: Shamai A. Grossman

Acute Coronary Syndrome: Unstable Angina

Clinical Presentation

SIGNS AND SYMPTOMS

- Unstable angina is defined by either:
  - —New-onset symptoms
  - —Symptoms that occur at rest
  - —A change in the patient's usual pattern of angina
- Chest pain
  - —Most common presentation
  - —Substernal pressure
  - —Heaviness
  - —Squeezing
  - —Burning sensation
  - —Tightness
- Occasional anginal equivalents
  - —Abdominal pain
  - —Syncope
  - —Diaphoresis
  - —Nausea or vomiting
  - —Weakness
- Chest pain may localize or radiate to arms, shoulders, back, neck, or jaw
- May be associated with dyspnea, syncope, fatigue, diaphoresis, nausea, or vomiting
- Symptoms are usually reproduced by exertion, eating, exposure to cold, or emotional stress
- Symptoms commonly last 15 minutes or more
- Usually improved or relieved with rest or nitroglycerin
- Symptoms generally unchanged with position or inspiration
- Positive Levine sign or clenched fist over chest is suggestive of angina
- Blood pressure is usually elevated during symptoms
- Physical exam is usually unrevealing
- Occasional physical findings include:
  - —S3 or S4 due to LV systolic or diastolic symptoms
  - —Papillary muscle dysfunction resulting in mitral regurgitation
  - —Diminished peripheral pulses

MECHANISM/DESCRIPTION

- Imbalance in myocardial blood supply and oxygen requirements
- Canadian Cardiovascular Classification: class III: severe limitations of ordinary physical activity
- Class IV: inability to perform any activity without discomfort, symptoms may be present at rest

ETIOLOGY

- Atherosclerotic narrowing of coronary vessels
- Vasospasm, although this is usually at rest and considered unstable if new onset
- Microvascular angina or abnormal relaxation of vessels with diffuse vascular disease
- Plaque disruption
- Thrombosis
- Arteritis
  - —Lupus
  - —Takayasu's disease
  - —Kawasaki's disease
  - —Rheumatoid arthritis
- Anemia: hemoglobin <8 g/dL
- Hyperbarism or elevations in carboxyhemoglobin
- Structural abnormalities of coronary arteries
  - —Radiation fibrosis
  - —Aneurysms
  - —Ectasia
- Cocaine or amphetamine induced vasospasm
- Cardiac risk factors include:
  - —Hypercholesterolemia
  - —Diabetes mellitus
  - —Hypertension
  - —Smoking
  - —Family history
  - —Male, age >55
  - —Postmenopausal women

Pre-Hospital

- Intravenous access
- Aspirin
- Oxygen
- Cardiac monitoring
- Sublingual nitroglycerin for symptom relief

CAUTIONS

- All chest pain should be treated and transported as a possible life-threatening emergency

Diagnosis

ESSENTIAL WORKUP

- History is critical in differentiating stable and unstable angina
- EKG
  - —Will be normal approximately 50% of the time
  - —ST segment changes or T-wave inversions most often will be unchanged from previous tracings
  - —Must be compared to prior tracings if available
  - —New ST segment changes or T-wave inversions are suspicious for unstable angina
  - —Serial EKG tracings that remain unchanged may assist in differentiating stable from unstable angina
  - —1-mm depression of the ST segment below the baseline, 80 msec from the J point, is characteristic of angina
- EKG may be helpful in diagnosing other etiologies of chest pain
  - —Pericarditis is suggested by diffuse ST elevations followed by T-wave inversions and PR depression
  - —Pulmonary embolism is suggested by an S1, Q3, T3 pattern and unexplained tachycardia

LABORATORY

- Cardiac enzymes
- Hematocrit
- Coagulation profile
- Creatinine

IMAGING/SPECIAL TESTS

- Chest x-ray
  - —Usually normal
  - —May show cardiomegaly
  - —Congestive heart failure is suggestive of unstable angina
  - —May identify other etiologies of chest pain such as pneumonia
- Rest echocardiography may establish the diagnosis of acute coronary insufficiency (ACI)
  - —Has a sensitivity of 70% and specificity of 87% for ACI
- Technetium Tc-99 sestamibi (rest)
  - —Has a sensitivity of 81% and specificity of 73% for ACI
- Exercise stress testing may help establish the diagnosis of angina and provide prognostic information when the clinical presentation is equivocal
  - —Exercise stress testing with EKG alone has a sensitivity of 68% and specificity of 77%
  - —Exercise stress testing with echocardiography has a sensitivity of 85% and specificity of 77%
  - —Exercise stress testing with thallium-201 or technetium Tc-99m sestamibi has a sensitivity of 87% and specificity of 64%
  - —1-mm depression of the ST segment below the baseline, 80 msec from the J point, in three consecutive beats and two consecutive leads is characteristic of cardiac ischemia
  - —Early positive (within 3 minutes) stress tests are worrisome for unstable angina

DIFFERENTIAL DIAGNOSIS

- Anxiety
- Aortic dissection
- Biliary colic
- Costochondritis
- Esophageal reflux
- Esophageal spasm
- Herpes zoster
- Hiatal hernia
- Mitral valve prolapse
- Myocardial infarction
- Panic disorder
- Peptic ulcer disease
- Pneumonia
- Psychogenic
- Pulmonary embolus
- Unstable angina

Treatment

INITIAL STABILIZATION

- Intravenous access
- Oxygen
- Cardiac monitoring
- Oxygen saturation

ED TREATMENT

- Aspirin should be administered first to all patients with suspected unstable angina
- Sublingual nitroglycerin, nitro paste, or IV nitroglycerin
  - —Symptoms that persist after three sublingual nitroglycerins are strongly suggestive of unstable angina, acute myocardial infarction, or noncardiac etiology
- Beta-blockers should be administered if no contraindications, e.g., bradyarrhythmias or obstructive pulmonary disease, are present
- Morphine may be given to relieve pain and increase oxygen-carrying capacity
- Enoxaparin or heparin is generally appropriate as the next line of therapy
- If unstable angina is clearly the clinical diagnoses, a glycoprotein IIb/IIIa inhibitor should be started as well

MEDICATIONS

- Aspirin 160–325 mg
- Nitroglycerin: 0.4 mg sublingual
- Nitropaste 1–2 inches
- Nitroglycerin drip at 5–10 μg/min
- Morphine 2 mg i.v.
- Metoprolol 5 mg i.v. q 5–15 min followed by 25–50 mg PO starting dose as tolerated (Note: beta-blockers contraindicated in cocaine chest pain)
- Enoxaparin (Lovenox) 1 mg/kg SC q12h
- Heparin 80 units/kg i.v. bolus, then 18 units/kg/hr
- Glycoprotein IIb/IIIa inhibitors
  - —Eptifibatide (Integrilin) 180 μg/kg i.v. over 1 to 2 minutes, followed by continuous intravenous infusion of 2 mcg/kg/minute up to 72 hours
  - —Tirofiban (Aggrastat) 0.4 μg/kg/min for 30 minutes, then 0.1 μg/kg/min for 48–108 hours
  - —Abciximab (ReoPro) for use prior to PCI only: 0.25 mg/kg i.v. bolus

Disposition

ADMISSION CRITERIA

- Patients with unstable angina require hospital admission
- If the diagnosis is unclear, admission to the hospital or an ED observation unit may be useful for serial cardiac enzymes, EKGs, and exercise stress testing and/or cardiac catheterization

DISCHARGE CRITERIA

- No patient with unstable angina should be discharged from the ED

Miscellaneous

ICD9: 411.1

ICD10: I20.0

SUGGESTED READINGS

Boden WE, McKay RG. Optimal treatment of acute coronary syndromes—an evolving strategy. N Engl J Med 2001;344: 1939–1942.

Braunwald E, et al. ACC/AHA guidelines for the management of patients with unstable angina and non ST segment elevation myocardial infarction. J Am Coll Cardiol 2000;36:970–1062.

Cannon CP, et al. Comparison of early invasive and conservative strategies in patients with unstable coronary syndromes treated with the glycoprotein IIb/IIIa inhibitor tirofiban, the TACTICS-thrombolysis in myocardial infarction 18 investigators. N Engl J Med 2001;344: 1879–1887.

Lau J, Ioannidis JP, Balk EM, et al. Diagnosing acute cardiac ischemia in the emergency department: a systematic review of the accuracy and clinical effect of current technologies. Ann Emerg Med 2001;37(5):453–460.

Authors: Shamai A. Grossman; Leon Sanchez

Acute Necrotizing Ulcerative Gingivitis (ANUG)

Clinical Presentation

SIGNS AND SYMPTOMS

- Sudden onset of generalized mouth pain
- Malaise
- Low-grade fever is uncommon
- Foul breath
- Increased pain with chewing
- Generalized gingival inflammation with varying degrees of erythema
- Spontaneously bleeding gums
- Necrotic tissue in and about the gingival crest
- Gray-white pseudomembrane
  —Covers ulcerative lesions
  —Leaves a bleeding surface when removed
- Loss of gingival tissue especially interdental papillae
  —Pathognomonic for ANUG
- +/− lymphadenopathy
- Change in taste

MECHANISM/DESCRIPTION

- Periodontal disease
- Bacteria invade nonnecrotic tissue
  —Cause inflamed gingival with ulcerated and necrotic lesions
- Also know as trench mouth
- Not contagious
- Occurs in the young to middle aged
- Males affected more than females
- Cancrum oris (noma)-extension of ANUG to the lips and buccal mucosa
  —Mainly sub-Saharan Africa
- Predisposing factors
  —Poor oral hygiene
  —Local traumas
  —Emotional and physical stress
  —Smoking
  —Immunodeficiencies
  —Poor nutrition

ETIOLOGY

- An overgrowth of normal oral flora
  —Anaerobic fusiform bacilli
  —Spirochetes

Pre-Hospital

N/A

Diagnosis

ESSENTIAL WORKUP

- Clinical diagnosis
- Rule out systemic diseases when lesions have extended beyond the gingival tissue to
  —Buccal mucosa
  —Tongue
  —Palate
  —Pharynx

LABORATORY

- Laboratory tests not helpful
  —Gram stains show only normal flora

DIFFERENTIAL DIAGNOSIS

- Acute gingivitis
- Aphthous ulcers
- Traumatic ulcers
- Herpetic gingivostomatitis
- Squamous cell carcinoma
- Syphilis
- HIV
- Ulcers secondary to systemic disease
  —Diabetes mellitus
  —Uremia
  —Sickle cell disease
  —Blood dyscrasias
  —Connective tissue disorders

Treatment

INITIAL STABILIZATION

- 0.9% NS 500 cc (20 cc/kg) IV bolus for dehydration

ED TREATMENT

- Administer systemic and topical pain management
  —Narcotics
  —Viscous lidocaine
- Débride pseudomembrane
  —Use gauze or cotton-tip applicator soaked in H_2O_2
  —Removal of this membrane leaves a raw bleeding surface at ulcer base
  —Removal imperative for tissue healing
- Dilute hydrogen peroxide rinses
  —3% solution (dilute commercial solution)
- Indications for antibiotics (clindamycin or penicillin)
  —Extensive gingival involvement
  —Lymphadenopathy
  —Systemic signs

Outpatient Therapy

- Improve oral hygiene with daily brushing and flossing of teeth
- Perform dilute hydrogen peroxide rinses up to 12 times daily
- Chlorhexidine gluconate (Peridex) 15 mL swish/spit b.i.d.
- Use analgesics for pain control
- Remove predisposing factors
- Avoid irritants (spicy foods, hot beverages)
- Adequate nutrition
- Relief should occur 24 hours after start of antibiotics
- Follow-up with a dentist to avoid recurrence

Complications

- Periodontal disease from soft tissue
- Alveolar bone destruction
- Extension to face (noma)

MEDICATIONS

- Hydrogen peroxide (50% solution of 3%)
- Lidocaine (viscous 2%): 15 mL PRN (peds: 5 mL PO q3h for a 20-kg child) PO q3h
- Metronidazole: 250–750 mg (peds: 30/kg/24 hours) PO q.i.d. × 7 days
- Penicillin VK: 500 mg (peds: under age 12: 25–50 mg/kg/24 hours) PO q.i.d. × 10 days
- Tylenol with codeine #3: 1–2 tabs (peds: 3–6 years old: 10 mL) PO q4h PRN
- Clindamycin 300 mg PO (peds: 6–8 mg/kg/24 hours) t.i.d.
- Chlorhexidine gluconate (Peridex) 15 mL swish/spit b.i.d.
- Ibuprofen 600 mg (peds: 20 mg/kg/24 hours) q6h

Disposition

ADMISSION CRITERIA

- Extensive disease with systemic signs
- Children under 12 years old
- Severely immunocompromised patient requiring IV antibiotic treatment
- Severe dehydration
- Noma (cancrum oris) infection mouth/face
  —70% mortality with no Rx

DISCHARGE CRITERIA

- Able to maintain hydration

Miscellaneous

ICD9: 523.0

ICD10: A69.1

SUGGESTED READINGS

American Academy of Periodontology. Parameter on acute periodontal diseases. J Periodont 2000;71[5 suppl]:863–866.

Avendor TM. Seasonal variation of acute necrotising ulcerative gingivitis in South Africans. Oral Dis 2001;7(3):150–154.

Enwonwu CO. Oro-facial gangrene (noma/cancrum oris): pathogenetic mechanisms. Crit Rev Oral Biol Med 2000;11(2):159–171.

Rakel. Conn's current therapy, 54th ed. Philadelphia: W.B. Saunders, 2002.

Author: Forrest D. Holden

Adrenal Insufficiency

Clinical Presentation

SIGNS AND SYMPTOMS

Symptoms

- Depression
- Lethargy
- Malaise
- Myalgias
- Anorexia
- Abdominal pain
- Nausea
- Vomiting
- Dehydration (primary adrenal insufficiency only)
- Salt craving

Signs

- Fever or hypothermia
- Mental status changes
- Tachycardia
- Orthostatic blood pressure changes or frank shock
- Weight loss
- Goiter
- Hypogonadism
- Hyperkalemia
- Sodium depletion
- Eosinophilia
- Hyperpigmentation (primary adrenal insufficiency only)
- Vitiligo

Addisonian Crisis

- Hypotension and shock
- Hyponatremia
- Hyperkalemia
- Hypoglycemia

MECHANISM/DESCRIPTION

- Inadequate hydrocortisone secretion to meet body stress requirement
- Adrenal deficiency
  —Inadequate cortisol
  —ACTH stimulation unresponsive
- Functional hypoadrenalism
  —Inadequate cortisol
  —ACTH stimulation partial responsiveness

Addisonian Crisis (acute adrenal insufficiency)

- Life-threatening emergency
- Precipitated by intensification of
  —Chronic adrenal insufficiency
  —Acute adrenal hemorrhage
  —Rapid steroid withdrawal
  —Treatment of hypothyroidism with unrecognized adrenal disease
  —Steroid dependent patient under stress due to pregnancy, surgery, trauma, infection, or dehydration

ETIOLOGY

Primary Adrenal Failure

- Adrenal dysgenesis/impaired steroidogenesis
  —Congenital hypoplasia
  —Allgrove syndrome (ACTH resistance, achalasia, alacrima)
  —Glycerol kinase deficiency (psychomotor retardation, hypogonadism, muscular dystrophy)
  —Congenital hyperplasia
  —Aldosterone synthetase deficiency
  —Mitochondrial disease
- Adrenal destruction
  —Autoimmune
    -Autoimmune polyglandular syndrome type 1, 2 (alopecia universalis, chronic mucocutaneous candidiasis, hypoparathyroid, thyroid autoimmunity, diabetes, celiac disease, pernicious anemia)
    -Adrenoleukodystrophy
  —Infectious
    -Granulomatous: tuberculosis
    -Protozoal and fungi: histoplasmosis, coccidioidomycosis, candidiasis
    -Viral: CMV, HSV, HIV
    -Bacterial
  —Infiltration
    -Sarcoid
    -Neoplasm
    -Hemochromatosis
    -Amyloidosis
    -Iron depletion
- Postadrenalectomy
- Hemorrhage
  —Sepsis: particularly meningococcemia, *Pseudomonas*
  —Birth trauma/anoxia
  —Pregnancy
  —Seizures
  —Anticoagulants
  —Rhabdomyolysis
- Pharmacologic inhibition
  —Etomidate
  —Herbal medications
  —Ketoconazole
  —Metyrapone
  —Suramin

Secondary Adrenal Failure

- Pituitary insufficiency
  —Sepsis
  —Head trauma
  —Hemorrhage
  —Infarction (Sheehan's syndrome)
  —Infiltration: neoplasm, amyloid, sarcoid, hemachromatosis
  —ACTH deficiency
  —Pharmacologic: glucocorticoid administration, herbal medicines

Tertiary Adrenal Failure

- Hypothalamus insufficiency
- Sepsis
- Infiltrative: neoplasm, amyloid, sarcoid, hemachromatosis
- Head trauma

Pre-Hospital

N/A

Diagnosis

ESSENTIAL WORKUP

- Laboratory confirmation of the diagnosis not possible in the ED
- Adrenal crisis—life-threatening condition
  —High degree of suspicion should prompt the initiation of therapy before definitive diagnosis
- Plasma cortisol
  —Level $<20\ \mu g/dL$ in the setting of shock suggests adrenal insufficiency
- Electrolytes
  —K^+
  —Na^+
- BUN, Cr
  —Elevated due to dehydration
- Serum glucose
  —May be low

LABORATORY

- CBC with differential
  —Anemia
  —Eosinophilia
  —Lymphocytosis
- Arterial blood gases
  —Hypoxemia
  —Acidosis
- Cosyntropin stimulation test
  —Adrenal deficiency
    -Random serum cortisol $<20\ \mu g/dL$ (while stressed)
    -ACTH stimulation unresponsive
  —Functional hypoadrenalism
    -Random serum cortisol $= 20\ \mu g/dL$ (while stressed)
    -Post-ACTH stimulation 60 minutes $<30\ \mu g/dL$ or delta cortisol (60 min − baseline) $= 9\ \mu g/dL$
- Search for underlying infection

IMAGING/SPECIAL TESTS

- EKG
- CXR

DIFFERENTIAL DIAGNOSIS

- Sepsis
- Shock from any etiology
- Acute abdominal emergency

Treatment

INITIAL STABILIZATION

- ABCs
- Cardiac monitor
- Blood pressure support for hypotension
  - —0.9% NS IVF 500 cc–1 L (peds: 20 cc/kg) bolus
  - —Avoid pressors (if possible)
    - -May precipitate dysrhythmias
- Supplemental oxygen to meet metabolic needs
- Correct hyperthermia
  - —Initiate cooling measures

ED TREATMENT

- Glucocorticoid replacement
  - —IV hydrocortisone or dexamethasone
  - —Dexamethasone will not interfere with the results of the cosyntropin stimulation tests
- Volume expansion
  - —D5W 0.9% NS at a rate of 500–1,000 mL/hr for the first 3–4 hours
  - —Care should be taken to note the patient's age, volume, and cardiac and renal function
- For hypoglycemia
  - —Dextrose—D50W
- Treat life-threatening dysrhythmias secondary to hyperkalemia with calcium, bicarbonate, insulin/glucose
- Identification and correction of the underlying precipitant

MEDICATIONS

- Dexamethasone: 4 mg (peds: 0.15 mg/kg/dose) q12h
- Dextrose: 50–100 cc D50 (peds: 2 cc/kg of D10 over 1 min) i.v.
- Hydrocortisone: 100 mg (peds: 1–2 mg/kg/dose) i.v. q6h
- Insulin (regular): 10 units IVP
- Sodium bicarbonate: 1–2 mEq/kg i.v.

Disposition

ADMISSION CRITERIA

- Admit all patients with acute adrenal insufficiency
- ICU admission for unstable or potentially unstable

DISCHARGE CRITERIA

- Normal laboratory evaluation with treated adrenal insufficiency

Miscellaneous

ICD9: 255.4

ICD10: E27.4

SUGGESTED READINGS

Chang SS, Liaw SJ, Bullard MJ, et al. Adrenal insufficiency in critically ill emergency department patients: a Taiwan preliminary study. Acad Emerg Med 2001;8(7):761–764.

Oelkers W. Adrenal insufficiency. N Engl J Med 1996;355:1206–1212.

Rivers E, et al. Adrenal dysfunction in hemodynamically unstable patients in the emergency department. Acad Emerg Med 1999;6(6):626–630.

Rivers E, et al. Clinical investigations in critical care, adrenal insufficiency in high risk surgical ICU patients. Chest 2001; 119(3):889–896.

Ten S, New M, Noel M. Clinical review 130 Addison's disease 2001. J Clin Endocrinol Metab 2001;86(7):2909–2922.

Authors: Rita Cydulka; Michael Policastro

Airway Management

Clinical Presentation

SIGNS AND SYMPTOMS

Clinical Conditions Requiring Airway Management

- Failure to maintain or protect the airway
  - —Stridor
  - —Oropharyngeal swelling
  - —Absence of gag reflex
  - —Inability to clear secretions
- Hypoxia or ventilatory failure
  - —Shortness of breath
  - —Cyanosis
  - —Altered mental status
  - —Status epilepticus
- Ventilation control
  - —Head injury
  - —Tricyclic overdose
- Sedation for diagnostic procedures in agitated patients
- Early management if the prognosis suggests that the airway will soon be compromised

Recognition of a Difficult Airway

- Anatomic considerations
  - —Mallampati criteria—increasing difficulty
    - -Class I—soft palate, uvula, fauces, pillars visible
    - -Class II—soft palate, uvula, fauces visible
    - -Class III—soft palate visible
    - -Class IV—hard palate only
  - —Rule of 3, 3, 2—difficult airway if met
    - -Mouth opens >3 fingerbreadths
    - -Horizontal length of mandible >3 fingerbreadths
    - -Thyromental distance <2 fingerbreadths
  - —Congenital syndromes
  - —Goiter
  - —Obesity
  - —Acromegaly
  - —Arthritis
  - —Tumor
- Acquired conditions
  - —Angioedema
  - —Infection
    - -Epiglottitis
    - -Supraglottitis
    - -Croup
    - -Abscess (intraoral, retropharyngeal)
    - -Ludwig's angina
  - —Trauma
    - -Facial injury
    - -Penetrating neck trauma
    - -Cervical spine injury
    - -Laryngeal-tracheal injury
    - -Burns
  - —Laryngeal-tracheal tumors
  - —History of radiation therapy to the neck
  - —Rheumatoid arthritis and other arthropathies that decrease cervical spine mobility
  - —Profuse upper gastrointestinal hemorrhage

MECHANISM/DESCRIPTION

- Oral and nasopharyngeal airways
  - —Lift the tongue off hypopharynx
  - —Facilitate bag-valve-mask (BVM) ventilation
  - —Insert when gag reflex is absent
- Oral rapid sequence intubation (RSI)
  - —Preferred method—minimizes aspiration risk
  - —Induction of anesthesia and paralysis
  - —Method of choice for suspected head injury
  - —Contraindicated in patients who should not be paralyzed
- Oral awake intubation
  - —Oral intubation with sedation only
  - —Ketamine is the most common agent used for this purpose
    - -Dissociative anesthesia
    - -Contraindicated in head injury (may elevate ICP)
    - -Use with benzodiazepines
    - -Indicated when paralysis is hazardous due to airway distortion
- Gum elastic bougie
  - —Airway adjunct used when vocal cords are not well visualized
  - —Placement confirmed by feeling bougie bump against tracheal rings
  - —Slide endotracheal (ET) tube over the bougie, then remove bougie
- Fiberoptic intubation
  - —ET tube placed over the bronchoscope
  - —Nasotracheal or orotracheal approach
  - —Indications
    - -Anatomic limitations to glottis visualization
    - -Limited movement of mandible or cervical spine
    - -Unstable cervical spine injury
  - —Contraindications
    - -Need for immediate airway management
    - -Significant airway hemorrhage
- Lighted stylet
  - —Used to transilluminate the neck and guide tube placement
  - —Alternative to laryngoscopic intubation
  - —Indications
    - -Blood in the oropharynx
    - -Failed airway
- Laryngeal mask airway (LMA)
  - —Inserted blindly into oropharynx and inflated
  - —Patient ventilated through tube connected to the mask
  - —Used to ventilate until definitive airway is established
  - —Less protection against aspiration compared to ET intubation
  - —Intubating LMA can be used to place an ET tube blindly
- Blind nasotracheal intubation
  - —Indications
    - -Oral access impaired (angioedema)
    - -Unsuccessful oral intubation
    - -Neuromuscular blockade is contraindicated
    - -Limited cervical mobility (rheumatoid arthritis)
  - —Contraindications
    - -Apnea
    - -Anticoagulation
    - -Massive facial, nasal, or head trauma
    - -Upper airway abscess
    - -Acute epiglottitis
    - -Penetrating neck trauma
- Cricothyrotomy
  - —Incision in cricothyroid membrane
  - —Shiley tracheostomy tube is inserted in the airway
  - —Indications
    - -Other airway attempts have failed
    - -Massive facial trauma
    - -Total upper airway obstruction
  - —Contraindications
    - -Laryngeal crush injury
    - -Expanding zone II or III hematoma
- Percutaneous translaryngeal ventilation
  - —A temporizing measure until definitive airway is established
  - —Percutaneous placement of 12- or 14-gauge catheter through cricothyroid membrane
  - —Intermittent ventilation via high-pressure oxygen source
  - —Indications
    - -Failed oral or nasal intubation until cricothyrotomy is complete
  - —Contraindications
    - -Upper airway obstruction that prevents expiration
- Retrograde tracheal intubation
  - —A technique available when all others have failed
  - —Retrograde advancement of guidewire through translaryngeal catheter
  - —ET tube advanced over wire once it comes out of the mouth

ETIOLOGY

N/A

PEDIATRIC CONSIDERATIONS

- Estimation of ET tube size: 4 + age/4
- Uncuffed ET tubes should be used in patients <8 years old
- Straight Miller blade is preferred in patients <3 years old
- Preferred surgical airway is PTV for patients <12 years old

Pre-Hospital

CONTROVERSIES

- Use of facilitated intubation (paralysis and sedation) is controversial for urban EMS systems with short transport times
- RSI used primarily by flight crews

CAUTIONS

- Basic life support providers use only BVM ventilation
- Options for patients in respiratory arrest for ALS providers:
  - —BVM ventilation followed by definitive airway management in the ED
  - —Orotracheal intubation
  - —Pharyngotracheal lumen airway, e.g., the Combitube
    - -A device with two tubes and two balloons
    - -Ventilates either with tracheal or esophageal intubation
    - -Functions as an ET tube or esophageal obturator depending on placement
    - -Indicated when ET intubation is not available
  - —Contraindications
    - -Children
    - -Caustic ingestions
    - -Esophageal disease
    - -Presence of gag reflex

Diagnosis

ESSENTIAL WORKUP

- Verification of correct tube placement
  - —Auscultate over stomach, axillae, and anterior lung fields
  - —Observe chest wall movement
  - —Condensation in the tube during ventilation
  - —End-tidal CO_2 colorimetric device
    - -Changes color if CO_2 is sensed, indicating tracheal placement
    - -Color change may not be seen in cardiac arrest

LABORATORY

- Pulse oximetry should rise after tracheal intubation
- Arterial blood gas to manage ventilator settings after intubation

IMAGING/SPECIAL TESTS

- Syringe aspiration technique
  - —Detects esophageal intubation
  - —Catheter-tipped 60-cc syringe is inserted at proximal end of the ET tube
  - —Resistance to aspiration indicates esophageal placement
- Chest radiography
  - —To exclude mainstem bronchus intubation or pneumothorax
  - —May not rule out esophageal intubation, as the tube may appear to be in the trachea

DIFFERENTIAL DIAGNOSIS

- Esophageal intubation
- Right or left mainstem bronchus intubation
- Extratracheal placement through tear in pyriform sinus or trachea
- Pneumothorax

Treatment

INITIAL STABILIZATION

- Maintain in-line cervical spine immobilization
- Check equipment
  - —Suction
  - —Oxygen
  - —BVM
  - —Various sizes of ET tubes
  - —Laryngoscope blades
  - —Stylets
  - —Medications

ED TREATMENT

- Rapid sequence intubation
- Preoxygenation
  - —100% FIO_2 for 5 minutes
- Premedication
  - —Performed 2–3 minutes prior to paralytic
  - —Defasciculating dose of vecuronium or pancuronium
  - —Fentanyl and lidocaine minimize the rise in ICP in head-injured patients
  - —Lidocaine decreases airway irritability in reactive airway disease
  - —Atropine attenuates the vagal effect in children
- Apply cricoid pressure (Sellick's maneuver) to occlude esophagus and prevent aspiration
- Avoid mask ventilation after preoxygenation to reduce aspiration risk
- Induction/paralysis
  - —Administration of induction agent (e.g., etomidate or thiopental)
  - —Administration of paralytic agent (e.g., succinylcholine)
  - —Thiopental
    - -Contraindicated in hypovolemic or hypotensive patients
  - —Succinylcholine
    - -Relative contraindications
      - *Anticipated difficult oral intubation
      - *Open globe injury
      - *Organophosphate poisoning
      - *Burns >3 days old
- Intubation
  - —After muscle tone is lost (45–60 seconds after succinylcholine chloride (SCh) administration)
  - —Use a stylet with the ET tube
  - —Inflate cuff once the tube is placed before ventilating
  - —Confirm correct ET tube placement
- Postintubation
  - —Benzodiazepines and opiates used for continued sedation
  - —Vecuronium may be used for continued paralysis

PEDIATRIC CONSIDERATIONS

- Use atropine to reduce secretions from ketamine
- A defasciculating neuromuscular blocking agent is not needed for children <5 years old

MEDICATIONS

- Atracurium: 0.4–0.5 mg/kg i.v.
- Atropine: 0.02 mg/kg i.v.
- Diazepam: 2–10 mg i.v. (peds: 0.2–0.3 mg/kg)
- Etomidate: 0.3 mg/kg i.v.
- Fentanyl: 3 μg/kg i.v.
- Ketamine: 1–2 mg/kg i.v. or 4–7 mg/kg i.m.
- Lidocaine: 1.5 mg/kg i.v.
- Midazolam: 1–5 mg i.v. (0.07–0.30 mg/kg for induction)
- Propofol: 2–2.5 mg/kg i.v.
- Pancuronium: 0.01 mg/kg i.v. (defasciculating dose); 0.1 mg/kg i.v. (paralyzing dose)
- Succinylcholine: 1.5 mg/kg i.v. (peds: 2 mg/kg); 2.5 mg/kg i.m. or s.c.; 0.15 mg/kg i.v. (defasciculating pretreatment dose)
- Thiopental: 3 mg/kg i.v.
- Vecuronium: 0.01 mg/kg i.v. (defasciculating dose); 0.1 mg/kg i.v. (paralyzing dose)

Disposition

ADMISSION CRITERIA

- All intubated patients should be admitted to an ICU

DISCHARGE CRITERIA

- Certain ED patients who have been intubated for airway protection or to facilitate diagnostic workup may be extubated in the ED after a period of observation, and then discharged

Miscellaneous

ICD-9: N/A

ICD10: N/A

SEE ALSO: RAPID SEQUENCE INTUBATION

SUGGESTED READINGS

Clinton JE, McGill JW. Basic airway management and decision-making. In: Roberts JR, Hedges JR, eds. Clinical procedures in emergency medicine, 3rd ed. Philadelphia: WB Saunders, 1998:1–14.

Levitan R, Ochroch EA. Airway management and direct laryngoscopy. A review and update. Crit Care Clin 2000;16(3):373–388.

Reed AP. The unanticipated difficult airway. Anesth Clin North Am 1996;14(3):443–469.

Wadbrook PS. Advances in airway pharmacology. Emerging trends and evolving controversy. Emerg Med Clin North Am 2000;18(4):767–788.

Walls RM. Airway. In: Marx JA, et al., eds. Rosen's emergency medicine: concepts and clinical practice, 5th ed. St. Louis: Mosby, 2002:2–21.

Authors: Scott G. Weiner; Carlo L. Rosen

Alcohol, Poisoning

Clinical Presentation

SIGNS AND SYMPTOMS

Acute Alcohol Intoxication

- Sedation
- Relaxation
- Euphoria
- Memory loss
- Impaired judgment
- Ataxia
- Slurred speech
- Nausea/vomiting
- Obtundation/coma

Alcohol Withdrawal Syndrome

Early or Minor Withdrawal

- <8 hours after last drink (blood alcohol level becomes zero)
  —Symptoms of a hangover
  —Headache
  —Nausea/vomiting
- 12 hours after last drink
  —Mild tremors/anxiety
  —Anorexia, nausea, vomiting
  —Weakness
  —Myalgias
  —Vivid dreams/nightmares
- 12–36 hours after last drink
  —Irritability/agitation
  —Tachycardia/hypertension
  —Tremors in hands and tongue
- Alcohol hallucinosis
  —24 hours after last drink
  —Visual most common (bug crawling)
  —Auditory (buzz, clicks)
  —Present in minor and major withdrawal
- Alcoholic withdrawal seizures
  —8–12 hours after last drink
  —Brief, spontaneously abating tonic-clonic activity
  —Precedes delirium tremens (DTs)

Late Alcohol Withdrawal or Major Withdrawal

- 48 hours after last drink
- DTs
  —Clouded consciousness and delirium (hallmark)
  —Confusion/disorientation
  —Agitation/combativeness
  —Tachycardia/hypertension
  —Hyperpyrexia
  —Diaphoresis

MECHANISM/DESCRIPTION

Alcohol Intoxication

- Direct CNS depressant effect
- Blood alcohol levels drop by 15–40 mg/dL/hr depending on individual variables and chronicity of alcohol use

Alcohol Withdrawal

- Occurs after partial or complete alcohol abstinence in a chronic alcoholic
- CNS excitation
- Increased autonomic catecholamine release
- Decreased inhibitory activity

PEDIATRIC CONSIDERATION

- Coma from intoxication more common in adolescents at a lower alcohol level than adults
- Hypoglycemia may occur in acutely intoxicated children

Pre-Hospital

CAUTIONS

- Do not induce emesis because of aspiration risk
- Administer benzodiazepines for seizures
- Administer coma cocktail for mental status changes

Diagnosis

ESSENTIAL WORKUP

- Investigate for life-threatening causes of seizures
  —Hypoglycemia
  —Intracranial hemorrhage
  —CNS infection
  —Electrolyte abnormalities
- Obtain accurate alcohol drinking/abstinence history
- Evaluate for occult trauma

LABORATORY

- Alcohol level if abnormal mental status
- Toxicology screen to exclude common co-ingestants
- Electrolytes, BUN, creatinine, and glucose
- CBC
- Magnesium, calcium, and phosphate
- PTT, PT/INR if coagulopathy suspected
- Liver function tests if liver disease suspected
- Ammonia level if hepatic encephalopathy suspected

IMAGING/SPECIAL TESTS

- CT of head if
  —Altered mental status in greater proportion to intoxication
  —Suspected head trauma
  —Signs of increased intracranial pressure or focal findings on neurologic exams
  —Partial (focal) seizures
  —New-onset seizure
  —Unimproved or deteriorating level of consciousness
- EEG differentiates alcohol withdrawal seizures from idiopathic epilepsy
- CXR if suspected pneumonia

DIFFERENTIAL DIAGNOSIS

Acute Alcohol Intoxication

- Hypoglycemia
- Carbon dioxide narcosis
- Mixed-drug overdose
- Ethylene glycol, methanol, isopropanol poisoning
- Hepatic encephalopathy
- Psychosis
- Severe vertigo
- Psychomotor seizure

Alcohol Withdrawal–Related Seizures

- Sedative-hypnotic withdrawal
- Acute intoxication or poisoning
  —Carbon monoxide
  —Isoniazid
  —Amphetamine
  —Anticholinergic
  —Cocaine
- Idiopathic epilepsy
- Infection
  —Meningitis
  —Encephalitis
  —Brain abscess
- Trauma
- Intracranial hemorrhage
- CVA
- Tumor
- Anticonvulsant noncompliance

Treatment

INITIAL STABILIZATION

- ABCs
- Evaluate C-spine if suspected trauma
- IV rehydration with D5.9% NS
- Administer naloxone, thiamine, and glucose (or Accucheck) if altered mental status

ED TREATMENT

Alcohol Withdrawal Syndrome

- Benzodiazepine is agent of choice (diazepam, lorazepam, chlordiazepoxide)
  —Cross-tolerant with alcohol
  —Increases $GABA_A$-mediated transmission
  —Anticonvulsant effect
  —Large doses required with significant withdrawal
  —May halt progression to DTs
- Barbiturates (phenobarbital)
  —Cross-tolerant with alcohol
  —Anticonvulsant effect
  —Useful if severe withdrawal or DTs refractory to large doses of benzodiazepines
- Beta-blocker (propranolol and atenolol)
  —Normalizes vital sign abnormalities
  —Does *not* treat CNS complications of alcohol use or withdrawal
- α-Agonist (clonidine)
  —Centrally acting α_2-adrenergic agonist
  —Normalizes vital sign abnormalities
  —Does *not* treat CNS complications of alcohol use or withdrawal
- Phenytoin
  —Not indicated in alcohol withdrawal seizures
  —Indicated if seizures secondary to idiopathic epilepsy, posttraumatic, or status epilepticus

Fluid and Electrolyte Disturbances

- Replete magnesium if
  —Hypomagnesemia
  —Clinical signs of
    -Ataxia
    -Vertigo
    -Hyperactive reflexes
    -Tremors
    -Athetoid and choreiform movements
    -Babinski sign
    -Hyperacusis
  —Hypokalemia
- Correct hyponatremia
- Correct hypokalemia
- Alcoholic ketoacidosis
  —Aggressive rehydration with D5.9% NS
  —Exclude other causes of acidosis

MEDICATIONS

- Chlordiazepoxide (Librium): 25–100 mg, PO or i.v. q6h
- Dextrose: D50W 1 amp (50 mL or 25 g) (peds: D25W 2–4 mL/kg) i.v.
- Diazepam: 5–10 mg i.v. q 5–10 min until patient calm
- Lorazepam: 0.5–4 mg i.v./i.m. q 5–10 min until patient calm
- Naloxone (Narcan): 0.4–2 mg (peds: 0.1 mg/kg) i.v. or i.m. initial dose
- Phenobarbital: 10–20 mg/kg i.v. (loading dose)
- Phenytoin: 15–18 mg/kg at 50 mg/min i.v.
- Thiamine (vitamin B_1): 100 mg (peds: 50 mg) i.v. or i.m.

Disposition

ADMISSION CRITERIA

- Hepatic failure, infection, dehydration, malnutrition, cardiovascular collapse, cardiac dysrhythmia, trauma
- Hallucinations, tachycardia >100/min, severe tremors, extreme agitation
- Wernicke's encephalopathy
- Confusion or delirium

DISCHARGE CRITERIA

- Clinically sober
- Seizure free for 6 hours (with negative workup if first seizure)

Miscellaneous

ICD9: 980.0

ICD10: T51.9

SEE ALSO: ETHYLENE GLYCOL, POISONING METHANOL, POISONING

SUGGESTED READINGS

Chang PH, Steinberg MB. Alcohol withdrawal. Med Clin North Am 2001;85(5):1191–1212.

Chiang C, Wax P. Withdrawal syndromes. In: Ford MD, Delaney KA, Ling LJ, et al., eds. Clinical toxicology. Philadelphia: WB Saunders, 2001:582–586.

D'Onofrio G, Rathlev NK, Ulrich AS, et al. Lorazepam for the prevention of recurrent seizures related to alcohol. N Engl J Med 1999;340(12):915–919.

Mayo-Smith MF. Pharmacological management of alcohol withdrawal. JAMA 1997;278(2):144–151.

McMicken DB, Freedland ES. Alcohol-related seizures. Emerg Med Clin North Am 1994;12(4):1057–1079.

Author: Mark B. Mycyk

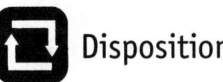

Alcoholic Ketoacidosis

Clinical Presentation

SIGNS AND SYMPTOMS

- Dehydration
- Fever absent unless there is an underlying infection
- Tachycardia due to
  - —Dehydration with associated orthostatic changes
  - —Concurrent alcohol withdrawal
- Tachypnea
  - —Common
  - —Deep, rapid, Kussmaul respirations frequently present
- Nausea and vomiting
- Abdominal pain
  - —Usually diffuse with nonspecific tenderness
  - —Rebound tenderness, abdominal distention, hypoactive bowel sounds uncommon
    - -Mandates a search for an alternative, coexistent illness
- Decreased urinary output from hypovolemia
- Mental status
  - —Minimally altered as a result of hypovolemia and possibly intoxication
  - —Altered mental status mandates a search for other associated conditions such as
    - -Head injury, CVA, intracranial hemorrhage
    - -Hypoglycemia
    - -Alcohol withdrawal

MECHANISM/DESCRIPTION

- Increased production of ketone bodies due to
  - —Malnourished and hypovolemic patient
  - —Depleted glycogen stores in the liver
  - —Elevated ratio of NADH/NAD due to ethanol metabolism
  - —Increased free fatty acid production
- Elevated NADH/NAD ratio leads to the predominate production of β-hydroxybutyrate (BHB) over acetoacetate (AcAc)

ETIOLOGY

- Malnourished, chronic alcohol abusers following a recent episode of heavy alcohol consumption
  - —Develop nausea/vomiting/abdominal pain
  - —Leading to the cessation of alcohol ingestion
  - —In combination with decreased caloric intake over the preceding several days
- Presentation usually occurs within 12–72 hours

Pre-Hospital

CAUTIONS

- Supportive measures including IV access with 0.9 NS, oxygen, and cardiac monitoring
- Search for historical clues that may suggest other etiologies such as toxic ingestions or diabetic history
- Attend to other possible coexistent illnesses such as GI bleeding

Diagnosis

ESSENTIAL WORKUP

- Presence of an increased anion gap metabolic acidosis secondary to the presence of ketones
- Recent history of alcohol consumption

LABORATORY

Acid–Base Disturbance

- Increased anion gap metabolic acidosis hallmark
- Mixed acid-base disturbance common
  - —Respiratory alkalosis
  - —Metabolic alkalosis secondary to vomiting and dehydration
  - —Hyperchloremic acidosis
- Mild lactic acidosis common
  - —Due to dehydration and the direct metabolic effects of ethanol
  - —Profound lactic acidosis should prompt a search for other disorders such as seizures, hypoxia, and shock
- Positive urine and serum nitroprusside reaction tests
  - —May not reflect the severity of the underlying ketoacidosis since BHB predominates and is not measured by this test
  - —May become misleadingly more positive during treatment as more AcAc is produced

Electrolytes

- Decreased serum bicarbonate
- Hypokalemia due to vomiting
- Hypocalcemia
- Hypophosphatemia
- Glucose
  - —Usually mildly elevated
  - —Hypoglycemia may be present
- BUN and creatinine mildly elevated due to dehydration

CBC

- Mild leukocytosis
- Thrombocytopenia and anemia commonly due to chronic alcoholism

Urinalysis

- Ketonuria without glucosuria

Amylase/Lipase

- Elevated with associated pancreatitis

Liver Function Tests

- Mildly elevated LFT

Osmolal Gap

- May be mildly elevated
- A level over 20 mOsm/kg should prompt evaluation for other ingestions (methanol and ethylene glycol)

IMAGING/SPECIAL TESTS

- CXR if suspect associated pneumonia
- Abdominal films for free air if an acute abdomen is present
- CT scan of the head if associated trauma or unexplained altered mental status

DIFFERENTIAL DIAGNOSIS

- Increased anion gap metabolic acidosis
  - —Lactic acidosis
  - —Carbon monoxide poisoning
  - —Aspirin
  - —Methanol
  - —Ethylene glycol
  - —Paraldehyde
  - —Isoniazid
  - —Diabetic ketoacidosis—more severe hyperglycemia/diabetic history
  - —Uremia
- Hypovolemia
  - —GI bleeding
  - —Sepsis
- Abdominal pain
  - —Pancreatitis
  - —GI bleeding
  - —Gastritis
  - —Hepatitis
  - —Perforated ulcer
  - —Alcohol withdrawal

Treatment

INITIAL STABILIZATION

- Cardiac monitor and supplemental oxygen
- Naloxone, thiamine, and dextrose if altered mental status
- IV: 0.9% NS
  —500 cc—1 L bolus
  —Promotes renal excretion of ketone bodies

ED TREATMENT

- Antiemetic for vomiting—promethazine or prochlorperazine
- Benzodiazepines for symptoms of alcohol withdrawal
- Start dextrose containing solutions (D5W 0.9% NS)
  —Avoid with significant hyperglycemia
  —Repletes glycogen stores
  —Decreases production of ketone bodies by stimulating the production of endogenous insulin
  —More rapid resolution of the metabolic abnormalities than saline alone
- Thiamine repletion prior to glucose administration to avoid precipitating Wernicke's encephalopathy
- Sodium bicarbonate rarely indicated
  —Consider in severe acidosis with associated cardiovascular dysfunction or irritability
- Electrolyte replacement
  —Hypokalemia occurs with treatment and should be anticipated
  —Hypophosphatemia may occur with treatment
  —Magnesium replacement as indicated
- Insulin is not indicated and may precipitate hypoglycemia
- Treatment of associated disorders is usually indicated

MEDICATIONS

- D50W: one ampule of 50% dextrose (25 g) IVP
- Lorazepam (benzodiazepine): 2 mg i.v. and titrate to effect
- Naloxone: 2 mg IVP
- Prochlorperazine: 5–10 mg IVP
- Promethazine: 12.5–25 mg IVP
- Thiamine: 100 mg IVP

Disposition

ADMISSION CRITERIA

- Persistent metabolic acidosis
- Persistent orthostatic hypotension
- Persistent nausea and vomiting
- Abdominal pain of uncertain etiology
- Comorbid illness requiring admission for treatment
- Monitored bed due to electrolyte abnormalities requiring continued treatment

DISCHARGED CRITERIA

- Many patients can be managed in observation unit over 12 hours
- Tolerating oral fluids well
- Resolution of metabolic abnormalities
- No other associated illnesses requiring additional therapy

Miscellaneous

ICD9: 276.2

ICD10: E87.2

SEE ALSO: DIABETIC KETOACIDOSIS, ACIDOSIS

SUGGESTED READINGS

Adams SL. Alcoholic ketoacidosis. Emerg Med Clin North Am 1990;8(4):749–760.

Godet C, Hira M, Adoun M, et al. Rapid diagnosis of alcoholic ketoacidosis by proton NMR. Intensive Care Med 2001;27(4):785–786.

Hoger J. Severe metabolic acidosis in the alcoholic: differential diagnosis and management. Hum Exp Toxicol 1996;15(6): 482–488.

Smith D, Kelly D, Daly A, et al. Alcoholic ketoacidosis presenting as diabetic ketoacidosis. Ir J Med Sci 1999;168(3):186–188.

Wrenn KD, Slovis CM, et al. The syndrome of alcoholic ketoacidosis. Am J Med 1991;91(2):119–128.

Author: Jefferson Bracey

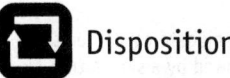

Altered Mental Status

Clinical Presentation

SIGNS AND SYMPTOMS

Confusion

- Difficulty in maintaining a coherent stream of thinking and mental performance
  —Remember to consider the level of education and language and possible learning disabilities
- Inattention
- Memory deficit
  —Inability to recall any of the following
    -The date, inclusive of month, day, year, and day of week
    -The precise place
    -Items of universally known information
    -Why the patient is in the hospital
    -Address, telephone number, or Social Security number
- Impaired mental performance
  —Difficulty retaining seven digits forward and four backward
  —Difficulty naming ordinary objects
  —Serial calculations
    -Holding the result of one calculation in a working memory in order to pursue the next step
    -Serial 3-from-30 subtraction test
- Disorganized and rambling language
  —May be mistaken for aphasia

Findings that Suggest an Underlying Cause

- Fever
  —Infectious etiologies, drug toxicities, endocrine disorders, heat stroke
- Severe hypertension and decreased heart rate (Cushing's reflex)
  —Suggestive of an intracranial structural lesion
- Hypotension
  —Infectious and toxicologic etiologies, decreased cardiac output
- Hypothermia
  —Hypoglycemia, environmental factors, Addisonian crisis
- Eye resting position
  —Dysconjugate gaze in horizontal plane occurs with drowsiness
  —Dysconjugate gaze in vertical plane occurs with pontine or cerebellar lesions
  —Sustained conjugate downward eye deviation occurs with a variety of neurologic disorders
  —Sustained conjugate upward gaze occurs with hypoxic encephalopathy
  —Eyes fluttering upwards (Bell's phenomenon) occurs with psychogenic coma
  —Ocular bobbing
    -Cyclical brisk conjugate caudal jerks of the globes followed by a slow return to midposition
    -Bilateral pontine damage, metabolic derangement, and brainstem compression
  —Ocular dipping
    -Slow, cyclical, conjugate, downward movement of the eyes followed by a rapid return to midposition
    -Diffuse cortical anoxic damage
- Pupillary examination
  —Normal size, shape, and response to light indicates intact midbrain function
  —Nearly all toxic and metabolic causes of coma leave the pupillary reflexes sluggish but bilaterally intact
- Focal findings
  —Hemiparesis
  —Hemianopsia
  —Aphasia
  —Myoclonus
  —Convulsions
- Asterixis
  —Arrhythmic flapping tremor (almost always bilateral)
  —Caused by metabolic encephalopathy
    -Hepatic failure or severe renal failure
    -Anticonvulsant drug ingestion
- Myoclonic jerking and tremor
  —Uremic encephalopathy
  —Antipsychotic drug ingestion

MECHANISM/DESCRIPTION

- Dysfunction in either the reticular activating system in the upper brainstem or a large area of one of the cerebral hemispheres
- Definitions
  —Confusion: a behavioral state of reduced mental clarity, coherence, comprehension, and reasoning
  —Drowsiness: the patient cannot be easily aroused by touch or noise and cannot maintain alertness for some time
  —Lethargy: depressed mental status in which the patient may appear wakeful but has depressed awareness of self and environment globally; cannot be aroused to full function
  —Stupor: the patient can be awakened only by vigorous stimuli, and an effort to avoid uncomfortable or aggravating stimulation is displayed
  —Coma: the patient cannot be aroused by stimulation and no purposeful attempt is made to avoid painful stimuli

ETIOLOGY

- Hypoxic
  —Severe pulmonary disease
  —Anemia
  —Shock
  —Intracardiac shunting (especially in pediatrics)
- Metabolic
  —Hypoglycemia
  —Diabetic ketoacidosis
  —Nonketotic hyperosmolar coma
  —Thiamine deficiency
  —Hyperammonemia
  —Uremia
  —CO_2 narcosis
  —Hyperglycemia
  —Hyponatremia; hypernatremia
  —Hypocalcemia; hypercalcemia
  —Hypomagnesemia; hypermagnesemia
  —Hypophosphatemia
  —Acidosis; alkalosis
- Toxicologic
  —Ethanol
  —Isopropyl alcohol
  —Methanol
  —Ethylene glycol
  —Salicylates
  —Sedatives and narcotics
  —Anticonvulsants
  —Psychotropics
  —Isoniazid
  —Heavy metals
  —Carbon monoxide
  —Cyanide
- Endocrine
  —Myxedema coma
  —Thyrotoxicosis
  —Hypothyroidism
  —Addison's disease
  —Cushing's disease
  —Pheochromocytoma
  —Hyperparathyroidism
- Environmental
  —Hypothermia
  —Heat stroke
  —Neuroleptic malignant syndrome
  —Malignant hyperthermia
- Intracranial hypertension
- Hypertensive encephalopathy
- Pseudotumor cerebri
- CNS inflammation
- Meningitis
- Encephalitis
- Encephalopathy
- Cerebral vasculitis
- TTP
- Subarachnoid hemorrhage
- Carcinoid meningitis
- Traumatic axonal shear injury
- Primary neuronal or glial disorders
  —Creutzfeldt-Jakob disease
  —Marchiafava-Bignami disease
  —Adrenoleukodystrophy
  —Gliomatosis cerebri
  —Progressive multifocal leukoencephalopathy
- Seizures and postictal state
- Supratentorial lesions
  —Hemorrhage
  —Infarction
  —Tumors
  —Abscess

- Subtentorial lesions
  - —Cerebellar hemorrhage
  - —Posterior fossa subdural or extradural hemorrhage
  - —Cerebellar infarct
  - —Cerebellar tumor
  - —Cerebellar abscess
  - —Basilar aneurysm
  - —Pontine hemorrhage
  - —Brainstem infarct
  - —Basilar migraine
  - —Brainstem demyelination

Pre-Hospital

CAUTIONS

- Airway management if loss of airway patency
- IV access, supplemental oxygen, cardiac monitor
- Bag-mask ventilation with cricoid pressure
- Endotracheal intubation if no response to coma cocktail
- Coma cocktail
  - —Dextrose
  - —Naloxone
  - —Thiamine
- Look for signs of an underlying cause
  - —Medications
  - —Medic alert bracelets
  - —Document a basic neurologic examination
  - —GCS
  - —Pupils
  - —Extremity movements
  - —Gross signs of trauma
  - —Talk with family/pre-hospital personnel for information

CONTROVERSIES

- Empirical dextrose should not be withheld or delayed if Dextrostix is not available
  - —Glucose can be safely administered before thiamine
  - —Glucose does not worsen outcome in patients with stroke
- Administration of charcoal by pre-hospital personnel

Diagnosis

ESSENTIAL WORKUP

LABORATORY

- Dextrostix and glucose
- CBC
- Electrolytes (including calcium)
- BUN, creatinine
- Arterial blood gases
- Toxicologic screen (including toxic alcohols)
- EKG
- UA
- Consider LFTs, ammonia, serum osmolarity

IMAGING/SPECIAL TESTS

- Caloric stimulation of the vestibular apparatus
  - —Indicated to assess unresponsive patients
  - —Contraindications include tympanic membrane perforation and cerumen impaction
  - —Irrigate the external auditory canal with 10 cc of ice-cold water after elevating the head to 30 degrees
  - —Bilateral tonic deviation of the eyes toward the stimulus indicates an intact brainstem
  - —Nystagmus-like quick corrective phases indicates intact cerebral hemispheres
  - —A normal response in an unresponsive patient raises the suspicion of psychogenic coma
- CT scan
  - —Noncontrast only to rule out hemorrhage and mass effect
- Lumbar puncture (LP)
  - —Indicated when the etiology remains unclear after laboratory and CT scan
  - —Empiric antibiotics should be given before LP to avoid any delay in therapy in patients with suspected meningitis[1]

DIFFERENTIAL DIAGNOSIS

- Locked in syndrome
  - —Rare disorder caused by damage to the corticospinal, corticopontine, and corticobulbar tracts resulting in quadriplegia and mutism with preservation of consciousness
  - —Communication may be established through eye movements (maintain vertical eye movements)
- Psychogenic unresponsiveness
  - —Conversion reactions
  - —Catatonia
- Malingering
- Akinetic mutism (abulic state)
- Dementia
  - —The mental status waxes and wanes
  - —Attention is preserved in the early stages

Treatment

INITIAL STABILIZATION

- Intravenous D50
- Naloxone
- Thiamine

ED TREATMENT

- Consider empiric use of antibiotics for altered mental status of undetermined etiology
  - —Broad spectrum with good CSF penetration such as ceftriaxone and vancomycin
- Empiric treatment if a toxic ingestion is suspected
  - —Activated charcoal
  - —Alcohol drip if methanol or ethylene glycol is suspected
- Correct body temperature
  - —Warmed humidified O_2 and IV fluids if hypothermic
  - —Ice packs and forced air movement over exposed moistened skin if severe hyperthermia
- Specific therapy directed at underlying cause

MEDICATIONS

- Ceftriaxone: 2 g i.v.
- Dextrose: 1–2 mL/kg of D50W (peds: 2–4 mL/kg D25W) i.v.
- Diazepam: 0.1–0.3 mg/kg slow i.v. (max 10 mg/dose) q 10–15 min × 3 doses
- Lorazepam: 0.05–0.1 mg/kg i.v. (max 4 mg/dose q 10–15 min)
- Naloxone: 0.01 to 0.1 mg/kg i.v./i.m./s.c./ET
- Thiamine: 100 mg i.m. or 100 mg thiamine in 1,000 mL of intravenous fluid wide open

Disposition

ADMISSION CRITERIA

- All patients with acute changes in mental status require admission

DISCHARGE CRITERIA

- Treated hypoglycemia related to insulin therapy with resolved symptoms
- Chronic altered mental status (e.g., dementia) without change from baseline

Miscellaneous

ICD9: 293.0, 293.81, 293.82, 294.1, 294.8

ICD10: F99

SEE ALSO: COMA

SUGGESTED READINGS

Hoffman RS, Goldfrank LR. The poisoned patient with altered consciousness. Controversies in the use of a "coma cocktail." JAMA 1995;274:562–569.

Samuels MA. The evaluation of comatose patients. Hosp Pract 1993;28:165–182.

Thakore S, Murphy N. The potential role of prehospital administration of actival charcoal. Emerg Med J 2002;19(1):63–65.

Authors: Kriti Bhatia; David F. M. Brown

[1] What is the place for MRI? Notably in patients with focal findings some centers will use MRI as the primary imaging study with the consideration of thrombolysis if ischemic stroke seen and time frame acceptable.

Amebiasis

Clinical Presentation

SIGNS AND SYMPTOMS

Intestinal Disease

- Onset 1 week to 1 month postexposure
- Acute diarrhea
  - —1–4 weeks' duration
  - —Afebrile
  - —Occult blood present in stool
  - —Benign abdominal exam
- "Classic" dysentery
  - —1–4 weeks' duration
  - —Bloody mucoid diarrhea
  - —Abdominal pain
  - —Bloating
  - —Tenesmus
  - —Weight loss
  - —Fever
  - —Benign abdominal exam
- Fulminant colitis
  - —Toxic-appearing patient
  - —Rigid abdomen in 25% of patients
  - —Fever
  - —Severe bloody diarrhea
  - —Rapid progression to perforated viscus and frank peritonitis
  - —High mortality (>50%)
  - —Children, pregnant women, and immunosuppressed patients at higher risk
- Toxic megacolon
  - —Toxic-appearing patient
  - —Profuse diarrhea (>10 stools per day)
  - —Fever
  - —Tachycardia
  - —Distended, tympanitic abdomen with signs of peritonitis
  - —Associated with administration of corticosteroids to patients with amebiasis
  - —High mortality
- Ameboma
  - —Intraluminal granulated mass
  - —Most common in the cecum, ascending colon, and rectosigmoid colon
  - —Tender palpable mass on exam
- Amebic strictures
  - —Due to chronic inflammation and scarring
  - —Most common in the anus, rectum, or sigmoid colon
  - —May lead to partial or complete bowel obstruction
  - —Crampy abdominal pain
  - —Nausea and vomiting (may be feculent)
  - —Inability to pass stool or flatus if obstruction is complete
  - —Distended, tender abdomen with high-pitched bowel sounds
- Chronic amebic colitis
  - —Mild recurrent episodes of bloody diarrhea, abdominal cramping, tenesmus
  - —Weight loss
  - —May persist for years

Extraintestinal Disease

- Amebic liver abscess
  - —Most frequent extraintestinal manifestation
  - —Single abscess in right lobe (80%)
  - —Symptomatic within 5 months of exposure (median of 3 months)
  - —Fever
  - —Cough
  - —Right upper quadrant pain
  - —Hepatomegaly with point tenderness
  - —Rales at right lung base
  - —Concurrent diarrhea unusual (20–33% of patients)
  - —Complication: rupture into pleural cavity (10–20%), peritoneum (2–7%) or pericardium (rare)
- Extrahepatic amebic abscess
  - —Hematologic spread
  - —Brain
  - —Lung
  - —Perinephric
  - —Splenic
  - —Vaginal/cervical/uterine
- Cutaneous amebiasis
  - —Perineum and genitalia
  - —Well-defined, irregularly shaped friable ulcers
  - —Purulent exudate
  - —Painful

MECHANISM/DESCRIPTION

- Endemic in developing countries
- Fecal-oral transmission
  - —Humans are sole reservoir
- Populations at risk:
  - —Travelers to and immigrants from endemic areas
  - —Institutionalized persons
  - —Practitioners of anal sexual activity
- Risk factors for increased severity of disease and complications:
  - —Corticosteroid use
  - —Malignancy
  - —Malnutrition
  - —Pregnancy/postpartum state
  - —Children and neonates
- Biphasic life cycle:
  - —Ingested as cysts
  - —Cysts become trophozoites, which cause an invasive colitis
  - —Create multiple flask-shaped ulcers in the colonic mucosa and muscularis
  - —Extraintestinal spread is hematogenous

ETIOLOGY

- *Entamoeba histolytica*, a nonflagellated protozoa

PEDIATRIC CONSIDERATIONS

- Children more likely than adults to present with severe colitis

Pre-Hospital

CAUTIONS

- Universal precautions
  - —Avoid contact with fecal matter or contaminated items
  - —Wear gloves
  - —Strict hand washing

Diagnosis

ESSENTIAL WORKUP

- History
  - —Possible sources of exposure
  - —Membership in high-risk group
- Physical exam
  - —Identify evidence of peritonitis, sepsis, or shock
  - —Tender abdominal mass mandates workup for liver abscess or ameboma
  - —Digital rectal exam shows gross or occult blood in >70% of patients
- Stool sample for *E. histolytica*-specific antigen
  - —World Health Organization standard
  - —Stool microscopy is insensitive and no longer the test of choice
- Fecal leukocytes and culture
  - —Rule out infection due to enteroinvasive bacteria
  - —Negative in amebiasis

LABORATORY

- Serum for anti-*E. histolytica* antibodies
  - —Essential if suspecting liver abscess as these patients rarely shed parasites in their stool
  - —90–100% sensitive in amebic liver abscess
  - —70–90% sensitive in amebic colitis
- CBC
  - —Leukocytosis in amebic liver abscess and peritonitis
- Alkaline phosphatase
  - —Elevated in amebic liver abscess
- Serum electrolytes, BUN/Cr if prolonged diarrhea or evidence of dehydration

IMAGING/SPECIAL TESTS

- Colonoscopy with biopsy
  - —Provides definitive diagnosis of amebic dysentery, colitis, ameboma, and amebic stricture
- Abdominal ultrasound
  - —First-line screen for liver abscess
  - —Abscess is a well-defined, inhomogeneous cystic mass
  - —Evaluate abscess for risk of rupture (location, size)

- Abdominal CT or MRI
  - —Equivalent to ultrasound for delineating liver abscesses
  - —Superior to ultrasound for detecting abscesses in other organs
- Percutaneous fine-needle aspiration of liver abscess
  - —Indicated to exclude bacterial abscess if high suspicion for this entity (elderly patient, nondiagnostic serology, failure of antiamebic therapy)
- Head CT or MRI
  - —Suspect amebic brain abscess if patient with known amebiasis presents with altered mental status or focal neurologic findings
  - —Irregular nonenhancing lesions
- Chest x-ray
  - —Elevated right hemidiaphragm and/or right pleural effusion in liver abscess

DIFFERENTIAL DIAGNOSIS

Intestinal Amebiasis

- Enteroinvasive bacterial infection *(Staphylococcus, E. coli, Shigella, Salmonella, Yersinia, Campylobacter)*
- Inflammatory bowel disease
- Ischemic colitis
- Arteriovenous malformation
- Abdominal aortic aneurysm
- Perforated duodenal ulcer
- Intussusception
- Diverticulitis
- Pancreatitis
- Colorectal carcinoma

Amebic Abscess

- Bacterial abscess
- Tuberculous cavity
- Echinococcal cyst
- Malignancy
- Cholecystitis

Cutaneous Amebiasis

- Carcinoma
- Sexually transmitted diseases (condyloma acuminata, chancroid, syphilis)

Treatment

INITIAL STABILIZATION

- ABCs
- IV 0.9 NS if signs of significant dehydration or shock

ED MANAGEMENT

- Oral fluids for mild dehydration
- Avoid antidiarrheal agents
- Correct any serum electrolyte imbalances
- Stool sample for *E. histolytica*-specific antigen *plus* serology for anti-*E. histolytica* antibodies
- If stool or serum is positive for *E. histolytica*:
  - —Metronidazole is first-line drug for systemic amebiasis
  - —90% cure rate
  - —Use with caution in first-trimester pregnancy but do not withhold if patient has fulminant colitis or amebic abscess
  - —Erythromycin for mild dysentery in first-trimester pregnancy
  - —Tetracycline for mild dysentery in metronidazole-intolerant patients but will not eradicate hepatic infection
  - —Dehydroemetine if metronidazole fails
    - -Must admit all dehydroemetine patients to a monitored setting because of the potential for cardiac toxicity and dysrhythmia
  - —Always follow systemic therapy with a luminal amebicidal agent to eradicate intestinal colonization (diloxanide furoate, paromomycin, or iodoquinol)
- If stool or serum is negative for *E. histolytica*:
  - —Refer to gastroenterologist for colonoscopy with biopsy
  - —Repeat serology in 7 days
  - —Consider empiric course of metronidazole if high suspicion for amebiasis and patient is critically ill
- If evidence of peritonitis or sepsis:
  - —Add IV antibiotic directed against anaerobic and gram-negative bacteria
  - —Surgical consult
  - —Conservative medical management
  - —Surgery if toxic megacolon or colonic perforation
- If liver abscess is suspected:
  - —Ultrasound of hepatobiliary system with concurrent amebic serology
  - —Abdominal CT scan if ultrasound is equivocal
  - —If imaging demonstrates an abscess but serology is negative, treat with amebicidals as above and repeat serology in 7 days
  - —Consult surgery for drainage of extremely large and left lobe abscesses (risk of rupture)
  - —If symptoms do not improve after 3–5 days of empiric amebicidal therapy, consider fine-needle aspiration to rule out bacterial liver abscess or hepatoma

MEDICATIONS

- Dehydroemetine: 90 mg (peds: 1–1.5 mg/kg/24 hr) i.m. q24h × 5 days
- Diloxanide furoate: 500 mg (peds: 20 mg/kg/24 hr) PO q8h × 10 days
- Erythromycin: 500 mg (peds: 30–50 mg/kg/24 hr) PO q6h × 10 days
- Iodoquinol: 650 mg (peds: 30–40 mg/kg/24 hr) PO q8h × 20 days
- Metronidazole: 750 mg (peds: 30–50 mg/kg/24 hr) PO q8h or 500 mg (peds: 15 mg/kg load then 7.5 mg/kg/24 hr) i.v. q6h × 10 days
- Paromomycin: 25–30 mg/kg/24 hr PO q8h × 7–10 days
- Tetracycline: 250 mg PO q8h × 10 days

Disposition

ADMISSION CRITERIA

- Shock, sepsis or peritonitis
- Hypotension or tachycardia unresponsive to IV fluids
- Children with >10% dehydration
- Severe electrolyte imbalance
- Patients unable to maintain adequate oral hydration
  - —Extremes of age, cognitive impairment, significant comorbid illness
- Fulminant colitis
- Liver abscesses requiring surgical drainage
- Extrahepatic abscesses
- Failure of outpatient regimen
- Dehydroemetine therapy

DISCHARGE CRITERIA

- Nontoxic presentation of acute or chronic dysentery
- Able to maintain adequate oral hydration
- Dehydration responsive to IV fluids

Miscellaneous

ICD 9: 006.0

ICD 10: A06.9

SEE ALSO: DIARRHEA, GASTROENTERITIS

SUGGESTED READINGS

Adachi JA, Backer HD, Dupont HL. Infectious diarrhea from wilderness and foreign travel. In: Auerbach PS, ed. *Wilderness medicine,* 4th ed. St. Louis: Mosby, 2001:1237–1270.

Li E, Stanley SL. Protozoa: amebiasis. Gastroenterol Clin North Am 1996;25: 471–491.

Petri WA, Singh U. Diagnosis and management of amebiasis. Clin Infect Dis 1999;29:1117–1125.

Ravdin JI. Amebiasis. Clin Infect Dis 1995;20:1453–1466.

Author: Ann Nguyen

Amenorrhea

Clinical Presentation

SIGNS AND SYMPTOMS

- Absence of menstruation
- Low estrogen: atrophic vaginal mucosa, mood swings, and irritability
- High androgen: truncal obesity, hirsutism, acne, male-pattern baldness

MECHANISM/DESCRIPTION

- Primary: no spontaneous uterine bleeding by age 14 in the absence of the development of secondary sexual characteristics or by age 16 with otherwise normal development
- Secondary: absence of menstrual bleeding for 6 months in a woman with prior regular menses or for 12 months in a woman with prior oligomenorrhea

ETIOLOGY

- Pregnancy
- Menopause, ovarian failure
- Asherman's syndrome (intrauterine adhesions)
- Dysfunction of the hypothalamic-pituitary-ovarian axis
- Endocrinopathies
- Gonadal dysgenesis
- Obesity, starvation, intense exercise
- Drugs: oral contraceptives, antipsychotics, antidepressants, calcium channel blockers, chemotherapeutic agents, digitalis, marijuana
- Chromosomal abnormalities
- Autoimmune disorders

Pre-Hospital

- If amenorrhea is the result of pregnancy, stabilize patient according to specific abnormalities of pregnancy

Diagnosis

ESSENTIAL WORKUP

- Pregnancy test

LABORATORY

- If pregnancy test is negative, no further testing needed emergently
- May send TSH, prolactin, LH, FSH for follow-up by gynecology or private MD

IMAGING/SPECIAL TESTS

- None needed emergently

DIFFERENTIAL DIAGNOSIS

- Pregnancy

Treatment

INITIAL STABILIZATION

N/A

ED TREATMENT

- Reassurance and referral to gynecology or private MD

MEDICATIONS

- Defer for gynecology evaluation

Disposition

ADMISSION CRITERIA

- No need for admission

DISCHARGE CRITERIA

- All patients can be discharged with appropriate referral

Miscellaneous

ICD9: 626.0

ICD10: N91.2

SUGGESTED READINGS

Kiningham RB, Apgar BS, Schwenk TL. Evaluation of amenorrhea. Am Fam Physician 1996;53(4):1185–1194.

Warren MP. Evaluation of secondary amenorrhea. J Clin Endocrinol Metab 1996;81(2):437–442.

Author: Christy Rosa Mohler

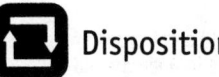

Amphetamine, Poisoning

Clinical Presentation

SIGNS AND SYMPTOMS

Central Nervous System (CNS)

- Agitation
- Delirium
- Hyperactivity
- Tremors
- Dizziness
- Mydriasis
- Headache
- Choreoathetoid movements
- Hyperreflexia
- Cerebrovascular accident
- Seizures and status epilepticus
- Coma

Psychiatric

- Euphoria
- Increased aggressiveness
- Anxiety
- Hallucinations (visual, tactile)
- Compulsive repetitive actions

Cardiovascular

- Palpitations
- Hypertensive crisis
- Tachycardia or (reflex) bradycardia
- Dysrhythmias (usually tachydysrhythmias)
- Cardiovascular collapse

Other

- Rhabdomyolysis
- Myoglobinuria
- Acute renal failure
- Anorexia
- Diaphoresis
- Disseminated intravascular coagulation (DIC)

DESCRIPTION/MECHANISM

- Increased release of norepinephrine, dopamine, serotonin
- Decreased catecholamine reuptake
- Direct effect on α- and β-adrenergic receptors

ETIOLOGY

- Prescription drugs
  —Amphetamine (benzedrine)
  —Dextroamphetamine (Dexedrine)
  —Diethylpropion (Tenuate)
  —Fenfluramine (Pondimin)
  —Methamphetamine
  —Methylphenidate (Ritalin)
  —Phenmetrazine (Preludin)
  —Phentermine
- "Designer drugs"
  —Variants of illegal parent drugs
  —Often synthesized in underground laboratories
  —"Ice"
    -Crystalline methamphetamine hydrochloride
    -Smoked, insufflated, or injected
    -Rapid onset; duration several hours
  —"Crank"
  —"Ecstasy" (3,4,-methylenedioxy-methamphetamine, MDMA, XTC)
    -Often used at dances and "rave" parties
    -Dehydration can lead to hyperthermia, hyponatremia, fatality
  —MDA (3,4,-methylenedioxyamphetamine)
  —Methcathinone ("cat," "Jeff," "mulka")
    -Derivative of cathinone, found in the evergreen tree *Catha edulis*
    -Frequently synthesized in home laboratories
    -Does not show up on urine toxicology screens

Pre-Hospital

CAUTIONS

- Patient may be uncooperative or violent
- Secure IV access
- Protect from self-induced trauma

Diagnosis

ESSENTIAL WORKUP

- Vital signs
  —Temperature
    -Rectal temperature most reliable
    -Temperature >40°C indication for urgent cooling
  —Blood pressure
    -Severe hypertension can lead to cardiac and neurologic abnormalities
    -Late in course, hypotension may supervene
- EKG
  —Ventricular tachydysrhythmias
  —Reflex bradycardia

LABORATORY

- Urinalysis
  —Blood
  —Myoglobin
- Electrolytes, BUN/Cr, glucose
  —Hypoglycemia may contribute to altered mental status
  —Acidosis may accompany severe toxicity
  —Rhabdomyolysis may cause renal failure
  —Hyperkalemia—life-threatening consequence of acute renal failure
- Coagulation profile
  —INR, PT, PTT, platelets
  —For DIC
- CPK
  —Markedly elevated in rhabdomyolysis
- Urine toxicology screen
  —For other toxins with similar effects (e.g., cocaine)
  —Some amphetamine-like substances (e.g., methcathinone) may not be detected
- ABG

IMAGING/SPECIAL TESTS

- CXR for
  —Adult respiratory distress syndrome
  —Noncardiogenic pulmonary edema
- CT (head)
  —Indications
    -Significant headache
    -Altered mental status
    -Focal neurologic signs
  —For subarachnoid hemorrhage, intracerebral bleed
- Lumbar puncture
  —Indications
    -Suspected meningitis (headache, altered mental status, hyperpyrexia)
    -Suspected subarachnoid hemorrhage
  —Indicated if subarachnoid hemorrhage suspected and CT normal

DIFFERENTIAL DIAGNOSIS

Drugs that Cause Delirium

- Anticholinergics
  —Belladonna alkaloids
  —Antihistamines
  —Tricyclic antidepressants
- Cocaine
- Ethanol withdrawal
- Sedative/hypnotic withdrawal
- Hallucinogens
- Phencyclidine

Drugs that Cause Hypertension and Tachycardia

- Sympathomimetics
- Anticholinergics
- Ethanol withdrawal
- Phencyclidine
- Caffeine
- Phenylpropanolamine
- Ephedrine
- Monoamine oxidase inhibitors
- Theophylline
- Nicotine

Drugs that Cause Seizures

- Carbon monoxide
- Carbamazepine
- Cyanide
- Cocaine
- Cholinergics (organophosphate insecticides)
- Camphor
- Chlorinated hydrocarbons

- Ethanol withdrawal
- Sedative/hypnotic withdrawal
- Isoniazid
- Theophylline
- Hypoglycemics
- Lead
- Lithium
- Local anesthetics
- Anticholinergics
- Phencyclidine
- Phenothiazines
- Phenytoin
- Propoxyphene
- Salicylates
- Strychnine

Treatment

INITIAL STABILIZATION

- ABCs
- Establish IV 0.9% NS access
- Cardiac monitor
- Naloxone, dextrose (or Accucheck) and thiamine if altered mental status

ED TREATMENT

Decontamination

- Gastric lavage
  - —Consider if recent (1–2 hours) or life-threatening ingestion
  - —Instill activated charcoal through large-bore orogastric tube both before and after lavage
- Administer activated charcoal with sorbitol

Hypertensive Crisis

- Initially administer benzodiazepines if agitated
- Alpha-blocker (phentolamine) as second-line agent
- Nitroprusside for severe, unresponsive hypertension

Agitation, Acute Psychosis

- Administer benzodiazepines

Hyperthermia

- Benzodiazepines if agitated
- Emergent cooling if temperature >40°C
  - —Tepid water mist
  - —Evaporate with fan
  - —Paralysis
    - -Indicated if muscle rigidity and hyperactivity contributing to persistent hyperthermia
    - -Nondepolarizing agent (e.g., pancuronium)
    - -Avoid succinylcholine
    - -Intubation; mechanical ventilation
  - —Administer acetaminophen
  - —Apply cooling blankets

Rhabdomyolysis

- Administer benzodiazepines
- Hydrate with 0.9% NS
- Maintain urine output at 1–2 mL/min
- Hemodialysis (if acute renal failure and hyperkalemia occur)

Seizures

- Maintain airway
- Administer benzodiazepines
- Phenobarbital if unresponsive to benzodiazepines
- Phenytoin contraindicated

MEDICATIONS

- Activated charcoal slurry: 1–2 g/kg up to 90 g PO
- Dextrose: D50W 1 amp (50 mL or 25 g) (peds: D25W 2–4 mL/kg) i.v.
- Diazepam (benzodiazepine): 5–10 mg (peds: 0.2–0.5 mg/kg) i.v.
- Lorazepam (benzodiazepine): 2–6 mg (peds: 0.03–0.05 mg/kg) i.v.
- Nitroprusside: 1–8 μg/kg/min i.v. (titrated to blood pressure)
- Phenobarbital: 15–20 mg/kg at 25–50 mg/min until cessation of seizure activity
- Phentolamine: 1–5 mg i.v. over 5 minutes (titrated to blood pressure)
- Sorbitol: 1–2 g/kg to a max of 100 g PO mixed in the activated charcoal slurry (peds: >1-year-old: 1–1.5 g/kg as a 35% solution to a max of 50 g); avoid repeat doses of sorbitol

Disposition

ADMISSION CRITERIA

- Hyperthermia
- Persistent altered mental status
- Hypertensive crisis
- Seizures
- Rhabdomyolysis
- Persistent tachycardia

DISCHARGE CRITERIA

- Asymptomatic after 6 hours observation
- Absence of above admission criteria

Miscellaneous

ICD9: 969.7

ICD10: T43.6

SUGGESTED READINGS

Callaway CW, Clark RF. Hyperthermia in psychostimulant overdose. Ann Emerg Med 1994;24:68–75.

Chan P, Chen JH, Lee MH, et al. Fatal and nonfatal methamphetamine intoxication in the intensive care unit. Clin Toxicol 1994;32:147–155.

Derlet RW, Rice P, Horowitz BZ, et al. Amphetamine toxicity: Experience with 127 cases. J Emerg Med 1989;7: 157–161.

Doyon S. The many faces of ecstasy. Curr Opin Pediatr 2001;13:170–176.

Kalant H. The pharmacology and toxicology of "ecstasy" (MDMA) and related drugs. Can Med Assoc J 2001;165:917–928.

Author: Leon Gussow

Amputation, Traumatic/Reimplantation

Clinical Presentation

SIGNS AND SYMPTOMS

- Amputations are visually striking injuries
- Signs of neurovascular compromise in partial/incomplete amputations include:
  - —Distal part dusky and cyanotic
  - —Decreased sensation and two-point discrimination
  - —Delayed capillary refill, diminished or absent pulses
- Time from amputation and temperature are critical to reimplantation success
  - —*Warm ischemia time:* approximately 6 hours; longer for digits
  - —*Cold ischemia time:* up to 12 hours for parts containing muscle; up to 30 hours for digits

MECHANISM/DESCRIPTION

- Traumatic amputations commonly result from motor vehicle accidents, crush injuries, injuries from heavy equipment or high-speed tools, degloving injuries to digits (ring avulsions), and mammalian bites

Pre-Hospital

- Collect all amputated parts, including pieces of bone, tissue, skin
- See Initial Stabilization, below, for care of amputated parts
- Transport to the nearest microvascular reimplantation center
- Time is of the essence and air transport from remote locations may be indicated

Diagnosis

ESSENTIAL WORKUP

- A general assessment of circulation, sensation, and function should be performed
  - —Pulses, capillary refill (delayed if more than 2 seconds)
  - —Two-point discrimination tests (abnormal if greater than 5 mm on the hand)
  - —Allen test for hand injuries: compress either radial or ulnar artery firmly at the wrist while patient clenches fist and then relaxes; persistence of pallor indicates disruption of circulation from the uncompressed artery
- Pulse oximetry of a partially amputated part may be helpful

LABORATORY

- Laboratory tests should be directed by patient's condition, other medical issues, and amount of estimated blood loss

IMAGING/SPECIAL TESTS

- Radiograph amputated part and stump to assess bony injury and foreign body contamination

DIFFERENTIAL DIAGNOSIS

- Diagnostic considerations deal primarily with neurovascular integrity and potential for reimplantation/revascularization

Treatment

INITIAL STABILIZATION

- Goals of ED treatment
  - —Control hemorrhage
  - —Avoid further damage to the injured part
  - —Limit ischemia of the amputated part
  - —Immediate consultation by appropriate surgical specialist
- Control hemorrhage
  - —Apply direct pressure (bulky pressure dressing) and elevate the proximal stump
  - —If ineffective, apply pressure to pressure points
  - —As last resort, use tourniquet (blood pressure cuff preferable) and tighten just enough to stop bleeding
  - —Avoid hemostats, cautery, or vessel ligation
- Maintain normal blood volume with intravenous fluids
- *Care of amputated part* (complete or partial)
  - —Gently irrigate with isotonic fluid (no antiseptics or scrubbing)
  - —Wrap in gauze or cloth moistened with isotonic fluid
  - —Place in clean, dry plastic bag
  - —Place sealed bag in wet ice or refrigerator at 4°C
  - —*Never place directly on ice*

ED TREATMENT

- Assume patient is a candidate for reimplantation until qualified surgical consultation is obtained
- Considerations in the decision to reimplant include
  - —Age (younger favors improved outcome)
  - —Occupation
  - —Patient motivation
  - —General physical condition/other underlying diseases
  - —Mechanism of injury (clean laceration more successful than crush or avulsion)
  - —Location/level of amputation
  - —Condition of the amputated part
  - —Length of time from amputation
- *General indications for reimplantation*
  - —Thumb
  - —Multiple digits
  - —Individual digit distal to flexor digitorum superficialis (FDS) insertion
  - —Metacarpal (palm), wrist, or forearm
  - —Elbow or proximal arm (if sharp or moderately avulsed; ischemia time critical)
  - —Almost all pediatric amputations
- General contraindications to reimplantation
  - —Severely crushed or mangled parts
  - —Multiple level amputations
  - —Unstable patients with other serious injuries or diseases
  - —Extreme age
  - —Single-digit amputations proximal to FDS insertion in adults
  - —Prolonged warm ischemia time

- Tetanus prophylaxis
- Prophylactic antibiotics: recommended if devitalized tissue or contamination is present; combination of penicillin G and antistaphylococcal antibiotic or first-generation cephalosporin
- Keep patient NPO
- Provide adequate analgesia
- Traumatic ischemia is an accepted indication for hyperbaric oxygen therapy after reimplantation or grafting (may prevent reperfusion injury)

Fingertip Injuries

- Defined as distal to the insertion of the flexor and extensor tendons
- Primary goal is a painless fingertip with durable and sensate skin
- *Soft tissue loss without exposed bone;* options include:
  - —Cover defect with nonadherent dressing and allow to heal by secondary intention (best for small to moderate-sized defects)
  - —Apply a skin or composite graft
- *Soft tissue loss with exposed bone;* options include:
  - —Shorten bone below level of the skin and close primarily
  - —Cover defect with local or regional flap
  - —Microsurgical reimplantation [thumbs, fingers at or proximal to the distal interphalangeal (DIP) joint]
- Thumb amputations should be reimplanted if possible, even if distal to the DIP joint (functional importance)
- Treat nail-bed injuries and subungual hematomas

MEDICATIONS

- Penicillin G: 10–12 million U daily divided q4–6h (peds: 100,000–150,000 U/kg/day divided q4–6h)
- Cefazolin: 0.5–1.5 g i.v./i.m. q6–8h (peds: 25–50 mg/kg/day divided q6–8h)

PEDIATRIC CONSIDERATIONS

- Reimplantation almost always attempted in children
- Conservative management preferred in fingertip injuries
  - —Spontaneous regeneration of fingertip occurs in children under 12 years
  - —Nonmicrosurgical reattachment of the cleanly amputated fingertip as a composite graft can be successful

Disposition

ADMISSION CRITERIA

- Hospitalization is required for all but trivial amputations and degloving injuries

DISCHARGE CRITERIA

- Minor injuries (e.g., fingertip amputations or mild degloving injuries with stable vascular supply) can be discharged with orthopedic or surgical follow-up

Miscellaneous

ICD9: 886.0

ICD10: T14.7

SUGGESTED READINGS

Antosia L. Hand. In: Rosen P, et al., eds. Emergency medicine: concepts and clinical practice, 4th ed. St. Louis: CV Mosby, 1998:658–661.

Fassler P. Fingertip injuries: evaluation and treatment. J Am Acad Orthop Surg 1996;4:84–92.

Strauss M. Crush injury and other acute traumatic peripheral ischemias. In: Kindwall E, ed. Hyperbaric medicine practice. Flagstaff, AZ: Best, 1994.

Verdile V, et al. Hand and Wrist Injuries. In: Ferrara P, et al., eds. Trauma management: an emergency medicine approach. St. Louis: Mosby, 2001:392–393.

Author: Mary Anne Fuchs

Amyotrophic Lateral Sclerosis

Clinical Presentation

SIGNS AND SYMPTOMS

- Weakness (bilateral) with eventual muscle wasting is the most common presentation of amyotrophic lateral sclerosis (ALS)
- Both lower motor neuron (weakness and wasting with fasciculation) and upper motor neuron signs (Babinski's sign with hyper-reflexia)
- May begin in either the arms or the legs; later all limbs are affected
- Dysphagia or facial dysarthrias (drooling, dysphagia) occur, but are rarely the presenting symptoms
- Respiratory muscles and the vocal cords are affected late
- Muscle cramps and weight loss
- Muscle fasciculation is common but may not be apparent to the patient
- Extraocular muscles, sphincters, cognition, and sensation are spared
- 80% of cases begin between ages 40 and 70 years
- Death (usually from respiratory paralysis) occurs within 3–5 years of the diagnosis
- Musculoskeletal pain is common late in the disease and is related to complications, not the primary disease

DISEASE DESCRIPTION

- A progressive disease of adults usually manifests by muscle weakness, wasting, fasciculations, Babinski's sign, and hyperreflexia; partial or incomplete forms in which upper or lower motor neuron manifestations predominately also occur

ETIOLOGY

- The etiology of ALS is unknown
- Pathologically, there is loss of both upper and lower motor neuron cells with a striking predilection for the motor system and sparing of other neurons

Pre-Hospital

CONTROVERSIES

- Many patients will have advanced directives
  - —Unless immediate intervention is essential, intubation should be avoided until directives have been ascertained
  - —Noninvasive means of ventilatory support may be tried first

Diagnosis

ESSENTIAL WORKUP

Previously Undiagnosed ALS

- The diagnosis of ALS is clinical and rarely made in the ED; recognition of the possibility of this disease is sufficient and mandates referral for workup
- If ALS is suspected, forced vital capacity (FVC) should be performed

Known ALS Patient

- Patients with known disease and progressive symptoms:
  - —Evaluate potentially treatable complications with lab and imaging studies
- FVC is a sensitive indicator of respiratory muscle weakness
  - —FVC <50% of predicted is considered a sign of advanced disease
  - —Compare with the patient's own previous baseline
- Chest radiography may reveal evidence of aspiration or pneumonia or comorbid conditions such as CHF
- Pulse oximetry and blood gas analysis aid in the diagnosis of respiratory failure
- Electrolytes and other blood chemistry tests may reveal a treatable cause of increasing weakness
- Cervical spine, other skeletal radiography, or head CT may be needed in case of falls (common in ALS)

LABORATORY AND SPECIAL TESTING

- Electromyography (EMG) may help confirm the diagnosis

DIFFERENTIAL DIAGNOSIS

- Cervical cord compression (tumor, spondylosis with osteophytes, others)
  - —Similar symptoms but usually acute onset with pain and sensory changes
  - —Spinal MRI or myelography is used for diagnosis
- Thyrotoxicosis may mimic ALS
  - —It is usually associated with marked systemic symptoms
  - —TSH is best screening test
- Heavy metal poisoning (lead, mercury, arsenic)
- Syphilis and Lyme disease
- Lymphoma may have an associated lower motor neuron syndrome, which mimics ALS

Treatment

- There is no specific therapy for ALS
- Treatment issues in the ED revolve around symptomatic therapy and identification and treatment of complications

INITIAL STABILIZATION

- Respiratory insufficiency or failure
  —Ascertain any advanced directives
  —Noninvasive ventilatory support
  —Intubation as indicated
- Weaning off the ventilator is very difficult
  —Average survival after institution of ventilation is 19 months (range: 1–61 months)

ED TREATMENT

- Sedation and pain control as indicated
  —Joint pain may respond to NSAIDs
- Insomnia from pressure pain (due to immobility) may respond to diphenhydramine or amitriptyline
- Aspiration or drooling may be treated with amitriptyline (dries secretions)
- Muscle cramps may respond to baclofen
- Constipation is related to immobility and diet and is treated with laxatives, stool softeners, and dietary changes

MEDICATIONS

- Amitriptyline: 25–50 mg PO qhs
- Baclofen: 10–25 mg PO t.i.d.
- Diphenhydramine: 25–50 mg PO qhs

Disposition

ADMISSION CRITERIA

- Need for respiratory support
- Dehydration, inanition
- Unable to be cared for at home due to progression of illness
- Complications (e.g., infection) that require admission

DISCHARGE CRITERIA

- *Suspected ALS:* refer for outpatient evaluation if general condition permits and other serious conditions requiring admission are ruled out
- *Complication of known ALS:* discharge if effective outpatient treatment available

Miscellaneous

ICD9: 335.20

ICD10: G12.2

SUGGESTED READINGS

Appel SH, Appel LV. Treatment of amyotrophic lateral sclerosis. In: Calne D, ed. Neurodegenerative diseases, 1st ed. Philadelphia: WB Saunders, 1994: 523–542.

Brooks BR. Natural history of ALS: symptoms, strength, pulmonary function, and disability. Neurology 1996;47[suppl 2]:S71–S81.

Caroscio JT. Amyotrophic lateral sclerosis: a guide to patient care. New York: Thieme Medical, 1986.

Festoff BW. Amyotrophic lateral sclerosis: current and future treatment strategies. Drugs 1996;51(1):28–44.

Rowland LP. Natural history and clinical features of amyotrophic lateral sclerosis and related motor neuron diseases. In: Calne D, ed. Neurodegenerative diseases, 1st ed. Philadelphia: WB Saunders, 1994:507–521.

Author: Richard S. Krause

Anal Fissure

Clinical Presentation

SIGNS AND SYMPTOMS

- Bright red blood per rectum usually on toilet paper
- Sharp, cutting, or burning pain with bowel movement
  —May last for hours
- Constipation, unable to pass stool secondary to pain

MECHANISM/DESCRIPTION

- Hard stool passes and "cuts" anoderm
- Linear tear from dentate line to anoderm
  —95% posterior midline
  —5% anterior midline
  —Externally = skin tag or sentinel pile
  —Internally = hypertrophied anal papilla
  —Chronic fissure may reveal fibers of internal sphincter with sentinel pile

ETIOLOGY

- Stress or a tight anal sphincter leads to ischemia of posterior anoderm
- Diarrhea or hard bowel movement tears anoderm
- Anal intercourse, sexual abuse
- Lateral fissures indicate underlying systemic disease
  —Crohn's
  —Anal cancer
  —Leukemia
  —Syphilis
  —Previous anal surgery

PEDIATRIC CONSIDERATIONS

- Most common cause of rectal bleeding in infants
- May indicate sexual abuse

Pre-Hospital

N/A

Diagnosis

ESSENTIAL WORKUP

- History of
  —Passage of hard stool
  —Episode of diarrhea
- Examination of anus
  —Gently retracting the buttocks and having the patient bear down to visualize the fissure
  —Severe pain usually prevents a digital exam
  —Use lidocaine jelly or ELA-Max5 prior to digital rectal exam

LABORATORY

- HCT if severe bleeding by history

IMAGING/SPECIAL TESTS

N/A

DIFFERENTIAL DIAGNOSIS

- Crohn's disease
- Chronic ulcerative colitis
- Anorectal carcinoma
- Perirectal abscess
- Thrombosed hemorrhoid
- Sexual abuse
- Tuberculosis
- Syphilis
- Lymphoma
- Leukemia
- Previous anal surgery

PEDIATRIC CONSIDERATIONS

- A clear test tube may be used as an anoscope to visualize the anal canal/fissure

Treatment

INITIAL STABILIZATION

N/A

ED TREATMENT

- Oral pain medication
  - —NSAID
  - —Cox-2 inhibitor
- Topical anesthetics
  - —ELA-Max5
  - —Lidocaine jelly
- Sitz baths to relieve sphincter spasm
  - —Warm water only
- Oral muscle relaxants or Valium to relieve sphincter spasm
- High-fiber diet instruction
- Encourage 10–12 glasses of water per day

MEDICATIONS

- Cyclobenzaprine (Flexeril): 10 mg (peds: not indicated) PO t.i.d.
- Diazepam (Valium): 5 mg (peds: 0.12–0.8 mg/kg/day) PO t.i.d. PRN spasm
- Docusate sodium (Colace): 50–200 mg (peds: <3 years = 10–40 mg/day; 3–6 years = 20–60 mg/day; >6–12 years = 40–150 mg/day) PO q12h
- ELA-Max5 (5% lidocaine anorectal cream): apply to perianal area q4h PRN pain (peds: not for <12 years of age)
- Fiber/bran: 20 g/day
- Ibuprofen: 400–600 mg (peds: 40 mg/kg/day) PO q6h
- Nitroglycerin ointment 0.2%: apply to fissure b.i.d. (peds: not indicated)
- Psyllium seeds: 1–2 tsp (peds: 0.25–1 tsp/day) PO q24h

Disposition

ADMISSION CRITERIA

None

DISCHARGE CRITERIA

- Initial treatment is conservative therapy for acute anal fissures as an outpatient
- Operative referral for chronic fissure

Miscellaneous

ICD9: 565.0

ICD10: K60.2

SEE ALSO: HEMORRHOID

SUGGESTED READINGS

Hananel N, Gordon PH. Re-examination of clinical manifestations and response to therapy of fissure-in-ano. Dis Colon Rectum 1997;40:229–233.

Mazier WP. Hemorrhoids, fissures and pruritus. Ann Surg Clin North Am 1994;74(6):1277–1291.

Author: Julia Sone

Anaphylaxis

Clinical Presentation

SIGNS AND SYMPTOMS

- Symptoms begin within seconds to minutes after contact with an offending antigen
- Some patients may have an initial sensation of impending doom followed by more clearly definable symptomatology
- Respiratory: bronchospasm, laryngeal edema
- Cardiovascular: hypotension, dysrhythmias, myocardial ischemia
- Gastrointestinal: nausea, vomiting, diarrhea
- Cutaneous: urticaria, angioedema
- Hematologic: activation of intrinsic coagulation pathway sometimes leading to DIC, thrombocytopenia
- Neurologic: seizures
- Death can occur from airway obstruction or circulatory collapse

MECHANISM/DESCRIPTION

- An acute, widely distributed form of shock that occurs within minutes of exposure to antigen in a sensitized individual
- There are approximately 400–800 deaths annually in the U.S. attributed to anaphylaxis
- Release of bioactive molecules such as histamine, leukotrienes, and prostaglandins from inflammatory cells
  —Mediator release results in increased vascular permeability, vasodilation, smooth-muscle contractions, and increased epithelial secretion
  —Physiologically this is manifested in a decrease in total peripheral resistance, venous return and cardiac output, as well as intravascular volume depletion

ETIOLOGY

- IgE-mediated
  —Antibiotics, particularly penicillin family
  —Venoms, especially bee and wasp
  —Latex
  —Vaccines
  —Foodstuffs (shellfish, soybeans, peanuts, tree nuts, wheat, milk, eggs, nitrates/nitrites)
- Non-IgE mediated
  —Iodine contrast media
  —Opiates
  —Vancomycin
  —Quaternary ammonium muscle relaxants

Pre-Hospital

CAUTIONS

- **Early intubation is paramount as laryngeal edema and spasm can progress rapidly**
- **Laryngeal edema can be managed with racemic epinephrine prior to intubation**
- **Subcutaneous epinephrine (0.5 mg of 1:1,000 solution) can be administered en route even prior to establishment of an IV**

Diagnosis

ESSENTIAL WORKUP

- Diagnosis is made based on clinical symptoms
  —It is important not to underestimate the potential severity of an allergic reaction in its early stages
- EKG in patients with previous cardiac history or ischemic symptoms

LABORATORY

- While there are no specific tests necessary to make the diagnosis of anaphylaxis, an arterial blood gas may be helpful in evaluating ventilatory status
- These changes can be noted during anaphylaxis
  —Elevation of plasma histamine
  —Increase in hematocrit secondary to fluid extravasation

IMAGING/SPECIAL TESTS

- Hyperinflation on CXR
- EKG abnormalities including dysrhythmias, ischemic changes, infarction

DIFFERENTIAL DIAGNOSIS

- Pulmonary embolism
- Acute myocardial infarction
- Airway obstruction
- Asthma
- Tension pneumothorax
- NSAID reaction
- Vasovagal collapse
- Hereditary angioedema
- Serum sickness
- Systemic mastocytosis
- Pheochromocytoma
- Carcinoid syndrome

Treatment

INITIAL STABILIZATION

- ABCs
  - —Assure adequate ventilation
  - —Orotracheal intubation is the technique of choice
    - -This may be required but difficult because of laryngeal edema, spasm, or soft tissue swelling
  - —Consider blind nasotracheal intubation if soft tissue swelling prohibits an oral approach and there is absence of stridor
  - —Transtracheal jet insufflation or cricothyrotomy may be necessary to control the airway
- Epinephrine IV/SC or endotracheal administration
  - —Direct injection into the venous plexus at the base of the tongue is an option
- Volume resuscitation with crystalloids or colloids
- A tourniquet can be used to decrease venous return from the site of antigen entry

ED TREATMENT

- Continuous cardiac and vital sign monitoring until stable
- Persistent bronchospasm can be treated with β_2-agonist bronchodilators
- Hypotension should be treated with volume repletion
  - —Vasopressors, MAST garments, and Trendelenburg positioning are useful adjuncts
- Antihistamines (both H_1 and H_2 blockers) have been shown to be helpful in preventing histamine interactions with target tissues
- Corticosteroids help prevent the progression or recurrence of anaphylaxis
- Glucagon is particularly useful in epinephrine-resistant anaphylaxis from β-adrenergic blocking agents

MEDICATIONS

- Diphenhydramine: adult: 50 mg i.v.; peds: 1–2 mg/kg slow IVP
- Epinephrine: 0.3–0.5 mg (use 1:1,000 dilution for s.c. route, and 1:10,000 for i.v. route); peds: epinephrine 0.01 mg/kg s.c./i.v.
- Racemic epinephrine: 2.25% solution (0.5 mL placed in a nebulizer in 2.5 mL of normal saline)
- Glucagon: adult: 1 mg i.v.
- Hydrocortisone: adults: 500 mg i.v.; peds: 4-8 mg/kg/dose i.v.
- Methylprednisolone: adult: 125 mg i.v.; peds: 1–2 mg/kg i.v.
- Prednisone: adult: 60 mg PO; peds: 1 mg/kg PO
- Ranitidine: adult: 50 mg i.v. *or* cimetidine 300 mg i.v.

Disposition

ADMISSION CRITERIA

- Intubated patients or patients in respiratory distress should be admitted to an ICU setting
- A monitored bed may be necessary for the patient who has not had substantial response to initial therapy
- Patients with significant generalized reactions and persistent symptoms should be admitted for observation for 24 hours

DISCHARGE CRITERIA

- Patients with complete resolution of symptoms may be discharged after several hours of ED observation
- Patients with allergic reactions should have follow-up within 48 hours of discharge to evaluate effectiveness of outpatient therapy
- A follow-up visit with an allergist is also recommended
- Patients should be advised to carry some type of treatment that can be self-administered in the event of future reactions such as the prefilled syringe epi-pen
- Patients with a known trigger should be counseled on strict avoidance of that trigger

Miscellaneous

ICD9: 995.0

ICD10: T78.2

SEE ALSO: ANGIOEDEMA

SUGGESTED READINGS

Barach EM, et al. Epinephrine for the treatment of anaphylactic shock. JAMA 1984;251:2118.

Neugut AI, Ghatak AT, Miller RL. Anaphylaxis in the United States: an investigation into its epidemiology. Arch Intern Med 2001;161:15–21.

Muelleman RL, et al. Allergy, hypersensitivity and anaphylaxis. In: Rosen P, Barkin R, eds. Emergency medicine. St. Louis: CV Mosby, 1998:2759–2776.

Author: Sean-Xavier Neath

Anemia

Clinical Presentation

SIGNS AND SYMPTOMS

General

- Depends on
  - —Rapidity of onset and underlying disease
  - —Hemodynamic stability
  - —Severity and type of anemia
- Asymptomatic if mild and chronic
- Fatigue
- Decreased exercise intolerance
- Tachypnea
- Heme-positive stool

Cardiovascular

- Dyspnea on exertion
- Chest pain/angina
- Syncope
- Tachycardia, cardiomegaly, murmurs
- Postural hypotension

DERMATOLOGIC

- Skin
  - —Cool (vasoconstriction)
  - —Pallor
  - —Jaundice
  - —Purpura
  - —Telangiectasia
- Spoon-shaped nails (koilonychia)

CNS

- Neuropathy
- Altered mental status

Miscellaneous

- Bone or joint pain (with sickle cell disease)
- Hepatomegaly, splenomegaly
- Lymphadenopathy
- Findings reflect underlying disease

MECHANISM/DESCRIPTION

- Adult female: Hb <12 g/dL or Hct <37%
- Adult male: Hb <14 g/dL or Hct <42%
- Normal blood count values depend on age:
  - —Birth: mean Hb = 16.5, mean Hct = 51
  - —1 year old: mean Hb = 12, mean Hct = 36
  - —6 year old: mean Hb = 12.5, mean Hct = 37
  - —Adult male: mean Hb = 14, mean Hct = 42
  - —Adult female: mean Hb = 12, mean Hct = 37
- Hb depends on ambient oxygen pressure
  - —Increased Hb/Hct with neonates and people living above 4,000 feet

Etiology

- Excessive blood loss
  - —Trauma
  - —GI bleed
  - —Menstruation
- Hemolysis (i.e., increased destruction)
  - —Hypersplenism
  - —Autoimmune hemolytic anemia
  - —Mechanical trauma (prosthetic heart valves, vasculitis, TTP, HUS, DIC)
  - —Toxins
  - —Infections (malaria, clostridia)
  - —Membrane abnormalities
  - —Intracellular RBC abnormalities (G6PD, sickle cell anemia, thalassemia)
- Decreased RBC synthesis
  - —Hypochromic/microcytic
    - -Iron deficiency
    - -Thalassemia
    - -Sideroblastic
    - -Chronic disease
  - —Normochromic/macrocytic
    - -Hypothyroidism
    - -Folic acid deficiency
    - -B_{12} deficiency
    - -Liver disease
    - -Scurvy
  - —Normochromic/normocytic
    - -Aplastic anemia
    - -Chronic renal failure
    - -Malignancy
    - -Adrenal insufficiency
    - -Hyperparathyroidism
    - -Alcohol abuse

Pre-Hospital

CAUTIONS

- Administer high flow oxygen
- Ongoing blood losses require close assessment and rapid transport
- Place multiple large-bore IV catheters and infuse crystalloid if unstable

CONTROVERSIES

- Some current research suggests that rapid infusion of crystalloid may worsen hemorrhage in trauma

Diagnosis

ESSENTIAL WORKUP

- Bedside Hct
- Vital signs (including orthostatic)

LABORATORY

- CBC
- RBC indices
  - —MCV (normal: 80–95 μm^3)
  - —MCH (normal: 27–34)
  - —MCHC (normal: 30–35%)
- Platelet count
- Reticulocyte count
  - —Normal 0.5–1.5% (reticulocytes/1,000 RBCs)
  - —Falsely elevated in anemia if total RBC decreases
  - —Corrected reticulocyte count = reticulocyte count × Hct/45
- Reticulocyte index (RI) = [reticulocyte count (%) × Hct]/(2 × normal Hct)
  - —RI <2% implies inadequate RBC production
  - —RI >2% implies excessive RBC destruction or loss
- Stool for occult blood for GI bleed
- Electrolytes, BUN, Cr, glucose
  - —For chronic renal failure
- Urinalysis
  - —Hematuria
  - —Hemoglobinuria in hemolytic anemia

Workup Strategy

- Hypochromic/microcytic anemias
  - —Iron
  - —Transferrin
  - —Ferritin
- Macrocytic anemias
  - —Folate
  - —Vitamin B_{12}
  - —Liver function tests
  - —Thyroid function tests
- Hemolytic anemia
  - —Coombs test
  - —Serum bilirubin—increased unconjugated
  - —Urinalysis for hemoglobinuria
  - —Plasma for free hemoglobin
  - —LDH

IMAGING/SPECIAL TESTS

- Peripheral smear
- Hb electrophoresis for sickle cell anemia/thalassemia
- Coombs' test—positive in autoimmune hemolytic anemia
- Iron, iron binding capacity, transferrin, ferritin
  - —Iron deficiency
    - -Iron—decreased
    - -Iron-binding capacity—increased
    - -Ferritin—decreased
  - —Chronic disease
    - -Iron—decreased
    - -Iron-binding capacity—decreased
    - -Ferritin—normal/increased
  - —Thalassemia
    - -Iron—normal
    - -Iron-binding capacity—normal
    - -Ferritin—normal
  - —Sideroblastic anemia
    - -Iron—increased
    - -Iron-binding capacity—normal
    - -Ferritin—increased
- Bone marrow biopsy to exclude
  - —Leukemia, lymphomas, pancytopenia, agranulocytosis

Differential Diagnosis

- Dilutional anemia
- Increased plasma volume
- Fluid overload
- Congestive heart failure
- Acquired vs. inherited anemia
- Blood loss
- Nutritional deficiency/malabsorption
- Hemolysis
- Toxin causing bone marrow suppression
- Malignancy
- Chronic disease

PEDIATRIC CONSIDERATIONS

- Hemolytic anemia of the newborn due to Rh antibody crossing placenta when Rh-negative mother has Rh-positive child

Treatment

INITIAL STABILIZATION

- ABCs
- Oxygen
- IV fluid resuscitation with 0.9% NS if ongoing loss/hypotension

ED TREATMENT

- Depends on severity of anemia and acuteness of onset
- Transfusion for hemorrhage with unstable vital signs
- Most anemias seen in ED are chronic and do not require immediate intervention

Therapy for Specific Anemia

- Iron deficiency
  - —$FeSO_4$ 300 mg PO t.i.d.
  - —Investigate underlying cause
  - —Increase Hb expected in 2–3 weeks
- Renal failure
  - —Recombinant erythropoietin when no endogenous erythropoietin produced
- Autoimmune hemolytic anemia
  - —Corticosteroids (prednisone 60 mg/d until response)
  - —Immunosuppressive agents
  - —Plasmapheresis
  - —Splenectomy if splenic sequestration
- Drug-induced hemolytic anemia: stop offending agent
- Anemia of chronic disease: treat underlying disease
- Vitamin B_{12} deficiency
  - —B_{12} 1,000 μg i.m. daily for 1 week, then weekly for 1 month, then monthly
  - —Hematologic parameters normalize within 2 months
  - —Neurologic symptoms present >6 months may be permanent
- Folate deficiency
  - —Folic acid 1 mg PO qd
- Aplastic anemia
  - —Antithymocyte globulin
  - —Bone marrow transplantation
- Sickle cell anemia
  - —Supportive care with oxygen, rehydration, analgesia
  - —Treat precipitating cause
- Marrow replacement for
  - —Leukemia

Disposition

ADMISSION CRITERIA

- Unstable vital signs
- Ongoing blood losses
- Symptomatic anemia—worsening angina/dyspnea/syncope
- Pancytopenia
- Need for transfusion
- Need for aggressive evaluation

DISCHARGE CRITERIA

- Discharge vast majority of stable patient for outpatient workup

Miscellaneous

ICD9: 285.9

ICD10: D64.9

SEE ALSO: SICKLE CELL DISEASE

SUGGESTED READINGS

Beutler E. The common anemias. JAMA 1988;259:2433–2437.

Braunwald E, Isselbacher K, et al., eds. Harrison's principles of internal medicine, 15th ed. New York: McGraw-Hill, 2001.

Colon-Otero G, Menke D, Hook CC. A practical approach to the differential diagnosis and evaluation of the adult patient with macrocytic anemia. Med Clin North Am 1992;76:581–597.

Hoffman R, Benz E, Shattil S, et al., eds. Hematology: basic principles and practice, 3rd ed. New York: Churchill-Livingstone, 2000.

Scott R. Common blood disorders: a primary care approach. Geriatrics 1993;48:72–80.

Author: Marc Gelman

Angioedema

Clinical Presentation

SIGNS AND SYMPTOMS

- Edema of the airway, face, or extremities
- Abdominal pain associated with nausea, vomiting, and diarrhea
- Attacks of hereditary angioedema are not associated with hives
- Emotional stress or physical trauma can trigger attacks
- The lesions of angioedema are large swollen and nonpitting wheals
- The eyelids and lips are frequently involved
  —Involvement of the pharynx and larynx may cause airway obstruction

MECHANISM/DESCRIPTION

- Nonpruritic, well-demarcated, nonpitting edema of the dermis
- Primarily involves the periorbital and perioral regions
- Similar in pathologic basis to urticaria except that affected tissue lies deeper
  —Urticaria affects superficial tissue and causes irritation to mast cells and nerves in the epidermis leading to intense itching
  —Angioedema occurs in deeper layers, which have fewer mast cells and nerves, therefore causing less itching
- There are two types of angioedema: the classic hereditary form and the acquired forms
  —Hereditary angioedema is an autosomal-dominant disorder caused by a deficiency of C1 esterase inhibitor (C1-INH), which leads to the formation of bradykinin resulting in angioedema
  —The acquired forms demonstrate normal quantities and function of C1-INH, but it becomes bound to circulating antibodies that inactivate it
  —Absolute or functional deficiency of C1-INH from either type results in unopposed activity of the first component of the complement cascade, resulting in higher levels of bradykinin, which incites the formation of angioedema

ETIOLOGY

- Typical triggers include:
  —Food additives
  —Food allergies
  —Drug allergies
  —Insect stings
  —Exposure to heat or cold
  —Exercise
  —Thyroid disease
  —Diabetes
  —Lupus
  —Infections
  —Contact allergies
  —ACE inhibitors

Pre-Hospital

- Early intubation may be necessary before airway edema becomes too severe

Diagnosis

ESSENTIAL WORKUP

- Diagnosis is made based on clinical presentation of large nonpitting, nonpruritic wheals
- A family history need not be present to diagnose the disease

LABORATORY

- CBC with differential, ESR, ANA, rheumatoid factor
- Skin biopsy if urticarial lesion is accessible

IMAGING/SPECIAL TESTS

- Measurement of C1-INH levels
  —Patients affected with hereditary angioedema have very low levels, carriers will have half-normal levels
- C4 and C2 levels are low during attacks in both hereditary and acquired forms
- These levels not routinely available in ED

DIFFERENTIAL DIAGNOSIS

- Primary angioedema
  —IgE-mediated allergic reactions
  —Drug reactions
  —Food allergies
  —Inhalation, ingestion, or contact with allergens
  —Panic attacks, globus hystericus
- Secondary angioedema
  —Physical urticaria such as cold, pressure, solar
  —Systemic mastocytosis
  —Familial cold urticaria
  —C3b inactivator deficiency
  —Amyloidosis
  —Exercise-induced anaphylaxis
  —Transfusion reaction
  —Collagen vascular disease
  —ACE-inhibitor reaction

PEDIATRIC CONSIDERATIONS

- Recurrent angioedema presenting around puberty should raise suspicion of hereditary angioedema
- The patient should be referred to an allergist/immunologist if there is a family history of angioedema, or if the angioedema is accompanied by abdominal pain, or triggered by trauma

Treatment

INITIAL STABILIZATION

- Active airway management and supportive measures are the primary goals of emergency treatment
- Early intubation may be necessary in severe cases
  - —Orotracheal intubation is the technique of choice
    - -This may be required but difficult because of laryngeal edema, spasm, or soft tissue swelling
  - —Consider blind nasotracheal intubation if soft tissue swelling prohibits an oral approach and there is absence of stridor
  - —Transtracheal jet insufflation or cricothyrotomy may be necessary to control the airway
- Epinephrine, antihistamines, and steroids in obstructive airway swelling, though response is variable

ED TREATMENT

- A C1-INH concentrate is available, which is useful during acute attacks
- Fresh frozen plasma as a replacement source for C1-INH is controversial and should be used only as a last resort
- Attenuated androgens such as danazol are used in the long-term prophylactic treatment
- Angioedema associated with ACE inhibitors (ACEIs) occurs in 0.1–0.2% of cases and requires immediate withdrawal of the ACEI and replacement with another antihypertensive medication

MEDICATIONS

- C1-INH concentrate given in 5% dextrose over 10–45 minutes or fresh frozen plasma (if C1-INH is unavailable)
- Cimetidine 300 mg i.v.
- Diphenhydramine: adult: 50 mg i.v.; peds: 1–2 mg/kg slow IVP
- Epinephrine: 0.3–0.5 mg (use 1:1,000 dilution for s.c. route, and 1:10,000 for i.v. route); peds: epinephrine 0.01 mg/kg s.c./i.v.
- Racemic epinephrine: 2.25% solution (0.5 mL placed in a nebulizer in 2.5 mL of normal saline)
- Glucagon: adult: 1 mg i.v.
- Hydrocortisone: adult: 500 mg i.v.; peds: hydrocortisone 4–8 mg/kg/dose i.v.
- Methylprednisolone: adult: 125 mg i.v.; peds: 1–2 mg/kg i.v.
- Prednisone: adult: 60 mg PO; peds: 1 mg/kg PO
- Ranitidine: adult: 50 mg i.v.

PEDIATRIC CONSIDERATIONS

- Because the prophylactic treatment currently available is anabolic steroids, careful consideration must be made before the use of danazol or stanozolol in children

Disposition

ADMISSION CRITERIA

- Patients with systemic symptoms that do not resolve completely will need to be hospitalized for observation
- A monitored bed is recommended for those with airway involvement

DISCHARGE CRITERIA

- Patients without systemic symptoms who are stable for discharge should been seen in outpatient follow-up in a few days
- Patients should be evaluated by an allergist/immunologist after the initial presentation

Miscellaneous

ICD9: 995.1

ICD10: T78.3

SEE ALSO: ANAPHYLAXIS

SUGGESTED READINGS

Alsenz J, Bork K, Loos M. Autoantibody-mediated acquired deficiency of C1 inhibitor. N Engl J Med 1987;316:1360.

Grattan C, Powell S, Humphreys F. Management and diagnostic guidelines for urticaria and angio-oedema. Br J Dermatol 2001;144:708–714.

Nadel ES, Brown DF. Angioedema. J Emerg Med 1988;16(3):477–479.

Nzeako UC, Frigas E, Tremaine WJ. Hereditary angioedema. Arch Intern Med 2001;161:2417–2429.

Author: Sean-Xavier Neath

Ankle Fracture/Dislocation

Clinical Presentation

SIGNS AND SYMPTOMS

- History of trauma
- Local ankle pain, swelling, deformity
- Inability to bear weight
- Soft tissue injury, swelling, ecchymosis, skin tenting, skin blanching
- Neurovascular compromise, diminished capillary refill, diminished posterior tibialis (PT) or dorsalis pedis (DP) pulses
- Diminished range of motion

MECHANISM/DESCRIPTION

- Common mechanisms and injury patterns of the ankle

Mechanism of Injury

- *Inversion injury*
  - —Avulsion fracture of the lateral malleolus
  - —Oblique fracture of the medial malleolus
- *Eversion injury*
  - —Avulsion fracture of the medial malleolus
  - —Oblique fracture of the fibula
- *External rotation injury*
  - —Disruption of the tibiofibular syndesmosis, or a fibular fracture above the plafond
  - —Anterior or posterior tibial fracture with separation of the distal tibia and fibula (unstable fracture)
- *Inversion and external rotation (Maisonneuve fracture)*
  - —Medial malleolus avulsion fracture or deltoid ligament tear, disruption of the tibiofibular syndesmosis, and an oblique fracture of the proximal fibula

PEDIATRIC CONSIDERATIONS

- Ankle fractures in children often involve the *physis* (growth plate)
  - —May cause chronic deformity from growth plate injury
  - —In children younger than 10 years of age, growth plate is weaker than physis and more likely site of injury
- *Tillaux fracture:* Salter-Harris type III injury of the lateral tibial epiphysis caused by eversion and lateral rotation
- *Triplane fracture:* unusual fracture of distal tibia with fracture lines in three distinct planes (coronal, transverse, sagittal)

Pre-Hospital

- Immobilize with soft splint to reduce pain, bleeding, and further soft tissue injury

CAUTIONS

- Traction devices are usually unnecessary
  - —Contraindicated with open injuries
- Protruding bone should not be reduced; the wound should be covered with a clean dressing

Diagnosis

ESSENTIAL WORKUP

Physical Examination

- *Ottawa ankle rule:* decision rules for ordering radiographs in patients with suspected injury to the ankle and midfoot.
  - —Malleolar zone (if either finding is present, then *ankle* radiographs are indicated):
    - -1. Bony tenderness at the posterior edge or distal 6 cm of either malleoli
    - -2. Inability to bear weight for four consecutive steps either immediately after the injury or in the ED
  - —Midfoot zone (if either finding is present, then *foot* radiographs are indicated):
    - -1. Bony tenderness at the base of the fifth metatarsal
    - -2. Bony tenderness of the navicular medially
- Assess the skin for disruption or ischemia
- Careful evaluation of distal neurovascular status
  - —Capillary refill
  - —Palpation or Doppler of dorsalis pedis and posterior tibialis pulses
- Palpate proximal fibula for tenderness especially when medial malleolus or deltoid ligament tenderness is present
  - —The peroneal nerve is at risk for injury as it wraps around the fibular head; test the anterior tibialis and extensor hallucis longus; also assess sensation in first webspace

Radiography

- Anteroposterior (AP), lateral, and mortise (leg internally rotated 20 degrees) views of the ankle if tenderness is elucidated in the malleolar zone
- Evaluate the mortis view for widening of the medial clear space >4 mm and tibiofibular clear space >6 mm
- Consider radiographs for the following special circumstances:
  - —Altered sensorium or diminished distal limb sensation
  - —Multiple painful and distracting injuries
  - —Injuries that occurred 10 days prior to evaluation

IMAGING/SPECIAL TESTS

- Unstable ankle fractures or dislocations require postreduction radiographs in all three planes after splinting
- AP and lateral radiographs of the tibia and fibula are indicated if a Maisonneuve fracture is suspected clinically
- Stress-testing the ligaments in a painful ankle is unnecessary in the ED if the patient will be reexamined in 3–5 days
- Stress radiographs of the ankle are usually unnecessary acutely
- CT scan or MRI may be useful to assess the degree of injury to the tibial plafond, intraarticular pathology, ligamentous injuries, and pediatric epiphyseal injuries

DIFFERENTIAL DIAGNOSIS

- Ankle sprain
- Achilles tendon injury
- Os trigonum fracture
- Fifth metatarsal fracture (Jones fracture)
- Peroneal tendon dislocation or injury
- Talar fractures
- Talar-dome fracture
- Subtalar dislocations
- Calcaneal fractures
- Foot fractures
- Ankle diastasis

PEDIATRIC CONSIDERATIONS

- Injury to the growth plates may not be apparent on plain radiographs
- Consider immobilization, non-weight-bearing status, and orthopedic referral if clinical suspicion warrants even in the setting of negative radiographs
- CT scan or MRI may be warranted to delineate the extent of the injury
- Inform parents of the possibility of growth abnormalities in patients with injury to the physis

Treatment

INITIAL STABILIZATION

- Avoid weight bearing
- Ice
- Compression
- Elevation

ED TREATMENT

Ankle Fracture

- *All ankle fractures or dislocations require orthopedic consultation or referral*
- Open ankle fractures
  - —Remove contaminants
  - —Apply moist sterile dressing
  - —Assess tetanus immunity
  - —Antibiotics
  - —Emergent orthopedic consultation
- Closed ankle fractures
  - —Closed reduction, if necessary
  - —Immobilize with a posterior splint
  - —*Posterior splint* immobilizes the foot at a 90-degree angle with the application of bulky dressings and covered by volar (posterior) and coaptation (U-shaped stirrup) splinting material
- *Stable injury* (injury to only one side of the ankle)
  - —Isolated injury to the lateral malleolus without medial involvement is virtually always stable
  - —Apply posterior splint
- *Unstable injury* (both sides of the ankle are injured)
  - —Urgent orthopedic consultation
  - —Posterior splint as in stable injuries
  - —May require open reduction and internal fixation (ORIF) emergently before significant swelling develops
- *Neurovascular injury* requires emergent orthopedic consultation

Ankle Dislocations

- Closed reduction should be performed as rapidly as possible to minimize ischemia to the skin and reduce the risk of avascular necrosis of the talus
- Skin tenting and evidence of neurovascular compromise are indications for immediate reduction, even prior to radiographs
- Most ankle dislocations require ORIF
- After reduction place a posterior splint

MEDICATIONS

- Closed fractures
  - —Primarily analgesics (opioids)
- Dislocations or displaced fractures requiring closed reduction
  - —Short-acting benzodiazepine (midazolam 0.05–0.1 mg/kg i.v.) or barbiturate (methohexital 1–1.5 mg/kg i.v.) with opioid analgesic
- Open fractures
  - —Cefazolin: 2 g i.v. loading dose (50 mg/kg pediatric dose)
  - —Gentamicin: 5–7 mg/kg i.v. (2.5 mg/kg pediatric dose)
  - —Vancomycin: 1 g i.v. loading dose (10 mg/kg in children) if penicillin allergic
  - —Tetanus toxoid if indicated

Disposition

ADMISSION CRITERIA

- Unstable ankle fractures require urgent orthopedic consultation and may require admission
- Open ankle fractures and dislocations should be admitted for débridement, irrigation, and IV antibiotics
- Ankle dislocations that are treated with either open or closed reduction
- Concern for compartment syndrome or neurovascular injury

DISCHARGE CRITERIA

- Simple nondisplaced stable ankle fractures without neurovascular compromise may be discharged following splinting

Miscellaneous

ICD9: 824.8, 837.0

ICD10: S82.8; S92.1; S93.0

SUGGESTED READINGS

Duchesneau S, Fallat LM. The Maisonneuve fracture. J Foot Ankle Surg 1995;34(5): 422–428.

Marsh JL, Saltzman CL. Ankle fractures. In: Bucholz RW, Heckman JD, eds. Rockwood and Green's fractures in adults, 5th ed. Philadelphia: Lippincott Williams & Wilkins, 2001:201–283.

Moehring HD, Tan RT, Marder RA, et al. Ankle dislocation. J Orthop Trauma 1994;8:167–172.

Plint AC, Bulloch B, Osmond MH, et al. Validation of the Ottawa Ankle Rules in children with ankle injuries. Acad Emerg Med 1999;6(10):1005–1009.

Stiell IG, McKnight RD, Greenberg GH, et al. Decision rules for use of radiography in acute ankle injuries: refinement and prospective validation. JAMA 1993;269: 1127–1132.

Author: Binh T. Ly

Ankle Sprain

Clinical Presentation

SIGNS AND SYMPTOMS

- Grade I (mild)
  - —Pain
  - —Minimal to no difficulty in ambulation
  - —Localized edema absent to slight
  - —No ligamentous instability (see Diagnosis, below)
- Grade II (moderate)
  - —Pain
  - —Moderate difficulty with ambulation
  - —Localized edema moderate to significant
  - —Ecchymosis may be present
  - —Ligamentous weakness (see Diagnosis, below)
- Grade III (severe)
  - —Pain
  - —Unable to ambulate
  - —Joint instability to exam (see Diagnosis, below)
  - —Marked edema
  - —Ecchymosis usually present
  - —Ligamentous weakness

MECHANISM/DESCRIPTION

- Ankle sprains are injuries to the ligamentous supports of the ankle
  - —The ankle joint is a hinge joint composed of the tibia, fibula, and talus
  - —The injury may range from stretching with only microscopic damage (grade I) to partial disruption (grade II) to complete disruption (grade III)
- 85–90% of all ankle sprains involve the lateral ligaments [anterior talofibular (ATFL), posterior talofibular (PTFL), and calcaneofibular (CFL)], and are usually the result of an inversion injury
  - —The ATFL is the most commonly injured
  - —If the ankle is injured in a neutral position, the CFL is often injured
  - —The PTFL is rarely injured in the absence of disruption of both of the other lateral ligaments
- Injury to the deltoid ligament (connecting the medial malleolus to the talus and navicular bones) is usually the result of an eversion injury
  - —Often associated with avulsion at the medial malleolus or talar insertion
  - —It is rarely found as an isolated injury, and, when found, one should suspect an associated lateral malleolus fracture, or fracture of the proximal fibula (Maisonneuve fracture)
- Syndesmosis sprains (injury to the tibiofibular ligaments or the interosseous ligament of the leg) occur most commonly in collision sports
  - —Syndesmosis injuries (a.k.a., "high ankle sprains") have a higher morbidity and potential for long-term complications

PEDIATRIC CONSIDERATIONS

- Children under age 10 with traumatic ankle pain and no radiologic evidence of fracture most likely have a Salter-Harris I fracture
  - —The ligaments are actually stronger than the open epiphysis

Pre-Hospital

- Immobilize ankle as necessary

Diagnosis

ESSENTIAL WORKUP

- History may predict the type of injury found and should include:
  - —Time of injury
  - —Mechanism
  - —The presence of a "pop" or "crack"
  - —History of previous trauma
  - —Relevant medical conditions (e.g., bone or joint disease)
  - —Treatments attempted prior to arrival
  - —Ability to bear weight subsequent to the injury
- The physical exam is aimed at detecting joint instability and other injuries
  - —Note the presence or absence of bony tenderness at the medial and lateral malleoli as well as at the base of the fifth metatarsal
  - —Document neurovascular status distal to the injury
  - —Assess range of motion and compare it to the uninjured side
  - —Stress testing in the ED is often limited by pain and may impair detection of ligament injury
  - —The squeeze test helps identify syndesmosis injuries: squeeze the tibia and fibula together at the midcalf; pain felt in the ankle indicates a positive test

IMAGING/SPECIAL TESTS

- Ankle injuries should be radiographed if there is concern for fracture
- The *Ottawa Ankle Rules,* a selective strategy for obtaining ankle x-rays in adults under age 55, suggest that foot or ankle x-rays are unnecessary except when any of the following are present:
  - —Bony tenderness at the posterior edge of the distal 6 cm or tip of either malleolus
  - —Bony tenderness along the base of the fifth metatarsal or navicular bone
  - —Inability to take four unassisted steps both immediately after the injury and in the ED
- The rules have been prospectively validated by the original authors as well as independently by groups in the U.S., U.K., France, and other countries
- Stress radiographs are rarely useful in the ED and should not be routinely ordered unless requested by a consultant

DIFFERENTIAL DIAGNOSIS

- Ankle fracture (lateral, medial, or posterior malleolus) or dislocation
- Achilles tendon injury
- Maisonneuve fracture
- Os trigonum fracture
- Fifth metatarsal fracture (Jones fracture)
- Transchondral talar dome fracture
- Peroneal tendon dislocation or injury

Treatment

INITIAL STABILIZATION

- Prevent further injury; avoid weight-bearing if painful
- RICE (rest, ice, compression, elevation)

ED TREATMENT

- The goal of treatment is reduction of pain and the return to normal activity without long-term pain or joint laxity
- Existing evidence supports early mobilization and functional treatment
  —Unstable ankles (i.e., grade III) or those with severe pain may benefit from brief immobilization followed by early return to functional treatment
- Grade I or II sprains can be treated with functional support (elastic bandage, air splint, gel splint, etc.)
- Grade III sprains can be treated by immobilization (sugar tong with posterior splint or bulky Jones dressing) and early orthopedic consultation or referral
- Crutches may be needed initially for comfort, but encourage weight-bearing as tolerated
- NSAIDs are useful for treating pain
- Once the acute pain and swelling have resolved, strengthening exercises and proprioceptive training improve ankle strength and function
- Full sports activities may be resumed only when running and turning are pain-free
- Ankle taping, air-splints, or gel-splints reduce the risk of recurrent injury in high-risk sports such as basketball, volleyball, soccer, and cross-country running

Disposition

ADMISSION CRITERIA

- An isolated ankle sprain should not require admission

DISCHARGE CRITERIA

- Grade I and II sprains should be instructed to follow up with the primary care physician in 1–2 weeks
- Grade III sprains and syndesmosis injuries should be referred to an orthopedic surgeon or sports medicine specialist within 7–10 days

Miscellaneous

ICD9: 845.00

ICD10: S93.4

SUGGESTED READINGS

Geppert MJ. Soft tissue injuries of the ankle. In: Orthopedic knowledge update: foot and ankle 2, 2nd ed. Rosemont: American Academy of Orthopedic Surgeons, 1998:229–242.

Ho K, Abu-Laban RB. Ankle and foot. In: Marx JA, ed. Rosen's Emergency medicine: concepts and clinical practice, 5th ed. St. Louis: Mosby, 2002:706–735.

Michael JA, Stiell IG. Ankle injuries. In: Tintinalli JE, Kelen GD, Stapczynski JS, eds. Emergency medicine: a comprehensive study guide, 5th ed. New York: McGraw-Hill, 2000:1825–1833.

Renstrom PA, Konradsen L. Ankle ligament injuries. Br J Sports Med 1997;31:11–20.

Stiell IG, McKnight RD, Greenberg GH, et al. Decision rules for use of radiography in acute ankle injuries: refinement and prospective validation. JAMA 1993;269:1127–1132.

Author: Taylor Y. Cardall

Ankylosing Spondylitis

Clinical Presentation

SIGNS AND SYMPTOMS

- *Low back pain,* especially *sacroiliitis,* is the most common presentation; it is exacerbated by rest and improved with mild activity or stooping forward
- *Paralysis* from minor spinal trauma or manipulation
- May present with *cauda equina syndrome*
- Enthesitis (inflammation at tendon or ligament insertion) is common
  - —*Achilles tendonitis* or *plantar fasciitis*
- May have *asymmetric arthritis* of large joints of lower extremities
- *Uveitis* may precede onset of arthritis
- May have *aortic valve regurgitation*
- Restrictive lung disease

ETIOLOGY

- Genetic predisposition: prior trauma, infection, or neuroendocrine-immune system may play a role
- HLA-B27 genetic susceptibility

MECHANISM/DESCRIPTION

- Spinal predilection
- Onset before 40 years of age
- Male to female ratio is 3:1
- Inflammation at the bony insertions of ligaments or tendons (entheses)
- May have systemic inflammatory manifestations such as uveitis
- *Spondylitis* of ankylosing spondylitis (AS) begins at the insertions of the outer fibers of the annulus fibrosis (enthesitis) of the vertebrae
  - —Begin to ossify and may lead to complete fusion, *ankylosis,* of the vertebrae
- The fused spine is dangerously brittle: significantly increases the risks for *fracture* and *paralysis*

PEDIATRIC CONSIDERATIONS

- Juvenile ankylosing spondylitis (JAS) may mimic a septic process with fever and systemic signs
- Onset of JAS is late childhood or adolescence (usually before age 16) primarily boys
- JAS may initially present as aortic regurgitation with fulminant aortitis
- JAS has a much greater predilection for *extraspinal* joints and entheses of the lower extremities; examine for:
  - —*Asymmetrical arthritis* of the joints of the lower extremities, especially hip
  - —*Enthesitis* of the Achilles tendon attachment at the heel, the plantar fascia attachments to the sole of the foot, the patellar ligament attachment to the tibial tuberosity, and the quadriceps tendon attachments to the patella

Pre-Hospital

CAUTIONS

- There is an increased risk of traumatic spinal injury from even minor injuries
- Intubation difficulty and restrictive lung disease if thoracic involvement

Diagnosis

ESSENTIAL WORKUP

- Exclude fracture or nerve injury in any new spinal pain of a patient suspected of AS
- Exclude sepsis or septic joint
- Evaluate for sacroiliitis with *pelvic rock* test (compression) or *Patrick test* (sacroiliac distraction)

LABORATORY

- ESR may be elevated
- CBC may show mild leukocytosis with slight to moderate anemia and thrombocytosis
- BUN, creatinine, and electrolytes may be useful to assess renal involvement

IMAGING/SPECIAL TESTS

- Pelvic x-ray: should be done in any adult patient suspected of ankylosing spondylitis
  - —Sacroiliitis is essential to the diagnosis of AS; this is seen initially as subchondral bony erosions on the iliac side of the SI joint, which later manifest as bony proliferation and sclerosis
- Lumbar, thoracic, and cervical spine x-rays to exclude fracture for complaint of *new pain to these areas with or without trauma*
- CT should be performed to further evaluate possible fractures on plain radiographs
- MRI should be performed emergently on any patient with *neurologic deficit*
- Chest x-ray may show findings similar to TB with patchy inflammatory infiltrates

DIFFERENTIAL DIAGNOSIS

- *Mechanical* low back pain is generally improved with rest and exacerbated by exercise without signs of systemic inflammatory process
- *Infectious* low back pain is more constant, unremitting, and associated with fever
- *Neoplastic* low back pain is more typical in patients over the age of 40 and more constant and unremitting
  - —Night pain is a characteristic symptom
- *Septic arthritis* should be excluded by arthrocentesis if single joint involvement
- *Psoriatic arthritis* usually presents in a patient with known psoriasis and has much greater predilection for the *hands and feet*
- *Reiter's disease:* the classic triad of arthritis, urethritis, and conjunctivitis: symptom onset about 1 month after an episode of urethritis or enteritis
- Arthritis associated with inflammatory bowel disease occurs in patients with Crohn's disease or ulcerative colitis
  - —Primarily involves knee, elbow, ankle, or wrist, and usually exacerbated by flares of the bowel disease

PEDIATRIC CONSIDERATIONS

- Juvenile *rheumatoid* arthritis has a greater predilection for the small joints of the hands

Treatment

INITIAL STABILIZATION

- Trauma: ABCs while maintaining immobilization (including in-line spinal stabilization if intubation required)
- Acute paralysis: methylprednisolone IV and immediate neurosurgical evaluation

ED TREATMENT

- Control pain and inflammation with NSAIDs; steroids may be useful in severe refractory cases
- Exclude infection by clinical presentation, laboratory analysis, and possibly arthrocentesis
- Exclude spinal fracture (use CT for equivocal findings on plain radiographs)

MEDICATIONS

- NSAIDs
  - —Ibuprofen: 35 mg/kg/day divided t.i.d.-q.i.d. with food, adult 400–600 mg PO q.i.d.
  - —Indomethacin: 1–2 mg/kg/day divided t.i.d. with food, adult 25 mg PO t.i.d.
  - —Naproxen: 10–20 mg/kg/d divided b.i.d. with food, adult 250–500 mg PO b.i.d.
  - —Tolmetin sodium: 20–30 mg/kg/d divided t.i.d. with food, 200–600 mg PO t.i.d.

(Note: if NSAIDS are poorly tolerated, ineffective, or contraindicated, consider opioid analgesics, muscle relaxants, or low dose steroids)

- Steroids
  - —Methylprednisolone: high-dose protocol for acute paralysis: 30 mg/kg bolus, then 5.4 mg/kg/hr for 24 hours total; severe refractory pain: 1,000 mg i.v. single dose (controversial)

PEDIATRIC CONSIDERATIONS

- Indomethacin is generally considered second-line therapy due to side effects

Disposition

ADMISSION CRITERIA

- Sepsis or septic joint cannot be excluded
- Pain is intractable
- Acute neurologic impairment

DISCHARGE CRITERIA

- No serious injuries or neurologic deficit
- Pain controlled

SPECIAL PEDIATRIC DISPOSITION DECISIONS

- Referral for physiotherapy
- Resting splints for inflamed joints
- Orthoses for inflamed entheses (such as heel cushion inserts to rest Achilles tendon attachment)

Miscellaneous

ICD9: 720.0

ICD10: M45

SUGGESTED READINGS

Banares A, Hernandez-Garcia C, Fernandez-Guttierez B, et al. Eye involvement in the spondyloarthropathies. Rheumatol Dis Clin North Am 1998;24:663–676.

Burgos-Vargas R, Petty RE. Juvenile ankylosing spondylitis. Rheum Dis Clin North Am 1997;23:569–598.

Karasick D, Schweitzer ME, Abidi NA, et al. Fractures of the vertebrae with spinal cord injuries in patients with ankylosing spondylitis: imaging findings. AJR 1995;165:1205–1208.

Lee-Chang TL Jr. Pulmonary manifestations of ankylosing spondylitis and relapsing polychondritis. Clin Chest Med 1998;19:747–757.

van der linden S, vander Heijde D. Ankylosing spondylitis. Rheumatol Dis Clin North Am 1998;24:663–676.

Author: Paul L. DeSandre

Anterior Cruciate Ligament Injury

Clinical Presentation

SIGNS AND SYMPTOMS

- Feeling knee "give way," hearing a "pop," or feeling a tearing sensation at the time of injury
- Pain most common complaint with anterior cruciate ligament (ACL) rupture
  - —Partial injury may not be particularly painful due to paucity of pain fibers in ACL itself
- Most patients report immediate knee dysfunction and loss of ability; some may ambulate despite a complete ACL rupture because of stability from supporting structures
- *Immediate effusion* (hemarthrosis within 2–3 hours) usually indicates a significant intraarticular injury
  - —About 70% of acute knee hemarthroses are due to ACL injury
  - —Lack of hemarthrosis does not rule out ACL injury: capsular disruption may allow extravasation of intraarticular blood
- "Locking" may occur due to interposition of torn cruciate, or associated torn menisci, or loose body; pseudo-locking may be present from pain, effusion, or spasm
- Stress testing—*always compare the injured to the uninjured side: asymmetry is more reliable than absolute degree of laxity*
  - —*Lachman test* is most reliable
  - —Knee flexed 20 degrees, patient supine with thigh supported; tibia is brought forward on the femur, one hand holding proximal tibia, the other stabilizing the femur just above the patella
  - —Pain with no motion is probable grade 1 injury
  - —Pain with motion indicates partial tear or disruption
  - —Firm end point of motion suggests partial tear
  - —*Pivot shift test:* more specific for ACL injury but unreliable without anesthesia; use cautiously in acutely injured knee
  - —Patient supine, knee in full extension
  - —Internal rotation of tibia via a hand on foot is applied simultaneously with valgus stress form the other hand
  - —With knee flexion to 20–30 degrees, the examiner notices a jerk at the anterolateral corner of the proximal tibia
  - —*Anterior drawer sign:* not as sensitive or specific as Lachman test
  - —Knee flexed 90 degrees, patient supine, hip flexed 45 degrees, foot neutral and stabilized
  - —Anterior motion is positive

ETIOLOGY

- The ACL is the most commonly injured ligament of the knee
- Most injuries to the ACL are sports related, especially skiing and football
  - —Noncontact injury is common: "plant and pivot" or "stop and jump" mechanism

MECHANISM/DESCRIPTION

- The ACL inserts anterolaterally to the anterior tibial spine and to the posterior aspect of the lateral femoral condyle; portions of the tendon are under tension (i.e., at risk) in both flexion and extension
- The ACL prevents excessive anterior movement, excessive internal rotation of the tibia on the femur, or hyperextension of the knee
- Mechanism of injury is often deceleration with flexion and rotation; also common is hyperextension

PEDIATRIC CONSIDERATIONS

- The ACL is the most frequently injured knee ligament in children

Pre-Hospital

CAUTIONS

- The knee must be adequately immobilized to prevent complete rupture of the ACL

Diagnosis

ESSENTIAL WORKUP

- Neurovascular evaluation, exclusion of fractures/dislocations, valgus/varus stress at 20-degree flexion, Lachman test, extensor mechanism function
- The Lachman test (as described above) is the most important and sensitive test for ACL injury
- Look for signs of associated ligament or meniscus injury, present in about half of patients with ACL injury

LABORATORY

- If the cause of a knee effusion is uncertain, synovial aspirate can be sent for cell count, Gram stain, and culture and crystals; fat globules in the aspirate suggest a fracture
  - —Arthrocentesis usually not indicated with an ACL injury

IMAGING/SPECIAL TESTS

- Plain films have a low rate of positive findings: clinical decision rules limit the number of negative plain films obtained
- The Ottawa knee rules (apply to adults): plain films required for patients with any of five findings:
  - —1. Age 55 or older
  - —2. Isolated tenderness of patella
  - —3. Tenderness at head of fibula
  - —4. Inability to flex 90 degrees
  - —5. Inability to bear weight both immediately and in the ED (four steps)
- The *lateral capsular sign* is a lateral tibial plateau avulsion fracture, just below the joint line; is diagnostic for an ACL rupture but present in <10% of ACL injuries
- MRI is replacing arthroscopy for definitive images of the cruciate ligaments, but is rarely indicated emergently

DIFFERENTIAL DIAGNOSIS

- Meniscal injury
- Collateral ligament injury
- Tibial plateau injury

PEDIATRIC CONSIDERATIONS

- Tears of the ACL in children often occur at the insertion site of the ligament
- Children and adolescents show more laxity on exam than adults
- Ottawa knee rules do not apply to children

Treatment

INITIAL STABILIZATION

- Establish integrity of neurovascular function
- Immobilize the knee, ice, elevate

ED TREATMENT

- Injury is graded by severity
  - —Grade 3 is complete disruption of the ligament
  - —Grade 2 represents severe stretching with partial tear of the ligament
  - —Grade 1 is microscopic ligamentous damage with no clinical instability
- General care
  - —Immobilization/non-weight-bearing
  - —Ice for first 48 hours, elevation
  - —Analgesic
  - —First-degree injury may be treated with compressive wrap and weight-bearing as tolerated
  - —Orthopedic referral within 1–2 weeks is necessary if significant ligamentous injury (grade 2 or 3) is present
  - —Reexamination is recommended at 48 hours if the ED exam is inconclusive or if history suggests a more significant injury than the initial exam demonstrates (i.e., severe symptoms, hearing a pop)
  - —Aspiration of a tense hemarthrosis may relieve pain

MEDICATIONS

- NSAIDs or narcotic pain medications are the mainstay
- Motrin 400–600 mg PO q.i.d. PRN

PEDIATRIC CONSIDERATIONS

- Surgical repair is generally recommended for adolescents with grade 3 injury

Disposition

ADMISSION CRITERIA

- Isolated ACL injury rarely requires emergent hospitalization; for suspected complete ruptures, definitive therapy is often surgical, and orthopedic consultation is appropriate
- Controversy remains in the orthopedic literature as to whether conservative versus surgical treatment yields the best long-term results

DISCHARGE CRITERIA

- Most patients can be managed as outpatients with appropriate referral

Miscellaneous

ICD9: 959.7

ICD10: S83.5

SUGGESTED READINGS

Gersoff WK, Clancy WG Jr. Diagnosis of acute and chronic anterior cruciate ligament tears. Clin Sports Med 1988;7(4):727.

Solomon DH, Simel DL, et al. Does this patient have a torn meniscus or ligament of the knee? Value of the physical examination. JAMA 2001;286(13):1610.

Stiell IG, Greenberg GH, et al. Prospective validation of a decision rule for the use of radiography in acute knee injuries. JAMA 1996;275:611.

Swenson TM, Hamer CD. Knee ligament and meniscal injuries. Orthop Clin North Am 1995;26:529.

Zarins B, Adams M. Knee injuries in sports. N Engl J Med 1988;318(15):950.

Author: Moss Mendelson

Anthrax

Clinical Presentation

SIGNS AND SYMPTOMS

Inhalation Anthrax

- Fever, chills
- Fatigue, malaise, lethargy
- Cough, usually dry or minimally productive
- Nausea or vomiting
- Dyspnea
- Diaphoresis (often described as "drenching sweats")
- Chest pain or discomfort
- Myalgias
- Tachycardia (>100/min)
- Fever
- Meningeal signs (headache, confusion)

Cutaneous Anthrax

- Skin lesion
  —Painless pruritic papule
  —Turning into a vesicle that ruptures forming a necrotic ulcer
- Black eschar
- Surrounding gelatinous nonpitting edema

MECHANISM/DESCRIPTION

Inhalation Anthrax

- Incubation period usually 1–6 days, but can be as long as 42 days or more
- Onset gradual and nonspecific, similar to a flu-like or viral syndrome
- After several days of mild symptoms, patient rapidly deteriorates
  —Increasing severe dyspnea
  —Stridor
  —Cyanosis
  —Shock
- Patients can develop hemorrhagic meningitis
- Mortality rate
  —Approximately 100% if untreated
  —In recent cases from deliberate exposure through the U.S. mail in the fall of 2001, 6 of 11 patients survived with treatment (mortality rate 45%)
- Anthrax spores are robust and resistant to destruction by heat, light, or drying
- Spores deposited in pulmonary alveoli, engulfed by macrophages and transported to mediastinal lymph nodes
- In lymph nodes, spores germinate, multiply, and then spread in blood throughout body
- Inhalation anthrax is *not* contagious person-to-person

Cutaneous Anthrax

- Over 95% of naturally occurring anthrax cases seen today are cutaneous
- Incubation period 1–5 days
- Mortality rate
  —20% untreated
  —1% if treated with antibiotics
- Anthrax spore does not penetrate intact skin
- Spore enters through cut, abrasion, or break in skin
- Engulfed by macrophages and taken to regional lymph nodes
- Can spread throughout body if untreated

ETIOLOGY

- *Bacillus anthracis*
  —Rod-shaped
  —Gram-positive
  —Spore-forming
  —Zoonotic disease of animals (goats, sheep, cattle, horses)
  —"Wool-sorter's disease" (inhalation anthrax)
    -Occupational hazard for those who worked with animal skins and products)
    -Rarely seen now that many animals are vaccinated for anthrax

Pre-Hospital

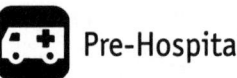

- Symptomatic patients are not contagious person-to-person
- Standard universal infectious precautions

Diagnosis

ESSENTIAL WORKUP

- Suspect bioterrorism event if multiple cases of relatively young, healthy patients who present with a flu-like syndrome, and within days deteriorate rapidly

LABORATORY

- Blood cultures
  —Often turn positive within 12–24 hours, even in early stages
- CBC
  —White blood count can be normal or minimally elevated
  —Neutrophilia (>70%)
  —Left shift (neutrophil bands >5%)
- ABG
  —Hypoxemia
- Lumbar puncture
  —Indicated if meningeal signs and symptoms
  —Up to 50% of patients with inhalation anthrax may develop hemorrhagic meningitis
  —May see *B. anthracis* on Gram stain of CSF

IMAGING/SPECIAL TESTS

- CXR
  —Mediastinal widening
  —Pulmonary infiltrate/consolidation
  —Pleural effusion
- CT chest
  —Good follow-up test if suspect anthrax and CXR normal or equivocal
  —Pleural effusion
  —Mediastinal lymphadenopathy
- Pleurocentesis
  —Culture of pleural fluid often positive for *B. anthracis*
  —May see organism on specimen from pleural biopsy
- Skin punch biopsy of cutaneous lesion

DIFFERENTIAL DIAGNOSIS

Inhalation Anthrax

- Early presentation similar to influenza or viral syndrome
- Bacterial pneumonia
- Bacterial meningitis

Cutaneous Anthrax

- Brown recluse spider bite
- Tularemia
- Streptococcal or staphylococcal skin infection

Treatment

INITIAL STABILIZATION

- Fluid resuscitation
- Supplemental oxygen, intubation, supported ventilation as indicated

ED TREATMENT

Inhalation Anthrax

- Specific treatment recommendations are evolving as experience with anthrax increases
- Victims of inhalation anthrax in the fall of 2001 outbreak were treated with at least two, and usually three, different antibiotics
  - —Ciprofloxacin
  - —Doxycycline
  - —Rifampin
  - —Clindamycin
  - —Vancomycin
- All treatment of inhalation anthrax should be done in consultation with local or national public health officials
- Antibiotic choice may depend on susceptibility profile of the specific anthrax strain involved
- Duration of treatment: 60 days
- Can switch to fewer oral antibiotics as patient improves

Cutaneous Anthrax

- Ciprofloxacin or doxycycline
  - —Uncomplicated cases can be treated with oral antibiotic
  - —Intravenous therapy if extensive edema, lesion on head or neck, or systemic signs or symptoms
  - —Duration of therapy
    - -Naturally acquired cutaneous anthrax is treated for 2 weeks
    - -If acquired from deliberate release or bioterrorist event, treat for 60 days to protect against possibility of inhalation exposure

MEDICATIONS

- Ciprofloxacin: 400 mg i.v. q12h
- Clindamycin: 900 mg i.v. q12h
- Doxycycline: 100 mg i.v. q12h
- Rifampin: 10 mg/kg i.v. single daily dose, not to exceed 600 mg/day
- Vancomycin: 1 g i.v. q12h

PEDIATRIC CONSIDERATIONS

- Medication use
  - —Although some of the medications used to treat anthrax can have adverse effects in children (e.g., ciprofloxacin, doxycycline), it is often recommended that these be used even in pediatric cases
  - —Institute in consultation with public health officials

Disposition

ADMISSION CRITERIA

- Known or suspected symptomatic inhalation anthrax
- Cutaneous anthrax with significant signs and symptoms
  - —Extensive edema
  - —Head or neck lesions
  - —Dyspnea
  - —Systemic manifestations

DISCHARGE CRITERIA

- Localized cutaneous anthrax without significant signs or symptoms (as outlined above)

Miscellaneous

ICD 9: 022

ICD10: A22.9

SEE ALSO: HAZMAT

SUGGESTED READINGS

Centers for Disease Control and Prevention. Recommendations for antimicrobial prophylaxis for children and breastfeeding mothers and treatment of children with anthrax. JAMA 2001;286(21):2663–2664.

Inglesby TV, Henderson DA, Bartlett JG, et al. Anthrax as a biological weapon: medical and public health management. Working Group on Civilian Biodefense. JAMA 1999;281(18):1735–1745.

Jernigan JA, Stephens DS, Ashford DA, et al. Bioterrorism-related inhalational anthrax: the first 10 cases reported in the United States. Emerg Infect Dis 2001;7:933–944.

Swartz MN. Recognition and management of anthrax—an update. N Engl J Med 2001;345(22):1621–1626.

Author: Leon Gussow

Anticholinergic, Poisoning

Clinical Presentation

SIGNS AND SYMPTOMS

Classic Toxidrome

- "Mad as a hatter"—altered mental status
- "Hot as a hare"—hyperthermia
- "Red as a beet"—flushed skin
- "Dry as a bone"—dry skin and mucous membranes
- "Blind as a bat"—blurred vision secondary to mydriasis

General

- Hyperthermia
- Altered mental status

Ocular

- Unreactive mydriasis
- Inability to accommodate

Cardiovascular

- Sinus tachycardia
- Dysrhythmias (rare except in massive ingestions)
- Hypo- or hypertension
- Cardiogenic pulmonary edema

Pulmonary

- Tachypnea
- Respiratory failure

GI

- Decreased/absent bowel sounds
- Dysphagia
- Decreased GI motility
- Decreased salivation

GU

- Urinary retention

Integument

- Decreased sweating
- Flushed skin
- Dry skin and mucous membranes

CNS

- Altered mental status
- Auditory or visual hallucinations
- Coma
- Seizures

MECHANISM

- Central and peripheral cholinergic blockade
- Depending on the drug involved, antagonism of muscarinic (most common), nicotinic, or both receptors

ETIOLOGY

- Many drugs contain *anticholinergic properties*
  —Mild at therapeutic doses
  —Life-threatening in overdose
- Anticholinergic substances
  —Antihistamines
  —Belladonna alkaloids, synthetic congeners
  —Antiparkinsonian drugs
  —Cyclic antidepressants
  —Antipsychotics
  —Mydriatics
  —Skeletal muscle relaxants (orphenadrine, cyclobenzaprine)
  —Antispasmodics
  —Mushrooms—*Amanita muscaria, A. pantherina*
  —Plants—deadly nightshade, mandrake, henbane
  —Jimson weed—smoked or ingested

Pre-Hospital

CAUTIONS

- Transport all pills/pill bottles involved in overdose for identification in ED
- Scopolamine eyedrops have been added to beverages to rob unsuspecting victims
- Jimson weed
  —Common adolescent ingestion
  —Consider in a young adult with unexplained visual difficulty, dilated pupils, and delirium
  —50–100 seeds contain the equivalent of 3–6 mg atropine

Diagnosis

ESSENTIAL WORKUP

- Diagnosis based on clinical presentation and an accurate history

LABORATORY

- Toxicologic screen excludes other ingestions
- Electrolytes, BUN, Cr, glucose
- CBC
- Creatine kinase if suspected rhabdomyolysis
- Acetaminophen level
  —Detects occult ingestion (e.g., Tylenol PM)

IMAGING/SPECIAL TESTS

- EKG
  —Sinus tachycardia most common
  —QRS prolongation
  —AV dissociation
  —Bundle branch block
  —Dysrhythmias

DIFFERENTIAL DIAGNOSIS

- Sympathomimetic intoxication
- Withdrawal syndrome
- Acute psychiatric disorders
- Sepsis

Treatment

INITIAL STABILIZATION

- ABCs
  - —Airway control essential
  - —Administer supplemental oxygen
  - —IV access
  - —Cardiac monitor and pulse oximetry
- Naloxone, thiamine, D50 (or Accucheck) if altered mental status

ED TREATMENT

Decontamination

- Avoid ipecac because of aspiration risk
- Administer activated charcoal
- Ocular lavage for eyedrop exposure
- Jimson weed considerations
  - —Gastric decontamination recommended up to 12–24 hours after the ingestion of seeds from slowed GI motility
  - —Consider polyethylene glycol electrolyte solution (GoLytely) for seed ingestions if no evidence of obstruction

Physostigmine

- Reversible acetylcholinesterase inhibitor that crosses the blood-brain barrier
- Reverses both central and peripheral anticholinergic effects
- Use with caution due to risk of dysrhythmias (especially asystole), seizures, and cholinergic crises
  - —Place on cardiac monitor
  - —Observe for cholinergic symptoms
- Indicated in the presence of peripheral anticholinergic signs and the following:
  - —Seizures unresponsive to conventional therapy
  - —Uncontrollable agitation
  - —Hemodynamically unstable arrhythmias unresponsive to conventional therapy
  - —Hypertension uncontrolled by standard treatment
- Contraindications
  - —Cyclic antidepressant overdose (potentiates toxicity)
  - —Cardiovascular disease
  - —Asthma/bronchospasm
  - —Intestinal obstruction
  - —Heart block
  - —Peripheral vascular disease
  - —Bladder obstruction

Treat Complications

- Standard cooling measures for hyperthermia
- Treatment of hypertension usually unnecessary
  - —Conventional therapy for severely elevated BP
- Treat seizures with benzodiazepines and barbiturates
- Dysrhythmias
  - —Use standard antidysrhythmics
  - —Avoid class Ia antidysrhythmic due to the quinidine-like effect of many anticholinergic drugs
  - —Sodium bicarbonate may reverse the quinidine-like effects
- Use benzodiazepines for treatment of agitation
  - —Avoid phenothiazines due to anticholinergic effects

MEDICATIONS

- Activated charcoal slurry: 1–2 g/kg PO
- Dextrose: D50W 1 amp (50 mL or 25 g) (peds: D25W 2–4 mL/kg) i.v.
- Diazepam (benzodiazepine): 5–10 mg (peds: 0.2–0.5 mg/kg) i.v.
- Naloxone (Narcan): 0.4–2 mg (peds: 0.1 mg/kg) i.v. or i.m. initial dose
- Phenobarbital: 10–20 mg/kg i.v. (loading dose)
- Polyethylene glycol-electrolyte solution (CoLyte, GoLytely): 2 L/hr (peds: 25–40 mL/kg/hr) PO or per NGT until rectal effluent clear
- Physostigmine: 0.5–2.0 mg (peds: 0.02 mg/kg) i.v. over 5 minutes, repeat if necessary in 30–60 minutes
- Thiamine (vitamin B_1): 100 mg (peds: 50 mg) i.v. or i.m.

Disposition

ADMISSION CRITERIA

- ICU admission for moderate to severe anticholinergic symptoms (agitation control, temperature control, and observation for seizures or dysrhythmias)
- Any patient receiving physostigmine

DISCHARGE CRITERIA

- Mild and improving symptoms of anticholinergic toxicity after 6–8 hours of ED observation

Miscellaneous

ICD9: 971.1

ICD10: T44.3

SUGGESTED READINGS

Burns MJ, Linden CH, Graudins A, et al. A comparison of physostigmine and benzodiazepines for the treatment of anticholinergic poisoning. Ann Emerg Med 2000;35:374–381.

Ceha LJ, Presperin C, Young E, et al. Anticholinergic toxicity from nightshade berry poisoning responsive to physostigmine. J Emerg Med 1997;15: 65–69.

Delaney KA. Anticholinergics and antihistamines (H1 antagonists). In: Ford MD, Delaney KA, Ling LJ, et al., eds. Clinical toxicology. Philadelphia: WB Saunders, 2001:472–477.

Hidalgo HA, Mowers RM. Anticholinergic drug abuse. Ann Pharmacother 1990;24:40.

Reilly KM, Chan L, Mehta NJ, et al. Systemic toxicity from ocular homatropine. Acad Emerg Med 1996;3:868–871.

Author: Mark B. Mycyk

Aortic Dissection, Thoracic

Clinical Presentation

SIGNS AND SYMPTOMS

- Chest pain
  - —May be absent in as many as 15% of patients
  - —Substernal if type A dissection
  - —Interscapular if descending thoracic
  - —Lumbar if abdominal aorta is involved
  - —Starts abruptly
  - —Usually described as sharp more than tearing
  - —Most severe at onset
  - —May be mild or pressure-like
- Back pain
  - —Commonly interscapular or lumbar
- Combination of chest, back, and abdominal pain
- Pulse deficits
  - —Discrepancies in blood pressure between limbs
  - —Usually in the upper extremities
- Neurologic deficits
  - —CVA
  - —Visual changes
- Nausea, vomiting
- Hypertension
  - —35–40% may be normotensive
- Spinal cord deficits
- Murmur of aortic regurgitation
  - —Occurs in up to 31% of patients
  - —Musical, vibrating quality with variable intensity

COMPLICATIONS

- Myocardial infarction
- Cardiac tamponade
- Stroke
- Hemothorax
- Congestive heart failure
- Limb ischemia
- Spinal cord ischemia
- Renal failure
- Bowel ischemia/infarction

MECHANISM/DESCRIPTION

- Aortic dissection begins when a jet of blood induces an intimal tear
- Blood then dissects through the media under aortic systolic pressure
- It is thought that hypertension is a major factor in the dissection process
- Dissections can start proximally at the root and dissect distally to involve any or all branches of the aorta such as the carotid and subclavian arteries
- The dissection process can also proceed proximally to involve the aortic root, the coronary ostia, and the pericardium
- Dissection that progresses proximally may lead to occlusion of the coronary ostia, aortic valve incompetence, or cardiac tamponade

CLASSIFICATION

- Two classification schemes: Debakey and Stanford
- Stanford classification being used more commonly
- Stanford classification
  - —Type A: any dissection involving the proximal aorta (aortic root)
  - —Type B: dissection distal to the ascending aorta
- Debakey classification
  - —Debakey I: intimal tear in aortic arch (may involve root)
  - —Debakey II: tear confined to the aortic root (ascending aorta)
  - —Debakey III: tear distal to the takeoff of the left subclavian artery

INCIDENCE

- Incidence is 5 per million population per year
- Men are affected more commonly than women
- Most cases occur between the ages of 40 and 80

MORBIDITY/MORTALITY

- Aortic dissection has a high morbidity and mortality
- Overall mortality of aortic dissection is 20–30%

ETIOLOGY

- Any process that affects the mechanical properties of the aortic wall can lead to dissection
  - —Hypertension
  - —Congenital heart disease (bicuspid aortic valve, coarctation)
  - —Aortic wall connective tissue abnormalities (cystic medial necrosis)
  - —Connective tissue disease
    - -Marfan's disease
    - -Ehlers-Danlos
  - —Pregnancy
  - —Infectious/inflammatory conditions of the aorta
    - -Lupus
    - -Syphilis
    - -Endocarditis
    - -Giant cell arteritis
  - —Cigarette use

Pre-Hospital

- Monitor
- Intravenous access

CAUTION/CONTROVERSY

- Therapies such as heparin or thrombolytic agents may be harmful and potentially lead to patient demise if a thoracic dissection is present
- Proper risk factor analysis may help aid in the diagnosis in atypical cases

Diagnosis

ESSENTIAL WORKUP

- EKG
  - —Useful in ruling in or out ST-elevation myocardial infarction or ischemia
  - —Dissection may involve coronary ostia and cause myocardial infarction
  - —Inferior MI (RCA lesion) is more common than LCA involvement
  - —Useful for evaluating the presence of left ventricular hypertrophy
  - —A normal EKG in the presence of severe, acute-onset chest/back pain should heighten one's suspicion of an aortic dissection
  - —Electrical alternans may be present if the dissection involves the pericardium (tamponade)

LABORATORY

- Leukocytosis
- Hematuria
- Elevated BUN and creatinine
- Elevated amylase secondary to bowel ischemia
- Cardiac enzymes should be checked to evaluate for myocardial infarction

IMAGING/SPECIAL TESTS

- Chest x-ray
  - —Useful in excluding other etiologies such as pneumothorax and pneumonia
  - —In dissection, there may be a widened mediastinum or abnormal aortic contour
  - —An enlarged heart secondary to pericardial fluid (blood) may be present
  - —Chest x-ray is estimated to be completely normal in as many as 12–18% of cases
- Echocardiogram—transthoracic or transesophageal
  - —Transthoracic
    - -Not very helpful in the diagnosis of aortic dissection
    - -May be used to evaluate for complications of a known dissection, such as tamponade, valvular incompetence, or MI (from ostial occlusion)
  - —Transesophageal
    - -May be performed in the ED
    - -Patients may require intubation in order to be imaged
    - -Provides information regarding extent of dissection and complications
- Computed tomography
  - —Very useful in defining extent of dissection
  - —May also be used in diagnosing clinical entities such as pulmonary embolism
  - —Has a high sensitivity for the diagnosis of aortic dissection, and is the diagnostic modality of choice in many centers
- MRI
  - —Highly sensitive and specific
  - —Requires patient transport out of the ED
  - —Time delays required to perform the procedure may not be an option
  - —Study of choice in the presence of renal insufficiency or dye allergy
- Aortography
  - —High sensitivity and specificity
  - —Helps in preoperative planning
  - —Difficult to obtain in many centers
- Cardiac catheterization
  - —Some patients may have diagnosis of aortic dissection made by cardiac catheterization
  - —Since a small percentage of patients with dissection may present with a myocardial infarction, the diagnosis may become apparent when an intimal flap is discovered at the time of catheterization

DIFFERENTIAL DIAGNOSIS

- Myocardial infarction
- Unstable angina
- Pneumothorax
- Esophageal rupture
- Pulmonary embolism
- Pericarditis
- Pneumonia
- Musculoskeletal chest wall pain

Treatment

INITIAL STABILIZATION

- Two large-bore intravenous lines
- Continuous cardiac monitoring
- Pulse oximetry
- Oxygen
- Type and cross

ED TREATMENT

- Blood pressure reduction to reduce shear forces and slow down the dissection process
- Medications: intravenous beta-blockade and nitroprusside
  - —Medications are used to control hypertension and decrease shear forces within the aortic wall
  - —Intravenous beta-blockers decrease contractility and shear forces
  - —Esmolol (i.v.): 500-μg/kg bolus followed by 25–50 μg/kg drip or labetalol
    - -Contraindications: bradycardia, COPD, hypotension
  - —Nitroprusside (commonly used in conjunction with IV beta-blocker); start drip at 0.5 μg/km/min, titrate to lower BP
  - —Caution should be used when using these two agents together; to prevent an increase in shear force IV beta-blocker therapy should be started before nitroprusside
- Emergent surgery
  - —Treatment of choice for type A dissection
  - —Treatment of type B dissections if failed medical therapy
- Medical management
  - —Treatment of choice for stable type B dissections

MEDICATIONS

- Esmolol 500-μg/kg bolus, then 25–50 μg/kg/min
- Labetalol 10–20 mg i.v. every 10–15 minutes, drip 2–4 mg/hour
- Nitroprusside: start drip at 0.5 μg/kg/min and titrate up to effect

Disposition

ADMISSION CRITERIA

- All patients with thoracic aortic dissection should be admitted to ICU
- Emergent cardiothoracic surgical consultation should be obtained, especially in cases of type A Stanford dissection

DISCHARGE CRITERIA

N/A

Miscellaneous

ICD9: 441.01

ICD10: I71.0

SUGGESTED READINGS

Braverman AC, et al. Aortic dissection. Curr Opin Cardiol 1997;12(4):389–390.

Dmowski AT, Carey MJ. Aortic dissection. Am J Emerg Med 1999;17(4):372–375.

Erbel R, Alfonso F, Boileau C, et al. Diagnosis and management of aortic dissection. Eur Heart J 2001;22(18): 1642–1681.

Ghosh AK. Clinical diagnosis of acute aortic dissection. Arch Intern Med 2001;12:161.

Hagan PG, Neinaber CA, Isselbacher EM, et al. The International Registry of Acute Aortic Dissection (IRAD): new insights into an old disease. JAMA 2000;283(7): 897–903.

Authors: Robert L. Rogers; Jonathan Olshaker

Aortic Rupture, Traumatic

Clinical Presentation

SIGNS AND SYMPTOMS

- Substernal chest pain, midscapular pain
- Shortness of breath, dyspnea, dysphagia, stridor, hoarseness (from expanding hematoma)
- Harsh precordial or midscapular systolic murmur
- *Acute coarctation syndrome:* hypertension of upper extremity; increased pulse amplitude of upper extremities, decreased in lower extremities; cyanosis of lower extremities
- Paraplegia, anuria, or ischemic extremity pain, due to impaired spinal blood supply
- Swelling of neck (extravasation of blood)
- Back pain with acute abdomen

MECHANISM/DESCRIPTION

- Several theories:
  - —Shear forces from unequal rates of deceleration of more fixed descending aorta and more mobile arch
  - —"Bending" stress created by lateral impact
  - —Twisting of the arch, forcing it superiorly causing stretch
  - —*Osseous pinch:* bony compression of thoracic cage causing tearing of major vessels
  - —*Water-hammer pulse wave:* sudden increase in intraluminal pressure in compressed vessels
- Most common location is the isthmus at the ligamentum arteriosum
- Brachiocephalic vessels may also be injured
- Innominate artery most common branch of aorta injured
- Most tears are transverse, not longitudinal
- Tears may be partially or completely circumferential

ETIOLOGY

- Most commonly due to motor vehicle accidents (MVA)
- Other mechanisms: auto vs. pedestrian, airplane crashes, falls from heights, crush and blast injuries, direct blow to chest
- Cause of death in up to 20% of victims of lethal MVA
- Approximately 85% of patients with traumatic aortic injury (TAI) die before reaching the hospital
- Of those patients with TAI who survive the initial event, 71–84% will survive with prompt diagnosis and treatment, whereas up to 90% will die without treatment
- Drivers are 50% more likely to sustain TAI than passengers
- Ejection doubles the risk of TAI

PEDIATRIC CONSIDERATIONS

- Rare in patients <15 years
- Children may be protected by more compliant chest wall

Pre-Hospital

- Important information about the scene:
  - —Rate of speed, direction of impact
  - —Damage to steering wheel
  - —Ejection from vehicle
  - —Restraints used
  - —Driver or passenger
- Immediate transport of any patient with suspected TAI to trauma center

Diagnosis

ESSENTIAL WORKUP

- *Plain chest radiograph* is the primary screening tool

LABORATORY

- CBC
- Electrolytes
- PT/PTT
- Type and crossmatch

IMAGING/SPECIAL TESTS

- *Plain chest radiograph:* findings consistent with mediastinal hemorrhage, hematoma, or associated injuries, rather than direct evidence of TAI
  - —Widened mediastinum (>8 cm AP supine at level of aortic arch, >6 cm PA upright, or >0.25 mediastinum-width to chest-width ratio)
  - —Obliteration of aortic knob
  - —Obscured descending aorta
  - —Opacification of aortopulmonary window
  - —Left apical capping
  - —Deviation of trachea to right
  - —Depression of left mainstem bronchus
  - —Displacement of nasogastric tube to right
  - —Widened left paraspinal stripe without spinal fracture
  - —Left hemothorax, pleural effusion, pneumomediastinum
  - —Fracture of sternum, or first or second ribs
- 12–28% may have normal chest radiograph
- *Aortography:* still considered the gold standard
  - —Shows location and extent of injury
  - —Also diagnoses nonaortic great vessel injuries
  - —Can have false-negative with thrombosis of a false lumen
- CT
  - —May be considered in hemodynamically stable patients with low suspicion but suggestive chest film
  - —Mediastinal hematoma is indication for angiography
- Spiral CT
  - —Recent studies have shown advantages over conventional CT
  - —Artifact and slice thickness may miss a small tear
  - —Aortography often needed to confirm findings

- Transesophageal echocardiography
  —Can be done rapidly in the ED
  —Demonstrates the isthmus well
  —May not visualize distal ascending aorta or arch well
  —Patients with cervical fractures, maxillofacial, or esophageal injuries are not candidates
  —Can detect other cardiac injuries, e.g., cardiac contusion, pericardial effusion, etc.
- MRI
  —High accuracy, but many limitations
  —Limited availability, lengthy study time
  —Difficulty monitoring patients
  —Trauma patients often have support devices that cannot enter the magnetic field
  —Not widely used in the diagnosis of TAI
- Note: Patients at very high risk for TAI by clinical suspicion should undergo aortography even if other studies are negative

DIFFERENTIAL DIAGNOSIS

- Mediastinal hematoma due to other causes
- Mediastinal lymphadenopathy
- Redundant aorta due to hypertension

PEDIATRIC CONSIDERATIONS

- Presence of large thymus may make diagnosis of widened mediastinum difficult

Treatment

INITIAL STABILIZATION

- Follow trauma care protocols
- In addition to usual resuscitative measures, avoid maneuvers that may result in Valsalva (e.g., gagging, straining)

ED TREATMENT

- *Emergent surgical/trauma consult*
- *Medical therapy of hypertensive patient* to lower risk of rupture of pseudoaneurysm
  —Negative inotropes, e.g., beta-blockers (esmolol or labetalol) to target heart rate 60 ± 5 bpm, SBP 100–120 mm Hg, MAP 70–80
  —In patients where beta-blockade is contraindicated (sinus bradycardia, second- or third-degree A-V block, CHF, bronchospasm) calcium channel blockers may be used
  —Add vasodilators (e.g., nitroprusside sodium) as needed after negative inotropes
  —For significant hypotension, rapid volume expansion, including blood, should be given
  —For refractory hypotension requiring vasopressors, norepinephrine or phenylephrine are preferred, with dopamine used to improve renal perfusion
- Central venous catheter
- Arterial pressure monitoring catheter
- *Acute coarctation syndrome* is a relative contraindication to antihypertensive therapy
- Peritoneal injuries take precedence. Patients with suspected intraabdominal injuries should have diagnostic peritoneal lavage/ultrasound done in the ED
- Concomitant workup of other injuries

MEDICATIONS

- Diltiazem 20 mg (0.25 mg/kg) i.v. over 2 min; rebolus 25 mg (0.35 mg/kg) in 15 min if needed; infusion 5–15 mg/hr
- Esmolol: 500–1000 μg/kg (peds 100–500 μg/kg over 1 minute) i.v. load; infusion 50–150 (peds 25–100) μg/kg/min; repeat load, increase drip 50 (peds 25) μg/kg/min q 5 min; max 300 (peds 200) μg/kg/min
- Labetalol: 20 mg i.v. over 2 min, followed by additional doses of 40–80 mg (peds 0.2–10 mg/kg/dose, max 20 mg/dose) i.v. q 10–15 min, max 300 mg total; start infusion at 2 mg/min and titrate up to 10 mg/min (peds infusion 0.4–1 mg/kg/hr, max 3 mg/kg/hr)
- Nitroprusside: start at 0.3 μg/kg/min; maximum 10 mcg/kg/min
- Norepinephrine 8–12 μg/min i.v. (peds start 0.05–0.1 μg/kg/min, max 2 μg/kg/min)
- Phenylephrine 50 μg (peds 5–20 μg/kg/dose) boluses i.v. q 10–15 min PRN; infusion 100–180 μg/min i.v. (peds 0.1–0.5 μg/kg/min)

Disposition

ADMISSION CRITERIA

- All patients with aortic injuries must be admitted to the ICU if not taken directly to the operating room

DISCHARGE CRITERIA

N/A

Miscellaneous

ICD9: 901.0, 902.0

ICD10: S25.0, S35.0

SUGGESTED READINGS

Britt LD, Weireter LJ Jr, Cole FJ Jr. Newer diagnostic modalities for vascular injuries. The way we were, the way we are. Surg Clin North Am 2001;81(6):1263–1279.

Fabian TC, et al. Prospective study of blunt aortic injury: multicenter trial of the American Association for the Surgery of Trauma. J Trauma 1997;42(3):374–380.

Feliciano DV. Trauma to the aorta and major vessels. Chest Surg Clin North Am 1997;7(2):305–323.

Gavant ML. Helical CT grading of traumatic aortic injuries. Impact on clinical guidelines for medical and surgical management. Radiol Clin North Am 1999;37(3):553–574.

Greenberg MD, Rosen CL. Evaluation of the patient with blunt chest trauma: an evidence based approach. Emerg Med Clin North Am 1999;17(1):41–62.

Lowe LH, et al. Traumatic aortic injury in children: Radiologic evaluation. AJR 1998;170(1):39–42.

White CS, et al. Pictorial review: imaging of traumatic aortic injury. Clin Radiol 1995;50(5):281–287.

Author: Elizabeth L. Lynch

Aphthous Ulcers

Clinical Presentation

SIGNS AND SYMPTOMS

- Minor aphthous ulcers (70–90% of all aphthae)
  - —<10 mm diameter, can see 1–5 at a time
  - —Painful, shallow ulcers
  - —Necrotic centers
  - —Raised margins and erythematous halos
  - —Gray-white pseudomembrane
  - —Found on nonkeratinized mucosa of anterior mouth
  - —Labial mucosa, maxillary and mandibular sulci, nonattached gingiva
  - —Floor of mouth
  - —Ventral surface of tongue
  - —Last for 5–14 days; do not scar
  - —Fever is rare
- Major aphthous ulcers (10–15%)
  - —Similar in appearance and pain to minor
  - —>10 mm in diameter, 1–10 ulcers at a time
  - —Deeper than minor form
  - —Involve all areas of oropharynx including pharynx, soft palate, tonsillar fauces
  - —Last for weeks to months, heal with scarring
  - —Often underlying disease
  - —Fever is rare
- Herpetiform aphthous ulcers (7–10%)
  - —Multiple small clusters
  - —1- to 3-mm diameter, 10–100 at any time
  - —Herpetiform in nature, but HSV cannot be cultured from lesions
  - —Last for 7–30 days; scarring could occur
  - —Fever is rare

ETIOLOGY

- Single etiology: unknown
- Etiology likely multifactorial with correlation with the following:
  - —Immunologic dysfunction
  - —Infection
  - —Food hypersensitivities
  - —Vitamin deficiency
  - —Pregnancy
  - —Menstruation
  - —Psychiatric and genetic factors
- Risk factors: trauma, stress, vitamin deficiency, immunodeficiency
- Epidemiology: usually occurs in children and young adults (10–30 years old)

Pre-Hospital

N/A

Diagnosis

ESSENTIAL WORKUP

- Diagnosis is made by history and clinical presentation
- Rule out oral manifestation of systemic disease
- Focus on symptoms of eye, mouth, genitalia, skin, GI tract, allergy, and diet history

LABORATORY

- Needed only when other etiologies causing ulcers are suspected
- CBC
- RPR/FTA
- ANA
- Tzank stain
  - —Inclusion giant cells (herpes)
- Biopsy
  - —Multinucleated giant cells (cytomegalovirus)
- Fungal cultures
  - —Cryptosporidium

DIFFERENTIAL DIAGNOSIS

- Trauma
  - —Biting
  - —Dentures
- Infection
  - —Herpesvirus
    - -Vesicular lesions
    - -Ulcers on attached mucosa
  - —Cytomegalovirus
    - -Immunocompromised
  - —Varicella
    - -Characteristic skin lesions
  - —Coxsackie virus
    - -Ulcers preceded by vesicles
    - -Hand, foot, buttock lesions
  - —Syphilis
    - -Other skin or genital lesions
  - —Erythema multiforme
    - -Lip crusting
    - -Lesions on attached and unattached mucosa skin lesions
  - —Cryptosporidium, mucormycosis, histoplasmosis
    - -Immunocompromised patient
  - —Necrotizing gingivitis
- Underlying disease
  - —Behçet's syndrome
    - -Genital ulceration
    - -Uveitis
    - -Retinitis
  - —Reiter's syndrome
    - -Uveitis
    - -Urethritis
    - -HLA-B27 arthritis
  - —Inflammatory bowel disease
    - -Bloody or mucous diarrhea
    - -GI ulcerations
  - —Lupus erythematosus
    - -Malar rash
  - —Bullous pemphigoid/pemphigoid vulgaris
    - -Vesiculobullous lesions on attached and unattached mucosa
    - -Diffuse skin involvement
  - —Cyclic neutropenia
    - -Periodic fever
  - —Squamous cell carcinoma
    - -Chronicity
    - -Head/neck adenopathy
- Immunocompromised patient
  - —HIV
  - —Agranulocytosis

Treatment

INITIAL STABILIZATION

N/A

ED TREATMENT

- Symptomatic pain relief with analgesics: can use the following for initial pain relief
  - —Viscous lidocaine 2%: apply to ulcer as needed q.i.d.
  - —Sucralfate: 10 mL: swish and swallow or swish and spit q.i.d.
  - —Magnesium hydroxide/diphenhydramine hydrochloride 5 mg/5 mL in 1/1 mix swish and swallow qid
  - —Dyclonine HCL 1% solution: 5 mL rinse q.i.d.
  - —5-aminosalicylic acid 5% cream: t.i.d. for 2 weeks
  - —Topical OC preps; Orabase, Anusol, etc.

MEDICATIONS

- Analgesia
  - —5-Aminosalicylic acid 5% cream: t.i.d. for 2 weeks
  - —Dyclonine HCL 1% solution: 5 mL rinse q.i.d.
  - —Magnesium hydroxide/diphenhydramine hydrochloride 5 mg/5 mL in 1/1 mix swish and swallow q.i.d.
  - —Sucralfate: 10 mL: swish and swallow or swish and spit q.i.d.
  - —Viscous lidocaine 2%: apply to ulcer as needed q.i.d.
- Promote ulcer healing/prevent recurrence (first-line agents)
  - —Amlexanox 5% paste—0.5 cm applied to ulcer q.i.d. after meals
  - —Clobetasol 0.05%—0.5 cm applied to ulcer qd/b.i.d.
  - —Fluocinonide 0.05% gel: 0.5 cm applied to ulcer up to 5× a day
  - —Triamcinolone 0.1% in Orabase: apply to ulcer b.i.d.–q.i.d. until healed
- Second-line agents:
  - —Prednisone tablets 40 mg PO qd × 7 days
  - —Thalidomide: 200 mg PO qd × 4 weeks

Disposition

ADMISSION CRITERIA

- Unable to eat or drink after appropriate analgesia

DISCHARGE CRITERIA

- Tolerating fluids
- Follow-up with PCP if lesions have not resolved in 2 weeks

Miscellaneous

PREVENTION

- Well-balanced diet
- Good oral hygiene
- Stress reduction
- Zinc lozenges: suck one lozenge 4–6 times a day
- Vitamin C, 500 mg 1 PO t.i.d./q.i.d.
- Vitamin B complex, 1 PO t.i.d./q.i.d.

ICD9: 528.2

ICD10: K12.0

SUGGESTED READINGS

McBride DR. Management of aphthous ulcers. Am Fam Physician 2000;62(1): 149–154.

Shashy RG, Ridley MB. Aphthous ulcers: A difficult clinical entity. Am J Otolaryngol 2000;21(6):389–393.

Ship JA, Chavez EM, Doerr PA, et al. Recurrent aphthous stomatitis. Quintessence Int 2000;31(2):95–112.

Sook BW, Sonis ST. Recurrent aphthous ulcers: a review of diagnosis and treatment. J Am Dent Assoc 1996;127(8):1202–1213.

Author: Ryan Friedberg

Apnea

Clinical Presentation

SIGNS AND SYMPTOMS

- Prolonged cessation of airflow
  - —Often occurs during sleep
  - —Duration may be short (<15 seconds) or prolonged (= 20 seconds)
- Periodic breathing
  - —Three or more respiratory pauses of greater than 3 seconds' duration with less than 20 seconds of respiration between pauses
- Associated findings after an event suggest severity
  - —Need for assisted ventilation
  - —Fever or hypothermia
  - —Tachypnea
  - —Shock
  - —Bradycardia

Pathologic Apnea

- Respiratory pause >20 seconds
- Cyanosis
- Marked pallor
- Hypotonia
- Bradycardia

Apparent Life-Threatening Event (ALTE)

- Frightens the observer
- Combination of any of the following
  - —Apnea
  - —Color change
  - —Marked change in muscle tone

Apnea of Prematurity

- Periodic breathing in a premature infant
- Usually ceases by 37 weeks, gestational age

Apnea of Infancy

- Unexplained cessation of breathing for 20 seconds or longer
- Shorter respiratory pause associated with one of the following
  - —Bradycardia
  - —Cyanosis
  - —Pallor
  - —Marked hypotonia

MECHANISM/DESCRIPTION

- Cessation of airflow
  - —Central or diaphragmatic (absence of respiratory effort)
  - —Obstructive (usually upper airway)
  - —Mixed
- Occurs in 0.5–6% of all infants
- Mean age of presentation between 8 and 14 weeks of age
- Male predominance

ETIOLOGY

- Central apnea
  - —Seizure
  - —Brainstem tumor
  - —Increased intracranial pressure
  - —CNS immaturity
- Obstructive apnea
  - —Stridor
    - -Vascular ring
    - -Vascular cord paralysis
    - -Foreign body
    - -Croup
    - -Epiglottitis
    - -Laryngeal web
    - -Tracheostomy plug
    - -Subglottic stenosis
  - —Premature infants
    - -Positional
    - -Laryngomalacia
    - -Tracheomalacia
  - —Abnormal airway
    - -Choanal atresia/stenosis
    - -Tracheoesophageal fistula
    - -Craniofacial abnormalities
    - -Enlarged tonsils
  - —Mixed apnea
    - -Dysrhythmias
    - -QT prolongation
    - -Pneumonia
    - -Bronchopulmonary dysplasia
    - -Sepsis
    - -Pertussis
    - -Meningitis
    - -Encephalitis
    - -Hypoglycemia
    - -Seizure
    - -Intracranial hypertension
    - -Shock
    - -Anemia
    - -Poisoning
    - -Neuromuscular disorders
- Suspected etiologies leading to near SIDS or ALTE
  - —Suffocation
  - —Electrolyte abnormality
  - —Gastroesophageal reflux
  - —Mineral deficiencies
  - —Cardiac dysrhythmias
  - —Amino acid deficiencies
  - —Abnormal ventilatory response to hypoxia/hypercarbia
  - —Occult trauma

Pre-Hospital

- All infants with an apneic event or ALTE should be transported to the ED
- Ventilatory support during apnea
- All cardiac arrests should be assumed to be secondary to respiratory arrest in children

Diagnosis

ESSENTIAL WORKUP

- Duration of apnea
- Position of sleep
  - —Prone position is inadvisable
- Determine if the event occurred when the child was awake or asleep
- Presence and order of color changes
- Description of movements and muscle tone
- Assess for risk factors for SIDS
  - —Term infant
  - —Premature infant with low birth weight
  - —Male sex
  - —Low socioeconomic class

LABORATORY

- Electrolytes
- Glucose
- BUN/creatinine
- Stool samples for clostridia and botulinum testing
- Suspicion of a serious infection
  - —Pan cultures
  - —Pertussis and chlamydia cultures

IMAGING/SPECIAL TESTS

- EKG
- CXR
  - —Anteroposterior and lateral soft tissue neck films
  - —Obstructive apnea
  - —Stridor
- Lumbar puncture indicated with signs of infection

DIFFERENTIAL DIAGNOSIS

- Munchausen syndrome by proxy
- Breath-holding spell
- Gastroesophageal reflux
- Seizure

Treatment

INITIAL STABILIZATION

- Intubate and assist in ventilation as needed for persistent apnea
- Initiate CPR and PALS algorithms if arrest or near arrest
- Supplemental oxygen
- Intravenous access
- Cardiac monitoring
- Pulse oximetry

ED TREATMENT

- Theophylline or caffeine
  —Indicated for apnea of prematurity
  —Reduces periodic breathing

MEDICATIONS

- Caffeine 10 mg/kg (loading dose) 2.5 mg/kg qd PO
- Dextrose 25: 2–4 mL/kg i.v.
- Theophylline: 6 mg/kg/d

Disposition

ADMISSION CRITERIA

- Pediatric ward with apnea/bradycardia monitor
  —Primary apnea
  —Any child who meets criteria for ALTE
- Pediatric ICU
  —Any field or ED resuscitation

DISCHARGE CRITERIA

N/A

Miscellaneous

ICD9: 770.8

ICD10: R06.8

SUGGESTED READINGS

Brooks JG. Apparent life-threatening events and apnea of infancy. Clin Perinatol 1992;19(4):809.

Marcus CL, et al. Clinical practice guideline: diagnosis and management of childhood obstructive sleep apnea syndrome. Pediatrics 2002;109(4):704–712.

Steinschneider A, Richmond C, Ramaswamy V, et al. Clinical characteristics of an apparent life-threatening event (ALTE) and the subsequent occurrence of prolonged apnea or prolonged bradycardia. Clin Pediatr (Phila) 1998;37(4):223–229.

Torrey SB. Apnea. In: Fleisher GR, et al., eds. Textbook of pediatric emergency medicine, 3rd ed. Baltimore: Williams & Wilkins, 1993:107–111.

Author: Hartwel Lin

Appendicitis

Clinical Presentation

SIGNS AND SYMPTOMS

- Abdominal pain: the primary symptom
  —Normal location:
    -Right lower quadrant (RLQ) pain
    -35% of patients have appendix located within 5 cm of "normal" location
  —Retrocecal appendix (28–68%):
    -Back pain
    -Flank pain
    -Testicular pain
  —Pelvic appendix (27–53%):
    -Suprapubic pain
  —Long appendix (<0.2%):
    -Inflamed tip may cause pain in RUQ or LLQ
- Anorexia
- Vomiting
- Change in bowel habits: diarrhea (33%), constipation (9–33%)
- Fever: normal to mild elevation (<1 degree) initially, increases with perforation
- Classic presentation (<75% of adults)
  —Initially periumbilical pain
  —Followed by anorexia (first symptom in 95%) and nausea
  —Localizes to RLQ (1-12 hours after onset)
  —Finally, vomiting with fever
- Patient position
  —Supine or decubitus with legs (particularly the right) drawn up
  —Prefer not to move
  —Shuffling gait
- Abdominal exam
  —Tenderness at McBurney's point (one third of the distance from the right anterior superior iliac spine to the umbilicus)
  —Guarding
    -Voluntary guarding early due to muscular resistance to palpation
    -Involuntary guarding (rigidity) later as inflammation progresses and perforation occurs
  —Rebound
    -Pain with *any* rapid movement of the peritoneum (bumping stretcher)
    -Best assessed by gently percussing the area (particularly in children)
  —Rectal exam is of little value (may localize tenderness/mass to RLQ)
- Specific signs (less useful in pediatric patients)
  —*Rovsing's sign:* pain in the *right* lower quadrant when palpating the *left* lower quadrant
  —*Psoas sign:* increased pain on extension of right hip with the patient lying on the left side, due to the inflamed appendix touching the iliopsoas muscle
  —*Obturator sign:* pain elicited by passive internal rotation and flexion at the right hip

Considerations in the Pregnant Patient

- Enlarging uterus displaces the appendix upwardly and laterally
- Hyperemesis gravidarum and other nonsurgical causes of vomiting should not cause abdominal tenderness

Considerations in the Elderly Patient

- Three times more likely to have a perforated appendix (due to anatomic changes)
- Delayed diagnosis due to minimally abnormal tests and atypical presentations

ETIOLOGY

- Luminal obstruction of the appendix (usually by a fecalith)
- Appendiceal lumen becomes distended, inhibiting lymphatic and venous drainage
- Bacterial invasion of the wall, with edema and blockage of arterial blood flow
- Perforation and spillage of contents into the peritoneal cavity causing peritonitis (usually 24-36 hours from onset)
- May wall off and form an abscess

MECHANISM/DESCRIPTION

Pain Migration

- Periumbilical pain: appendiceal distention stimulates stretch receptors, which relay pain via *visceral* afferent pain fibers to the 10th thoracic ganglion
- Localization of pain: as the inflammation extends to surrounding tissues, pain occurs due to stimulation of *parietal* nerve fibers and localizes to the position of the appendix

PEDIATRIC CONSIDERATIONS

- 28–57% misdiagnosis in patients <12 years old (nearly 100% in patients <2 years old)
- 70–94% perforation rate in young children (<2 years old)
- Presentations often nonspecific and difficult to localize (<50% have classic presentation)
- Anorexia, vomiting, and diarrhea more common (half-eaten meal hours before complaints of pain may more accurately indicate the duration of symptoms)
- Observe the child *before* the examination for subtle indications of local inflammation
  —Limping gait
  —Hesitation to move or climb
  —Flexed right hip

Pre-Hospital

N/A

Diagnosis

ESSENTIAL WORKUP

- Suggestive history and physical exam sufficient to establish a preoperative diagnosis and warrant surgical consultation
- The tests listed below may be used to assist in the diagnosis
- In atypical cases, repeat serial exams in conjunction with some of the tests listed below have been shown to be effective, with decreased rates of negative appendectomies and no increase in rates of perforation

LABORATORY

- CBC
  —WBC >10,000, with left shift (80–90%)
  —Normal WBC does *not* exclude the diagnosis
- C-reactive protein
  —Overall sensitivity 62%, specificity 66%
  —May not be elevated early
  —Increased sensitivity with serial measurements
- Urinalysis
  —Generally normal
  —Mild pyuria, bacteriuria, or hematuria (20–40%)
  -Pyuria present if the inflamed appendix lies near the ureter or bladder
- Pregnancy test for females of child-bearing age

IMAGING/SPECIAL TESTS

- Not necessary unless the diagnosis is unclear
- Plain abdominal radiographs not recommended
  —Normal in >50%
  —Radiopaque fecalith <10%
- Ultrasound: sensitivity 75–90%; specificity 85–95%
  —Noncompressible appendix of 7-mm AP diameter
  —Presence of an appendicolith
  —Interruption of continuity of echogenic submucosa
  —Periappendiceal fluid/mass
  —Limited by obesity, bowel gas, retrocecal appendix, and operator
  —Negative study of limited use
- CT: sensitivity 87–100%; specificity 89–98%
  —Highest yield using oral and colonic contrast with a focused appendiceal CT technique (5-mm cuts starting 3 cm above the cecum and extending distally 12–15 cm)
  —Fat streaking (100%)
  —6 mm in diameter (93%)
  —Focal cecal apical thickening (69%)
  —Defines appendiceal masses (phlegmon vs. abscess)
  —More likely to find alternative diagnoses than ultrasound
- Laparoscopy
  —May be used diagnostically
  —Gross inflammation often absent in the presence microscopic findings

DIFFERENTIAL DIAGNOSIS

- Gastroenteritis
- Meckel's diverticulum
- Crohn's disease
- Diverticulitis
- Urinary tract infection
- Pelvic inflammatory disease
- Ovarian cyst/torsion
- Tubo-ovarian abscess
- Renal stone
- Testicular torsion
- Sickle cell disease (especially in black children)
- Mesenteric adenitis
- Henoch-Schönlein purpura
- Diabetic ketoacidosis
- Cholecystitis

Treatment

INITIAL STABILIZATION

- ABCs
- Fluid resuscitation with LR or 0.9% NS

ED TREATMENT

- Immediate surgical consult for convincing history and physical exam
  —Laparoscopic vs. open techniques performed
  —Negative appendectomy rate of 10% in males and 20% in females
  —Percutaneous drainage, IV antibiotics, and possible interval appendectomy in appendiceal abscesses
- Preoperative antibiotics (cefoxitin or ampicillin/sulbactam)
- NPO
- Order CT if a palpable mass is present in the RLQ to define phlegmon vs. abscess
- If diagnosis is uncertain, send serial labs, observe and repeat exams (6–10% negative appendectomy rate with observation protocols)
- Analgesics
  —Administration of analgesics, including narcotics, does not adversely affect the abdominal exam or mask pathology)

MEDICATIONS

- Ampicillin/sulbactam (Unasyn): 3 g (peds: 100–200 mg ampicillin/kg/24 hours) q6h i.v.
- Cefoxitin (Mefoxin): 2 g (peds: 80–100 mg/kg/24 hours) q6h i.v.

Disposition

ADMISSION CRITERIA

- Surgical intervention of acute appendicitis
- Observation or further diagnostic workup if diagnosis is uncertain

DISCHARGE CRITERIA

- Patients with abdominal pain thought not to be appendicitis may be discharged if
  —Resolved or resolving symptoms
  —Minimal or no abdominal tenderness
  —No laboratory/radiologic abnormalities
  —Able to tolerate PO intake
  —Adequate social support and able to return if symptoms worsen

Miscellaneous

ICD9: 540.9, 540.0, 540.1

ICD10: K37

SUGGESTED READINGS

Birnbaum BA, Wilson SR. Appendicitis at the millennium. Radiology 2000;215(2):337–348.

Graffeo CS, Counselman FL. Appendicitis. Emerg Med Clin North Am 1996;14:653–671.

Jones PF. Suspected acute appendicitis: trends in management over 30 years. Br J Surg 2001;88(12):1570–1577.

Rothrock SG, Pagane J. Acute appendicitis in children: emergency department diagnosis and management. Ann Emerg Med 2000;36(1):39–51.

Wolfe JM, Henneman PL. Acute appendicitis. In: Marx JA. Rosen's emergency medicine: concepts and clinical practice, 5th ed. St. Louis: Mosby, 2002.

Author: Harsh Sulé

Clinical Presentation

SIGNS AND SYMPTOMS

Gastrointestinal
- Dry burning sensation in mouth and throat
- Garlicky odor: *stools and breath*
- Nausea, vomiting
- Abdominal pain
- Watery (rice water) diarrhea
- Hemorrhagic gastroenteritis due to diffuse capillary damage

Cardiopulmonary
- Tachycardia
- Cardiogenic and noncardiogenic pulmonary edema
- Conduction abnormalities
  —QT prolongation
  —Broadening QRS
  —Flat T waves
  —ST depression
- Ventricular tachycardia/fibrillation
- Torsades de pointes
- Circulatory collapse

Neurologic
- Headache
- Delirium
- Encephalopathy
- Seizures
- Coma
- Early painful dysesthesias
- Delayed sensorimotor peripheral neuropathy 2–6 weeks, post-acute exposure

Hematologic
- Pancytopenia
- Leukopenia reaches nadir 1–3 weeks
- Basophilic stippling
- Hematologic anemia
- Eosinophilia
- Hemolysis
  —4–6 hours after onset of symptoms
  —Dark red urine

Dermatologic
- Hyperpigmentation (rain drop) distribution
- Aldrich-Mees lines (5%) on nails 2–3 weeks, postingestion
- Patchy alopecia
- Toxic erythroderma

Hepatic
- Hepatic transaminase elevation
- Jaundice
- Noncirrhotic portal hypertension

Oncologic
- Basal cell
- Squamous cell carcinoma
- Bronchogenic carcinoma
- Hepatocellular carcinoma
- Bowen's disease of the skin

MECHANISM
- Disrupts enzymatic reaction by binding to sulfhydryl groups (trivalent arsenic) or substituting for phosphate (pentavalent arsenic)
- Combines with globin chain of hemoglobin
- Trivalent arsenic 5–10 times more toxic than pentavalent arsenic
- Soluble arsenic compounds are well absorbed after inhalation or ingestion

ETIOLOGY
- By-product of copper, lead, zinc, and coal
- Pesticides
- Chinese and Korean herbicides, kelp supplements
- Wells from watersheds near old mines, lumbar preservatives
- Food additive to poultry and livestock feed

Pre-Hospital

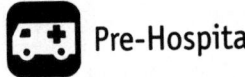

- Secure ABCs and remove exposure

Diagnosis

ESSENTIAL WORKUP
- Urine arsenic level
- CBC

LABORATORY

Arsenic Level
- Spot urine arsenic level >1,000 μg/L
  —Peak in 10–50 hours, postexposure
  —May be elevated for up to 1–2 weeks, postexposure
- Blood arsenic levels
  —Highly variable and of little use
  —Arsenic present in blood during first 2–4 hours postingestion
- Elevated arsenic levels in hair and nails persists for months

Other Tests
- CBC for
  —Anemia
  —Leukopenia
  —Leukocytosis
  —Basophilic stippling
- Electrolytes, BUN/Cr, glucose
- Urinalysis dipstick for occult blood (myoglobin)

IMAGING/SPECIAL TESTS
- Cranial CT/lumbar puncture for altered mental status as indicated

DIFFERENTIAL DIAGNOSIS
- Other heavy metal intoxications
- Cyclic antidepressants
- Encephalopathy/Korsakoff's syndrome
- Hyperemesis gravidarum
- Shock
- Guillain-Barré syndrome
- Addison's disease
- Cholera

Treatment

INITIAL STABILIZATION

- Secure ABCs and monitoring
- D50W, thiamine, naloxone, and oxygen for altered mental status
- Avoid type Ia antiarrhythmics in treating dysrhythmias secondary to prolonged QT
- Administer 0.9% NS bolus followed by vasopressors for hypotension/shock

ED TREATMENT

Decontamination

- For acute oral ingestions
  —Gastric lavage if recent (<1–2 hours) ingestion
  —Activated charcoal
  —Whole bowel irrigation (if lead-containing material visible on x-ray after initial treatment)
- Dermal exposure
  —If stable, decontaminate in the ED decontamination room prior to further evaluation

Chelation Therapy

- In symptomatic patients, administer BAL (dimercaprol) 3 mg/kg deep i.m. every 4–6 hours for 2 days, then every 12 hours for 7–10 days
- In stable patients or those with chronic exposure, administer oral DMSA (succimer) 10 mg/kg every 8 hours or 5 days, then same dose every 12 hours for 14 days

Hemodialysis

- For massive acute ingestions
- For hypotension in spite of fluid resuscitation
- For oliguria/progressive acidosis
- Administer BAL concurrently with hemodialysis

Alkalinization

- Administer sodium bicarbonate if evidence of acute hemolysis (positive urine dipstick for blood without urine RBCs on microscopy)
- Follow electrolytes/renal function closely

MEDICATIONS

- Dextrose: D50W 1 amp (50 mL or 24 g) (peds: D25W 2–4 mL/kg) i.v.
- Naloxone (Narcan): 2 mg (peds: 0.1 mg/kg) i.v. or i.m. initial dose
- Sodium bicarbonate: 1–2 mEq/kg added to 1 L of D5W
- Thiamine (vitamin B_1): 100 mg (peds: 50 mg) i.v. or i.m.

Disposition

ADMISSION CRITERIA

- Symptomatic patients

DISCHARGE CRITERIA

- Asymptomatic and urine level below 50 μg/L

Miscellaneous

ICD9: 985.1

ICD10: T57.0

SUGGESTED READINGS

Ellenhorn MJ, Schoonwald S, Ordog G, et al. Arsenic. In: Ellenhorn's medical toxicology, 2nd ed. Baltimore: Williams & Wilkins, 1997:1538–1543.

Ford M. Arsenic-Goldfrank's toxicologic emergencies, 6th ed. Norwalk, CT: Appleton & Lange, 1998:1011–1028.

Trepka MJ, et al. Arsenic burden among children in industrial areas of Eastern Germany. Sci Total Environ 1996;180(2):95–105.

Authors: Meika Neblett; Lisandro Irizarry

Arterial Gas Embolism

Clinical Presentation

SIGNS AND SYMPTOMS

Cerebral

- Dive-related stroke
- Second leading cause of dive-related death (after drowning)
- Two main presentations
  - —Apnea and full cardiopulmonary arrest
  - —Any combination of neurologic deficits
- Presentation depends on the arterial distribution of the gas embolism
  - —Change in level of consciousness (40%)
  - —Sensory loss (20%)
  - —Motor deficit (20%)
  - —Paraplegia (10%)
  - —Seizure (4%)
  - —Visual changes
  - —Aphasia
  - —Paresthesias
- Rapid onset
  - —8.6% during the ascent
  - —83.6% <5 minutes after surfacing
  - —7.8% between 5 and 10 minutes after surfacing
- Spontaneous improvement minutes after the initial deficits may occur
  - —High incidence of relapse
  - —Improvement may be transiently related to postural changes that affect the distribution of the bubbles flowing to the brain

Pulmonary

- Shortness of breath
- Bloody, frothy sputum
- Subcutaneous air

Cardiac

- Myocardial infarction due to air in the coronary vessels
- Reduced cardiac output due to air trapped in ventricle
- Hamman's sign: crepitus on auscultation of the heart

Renal

- Renal infarction due to air embolism

MECHANISM/DESCRIPTION

- Extreme manifestation of pulmonary barotrauma
- Overpressurization of lung tissue causing pleural tear with air entering the vascular circulation
  - —Air bubbles tend to rise and enter the cerebral vessels where they occlude vascular flow
  - —Boyle's law: pressure inversely related to volume
  - —As pressure increases/decreases, volume decreases/increases
  - —Trapped air (in lungs with closed glottis) expands on diver ascent
- Arterial embolism can also occur via pulmonary AV shunts, or as paradoxical embolism via a patent foramen ovale (up to 30% of the adult population)

ETIOLOGY

- Breath-holding during ascent
  - —Symptoms attributable to a shower of bubbles and multiple blood vessel involvement
- Iatrogenically during placement of CVP lines, cardiothoracic surgery, or hemodialysis
- Penetrating injuries to heart with emergent repair of cardiac wound

Pre-Hospital

CONTROVERSIES

- Trendelenburg positioning patients with suspected arterial gas embolism (AGE) is not effective
  - —Hypothesized that elevation of the legs could cause the air bubbles to migrate away from the cerebral circulation and that increased hydrostatic pressure in brain will shrink bubbles
  - —Trendelenburg positioning may in fact increase injury by increasing the intracerebral pressure

CAUTIONS

- Patients who experience sudden neurologic recovery can relapse quickly as bubble positions change

Diagnosis

ESSENTIAL WORKUP

- Recognize AGE as potential diagnosis
  - —Altered mental status within 10 minutes of surfacing from compressed air dive
  - —Sudden neurologic decompensation following placement of central line
- Inquire as to unusual circumstances during ascent
  - —Breath-holding
  - —Panic/out of air situation
- Thorough neurologic exam must carefully document the extent of the deficits to the motor, sensory, cerebellar, and cranial nerves

LABORATORY

- Serum creatinine kinase activity has been shown to be a marker of the severity of cerebral AGE
- CBC
- Electrolytes, BUN, Cr, glucose
- ABG when respiratory symptoms present

IMAGING/SPECIAL TESTS

- CXR
  - —For evidence of pneumothorax or mediastinal emphysema (both rare)
- EKG
- Echocardiogram
  - —Looking for evidence of patent foramen ovale
- CT head
  - —For altered mental status
  - —Do not delay recompression for CT when AGE almost certain clinically

DIFFERENTIAL DIAGNOSIS

- CVA from causes unrelated to gas embolism
- Neurologic deficits due to decompression sickness

Treatment

INITIAL STABILIZATION

- ABCs
  - —100% oxygen by tight-fitting mask
  - —Intubation for ventilation/protection of airway required
  - —IV access with volume augmentation

ED TREATMENT

- Hyperbaric oxygen recompression therapy (see Hyperbaric Oxygen Therapy)
  - —For all AGE
  - —Arrange transportation to nearest hyperbaric facility
  - —Aircraft capable of cabin pressurization below 1,000 feet barometric pressure best suited for transfers
  - —Prophylactic chest tube for simple pneumothorax to prevent conversion to tension pneumothorax during recompression
  - —Fill endotracheal and Foley catheter balloons with water or saline to avoid shrinkage/damage during recompression
- Divers Alert Network (DAN)
  - —Based at Duke University Medical Center
  - —Provides a 24-hour emergency hotline for medical consultation on the treatment of dive-related injuries and for referrals to hyperbaric chambers (telephone: 1-919-684-8111)

Disposition

ADMISSION CRITERIA

- Admit all following initial hyperbaric therapy for observation and reexamination

DISCHARGE CRITERIA

- None should be discharged from the emergency department

Miscellaneous

ICD9: 958.0

ICD10: T79.0

SEE ALSO: DECOMPRESSION SICKNESS; HYPERBARIC OXYGEN THERAPY; AND BAROTRAUMA

SUGGESTED READINGS

Beckman TJ. A review of Decompression Sickness and Arterial Gas Embolism. Arch Fam Med 1997;6(5):491–494.

Edmonds C, Lowry C, Pennefather J. Diving and subaquatic medicine. Oxford: Butterworth-Heinemann, 1992.

Jerrard DA. Diving medicine. Emerg Med Clin North Am 1992;10(2):329–338.

Smith RM, Neuman TS. Elevation of serum creatine kinase in divers with arterial gas embolism. N Engl J Med 1994;330:19–24.

Author: Jeffrey Gordon

Arterial Occlusion

Clinical Presentation

SIGNS AND SYMPTOMS

The 6 P's

- Pain
- Pallor
- Paresthesias
- Paralysis
- Pulseless
- Poikilothermia

Chronic

- Claudication
- Decreased pulses after activity
- Hair-free atrophic skin
- Poorly healing wounds or ulcers
- Ankle-brachial index (ABI) measurements
  —Use a Doppler probe
  —Inflate a blood pressure cuff on the arm until the radial pulse is no longer heard
  —Release the valve and note the pressure at which the radial pulse returns
  —Repeat this procedure with the cuff around the calf and note the return of the dorsalis pedis and posterior tibialis pulse
  —The ratio of the ankle pressure/radial pressure = ABI
  -Normal: 1 or greater
  -Typical claudicant: 0.5–0.8
  -Rest pain/impending tissue injury: <0.3

ETIOLOGY

Thrombotic

- Low flow and hypercoagulable states

Embolic

- Atrial fibrillation
- Myocardial infarction
- Valvular disease
- Endocarditis
- Proximal arterial aneurysm
- Atherosclerotic plaques

Pre-Hospital

- Recognition of a potentially limb-threatening emergency

CAUTIONS

- Do not elevate, ice, or warm the affected extremity

Diagnosis

- Peripheral ischemic syndromes often result in changes in acid–base status (acidemia) and electrolyte derangement (hyperkalemia), which are acutely exacerbated upon reperfusion

ESSENTIAL WORKUP

- Acute arterial occlusion is a clinical diagnosis

LABORATORY

- Electrolytes/anion gap
- BUN, creatinine
- CBC
- CPK
- Specimen for type and screen

IMAGING/SPECIAL TESTS

- EKG
- Duplex ultrasound
- Angiography

DIFFERENTIAL DIAGNOSIS

- Lumbar spine disorders
- Venous thrombosis
- Decreased cardiac output in the setting of advanced atherosclerotic disease
- Frostbite
- Peripheral neuropathy
- Fractures and sprains
- Muscle strains

Treatment

ED TREATMENT

- Prompt vascular surgery consultation
- Surgical options
- Fogarty catheter
- Mechanical thrombectomy
- Percutaneous aspiration thrombectomy
- Bypass grafting
- PTCA
- Intraarterial agents (urokinase plus abciximab)
- Intravenous thrombolysis is not recommended
- Aspirin
- Heparin

MEDICATIONS

- Aspirin: 325 mg PO; four chewable baby aspirin
- Heparin: 80 IU/kg loading bolus; 18 IU/kg/hr

Disposition

ADMISSION CRITERIA

- All patients with critical arterial occlusion should be admitted with an emergent vascular surgery consult

DISCHARGE CRITERIA

- Patients with chronic occlusive disease, resolved pain and stable ABI measurements
- No other acute medical issues (such as new atrial fibrillation)
- Vascular surgical follow-up can be assured
- Patients should be instructed to return for any recurrent or progressive symptoms

Miscellaneous

ICD9: 444.9

ICD10: I74.9

SEE ALSO: PERIPHERAL VASCULAR DISEASE

SUGGESTED READINGS

Bassiouny HS. Noninvasive evaluation of the lower extremity arterial tree and graft surveillance. Surg Clin North Am 1995;75:593–606.

Cooke JP, Ma AO. Medical therapy of peripheral artery occlusive disease. Surg Clin North Am 1995;75:569–579.

Jackson MR. Antithrombotic therapy in peripheral arterial occlusive disease. Chest 2001;119[1 suppl]:283S–299S.

Morgan R, Belli AM. Percutaneous thrombectomy: a review. Eur Radiol 2002;12(1):205–217.

Working Party on Thrombolysis in the Management of Limb Ischemia. Thrombolysis in the management of limb ischemia. J Intern Med 1996;240:343–355.

Author: Chris Lipinski

Clinical Presentation

SIGNS AND SYMPTOMS

- Patients usually over age 60
- Chronic progressive joint pain, worse with weight bearing/improved with rest
- Asymmetric joint involvement
- Increased joint stiffness after rest
- Commonly involves hands, knees, hips, spine, and metatarsophalangeal joints
- Patellofemoral joint commonly exhibits crepitus and varus or valgus deformity
- *Absence of systemic symptoms*

MECHANISM/DESCRIPTION

- Multifactorial with mechanical and inflammatory components
- Loss of articular cartilage with reactive changes at joint margins and subchondral bone

PEDIATRICS CONSIDERATIONS

- Osteoarthritis is not seen in the pediatric population

Pre-Hospital

CAUTIONS

- Acute or increased joint pain following trauma should be regarded as fractured —Immobilize as necessary
- Patients with cervical spine arthritis may be difficult to fit with cervical collars; tape and sandbags should be used

Diagnosis

ESSENTIAL WORKUP

- Joint exam, especially range of motion and functional ability
- With effusion and warmth or erythema, synovial fluid exam can differentiate osteoarthritis from gout or septic arthritis

LABORATORY

- Synovial fluid exam for cell count and differential, crystal analysis, Gram stain, and culture, if clinically indicated

IMAGING/SPECIAL TESTS

- Radiographs not routine unless in setting of trauma
- X-rays may reveal joint space narrowing, osteophyte formation, marginal erosions, or sclerosis of periarticular bone

DIFFERENTIAL DIAGNOSIS

- Rheumatoid arthritis, septic arthritis, and gout

Treatment

INITIAL STABILIZATION

- Immobilize affected joint in the setting of trauma until fracture ruled out

ED TREATMENT

- Pain management with NSAIDs or acetaminophen
- Avoid unnecessary joint immobilization

MEDICATIONS

- Acetaminophen: 650–1,000 mg PO q4h
- Enteric-coated aspirin: 325–650 mg PO q6h
- Hydrocodone (rarely): 5–10 mg PO q6h
- Ibuprofen: 600 mg PO q6h

Disposition

ADMISSION CRITERIA

- Admission rarely required without associated trauma

DISCHARGE CRITERIA

- Ambulatory and capable of activities of daily living
- Instructions for gentle stretching exercises and joint range of motion

Miscellaneous

ICD9: 715.90

ICD10: M19.9

SUGGESTED READINGS

Dearborn JT, Jergesen HE. The evaluation of and initial management of arthritis. Prim Care 1996;23:215.

Fife RS. Osteoarthritis: epidemiology, pathology, and pathogenesis. In: Klippel JH, ed. Primer on the rheumatic diseases, 11th ed. Atlanta: Arthritis Foundation, 1997.

Hochberg MC. Osteoarthritis: clinical features and treatment. In: Klippel JH, ed. Primer on the rheumatic diseases, 11th ed. Atlanta: Arthritis Foundation, 1997.

Author: Michael K. Doney

Arthritis, Juvenile Idiopathic (formerly Juvenile Rheumatic Arthritis)

Clinical Presentation

SIGNS AND SYMPTOMS

Systemic Onset

- Diurnal spiking fever
- Macular/papular salmon colored rash
  —Trunk and axilla
  —Fades with resolution of fever
- Ill appearance during temperature spike
- Polyarthralgia
  —May show up weeks to months after onset of fever and rash
- Systemic symptoms: hepatosplenomegaly, lymphadenopathy, pleural effusion, pericardial effusion

Pauciarticular

- Asymmetrical arthritis
  —Involves larger joints *but hip rarely affected*
  —Symptoms worse in the morning
  —Joints swollen, mildly tender, with decreased range of motion (ROM)
  —Leg length discrepancy
- Uveitis common
- Child looks healthy

Polyarticular

- Arthritis often symmetrical
  —Small or large joints
  —Soft tissue swelling and tender joints
  —Decreased ROM of cervical and lumbar spine and TMJ

Psoriatic

- Psoriasis
- Dactylitis
- Nail abnormalities
- Arthralgias of back and sacroiliac (SI) pain

Enthesitis Related

- Arthritis; asymmetric large joints of lower extremities
- SI joint tenderness
- Spinal pain with limited flexion of lumbar spine
- Uveitis
- *Child with severe pain and red hot joint probably does not have JAI*

MECHANISM/DESCRIPTION

- Group of nonhomogeneous syndromes characterized by persistent unexplained arthritis lasting greater than 6 weeks in children under 16 years old
- Affects approximately 60,000–250,000 children
- Previously called juvenile rheumatic arthritis (JRA)
- "Durban criteria"
  —Slowly replacing traditional systemic, pauciarticular, and polyarticular categorization
  —Seven-tiered classification system
    -Systemic
    -Polyarticular rheumatoid factor (RF) positive
    -Polyarticular RF negative
    -Pauciarticular
    -Psoriatic
    -Enthesitis related
    -Other: fit into more than one category or no category
  —Further classified by age, duration, number, and distribution of joint involvement, family history, and presence or absence of uveitis and laboratory values: antinuclear antibody (ANA), RF, and HLA-B27
- Systemic onset
  —10% of cases with equal male to female ratio
  —High fever of at least 2 weeks' duration
  —Accompanied by at least one of the following: rash, arthritis, lymphadenopathy, or hepatosplenomegaly
  —Increased risk of disseminated intravascular coagulation
  —Up to 50% go on to develop chronic arthritis with increased incidence of micrognathia and cervical spine fusion
- Pauciarticular onset
  —50% of cases, female predominance
  —Four or fewer joints are involved at presentation with monoarticular involvement common
  —Peak incidence 2–3 years old
  —No evidence of systemic involvement
  —Uveitis in about 20%
  —Labs with possible exception of an ANA usually normal
  —Those with no joint progression and normal ESR and red cell count have an excellent prognosis
- Enthesitis related
  —Older age (>8 years)
  —Male dominance associated with SI joint, back pain, or positive HLA-B27
  —Spondyloarthropathy
- Polyarticular
  —40% of JAI
  —Female predominance
  —Five or more joints involved
  —Two peaks: 2–5 years old and 10–14 years old
  —Older children are more likely to be RF positive and to have early onset of adult rheumatoid arthritis
  —Systemic involvement rare except for fatigue and anemia
- Psoriatic arthritis
  —Associated with skin changes, finger or nail involvement, or positive family history of psoriasis
- Long-term prognosis of JAI based on type, duration, and severity
- 30–50% of patients with JAI have long-term complications with systemic, polyarticular, and progressive pauciarticular having worst prognosis

ETIOLOGY

- Unknown—may be viral with a strong genetic component

Pre-Hospital

CAUTIONS

- Splint the affected joint if trauma is a concern

Diagnosis

ESSENTIAL WORKUP

- Clinical diagnosis after exclusion of other identifiable diseases that cause joint inflammation

LABORATORY

- CBC
  —WBC may be elevated
  —Anemia and thrombocytosis are common
- Sedimentation rate may be elevated (common in systemic)
- RF positive in about 20% of cases (rare in systemic and pauciarticular)
- ANA
  —Positive in 30–40% of children
  —Mostly seen in young girls with pauciarticular disease and polyarticular RF-positive disease
- HLA subtyping and specific allele identification
  —May be positive in those with enthesitis related or psoriatic arthritis
- Lyme's titer if concern of tick exposure

IMAGING/SPECIAL TESTS

- Joint radiograph
  —Early presentation: soft tissue swelling, joint effusion
  —Late presentation: osteoporosis, joint destruction, early growth plate closure
- Arthrocentesis: indicated if concern for septic arthritis
  —5,000–8,000 WBC/mm^3
  —Negative Gram stain and culture

DIFFERENTIAL DIAGNOSIS

- Trauma
- Infection
  —Septic arthritis, toxic viral synovitis, Lyme disease, rheumatic fever, tuberculosis, subacute endocarditis
- Other rheumatic/connective tissue diseases
  —Systemic lupus erythematosus, polyarteritis nodosa, Henoch-Schönlein purpura, fibromyalgia
- Neoplasm
  —*Be suspicious of neoplasm in severely uncomfortable child with midshaft bone pain*
- Hematologic disease
  —Sickle cell disease, hemophilia
- Drug reactions

Arthritis, Juvenile Idiopathic (formerly Juvenile Rheumatic Arthritis)

Treatment

INITIAL STABILIZATION

- Toxic-appearing children
  - —Intravenous access
  - —Supplemental oxygen

ED TREATMENT

- NSAIDs
  - —May be all that is required in those with mild JAI
  - —Children respond differently to different subsets of NSAIDs; several should be tried before class is considered ineffective
- Steroids in conjunction with pediatrician or rheumatologist
  - —Systemic steroids used judiciously due to long-term complications but may be needed in acute
  - —Intraarticular steroids may provide long-term relief in patients with mono- and pauciarticular disease
- Methotrexate
  - —Commonly used as second-line therapy
  - —Supplement with folic acid
- Anticytokine therapy
  - —Etanercept, which binds tissue necrosis factor-α, has been used successfully for polyarticular disease
- Other therapies less commonly used
  - —Gold, hydroxychloroquine, sulfasalazine, cyclosporine, and cytotoxic agents
- Antibiotics not indicated for JIA
  - —Toxic children with suspicion of sepsis, septic arthritis, Lyme disease

MEDICATIONS

- Ibuprofen: 30–50 mg/kg divided q.i.d. up to 3,200 mg
- Methotrexate: 15–20 mg/m^2 orally once per week
- Methylprednisone: 30 mg/kg qd i.v. up to 1 g for 1–5 days for high-dose pulse steroids
- Naprosyn: 10–20 mg/kg divided b.i.d. up to 1,250 mg
- Prednisone: 0.5–2 mg/kg PO
- Sulfasalazine: 40–60 mg/kg/d divided t.i.d. or q.i.d.
- Tolmetin: 25 mg/kg/d divided q.i.d.
- Triamcinolone: 10–40 mg given intraarticularly to large joints

Disposition

ADMISSION CRITERIA

- Unclear diagnosis, poor follow-up
- Severe pain
- Ill-appearing child

DISCHARGE CRITERIA

- No evidence of septic joint
- Patient appears comfortable
- Appropriate follow-up has been arranged

Miscellaneous

- Children with JAI, especially those with a positive ANA, should have frequent eye exams to rule out asymptomatic uveitis

ICD9: 714.3

ICD10: M08.9

SUGGESTED READINGS

Cassidy J. Medical management of children with juvenile rheumatoid arthritis. Drugs 1999;58(5):831–850.

Hofer M, Mouy R, Prieur A. Juvenile idiopathic arthritides evaluated prospectively in a single center according to the Durban criteria. J Rheumatol 2001;28:1083–1090.

Lehman T. Polyarticular onset juvenile rheumatic arthritis. UpToDate version 9.3, 2002 Available at: *www.update.com.*

Petty RE, Southwood TR, Baum J, et al. Revision of the proposed classification criteria for juvenile idiopathic arthritis: Durban, 1997. J Rheumatol 1998;25(10):1991–1994.

Zak M, Pedersen FK. Juvenile chronic arthritis into adulthood: a long term follow-up study. Rheumatology 2000;39:198–204.

Author: Jeannette Wolfe

Arthritis, Monoarticular

Clinical Presentation

SIGNS AND SYMPTOMS

- Symptoms located to one joint
  - —Pain
  - —Swelling
  - —Warmth
  - —Erythema
  - —Decreased range of motion
  - —Hyperacute presentation most typical, with infectious and crystalline etiologies
- Infectious (septic) arthritis
  - —Fever, chills, systemically ill
  - —Large joints affected more often
  - —Adults: knee > hip = shoulder > ankle > wrist
  - —Gonorrhea: abdominal pain, genital discharge
  - —Lyme disease: knees or shoulders most common, nonspecific constitutional symptoms, centrally clearing expanding skin eruption
- Crystalline
  - —Recurrent, self-limited inflammatory attacks, often of same joint
  - —Tissue extension identical to cellulitis, septic arthritis
  - —Gout: First metatarsophalangeal joint ("podagra") > ankle > tarsal joints > knee
  - —Pseudogout: Knee > wrist > ankle = elbow
  - —Tophi: crystalline granulomas overlying affected joints
- Inflammatory
  - —Inflammatory bowel disease: abdominal pain, bloody diarrhea with mucus, weight loss
  - —Reiter's syndrome: conjunctivitis, urethritis, balanitis
  - —Psoriatic arthritis: characteristic skin plaques, "sausage digits"
  - —Chronic: infections (tuberculosis, fungi), tumors
- Noninflammatory
  - —Osteoarthritis: stiffness in morning, after activity (gelling), pain relieved by rest
  - —Congenital hip dysplasia: hip pain in young
  - —Neuropathic: Charcot joint, swelling, effusion, little pain
  - —Trauma: pain, swelling

MECHANISM/DESCRIPTION

- Affects and remains localized to one joint
- *Presence of one etiology does not exclude another*
- Infectious (septic) arthritis
  - —Hematogenous spread, contiguous extension (cellulitis, osteomyelitis), direct inoculation (puncture wound, joint surgery)
  - —Predisposing factors: immunosuppression, IV drug use, chronic illness, local pathology (inflammatory arthritis, trauma, prosthetic joint)
- Crystalline: crystal deposition in, around joint
  - —Gout: uric acid crystals secondary to overproduction, underexcretion
  - —Alcoholism, loop diuretics, renal failure, males 40–50, women over 60
  - —Pseudogout: calcium pyrophosphate dihydrate (CPPD) crystals
  - —Most common monoarthritis in elderly; peak incidence females 60–70
  - —Increased incidence: elderly, trauma, surgery, hyperparathyroidism, hemochromatosis, hypothyroidism
- Noninflammatory
  - —Osteoarthritis: nonspecific, destructive process cartilage or bone, loss of articular cartilage with reactive changes at joint margins
  - —Greater incidence in men than in women until 60 years of age, then ratio reverses
  - —Morbidly obese
  - —Congenital hip dysplasia: hip pain in young
  - —Trauma: fracture, Charcot joint

Etiology

- Infectious, bacterial
  - —*Neisseria gonorrhea*
  - —*Staphylococcus aureus:* trauma, IV drug use
  - —Salmonella: sickle cell disease
  - —Gram-negative organisms, anaerobes: immunocompromised
- Infectious, spirochetal
  - —Tuberculosis
  - —Lyme disease
- Infectious, viral
  - —More commonly polyarticular
- Infectious, fungal
  - —More commonly chronic
- Crystalline
  - —Gout (urate)
  - —Pseudogout (CPPD)
- Inflammatory
  - —Inflammatory bowel disease
  - —Rheumatoid arthritis
  - —Psoriatic
  - —Reiter's syndrome (seronegative spondyloarthropathy)
- Noninflammatory
  - —Osteoarthritis: structural disease
  - —Trauma: fracture, internal derangement, neuropathic arthropathy
  - —Tumor: chronic effusion

PEDIATRIC CONSIDERATIONS

- Infectious (rare): hip = knee
  - —*Escherichia coli:* infants
  - —*Haemophilus influenzae:* 6–24 months
- Noninflammatory
  - —Congenital hip dysplasia
  - —Legg-Calvé-Perthes: spontaneous osteonecrosis femoral head, age 4–9, bilateral 10% cases
  - —Slipped capital femoral epiphysis: overweight adolescents

Pre-Hospital

- Physical immobilization of the joint, medication for pain control
- IV placement

Diagnosis

ESSENTIAL WORKUP

- Complete history; any joint disorder is capable of presenting as monoarthritis
  - —Trauma
  - —Surgery
  - —Medications
  - —Intravenous drug abuse
  - —Intraarticular injections
  - —Immunosuppression
- Establish truly monoarticular (vs. migratory); exacerbation vs. superimposed process
- Onset rapidity
  - —Seconds to minutes: trauma, internal derangement
  - —Hours to 2 days: inflammatory; bacterial infection, crystalline
- Complete physical examination

LABORATORY

- Arthrocentesis and joint fluid analysis
  - —The definitive procedure
  - —Culture is definitive study of the fluid
  - —WBC with differential, crystal analysis, Gram stain, glucose, viscosity
- Serology
  - —WBC with differential
  - —Blood cultures; panculture if suspected gonorrhea, sepsis
  - —Acute-phase reactant (ESR, CRP)
  - —Uric acid can be normal under all conditions; not helpful
  - —Consider glucose, chemistries, rheumatologic studies

IMAGING/SPECIAL TESTS

- Plain films
  - —Infectious: soft tissue swelling, osteoporosis, erosion, joint margin destruction
  - —Crystalline: asymmetric bone erosions, reactive bone formation, soft tissue calcification
  - —Bone and cartilage disorders: asymmetric joint narrowing, osteophytes, subchondral cysts, loose bodies, fracture
- MRI detects bone necrosis
  - —Study of choice occult fractures
- Nuclear medicine sensitive tool for deep joints difficult to examine, fibrocartilaginous joints, spine
- Ultrasound: presence of joint fluid, tissue perfusion, periarticular structures, aspiration guidance
- Synovial, bone biopsy
  - —Chronic, unexplained, monoarticular arthritis
  - —Gonococcal, mycobacterial disease is suspected and no fluid available

DIFFERENTIAL DIAGNOSIS

See Etiology, above

Treatment

INITIAL STABILIZATION

- None unless underlying illness or trauma mandates

ED TREATMENT

- Septic arthritis
  - —Empiric IV antibiotics for anticipated organism
  - —Gram-positive cocci: penicillinase-resistant penicillin, vancomycin (methicillin resistance)
  - —Gonorrhea: ceftriaxone or cefotaxime, ceftizoxime, nafcillin, oxacillin
  - —IV drug use: penicillinase-resistant antibiotic + aminoglycoside
  - —Gram-negative: antipseudomonal penicillin + aminoglycoside or third-generation cephalosporin
  - —Prosthetic joint, postoperative, postinjection: vancomycin + ciprofloxin or aztreonam, antipseudomonal aminoglycoside, cefepime
  - —Neonates, children under 2 years broad-spectrum antibiotics to cover ampicillin-resistant *H. influenzae, S. aureus*, group B streptococci
  - —Surgery: open vs. closed (daily) drainage
- Crystalline
  - —NSAIDs (indomethacin)
  - —Colchicine secondary choice to NSAIDs; local necrosis if extravasates
  - —Prednisone when NSAIDs, colchicine contraindicated
  - —ACTH for resistant cases, contraindication to NSAIDs
  - —Allopurinol decreases uric acid production; avoid in acute therapy
  - —Probenecid long-term; uricosuric
- Osteoarthritis
  - —NSAIDs, analgesics
  - —Physical support, rehabilitation

MEDICATIONS

- ACTH 40–80 IU i.m. then 40 IU i.m. q6–12h until improvement
- Allopurinol 200–600 mg qd
- Aztreonam 2 g i.v. b.i.d.
- Cefepime 2 g i.v. b.i.d.
- Cefotaxime 1 g i.v. t.i.d.
- Ceftriaxone 1 g i.v. qd
- Ceftizoxime 1 g i.v. t.i.d.
- Ciprofloxin 400 mg b.i.d.
- Colchicine 1–2 mg i.v. in 20 cc NS over 10 min; 0.5 mg PO q1h until asymptomatic, nausea diarrhea develop, or 10 doses
- Indomethacin 75–200 mg qd, divided dosages
- Nafcillin 2 g i.v. q4h
- Oxacillin 2 g i.v. q4h
- Prednisone 20–40 mg PO qd × 3–4 days
- Probenecid 250 mg b.i.d. starting; maximum 3 g qd
- Vancomycin 1 g i.v. b.i.d.

Disposition

ADMISSION CRITERIA

- All septic arthritis
  - —General medical/surgical bed
  - —ICU if generalized sepsis
- Crystalline
  - —Intractable pain
  - —Intractable nausea, vomiting (colchicine)
  - —Septic joint superimposed on other arthritides
- Traumatic joint requiring surgical intervention

DISCHARGE CRITERIA

- Crystalline tolerating oral NSAIDs
- Inflammatory unless admission required by overall disease manifestations
- Osteoarthritis
- Medication compliance
- Timely follow-up arranged

Miscellaneous

ICD9: 716.6

ICD10: M13.1

SUGGESTED READINGS

Gilbert DN, Moellering RC, Sande MA, eds. The Sanford guide to antimicrobial therapy, 32nd ed. Hyde Park, VT: Antimicrobial Therapy, 2002:21–22.

McCune WJ, Golbus J. Monoarticular arthritis. In: Ruddy S, Harris ED, Sledge CB, eds. Kelly's textbook of rheumatology, vol 1, 6th ed. Philadelphia: WB Saunders, 2001:367–377.

Schumacher HR. Synovial fluid analysis and synovial biopsy. In: Ruddy S, Harris ED, Sledge CB, eds. Kelly's textbook of rheumatology, vol 1, 6th ed. Philadelphia: WB Saunders, 2001:605–619.

Till SH, Snaith ML. Assessment, investigation, and management of acute monoarthritis. J Acc Emerg Med 1999;16(5):355–361.

Towheed TE, Hochberg MC. Acute monoarthritis: a practical approach to assessment and treatment. Am Fam Physician 1996;54(7):2239–2243.

Author: Paul Blackburn

Clinical Presentation

SIGNS AND SYMPTOMS

- Malaise, fatigue, generalized musculoskeletal pain
- After a period of weeks to months patients develop swollen, warm, painful joints
  - —Often worse in the morning
- Joint involvement usually symmetric and polyarticular
  - —Starting in the small joints of the hands and feet, later wrists, elbow, and knees
- The DIP joints of the hand are generally not involved; presence of swelling in these joints should suggest another type of arthritis
- Synovitis is typically gradual
- Extraarticular complications include subcutaneous nodules, vasculitis, pericarditis, myocarditis, pulmonary fibrosis, pneumonitis, Sjögren's syndrome, and mononeuritis multiplex
  - —Evidence of mild pericarditis on echocardiogram is found in up to one third
- In long-standing disease, there are classic joint findings, which may include MCP swelling with ulnar deviation, swan neck, and boutonniere deformities
- Patients usually present to the ED due to exacerbations of the disease or a complication in other organ systems

Complications of Rheumatoid Arthritis (RA) that Precipitate Presentation to the ED

- Exacerbations of the disease with joint pain and stiffness
- Airway obstruction from cricoarytenoid arthritis or laryngeal nodules
- Heart block, constrictive pericarditis, or myocarditis
- Pulmonary fibrosis, pleuritis, intrapulmonary nodules, or pneumonitis
- Hepatitis
- Neurologic findings may result from cervical spine subluxation or ocular manifestations such as scleritis and episcleritis
- Patients can present with infectious complications of chronic steroid use or with fractures resulting from steroid-induced osteopenia
- Patients may present with side effects related to chronic salicylate or NSAID use such as GI bleeding
- Drugs such as methotrexate, gold, or d-penicillamine also have toxic side effects, most commonly gastrointestinal

MECHANISM/DESCRIPTION

- RA is a chronic systemic inflammatory disorder that attacks the joints
  - —RA causes a nonsuppurative, proliferative synovitis, progressing to destruction of the articular cartilage and ankylosis of the joint
- Involvement of the knee is common; Baker's cysts may be seen in chronic disease
- Involvement of the spine is limited to the cervical region and may cause atlantoaxial subluxation, which rarely results in cord compression

ETIOLOGY

- Etiology is unknown
- Prevalence is about 1% of both the U.S. and world population
  - —Female to male ratio is 3:1
  - —Typical age of onset is between 30 and 50
- Genetic predisposition is related to HLA-DR4 haplotype
- Other possible triggers include infection and autoimmune response

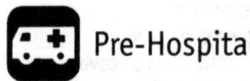

Pre-Hospital

CAUTIONS

- Cervical spine immobilization and airway support for the rare cases in which patients develop respiratory or cervical spine problems related to RA

Diagnosis

ESSENTIAL WORKUP

- Primary diagnosis of RA is rarely made in the ED
- Synovitis should be present for at least 6 weeks; a minimum of four of the following seven criteria as established by the American Rheumatism Association must be met to make the diagnosis:
  - —Stiffness of the involved joints in the morning for at least an hour
  - —Arthritis in three or more joints with effusion or soft tissue swelling
  - —Arthritis of joint in hand (wrist, MCP, or PIP)
  - —Symmetric arthritis
  - —Rheumatoid nodules on extensor surfaces or juxtaarticular surfaces
  - —Significantly elevated rheumatoid factor
  - —Characteristic x-ray changes include erosions and decalcification (not attributable to osteoarthritis)
  - —Other pertinent history: malaise, weakness, weight loss, myalgias, bursitis, tendonitis, fever of unknown etiology
- Initial workup should focus on demonstrating that other causes of arthritis are not present, especially septic arthritis, reactive arthritis, or gout
  - —Arthrocentesis of a joint effusion may be required
- EKG, chest x-ray, C-spine or extremity x-ray, and hemoglobin testing are essential if the patient presents with complications of RA

LABORATORY

- CBC: mild anemia with leukocytosis and thrombocytosis
- ESR: often greater than 30
- Rheumatoid factor: elevated in about 70% of cases
- Joint fluid analysis: typically between 4,000 and 50,000 white cells with 75% neutrophils; microscopic Gram stain of fluid should show no organisms and no crystals
- EKG: conduction defects are rare but heart block may be seen

IMAGING/SPECIAL TESTS

- Joint x-ray with joint effusion, juxtaarticular erosions and decalcification, narrowing of joint space, and loss of cartilage
- Chest film may reveal pulmonary fibrosis, pleural changes, nodular lung disease, or pneumonitis; cardiac silhouette may show changes related to myocarditis
- Cervical spine x-ray: atlantoaxial joint subluxation may occur

DIFFERENTIAL DIAGNOSIS

- Osteoarthritis
- Septic arthritis
- Reactive arthritis
- Gonococcal arthritis
- Lyme disease
- Gout
- Connective tissue disorders
  —SLE, dermatomyositis, polymyositis, vasculitis, Reiter's syndrome, and sarcoid
- Rheumatic fever
- Malignancy

PEDIATRIC CONSIDERATIONS

- *Juvenile rheumatoid arthritis* (JRA) is a distinct entity (see Arthritis, Juvenile Idiopathic)

INITIAL STABILIZATION

- ABCs
  —Manage airway with attention to C-spine immobilization during intubation
  —Treat complications of RA as appropriate

ED TREATMENT

- Salicylates or NSAIDs are first-line treatment for RA
  —If one NSAID fails, another NSAID from a different chemical class may work better
  —Early treatment of RA is important as joint changes may be most progressive during the first 18 months
- Glucocorticoids, methotrexate, and other second-line therapies should be initiated by a rheumatologist

MEDICATIONS

- Aspirin (ECASA): adult: 900 mg PO q.i.d. (2.6–5.4 g/d); peds: 60–90 mg/kg/d q.i.d. up to 3.6 g
- Auranofin: adult: 3–9 mg/d divided b.i.d.; peds: 0.15 mg/kg/d up to 9 mg divided b.i.d.
- Celecoxib (Celebrex): 100–200 mg PO b.i.d.; peds: N/A
- Hydroxychloroquine: adult: 200–600 mg/d divided b.i.d.; peds: 6 mg/kg/d up to 600 mg per day
- Ibuprofen (Ibuprin, Advil, Motrin): 200–800 mg PO q6h; peds: 10 mg/kg PO q6h
- Leflunomide (Arava): 100 mg PO qd for 3 days, then maintenance dose of 10–20 mg PO qd; peds: N/A
- Methotrexate (Rheumatrex): 0.2–0.4 mg/kg PO per week single dose
- Prednisone: maintenance: 5–10 mg PO qd; acute exacerbations: 20–50 mg PO qd; peds: maintenance: 0.1 mg/kg/d PO, acute exacerbations: 2–5 mg/kg/d PO
- Rofecoxib (Vioxx) 25 mg PO qd; peds: N/A
- Sulfasalazine: adult: 500–1000 mg PO b.i.d.; peds: 30–60 mg/kg/d q.i.d. up to 2 g
- Valdecoxib (Bextra): 10 mg PO qd; peds: N/A

Disposition

ADMISSION CRITERIA

- Patients with severe or life-threatening presentations of RA and its complications should be admitted to the hospital
- Admission is warranted when the diagnosis is unclear and serious illnesses such as septic joint or systemic vasculitis may be present
- Admission may be required for pain control or if the patient has inadequate social supports and self-care isn't likely
- Pediatric patients with fever and arthritis should be strongly considered for admission

DISCHARGE CRITERIA

- Patients without serious complications may be managed as outpatients with appropriate follow-up

Miscellaneous

ICD9: 714.0

ICD10: M06.9

SUGGESTED READINGS

Anaya J, Diethelm L, Ortiz L, et al. Pulmonary involvement in rheumatoid arthritis. Semin Arthritis Rheum 1995;24(4):242–254.

Bingham CO. Development and clinical application of COX-2 selective inhibitors for the treatment of osteoarthritis and rheumatoid arthritis. Cleve Clin J Med 2002;69[suppl 1]:Si5–12.

Ilowite NT. Current treatment of juvenile rheumatoid arthritis. Pediatrics 2002;109(1):109–115.

Jain R, Lipsky P. Treatment of rheumatoid arthritis. Adv Rheum 1997;81(1):57–84.

King R. Arthritis, rheumatoid. *emedicine.com* 2002(January 4).

Leicht M, Harrington T, Davis D. Cricoarytenoid arthritis: a cause of laryngeal obstruction. Ann Emerg Med 1987;16(8):885–888.

Sanders S, Harisdangkul V. Leflunomide for the treatment of rheumatoid arthritis and autoimmunity. Am J Med Sci 2002;323(4):190–193.

Smith JB, Haynes MK. Rheumatoid arthritis: a molecular understanding. Ann Intern Med 2002;136(12):908–922.

Weyand C, Goronzy J. Pathogenesis of rheumatoid arthritis. Adv Rheum 1997;81(1):29–55.

Author: Hagop Isnar

Arthritis, Septic

Clinical Presentation

SIGNS AND SYMPTOMS

- Septic arthritis (SA) presents abruptly as a single painful, swollen, warm, and tender joint
- Common findings include:
  —Fever
  —A separate source of infection (e.g., skin) (~50%)
  —Extremely painful joint motion in all planes
  —A joint effusion (less evident in sacroiliac, hip, and shoulder)
- Any joint can be involved
- Most commonly knee than hip
- Commonly seen in intravenous drug abuse (IVDA): sacroiliac and sternoclavicular joints
  —Vertebral involvement such as lumbar facets possible
- Polyarticular involvement in 10–20%:
  —Mostly with rheumatoid arthritis; delay in diagnosis is secondary to low suspicion and more subtle presentations (fever in only 50%)
  —Patients with sepsis
- Gonococcal (GC) SA features:
  —Develops in 1–3% of untreated gonorrhea
  —Typically monoarticular but commonly polyarticular
  —Migratory polyarthralgia, tenosynovitis, and dermatitis
  —Involves small joints (e.g., wrist, elbow, ankle)
  —Signs of urethral or vaginal GC infection may be present
  —Painless maculopapular lesions on trunk, arms, and legs

ETIOLOGY

- Risk factors
  —Old age, infancy
  —IVDA, endocarditis
  —Females (GC)
  —Immunosuppression (AIDS, diabetes, chemotherapy)
  —Repeated joint injections, preexisting joint diseases, trauma, or prosthesis
- No bacterial pathogen is identified in 10–20%
- Most common organisms:
  —*Staphylococcus aureus* in adults, hip infections (80%), and patients with rheumatoid arthritis or diabetes
  —*Neisseria gonorrhea* (GC) most common in young, healthy, and sexually active patients
  —Other common pathogens: group A β-hemolytic, B, C, and G streptococci
  —Gram-negative rods (e.g., *H. influenzae, E. coli*) in old age, infancy, immunosuppression, and IVDA (*Pseudomonas*)
  —Anaerobes: diabetes, prosthetic joints
  —Mycobacterial and fungal etiologies: atypical (e.g., in HIV); more indolent course

MECHANISM/DESCRIPTION

- Bacteria can be introduced into a joint by:
  —Hematogenous spread (most common)
  —Invasive procedures
  —Contiguous infection (e.g., osteomyelitis, cellulitis)
  —Direct inoculation such as plant thorns or nails
- Acute inflammatory process results in WBC migration into joint
- Synovial hyperplasia, cartilage damage, and formation of a purulent effusion
- Irreversible loss of function in up to 50% of cases

PEDIATRIC CONSIDERATIONS

- Hip infections are most common
  —Commonly in patients with otitis media or upper respiratory tract infections
  —Complications of SA of hip in children: avascular necrosis, epiphyseal separation, pathologic dislocation, and arthritis
- 50% occur in children less than 3 years old
- Infants present with irritability, fever, and loss of appetite
- Older children present with a limp or refusal to bear weight or use joint

Pre-Hospital

No specific considerations

Diagnosis

ESSENTIAL WORKUP

Arthrocentesis

- Perform joint aspiration in any suspected case of SA
- Send fluid for protein and glucose, cell count, Gram stain, and culture
- Typical SA findings:
  —A turbid, purulent, or serosanguinous fluid
  —A leukocytosis (50,000–150,000/mm^3) with a polymorphonuclear predominance (>75%)
  —Often a depressed glucose and an elevated protein level
- The appearance of crystals does not rule out SA
- Use special stain or culture media when indicated (e.g., GC, anaerobes, fungus, mycobacterium)
- Intraarticular lidocaine reduces the sensitivity of subsequent cultures, immediate emptying of aspirated sample into a blood culture flask increases the yield
- In non-GC SA, Gram stain and culture are positive in 50% and 90% of cases, respectively
  —Drops to nearly 10% and 50% in GC SA, respectively
- Fluoroscopic, sonographic, or CT guidance can be used in technically difficult aspirations
- Arthrocentesis is contraindicated whenever there is an underlying joint prosthesis or an overlying skin infection
  —If cellulitis present, use an alternate approach through normal skin

LABORATORY

- Nonspecific serum leukocytosis, left shift, and ESR elevation are usually present
- Urinalysis and culture can reveal a urologic source for the pathogen
- Blood cultures may be useful: positive in 50–70% of non-GC SA
- Culture any potential focus of infection (pharynx, urine, cervix, or anus), particularly when suspecting GC

IMAGING/SPECIAL TESTS

- Plain radiographs to identify
  - —Effusion
  - —Baseline status of the joint
  - —Contiguous osteomyelitis
  - —Concurrent rheumatologic diseases
  - —Fractures or foreign body
  - —Joint loosening (a late and nonspecific sign)
- Ultrasound, CT, and MRI are more sensitive
  - —Ultrasound may be used to guide aspiration of some joints (e.g., hip) and detecting joint effusions, decreasing the incidence of unsuccessful aspirations
- Scintigraphic techniques are increasingly sensitive, specific, and useful in diagnosis of SA; they determine the site and distribution of joint infection
- Other tests
  - —Bacterial DNA amplification techniques in early detection of organisms

DIFFERENTIAL DIAGNOSIS

- Viral arthritis
- Rheumatoid arthritis
- Gout or pseudogout
- HIV-associated arthritis
- Reactive arthritis
- Lyme disease
- Osteomyelitis
- Endocarditis
- Trauma
- In children:
  - —Juvenile rheumatoid arthritis
  - —Slipped capital femoral epiphysis
  - —Legg-Calvé-Perthes
  - —Metaphyseal osteomyelitis
  - —Transient synovitis

PEDIATRIC CONSIDERATIONS

- Due to vaccine, *H. influenzae* is no longer most common
- *S. aureus* is most common
- Group B streptococcus, enterobacteria, and gram-negative rods in the newborn

Treatment

INITIAL STABILIZATION

- Patient may be septic and require resuscitation
- If patient is toxic, do not delay antibiotics for aspiration results

ED TREATMENT

- Promptly aspirate joint fluid
- Obtain cultures
- Start empiric antibiotics: staphylococcal, streptococcal, and Gram-negative coverage; duration of treatment recommended is 2–4 weeks
  - —Combine β-lactamase-resistant penicillin (e.g., nafcillin) with an aminoglycoside (e.g., gentamicin) or a third-generation cephalosporin (e.g., ceftriaxone)
  - —Initial guidance by Gram stain, patient's age, risk factors, and comorbid illness is appropriate
  - —When suspecting GC, use a third-generation cephalosporin or a quinolone (e.g., ceftriaxone, ciprofloxacin)
  - —Intraarticular antibiotics are contraindicated
- Early orthopedic consultation to evaluate eligibility for surgical drainage
- Pain control: narcotics and moderately flexed splinting
- Immunologic therapies are experimental at this point
- Prosthesis: some may try to preserve it unless it is loose on plain films

MEDICATIONS

- Cefotaxime: 1 g i.v. q8h; peds: 50 mg/kg q12h
- Ceftriaxone: 1 g i.v. qd; peds: 50 mg/kg
- Ciprofloxacin: 400 mg i.v. q12h
- Gentamicin: 2–5 mg/kg i.v. load
- Nafcillin: 2 g i.v. q4h; peds: 25 mg/kg q6h
- Piperacillin: 4 g i.v. q6h
- Tobramycin: 1 mg/kg i.v. q8h; peds: 2.5 mg/kg q8h
- Vancomycin: 1 g i.v. q12h; peds: 10 mg/kg q6h

PEDIATRIC CONSIDERATIONS

- Open surgical drainage is the method of choice in pediatric hip SA
- Cover *H. influenzae* type B if prior immunization cannot be established

Disposition

ADMISSION CRITERIA

- All patients with suspected SA should be admitted unless SA is ruled out
- May undergo drainage of their joint as indicated, by serial aspirations, arthroscopy, or arthrotomy; method used depends on the joint location, patient's age, joint fluid thickness, and surgical preference

DISCHARGE CRITERIA

- Cases where suspected SA has been adequately ruled out

Miscellaneous

ICD9: 711.00

CORE CONTENT CODE: 10.2.1.1

ICD10: M00.9

SUGGESTED READINGS

Baker D, Schumacher HR. Acute monoarthritis. N Engl J Med 1993;329(14):1013–1019.

Deng GM, Tarkowski A. The role of bacterial DNA in septic arthritis. Int J Mol Med 2000;6:29–33.

Donatto KC. Orthopedic management of septic arthritis. Rheum Dis Clin North Am 1998;24(2):275–286.

Dubost JJ, Soubrier M. Pyogenic arthritis in adults. Joint, bone, spine. Rev Rhum 2000;67(1):11–21.

Goldenberg D. Septic arthritis. Lancet 1998;35:197–202.

Greenspan A, Tehranzadeh J. Imaging of infectious arthritis. Radiol Clin North Am 2001;39(2):267–276.

Ho G. Bacterial arthritis. Curr Opin Rheumatol 2001;1:310–314.

Malleson P. Management of childhood arthritis. Part 1: acute arthritis. Arch Dis Child 1997;76:460–462.

Ryan M, Kavanagh R, Wall P, et al. Bacterial joint infections in England and Wales: analysis of bacterial isolates over a four year period. Br J Rheumatol 1997;36:370–373.

Smith J, Piercy E. Infectious arthritis. Clin Infect Dis 1995;20:225–231.

Authors: Ziad Kazzi; A. Antoine Kazzi

Ascites

Clinical Presentation

SIGNS AND SYMPTOMS

- Abdominal distention and discomfort
- Weight gain; less frequently weight loss
- Dyspnea and orthopnea
- Lower extremity edema
- Sacral, scrotal, and penile edema
- Abdominal wall hernias and muscle wasting
- Shifting dullness, flank fullness, fluid wave, and puddle sign
- Symptoms and signs of the underlying etiology

ETIOLOGY

- Parenchymal liver disease
  —Cirrhosis and alcoholic hepatitis
    -Account for 80% of adult patients
  —Fulminant hepatic failure
- Hepatic congestion
  —Congestive heart failure
  —Constrictive pericarditis
  —Tricuspid insufficiency or stenosis
  —Veno-occlusive disease and Budd-Chiari syndrome
- Malignancies
  —Peritoneal carcinomatosis
  —Hepatocellular carcinoma or metastatic disease
- Infections
  —Tuberculous or fungal peritonitis
  —Bacterial peritonitis
- Hypoalbuminemic states
  —Nephrotic syndrome
  —Severe malnutrition with serum albumin <2.0 g/dL
  —Protein-losing enteropathy
- Other conditions
  —Pancreatic ascites
  —Biliary ascites
  —Nephrogenous ascites
  —Benign ovarian tumors
  —Chylous ascites from lymphatic leak or obstruction
  —Connective tissue disease
  —Myxedema
  —Granulomatous peritonitis

MECHANISM

- Salt and water retention associated with *arterial vasodilation,* expansion of plasma volume, and *decreased effective plasma volume*
- Percolation of lymph from hepatic capsule due to disturbed Sterling's forces from sinusoidal portal hypertension >8 mm Hg
- Decreased plasma oncotic pressure from hypoalbuminemia
- Peritoneal irritation due to an infectious, inflammatory, or malignant process
- Damage to intraabdominal lymphatics, veins, or arteries

PEDIATRIC CONSIDERATION

- Majority of pediatric cases due to
  —Malignancy (e.g., Burkitt lymphoma and rhabdomyosarcoma)
  —Nephrotic syndrome
  —Malnutrition

Pre-Hospital

CAUTION

- Sudden increase in abdominal girth, pain, or fever requires urgent evaluation for possible complicating factor such as
  —Infection
  —Hepatoma
  —Obstruction of hepatic outflow
  —Decompensated liver function
- Ambulance transport for extreme weakness, dizziness, or respiratory distress

Diagnosis

ESSENTIAL WORKUP

- Thorough search for liver disease, congestive heart failure, tuberculosis, malignancy, and other systemic disorders
- Abdominal paracentesis
  —Mandatory in new-onset ascites, worsening encephalopathy, presence of fever, or abdominal pain/tenderness
- Test ascitic fluid for
  —Cell count and differential
  —Albumin/total protein
  —Gram stain, and culture in blood culture bottles ×2
  —LDH
  —Glucose
  —TB culture
  —Amylase
  —Triglyceride
  —Cytology
  —Bilirubin

LABORATORY

- CBC
- Electrolytes, BUN, Cr, glucose
- Liver function tests/liver enzymes
- PT, PTT
- ABGs or pulse oximeter
- Urinalysis
- Spot urine for sodium
- Viral hepatitis serology
- Amylase/lipase
- α-Fetoprotein
- TSH

IMAGING/SPECIAL TESTS

- CXR: signs of CHF, pleural effusion, and cavitary or mass lesion
- Abdominal ultrasound
  —Confirmation of ascites, especially if <2 L, and evaluation of the liver, pancreas, spleen, and ovaries
  —May guide paracentesis
- Doppler study: evaluation of hepatic blood flow
- Abdominal CT scan
- Echocardiogram
- Peritoneoscopy: ascites of unknown etiology; especially TB

DIFFERENTIAL DIAGNOSIS

- Ascites is one of the five "F" causes of abdominal swelling:
  —Fluid (including cystic lesion in solid organ)
  —Fat
  —Flatus
  —Fetus
  —Feces
  —Other causes include massive organomegaly
- *Serum-ascites albumin gradient (SAAG)* = ascitic albumin − serum albumin
  —Superior to ascitic fluid total protein in the differential diagnosis of ascites
  —SAAG $\geq$ 1.1 g/dL
    -97% accurate in predicting portal hypertension
    -Cirrhosis
    -Alcoholic hepatitis
    -Cardiac
    -Massive liver metastases
    -Fulminant hepatic failure
    -Portal vein thrombosis
    -Veno-occlusive disease
    -Myxedema
    -Fatty liver of pregnancy
    -Spontaneous bacterial peritonitis
  —SAAG <1.1 g/dL
    -Peritoneal carcinomatosis
    -Tuberculosis
    -Pancreatic ascites
    -Nephrotic syndrome
    -Bowel obstruction or infarction
    -Vasculitis
    -Postoperative lymphatic leak
  —Protein is high in CHF and low in Budd-Chiari

PEDIATRIC CONSIDERATION

- Malignancy and nephrotic syndrome most common etiology

Treatment

INITIAL STABILIZATION

- Symptomatic hypotension: administer volume expander (100 g albumin in 500 mL of 0.9% NS)

ED TREATMENT

- Early detection of the following complications is necessary
  - —Spontaneous bacterial peritonitis
    - -High degree of suspicion
    - -Low threshold for paracentesis and prompt therapy
  - —Tense ascites and hydrothorax
    - -Provide supplemental oxygen
    - -Perform therapeutic paracentesis (usually 1–2 L) or serial thoracocenteses (not chest tube) to relieve respiratory distress
  - —Abdominal wall hernias
    - -Watch for incarceration, ulceration, or rupture
    - -Perform therapeutic paracentesis and obtain an emergent surgical consultation
  - —Persistent leak at paracentesis site
    - -Remove more fluid
    - -If necessary, use stomal barrier device
  - —*Meralgia paresthetica*
    - -Due to pressure on the lateral femoral cutaneous nerve
    - -Relieve the pressure by paracentesis or diuresis
- Large-volume paracentesis
  - —5–10 L (100 mL/kg)
  - —Can be performed safely in the ED in patients with stable hemodynamics
  - —Replace with IV albumin (8 g/L fluid removed)
  - —Monitor the patient for 8 hours prior to discharge
- Nonparacentesis reduction of ascites
  - —Strict sodium restriction
    - -<1 g/day
    - -Restrict water only if serum sodium <125 mEq/L
  - —Spironolactone
    - -Works best for cirrhotic ascites
    - -Alternative agents: amiloride or triamterene
  - —Furosemide
    - -Works best for other causes of ascites
    - -Add to spironolactone in cirrhotics at spironolactone/furosemide ratio of 100 mg/40 mg
    - -Add metolazone for less responsive cases
  - —Diuretic principles
    - -Administer diuretics as a single morning dose for better effect and compliance
    - -Obtain spot-urine sodium to evaluate response
    - -Urinary Na >10 mEq/L are more responsive to diuretics
    - -Diuretic-induced weight loss should not exceed 2 lbs/d in patients without edema and 5 lbs/d in patients with edema
    - -Monitor electrolytes and renal function
  - —*Refractory ascites*
    - -Accounts for 10%
    - -Assure compliance with diet and medications
    - -NSAIDs diminish response to diuretics
    - -Implement peritoneovenous shunt or surgical or transjugular intrahepatic portosystemic shunt *only if* program of therapeutic large volume paracentesis fails
    - -Liver transplantation provides a cure
  - —*Treatment of the underlying etiology* for ascites caused by conditions other than cirrhosis (e.g., antituberculous agents and treatments of CHF)

MEDICATIONS

- Amiloride: 10–40 mg/day PO
- Furosemide: 40–160 mg/day (peds: 1–3 mg/kg) PO
- Metolazone: 5 mg/day
- Spironolactone: 100–400 mg/day (peds: 1–6 mg/kg) PO
- Triamterene: 100–300 mg/day PO

Disposition

ADMISSION CRITERIA

- Decompensated CHF
- Fulminant liver failure
- Hepatic encephalopathy
- Spontaneous bacterial peritonitis
- Hepatorenal syndrome
- GI bleeding
- Refractory or tense ascites not responding to ED treatment

DISCHARGE CRITERIA

- Patients responding to ED management

Miscellaneous

ICD9: 789.5

ICD10: R18

SUGGESTED READINGS

Bataller R, Gines P. Practical recommendations for the treatment of ascites and its complications. Drugs 1997;54:571.

Runyon BA. Treatment of patients with cirrhosis and ascites. Semin Liver Dis 1997;17:249.

Runyon BA, Montano AA, Akriviadis EA, et al. The serum-ascites albumin gradient is superior to the exudate-transudate concept in the differential diagnosis of ascites. Ann Intern Med 1992;117:215.

Runyon BA. Care of patient with ascites. N Engl J Med 1994;330:337.

Runyon BA. Management of adult patients with ascites caused by cirrhosis. Hepatology 1998;27(1):264–272.

Author: Stuart Feldman
First edition author: Abbas Zagnoon

Asthma, Adult

Clinical Presentation

SIGNS AND SYMPTOMS

- Wheezing
- Dyspnea
- Chest tightness
- Cough
- Tachypnea
- Tachycardia
- Respiratory distress
  - —Posture sitting upright or leaning forward
  - —Use of accessory muscles
  - —Inability to speak in full sentences
  - —Diaphoresis
  - —Poor air movement
  - —Altered mental status

MECHANISM/DESCRIPTION

- Increased expiratory resistance
  - —Bronchospasm
  - —Airway inflammation
  - —Mucosal edema
  - —Mucous plugging
- Consequences
  - —Air trapping
  - —Increased dead space
  - —Hyperinflation
- Risk factors for life-threatening disease
  - —Prior intubations
  - —Intensive care unit admissions
  - —Chronic steroid use
  - —Hospital admission for asthma during the past year
  - —Inadequate medical management
  - —Increasing age
  - —Ethnicity (African Americans)
  - —Lack of access to medical care

ETIOLOGY

- Pollen
- Dust mites
- Molds
- Animal dander
- Other environmental allergens
- Viral upper respiratory infections
- Occupational chemicals
- Tobacco smoke
- Environmental change
- Cold air
- Exercise
- Emotional factors
- Drugs
  - —Aspirin
  - —NSAIDs
  - —Beta-blockers

Pre-Hospital

- Recognize the "quiet chest" as respiratory distress
- Supplemental oxygen
- Continuous nebulized β-agonist
- Administration of subcutaneous epinephrine
  - —Severe disease with decreased breath sounds

Diagnosis

ESSENTIAL WORKUP

- Primarily a clinical diagnosis
- Measure and follow severity with peak expiratory flow rate (PEFR)
- Assess for underlying disease
  - —Pneumonia
  - —Pneumothorax

LABORATORY

- Arterial blood gas
  - —Not helpful during the initial evaluation
  - —The decision to intubate should be based on clinical criteria
  - —Mild-moderate asthma: respiratory alkalosis
  - —Severe airflow obstruction and fatigue: respiratory acidosis
- Pulse oximetry
  - —Less than 90% is indicative of severe respiratory distress
  - —Patients with impending respiratory compromise may still maintain a saturation above 90% until sudden collapse
- WBC
  - —Leukocytosis is nonspecific
  - —Pneumonia
  - —Chronic steroid use
  - —Stress of an asthma exacerbation
  - —Demargination occurs after administration of epinephrine and steroids

IMAGING/SPECIAL TESTS

- Peak expiratory flow rate
  - —Estimates the degree of airflow obstruction
    - -Normal peak flow in an adult is 400–600
    - -Between 100 and 300 indicates moderate airway obstruction
    - -<100 is indicative of severe airway obstruction
    - -Use serially as an objective measure of the response to therapy
- Forced expiratory volume (FEV)
  - —More reliable measure of lung function than PEFR
  - —More operator dependent
  - —Difficult to use as a screening tool
  - —Often unavailable in the ED
  - —Severe airway obstruction: FEV_1 less than 30–50%
- Chest radiograph
  - —Indications
    - -Fever
    - -Suspicion of pneumonia
    - -Suspicion of pneumothorax or pneumomediastinum
    - -Foreign body aspiration
    - -First episode of asthma
    - -Comorbid illness
    - -Diabetes
    - -Renal failure
    - -AIDS
    - -Cancer
  - —Findings
    - -Hyperinflation
    - -Scattered atelectasis
- EKG
  - —Indicated in patients at risk for cardiac disease
    - -Dysrhythmias
    - -Myocardial ischemia
  - —Transient changes in severe asthma
    - -Right axis deviation
    - -Right bundle branch block
    - -Abnormal p waves
    - -Nonspecific ST-T wave changes

DIFFERENTIAL DIAGNOSIS

- Congestive heart failure
- Myocardial ischemia
- Pulmonary embolus
- Pneumonia
- Bronchitis
- Bronchiolitis
- Croup
- Foreign body aspiration
- Upper airway obstruction
- Angioedema
- Allergic reaction
- Chronic obstructive pulmonary disease (COPD)
- Chronic cor pulmonale
- Chemical pneumonitis
- Carcinoid tumors
- Smoke inhalation
- Immersion injury
- Venous air embolus

Treatment

INITIAL STABILIZATION

- Immediate initiation of inhaled β-agonist treatment
- Intubate for fatigue and respiratory distress
- Steroids

ED TREATMENT

β-Adrenergic Agonist

- Mild-moderate asthmatic
  - —Administer every 20 minutes
- Severe asthmatic
  - —Continuous nebulized treatment
- Selective β_2-agonists (albuterol)
- Subcutaneous β-agonist
  - —Severe exacerbations
  - —Limited inhalation of aerosolized medicine
  - —More side effects because of systemic absorption
    - -Tachycardia
    - -Tremors
  - —Relative contraindications: age >40 and coronary disease
- Corticosteroids
  - —Reduce airway wall inflammation
  - —Administered early
  - —Onset of action may take 4–6 hours
  - —Administer intravenously or orally
  - —Intravenous Solu-Medrol in the treatment of severe asthma exacerbation
  - —Mild-moderate exacerbations may be treated with oral prednisone
  - —Inhaled corticosteroids are currently not recommended as initial therapy
- Oxygen
  - —Maintain an oxygen saturation above 90%
- Aminophylline
  - —Rare utility in acute management
  - —Toxicity
    - -Nausea
    - -Tremor
    - -Anxiety
    - -Palpitations
    - -Tachycardia
- Anticholinergic agents
  - —If minimal response to initial β-agonist treatment
  - —Severe airflow obstruction
  - —Inhaled anticholinergic agents should be used in conjunction with β-agonists
- Magnesium sulfate
  - —No benefit in mild-moderate asthma
  - —Benefit of magnesium remains unclear in severe asthma
- Heliox
  - —Mixture of helium and oxygen (80:20, 70:30, 60:40)
  - —Less dense than air
  - —Decrease airway resistance
  - —Decrease in respiratory exhaustion
  - —Not currently recommended for routine use
    - -Consider in severe asthma
- Ketamine
  - —Bronchodilator and an anesthetic agent
  - —Useful as an induction agent during intubation
  - —Contraindications
    - -Hypertension
    - -Coronary disease
    - -Preeclampsia
    - -Increased intracranial pressure
- Halothane
  - —Inhalation anesthetics are potent bronchodilators
  - —Refractory asthma in intubated patients
- Intubation of the asthmatic patient
  - —Rapid sequence intubation
    - -Lidocaine to attenuate airway reflexes
    - -Etomidate or ketamine as an induction agent
    - -Succinylcholine should be administered to achieve paralysis
    - -A large endotracheal tube >7 mm should be used to facilitate ventilation
    - -May need to mechanically exhale for the patient
    - -Permissive hypercapnia

MEDICATIONS

- β-agonists
  - —Albuterol: adult: 2.5 mg in 2.5 mL normal saline q 20 min inhaled; peds: 0.1–0.15 mg/kg/dose q 20 min (minimum dose 1.25 mg)
  - —Epinephrine: adult: 0.3 mg (1:1,000) s.c. q 0.5–4.0 h × 3 doses; peds: 0.01 mg/kg up to 0.3 mg s.c.
  - —Terbutaline: adult: 0.25 mg s.c. q 0.5 h × 2 doses; peds: 0.01 mg/kg up to 0.3 mg s.c.
- Corticosteroids
  - —Methylprednisolone: adult: 60–125 mg i.v.; peds: 1–2 mg/kg/dose i.v. or PO q6h × 24 hours
  - —Prednisone: adult: 40–60 mg PO; peds: 1–2 mg/kg/day in single or divided doses
- Anticholinergics
  - —Glycopyrrolate: 2 mg in NS q1h × 3
  - —Ipratropium bromide: 0.5 mg in 3 mL NS q1h × 3 doses
- Magnesium: 2 g i.v. over 20 minutes
- Aminophylline: 0.6 mg/kg/h i.v. infusion
- Rapid sequence intubation
  - —Etomidate: 0.3 mg/kg *or* ketamine: 1–1.5 mg/kg
  - —Lidocaine: 1–1.5 mg/kg
  - —Succinylcholine: 1.5 mg/kg

Disposition

ADMISSION CRITERIA

Intensive Care Unit

- Persistent respiratory distress
- PEFR <100 and minimal air movement
- Intubated patients

Medical Wards or Observation Unit

- PEFR <40% of predicted
- Patients without subjective improvement
- Patients with continued wheeze and diminished air movement
- Patients with moderate response to therapy and no respiratory distress
  - —Factors that should favor admission
    - -Prior intubation
    - -Recent emergency department visit
    - -Multiple emergency department visits or hospitalizations
    - -Symptoms for more than 1 week
    - -Failure of outpatient therapy
    - -Use of steroids
    - -Inadequate follow-up mechanisms
    - -Psychiatric illness
- Complications
  - —Pneumothorax
  - —Pneumomediastinum
  - —Pneumonia
  - —Fatigue

DISCHARGE CRITERIA

- Patient reports subjective improvement
- Clear lungs with good air movement
- PEFR or FEV_1 greater than 70% of predicted
- Peak flow should be greater than 300
- Adequate follow-up within 48–72 hours

Miscellaneous

ICD9: 493

ICD10: J45.9

SUGGESTED READINGS

Corbridge TC, Hall JB. The assessment and management of adults with status asthmaticus. Am J Respir Crit Care Med 1995;151:1296–1316.

Guidelines for the diagnosis and management of asthma: National Asthma Education Program Expert Panel Report. NIH publication no. 91-3042. Bethesda, MD: Department of Health and Human Services, 1991.

Jagoda A, Shepherd SM, Spevitz A, et al. Refractory asthma, part 1: epidemiology, pathophysiology, pharmacologic interventions. Ann Emerg Med 1997;29:262–274.

Jagoda A, Shepherd SM, Spevitz A, et al. Refractory asthma, part 2. Airway interventions and management. Ann Emerg Med 1997;29:275–281.

Manthous CA. Management of severe exacerbations of asthma. Am J Med 1995;99:298–308.

Author: Eric S. Nadel

Asthma, Pediatric

Clinical Presentation

SIGNS AND SYMPTOMS

General

- Fatigue, somnolence
- Diaphoresis, agitation
- Hypoxia, cyanosis
- Tachycardia
- Dehydration
- Pulsus paradoxus

Respiratory

- Wheezing, rales, rhonchi
- Cough, acute or chronic
- Tachypnea
- "Tight chest"
- Dyspnea, shortness of breath with prolonged expiratory phase
- Retractions, accessory muscle use, nasal flaring
- Hyperinflation
- Often a history of recurrent episodes and chronic restrictions
- Complications
  —Recurrent pneumonia, bronchitis
  —Atelectasis
  —Pneumothorax, pneumomediastinum
  —Respiratory distress/failure/death

MECHANISM/DESCRIPTION

- 2.7 million children (<18 years) affected in the U.S.
- 850,000 ED visits per year in the U.S.
- Inflammatory events, usually viral, lead to bronchoconstriction
  —Compounded by hyperreactivity of airways
  —Mediators of the inflammatory cascade
- Airway obstruction produces increased airway resistance and gas trapping
  —Mucosal edema
  —Bronchospasm
  —Mucous plugging
- Infants more vulnerable to respiratory failure
  —Increased peripheral resistance
  —Decreased elastic recoil with early airway closure
  —Unstable rib cage
  —Mechanically disadvantaged diaphragm
- Family history of allergy and asthma
- Medical history of early injury to airway (bronchopulmonary dysplasia, pneumonia, intubation, croup, reflux, passive exposure to smoking), reactions to foods and drugs, other allergic manifestations
- Environmental exposures such as pets, smoke, carpets, dust

ETIOLOGY

Precipitating/Aggravating Factors

- Infection
  —Viral
  —Bacterial
- Allergic/irritant
  —Environment: pollens, grasses, mold, house dust mites, animal dander
  —Occupational chemicals: chlorine, ammonia
  —Irritants: smoke, pollutants, gases, aerosols
  —Food and additives
  —Exercise
  —Cold weather
  —Emotional: stress, phobia
  —Intoxication: beta-blockers, aspirin, NSAIDs

Pre-Hospital

- Oxygen and oxygen saturation monitoring
- Nebulized β-adrenergic agonist: albuterol
- Intubate for respiratory failure or severe fatigue
- Rapid transport and good communication with ED

Diagnosis

ESSENTIAL WORKUP

- Clinical diagnosis based primarily on physical exam and history; assess ventilation by auscultating air exchange
- Follow response to bronchodilator therapy with present illness and past episodes
- Exclude other differential considerations
- Pulse-oximetry
  —Initial SaO_2 <91% (sea level) associated with significant illness: admission, relapse, prolonged course
  —Peak flow meters in cooperative patients (usually >5 years old)
  —<50% of best or predicted suggests severe obstruction
  —50–70% predicts moderate to severe obstruction
  —>70–90% associated with mild to moderate obstruction
  —>90% considered normal

LABORATORY

- Arterial blood gas (ABG) may be an adjunct to pulse oximetry to measure oxygenation and clinical exam to assess ventilation; not mandatory or routinely done
- CBC as a nonspecific marker of infection
- Theophylline level: only for patients on theophylline (not recommended)

IMAGING/SPECIAL TESTS

- Chest x-ray in the following patients
  —<1 year of age to exclude foreign body or atelectasis
  —First episode of wheezing (suggested)
  —Increasing respiratory distress or minimal response to therapy
  —Respiratory distress/failure
  —Shortness of breath in the absence of wheezing

DIFFERENTIAL DIAGNOSIS

- Infection/inflammation
  —Bronchiolitis; clinically difficult to differentiate except by age and clinical history
  —Pneumonia: viral, bacterial, chemical, hypersensitivity
  —Aspiration
  —Lymphadenopathy
  —Anaphylactic reaction
- Anatomic
  —Pneumothorax
  —Foreign body
- Vascular disorder
  —Compression of trachea by vascular anomaly
  —Pulmonary edema
  —Pulmonary embolism
  —Congestive heart failure
- Congenital disease
  —Cystic fibrosis
  —Tracheoesophageal fistula
  —Bronchogenic cyst
- Intoxication: metabolic acidosis
- Neoplasm
- Vocal chord dysfunction

Treatment

INITIAL STABILIZATION

- Maintain SaO_2 >90–95%
- β-adrenergic nebulizer(s): albuterol
- Intubate for respiratory failure

ED TREATMENT

- Assess patient for signs of potential respiratory failure
  - —Cyanosis
  - —Severe anxiety or irritability
  - —Lethargy, somnolence, fatigue
  - —Persistent tachypnea
  - —Poor air entry, ventilation
  - —Severe retractions
- Monitor oxygenation; titrate oxygen saturation to SaO_2 >95% (sea level)
- β-adrenergic nebulizer: albuterol
  - —Frequent or continuous for severe asthma
- Levalbuterol may require less frequent dosing
- Ipratropium bromide may be added as adjunct to β-adrenergic agonists
- Steroid therapy
  - —Oral for moderate exacerbations in those able to take oral meds
  - —Intravenous for severe exacerbations or in those unable to take oral meds
- Subcutaneous epinephrine or terbutaline for severe or refractory asthma (rarely used)
- Magnesium sulfate may be useful in severe disease following standard therapy
- Intubate for respiratory failure
  - —Ketamine is a useful induction agent

MEDICATIONS

- Albuterol (0.5% solution or 5 mg/mL)
  - —Nebulizer: 0.015 mg (0.03 mL)/kg/dose, up to 5 mg/dose, q 15–30 min as needed
  - —Metered-dose inhaler (with spacer) (90 μg/puff) 2 puffs q 5–10 min, max 10 puffs
- Epinephrine (1:1,000) (1 mg/mL): 0.01 mg/kg s.c., up to 0.35 mL/dose, q 20 min for 2 doses
- Ipratropium bromide: nebulizer (0.02% inhaled sol 500 μg/2.5 mL), 250–500 μg/dose q6h
- Ketamine (for intubation): 1–2 mg/kg i.v. as induction agent
- Levalbuterol (0.63 and 1.25 mg vials) q6–8h by nebulizer
- Magnesium sulfate: 25 mg/kg/dose i.v. over 20 min; max 1.2–2 g/dose
- Methylprednisolone: 1–2 mg/kg/dose i.v. q6h; max 125 mg/dose
- Prednisolone: 1–2 mg/kg/dose PO q12h (available as 15 mg/5 mL)
- Prednisone: 1–2 mg/kg/dose PO q6–12h; max 80 mg/dose
- Terbutaline (0.01%): 0.01 mL/kg s.c. q 15–20 min up to 0.25 mL/dose, q 20 min for 2 doses

Disposition

ADMISSION CRITERIA

- Persistent respiratory difficulty
  - —Persistent wheezing
  - —Increased respiratory rate/tachypnea
  - —Retraction and use of accessory muscles
- SaO_2 <93% (sea level) on room air
- Peak expiratory flow rate (PEFR) <50–70% predicted levels
- Inability to tolerate oral medicines or liquids
- Prior ED visit in last 24 hours
- Comorbidity
  - —Congenital heart disease
  - —Bronchopulmonary dysplasia
  - —Cystic fibrosis
  - —Neuromuscular disease
- Concomitant illness
  - —Pneumonia
  - —Severe viral infection

Intensive Care Unit Criteria

- Severe respiratory distress
- SaO_2 <90% or PaO_2 <60 mm Hg on 40% oxygen
- $PaCO_2$ >40 mm Hg
- Significant complications
  - —Pneumothorax
  - —Dysrhythmia

DISCHARGE CRITERIA

- Good response to therapy—observe in ED 60 minutes after last treatment before discharging
  - —PEFR >70% predicted
  - —SaO_2 >93% on room air (sea level)
  - —Respiratory rate normal
  - —No retractions
  - —Clear or minimal wheezing
  - —No or minimal dyspnea
- Good follow-up and compliance

Discharge Treatment

- Intensive β-adrenergic regimen for 3–5 days
- Short course (3–5 days) of steroids (2 mg/kg/d) for those presenting with moderate symptoms
- Follow-up appointment 24–72 hours
- Instructions to return for shortness of breath refractory to home regimen
- Long-term therapy should be considered for children with recurrent episodes, persistent symptoms, or activity limitations

Miscellaneous

ICD9: 493.9

ICD10: J45.0

SEE ALSO: BRONCHIOLITIS

SUGGESTED READINGS

Baren JM, Zorc JJ. Contemporary approach to the emergency department management of pediatric asthma. Emerg Med Clin North Am 2002;20(1):115–138.

Markoff BA, MacMillan JF Jr, Kumra V. Discharge of the asthmatic patient. Clin Rev Allergy Immunol 2001;20(3):341–355.

Rowe BH, Brerzlaff JA, Bourdon C, et al. Intravenous magnesium sulfate treatment for acute asthma in the emergency department: a review of the literature. Ann Emerg Med 2000;36:181–190.

Scarfone RJ, Loiselle JM, Joffe MD, et al. A randomized trial of magnesium in the emergency department treatment of children with asthma. Ann Emerg Med 2000;36:572–578.

Smith SR, Strunk RC. Acute asthma in the pediatric emergency department. Pediatr Clin North Am 1999;46(6):1145–1165.

Szefler SJ. Asthma: the new advances. Adv Pediatr 2000;47:273–308.

Author: Nathan I. Shapiro

Asystole

Clinical Presentation

SIGNS AND SYMPTOMS

- Unresponsive patient
- Pulseless
- No spontaneous respirations

MECHANISM

- Absence of cardiac electrical activity
- End-stage cardiac rhythm

ETIOLOGY

- May occur after progressive dysrhythmia
  —Bradycardia
  —Prolonged ventricular fibrillation
  —Prolonged pulseless electrical activity
- Survival is extremely unlikely when asystole occurs in the pre-hospital setting
- Potentially reversible causes include:
  —Hypoxia
  —Acidosis
  —Hyperkalemia
  —Hypokalemia
  —Drug overdose
  —Hypothermia

Pre-Hospital

- No intervention for valid Do Not Resuscitate document
- No intervention in clearly deceased patient
  —Rigor mortis
  —Dependent livedo
  —Injury incompatible with life, e.g., decapitation

Diagnosis

ESSENTIAL WORKUP

- Confirm asystole in two limb leads to exclude ventricular fibrillation
- Confirm lead and cable connections
- Confirm monitor power is on
- Confirm monitor gain is up
- Identify reversible causes

DIFFERENTIAL DIAGNOSIS

- Ventricular fibrillation

Treatment

INITIAL STABILIZATION

- Initiate basic CPR
- Confirm asystole with defibrillator
- Place airway device and confirm placement
- Establish IV access
- Confirm asystole in two limb leads with monitor
- Consider early transcutaneous pacing
- Epinephrine and atropine every 3–5 minutes
- Treat potentially reversible causes
- Sodium bicarbonate if hyperkalemia or drug overdose suspected

ED TREATMENT

- Consider stopping resuscitation efforts if the following are met:
  —Adequate CPR
  —Tracheal intubation
  —Effective ventilation
  —IV access
  —Ventricular fibrillation excluded
  —Epinephrine and atropine given
  —Reversible causes corrected
  —Documented asystole despite 10 minutes of above interventions

MEDICATIONS

- Atropine 1 mg i.v. every 3–5 minutes
- Epinephrine 1 mg i.v. every 3–5 minutes
- Sodium bicarbonate 1 mEq/kg i.v.
  —Administer only if primary acidosis is suspected

Disposition

ADMISSION CRITERIA

- All patients with return of spontaneous circulation
- Intensive care unit for cardiac and blood pressure monitoring

DISCHARGE CRITERIA

N/A

Miscellaneous

ICD9: 427.5

ICD10: I46.9

SEE ALSO: CARDIAC ARREST

SUGGESTED READINGS

Cummins RO, Graves JR, Larsen MP, et al. Out-of-hospital transcutaneous pacing by emergency medical technicians in patients with asystolic cardiac arrest. N Engl J Med 1993;328:1377–1382.

Guidelines 2000 for Cardiopulmonary Resuscitation and Emergency Cardiovascular Care. Part 6: advanced cardiovascular life support: 7C: a guide to the International ACLS algorithms. The American Heart Association in collaboration with the International Liaison Committee on Resuscitation. Circulation 2000;102[8 suppl]:I142–157.

Authors: Benjamin Sun; David F. M. Brown

Ataxia

Clinical Presentation

SIGNS AND SYMPTOMS

- Inability to perform coordinated movements
- Altered hand coordination
  - —Abnormal finger-to-nose test with eyes closed
- Altered coordination in lower extremities
  - —Abnormal heel-to-shin coordination
- Impaired balance
  - —From dysfunction of two out of three of vision, vestibular sense, or proprioception
  - —Evaluated by Romberg test and tandem gait
  - —Positive Romberg sign = steady with eyes open but unsteady with eyes closed; suggests a sensory cause of ataxia
  - —Unsteady with eyes open and closed suggests a cerebellar cause of ataxia
- Impaired gait
- Intentional tremor
- Frontal lobe lesions
  - —Wide based gait
  - —Tendency to fall backward
  - —Motor perseveration
  - —Grasp and suck reflexes
  - —Urinary incontinence
  - —Slowness in thinking
  - —Headache
  - —Altered mental status
- Subcortical lesions
  - —Emotional lability
  - —Brisk reflexes
  - —Dysarthria
  - —Dementia
- Brainstem lesions
  - —Crossed motor or sensory findings
  - —Internuclear ophthalmoplegia
  - —Nystagmus
  - —Dysarthria
- Cerebellar lesions
  - —Truncal and gait ataxia if midline lesions
  - —Ipsilateral limb ataxia if hemispheric lesions
  - —Nystagmus
  - —Hypotonia
  - —Occipital headache
  - —Occipital gaze palsy
- Posterior column dysfunction
  - —Positive Romberg sign
  - —Neck and arm pain
  - —Positive Babinski sign
  - —Loss of vibration and position sense
- Peripheral neuropathy
  - —Loss of deep tendon reflexes
  - —Decreased strength

MECHANISM/DESCRIPTION

- Disorder of coordination and rhythm
- May result from dysfunction at different levels of the cerebellar circuit
  - —Cerebellum, spinocerebellar pathways, or vestibular sensory input, the integration of these inputs in the brainstem or cerebellum, or the motor output to the spinal neurons that control axial and proximal muscles
  - —Motor ataxia is caused by lesions of the cerebellum or contralateral frontal lobe or internal capsule; sensory pathways are intact, but integration of proprioceptive data is faulty
  - —Sensory ataxia is caused by lesions that affect the peripheral sensory fibers, dorsal root ganglia cells, posterior columns of the spinal cord, lemniscal system in the brainstem, thalamus, or parietal cortex; proprioceptive data sent to the cerebellum are faulty
- Different types of ataxia should be distinguished
  - —Vertiginous ataxia due to dizziness
  - —Cerebellar ataxia due to imbalance
  - —Spinal cord and muscular ataxia due to weakness

ETIOLOGY

- Acute symmetric
  - —Toxicologic
    - -Alcohol
    - -Lithium
    - -Diphenylhydantoin
    - -Barbiturates
  - —Acute viral cerebritis
  - —Meningitis
  - —Hydrocephalus
  - —Postinfection syndrome
  - —Hyponatremia
  - —Hypothyroidism
- Acute focal
  - —Anterior cerebral artery syndrome
  - —Cerebellar infarction
  - —Cerebellar hemorrhage
  - —Subdural hematoma of the posterior fossa
  - —Cerebellar abscess
- Subacute symmetric
  - —Mercury
  - —Hydrocarbons
  - —Toluene
  - —Vitamin B_1 or B_{12} deficiency
  - —Lyme disease
  - —AIDS
  - —Toxoplasmosis
  - —Mycoplasma
  - —Legionella
  - —Bacterial abscesses
  - —Creutzfeldt-Jakob disease
- Subacute focal
  - —Cerebellar glioma
  - —Metastatic tumors
  - —Paraneoplastic syndromes
    - -Breast cancer
    - -Hodgkin's disease
    - -Children with neuroblastomas
  - —Multiple sclerosis
  - —AIDS-related multifocal leukoencephalopathy
  - —Lymphoma
  - —Cervical spondylosis
  - —Syringomyelia
  - —Guillain-Barré syndrome
- Chronic
  - —Stable gliosis
  - —Inherited and developmental ataxias
    - -Friedreich ataxia and other recessive ataxias
    - -Ataxia-telangiectasia
    - -Autosomal-dominant cerebellar ataxia
    - -Cerebellar hypoplasia
    - -Hartnup disease
    - -Niemann-Pick disease
    - -Pyruvate decarboxylase deficiency
    - -Dandy-Walker and Arnold-Chiari malformation
    - -Joubert and Gillespie syndromes

Pre-Hospital

CAUTIONS

- Acute onset of ataxia may be due to stroke or hemorrhage
  - —Monitor
  - —Supplemental oxygen
  - —IV access
  - —Observe mental status carefully as deterioration may warrant field endotracheal intubation

Diagnosis

ESSENTIAL WORKUP

- A careful history and physical are essential to classify the ataxia and determine the etiology
  - —Onset
    - -Hours to days—acute
    - -Weeks to months—subacute
    - -Years—chronic
  - —Bilateral, symmetrical, or focal involvement
  - —Truncal or limb ataxia
  - —Motor or sensory ataxia
- Neurologic exam
  - —Mental status
  - —Motor sensory
  - —Finger-to-nose
  - —Heel-to-shin
  - —Romberg
  - —Gait (if possible)
  - —Speech
  - —Cranial nerves
  - —Babinski
- Assess for associated signs or symptoms of acute, life-threatening disorders
  - —Altered mental status
  - —Headache
  - —Focal weakness, numbness, tingling
  - —Nausea/vomiting
  - —Slurred speech
  - —Incontinence

LABORATORY

- Electrolytes
- Blood glucose level
- Toxicology screen
- Anticonvulsant drug screen
- CBC, consider lumbar puncture if infection, abscess suspected
- TSH, free T_4 if hypothyroidism suspected

IMAGING/SPECIAL TESTS

- Head CT scan
  - —Identifies supratentorial masses, hemorrhage, or evidence of hydrocephalus
  - —If MRI is unavailable, obtain both contrast and noncontrast studies
- MRI
  - —Diagnostic study of choice to assess the posterior fossa
  - —MR angiogram may be indicated if a vertebral basilar artery insufficiency is suspected
- Lumbar puncture
  - —Rarely indicated unless fever or mental status changes suggest an infectious etiology
  - —Indicated in the evaluation for possible Lyme disease although may be done in this setting as an outpatient
- Electromyography
  - —Not indicated as part of the emergency workup
  - —Assesses for denervation of peripheral nerves

DIFFERENTIAL DIAGNOSIS

See Etiology, above

Treatment

INITIAL STABILIZATION

- ABCs
- IV access, cardiac monitor if altered mental status or cerebellar hemorrhage suspected
- Naloxone, dextrose (or rapid fingerstick glucose) if altered mental status
- Empiric thiamine in chronic alcoholics and poorly nourished patients

ED TREATMENT

- Treatment should be determined by the underlying cause

MEDICATIONS

- Dextrose: D50W 1 amp (50 mL or 25 g) (peds: D25W 2–4 mL/kg) i.v.
- Naloxone (Narcan): 2 mg (peds: 0.1 mg/kg up to 2 mg) i.v. or i.m. initial dose
- Thiamine (vitamin B_1): 100 mg i.m. or 100 mg thiamine in 1,000 mL of intravenous fluid wide open

Disposition

ADMISSION CRITERIA

- Acute and subacute ataxia if an underlying etiology cannot be established
- Patients who cannot ambulate safely without home support
- Patients with cerebellar hemorrhage should be admitted to the ICU

DISCHARGE CRITERIA

- Reversible acute and subacute causes or chronic causes if patient's mental status OK and can ambulate without risk of injury
  - —Alcohol, medications
- Cerebellar atrophy

Miscellaneous

ICD9: 334.0, 334.2, 334.3, 334.8

ICD10: R27.0

SEE ALSO: DIZZINESS

SUGGESTED READINGS

Baloh RW. Approach to the dizzy patient. In: Baloh RW, ed. Neurotology. Baillieres Clin Neurol 1994;3:453.

Huff JS. Ataxia and Gait Disturbances. In: Tintinalli JE, et al., eds. Emergency medicine: a comprehensive study guide, 5th ed. New York: McGraw-Hill, 2000:1449–1452.

Rosenberg RN. Ataxic disorders. In: Fauci AS, et al., eds. Harrison's principles of internal medicine. Philadelphia: McGraw-Hill, 1998:2363–2368.

Author: Sean P. Kelly

Atrial Fibrillation

Clinical Presentation

SIGNS AND SYMPTOMS

- Palpitations
- Dyspnea
- Weakness
- Light-headedness
- Syncope
- Irregularly irregular pulse
- Intermittent loss of a pulse with a QRS complex on the monitor
- S_1 of variable intensity
- Loss of A waves in the jugular pulse
- Signs of instability
  —Hypotension
  —Persistent angina
  —Pulmonary edema
  —Altered mental status
  —Acute neurologic injury

MECHANISM/DESCRIPTION

- Chaotic atrial electrical activity
  —Rate of 350–600
  —Loss of mechanically effective atrial contractions
- AV node limits the number of impulses reaching the ventricles
  —Typical ventricular rate 160–200 if the AV node is healthy
- Loss of organized atrial contractions and rapid ventricular rate
  —Decrease in stroke volume
  —Decrease in cardiac output
- Affects over 1 million Americans each year
- Most common dysrhythmia requiring intervention
- Rare in those less than 35 years of age
- Occurs in 5% of people over 70
- Spontaneously converts in 24 hours in patients with new-onset atrial fibrillation
- Sinus rhythm is maintained in 30% without medical therapy
- Mortality is twice that of the general population
- Complications
  —CVA in 35% of patients
    -Embolic, especially on conversion
    -Hemorrhagic after anticoagulation
  —Mesenteric ischemia
  —Syncope
  —Angina

ETIOLOGY

- Predisposing conditions
  —Hypertension
  —Coronary artery disease
  —Hypothyroidism
  —Heavy alcohol intake
  —Mitral valve disease
  —Chronic pulmonary disease
  —Pulmonary embolus
  —Wolff-Parkinson-White (WPW) syndrome
  —Hypoxia
  —Digoxin toxicity
  —Chronic pericarditis
  —Idiopathic atrial fibrillation

Pre-Hospital

CAUTIONS

- Intravenous access
- Monitor
- Oxygen

CONTROVERSIES

- Cardioversion
  —Unstable patients
  —Rarely required

Diagnosis

ESSENTIAL WORKUP

- EKG to determine rhythm
  —Irregularly irregular R-R intervals, no identifiable P waves, low amplitude undulations (f waves)
  —Slow the rate transiently when in doubt of the underlying rhythm
- Ordering of ancillary studies should be based on the individual presentation

LABORATORY

- Pulse oximetry
- CBC
- Electrolytes
- Cardiac enzymes
- Thyroid function
  —Yield is very low without other signs of hyperthyroidism

IMAGING/SPECIAL TESTS

- Echocardiogram
  —Inpatient study
  —Transthoracic or transesophageal
  —Assess for atrial enlargement as an etiology
  —Assess for atrial thrombus and the need for immediate anticoagulation

DIFFERENTIAL DIAGNOSIS

- Atrial flutter with variable AV block
- Multifocal atrial tachycardia
- Sinus rhythm with frequent premature atrial contractions
- Atrial tachycardia with variable AV block

Treatment

INITIAL STABILIZATION

- Oxygen
- Monitor
- Intravenous access
- Unstable patients
  —Immediate synchronized cardioversion starting at 100 J

EMERGENCY DEPARTMENT MANAGEMENT

- Stable patients with a narrow complex tachycardia—if pulse <100 beats/min, no treatment is needed in the ED
  —If pulse is 100–120 beats/min, rate control in the ED may be appropriate
  —Control rate if pulse >120 beats/min
  —Calcium channel blockers:
    -Diltiazem is preferred over verapamil due to a lower incidence of hypotension
    -Parenteral or oral routes
  —Beta-blockers
  —Digoxin
    -Use in the setting of preexistent CHF
  —Procainamide
    -If rate control is recalcitrant to other agents or in the case of possible WPW
  —Cardioversion
    -Should only be considered in stable patients when they have been in Afib for less than 48 hours
    -No clinically significant LV dysfunction, mitral valve disease, or previous embolism
    -Beyond 48 hours anticoagulation is required before cardioversion in stable patients
  —Cardioversion is possible if thrombus absent by transesophageal echocardiogram (TEE) even if Afib >48 hours (with heparin drip, no bolus, for anticoagulation)
  —Synchronized DC cardioversion with sedation starting at 100 J
  —Ibutilide
    -Requires a normal QTc, no history of torsades, and correction of hypokalemia
    -Posttreatment monitoring for at least 4 hours for possible torsades des pointes
  —Procainamide
- Wide complex irregular tachycardia
  —WPW syndrome may be the underlying cause
  —Avoid all calcium channel blockers, beta-blockers, and digoxin
  —Stable patients should be treated with procainamide
  —Unstable patients should be cardioverted

MEDICATIONS

- Digoxin: 0.5 mg i.v. initially, then 0.25 mg i.v. q4h until desired effect
- Diltiazem: 0.25 mg/kg i.v. over 2 min; if unsuccessful, repeat in 15 min as 0.35 mg/kg i.v. over 2 min
- Esmolol: 0.5 mg/kg over 1 min; maintenance infusion at 0.05 mg/kg/min over 4 min, then 0.1–0.2 mg/kg/min continuously
- Heparin: load 80 IU/kg i.v.; infusion at 18 IU/kg/h
- Ibutilide (Corvert): 1 mg i.v. for patients >60 kg; 0.01 mg/kg i.v. for patients <60 kg infused over 10 min; dose can be repeated once if NSR not restored within 10 min after infusion; patients must be monitored for 4 hours afterward for QT prolongation and torsades
- Metoprolol: 5–10 mg slow i.v. push at 5-min intervals to total of 15 mg
- Procainamide: 6–13 mg/kg i.v. at 0.2–0.5 mg/kg/min until dysrhythmia controlled up to a total dose of 1,000 mg, then 2–6 mg/min
- Propranolol: 0.1 mg/kg divided into equal doses at 2- to 3-min intervals
- Quinidine gluconate: 324–648 mg PO q8–12h
- Verapamil: 2.5–5 mg i.v. bolus over 2 min; may repeat with 5–10 mg every 15–30 min to max of 20 mg

Disposition

ADMISSION CRITERIA

- Hypotension
- Chest pain suggestive of cardiac ischemia or EKG evidence of myocardial injury
- New-onset or worsening congestive heart failure
- Persistent or recurrent rapid ventricular rate
- Age over 65 years or significant concomitant medical problems
- Hemodynamic dependence on atrial contraction
  —Significant mitral or aortic stenosis
- Hypertrophic cardiomyopathy
- New-onset atrial fibrillation
  —Intravenous anticoagulation
  —Cardioversion or chemical conversion planned on an inpatient basis

DISCHARGE CRITERIA

- Patients who convert to sinus rhythm
- Patients in chronic atrial fibrillation with adequate ventricular rate control
- New-onset atrial fibrillation
  —Outpatient anticoagulation with Lovenox
  —Rate is first controlled
  —Close follow-up arranged

Miscellaneous

ICD9: 427.3

ICD10: I48

SUGGESTED READINGS

Cunningham R, Mikhail MG. Management of patients with syncope and cardiac arrhythmias in an emergency department observation unit. Emerg Med Clin North Am 2001;19(1):105–121.

Deantonio HJ, Movahed A. Atrial fibrillation: current therapeutic approaches. Am Fam Physician 1992;45(6):2576–2584.

Falk RH. Atrial fibrillation. N Engl J Med 2001;344(14):1067–1078.

Golzari H, Cebul RD, Bahler RC. Atrial fibrillation: restoration and maintenance of sinus rhythm and indications of anticoagulation therapy. Ann Intern Med 1996;125:311–323.

Havranek EP. The management of atrial fibrillation: current perspectives. Am Fam Physician 1994;50(5):959–968.

National Heart, Lung, and Blood Institute Working Group on Atrial Fibrillation. Current understanding and research imperatives. J Am Coll Cardiol 1993;22:1830–1834.

Zipes DP. Specific arrhythmias: diagnosis and treatment. In: Braunwald E, ed. Heart disease: a textbook of cardiovascular medicine, 5th ed. Philadelphia: WB Saunders, 1997:640–704.

Authors: Chirag Patel; Kevin Curtis

Atrial Flutter

Clinical Presentation

SIGNS AND SYMPTOMS

- Palpitations
- Syncope/presyncope
- Fatigue
- Dyspnea
- Poor exercise capacity
- Tachycardia
  - —Most often with a regular pulse
- Signs of instability
  - —Hypotension
  - —Chest pain
  - —Heart failure
  - —Heart rate >150 bpm

MECHANISM/DESCRIPTION

- Atrial dysrhythmia characterized by several electrocardiographic findings
  - —Regular atrial rate between 250 and 350
  - —Beat to beat uniformity
  - —Sawtooth flutter waves
- A reentrant circuit in the right atrium is thought to be the underlying mechanism
- Most sensitive rhythm to cardioversion
- Seldom occurs in absence of organic heart disease
- Less common than SVT or atrial fibrillation
- Typically paroxysmal, lasting seconds to hours
  - —Often reverts to sinus rhythm or atrial fibrillation

PEDIATRIC CONSIDERATIONS

- Infants do not tolerate atrial flutter well
  - —The AV node is capable of very rapid conduction
  - —Extremely rapid ventricular rates can lead to shock or congestive heart failure
- Atrial flutter can occur in the fetus and young infant without associated cardiac defects
  - —Often does not recur beyond neonatal period
- Most older children have an underlying cardiac abnormality
  - —More likely to recur, more difficult to control

ETIOLOGY

- Ischemic heart disease
- Valvular heart diseases
- Congestive heart failure
- Myocarditis
- Cardiomyopathies
- Pulmonary embolus
- Other pulmonary disease
- Electrolyte abnormalities
- Postoperative following cardiac surgery (often in first postoperative week)
- Thyrotoxicosis

Pre-Hospital

CAUTIONS

- Intravenous access
- Supplemental oxygen
- Cardiac monitoring
- Transport to the nearest facility
- Unstable patients should be cardioverted in the field
  - —Immediate synchronized cardioversion
  - —Start with 50 J, then 100 J, 200 J, 300 J, and 360 J

CONTROVERSIES

- Adenosine
  - —Used in some systems in the field for SVT
  - —Unlikely to break atrial flutter
  - —May aid in the diagnosis of atrial flutter by unmasking the flutter waves

Diagnosis

ESSENTIAL WORKUP

- EKG to determine rhythm and suggest underlying cause
  - —Slow the rate when in doubt of the underlying rhythm
- Ancillary studies are based on the clinical examination to determine underlying causes

LABORATORY

- CBC
- Electrolytes
- Cardiac enzymes
- Thyroid function

IMAGING/SPECIAL TESTS

- EKG
  - —Regular atrial rate between 250 and 350
  - —Beat to beat uniformity of cycle length, polarity, and amplitude
  - —Sawtooth flutter waves directed superiorly and most visible in leads II, III, aVF
  - —AV block usually 2:1, but occasionally greater or irregular
  - —If rhythm is equivocal, slow the rate to show the presence of flutter waves
    - -Vagal maneuvers
    - -Adenosine
- CXR
  - —Left atrial enlargement
  - —Cardiomegaly
  - —Heart failure
- Transesophageal echocardiogram (TEE)
  - —Consider before pharmacoconversion or cardioversion

DIFFERENTIAL DIAGNOSIS

- SVT
- Sinus tachycardia
- Atrial fibrillation
- Multifocal atrial tachycardia
- Ventricular tachycardia

Treatment

INITIAL STABILIZATION

- Immediate synchronized cardioversion starting at 50 J-min if the patient is unstable
- Oxygen
- Monitor
- Intravenous access

ED TREATMENT

- Pharmacoconversion or cardioversion if the onset is within 48 hours
- Rate control prior to conversion to sinus rhythm if the onset is greater than 48 hours
- Anticoagulation
  - —Controversial
    - -Atrial activity remains organized therefore risk of thrombus formation is lower than with atrial fibrillation
    - -Higher risk of thromboembolism than previously believed (rates vary from 0–7%)
  - —Patients at higher risk for thromboembolism include:
    - -Patients who go back and forth between atrial fibrillation and flutter
    - -Valvular heart disease
    - -Left ventricular dysfunction
    - -Prior stroke or thromboembolism
    - -Longer symptom duration (>48 hours)
    - -Anticoagulation prior to cardioversion should be considered in these patients
- Rate control
  - —Rate control should be instituted prior to giving an antidysrhythmic to avoid risk of a 1:1 AV conduction ratio and hemodynamic collapse
  - —ACLS recommendations for rate control
  - —Cardiac function preserved
  - —Calcium channel blockers
  - —Beta-blockers
  - —Digoxin
  - —Cardiac function impaired (EF <40% or CHF)
  - —Digoxin
  - —Diltiazem
  - —Amiodarone
  - —Preexcited [Wolff-Parkinson-White (WPW) syndrome] and normal LV function
  - —Amiodarone
  - —Flecainide
  - —Procainamide
  - —Propafenone
  - —Sotalol
  - —Preexcited (WPW) and LV dysfunction (CHF)
  - —Amiodarone
- Pharmacoconversion
  - —Cardiac function preserved (*use only one*)
    - -Amiodarone
    - -Ibutilide
    - -Flecainide
    - -Propafenone
    - -Procainamide
  - —Cardiac function impaired (EF <40% or CHF)
    - -*Consider cardioversion*
    - -Amiodarone
  - —Preexcited (WPW) and normal LV function
    - -Amiodarone
    - -Flecainide
    - -Procainamide
    - -Propafenone
    - -Sotalol
  - —Preexcited (WPW) and LV dysfunction (CHF)
    - -Amiodarone
    - -*Consider cardioversion*
    - -Note: In WPW adenosine, beta-blockers, calcium channel blockers, and digoxin are class III (can be harmful)
    - -Can cause increased ventricular response, which can deteriorate to ventricular fibrillation
- Cardioversion
  - —50–360 J
  - —Sedation when possible
  - —Safest and most effective means of restoring sinus rhythm
  - —In most patients, it can be accomplished with 25–100 J

PEDIATRIC CONSIDERATIONS

- Verapamil is not recommended in infants and young children as it is associated with a low cardiac output and serious cardiovascular compromise
- Digoxin is the first-line drug therapy for pediatric atrial flutter
  - —Consider cardioversion as first-line therapy in neonates
- Beta-blockers, class IA antiarrhythmics (procainamide, quinidine) or amiodarone are alternatives

MEDICATIONS

- Amiodarone: 150 mg i.v. over 10 min, then continuous infusion at 1 mg/min for 6 hours, then 0.5 mg/min; supplemental 150-mg infusions can be dosed PRN to a maximum daily dose of 2 g; peds: 5 mg/kg i.v. loading dose, divided into 1-mL/kg boluses over 5–10 min; 10–15 mg/kg/d as continuous infusion
- Atenolol: 5 mg i.v. over 5 min, may repeat in 10 min if tolerated, then 50 mg PO q12h
- Digoxin: 0.5 mg i.v. initially, then 0.25 mg i.v. q1–2h until desired effect, side effects, or total dose of 1.5 mg peds: 8–15 μg/kg/d divided qd–b.i.d.
- Diltiazem: 0.25 mg/kg i.v. over 2 min followed in 15 min by 0.35 mg/kg i.v. over 2 min
- Esmolol: 0.5 mg/kg over 1 min; maintenance infusion at 0.05 mg/kg/min; can repeat loading dose and increase in increments of 0.05 mg/kg/min q 4 min up to 0.3 mg/kg/min
- Flecainide: 2 mg/kg i.v. at 10 mg/min
- Ibutilide (Corvert): 1 mg i.v. over 10 minutes for patients >60 kg; 0.01 mg/kg i.v. for patients <60 kg infused over 10 min; dose can be repeated once if NSR not restored within 10 min after infusion; patients must be monitored for 4–6 hours afterward for QT prolongation and VT
- Metoprolol: 5 mg i.v. push over 5 min at 5-min intervals to total of 15 mg, then 50 mg PO b.i.d.
- Procainamide: 20 mg/min until arrhythmia suppressed, hypotension, QRS prolongation of 50%, or total of 17 mg/kg; may be given at rate up to 50 mg/min; peds: 10–15 mg/kg loading dose; 20–80 μg/kg/min infusion
- Propafenone: 1–2 mg/kg i.v. at 10 mg/min
- Propranolol: 0.1 mg/kg in 3 equal doses by slow i.v. push at 2- to 3-min intervals; not faster than 1 mg/min; peds: 0.01–0.15 mg/kg/dose q6–8h
- Quinidine gluconate: 324–648 mg PO q8–12h
- Sotalol: not available i.v. in U.S.
- Verapamil: 2.5–5.0 mg i.v. bolus over 2 min; may repeat with 5–10 mg every 15–30 min to max of 20 mg

Disposition

ADMISSION CRITERIA

- New-onset atrial flutter requiring antidysrhythmics
- Symptomatic (i.e., chest pain that warrants a rule out or cardioversion)
- Congestive heart failure

DISCHARGE CRITERIA

- Chronic atrial flutter with good rate control

Miscellaneous

ICD9: 427.32

ICD10: I48

SUGGESTED READINGS

Elhendy A, Gentile F, et al. Thromboembolic complications after electrical cardioversion in patients with atrial flutter. Am J Med 2001;111(6):433–438.

International Guidelines 2000 for Cardiopulmonary Resuscitation and Emergency Cardiovascular Care. Part 6: Advanced cardiovascular life support. Section 5: Pharmacology I: Agents for arrhythmias. Circulation 2000;102 [suppl I]:I112–I128.

Luedtke SA, Kuhn RJ, McCaffrey FM. Pharmacologic management of supraventricular tachycardias in children. Part 2: atrial flutter, atrial fibrillation, and junctional and atrial ectopic tachycardia. Ann Pharmacother 1997;31: 1347–1359.

Niebauer MJ, Chung MK. Management of atrial flutter. Cardiol Rev 2001;9(5): 253–258.

Waldo AL. Treatment of atrial flutter. Heart 2000;84(2):227–232.

Author: Liesl Curtis

Atrioventricular Blocks

Clinical Presentation

SIGNS AND SYMPTOMS

- First-degree AV block
  - —Asymptomatic
- Type I second-degree AV block
  - —Regularly irregular pulse
- Type II second-degree AV block and third-degree block
  - —Palpitations
  - —Irregular pulse
  - —Chest pain
  - —Hypotension
  - —Presyncope/syncope
  - —Altered mental status
  - —Dyspnea
  - —Rales
  - —Cyanosis
  - —Jugular venous distention

MECHANISM/DESCRIPTION

- Impaired conduction through the AV node or His-Purkinje system
- First-degree AV block
  - —Prolonged conduction through the AV node >0.20 seconds
  - —Ventricular impulses are not lost
- Second-degree AV block
  - —Marked by a failure of some atrial impulses to reach ventricles
  - —Type I (Wenckebach)
    - -Progressive prolongation of the PR interval until there is a nonconducted P wave and a dropped QRS complex
    - -Usually secondary to conduction deficit in AV node
    - -Generally benign
    - -May be a complication of an inferior wall myocardial infarction
  - —Type II
    - -PR intervals are constant until a single or multiple beats are dropped
    - -Less common than type I
    - -Conduction deficit is usually below the level of the AV node
    - -High likelihood of progression to complete heart block
    - -Worse prognosis if associated with an acute myocardial infarction
- Third-degree AV block
  - —Also know as complete heart block
  - —All atrial impulses are unable to reach the ventricular conducting system; a ventricular escape pacemaker then takes over, resulting in AV dissociation
  - —Constant PP and RR intervals with variable PR intervals because PP and RR intervals are independent of each other
  - —More severe symptoms occur when the block is lower in the conducting system
  - —If secondary to toxicologic agents, often resolves upon omission of offending toxin
  - —Never a benign condition

ETIOLOGY

- Essentially due to:
  - —A structural lesion
  - —Increase in inherent refractory period
  - —Marked shortening of the supraventricular cycle
- Myocardial infarction
  - —First-degree block and type I second-degree AV block may be associated with an inferior wall MI
  - —Type II second-degree AV block may be associated with an anterior wall MI
- Toxicologic
  - —Digoxin
  - —Beta-blockers
  - —Calcium channel blockers
  - —Amiodarone
  - —Procainamide
  - —Class 1C agents: propafenone, encainide, flecainide
  - —Clonidine
- Congenital
- Valvular heart disease
- Surgical trauma
- Increased vagal tone
- Infectious
  - —Syphilis
  - —Diphtheria
  - —Chagas' disease
  - —Tuberculosis
  - —Toxoplasmosis
  - —Lyme disease
  - —Myocarditis
  - —Endocarditis
  - —Rheumatic fever
- Collagen vascular diseases
- Infiltrative diseases
  - —Sarcoidosis
  - —Amyloidosis
  - —Hemachromatosis
- Cardiomyopathy
- Electrolyte disturbances
  - —Hyperkalemia
- Myxedema
- Hypothermia

PEDIATRIC CONSIDERATIONS

- Occurs in children, but is often asymptomatic
- Associated mortality is highest in the neonatal period
- Associated with:
  - —Congenitally acquired maternal antibodies
  - —Congenital heart disease
  - —Infectious etiologies, such as rheumatic fever or myocarditis

Pre-Hospital

- Transcutaneous pacing for unstable type II second-degree block or third-degree block

CAUTIONS

- Atropine
  - —Avoid with type II second-degree block because it may precipitate complete heart block
  - —Contraindicated in third-degree heart block with a widened QRS complex
- Attempts should be made at preventing increases in vagal tone

Diagnosis

ESSENTIAL WORKUP

- A 12-lead EKG to determine the type of block and identify evidence of infarction or drug toxicity
  - —First-degree AV block
    - -PR interval >0.20 seconds
  - —Second-degree AV block
    - -Type I: progressive prolongation of PR interval until there is a nonconducted P wave and a dropped QRS; occurs in repeated cycles; QRS is usually narrow
    - -Type II: PR interval remains constant; atrial impulses are not conducted intermittently, giving the appearance of an occasionally dropped ventricular beat; QRS may be prolonged depending on the level of the lesion
  - —Third-degree AV block
    - -Complete electrical dissociation: atria and ventricles beat at separate, unrelated rates; constant PP and RR intervals with variable PR intervals
    - -QRS duration depends on the level of the pacemaker: pacemakers above the level of the His-Purkinje system result in narrow QRS complexes, pacemakers below this level produce wide QRS complexes

LABORATORY

- Electrolytes
- Calcium, magnesium
- Cardiac enzymes
  - —Especially for type II second-degree and third-degree blocks
- Digoxin level

IMAGING/SPECIAL TESTS

- Chest radiograph
  - —May identify cardiomyopathy or congestive heart failure
- Echocardiogram
  - —May identify regional wall motion abnormalities or valvular dysfunction

DIFFERENTIAL DIAGNOSIS

- Accelerated junctional rhythm
- Idioventricular rhythm
- Sinus bradycardia

Treatment

INITIAL STABILIZATION

- Transcutaneous pacemaker
  - —Profound bradycardia and chest pain
  - —Shortness of breath
  - —Hypotension
  - —Mild sedation is recommended beforehand
- Atropine
  - —Complete heart block and narrow QRS
  - —If symptomatic bradycardia

ED TREATMENT

- First-degree AV block
  - —No treatment required
  - —Close monitoring to ensure it does not progress to higher level AV block
  - —Evaluate for associated MI, electrolyte abnormalities, medication excess
- Type I second-degree AV block
  - —Usually no treatment needed
  - —If symptomatic, atropine will enhance AV conduction
- Type II second-degree AV block
  - —Temporary transcutaneous or transvenous pacemaker
  - —Atropine and isoproterenol are not effective
- Third-degree AV block
  - —May transiently respond to atropine
  - —Emergent pacemaker
  - —Digoxin-specific antibodies
    - -Digoxin overdose with a complete heart block
  - —Glucagon
    - -If beta-blocker or calcium channel overdose
  - —Calcium
    - -If calcium channel blocker overdose

MEDICATIONS

- Atropine: 0.5–1.0 mg i.v. every 5 minutes as necessary
- Calcium chloride: 250–500 mg (2.5–5 cc) i.v.
- Glucagon: 5–10 mg i.v. over 5 minutes
- Isoproterenol: begin infusion at 2 μg/min and titrate to a max 10 μg/min
- Digoxin-specific antibodies:
  - —Serum level × weight (kg) = number of vials to be administered

PEDIATRIC CONSIDERATIONS

- Atropine: 0.01–0.03 mg/kg i.v./ETT
- Calcium chloride: 20 mg/kg i.v.
- Glucagon: 50 μg/kg i.v. over 5 minutes
- Isoproterenol: begin infusion at 0.1 μg/kg/min and titrate to a max of 1.5 μg/kg/min
- Digoxin-specific antibodies:
- Serum level × weight (kg) = number of vials to be administered

Disposition

ADMISSION CRITERIA

- Monitored bed
  - —Type II second-degree block
  - —Third-degree block

DISCHARGE CRITERIA

- Asymptomatic first-degree and type I second-degree blocks
- Assure follow-up for further outpatient workup

Miscellaneous

ICD9: 426.0, 426.1

ICD10: I44.3

SUGGESTED READINGS

Barold SS, Serge S, Hayes DL. Second-degree atrioventricular block: a reappraisal. Mayo Clin Proc 2001; 76(1):44–57.

Brady WJ, Harrigan RA. Diagnosis and management of bradycardia and atrioventricular block associated with acute coronary ischemia. Emerg Med Clin North Am 2001;19:371–384.

Haushik V, Leon A, Forrester JS, et al. Bradyarrhythmias, temporary and permanent pacing. Crit Care Med 2001;28(10):N121–N128.

Olgin JE, Zipes DP. Specific arrhythmias: diagnosis and treatment. In: Brunwald E, ed. Heart disease: a textbook of cardiovascular medicine, 6th ed. Philadelphia: WB Saunders, 2001:872–876.

Authors: Colleen N. Roche; James Scott

Babesiosis

Clinical Presentation

SIGNS AND SYMPTOMS

- Common symptoms
  - —Fatigue, malaise, weakness
  - —Fever
  - —Shaking chills
  - —Diaphoresis
  - —Nausea, anorexia
- Less common symptoms
  - —Headache
  - —Myalgias
  - —Cough
  - —Weight loss
  - —Arthralgias
  - —Abdominal pain
  - —Shortness of breath
  - —Light-headedness, dizziness
  - —Vomiting
  - —Dark urine
  - —Rash
  - —Diarrhea
- Physical findings
  - —May be normal
  - —Fever
  - —Relative bradycardia
  - —Jaundice
  - —Heart murmur
  - —Hepatosplenomegaly
  - —Rash uncommon
- Petechial or purpuric rash may be seen with severe thrombocytopenia
- Erythema migrans may represent concurrent Lyme disease
- More severe disease tends to occur in immunocompromised patients (splenectomy, HIV, immunosuppressive therapy), and patients older than 50 years
- Severe hemolytic anemia
  - —CHF, pulmonary edema
  - —ARDS
  - —Renal insufficiency
  - —Shock
  - —Myocardial infarction
  - —Disseminated intravascular coagulation (DIC)
- Asymptomatic infection is common
  - —Seroprevalence rates of 4–7% among blood donors in endemic areas

DESCRIPTION/ETIOLOGY/MECHANISM

- Malaria-like illness characterized by fever, hemolysis, and hemoglobinuria
- Caused by intraerythrocytic parasitic infection by protozoa of the genus *Babesia*
- Zoonotic disease requiring transmission from animal reservoir to humans via a tick vector
  - —Most common animal reservoir in U.S. is white-footed mouse *(Peromyscus leucopus)*; tick vector is deer tick *(Ixodes scapularis)*
  - —Three developmental stages of tick (larva, nymph, adult): each requires blood meal to mature to next stage; all stages can transmit disease; nymph is primary vector in humans
  - —Engorged nymph only 2 mm in diameter; most patients do not recall a tick bite
  - —Peak period of clinical infection (June through August) corresponds with nymph feeding period
  - —Most common in northeast coastal region of the U.S., although cases have also been reported from midwest and western regions of the U.S., Europe, Asia, Africa, and South America
  - —*I. scapularis* also vector for Lyme disease, possibly ehrlichiosis: up to 25% of patients with babesiosis co-infected with Lyme disease *(Borrelia burgdorferi)*; concurrent ehrlichiosis reported in babesiosis patients
- Protozoa pass from tick salivary glands to mammalian bloodstream; erythrocytes are penetrated and infected
  - —Parasites mature inside RBCs; divide into daughter cells
  - —Infected RBCs become less deformable predisposing to capillary blockage with lung, renal, liver, and spleen involvement; infected cells also more easily cleared by spleen; thus, more mild disease if spleen intact
  - —As parasites exit erythrocyte, membrane is damaged (perforations, protrusions, and inclusions), leading to hemolysis and hemoglobinuria
- Clinical presentation varies by region
  - —North American (most common): mild or subclinical disease, may be self-limited, rodent strain *(Babesia microti)*, 95% of patients with intact spleens
  - —European (less common): fulminant disease, frequently fatal, bovine strain *(Babesia divergens)*, 80% of patients s/p splenectomy
- Incubation period: 1–4 weeks after tick bite; 6–9 weeks after transfusion
- Mortality among hospitalized patients in U.S. reported to be 6.5%
- When left untreated, silent babesial infection may persist for months or even years
- Many case reports of transmission via PRBC/platelets; risk of transmission via PRBCs reported to be 0.17% in endemic areas

PEDIATRIC CONSIDERATIONS

- Transplacental and/or perinatal transmission of the disease has been described

Pre-Hospital

CAUTIONS/CONTROVERSIES

- Acute respiratory failure, shock, and myocardial infarction reported as complications of babesiosis
  - —Ensure a patent airway
  - —Provide supplemental oxygen and ventilatory assistance as needed
  - —If patient appears to be in shock, establish IV access and administer a fluid bolus of 0.9% NS 500 mL (peds: 20 mL/kg) i.v.

Diagnosis

ESSENTIAL WORKUP

- Consider in any febrile patient from an endemic area during tick season, and as part of differential diagnosis of posttransfusion infections, especially in endemic regions
- Microscopic examination of Giemsa- or Wright-stained thick and thin peripheral blood smears
  - —Parasites within RBCs vary in appearance and can be round, oval, or pear shaped
  - —Most common appearance is round (ring forms) to oval (pyriform) rings with pale blue cytoplasm and red-staining nucleus; extracellular parasites may also be seen
  - —Parasites in budding tetrad formation (Maltese cross) are highly suggestive of babesiosis but are a rare finding
  - —Malaria may be excluded by absence of intracellular brownish pigment granules (hemozoin) and synchronous stages (schizonts and gametocytes)
  - —Level of parasitemia can range from <1% to >85%; higher levels more common in splenectomized patients
  - —With low-level parasitemia, examination of multiple smears over several days may be necessary to make diagnosis

LABORATORY

- Serologic testing for other concurrent tick-borne diseases (Lyme disease, ehrlichiosis)
- CBC (anemia, thrombocytopenia, mild leukopenia, atypical lymphocytosis)
- Elevated ESR
- Elevated reticulocyte count
- Decreased serum haptoglobin
- Urinalysis (hemoglobinuria, proteinuria)
- Liver function studies (elevated bilirubin, serum LDH, alkaline phosphatase, transaminases)
- Blood and urine cultures if presentation consistent with sepsis
- CSF analysis if presentation suggestive of CNS infection

IMAGING/SPECIAL TESTS

- Indirect immunofluorescent antibody assay
  - —Serum antibody titer usually rises within a few weeks of infection; falls off slowly over months
  - —Titers of 1:256 or more are indicative of active infections; most patients develop titers of 1:1,024 or more within a few weeks
  - —Titers of 1:32 or lower indicate prior infection
- PCR-based diagnostic assay may be useful in detecting early cases with very low levels of parasitemia
- Chest radiograph indicated for respiratory complaints or evidence of hypoxia
- EKG indicated for ischemic symptoms

DIFFERENTIAL DIAGNOSIS

- Malaria
- Other tick-borne diseases
  - —Lyme disease
  - —Ehrlichiosis
  - —Rocky Mountain spotted fever
  - —Colorado tick fever
  - —Q fever
  - —Tularemia
  - —Relapsing fever
- Typhoid fever

Treatment

INITIAL STABILIZATION

- ABCs
- Pulse oximetry: hypoxia may be present in patients with severe disease
- Airway management, ventilatory support for patients with acute respiratory failure
- Intravenous access should be established in patients with evidence of or risk factors for severe disease
- Intravenous fluids; pressor support for patients in shock

ED TREATMENT

- Institute antibiotic therapy in patients with significant symptoms, especially if immunocompromised, s/p splenectomy or elderly
  - —Combination therapy with clindamycin PLUS quinine is the standard of care, but adverse effects or treatment failure may limit use
  - —Combination therapy with atovaquone PLUS azithromycin has comparable efficacy to clindamycin-quinine (65% vs. 73%) with fewer adverse effects (12% vs. 67%) and may be used as an alternative
- Consider admission for exchange transfusion (two to three blood volumes) as adjunctive therapy to rapidly reduce level of parasitemia and remove toxic erythrocyte, babesial, or macrophage-produced factors in patients with severe symptoms of or risk factors for severe disease:
  - —Immunodeficiency (f.ex. HIV)
  - —S/p splenectomy
  - —Severe hemolysis
  - —*B. divergens* infection
  - —High-level parasitemia (>10%)
- Consider antibiotic therapy in confirmed cases, even if mild or asymptomatic, due to risk of transmission via blood transfusion and/or recrudescence, particularly if subsequent splenectomy or immunosuppression occurs
- Hemodialysis may be indicated for patients with acute renal failure
- Treat fever with antipyretics

MEDICATIONS

- Acetaminophen: 325–1,000 mg (peds: 40–60 mg/kg/24 hr) PO/PR q4–6h PRN
- Atovaquone: 750 mg (peds: 40 mg/kg/24 hr) PO b.i.d. × 7 days
- Azithromycin: 500 mg (peds: 10 mg/kg up to max 500 mg) PO on day 1, followed by 250 mg (peds: 5 mg/kg up to max 250 mg) PO q.d. × 6 days
- Clindamycin: 300–600 mg (peds: 20 mg/kg/24 hr) i.v./i.m. q6h × 7–10 days
- Ibuprofen: 200–400 mg (peds: 20–40 mg/kg/24 hr) PO q6–8h PRN
- Quinine: 650 mg (peds: 25 mg/kg/24 hr) PO q8h × 7–10 days
  - —Quinine is contraindicated in pregnancy

Disposition

ADMISSION CRITERIA

- Patients requiring exchange transfusion
- Patients with severe disease
  - —Severe, symptomatic anemia
  - —Jaundice
  - —Renal insufficiency
  - —Respiratory distress
  - —DIC
  - —Shock
- Patients at risk of developing severe disease
  - —Immunodeficiency (e.g., HIV)
  - —S/p splenectomy
  - —*B. divergens* infection
  - —High-level parasitemia (>10%)

DISCHARGE CRITERIA

- Patients with asymptomatic or mild disease
- Intact spleen

Miscellaneous

ICD9: 08882

ICD10: B60.0

SUGGESTED READINGS

Boustani MR, Gelfand JA. Babesiosis. Clin Infect Dis 1996;22:611–615.

Boustani MR, Lepore TJ, Gelfand JA, et al. Acute respiratory failure in patients treated for babesiosis. Am J Respir Crit Care Med 1994;149:1689–1691.

Dacey MJ, Martinez H, Raimondo T, et al. Septic shock due to babesiosis. Clin Infect Dis 2001;33:E37–E38.

Dobroszycki J, Herwaldt BL, Boctor F, et al. A cluster of transfusion-associated babesiosis cases traced to a single asymptomatic donor. JAMA 1999;281:927–930.

Dorman SE, Cannon ME, Telford SR III, et al. Fulminant babesiosis treated with clindamycin, quinine, and whole-blood exchange transfusion. Transfusion 2000;40:375–380.

Homer MJ, Aguilar-Delfin I, Telford SR III, et al. Babesiosis. Clin Microbiol Rev 2000;13:451–469.

Krause PJ, Lepore T, Sikand VK, et al. Atovaquone and azithromycin for the treatment of babesiosis. N Engl J Med 2000;343:1454–1458.

Krause PJ, Spielman A, Telford SR III, et al. Persistent parasitemia after acute babesiosis. N Engl J Med 1998;339:160–165.

McQuiston JH, Childs JE, Chamberland ME, et al. Transmission of tick-borne agents of disease by blood transfusion: a review of known and potential risks in the United States. Transfusion 2000;40:274–284.

White DJ, Talarico J, Chang HG, et al. Human babesiosis in New York State: review of 139 hospitalized cases and analysis of prognostic factors. Arch Intern Med 1998;158:2149–2154.

Author: Philip Anderson

Back Pain

Clinical Presentation

SIGNS AND SYMPTOMS

- Musculoligamentous
  - —Poorly localized and dull back/gluteal pain without radiation past the knee
  - —Usually there are no objective neurologic signs
  - —Back spasm is a variable and poorly reproducible finding
- Sciatica
  - —Sharp, shooting, well-localized pain
  - —Leg complaints often greater than back
  - —May present with
    - -Asymmetric deep tendon reflexes
    - -Decreased sensation in a dermatomal distribution
    - -Objective weakness
- Massive central disc herniation (cauda equina syndrome)
  - —Decreased perineal sensation
  - —Urinary retention
  - —Fecal incontinence
- Infectious processes
  - —Fever
  - —Localized percussion tenderness of the vertebral bodies
- Bony lesion
  - —Continuous pain that does not change with rest
  - —Constitutional symptoms
- Vascular etiology
  - —Severe, often "ripping or tearing" pain
  - —May be associated with cold or insensate extremities

MECHANISM/DESCRIPTION

- Low back pain (LBP)
  - —Refers to pain in the area between the lower rib cage and the gluteal folds, often with radiation into the thighs
- Sciatica
  - —Pain in the distribution of the lower lumbar spinal roots
  - —Often accompanied by neurosensory and motor deficits
- Pain classification
  - —Acute if 0–6 weeks
  - —Subacute if 6–12 weeks
  - —Chronic if >12 weeks

ETIOLOGY

- Nonspecific musculoligamentous source (great majority)
- Herniation of the nucleus pulposus
- Degenerative joints or discs
- Spinal stenosis
- Anatomic abnormalities—especially spondylolisthesis
- Fractures from trauma and osteoporosis
- Underlying systemic diseases
  - —Neoplasm
  - —Infections
  - —Vascular
    - -Aneurysmal
    - -Dissection
  - —Renal

Pre-Hospital

CAUTIONS

- Trauma patients with acute back pain should be immobilized on a backboard until an unstable fracture can be ruled out
- Rapid transport with IV access for any patient with concerns of vascular etiology

Diagnosis

ESSENTIAL WORKUP

- Thorough history and physical including detailed neurologic and vascular examination
- No specific tests are needed for uncomplicated musculoligamentous or sciatic pain without complicating factors
- Rapid diagnostic testing and vascular consultation for pain concerning aortic etiology

LABORATORY

- Urinalysis for suspected
  - —Urinary tract infection
  - —Pyelonephritis
  - —Prostatitis
- ESR
  - —Very sensitive, though nonspecific for infectious etiologies
  - —Used for screening if suspicion exists

IMAGING/SPECIAL TESTS

- Lumbosacral radiograph
  - —Significant trauma
  - —Age older than 50 years
  - —History or signs/symptoms of cancer
  - —Fever
  - —IV drug user
  - —Pain at rest
  - —Suspicion of ankylosing spondylitis
  - —Pain that does improve after 4 weeks
- MRI
  - —Suspicion of abscess
  - —Rapidly progressing neurologic symptoms or urinary retention or fecal incontinence associated with back pain
- Abdominal CT or bedside US
  - —Suspicion of abdominal aortic aneurysm (AAA)
- Chest CT or TEE
  - —Suspicion of aortic dissection or aneurysm

DIFFERENTIAL DIAGNOSIS

- Spinal origins
  - —Musculoligamentous
  - —Discogenic
  - —Fracture
  - —Spondylolisthesis
  - —Ankylosing spondylitis
  - —Osteomyelitis
  - —Epidural abscess/hematoma
  - —Neoplasm
- Nonspinal causes
  - —AAA
  - —Prostatitis
  - —Upper urinary tract infection
  - —Abdominal neoplasm
  - —Renal colic
  - —Aortic dissection

Treatment

INITIAL STABILIZATION

- IV fluid/blood products resuscitation if hypotension/leaking AAA
- Heart rate, then BP, control for aortic dissection

ED TREATMENT

- Acute uncomplicated back pain
  - —*Short course* of bed rest: 24–48 hours followed by early mobilization
  - —Return to regular activity within limits

MEDICATIONS

- NSAIDs for musculoligamentous pain, renal colic
  - —Treatment of choice
  - —No agent has definitive benefits over others
  - —Recommend using cost and dosing schedules as guide
- Muscle relaxants helpful in LBP
  - —Cyclobenzaprine
  - —Metaxalone
  - —Methocarbamol
- Limited course of narcotic analgesics for severe pain not relieved by antiinflammatory agents or renal colic
- Spinal manipulation
  - —A short course (<2 weeks) may be helpful in acute LBP without sciatica
- Physical therapy/exercise
  - —No clear consensus for indications
  - —May be helpful in preventing further episodes
- Expected recovery to pain-free state
  - —33%: within 1 week
  - —75%: within 3 weeks
  - —90%: within 2 months
- ED management of aortic dissection geared toward preventing progression of the dissection
- Reducing the pressure gradient or the force of contraction (dP/dt), by controlling the heart rate and mean arterial blood pressure
- Initial control of heart rate with β-blockade followed by control of mean arterial pressure with sodium nitroprusside or combination therapy with labetalol

MEDICATIONS

Pain Control

- Acetaminophen: 650–1,000 mg PO q4–6h
- Cyclobenzaprine: 10 mg PO t.i.d.
- Hydrocodone/acetaminophen: 5/500 mg PO q4–6h
- Ibuprofen: 600–800 mg PO q6–8h
- Metaxalone: 800 mg PO q6–8h
- Methocarbamol: 1,000–1,500 mg PO q6h
- Naproxen: 250–500 mg PO q12h
- Oxycodone/acetaminophen: 5/500 mg PO q4–6h

BLOOD PRESSURE/HEART RATE CONTROL

- Esmolol: 500 μg/kg followed by an infusion of 50–200 μg/kg/min
- Labetalol: has both α-blocking and β-blocking activity and can be used as monotherapy; 20 mg i.v. bolus every 5–10 minutes, incrementally increased to 80 mg until heart rate of 60–80 beats/min has been reached or a total of 300 mg is given
- Sodium nitroprusside: 0.3–10 μg/kg/min titrate to BP of 100–120 systolic

Disposition

ADMISSION CRITERIA

- Severe pain with inability to ambulate
- Progressive neurologic deficits
- Signs of cauda equina syndrome
- Evidence of infectious, vascular, or neoplastic etiologies

DISCHARGE CRITERIA

- Uncomplicated presentation with ability to control pain and ambulate

Miscellaneous

ICD9: 724.2

ICD10: M59.9

SUGGESTED READINGS

Brody M. Low back pain. Ann Emerg Med 1996;27(4):454–456.

Deyo RA, Rainville J, Kent DL. What can the history and physical tell us about low back pain? JAMA 1992;268:760–765.

Frymoyer JW. Back pain and sciatica. N Engl J Med 1988;318:291–299.

Hagan PG, Nienaber MB, Christoph A, et al. The International Registry of Acute Aortic Dissection (IRAD): new insights into an old disease. JAMA 2000;283(7):897–903.

Malmivaara A, Hakkinen U, Aro T, et al. The treatment of acute low back pain—bed rest, exercises, or ordinary activity? N Engl J Med 1995;332:351–355.

Author: Eric Legome

Bacterial Tracheitis

Clinical Presentation

SIGNS AND SYMPTOMS

- Usually preceding viral infection with acute change in course of illness
- General
  - —Toxic appearance
  - —Fever
  - —Hoarseness
  - —Sore throat/neck pain
  - —Dysphonia
    - -Drooling uncommon
- Respiratory
  - —Respiratory distress
  - —Cyanosis
  - —Dyspnea
  - —Inspiratory/expiratory stridor
  - —Retractions
  - —Nasal flaring
  - —Barking/brassy cough
  - —Wheezing/rhonchi
- Complications
  - —Respiratory
    - -Airway obstruction
    - -Subglottic stenosis
    - -Pulmonary edema
    - -Pneumothorax
    - -ARDS
    - -ETT plugging
  - —Infection
    - -Septic shock
    - -Toxic shock syndrome
    - -Pneumonia
    - -Retropharyngeal cellulitis
  - —Cardiopulmonary arrest

MECHANISM/DESCRIPTION

- Usually secondary bacterial infection of damaged trachea from an antecedent viral infection or instrumentation
- Potentially fatal (0–20% mortality rate)
- Tracheal membrane formation, purulent discharge, subglottic edema, erosions, with normal epiglottis
- Classically acute in onset, may be gradual
- Slight male predominance
- Mean age 5 years; rarely occurs in adults
- Recently more common than epiglottitis presumably due to success of *Haemophilus influenzae* immunization
- More frequent August through December

ETIOLOGY

- *Staphylococcus aureus*
- *Moraxella catarrhalis*
- *Streptococcus pneumoniae*
- *Haemophilus influenzae* type B
- Group A streptococcal species
- Anaerobes
- *Klebsiella pneumoniae*
- *Pseudomonas aeruginosa*
- Nocardia
- Associated with influenza A and parainfluenza
- Aspergillus, HSV in immunocompromised hosts (HIV)

Pre-Hospital

- Assess airway/breathing
  - —Supplemental oxygen
  - —Racemic epinephrine aerosol if easily tolerated
  - —Reassurance; avoid agitating child
- Bag-valve-mask (BVM) ventilation if in respiratory failure
- Intubate if unable to maintain airway
- Immediate transport
- Notify receiving ED of airway status

Diagnosis

ESSENTIAL WORKUP

- Clinical assessment and management of airway takes priority over diagnostic workup; secure airway, optimally in OR under controlled conditions
- Ensure adequate oxygenation before proceeding
  - —Pulse oximetry

LABORATORY

- WBC variably elevated
- Blood cultures usually negative
- Request tracheal cultures from endoscopist/surgeon

IMAGING/SPECIAL TESTS

- Flexible fiberoptic laryngoscopy
  - —Permits direct visualization of epiglottis
  - —Mucosal edema
  - —Subglottic edema, secretions, membrane
- Bronchoscopy
  - —Direct visualization of trachea
  - —Laryngotracheal inflammation and erosions
  - —Mucopurulent secretions
  - —Membranes
  - —Therapeutic stripping of membranes
  - —Enables direct culture of material
- Radiographs of neck soft tissue
  - —Do in ED, if done; accompany at all times
  - —Intratracheal membranes
  - —Tracheal margin irregularities
  - —Subglottic narrowing
  - —Clouding of tracheal air column
  - —Irregular intratracheal densities
  - —Normal epiglottis

DIFFERENTIAL DIAGNOSIS

- Infection
  - —Epiglottitis
  - —Croup
  - —Peritonsillar abscess
  - —Retropharyngeal abscess
  - —Uvulitis
  - —Laryngeal diphtheria
- Angioedema
- Intraluminal obstruction
  - —Foreign body aspiration
- Caustic ingestion
- Trauma

Treatment

ED TREATMENT

- Airway management
  - —Anticipate difficult airway
  - —Intubation required in 57–83%
  - —Intubation should ideally be performed in the OR with surgical airway backup
  - —Select an ETT one to two sizes smaller than usual for age/size
  - —Meticulous ETT care and suctioning
  - —If BVM ventilation needed, use appropriately sized mask with two-hand seal
  - —Supplemental oxygen
  - —Humidification
- Bronchoscopy if not rapidly deteriorating
  - —Assess need for intubation
  - —Therapeutic stripping of membranes
- IV antibiotics to cover typical pathogens
  - —Cefuroxime and nafcillin or vancomycin
  - —Clindamycin and chloramphenicol for penicillin-allergic patients

MEDICATIONS

- Cefuroxime: 50 mg/kg i.v.; max 3 g
- Chloramphenicol: 20 mg/kg i.v. loading dose
- Clindamycin: 10 mg/kg i.v.; max 1 g
- Nafcillin: 50 mg/kg i.v.; max 2 g
- Racemic epinephrine: 2.25% solution diluted 1:8 with water in doses of 2–4 mL via aerosol
- Vancomycin: 15 mg/kg i.v.; max 1 g

Disposition

ADMISSION CRITERIA

- All patients with suspected or documented bacterial tracheitis
  - —Admit to ICU
  - —Mean ICU length of stay is 2.8 days

DISCHARGE CRITERIA

- None

Miscellaneous

ICD9: 464.11, 464.10

ICD10: J04.1

SEE ALSO: EPIGLOTTIS, PEDIATRIC

SUGGESTED READINGS

Bernstein T, Brilli R, Jacobs B. Is bacterial tracheitis changing? A 14-month experience in a pediatric intensive care unit. Clin Infect Dis 1998;27:458–462

Britto J, Habibi P, Walters S, et al. Systemic complications associated with bacterial tracheitis. Arch Dis Child 1996;74:249–250.

Brook I. Aerobic and anaerobic microbiology of bacterial tracheitis in children. Pediatr Emerg Care 1997;13(1): 16–18.

Donnelly BW, McMillan JA, Weiner LB. Bacterial tracheitis: Report of eight new cases and review. Rev Infect Dis 1990;12:729–735.

Gallagher PG, Myer CM III. An approach to the diagnosis and treatment of membranous laryngotracheobronchitis in infants and children. Pediatr Emerg Care 1991;7(6):337–342.

Author: Gary Bubly

Barbiturates, Poisoning

Clinical Presentation

SIGNS AND SYMPTOMS

CNS

- Lethargy
- Slurred speech
- Incoordination
- Ataxia
- Coma (mimicking death)
- Loss of reflexes

Cardiovascular

- Hypotension
- Bradycardia (direct myocardial depressant)

Ophthalmologic

- Miosis (generally associated with deep coma)
- Nystagmus
- Disconjugate gaze

Other

- Respiratory depression (inhibition of neurogenic respiratory drive)
- Hypothermia
- Bullae or "barb blisters" (not always present)

MECHANISM

- Increases γ-aminobutyric acid (GABA) activity
- Direct myocardial depression
- Inhibition of vascular smooth muscle

Pre-Hospital

CAUTIONS

- Moderate to severe poisonings require paramedic transport
- Intubation often necessary because of respiratory depression or loss of gag reflex
- Hypotension often requires IV fluids, inotropic support, and vasopressors

Diagnosis

ESSENTIAL WORKUP

- Obtain vital signs, check gag reflex, finger stick glucose
- Oxygen saturation monitor/ABG
- EKG/continuous cardiac monitoring
- Barbiturate poisoning can mimic death
  - —Cannot pronounce patient until barbiturate poisoning has been ruled out in patients in whom it is suspected

LABORATORY

- Electrolyte, BUN/Cr, glucose
  - —Patients down for a long period may be hyperkalemic from skeletal muscle breakdown and at risk of rhabdomyolysis
  - —To assess renal function, potassium, bicarbonate, calcium, magnesium
  - —Calculate anion gap
- Urinalysis
  - —For myoglobin
  - —Toxic alcohols, primidone can cause crystalluria
- CPK for rhabdomyolysis
- Urine toxicology screen
- Obtain serum phenobarbital level (if known or suspected)
- Acetaminophen and salicylate levels if suspected suicide
- CBC for other etiologies for altered mental status

IMAGING/SPECIAL TESTS

- CT scan of head for altered mental status
- CXR for aspiration
- Lumbar puncture for altered mental status workup
- Thyroid function tests

DIFFERENTIAL DIAGNOSIS

- Sedative-hypnotic poisoning (including toxic alcohols)
- Carbon monoxide poisoning
- CNS infections
- Space-occupying lesions of the head
- Hypoglycemia
- Uremia
- Electrolyte imbalance (i.e., hypermagnesemia)
- Postictal state following seizure
- Hypothyroidism
- Liver failure
- Psychiatric illness

Treatment

INITIAL STABILIZATION

- ABCs
  - —Administer supplemental oxygen
  - —Severe poisonings usually require endotracheal intubation
- 0.9% NS
  - —Hypotensive patients require 1–2 L i.v. fluid resuscitation and other IV medications
- Activated charcoal effectively binds barbiturates and may decrease systemic absorption

ED TREATMENT

- Administer one dose of activated charcoal
  - —Initiate "gut dialysis" with repeated dose activated charcoal (without sorbitol) given q2–4h (as long as bowel sounds are present)
- Rewarm patient if hypothermic (see hypothermia chapter)
- Treat hypotension resistant to IV fluid bolus with cardiac inotropic agents such as dopamine or dobutamine
- Trap phenobarbital ions in urine by administering sodium bicarbonate as an infusion to maintain blood pH at 7.45
- Treat hyperkalemia (from muscle breakdown) with calcium, sodium bicarbonate, insulin and glucose, and/or potassium-binding agents
- Consider hemodialysis if patient has
  - —Decreased or no renal function
  - —Prolonged coma
  - —Serum phenobarbital level >100 mg/dL
- Repeat phenobarbital level 2–4 hours after initial level if the patient is symptomatic or to determine whether level is increasing

MEDICATIONS

- Activated charcoal: 1 g/kg PO
- Dobutamine: 10 μg/kg/min titrating to desired effect (to max of 20 μg/kg/min)
- Dopamine: 5–10 μg/kg/min titrating to desired effect (to max of 20 μg/kg/min)
- Sodium bicarbonate
  - —Bolus: 1–3 ampules (44 mEq/ampule) i.v. over 20–30 minutes (peds: 1–2 mEq/kg/dose)
  - —1–2 ampules (45–50 mEq) in D5W 0.45% NS to achieve a blood pH of about 7.45 and maintain a good urine output (monitor serum potassium closely)

Disposition

ADMISSION CRITERIA

- ICU admission for
  - —Ataxia
  - —Drowsiness
  - —Coma
  - —Respiratory depression
  - —Hypotension
  - —Hypothermia
  - —Rhabdomyolysis

DISCHARGE CRITERIA

- Asymptomatic after minimum of 6 hours of observation with two consecutive subtoxic phenobarbital levels (if applicable) before discharge

Miscellaneous

ICD9: 967.0

ICD10: T42.3

SEE ALSO: BENZODIAZEPINE, POISONING; HYPOTHERMIA

SUGGESTED READINGS

Ellenhorn MJ, Schoonwald S, Ordog G, et al. Sedative-hypnotic drugs. In: Ellenhorn MJ, et al, eds. Ellenhorn's medical toxicology, 2nd ed. Baltimore: Williams & Wilkins, 1997:684–711.

Frenia ML, Schauben JL, Wears RL, et al. Multiple-dose activated charcoal compared to urinary alkalinization for the enhancement of phenobarbital elimination. J Toxicol Clin Toxicol 1996;34:169–175.

Osborn HH. Sedative-hypnotic agents. In: Goldfrank LR, et al, eds. Goldfrank's toxicologic emergencies, 6th ed. Stamford: Appleton & Lange, 1998:1001–1016.

Pond SM, Olson KR, Osterloh J, et al. Randomized study of the treatment of phenobarbital overdose with repeated doses of activated charcoal. JAMA 1984;251:3104–3108.

Schiebel N, Vilas I. Barbiturates. In: Ford MD, et al, eds. Clinical toxicology, 1st ed. Philadelphia: WB Saunders, 2001:569–574.

Authors: Sean Patrick Nordt; Richard F. Clark

Barotrauma

Clinical Presentation

SIGNS AND SYMPTOMS

- Middle ear (barotitis media)
  - —Begins as a clogged sensation
  - —Increasingly painful as the pressure differential increases across the tympanic membrane (TM)
  - —Progresses to rupture of the TM
  - —TM appearance
    - -Progresses from TM congestion to edema to hemorrhage to TM rupture
- External ear
  - —May result from tight-fitting hood, earplug or earwax occluding canal
  - —Auditory canal mucosa becomes edematous, then hemorrhagic, and ultimately tears
- Inner ear
  - —Sudden, severe vertigo
  - —Tinnitus
  - —Sensineural hearing loss in the affected ear
- Paranasal sinuses
  - —Sinus congestion
  - —Pain
  - —Epistaxis
- Facial
  - —Occlusive dive mask: conjunctival hemorrhage, facial edema, and swelling
- Extremities
  - —Tight-fitting dive suit: edema and erythema of the skin at locations of air pockets
- Teeth (barodontalgia)
  - —Severe tooth pain: possible air trapped in fillings
- GI (aerogastralgia)
  - —Excessive belching
  - —Flatulence
  - —Abdominal distention
- Pulmonary
  - —Dyspnea: "the chokes"
  - —Cough with a frothy red sputum
  - —Subcutaneous emphysema
  - —Delayed symptoms include bull neck appearance, dysphagia, changes in voice character

MECHANISM/DESCRIPTION

- Boyle law: at a constant temperature, pressure (P) is inversely related to volume (V)
  - —$PV = K$ (constant) or $P_1V_1 = P_2V_2$
  - —Increase of pressure mandates a reduction of volume by same factor
- Injury to body as result of the expansion and contraction of gas in an enclosed space
  - —Tissue damage when a gas-filled space does not equalize its pressure with external pressure
- Gas-filled cavities in the body are subject to expansion/contraction
  - —Lung
  - —Middle ear
  - —Sinus
- Solid and liquid-filled spaces distribute pressure equally
- Volume changes experienced during diver ascent are greatest in the few feet nearest the surface

ETIOLOGY

- Middle ear
  - —Barotrauma of descent
  - —Most common type of barotrauma
  - —Seen in 30% of inexperienced divers and 10% of experienced divers
  - —Inadequate equalization of pressure between the middle ear and external ear canal
  - —Eustachian tube provides sole route of pressure equalization for the middle ear
  - —Inadequate clearance via eustachian tube leads to increasingly negative pressure gradient across TM
- External ear
  - —Barotrauma of descent
  - —Pressure cannot equalize throughout the canal because of blockage and a relative intracanal vacuum is created as pressure differential across the obstruction increases
- Inner ear
  - —Barotrauma of descent
  - —Results from forceful attempts at equalizing middle ear pressure (Valsalva, Frenzel maneuvers)
  - —Increased middle ear pressure can raise intracranial pressure and cause rupture of the round or labyrinth windows, allowing perilymph to enter the middle ear
- Paranasal sinus
  - —Barotrauma of descent
  - —Nasal ostia act as a valve to regulate sinus pressure
  - —If the ostia fail to allow pressure equalization, congestion, edema, and hemorrhage can occur
- External objects
  - —Air pockets in dive suit/mask expand and contract
- Teeth
  - —Air trapped inside a filling
- GI
  - —Barotrauma of ascent
  - —Swallowed air in the GI tract expands as external pressure decreases
- Pulmonary barotrauma (PBT, or pulmonary overpressurization syndrome)
  - —Barotrauma of ascent
  - —Lungs expand against a closed glottis (breath-holding)
  - —Can lead to pulmonary rupture
  - —Potential arterial gas embolism (see gas embolism chapter)
  - —Divers with decreased lung compliance/increased lung volumes at increased risk (COPD, asthma)

Pre-Hospital

CAUTIONS

- For barotrauma of descent, unless an air-filled cavity has ruptured, no progression of the disease upon return to normal atmospheric pressure expected
- If patient transport requires air evacuation, maintain air cabin pressure at 1 atm or fly below 1,000 feet to avoid aggravating barotrauma

Diagnosis

ESSENTIAL WORKUP

- HEENT exam with particular attention paid to the TM and auditory canal to determine if rupture has occurred
- Pulmonary exam looking for signs of subcutaneous emphysema and pneumothorax
- Neurologic exam looking for signs of inner ear pathology

LABORATORY

- ABG for pulmonary symptoms

IMAGING/SPECIAL TESTS

- Sinus imaging
  —CT
  —Plain films
- CXR for pneumothorax
- Abdominal series (upright, decubitus) for free air from a ruptured viscus

DIFFERENTIAL DIAGNOSIS

- Decompression sickness
- Otitis media
- Otitis externa
- Sinusitis

Treatment

INITIAL STABILIZATION

- ABCs
  —100% oxygen for ill-appearing patients
  —Intubation for patients with subcutaneous emphysema of the neck
  —Immediate needle thoracostomy for evidence of tension pneumothorax

ED TREATMENT

- Establish IV access for unstable patients
- Control bleeding from the ear or nose
- Oral decongestants for middle ear or sinus congestion
- Antibiotics with TM or sinus rupture
- Analgesics

MEDICATIONS

- Amoxicillin: 250–500 mg (peds: 40 mg/kg/24 hr) PO t.i.d.
- Bactrim DS: 1 tablet (peds: 40/200 per 5–5 mL/10 kg/dose) PO b.i.d.
- Pseudoephedrine (Sudafed): 60 mg (peds: 6–12 years old, 30 mg; 2–5 years old, 15 mg/dose) PO q4–6h

Disposition

ADMISSION CRITERIA

- PBT
- Inner ear barotrauma with round window rupture or severe vertigo

DISCHARGE CRITERIA

- Most non-PBT
- ENT follow-up for severe TM or sinus pathology

Miscellaneous

ICD9: 993.2

ICD10: T70.2

SEE ALSO: ARTERIAL GAS EMBOLISM; DECOMPRESSION SICKNESS; HYPERBARIC OXYGEN

SUGGESTED READINGS

Becker GD, Parell GJ. Barotrauma of the ears and sinuses after scuba diving. Eur Arch Otorhino 2001;258(4):159–163.

Bradley ME. Pulmonary barotrauma. In: Bove AA, Davis JC. Diving medicine, 2nd ed. Philadelphia: WB Saunders, 1990:188–191.

Jerrard DA. Diving medicine. Emerg Med Clin North Am 1992;10(2):329–338.

Raymond LW. Pulmonary barotrauma and related events in divers. Chest 1995;107: 1648–1652.

Tetzlaff K, et al. Risk factors for pulmonary barotrauma in divers. Chest 1997;112(3): 654–659.

Author: Jeffrey Gordon

Bartholin's Abscess

Clinical Presentation

SIGNS AND SYMPTOMS

- Swollen, painful labia
- Tender, fluctuant mass on posterolateral margin of vestibule of vagina
- Warmth, erythema

DESCRIPTION

- Bartholin's glands are located inferiorly on either side of vaginal opening. Ducts open on sides of vestibule
- Obstruction of duct results in cyst, usually painless; infection of cyst results in abscess
- Most common in women aged 20–40 years

ETIOLOGY

- Anaerobic and aerobic microflora normally found in vagina, e.g., *Bacteroides* species, *Peptostreptococcus* species, *Escherichia coli*, other gram-negative organisms
- Occasionally *Neisseria gonorrhoeae* and *Chlamydia trachomatis*

Pre-Hospital

N/A

Diagnosis

ESSENTIAL WORKUP

- Diagnosis based on findings of tender, localized, fluctuant mass in region of Bartholin's gland

LABORATORY

- Culture material from abscess for GC and chlamydia
- Culture cervix for GC and chlamydia

DIFFERENTIAL DIAGNOSIS

- Bartholin's cyst
- Carcinoma of Bartholin's gland (rare)
- Perineal hernia

Treatment

ED MANAGEMENT

- Prompt incision and drainage (I&D) using local anesthesia in lithotomy position
- Narcotic analgesia for patient comfort
- Alternative approaches include
  —Simple I&D
  —Word catheter method
  —Marsupialization
- Antibiotics not necessary after I&D; if mild cellulitis is present or patient is immunocompromised, broad-spectrum coverage may be started; if STD suspected, treat with antibiotics
- Simple I&D
  —After local anesthesia, palpate abscess between thumb and index fingers; spread vulva apart and make stab incision on *mucosal* surface of abscess, parallel to hymenal ring
  —When incising abscess, two tissue layers must be penetrated; first labial mucosa and then abscess wall; free flow of pus indicates penetration of abscess wall
  —Pack wound with iodoform gauze
  —Follow up in 24–48 hours for removal of packing
  —Start sitz baths after 24 hours
  —Consider referral for marsupialization to avoid recurrence

- Word catheter method
  —Use small, inflatable, bulb-tipped Word catheter to treat abscess; may avoid recurrence and make marsupialization unnecessary
  —A stab wound is made as with simple I&D; it should be just large enough to easily admit catheter so that balloon does not fall out after inflation
  —After inserting bulb tip of catheter, inflate balloon by injecting 2–4 mL water using 25-gauge needle (to minimize size of puncture); overinflation may cause patient discomfort; this may be remedied by withdrawing some water from balloon
  —Sitz baths may be started after 24 hours
  —Follow up in 2–4 days
  —Leave catheter in place for 6–8 weeks until epithelialization is complete; after device is removed, gland resumes normal function; common for catheter to fall out prematurely; if this occurs, catheter may be reinserted or abscess can heal as with simple I&D
- Marsupialization
  —Procedure allows for a permanent fistula by suturing wound edges of abscess cavity to edges of labial mucosa; may be technically more challenging in ED and best reserved for specialist
  —Excise an ellipse of labial mucosa that overlays cyst cavity
  —I&D abscess
  —Evert edges of abscess and suture them to labial epithelium using absorbable suture such as polyglactin; opening will shrink but remain patent; packing is not needed
  —Start sitz baths in 24–48 hours
  —Follow up within 1 week

MEDICATIONS

Broad-spectrum Coverage

- Amoxicillin/clavulanic acid: 875 mg PO b.i.d. for 5 days with metronidazole 500 mg PO b.i.d. for 5 days
- Ciprofloxacin: 500 mg PO b.i.d. for 5 days with metronidazole 500 mg PO b.i.d. for 5 days

Disposition

ADMISSION CRITERIA

- Sepsis
- Significant cellulitis
- Evidence of necrotizing infection

DISCHARGE CRITERIA

- Nontoxic patients may be discharged with a designated follow-up plan

Miscellaneous

ICD9: 616.3

ICD10: N75.1

SUGGESTED READINGS

Aghajanian A. Bartholin's duct abscess and cyst: a case control study. South Med J 1994;87:26–29.

Brook I. Aerobic and anaerobic microbiology of Bartholin's abscess. Surg Gynecol Obstet 1989;169:32–34.

Van Bogaert LJ. Management of Bartholin's abscess. World Health Forum 1997;18(2): 200–201.

Word B. Office treatment of cyst and abscess of Bartholin's gland duct. South Med J 1968;61:514–518.

Authors: Marilyn Althoff; Mark Mandell

Bell's Palsy

Clinical Presentation

SIGNS AND SYMPTOMS

- Sudden onset of unilateral facial droop, incomplete eyelid closure, and loss of forehead muscle tone
  - —Maximal deficit by 5 days in almost all cases (2 days in 50%)
- If forehead muscle tone is *not* lost, a central lesion is strongly implied (i.e., this is *not* Bell's palsy)
- Tearing (68%) or dryness of the eye (16%) and less frequent blinking on the affected side
- Bell's phenomenon (upward rolling of the eye on attempted lid closure) may be seen
- Subjective "numbness" of the affected side, abnormal taste, drooling, hyperacusis (sensitivity to loud sounds)
- Fullness or pain behind mastoid
- Viral prodrome frequently reported

Pre-Hospital

MECHANISM/DESCRIPTION

- Bell's palsy refers to acute, *idiopathic* peripheral palsy of CN VII (facial nerve)
- Complete recovery in 85% of the cases without treatment
- Degree of deficit correlates with prognosis
  - —Complete lesions have the poorest prognosis
  - —Partial lesions almost always have excellent results
- Recovery usually begins within 2 weeks (often taste returns first) and is complete by 2–3 months
  - —Advanced age and slow recovery are poor prognosticators
- Affects men and women equally
- Age predominance between the third and fifth decade (may occur at any age)
- Incidence 15–40/100,000/year

ETIOLOGY

- Innervation to each side of the forehead is from both motor cortices; unilateral cortical processes do *not* completely disrupt motor activity of the forehead; therefore, only a peripheral or brainstem lesion can interrupt motor function of just one side of the forehead
- Idiopathic by definition, but a viral cause (particularly herpes simplex) suspected
- Lyme disease, infectious mononucleosis (Epstein-Barr virus [EBV] infection), varicella-zoster infections, and others may cause peripheral seventh nerve palsy
- Mechanism: edema and nerve degeneration within the stylomastoid foramen

Diagnosis

ESSENTIAL WORKUP

- Diagnosis is clinical and based on the history and physical exam
- Motor weakness isolated to the seventh nerve distribution and involves both the upper and the lower face
- An otherwise *normal* neurologic exam including all cranial nerves and extremity motor function

LABORATORY

- Not helpful in the diagnosis of Bell's palsy
- Lyme titers are useful when Lyme disease is suspected or in an endemic area
- Tests for mononucleosis (CBC, Monospot) if EBV infection suspected

IMAGING/SPECIAL TESTS

- Not helpful in the diagnosis of Bell's palsy; CNS imaging (CT, MRI) useful if CNS pathology is suspected

DIFFERENTIAL DIAGNOSIS

- Brainstem events (mass, bleed, infarct) affecting CN VII almost always involve CN VI (abnormal EOM) and may affect the long motor tracts
- Lyme disease: history of tick bite, erythema migrans rash, or endemic area
- Zoster (Ramsay-Hunt syndrome): look for herpetic vesicles, inquire about tinnitus or vertigo
- Infectious mononucleosis: look for pharyngitis, posterior cervical adenopathy
- Tumors: look for parotid, bone, or metastatic masses, acoustic neuroma (deafness)
- Trauma: skull fracture or penetrating facial injury may damage CN VII
- Middle ear or mastoid surgery or infection, cholesteatoma
- Meningeal infection
- Guillain-Barré syndrome: other neurologic deficits (e.g., ascending motor weakness or diminished DTRs) present
- Basilar artery aneurysm; other CN deficits should be present
- Bilateral peripheral CN VII palsy: consider multiple sclerosis, sarcoid, leukemia, and Guillain-Barré; idiopathic (Bell's) palsy may be bilateral in rare cases
- Bell's palsy may reoccur; treatment is unchanged

Treatment

INITIAL STABILIZATION

- Patients with an isolated peripheral CN VII palsy are stable

ED TREATMENT

- High-dose oral steroids may hasten recovery if started within 1 week of onset
  - —Complications of therapy are rare and treatment is recommended unless contraindicated
- Corneal damage may result from incomplete eyelid closure
  - —Lubricating and hydrating ophthalmic preparations and eyelid taping at night are *essential*
- Acyclovir with prednisone may be effective in improving functional nerve recovery
  - —Initiate within 72 hours of symptom onset
- Suspected Lyme disease should be treated with doxycycline or amoxicillin
- Surgical decompression may be indicated for complete lesions that do not improve; this is controversial

MEDICATIONS

- Acyclovir: 400 mg 5 times/day PO × 7 days (peds: no data to support its use)
- Lacri-Lube: q.h.s. and PRN; dryness/irritation in the affected eye (or equivalent)
- Prednisone: 30–40 mg PO b.i.d. (or 60 mg PO q.d.) × 5 days then taper over 5 days; total 10 days of therapy (peds: 2 mg/kg/day PO [max 60 mg])

Disposition

ADMISSION CRITERIA

- Isolated peripheral CN VII palsy does not require admission

DISCHARGE CRITERIA

- Isolated peripheral CN VII palsy may be treated on an outpatient basis
- Follow-up should be within 1 week

Miscellaneous

ICD9: 351.0

ICD10: G51.0

SUGGESTED READINGS

Adour K, et al. Bell's palsy treatment with acyclovir and prednisone compared with prednisone alone. Ann Otol Rhinol Laryngol 1996;105:371–378.

Austin JR, et al. Idiopathic facial nerve paralysis: a randomized double blind controlled study of placebo versus prednisone. Laryngoscope 1993;103: 1326–1333.

Grogan PM, et al. Practice parameter: steroids, acyclovir, and surgery for Bell's palsy (an evidence-based review). Neurology 2001;56(7):830–836.

Ramsey JR, et al. Corticosteroid treatment for idiopathic facial nerve paralysis: a meta-analysis. Laryngoscope 2000;110:335–341.

Authors: Robert F. McCormack; Richard S. Krause

Benzodiazepine, Poisoning

Clinical Presentation

SIGNS AND SYMPTOMS

- CNS
  —Sedation/drowsiness
  —Slurred speech
  —Coma
  —Delirium
  —Mid-position to small pupils
- Neuromuscular
  —Incoordination
  —Slowed voluntary movements
  —Ataxia
  —Hypotension
  —Hyporeflexia/areflexia
- Cardiovascular
  —Mild depression
  —Rare fatality
- Respiratory
  —Mild depression
  —Less depression versus barbiturates
  —Short acting and IV may produce depression
- GI
  —Nausea, vomiting, diarrhea
- Other
  —Hypothermia
  —Complications may include cerebral hypoxia, rhabdomyolysis, pressure-induced neuropathies
  —No long-term organ toxicity

MECHANISM

- Potentiates activity of γ-aminobutyric acid (GABA) (major inhibitory neurotransmitter) by binding to its own specific site
- Facilitates GABA binding to its site
- Results in chloride influx, membrane hyperpolarization, and inhibition of cellular excitation
- Pharmacologic profile
  —Highly protein bound
  —Large V_d
  —Hepatic metabolism
- Duration of action is inversely proportional to lipophilicity
  —Duration of lorazepam > diazepam > midazolam

Pre-Hospital

CAUTIONS

- Attention to airway and breathing
- Cardiac monitor
- IV access
- Rapid glucose determination
- Bring in pill bottles/pills in suspected overdose

Diagnosis

ESSENTIAL WORKUP

- Diagnosis based on
  —History of ingestion or recent injection
  —Clinical findings associated with CNS depression
  —No response to naloxone

LABORATORY

- Pulse oximetry
- Electrolytes, BUN, Cr, serum glucose
- UA for myoglobin when coma present
- Core body temperature
- ABG
- Qualitative urine screen
  —Confirms exposure many times but does not indicate or measure intoxication
  —False-negative test results reported
  —Qualitative immunoassays detect only benzodiazepines (BZs) that are metabolized to oxazepam
  —Those that do not produce this metabolite (clonazepam, lorazepam, midazolam, alprazolam) are not detected on the qualitative screen
  —Do not correlate with the clinical state
  —Serum levels not acutely practical
  —Clinical signs and symptoms more important than theoretic LD_{50} or serum levels
- Alcohol(s) level
- Barbiturate level
- Acetaminophen and salicylate levels
- Pregnancy test

IMAGING/SPECIAL TESTS

- EKG
- CXR for aspiration pneumonia

DIFFERENTIAL DIAGNOSIS

- Drugs and toxins causing decreased level of consciousness
  —Hypoglycemics
  —Other sedative-hypnotics (barbiturates)
  —Antidepressant-antipsychotic
  —Narcotics
  —Anticonvulsants
  —Carbon monoxide/cyanide
  —Alcohols
- Nontoxic medical condition
  —Hypoxemia
  —Hypothermia
  —Head trauma (intracranial bleeding)
  —Infection (meningitis or encephalitis)
  —Electrolyte and metabolic disturbances

Treatment

INITIAL STABILIZATION

- ABCs
  - —Secure airway and assist ventilation with supplemental oxygen to prevent hypoxemia and shock
  - —IV access with 0.9% NS
  - —Cardiac monitor
- Administer naloxone, thiamine, and dextrose if altered mental status

ED TREATMENT

- *Gastric emptying* (i.e., emesis, lavage): not necessary in pure BZ ingestion if activated charcoal (AC) is given promptly
- Gastric lavage considered only if presents within 1 hour of a life-threatening ingestion with protected airway
- AC PO or via NGT
- No role for diuresis, dialysis, or charcoal hemoperfusion
- Flumazenil (FZ)
  - —Competitive BZ-receptor inhibitor: rapidly reverses BZ-induced coma and respiratory depression
  - —Onset within 1–2 minutes; peak at 6–10 minutes; duration 1–2 hours (repeated dosing may be indicated)
  - —Efficacy dependent on the dose of BZ being antagonized and the dose of FZ used
  - —Do not administer empirically as part of any standard protocol therapy or in unknown poisoned patient
  - —Might help avert need of airway intubation
  - —May be beneficial in shortening hospital stay
  - —Indications include isolated BZ overdose in nonhabituated user
  - —Useful to reverse iatrogenic poisoning (conscious sedation)
  - —Contraindications include
    - -Co-ingestions that might lower seizure threshold (TCAs)
    - -Seizure activity
    - -Allergy
    - -Neuromuscular blockade
  - —Do not use if hypotension, hypoxia, dysrhythmias, or increased intracranial pressure
  - —May precipitate withdrawal state

MEDICATIONS

- AC: 1–2 g/kg PO/n.g. (ideal 10:1 ratio)
- Dextrose: D50W 1 ampule (50 mL or 25 g) (peds: D25W 2–4 mL/kg) i.v.
- FZ (Romazicon)
  - —Initial: 0.2 mg i.v. over 30 seconds (adult)
  - —If no response: 0.3 mg i.v. after 30 seconds
  - —If still no response: 0.5 mg i.v. and repeat every 1 minute if needed, to maximum dose of 3 mg
  - —Continuous infusion at 0.2–1.0 mg/hr if multiple repeated doses required to maintain response
  - —Peds: dosing not established, recommended starting dose is 0.01 mg/kg i.v., titrate to maximum dose of 1 mg, continuous infusion at 0.005–0.01 mg/kg/hr
- Naloxone (Narcan): 2 mg (peds: 0.1 mg/kg) i.v. or i.m. initial dose
- Thiamine (vitamin B_1): 100 mg i.v. or i.m.

Disposition

ADMISSION CRITERIA

- Persistent or profound CNS depression
- Cardiovascular or respiratory compromise
- Co-ingestants with potential delayed toxicity

DISCHARGE CRITERIA

- Discharge after 4–6-hour observation period if no signs or symptoms of BZ poisoning develop
- If FZ used, observe for additional 2–4 hours for recurrent sedation

Miscellaneous

ICD9: 969.4

ICD10: T42.4

SUGGESTED READINGS

Farrell SE. Benzodiazepines. In: Ford MD, Delaney KA, Ling LJ, et al, eds. Clinical toxicology. Philadelphia: WB Saunders, 2001.

Leikin J, Paloucek F. Benzodiazepines, qualitative, urine. In: Poisoning and toxicology handbook, Hudson, OH: Lexi-comp, 2002.

Osborn HH. Sedative-hypnotic agents. In: Goldfrank LR, ed. Goldfrank's toxicologic emergencies. Stamford, CT: Appleton & Lange, 1998.

Rasanan I, Ojanpera I, Vuori E. Quantitative screening for benzodiazepines in blood by dual-column gas chromatography and comparison of the results with urine immunoassay. J Anal Toxicol 2000; 24:46–53.

Spivey WH. Flumazenil and seizures: analysis of 43 cases. Clin Ther 1992; 14:292.

Spivey WH, Roberts JR, Derlet RW. A clinical trial of escalating doses of flumazenil for reversal of suspected benzodiazepine overdose in the emergency department. Ann Emerg Med 1993;22: 1813–1821.

Weinbroum A, et al. The use of flumazenil in the management of acute drug poisoning—a review. Intensive Care Med 1991;17:32–38.

Author: Sean Bryant

β-Blocker, Poisoning

Clinical Presentation

SIGNS AND SYMPTOMS

- Cardiovascular
  - —Hypotension
  - —Bradycardia
  - —Cardiac conduction delays
  - —Heart block
  - —Heart failure
  - —Electrical mechanical dissociation
- Neurologic
  - —Coma
  - —Seizures
- Pulmonary
  - —Bronchospasm
  - —Pulmonary edema
- Metabolic
  - —Hypoglycemia

MECHANISM

- Normal physiology
  - —Cardiovascular: β_1-receptors
    - -ATP converted to cAMP by adenyl cyclase with stimulation of β-receptors
    - -cAMP activates protein kinase, which phosphorylates proteins of the sarcoplasmic reticulum
    - -Sarcoplasmic reticulum releases calcium
    - -Excitation–contraction coupling occurs
- Effects of β-blockers
  - —Cardiovascular
    - -Decreased excitation/contraction
    - -Sodium channel blockade causes a prolongation of the QRS complex (with some agents)
    - -Prolongation of QTc interval leading to ventricular dysrhythmias (with some agents)
  - —Neurologic
    - -CNS effects with the lipophilic agents (propranolol, metoprolol, labetalol)

Pre-Hospital

CAUTIONS

- Transport pills and pill bottles when overdose suspected

Diagnosis

ESSENTIAL WORKUP

- With unknown ingestion: suspect β-blocker poisoning with bradycardia/hypotension
- EKG
  - —Conduction delays
  - —First-, second-, or third-degree heart block
  - —Bradycardia

LABORATORY

- CBC
- Electrolytes, BUN, Cr, glucose

DIFFERENTIAL DIAGNOSIS

- Calcium channel blocker toxicity
- Clonidine toxicity
- Digoxin toxicity
- Acute myocardial infarction with heart block

Treatment

INITIAL STABILIZATION

- ABCs
  - —Airway protection as indicated by mental status
  - —Supplemental oxygen as needed
  - —0.9% NS IV access
  - —Close hemodynamic monitoring
- Naloxone and thiamine if altered mental status
- Accucheck and treat hypoglycemia with D50W
- Treat prolonged seizures with benzodiazepines

ED TREATMENT

Goals

- Heart rate >60 beats/minute
- Systolic BP >90 mm Hg
- Adequate urine output
- Improving level of consciousness

GI Decontamination

- Syrup of ipecac is contraindicated in the emergency department
- Consider lavage with Ewald tube if ingestion within 1 hour
  - —Propranolol may cause esophageal spasm producing difficulty with passage and removal of gastric lavage tube
- Activated charcoal helpful especially in the presence of co-ingestants

Bradycardia/Hypotension

- Atropine
  - —Initial agent
  - —Low success rate
- Glucagon
  - —Administer if atropine does not increase heart rate
  - —Promotes cAMP production through a receptor site other than the β-receptor
  - —May cause nausea and vomiting
  - —Mix with NS or D5W
    - -Do not use the phenol diluent that comes with glucagon
- IV fluids
  - —Administer cautiously in the hypotensive patient
  - —Swan-Ganz catheter or CVP monitoring to help follow volume status
- Amrinone
  - —Use in conjunction with glucagon to treat symptomatic sustained bradycardia

- Pressor agents
  - —Initiate when symptomatic hypotension/bradycardia persists after atropine/glucagon
  - —Use invasive monitoring to help guide therapy
  - —Utility may be limited due to β-blockade: higher doses may be required
  - —Isoproterenol (nonselective β-agonist)
    - -Titrate for BP and heart rate
  - —Epinephrine (potent α- and β-receptor agonist)
    - -BP increases as a result of direct myocardial stimulation, increase in heart rate, and vasoconstriction
    - -Use if no BP response with isoproterenol
  - —High-dose dopamine
- Sodium bicarbonate
  - —In theory, this is used if there is evidence of prolongation of QRS >100 ms due to some of the β-blockers also causing sodium channel blockade leading to a prolonged QRS
  - —Not routinely administered for all β-blocker toxicities
- Electrical pacing: when other treatment options have failed
- Insulin
  - —Potential for treatment in the future

Enhanced Elimination

- Hemodialysis helpful with water-soluble β-blocking agents
  - —Nadolol
  - —Atenolol
  - —Sotalol

MEDICATIONS

- Activated charcoal: 1 g/kg PO
- Amrinone: loading dose 0.75 mg/kg; maintenance drip 2–20 μg/kg/min; titrate for effect
- Atropine: 0.5 mg (peds: 0.02 mg/kg) i.v.; repeat 0.5–1.0 mg i.v. (peds: 0.04 mg/kg)
- Dopamine: 2–20 μg/kg/min i.v.
- Dextrose: D50W 1 ampule (50 mL or 25 g) (peds: D25W 2–4 mL/kg) i.v.
- Epinephrine: 2 μg/min (peds: 0.1 μg/kg/min); titrate to effect
- Glucagon: 3.5–5 mg i.v. (peds: 0.03–0.1 mg/kg) bolus followed by 70-μg/kg/hr infusion
- Isoproterenol: 5 μg/min i.v. and titrate for heart rate effect
- Naloxone (Narcan): 2 mg (peds: 0.1 mg/kg) i.v. or i.m. initial dose
- Sodium bicarbonate: 1 mEq/kg IVP
- Thiamine (vitamin B_1): 100 mg (peds: 50 mg) i.v. or i.m.

Disposition

ADMISSION CRITERIA

- ICU admission for decreased level of consciousness or hemodynamic instability (bradycardia, conduction delays, hypotension)
- Observation and monitoring for 24 hours for long-acting or sustained-release preparations due to the potential delay in symptoms

DISCHARGE CRITERIA

- Asymptomatic 8–10 hours after ingestion of short- or immediate-release preparation

Miscellaneous

ICD9: 977.9

ICD10: T44.7

SUGGESTED READINGS

Kerns W, Kline J, Ford MD. β-Blocker and calcium channel blocker toxicity. Emerg Med Clin North Am 1994;12:365–390.

Kerns W, Schroeder D, Williams C, et al. Insulin improves survival in a canine model of acute beta-blocker toxicity. Ann Emerg Med 1997;29:748–757.

Love J. Acebutolol overdose resulting in fatalities. J Emerg Med 2000;18:341–344.

Love J, Howell J. Glucagon therapy in the treatment of symptomatic bradycardia. Ann Emerg Med 1997;29:181–183.

Author: Janet Eng

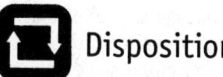

Bipolar Disorder

Clinical Presentation

SIGNS AND SYMPTOMS

- Appearance
  - —Hyperactive, if not agitated
  - —Talkative, often with loud, rapid or, "pressured" speech
- Affect
  - —Irritable
  - —Argumentative
  - —Often multiple recent arguments or fights
  - —Less commonly euphoric or expansive
  - —Often labile with depressed or tearful intervals (may confound diagnosis)
  - —Patient likely to describe mood as tense, irritable, or depressed rather than euphoric
- Neurovegetative
  - —Increased energy
  - —Engaged in multiple goal-directed activities many hours per day
  - —Feelings of energy
  - —Racing thoughts
  - —Decreased sleep
- Thought process
  - —Rapid, distractible, may be incoherent, delirious
- Thought content
  - —Psychosis possible
  - —Mood congruent (such as delusions of grandeur or power)
  - —Mood incongruent (may be indistinguishable from other psychotic disorders)
- Judgment
  - —Inflated self-esteem, perhaps to grandiose or psychotic extent
  - —Uncharacteristic, irresponsible behavior, such as financial or sexual indiscretions, with inability to recognize negative consequences of actions
  - —Substance abuse frequent during mania
- Sensorium
  - —Typically normal
  - —Confusion or delirium possible

MECHANISM/DESCRIPTION

- Mania
  - —Presentation is diverse, from simple irritability or cheerfulness to psychosis, delirium, or agitation, which may be difficult to recognize as mania
  - —Full extent of pathology often revealed only by outside informants
  - —Onset gradual or acute, duration several weeks or months, rarely chronic
- Hypomania
  - —Milder symptoms without marked impairment
- Mixed mood
  - —Simultaneous symptoms of mania and depression
  - —Treat in ED as for mania
- Bipolar (formerly *manic depressive*) disorder
  - —Defined as one or more episodes of hypomanic, manic, or mixed mood
  - —Possibly with episodes of depressed mood
  - —Typically beginning in the teens or twenties
  - —Episodes of abnormal mood may be mild or severe, brief or prolonged, infrequent or chronic, chiefly elevated or chiefly depressed in character
  - —Bipolar disorder may be readily treatment responsive or nearly intractable
- Schizoaffective disorder also characterized by episodes of altered mood, but psychotic features present even when mood is normal

Diagnosis

ESSENTIAL WORKUP

- Psychiatric history
  - —Recent symptoms of mania (often collateral sources critical)
  - —Past mania or depression
  - —Noncompliance with mood stabilizer
  - —Recent initiation or discontinuation of antidepressant may trigger elevated mood
  - —Recent substance abuse
  - —Bipolar family history
- Medical history
  - —Especially endocrine, metabolic, or neurologic disorders
  - —Particularly likely to be secondary to medical condition if first episode, age older than 40 years, atypical or mixed presentation, and abnormal sensorium
  - —Current or recent medications
- Physical and neurologic exam; vital signs
- Mania may present as delirium, and need workup of full differential diagnosis of delirium

LABORATORY

- Toxicologic screen (urine or serum)
- Electrolytes
- Blood glucose
- CBC
- TSH
- Lithium, carbamazepine, valproate serum levels if relevant
- Other tests as suggested by history or exam

IMAGING/SPECIAL TESTS

- Head imaging only with suspicion of neurologic etiology

DIFFERENTIAL DIAGNOSIS

- Primary mania of bipolar or schizoaffective disorder
- Psychosis
- Agitated depression
- Personality disorders (borderline, narcissistic, antisocial)
- Attention deficit disorder
- Conduct or intermittent explosive disorders
- Organic brain syndrome
- Intoxication or withdrawal from alcohol or sedative-hypnotics
- Intoxication with cocaine, amphetamines, or phencyclidine
- Accidental or deliberate toxic overdose
- Treatment with antidepressants or ECT in susceptible individuals
- Corticosteroid or thyroid hormones
- Anticholinergics
- Sympathomimetics
- Treatments of parkinsonism
- Cyclobenzaprine (Flexeril)
- Recent discontinuation of antidepressant medication
- Endocrine or metabolic disorders (particularly thyroid disease)
- Encephalitis
- Meningitis
- Postictal states
- Multiple sclerosis
- Post-CVA
- CNS tumors
- CNS vasculitis
- General paresis

Treatment

INITIAL STABILIZATION

- High violence potential
  - —Quiet environment
  - —Prompt evaluation
  - —Nonconfrontational manner
  - —Adequate security backup
  - —Physical restraint and sedation as needed
- For cooperative patient
  - —PO neuroleptics (e.g., haloperidol, consider chlorpromazine as alternate) or benzodiazepines (e.g., lorazepam)
- For severe agitation
  - —Synergistic combination of i.m., IV, or PO haloperidol and lorazepam
  - —Benztropine for prevention of acute dystonic reaction to haloperidol is not usually required when concurrent benzodiazepine is given
  - —Consider chlorpromazine i.m. as alternative

ED TREATMENT

Outpatient Management

- Consider neuroleptics for symptomatic treatment
- Agents for sleep
- Initiation or restart of mood stabilizer therapy
  - —Action of mood-stabilizing agents requires days or weeks, even after full serum level attained

Inpatient Management

- Consider sedation or initiation of mood stabilizer in consultation with admitting psychiatrist

MEDICATIONS

Acute Agitation

- Lorazepam: 2 mg PO (lower dose in mild agitation or in frail or elderly); may repeat every 30 minutes, generally not to exceed 12 mg/24 hr
- Haloperidol: 5 mg PO (lower dose in mild agitation or in frail or elderly); may repeat every 30 minutes, generally not to exceed 20 mg/24 hours (consider benztropine 1–2 mg PO b.i.d. prophylaxis of dystonic reaction, particularly in continued neuroleptic treatment without benzodiazepine or in patients with history of dystonia); consider chlorpromazine 50–100 mg PO as alternative to haloperidol
- Synergistic combination of haloperidol, 5–10 mg i.m./i.v./PO plus lorazepam 1–2 mg i.m./i.v./PO, repeat every 30 minutes as required (doses may be smaller in elderly or frail patients)
- Chlorpromazine: 50 mg i.m. may be useful alternative (lower dose in frail or elderly; avoid if hypotensive)

Typical Outpatient Medications

- Benztropine: 1 mg PO b.i.d.
- Carbamazepine: 400–2,000 mg/day (often in divided doses or in sustained release dose forms)
- Clonazepam: 0.5–2 mg PO q.h.s. or 0.5–2 mg PO b.i.d.
- Haloperidol: 0.5–5 mg PO b.i.d.
- Lithium: 600–3,000 mg/day (often in divided doses or in sustained release dose forms; in acute mania, initiate at 300 mg PO t.i.d.)
- Olanzapine: 1.25–30 mg/day, q.h.s. or in divided doses
- Perphenazine: 4–16 mg PO b.i.d.
- Risperidone: 0.5–3 mg PO b.i.d.
- Valproate (e.g., Depakote): 750–3,000 mg/day (often in divided doses; in acute mania, initiate at 250 mg PO t.i.d.)

Disposition

ADMISSION CRITERIA

- Involuntary hospitalization is required by danger to self
  - —Suicidal risk, especially if mixed or labile mood or psychotic
  - —Unsafe behaviors due to impaired judgment
  - —Medically unstable
  - —Hospitalization diagnostically required
- Involuntary hospitalization also required by
  - —Risk of behaviors dangerous to others or assaultiveness
  - —Inability to care for self (unable to obtain basic needs, such as food, clothing, or shelter)

DISCHARGE CRITERIA

- Patients with mild symptoms may be discharged on medications as above if
  - —Necessary supports to ensure safety
  - —Patient compliant with treatment plan
  - —Consultation with outpatient psychiatrist is available within 1–3 days
- Some patients who are not legally committable may refuse treatment
  - —Explain availability of treatment in future to patient and any involved friends or family

Miscellaneous

ICD9: 296.4, 296.5, 296.6, 296.7, 295.7

ICD10: F31.9

SUGGESTED READINGS

Allen MH, Currier GW, Hughes DH, et al. The Expert Consensus Guideline Series. Treatment of behavioral emergencies. Postgrad Med 2001;Spec No:1–88.

Muller-Oerlinghausen B, Berghofer A, Bauer M. Bipolar disorder. Lancet 2002; 359(9302):241–247.

Sachs GS. Bipolar mood disorders: practical strategies for acute and maintenance treatment. J Clin Psychopharmacol 1996;16[Suppl 1]:32S–47S.

Sachs GS, Printz DJ, Kahn DA, et al. The Expert Consensus Guideline Series: medication treatment of bipolar disorder 2000. Postgrad Med 2000;Spec No:1–104.

Authors: Paul H. Desan; Gary S. Sachs

Bite, Human

Clinical Presentation

SIGNS AND SYMPTOMS

- Third most common bite (after dogs and cats)
- Most bites (up to 75%) occur during aggressive acts
- 15–20% are related to sexual activity (love nips)
- Location
  - —Upper extremities (60–75%)
  - —Head and neck (15–20%)
  - —Trunk (10–20%)
  - —Lower extremities (about 5%)
- Two types of bites
  - —Occlusional bites: Laceration or crush injury to affected body part
  - —*Clenched-fist injuries* (CFIs) (most serious type): present as small wounds over metacarpophalangeal joints in dominant hand (fight bites)
- Frequent complications
  - —Cellulitis
  - —Serious deep-space infections (septic arthritis and osteomyelitis)
  - —Fractures and tendon injuries
  - —Hand bites have highest rates of infection

MECHANISM/DESCRIPTION

Occlusional Bites

- Occurs when human teeth bite into the skin
- Same risk of infection as other wounds

Clenched-fist Injuries

- Sustained from a clenched fist striking the mouth and teeth of another person
- With joint relaxation from the clenched position
  - —Puncture site sealed
  - —Oral bacteria inoculated in the anaerobic setting within the joint
- Bacterial inoculation carried by the tendons deeper into the potential spaces of the hand
  - —Increases chances for a more extensive infection

ETIOLOGY

- Aerobic and anaerobic organisms
  - —Most common
    - -*Streptococcus*
    - -*Staphylococcus*
  - —Anaerobes (about 50%)
    - -*Eikenella corrodens*
    - -*Haemophilus influenzae*
    - -*Neisseria* species
    - -*Corynebacterium*
- *E. corrodens* exhibits synergism with *Streptococcus, Staphylococcus aureus, Bacteroides,* and gram-negative organisms

PEDIATRIC CONSIDERATIONS

- Human bite marks rarely occur accidentally; good indicators of inflicted injury

Pre-Hospital

N/A

Diagnosis

ESSENTIAL WORKUP

History

- Time of injury
- Patient allergies
- Relevant medical history (immune status)
- Last tetanus shot

Physical Examination

- Record the location and extent of all injuries
- Document any swelling, crush injuries, or devitalized tissue
- Note the range of motion of affected areas
- Note the status of tendon and nerve function
- Document any signs of infection, including regional adenopathy
- Document any joint or bone involvement

LABORATORY

- Aerobic and anaerobic cultures from any infected bite wound
- Cultures not indicated if wounds not clinically infected

IMAGING/SPECIAL TESTS

- Plain radiograph indications
  - —Fracture
  - —Suspect foreign body, e.g., tooth
  - —Baseline film if a bone or joint space has been violated in evaluating for osteomyelitis
  - —For infection in proximity to a bone or joint space

DIFFERENTIAL DIAGNOSIS

- Bite injuries from animals
  - —Sharper teeth cause more punctures and lacerations than human teeth, which usually cause more crush-type injuries

PEDIATRIC CONSIDERATIONS

- In suspected sexual abuse
  - —Check for a central area of bruising or "hickey" from suction
- Linear abrasions or bruises on both the dorsal and palmar/plantar surfaces of the hand or foot
  - —Highly suggestive of bite marks
  - —Lesions on one extremity should prompt a search for lesions on the other extremities
- An intercanine distance of >3 cm indicates permanent dentition (present only if the attacker is older than 8 years)
- If abuse suspected
  - —Rub a saline-moistened swab in the wound to collect any saliva and then place in a paper envelope for analysis
  - —Obtain photographs

Treatment

INITIAL STABILIZATION

- ABCs: ensure patent airway and adequate peripheral tissue perfusion

ED TREATMENT

- Wound irrigation
  - —Copious volumes of NS with an 18-gauge needle or plastic catheter tip aimed in the direction of the puncture
  - —Care should be taken not to inject fluid into the tissues
- Débridement
  - —Remove any foreign material, necrotic skin tags, or devitalized tissues
  - —Do not débride puncture wounds
  - —Remove any eschar present so that underlying pus may be expressed and irrigated
- Closed-fist injuries
  - —Immobilize
  - —Splint in a position of function that maintains the maximal length of ligaments and intrinsic muscles
  - —Use a bulky hand dressing
  - —Consultation with hand surgeon regarding operative irrigation/exploration of wound
  - —Elevation for several days until any edema resolved
  - —Sling for outpatients
  - —Place the hand in a tubular stockinette attached to an IV pole for inpatients
- Do not perform primary repair of avulsion wounds
- Wound closure
  - —Do not suture infected wounds or wounds >24 hours after injury
  - —Repair of wounds >8 hours after bite: controversial
  - —Close facial wounds up to 24 hours after bit (warn patient of high risk of infection)
  - —Infected wounds and those presenting >24 hours should be left open
  - —May approximate the wound edges with Steri-Strips and perform a delayed primary closure
  - —Do not suture closed-first injuries
- Prophylactic antibiotics controversial for low-risk bites
- Antibiotics for outpatients with
  - —Moderate to severe injuries with crush injury or edema
  - —Involvement of the bone or a joint
  - —Hand bites
  - —Wounds near a prosthetic joint
  - —Underlying disease (diabetes, prior splenectomy, or immunosuppression) that increases the risk of developing a more serious infection
- Tetanus prophylaxis
- Refer for possible testing/surveillance for HIV infection

MEDICATIONS

- Amoxicillin/clavulanic acid (Augmentin): 500/125 mg (peds: 40 mg/kg/24 hr) q8h PO
- Cefoxitin (Mefoxin): 1–2 g (peds: 80–160 mg/kg/24 hr) q6h i.v.
- Ciprofloxacin (Cipro): 500–750 mg q12h PO or 400 mg q12h i.v.
  - —Poor anaerobic coverage
- Clindamycin (Cleocin): 150–450 mg (peds: 8–20 mg/kg/24 hr) PO q6h or 600–900 mg (peds: 20–40 mg/kg/24 hr) i.v. q8h
  - —No coverage against *E. corrodens*
- Dicloxacillin (Pathocil): 500 mg (peds: 50 mg/kg/24 hr) PO q6h
- Penicillin (Penicillin VK): 500 mg (peds: 50 mg/kg/24 hr) PO q6h
- Ticarcillin/clavulanic acid (Timentin): 3.1 g q4–6h
- Trimethoprim-sulfamethoxazole (Septra DS): 1 tablet q12h (peds: 8 mg/kg trimethoprim and 40 mg/kg sulfamethoxazole per day divided into two daily doses) PO
  - —Poor anaerobic coverage

Disposition

ADMISSION CRITERIA

- Infected wounds at presentation
- Severe/advancing cellulitis/lymphangitis
- Signs of systemic infection
- Infected wounds that have failed to respond to outpatient (oral) antibiotics

DISCHARGE CRITERIA

- Healthy patient with localized wound infection: discharge on antibiotics with 24-hour follow-up
- 48-hour follow-up for noninfected wounds

Miscellaneous

ICD9: 879.8

ICD10: T14.1

SEE ALSO: BITE, MAMMAL

SUGGESTED READINGS

Bunzli WF, et al. Current management of human bites. Pharmacotherapy 1998;18(2):227–234.

Galloway RE. Mammalian bites. J Emerg Med 1998;6:325–331.

Goldstein EJ. Bite wounds and infection. Clin Infect Dis 1992;14:633–640.

Griego RD, et al. Dog, cat, and human bites: a review. J Am Acad Dermatol 1995;33:1019–1029.

Presutti RJ. Bite wounds. Postgrad Med 1997;101(4):243–254.

Smith PF, et al. Treating mammalian bite wounds. J Clin Pharm Ther 2000;25:85–99.

Author: Daniel Wu

Clinical Presentation

SIGNS AND SYMPTOMS

- Distribution of mammalian bites
- Dog bites represent 80–90% of all bites
- Cat bites represent 5–15% of all bites
- Human bites represent 2–5% of all bites (see human bite chapter)
- Rat bites represent 2–3% of all bites

Dog Bites

- Appearance
  - —Crush injuries (most common), tears, avulsions, punctures, and scratches
- Low rates of infection compared with cat and human bites
- Infections usually present with
  - —Cellulitis
  - —Malodorous gray discharge
  - —Fever
  - —Lymphadenopathy

Cat Bites

- Appearance
  - —Puncture wounds (most common)
  - —Abrasions
  - —Lacerations
- High infection rates (30–50%) due to deeper puncture wounds

Cat-scratch Disease

- From the bite/scratch of a cat, dog, or monkey
- Small macule or vesicle that progresses to a papule
  - —Begins several days (3–10) after inoculation
  - —Resolves within several days or weeks
- Regional lymphadenopathy occurs 3 weeks postinoculation
  - —Tender
  - —Nonsuppurative
  - —Resolves after 2–4 months
- Low-grade fever, malaise, headache

Complications of Mammalian Bites

- Cellulitis
- Abscess formation
- Septic arthritis
- Osteomyelitis
- Sepsis
- Rat-bite fever (rare)

MECHANISM/DESCRIPTION

- Most bites are from provoked animals

Dog Bite Wounds

- Large dogs inflict the most serious wounds (pit bulls cause the most human fatalities)
- Most fatalities in children (70%) due to bites to face/neck
- Dogs of family or friends account for most bites

Cat Bite Wounds

- Majority from pets known to victim
- 30–50% infection rate in those seeking care
- Puncture wounds most frequent due to sharp thin teeth causing deep inoculation of bacteria

Cat-scratch Disease

- Three of the following four criteria
  - —Cat contact, with presence of scratch or inoculation lesion of the skin, eye, or mucous membrane
  - —Positive CSD skin test result
  - —Characteristic lymph node histopathology
  - —Negative results of laboratory studies for other causes of lymphadenopathy

Rat Bite Wounds

- Occur in laboratory personnel or children of low socioeconomic class
- 10% infection rate
- Rat bites rarely transmit rabies and prophylaxis not routine

ETIOLOGY

Dog and Cat Bites

- *Pasteurella multocida* is the major organism in both
  - —Twice as likely to be found in cat bites than dog bites
  - —Gram-negative aerobe found in up to 80% of cat infections
  - —Infection appears <24 hours
- *Staphylococcus* or *Streptococcus*
  - —Infection appears >24 hours
- Other organisms include anaerobes and *Capnocytophaga canimorsus* (dogs)

Cat-scratch Disease

- Caused by *Bartonella henselae*

Rat Bites

- Caused by *Spirillum minus* and *Streptobacillus moniliformis*

Pre-Hospital

N/A

Diagnosis

ESSENTIAL WORKUP

History

- Animal's behavior, provocation, location, ownership
- Time since attack
- Past medical history: conditions compromising immune function, allergies, and tetanus status

Physical Examination

- Record the location and extent of all injuries
- Document any swelling, crush injuries, or devitalized tissue
- Note the range of motion of affected areas
- Note the status of tendon and nerve function
- Document any signs of infection, including regional adenopathy
- Document any joint or bone involvement

LABORATORY

- Aerobic and anaerobic cultures from any infected bite wound
- Cultures not routinely indicated if wounds not clinically infected

Cat-scratch Disease

- Presence of elevated titers of *Bartonella (Rochalimaea) henselae,* or
- Positive reaction to cat-scratch antigen (CSA)
  - —Inject 0.1 mL CSA intradermally
  - —Induration at the site 48–72 hours later equal to or exceeding 5 mm is positive

IMAGING/SPECIAL TESTS

- Plain radiograph indications
  - —Fracture
  - —Suspect foreign body, e.g., tooth
  - —Baseline film if a bone or joint space has been violated in evaluating for osteomyelitis
  - —For infection in proximity to a bone or joint space

DIFFERENTIAL DIAGNOSIS

- Human bite injuries: human teeth cause crush injuries and animal teeth cause more punctures and lacerations
- Bite injuries from other animals

CSD-caused Lymphadenopathy

- Reactive hyperplasia (leading cause of lymphadenopathy in children younger than 16 years)
- Infection, chronic lymphadenitis, drug reaction, malignancy, and congenital conditions

Treatment

ED TREATMENT

- Wound irrigation
  - —Copious volumes of normal saline irrigation with an 18-gauge plastic catheter tip aimed in the direction of the puncture
  - —Avoid injection of saline through tissue planes due to force of irrigation
- Débridement
  - —Remove foreign material, necrotic skin tags, or devitalized tissues
  - —Do not débride puncture wounds
  - —Remove any eschar present so underlying pus may be expressed and irrigated
- Wound closure
  - —Do not suture infected wounds or wounds >24 hours after injury
  - —Repair of wounds >8 hours: controversial
  - —Close facial wounds (warn patient of high risk of infection)
  - —Infected wounds, those presenting >24 hours, and deep hand wounds should be left open
  - —May approximate the wound edges with Steri-Strips and perform a delayed primary closure
- Antibiotic indications
  - —Infected wounds
  - —Cat bites
  - —Hand injuries
  - —Severe wounds with crush injury
  - —Puncture wounds
  - —Full-thickness puncture of hand, face, or lower extremity
  - —Wounds requiring surgical dibridement
  - —Wounds involving joints, tendons, ligaments, or fractures
  - —Immunocompromised patients
  - —Wounds presenting >8 hours after the event
- Antibiotic choices
  - —Oral
    - -Amoxicillin/clavulanic acid (Augmentin) first line
    - -Cefuroxime axetil (Ceftin)
    - -Clindamycin (Cleocin)
    - -Ciprofloxacin (Cipro)
    - -Doxycycline (Vibramycin)
    - -Trimethoprim-sulfamethoxazole (Bactrim)
  - —IV
    - -Ampicillin/sulbactam (Unasyn)
    - -Cefoxitin (Mefoxin)
    - -Clindamycin (Cleocin)
    - -Ciprofloxacin (Cipro)
    - -Imipenem/cilastatin (Primaxin)
    - -Piperacillin/tazobactam (Zosyn)
    - -Ticarcillin/clavulanic acid (Timentin)
- Elevate injured extremity
- Tetanus prophylaxis

Rabies Immunoprophylaxis

- Not required if rabies not known or suspected
- Rodents (squirrels, hamsters, rats, mice) and rabbits rarely transmit the disease
- Skunks, raccoons, bats, and foxes represent the major reservoir for rabies
- Recommended in following situations
  - —Dog or cat in rabies-known area unable to be quarantined for 10 days
  - —Previously healthy dog or cat becomes ill while being quarantined (and awaiting results of rabies fluorescent antibody test)
  - —An ill dog or cat while awaiting rabies test results (to be continued or halted based on results of rabies test)
- Active immunization
  - —Human diploid cell vaccine (HDCV): 1 mL i.m. on days 1, 3, 7, 14, and 28 after exposure
- Passive immunization
  - —Human rabies immune globulin (HRIG): 20 IU/kg
  - —Up to one half in area around wound with the rest i.m.

Cat-scratch Disease

- Analgesics
- Apply local heat to affected nodes
- Avoid lymph node trauma
- Disease usually self-limiting
- Antibiotics controversial, consider if severe disease is present or immunocompromised victim

MEDICATIONS

- Amoxicillin/clavulanic acid (Augmentin): 500 mg (peds: 40 mg/kg/24 hr) PO t.i.d. (first line for all three animals)
- Ampicillin/sulbactam (Unasyn): 1.5–3.0 g i.v. q6h
- Cefoxitin (Mefoxin): 2.0 g i.v. q8h
- Cefuroxime axetil (Ceftin): 500 mg PO b.i.d.
- Clindamycin (Cleocin): 300 mg PO q6h; 900 mg i.v. q8h
- Ciprofloxacin (Cipro)500 mg PO/b.i.d.; 400 mg i.v. q12h
- Doxycycline (Vibramycin): 100 mg PO b.i.d.
- Imipenem/cilastatin (Primaxin): 0.5–1.0 g (peds: 50 mg/kg/24 hr) i.v. q6h
- Piperacillin/tazobactam (Zosyn): 3.375 g i.v. q6h
- Ticarcillin/clavulanic acid (Timentin): 3.1 g i.v. q6h
- Trimethoprim-sulfamethoxazole (Bactrim): 1 tablet (peds: 6–12 mg TMP, 30–60 mg SMX/kg/24 hr) PO b.i.d.

Disposition

ADMISSION CRITERIA

All Bites

- Infected wounds at presentation
- Severe/advancing cellulitis/lymphangitis
- Signs of systemic infection
- Infected wounds that have failed to respond to outpatient (PO) antibiotics

Cat-scratch Disease

- Prolonged fever, systemic symptoms, and/or marked lymphadenopathy

DISCHARGE CRITERIA

- Healthy patient with localized wound infection: discharge on antibiotics with 24-hour follow-up
- 48-hour follow-up for noninfected wounds

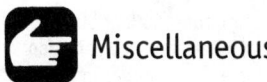

Miscellaneous

ICD9: 879.8

ICD10: T14.1

SEE ALSO: RABIES

SUGGESTED READINGS

Chen SCA, Gilbert GL. Cat scratch disease: past and present. J Paediatr Child Health 1994;30:467–469.

Galloway RE. Mammalian bites. J Emerg Med 1998;6:325–331.

Goldstein EJ. Bite wounds and infection. Clin Infect Dis 1992;14:633–640.

Griego RD, et al. Dog, cat, and human bites: a review. J Am Acad Dermatol 1995;33:1019–1029.

Klein JD. Cat scratch disease. Pediatr Rev 1994;15(9):348–353.

Smith PF, et al. Treating mammalian bite wounds. J Clin Pharm Ther 2000;25:85–99.

Willey JF. Mammalian bites: review of evaluation and management. Clin Pediatr 1990;29(5):283–287.

Author: Daniel Wu

Bladder Injury

Clinical Presentation

SIGNS AND SYMPTOMS

- Abdominal or pelvic pain, difficulty voiding
- Hypotension, low urine output, gross or microscopic hematuria

MECHANISM/DESCRIPTION

- Blunt and less frequently penetrating trauma are the most common causes
  - —10–15% of pelvic fractures have associated bladder injury
  - —95% of bladder ruptures have an associated pelvic fracture
- Iatrogenic manipulation
- Spontaneous injury from another process: neoplasm, urethral obstruction, tuberculosis, radiation damage, occult trauma

ETIOLOGY

- Bladder rupture
  - —Intraperitoneal rupture (60% of bladder ruptures) occur by hydraulic compression
  - —Compressive forces cause a tear in the bladder dome, the weakest portion *in situ*
  - —Occurs more frequently with a distended bladder
  - —Extraperitoneal bladder rupture (30% of bladder ruptures)
  - —Damage from fracture fragments
  - —Shearing forces from ligaments attached to the bladder
  - —Extraperitoneal bladder rupture can occur with rising blood pressure
  - —Combined extraperitoneal and intraperitoneal rupture occurs in 10% of bladder ruptures
  - —Bladder contusion is more common (50–65% of all bladder injuries)
  - —Damage to the endothelial lining or the muscularis layer with an intact bladder wall
  - —It is a diagnosis of exclusion and usually resolves without intervention

Potential Complications

- Peritonitis
- Sepsis
- Incontinence
- Infected pelvic hematoma
- Fistulae

PEDIATRIC CONSIDERATIONS

- Intraperitoneal rupture is more common in children than in adults, because the bladder is an abdominal organ in pediatric patients
- Bladder injury is more common in children than in adults, because the pediatric bony pelvis is less rigid and transmits more force to adjacent structures

Pre-Hospital

CAUTIONS

- Do not attempt bladder catheterization in the field

Diagnosis

ESSENTIAL WORKUP

- Meticulous physical examination of perineum and pelvis
- Radiographic evaluation (retrograde urethrogram [RUG], cystography, see later discussion)

LABORATORY

- Urinalysis
  - —Gross hematuria is noted in approximately 90% of patients with significant bladder or urethral trauma
  - —Microscopic hematuria is noted in <2%
- BUN and creatinine
  - —The BUN can be elevated secondary to resorption of urine from an intraperitoneal rupture
- Electrolytes
  - —Hyperkalemia and hypernatremia may result from resorption of urine within the peritoneum

IMAGING/SPECIAL TESTS

- Excretory urethrography may demonstrate bladder rupture or urethral injury in 15% of cases
- *Cystography* is the criterion standard for bladder evaluation
  - —Performed immediately unless other surgical or medical emergencies have greater priority
  - —A scout film (KUB) is initially obtained
  - —The first 100 mL of water-soluble contrast is infused by a Foley catheter into the bladder
- The plain film is repeated to evaluate for early extravasation
  - —If results are normal, an additional 200–300 mL of contrast is infused
  - —Cystogram films are now taken in the AP, lateral, and oblique planes to rule out a bladder injury
  - —Outlining of bowel or contrast within the paracolic gutters is indicative of an intraperitoneal rupture
  - —A teardrop- or star-shaped form are noted with extraperitoneal ruptures
  - —After drainage of the contrast, a postdrainage film is taken, which will occasionally demonstrate extravasated contrast not visible with a distended bladder
- CT scan is not sensitive enough to evaluate bladder injuries

DIFFERENTIAL DIAGNOSIS

- Perineal trauma
- Urethral trauma
- Renal or ureteric trauma

PEDIATRIC CONSIDERATIONS

- When cystography occurs, 3–5 mL/kg of total contrast material should be used

Treatment

INITIAL STABILIZATION

- ABCs of trauma care
- Early urologic consultation

ED TREATMENT

- Immediate surgical exploration for intraperitoneal ruptures and many extraperitoneal ruptures
- Extraperitoneal ruptures may be managed solely by catheter drainage if contraindications to surgical repair exist
- No specific interventions are required for bladder contusions

Disposition

ADMISSION CRITERIA

- Concurrent closed head injury, blunt abdominal trauma, or pelvic fracture requiring admission and observation
- Need for operative management of bladder or other injuries

DISCHARGE CRITERIA

- After thorough urologic evaluation, patients without significant bladder injury may be considered for outpatient management
  - —Patients who are unable to void may require urinary catheter and leg bag

Miscellaneous

ICD9: 867.0

ICD10: S37.2

SUGGESTED READINGS

Corriere JN Jr. Diagnosis and management of lower urinary tract injuries, AUA Update Series, lesson 16, vol VII. Houston, TX: AUA Office of Education Houston, 1988: 121–127.

Harwood-Nuss AL, Sandler CM. Genitourinary trauma. In: Rosen P, Doris PE, Barkin RM, et al, eds. Diagnostic radiology in emergency medicine. St. Louis: Mosby-Year Book, 1992.

Sandler CM, et al. Lower urinary tract trauma. World J Urol 1988;16:69–75.

Thomas CL, McAninch JW. Bladder trauma, AUA Update Series, lesson 31, vol VIII. Houston, TX: AUA Office of Education, 1989:241–247.

Author: Kenneth Bramwell

Blow Out Fracture

Clinical Presentation

SIGNS AND SYMPTOMS

- Periorbital tenderness, swelling, ecchymosis
- Impaired ocular mobility or diplopia
  - —Upward gaze due to inferior rectus entrapment
  - —Ipsilateral lateral gaze with medial rectus entrapment
- Infraorbital hypoesthesia
  - —Due to compression/contusion of infraorbital nerve
- Enophthalmos
  - —Due to herniation of orbital fat through fracture
- Periorbital emphysema
  - —From the ethmoid or maxillary sinus
- Normal visual acuity (unless associated ocular injury)
- Epistaxis

Associated Injuries

- Ocular injuries
  - —Ruptured globe
    - -Incidence 5–10% of blow out fractures
    - -Ophthalmologic emergency
  - —Subconjunctival hemorrhage
  - —Corneal abrasion/laceration
  - —Hyphema
  - —Iridodialysis
  - —Traumatic iridocyclitis (uveitis)
  - —Traumatic mydriasis
  - —Retinal detachment
  - —Vitreous hemorrhage
  - —Compressive orbital emphysema
  - —Retrobulbar hemorrhage
  - —Optic nerve injury
- Facial fractures
  - —Nasal bones
  - —Zygomatic arch fracture
- Neck injuries
- Intracranial injury

Late Complications

- Sinusitis
- Orbital infection
- Permanent restriction of extraocular movement
- Enophthalmos

MECHANISM/DESCRIPTION

- Defined as an orbital floor fracture without orbital rim involvement
- Caused by blunt trauma to the orbit
- Force transmitted through the orbital structures to the weakest structural point: the orbital floor
  - —Results in fracture of the orbital floor
- Orbital floor serves as roof to air-filled maxillary and ethmoid sinuses
  - —Communication between the spaces results in orbital emphysema
- Orbit contains fat, which holds the globe in place
  - —Orbital floor fracture may result in herniation of the fat on the inferior orbital surface into the maxillary or ethmoid sinuses
  - —Leads to enophthalmos due to orbital volume loss
  - —Sinus congestion and fluid collection occur secondary to edema
- Infraorbital nerve runs through the bony canal 3 mm below the orbital floor
  - —Injury results in hypoesthesia of the ipsilateral cheek
  - —Distinguished from hypoesthesia due to swelling by testing for decreased sensation on the ipsilateral gingiva, which is within the infraorbital nerve distribution
- Inferior rectus and the inferior oblique muscle run along the orbital floor
  - —Restriction of these extraocular muscles occurs due to entrapment within the fracture, contusion, or cranial nerve dysfunction
  - —Diplopia on upward gaze
  - —Inability to elevate the affected eye normally on exam
- Medial rectus located above the ethmoid sinus
  - —Less commonly entrapped
  - —Diplopia on ipsilateral lateral gaze

ETIOLOGY

- Most commonly caused by handballs, baseballs, or fists

PEDIATRIC CONSIDERATIONS

- Orbital floor fractures: extremely unlikely before 7 years of age
- Lack of pneumatization of the paranasal sinuses; therefore, orbital floor is not as weak a point in the orbit
- Orbital roof fractures with associated CNS injuries more common

Pre-Hospital

- Metal protective eye shield if possible globe injury
- Place in supine position

Diagnosis

ESSENTIAL WORKUP

- Thorough ophthalmologic examination
  - —Visual acuity (should not be affected)
  - —Test extraocular movements for disconjugate gaze or diplopia
  - —Palpate bony structures for evidence of step off
  - —Test sensation in inferior orbital nerve distribution
  - —Examine lid and adnexa
  - —Careful attention not to place pressure on the globe until ruptured globe excluded
  - —Slit-lamp and funduscopic examination to identify associated injuries

LABORATORY

- Preoperative laboratory studies if indicated

IMAGING/SPECIAL TESTS

- Plain radiographs
  - —Facial films
  - —Orbits
  - —Water's view and exaggerated Water's view
    - -Classic "teardrop sign" illustrates herniated mass of orbital contents in the ipsilateral maxillary sinus
    - -Opacification of or air fluid level in the ipsilateral maxillary sinus (less specific)
    - -Orbital floor bony fracture
    - -Lucency in orbits consistent with orbital emphysema
  - —Diagnostic in up to 97%
  - —10% false-positive and false-negative rate
- CT orbits: excellent alternative
  - —If diagnosis in question and for follow-up
  - —Defines involved anatomy
  - —Obtain 1.5-mm cuts
- Forced duction test
  - —Distinguishes nerve dysfunction from entrapment
  - —Topical anesthesia applied to the conjunctiva on the opposite side and the globe is pulled away from the expected point of entrapment; if the globe is not mobile, the test is positive

DIFFERENTIAL DIAGNOSIS

- Retrobulbar hemorrhage
- Periorbital contusion/ecchymosis
- Cranial nerve palsy
- Ruptured globe
- Orbital cellulitis
- Periorbital cellulitis

PEDIATRIC CONSIDERATIONS

- Immature facial skeleton with lack of pneumatization of the paranasal sinuses makes plain radiographs of limited value
- Orbital CT: study of choice

Treatment

INITIAL STABILIZATION

- Initial approach and immediate concerns
  - —Rule out ruptured globe
  - —Assess for associated intracranial or cervical spine injuries
  - —Test visual acuity
    - -Decreased visual acuity suggestive of associated ocular injury

ED TREATMENT

- Apply cool compresses for the first 24–48 hours to decrease swelling to minimize or reverse herniation and avoid surgical intervention
- Avoid Valsalva's maneuvers and nose blowing to prevent compressive orbital emphysema
- Prophylactic antibiotics to prevent infection
- Nasal decongestants
- Analgesics
- Tetanus prophylaxis

MEDICATIONS

- Amoxicillin: 250–500 mg PO t.i.d. × 10–14 days
- Cephalexin: 250–500 mg PO q.i.d. × 10–14 days
- Erythromycin: 250–500 mg PO q.i.d. × 10–14 days
- Phenylephrine nasal spray: b.i.d. × 10–14 days

Disposition

ADMISSION CRITERIA

- Rarely indicated except with
  - —Severe herniation of orbital contents threatening vision
  - —Cosmetically enophthalmos typically >5 mm
  - —Associated injuries that mandate admission

DISCHARGE CRITERIA

- Consultation with facial trauma service
  - —Arrange follow-up evaluation within 1-2 weeks of injury and to determine need for surgery
- Immediate ophthalmology evaluation if patient has evidence of visual loss or within 24 hours for complete retinal evaluation
- Need for surgical intervention
  - —Rarely indicated immediately
  - —85% resolve without surgical intervention
  - —Typically observe for 10–14 days until swelling resolves
  - —Surgery indications
    - -Persistent diplopia
    - -Restricted extraocular movements
    - -Cosmetically significant enophthalmos

Miscellaneous

ICD9: 829.0

ICD10: S02.3

SUGGESTED READINGS

Anderson PJ, Poole MD. Orbital floor fractures in young children. J Craniomaxillofac Surg 1995;23(3): 151–154.

Bains RA, Rubin PA. Blunt orbital trauma. Int Ophthalmol Clin 1995;35(1):37–46.

Hatton MP, Watkins LM, Rubin PA. Orbital fractures in children. Ophthalmol Plast Reconstr Surg 2001;17(3):174–179.

Joondeph BC. Blunt ocular trauma. Emerg Med Clin North Am 1988;6(1):151.

Koltai PJ, Amjad I, Meyer D. Orbital fractures in children. Arch Otolaryngol Head Neck Surg 1995;121(12): 1375–1379.

Linden JA, Renner GS. Trauma to the globe. Emerg Med Clin North Am 1995;13(3): 581–605.

Author: Shari Schabowski

Boerhaave's Syndrome

Clinical Presentation

SIGNS AND SYMPTOMS

- Mackler triad
  - —Vomiting
  - —Chest pain
  - —Subcutaneous emphysema
- Retrosternal chest pain present in most patients
  - —Often pleuritic
  - —Radiates to the back
  - —Worsened with swallowing
- Dyspnea with mediastinitis
- Diaphoresis
- Voice changes
- Subcutaneous emphysema in neck and chest wall
- Mediastinal crackling on auscultation (Hamman's sign)
- Fever
- Shock in severe cases
- If untreated, mediastinitis with abscess formation
- Not usually associated with bleeding

MECHANISM/DESCRIPTION

- Spontaneous esophageal rupture
- Sudden increase in intraabdominal pressure
  - —Causes complete, full thickness, longitudinal tear in the distal esophagus at the left posterolateral aspect
- Esophagus has no serosal layer (which normally contains collagen and elastic fibers)
  - —Results in a weak structure vulnerable to perforation and mediastinal contamination
  - —Esophageal wall is further weakened by conditions that damage the mucosa such as esophagitis of various causes
- Significant morbidity/mortality
  - —Due to explosive nature of the tear
  - —Almost instant contamination of the mediastinum with intraesophageal contents

ETIOLOGY

- Associated with forceful vomiting and retching
- Reported with heavy lifting, seizures, childbirth, blunt trauma, induced emesis, and laughing
- Common in middle-aged men
- Alcohol consumption and ingesting large meals are predisposing factors

PEDIATRIC CONSIDERATIONS

- Described but rare in neonates

Pre-Hospital

CAUTIONS

- Airway control if unresponsive or airway patency in jeopardy
- Establish one large-bore IV catheter and treat hypotension with 0.9% NS solution
- Avoid analgesics until patient in the ED to avoid the complication of hypotension

Diagnosis

ESSENTIAL WORKUP

- Upright CXR (preferably posteroanterior and lateral views if tolerated) evaluating for
  - —Pneumomediastinum
  - —Subcutaneous emphysema
  - —Pleural effusion (left side)
  - —Pneumothorax
  - —Widened mediastinum
  - —Hydropneumothorax
  - —Empyema
- *Esophagram* identifies leak in esophagus
  - —Initially use water-soluble contrast material
  - —If the esophagus is intact, use barium contrast for better detail

LABORATORY

- CBC
- PT/PTT
- Blood cultures
- Pleural effusion amylase content

IMAGING/SPECIAL TESTS

- EKG
- Endoscopy
  - —Useful for diagnosis
  - —Operator dependent
- CT chest
  - —Sensitive for identifying free air but can not isolate the lesion
  - —Indicated if esophagram cannot be obtained
  - —Evaluates other intrathoracic structures

DIFFERENTIAL DIAGNOSIS

- Myocardial infarction
- Pneumothorax
- Pericarditis
- Pneumonia
- Pancreatitis
- Ruptured abdominal viscus
- Dissecting aortic aneurysm
- Pulmonary thromboembolism
- Mesenteric thrombosis
- Cholecystitis
- Spontaneous pneumomediastinum (clinically benign)

Treatment

INITIAL STABILIZATION

- ABCs
  —Airway control: 100% oxygen or intubate if unresponsive or airway patency is in jeopardy
  —Establish IV access with at least one large-bore catheter or more if unstable
  —Treat hypotension
    -Administer 1-L (20-mL/kg) bolus with 0.9% NS (or lactated Ringer's solution)
    -Initiate dopamine if BP does not respond to fluids
    -Central catheter placement if unstable for more efficient delivery of fluids and monitoring of CVP

ED TREATMENT

- NPO
- Careful placement of a NGT to decompress the stomach
- Bladder catheter to monitor urine output
- Expedient diagnosis to decrease incidence of morbidity/mortality
- Prompt surgical consultation
- Definitive treatment
  —Surgical repair of the perforation
  —Adequate drainage
- Initiate broad-spectrum antibiotics directed against oral microflora and GI pathogens
  —Ampicillin/sulbactam plus gentamicin

MEDICATIONS

- Ampicillin/sulbactam: 3.0 g IVPB q6h
- Dopamine: 2–20 μg/kg/min IVPB
- Gentamicin: 2 mg/kg load then 1.7 mg/kg IVPB q8h or 5.1 mg/kg IVPB q.d. (assuming normal renal function)

Disposition

ADMISSION CRITERIA

- All cases of Boerhaave's syndrome must be admitted to the surgical ICU after definitive surgical repair of the lesion
- Surgery should be performed directly from the ED without delay

DISCHARGE CRITERIA

N/A

Miscellaneous

ICD9: 520.4

ICD10: K22.3

SUGGESTED READINGS

Jagminas L, et al. Boerhaave's syndrome presenting with abdominal pain and right hydropneumothorax. Am J Emerg Med 1996;14(1):53–55.

Ma G, et al. Spontaneous esophageal rupture. J Emerg Med 2000;18(2): 257–258.

Troum S, et al. Surviving Boerhaave's syndrome without thoracotomy. Chest 1994;106(1):297–298.

Younes Z, et al. The spectrum of spontaneous and iatrogenic esophageal injury: perforations, Mallory-Weiss tears, and hematomas. J Clin Gastroenterol 1999;29(4):306–317.

Author: Dino P. Rumoro

Botulism

Clinical Presentation

SIGNS AND SYMPTOMS

Food-borne Botulism (Classic Botulism)

- Most common
  - —Diplopia
  - —Blurred vision
  - —Bulbar weakness: dysphagia, dysarthria, dysphonia
- Subsequent symmetric, descending weakness or paralysis of the extremities (hallmark of the disease)
- No sensory deficit
- Remains awake/alert; mentation unaffected
- Ventilatory insufficiency from weakness of respiratory muscles
- Autonomic dysfunction (sympathetic and parasympathetic)
  - —Dry mouth
  - —Blurred vision
  - —Orthostatic hypotension
  - —Constipation
  - —Urinary retention
- Nausea and vomiting with food-borne botulism only
- Afebrile

Infantile Botulism

- Constipation
- Weakness
- Poor suck
- Lethargy
- Hypotonia
- Flaccid facial expression
- Respiratory difficulty

Wound Botulism

- Finding similar to food-borne botulism
- May be febrile

MECHANISM/DESCRIPTION

- Caused by a polypeptide, heat-labile exotoxin produced by *Clostridium botulinum*
  - —Most potent poison known
- Toxin blocks neuromuscular transmission in cholinergic nerve fibers
- Symptoms occur by inhibition of acetylcholine release from presynaptic nerve membranes
  - —Damage is permanent
  - —Recovery is by formation of new synapses through sprouting from the axon
- Onset: 12–36 hours after exposure
  - —Death can occur in 24 hours
- Slow recovery; symptoms often persist for months
- Mortality
  - —Untreated: 60–70%
  - —With supportive care: 10–15%
- Three major types: *food-borne botulism, wound botulism,* and *infantile botulism* (see Pediatric Considerations)
- Food-borne botulism
  - —Occurs by ingestion of preformed toxin; improperly canned food facilitates the necessary anaerobic conditions
  - —Conditions required for exposure
    - -Food product contaminated with *C. botulinum* bacilli or spores
    - -Proper conditions for germination of spores exist
    - -Time and conditions permit production of toxin before eating
    - -Food not heated sufficiently to destroy botulism toxin
    - -Toxin containing food ingested by susceptible host
- Wound botulism
  - —Clinical evidence of botulism after trauma with a resultant infected wound and no history suggestive of food-borne illness
  - —*Botulinum* isolated in about 50%
  - —Wounds usually contaminated with soil
  - —Seen rarely in chronic drug abusers
- Other types
  - —Hidden botulism is an adult variant of infantile botulism seen in compromised hosts (rare)
  - —Inadvertent botulism seen rarely from reactions to botulism toxin used therapeutically
    - -Symptoms similar to those of classic botulism

ETIOLOGY

- *C. botulinum* is a large spore-forming, usually gram-positive, strictly anaerobic bacilli ubiquitous in nature
- Each strain produces antigenically distinct toxins, designated types A through G
  - —Types A, B, and E are responsible for most human cases

PEDIATRIC CONSIDERATIONS

- *Infantile botulism* occurs from the ingestion of *C. botulinum* spores, which germinate in the gut and produce the toxin
- 90% occur in children younger than 6 months
- Progresses for 1–2 weeks then stabilizes for 2–3 weeks before receding
  - —Usually subacute presentation with low mortality
- Slower onset is attributed to the toxin being produced locally, as opposed to being ingested in one dose
- *C. botulinum* spores found in honey
  - —Honey not recommended for children younger than 6 months

Pre-Hospital

CAUTIONS

- Death is invariably from progressive ventilatory failure
  - —Intubate as soon as respiratory insufficiency noted

Diagnosis

ESSENTIAL WORKUP

- Clinical diagnosis
- Workup focuses on differentiation from other conditions causing general paralysis
- Notify public health officials of diagnosis

LABORATORY

- CBC
- Electrolytes, BUN/Cr, glucose
  - —Check for hypokalemia
- ABG
  - —For signs of respiratory insufficiency
- Toxin detection in
  - —Blood
  - —Feces
  - —Gastric contents
  - —Suspected food and containers
- Anaerobic blood cultures

IMAGING/SPECIAL TESTS

- CSF testing
  - —Normal
  - —Helps differentiate from Guillain-Barré syndrome
- Electrophysiologic studies: normal nerve conduction with diminished evoked muscle action potential
- Edrophonium testing may be positive, but not to the degree seen in myasthenia gravis

DIFFERENTIAL DIAGNOSIS

- Myasthenia gravis (less acute)
- Lambert-Eaton myasthenic syndrome (less acute)
- Polio (fever and asymmetric)
- Guillain-Barré (simultaneous sensory findings and elevated spinal fluid protein)
- Tick paralysis
- Magnesium intoxication
- Hypokalemic periodic paralysis
- Diphtheritic neuropathy

PEDIATRIC CONSIDERATIONS

- Often misdiagnosed as dehydration, sepsis, or Reye's syndrome

Treatment

INITIAL STABILIZATION

- Early intubation and ventilatory support is the key to survival
- Respiratory difficulties occur rapidly

ED TREATMENT

- Trivalent ABE antitoxin
  —IV administration as soon as the diagnosis is made, without waiting for laboratory confirmation
  —Use should be preceded by testing for hypersensitivity to horse serum
- NG suctioning if ileus is profound
- With *wound botulism,* perform wound débridement even if it appears to be healing
- Antibiotics for specific infectious complications

MEDICATIONS

- Trivalent botulism antitoxin: 2 vials (approximately 10,000 IU each of types A, B, and E) i.v.

PEDIATRIC CONSIDERATIONS

- Antitoxin is rarely indicated for *infantile botulism*
- Antibiotics
  —Ineffective in eradicating organism from the intestine
  —Release of toxin in the gut through bacterial cell lysis may worsen neurologic symptoms

Disposition

ADMISSION CRITERIA

- Admit suspected botulism poisoning to monitored bed
  —ICU admission for any respiratory deficiency

DISCHARGE CRITERIA

- Clinical course of botulism poisoning is unpredictable; it can become rapidly progressive and fatal
  —Discharge only patients with a prolonged period of progressive recovery from symptoms

Miscellaneous

ICD9: 005.1

ICD10: A05.1

SUGGESTED READINGS

Bleck TP. Clostridium botulinum. In: Mandell GI, Bennett JE, Dolin R, eds. Mandell, Douglas, and Bennett's principles and practice of infectious diseases, 4th ed. New York: Churchill-Livingstone, 1995.

Cherington M. Clinical spectrum of botulism. Muscle Nerve 1998(June): 701–710.

Hatheway CL. Botulism: the present status of the disease. Curr Top Microbiol Immunol 1995;195:55–75.

Mechem CC, Walter FG. Wound botulism. Vet Hum Toxicol 1994;36:233–237.

Midura TF. Update: infant botulism. Clin Microbiol Rev 1996(Apr):119–125.

Wigginton JM, Thill P. Infant botulism: a review of the literature. Clin Pediatr 1993;32:669–674.

Author: Philip Shayne

Bowel Obstruction

Clinical Presentation

SIGNS AND SYMPTOMS

- Abdominal pain
  - —Intermittent early
  - —Constant with strangulated obstruction
- Vomiting
  - —Bile-stained emesis with proximal obstruction
  - —Feculent emesis with distal obstruction
- Obstipation
- Vital signs
  - —Usually normal
  - —Tachycardia
  - —Hypotension with significant fluid loss
  - —Fever with strangulation or perforation
  - —Hypothermia with sepsis
- Hyperactive and high-pitched bowel sounds
- Abdomen examination
  - —Diffuse tenderness
  - —Pain out of proportion to findings suggests ischemic or gangrenous bowel
  - —Peritoneal signs (rebound/guarding) indicates strangulation or perforation
- Rectal exam
  - —Rectal mass
  - —Occult blood in stool
- Hernias
  - —Inguinal
  - —Femoral
  - —Ventral hernia

MECHANISM/DESCRIPTION

- Obstruction of normal flow of intestinal contents due to mechanical or nonmechanical causes
- Obstruction leads to rapid increase in both anaerobic and aerobic bacteria with resultant increase in methane and hydrogen production
- Distended bowel becomes progressively edematous and increased intestinal secretions cause further distention
- Retrograde peristalsis causes vomiting

ETIOLOGY

Small Bowel

- Adhesions: most common
- Hernias
- Neoplasms
- Stricture: inflammatory bowel disease
- Trauma: bowel wall hematoma
- Ascaris infection

Large Bowel

- Carcinoma
- Volvulus
- Diverticular disease
- Inflammatory bowel disease
- Ischemic colitis

PEDIATRIC CONSIDERATIONS

- Intussusception
  - —Leading cause of intestinal obstruction in infants
  - —Most common between 3 and 12 months of age
- Incarcerated inguinal/umbilical hernia
- Malrotation with volvulus
  - —Can occur as early as 3–7 days of age
  - —Double bubble often seen on upright abdominal radiograph due to partial obstruction of duodenum, resulting in air in stomach and in first part of duodenum
- Pyloric stenosis
  - —Progressive, projectile nonbilious vomiting often after feeding
  - —Male/female ratio: 5:1 incidence
  - —Onset usually 2–5 weeks of age

Pre-Hospital

CAUTIONS

- Abdominal pain, nausea/vomiting: very common symptoms in elderly patients with acute myocardial infarctions
  - —Abdominal distention, obstipation, and colicky pain suggests a GI etiology

Diagnosis

ESSENTIAL WORKUP

- Plain radiographs of chest and abdomen
  - —Upright CXR
  - —Evaluate lung for pathology
  - —Check for free air beneath diaphragm
  - —Upright and supine abdomen: obstructive findings
    - -Distended loops of bowel (normal small bowel <3 cm in diameter)
    - -Dilation of cecum >13 cm indicates potential rupture
    - -Air fluid levels
    - -Nearly completely fluid-filled small bowel loops may produce "string of pearls" sign
- Careful examination for hernias
- Heme test stool

LABORATORY

- CBC
  - —Leukocytosis common
- Electrolytes, BUN/Cr, glucose
  - —Hypochloremia and hypokalemia with vomiting in proximal obstructions
  - —Prerenal azotemia with significant dehydration
- Amylase/lipase
- Urinalysis

IMAGING/SPECIAL TESTS

- CT abdomen, barium enema, or upper GI
  - —If carcinoma or other mass lesion suspected as cause for obstruction

DIFFERENTIAL DIAGNOSIS

- Perforated ulcer
- Pancreatitis
- Cholecystitis
- Colitis
- Paralytic ileus
- Mesenteric ischemia
- Uremia

Treatment

INITIAL STABILIZATION

- ABCs
- 0.9% NS IV fluid resuscitation when
  - —Significant volume depletion
  - —Strangulated or perforated bowel

ED TREATMENT

- NGT suction
- Foley catheter to monitor urine output
- Surgical consultation
- Administer antibiotics (cefoxitin) for suspected strangulated/perforated bowel
- Administer analgesic as needed after surgical consultation

MEDICATIONS

- Cefoxitin: 1–2 g q6–8h (peds: 0–7 days 40 mg/kg/24 hr q12h; >7 days 80–160 mg/kg/24 hr q6h) IVPB
- Demerol: 25-mg increments (peds: 1 mg/kg) i.v. PRN
- Morphine sulfate: 2–4-mg increments (peds: 0.1 mg/kg) i.v. PRN

Disposition

ADMISSION CRITERIA

- All patients with suspected/confirmed intestinal obstruction should be admitted with early surgical consultation obtained

DISCHARGE CRITERIA

N/A

Miscellaneous

ICD9: 560.9

ICD10: K57.6

SUGGESTED READINGS

Holder W. Intestinal obstruction. Gastroenterol Clin North Am 1988;17(2):317.

Kimura K, Loening-Baucke V. Bilious vomiting in the newborn: rapid diagnosis of intestinal obstruction. Am Fam Physician 2000;61(9):2791–2798.

Marx JA. Rosen's emergency medicine: concepts and clinical practice, 5th ed. St. Louis: Mosby, 2002:1283–1293, 1332–1337.

Sanson TG, O'Keefe KP. Evaluation of abdominal pain in the elderly. Emerg Med Clin North Am 1996;14(3):615–627.

Sivit C. Gastrointestinal emergencies in older infants and children. Radiol Clin North Am 1997;35(4):865.

Author: Julio Silva

Bradyarrhythmias

Clinical Presentation

SIGNS AND SYMPTOMS

- Asymptomatic/none
- Syncope
- Near syncope
- Dizziness
- Bradycardia
- Low BP

MECHANISM/DESCRIPTION

- Pulse <60 beats/minute
- Two mechanisms
  - —Depression of the pacemaker in the sinus node
  - —Conduction system block with a subsidiary pacemaker

ETIOLOGY

- Sinus bradycardia
  - —Normal variant
  - —Overstimulation of the vagus nerve
  - —Prolongation of sinus node refractory period
  - —Acute inferior wall ischemia
  - —Myxedema
  - —Carotid sinus oversensitivity
  - —Eye manipulation
  - —Increased intracranial pressure
  - —Hypothermia
  - —Hypoglycemia
  - —Hypoxia
  - —β-Blocker or calcium channel blocker toxicity
  - —Amiodarone toxicity
  - —Clonidine toxicity
  - —Organophosphate toxicity
  - —Cimetidine
  - —Ranitidine
  - —Nitrates
  - —Guanethidine
  - —Acetylcholine
- Junctional bradycardia
  - —Loss of atrial rhythm, AV pacemaker takes over at 45–60 impulses/minute
  - —β-Blocker or calcium channel blocker toxicity
  - —Digitalis toxicity
  - —Cardiac ischemia
- Idioventricular bradycardia
  - —Loss of both SA and AV nodal activity; bundle branch or Purkinje network takes over at 30–40 impulses/minute
  - —Myocardial infarction
  - —Cardiac tamponade
  - —Exsanguinating hemorrhage
  - —Severe acidemia
  - —Preterminal rhythm
- Second-degree heart block: Mobitz type I (Wenckebach)
  - —Increased refractory period in the AV node
  - —β-Blocker or calcium channel blocker toxicity
  - —Digitalis
  - —Inferior wall ischemia
  - —Increased vagal tone
  - —Myocarditis
  - —May be present during sleep in normal individuals
- Second-degree heart block: Mobitz type II
  - —Prolongation of refractory period in His-Purkinje system
  - —Anteroseptal ischemia
  - —Sclerodegenerative disease
  - —Risk of third-degree heart block
- Third-degree heart block
  - —Complete loss of conduction of rhythm from working atrial pacemaker; ventricular pacemaker takes over
  - —Cardiac ischemia
  - —Severe β-blocker or calcium channel blocker toxicity
  - —Digitalis toxicity
- Sick sinus syndrome (tachy/brady rhythm)
  - —Impaired supraventricular impulse generation or conduction leading to intermittent bradycardia (sinus bradycardia, prolonged sinus arrest, or SA block) and intermittent tachycardias (SVT, junctional tachycardia, atrial fibrillation, and atrial flutter)
  - —Medications given to limit the fast rate may exacerbate bradyarrhythmias
  - —Autonomic dysfunction
  - —Acute pain
  - —Quinidine
  - —Procainamide
  - —Disopyramide
  - —Sotalol
  - —Systemic infection
    - -Myocarditis
    - -Acute rheumatic fever
    - -EBV
    - -Infiltrating myocardiopathies: amyloidosis, sarcoidosis
    - -Paraneoplastic syndrome
- Renal failure may potentiate drug toxicity inducing bradyarrhythmias

PEDIATRIC CONSIDERATIONS

- Most common cause is hypoxemia

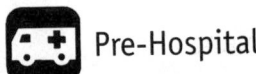

Pre-Hospital

CAUTIONS

- Treat the patient not the rate
- Epinephrine/atropine
  - —May increase the rate but can lead to increased ischemia
  - —Should be used only for patients with evidence of hypoperfusion
  - —Atropine does not affect the rate in third-degree heart block
- External pacing
  - —Initiated for poor perfusion that cannot be corrected by other means
  - —Must obtain ventricular capture; demonstrated by a palpable pulse
- Hypothermia: avoid medication or pacing
- Pediatrics: correct hypoxemia before attempting to increase the heart rate

Diagnosis

ESSENTIAL WORKUP

- 12-lead EKG and continuous cardiac monitoring
- Pulse oximetry
- BP monitoring

LABORATORY

- Serum glucose
- Serum potassium
- BUN and creatinine
- Cardiac enzymes
- Digoxin level if relevant
- Thyroid function tests

DIFFERENTIAL DIAGNOSIS

- Sinus bradycardia
  - —Normal P waves with narrow QRS complex
  - —Sinus arrhythmia may be present
- Junctional bradycardia
  - —Narrow QRS complex arises from AV node
  - —No normal P waves; retrograde P waves may be visible
  - —Rate 40–60
- Idioventricular bradycardia
  - —QRS complex wide, >0.16 seconds
  - —Rate usually <40
  - —No P waves visible
- Second-degree heart block: Mobitz type I (Wenckebach)
  - —Progressive prolongation of PR interval until a P fails to conduct
  - —Pause less than fully compensatory
  - —PR interval resets after dropped systole
  - —Narrow QRS complex unless associated with a bundle branch block (BBB)
  - —Progression to complete heart block is rare
  - —Often adequate for perfusion
- Second-degree heart block: Mobitz type II
  - —Sudden failure of AV conduction without preceding prolongation of the PR interval
  - —Often associated with prolonged QRS complex (BBB)
  - —High incidence of progression to complete heart block
  - —May be adequate for perfusion
- Third-degree (complete) heart block
  - —Normal P waves dissociated from ventricular beats
  - —If ventricular beats originate in AV node: QRS complex narrow, rate 40–60
  - —If ventricular beats originate below AV node: QRS complex wide, rate <40
- Sick sinus syndrome
  - —Intermittent bradycardia: sinus bradycardia, prolonged sinus arrest, SA block
  - —Intermittent tachycardia: SVT, junctional tachycardia, atrial fibrillation, atrial flutter
- Sinus arrest
  - —Prolonged sinus recovery causing periods of asystole
  - -Greater than 3 seconds
- Atrial fibrillation with slow ventricular response
  - —Unorganized atrial beats irregularly conducted through AV node
  - —Narrow ventricular beats unless associated with a BBB

Treatment

INITIAL STABILIZATION

- IV access
- Supplemental oxygen
- Airway control as needed
- Atropine and/or epinephrine for bradyarrhythmias caused by overstimulation of the vagal nerve
- External pacing in third-degree heart block, severe sinus arrest, idioventricular rhythms, or failure of medication
  - —Follow with early placement of a transvenous pacemaker
- Isoproterenol may be required for continuous rate and BP support
- Digitalis toxicity
  - —Treat hypokalemia or hyperkalemia
  - —If no improvement, treat with digoxin-specific antibodies
- β-Blocker toxicity
  - —Glucagon drip
  - —Wean the infusion as the β-blockade wears off
- Calcium channel toxicity
  - —Calcium chloride until the bradyarrhythmia resolves or normal perfusion is restored
- Organophosphate toxicity
  - —Atropine until tachycardic
  - —May require >40 mg of atropine

ED TREATMENT

- Initiate treatment of ischemia associated with the bradyarrhythmia
- Correct acid-base disturbances

MEDICATIONS

- Atropine: 0.5 mg i.v.; repeat every 5 minutes PRN; maximum dose of 0.04 mg/kg (peds: 0.02 mg/kg, minimum 0.1 mg)
- Calcium chloride: 10–20 mL (peds: 20 mg/kg i.v.) i.v. 10% solution bolus
- Dopamine: 2–5 μg/kg/min i.v.; maximum 20 μg/kg/min
- Epinephrine: 2 μg/min; maximum 10 μg/min (peds: 0.01-mg/kg bolus; 0.2–2-μg/kg/min infusion)
- Glucagon: 50-μg/kg bolus followed by 3–5 μg/kg/min
- Isoproterenol: 2–10 μg/min (peds: 0.1–0.25-μg/kg/min infusion), titrate to heart rate

Disposition

ADMISSION CRITERIA

- ICU
  - —New-onset bradyarrhythmias with hypoperfusion
  - —Patients requiring transvenous pacemakers
  - —Patients requiring perfusion support
  - —Acute ischemic disease
  - —After/ongoing emergent antidote treatment
- Admit others with symptomatic bradyarrhythmias to telemetry

DISCHARGE CRITERIA

- Asymptomatic sinus bradycardia or Mobitz type I (Wenckebach) second-degree heart block
- Asymptomatic, congenital third-degree heart block

Miscellaneous

ICD9: 427.8

ICD10: I49.8

SUGGESTED READINGS

Brady WJ Jr, Harrigan RA. Diagnosis and management of bradycardia and atrioventricular block associated with acute coronary ischemia. Emerg Med Clin North Am 2001;19(2):371–384, xi–xii.

Gibler WB. Arrhythmias and antiarrhythmic therapy. In: Gibler WB, Aufderheide TP, eds. Emergency cardiac care. St. Louis: Mosby-Year Book, 1994:345–384.

Kaushik V, Leon AR, Forrester JS Jr, et al. Bradyarrhythmias, temporary and permanent pacing. Crit Care Med 2000;28[10 Suppl]:N121–N128.

Lampert R, Ezekowtiz MD. Management of arrhythmias. Clin Geriatr Med 2000;16(3):593–618.

Author: Mary Patricia McKay

Bronchiolitis

Clinical Presentation

SIGNS AND SYMPTOMS

- Age younger than 2 years
- Nasal congestion
- Cough
- Wheezing
- Crackles
- Respiratory distress manifested by nasal flaring, retractions, grunting
- Fever usually <39.5°C
- Cyanosis (rare)

MECHANISM/DESCRIPTION

- Lower respiratory tract infection by airway inflammation and bronchoconstriction with wheezes/tachypnea and respiratory distress and upper respiratory prodrome

ETIOLOGY

- Respiratory syncytial virus (RSV) in 85–90% of cases
- Influenza
- Parainfluenza
- Adenovirus

Pre-Hospital

CAUTIONS

- Young infants have limited respiratory reserve and decompensate rapidly with little warning
- Monitor cardiorespiratory status and oxygenation
- Supplemental oxygen if saturation 92% and/or severe distress
- Watch for apneic pauses
  —Greatest risk in children younger than 6 months, premature
- Bag-mask ventilation if recurrent apneas

Diagnosis

ESSENTIAL WORKUP

- Clinical diagnosis
- Defining viral etiology may be useful for cohorting in hospital if admitted
- Assess ventilation clinically
- Pulse oximetry
  —Confirms proper oxygenation on continuing basis
  —Follows trends over the course of illness

LABORATORY

- Most patients need no specific tests beyond oximetry
- Nasopharyngeal aspirate/wash
  —Viral cultures
  —Fluorescent antibodies
  —Commercial kits are available
  —Consider when
    -Clinical symptoms suggestive of other etiology (pertussis, chlamydia)
    -Critically ill child
    -Coexisting signs suggesting bacterial sepsis
    -Bronchopulmonary dysplasia or chronic lung disease
    -Coexistent cardiac disease
    -Prematurity
    -Other conditions warranting antiviral therapy (rare)

IMAGING/SPECIAL TESTS

- CXRs
  —Usually hyperventilation, airway disease, atelectasis, variable infiltrate, isolated consolidation rare
  —Useful for monitoring course, rarely changes management acutely
  —Consider when
    -Need to exclude other diagnoses such as CHF, aspiration, congenital airway anomaly (rare)
    -Chronic course with lack of resolution over 7–10 days
    -Critically ill infants with impending respiratory failure
    -Atypical presentation in toxic or deteriorating child

DIFFERENTIAL DIAGNOSIS

- Asthma: recurrent episodes of "bronchiolitis," common in those with severe initial exacerbation
- Pertussis: no respiratory distress between coughing spasms, no wheezing
- Bacterial pneumonia: often toxic appearance, no wheezing, isolated airspace disease (consolidation) with no airway abnormality on CXR
- Foreign body: sudden onset of symptoms, usually afebrile
- CHF: preexisting clinical red flags (FTT, feeding problems)

Treatment

INITIAL STABILIZATION

- Pediatric advanced life support
- Emergent intubation if recurrent apneas, impending respiratory failure

ED TREATMENT

- Supplemental oxygen if oxygen saturation 92% (sea level)
- Parenteral hydration if dehydration or severe respiratory distress
- Bronchodilators (albuterol, racemic epinephrine, L-epinephrine)
  —Indicated in all but mildest cases; 60% response rate
  —Trial of two to three consecutive treatments
  —Continue if clear response to trial decreases respiratory distress
  —Racemic epinephrine or L-epinephrine may be useful in moderate to severe distress if poor response to albuterol
- Steroids
  —Dexamethasone
  —Controversial
  —Recent ED study suggests superior clinical efficacy and $2\frac{1}{2}$ times lower hospitalization rate 4 hours after treatment in children with moderate or severe disease; optimal duration of therapy is unknown
- Antibiotics
  —Almost never indicated since viral etiology
  —Consider if associated signs of focal bacterial disease (otitis), radiographic evidence of isolated lobar consolidation without airway disease, significant toxicity, sepsis
- Ribavirin
  —May rarely be indicated in the early course of hospitalization in children with severe underlying chronic disease
  —No role in ED management

MEDICATIONS

- Albuterol: 0.03 mL/kg/dose; may also dose as 2.5 mg (0.5 mL/dose) via nebulizer with 3 mL NS every 20–30 minutes
- Dexamethasone: 0.6 mg/kg/dose PO; may be given parenterally if not tolerated orally
- L-Epinephrine: 2.5 mL (1:1,000 solution) via nebulizer in 2 mL NS
- Racemic epinephrine: 0.25–0.75 mL via nebulizer in 3 mL NS
- Ribavirin (Virazole): continuous inhalation 12–20 hh/24 hr for 3–5 days

Disposition

ADMISSION CRITERIA

- Need for supplemental oxygen
- Inability to self-hydrate
- Apnea
- Severe underlying chronic lung disease or cardiac disease
- Persistent significant respiratory distress after several doses of β_2-agonists therapy or 4 hours after corticosteroids
- Suspicion of comorbidity/alternative diagnosis/underlying systemic disease/immunodeficiency or immunosuppressive therapy
- Strongly consider in infants younger than 8 weeks

DISCHARGE CRITERIA

- Feeding well
- Acceptable room air saturation
- Absence of significant respiratory distress
- Follow-up available within 24 hours

Miscellaneous

ICD9: 466.1.9

ICD10: J21.9

SEE ALSO: ASTHMA, PEDIATRIC

SUGGESTED READINGS

Dawson KP, Long A, Kennedy J, et al. The chest radiograph in acute bronchiolitis. J Paediatr Child Health 1990;26:290–311.

Gadomski AM, Lichensttein R, Horton L, et al. Efficacy of albuterol in the management of bronchiolitis. Pediatrics 1994;93:907–912.

Kellner JD, Ohlsson A, Gadomski AM, et al. Efficacy of bronchodilator therapy in bronchiolitis. A meta-analysis. Arch Pediatr Adolesc Med 1996;150(11):1166–1167.

Menon K, Sutcliffe T, Klassen TP. A randomized trial comparing the efficacy of epinephrine with salbutamol in the treatment of acute bronchiolitis. J Pediatr 1995;126:1004–1007.

Reionen T, Korppi M, Pitkakangas S, et al. The clinical efficacy of nebulized racemic epinephrine and albuterol in acute bronchitis. Arch Pediatr Adolesc Med 1995;149:686–692.

Roosevelt G, Sheehan K, Grupp-Phelan J, et al. Dexamethasone in bronchiolitis: a randomized controlled trial. Lancet 1996;348:292–295.

Schuh S, Coates AL, Binnie R, et al. Efficacy of oral dexamethasone in outpatients with acute bronchiolitis. J Pediatr 2002;140:27–32.

Author: Suzanne Schuh

Bronchitis

Clinical Presentation

SIGNS AND SYMPTOMS

- Complaints that may precede upper respiratory tract infection (URTI) symptoms
  - —Malaise
  - —Chills
  - —Myalgias
  - —Coryza
  - —Sore throat
- Onset of URTI symptoms
  - —Cough, initially dry and nonproductive
  - —Cough, later becomes mucoid or mucopurulent
  - —Fever, not usually above 102°F (38.5°C)
  - —Chest pain or burning related to cough
  - —Dyspnea may be present
  - —Mild hemoptysis
  - —Wheezing
  - —Rales
  - —Scattered rhonchi
  - —Initial symptoms improve after 3–5 days, with 1–2 weeks of residual cough and malaise

MECHANISM/DESCRIPTION

- Hyperemia and edema of the mucous membranes
- Production of mucopurulent exudates
- Impairment of the productive function of the cilia, lymphatics, and phagocytes
- Airway obstruction from
  - —Edema
  - —Secretions
  - —Bronchial muscle spasm

ETIOLOGY

- Viral infections are the primary cause of bronchitis
  - —Parainfluenza
  - —Influenza A and B
  - —Respiratory syncytial virus (RSV)
  - —Echovirus
  - —Coronavirus
  - —Adenovirus
  - —Coxsackievirus
  - —Rhinovirus
  - —Measles and herpes viruses (can cause severe viral bronchitis)
- Particularly severe or long-lasting bronchitis
  - —*Mycoplasma pneumoniae*
  - —*Chlamydia pneumoniae*
  - —*Bordetella pertussis*
- Rates of pertussis are increasing, even in the fully immunized population (little protection remains after 10 years)
- Other bacteria have not been conclusively proven to cause bronchitis except in those with chronic lung disease

Pre-Hospital

- Maintain adequate oxygenation
- Bronchodilators if wheezing is present

Diagnosis

ESSENTIAL WORKUP

- Pulse oximetry to assess oxygenation
- Exclude other respiratory disorders
- The diagnosis is clinical; however, influenza A and B testing is available to confirm these organisms are the cause of symptoms
- More involved workup may be considered if symptoms last beyond expected time frame
- Pertussis may be considered in the patient with an acute cough illness lasting 14 days or more in a person with at least one pertussis-associated symptom (paroxysmal cough, posttussive vomiting, inspiratory whoop) or 14 days or more of cough in a person within an outbreak setting

LABORATORY

- Influenza A and B testing may help immediately confirm clinical suspicion
- In most cases, no specific test will help make the diagnosis immediately
- Viral or bacterial cultures are rarely helpful
- CBC may show leukocytosis, but this is a nonspecific finding
- Pertussis may be confirmed using PCR testing, but diagnosis will be delayed

IMAGING/SPECIAL TESTS

- CXR
  - —No evidence of consolidation
  - —Indications
    - -Shortness of breath
    - -Hypoxia
    - -Chest pain
    - -Heart rate >100 beats/minute
    - -Respiratory rate ≥24 breaths/minute
    - -Temperature ≥38°C
    - -Focal findings on chest examination
    - -Elderly patient with multiple comorbid conditions

DIFFERENTIAL DIAGNOSIS

- Influenza causing bronchitis
- Pneumonia
- Reactive airway disease
- Aspiration
- Acute sinusitis
- Bronchiectasis
- Bacterial tracheitis
- Chronic bronchitis or COPD exacerbation in those with underlying chronic lung disease

PEDIATRIC CONSIDERATIONS

- Differential diagnosis includes
  - —Retained foreign body
  - —Cystic fibrosis
  - —Allergic respiratory disease

Treatment

INITIAL STABILIZATION

- Aggressive initial management of these patients is seldom required
- Administer oxygen if the patient is hypoxic
- Fluids may be administered if the patient is dehydrated

ED TREATMENT

- Bronchitis is usually a viral process, treatment is symptomatic
- Cough suppressants may be considered
- β-Adrenergic inhaler for patients with severe cough or wheezing
- Amantadine may be used in known outbreaks of influenza A
- Oseltamivir (Tamiflu) and zanamivir (Relenza) may be considered in patients with recent onset of influenza
- Antibiotics
  —Generally, antibiotics are not indicated
  —Antibiotics do not improve symptoms more quickly
  —Consider use in those patients who have recurrence of fever after initial improvement
- Symptomatic control with antipyretics and analgesics
- Although patients should be encouraged to stop smoking, the use of tobacco is not an indication for antibiotics unless the patient has a known history of emphysema

MEDICATIONS

- Albuterol: 0.5 mL in a 0.5% solution nebulized every 6 hours
- Amantadine: 100 mg PO q.d., must be given within 48 hours of symptom onset
- Oseltamivir (Tamiflu) and zanamivir (Relenza) within 48 hours of symptom onset for influenza-related bronchitis
  —Zanamivir: 10 mg inhalation q12h × 5 days (no pediatric dosing)
  —Oseltamivir: 75 mg PO b.i.d. (peds: 2 mg/kg) × 5 days
- Erythromycin should be given to proven cases of pertussis and to household contacts of those with proven pertussis
- Yearly influenza vaccinations should be encouraged in health care providers and in the high-risk population (elderly, immunocompromised, chronic lung disease)

PEDIATRIC CONSIDERATIONS

- Use of acetaminophen rather than aspirin for analgesia
- Repeated bouts in children should lead to referral for complete evaluation of the respiratory tract

Disposition

ADMISSION CRITERIA

- Underlying significant cardiopulmonary compromise
- Significant hypoxia
- Ill patient with unclear diagnosis

DISCHARGE CRITERIA

- No pulmonary compromise should be present
- Instruct patients, particularly high-risk patients, to return if no improvement or worsening of symptoms occurs
- Bed rest
- Fluids
- Aspirin or acetaminophen

Miscellaneous

ICD10: 466, 490

ICD10: J40

SEE ALSO: COUGH

SUGGESTED READINGS

Gonzales R, Bartlett JG, Besser RE, et al. Principles of appropriate antibiotic use for treatment of uncomplicated acute bronchitis: background. Ann Intern Med 2001;134:521–529.

Gonzales R, Sande MA. Uncomplicated acute bronchitis. Ann Intern Med 2000;133:981–991.

Karras DJ. Update on emerging infections: news from the Centers for Disease Control and Prevention. Ann Emerg Med 2002;40:115–119.

MacKay DN. Treatment of acute bronchitis in adults without underlying lung disease. J Gen Intern Med 1996;11:557–562.

Orr PH, Scherer K, Macdonald A, et al. Randomized placebo-controlled trials of antibiotics for acute bronchitis. A critical review of the literature. J Fam Pract 1993;36:507–512.

Author: Robin R. Hemphill

Bundle Branch Blocks

Clinical Presentation

SIGNS AND SYMPTOMS

- Asymptomatic
- Right bundle branch block (RBBB): split S_2 that persists with expiration
- Left bundle branch block (LBBB): reversed/paradoxic split S_2
- Syncope (ventricular tachycardia in 20–30%)
- Chest pain

MECHANISM/DESCRIPTION

- Blockage of intraventricular electrical impulses through the right and left bundles
- Complete BBB
  - —Absence or delay of conduction down one bundle, with normal conduction down the other bundle
  - —Affected ventricle depolarizes from muscle to muscle in slower and more disorganized fashion
  - —QRS complex $\geq$120 ms
- Incomplete BBB
  - —Delayed depolarization but less than complete BBB
  - —120 ms > QRS complex $\geq$100 ms
- RBBB
  - —Delayed depolarization of the right ventricle
- LBBB
  - —Delayed depolarization of the left ventricle
  - —LBBB can be caused by delay of conduction in main left bundle or delay in both fascicles of the left bundle
  - —Causes early activation of the right side of the septum and the right ventricular myocardium (so loss of "septal Q" on EKG)
  - —Left bundle branches into two fascicles
    - -Left anterior fascicle (LAF): initial septal activation proceeds inferiorly, anteriorly, and to the right
    - -Left posterior fascicle (LPF): rare; activation begins in the mid septum and finishes in inferior and posterior walls
- Bifascicular block
  - —RBBB with concomitant block of the LAF or LPF

ETIOLOGY

- Myocardial infarction
- Cardiomyopathy
- Hypertension
- Age-related fibrosis of Purkinje fibers
- Valvular disease
- Exercise induced
- Congenital/atrial septal defect
- Brugada's syndrome (RBBB): cause of sudden cardiac death in otherwise healthy patients
- Chagas' disease (especially Central/South America)
- Postoperative, following cardiac surgery
- Drugs
  - —β-Blockers
  - —Calcium blockers
  - —TCAs
  - —Type Ia and Ic antiarrhythmics
  - —Digitalis

Pre-Hospital

CAUTIONS

- Monitor: difficult to diagnose from single lead
- Avoid confusing with ventricular tachycardia or ischemia
- Treat patient; BBB requires no specific therapy

Diagnosis

ESSENTIAL WORKUP

- EKG
  - —RBBB
    - -Complete: QRS complex $\geq$0.12 seconds; incomplete: $\leq$0.10 seconds QRS complex $\leq$0.12 seconds
    - -rsr′, rsR′, rSR′ in V_1 or V_2 (M shape)
    - -wide and deep S wave in V_5 through V_6
    - -Brugada's syndrome: RBBB and ST-segment elevation in V_1 through V_3
  - —LBBB
    - -Broad slurred R waves in leads V_5 through V_6, aVL, and I
    - -Small/absent r wave in V_1 through V_2 and deep S waves
    - -Absence of normal q waves in leads V_5 through V_6 and I
  - —LAF block
    - -QRS complex <120 ms, axis −45 to −90
    - -Deep S wave in leads II, III, aVF, qR in leads aVL and I
  - —LPF block
    - -QRS <120 ms, axis $\geq$120
    - -RS waves in leads I and aVL, qR in leads II, III, and aVF
    - -Exclusion of other things causing right axis deviation (RV overload, RVH, lateral infarction)

LABORATORY

- Potassium if hyperkalemia is suspected
- Cardiac enzymes if ischemia is suspected

IMAGING/SPECIAL TESTS

- CXR
  - —May reveal cardiac enlargement or CHF
- Electrophysiologic testing
  - —Especially for unexplained syncope in patient with structural heart disease, as part of inpatient workup

DIFFERENTIAL DIAGNOSIS

- Ventricular tachycardia
- Myocardial infarction
  - —Criteria for diagnosing myocardial infarction with LBBB: ST-segment elevation $\geq$1 mm concordant with QRS
    - -ST-segment elevation $\geq$5 mm discordant with QRS
    - -ST-segment depression $\geq$1 mm in leads V_1 through V_3
- Hyperkalemia
- Ventricular hypertrophy
- Drug effects (see Etiology section)

Treatment

INITIAL STABILIZATION

- Standard treatment for symptoms of ischemia, shortness of breath, and syncope
- Bifascicular block and symptomatic high-degree AV block
  - —Apply transcutaneous pacing pads to back and chest
  - —IV sedation and analgesia
  - —Gradually increase current until capture is achieved

ED TREATMENT

- Asymptomatic: none
- Thrombolysis for symptoms suggestive of myocardial infarction and new BBB
- Transvenous pacemaker indications
  - —Bifascicular block and symptomatic type II second-degree or third-degree (i.e., advanced) AV block
  - —Bifascicular block and asymptomatic advanced AV block in the setting of myocardial infarction

MEDICATIONS

N/A

Disposition

ADMISSION CRITERIA

- Concern for myocardial ischemia
- Syncope
- BBB with advanced AV block or complete heart block

DISCHARGE CRITERIA

- Asymptomatic or incidental finding of BBB
- Refer for further evaluation of underlying cardiac disease

Miscellaneous

ICD9: 426.2-426.5

ICD10: I45.4

SUGGESTED READINGS

Brignole M, Menozzi C, Moya A, et al. Mechanism of syncope in patients with bundle branch block and negative electrophysiological test. Circulation 2001;104:2045–2050.

Brugada J, Brugada R, Brugada P. Right bundle-branch block and ST-segment elevation in leads V_1 through V_3: a marker for sudden death in patients without demonstrable structural heart disease. Circulation 1998;97:457–460.

Sgarbossa EB, Pinski SL, Barbagelata A, et al. Electrocardiographic diagnosis of acute myocardial infarction in the presence of left bundle-branch block. N Engl J Med 1996;334:481–487.

Authors: Keith Boniface; James Scott

Burns

Clinical Presentation

SIGNS AND SYMPTOMS

- First-degree burns (involve epidermis only): local erythema and pain only; healing occurs in several days
- Second-degree burns (involve the epidermis and dermis, sparing portion of dermal appendages)
  - —Skin is erythematous, moist, often with blisters and bullae
  - —Deep partial-thickness burns may have blanched, white areas and thick-walled blisters
  - —Sensation is intact; heal via epithelialization within 2–6 weeks, depending on depth
- Third-degree burns (destroy epidermis and dermis, including dermal appendages): appear white and leathery; thrombosed blood vessels or skin charring may be visualized; the wounds are insensate
- Inhalation injury
  - —Facial burns
  - —Carbonaceous sputum
  - —Pharyngeal injection
  - —Wheezing
  - —Hoarseness
- Carbon monoxide poisoning: suspect with a history of an exposure to combustion
- Cyanide poisoning should be suspected from burning wool, silk, nylon, and polyurethane found in furniture and paper

Pre-Hospital

CAUTIONS

- Remove smoldering clothes/jewelry
- Cool injury with cloth or gauze soaked in cool water
- Immobilize spine if decreased sensorium or trauma
- Reevaluate airway frequently for signs of inhalation injury and airway swelling
  - *—Intubate early for signs of respiratory distress*
- Initiate early IV fluid therapy
- Transport to burn center (for major burns) if transport time shorter than 30 minutes

Diagnosis

ESSENTIAL WORKUP

- Measure extent of second- and third-degree burns in terms of total body surface area (TBSA) percentage
- "Rule of nines"
  - —TBSA of body parts is estimated by multiples of 9%, applies to adults only
  - —In infants and children, the head contributes more to the percentage of TBSA and legs contribute less
- Estimates of percentage of TBSA
  - —Adults
    - -Head and neck, 9
    - -Arms: right, 9; left, 9
    - -Legs: right, 18; left, 18
    - -Trunk: front, 18; back, 18
    - -Perineum, 1
  - —Infants/children
    - -Head and neck, 20/10*
    - -Arms: right, 10; left, 10
    - -Legs: right, 10/15*; left, 10/15*
    - -Trunk: front, 20; back, 20
- The patient's palm is approximately 1% of TBSA and is helpful in assessing smaller, scattered burns
- Blood gas with carbon monoxide level for closed space or inhalation exposures
- Fiberoptic bronchoscopy is a safe way to assess inhalation injury
- For severe burns, obtain CBC, serum electrolytes, glucose, BUN, creatinine, and PT/PTT

IMAGING/SPECIAL TESTS

- Initial CXR film is usually normal

DIFFERENTIAL DIAGNOSIS

- Electrical injury
- Chemical injury
- Associated trauma or intoxication

*Use the first percentage for infants and younger children.

Treatment

INITIAL STABILIZATION

- ABCs
  - —Early intubation for patients with signs of upper airway injury, significant nasolabial burns, or circumferential neck burns
- IV access, supplemental 100% oxygen
- Evaluation for trauma
- Provide adequate analgesia (morphine preferred)

ED TREATMENT

Fluid Resuscitation: Second- and Third-degree Burns

- *Parkland formula:* 2–4 mL of lactated Ringer's solution or NS per kilogram per percentage of BSA burned; one half of this total is given in the first 8 hours and the remaining half over the next 16 hours
- For example: a 90-kg patient with a 40% TBSA burn would requires 2–4 mL $\times$ 90 kg $\times$ 40% = 7,200–14,400 mL over 24 hours, with 3,600–7,200 mL over the first 8 hours or 450–900 mL/hr
- For burns >20% TBSA, IV fluid therapy is guided by urine output using a bladder catheter; maintain urine output of 0.5–1.0 mL/kg/hr for adults and 1.0–1.5 mL/kg/hr for children

Escharotomy

- Circumferential burn eschar of the extremities may lead to neurovascular compromise
  - —Monitor pulses
  - —Elevate burned extremity
  - —If circulation is compromised, escharotomy incisions on extremities should be made medially and laterally along the long axis of the limb just to the subcutaneous layer through the entire length of the burn eschar
- A circumferential burn of the chest wall may prevent adequate ventilation unless escharotomy is performed
  - —Make longitudinal incisions along each midclavicular line from 2 cm below the clavicle to the tenth rib; connect with two transverse incisions across the chest, forming a square

Wound Care

- Sterile technique
- If admitted to a burn unit, simple coverage of the wounds with sterile moist dressings is appropriate
- If disposition is delayed, cleanse with sterile saline or poloxamer 188 product (e.g., Shur-Clens), debride blisters except those on palms or soles, and apply topical antibacterial agent (e.g., silver sulfadiazine)
- Do not delay transfer to burn unit for wound care
- Prophylactic antibiotics not indicated

Outpatient Management of Minor Burns

- Sterile technique for cleansing and débridement
- Remove loose, necrotic skin; débride broken, tense, or infected blisters
- *Topical antibacterial agents:* (e.g., silver sulfadiazine, povidone-iodine, mafenide acetate) recommended in deep partial-thickness or full-thickness burns only
- *Burn dressings* should keep the wound moist and absorb exudate
  - —Inner layer should be nonadherent porous mesh gauze saturated with a non-petroleum–based lubricant, or use a mild ointment (e.g., bacitracin or Polysporin) under a nonadherent porous gauze
  - —The next layer should be fluffed course mesh gauze
  - —The outer wrap should keep the dressing in place without constricting
- Dressings should be changed at least daily
- Tetanus prophylaxis

MEDICATIONS

- Mafenide acetate cream: apply to wound 1–2 times/day, thickness of 1⁄16 inch (Sulfamylon)
- Morphine: 0.1–0.2 mg/kg titrated to effect for pain control after shock
- Povidone-iodine ointment: apply to wound 1–2 times/day to a thickness of 1⁄16 inch
- Silver sulfadiazine cream: apply to wound 1–2 times/day to a thickness of 1⁄16 inch

PEDIATRIC CONSIDERATIONS

- *Parkland formula* underestimates fluid requirements in children; the *Galveston formula* may be used instead: 5,000 mL/m^2 BSA burned plus 2,000 mL/m^2
- TBSA of 5% dextrose in lactated Ringer's solution i.v. over the first 24 hours, half in the first 8 hours and the other half over the next 16 hours
- Consider nonaccidental trauma, particularly with burns on the back of hands or feet, buttocks, the perineum, and the legs
- Avoid hypothermia
  - —Children have greater BSA/mass ratio and lose heat more rapidly
- Avoid hypoglycemia
  - —Children are more prone to hypoglycemia due to limited glycogen stores

Disposition

ADMISSION CRITERIA

Injuries Requiring Admission

- Partial-thickness burns of noncritical areas (not the eyes, ears, face, hands, feet, or perineum) involving 10–20% of BSA in adults (older than 10 years and younger than 50 years)
- Partial-thickness burns of noncritical areas involving 5–10% of BSA in children younger than 10 years
- Suspicion of nonaccidental trauma
- Patients unable to care for wounds in outpatient setting (e.g., homeless patients)

Injuries Requiring Transfer and Admission to a Burn Center

- Second- and third-degree burns involving ≥10% of BSA in patients younger than 10 or older than 50 years
- Second- and third-degree burns over >20% of BSA in any patient
- Third-degree burns involving >5% of BSA
- Significant burns of face, hands, feet, genitalia, perineum, or major joints
- Significant electrical injury
- Significant chemical injury
- Significant inhalation injury, concomitant mechanical trauma, or preexisting medical disorders (e.g., immunosuppressed patients, diabetes, AIDS, cancer, or alcoholism)

DISCHARGE CRITERIA

- Patients with burns that do not meet the aforementioned admission criteria; in general, partial-thickness burns of <15% of BSA in adults (<10% in children) involving noncritical areas only and in patients able to manage wounds as an outpatient and follow up reliably

Miscellaneous

ICD9: 949.0

ICD10: T30.0

SUGGESTED READINGS

Dimrick AR, Wagner RG. Burns. In: Schwartz GR, Hanko BK, Mayer TA, eds. Principles and practice of emergency medicine, 4th ed. Baltimore: Williams & Wilkins, 1999.

Edlich RF. Thermal burns. In: Rosen P, Barkin R, eds. Emergency medicine: concepts and clinical practice, 5th ed. St. Louis: Mosby, 2000:941.

Schwartz LR. Thermal burns. In: Tintinalli JE, Ruiz E, Krome R, eds. Emergency medicine: a comprehensive study guide, 4th ed. New York: McGraw-Hill, 1996: 893.

Yowler CJ, Fratianne RB. Current status of burn resuscitation. Clin Plastic Surg 2000;27:1–10.

Author: Mary Anne Fuchs

Bursitis

Clinical Presentation

SIGNS AND SYMPTOMS

- Localized pain that worsens with movement of structures adjacent to affected bursae
- Often reduced active range of motion (ROM) with preserved passive ROM
- Localized swelling may be present with superficial bursal involvement
- Usually presents with acute onset but may be chronic (especially in hip)
- Overlying erythema, warmth, or skin trauma may be present with infectious bursitis
- May have low-grade temperature

MECHANISM/DESCRIPTION

- Bursae are sacs lined with synovial membrane
  - —Approximately 150 are located at sites of friction between bones, ligaments, tendons, muscles, and skin
  - —They provide lubrication for movement
- Bursitis is inflammation of a bursae caused by trauma (acute or chronic), repetitive use, infection, crystal deposition, or systemic disease

ETIOLOGY

- Trauma (most common cause) following either a specific traumatic event or repetitive use of related joints
- Infection: may be obvious or microscopic
  - —Higher risk with diabetes, chronic alcohol abuse, uremia, gout, and immunosuppression
  - —Staphylococci cause 90%
- Crystal deposition: calcium phosphate, urate
- Systemic disease: rheumatoid, gout, ankylosing spondylitis, psoriatic arthritis, lupus, rheumatic fever

Affected Joints

- Potentially any bursa may be affected
- Commonly affected joints
  - —Shoulder
  - —Elbow: usually secondary to trauma, high incidence of infection
  - —Wrist and hand
  - —Hip: more common in older women
  - —Knee: often secondary to chronic trauma or arthritis
  - —Foot: calcaneal bursitis is almost always from improper shoes/high heels

Pre-Hospital

CAUTIONS

- May be difficult to distinguish from fractures; suspicious joints should be immobilized, particularly in the setting of trauma

Diagnosis

ESSENTIAL WORKUP

- Full assessment of adjacent musculoskeletal structures
- Any suspicion of infection warrants aspiration of bursae (especially olecranon and prepatellar bursae)
- Aspiration of hip and other deep bursae should be deferred to orthopedics or rheumatology or may be guided in ED by US

LABORATORY

- Serum labs
  - —Suspected infection: CBC with differential
  - —Evaluation of related systemic disease (e.g., uric acid level for gout)
  - —Send serum glucose if bursal fluid aspiration is done
- Bursal fluid analysis
  - —Analysis of bursa fluid: cell count with differential, glucose and total protein, crystal determination, Gram stain, culture
  - —Because infection and inflammation may be difficult to differentiate, cultures must always be sent
  - —Normal fluid is clear yellow and has 0–200 WBCs; 0 RBCs; low protein and glucose is same as serum
  - —Traumatic bursitis: fluid is bloody/xanthochromic and has <1,200 WBCs; many RBCs; low protein and normal glucose
  - —Infective bursitis: fluid is yellow, cloudy, and has >50,000 WBCs; few RBCs; slightly increased protein and decreased glucose; bacteria on Gram stain
  - —Rheumatoid and microcrystalline inflammation: fluid is yellow to cloudy and has 1,000–40,000 WBCs; few RBCs; slightly increased protein and variable glucose; use polarizing microscope to identify crystals

IMAGING/SPECIAL TESTS

- X-rays may demonstrate chronic arthritic changes or calcium deposits; recommended when trauma is involved to rule out fracture or foreign body
- MRI and US may aid in diagnosis of deep bursitis and in defining the extent of infectious bursitis

DIFFERENTIAL DIAGNOSIS

- Arthritis, gout
- Tendonitis
- Fracture, tendon/ligament tear, contusion, sprain
- Also in hips: neuritis, lumbar spine disease, sacroiliitis

Treatment

INITIAL STABILIZATION

- Immobilize joint if pain severe
  —Shoulders should not be immobilized for >2–3 days because of the risk of adhesive capsulitis

ED TREATMENT

- Non-infectious bursitis
  —Rest and removal of aggravating factors (e.g., avoid direct pressure and repetitive use)
  —Ice-affected areas for 10 minutes, 4 times/day until improved; may alternate with heat
  —NSAIDs for at least 7 days; best if continued for 5 days after improvement to help prevent recurrence
  —If no improvement within 5–7 days and infection has been ruled out (by culture), injection of lidocaine and steroids may be considered
  —Mix 2 mL of 2% lidocaine with 20–40 mg of depoglucocorticoid and inject 1–3 mL of this mixture into the bursae using sterile technique
  —Steroid injections should not be repeated until at least 4 weeks have passed and no more than two injections into one joint should be performed without rheumatologic or orthopedic consultation
- Septic bursitis
  —Should be treated with antibiotics and drainage of bursae
  —Base antibiotic choice on the Gram stain
  —Penicillinase-resistant antistaphylococcal drug may be used if Gram stain result is negative or shows gram-positive cocci
  —If gram-negative organisms are found, blood cultures should be done and another primary source for the infection should be sought
  —Antibiotics should be continued for 5–7 days beyond the sterilization of bursal fluid
- Treat associated diseases as needed (e.g., gout)

MEDICATIONS

- NSAIDs (many choices, a few are listed here)
  —Diclofenac: 50 mg PO b.i.d./t.i.d.
  —Ibuprofen: 600 mg PO q6h (peds: 5–10 mg/kg PO q6h)
  —Ketorolac: 30 mg i.v./i.m. q6h or 10 mg PO q4–6h
  —Piroxicam: 20 mg PO q.d.
- Corticosteroids
  —Methylprednisolone acetate: 20–40 mg single intrabursal injection
  —Triamcinolone acetonide: 20–40 mg single intrabursal injection

Disposition

ADMISSION CRITERIA

- Patients with high fevers, chills/rigors, large surrounding cellulitis, unable to take oral antibiotics, failed outpatient therapy, or immunosuppressed
- Unusual organisms, extrabursal primary site, or deep bursal involvement

DISCHARGE CRITERIA

- Most patients may be treated as outpatients

Follow-Up

- Most patients respond to therapy in 3–4 days and may follow up with PCP within a week
- Septic bursitis requires repeated bursal aspiration every 3–5 days until sterile
- Rheumatology or orthopedic referral is recommended for patients who do not respond to intrabursal steroids or recurrent bursitis

Miscellaneous

ICD9: 727.3

ICD10: M71.9

SUGGESTED READINGS

Butcher JD, et al. Lower extremity bursitis. Am Fam Physician 1996;53(7): 2317–2324.

Greene WB, ed. Essentials of musculoskeletal care, 2nd ed. Rosemont, IL: American Academy of Orthopedic Surgeons, 2001:20–23; 368–370; 402–403;335–337.

Kopicky-Burd J. Nonarticular rheumatic disorders. In: Barker LR, ed. Principles of ambulatory medicine, 3rd ed. Baltimore: Williams & Wilkins, 1991:827–835.

Larsson L, Baum J. The syndromes of bursitis. Bull Rheum Dis 1986;36(1).

Talbot-Stern JK. Arthritis, tendonitis, and bursitis. In: Rosen P, ed. Emergency medicine, 3rd ed. St. Louis: Mosby–Year Book, 1992:822–826.

Author: Kelly Pettit

Calcium Channel Blocker, Poisoning

Clinical Presentation

SIGNS AND SYMPTOMS

- Cardiovascular
  - —Hypotension
  - —Bradycardia
  - —Reflex tachycardia (dihydropyridine)
  - —Conduction abnormalities/heart blocks
- Neurologic
  - —CNS depression
  - —Coma
  - —Seizures
- Metabolic
  - —Hyperglycemia

MECHANISM/DESCRIPTION

Three Classes of Calcium Channel Blockers

- Phenylalkylamines (verapamil)
  - —Vasodilation resulting in a decrease in BP
  - —Negative chronotropic and inotropic effects: reflex tachycardia not seen with a drop in BP
- Dihydropyridine (nifedipine)
  - —Decreased vascular resistance resulting in a drop in BP
  - —Little negative inotropic effect: reflex tachycardia occurs
- Benzodiazepine (diltiazem)
  - —Decreased peripheral vascular resistance leading to a decrease in BP
  - —Heart rate (HR) and cardiac output initially increased
  - —Direct negative chronotropic effect, which leads to a fall in HR

Effects of Calcium Channel Blockade

- Calcium plays key role in cardiac and smooth muscle contractility
- Calcium channel blockers (CCBs) prevent
  - —The entry of calcium, resulting in a lack of muscle contraction
  - —The normal release of insulin from pancreatic islet cells, resulting in hyperglycemia

Pre-Hospital

CAUTIONS

- Transport pill/pill bottles to ED
- Calcium for bradycardic/unstable patient with confirmed CCB overdose

Diagnosis

ESSENTIAL WORKUP

- EKG
  - —Bradycardia (tachycardia with nifedipine)
  - —Conduction delays: QRS-complex prolongation
  - —Heart blocks

LABORATORY

- Ionized calcium level when administering calcium
- Digoxin level if patient taking digoxin (dictate safety of calcium administration)
- CBC
- Electrolytes, BUN, creatinine, glucose
  - —Hyperglycemia/metabolic acidosis may occur
- Toxicology screen if co-ingestants suspected

DIFFERENTIAL DIAGNOSIS

- β-Blocker toxicity
- Clonidine toxicity
- Digitalis toxicity
- Acute myocardial infarction with heart block

Treatment

INITIAL STABILIZATION

- ABCs
  - —Airway protection as indicated
  - —Supplemental oxygen as needed
  - —0.9% NS IV access
  - —Hemodynamic monitoring

ED TREATMENT

Goals

- Heart rate >60 beats/minute
- Systolic BP >90 mm Hg
- Adequate urine output
- Improving level of consciousness

GI Decontamination

- Syrup of ipecac: contraindicated in the ED
- Activated charcoal
  - —May be helpful especially in the presence of co-ingestants
- Whole bowel irrigation
  - —Beneficial with ingestion of sustained-release preparations
  - —Contraindicated in hemodynamically unstable patients

Calcium

- First-line agent for CCB toxicity
- Calcium chloride (10%)
- Contains 1.36 mEq Ca^{2+}/mL (3 times more calcium than calcium gluconate)
- Can cause tissue necrosis and sloughing with extravasation
- Very irritating to veins
- Calcium gluconate (10%)
  - —Contains 0.45 mEq Ca^{2+}/mL
  - —Does not cause tissue necrosis like calcium chloride
  - —Calcium gluconate: preferred agent in an acidemic patient
- Follow serum calcium levels if repeated doses of calcium administered
- Contraindicated in digoxin toxicity because calcium can produce serious adverse effects in digoxin toxicity

Bradycardia/Hypotension

- IV fluids
  - —Administer cautiously in the hypotensive patient
  - —Swan-Ganz catheter or CVP monitoring to help follow volume status
- Atropine usually ineffective
- Pressor agents
  - —No clear evidence that one agent is more effective than another
  - —Institute invasive monitoring to help guide treatment
  - —Dopamine
    - -β_1-Receptor agonist at low doses, which causes a positive inotropic effect on the myocardium
    - -α-Receptor agonist at higher doses, which leads to vasoconstriction
  - —Epinephrine
    - -Potent α- and β-receptor agonist
- Glucagon
  - —Promotes cAMP production through a receptor site other than the β-receptor
  - —May cause nausea and vomiting
  - —Mix with NS or 5% dextrose in water
    - -Do not use the phenol diluent that comes with glucagon
- Amrinone
  - —Selective phosphodiesterase III inhibitor
  - —Indirectly increases cAMP
- Electrical pacing: when other treatment options have failed
- Insulin
  - —Potential for treatment in the future

MEDICATIONS

- Amrinone: loading dose 0.75 mg/kg; maintenance drip 2–20 μg/kg/min; titrate for effect
- Atropine: 0.5 mg (peds: 0.02 mg/kg) i.v.; repeat 0.5–1.0 mg i.v. (peds: 0.04 mg/kg)
- Calcium chloride: 10 mL of 10% solution slow IVP (peds: 0.2–0.25 mL/kg; repeat in 10 minutes if necessary) followed by infusion 20–50 mg/kg/hr
- Calcium gluconate: 10 mL of 10% solution slow IVP (peds: 1 mL/kg; may repeat in 10 minutes if necessary)
- Dopamine: 2–20 μg/kg/min; titrate to effect
- Epinephrine: 2 μg/min (peds: 0.1 μg/kg/min); titrate to effect
- Glucagon: 3.5–5 mg (peds: 0.03–0.1 mg/kg) i.v. bolus followed by 70 μg/kg/hr infusion
- GoLYTELY WBI: 2 L/hr PO or by NGT for 4–6 hours or until rectal effluent is clear (peds: 40 mL/kg/hr)

Disposition

ADMISSION CRITERIA

- Admit symptomatic patients to a monitored bed for hemodynamic monitoring
- Admit all ingestions of sustained-release CCBs for 24 hours of observation and monitoring due to the potential delay in symptoms

DISCHARGE CRITERIA

- Discharge asymptomatic patients 8 hours after ingestion of immediate-release preparation

Miscellaneous

ICD9: 977.9

ICD10: T46.1

SEE ALSO: β-BLOCKER, POISONING

SUGGESTED READINGS

Haddad LM. Resuscitation after nifedipine overdose exclusively with intravenous calcium chloride. Am J Emerg Med 1996;14:602–603.

Kalman S, Berg S, Lisander B. Combined overdose with verapamil and atenolol: treatment with high doses of adrenergic agonists. Acta Anaesthesiol Scand 1998;45:379–382.

Kline JA, Leonova E, Raymond RM. Beneficial myocardial metabolic effects of insulin during verapamil toxicity in the anesthetized canine. Crit Care Med 1995;23:1251–1263.

Author: Janet Eng

Candidiasis, Oral

Clinical Presentation

SIGNS AND SYMPTOMS

- Pseudomembranous candidiasis (thrush)
  —Painless white mucosal plaques
  —Adherent but removable
  —Erythematous base
  —May become confluent and curdlike
- Atrophic candidiasis (denture stomatitis)
  —Burning sensation in mouth or on tongue
  —Erythematous with few, if any, white patches
  —Usually limited to the denture-bearing mucosa
- Angular cheilosis
  —Cracking and erythema at the corners of the mouth
  —Lesion can be asymptomatic, itching, or painful
- Hyperplastic candidiasis
  —Chronic, invasive ulcers
  —Typically on lateral borders of tongue or buccal mucosa
  —Plaques cannot be easily removed

MECHANISM/DESCRIPTION

- Candida organisms are normally present as oral flora in 20–60% of the healthy population and up to 80% of elderly or those in hospice or long-term care facilities
- Overgrowth of candida albicans from alterations in the intraoral environment
  —Antimicrobial activity
  —Changes in salivary flow (anticholinergic medications, steroid inhalers, psychotropics, and others)
  —Presence of dentures or other orthodontic appliances
- Fungal proliferation from reduced host defenses
  —Interruption of the epithelial barrier (cheek biting)
  —Endocrinopathies (diabetes, hypothyroidism)
  —Immunosuppression (iatrogenic, congenital, or acquired)

ETIOLOGY

- General
  —Varies in severity from superficial and local to severe systemic disease with 50% mortality
  —In immunocompetent individuals, a benign course is the norm
  —Often recurrent in immunocompromised patients
  —Early manifestation of AIDS in HIV-infected patients
- Acute pseudomembranous candidiasis (thrush)
  —Commonly seen in infancy, old age, and with other serious underlying conditions (diabetes, leukemia, AIDS)
  —Frequently medication induced in immunocompetent
- Acute and chronic atrophic candidiasis
  —Has been described in up to 60% of denture wearers
  —Most common form of oral candidiasis in older adults
- Angular cheilosis
  —Usually associated with intraoral candidal infection
  —Common in elderly secondary to facial wrinkling
  —Often superinfected with *Staphylococcus epidermidis*
- Hyperplastic candidiasis
  —Immunosuppressed individuals
  —High incidence with frequent malignant degeneration in tobacco users

PEDIATRIC CONSIDERATIONS

- Signs and symptoms
  —Oral thrush, anorexia, and discomfort
- Mechanism/description
  —The susceptibility of infants is likely due to the immaturity of their immune system and lack of mature oral flora
  —Rare in first week of life, peak prevalence at 4 weeks
- Etiology
  —The source of infection is believed to be the maternal birth canal

Pre-Hospital

N/A

Diagnosis

ESSENTIAL WORKUP

- Determine whether there is an etiology for a breakdown of host factors
- If no reason is found, evaluation for possible HIV infection or diabetes
- Exclude a systemic infection

LABORATORY

- CBC
  —Exclude neutropenia in patients undergoing chemotherapy
  —In the patient without predisposing conditions to assess immunocompetence
- Biopsy
- Fungal scrapings with potassium hydroxide preparation
- Culture on blood or Sabouraud's agar
  —Positive result may be due to normal flora

DIFFERENTIAL DIAGNOSIS

- Hairy leukoplakia
- Hyperkeratosis
- Lichen planus
- Squamous cell carcinoma
- Adherent food/milk

Treatment

INITIAL STABILIZATION

N/A

ED TREATMENT

- Topical antifungal medications
  - —Clotrimazole
  - —Itraconazole
  - —Nystatin
  - —Combine with topical steroid for angular cheilosis
- Systemic agents should be reserved for those with disease resistant to topical therapy
  - —Fluconazole
  - —Itraconazole
  - —Ketoconazole
- Analgesia
  - —"Magic mouthwash"

MEDICATIONS

- Topical
  - —Clotrimazole: 10 mg troche 5 times/day for 14 days
  - —Itraconazole: 10 mL solution, swish and swallow q.d. × 14 days
  - —Nystatin: 10 mL oral suspension (peds: infants, 200,000 units q.i.d.; children, 400,000–600,000 units q.i.d.), swish and swallow q.i.d. × 14 days
  - —Nystatin troche: 1–2 lozenges 4–5 times/day × 14 days
  - —Nystatin/triamcinolone acetonide ointment: apply b.i.d. × 14 days
- Systemic
  - —Fluconazole: 200 mg day 1, then 100 mg (peds: 6 mg/kg, then 3 mg/kg) PO q.d. × 14 days; resistance is developing
  - —Itraconazole solution: 200 mg PO q.d. × 14 days
  - —Ketoconazole: 200 mg (peds: 3.3 mg/kg/24 hr) PO q.d. × 14 days
  - —Nystatin: 500,000 units, 2 tabs t.i.d. × 14 days

PEDIATRIC CONSIDERATIONS

- Dissolve troche in nipple of bottle
- Mix suspensions with fruit juice and freeze into popsicle
- Apply suspensions to affected areas with cotton-tipped swab

Disposition

ADMISSION CRITERIA

- Inability to tolerate oral intake due to discomfort
- Newly diagnosed immunocompromised state
- Systemic infection

DISCHARGE CRITERIA

- Patients with candidiasis that does not threaten the patient's hydration status may be discharged with close follow-up

Miscellaneous

ICD9: 112.0

ICD10: B37.0

SUGGESTED READINGS

Fotos PG, Lilly JP. Clinical management of oral and perioral candidosis. Dermatol Clin 1996;14:273–280.

Glick M. Viral and fungal infections of the oral cavity in immunocompetent patients. Infect Dis Clin North Am 1999;13(4):817–831.

Greenspan D. Treatment of oropharyngeal candidiasis in HIV-positive patients. J Am Acad Dermatol 1994;31:S51–S55.

Hoppe JE. Treatment of oropharyngeal candidiasis and candidal diaper dermatitis in neonates and infants; review and reappraisal. Pediatr Infect Dis J 1997;16(9):885–894.

Mooney MA, Thomas I, Sirois D. Oral candidosis. Int J Dermatol 1995;34:759–765.

Shay K, Truhlar MR, Renner RP. Oropharyngeal candidosis in the older patient. J Am Geriatr Soc 1997;45(7):863–870.

Authors: Kristine M. Thompson; Deepi G. Goyal

Carbamazepine, Poisoning

Clinical Presentation

SIGNS AND SYMPTOMS

- Neurologic manifestations common
- Cardiotoxicity rare, except in massive overdose

CNS

- Ataxia
- Dizziness
- Drowsiness
- Nystagmus
- Hallucinations
- Combativeness
- Coma
- Seizures

Respiratory System

- Respiratory depression
- Aspiration pneumonia

Cardiovascular System

- Hypotension
- Conduction disturbances (mostly in elderly)
- Supraventricular tachycardia
- Sinus tachycardia or bradycardia
- EKG changes
  - —Prolongation of PR, QRS, and QTc intervals
  - —T-wave changes

Miscellaneous

- Anticholinergic manifestations
  - —Decreased bowel sounds
  - —Mydriasis
  - —Flushing
  - —Urinary retention
- Neuromuscular changes
  - —Tremor
  - —Slurred speech
  - —Myoclonus
  - —Choreiform and choreoathetoid movements

MECHANISM/DESCRIPTION

- Anticholinergic
- Similarities to phenytoin and TCAs
- Sodium channel blocker
- Decreases synaptic transmission

Pre-Hospital

CAUTIONS

- Do *not* administer ipecac
- Intubate if significant respiratory depression or airway compromise
- Secure IV access
- Get complete information about all products potentially ingested

Diagnosis

ESSENTIAL WORKUP

- Continuous cardiac monitor
- Serum carbamazepine level
  - —Therapeutic, 6–12 μg/L
  - —Levels >25–40 μg/mL associated with serious toxicity
    - -Coma
    - -Seizures
    - -Respiratory failure
    - -Conduction defects
  - —Serum levels do not clearly predict clinical toxicity
    - -Active metabolite carbamazepine epoxide not measured
    - -Neurologic manifestations depend on CNS (not serum) level
- EKG
  - —Conduction delays
    - -Increased QRS interval
    - -Increased PR interval
  - —Dysrhythmias
    - -Sinus tachycardia (massive carbamazepine overdose)
    - -Bradydysrhythmia (often seen in elderly with mild increase in carbamazepine level)
- Serum acetaminophen level

LABORATORY

- CBC
  - —Leukopenia or leukocytosis
- Electrolytes, BUN/Cr, glucose
  - —Hyperglycemia
  - —Hypokalemia
  - —Hyponatremia
- ABGs
- Urinalysis
  - —Glucosuria
  - —Ketonuria
- Pregnancy test
- ALT, AST, bilirubin, alkaline phosphatase
  - —May be mildly elevated
  - —Usually not clinically significant

IMAGING/SPECIAL TESTS

- CXR for
  - —Aspiration pneumonia
  - —Pulmonary edema

DIFFERENTIAL DIAGNOSIS

Drugs that Cause Decreased Mental Status

- Alcohol
- Anticholinergics
- Barbiturates
- Benzodiazepines
- Lithium
- Opiates
- Phenothiazines

Drugs that Cause Seizures

- Alcohol withdrawal
- Anticholinergics
- Camphor
- Isoniazid
- Lithium
- Phenothiazines
- Sympathomimetics
  - —Amphetamine
  - —Cocaine
- TCAs

Drugs that Cause Abnormal Movement

- Antihistamines
- Butyrophenones
- Caffeine
- Cocaine
- Levodopa
- Meperidine
- Phencyclidine
- Phenothiazines
- Phenytoin
- TCAs

Treatment

INITIAL STABILIZATION

- ABCs
- Establish IV access with 0.9% NS
- Oxygen
- Cardiac monitor
- Naloxone, thiamine, D50W (or Accu-Chek) if altered mental status

ED TREATMENT

General Management

- Gastric lavage
  - —Consider if recent ingestion (<1–2 hours) and significantly decreased mental status
  - —Few patients will need gastric lavage
  - —Instill activated charcoal through orogastric tube before and after lavage
- Activated charcoal
  - —Administer sorbitol with first dose (only) of activated charcoal
  - —Administer with caution if GI activity is decreased
  - —Contraindicated if bowel sounds are absent
- Multidose activated charcoal
  - —Decreases mean half-life of carbamazepine
  - —Binds unabsorbed drug in GI tract
  - —Interrupts enterohepatic circulation
  - —Do not give additional sorbitol
- Charcoal hemoperfusion
  - —Removes only small amount of ingested dose
  - —Patients usually do well with supportive care without hemoperfusion
  - —Indicated in cases of clinical deterioration or lack of improvement with good supportive care
- Psychiatric consultation

Respiratory Depression

- Intubation
- Ventilatory support

Hypotension

- 0.9% NS IV fluid resuscitation with 1 L initial fluid bolus
- Norepinephrine if unresponsive to IV fluids

Seizures

- Diazepam (drug of choice)
- Phenobarbital (if diazepam ineffective)
- Phenytoin not effective in most toxic seizures

MEDICATIONS

- Activated charcoal (initial bolus): slurry 1–2 g/kg up to 100 g PO mixed with sorbitol (below)
- Dextrose: D50W 1 ampule (50 mL or 25 g) (peds: D25W 2–4 m/kg) i.v.
- Diazepam: 5–10 mg (peds: 0.2–0.5 mg/kg) i.v.
- Multidose activated charcoal: 25 g (peds: 0.25 g/kg) q2h PO after bolus dose (above)
- Naloxone (Narcan): 2 mg (peds: 0.1 mg/kg) i.v. or i.m. initial dose
- Norepinephrine: 4–12 μg/min (peds: 0.05–0.1 μg/kg/min) i.v. titrated to effect
- Sorbitol: 1–2 g/kg to max 100 g (peds: older than 1 year old, 1–1.5 g/kg as a 35% solution to max 50 g) PO mixed with activated charcoal slurry (first dose only)

Disposition

ADMISSION CRITERIA

- Decreased mental status at any time, even if resolving
  - —Observe at least 24 hours for late relapse
- Seizures
- Cardiac dysrhythmias
- Lack of psychiatric clearance after suicidal ingestion

DISCHARGE CRITERIA

- Asymptomatic after 6 hours of observation
- Normal mental status
- Normal or baseline EKG
- GI motility present
- Psychiatric clearance (after suicidal ingestion)

Miscellaneous

ICD9: 966.3

ICD10: T42.1

SUGGESTED READINGS

Deshpande G, Meert KL, Valentini RP. Repeat charcoal hemoperfusion treatments in life threatening carbamazepine overdose. Pediatr Nephrol 1999;13: 775–777.

Hojer J, Malmlund H, Berg A. Clinical features in 28 consecutive cases of laboratory confirmed massive poisoning with carbamazepine alone. Clin Toxicol 1993;31:449–458.

Schmidt S, Schmitz-Buhl M. Signs and symptoms of carbamazepine overdose. J Neurol 1995;242:169–173.

Seymour JF. Carbamazepine overdose: features of 33 cases. Drug Safety 1993;8:81–88.

Wason S, Baker RC, Carolan P, et al. Carbamazepine overdose—the effects of multiple dose activated charcoal. Clin Toxicol 1992;30:39–48.

Author: Leon Gussow

Carbon Monoxide, Poisoning

Clinical Presentation

SIGNS AND SYMPTOMS

CNS

- Headache
- Dizziness
- Ataxia
- Confusion
- Acute encephalopathy
- Syncope
- Seizures
- Coma

GI

- Nausea
- Vomiting

Cardiovascular

- Chest pain
- Palpitations
- Tachycardia
- Premature ventricular contractions
- Dysrhythmias
- Myocardial ischemia/infarction

Respiratory

- Dyspnea
- Tachypnea
- Respiratory alkalosis
- Noncardiogenic pulmonary edema

Ophthalmologic

- Decreased vision
- Retinal hemorrhage

Other

- Rhabdomyolysis
- Lactic acidosis

MECHANISM/DESCRIPTION

- Formation of carboxyhemoglobin
  —Decreases oxygen-carrying capacity
  —Shifts oxyhemoglobin dissociation curve to left, decreasing oxygen release to tissues
- Binding to intracellular heme proteins (cytochrome oxidase, cytochrome P-450)
  —Interrupts cellular respiration and oxygen use
  —Causes lactic acidosis
- Binding to myoglobin
  —Decreases oxygen extraction
  —Impairs function of skeletal and cardiac muscle

ETIOLOGY

- Endogenous (natural hemoglobin turnover)
- Incomplete combustion of carbon-containing compounds
  —Internal combustion engines
  —Natural gas
  —Space heaters
  —Kerosene heaters
  —Charcoal
  —Sterno
  —Indoor hibachis
  —Accidental fires
  —Fireplaces
  —Furnaces
  —Smoking (causes carboxyhemoglobin levels up to 10–15%)
- Methylene chloride
  —Found in some solvents and furniture-stripping compounds
  —Slowly released from tissues and metabolized by liver to carbon monoxide
  —Peak carboxyhemoglobin level delayed after exposure
  —Half-life approximately two times that of inhaled carbon monoxide

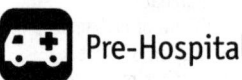

Pre-Hospital

CAUTIONS

- Remove patient from contaminated environment
- Assess for smoke inhalation or thermal injury
- Assess airway and ventilation to determine need for intubation
- Administer 100% oxygen to all patients suspected of having carbon monoxide toxicity

Diagnosis

ESSENTIAL WORKUP

- History
  —May present with mild, nonspecific symptoms
  —Question for
    -Similar symptoms in other household members
    -Malfunctioning furnaces
    -Use of space heaters or open ovens for supplemental heat
    -Ill pets
- ABGs
  —Normal Po_2 and calculated oxygen saturation
  —Measured oxygen saturation will be low
  —Metabolic acidosis with severe exposure
- Carboxyhemoglobin level
  —*Caution:* patient may be critically ill from carbon monoxide despite an unimpressive carboxyhemoglobin level
  —Measure as soon as possible
  —Normal 0–3% (up to 10% in cigarette smokers)
  —Misleadingly low if a significant time has passed since exposure or if supplemental oxygen administered
  —May not reflect clinical severity
    -Calibrate breathalyzers carefully
    -Less accurate than direct measurement

LABORATORY

- Electrolytes, BUN/Cr, glucose
  —Metabolic acidosis and increased anion gap associated with increased clinical severity
- Urinalysis
  —Myoglobin with rhabdomyolysis
- Cardiac enzymes
  —Draw serial enzymes if suspect myocardial ischemia or infarction
- Acetaminophen level
  —For suicidal exposures
- Salicylate level
  —For increased anion gap metabolic acidosis
- Pregnancy test

IMAGING/SPECIAL TESTS

- Pulse oximetry
  - —Pulse oximeter reads carboxyhemoglobin as oxyhemoglobin
  - —False elevated reading
- EKG
  - —Carbon monoxide can precipitate myocardial ischemia or infarction
  - —Dysrhythmias
  - —Nonspecific ST-T changes
- CXR (aspiration, pulmonary edema)
- CT head
  - —White matter changes are typical of carbon monoxide poisoning and associated with poor long-term neurologic outcome
  - —Low-density lesions in the globus pallidus may be clue to diagnosis in occult cases
  - —Rule out intracranial causes of altered mental status

DIFFERENTIAL DIAGNOSIS

- Viral illness
- Meningitis
- Encephalitis
- Intracranial bleed
- Influenza or viral syndrome
- Gastroenteritis
- Migraine
- Tension headache
- Ethanol intoxication
- Opiates
- Sedative-hypnotic overdose
- Cyanide poisoning
- Salicylate overdose
- Toxic alcohol exposure

Treatment

INITIAL STABILIZATION

- ABCs
- 0.9% NS IV
- Oxygen (100%)
- Cardiac monitor
- Naloxone, dextrose (or Accu-Chek), and thiamine if altered mental status

ED TREATMENT

Oxygen

- Administer 100% normobaric oxygen
  - —Via mask or ETT
- Continue until carboxyhemoglobin level <5–10%
- Half-life of carboxyhemoglobin
  - —Room air about 300 minutes
  - —100% normobaric oxygen about 90 minutes
  - —Hyperbaric oxygen (3 atm) about 20 minutes

Hyperbaric Oxygen

- Dose
  - —100% at 3 atm for 45 minutes
  - —May be repeated
- Benefits
  - —Decreases half-life of carboxyhemoglobin
  - —Increases dissolved oxygen
  - —May clear carbon monoxide from mitochondria and myoglobin
  - —Decreases lipid peroxidation
  - —Decreases incidence of cerebral edema
  - —May decrease mortality and long-term neurologic morbidity in selected cases
- Potential adverse effects
  - —Ear discomfort and tympanic membrane rupture
  - —Pneumothorax
  - —Seizure
  - —Risk of transporting unstable patient
- Indications
  - —History of coma at any time during or after exposure
  - —Significant persistent neurologic deficits
  - —Cardiac instability (must weigh potential benefit against risk of transfer)
  - —Persistent metabolic acidosis
  - —Carboxyhemoglobin level >40%
  - —Carboxyhemoglobin level >15% in pregnant patient

Special Considerations in the Pregnant Carbon Monoxide Victim

- Fetal carboxyhemoglobin levels 10–15% higher than maternal
- Fetal carboxyhemoglobin clearance delayed compared with maternal clearance
- Treat pregnant carbon monoxide victims with 100% oxygen for five times as long as it takes to get the maternal level <10%
- Hyperbaric oxygen if level >15%

MEDICATIONS

- Dextrose: D50W 1 ampule (50 mL or 25 g) (peds: D25W 2–4 mL/kg) i.v.
- Naloxone (Narcan): 2 mg (peds: 0.1 mg/kg) i.v. or i.m. initial dose
- Thiamine (vitamin B_1): 100 mg (peds: 50 mg) i.v. or i.m.

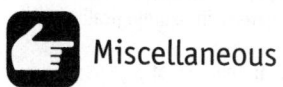

Disposition

ADMISSION CRITERIA

- Persistent symptoms after 4 hours of treatment
- Evidence of myocardial ischemia or cardiac instability
- Seizures
- Persistent metabolic acidosis
- Syncope
- Rhabdomyolysis

DISCHARGE CRITERIA

- Asymptomatic after 4 hours of observation
- Absence of aforementioned admission criteria
- Psychiatric clearance (if suicidal exposure)

Miscellaneous

ICD9: 986

ICD10: T58

SEE ALSO: HYPERBARIC OXYGEN

SUGGESTED READINGS

Hampson NB, Zmaeff JL. Outcome of patients experiencing cardiac arrest with carbon monoxide poisoning treated with hyperbaric oxygen. Ann Emerg Med 2001;38:36–41.

Raphael JC, Elkharrat D, Jars-Guincestre MC, et al. Trial of normobaric and hyperbaric oxygen for acute carbon monoxide intoxication. Lancet 1989;2:414.

Scheinkestel CD, Bailey M, Myles PS, et al. Hyperbaric or normobaric oxygen for acute carbon monoxide poisoning: a randomised controlled clinical trial. Med J Aust 1999;170:203–210.

Sloan EP, Murphy DG, Hart R, et al. Complications and protocol considerations in carbon monoxide-poisoned patients who require hyperbaric oxygen therapy: report from a ten-year experience. Ann Emerg Med 1989;18:629.

Weaver LK. Carbon monoxide poisoning. Crit Care Clin 1999;15:297–317.

Author: Leon Gussow

Cardiac Arrest

Clinical Presentation

SIGNS AND SYMPTOMS

- Unresponsiveness
- Pulselessness
- Shallow, gasping respirations may persist for a few minutes
- Occasionally preceded by
  - —Chest pain
  - —Dyspnea
  - —Palpitations
  - —Seizure activity
- Immediately before arrest
  - —Shock or hypotension
  - —Impaired mentation

MECHANISM/DESCRIPTION

- Sudden death
  - —Death within 24 hours of symptom onset
  - —Initial presentation in 50% of patients with cardiovascular disease
- Return of spontaneous circulation (ROSC) achieved in 9–65%
- 1–20% of patients survive to discharge
- Factors affecting survival
  - —Initial rhythm
  - —Time to successful defibrillation
- Incidence of rearrest in neurologically intact survivors
  - —30% at 1 year and 60% at 5 years

ETIOLOGY

- Acute coronary ischemia
  - —Underlying etiology in 50% of arrests
  - —Myocardial irritability leads to ventricular fibrillation
- Primary dysrhythmia
  - —Congenital and acquired electrical abnormalities
  - —Hypertrophic/dilated cardiomyopathy
  - —Myocarditis
- Cardiac rupture
- Pericardial tamponade
- Metabolic abnormalities
- Noncardiac etiologies
  - —Consider especially in cases of pulseless electrical activity
  - —Tension pneumothorax
  - —Hemorrhage
  - —Massive pulmonary embolus
  - —Sepsis
  - —Severe acidosis
- Drugs or toxins
  - —Antidysrhythmics
  - —Digoxin
  - —Beta-blockers
  - —Calcium channel blockers
  - —Tricyclic antidepressants
  - —Cocaine
  - —Heroin

Pre-Hospital

- Prompt initiation of CPR
- Confirm underlying rhythm
- Early defibrillation of VT or VF
  - —Automated external defibrillator
    - -EMT-D or layperson
- Secure airway and provide adequate respirations
  - —Endotracheal intubation
  - —Laryngeal mask airway
- Postresuscitation care
  - —Identify cause of arrest
  - —12-Lead EKG
  - —Monitor vital signs
- Transport to the closest facility
  - —If return of spontaneous circulation, consider transport to center equipped for interventional cardiac care
    - -Pediatric critical care center for children
- Termination of resuscitative efforts
  - —Persistent, confirmed asystole
  - —Prolonged arrest

Diagnosis

ESSENTIAL WORKUP

- "Quick look" using paddles of a cardiac defibrillator
- Determine rhythm

LABORATORY

- Indicated only when successful ROSC is achieved
  - —Electrolytes
  - —BUN/creatinine
  - —Creatinine kinase with isoenzymes, cardiac troponin
  - —Arterial blood gas (avoid arterial puncture in thrombolysis candidates)
  - —Complete blood count
  - —Therapeutic drug levels
  - —Toxicologic testing

IMAGING/SPECIAL TESTS

- Electrocardiogram
  - —Establish or rule out acute coronary syndrome
- Chest radiograph
  - —Endotracheal tube position
  - —Cardiac silhouette
  - —Pneumothorax
- Echocardiogram
  - —Pericardial effusion
  - —Wall motion abnormality
  - —Valvular dysfunction

DIFFERENTIAL DIAGNOSIS

- Sudden loss of consciousness with a palpable pulse
  - —Syncope
  - —Seizure
  - —Acute stroke
  - —Hypoglycemia
  - —Acute airway obstruction
  - —Head trauma
  - —Toxins

Treatment

INITIAL STABILIZATION

- Initiate advanced cardiac life support (ACLS)
- Perform CPR as long as no pulse is palpable
  —Stop CPR only briefly to check cardiac rhythm or intubate
- Secure the airway
- Obtain intravenous access
- Cardiac monitor
- Therapy based on the underlying rhythm according to ACLS protocols

ED TREATMENT

Pulseless VT or VF

- Immediate defibrillation with up to three countershocks
  —200 J
  —200–300 J
  —360 J
- If defibrillation is unsuccessful
  —Epinephrine, *or*
  —Vasopressin
- If refractory to defibrillation and epinephrine
  —Amiodarone
  —Lidocaine
  —Procainamide
  —Magnesium for torsades de pointes

Asystole

- Dismal prognosis if this is the presenting rhythm
- Confirm in two or more leads
- Epinephrine
- Atropine
- Consider transcutaneous pacing for severe brady-asystolic rhythm

Pulseless Electrical Activity (PEA)

- Epinephrine
- Atropine
- Treat for reversible cause of PEA as indicated
  —Pneumothorax
  —Cardiac tamponade
  —Hypoxia
  —Pulmonary embolus
  —Hypovolemia (hemorrhage)

Postresuscitation

- Treat the underlying cause of the arrest
- EKG to establish presence of acute coronary syndrome
- Ventilatory support
- Continue antidysrhythmic therapy
- Correct electrolyte abnormalities
- Initiate volume resuscitation and provide inotropic support as needed

MEDICATIONS

- Amiodarone: 300 mg (peds: 5 mg/kg) IVP
- Atropine: 1 mg (peds: 0.02 mg/kg) i.v. every 3–5 minutes up to 0.04 mg/kg
- Epinephrine: 1 mg (peds: 0.01 mg/kg) IVP every 3–5 minutes
- Lidocaine: 100 mg (peds: 1 mg/kg) IVP, then 2–4 mg/min (peds: 20–50 μg/min) i.v. continuous infusion
- Magnesium : 1–2 g (peds: 25–50 mg/kg) slow i.v.
- Procainamide: 20 mg/min slow i.v. to a total of 1 g or until arrhythmia is suppressed; maintenance infusion 1–4 mg/min (peds: 15 mg/kg over 30 min, then 20–80 μg/kg/min i.v.)
- Sodium bicarbonate: 1 mEq/kg slow i.v.
- Vasopressin: 40 U IVP (adults with VT/VF only)

Disposition

ADMISSION CRITERIA

- Return of spontaneous circulation
  —Coronary care unit or ICU
  —Postresuscitation care

DISCHARGE CRITERIA

N/A

Miscellaneous

ICD9: 798

ICD10: 146.9

SUGGESTED READINGS

American Heart Association. Guidelines 2000 for cardiopulmonary resuscitation and emergency cardiovascular care. Circulation 2000;102(Suppl):I-1–I-384.

Dorian P, Cass D, Schwartz B, et al. Amiodarone as compared with lidocaine for shock-resistant ventricular fibrillation. N Engl J Med 2002;346:884–890.

Kouwenhoven W, Jude JR, Knickerbocker GG. Closed-chest cardiac massage. JAMA 1960;173:1064–1067.

Safar P, Escarraga LA, Elam JO. A comparison of the mouth-to-mouth and mouth-to-airway methods of artificial respiration with the chest-pressure arm-lift methods. N Engl J Med 1958;258: 671–677.

Stiel IG, Hebert PC, Wells GA, et al. Vasopressin versus epinephrine for inhospital cardiac arrest: a randomised controlled trial. Lancet 2001;358: 105–109.

Zoll PM, Linenthal AJ, Gibson W, et al. Termination of ventricular fibrillation in man by externally applied electric countershock. N Engl J Med 1956;254: 727–732.

Author: Todd Rothenhaus

Cardiac Pacemakers

Clinical Presentation

SIGNS AND SYMPTOMS

- Pacemaker failure
  - —Bradycardia
  - —Syncope
  - —Hypotension, progressive to shock and hemodynamic collapse
  - —Fatigue and weakness
  - —Dyspnea on exertion or shortness of breath secondary to congestive heart failure
  - —Ischemic chest pain
  - —Altered level of consciousness
- Pacemaker-induced tachycardia
  - —Dyspnea
  - —Ischemic chest pain
  - —Lightheadedness
  - —Syncope
- Pacemaker syndrome
  - —Symptoms related to asynchronous AV contractions
  - —Lightheadedness
  - —Dyspnea
  - —Palpitation
  - —Syncope

MECHANISM/DESCRIPTION

Equipment

- Permanent, implanted pacemaker has three components
  - —A battery-powered energy source
    - -Lithium batteries last 7–10 years
  - —Generator
    - -A sophisticated computer with many programmable parameters
  - —Leads connected to the right ventricle or the right atrium
    - -These typically sense electrical activity and pace
- Pacemaker magnet
  - —Placed over pulse generator
  - —Converts pacer to asynchronous mode
  - —Useful if no pacer spikes on presenting rhythm
  - —A depleted battery will result in decrease in magnet rate by 10%

Pacemaker Terminology

- Fixed mode
  - —The pacemaker is set to fire at a set rate regardless of patient's underlying rhythm
  - —Commonly seen in very old pacers
- Demand mode
  - —The pacemaker fires only when necessary
  - —It senses the underlying rhythm
  - —It will only pace the atria or ventricle if the intrinsic rhythm is absent
- Sensing
  - —Refers to the pacemaker's ability to determine whether the atria or ventricle is being intrinsically paced
- All pacemakers have a five-letter code to describe their function
- For emergency department purposes, only the first three letters of the code are necessary
- Pacemaker code describes pacemaker components and function
  - —First letter in code indicates chamber being sensed by pacemaker
    - -**A** = Atria
    - -**V** = Ventricle
    - -**D** = Dual (both chambers)
  - —Second letter in code indicates chamber that can be paced
    - -**A** = Atria
    - -**V** = Ventricle
    - -**D** = Dual (both chambers)
  - —Third letter in code describes pacemaker's response to sensed intrinsic complex
    - -**T** = trigger (a sensed beat results in a pacing response as when a sensed atrial beat provokes a subsequent ventricular beat)
    - -**I** = inhibit (a sensed beat precludes pacemaker function)
    - -**D** = dual (a pacemaker is capable of both functions)
    - -**O** = no response
  - —Most common pacemakers are VVI (single lead) and DDD (two leads)

Pacemaker-Associated Complications

- Pacemaker-associated infection
  - —Infection of pacemaker components often associated with endocarditis
  - —*Staphylococcus epidermidis* and *Staphylococcus aureus* account for > 90% of infections
  - —Transesophageal echo is preferred diagnostic method
- Venous thrombosis
  - —Very common (overall incidence 30–50%)
  - —Symptomatic, acute obstruction is rare (<3%)
  - —Pulmonary embolism is rare
- Pacemaker failure to pace or discharge impulse
  - —Component failure is rare
  - —Battery depletion is rare with routine checks, not abrupt
  - —Lead fracture or disconnection
  - —Oversensing of muscular activity or external electrical interference
- Pacemaker failure to capture myocardium
  - —Lead dislodgment
    - -Most common cause
    - -Change in cardiac signal or QRS morphology
  - —Twiddler's syndrome
    - -Unintentional manipulation of pacemaker generator causing lead to dislodge from myocardium
  - —Elevated myocardial threshold
    - -Hyperkalemia
    - -Ischemia
  - —Failure to sense intrinsic depolarization
- Pacemaker-mediated tachycardia
  - —Occurs with dual-chamber pacemakers
  - —A reentry rhythm using generator and intrinsic conduction system
  - —Maximum rate typically 140 beats/min due to built-in safeguards
- Runaway pacemaker
  - —Rare, triggered by battery depletion or component failure
  - —Often rapid rates (>200 beats/min) with hemodynamic compromise

Pre-Hospital

N/A

Diagnosis

ESSENTIAL WORKUP

- 12-Lead EKG to assess whether there are any obvious evidence of pacemaker failure
- Metabolic workup to determine whether an acquired medical condition led to an elevated myocardial threshold

LABORATORY

- Serum potassium
- Arterial blood gas
- Serum levels of antidysrhythmic drugs

IMAGING/SPECIAL TESTS

- EKG with pacer magnet
  - —Assess magnet rate
    - -Particularly useful when the baseline EKG does not reveal pacer spikes
    - -The magnet activates asynchronous pacing mode
    - -Produces pacer spikes at a preprogrammed rate—regardless of the intrinsic rhythm
    - -If the magnet rate equals the preprogrammed rate set at implantation, the pacer is OK
    - -If the magnet rate is > 10% slower than at implantation, the battery is depleted
    - -If there are no pacer spikes, there is significant pacemaker malfunction
- Chest radiograph
  - —Evaluate problem with pacer lead(s) and position
    - -Fractured lead
    - -Lead dislodgment
    - -Perforation

DIFFERENTIAL DIAGNOSIS

N/A

Treatment

INITIAL STABILIZATION

- Oxygen administered via 100% non-rebreather
- Intubation as needed
- Intravenous access
- Advanced cardiac life support (ACLS) drugs as per usual protocol
- Defibrillation: avoid placing paddles over generator
- Transcutaneous pacemaker in hemodynamically unstable patients with pacemaker failure

ED TREATMENT

- Pacemaker failure
  - —Transcutaneous pacemaker
  - —Temporary transvenous pacemaker
    - -Obtain central intravenous access with a Cortiss introducer
    - -Perform the procedure under fluoroscopy if possible
    - -Set the pulse generator to asynchronous mode
    - -Turn the output dial all the way up
    - -Advance the catheter through the central venous access Cortiss until you see a QRS complex on the monitor
    - -Check the femoral pulse
    - -If you have a pulse and see a QRS complex, the pacer is "capturing"
    - -Slowly turn the output dial down until you lose the QRS complex (capture threshold)
    - -Turn the output dial up to 2 or 3 times the capture threshold
    - -Continuous EKG monitoring facilitates correct placement
- Treat hyperkalemia (see Hyperkalemia)
- Runaway pacemaker
  - —AV node blocking or reprogramming
  - —In extreme situation, may need to disconnect lead from generator surgically

MEDICATIONS

- Adenosine: 6 mg i.v. bolus

Disposition

ADMISSION CRITERIA

- Permanent pacemaker failure
- Suspicion of infection involving pacemaker components

DISCHARGE CRITERIA

- Asymptomatic pacemaker malfunction
- A cardiologist has interrogated the pacemaker

Miscellaneous

ICD9: 429.4

ICD10:

SUGGESTED READINGS

Cardall TY, Brady WJ, Chan TC, et al. Permanent cardiac pacemakers: issues relevant to the emergency physician, parts I and II. J Emerg Med 1999;17: 479–489,697–709.

Griffin J, Smithline H, Cook J. Runaway pacemaker: a case report and review. J Emerg Med 2000;19:177–181.

Kusumoto FM, Goldschlager N. Cardiac pacing. N Engl J Med 1996;334:89–98.

Author: Susan P. Torrey; Jill Griffin

Cardiac Testing

Clinical Presentation

SIGNS AND SYMPTOMS

- Chest pain
  - —Substernal pressure
  - —Heaviness
  - —Squeezing
  - —Burning sensation
  - —Tightness
  - —May localize or radiate to arms, shoulders, back, neck, or jaw
- Associated findings
  - —Dyspnea
  - —Syncope
  - —Fatigue
  - —Diaphoresis
  - —Nausea or vomiting
- Usually reproduced by exertion, eating, exposure to cold, or emotional stress
- Anginal symptoms last less than 20 minutes but more than a few seconds
- Myocardial infarction should be considered if symptoms last longer than 20 minutes
- Usually relieved with rest or nitroglycerin
- Symptoms generally unchanged with position or inspiration
- Occasional anginal equivalents include
  - —Abdominal pain
  - —Dyspnea
  - —Syncope
  - —Diaphoresis
  - —Nausea or vomiting
  - —Weakness
- Positive Levine sign or clenched fist over chest is suggestive of angina
- Blood pressure is usually elevated during symptoms
- Physical exam is usually unrevealing
- Occasional physical findings include
  - —S3 or S4 due to LV systolic or diastolic symptoms
  - —Mitral regurgitation or pansystolic murmur
  - —Diminished peripheral pulses

MECHANISM/DESCRIPTION

- Indicated for emergency patients who present with undifferentiated chest pain
- Acute cardiac ischemia (ACI) encompasses a spectrum of disease processes, including acute myocardial infraction (AMI) and unstable angina pectoris (UAP)
- Syndromes of ACI are a leading cause of death in the United States and worldwide
- About 10% of ED visits are cardiac related, most with chest pain
  - —10% of ED malpractice claims are due to missed diagnosis of AMI
  - —2–8% of patients presenting to the ED with chest pain are sent home with AMI
  - —History, physical exam, and EKG miss 1–4% of all AMIs
- Various approaches to differentiation of chest pain may be employed
  - —History is the critical component
  - —All modalities beyond history and EKG are adjuncts to diagnosing the etiology of chest pain

ETIOLOGY

- Cardiac risk factors include
  - —Hypercholesterolemia
  - —Diabetes mellitus
  - —Hypertension
  - —Smoking
  - —Family history
  - —Men > 35 years old
  - —Postmenopausal women
- Atherosclerotic narrowing of coronary vessels
- Vasospasm, although this is usually at rest and considered unstable if new onset
- Microvascular angina or abnormal relaxation of vessels with diffuse vascular disease
- Anemia: hemoglobin < 8 g/dL
- Hyperbarism or elevations in carboxyhemoglobin
- Medication-induced vasospasm

Pre-Hospital

- Intravenous access
- Oxygen
- Cardiac monitoring
- Out-of-hospital EKG
  - —Alone has a sensitivity of 76% and specificity of 88% for ACI
  - —Alone has a sensitivity of 68% and specificity of 97% for AMI
- Sublingual nitroglycerin for symptom relief

CAUTIONS

- All chest pain should be treated and transported as a possible life-threatening emergency

Diagnosis

ESSENTIAL WORKUP

- History is critical in differentiating stable and unstable angina
- Single EKG
  - —Normal in most cases of ACI
  - —ST-segment changes or T-wave inversions most often are unchanged from previous tracings
  - —Must be compared with prior tracings if available
  - —New ST-segment changes or T-wave inversions are suspicious for unstable angina
  - —1-mm depression of the ST segment below the baseline, 80 milliseconds from the J point, is characteristic of angina
- Continuous or serial EKG
  - —Alone has a sensitivity of 21–25% and specificity of 92–99% for ACI
  - —Alone has a sensitivity of 39% and specificity of 88% for AMI
- EKG may be helpful in diagnosing other etiologies of chest pain
  - —Pericarditis is suggested by diffuse ST-segment elevations followed by T-wave inversions and PR depression
  - —Pulmonary embolism is suggested by an S1, Q3, T3 pattern and unexplained tachycardia

LABORATORY

- Cardiac enzymes
  - —Indicated if the history is suspicious for acute myocardial infarction
  - —Should not be abnormal in unstable angina
  - —Should not be elevated and are not indicated in stable angina
  - —Creatine kinase
    - -Single value on presentation has sensitivity of 37% and specificity of 87% for AMI
    - -Serial values have sensitivity of 66–99% and specificity of 68–84% for AMI
  - —CK-MB
    - -Single value on presentation has sensitivity of 42% and specificity of 97% for AMI
    - -Serial values have sensitivity of 79% and specificity of 96% for AMI
  - —Myoglobin
    - -Single value on presentation has sensitivity of 49% and specificity of 91% for AMI
    - -Serial values have sensitivity of 89% and specificity of 87% for AMI
  - —Troponin I
    - -Single value on presentation has sensitivity of 39% and specificity of 93% for AMI
    - -Serial values have sensitivity of 90–100% and specificity of 83–96% for AMI

—Troponin T
-Single value on presentation has sensitivity of 39% and specificity of 93% for AMI
-Serial values have sensitivity of 93% and specificity of 85% for AMI

IMAGING/SPECIAL TESTS

- Chest x-ray
  —Usually normal
  —May show cardiomegaly
  —Congestive heart failure is suggestive of unstable angina
  —May identify other etiologies of chest pain such as pneumonia
- Echocardiography may establish the diagnosis of ACI
  —Rest echocardiography has a sensitivity of 70% and specificity of 87% for ACI
  —Rest echocardiography has a sensitivity of 93% and specificity of 66% for AMI
- Technetium-99m sestamibi (rest)
  —Has a sensitivity of 81% and specificity of 73% for ACI
  —Has a sensitivity of 92% and specificity of 67% for AMI
- Exercise stress testing may help establish the diagnosis of angina and provide prognostic information
  —1-mm depression of the ST segment below the baseline, 80 milliseconds from the J point, in three consecutive beats and two consecutive leads is characteristic of cardiac ischemia
  —Early positive (within 3 minutes) stress tests are worrisome for unstable angina
  —Six minutes of exercise using a standard Bruce protocol suggests an excellent prognosis
  —Exercise stress testing with EKG alone has a sensitivity of 68% and specificity of 77%
  —Exercise stress testing with echocardiography has a sensitivity of 85% and specificity of 77%
  —Exercise stress testing with thallium-201 or technetium-99m sestamibi has a sensitivity of 87% and specificity of 64%

DIFFERENTIAL DIAGNOSIS

- Aortic dissection
- Anxiety
- Biliary colic
- Costochondritis
- Esophageal spasm
- Esophageal reflux
- Herpes zoster
- Hiatal hernia
- Mitral valve prolapse
- Myocardial infarction
- Peptic ulcer disease
- Psychogenic
- Panic disorder
- Unstable angina
- Pneumonia
- Pulmonary embolus

Treatment

INITIAL STABILIZATION

- Intravenous access
- Oxygen
- Cardiac monitoring
- Oxygen saturation

ED TREATMENT

- See Acute Coronary Syndrome: Stable Angina; Acute Coronary Syndrome: Unstable Angina; and Acute Coronary Syndrome: Myocardial Infarction for more detail

GUIDELINES FOR CARDIAC TESTING

- History suggestive of acute cardiac syndrome
  —Obtain EKG and first set of cardiac enzymes
- EKG or first set of cardiac enzymes abnormal
  —Admit patient; consider cardiology consult
- Ongoing chest pain or pressure
  —Obtain pain sestamibi or echocardiogram
- Pain sestamibi or echocardiogram abnormal
  —Admit patient; consider cardiology consult
- Second set of cardiac enzymes abnormal
  —Admit patient; consider cardiology consult
- History suggestive of acute cardiac syndrome, EKG nondiagnostic, enzymes normal
  —Ancillary testing
  -Standard endotracheal tube (ETT)
  -Stress echocardiogram or sestamibi (abnormal or uninterpretable EKG)
  -Pharmacologic ETT (i.e., dobutamine echocardiogram or dipyridamole [Persantine] sestamibi (patient unable to exert)
  —Ancillary testing abnormal
  -Admit patient or cardiology consult

MEDICATIONS

- Patient should not be started on new antianginal medication before stress testing in the ED

Disposition

ADMISSION CRITERIA

- History suggestive of cardiac etiology for chest pain
- Abnormal or changed EKG
- Positive cardiac enzymes
- Positive rest imaging
- If the diagnosis is unclear, admission to the hospital or an ED observation unit may be useful for serial cardiac enzymes, EKGs, and exercise stress testing
- Early positive stress test
- If the patient has an otherwise positive stress test, the decision for admission should be made in consultation with the primary care physician or cardiologist

DISCHARGE CRITERIA

- Patients who meet the following criteria are safe to discharge
  —History not suggestive of cardiac etiology for chest pain
  —Normal EKG
  —Normal cardiac testing

Miscellaneous

ICD9: N/A

ICD10: N/A

SUGGESTED READINGS

Braunwald E, Antman EM, Beasley JW, et al. ACC/AHA guidelines for the management of patients with unstable angina: a report of the American College of Cardiology/American Heart Association Task Force on Practice Guidelines. J Am Coll Cardiol 2000;36:970–1062.

Ioannidis JPA, Salem D, Chew PW, et al. Accuracy and clinical effect of out-of-hospital electrocardiography in the diagnosis of acute cardiac ischemia: a meta-analysis. Ann Emerg Med 2001;37: 461–470.

Ioannidis JPA, Salem D, Chew PW, et al. Accuracy of imaging technologies in the diagnosis of acute cardiac ischemia in the emergency department: a meta-analysis. Ann Emerg Med 2001;37:471–477.

Lau J, Ioannidis JPA, Balk EM, et al. Diagnosing acute cardiac ischemia in the emergency department: a systematic review of the accuracy and clinical effect of current technologies. Ann Emerg Med 2001;37:453–460.

Authors: Shamai A. Grossman; Rick G. Kulkarni

Cardiac Transplantation Complications

Clinical Presentation

SIGNS AND SYMPTOMS

Acute Rejection

- Nonspecific symptoms predominate because the heart is usually denervated
  - —Fatigue
  - —Dyspnea
  - —Low-grade fever
  - —Nausea
  - —Vomiting
- Signs of heart failure
  - —Tachypnea
  - —Rales
  - —Hypoxia
  - —S3
  - —Murmur
  - —Edema

Allograft Vasculopathy

- As early as 3 months after transplantation (20–50% incidence at 5 years)
- Insidious onset
  - —Fatigue
  - —Cough
  - —Dyspnea
- Acute onset
  - —Heart failure
  - —Sudden death
  - —Infarction
- Denervated hearts do not present with typical angina

Infection (Opportunistic and Conventional)

- Fever > 37.5°C
- Skin lesions (zoster)
- Cytomegalovirus (CMV)
  - —Mild (flu-like illness)
    - -Fever
    - -Nausea
    - -Malaise
  - —Severe
    - -Pneumonitis (13–50% mortality)
    - -Hepatitis
    - -Gastroenteritis
    - -Profound leukopenia

Pediatric Considerations

- Irritability
- Poor feeding
- Changes in sleep patterns

MECHANISM/DESCRIPTION

- More than 40,000 transplantations to date worldwide (2,000 per year in U.S.)
- 1-year survival 85%; 5-year, 69%
- Immunosuppression decreases rejection
- Frequent biopsies initially to evaluate rejection; echocardiography in children
- Substantial evidence indicates heart eventually reinnervates
- Maintenance immunosuppression with three-drug regimen
- Prednisone (children weaned off quickly, adults slowly)
- Cyclosporine (Neoral, a second-generation cyclosporine) or tacrolimus (Prograf)
- Azathioprine (Imuran) or mycophenolate mofetil (CellCept)
- Complications occur most commonly in the first 6 weeks after cardiac transplantation
  - —Period of heaviest immunosuppression

ETIOLOGY

- Acute rejection
  - —Lymphocyte infiltration and myocyte destruction
  - —Most common in first 6 weeks (although may occur any time)
  - —75% prevalence
- Allograft vasculopathy
  - —Limits long-term survival
  - —Immune-mediated atherosclerosis
  - —Obliterative diffuse concentric lesions of small to medium arteries with superimposed focal plaques and thrombosis
  - —20–50% incidence at 5 years
- Infections
  - —First month
    - -Nosocomial bacterial infections
    - -Pneumonia (*Pseudomonas*, *Legionella*, other gram-negative organisms)
    - -Mediastinitis (0.4–4.5% incidence)
    - -Urinary tract infection (UTI)
  - —First year
    - -Opportunistic and conventional infections
    - -CMV (occurs in 73–100% patients)
    - -Herpes simplex virus (HSV)
    - -*Legionella*
    - -Fungal infections
    - -*Pneumocystis carinii*
  - —Pediatric considerations
    - -Once off steroids, bacteremia risk is similar to that in the general population
    - -High incidence of pneumonia
    - -Patients on steroids may not show meningeal signs
- Medication toxicity
  - —Cyclosporine
    - -Nephrotoxicity
    - -Hepatotoxicity
    - -Neurotoxicity (tremor, paresthesias, seizure)
  - —Azathioprine
    - -Bone marrow suppression
    - -Leukopenia
  - —Steroids
    - -Osteoporosis
    - -Cushing's disease
- Neoplasms in immunosuppressed cardiac transplant recipients
  - —Threefold increase in incidence versus general population
  - —Skin and lip cancer
  - —Non-Hodgkin's lymphoma
  - —Kaposi's sarcomas
  - —Uterine, cervical, and vulval neoplasms
  - —No increase in adenocarcinomas (breast, lung, prostate, colon)

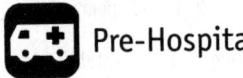

Pre-Hospital

N/A

Diagnosis

ESSENTIAL WORKUP

- Assess for signs of rejection, cardiac dysfunction, and infarction
  - —EKG
  - —Cardiac enzymes
  - —Chest radiograph
  - —Echocardiography
- Blood and urine cultures if any sign of infection
- Electrolytes should be obtained to assess for cyclosporine toxicity

LABORATORY

- Electrolytes
  - —Cyclosporine effects
    - -Increased BUN, creatinine
    - -Hyperkalemia
    - -Metabolic acidosis
    - -Hyponatremia
- Fever
  - —Blood and urine culture
  - —Lumbar puncture (LP) if seizures, altered mental status, or severe headache
- CMV titers or polymerase chain reaction (PCR)
- Buffy coat
- Urine antigen test
- Cyclosporine level trough
  - —Do not order random level

IMAGING/SPECIAL TESTS

- EKG
  - —New atrial arrhythmia
  - —Tachycardia
  - —20% decrease in total voltage (nonsensitive)
  - —Note that normal rhythm for denervated heart is sinus 90–110 beats/min
  - —Expect two P waves (native and donor heart); native P waves do not correspond to QRS
- Chest x-ray
  - —Cardiomegaly
  - —Pulmonary edema
  - —Pleural effusions
  - —Compare with previous (healthy donor heart may be appear large in small recipient)
- Echocardiography
  - —Decreased mitral deceleration time
  - —Initial diastolic dysfunction
  - —Biventricular enlargement
  - —Mitral/tricuspid regurgitation
  - —Echocardiography in pediatrics
- Possible rejection requires biopsy

DIFFERENTIAL DIAGNOSIS

- Rejection
- Cyclosporine toxicity
- Ischemia
- CMV
- Sepsis
- Viral illness
- Malignancy

PEDIATRIC CONSIDERATIONS

- Evaluate fever in standard manner *plus* chest x-ray and EKG
- If on steroids, then LP

Treatment

INITIAL STABILIZATION

- IV access
- Oxygen
- Monitor
- Intubation
- Defibrillation/pacing
- Vasopressors as required
- Arrhythmias
  - —Advanced cardiac life support (ACLS)
  - —Bradycardia does not respond to atropine—use isoproterenol

ED TREATMENT

- Hemodynamically significant rejection
  - —Methylprednisolone
  - —May also require OKT3 anti-T-cell antibodies or antithymocyte immunoglobulin (by transplantation team)
- Infarct/vasculopathy
  - —Aspirin
  - —Heparin
  - —Possible angioplasty
  - —Likely need retransplantation
- CMV
  - —Empiric IV ganciclovir
- HSV
  - —Oral or IV acyclovir
- Gastroenteritis
  - —Search for CMV infection with culture, serology
- Diarrhea in pediatrics
  - —Increase cyclosporine 25–50% in consultation with transplantation team
- Fever without a source
  - —Consult infectious disease or transplantation team
- Headache
  - —Threshold for CT scan and LP should be low (meningitis, abscess)
- Serious illness/trauma/operation
  - —Steroid burst

MEDICATIONS

- Acyclovir: 5–10 mg/kg i.v. q6h (dose over 1 hour); genital herpes: 400 mg PO t.i.d. × 7–10 days; varicella: 20 mg/kg up to 800 mg PO q.i.d. for 5 days (limits further spread even if begun after three days of symptoms)
- Ceftriaxone: 50 mg/kg i.m.
- CellCept: per transplantation team
- Cyclosporine: based on *trough* levels, changed only by transplantation team
- Ganciclovir: 5 mg/kg b.i.d. for 2–3 weeks (adjust for renal function)
- Imuran: per transplantation team
- Isoproterenol: 1–4 μg/min, titrate to effect; max, 10 μg/min
- Methylprednisolone: 1 g i.v.; peds: 10–20 mg/kg i.v.
- Neoral: per transplantation team

Disposition

ADMISSION CRITERIA

- Hemodynamically significant rejection
- Vasculopathy/ischemia
- New dysrhythmia
- Poorly controlled hypertension
- Congestive heart failure (CHF)
- Dyspnea
- Hypoxia
- Temperature >38°C in adult or child on steroids
- Suspected CMV (unexplained fever, gastroenteritis, or interstitial pneumonitis)
- Not tolerating oral medicines
- Syncope

DISCHARGE CRITERIA

- Mild rejection
- Only in consultation with transplantation team
- Fever in nontoxic child
  - —Do not give children stress dose steroids
- Limit NSAID use because risk for renal insufficiency from acyclovir and tacrolimus

Miscellaneous

ICD9: N/A

ICD10: N/A

SEE ALSO: TRANSPLANT REJECTION

SUGGESTED READINGS

Chinnock R, Sherwin T, Robie S, et al. Emergency department presentation and management of pediatric heart transplant recipients. Pediatr Emerg Care 1995;11(5):355–360.

Johnson MR. Clinical follow-up of the heart transplant recipient. Curr Opin Cardiol 1995;10:180–192.

Mill MR, Grady MS. Cardiac transplantation. In: Tintinalli JE, Kelen GD, Stapczynski JS, eds. Emergency medicine: a comprehensive study guide, 5th ed. San Francisco: McGraw-Hill, 1999:422–428.

Miniati DN, Robbins RC, Reitz BA. In: Braunwald E, ed. Heart disease: a textbook of cardiovascular medicine, 6th ed. Philadelphia: WB Saunders, 2001:615–631.

Authors: Benjamin D. Vanlandingham; Samuel M. Keim

Cardiogenic Shock

Clinical Presentation

SIGNS AND SYMPTOMS

General

- Anxiety
- Hypotension
  - —Systolic blood pressure < 90 mm Hg
  - —Decline by at least 30 mm Hg below baseline level
- Cyanosis
- Pallor
- Diaphoresis
- Dulled sensorium
- Decrease in body temperature
- Urine flow of less than 20 mL/h

Neck

- Jugular venous distention

Respiratory

- Dyspnea
- Increased respiratory rate
- Rales

Cardiac

- Ischemic chest pain
- Tachycardia
- Weak, thready pulse
- Systolic apical blowing murmur
- Gallop rhythm
  - —S3 reflects severe myocardial dysfunction
  - —S4 is present in 80% patients in sinus rhythm with acute myocardial infarction (AMI)
- Systolic click
  - —Suggests rupture of the chordae tendineae

Abdominal

- Epigastric pain
- Nausea and vomiting

Extremities

- Cold, moist skin

Neurologic

- Obtundation

MECHANISM/DESCRIPTION

- Circulatory failure and shock due to a prior deficiency in the heart"s ability to function as a pump
- Three possible underlying causes
  - —Necrosis of more than 40% of the left ventricular mass
  - —Right ventricular infarct
  - —Rupture of papillary muscles or the ventricular wall
- 7–15% of patients hospitalized with AMI develop cardiogenic shock

ETIOLOGY

- AMI
- Myocarditis
- Cardiomyopathy
- Valvular heart disease
- Dysrhythmias
- Drugs/toxins
  - —Beta-blockers
  - —Calcium channel blockers
  - —Adriamycin

Pre-Hospital

CAUTIONS

- Supplemental oxygen
  - —100% O_2 by face mask
- Intravenous access
- Consider a small bolus of crystalloid if rales are absent
- Endotracheal intubation if loss of airway patency

CONTROVERSIES

- Transport only to a chest pain center capable of emergent catheterization

Diagnosis

ESSENTIAL WORKUP

- A careful history and physical examination are needed to exclude other causes of shock
- Ancillary studies further define the type and degree of cardiac injury and determine the indications for emergent catheterization or surgical intervention

LABORATORY

- CBC
  - —Leukocytosis is common
- Pulse oximetry
  - —Used to help predict the need for airway management
- Electrolytes
  - —Hyperkalemia is rarely associated with massive muscle destruction
- Cardiac enzymes

IMAGING/SPECIAL TESTS

- Electrocardiogram
  - —Similar findings to acute myocardial infarction
  - —May also occur in 2–4% of patients with either
    - -Unstable angina, *or*
    - -Non-ST-segment myocardial infarction
- Echocardiography
  - —Akinetic ventricle
  - —Incompetent valve
  - —Ruptured septum, papillary muscle, or ventricular wall

DIFFERENTIAL DIAGNOSIS

- Obstructive shock
  - —Myocardial infarction
  - —Right ventricular infarction
  - —Myocarditis
  - —Cardiomyopathy
  - —Drugs
    - -Beta-blockers
    - -Calcium channel blockers
    - -Adriamycin
  - —Tension pneumothorax
  - —Cardiac tamponade
    - -Retrograde aortic dissection
    - -Constrictive pericarditis
  - —Pulmonary embolus
  - —Septal rupture
  - —Acute valvular incompetence
    - -Ischemia
    - -Endocarditis
  - —Spontaneous esophageal rupture
  - —"Cold" septic shock
  - —Air embolus
- Addisonian crisis
- Ruptured esophagus
- Hypovolemic shock
- Vasogenic shock

Treatment

INITIAL STABILIZATION

- Intravenous access
- Monitor
- Endotracheal intubation
- —Rapid-sequence intubation using an induction agent with minimal cardiac effects
  - -Etomidate
  - -Fentanyl

ED TREATMENT

- Myocardial ischemia
  - —Aspirin
  - —Heparin
- Pulmonary edema
  - —Adequate blood pressure
    - -Vasodilators: nitroprusside; dobutamine; IV nitroglycerin
    - -Furosemide
    - -Amrinone if no improvement
  - —Hypotension
    - -Norepinephrine
- Right ventricular infarct
  - —Volume load
  - —Dobutamine
  - —Avoid diuretics
    - -Decrease preload, worsen already poor cardiac output
  - —Avoid dopamine
    - -Increases pulmonary vascular resistance
- Consult cardiology and/or cardiovascular surgery early
  - —Early revascularization is the single most important factor in the decline in the mortality rate of this disease during the past 8 years

MEDICATIONS

- Amrinone: 0.75 mg/kg, then 5–10 μg/kg/min
- Dobutamine: 2–10 μg/kg/min
- Furosemide: 20–100 mg i.v.
- Nitroglycerin: begin at 10 μg/min and increase 10 μg/min
- Nitroprusside: 1–50 μg/kg/min
- Norepinephrine: begin at 8–12 μg/min and increase infusion as needed

Disposition

ADMISSION CRITERIA

- All patients in cardiogenic shock require admission to a critical care unit

DISCHARGE CRITERIA

N/A

Miscellaneous

ICD9: 785.51

ICD10: R57.0

SEE ALSO: SHOCK

SUGGESTED READINGS

Carnendran L, Abboud R, Sleeper LA, et al. Trends in cardiogenic shock: report from the SHOCK study. Should we emergently revascularize occluded coronaries for cardiogenic shock? Eur Heart J 2001;22(6):444–445.

Dauerman HL, Goldberg RJ, Gore JM. Treatment options for acute myocardial infarction complicated by cardiogenic shock. Cardiol Rev 2000;8(4):207–215.

Hasdai D, Topol EJ, Califf RM, et al. Cardiogenic shock complicating acute coronary syndromes. Lancet 2000;356(9231):749–756.

Author: Thomas Lemke

Cardiomyopathy

Clinical Presentation

SIGNS AND SYMPTOMS

Dilated Cardiomyopathy

- General
  - —Fatigue
  - —Weakness
- Respiratory
  - —Dyspnea on exertion
  - —Orthopnea
- Cardiac
  - —Chest pain
  - —S4 gallop is almost always present
  - —S3 gallop only after cardiac decompensation occurs
  - —Jugular venous distention (JVD)
  - —Dysrhythmias
  - —Mitral or tricuspid regurgitation
- Abdomen
  - —Enlarged, pulsatile liver
- Extremities
  - —Peripheral edema
  - —Systemic emboli

Hypertrophic Cardiomyopathy

- See Cardiomyopathy, Hypertrophic

Restrictive Cardiomyopathy

- General
  - —Exercise intolerance
  - —Weakness
- Respiratory
  - —Dyspnea
  - —Pulmonary congestion
- Cardiac
  - —Exertional chest pain is usually absent
  - —JVD with Kussmaul's sign (rise with inspiration)
  - —Apex is usually easily palpated
  - —Mitral regurgitation
- Abdominal
  - —Increased abdominal girth
  - —Right upper-quadrant pain
  - —Ascites
  - —Hepatomegaly
- Extremities
  - —Edema
  - —Peripheral edema

Arrhythmogenic Right Ventricular Cardiomyopathy

- Dizziness
- Near syncope and syncope
- Palpitations
- Sudden death
- Ventricular arrhythmias

MECHANISM/DESCRIPTION

- Diseases of the myocardium associated with cardiac dysfunction
- Classification is by dominant pathophysiology or specific disease with associated heart muscle abnormalities
  - —Dilated cardiomyopathy
    - -Dilated and impaired contraction of the left or both ventricles
    - -Idiopathic dilated cardiomyopathy accounts for 25% of all cases of heart failure
  - —Hypertrophic cardiomyopathy
    - -Left or right asymmetric ventricular hypertrophy
    - -Usually involves the interventricular septum
  - —Restrictive cardiomyopathy
    - -Restrictive filling and reduced volume of either or both ventricles
    - -Normal or near-normal systolic function
  - —Arrhythmogenic right ventricular cardiomyopathy
    - -Progressive fibrofatty replacement of the right ventricular myocardium
    - -Relative sparing of the septum
  - —Unclassified cardiomyopathy
    - -Disorders such as fibroelastosis that do not fit into a dominant pattern
  - —Specific cardiomyopathy
    - -Heart muscle disease associated with a systemic disease or condition

Pediatric Considerations

- Genetic 20–30%
- Acquired
- Idiopathic

ETIOLOGY

- Dilated
  - —Idiopathic
  - —Viral
  - —Genetic/toxic
  - —Immune
- Hypertrophic
  - —Familial disease with autosomal dominance
- Restrictive
  - —Idiopathic
  - —Amyloid
- Arrhythmogenic right ventricular
  - —Familial disease with dominant and recessive patterns
- Specific
  - —Infectious
    - -Lyme disease
    - -Viral
    - -Chagas' disease
    - -HIV
  - —Toxic agents
    - -Alcohol
    - -Chemotherapeutic agents
  - —Peripartum period
  - —Metabolic
    - -Hyperthyroidism
    - -Pheochromocytoma
  - —General systems diseases
    - -Lupus
    - -Scleroderma

Pre-Hospital

- Monitor
- Oxygen
- Avoid or use a lower dose of nitroglycerine
  - —History or suspicion of hypertrophic cardiomyopathy
- Cardioversion if with acute deterioration due to atrial fibrillation
- Left ventricular heart failure
  - —Oxygen
  - —Nitroglycerine spray
  - —Furosemide
  - —Morphine

Diagnosis

ESSENTIAL WORKUP

- Antecedent illness or exposure
  - —Chemotherapy
  - —HIV
  - —Lyme disease
  - —Viral
- Underlying systemic condition
  - —Hemochromatosis
  - —Sarcoidosis
  - —Pregnancy
- Family history
  - —Familial sudden death
  - —Exertional complaints (syncope, dyspnea)

LABORATORY

- CBC
- Erythrocyte sedimentation rate (ESR)
- Cardiac enzymes
- BNP: level >80 pg/mL has a sensitivity of 98% and a specificity of 93% for CHF
- Serologies
  - —Not useful in the emergency department

IMAGING/SPECIAL TESTS

- Chest x-ray
  - —Dilated cardiomyopathy
    - -Cardiomegaly
    - -Pulmonary congestion
    - -Pleural effusions
  - —Hypertrophic cardiomyopathy
    - -Normal to markedly increased cardiac silhouette
    - -Left atrial enlargement
  - —Restrictive cardiomyopathy
    - -Normal cardiac silhouette
    - -Pulmonary congestion
- EKG
  - —Hypertrophic cardiomyopathy
    - -LV hypertrophy
    - -Abnormal septal Q waves
  - —Dilated, Lyme, Chagas', and toxic cardiomyopathies
    - -Atrial fibrillation
    - -Heart block
    - -Conduction abnormalities
- Emergency transthoracic 2D echocardiogram
  - —Depressed LV ejection fraction
  - —Excludes pericardial tamponade
- Formal transthoracic Doppler echocardiography
  - —Study of choice in patients with cardiomyopathy
  - —Identification of underlying disease
- Nuclear scintigraphy
  - —Indicated when EKG is indeterminate
  - —Direct determination of the thickness of the septum and free wall
  - —Alternative assessment to echo of
- CT and MRI distinguish between constrictive pericarditis and restrictive cardiomyopathy
- Cardiac catheterization
  - —Dilated cardiomyopathy
    - -Suspicion of ischemia
    - -Treatable systemic disease
  - —Hypertrophic cardiomyopathy
    - -Assessment of hemodynamic abnormalities

DIFFERENTIAL DIAGNOSIS

- Other causes of dyspnea
  - —Chronic obstructive pulmonary disease (COPD)
  - —Anemia
  - —Asthma
  - —Interstitial lung disease
  - —Pulmonary embolism
  - —Pericardial tamponade
    - -Valvular heart disease
  - —Ischemic heart disease
  - —Hypothyroidism
  - —Constrictive pericarditis, commonly confused with restrictive cardiomyopathy
- Other causes of syncope
  - —Hypovolemia
  - —Heat disorder
  - —Hypoglycemia

Treatment

- Inotropic and mechanical support with an intraaortic balloon
  - —Indicated for fulminant dilated myopathy
- Anticoagulation
  - —Dilated cardiomyopathy
  - —Atrial fibrillation
  - —Systemic embolization
- Limited ED experience with agents effective in hypertrophic cardiomyopathy
  - —Disopyramide to reduce obstruction
  - —Amiodarone to convert and maintain sinus rhythm
- Standard treatment of CHF
- Standard treatment of atrial or ventricular dysrhythmias

MEDICATIONS

- Amiodarone: 5 mg/kg over 10 minutes
- Carnitine (peds: 50–300 mg/kg/d PO or i.v.)
- Digoxin: start 0.125 mg PO (peds: neonates, 4–6 μg/kg/d i.v. divided q12 load 20–20 μg/kg; 1 mo–2 yr, 7.5–12 mcg/kg/d i.v. divided q12 load 30–50 μg/kg; 2–5 yr, 6–9 μg/kg/d divided q12 load 25–35 μg/kg; 5–10 yr, 4–8 μg/kg/d i.v. divided q12 load 8–12 μg/kg; >10 yr, 2–3 μg/kg/d i.v.: start 8–12 μg/kg; give half of loading dose $\times$ 1; divide remainder into 2 doses q6–12h; obtain EKG after each loading dose)
- Disopyramide: 100–200 mg PO q6h
- Furosemide: 20–40 mg i.v. to a max of 200 mg on subsequent doses (peds: 1 mg/kg i.v. q12–24h)
- Heparin: Load 80 IU/kg i.v.; then 18 IU/kg/h
- Milrinone: Bolus 50 μg/kg i.v. over 10 minutes, then 0.375–0.75 μg/kg/min i.v.
- Morphine: 2–5 mg i.v.
- Nesiritide: Bolus 2 μg/kg i.v., then 0.01 μg/kg/min i.v. with a maximum of 0.03 μg/kg/min
  - —Do not run through same IV simultaneously as furosemide, hydralazine, or heparin because of risk for precipitation
- Nitroglycerine: 5 μg/min i.v.
- Verapamil: 2.5–10 mg i.v. over 2 minutes; max 20 mg (peds: <1 yr, 0.1–0.2 mg/kg i.v. over 2 minutes; may repeat $\times$ 1 in 30 minutes. Use continuous EKG monitoring; 1–15 yr, 0.1–0.3 mg/kg over 2 minutes; max 5 mg first dose; may give second dose up to 10 mg at 30 minutes)

Disposition

ADMISSION CRITERIA

- New or suspected cardiomyopathy
- Syncope where dysrhythmias or HCM are possible etiologies
- Familial history of premature sudden death
- Cardiogenic shock
  - —Consider transfer to a cardiac center capable of mechanical support and cardiac transplantation

Pediatric Considerations

- All

DISCHARGE CRITERIA

- Diagnosed cardiomyopathy with mild CHF that improves with ED therapy
- Restrictive or hypertrophic cardiomyopathy
  - —Cardiology consultation for discharge planning

Miscellaneous

ICD9: 425.4

ICD10: I42.9

SUGGESTED READINGS

Douglas WE, et al. Hypertrophic cardiomyopathy: Clinical spectrum and treatment. Circulation 1995;92: 1680–1692.

Pisani B, Taylor DT, Mason JW. Inflammatory myocardial diseases and cardiomyopathies. Am J Med 1997;102:459–469.

Wynne J, Braunwald E. The cardiomyopathies and myocarditises. In: Braunwald E, ed. Heart disease: a textbook of cardiovascular medicine, 6th ed. Philadelphia: WB Saunders, 2001.

Authors: Elizabeth Temin; James Feldman

Cardiomyopathy, Hypertrophic

Clinical Presentation

SIGNS AND SYMPTOMS

General

- Symptoms correlate with exertion, Valsalva maneuver, or suddenly assuming upright position
- Severity depends on the location and degree of ventricular wall thickening
- Shortness of breath
- Dyspnea on exertion
- Exertional or postprandial angina
- Presyncope
- Syncope
- Congestive heart failure (CHF)
- Cardiovascular collapse
- Dysrhythmias
  - —Paroxysmal atrial fibrillation (Afib)
    - -Often leads to significant, rapid clinical deterioration when present with CHF
  - —Supraventricular tachycardia
  - —Nonsustained ventricular tachycardia (VT) occurs in young adults
  - —Bradydysrhythmias less common
  - —VT or ventricular fibrillation may lead to sudden death
- No or subtle physical findings
- Double apical cardiac impulse at the mid to upper sternum
- Loud, left-sided S4
- Murmur
  - —Crescendo-decrescendo midsystolic murmur at the apex
    - -Increasing in intensity with Valsalva maneuver or standing up
    - -Quieter with recumbency, swatting, or handgrips
  - —With more severe obstruction, a more apparent murmur with radiation to the left sternal border
  - —Radiation to the axilla if there is associated mitral insufficiency

MECHANISM/DESCRIPTION

- Hypertrophic cardiomyopathy (HCM)
  - —Hypertrophied, nondilated left ventricle in the absence of another cause of LV hypertrophy such as hypertension or aortic stenosis
  - —Predominant abnormality identified (one third of cases) in young (<35 years old) athletes suffering sudden atraumatic death
  - —Occurs in all ages from neonate to elderly
    - -Average age of diagnosis is 30–40 years old
- Structural abnormality
  - —Irregular, marked ventricular wall thickening with disarray of myofibrils in the thickened regions and fibrin deposition
  - —Thickening usually asymmetric involving the septum to a greater extent than the free ventricular wall
  - —Atrial dilation

Four Clinical Patterns

- Diastolic dysfunction
  - —Due to impaired relaxation, with normal to supranormal systolic function until end-stage disease
    - -Accounts for a loud S4
  - —Ultimately leads to atrial overload and dilation, with associated atrial fibrillation
  - —Frequently provokes CHF because of the diastolic filling dependence on atrial contribution
- Ischemia
  - —Usually due to phenomena affecting small intramural vessels with normal coronary arteries
- Subaortic obstruction
- Systolic dysfunction

ETIOLOGY

- Autosomal dominantly inherited disorder of cardiac muscle with variable phenotypic expression
- Prevalence about 1 in 500
- Hypertrophied, nondilated left ventricle in the absence of clinical settings can lead to ventricular hypertrophy (systemic hypertension [HTN], aortic stenosis [AS], or "athlete's heart")

PEDIATRIC CONSIDERATIONS

- Prepubescent manifestation is generally much more severe
- Infants present with severe, progressive CHF
- Marked progression often occurs during the rapid growth years of 12 to 18

Pre-Hospital

CAUTIONS

- Consider HCM in patients who decompensate during standard treatments for CHF, ischemia, or supraventricular tachycardia, and in young athletes who collapse during or just after exertion

Diagnosis

ESSENTIAL WORKUP

- Transthoracic cardiac echo/Doppler establishes the diagnosis of HCM
- EKG findings
  - —Normal in 15% of patients
  - —LV hypertrophy with strain
  - —Large Q waves or deep inverted T waves, particularly with apical hypertrophy
  - —Apical infarction
- Chest radiography findings
  - —Normal
  - —Bulge along left heart border representing hypertrophy of free wall of left ventricle
  - —Right or left atrial enlargement
  - —Pulmonary vascular redistribution

IMAGING/SPECIAL TESTS

- Nuclear angiography assesses systolic and diastolic function
- Stress thallium and positron emission tomography evaluate ischemia
- Nuclear magnetic resonance imaging supplements indeterminate echocardiography

DIFFERENTIAL DIAGNOSIS

- Aortic stenosis
- Pulmonic stenosis
- Ventricular septal defect
- Mitral regurgitation
- Mitral valve prolapse
- Arteriosclerotic coronary vascular disease
- Differentiate in patients presenting with CHF or angina
- Vagal and other causes of syncope and presyncope (if HCM is considered, it must be ruled out because it is much more likely to be fatal with repeat episodes)
- More ominous in the setting of HCM

Treatment

INITIAL STABILIZATION

- ABCs
- Intravenous catheterization
- Supplemental oxygen
- Cardiac monitor
- Pulse oximetry

ED TREATMENT

- Do *not* place in seated or Fowler's position
  —Patient may need to remain supine
- Standard CHF or anginal vasodilator therapy may lead to cardiovascular collapse; if this occurs, treat with fluid bolus
- Control heart rate and improve diastolic filling (underlying principle in treating HCM-associated CHF and angina)
  —Beta-blockers
    -Mainstay of therapy
    -Decrease dysrhythmias and lower elevation of pressure gradient across the LV outflow tract
  —Calcium channel blockers
    -Verapamil reduces obstruction by decreasing contractility and improving diastolic relaxation and filling
    -Nifedipine relatively contraindicated
  —Standard CHF or anginal vasodilator therapy may lead to cardiovascular collapse
- Administer anticoagulants for recurrent paroxysmal atrial fibrillation
- Dysrhythmia management
  —Beta-blockers and calcium channel blockers first line for supraventricular dysrhythmias
  —Amiodarone
    -Drug of choice for ventricular dysrhythmias
    -Used when beta-blockers and calcium channel blockers fail
  —Disopyramide
    -Effective for supraventricular and ventricular dysrhythmias
  —Electrical cardioversion
    -Used early in HCM with atrial fibrillation and CHF

LONG-TERM AND DEFINITIVE TREATMENTS

- Surgical therapy
  —Septal myomectomy for patients with large systolic gradients that do not respond to drug therapy
  —Relatively high operative mortality
- Nonsurgical therapy
  —Alcohol injection to sclerose first major septal artery leading to decreased septal tissue

MEDICATIONS

- Amiodarone: 150 mg over 10 minutes, then 360 mg over 6 hours, then 540 mg over next 18 hours (peds: 5 mg/kg i.v. over 1 hour, with a starting-maintenance dose of 5 μg/kg/min)
- Diltiazem: 0.25 mg/kg i.v. over 2 minutes; may repeat in 15 minutes at 0.35 mg/kg
- Disopyramide: 100 mg i.v. over 10 minutes (10 mg every 3 minutes)—dysrhythmias and CHF
- Esmolol: 500 μg/kg/min load over 1 minute, then 50 μg/kg/min for 4 minutes, titrate up to 200 μg/kg/min depending on response
- Propranolol: 1–3 mg slow i.v. bolus
- Verapamil: 2.5 mg i.v. bolus over 1–2 minutes, may repeat as 5.0 mg in 15–30 minutes

Disposition

ADMISSION CRITERIA

- Telemetry admission for dysrhythmia
- ICU admission
  —Syncopal episodes
  —CHF
  —Angina
  —Hemodynamically significant tachydysrhythmias

DISCHARGE CRITERIA

- When HCM is an incidental finding during the ED evaluation for another presentation
  —Need urgent follow-up with a cardiologist
  —Counsel against any activities that may decrease diastolic filling pending follow-up

Miscellaneous

ICD9: 425.4

ICD10: I42.2

SUGGESTED READINGS

Maron BJ, Pelliccia A, Spirito P. Cardiac disease in young trained athletes. Insights into methods for distinguishing athlete's heart from structural heart disease, with particular emphasis on hypertrophic cardiomyopathy. Circulation 1995;91(5):1596–1601.

McKenna WJ, Sadoul N, Slade AK, et al. The prognostic significance of nonsustained ventricular tachycardia in hypertrophic cardiomyopathy. Circulation 1994;90(6):3115–3117.

Spirito P, Rapezzi C, Autore C, et al. Prognosis of asymptomatic patients with hypertrophic cardiomyopathy and nonsustained ventricular tachycardia. Circulation 1994;90:2743–2747.

Spirito P, Seidman CE, McKenna WJ, et al. The management of hypertrophic cardiomyopathy. N Engl J Med 1997;336(11):775–785.

Wigle ED, Rakowski H, Kimball BP, et al. Hypertrophic cardiomyopathy. Clinical spectrum and treatment. Circulation 1995;92(7):1680–1692.

Author: L. Kristian Arnold

Cardiomyopathy, Peripartum

Clinical Presentation

SIGNS AND SYMPTOMS

- Dyspnea
- Chest pain
- Orthopnea
- Cough
- Paroxysmal nocturnal dyspnea
- Anorexia
- Fatigue
- Jugular venous distention
- Gallop rhythm
- Mitral regurgitation murmur
- Loud P2
- Pulmonary rales
- Peripheral edema
- Ascites
- Hepatomegaly
- Hepatojugular reflux

DESCRIPTION/MECHANISM

- Onset of myocardial failure during last month of pregnancy or first 5 months after delivery
  - —Absence of a specific etiology
  - —Absence of a history of cardiac disease
- Occurs in 1 of every 3,000 to 15,000 pregnancies
- Classified as a form of dilated cardiomyopathy
- About 50% resolve spontaneously
- Mortality ranges between 18% and 56%
- Risk factors
  - —Older women
  - —Multiparous
  - —Twin births
  - —Prolonged tocolytic therapy

ETIOLOGY

- A variety of etiologies are suspected but unproven
  - —Viral infection leading to myocarditis, favored by immunosuppression during pregnancy
  - —Immunologic response to an unknown maternal or fetal antigen
  - —Maladaptive response to the hemodynamic stresses of pregnancy
  - —Stress-activated cytokines
  - —Prolonged tocolysis

Pre-Hospital

CAUTIONS

- Differentiate pulmonary edema from acute reactive airway disease

Diagnosis

ESSENTIAL WORKUP

- Chest x-ray
  - —Pulmonary venous congestion
  - —Cardiomegaly
- EKG
  - —Nonspecific
  - —Left ventricular hypertrophy
  - —Left atrial enlargement
  - —T-wave flattening or inversion
  - —Arrhythmias
  - —Ventricular ectopy (40%)
  - —Atrial fibrillation (20%)

LABORATORY

- Electrolytes, BUN, creatinine
- Creatine kinase with muscle and brain fraction

IMAGING/SPECIAL TESTS

- EKG
  - —Demonstrates chamber enlargement and decreased ejection fraction
- Endomyocardial biopsy
  - —Indicated to assess for myocarditis and steroid therapy

DIFFERENTIAL DIAGNOSIS

- Other causes of congestive heart failure
  - —Ischemia
  - —Infarction
  - —Myocarditis
  - —Valvular rupture or disease
  - —Decreased contractile efficiency
    - -Drug related
- Pulmonary embolism
- Pneumonia
- Asthma
- Cardiac ischemia
- Anemia
- Hyperthyroidism
- Constrictive pericarditis
- Pericardial tamponade
- Right-sided congestive heart failure (CHF)
- Nephrotic syndrome
- Cirrhosis

Treatment

INITIAL STABILIZATION

- ABCs
  - —Prompt evaluation of respiratory and hemodynamic status
  - —Control airway as needed
  - —Supplemental oxygen
  - —Continuous positive airway pressure as needed

ED TREATMENT

Prepartum Therapy

- Amlodipine
  - —A dihydropyridine calcium channel blocker that has been shown to improve survival in nonischemic cardiomyopathy patients
- Nitrates
- Intravenous furosemide
- Digoxin to control rate due to atrial fibrillation

Postpartum Therapy

- Add angiotensin-converting enzyme inhibitors (enalapril) or angiotensin II receptor blockers
- Anticoagulation therapy often recommended
  - —30% cases complicated by systemic or pulmonary embolism
  - —During pregnancy, use subcutaneous heparin rather than warfarin, which causes birth defects
- For severe symptoms or lack of response to standard therapy
  - —Dobutamine
  - —Dopamine
  - —Nitroprusside

MEDICATION

- Amlodipine: 2.5–10 mg PO daily
- Amrinone: 0.75 mg/kg i.v. load; 5–10 μg/kg/min i.v.
- Bumetanide: 0.5–2.0 mg i.v.
- Digoxin: 1 mg i.v. load over 1 day; 0.125–0.375 mg/day PO
- Dobutamine: 2–10 μg/kg/min i.v.
- Dopamine: 2–20 μg/kg/min i.v.
- Enalapril: 0.625–1.25 mg i.v.; 2.5–20 mg/d PO
- Furosemide: 20–100 mg i.v.
- Metoprolol: 12.5 mg b.i.d. PO
- Morphine sulfate: 2–4 mg i.v. every 5 minutes
- Nitroglycerin: 0.4 mg sublingual; 1–2 inches of nitro paste; 5–20 μg/min i.v., max of 100–200 μg/min i.v.
- Nitroprusside: 0.5–10 μg/kg/min i.v.

Disposition

ADMISSION CRITERIA

- Patients with pulmonary edema, cardiogenic shock, or evidence of ischemia should be admitted to an ICU setting
- All symptomatic patients with new onset of peripartum cardiomyopathy should be admitted

DISCHARGE CRITERIA

- Mild LV dysfunction
- Established history of peripartum cardiomyopathy
  - —Mild fluid overload attributable to excessive salt intake
  - —Complete resolution of symptoms following ED treatment
  - —No evidence of cardiac ischemia

Miscellaneous

ICD9: 674.8

ICD10: 090.3

SUGGESTED READINGS

Brown CS. Peripartum cardiomyopathy: a comprehensive review. Am J Obstet Gynecol 1998;178(2):409–414.

Pearson GD, et al. Peripartum cardiomyopathy. National Heart, Lung, and Blood Institute and Office of Rare Diseases (National Institutes of Health) Workshop Recommendations and Review. JAMA 2000;283:1183–1188.

Author: Richard Wolfe

Carpal Fractures

Clinical Presentation

SIGNS AND SYMPTOMS

- Local pain in wrist, particularly in radial anatomic "snuffbox"
- Swelling
- Decreased range of motion of the wrist

MECHANISM

- Crush injury or direct blow
- Fall on an outstretched hand (FOOSH)

PEDIATRIC CONSIDERATIONS

- These injuries are rare in children, but the bones are incompletely calcified in children, and fractures may be more difficult to detect

Pre-Hospital

CAUTIONS

- Any patient with a wrist injury should be referred to a physician or ED because fractures may be easily missed on initial screening
- Any patient with swelling or significant pain at the wrist should be splinted to the elbow, the extremity elevated, and ice applied

Diagnosis

ESSENTIAL WORKUP

- A complete physical examination of the entire upper extremity and shoulder girdle is important so that associated injuries are not missed
- A set of wrist x-rays is essential

IMAGING/SPECIAL TESTS

- Special views (e.g., "scaphoid views") may be obtained for most of the carpals if physical examination is suspicious
- This is one area in which comparison with a good radiographic atlas may be very helpful to the less-experienced physician

DIFFERENTIAL DIAGNOSIS

- Scaphoid (carpal navicular) is the most commonly fractured carpal
- Metacarpal base fracture
- Distal radius or ulna fracture
- Lunate or perilunate dislocation

PEDIATRIC CONSIDERATIONS

- Be wary of epiphyseal injuries of the distal radius; children rarely get simple sprains or fractures of the wrist

Treatment

INITIAL STABILIZATION

- Assess for other, more serious injuries
- Immobilize the involved extremity pending definitive evaluation
- Intermittent ice application, elevation
- Prevent contamination of any lacerations overlying the area

ED TREATMENT

- Isolated fractures of the carpals (except the scaphoid) are very rare; if present, they should be treated with sugar-tong splinting from the forearm to the distal hand
- Even suspected scaphoid fractures (snuffbox tenderness but negative initial x-ray) require immobilization by splint of the forearm, wrist, thumb, and hand (thumb spica splint)
  —Immobilize for 10 days to 2 weeks, then repeat x-ray
- Chip fractures off the dorsal aspect of the triquetrum are treatable with simple immobilization splinting
- Associated injuries such as lunate or perilunate dislocation should be sought
- Hamate fractures are rare but may be associated with ulnar artery injury; thus, an Allen test of hand circulation is imperative in a patient with this fracture
- Any open carpal fracture requires parenteral antibiotics and immediate orthopedic consultation

MEDICATIONS

- Mild oral analgesics, NSAIDs, or hydrocodone is important for patient comfort
  —Motrin: 400–600 mg PO q.i.d.
- Proper splinting will relieve most of the pain for these injuries

Disposition

ADMISSION CRITERIA

- Open fractures are admitted for early operative irrigation and débridement
- Patients with injuries requiring surgical management (open reduction) frequently are admitted for early intervention

DISCHARGE CRITERIA

- Closed, nondisplaced carpal fractures treated with adequate splinting of entire forearm may be discharged to have orthopedic follow-up in several days

Miscellaneous

ICD9: 814.00, 814.01

ICD10: NEC S62.1

SUGGESTED READINGS

American Society for Surgery of the Hand. The hand: examination and diagnosis, 3rd ed. New York: Churchill Livingstone, 1990.

American Society for Surgery of the Hand. The hand: primary care of common problems, 2nd ed. New York: Churchill Livingstone, 1990.

Eisenhauer MA. Wrist and forearm. In: Marx JA, et al, eds. Rosen's emergency medicine: concepts and clinical practice, 5th ed. St. Louis: Mosby, Inc., 2002:538–542.

Hart RG, Uehara DT, Wagner MJ. Emergency and primary care of the hand. Dallas: American College of Emergency Physicians, 2001.

Author: Matthew Walsh

Carpal Tunnel Syndrome

Clinical Presentation

SIGNS AND SYMPTOMS

- Pain
  - —Location: wrist or hand, sometimes radiating to elbow, forearm, or shoulder
  - —Often worse at night—relieved by "shaking out" the hand
  - —Exacerbated by repetitive wrist movement and by activities in which the wrist is flexed (e.g., driving)
- Numbness/paresthesias in median nerve distribution (thumb, index, middle, and radial aspect of ring finger)
- Weakness of the abductor pollicis brevis and opponens muscles, which are innervated by the recurrent branch of the median nerve; patient may complain of dropping things or having decreased fine motor control
- Atrophy of thenar muscles (late finding)
- Loss of two-point discrimination (late finding)

ETIOLOGY

- Trauma
- Pregnancy, birth control pills
- Granulomatous disease: tuberculosis, sarcoidosis
- Mass lesions with median nerve compression
- Osteophytes
- Amyloid
- Multiple myeloma
- Rheumatoid arthritis
- Occupational/overuse syndromes—high impact, heavy repetition
- Endocrine disorders: hypothyroidism, diabetes mellitus, acromegaly
- Chronic hemodialysis
- Idiopathic

MECHANISM/DESCRIPTION

- The median nerve, flexor digitorum profundus, flexor digitorum superficialis, and flexor pollicis longus are located in the carpal tunnel—an area bound by the carpal bones and the transverse carpal ligament. Compression of the median nerve causes symptoms

PEDIATRIC CONSIDERATIONS

- Idiopathic carpal tunnel syndrome is rare in children; most cases have an underlying, correctable etiology including
- Trauma
- Mucolipidosis
- Hamartoma of the median nerve
- Anomalous flexor digitorum superficialis (FDS)
- Hemophilia with hematoma

Pre-Hospital

N/A

Diagnosis

ESSENTIAL WORKUP

- History of characteristic nocturnal pain and paresthesias in the median nerve distribution are essential to making the diagnosis. Muscle weakness and thenar wasting are later findings
- Provocative testing
  - —Tinel's sign: gentle tapping over the median nerve at the wrist produces tingling in the fingers in the median nerve distribution (sensitivity, 64%; specificity, 55%)
  - —Phalen's test: wrist flexion for 60 seconds produces numbness or tingling in the median nerve distribution (sensitivity ranges from 40–88%, with a specificity of 80–88%)
  - —Tourniquet test: BP cuff inflated to 200 mm Hg for 2 minutes produces paresthesias in the median nerve distribution

LABORATORY

- Not indicated in most cases
- Thyroid function studies; rheumatoid factor and immune panel if indicated by history and physical exam

IMAGING/SPECIAL TESTS

- Nerve conduction studies and electromyography are criterion standard tests
- Wrist radiograph if trauma or degenerative arthritis suspected
- CT in select cases—may show encroachment of carpal tunnel
- MRI—displays the soft tissues well but has questionable value owing to cost
  - —Findings: palmar bowing of transcarpal ligament, flattened median nerve, median nerve or synovial swelling, fluid in carpal tunnel, signal abnormality of median nerve
- Ultrasound can be diagnostic
  - —Findings: median nerve swelling at proximal canal, median nerve flattening at distal canal, bowing of transcarpal ligament

DIFFERENTIAL DIAGNOSIS

- Cervical nerve root compression—origin of median nerve is at the sixth and seventh cervical roots; symptoms aggravated by erect posture and neck movement
- Hand-arm vibration syndrome characterized by Raynaud's, numbness and tingling in ulnar and median nerve distributions when exposed to cold or vibration, weakened grip, and upper extremity myalgias; associated with prolonged exposure to vibration
- Thoracic outlet obstruction
- Osteoarthritis of the first carpometacarpal joint
- Brachial plexitis
- Generalized neuropathy
- Syringomyelia

Treatment

INITIAL STABILIZATION

- None necessary

ED TREATMENT

- Splint wrist in neutral or slightly extended position
- Aspirin or NSAIDs
- Avoidance of repetitive wrist movement
- Referral to occupational medicine for ergometric testing if due to repetitive motion
- Wrist splint to be worn at night until follow-up with hand surgeon
- May need referral to a hand surgeon for consideration of surgical release of transverse carpal ligament using either open or endoscopic technique

MEDICATIONS

- NSAIDs (there are many choices, a few are listed below)
  —Diclofenac: 50 mg PO b.i.d. or t.i.d.
  —Ibuprofen
    -Adult: 600 mg po q6h
    -Pediatric: 5–10 mg/kg PO q6h
  —Ketorolac: 30 mg i.v. or i.m. q6h or 10 mg PO q4–6h
  —Piroxicam: 20 mg PO daily
- Local corticosteroid injection provides transient relief in two thirds of patients (many different regimens)
  —Hydrocortisone: 25–100 mg
  —Methylprednisolone: 40 mg
  —Prednisolone suspension: 20–40 mg
  —Triamcinolone: 20 mg

Disposition

ADMISSION CRITERIA

N/A

DISCHARGE CRITERIA

- Discharge to home with appropriate follow-up with primary physician, occupational medicine, or hand surgeon

Miscellaneous

ICD9: 354.0

ICD10: G56.0

SUGGESTED READINGS

Al-Qattan MM, Thompson HG, Clarke HM. Carpal tunnel syndrome in children and adolescents with no history of trauma. J Hand Surg 1996;21B(1):108–111.

Kanaan N, Sawaya RA. Carpal tunnel syndrome: modern diagnostic and management techniques. Br J Gen Pract 2001;51:311–314.

O'Gradaigh D, Merry P. Corticosteroid injection for the treatment of carpal tunnel syndrome. Ann Rheum Dis 2000;59: 918–919.

Sternbach G. The carpal tunnel syndrome. J Emerg Med 1999;17:519–523.

Whitley JM, McDonnell DE. Carpal tunnel syndrome a guide to prompt intervention. Postgrad Med 1995;97(1):89–96.

Authors: Matthew Spencer; Linda Spillane

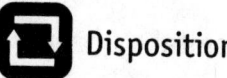

Cauda Equina Syndrome

Clinical Presentation

SIGNS AND SYMPTOMS

- Low back pain
- Sciatica (unilateral or bilateral)
- Bladder and rectal dysfunction
  - —Retention or incontinence
- Saddle hypalgesia or anesthesia
- Lower extremity sensory deficits
  - —May be asymmetric
- Lower extremity motor deficits
  - —Decreased foot dorsiflexion strength
  - —Decreased quadriceps strength
  - —Difficulty ambulating owing to weakness or pain
- Decreased deep tendon reflexes

MECHANISM/DESCRIPTION

- Compression of the lumbar and sacral nerve fibers in the cauda equina in the spinal canal, that is, the nerve fibers below the conus medullaris, which ends at the L1-2 interspace
- Controversy exists regarding the urgency of decompression, and recommendations range from within 6 hours of symptom onset to within 24 hours

ETIOLOGY

- Herniated disc most common
  - —L4 to L5 discs → L5 to S1 → L3 to L4
  - —Most common in fourth and fifth decades of life
- Blunt trauma
- Penetrating trauma
- Mass effect from
  - —Myeloma, lymphoma, sarcoma, meningioma, neurofibroma
  - —Spine metastases (breast, lung, prostate, thyroid, renal)
  - —Epidural abscess (especially in IV drug users), hematoma

Pre-Hospital

- ABCs and cervical spine
- If evidence of trauma, the patient should be transported with full spine immobilization

CAUTIONS

- Even in the nontrauma patient, spinal immobilization is important given the possibility of an unstable lesion

Diagnosis

ESSENTIAL WORKUP

- Neurologic exam most essential
  - —Perineal sensation
  - —Rectal tone
  - —Straight-leg raise
  - —Laségue's sign: with patient supine, flex hip and dorsiflex foot; pain or spasm in posterior thigh indicates lumbar root or sciatic nerve irritation
  - —Anal wink: reflex contraction of external anal sphincter with gentle stroking of skin lateral to anus
- Catheterization for postvoid residual volume
  - —Greater than 50–100 mL is considered abnormal; residual increases with age
  - —Diagnosis unlikely if normal

LABORATORY

- Based on differential diagnoses
- CBC, urinalysis, erythrocyte sedimentation rate (ESR)

IMAGING/SPECIAL TESTS

- X-rays of the lumbosacral (LS) spine
- MRI of spine is definitive study; CT myelogram if MRI unavailable

DIFFERENTIAL DIAGNOSIS

- Conus medullaris or higher cord compression
- Osteoarthritis, LS strain, sciatica
- Ankylosing spondylitis, spinal stenosis
- Vertebral fracture (pathologic and nonpathologic)
- Osteomyelitis
- Spinal epidural abscess
- Abdominal aortic aneurysm
- Vascular claudication
- Hip pathology
- Acute transverse myelitis

Treatment

INITIAL STABILIZATION

- ABCs
- Spine immobilization if trauma or unstable spine lesion suspected
- Analgesia
- NPO until evaluated by neurosurgery

ED TREATMENT

- Repeat neurologic exams to detect progression
- For acute spinal cord trauma (<8 hours), begin high-dose methylprednisolone protocol
- Immediate neurosurgical consultation in all cases

MEDICATIONS

- High-dose steroid protocol
  —Methylprednisolone: 30 mg/kg i.v. bolus, then 5.4 mg/kg/h infusion over next 23 hours
- Morphine sulfate: adult: 2–4 mg i.v. every 5 minutes; peds: 0.1 mg/kg/dose every 5 minutes; max, 15 mg
- Promethazine HCl: adult: 25–50 mg i.v. q4h; peds: 0.25 mg/kg/dose q4h, max, ½ adult dose

Disposition

ADMISSION CRITERIA

- All patients with acute cauda equina syndrome must be admitted to the neurosurgical service
  —Patients have good prognosis with rapid surgical decompression
  —Treatment should not be delayed
- Patients presenting late (>48 hours) also benefit from surgical decompression

DISCHARGE CRITERIA

- Patients with established cauda equina syndrome with prior complete evaluation and no new neurologic deficits may be discharged with close follow-up with their neurosurgeon

Miscellaneous

ICD9: 344.60

ICD10: G83.4

SUGGESTED READINGS

Campana BA. Soft tissue spine injuries and back pain. In: Rosen P, et al., eds. Emergency medicine: Concepts and clinical practice, 4th ed. St. Louis: CV Mosby, 1998:878–905.

Della-Giustina DA. Emergency department evaluation and treatment of back pain. Emerg Med Clin North Am 1999;27(4):877–893.

Green BA, et al. Spinal cord injury in adults. In: Youmans JR, et al., eds. Neurological surgery, 4th ed. Philadelphia: WB Saunders, 1996:1969–1940.

Kostuik JP, Harrington I, Alexander D, et al. Cauda equina syndrome and lumbar disc herniation. J Bone Joint Surg 1986;68A:386–391.

Miller DW, et al. General methods of clinical examination. In: Youmans JR, et al., eds. Neurological surgery, 4th ed. Philadelphia: WB Saunders, 1996:40.

Shapiro S. Medical realities of cauda equina syndrome secondary to lumbar disc herniation. Spine 2000;25(3):348–352.

Author: Kyan Berger

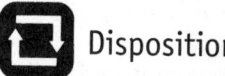

Caustic Ingestion

Clinical Presentation

SIGNS AND SYMPTOMS

Oropharyngeal

- Pain
- Erythema
- Burns
- Erosions
- Ulcers
- Drooling
- Hoarseness
- Stridor
- Aphonia
- Absence of visible lesions in the oropharynx does *not* exclude visceral injuries

Pulmonary

- Tachypnea
- Cough
- Pneumonitis if aspirated

Gastrointestinal

- Pain
- Emesis or hematemesis
- Melena, dysphagia
- Odynophagia
- Peritonitis due to perforation
- Esophageal or gastric perforation

Cardiovascular

- Tachycardia
- Hypotension
- Orthostatic changes

Hematologic

- Acid ingestion can cause RBC hemolysis

Dermatologic

- Pain
- Erythema
- First-, second-, or third-degree burns

Ocular

- Pain
- Erythema
- Injection
- Corneal burns
- Full-thickness corneal damage

Metabolic

- Metabolic acidosis

ETIOLOGY

- Direct chemical injuries
- Injuries occur secondary to acid and alkali exposures
- Many caustic agents (acids and alkalis) are found in common household and industrial products
- Caustic substances:
  —Ammonia hydroxide
  —Formaldehyde
  —Hydrochloric acid
  —Hydrofluoric acid
  —Iodine
  —Phenol
  —Sodium hydroxide
  —Sodium borates, carbonates, phosphates, and silicates
  —Sodium hypochlorite
  —Sulfuric acid

MECHANISM/DESCRIPTION

Alkalis

- Dissociate in the presence of H_2O to produce hydroxy (OH^-) ions, which leads to liquefaction necrosis
- Postingestion—more commonly damages the esophagus than the stomach
- Esophageal damage (in the order of increasing damage) consists of
  —Superficial hyperemia
  —Mucosal edema
  —Superficial blisters
  —Exudative ulcerations
  —Full-thickness necrosis
  —Perforation
  —Fibrosis with resulting esophageal strictures
- Do *not* directly produce systemic complications

Acids

- Dissociate in the presence of H_2O to produce hydrogen (H^+) ions, which leads to a coagulation necrosis with eschar formation
- Postingestion—more commonly damage the stomach because of rapid transit time through esophagus
- Gastric damage (in the order of increasing damage) consists of
  —Edema
  —Inflammation
  —Immediate or delayed hemorrhage
  —Full-thickness necrosis
  —Perforation
  —Fibrosis with resulting gastric outlet obstruction
- Well-absorbed and can cause hemolysis of RBCs and a systemic metabolic acidosis

Pre-Hospital

CAUTIONS

- For oral burns or symptoms: rinse mouth liberally with water or milk
- Water or milk can be given to patients who are able to drink, are not complaining of significant abdominal pain, and do not have airway compromise or vomiting
- Copious irrigation for ocular or dermal exposure

Diagnosis

ESSENTIAL WORKUP

- History of or signs and symptoms of an exposure
- Absence of oropharyngeal lesions does *not* exclude visceral injury

LABORATORY

- CBC
- Electrolytes, BUN, creatinine, glucose
- Arterial blood gas
- Blood cultures
  —If mediastinitis or peritonitis suspected
- Type and cross-match

IMAGING/SPECIAL TESTS

- Chest and abdominal radiographs for
  —Esophageal or gastric perforation
- Esophageal and gastric endoscopy
  —For symptomatic patients to determine the extent of injury
  —Perform within the first 12–24 hours after ingestion
  —Not recommended in the presence of respiratory distress without proper airway management
  —Not recommended in the presence of severe pharyngeal damage
- Radiographic oral contrast imaging not recommended acutely
  —May be used in follow-up for strictures

DIFFERENTIAL DIAGNOSIS

- Chemical injuries from corrosives, acids, alkalis, desiccants, vesicants, and oxidizing and reducing agents
- Foreign body ingestion
- Upper airway infection or angioedema

Treatment

INITIAL STABILIZATION

- ABCs
  - —Prophylactic intubation if there is any evidence of respiratory compromise
  - —Blind nasotracheal intubation contraindicated
- Treat hypotension with 0.9% NS IV fluid resuscitation

ED TREATMENT

Decontamination

- Dermal or ocular exposure
  - —Immediate and thorough irrigation with water or 0.9% NS until physiologic pH attained
  - —Alkalis require more irrigation than acids
- Ipecac, activated charcoal, gastroesophageal lavage, and a neutralizing acid or base are all contraindicated with caustic ingestions
- Dilution
  - —Water or milk in the first 30 minutes of ingestion
  - —Especially useful for solid caustic alkali ingestions
  - —Excessive intake may induce vomiting and worsen esophageal damage
  - —If respiratory distress, intubate before dilution
  - —Contraindicated if esophageal or gastric perforation suspected

ADDITIONAL THERAPY

- NPO if oral exposure
- Broad-spectrum antibiotics if mediastinitis or peritonitis suspected
- Antiemetics for nausea and vomiting
- Treat dermal exposures according to standard burn recommendations
- Detailed examination for ocular exposures
- Intravenous H_2 blockers for symptomatic relief
- Gastroenterology and surgical consultation
- Benefit of corticosteroids following esophageal damage is controversial
  - —May prevent the formation of esophageal stricture
  - —May promote bacterial invasion, immune suppression, and tissue softening
  - —The decision to initiate corticosteroids requires input from entire team caring for patient
  - —Initiate broad-spectrum antibiotics if corticosteroids are given
- Laparoscopy or laparotomy for perforation and full-thickness necrosis
- Topical hydrofluoric acid exposure (options depend on severity and location)
  - —Intradermal injection of 5% calcium gluconate (0.5 mL/cm^2 of skin with 30-gauge needle)
  - —Intraarterial infusion of 10 mL of 10% calcium gluconate in 40 mL D5W over 4 hours

MEDICATIONS

- Methylprednisolone: 40 mg q8h i.v. (peds: 2 mg/kg/d i.v.); the course of therapy is 14–21 days followed by a corticosteroid taper
- Ranitidine (Zantac): 50 mg i.v. q6–8h

Disposition

ADMISSION CRITERIA

- All symptomatic patients
- Nonaccidental ingestion

DISCHARGE CRITERIA

- Asymptomatic patients who accidentally ingested and are able to swallow without difficulty
- Minimal oropharyngeal pain with a corresponding visible lesion; no drooling; no respiratory compromise; no deep throat, chest, or abdominal pain; and able to swallow without difficulty

Miscellaneous

ICD9: 983.2, 983.1

ICD10: T54.9

SUGGESTED READINGS

Anderson KD, Rouse TM, Randolph JG. A controlled trial of corticosteroids in children with corrosive injury of the esophagus. N Engl J Med 1990;323:10:637–640.

Homan CS, Singer AJ, Henry MC, et al. Thermal effects of neutralization therapy and water dilution for acute alkali exposure in canines. Acad Emerg Med 1997;4:1:27–32.

Rao RB, Hoffman RS. Caustics and batteries. In Goldfrank LR, Flomenbaum NE, Lewin NA, et al., eds. Goldfrank's toxicologic emergencies, 6th ed. Stamford, CT: Appleton & Lange, 1998:1399–1420.

Author: Paul Kolecki

Cavernous Sinus Thrombosis

Clinical Presentation

SIGNS AND SYMPTOMS

Symptoms

- Headache
- Deep retrobulbar pain
- Fever
- Eyelid and facial swelling
- Dysesthesias of the forehead and cheek
- Diplopia or decreased visual acuity
- Progressive confusion and lethargy

Signs

- Ptosis
- Chemosis
- Periorbital and facial edema
- Ophthalmoplegia or nonreactive pupil
- Retinal edema and hemorrhage or papilledema
- Confusion, lethargy, coma
- Cardiovascular collapse

MECHANISM/DESCRIPTION

Anatomy

- Cavernous sinuses lie superolateral to the sphenoid sinus and surround the sella
- Cranial nerves (CN) III, IV, V1, and V2 traverse the lateral wall of the sinus
- CN VI and the internal carotid artery occupy the medial portion of the sinus

Pathophysiology

- Local head and neck infections seed the cavernous sinuses via the superior ophthalmic veins
- Static flow through the sinuses favors bacterial growth that incites an inflammatory response, leads to fibrin formation and platelet aggregation, and culminates in thrombosis
- Once thrombosed, the obstructive signs and symptoms that define the cavernous sinus syndrome rapidly evolve
- Fulminant infection may seed the meninges or spread systemically
- Obstruction of the superior ophthalmic, facial, and retinal veins gives rise to chemosis, periorbital and facial edema, and retinal engorgement and hemorrhage
- Inflammation of the cranial nerves leads to
  —Ophthalmoplegia (CN III, IV, VI)
  —Pupillary fixation (CN III)
  —Dysesthesias of the forehead and cheek (CN V1, V2)
  —Loss of the corneal reflex (CN V1)
- Local extension may cause pituitary necrosis and hypopituitarism
- Intracranial extension may cause meningitis, subdural empyema, and intracerebral abscesses
- Extension to the internal carotid artery can cause thrombosis with hemiplegia, or erosive hemorrhage
- Blindness may result from
  —Central retinal artery occlusion
  —Central retinal vein occlusion
  —Septic emboli
  —Arteritis
  —Ischemic optic neuritis
  —Glaucomatous optic atrophy
  —Corneal ulceration from loss of corneal reflex
- Septic emboli may cause distant abscesses, sepsis, and death
- Mortality: 12–30%
- Morbidity: cranial neuropathies, blindness, seizures, vascular steal syndrome, hypopituitarism, and hemiparesis

ETIOLOGY

- *Septic* cavernous sinus thrombosis begins with
  —Localized infection of the midface or sinuses (most common)
  —Pharyngitis, otitis, odontogenic infections, head and neck surgery, and facial trauma
  —Leading organism: *Staphylococcus aureus*
- *Aseptic* cavernous sinus thrombosis is rare
  —Granulomatous conditions (TB)
  —Inflammatory disorders
  —From mass effect (tumors at base of skull, aneurysms)
  —Hypercoagulable states (postoperation, malignancy, pregnancy, oral contraceptives)

Pre-Hospital

N/A

Diagnosis

ESSENTIAL WORKUP

- Clinical diagnosis based on Eagleton's criteria
  —Symptoms of venous obstruction
  —Ophthalmoplegia
  —Sepsis or meningitis
  —Symptoms that begin unilateral and spread to become bilateral are diagnostic

LABORATORY

- CBC—leukocytosis, sometimes anemia
- Electrolytes, BUN, creatinine, glucose
- Prothrombin time (PT), partial thromboplastin time (PTT), platelets
- Blood cultures—usually positive if septic
- CSF examination—may reveal a parameningeal infection or meningitis

IMAGING/SPECIAL TESTS

- MRI
  —Leading modality for visualization of the dural venous sinuses
  —Capable of visualizing thrombus at any stage
- Dynamic helical CT
  —Bolus contrast infusion and rapid serial thin coronal sectioning has made CT competitive with MRI
  —Findings include delayed filling of the involved sinus, a filling defect (thrombus), and a dilated superior ophthalmic vein
- Conventional CT
  —Useful to detect cerebral hemorrhage or abscess
  —Distinguishes between orbital cellulitis and early cavernous sinus thrombosis
- Orbital venography and carotid arteriography
  —Replaced by less invasive technology
  —Useful when CT is nondiagnostic and MRI is unavailable
- 2D time-of-flight magnetic resonance angiography (MRA) flow studies and gadolinium-DTPA-enhanced MRI are promising modalities that may be of use in the future
- Chest x-ray
  —Indicated as with all toxic patients
  —May demonstrate septic pulmonary emboli or adult respiratory distress syndrome (ARDS)

DIFFERENTIAL DIAGNOSIS

- Distinguish *septic* from *aseptic* thrombosis
- Early presentation of periorbital edema and chemosis may mimic allergic blepharitis
- Orbital cellulitis: unilateral and has a less toxic course
- Tolosa-Hunt syndrome (superior orbital fissure syndrome, idiopathic granulomatous inflammation of the cavernous sinus) has similar signs but is slowly progressive and nontoxic

Treatment

INITIAL STABILIZATION

- IV fluids and empiric antibiotics as soon as diagnosis is suspected

ED TREATMENT

- Antibiotics
  —Nafcillin with metronidazole or chloramphenicol
  —If penicillin allergic, substitute vancomycin for nafcillin
- Anticoagulation
  —Significantly improves morbidity and may improve survival
  —Initiate only after CT shows absence of hemorrhage
- Drainage of any focal source of infection (sinus, mastoid) should be considered
  —Emergent consultation with a head and neck surgeon
- Eye protection to avoid corneal ulceration
- Steroids in aseptic thrombosis or in septic thrombosis complicated by hypotension from pituitary insufficiency
- Fibrinolytics (urokinase, streptokinase) have been used anecdotally

MEDICATIONS

- Chloramphenicol: 1.0 g (peds: 50–100 mg/kg/24h) i.v. q6h
- Heparin: titrated to PTT 1.5–2.0 control
- Methylprednisolone: 125 mg (peds: 1–2 mg/kg) i.v.
- Metronidazole: 1.0 g (peds: 15 mg/kg) load, followed by 500 mg (7.5 mg/kg) i.v. q6h
- Nafcillin: 1.5 g (peds: 100 mg/kg/24h) i.v. q4h
- Vancomycin: 500 mg (peds: 10 mg/kg) i.v. q6h

Disposition

ADMISSION CRITERIA

- Admit all patients with suspected septic cavernous sinus thrombosis

DISCHARGE CRITERIA

N/A

Miscellaneous

ICD9: 607.2/325

ICD10: G08

SUGGESTED READINGS

Eustis HS, et al. MR imaging and CT of orbital infections and complications in acute rhinosinusitis. Radiol Clin North Am 1998;36(6):1165–1183.

Gallagher RM, et al. Suppurative intracranial complications of sinusitis. Laryngoscope 1998;108:1635–1642.

Schuknecht B, et al. Tributary venosinus occlusion and septic cavernous sinus thrombosis: CT and MR findings. Am J Neuroradiol 1998;19(4):617–626.

Southwick FS, et al. Septic thrombosis of the dural venous sinuses. Medicine (Baltimore) 1986;65(2):82–106.

Author: Karen S. Cosby

Cellulitis

Clinical Presentation

SIGNS AND SYMPTOMS

- Common to all syndromes:
  - —Pain, tenderness, warmth
  - —Erythema
  - —Edema or induration
  - —Tender regional lymphadenopathy
  - —Lymphangitis
  - —Accompanying subcutaneous abscess possible
  - —Superficial vesicles
- Facial cellulitis in adults
  - —Local erythema and swelling usually secondary to skin trauma
  - —Odontogenic cases more serious
    - -Toothache, sore throat, or facial swelling
    - -Progressive extension into soft tissues of neck with fever, erythema, neck swelling, and dysphagia

Pediatric Presentations

- Facial cellulitis in children
  - —Erythema and swelling of the cheek and eyelid
  - —Rapidly progressive
  - —Usually unilateral
  - —Upper respiratory tract symptoms
  - —Risk for cavernous sinus thrombosis and permanent optic nerve injury
- Perianal cellulitis
  - —Erythema and pruritus extending from the anus several centimeters onto adjacent skin
  - —Pain on defecation
  - —Blood-streaked stools

MECHANISM/DESCRIPTION

- Acute, spreading erythematous superficial infection of the skin and subcutaneous tissues
  - —Variety of pathogens
- Progressive spread of erythema, warmth, pain, and tenderness
- Predisposing factors:
  - —Lymphedema
  - —Tinea pedis
  - —Open wounds
  - —Preexisting skin lesion (furuncle)
  - —Prior trauma or surgery
  - —Retained foreign body
  - —Vascular or immune compromise
  - —Injection drug use

ETIOLOGY

- Simple cellulitis
  - —Group A streptococci
  - —*Staphylococcus aureus*
- Extremity cellulitis after lymphatic disruption
  - —Non-group A β-hemolytic streptococci (groups C, B, G)
- Cellulitis in diabetic patients
  - —Can be polymicrobial with *S. aureus*, streptococci, gram-negative bacteria, and anaerobes, especially when associated with skin ulcers
- Facial cellulitis
  - —Streptococcal species
  - —*Haemophilus influenzae* type B
  - —*S. aureus*, associated with trauma
  - —Anaerobic oral flora, associated with intraoral laceration or dental abscess
- Facial cellulitis in children
  - —*Streptococcus pneumoniae*
  - —*H. influenzae* type B, although incidence declining since introduction of HIB vaccine
- Less common causes
  - —Clostridia
  - —Anthrax
  - —*Pasteurella multocida*—common after cat and dog bites
  - —*Eikenella corrodens*—human bites
  - —*Pseudomonas aeruginosa*
    - -Hot-tub folliculitis—self-limited
    - -Foot puncture wound
    - -Ecthyma gangrenosum in neutropenic patients
  - —*Erysipelothrix* species—raw fish, poultry, meat or hide handlers
  - —*Aeromonas hydrophila*—fresh-water swimming
  - —*Vibrio* species—seawater or raw seafood

Pediatric Considerations

- Perianal cellulitis
  - —Group A streptococci
  - —Associated or antecedent pharyngitis or impetigo
- Neonates—group B streptococci

Pre-Hospital

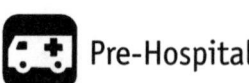

- No specific considerations

Diagnosis

ESSENTIAL WORKUP

- Cellulitis is a *clinical diagnosis*

LABORATORY

- White blood count unnecessary
- Gram stain and culture may focus antimicrobial selection
  - —Aspiration and culture of the leading edge are not helpful, except under these circumstances:
    - -Unusual pathogens suspected
    - -Fluctuant area detected
    - -Treatment failure
  - —Blood cultures usually negative

IMAGING/SPECIAL TESTS

- Plain radiographs may reveal abscess formation, subcutaneous gas, or foreign bodies
  - —Extension to bone (osteomyelitis) not visualized early on plain radiographs
- Extremity vascular imaging (Doppler ultrasound) can help rule out deep venous thrombosis

DIFFERENTIAL DIAGNOSIS

- Lymphangitis or lymphadenitis
- Thrombophlebitis or deep venous thrombosis (DVT)
  - —Differentiation from cellulitis
    - -Absence of an initial traumatic or infectious focus
    - -No regional lymphadenopathy
    - -Presence of risk factors for DVT
- Insect bite
- Allergic reaction
- Acute gout or pseudogout
- Fasciitis or myositis
- Ruptured Baker's cyst
- Herpetic whitlow
- Neoplasm
- Phytophotodermatitis
- Differential diagnosis of *facial cellulitis*
  - —Allergic angioedema
  - —Conjunctivitis
  - —Contusion

PEDIATRIC CONSIDERATIONS

- Differential diagnosis of *perianal cellulitis*
  - —Candida intertrigo
  - —Psoriasis
  - —Pinworm infection
  - —Child abuse
  - —Behavioral problem
  - —Inflammatory bowel disease

Treatment

INITIAL STABILIZATION

- Airway compromise possible with deep extension of facial cellulitis

ED TREATMENT

- Simple cellulitis
  —Outpatient: oral dicloxacillin: 7–10 days
  —Alternatives: oral macrolide, cephalexin, or levofloxacin
  —Inpatient: IV nafcillin or equivalent
- Extremity cellulitis after lymphatic disruption
  —Same as simple cellulitis
- Cellulitis in diabetic patients
  —Outpatient: oral amoxicillin clavulanate or clindamycin
  —Inpatient: IV cefoxitin plus gentamicin (or other aminoglycoside, or imipenem cilastatin)
- Facial cellulitis in adults
  —Outpatient: oral amoxicillin clavulanate, azithromycin, or clarithromycin
  —Inpatient: IV cefoxitin or levofloxacin
  —Odontogenic source
  -Drainage essential
  -Coverage for anaerobes: clindamycin
- Facial cellulitis in children
  —IV ceftriaxone
- Perianal cellulitis
  —Penicillin
- Animal or human bite
  —Oral amoxicillin clavulanate
- Foot puncture wound
  —Oral or IV ciprofloxacin or IV ceftazidime
- Cool compresses for comfort
- Analgesics
- Extremity elevation

MEDICATIONS

- Amoxicillin clavulanate: 500–875 mg (peds: 45 mg/kg/24 h) PO b.i.d. or 250–500 mg (peds: 40 mg/kg/24 h) PO t.i.d.
- Azithromycin: (adults and peds) 10 mg/kg up to 500 mg PO on day 1, followed by 5 mg/kg up to 250 mg PO qd to complete 5 days
- Cefazolin: 1–2 g (peds: 50–100 mg/kg/24 h) i.v. q6–8h
- Cefoxitin: 1–2 g (peds: 80–160 mg/kg/24 h; max, 12 g/24 h) i.v. q6h
- Ceftazidime: 500–1,000 mg (peds: 100–150 mg/kg/24 h; max, 6 g/24 h; use sodium formulation in peds) i.v. q8h
- Ceftriaxone: 1–2 g (50–75 mg/kg/24 h) i.v. qd
- Cephalexin: 500 mg PO q.i.d. (peds: 50–100 mg/kg/24 h q.i.d.)
- Ciprofloxacin: (adult only) 500–750 mg PO b.i.d. or 400 mg i.v. q8–12h
- Clarithromycin: 250 mg (peds: 7.5 mg/kg) PO b.i.d.
- Clindamycin: 450–900 mg (peds: 20–40 mg/kg/24 h) PO or i.v. q8h
- Dicloxacillin: 125–500 mg (peds: 12.5–25 mg/kg/24 h) PO q6h
- Erythromycin base: (adult) 250–500 mg PO q.i.d. or 333 mg PO t.i.d.
- Gentamicin: load 2–5 mg/kg i.v., then 1–1.5 mg/kg/24 h i.v. q8h; dose adjustments for neonates/infants, renal insufficiency, and based on serum levels
- Imipenem cilastatin: 500–1,000 mg (peds: 25 mg/kg) i.v. q6h
- Levofloxacin: (adult only) 500–750 mg PO or i.v. qd
- Nafcillin: (adult only) 1–2 g i.v. q4h
- Procaine penicillin G: (peds) 25–50,000 Us/kg/24 h i.m. q12h, followed by penicillin VK, 25–50 mg/kg/24 h PO q.i.d.; if toxic appearing, 100,000–400,000 U/kg/24 h i.v. q6h
- Vancomycin: 1 g i.v. q12h (peds: 10–15 mg/kg i.v. q6h, dosing adjustments required under age 5 years); check serum levels

Disposition

ADMISSION CRITERIA

- Toxic appearing
- Tissue necrosis
- History of immune suppression
- Concurrent chronic medical illnesses
- Unable to take oral medications
- Unreliable patients

DISCHARGE CRITERIA

- Mild infection in a non-toxic-appearing patient
- Able to take oral antibiotics
- No history of immune suppression or concurrent medical problems
- No hand or face involvement
- Has adequate follow-up within 24–48 hours

Miscellaneous

ICD9: 682.9

ICD10: L03.9

SUGGESTED READINGS

Abyad A. Cellulitis. In: Dambro M, ed. Griffith's 5-minute clinical consult. Philadelphia: Lippincott Williams & Wilkins, 2001:190–191.

Givner LB, Mason EO, Barson WJ, et al. Pneumococcal facial cellulitis in children. Pediatrics 2000;106(5):e61.

Magnussen CR. Skin and soft-tissue infections. In: Reese RE, Betts RF, eds. A practical approach to infectious diseases, 4th ed. Boston: Little, Brown, 1996:96–132.

Stevens DL. Infections of the skin, muscle and soft tissues. In Brunwald E, Fauci AS, Kasper DL, et al., eds. Harrison's principles of internal medicine, 15th ed. New York: McGraw-Hill, 2001:821–825.

Swartz MN. Cellulitis and subcutaneous tissue infections. In: Mandell GL, Bennett JE, Dolin R, eds. Mandell, Douglas and Bennett's principles and practice of infectious diseases, 5th ed. New York: Churchill Livingstone, 2000:1037–1057.

Authors: John Mahoney; Dolores Gonthier

Cerebral Aneurysm

Clinical Presentation

SIGNS AND SYMPTOMS

- Commonly asymptomatic before rupture
- Sentinel headaches occur in 30—60% of patients before rupture; can be unilateral
- Seizures, syncope, or altered level of consciousness
- Compression of adjacent structures may cause neurologic symptoms
  - —Anterior communicating artery (ACA) aneurysms
    - -Optic tract: altitudinal field cut or homonymous hemianopsia
    - -Optic chiasm: bitemporal hemianopsia
    - -Optic nerve: unilateral amblyopia
  - —Aneurysms at the internal carotid-posterior communicating artery (PCA) junction
    - -Oculomotor nerve: fixed and dilated pupil, ptosis, diplopia, and temporal deviation of the eye with an inability to turn the eye upward, inward, or downward
    - -Aneurysms in the cerebral cortex may produce focal deficits, including hemiparesis, hemisensory loss, visual disturbances, aphasia, and seizures
- Rupture results in subarachnoid hemorrhage (SAH)
  - —Headache; severe ("worst headache ever") with sudden onset ("thunderclap"); different from prior headaches; classically without focal deficits
  - —Nuchal rigidity (most common sign) secondary to blood in CSF

DESCRIPTION

- An abnormal, localized dilation or outpouching of the wall of a cerebral artery occurring in 5–10% of the population
- Rupture of saccular aneurysms account for 5–15% of strokes
- Of those that rupture, 40% occur at the ACA, 30% at the internal carotid, 20% in the middle cerebral artery (MCA), and 5–10% in the vertebrobasilar system

ETIOLOGY

- "Congenital," saccular, or berry aneurysms are the most common (90%)
  - —Develop at weak points in the arterial wall and occur at bifurcations of major cerebral arteries
  - —Incidence increases with age
  - —Multiple in 20–30%
  - —Increased incidence with polycystic kidney disease, cerebral arteriovenous malformation (AVM), type III collagen deficiency, fibromuscular dysplasia, Ehlers-Danlos syndrome, Marfan's syndrome, pseudoxanthoma elasticum, neurofibromatosis, moyamoya, coarctation of the aorta, tuberous sclerosis, sickle cell, Osler-Weber-Rendu, α_1-antitrypsin deficiency, system lupus erythematosus (SLE)
- Arteriosclerotic, fusiform or dolichoectatic (7%)
  - —More common in peripheral arteries
- Inflammatory (mycotic)
  - —10% of patients with bacterial endocarditis
- Traumatic, associated with severe closed head injury
- Neoplastic, embolized tumor fragments

PEDIATRIC CONSIDERATIONS

- Although rare in children, they are more likely to be giant (>25 mm) and occur in the posterior circulation
- Aneurysms in children have a high rate of hemorrhage and should be repaired early

Pre-Hospital

CAUTIONS

- Neurologic examination in the field can be extremely helpful. Assess level of consciousness, Glasgow Coma Scale score, gross motor deficits, speech abnormalities, gait disturbance, facial asymmetry, and other focal deficits
- Patients with subarachnoid hemorrhage (SAH) may need emergent intubation from rapidly deteriorating level of consciousness
- Patients must be transported to a hospital with emergent CT scanning and ICU-level treatment

Diagnosis

ESSENTIAL WORKUP

- Complete neurologic examination
- Emergent noncontrast head CT scan will diagnose 90–95% of SAHs
- Lumbar puncture with CSF analysis if CT scan is negative

LABORATORY

- Coagulation studies
- Baseline CBC with platelets and differential, electrolytes, renal and liver function tests, and arterial blood gases (ABGs)

IMAGING/SPECIAL TESTS

- Chest x-ray for pulmonary edema
- Four-vessel cerebral angiography remains the gold standard
- Magnetic resonance angiography (MRA)
- Helical CT scanning may be useful in detecting aneurysms > 3 mm
- Transcranial Doppler ultrasound may be useful to detect vasospasm

DIFFERENTIAL DIAGNOSIS

- Neoplasm
- AVM
- Optic neuritis
- Migraine
- Meningitis
- Encephalitis
- Hypertensive encephalopathy
- Hyperglycemia or hypoglycemia
- Temporal arteritis
- Acute glaucoma
- Subdural hematoma
- Epidural hematoma
- Intracerebral hemorrhage
- Thromboembolic stroke
- Air embolism
- Sinusitis

Treatment

INITIAL STABILIZATION

- ABCs for patients with SAH
  - —Supplemental oxygen
  - —Rapid-sequence intubation may be required for airway protection or for controlled ventilation
  - —Continuous cardiac monitoring and pulse oximetry
- For altered mental status, check blood glucose immediately, give naloxone, D_{50}, thiamine
- Management of acute hypertension is essential; this may be accomplished with labetalol, nitroprusside, or hydralazine
- Prevention of acute increases in intracranial pressure from vomiting should be accomplished with antiemetics
- Seizures should be managed acutely with intravenous benzodiazepines and phenytoin

ED TREATMENT

- Following initial stabilization, the major goals of early treatment of ruptured or leaking aneurysms are to prevent re-rupture, cerebral vasospasm, and hydrocephalus; see Subarachnoid Hemorrhage

Definitive Therapy for Aneurysm

- Optimal timing for angiography and surgery remain controversial, but there is a trend toward early surgery to decrease the incidence of rebleeding and cerebral vasospasm. Some patients may be candidates for interventional neuroradiologic treatment with detachable balloons or coils

MEDICATIONS

- Diazepam: 5–10 mg i.v. every 10–15 minutes; max, 30 mg (peds: 0.2–0.3 mg/kg every 5–10 minutes; max, 10 mg)
- Docusate sodium: 100 mg PO b.i.d.
- Hydralazine: 10–20 mg i.v. every 30 minutes
- Labetalol: 20–30 mg/min i.v. bolus, then 40–80 mg every 10 minutes; max, 300 mg; follow with continuous infusion 0.5–2 mg/min
- Lorazepam: 2–4 mg i.v. every 15 minutes PRN; peds: 0.03–0.05 mg/kg/dose, max, 4 mg/dose
- Nimodipine: 60 mg PO/NG q4h
- Nitroprusside: 0.25–10 μg/kg/min (adult and peds)
- Phenytoin: 15–20 mg/kg i.v. load at max 50 mg/min; max, 1.5 g (adult and peds); maintenance 4–6 mg/kg/d i.v./i.m.
- Prochlorperazine: 5–10 g i.v./i.m. q6–8h; peds: 0.2 mg/kg/d i.m. in 3–4 divided doses; max, 40 mg/d

Disposition

ADMISSION CRITERIA

- Any patient with an acute aneurysmal subarachnoid hemorrhage should be admitted, preferably to an ICU
- Any patient with a symptomatic unruptured aneurysm should receive admission and urgent neurosurgical consultation given the high rate of rupture

DISCHARGE CRITERIA

- Patients with incidentally discovered asymptomatic intracranial aneurysms may be discharged with close neurosurgical follow-up
- Note that the overall risk of rupture is 1–2% per year and that the critical size at which the risk for rupture outweighs the risk for surgery is controversial (classically 10 mm, but probably in the 4- to 8-mm range)

Miscellaneous

ICD9: 437.3

ICD10: I67.1

SEE ALSO: SUBARACHNOID HEMORRHAGE

SUGGESTED READINGS

Cerebrovascular diseases. In: Adams RD, Victor M, eds. Principles of neurology, 5th ed. New York: McGraw-Hill, 1993.

Barrow DL, Reisner A. Natural history of intracranial aneurysms and vascular malformations. Clin Neurosurg 1993;40:3–39.

Barsan WG, Kothari R. Stroke. In: Rosen P, et al., eds. Emergency medicine: concepts and clinical practice, 4th ed. St. Louis: CV Mosby, 1997:2184–2197.

Becker KJ. Epidemiology and clinical presentation of aneurysmal subarachnoid hemorrhage. Neurosurg Clin North Am 1998;9:435–444.

Bederson JB, Awad IA, Wiebers DO, et al. Recommendations for the management of patients with unruptured intracranial aneurysms: a statement for healthcare professionals from the Stroke Council of the American Heart Association. Stroke 2000;31:2742–2750.

Meyer FB, Morita A, Puumala MR, et al. Medical and surgical management of intracranial aneurysms. Mayo Clin Proc 1995;70(2):153–172.

White PM, Wardlaw JM, Easton V. Can noninvasive imaging accurately depict intracranial aneurysms? A systematic review. Radiology 2000;217:361–370.

Authors: Veronique Au; Rebecca Smith Coggins

Cerebral Vascular Accident

Clinical Presentation

SIGNS AND SYMPTOMS

- Aphasia
- Hemiparesis, hemiplegia
- Hemisensory loss
- Dysarthria, dysphagia
- Facial droop
- Ataxia, clumsiness
- Visual loss, photophobia, diplopia
- Headache
- Nausea, vomiting
- Vertigo, dizziness
- Altered level of consciousness, confusion, agitation
- Cardiac dysrhythmias, murmurs
- Cheyne-Stokes breathing, apnea
- Hypertension
- Transient ischemic attacks (TIAs), focal neurologic deficits that completely resolve in < 24 hours, precede most thrombotic cerebral vascular accidents (CVAs)

Anterior Cerebral Artery

- Contralateral hemiplegia (lower $\rightarrow$ upper), hemisensory loss, apraxia, confusion, impaired judgment

Middle Cerebral Artery

- Contralateral hemiplegia (upper $\rightarrow$ lower), hemisensory deficits, homonymous hemianopsia, dysphasia, dyslexia, agnosia

Posterior Cerebral Artery

- Cortical blindness in half the visual field, visual agnosia, altered mental status, impaired memory, third nerve palsy, hemiballismus

Vertebrobasilar System

- Impaired vision, visual field defects, nystagmus, diplopia
  - —Vertigo, dizziness
  - —Facial paresthesia, dysarthria, cranial nerve palsies, contralateral pain, and temperature deficits

DESCRIPTION

- An interruption of the blood flow to a specific region of the brain
  - —Neurologic findings determined by the specific area affected
  - —The onset may be sudden and complete, or stuttering and intermittent

ETIOLOGY

- CVAs may be ischemic (thrombotic or embolic) or hemorrhagic (intracranial or subarachnoid hemorrhage)
- Risk factors include diabetes, smoking, hypertension, coronary artery disease, peripheral vascular disease, oral contraceptive use, polycythemia vera, sickle cell anemia, and deficiencies of antithrombin III, protein C, or protein S
- *Thrombotic stroke* is caused by occlusion of blood vessels
  - —Clot formation at an ulcerated atherosclerotic plaque is most common
  - —Sludging (sickle cell anemia, polycythemia vera, protein C deficiency), arterial dissection, arteritis, or fibromuscular dysplasia
- *Embolic stroke* is caused by acute blockage of a cerebral artery by a piece of foreign material from outside the brain, including
  - —Cardiac mural thrombi associated with mitral stenosis, atrial fibrillation, cardiomyopathy, congestive heart failure (CHF), or myocardial infarction (MI)
  - —Prosthetic heart valves or abnormal native valves
  - —Atherosclerotic plaques in the aortic arch or carotid arteries
  - —Atrial myxoma
  - —Ventricular aneurysms with ventricular thrombi

PEDIATRIC CONSIDERATIONS

- CVAs in childhood are usually attributable to an underlying disease process such as sickle cell anemia, leukemia, or a blood dyscrasia

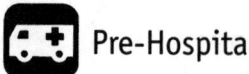

Pre-Hospital

CAUTIONS

- Patients may have difficulty moving or communicating after CVA
- Neurologic examination in the field is helpful and should include assessment of level of consciousness, Glasgow Coma Scale score, gross motor deficits, speech abnormalities, gait disturbance, facial asymmetry, and other focal deficits
- Hyperglycemia may exacerbate an ischemic insult; perform rapid blood glucose testing before administration of glucose containing fluids

Diagnosis

ESSENTIAL WORKUP

- Emergent noncontrast head CT scan to distinguish ischemic from hemorrhagic events; may be normal in the first 24–48 hours of ischemic stroke
- If CT is normal and subarachnoid hemorrhage is suspected, emergent lumbar puncture is indicated
- Electrocardiogram to evaluate for dysrhythmias and the presence of MI

LABORATORY

- Baseline CBC, electrolytes, renal function tests, liver function test (LFT), prothrombin time (PT), partial thromboplastin time (PTT)
- Urinalysis—hematuria is seen in subacute bacterial endocarditis (SBE) with embolic stroke
- Sedimentation rate—elevated in SBE, vasculitis, hyperviscosity syndromes
- Cardiac enzymes

IMAGING/SPECIAL TESTS

- Noncontrast head CT
- Chest x-ray
- Echocardiography
- Carotid ultrasonography
- MRI can detect ischemia < 2 hours after onset

DIFFERENTIAL DIAGNOSIS

- Intracranial bleeding
- Hypoglycemia
- Seizure disorder
- MI or CHF
- Panic attacks, depression
- Head trauma
- Meningitis
- Migraine
- Air embolism
- TIA
- Hypertensive encephalopathy
- Neoplasm
- Subdural hematoma
- Giant cell arteritis

Treatment

INITIAL STABILIZATION

- ABCs
  - —Supplemental oxygen 2-4 L via nasal cannula
  - —IV access
  - —Cardiac monitoring and pulse oximetry
  - —Rapid-sequence intubation may be required for airway protection or controlled ventilation to decrease intracranial pressure (ICP)
- For altered mental status, give naloxone and thiamine and check blood glucose

ED TREATMENT

- Treat elevated blood pressure if systolic BP > 220–240 or diastolic BP >130–150 on repeated measurements, or if indicated for other concurrent problems (MI, aortic dissection, CHF, hypertensive encephalopathy)
- Control seizures with benzodiazepines then phenytoin
- Maintain euvolemia and normothermia
- *Thrombolytics*
  - —Ischemic stroke only; administer within 3 hours of symptom onset (see Reperfusion Therapy, Cerebral)
  - —Contraindications: hemorrhage on CT, recent stroke, severe head trauma, systolic BP > 185, diastolic BP > 110, active internal bleeding, bleeding diathesis, anticoagulation, intracranial neoplasm
  - —Avoid anticoagulants and antiplatelet drugs for 24 hours
- Treat increased ICP and cerebral edema
  - —Elevate head of bed 30 degrees
  - —Controlled ventilation to keep PCO_2 35–40 mm Hg
  - —Mannitol
- Urgent neurosurgical decompression may be required in the presence of brainstem compression
- In patients with completed or minor strokes, aspirin may prevent recurrence

MEDICATIONS

- Aspirin: 81 mg PO qd
- Clopidogrel: 75 mg PO qd
- Diazepam: 5 mg i.v. every 5–10 minutes; max, 20 mg
- Enalapril: 0.675–1.25 mg i.v.
- Hydralazine: 10–20 mg i.v. every 30 minutes
- Labetalol: 15–20 mg/min i.v. bolus, then 40–80 mg every 10 minutes; max, 300 mg; follow with continuous infusion 0.5–2 mg/min
- Mannitol (15–25% solution): 0.5–2 g/kg i.v. over 5–10 minutes, then 0.5–1 g/kg q4–6h (adult and peds)
- Nitroprusside: 0.25–10 μg/kg/min (adult and peds)
- Trimetaphan: 1–4 mg/min
- Tissue plasminogen activator: 0.9 mg/kg i.v.; max, 90 mg, with 10% of dose given as a bolus and the remainder infused over 60 minutes

Disposition

ADMISSION CRITERIA

- Patients with acute CVA should be admitted to the hospital; patients with severely decreased level of consciousness, hemodynamic instability, life-threatening cardiac dysrhythmias, or significantly increased ICP should be treated in an ICU

DISCHARGE CRITERIA

- Patients who present with completed strokes that are days to weeks old may be discharged if they are able to function independently or have adequate social support
- Patients with multiple prior strokes who experience relatively minor new episodes may also be treated on an outpatient basis if similar criteria are met and stroke completed

Miscellaneous

ICD9: 436

ICD10: I64

SUGGESTED READINGS

Adams HP, Brott TG, Furlan AJ, et al. Guidelines for thrombolytic therapy for acute stroke: a supplement to the guidelines for the management of patients with acute ischemic stroke. A statement for healthcare professionals from a Special Writing Group of the Stroke Council, American Heart Association. Circulation 1996;94:1167–1174.

Barsan WG, Kothari R. Stroke. In: Rosen P, et al., eds. Emergency medicine: concepts and clinical practice, 4th ed. St. Louis: CV Mosby, 1997:2184–2197.

Brott TG, Clark WM, Fagan SC, et al. Stroke: the first hours. Guidelines for acute treatment. Englewood, CO: National Stroke Association, 2000.

Hacke W, Kaste M, Fieschi C, et al. Randomised double-blind placebo-controlled trial of thrombolytic therapy with intravenous alteplase in acute ischaemic stroke (ECASS II). Lancet 1998;352:1245–1251.

Naradzay JFX, Gaasch WR. Acute stroke. Emerg Med Clin North Am 1995;14(1):197–216.

NINDS rt-PA Stroke Study Group. Tissue plasminogen activator for acute ischemic stroke. N Engl J Med 1995;333:1581–1587.

Authors: Veronique Au; Rebecca Smith Coggins

Cervical Adenitis

Clinical Presentation

SIGNS AND SYMPTOMS

- Enlarged, tender cervical lymph node
- Usually unilateral and solitary
- Warmth and erythema of overlying skin
- Early in course firm but later possibly fluctuant node
- With or without fever
- Malaise
- Irritability in infants and children
- Usually a concurrent head and neck infection
  - —Pharyngitis, tonsillitis, peritonsillar abscess
  - —Otitis media, otitis externa
  - —Dental infection
  - —Impetigo, scalp infection

MECHANISM/DESCRIPTION

- An acute bacterial infection of a cervical lymph node, usually following bacterial invasion of the head or neck area
- This should be differentiated from lymphadenopathy caused by regional or systemic infection that involves inflammation of the node *but not bacterial infection* of the node itself
- Any cervical node can become infected; cervical nodes act as the final common pathway for lymph to drain from all areas of the head and neck
- The causative bacteria invade regional areas of the head and neck causing local lymph nodes to swell secondary to hyperplasia of sinusoidal cells and infiltration of lymphocytes (lymphadenopathy)
- If the reaction is not contained, the bacteria enter the lymph system and proliferate (lymphadenitis)
- Pus forms when neutrophils are incited, and abscess develops when host defenses are unable to clear infection
- Primarily a pediatric disease
  - —70–80% of patients are in the 1- to 4-year-old age group
- Becoming more common in adults owing to immunocompromised states such as HIV

ETIOLOGY

- 50–80% of cases are due to group A β-hemolytic streptococcus and *Staphylococcus aureus*
- Mycobacteria tuberculosis
  - —Scrofula or tuberculous lymphadenitis
  - —Rarely seen
  - —Usually a chronic lymphadenitis in the posterior cervical nodes
  - —PPD usually strongly reactive
  - —Treatment medical
- Atypical mycobacteria (nontuberculous)
  - —More commonly seen
  - —Usually a chronic lymphadenitis in the submandibular or anterior cervical nodes
  - —PPD unreliable
  - —Treatment is primarily surgical
- *Bartonella henselae* (cat-scratch disease)
  - —A subacute lymphadenitis
  - —Has indolent course but usually spontaneously resolves
- Anaerobes
  - —Consider in lymph nodes draining infections of the teeth or gingiva
- Rarer organisms
  - —*Haemophilus influenzae*
  - —*Yersinia pestis*
  - —*Nocardia* species
  - —*Francisella tularensis*
  - —*Brucella melitensis*
  - —*Mycoplasma pneumoniae*
  - —*Treponema pallidum*
  - —*Actinomyces israelii*

PEDIATRIC CONSIDERATIONS

- One of the most common causes of a neck mass in a child
- Overall group A β-streptococcus and *S. aureus* most common causes
- In neonates, group B streptococcus and *S. aureus* most common
- Group B streptococcal cellulitis-adenitis syndrome
  - —Neonates with fever, submandibular or facial cellulitis, and an ipsilateral otitis
  - —94% incidence of concurrent bacteremia
- *S. aureus* associated with more indolent course and higher frequency of suppuration

Pre-Hospital

N/A

Diagnosis

ESSENTIAL WORKUP

- Cervical adenitis is a clinical diagnosis
- Identify primary source of infection in head and neck area (e.g., otitis, tonsillitis)
- If no primary inflammatory source of infection in head and neck
  - —Address possible tuberculosis exposure with PPD
  - —Look for signs of systemic disease and viral illness

LABORATORY

- Unnecessary if there is a primary source of infection to treat
- Blood cultures in toxic-appearing patients
- Sepsis workup in neonates
- If the etiology is unclear, the following may help to discern a nonbacterial cause (see Differential Diagnosis)
  - —WBC with differential
  - —Monospot
  - —Throat cultures
  - —Antibody titers (e.g., Epstein-Barr virus [EBV], cytomegalovirus [CMV], toxoplasmosis)

IMAGING/SPECIAL TESTS

- Needle aspiration
  - —All fluctuant nodes should be aspirated
  - —Send for Gram stain, acid-fast stains, aerobic and anaerobic cultures, mycobacteria, and fungi
  - —If any suspicion of tuberculous lymphadenitis, the node should not be aspirated owing to risk for sinus development and chronic drainage
- Intradermal skin testing
  - —Mycobacteria, cat-scratch disease
- Chest x-ray, lateral neck, or Panorex
  - —Helpful if source of infection unclear or to rule out a deep space infection
  - —Chest x-ray to screen for tuberculosis
- CT or MRI of neck
  - —Helpful in delineating embryonic developmental masses or ruling out deep space infections
- Ultrasound
  - —Can differentiate cystic from solid structures but other findings nonspecific
  - —Can identify deep cavity abscess if not palpable on exam
- Excisional biopsy

DIFFERENTIAL DIAGNOSIS

- Lymphadenopathy (inflammation of node *but no bacterial infection*) can be a sign of many systemic diseases; usually these nodes are multiple and bilateral
- Viral infections are a common cause
  —Respiratory viruses (adenoviruses, rhinoviruses, enteroviruses)
  —EBV, herpes simplex virus (HSV), varicella-zoster virus (VSV), CMV
  —Mumps, rubella, rubeola
- Specific pediatric diseases with cervical adenitis in their diagnostic criteria
  —Kawasaki disease
  —Kikuchi's disease
  —PFAPA (periodic fever, aphthous stomatitis, pharyngitis, and cervical adenitis)
- Toxoplasmosis
- Congenital cysts
  —Brachial cleft cysts, thyroglossal duct cysts, cystic hygromas
- Malignancies
  —Leukemia, lymphoma, rhabdomyosarcoma, thyroid carcinoma
  —Rare as the etiology of a nonspecific lump in children (less than 2% overall)
- Other systemic diseases
  —Lupus, sarcoidosis

Treatment

INITIAL STABILIZATION

- Airway management
  —Rare cases of airway compromise

ED TREATMENT

- Treatment directed toward the primary source of infection in the head and neck
  —If unsure of etiology, cover group A streptococcus and *S. aureus*
- Aspirate all fluctuant nodes
- Many oral antibiotics are effective
  —Cephalexin
  —Dicloxacillin
  —Amoxicillin-clavulanic acid
  —Erythromycin (not as effective against *S. aureus*)
- Patients with suspected dental, periodontal, or anaerobic etiology
  —Clindamycin
  —Penicillin V
  —Amoxicillin-clavulanic acid
- Treatment should be for at least 10 days even if symptoms resolve sooner
- Warm, moist compresses
- Analgesics as needed

MEDICATIONS

- Amoxicillin-clavulanic acid: 250–500 mg (peds: 20–40 mg/kg/24 h) PO q8h
- Cefazolin: 1–2 g (peds: 25–50 mg/kg/24 h) i.v. q8h
- Cephalexin: 250–500 mg (peds: 25–50 mg/kg/24 h) PO q6h
- Clindamycin: 300 mg (peds: 8–25 mg/kg/24 h) PO q6h
- Clindamycin: 600–900 mg (20–40 mg/kg/24 h) i.v. q8h
- Dicloxacillin: 250–500 mg (peds: 25–50 mg/kg/24 h) PO q6h
- Erythromycin: 250–500 mg (peds: 40 mg/kg/24 h) PO q6h
- Nafcillin: 1–2 g (peds: 50–200 mg/kg/24 h) i.v. q4–6h
- Penicillin VK: 250–500 mg (peds: 25–50 mg/kg/24 h) PO q6h

Disposition

ADMISSION CRITERIA

- Neonates
- Toxic appearance
- Immunocompromised
- Inability to take PO
- Not improving on oral antibiotics

DISCHARGE CRITERIA

- Most patients can be discharged on oral antibiotics
- Close follow-up with a recheck in 2–3 days
- Ability to take PO antibiotics and fluids
- Return to the ED if
  —Worsening of symptoms
  —Development of abscess
  —Voice change
  —Dyspnea
  —Development of systemic symptoms

Miscellaneous

ICD9: 289.3

ICD10: I88.9

SUGGESTED READINGS

Chesney P. Cervical adenopathy. Pediatr Rev 1994;15(7):276–284.

Maraqa NF, Rathore MH. Lymphadenitis. In: Harwood-Nuss A, ed. The clinical practice of emergency medicine, 3rd ed. Philadelphia: Lippincott Williams & Wilkins, 2001:1284–1286.

Santamaria JP, Abrunzo TJ. Ear, nose and throat disorders. In: Pediatric emergency medicine, 2nd ed. St. Louis: Mosby, 1997:732–735.

Author: Kristine Reid

Cesarean Section, Emergency

Alert

The sole indication for an emergency physician to perform an emergent perimortem cesarean section is a gravid female (>24 weeks' gestation) in cardiopulmonary arrest who has not responded to initial resuscitative measures, regardless of the etiology.
The most important predictor of fetal survival is the length of time between the maternal cardiac arrest and the cesarean delivery.
Accordingly, the cesarean section should begin as soon as possible (within 4 minutes of the maternal arrest) with the goal of delivering the fetus within 1 minute.
Obtain STAT consultations from obstetrics, pediatrics (and surgery, if trauma related); however, do not defer or delay performing the procedure until the arrival of the respective consultants.
Do not perform the emergent cesarean section if patient is < 24 weeks' gestation.

Clinical Presentation

SIGNS AND SYMPTOMS

- Gravid female (>24 weeks gestation by fundal height) who is in cardiopulmonary arrest

ETIOLOGY

- Trauma (penetrating or blunt) is a major cause of maternal mortality
- Pulmonary embolus: thromboembolism is the number one cause of nontraumatic maternal mortality
- Cerebral vascular accident
- Amniotic fluid embolism
- Disseminated intravascular coagulation (DIC)
- Placenta previa
- Eclampsia
- Miscellaneous medical disorders
  —Asthma
  —Congestive heart failure
  —Infection

Pre-Hospital

CAUTIONS

- Time is of the essence; minimal scene time, "scoop and run"
- Place the patient in the left lateral decubitus position to avoid compression of the inferior vena cava by the gravid uterus (supine hypotension syndrome)
- If the patient has been traumatized and requires spinal immobilization, the uterus can be manually displaced to the left or the backboard can be wedged to keep the right hip elevated 45 degrees

Diagnosis

ESSENTIAL WORKUP

- Physical examination for apnea and pulselessness in the obviously gravid female
- Quickly evaluate for reversible causes of cardiopulmonary arrest
  —Tension pneumothorax
  —Pericardial tamponade
  —Supine hypotension syndrome
- Assess gestational age by fundal height
- Distance from pubis to fundus in centimeters is roughly equivalent to the gestational age in weeks
- Ultrasonography is beneficial if *immediately* available to assess the fetus

LABORATORY

- None immediately indicated

IMAGING/SPECIAL TESTS

- None are necessary to establish cardiopulmonary arrest
- Do *not* waste time by attempting to find fetal heart tones (FHTs)

DIFFERENTIAL DIAGNOSIS

- Cardiopulmonary arrest is a final common pathway; evaluate for underlying etiology

Treatment

INITIAL STABILIZATION

- ABCs
  —Emergency intubation, high-flow oxygen, cardiac and blood pressure monitoring, two large-bore peripheral intravenous lines, fluid resuscitation to include O-negative blood if indicated
- Fetal survival is dependent on maternal survival
- If the patient is <24 weeks' gestation, use advanced cardiac life support (ACLS) and advanced trauma life support (ATLS) protocols directed at maternal resuscitation; do *not* perform emergent cesarean section
- If the patient is >24 weeks' gestation, use the 4-minute rule
  —Perform ACLS or ATLS for 4 minutes; if no response, proceed to immediate emergent cesarean section
  —Goal is to deliver the fetus within 1 minute
  —If it is obvious there is no chance for maternal survival, begin perimortem cesarean section immediately

ED TREATMENT

- Call for STAT obstetrics, surgical, and pediatric consultations; but do not delay performing the procedure while waiting for consultants to arrive
- Ensure that a Foley catheter has been inserted to decompress the urinary bladder
- Perform a cesarean section
  —Use the linea nigra as a landmark for the vertical midline incision
  —Incise the abdominal wall from the pubic symphysis to the umbilicus
    -This incision should pass through the fascial and peritoneal layers
  —Retract the urinary bladder inferiorly against the pubic symphysis
  —Make a small vertical incision in the lower uterine segment, just cephalad to the urinary bladder
  —Extend the incision cephalad with scissors; inserting the free hand into the uterus and lifting the uterine wall away from the fetus will help to avoid injury to the fetus
  —Deliver the fetus, clamp the umbilical cord in two places, and cut the umbilical cord between the two clamps
  —Manually deliver the placenta
  —Perform neonatal resuscitation as indicated
  —Immediately reassess maternal vital signs because occasionally a return of spontaneous circulation may occur
  —Continue maternal resuscitation as appropriate
  —Suture the uterus

Disposition

ADMISSION CRITERIA

- The infant should be admitted to the neonatal intensive care unit
- If maternal resuscitation is successful, the patient should be admitted to the appropriate intensive care unit

DISCHARGE CRITERIA

- Neither the infant nor the mother should be discharged

Miscellaneous

ICD9: 669.73

ICD10: O82.1

SUGGESTED READINGS

Katz VL, Dotters DJ, Droegemueller W. Perimortem cesarean delivery. Obstet Gynecol 1986;68:571–575.

Lanoix R, Akkapedd V, Goldfeder B. Perimortem cesarean section: case reports and recommendation. Acad Emerg Med 1995;2:1063–1067.

Page-Rodriguez A, Gonzalez-Sanchez JA. Perimortem cesarean section of twin pregnancy: case review and review of the literature. Acad Emerg Med 1999;6:1072–1074.

Strong TH, Lowe RA. Perimortem cesarean section. Am J Emerg Med 1989;7:489–493.

Author: James Walker

Chancroid

Clinical Presentation

SIGNS AND SYMPTOMS

- Single erythematous pustule or papule
  - —Quickly erodes into 1–10 painful chancres (1–20 mm)
  - —Soft and friable with ragged, irregular borders
- Primary ulcer usually excavated
- Moist, granulation tissue at base
- Purulent or hemorrhagic secretion
- Location
  - —Male—penile shaft, glans, internal surface of foreskin, anus
  - —Female—cervix, vagina, vulva, perineum, anus
- Occurs 1 day to 2 weeks after exposure (median, 5–7 days)
- Inguinal adenopathy
  - —In 50% cases
  - —Appears 3–14 days after initial ulcer
  - —Unilateral (usually)
  - —Painful
  - —Suppurative large nodes (buboes)
  - —May rupture and form chronic draining sinuses
- Dysuria, dyspareunia secondary to contact with lesions
- Variants
  - —Phagedenic: secondary superinfection (esp. fusospirochetal) and rapid extensive tissue destruction
  - —Giant chancroid—very large, single ulcer
  - —Serpiginous ulcer—rapidly spreading, indolent, shallow ulcers in groin or thigh
  - —Follicular: multiple small ulcers with perifollicular distribution

MECHANISM/DESCRIPTION

- Sexually transmitted disease
- Increased risk for HIV infection

ETIOLOGY

- Causative agent: *Haemophilus ducreyi*

Pre-Hospital

N/A

Diagnosis

ESSENTIAL WORKUP

- Clinical diagnosis based on appearance (often inaccurate)

LABORATORY

- Confirm diagnosis with Gram stain or culture
  - —Obtain specimen from
    - -Base of ulcer
    - -Needle aspiration of inguinal node by placing needle through normal skin to avoid formation of fistula
    - -Do not incise node
  - —Gram stain unreliable (positive in 50–80%)
    - -Gram-negative coccobacilli: linear or school-of-fish pattern
  - —Culture difficult (positive in 0–80%)
  - —Polymerase chain reaction (PCR) assay: sensitive and specific, but not widely available
- Urinalysis for dysuria
- RPR for associated syphilis
- HIV, herpes simplex virus (HSV) testing
- Test for other sexually transmitted diseases

DIFFERENTIAL DIAGNOSIS

- Syphilitic chancre
  - —Usually painless, indurated, clean
- Herpes genitalis
  - —Vesicles
- Lymphogranuloma venereum
- Granuloma inguinale

Treatment

INITIAL STABILIZATION

- Wear gloves to examine suspicious lesions

ED TREATMENT

- Antibiotic choices
  - —Ceftriaxone: single IM dose
  - —Azithromycin: single PO dose
  - —Erythromycin
    - -Recommended for HIV-positive patients
  - —Ciprofloxacin
  - —Amoxicillin-clavulanic acid
- Needle aspiration of suppurative nodes (>5 cm diameter)
  - —To prevent chronic sinus drainage from spontaneous rupture
  - —Use 18-gauge needle through lateral intact skin
- Sexual abstinence or condom use until lesion healed
- Examine and treat sexual partner
- Recommend follow-up HIV testing
- Clinical course
  - —Symptoms improve within 3 days of treatment
  - —Ulcers improve within 7 days

MEDICATIONS

- Amoxicillin-clavulanic acid: 500 mg/125 mg PO t.i.d. × 7 days
- Azithromycin: 1 g PO
- Ceftriaxone: 250 mg i.m.
- Ciprofloxacin: 500 mg PO b.i.d. × 7 days
- Erythromycin: 500 mg PO × 7 days

Disposition

ADMISSION CRITERIA

N/A

DISCHARGE CRITERIA

- All patients

Miscellaneous

ICD9: 099.0

CORE CONTENT CODE: 19.4

ICD10: A57

SUGGESTED READINGS

Braunwald E, Fauci A, Isselbacher K, et al. Harrison's online chapter 149. New York: McGraw-Hill, 2002.

Mandell GL, Bennett JE, Douglas RG, et al. Principles and practice of infectious diseases, 5th ed. New York: Churchill Livingstone, 2000.

Shipkey G, Migala A, Holmes G. Chancroid. Med J 2001;2(7).

Authors: Norbert Elsner; Paul Gennis

Chemical Weapons Poisoning

Clinical Presentation

SIGNS AND SYMPTOMS

Blood Agents (Cyanide and Cyanogens)

Vital Signs

- Tachypnea and hyperpnoea (early); respiratory depression (late)
- Hypertension and tachycardia (early); hypotension and bradycardia (late)
- Death within seconds to minutes

CNS

- Headache
- Mental status changes
- Seizures
- Paralysis

Pulmonary

- Dyspnea
- Noncardiogenic pulmonary edema
- Cyanosis uncommon

GI

- Odor of bitter almonds
- Burning in mouth and throat
- Nausea, vomiting

Blister Agents (Mustards)

- Mortality, 2–3%; lethal exposure, 100 mg/kg, or 5- to 7-mL spread over 25% of the body

Dermatologic

- Skin erythema, edema, pruritus can appear 2–24 hours after exposure
- Necrosis and vesiculation appear 2–18 hours after exposure

HEENT

- Sore throat
- Sinusitis
- Eye pain
- Photophobia
- Lacrimation
- Blurred vision
- Blepharospasm
- Periorbital edema
- Conjunctival edema
- Corneal ulceration

Pulmonary

- Bronchospasm
- Tracheobronchitis
- Respiratory failure
- Hacking cough

GI

- Nausea, vomiting

Hematologic

- Leukopenia

Choking Agents, Lacrimators, Riot Control Agents (Chlorine, Phosgenes, Tear Gases)

HEENT

- Eye pain
- Lacrimation
- Blepharospasm
- Temporary blindness

Dermatologic

- Skin irritation
- Papulovesicular dermatitis (tear gas)
- Superficial burns

Pulmonary

- Cough
- Chest tightness
- Dry throat
- Sensation of suffocation

Delayed Toxicity (2–24 Hours)

- Severe dyspnea
- Pulmonary edema
- Foaming white or bloody sputum
- Cyanosis
- Pneumonitis
- GI
  —Hepatic and renal necrosis (phosgene)

Nerve Agents (Sarin, Tabun, Soman, VX)

S.L.U.D.G.E.B.A.M. Syndrome

- Salivation
- Lacrimation
- Urination
- Defecation
- GI cramps
- Emesis
- *Bronchorrhea, bronchoconstriction, bradycardia*
  —Most life threatening
- Abdominal upset
- Miosis

HEENT

- Miosis
- Hypersecretion by salivary, sweat, lacrimal, and bronchial glands

CNS

- Irritability
- Nervousness
- Giddiness
- Fatigue
- Lethargy
- Depression
- Ataxia
- Convulsions
- Coma

Pulmonary

- Bronchoconstriction
- Bronchorrhea

GI

- Nausea, vomiting
- Diarrhea
- Crampy abdominal pains
- Urinary and fecal incontinence

Musculoskeletal

- Fasciculations
- Skeletal muscle twitching
- Weakness
- Flaccid paralysis

MECHANISM

Blood Agents

- Inhibition of cellular respiration by binding to ferric ion in cytochrome oxidase A-A3

Blister Agents

- Alkylation and cross-linking of purine bases of DNA as well as alkylation of cysteine in proteins

Choking Agents, Lacrimators, Riot Control Agents

- Chlorine—forms hydrochloric and hydrochlorous acids, which form free radicals
- Phosgene
  —Irritant effects initially, then delayed pulmonary edema as late as 72 hours
  —Direct pulmonary damage from lipooxygenase-dependent arachidonate mediators, which permits capillary leakage of proteins, neutrophils, and fluid
- Lacrimators
  —Alkylating agents that bind to sulfhydryl groups of enzymes and coenzymes

Nerve Agents

- Anticholinesterase inhibition, which causes cholinergic overstimulation at muscarinic, nicotinic, and CNS sites

Pre-Hospital

CAUTIONS

- Avoid contamination
  —Use chemical protective overgarment (CPOG) with charcoal layer to absorb penetrating mustard
- For significant nerve agent exposure
  —Administer atropine even if tachycardic because the patient is most likely tachycardic from hypoxia

Diagnosis

ESSENTIAL WORKUP

- History and symptoms key to type of agent exposure
- Physical examination
  —Cyanide (bitter almonds)
  —Mustard (faint, sweet odor of mustard or garlic)
  —Check for S.L.U.D.G.E.B.A.M.
  —Lacrimators (eye irritation, lacrimation, blepharospasm)
  —Choking agents (dyspnea)

LABORATORY

- Arterial blood gases (ABGs)
  —Cyanide
    -decreased AV oxygen saturation gap; lactic acidemia with anion gap, arteralization of venous blood
- CBC
  —Leukopenia, thrombocytopenia, anemia with significant mustard exposure
- Electrolytes, BUN, creatinine, glucose
- Urinalysis

IMAGING/SPECIAL TESTS

- Chest x-ray for pulmonary edema
- Erythrocyte cholinesterase activity for nerve agents

DIFFERENTIAL DIAGNOSIS

- Asthma, chronic obstructive pulmonary disease (COPD) exacerbations
- Stevens-Johnson syndrome
- Toxic epidermal necrolysis
- Pemphigus vulgaris
- Scalded skin syndrome
- Organophosphate or carbamate pesticide poisoning
- Botulism
- Radiation poisoning
- Reactive airway disease
- Congestive heart failure (CHF)

Treatment

INITIAL STABILIZATION

- ABCs
- *Patient decontamination*
  —Brush off powder chemical
  —Irrigate skin and eyes with copious amounts of water or saline
  —Remove and dispose of clothing in double bags
- Protection for health care workers
  —Protective mask containing a charcoal filter
  —Chemical-resistant suit
  —Heavy rubber gloves and boots
- Administer oxygen
- Place on cardiac monitor and pulse oximetry
- Establish IV access with 0.9% NS

ED TREATMENT

Blood Agents

- 100% oxygen
- Sodium bicarbonate for acidosis
- Standard anticonvulsants as needed
- Lilly cyanide antidote kit
- Hydroxocobalamin and sodium thiosulfate

Blister Agents

- Supportive care
- Chloramine-T 0.2% in water over wounds, Fuller's earth, sulfadiazine
- Standard burn management
- Atropine to relieve eye pain
- Monitor fluids, electrolytes, CBC
- Experimental antidotes: sodium thiosulfate, vitamin E, *N*-acetylcysteine, vitamin C, thienamycin, L-carnitine (unproven)

Choking Agents, Lacrimators, Riot Control Agents

- Supportive care, bronchodilators
- Chest x-ray and careful monitoring for respiratory complications
  —Blurring of hila at 4–8 hours
  —High-dose steroids for pulmonary edema
- Phosgenes require monitoring of
  —CBC for polycythemia
  —Electrolytes, BUN, creatinine, and urinalysis for nephrotoxicity

Nerve Agents

- Supportive care
  —100% oxygen before atropine to minimize ventricular fibrillation
  —Frequent airway suctioning
- Atropine
  —Antagonizes muscarinic effects and some CNS but no effect on skeletal muscle weakness or respiratory failure
  —Pupillary response and heart rate are not useful measures of adequate atropinization
  —Stop atropine after patient regains consciousness and spontaneous ventilation (may need for periodic relapses); give as much as it takes to reverse respiratory compromise
- Pralidoxime chloride (2-PAM or Protopam)
  —Regenerates cholinesterase by reversing phosphorylation (unless aging has occurred)
  —Reduces abnormal skeletal muscle movements, improves skeletal muscle weakness, and reverses flaccid paralysis
  —May repeat first dose immediately if no response, but > 2 g qh may cause hypotension
  —If improvement from first dose, repeat 60–90 minutes later
- Diazepam—give for seizures if not relieved by above measures

MEDICATIONS

- Albuterol via nebulization: 2.5 mg in 2.5 mL NS (peds: 0.1–0.15 mg/kg/dose)
- Atropine: 2 mg i.m. or i.v. (6 mg in severely intoxicated patients) (peds: 0.02–0.08 mg/kg), then every 5–10 minutes titrate to clinical effect
- Diazepam: 5–10 mg i.v. over 3–5 minutes (peds: 0.2–0.4 mg/kg up to 10 mg over 2–3 minutes)
- Hydroxocobalamin/sodium thiosulfate: 5 g i.v. (available in France)
- Lilly Kit
  —Inhale amyl nitrite ampule for 30 seconds every minute until sodium nitrite given
  —Sodium nitrite: 10 mL of 3% solution i.v. over 3–5 minutes (peds: 0.15–0.33 mL/kg)
  —Monitor methemoglobin and stay below 30%
  —Sodium thiosulfate: 50 mL i.v. of 25% solution (peds: 1.65 mL/kg)
- Pralidoxime chloride (2-PAM, Protopam): 1–2 g i.v. over 20–30 minutes or 600 mg i.m. (diluted with water or saline to concentration of 300 mg/mL) given with first 3 atropine doses (peds: 25–50 mg/kg/dose i.v.), repeat in 2 hours if muscle weakness has not been relieved, and in 10- to 12-hour intervals if necessary
- Vitamin E: 20 mg/kg i.m.

Disposition

ADMISSION CRITERIA

- ICU admission for
  —Blood agents
  —Nerve agents
- Admit to watch for developing respiratory complications
  —Blister, choking, lacrimating agents

DISCHARGE CRITERIA

- Riot control exposures observe in ED for 6 hours and discharge if symptoms resolve

Miscellaneous

ICD9: N/A

ICD10: N/A

SEE ALSO: CYANIDE, POISONING; HAZMAT; POISONING; POISONING, ANTIDOTES; POISONING, TOXIDROMES

SUGGESTED READINGS

Davis K, Aspera G. Exposure to liquid sulfur mustard. Ann Emerg Med 2001;37: 653–656.

Ford M, Delaney K, Ling L, et al. Clinical toxicology, 1st ed. Philadelphia: WB Saunders, 2001 (Chap. 82, Inhalation: gases with immediate toxicity, 679–682; Chap. 83, Inhalation: gases with delayed toxicity, 683–694; Chap. 84, Lacrimating agents: tear gases and pepper spray, 695–698; Chap. 86, Cyanide, 705–711; Chap. 102, Organophosphates and carbamates, 819–828).

Leikin J, Paloucek F. Leikin and Paloucek's poisoning and toxicology handbook, 3rd ed. Lexi-Corp, Inc., 2002–869.

Author: Kirk Cumpston

Chest Pain

Clinical Presentation

SIGNS AND SYMPTOMS

Coronary Artery Disease

- Risk factors
  - —Male >40 years old
  - —Female >55 years old
  - —Postmenopausal
  - —Hypercholesterolemia
  - —Hypertriglyceridemia
  - —Hypertension
  - —Family history
  - —Diabetes
  - —Smoking
- Anxiety
- Shortness of breath
- Pressure
- Squeezing pain
- Radiation to arm, jaw
- Tachycardia or bradycardia
- Diaphoresis
- Nausea
- Vomiting
- Signs of congestive heart failure (CHF)

Aortic Dissection

- Risk factors
  - —Hypertension
  - —Connective tissue disorder
  - —Pregnancy
  - —Family history
  - —Coarctation of aorta
  - —Valvular disease
  - —Increasing age
- Sudden onset of pain with maximal intensity early
- Tearing pain
- Radiation to back
- Hypertension
- Differential pulses
- Associated neurologic changes

Pulmonary Embolism

- Risk factors
  - —Cancer
  - —Pregnancy, postpartum
  - —Oral contraceptives
  - —Postoperative
  - —Immobilization
  - —Family history
  - —Antithrombin III
  - —Protein S or C deficiency
  - —Factor V Leiden
  - —Increasing age
  - —Trauma
- Pleuritic pain
- Shortness of breath
- Anxiety
- Diaphoresis
- Tachypnea
- Tachycardia
- Low-grade fever
- Localized rales
- Wheezing

Acute Pericarditis

- Risk factors
  - —Trauma
  - —Cancer
  - —Collagen vascular disease
  - —Anticoagulants
  - —Recent myocardial infarction (MI) or surgery
  - —Drugs
  - —Recent viral infection
  - —Uremia
- Substernal pain
- Varies with respiration
- Increased with recumbency
- Relieved by leaning forward
- Anxiety
- Anorexia
- Fever
- Pericardial friction rub

MECHANISM/DESCRIPTION

- One of the most frequent chief complaints in the ED
- The primary consideration, diagnosis, and treatment of life-threatening etiologies
- The identification of nonlethal causes can often be investigated in an outpatient setting

ETIOLOGY

- Cardiac, vascular
  - —Acute ischemic coronary disease
  - —Acute pericarditis
  - —Aortic dissection
  - —Valvular disease
- Gastrointestinal
  - —Esophageal reflux
  - —Biliary colic
  - —Gastritis, peptic ulcer disease
  - —Esophageal rupture
- Pulmonary
  - —Pulmonary embolus
  - —Pleurisy
  - —Pulmonary hypertension
  - —Pneumothorax
  - —Pneumonia
- Other
  - —Musculoskeletal
  - —Herpes zoster (shingles)
  - —Functional, psychogenic

Pre-Hospital

- Intravenous access
- Cardiac monitoring
- Oxygen
- Pain control
  - —Nitrates
  - —Morphine
- All chest pain should be treated and transported as a possible life-threatening emergency

Diagnosis

ESSENTIAL WORKUP

- The history is the most important tool to distinguish between the various etiologies
- Have the patient define the key features
  - —Duration
  - —Location
    - -Retrosternal
    - -Subxiphoid
    - -Diffuse
  - —Frequency
    - -Constant
    - -Intermittent
    - -Sudden versus delayed onset
  - —Precipitating factors
    - -Exertion
    - -Stress
    - -Food
    - -Respiration
    - -Movement
  - —Quality
    - -Burning
    - -Squeezing
    - -Dull
    - -Sharp
    - -Tearing
    - -Heavy
  - —Associated symptoms
    - -Shortness of breath
    - -Diaphoresis
    - -Nausea
    - -Vomiting
    - -Jaw pain
    - -Back pain
    - -Radiation
    - -Palpitations
    - -Change to focal or generalized weakness
    - -Fatigue

EKG

- Inexpensive and available
- Cardiac ischemia
  - —Sensitivity for acute MI on initial tracing is less than 40%
  - —Certain signs increase suspicion
    - -T-wave inversion
    - -ST abnormalities
    - -New left bundle branch block
  - —Comparison with old tracings is often helpful and may be diagnostic
  - —Serial EKG
    - -Initial nondiagnostic pattern
    - -Change in symptoms
- Pulmonary embolism
  - —Classically associated with the S1, Q3, T3 pattern
    - -Sensitivity and specificity of this finding is poor
    - -Sinus tachycardia is seen in less than 50%
- Aortic dissection
  - —May present with an EKG consistent with inferior MI due to dissection into the right coronary artery

- Acute pericarditis
  - —Consistent although not universal pattern of EKG changes
    - -Diffuse ST elevations followed by T-wave inversions; not coexistent except in V1
    - -PR depression seen in a majority of acute pericarditis cases
- Noncardiac causes of chest pain
  - —Not usually associated with new abnormalities except sinus tachycardia

Chest X-Ray

- Pneumothorax
- Pneumonia
- A complication of ischemic heart disease such as CHF
- Aortic dissection
  - —Widened mediastinum seen in about 55–62% of patients
  - —A pleural effusion is found in about 20% of patients
  - —A normal chest x-ray is found in 12–15% of patients
- Acute pericarditis
  - —Usually normal unless massive effusion enlarges cardiac silhouette
- Esophageal rupture
  - —Usually will show mediastinal air
  - —May have left pleural effusion

LABORATORY

- Creatine kinase, with muscle and brain subunits (CK-MB) and troponin T or I
  - —They have a high positive predictive value
  - —If negative initially, they cannot be used to rule out MI
  - —Serial troponin studies rule out MI and significantly decrease the probability of significant ischemia
- D-Dimer
  - —Sensitive but poor specificity for physical examination
  - —Increased sensitivity with enzyme-linked immunosorbent assay (ELISA) methods
- Serum lipase
  - —If an atypical presentation of pancreatitis is suspected

IMAGING/SPECIAL TESTS

- Ultrasound
  - —Test of choice for pericardial and valvular disease
  - —May be helpful in acute ischemic coronary artery disease by showing wall motion abnormalities if there is no prior infarction.
  - —Transesophageal echocardiography can be used in diagnosis of aortic dissection, especially in unstable patients and those unable to tolerate contrast
  - —Right ventricular dilation and hypokinesia may suggest pulmonary embolus
- Stress echocardiogram
  - —Chest pain centers
  - —Stable patients in whom MI has been ruled out with serial enzymes and EKGs over 6–12 hours
- Helical CT scan
  - —Sensitive for aortic dissection
  - —Useful in stable patient
  - —Some centers are using in diagnosis of pulmonary embolus and in stable cardiac effusion
- V/Q scan
  - —Useful in pulmonary embolus
  - —Can rule in or out based on high probability or normal scan, in the patient with high or low pretest probability, respectively
  - —Otherwise, further testing based on clinical suspicion
- Angiography
  - —Useful in dissection, especially in stable patients
- MRI
  - —Mostly used to follow stable dissections or aneurysms over time

Treatment

INITIAL STABILIZATION

- Intravenous access
- Oxygen
- Cardiac monitoring
- Oxygen saturation
- Pain and severe hypertension or hypotension should be controlled

MEDICATIONS

- Aluminum and magnesium hydroxide: 15–30 mL PO q2–4h
- Aspirin: 160–325 mg PO
- Cimetidine: 300 mg i.v. or PO q6h
- Donnatal: 5–10 mL PO q6h
- Esmolol: 50 μg/kg bolus, then 50–200 μg/min drip
- Labetalol: 20 mg i.v. every 10 minutes up to 300 mg
- Metoprolol: 5 mg i.v. every 2 hours up to 15 mg
- Morphine sulfate: 2–4 mg every 5 minutes
- Nitroglycerin: 0.4 mg sublingual, or 1–2 inches of nitropaste, or drip at 5–10 μg/min and titrate to effect
- Nitroprusside: 0.3–10 μg/kg/min drip
- Propranolol: 1–2 mg i.v. every 2 minutes

Disposition

- Most patients may be admitted to a floor bed with telemetry if low-risk chest pain and a nondiagnostic EKG; high-risk patients are better served by an intensive care unit

ADMISSION CRITERIA

- Dependent on the risk for life-threatening cardiopulmonary etiologies
- Risk stratification
- Decisions are usually complex based on risk factors, symptoms, combinations of diagnostic interventions, and patient preference
- If a cardiopulmonary risk for chest pain is the diagnosis or a high probability, it is often prudent to admit the patient

DISCHARGE CRITERIA

- Very low risk for untoward event if discharge is planned
- Timely and appropriate follow-up must be ensured if discharge is planned

Miscellaneous

ICD9: 786.5

ICD10: R07.4

SUGGESTED READINGS

ACC/AHA guideline update for the management of patients with unstable angina and non–ST-segment elevation myocardial infarction. J Am Coll Cardiol 2000;36:970–1056; Executive Summary, Circulation 2000;102:1193–1209.

Gibler WB, Runyon JP, Levy R, et al. A rapid diagnostic and treatment center for patients with chest pain in the emergency department. Ann Emerg Med 1995;25:1–8.

Global Utilization of Streptokinase and t-PA for Occluded Coronary Arteries (GUSTO) Angiographic Investigators. The effects of tissue plasminogen activator, streptokinase, or both on coronary artery patency, ventricular function, and survival after acute myocardial infarction. N Engl J Med 1993;329:1615–1622.

Hagan PG, Nienaber C, Isselbacher E, et al., for the International Registry of Acute Aortic Dissection (IRAD). New insights into an old disease. JAMA 2000;283:897–903.

O'Gara PT, DeSanctis RW. Acute aortic dissection and its variants: toward a common diagnostic and therapeutic approach. Circulation 1995;92:1376–1378.

Pioped Investigators. Value of the ventilation perfusion scan in acute pulmonary embolism. Results of the prospective investigation of pulmonary embolism diagnosis (PIOPED). JAMA 1990;263:2753–2759.

Selker HP, Zalenski RJ, Antman EM, et al. An evaluation of technologies for identifying acute cardiac ischemia in the emergency department: executive summary of a National Heart Attack Alert Program Working Group Report. Ann Emerg Med 1997;29:1–12.

Author: Eric Legome

Chest Trauma, Blunt

Clinical Presentation

SIGNS AND SYMPTOMS

- Obvious contusion, wound, or other defect in the chest wall
- Crepitus or subcutaneous air in the chest wall
- Decreased or absent breath sounds
- Chest pain
- Tenderness to palpation on the chest wall
- Pain with deep inspiration or cough
- Dyspnea
- Usually occurs in combination with other injuries
- Hypotension
- Some patients with severe intrathoracic injuries, such as traumatic aortic disruption, may have *no* visible external signs of trauma

ETIOLOGY

- Common mechanisms include
  —Motor vehicle collisions
  —Motorcycle collisions
  —Pedestrians struck by a motor vehicle
  —Falls from great heights
  —Assaults
- Injuries can occur from direct blunt force to the chest or from rapid deceleration

Pre-Hospital

CAUTIONS

- All patients with any signs of life in the field should be transported to a trauma center
- Full spinal precautions
- Needle decompression may be necessary for tension pneumothorax
  —Unilaterally absent breath sounds
  —Hypotension
  —Jugular venous distention
  —Hyperresonance to percussion on involved side
- If large open pneumothorax exists, tape the dressing on three sides because a totally occlusive dressing can result in a tension pneumothorax

CONTROVERSIES

- Do not delay transport to hospital in order to obtain IV access; the load-and-go approach should be used and IV access established en route to the hospital

Diagnosis

ESSENTIAL WORKUP

- ABCs to determine the patient's stability
- A focused examination of the chest includes evaluation of respiratory effort and rate, chest wall excursion, crepitus, subcutaneous air, breath sounds, and heart sounds
- The presence of jugular venous distention should be noted
- Obtain a supine chest x-ray immediately; avoid an upright x-ray because of the potential for other injuries that may be exacerbated (especially spinal fractures)
- EKG and monitor to detect myocardial ischemia or dysrhythmias
- Baseline hemoglobin
- Pulse oximetry
- Arterial blood gas
- Serum lactate
- Type and screen

LABORATORY, IMAGING/SPECIAL TESTS

- If chest x-ray reveals widened mediastinum and patient is hemodynamically stable, repeat the x-ray in upright position when it is safe to do so
- If patient is unstable, an emergent thoracotomy may be necessary to repair a traumatic aortic disruption
- Chest CT with contrast, or aortic angiogram, is useful in identifying aortic and other large vessel injuries
- If there are signs of pericardial tamponade and patient is unstable, emergent pericardiocentesis may be necessary, followed by immediate transport to the OR for a pericardial window
- If there are signs of tamponade and patient is stable, perform an urgent echocardiogram
- Gastrografin swallow for possible esophageal injury (e.g., pneumomediastinum)
- Bronchoscopy for possible upper airway injuries (e.g., large persistent air leak after chest tube)
- EKG if sternal tenderness is present or abnormalities on cardiac monitor

DIFFERENTIAL DIAGNOSIS

- Simple pneumothorax
- Tension pneumothorax
- Open pneumothorax
- Hemothorax
- Rib fractures
- Flail chest
- Pulmonary contusion
- Myocardial contusion
- Myocardial rupture
- Pericardial tamponade
- Traumatic aortic disruption
- Esophageal injury
- Large vascular injury (subclavian, pulmonary artery)
- Tracheobronchial injury
- Diaphragmatic injury

PEDIATRIC CONSIDERATIONS

- Rib cage is very elastic in children and can withstand significant forces without overt signs of external trauma, but may have major internal injuries

Treatment

INITIAL STABILIZATION

- ABCs; intubate early if signs of respiratory insufficiency, shock, or altered mental status exist
- Resuscitation attempts should only be initiated in patients who arrive in the ED with vital signs
- Any patient who presents in blunt traumatic arrest is not likely to survive an emergency department thoracotomy, and therefore it is not indicated in this group
- If the patient is unstable and clinically has signs of a tension pneumothorax, perform a needle thoracostomy and place a chest tube immediately; do not wait to get a chest x-ray; place chest tube on the affected side or bilaterally if injury site is unclear
- Oxygen by non-rebreather face mask for stable patients
- Obtain vascular access, preferably 2 large IVs (>18 gauge)
- Maintain spinal immobilization

ED TREATMENT

- Notify trauma surgeon early of patients with significant injuries requiring surgical intervention or admission
- Tube thoracostomy if pneumothorax or hemothorax is identified (use at least a 36-French chest tube in an adult, largest that is practical for a child)
- Fluid resuscitation as necessary
  - —Aggressive fluid resuscitation may be harmful if severe pulmonary contusions exist
- Workup for associated intraabdominal injuries (e.g., with diagnostic peritoneal lavage [DPL], abdominal ultrasound, abdominal CT scan)
  - —Patients with chest trauma frequently have concomitant intraabdominal injuries (liver or spleen lacerations, diaphragm injury)
- Smalll doses of short-acting analgesics such as fentanyl as needed for pain control
- IV antibiotics if wounds are grossly contaminated
- Methylprednisolone for signs of spinal cord injury
- Tetanus booster if indicated

MEDICATIONS

- Fentanyl: 1–2 μg/kg
- Methylprednisolone: 30 mg/kg i.v. over 1 hour, followed by a continuous drip of 5.4 mg/kg/h for next 23 hours

Disposition

ADMISSION CRITERIA

- Patients with conduction blocks, frequent ectopy, or ischemic changes on EKG should be admitted to a monitored bed for possible myocardial contusion
- Hemodynamically unstable patients should go to the operating room emergently for a thoracotomy or laparotomy
- More than 1,000–1,500 mL of blood out of the chest tube upon initial insertion indicates probable need for thoracotomy; more than 200 mL of blood per hour from chest tube for several hours suggests the need for operative intervention to control hemorrhage
- Patients with significant rib fractures should be admitted for pain control, ideally with an epidural catheter
- Patients who lose their BP in the ED should undergo rapid open thoracotomy

DISCHARGE CRITERIA

- Patients with clinically insignificant chest wall contusions and an initial negative upright chest x-ray can be observed for 6 hours in the ED and have a repeat x-ray done; if the repeat x-ray reveals no pneumothorax, hemothorax, or pulmonary contusion and the patient is able to deep breathe and cough, the patient can be discharged home

Miscellaneous

ICD9: 862.8

ICD10: S29.9

SUGGESTED READINGS

Bodai BI, Smith JP, Blaidell FW. The role of emergency thoracotomy in blunt trauma. J Trauma 1982;22(6):487.

Calhoon JH, Grover FL, Trinkle JK. Chest trauma: approach and management. Clin Chest Med 1992;13:55.

Feliciano DV. The diagnostic and therapeutic approach to chest trauma. Semin Thorac Cardiovasc Surg 1992; 4:156.

Mansour KA, ed. Trauma of the chest. Chest Surg Clin North Am 1997;7.

Sheikh AA, Culbertson CB. Emergency department thoracotomy in children: rationale for selective application. J Trauma 1993;34(3):323.

Author: John Sakles

Chest Trauma, Penetrating

Clinical Presentation

SIGNS AND SYMPTOMS

- Impaled object in the chest wall
- Obvious wound in the chest wall with or without obvious bleeding
- Chest pain
- Dyspnea
- Respiratory distress
- Altered mental status from hypoxemia
- Absent or altered breath sounds on one or both sides
- Hypotension
- Jugular venous distention

ETIOLOGY

- Most commonly penetrating injuries result from gunshot wounds or stab wounds, but impalement from a fall is occasionally seen

Pre-Hospital

CAUTIONS

- All patients with any signs of life in the field per EMS should be transported to a trauma center
- Full spinal precautions should be maintained if there appears to be a risk for spinal injury
- Never remove impaled objects in the chest because exsanguination may follow
- Needle decompression may be necessary if tension pneumothorax exists (unilaterally absent breath sounds, hypotension, jugular venous distention)
- If large open pneumothorax exists, tape the dressing on three sides
  —A totally occlusive dressing can result in a tension pneumothorax

CONTROVERSIES

- Do not delay transport to hospital in order to obtain IV access; the load-and-go approach should be used and IV access established en route to the hospital

Diagnosis

ESSENTIAL WORKUP

- Perform a routine assessment of the ABCs
- Rapid examination evaluating respiratory effort and rate, chest excursion, crepitus, subcutaneous air, breath sounds, and heart sounds
- Upright chest x-ray is preferred for identifying a pneumothorax
  —Supine chest x-ray should be taken first if spinal precautions are maintained
- Baseline hemoglobin
- Pulse oximetry
- Arterial blood gas
- Serum lactate
- Type and screen

LABORATORY, IMAGING/SPECIAL TESTS

- With gunshot wounds (GSWs), other areas (e.g., abdomen, pelvis) should be imaged (the total number of wounds and bullets must equal an even number)
- Echocardiogram if signs of tamponade or if wound is close to the heart (the "box")
- Based on the location of wound, consider arteriogram of aortic arch, carotid arteries, or subclavian artery
- Esophageal Gastrografin swallow or endoscopy to identify esophageal perforation
- Bronchoscopy to identify tracheobronchial injuries

DIFFERENTIAL DIAGNOSIS

- Simple pneumothorax
- Tension pneumothorax
- Open pneumothorax
- Hemothorax
- Rib fractures
- Flail chest
- Pulmonary contusion
- Myocardial contusion
- Myocardial rupture
- Pericardial tamponade
- Traumatic aortic disruption
- Esophageal injury
- Large vascular injury (subclavian, pulmonary artery)
- Tracheobronchial injury
- Diaphragmatic injury
- Intraabdominal injury
- Spinal cord injury

Treatment

INITIAL STABILIZATION

- ABCs; intubate early if there are signs of serious chest injury, obvious respiratory distress, or hypotension
- Oxygen by non-rebreather face mask for stable patients
- Obtain vascular access, two peripheral large-bore IVs (>18 gauge), and fluid resuscitation as needed
- If the patient is unstable and clinically has signs of a tension pneumothorax, perform a needle thoracostomy and place a chest tube immediately; do not wait to get a chest x-ray
- If the patient is unstable and has signs of pericardial tamponade, perform an emergent pericardiocentesis, followed by rapid transport to the OR for a pericardial window
- Maintain spinal immobilization if indicated

ED TREATMENT

- Notify trauma surgeon of patient
- Tube thoracostomy if a pneumothorax or hemothorax is identified (use at least a 36-French chest tube in an adult)
- Fluid resuscitation as necessary; note that contused lung parenchyma will have leaky capillary beds, and aggressive crystalloid resuscitation may aggravate pulmonary dysfunction
- Any wound with an entry or exit site inferior to the nipple or posterior tip of the scapula should be considered to include an intraabdominal injury
  - —Work up with a diagnostic peritoneal lavage (DPL), ultrasound, CT scan, exploratory laparotomy or laparoscopy
- Describe the nature of the wounds accurately
  - —Retain any bullet fragments, clothes, or tissue removed from the wound
- Probing a chest wound is contraindicated because it can create a pneumothorax or worsen hemorrhage
- Impaled objects should be removed only in the OR, not in the ED
- Small doses of short-acting analgesics such as fentanyl or sedative agents such as midazolam as needed for pain control and sedation
- IV antibiotics if wound grossly contaminated
- For spinal cord injury, methylprednisolone
- Tetanus booster if indicated

MEDICATIONS

- Fentanyl: 1–2 μg/kg i.v.
- Methylprednisolone: 30 mg/kg i.v. over 1 hour, followed by a continuous drip of 5.4 mg/kg/h for 23 hours
- Midazolam: 0.05 mg/kg i.v.

Disposition

ADMISSION CRITERIA

- All patients with penetrating chest trauma should be admitted
- Any patient who has signs of life in the field but no blood pressure on ED arrival should have an emergent thoracotomy performed by the most experienced person present. If the source of bleeding is controlled and there are signs of cardiac activity, the patient should go to the OR for formal operative repair
- Hemodynamically unstable patients should go immediately to the OR
- Any patient with intrathoracic penetration should have a chest tube placed and should be admitted for observation
- More than 1,000–1,500 mL of blood out of the chest tube upon initial insertion indicates the need for thoracotomy; more than 200 mL of blood per hour from chest tube for several hours suggests the need for surgical intervention
- Patients with large, persistent air leaks usually require surgery
- Patients with significant rib fractures should be admitted and have an epidural catheter placed for pain control and pulmonary toilet

DISCHARGE CRITERIA

- Patients with isolated minor chest wounds and an initial negative chest x-ray can be observed for 6 hours in the ED and have a repeat x-ray performed; if repeat x-ray reveals no intrathoracic penetration, the patient can be discharged home

Miscellaneous

ICD9: 862.9

ICD10: S21.9

SUGGESTED READINGS

Baillot R, Dontigny L, Verdant A, et al. Penetrating chest trauma: a 20-year experience. J Trauma 1987;27(9):994.

Baxter BT, et al. Emergency department thoracotomy following injury: critical determinants for patient salvage. World J Surg 1988;12:671.

Calhoon JH, Grover FL, Trinkle JK. Chest trauma: approach and management. Clin Chest Med 1992;13:55.

Feliciano DV. The diagnostic and therapeutic approach to chest trauma. *Semin Thorac Cardiovasc Surg* 1992;4: 156.

Ivatury RR, Cayten CG, eds. The textbook of penetrating trauma. Baltimore: Williams & Wilkins, 1996.

Ivatury RR, Rohman M. Emergency department thoracotomy for trauma: a collective review. Resuscitation 1987;15:23.

Mansour KA, ed. Trauma of the chest. Chest Surg Clin North Am 1997;7.

Milham FH, Grindlinger GA. Survival determinants in patients undergoing emergency room thoracotomy for penetrating chest injury. J Trauma 1993;34(3):332.

Author: John Sakles

Chlamydia

Clinical Presentation

SIGNS AND SYMPTOMS

Female

- 3–5% asymptomatic carriers
- Cervicitis
  —Yellow, mucopurulent endocervical discharge
  —Cervical edema and friability
  —Vaginal bleeding
- Postcoital bleeding
- Vaginal itching
- Bartholin's cyst
- Pelvic inflammatory disease
  —Lower abdominal pain, tenderness
  —Vaginal discharge
  —Fever
  —Nausea and vomiting
- Pregnancy related
  —Preterm labor
  —Postpartum endometritis

Male

- Urethritis
  —Scant yellow-white mucoid discharge
  —Urinary tract infection symptoms
  -Dysuria usually less than with gonorrhea
  -Urgency
- Lymphogranuloma venereum
  —Small, shallow, painless vesicles or ulcer in genital region
  —May have rectal discharge or papule or stricture
  —Massive inguinal adenopathy (buboes) 2–12 weeks after symptoms start
  —Usually affects young males 20–40 years old
- Prostatitis
- Epididymitis
  —Unilateral scrotal pain, tenderness
- Proctitis
- Reiter's syndrome
  —Reactive arthritis
  —Urethritis
  —Conjunctivitis

Other

- Pharyngitis
- Pneumonia
- Conjunctivitis
  —Erythematous conjunctiva
  —Mucopurulent discharge
  —Photophobia
  —Pseudoptosis
  —Punctate keratitis

MECHANISM/DESCRIPTION

- Obligate intracellular parasite with features of both a virus and bacteria
  —Growth cycle alternates between two morphological forms
- Produce intracellular infection
  —Macrophage or nonmacrophage host cells support replication depending on species

ETIOLOGY

- Most common sexually transmitted disease in the United States
- Prevalence 3–5 times more than gonorrhea
- Major single cause of nongonococcal urethritis in heterosexual males
- Principal cause of infertility in females
- Number one cause of infectious blindness worldwide

PEDIATRIC CONSIDERATIONS

- Ophthalmia neonatorum—*Chlamydia trachomatis*
  —Bilateral conjunctivitis 5–13 days after birth
  —Corneal damage results in blindness if not treated
- Neonatal pneumonia
  —Subacute onset
  —Infants 1–4 months old
  —Staccato cough
  —Eosinophilia
  —Hypergammaglobulinemia

Pre-Hospital

N/A

Diagnosis

ESSENTIAL WORKUP

- Clinical diagnosis for chlamydia-related male sexually transmitted diseases (STDs)
- Vaginal examination for chlamydia-related female STDs

LABORATORY

- Gram stain of penile or vaginal discharge
  —10 or more polymorphonuclear leukocytes (PMNs) at 1,000 power without any gram-negative diplococci
  —Not sensitive or specific
- Identification of *Chlamydia trachomatis* by
  —Monoclonal antibodies
  —Antibody–antigen reaction
  —DNA detection by polymerase chain reaction and ligase chain reactions provide highest sensitivities (93–99%) and specificities (99–100%)
  —Plasmid DNA by direct probing
- Urinalysis for dysuria
  —WBC in males
- RPR for syphilis with STD
- Pulse oximetry or arterial blood gases (ABGs) for pneumonia

IMAGING/SPECIAL TESTS

- Chest x-ray for pneumonia

DIFFERENTIAL DIAGNOSIS

- Gonorrhea
- Trichomonas
- Syphilis

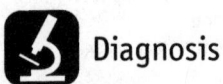

Treatment

INITIAL STABILIZATION

- ABCs—supplemental oxygen for pneumonia

ED TREATMENT

Urethritis/Cervicitis

- Antibiotic options
  - —Azithromycin PO 1 g × 1 dose
  - —Doxycycline PO 100 mg b.i.d. × 7 days
  - —Ofloxacin PO 300 mg b.i.d. × 7 days
  - —Erythromycin PO 500 mg q.i.d. × 7 days
  - —In pregnancy, options include:
    - -Amoxicillin PO 500 mg t.i.d. × 10 days
    - -Azithromycin PO × 1 dose
    - -Erythromycin PO 500 mg q.i.d. × 7 days
- Treat for concurrent gonorrhea
  - —Third-generation cephalosporin (cefixime, ceftriaxone)
- Recommend follow-up RPR for syphilis and HIV
- Condom use until symptoms resolve and partner treated
- Retesting not necessary after treatment except if symptoms persist or suspect reinfection
- Abstain from sexual intercourse for 7 days after single-dose treatment or until completion of 7-day therapy

Conjunctivitis

- Antibiotic options
  - —Doxycycline PO × 7 days
  - —Tetracycline PO × 7 days

Ophthalmia Neonatorum

- Erythromycin PO × 14 days
- Azithromycin PO × 3 days
- Ophthalmic ointment preparation containing tetracycline, erythromycin, and silver nitrate are not effective

Pneumonia

- Antibiotic options
  - —Doxycycline PO × 14 days
  - —Tetracycline PO × 14 days
  - —Erythromycin PO × 14 days

Lymphogranuloma Venereum

- Antibiotic options
  - —Doxycycline PO × 21 days
  - —Erythromycin PO × 21 days

MEDICATIONS

- Azithromycin: 1 g PO as single dose for adults (peds: 10 mg/kg as a single dose on the first day [not to exceed 500 mg/day], followed by 5 mg/kg on days 2–5 [not to exceed 250 mg/day])
- Cefixime (Suprax): 400 mg PO
- Ceftriaxone: 250 mg i.v.
- Doxycycline: 100 mg PO b.i.d.
- Erythromycin: 500 mg i.v. or PO q.i.d. (peds: 20–40 mg/kg/24 h)
- Ofloxacin: 300 mg PO
- Tetracycline: 500 mg PO q.i.d.

Disposition

ADMISSION CRITERIA

- Hypoxia with pneumonia

DISCHARGE CRITERIA

- Encourage treatment of partners within 60 days preceding symptoms, increased risk for ectopic pregnancy and infertility if untreated

Miscellaneous

ICD9: 78.88

ICD10: A74.9

SUGGESTED READINGS

Centers for Disease Control and Prevention. 1998 Guidelines for treatment of sexually transmitted diseases. MMWR 1998;47: RR1–116.

Drugs for sexually transmitted infections. Med Lett Drugs Ther 1999;41:85–90.

Kreipe RE. Sexually transmitted diseases in adolescents. Pediatr Infect Dis J 1998;17:921–922.

McKinzie J. Sexually transmitted diseases. Emerg Med Clin North Am 2001;19(3): 723–743.

Author: David Levine

Cholangitis

Clinical Presentation

SIGNS AND SYMPTOMS

- Charcot's triad
  - —Classic presentation of fever and chills; right upper quadrant (RUQ) pain and jaundice found in only 50–70%
  - —Addition of shock and altered mental status denotes a more advanced form of biliary sepsis known as *Reynold's pentad*
- Fever found in >90%
- Abdominal pain present in > 70%—localizing to RUQ
- Peritoneal findings found in 30%
- Clinically apparent jaundice may be absent in up to 40%
- AIDS sclerosing cholangitis presents with similar symptoms but with more chronic indolent course and near-normal serum bilirubin levels

MECHANISM/DESCRIPTION

- Partial or complete obstruction of the common bile duct due to gallstones, tumor, cyst, or stricture
- Increased intraluminal pressure in biliary tree
- Bacterial multiplication results in bacteremia and sepsis
- Purulent infection of biliary tree, which may involve the liver and gallbladder

ETIOLOGY

- Bacterial sources of infection include
  - —Ascending duodenal source
  - —Gallbladder infection
  - —Portal venous seeding
  - —Hematogenous spread with hepatic secretion
  - —Lymphatic spread
- Bacterial organisms include
  - —Anaerobes (*Bacteroides* and *Clostridium* species)
  - —Intestinal coliform (*Escherichia coli*)
  - —Enterococcus
- AIDS sclerosing cholangitis characterized by
  - —Papillary stenosis
  - —Sclerosing cholangitis
  - —Extrahepatic biliary obstruction
  - —Cytomegalovirus (MV), cryptosporidium, and microsporidia isolated but causal role not established

PEDIATRIC CONSIDERATIONS

- Extremely rare in childhood
- Clinical presentation similar
- Most commonly found after surgical correction for primary biliary atresia or choledochal cyst

Pre-Hospital

CAUTION

- Stabilize septic shock

Diagnosis

ESSENTIAL WORKUP

- EKG in patients at risk for coronary artery disease
- CBC
- Liver function test (LFT)
- Amylase, lipase
- Urinalysis
- Blood cultures
- Gallbladder ultrasound or HIDA scan

LABORATORY

- CBC
  - —Leukocytosis with left shift unless immunocompromised or severe sepsis
- LFTs consistent with cholestasis
  - —Elevated direct bilirubin and alkaline phosphatase
  - —Minimal elevation of transaminases (<200 IU/mL)
  - —Changes may lag symptom onset by 24–48 hours
- Amylase and lipase normal or mildly elevated
- Urinalysis positive for bilirubin

IMAGING/SPECIAL TESTS

- *Ultrasound* detects the level of ductal obstruction and the presence of gallstone etiology
- *Radionuclide scanning* (HIDA)
  - —Indicates obstruction when tracer not found in duodenum with 1 hour
  - —More sensitive than ultrasound in detecting obstruction in the first 24–48 hours before ductal dilation occurs
- *Abdominal radiograph and chest x-ray*
  - —Useful to rule out intestinal obstruction, perforation, or pneumonia
  - —20% gallstones radiopaque

DIFFERENTIAL DIAGNOSIS

- Acute cholecystitis
- Hepatitis or hepatic abscess
- Acute pancreatitis
- Right pyelonephritis
- Right lower lobe pneumonia or pulmonary embolism
- Perforated duodenal ulcer
- Appendicitis
- Sepsis with nonspecific elevation of LFTs
- Fitz-Hugh–Curtis syndrome

Treatment

INITIAL STABILIZATION

- Immediate IV fluid resuscitation for dehydration, hemodynamic compromise, and sepsis
- Vasopressors (dopamine) for hypotension refractory to volume replacement

ED TREATMENT

- Broad-spectrum antibiotics for coliforms, anaerobes, and enterococcus such as
  - —Ampicillin/sulbactam plus aminoglycoside (eg, gentamicin)
  - —Piperacillin/tazobactam plus aminoglycoside (eg, gentamicin)
  - —Substitute levofloxacin (Levaquin) (peds: clindamycin) and metronidazole in penicillin allergy
  - —Substitute aztreonam for aminoglycoside in renal insufficiency
- NPO
- NG suctioning if protracted vomiting or ileus
- IV fluid (0.9% NS) replacement and maintenance
- Narcotic analgesia if hemodynamically stable and diagnosis reasonably established
- Immediate surgical consultation
- Emergency invasive biliary drainage procedure (surgical, percutaneous, or endoscopic retrograde cholangiopancreatography [ERCP]) if no response to medical treatment in 12 to 24 hours

MEDICATIONS

- Ampicillin/sulbactam: 3.0 g (peds: 200 mg/kg/24 h) intravenous piggyback (IVPB) q6h
- Aztreonam: 2 g (peds: 120 mg/kg/24 h) IVPB q6h
- Clindamycin: 600–900 mg (peds: 25–40 mg/kg/24 h) IVPB q6–8h
- Dopamine: 2–20 μg/min IVPB titrate to maintain BP
- Gentamicin: 1.5–2.0 mg/kg (peds: 6–7 mg/kg/24 h) IVPB q8h; follow levels
- Levaquin: 500 mg IVPB q24h; contraindicated in peds
- Meperidine: 0.5 mg/kg IVP titrated up to 2.0 mg/kg for pain relief
- Metronidazole: 500 mg (peds: 30 mg/kg/24 h) IVPB q6h
- Piperacillin/tazobactam: 3.375 mg (peds: 300 mg/kg/24 h) IVPB q6h
- Promethazine: 12.5–25 mg (1–2 mg/kg/24 h) IVP q4–6h

Disposition

ADMISSION CRITERIA

- All patients with acute cholangitis should be admitted with immediate surgical and gastroenterologic consultation
- Admit patients with signs of septic shock to the ICU

DISCHARGE CRITERIA

- None

Miscellaneous

ICD9: 576.1

ICD10: K83.0

SEE ALSO: CHOLECYSTITIS; CHOLELITHIASIS

SUGGESTED READINGS

Hanau LH, Steigbigel NH. Cholangitis: pathogenesis, diagnosis and treatment. Curr Clin Top Infect Dis 1995;311:99–105.

Lai EC, Mok FP, Tan ES, et al. Endoscopic biliary drainage for severe acute cholangitis. N Engl J Med 1992;326:1582–1586.

Lipsett PA, Pitt HA. Acute cholangitis. Surg Clin North Am 1990;70:1297–1312.

Moscati RM. Cholelithiasis, cholecystitis and pancreatitis. In: Hunter DM, ed. Gastrointestinal emergencies, part II. Emerg Med Clin North Am 1996;14:719–737.

Mahajani RV, Uzer MF, Cholestasis: cholangiopathy in HIV-infected patients. Clin Liver Dis 1999;3:669–684.

Westphal JF, Brogard JM, Biliary tract infections: a guide to treatment. Drugs 1999;57:81–91.

Author: Robert Buckley

Cholecystitis

Clinical Presentation

SIGNS AND SYMPTOMS

Acute Calculous Cholecystitis

- Dull, aching, epigastric, or right upper quadrant (RUQ) pain
  - —Radiation to tip of right scapula, acromion, or thoracic spine
  - —Duration >6 hours more suggestive of cholecystitis than uncomplicated biliary colic
- As inflammation progresses, parietal peritoneal irritation leads to sharp, localized pain
- *Murphy's sign*
  - —Inspiratory arrest with gentle palpation of RUQ owing to increased pain
  - —Found in most cases
- Localized parietal peritoneal signs
  - —Percussion tenderness
  - —Rebound
  - —Found as the disease progresses
- Nausea, vomiting, fever, and chills often reported, but absent in most cases
- Jaundice in 20%
- History of prior attacks of biliary colic or known gallstones favors diagnosis

Acalculous Cholecystitis

- Occurs in critically ill patients (burns, sepsis, trauma, or postoperative)
- Localized pain and tenderness frequently absent
- Often presents with symptoms of generalized sepsis of unknown source

MECHANISM/DESCRIPTION

- Cholecystitis is defined as inflammation of the gallbladder

ETIOLOGY

- Acute calculous cholecystitis
  - —Due to bile stasis secondary to prolonged obstruction by a gallstone (see Cholelithiasis) in the gallbladder neck, cystic duct, or common bile duct
  - —Leads to increased intraluminal pressure and mucosal damage
  - —Release of inflammatory mediators results in distention, edema, and increased vascularity
  - —Coliforms and anaerobes lead to infection—primary causal role is controversial
- Acalculous cholecystitis
  - —10% of cases
  - —Underlying critical illness leads to biliary stasis and mucosal ischemia
  - —Subsequent mucosal inflammation and infection

PEDIATRIC CONSIDERATIONS

- *Acute calculous cholecystitis* extremely rare in childhood (see Cholelithiasis)
- *Acalculous cholecystitis* more common than calculous form in children
  - —Associated with systemic bacterial infections, scarlet fever, Kawasaki disease, and parasitic infections

Pre-Hospital

N/A

Diagnosis

ESSENTIAL WORKUP

- EKG in patients at risk for coronary artery disease
- CBC
- Liver function test (LFT)
- Amylase, lipase
- Urinalysis
- Human chorionic gonadotropin (hCG)
- Gallbladder ultrasound or HIDA scan

LABORATORY

- CBC
  - —WBC >12,000 cells/mm^3 supports diagnosis but may be normal in more than half of cases
- LFTs
  - —Transaminases, bilirubin, amylase, and lipase may be minimally elevated but are generally normal
  - —Disproportionate elevation of direct bilirubin and alkaline phosphatase compared with transaminases suspicious for common duct obstruction or cholangitis

IMAGING/SPECIAL TESTS

- Ultrasound
  - —Generally the first-line imaging procedure
  - —Positive findings include gallbladder wall thickening (>5 mm) or pericolic fluid—sensitivity, 90%; specificity, 80%
  - —Optimal if patient NPO >8 hours
- Radionuclide scanning (HIDA)
  - —Most useful when clinical suspicion remains high despite equivocal findings on ultrasound or when acalculous cholecystitis suspected
  - —Positive when tracer seen in small bowel but inflamed gallbladder fails to visualize
  - —Sensitivity, >95%; specificity, 90%
  - —False-positive results increase in nonfasting state
- Abdominal x-rays
  - —Exclude intestinal perforation or obstruction
  - —Air in the gallbladder wall consistent with emphysematous cholecystitis
  - —Gallstones radiopaque in up to 20%

DIFFERENTIAL DIAGNOSIS

- Biliary colic
- Hepatitis or hepatic abscess
- Cholangitis
- AIDS sclerosing cholangitis
- Pancreatitis
- Duodenal perforation
- Peptic ulcer disease
- Gastritis
- Duodenal perforation
- Right lower lobe pneumonia, pleurisy, or pulmonary infarction
- Myocardial infarction
- Abdominal aortic aneurysm
- Appendicitis
- Fitz-Hugh-Curtis syndrome
- Pyelonephritis

Treatment

INITIAL STABILIZATION

- IV, oxygen, cardiac monitoring until myocardial ischemic cause excluded
- Initiate IV fluid therapy for dehydration, hemodynamic compromise, or sepsis

ED TREATMENT

- Broad-spectrum antibiotics for coliforms, anaerobes, and enterococcus
  —Ampicillin/sulbactam
  —Piperacillin/tazobactam
  —Add aminoglycoside if sepsis or cholangitis suspected (see Cholangitis)
- Alternative antibiotics for penicillin allergic:
  —Adults: levofloxacin (Levaquin) and metronidazole
  —Peds: Clindamycin with aminoglycoside
- NPO
- IV fluid replacement and maintenance
- Antiemetics (promethazine) if vomiting
- NG suctioning if refractory vomiting or ileus
- Anticholinergics less useful than in simple biliary colic
- Narcotic analgesia (meperidine) once diagnosis firmly established
- Surgical consultation

MEDICATIONS

- Ampicillin/sulbactam: 3.0 g (peds: 200 mg/kg/24 h) intravenous piggyback (IVPB) q6h
- Clindamycin: 600–900 mg (peds: 25–40 mg/kg/24 h) IVPB q6–8h
- Gentamicin: 1.5–2.0 mg/kg (peds: 6–7 mg/kg/24 h) IVPB q8h; follow levels
- Glycopyrrolate (anticholinergic): 0.2 mg intravenous push (IVP) every 10 minutes up to 3 doses PRN pain
- Levaquin: 500 mg IVPB q24h; contraindicated in peds
- Meperidine: 0.5 mg/kg IVP titrated up to 2.0 mg/kg for pain relief
- Metronidazole: 500 mg (peds: 30 mg/kg/24 h) IVPB q6h
- Piperacillin/tazobactam: 3.375 mg (peds: 300 mg/kg/24 h) IVPB q6h
- Promethazine: 12.5–25 mg (1–2 mg/kg/24 h) IVP q4–6h

PEDIATRIC CONSIDERATIONS

- Therapy similar to adults

Disposition

ADMISSION CRITERIA

- All cases of cholecystitis should be admitted for parenteral antibiotics, analgesia, fluid replacement, and cholecystectomy in 24–72 hours
- Unstable patients (gallbladder perforation or sepsis) require immediate surgery

DISCHARGE CRITERIA

- None

Miscellaneous

ICD9: 575.10

ICD10: K81.9

SEE ALSO: CHOLANGITIS; CHOLELITHIASIS

SUGGESTED READINGS

Gruber PJ, Silverman RA, Gottesfeld S, et al. Presence of fever and leukocytosis in acute cholecystitis. Ann Emerg Med 1996;28:273–277.

Mahajani RV, Uzer MF. Cholestasis: cholangiopathy in HIV-infected patients. Clin Liver Dis 1999;3:669–684.

Moscati RM. Cholelithiasis, cholecystitis and pancreatitis. In: Hunter DM, ed. Gastrointestinal emergencies, part II. Emerg Med Clin North Am 1996;14:719–737.

Shea JA, Berlin JA, Escarce JJ, et al. Revised estimates of diagnostic test sensitivity and specificity in suspected biliary tract disease. Arch Intern Med 1994;154:2573–2581.

Silen W. Cholecystitis and other causes of acute pain in the right upper quadrant of the abdomen. In: Silen W, ed. Cope's early diagnosis of the acute abdomen, 20th ed. Oxford, UK: Oxford University Press, 2000:128–137.

Singer AJ, McCracken G, Henry MC, et al. Correlation among clinical, laboratory, and hepatobiliary scanning findings in patients with suspected acute cholecystitis. Ann Emerg Med 1996;28:267–272.

Author: Robert Buckley

Cholelithiasis

Clinical Presentation

SIGNS AND SYMPTOMS

- Dull, aching epigastric or right upper quadrant (RUQ) pain
  - —Arising over 2–3 minutes, continuous (rather than "colicky"), and lasting from 30 minutes to 6 hours before dissipating
  - —May radiate to the tip of right scapula, acromion, or thoracic spine
  - —Often correlated with ingestion of large, fatty meal
  - —Tenderness to deep palpation but without rebound
  - —*Murphy's sign* (inspiratory arrest during deep palpation of the RUQ) may be present during the episode of colic but should resolve when symptoms pass
- Anorexia
- Nausea and vomiting
- Afebrile
  - —Fever and chills suggest cholecystitis or cholangitis

MECHANISM

- Symptoms arise when gallstones pass through the cystic or common bile ducts leading to impedance of normal bile flow and gallbladder spasm
- Biliary dyskinesia produces symptoms identical to biliary colic in the absence of stones

ETIOLOGY

- Cholesterol stones
  - —Most common type of gallstone
  - —Form when solubility exceeded
- Pigment stones
  - —20%
  - —Composed of calcium bilirubinate
  - —Associated with clinical conditions such as hemolytic anemias that lead to increased concentration of unconjugated bilirubin
- Incidence increases with age and favors females to males 2:1
- Biliary sludge
  - —Nonstone, crystalline, granular matrix
  - —Associated with rapid weight loss, pregnancy, ceftriaxone or octreotide therapy, and organ transplantation
  - —May develop symptoms identical to cholelithiasis and its complications

PEDIATRIC CONSIDERATIONS

- Gallstones are exceedingly rare in childhood
- Most commonly associated with sickle cell disease, hereditary spherocytosis, or other hemolytic anemias that result in pigment stone formation

Pre-Hospital

N/A

Diagnosis

ESSENTIAL WORKUP

- Obtain EKG on those whose pain may be due to myocardial ischemia
- CBC
- Liver function tests (LFTs)
- Amylase, lipase
- Urinalysis
- Human chorionic gonadotropin (hCG)

LABORATORY

- CBC
  - —White blood cell count (WBC) usually normal but may elevate after vomiting
  - —Leukocytosis suggestive of cholecystitis or cholangitis
- LFTs
  - —Usually normal
  - —Elevation suggests common duct obstruction, cholangitis, cholecystitis, or hepatitis
- Amylase/lipase
  - —Normal or minimally elevated with passage of gallstone
  - —Elevation in context of severe persistent epigastric pain suggests pancreatitis
- Urinalysis
  - —Exclude nephrolithiasis or pyelonephritis
  - —Bilirubinuria suggests common duct obstruction or hepatitis

IMAGING/SPECIAL TESTS

- Ultrasound
  - —Detects gallstones with sensitivity and specificity >90%
  - —Dilation of common bile duct >10 mm indicates obstruction but may be normal with acute obstruction
  - —Gallbladder wall thickening >5 mm or pericolic fluid 90% sensitive and 80% specific for cholecystitis
  - —Accuracy enhanced in fasting patient with noncontracted gallbladder
- Radionuclide scanning (HIDA)
  - —Cannot detect gallstones
  - —Passage of tracer into small intestine without visualization of gallbladder highly diagnostic of cystic duct obstruction and cholecystitis; sensitivity and specificity roughly 95%
  - —Failure of tracer to pass into duodenum suggests common bile duct obstruction
- Plain x-rays
  - —Not helpful in diagnosing uncomplicated cholelithiasis
  - —Exclude intestinal perforation or intestinal obstruction
  - —Up to 20% of gallstones radiopaque
  - —Reveal rare complications such as air in gallbladder wall in emphysematous cholecystitis or air-filled gallbladder in biliary-enteric fistula

- CT scanning
  - —Less sensitive than ultrasound to detect gallstones
  - —Most useful to exclude other causes of upper abdominal pain such as aortic aneurysm, perihepatic abscess, or pancreatic pseudocyst

DIFFERENTIAL DIAGNOSIS

- Myocardial infarction
- Abdominal aortic aneurysm
- Acute cholecystitis, cholangitis, or choledocholithiasis
- Renal colic or pyelonephritis
- Duodenal ulcer perforation
- Acute pancreatitis
- Intestinal obstruction
- Peptic ulcer disease, gastritis, or gastroesophageal reflux
- Right lower lobe pneumonia, pleurisy, or pulmonary infarction
- Hepatitis or hepatic abscess
- Fitz-Hugh–Curtis syndrome

Treatment

INITIAL STABILIZATION

- IV access

ED TREATMENT

- IV hydration with 0.9% NS if vomiting
- NPO
- Anticholinergics (glycopyrrolate) commonly used despite lack of clinical trials proving benefit
- Parenteral NSAIDs (ketorolac) may lessen biliary spasm but may exacerbate peptic causes of pain
- Narcotic analgesics (meperidine) with antiemetic (promethazine)
  - —Administer for refractory pain once diagnosis is reasonably established
  - —Morphine sulfate may lead to spasm at sphincter of Oddi

MEDICATIONS

- Glycopyrrolate (anticholinergic): acutely, 0.2 mg intravenous push (IVP) every 10 minutes up to three doses until pain relieved, 2 mg PO t.i.d. for recurrent colic. (Use not well established for peds.)
- Ketorolac: 60 mg i.m. or 30 mg (peds: start 0.5 mg/kg for first dose up to 1 mg/kg/24 h) IVP q6h. In elderly: 30 mg i.m. or 15 mg IVP.
- Meperidine: 0.5 mg/kg IVP titrated to pain relief up to 2.0 mg/kg i.v.
- Promethazine: 12.5–25 mg (1–2 mg/kg/25 h) IVP q4–6h

PEDIATRIC CONSIDERATIONS

- Initial treatment strategy similar to adults

Disposition

ADMISSION CRITERIA

- Admission and surgical or gastroenterologic consultation for evidence of
  - —Acute cholecystitis
  - —Acute cholangitis
  - —Common duct obstruction
  - —Gallstone pancreatitis

DISCHARGE CRITERIA

- Lack of clinical, laboratory, or radiographic evidence of cholecystitis, cholangitis, common duct obstruction, or pancreatitis
- Resolution of all pain and tenderness
- Ability to tolerate oral fluids

Miscellaneous

ICD9: 572.4

ICD10: K80.2

SEE ALSO: CHOLANGITIS; CHOLECYSTITIS

SUGGESTED READINGS

Ahrendt SA, Pitt HA. Biliary tract: calculous biliary disease. In: Townsend CM Jr (ed). Sabiston textbook of surgery, 16th ed. Philadelphia: WB Saunders, 2001: 1083–1095.

Ko CW, Sekijima JH, Lee SP. Biliary sludge. Ann Intern Med 1999;130:301–311.

Moscati RM. Cholelithiasis, cholecystitis and pancreatitis. In: Hunter DM, ed. Gastrointestinal emergencies, part II. Emerg Med Clin North Am 1996;14:719–737.

Shea JA, Berlin JA, Escarce JJ, et al. Revised estimates of diagnostic test sensitivity and specificity in suspected biliary tract disease. Arch Intern Med 1994;154:2573–2581.

Silen W. The colics. In: Silen W, ed. Cope's early diagnosis of the acute abdomen, 20th ed. Oxford: Oxford University Press, 2000:142–149.

Author: Robert Buckley

Chronic Obstructive Pulmonary Disease

Clinical Presentation

SIGNS AND SYMPTOMS

- Dyspnea on exertion
- Barrel chest
- Cough
- Wheezing
- Retractions
- Low inspiratory-to-expiratory (I/E) ratio
- Cyanosis
- Poor air movement
- Orthopnea
- Leg edema
- Jugular venous distention
- S3 and S4 gallops

MECHANISM/DESCRIPTION

- A variety of processes, often present in the same patient, that result in large airway obstruction and impaired ventilation
  - —Emphysema: irreversible alveolar destruction decreases large airway elastic recoil
  - —Chronic bronchitis: airway inflammation without alveolar destruction
  - —Reactive airway disease: reversible bronchospasm, mucous plugging, and mucosal edema
- Chronic obstructive pulmonary disease (COPD) affects 15% of the U.S. population
- Prognosis depends on stage
- Poor prognosis for end-stage COPD (bedridden, baseline P_{CO_2} >60 mm Hg)
- Excellent prognosis for patients with early COPD (minor or no dyspnea on exertion, normal P_{CO_2}) with smoking abstinence

ETIOLOGY

- Smoking is the overwhelming cause
- α_1-Antitrypsin deficiency
- Air pollution
- Other pulmonary diseases

Pre-Hospital

- Supplemental oxygenation
  - —100% via non-rebreather
  - —Do not withhold for fear of CO_2 retention because this will only occur over a period of hours
- Initiate nebulized bronchodilator therapy

Diagnosis

ESSENTIAL WORKUP

LABORATORY

- Pulse oximetry
- Arterial blood gas analysis
  - —Timed to influence decision making
  - —Contemplating admission after maximal ED therapy
  - —Monitoring ventilatory response to oxygen therapy
  - —May not be necessary if room air oximetry >97%

IMAGING/SPECIAL TESTS

- Chest radiography
  - —Diagnosis of lobar collapse, pneumothorax, pneumonia, congestive heart failure (CHF)
- Spirometry
  - —Gold standard for diagnosing COPD
- Echocardiography
  - —Used to diagnose LV failure

DIFFERENTIAL DIAGNOSIS

- Pneumothorax
- CHF
- Pneumonia
- Pulmonary embolus
- Upper airway obstruction
- Restrictive lung disease

Treatment

INITIAL STABILIZATION

- Oxygen therapy
  - —Alert hypoxic patients
  - —Patients at risk for CO_2 narcosis
    - -Rare except in "blue bloaters" or end-stage COPD
    - -Monitor closely for ventilation suppression
    - -Regulate oxygen delivery to maintain oxygen saturation at 92%
  - —With mild altered mental status, an oxygen challenge is warranted
- Noninvasive ventilation
  - —May prevent intubation
  - —Not useful in pneumonia
- Intubation for airway control
  - —Ineffective ventilation
  - —CO_2 narcosis with pulse oximetry below 85%
- Ventilator settings
  - —Allow sufficient expiratory time to minimize air trapping and subsequent barotrauma, despite hypercapnia
- Bronchodilator therapy
  - —Anticholinergic and β-agonist medications
- Subcutaneous terbutaline
  - —If poor air movement precludes nebulized absorption
- Empiric antibiotics
  - —Controversial
- Steroid therapy

MEDICATIONS

- Albuterol: 2.5 mg via nebulizer every 10–30 minutes
- Ipratropium bromide: 0.5 mg via nebulizer q6h
- Methylprednisolone: 125 mg i.v. q6h
- Prednisone: 40 mg PO qd $\times$ 5 days
- Terbutaline: 0.25 mg SC every 30 minutes

Disposition

ADMISSION CRITERIA

- ICU admission
  - —Intubated patients
  - —CO_2 narcosis with oxygen saturation $<$90%
  - —Clinical tiring in the ED
  - —Severe ABG decompensation
  - —Severe cardiopulmonary disease
    - -Myocardial infarction
    - -Pulmonary edema
    - -Pulmonary embolism
- Admission to a regular hospital bed
  - —COPD patients with an additional pulmonary insult
    - -Pneumonia
    - -Lobar collapse
  - —Outpatient failure after maximal ED therapy
  - —Accessory muscle use
  - —Respiratory rate $>$40 breaths/min at rest
  - —Markedly decreased exercise tolerance

DISCHARGE CRITERIA

- Mild flare
- Complete resolution in the ED
- No underlying acute pulmonary disorders
- Outpatient course of steroids to prevent relapse

Miscellaneous

ICD9: 491.2

ICD10: J44.9

SUGGESTED READINGS

Barnes PJ. Chronic obstructive pulmonary disease. N Engl J Med 2000;343: 269–280.

Hotchkiss JR, Marini JJ. Noninvasive ventilation: an emerging supportive technique for the emergency department. Ann Emerg Med 1998;32:470–479.

Mandavia DP, Dailey RH. Chronic obstructive pulmonary disease. In: Marx J, et al. (eds). Rosen's emergency medicine: concepts and clinical practice, 5th ed. St. Louis: CV Mosby, 2002:956–969.

Witting MD, Lueck CH. The ability of pulse oximetry to screen for hypoxemia and hypercapnia in patients breathing room air. J Emerg Med 2001;20:341–348.

Author: Michael D. Witting

Cirrhosis

Clinical Presentation

SIGNS AND SYMPTOMS

- May be silent
- Insidious onset with nonspecific findings
  —Malaise
  —Fatigue
  —Anorexia
  —Nausea and vomiting
  —Weight loss
  —Pruritus
  —Hyperpigmentation
- Jaundice
- Hypotension
- Renal insufficiency
- Spider telangiectasias
- Palmar erythema
- Dupuytren's contractures
- Parotid and lacrimal gland enlargement
- Feminization
  —Testicular atrophy
  —Impotence
  —Loss of libido
  —Gynecomastia
- Ascites
- Amenorrhea
- Abdominal collateral circulation including caput medusae, hepatomegaly, splenomegaly
- Abdominal discomfort or tenderness
- Signs of complications
  —Hepatic encephalopathy (HE)
  —GI bleeding from esophageal varices
  —Portal hypertensive gastropathy or peptic ulcer disease
  —Fever

MECHANISMS/DESCRIPTION

- Dynamic process of inflammation, cellular injury and necrosis, diffuse fibrosis, and formation of regenerative nodules
- Progressive liver failure and loss of lobular and vascular architecture
- Intrahepatic portal hypertension due to increased resistance at the sinusoid, compression of the central veins, and anastomosis between the arterial and portal systems

ETIOLOGY

- Chronic viral hepatitis, C/C-GB or B (with or without hepatitis D)
- Chronic alcohol abuse
- Autoimmune hepatitis
- Biliary cirrhosis, primary (PBC) or secondary (sclerosing cholangitis)
- Metabolic
  —Hemochromatosis
  —Wilson's disease
  —Porphyria
- Drugs
  —Acetaminophen
  —Methotrexate
  —Amiodarone
  —α-Methyldopa
- Hepatic congestion
  —Right-sided heart failure
  —Pericarditis
  —Budd-Chiari syndrome (hepatic venous outflow obstruction)
- Infiltrative
  —Sarcoidosis
  —Amyloidosis
  —Nonalcoholic steatohepatitis
- Hepatocellular carcinoma, diffusely infiltrating
- Infections
  —Brucellosis

PEDIATRIC CONSIDERATIONS

- Etiology
  —*Congenital* (biliary atresia, arteriohepatic dysplasia)
  —*Metabolic* (cystic fibrosis, α_1-antitrypsin deficiency, fructosemia, tyrosinemia, galactosemia, and glycogen storage disease types III and IV)
  —*Infectious* (congenital hepatitis B could lead to cirrhosis during childhood)

Pre-Hospital

CAUTIONS

- Attention to active GI bleeding, encephalopathy, or tense infected ascites

Diagnosis

ESSENTIAL WORKUP

- Detailed historical and physical exam search for clues to liver disease

LABORATORY

- CBC
  —Anemia
  —Macrocytosis
  —Leukopenia
  —Thrombocytopenia
- Impaired liver function
  —High bilirubin
  —Low albumin
  —Prolonged prothrombin time (PT)
  —Hypoglycemia
- Increased liver enzymes
  —Aspartate transaminase (AST), alanine aminotransferase (ALT)—reflect injury
  —Alkaline phosphatase and 5′-nucleotidase reflect cholestasis
  —May be normal in inactive cirrhosis
- Electrolytes, BUN, and creatinine
  —Renal dysfunction and hepatorenal syndrome
- Arterial blood gases (ABGs) or pulse oximeter for
  —Suspected pneumonia
  —Congestive heart failure (CHF)
  —Hepatopulmonary syndrome: intrapulmonary vascular dilation and hypoxia, in association with liver disease
- Search for etiology as appropriate
  —Hepatitis B surface antigen
  —Hepatitis C antibody
  —Antinuclear antibody (ANA) and anti-smooth-muscle antibody (autoimmune hepatitis)
  —Antimitochondrial antibody (primary biliary cirrhosis)
  —Serum iron, transferrin saturation, and ferritin (hemochromatosis)
  —Ceruloplasmin (Wilson's disease)
  —Carbohydrate-deficient transferrin (a marker for alcoholism)
  —α_1-Antitrypsin (deficiency)
  —Serum immune electrophoresis (high immunoglobulin M [IgM] in PBC)
  —Cholesterol (chronic cholestasis)
  —α-Fetoprotein (hepatocellular cancer)

IMAGING/SPECIAL TESTS

- Chest x-ray for pleural effusion, cardiomegaly, and CHF
- Abdominal ultrasound for biliary obstruction, liver architecture, ascites, splenomegaly
- CT scan or MRI to explore abnormal finding on ultrasound
- Cholangiogram (endoscopic or radiologic) for suspected biliary obstruction
- Esophagogastroduodenoscopy (EGD) indicated for upper GI bleeding or variceal surveillance
- Liver biopsy to confirm diagnosis

DIFFERENTIAL DIAGNOSIS

- Ascites
  - —Increased right heart pressure
  - —Hepatic vein thrombosis
  - —Peritoneal malignancy/infection
  - —Pancreatic disease
  - —Thyroid disease
  - —Lymphatic obstruction
- Upper GI bleeding
  - —Peptic ulcer disease (PUD)
  - —Gastritis
- Encephalopathy
  - —Metabolic
  - —Toxic
  - —Intracranial process

Treatment

INITIAL STABILIZATION

- Treat complications such as active GI bleeding or hepatic encephalopathy
- Naloxone, dextrose (or Accucheck), and thiamine for altered mental status
- Reverse hypotension with IV fluids to prevent acute ischemic hepatic injury

ED TREATMENT

- For suspected variceal bleed
  - —Octreotide
  - —Reverse coagulopathy
    - -Fresh-frozen plasma 1 IU/h until bleeding is controlled
    - -Desmopressin (DDAVP)—improves bleeding time, and prolonged partial thromboplastin time (PTT)
  - —Balloon tamponade with Sengstaken-Blakemore tube or a variant for variceal compression (prophylactic intubation recommended)
  - —Endoscopic sclerotherapy
- Initiate broad-spectrum antibiotics in suspected sepsis or spontaneous bacterial peritonitis (SBP)
  - —Cefotaxime
  - —Ticarcillin-clavulanate
  - —Piperacillin-tazobactam
  - —Ampicillin-sulbactam
- Treat complicating conditions—ascites, hepatic encephalopathy (HE), SBP
- Treat pruritus with
  - —Cholestyramine, ursodeoxycholic acid, or rifampin
  - —Naloxone infusion 0.2 μg/kg/min for temporary relief for extreme cases
  - —Diphenhydramine 25 mg–50 mg i.m./i.v. q4h
- Consult gastroenterologist or transplantation coordinator whenever post-liver transplantation patient presents to the ED with liver dysfunction, suspected sepsis, or possible treatment-related complication
- For prolonged PT, administer vitamin K, 10 mg sq daily for 3 days
- Relieve biliary obstruction (e.g., stricture) by endoscopic, radiologic, or surgical means
- Provide nutritious diet; high in calorie and adequate in protein (1 g/kg), unless there is complicating HE
- Beta-blocker (propranolol) for large esophageal varices
  - —Titrated to pulse rate of 60% or 25% reduction of resting pulse

Specific Therapy

- Hemochromatosis: phlebotomy or deferoxamine (iron-chelating agent)
- Autoimmune hepatitis: prednisone with or without azathioprine (Imuran)
- Chronic hepatitis B or C: α-interferon (avoid in decompensated cirrhosis)
- Primary biliary cirrhosis: ursodeoxycholic acid
- Wilson's disease: penicillamine, trientine, or zinc oxide
- The only cure for most advanced cirrhosis is liver transplantation

MEDICATIONS

- Ampicillin-sulbactam: 1.5–3 g i.v. q6h (peds: 100–200 mg/kg/d div q6h) (renal dosing required)
- Azathioprine: 1–2 mg/kg PO
- Cefotaxime: 1–2 g q6–8h (peds: 50–180 mg/kg/d q6h) i.v.
- Cholestyramine: 4 g PO 1–6 times/day
- Desmopressin (DDAVP): 0.3 μg/kg in 50-mL saline infused over 15–30 minutes
- Dextrose: D-50-W 1 amp (50 mL or 25 g) (peds: D-25-W 2–4 mL/kg) i.v.
- Naloxone (Narcan): 0.2–2 mg (peds: 0.1 mg/kg) i.v. or i.m. initial dose
- Octreotide: 50–100 μg i.v. bolus followed by 50 μg i.v. infusion
- Piperacillin-tazobactam: 3.375 g i.v. q6h (peds: 100–400 mg/kg/d div q6–8h) (renal dosing required)
- Prednisone: 40 mg (peds: 1–2 mg/kg) PO qd
- Propranolol: 40 (initial)–240 mg (peds: 1–5 mg/kg/d) PO t.i.d.
- Rifampin: 600 mg (peds: 10–20 mg/kg) PO qd
- Thiamine: 100 mg (peds: 50 mg) i.v. or i.m.
- Ticarcillin-clavulanate: 3.1 g i.v. q4–6h (peds: 200–300 mg/kg/d div q4–6h) (renal dosing required)
- Ursodeoxycholic acid: 8–10 mg/kg/d t.i.d.

Disposition

ADMISSION CRITERIA

- Acute decompensation or complicating conditions
- Advanced grades HE, sepsis, active GI bleed, and hepatorenal and hepatopulmonary syndromes require ICU
- First presentation with clinically evident cirrhosis, unless close outpatient workup is possible

DISCHARGE CRITERIA

- Most patients with *compensated* cirrhosis can be treated as outpatients

Miscellaneous

ICD9: 571.5

ICD10: K74.6

SEE ALSO: VARICES; HEPATIC ENCEPHALOPATHY; HEPATITIS; SPONTANEOUS BACTERIAL PERITONITIS

SUGGESTED READINGS

Feldman S: Sleisenger and Fordtran's gastrointestinal and liver disease, 7th ed. Philadelphia: WB Saunders, 2002.

McGuire BM, Bloomer JR. Complications of cirrhosis. Postgrad Med 1998;103(2):209.

Munoz SJ. Long-term management of liver transplant recipient. Med Clin North Am 1996;80:1103.

Rosen HR, Shackleton CR, Martin P. Indications for and timing of liver transplantation. Med Clin North Am 1996;80:1069.

Author: Stuart Feldman

The author acknowledges the contribution of Abbas Zagnoon to this chapter.

Clavicle Fracture

Clinical Presentation

SIGNS AND SYMPTOMS

- Local pain, tenderness, and swelling over the fracture site
- Crepitus is often present owing to the clavicle's subcutaneous position
- Arm held in adduction against the chest wall with resistance to motion
- Shoulder displaced anteriorly and inferiorly

DESCRIPTION

- Clavicle fractures account for 5% of all fractures in all age groups
- 80% of clavicle fractures involve the middle third
- 15% occur in the distal third
- 5% occur in the medial third

CLASSIFICATION

- Group I: middle-third fractures
- Group II: distal-third fractures
  - —Type I: coracoclavicular ligaments are intact (nondisplaced)
  - —Type II: severing of the coracoclavicular ligaments (conoid)
  - —Type III: articular surface involvement of the acromioclavicular joint
- Group III: medial (proximal)-third fractures

MECHANISM

- Direct trauma to the clavicle
- Fall on the lateral shoulder
- Fall on the outstretched hand

PEDIATRIC CONSIDERATIONS

- Most common of all pediatric fractures
- May occur in newborns secondary to birth trauma

Pre-Hospital

CAUTIONS

- Medial-third fractures are frequently accompanied by other injuries owing to the severe force (intrathoracic injuries, sternal fractures, subluxation of the sternoclavicular joint)
  - —Consider spinal immobilization if appropriate
- Immobilize injured extremity

Diagnosis

ESSENTIAL WORKUP

- ABCs: look for other life-threatening injuries
- History: determine the mechanism of injury
- Physical exam
  - —Palpate the clavicle for tenderness, crepitus, and swelling
  - —Examine the humerus and shoulder joint for other fractures, dislocations, or subluxations
  - —Determine whether the fracture is *open* or *closed*
- Evaluate for associated injuries (often serious and life threatening) that must be excluded
  - —Skeletal injuries
    - -First rib fracture with underlying aortic injury
    - -Sternoclavicular joint separation/ fracture-dislocation
    - -Acromioclavicular joint separation/ fracture-dislocation
    - -Cervical spine injuries
  - —Vascular injuries
    - -Carefully check radial and ulnar pulses to assess for possible injury to the subclavian or internal jugular vessels
  - —Neurologic injuries
    - -A meticulous neurologic exam (both sensory and motor) is required to assess injury to the brachial plexus or any of its branches (including the ulnar, median, and radial nerves)
    - -The ulnar nerve is most frequently injured
  - —Pulmonary injuries
    - -Auscultate for equal bilateral breath sounds to rule out a concomitant pneumothorax or hemothorax

IMAGING/SPECIAL TESTS

- AP radiographs of both clavicles are mandatory and must include
  - —Upper third of the humerus
  - —Shoulder girdle (rule out other fractures)
  - —Upper lung fields (rule out pneumothorax)
- Oblique and apical lordotic views
  - —May be helpful, especially for medial and distal clavicle fractures that are not easily visualized on the AP view
- Stress views (weight-bearing) for *distal* clavicle fractures are no longer routinely recommended
- Angiography
  - —Should be performed if there is any evidence or suspicion of vascular injuries (most commonly *subclavian* vessels)

DIFFERENTIAL DIAGNOSIS

- Distal fractures: consider acromioclavicular separation
- Medial fractures: consider sternoclavicular separation
- Shoulder fracture-dislocation

Treatment

INITIAL STABILIZATION

- Ice packs to affected area
- Pain management using either narcotics or NSAIDs
- Immobilize affected side in a sling

ED TREATMENT

- Open fracture: uncommon occurrence, but usually requires open débridement and internal fixation (obtain immediate orthopedic referral)
- Closed fracture: if severely displaced, attempt closed reduction and immobilize depending on *type of fracture*
  - —Middle third
    - -If nondisplaced, a sling or shoulder immobilizer is enough to provide support
    - -Controversy exists as to whether closed reduction is necessary because the alignment is rarely maintained regardless of splinting technique
    - -To perform a closed reduction, 1% lidocaine should be injected into the fracture hematoma. The shoulders are pulled upward, outward, and backward, and the fracture is then manipulated into place
    - -Sedation may be given to alleviate pain or anxiety
    - -A figure-of-eight splint is then applied
    - -Ice should be applied for the first 24 hours
    - -Analgesia (narcotics or NSAIDs) for pain
  - —Distal third type I
    - -Ice for the first 24 hours
    - -Immobilization with a sling or shoulder immobilizer
    - -Orthopedic referral
    - -Analgesia (narcotics or NSAIDs) for pain
    - -Early range of motion
  - —Distal third type II
    - -Ice for the first 24 hours
    - -Immobilization with a sling or shoulder immobilizer
    - -Orthopedic referral (may require operative repair)
    - -Analgesia (narcotics or NSAIDs) for pain
  - —Distal third type III: same as type II
  - —Medial (proximal) third
    - -Ice for the first 24 hours
    - -Immobilization in a sling or shoulder immobilizer for support
    - -Analgesia (narcotics or NSAIDs) for pain
    - -Orthopedic follow-up
    - -Immediate referral if there are signs of neurovascular injury
- Reassess neurovascular status after all splints are applied

PEDIATRIC CONSIDERATIONS

- Children who do not cooperate with the figure-of-eight splint should be referred to an orthopedic surgeon for possible shoulder spica placement
- Most children will tolerate a shoulder immobilizer best

Disposition

ADMISSION CRITERIA

- Open fracture
- Associated injuries that are potentially life threatening

DISCHARGE CRITERIA

- Isolated closed clavicle fracture without other injuries
- Appropriate support services at home (especially for elderly patients)
- Orthopedic follow-up
- Adequate pain management

MEDICATIONS

- Acetaminophen: 500–1000 mg PO q6h PRN, peds: 15–20 mg/kg PO q6h PRN
- Ibuprofen: 600–800 mg PO q6h PRN with meals, peds: 5–10 mg/kg PO q6h PRN

Miscellaneous

ICD9: 810.00

ICD10: S42.0

SUGGESTED READINGS

Allman FL. Fractures and ligamentous injuries of the clavicle and its articulation. J Bone Joint Surg 1967;49A:774–784.

Heckman J, Bucholz R. Rockwood and Green's fractures in adults, 5th ed. Philadelphia: Lippincott Williams & Wilkins, 2001.

Heppenstall RB. Fractures and dislocations of the distal clavicle. Orthop Clin North Am 1975;6:477–486.

Neer CS. Fractures of the distal third of the clavicle. Clin Orthop 1968;58:43–50.

Post M. Current concepts in the treatment of fractures of the clavicle. Clin Orthop 1989;245:89–101.

Rowe CR. An atlas of anatomy and treatment of midclavicular fractures. Clin Orthop 1968;58:29–42.

Simon RR. Emergency orthopedics: the extremities. Norwalk, CT: Appleton and Lange, 1987.

Author: Jeffrey Manko

Cocaine, Poisoning

Clinical Presentation

SIGNS AND SYMPTOMS

- Sympathomimetic toxidrome

Cardiovascular

- Hypertension
- Tachycardia
- Chest pain (angina)

Respiratory

- Tachypnea
- Pleuritic chest pain
  - —Pneumomediastinum
  - —Pneumothorax
  - —Bronchitis
  - —Pulmonary infarction
- Cough

Central Nervous System

- Agitation
- Tremulousness
- Coma
- Seizures
- Stroke

Miscellaneous

- Hyperthermia (poor prognosis)
- Limb ischemia (inadvertent intraarterial injection)
- Corneal ulcerations (heavy crack smokers)
  - —Due to local chemical and thermal irritation causing disruption in corneal epithelium
- Rhabdomyolysis

MECHANISM/DESCRIPTION

- Sympathomimetic
- Inhibits neurotransmitter reuptake at the nerve terminal
- Metabolism
  - —Hepatic degradation
  - —Nonenzymatic hydrolysis
  - —Cholinesterase metabolism

ETIOLOGY

- IV, nasal, oral administration
- Oral ingestion
  - —Body stuffers
    - -Ingest hastily wrapped packets in attempt to evade police
  - —Body packers
    - -Ingest cocaine packets in order to smuggle the drug
    - -Cocaine wrapped carefully in packets containing large amounts of drug
    - -Oral, rectal, vaginal routes

Pre-Hospital

CAUTIONS

- Establish IV access
- Cardiac monitor
  - —Chest pain may be ischemic
  - —Benzodiazepines to control agitation
  - —Used as "speedball" (combination of heroin and cocaine)—administer naloxone increments to reverse coma

Diagnosis

ESSENTIAL WORKUP

- Recognition of the sympathomimetic toxidrome caused by cocaine
  - —Distinguish from anticholinergic toxidrome

Toxidrome Recognition

- Sympathomimetic:
  - —HR
  - —BP
  - —Moist skin
  - —Bowel sounds present
  - —Temperature
  - —No urinary retention
- Sympathomimetic:
  - —HR
  - —BP
  - —Dry skin
  - —Bowel sounds diminished
  - —Temperature
  - —Urinary retention present
- History of route of drug ingestion
  - —If oral ingestion, inquire how the packets were wrapped owing to leakage potential

LABORATORY

- CBC
- Electrolytes, BUN, creatinine, glucose
- Urinalysis dip for myoglobin
- Cardiac enzymes (troponin, creatine phosphokinase [CPK]) for
  - —Anginal chest pain
  - —Abnormal EKG
- CPK for evidence of myoglobinuria

IMAGING/SPECIAL TESTS

- EKG
  - —For anginal chest pain
  - —Consider possibility of myocardial infarction with cocaine chest pain
- Chest x-ray
  - —For chest pain or shortness of breath
  - —Check for pneumomediastinum, pneumothorax, aortic rupture
- KUB
  - —For body packers/stuffers
  - —Usually negative for stuffers because drug is loosely packed in cellophane
  - —Positive for packers because drug is densely packed and usually radiopaque
- CT of the abdomen with contrast
  - —When unreliable history of body packers/stuffers and KUB negative
- CT brain: when altered mental status/severe headache
  - —Cerebral ischemia/hemorrhage occurs

DIFFERENTIAL DIAGNOSIS

- Other agents with sympathomimetic effects
- Theophylline
- Caffeine
- Amphetamines
- Albuterol
- Tricyclic antidepressants
- Antihistamines
- PCP
- Thyrotoxicosis
- Neuroleptic malignant syndrome
- Hallucinogens

Treatment

INITIAL STABILIZATION

- ABCs
- IV access
- Cardiac monitor
- Naloxone (Narcan), thiamine, dextrose (or Accu-Chek) for altered mental status

ED TREATMENT

- Supportive care for mildly symptomatic patients
- Benzodiazepines
  —For agitation and tremor
  —Initial agents for hypertension and tachycardia
- Cooling measures for hyperthermia
  —Evaporative-convective method
- Treat rhabdomyolysis
  —0.9% NS hydration
  —Alkalinization with IV bicarbonate in severe cases

CARDIAC CHEST PAIN

- Aspirin
- Nitrates
- Oxygen
- Opiates
- Avoid beta-blockers because of unopposed alpha stimulation
- Angiography/angioplasty/thrombolysis for acute myocardial infarction

HYPERTENSION/TACHYCARDIA

- Benzodiazepine initial agent
- Use alpha-blocking agent (phentolamine) as sole agent or combine with beta-blocker (propranolol, esmolol) if unresponsive to benzodiazepine
  —Use labetalol cautiously (does not have equal alpha- and beta-blocking properties)
- IV nitroglycerin/nitroprusside for severe unresponsive hypertension

Body Packer/Stuffers

- Treat asymptomatic or minimally symptomatic body packers and body stuffers
  —With oral activated charcoal
  —Followed by whole-bowel irrigation with polyethylene glycol-electrolyte lavage solution (PEG-ELS)
- Surgical consultation for symptomatic body packers and stuffers
  —If toxicity is not easily managed with pharmacologic therapy (above), remove the packets intraoperatively

MEDICATIONS

- Activated charcoal slurry: 1–2 g/kg up to 90 g PO
- Dextrose: D50W 1 amp (50 mL or 25 g) (peds: D25W 2–4 mL/kg) i.v.
- Diazepam: 5 mg incremental doses i.v.
- Esmolol: 50–200 μg/kg/min i.v. infusion titrated to effect
- Lorazepam: 2 mg incremental doses i.v.
- Naloxone (Narcan): 2 mg (peds: 0.1 mg/kg up to 2 mg) i.v. or i.m. initial dose
- Nitroglycerin: 10–100 μg/min i.v. infusion
- Nitroprusside: 0.3 μg/kg/min i.v. (titrate to effect up to 10 μg/kg/min)
- Phentolamine: 5 mg i.v. every 15–20 minutes (titrate to clinical effect)
- Polyethylene glycol (GoLYTELY): 4 L PO over 4 hours until complete bowel evacuation
- Thiamine (vitamin B_1): 100 mg (peds: 50 mg) i.v. or i.m.

Disposition

ADMISSION CRITERIA

- Altered mental status
- Abnormal vital signs: HR >100 beats/min, diastolic BP >120 mm Hg, or hypotension
- Hyperthermia
- Cocaine-induced myocardial ischemia
- Body stuffers and body packers
- ICU admission for moderate to severe toxicity

DISCHARGE CRITERIA

- Mental status and vital signs normal after 6 hours of observation
- Body packers or stuffers with confirmed expulsion of packets and no clinical signs of toxicity after 12 hours of observation

Miscellaneous

ICD9: 968.5

ICD10: T40.5

SUGGESTED READINGS

Haim DY, Lippmann MI, Goldberg SK, et al. The pulmonary complications of crack cocaine. Chest 1995;107:233.

Hollander JE. The management of cocaine-associated myocardial ischemia. N Engl J Med 1995;33:1267.

Hollander JE, Hoffman RS: Cocaine. In Goldfrank LR, Flomenbaum NE, Lewin NA, et al (eds). Goldfrank's toxicologic emergencies, 6th ed. Stanford, CT: Appleton & Lange, 1998:1071–1089.

June R, Aks S, Keys N, et al. Medical outcome of cocaine bodystuffers. J Emerg Med 2000;18:221–224.

Lange RA, Hillis LD. Cardiovascular complications of cocaine use. N Engl J Med 2001;345:351–358.

Author: Steven Aks

Colon Trauma

Clinical Presentation

SIGNS AND SYMPTOMS

- Colon trauma is generally associated with other intraabdominal and extraabdominal injuries
- Injuries of significant severity may have *minimal early findings*
- It is not common to determine specific organ injury upon physical exam
- Retroperitoneal injuries are more likely to have a delayed presentation, but all colon injuries may present in a delayed manner
- On examination, assess for the following:
  - —Assess the abdomen for peritoneal signs
  - —Ecchymosis or hematoma on lower abdomen from lap-belt compression
  - —Ecchymosis on epigastric region from steering-wheel compression
  - —Grey Turner's sign from retroperitoneal hematoma
  - —Foreign bodies, blood, or heme-positive stool on rectal examination
  - —Bowel sounds are not helpful

MECHANISM/DESCRIPTION

- Trauma causing colon perforation will produce inflammation into the cavity in which it lies
- Peritoneal inflammation from hollow viscus perforation often requires hours to develop
- Mesenteric tears from blunt trauma cause hemorrhage and bowel ischemia
- Delayed perforation from ischemic or necrotic bowel may occur
- Peritonitis and sepsis may develop from the extravasated intraluminal flora
- Ascending and descending colon segments are retroperitoneal
- The left colon has a higher bacterial load than the right

ETIOLOGY

Penetrating Abdominal Trauma

- Much more common cause of colon trauma than blunt abdominal trauma
- Gunshot wounds have the highest incidence
- Transverse colon is most commonly injured

Blunt Abdominal Trauma

- Burst injury occurs from compression of a closed loop of bowel
- Direct compression as occurs when intestine is squeezed between a lap belt and the vertebral column
- Shearing forces may tear the bowel or its mesentery

Transanal Injury

- Iatrogenic endoscopic or barium enema injury
- Foreign bodies via sexual activities may reach and injure the colon
- Compressed air under high pressure such as at automobile repair facilities can perforate the colon even if the compressor is not inserted into the anus
- Swallowed sharp foreign bodies (e.g., toothpick) may penetrate the colon, particularly the cecum, appendix, and sigmoid.
  - —Most foreign bodies tend to pass the colon without complications

PEDIATRIC CONSIDERATIONS

- In contrast to adults, children have an equal frequency of blunt and penetrating colon injuries

Pre-Hospital

CAUTIONS

- Follow standard pre-hospital guidelines for trauma (i.e., ABCs)
- Do not remove penetrating foreign bodies
- Do not attempt to replace eviscerated bowel; cover with moist saline dressings
- Obtain history of mechanism of injury, vehicle damage, and seat-belt involvement

CONTROVERSIES

- Use of intravenous crystalloid resuscitation is still considered the standard of care

Diagnosis

- The diagnosis of colon injury remains a medical challenge secondary to the lack of sensitivity of both physical exam and diagnostic tests
  - —Colon trauma is most frequently diagnosed in the operating room
- Morbidity and mortality increase if the diagnosis of colon injury is delayed

ESSENTIAL WORKUP

- Hemodynamically unstable patients are diagnosed in the OR
- Serial abdominal examinations may be required because inflammation takes time to develop
- Abdominal CT with contrast is the best diagnostic study in stable patients
- Ultrasound and diagnostic peritoneal lavage (DPL) are more helpful in the potentially unstable patient

IMAGING/SPECIAL TESTS

- CT scanning with triple contrast allows intraperitoneal and retroperitoneal visualization
- CT may miss colon injuries, but the scans are usually not completely normal
- DPL or ultrasound in addition to CT will increase sensitivity
- Water-soluble enema with fluoroscopy is useful if above tests are inconclusive
- DPL will not detect retroperitoneal injuries
- Fecal or vegetable material on DPL analysis indicates hollow viscus injury
- Lavage white cell response may be negative secondary to delayed peritoneal inflammation
- In hollow viscus injuries, the lavage white blood cell count (WBC)-to-red blood cell count (RBC) ratio is higher than that typically seen with solid-organ (e.g., liver) injuries
- Lavage amylase levels are not helpful in the detection of colon injuries but are helpful in small bowel injuries
- See Abdominal Trauma, Blunt; Abdominal Trauma, Imaging; Abdominal Trauma, Penetrating for further DPL interpretations
- Plain abdominal radiographs can show indirect signs such as intraperitoneal and retroperitoneal free air

DIFFERENTIAL DIAGNOSIS

- Any intraabdominal organ injury should be entertained preoperatively
- A fractured pelvis may present similarly to intraperitoneal injuries in children

PEDIATRIC CONSIDERATIONS

- Children are often extremely frightened and may require rectal examination with anesthesia

Treatment

INITIAL STABILIZATION

- Refer to abdominal trauma section
- Airway, breathing, and circulation management should precede abdominal or colon evaluation
- Aggressive management with crystalloid and blood replacement is required because shock increases the mortality rate from colon injury

ED TREATMENT

- Early surgical consultation is necessary because surgery is the definitive treatment
- Eviscerated bowel should be covered in saline-soaked gauze in a nondependent position
- Administer broad-spectrum antibiotics to cover anaerobic and gram-negative bacteria if colon injury is suspected
- Tetanus prophylaxis should be ensured

MEDICATIONS

- Prophylactic antibiotic options (not exclusive)
- Aztreonam: 2 g i.v. (peds: 90–120 mg/kg/24 h div q6–8h i.v.) and clindamycin: 900 mg i.v. (peds: 25–40 mg/kg/24 h div q6–8h i.v.)
- Cefoxitin: 2 g i.v. (peds: 80–160 mg/kg/24 h div q4–6h i.v.)
- Gentamicin: 1.5 mg/kg i.v. (peds: 6–7.5 mg/kg/24 h div q8h) and clindamycin: 600 mg i.v. (peds: 25–40 mg/kg/24 h div q6–8h i.v.)

Disposition

ADMISSION CRITERIA

- Colon injuries require admission for surgical repair
- All foreign bodies that penetrate the colon require removal to prevent sepsis
- Patients with abdominal ecchymosis from seat-belt compression require admission and observation because of potential for undiagnosed hollow viscus injury

DISCHARGE CRITERIA

- Patients with mechanism that is not suspicious for serious abdominal injury, completely normal abdominal exam, normal hemodynamic status, and no other injury may be considered for discharge with appropriate precautions
- If there is any doubt about the possibility of colon injury, the patient should be admitted and observed

Miscellaneous

ICD9: 863.40

ICD10: S36.5

SUGGESTED READINGS

Asbun H, Irani H, Roe E, Bloch J. Intra-abdominal seatbelt injury. J Trauma 1990; 30:189–193.

Carrillo EH, Somberg LB, Ceballos CE, et al. Blunt traumatic injuries to the colon and rectum. J Am Coll Surg 1996;183: 548–552.

Stokes M, Jones D. ABC of colorectal diseases: colorectal trauma. BMJ 1992;305:303–306.

Authors: Blake Spirko; Fred Tilden

Coma

Clinical Presentation

SIGNS AND SYMPTOMS

General

- No spontaneous eye opening
- Lack of response to painful stimuli
- No motor activity
- Regular cardiorespiratory function
- Glasgow Coma Scale (GCS) scoring
  —Eye opening
    -Open
- Spontaneously: 4
- To verbal command: 3
- To pain: 2
- No response: 1
  —Best motor response
    -To verbal command
- Obeys: 6
  -To painful stimulus
- Localizes pain: 5
- Flexion—abnormal: 3
- Extension—abnormal: 2
- No response: 1
  —Best verbal response
    -Oriented and converses: 5
    -Disoriented and converses: 4
    -Verbalizes: 3
    -Vocalizes: 2
    -No response: 1
- Hypothermia
  —Infection, hypoglycemia, myxedema coma, alcohol and sedative-hypnotic poisoning
- Fever
  —Infection, thyrotoxicosis, anticholinergics, sympathomimetics, neuroleptic malignant syndrome, hypothalamic hemorrhage
- Hypertension
  —Structural lesion, hypertensive encephalopathy
- Hypotension
  —Systemic disease
  —Sepsis should be highly considered

HEENT

- Mydriasis
  —Organophosphates
- Miosis
  —Narcotics
  —Anticholinergics
  —Pontine lesion
- Loss of pupillary reflexes or unequal pupils
  —Structural lesions
- Evidence of head trauma
  —Contusions
  —Hematomas
  —Lacerations
  —Hemotympanum
- Neck
  —Nuchal rigidity
  —Meningitis
  —Subarachnoid hemorrhage

Neurologic

- Decorticate posturing
  —Flexion of elbows and wrists
  —Adduction and internal rotation of shoulders
  —Supination of the forearms
  —Suggests severe damage above the midbrain
- Decerebrate posturing
  —Extension of elbows and wrists
  —Adduction and internal rotation of shoulders
  —Pronation of the forearms
  —Suggests damage at the midbrain or diencephalon
- Asymmetric movements
  —Structural lesions
- Persistent twitching of an extremity
  —Status epilepticus

Coma

MECHANISM/DESCRIPTION

- Unresponsiveness
- Light coma
  - —Responds to noxious stimuli
- Deep coma
  - —Does not respond to pain
- Loss of either arousability or cognition
  - —Loss of arousal
  - —Arousal is primarily a brain-stem function
  - —Impairment of the reticular activating system
  - —Loss of cognition
  - —Requires dysfunction of both cerebral hemispheres
- Stupor
  - —Deep sleep, although not unconsciousness
  - —Exhibits little or no spontaneous activity
  - —Awaken with stimuli
  - —Little motor or verbal activity once aroused
- Obtundation
  - —Mental blunting with mild or moderate reduction in alertness
- Delirium
  - —Floridly abnormal mental status
  - —Irritability
  - —Motor restlessness
  - —Transient hallucinations
  - —Disorientation
  - —Delusions
- Clouding of consciousness
  - —Disturbance of consciousness
  - —Impaired capacity
  - —To think clearly
  - —To perceive, respond to, and remember current stimuli

ETIOLOGY

- Diffuse brain dysfunction (69%)
  - —Lack of nutrients
    - -Hypoglycemia
    - -Hypoxia
  - —Poisoning
    - -Ethanol
    - -Isopropyl alcohol
    - -Ethylene glycol
    - -Methanol
    - -Salicylates
    - -Sedative-hypnotics
    - -Narcotics
    - -Anticonvulsants
    - -Isoniazid
    - -Heavy metals
  - —Infection
    - -Bacterial meningitis
    - -Encephalitis
    - -Falciparum meningitis
    - -Rabies
  - —Hepatic encephalopathy
  - —Endocrine disorders
    - -Myxedema coma
    - -Thyrotoxicosis
    - -Addison's disease
    - -Cushing's disease
    - -Pheochromocytoma
  - —Electrolyte disorders
    - -Hypernatremia, hyponatremia
    - -Hypercalcemia, hypocalcemia
    - -Hypermagesemia, hypomagnesemia
    - -Hypophosphatemia
    - -Acidosis, alkalosis
  - —Temperature regulation
    - -Hypothermia
    - -Heat stroke
    - -Neuroleptic malignant syndrome
    - -Malignant hyperthermia
  - —Uremia
  - —Postictal state, status epilepticus
  - —Psychiatric
- Supratentorial lesions (19%)
  - —Hemorrhage (15%)
    - -Intraparenchymal hemorrhage
    - -Epidural hematoma
    - -Subdural hematoma
    - -Subarachnoid hemorrhage
  - —Infarction 2%
    - -Thrombotic arterial occlusion
    - -Embolic arterial occlusion
    - -Venous occlusion
  - —Tumor or abscess (2%)
    - -Hydrocephalus
    - -Herniation
    - -Hemorrhage from erosion into adjacent blood vessels
- Subtentorial lesions (12%)
  - —Infraction
  - —Hemorrhage
  - —Tumor
  - —Basilar migraine
  - —Brain-stem demyelination

Pre-Hospital

CAUTIONS

- Airway management if loss of airway patency
  - —Supplemental oxygen
  - —Bag-mask ventilation with cricoid pressure
  - —Endotracheal intubation if no response to coma cocktail
- Intravenous access
- Coma cocktail
  - —Dextrose
  - —Narcan
- Monitor patient
- Look for signs of an underlying cause
  - —Medications
  - —Medical alert bracelets
  - —Document a basic neurologic examination
  - —GCS
  - —Pupils
  - —Extremity movements

CONTROVERSIES

- Empiric dextrose should not be held or delayed if Dextrostix is not available
  - —Glucose can safely be administered before thiamine
  - —Glucose does not worsen outcome in patients with stroke
  - —Hypoglycemia is a much more likely cause of coma than a cerebrovascular accident (CVA)

Coma

ESSENTIAL WORKUP

- Detect and treat reversible causes
- Determine the underlying cause
- Immediate exclusion of coma-like states
  - —Noting resistance to passive opening of eyelids, fluttering of eyelids when stroked, abrupt eyelid closure, eye movements by saccadic jerks (rather than roving), or finding the eyes rolled back
  - —Provocation of nystagmus with ice-water caloric testing
  - —Before paralyzing a patient for intubation, an attempt should be made to detect a locked-in syndrome
  - —Demonstrating that the patient is able to blink on verbal command will establish this diagnosis
  - —Intubation is still indicated to prevent aspiration

LABORATORY

- Dextrostix
- CBC
- Electrolytes

IMAGING/SPECIAL TESTS

- Head CT scan
  - —Diagnosis of hemorrhage and midline shift
- Lumbar puncture
  - —All patients with coma of unknown etiology, particularly if fever is present
  - —Antibiotics may be administered before lumbar puncture
    - -This will have little effect on CSF cell count, differential, glucose, and protein for as long as 68 hours
  - —Control seizure first
  - —Noninvasive diagnostic studies such as CT scan should be performed before lumbar puncture in adults and children if there is evidence of increased intracranial pressure, a mass lesion, preexisting trauma, or focal findings
    - -Risk of tonsillar herniation in patients with a mass lesion is very small
- Electroencephalography
  - —Performed to rule out suspected seizure activities
  - —Little use in the emergency evaluation
    - -Status epilepticus should be treated empirically
    - -Rarely necessary to distinguish seizures from myoclonic movements
    - -Unlike electroencephalogram studies performed in a laboratory, lighting will cause artifacts

DIFFERENTIAL DIAGNOSIS

- Locked-in syndrome
- Psychogenic unresponsiveness

Treatment

INITIAL STABILIZATION

- Oxygenation
  - —Non-rebreather face mask
  - —Augment breaths with bag-valve mask
  - —Endotracheal intubation
- Empiric use of naloxone

ED TREATMENT

- Consider empiric use of antibiotics for coma of undetermined etiology
  - —Broad-spectrum with good CSF penetration such as ceftriaxone
- Administer mannitol if clinical or radiographic evidence of impending herniation
- Stop seizure activity with benzodiazepines
- Empiric treatment for a toxic ingestion
  - —Activated charcoal
  - —Alcohol drip if methanol or ethylene glycol suspected
- Correct body temperature
  - —Warmed humidified O_2 if hypothermic
  - —Ice packs and forced air movement over exposed wetted skin if severe hyperthermia
- Specific therapy directed at underlying cause once identified

MEDICATIONS

- Ceftriaxone: 100 mg/kg i.v.
- Dextrose: 1–2 mL/kg of D50W i.v.; neonate: 10 mL/kg D-10-W i.v.; peds: 4 mL/kg D25W i.v.
- Diazepam: 0.1–0.3 mg/kg slow i.v. (max: 10 mg/dose) every 10–15 minutes × three doses
- Lorazepam: 0.05–0.1 mg/kg i.v. (max: 4 mg/dose every 10–15 minutes)
- Mannitol: 0.25–1.0 g/kg i.v. over 20 minutes
- Naloxone: 0.01 mg/kg i.v./i.m./SC/ET
- Physostigmine: 0.06–0.08 mg/kg i.v.
- Thiamine: 100 mg i.m. or 100 mg thiamine in 1,000 mL of i.v. fluid wide open

Disposition

ADMISSION CRITERIA

- All patients who do not have a readily identifiable and completely reversible cause should be admitted

DISCHARGE CRITERIA

- Comatose patients with correctable hypoglycemia and opiate toxicity who respond completely to aggressive ED treatment

Miscellaneous

ICD9: 780.01

ICD10: R40.2

SEE ALSO: ALTERED MENTAL STATUS

SUGGESTED READINGS

Ellenhorn MJ, ed. Ellenhorn's medical toxicology: diagnosis and treatment of human poisoning. Baltimore: Williams & Wilkins, 1997:16–19

Ferrera PC, Chan L. Initial management of the patient with altered mental status. Am Fam Physician 1997:1773–1780.

Plum F, Posner J. The diagnosis of stupor and coma, 3rd ed. Philadelphia: FA Davis, 1986.

Wolfe R, Brown D. Coma. In: Marx J, ed. Rosen's emergency medicine: concepts and clinical practice, 5th ed. St. Louis: Mosby, 2002:137–144.

Authors: Gregory D. Jay; Linda C. Cowell

Compartment Syndrome

Clinical Presentation

SIGNS AND SYMPTOMS

- Severe, constant pain over the compartment that is disproportionate to extent of injury
- Pain increases with active contraction and passive stretching
- Muscle weakness
- Hypesthesia
- "6 Ps": *pain, pressure, paresis, paresthesia, and pulses present*

PATHOPHYSIOLOGY

- Elevated tissue pressure in closed spaces that compromises blood flow through capillaries supplying muscles and nerves
- Normal tissue pressure is less than 10 mm Hg
- Capillary blood flow in a compartment is compromised at pressures above 20 mm Hg
- Muscles and nerves can develop ischemic necrosis at pressures above 30 mm Hg
- When distal pulses are diminished on exam, muscle necrosis is probably present
- The four compartments of the leg are most frequently involved, but compartment syndrome can occur in the arm, forearm, hand, foot, shoulder, buttocks, and thigh

ETIOLOGY

- Decreased compartment size: circumferential cast, burn eschar, or mast trousers
- Increased compartment contents: compression of the compartment from edema or hematoma caused by direct trauma, fracture, overexertion of muscles, postischemic time, or limb compression during prolonged recumbency

Pre-Hospital

CAUTIONS

- Keep the extremity at the level of the heart to promote arterial flow but not diminish venous return
- Do not use ice if compartment syndrome is suspected—it may compromise microcirculation

Diagnosis

ESSENTIAL WORKUP

- The diagnosis is suggested by the above signs and symptoms and the appropriate clinical situation
- Palpation may or may *not* reveal tenseness and swelling

IMAGING/SPECIAL TESTS

- X-rays should be performed if fracture is suspected
- Diagnosis is aided by measurement of compartment pressures with a portable pressure monitoring system such as the Stryker IC pressure monitor system (Stryker Surgical, 420 East Alcott Street, Kalamazoo, MI 49001), which allows for intermittent pressure measurements using an 18-gauge needle or continuous pressure monitoring with the attachment for an indwelling catheter
- The technique for using the pressure monitoring system is as follows
  —Prep overlying skin with antiseptic solution
  —Local anesthetic can be infiltrated into the *subcutaneous tissue only,* taking care not to inject intramuscularly, which may artificially elevate intracompartmental tissue pressure measurements
  —The needle used for pressure measurements is advanced through the skin until a popping sensation is felt when the fascia is pierced
  —0.2 mL of saline is injected to clear the lumen of the needle, and the intracompartmental pressure measurement is then read
  —To ascertain correct placement of the needle within the compartment, external pressure may be applied over the muscle compartment, or the muscles can be passively stretched to increase the intracompartmental pressure transiently; once these maneuvers are discontinued, the pressure should drop to baseline and stabilize

DIFFERENTIAL DIAGNOSIS

- Chronic compartment syndrome
- Fascial hernia
- Stress fracture
- Arterial occlusion
- Neuropraxia
- Deep vein thrombosis
- Cellulitis
- Osteomyelitis
- Tenosynovitis
- Synovitis

Treatment

INITIAL STABILIZATION

- Acutely injured extremities that are casted should have the cast univalved and spread, and underlying cast padding should be cut
- Keep the extremity at the level of the heart

ED TREATMENT

- Acute compartment syndrome is a surgical emergency
- Mainstay of treatment is fasciotomy, particularly for compartment pressures higher than 30–40 mm Hg

MEDICATIONS

- There is no place for medications, including steroids or vasodilators, in the treatment of compartment syndrome
- Pain medication is essential after diagnosis is made or consultant evaluation is begun

Disposition

ADMISSION CRITERIA

- Emergent orthopedic or surgical consultation for compartment pressures higher than 30 mm Hg
- For compartment pressures higher than 20 mm Hg but lower than 30 mm Hg, surgical consultation should be sought and the patient admitted
- For compartment pressures between 15 and 20 mm Hg, serial measurement of pressures should be taken; if the patient cannot be relied on to return for repeat measurements, the patient should be admitted

DISCHARGE CRITERIA

- Compartment pressure less than 10–15 mm Hg: patients should be given symptomatic treatment and instructed to return for increased pain, swelling, development of paresthesias

Miscellaneous

ICD9: 958.8

ICD10: T79.6

SUGGESTED READINGS

Mabee JR. Compartment syndrome: a complication of acute extremity trauma. J Emerg Med 1994;12(5):651–656.

Mayeda DV. Knee and lower leg. In: Rosen P, ed. Emergency medicine: concepts and clinical practice, 3rd ed. St. Louis: CV Mosby, 1992.

Mubarak SJ, Hargens AR: Compartment syndromes and Volkman's contracture. Philadelphia: WB Saunders, 1981.

Author: Chet Shermer

Congenital Heart Disease, Acyanotic

Clinical Presentation

SIGNS AND SYMPTOMS

General

- Lethargy
- Poor feeding
- Dyspnea

Shock-Producing Congenital Heart Disease

- Hypotension
- Skin mottling
- Delayed capillary refill
- Diminished or absent femoral or dorsalis pedis pulses
- Cool and pale extremities
- Apical diastolic flow rumble
  —Significant left-to-right shunting

Congestive Heart Failure

- Gallop
- Rales or wheezing
- Hepatomegaly
- Splenomegaly
- Scalp edema
- Ascites

Syncope and Sudden Death

- Syncope with exercise
  —Hypertrophic obstructive cardiomyopathy
    -Family history of sudden death before age 50 years
    -Systolic ejection murmur along the lower left sternal border
    -Prominent peripheral pulses
  —Anomalous coronary artery syndrome
    -Asymptomatic
    -Chest pain
    -Nonspecific findings in infants: unexplained intermittent irritability; dyspnea; diaphoresis

MECHANISM/DESCRIPTION

- Aberrant embryonic development of the heart or great vessels
  —Left to right shunting leads to congestive heart failure (CHF) and shock
  —Conduction abnormalities and risk for dysrhythmias and sudden death
- Newborns with congenital heart disease (CHD)
  —A patent ductus arteriosus can compensate for the cardiac anomaly
    -Oxygenated pulmonary blood enters the systemic circulation
    -Systemic blood enters the pulmonary circulation
    -Closure of the ductus coincides with onset of symptoms
  —Symptoms usually present in the first 2 weeks of life
- Patients with CHD may present as older children and adults
  —Mild lesions
  —Multiple lesions counterbalance each other
  —Compensatory mechanisms
- Functional abnormalities with acyanotic CHD
  —Ventricular or atrial hypertrophy
  —Systemic or pulmonary hypertension
  —Left-to-right shunt
- CHD presenting as syncope or sudden death
  —Most causes of syncope are vasovagal in nature and are not life threatening
  —Hypertrophic obstructive cardiomyopathy (HOC)
    -Syncope during exercise
  —Anomalous coronary artery anatomy
    -Aberrant left coronary artery (LCA)
    -Anomaly most commonly associated with sudden death
    -The LCA travels between the aorta and the pulmonary artery
    -It becomes compressed between the two great vessels during exercise

ETIOLOGY

- Left-to right shunt
  —Atrial septal defect
  —Ventricular septal defect
  —Ruptured sinus of Valsalva aneurysm
  —Coronary arteriovenous fistula
  —Anomalous origin of the LCA
  —Aortopulmonary window
  —Patent ductus arteriosus
- Obstructing lesions causing shock
  —Hypoplastic left heart syndrome
  —Critical aortic stenosis
  —Coarctation of the aorta and interrupted aortic arch
- Syncope producing CHD
  —Hypertrophic obstructive cardiomyopathy
  —Aortic stenosis
  —Anomalous coronary artery
  —Congenital heart block

Pre-Hospital

CAUTIONS

- Avoid 100% non-rebreathers in cyanotic newborns
  —High oxygen tensions promote ductal closure

Diagnosis

ESSENTIAL WORKUP

- All children suspected of CHD require a chest radiograph and an EKG
- Exclude noncardiac causes of cyanosis, shock, and syncope in newborns
- Cardiology consult

LABORATORY

- Arterial blood gas (ABG) analysis
  —Helps to distinguish pulmonary disease from cardiac disease in the cyanotic newborn
- CBC
  —Erythrocytosis identifies chronically hypoxic patients

IMAGING/SPECIAL TESTS

- EKG
  —Usually abnormal
  —Left or right ventricular hypertrophy
  —Absent left ventricular forces
  —Absent anterior forces
  —Dysrhythmias
  —ST-T wave changes
- Chest radiograph
  —With normal pulmonary flow and right ventricular hypertrophy
    -Mitral or pulmonic stenosis
  —With normal pulmonary flow and left ventricular hypertrophy
    -Coarctation of the aorta
    -Aortic stenosis
  —With increased pulmonary flow and right ventricular hypertrophy
    -Atrial septal defect
  —With increased pulmonary flow and left ventricular hypertrophy
    -Ventricular septal defect
    -Patent ductus arteriosus

DIFFERENTIAL DIAGNOSIS

- Shock-producing CHD
  —Sepsis
  —Hypovolemia
  —Cardiomyopathy
  —Dysrhythmia
  —Adrenal insufficiency
- CHD

Treatment

INITIAL STABILIZATION

- Place air filters on the intravenous lines of all patients with CHD

ED TREATMENT

- Administer prostaglandin E_1 (PGE_1) to all symptomatic newborns
  - —Continuous intravenous infusion
  - —Promotes reopening of the ductus arteriosus
  - —Provides temporary compensation in most patients younger than 2 weeks of age
  - —Side effects of PGE_1
    - -Apnea
    - -Hypotension
    - -Fever
    - -Restlessness
  - —The overall benefits to most patients presenting in distress far outweigh the potential risks or side effects
- Treat apnea with ventilation and hypotension with fluids
  - —Provide supplemental oxygen if it does not agitate the patient
- Symptomatic patients with hypertrophic obstructive cardiomyopathy
  - —Give 10–20 mL/kg NS or i.v.
  - —Administer propranolol i.v.
- Inotropic support for shock caused by CHD
  - —Dobutamine or dopamine
- Administer antibiotics if sepsis or pneumonia is suspected
  - —Ampicillin and gentamicin

MEDICATIONS

- Acetaminophen: 15 mg/kg PO or PR
- Ampicillin: 50 mg/kg i.v.
- Dobutamine: 5–20 μg/kg/min i.v.
- Dopamine: 5–20 μg/kg/min i.v.
- Gentamicin: 2.5 mg/kg i.v.
- Ibuprofen: 10 mg/kg PO
- Morphine sulfate: 0.1–0.2 mg/kg SQ or i.v.
- Phenylephrine: 0.5–5 μg/kg/min i.v.
- Propranolol: 0.1 mg/kg i.v.
- Prostaglandin E_1: 0.05 μg/kg/min
- Sodium bicarbonate: 1–2 mEq/kg i.v.

Disposition

ADMISSION CRITERIA

- All newborns with suspected CHD
  - —Admit to PICU
  - —Surgical consultation for cardiac repair
- Known CHD with symptomatic or suspected respiratory syncytial virus
- Patients with worsening CHF

DISCHARGE CRITERIA

- Cardiology referral for syncope
  - —Syncope during exercise
  - —Absence of prodromal symptoms just before syncopal episode
  - —Family history of sudden death
  - —Abnormal EKG findings

Miscellaneous

ICD9: 745.1, 745.2, 745.3, 746.2, 746.85

ICD10: Q24.9

SUGGESTED READINGS

Friedman WF, Silverman N. Congenital heart disease in infancy and childhood. In: Braunwald E, ed. Heart disease, 6th ed. Philadelphia: WB Saunders, 2001:1505–1582.

McCollough M. Common complaints in the first 30 days of life. Emerg Med Clin North Am 2002;20(1):27–48.

Toepper WC. Cardiac disorders. In: Marx J, ed. Rosen's emergency medicine: concepts and current practices, 5th ed. St Louis: Mosby, 2002:2278–2295.

Author: Robert Woolard

Congenital Heart Disease, Cyanotic

Clinical Presentation

SIGNS AND SYMPTOMS

- Central cyanosis
  - —Visible in lips, nailbeds, mucosa, ears, and malar regions
  - —When due to right-to-left shunt
    - -Increases with agitation
    - -Associated with warm skin
    - -Minimal change with 100% O_2
- Peripheral cyanosis
  - —Nail beds and lips are blue
  - —Mucosa is pink
  - —Extremities are cool
- Differential cyanosis
  - —Always indicates the presence of congestive heard disease (CHD)
  - —Upper body pink, lower body blue
    - -Coarctation of the aorta or interruption of aortic arch
    - -Right to left flow through the ductus arteriosus
  - —Upper body blue, lower body pink
    - -Transposition of the great arteries and coarctation of the aorta
- Lethargy
- Poor feeding
- Dyspnea with exertion
- Clubbing
- Right-to-left shunting is not associated with a murmur
- Harsh continuous murmur of a patent ductus arteriosus at left sternal border
- Congestive heart failure
  - —Rales
  - —Hepatomegaly
  - —Scalp edema
  - —Ascites

Tetralogy of Fallot

- Hypercyanotic spells or "Tet spells"
  - —Follows events that decrease the systemic vascular resistance
    - -Wakening
    - -Feeding
    - -Defecation
- Systolic ejection murmur inversely proportional to severity
- Soft continuous murmur audible on auscultation of anterior and posterior chest

Pulmonary Valve Stenosis

- Jugular venous α waves
- Presystolic hepatic pulsations
- Systolic ejection murmur proportional to severity

Total Anomalous Pulmonary Venous Return

- Fixed, widely split second heart sound
- Soft, systolic ejection murmur along the left sternal border
- Mid-diastolic murmur along the lower left sternal border

MECHANISM/DESCRIPTION

- Aberrant embryonic development of the heart or great vessels
  - —Fixed right-to-left shunt at any level leads to central cyanosis
  - —Hypoperfusion and vasoconstriction cause peripheral cyanosis
- Certain conditions trigger cyanosis in older children and adults with CHD
  - —Cardiac shunt obstruction
  - —Pulmonary disease
  - —Decreased systemic vascular resistance
    - -Fever
    - -Dehydration

ETIOLOGY

- Tetralogy of Fallot
  - —RV outflow stenosis, right ventricular hypertrophy (RVH), ventricular septal defect (VSD), overriding aorta
- Transposition of great vessels
  - —A parallel circulatory system
  - —The aorta arises from the RV
  - —Two thirds have a patent ductus arteriosus; one third have a ventricular septal defect
  - —Presents from birth to the first week of life
- Truncus arteriosus
  - —A single great artery leaves the heart to provide systemic, pulmonary, and coronary circulations
  - —Total anomalous pulmonary venous return
    - -Pulmonary venous blood enters the systemic venous system or RA
- Tricuspid atresia
  - —No direct communication between the RA and RV
  - —The RV is not fully developed
  - —Presents in the first to fourth week of life
- Pulmonic valve stenosis
- Pulmonary atresia
  - —RV hypertrophy and cardiomegaly
  - —Right-to-left shunting through a patent foramen ovale
- Ebstein's anomaly
  - —Downward displacement of the tricuspid valve into the right ventricle due to an anomalous attachment of the tricuspid leaflets
  - —Resultant small RV
  - —Associated with pulmonary stenosis and a patent foramen ovale
  - —Presents in the first week of life
- Total anomalous pulmonary venous return
  - —All pulmonary venous flow returns to the RA, either directly or through the systemic venous system
  - —Symptoms generally appear before the first year of life
- Single ventricle states

Pre-Hospital

CAUTIONS

- Avoid 100% non-rebreathers in cyanotic newborns
  - —High oxygen tensions promote ductal closure

Diagnosis

ESSENTIAL WORKUP

- Differentiate central, peripheral, and differential cyanosis
- Chest radiograph to assess pulmonary blood flow
- EKG to assess for ventricular hypertrophy
- Exclude noncardiac causes of cyanosis in newborns
- Cardiology consult

LABORATORY

- Arterial blood gas (ABG) analysis
  - —Helps to distinguish pulmonary disease from cardiac disease in the cyanotic newborn
  - —Oxygen challenge test
    - -No response to 10 minutes of 100% oxygen by showing an increase in arterial Po_2
- CBC
  - —Erythrocytosis identifies chronically cyanotic patients

IMAGING/SPECIAL TESTS

- EKG
  - —Right axis deviation, RA hypertrophy
    - -Tetralogy of Fallot
    - -Total anomalous pulmonary venous congestion
    - -Hypoplastic left heart syndrome
    - -Transposition of the great vessels
    - -Pulmonary stenosis
    - -Tricuspid and pulmonary atresia
  - —LV hypertrophy
    - -Severe tricuspid atresia with atrial septal defect
  - —Biventricular hypertrophy
    - -Truncus arteriosus

- Chest radiograph
  - —With decreased pulmonary flow and RV hypertrophy
    - -Tetralogy of Fallot (boot-shaped heart)
  - —With decreased pulmonary flow and LV hypertrophy
    - -Severe tricuspid atresia with atrial septal defect
  - —With increased pulmonary flow and RV hypertrophy
    - -Hypoplastic left heart syndrome
    - -Transposition of the great vessels ("egg on a string")
    - -Total anomalous pulmonary venous return ("snowman sign")
  - —With increased pulmonary flow and biventricular hypertrophy
    - -Truncus arteriosus
  - —Box or funnel-shaped heart
    - -Ebstein's anomaly
- Echocardiogram
  - —Should be performed emergently in all infants with suspected and undiagnosed CHD

DIFFERENTIAL DIAGNOSIS

- Central cyanosis
  - —Primary lung disease of any kind
    - -Improves with oxygen and activity
    - -Pneumonia
    - -Pulmonary edema
    - -Pneumothorax
    - -Lung agenesis
    - -Bronchopulmonary dysplasia
    - -Chronic obstructive lung disease
  - —Hypoventilation
  - —CNS depression
    - -CNS trauma
    - -Drugs
    - -Sepsis, meningitis
  - —Upper airway obstruction
    - -Tracheal rings
    - -Epiglottitis
  - —Hypotonia
    - -Spinal cord insults
    - -Neuromuscular disease
    - -Drugs
  - —Abnormal or excessive hemoglobin
    - -Polycythemia
    - -Methemoglobinemia
    - -Sulfa-hemoglobinemia
- Peripheral cyanosis
  - —Shock
  - —Sepsis
  - —Hypothermia

Treatment

INITIAL STABILIZATION

- Cyanosis or hypotension in the neonate
  - —Endotracheally intubate all symptomatic patients
  - —The F_{IO_2} delivered should be no higher than 0.40 with ductal-dependent CHD
- Place air filters on the intravenous lines of all patients with CHD

ED TREATMENT

- Administer prostaglandin E_1 (PGE_1) to all symptomatic newborns
  - —Continuous IV infusion
  - —Promotes reopening of the ductus arteriosus
  - —Provides temporary compensation in most patients less than 2 weeks of age
  - —Not effective in managing total anomalous pulmonary venous return
  - —May exacerbate pulmonary and tricuspid valve regurgitation in patients with Ebstein's anomaly
  - —The overall benefits to most patients presenting in distress far outweigh the potential risks or side effects
- Cyanosis in the child or adult with known CHD
  - —Administer 10–20 mL/kg NS i.v. if dehydration seems likely
  - —Provide supplemental oxygen if pulmonary disease is suspected
  - —Treat fever with antipyretics
  - —Administer antibiotics if pneumonia is suspected
- Patients with "Tet spells"
  - —Provide a calming environment
  - —Place patient in the knee-chest position to increase SVR and promote left-to-right shunting
  - —Provide supplemental oxygen if it does not agitate the patient
- Inotropic support for shock caused by CHD
  - —Dobutamine or dopamine
- Administer antibiotics if sepsis or pneumonia is suspected
  - —Ampicillin and gentamicin

MEDICATIONS

- Acetaminophen: 15 mg/kg PO or PR
- Ampicillin: 50 mg/kg i.v.
- Dobutamine: 5–20 μg/kg/min i.v.
- Dopamine: 5–20 μg/kg/min i.v.
- Gentamicin: 2.5 mg/kg i.v.
- Ibuprofen: 10 mg/kg PO
- Morphine sulfate: 0.1–0.2 mg/kg SQ or i.v.
- Phenylephrine: 0.5–5 μg/kg/min i.v.
- Propranolol: 0.1 mg/kg i.v.
- Prostaglandin E_1: 0.05 μg/kg/min
- Sodium bicarbonate: 1–2 mEq/kg i.v.

Disposition

ADMISSION CRITERIA

- All newborns with suspected CHD
  - —Admit to PICU
  - —Surgical consultation for cardiac repair
- Children and adults with an acute worsening of cyanosis
- Known CHD with symptomatic or suspected respiratory syncytial virus
- Patients with worsening CHF

DISCHARGE CRITERIA

- Patients with tetralogy of Fallot who respond to minimal intervention
  - —Calming and knee-chest positioning
  - —Close follow-up

Miscellaneous

ICD9: 745.1, 745.2, 745.3, 746.2, 746.85

ICD10: Q24.9

SEE ALSO: CYANOSIS

SUGGESTED READINGS

Friedman WF, Silverman N. Congenital heart disease in infancy and childhood. In: Braunwald E, ed. Heart disease, 6th ed. Philadelphia: WB Saunders, 2001: 1505–1582.

McCollough M. Common complaints in the first 30 days of life. Emerg Med Clin North Am 2002;20(1):27–48.

Toepper WC. Cardiac disorders. In: Marx J (ed). Rosen's emergency medicine: concepts and current practices, 5th ed. St Louis: Mosby, 2002:2278–2295.

Author: Robert Woolard

Congestive Heart Failure

Clinical Presentation

SIGNS AND SYMPTOMS

- General
  —Fatigue
  —Weakness
  —Anxiety
- Left heart failure
  —Dyspnea
  —Orthopnea
  —Paroxysmal nocturnal dyspnea
  —Decreased exercise tolerance
  —Rales
  —Wheezes
  —Dullness at lung bases
  —S3 gallop
  —S4 may be present
- Right heart failure
  —Dyspnea on exertion
  —Jugular venous distention
  —Increased liver span
  —A positive abdominojugular reflex
  —Ascites
  —Dependent edema
- Severe impairment
  —Confusion
  —Tachypnea
  —Tachycardia
  —Mild hypotension
  —Cyanosis
  —Pulsus alternans
  —Frothy sputum
  —Cheyne-Stokes respirations

MECHANISM/DESCRIPTION

- Failure of the heart to pump blood at a rate sufficient to satisfy tissue metabolism
  —Low-output failure
    -Decreased cardiac output secondary to myocardial muscle failure
  —High-output failure
    -Cardiac output is normal or high
    -Output is insufficient to fulfill the requirement of metabolizing tissue
    -Hyperthyroidism
    -Severe asthma
- Acute congestive heart failure (CHF)
  —Rapidly progressive failure state
  —Usually caused by a precipitating event
  —The heart does not have the reserve to compensate for the added burden
- Chronic CHF
  —Slowly progressive failure state
- Left-sided failure
  —Hemodynamic burden placed on LV
  —Results in back up of pressure and fluid behind the involved chamber
  —Pulmonary congestion occurs
- CHF affects about 2% of the U.S. population
- Most common inpatient diagnosis over the age of 65
- The incidence of CHF increases twofold for each decade of life
- The presence of CHF increases the likelihood of mortality
  —Eight times for men
  —Five times for women

ETIOLOGY

- Decreased myocardial contractility
  —Ischemia
  —Infarction
  —Cardiomyopathy
  —Myocarditis
  —Decreased contractile efficiency
    -Drug related
    -Metabolic disorder
- Pressure overload states
  —Hypertension
  —Valvular abnormalities
  —Congenital heart disease
- Restricted cardiac output
  —Myocardial infiltrative disease
- Volume overload
- Thyrotoxicosis
- Severe anemia

Pre-Hospital

- Intravenous access
- Supplemental oxygen
  —100% non-rebreather mask
- Cardiac monitor
- Pulse oximetry
- Sublingual nitrates
- Furosemide
- Endotracheal intubation may be required in severe cases

CAUTIONS

- Administration of morphine, furosemide (Lasix), and nitrates
  —CHF can be difficult to distinguish from an acute exacerbation of chronic obstructive pulmonary disease (COPD), pneumonia, or asthma
  —Incorrect treatment may increase mortality

CONTROVERSIES

- Pre-hospital continuous positive airway pressure (CPAP)

Diagnosis

ESSENTIAL WORKUP

- The chest radiograph is essential in confirming the diagnosis and in assessing severity

LABORATORY

- Arterial blood gas
  —Rarely needed for emergency management when pulse oximetry is available
- Electrolytes
  —Generally normal before treatment
  —Hyperkalemia with severe low output states
- BUN and creatinine
  —Elevation in severe CHF
- Cardiac enzymes
  —May be useful if ischemia or infarction is presumed to be the underlying cause

IMAGING/SPECIAL TESTS

- Chest radiograph
  —Cardiomegaly
  —Three phases of pulmonary findings
    -Pulmonary redistribution
- Cephalization of vessels
  -Interstitial edema
- Effusions
- Kerley B lines
- Classic butterfly infiltrate
  -Frank alveolar infiltrates
- May be asymmetric and mistaken for pneumonia
- EKG
  —Assess for underlying cardiac ischemia
- Echocardiography
  —Acute valvular pathology
  —Pericardial tamponade

DIFFERENTIAL DIAGNOSIS

- Left-sided CHF
  —Acute exacerbation of COPD
  —Asthma exacerbation
  —Acute respiratory distress syndrome
  —Pneumonia
  —Bronchitis
  —Constrictive pericarditis
  —Pericardial tamponade
- Right-sided CHF
  —Nephrotic syndrome
  —Cirrhosis

Treatment

INITIAL STABILIZATION

- Intravenous access
- Supplemental oxygen
- Place patient in an upright position
- Cardiac monitor
- Pulse oximetry
- Control airway as needed
  - —CPAP
    - -Nasal Bi-PAP
    - -May decrease the need for intubation
  - —Endotracheal intubation for impending respiratory failure

ED TREATMENT

- Normotensive or hypertensive patients
  - —Rapid-acting nitrates
    - -Sublingual nitroglycerin
    - -Nitro paste
    - -IV nitroglycerin
- Pulmonary edema
- Failure of sublingual nitroglycerin and nitro paste to provide relief
  - —Morphine sulfate
  - —Intravenous diuretics
    - -Furosemide (Lasix) or bumetanide (Bumex)
    - -Sodium nitroprusside for afterload reduction may be required for severe persistent hypertension
- Hypotensive patients
  - —Avoid nitrates, morphine, and diuretics
  - —Agents that increase myocardial contractility
    - -Dopamine
    - -Dobutamine
    - -Amrinone
    - -Milrinone
- In less severe or chronic cases of low-output CHF
  - —Angiotensin-converting enzyme (ACE) inhibitors such as enalapril improve hemodynamic and increase exercise capacity
  - —Use in conjunction with other diuretics

MEDICATIONS

- Amrinone: 0.75 mg/kg i.v. load; 5–10 μg/kg/min i.v.
- Bumetanide (Bumex): 0.5–2.0 mg i.v.
- Digoxin: 1 mg i.v. load over 1 day; 0.125–0.375 mg/day PO
- Dobutamine: 2–10 μg/kg/min i.v.
- Dopamine: 2–20 μg/kg/min i.v.
- Enalapril: 0.625–1.25 mg i.v.; 2.5–20 mg/d PO
- Furosemide (Lasix): 20–100 mg i.v.
- Morphine sulfate: 2–4 mg i.v. every 5 minutes
- Nitroglycerin: 0.4 mg sublingual; 1–2 inches of nitro paste; 5–20 μg/min i.v., max of 100–200 μg/min i.v.
- Nitroprusside: 0.5–10 μg/kg/min i.v.

Disposition

ADMISSION CRITERIA

- Intensive care unit
  - —Pulmonary edema
  - —Cardiogenic shock
  - —Concomitant myocardial infarction or ischemia
- Medical wards
  - —New-onset CHF
  - —Symptoms not relieved by aggressive ED therapy

DISCHARGE CRITERIA

- Mild exacerbation of chronic CHF
  - —Responds to treatment
- Close follow-up should be arranged with continuation of diuretic, vasodilator, or ACE inhibitor therapy

Miscellaneous

ICD9: 428.0

ICD10: I50.0

SUGGESTED READINGS

Felker GM, O'Connor CM. Inotropic therapy for heart failure: an evidence based approach. Am Heart J 2001;142(3): 393–401.

Schamberger MS. Cardiac emergencies. Pediatr Ann 1996;25(6):339–344.

Smith TW, et al. Management of heart failure. In: Braunwald E, ed. Heart disease, 5th ed. Philadelphia: WB Saunders, 1997:492–514.

Authors: Robert Partridge; John F. Jardine

Conjunctivitis

Clinical Presentation

SIGNS AND SYMPTOMS

General

- Red eye (conjunctival irritation)
- Gritty, foreign body sensation
- Discharge
- Eyelid sticking (worse on arising)
- Conjunctival edema (chemosis) and eyelid edema
- Normal visual acuity, anterior chamber, and intraocular pressure

Bacterial—General

- Mucopurulent or purulent discharge
- Preauricular nodes

Gonococcal

- Hyperacute, copious purulent discharge—"pouring out" of the eye
- Severe chemosis and lid edema
- Inflammatory membranes
- Invade intact conjunctiva and cornea within 24 hours and cause ulcerations, scarring, and perforations leading to blindness

Chlamydia

- Lacrimation
- Mucopurulent discharge
- With or without photophobia
- Concomitant genital infection (>50%)
  —Transmission occurs via autoinoculation from genital secretions

Viral—General

- Watery, mucous discharge, lacrimation
- Foreign body sensation
- Pinpoint subconjunctival hemorrhages
- Inflammatory membranes

Herpes Simplex Virus (HSV)

- Acute follicular conjunctival reaction
- Skin lesions or vesicles along eyelid margin or periocular skin
- Corneal involvement—dendritic lesion

Herpes Zoster Virus (HZV)

- Associated with pain or paresthesias of the skin
- Rash or vesicles involving the distribution of cranial nerve V_1
- Dendritic characters on cornea
- Rarely vesicles or ulcers form on the conjunctiva

Allergic

- Hallmark: itching
- Either hyperemic or pale conjunctiva
- Watery discharge
- Papillary hypertrophy
- Frequent history of allergy, atopy, nasal symptoms

Contact Related

- Acute symptoms result of corneal ulceration

MECHANISM/DESCRIPTION

- Inflammation of the conjunctiva arising from a broad group of clinical causes

ETIOLOGY

Bacterial

Gonococcal

- Ophthalmic emergency
- *Neisseria gonorrhoeae* can invade intact conjunctiva and cornea within 24 hours and cause ulcerations, scarring, and perforations leading to blindness
- Often occurs in newborns

Chlamydia

- Transmission occurs via autoinoculation from genital secretions

Viral

- Adenovirus most common
- Frequently associated with recent upper respiratory infection symptoms or exposure to someone with a red eye

Herpes Simplex Virus

- Recurrent ocular infection occurs in 25% patients within 2 years
- Use of steroids is *contraindicated*

Allergic

- Frequent history of allergy, atopy, nasal symptoms

Contact Related

- Most vision-threatening cause of "red eye"
- May be due to chemical irritation, hypersensitivity from preservatives, medications
- *Pseudomonas* commonly implicated organism
- Anaerobes may be causative in patients using saliva to wet lenses

PEDIATRIC CONSIDERATIONS

- Often a manifestation of systemic disease in infants
- Neonates become infected during passage through the birth canal
  —Gonococcal, herpetic, chlamydial organisms most common
- Ophthalmia neonatorum is conjunctivitis within the first 4 weeks of life
- *Chlamydia trachomatis* is
  —Not eradicated by silver nitrate
  —Substantial percentage of infants treated with erythromycin still develop conjunctivitis

Pre-Hospital

N/A

Diagnosis

ESSENTIAL WORKUP

- History for:
  —Onset of inflammation
  —Environmental or work-related exposure
  —Ill contacts
  —Sexual activity, discharge, rash
  —Use of over-the-counter medicines or cosmetics
  —Systemic diseases
- Careful physical examination with slit-lamp including fluorescein staining

LABORATORY

- Bacteriologic studies
  - —Not indicated in routine cases
  - —Indications
    - -Ophthalmia neonatorum (except chemical)
    - -Suspected gonococcal ophthalmia
    - -Compromised host
    - -Signs and symptoms of systemic disease
    - -Refractory to treatment within 48–72 hours (with good compliance)
- Positive Gram stain for gram-negative intracellular diplococci
  - —Sufficient to initiate systemic and topical treatment for gonococcal disease
- RPR
  - —For suspected cases of sexually transmitted disease (STD)

DIFFERENTIAL DIAGNOSIS

- Dry eye
- Foreign body
- Corneal abrasion
- Allergies or hypersensitivity
- Nasolacrimal obstruction
- Anterior uveitis
- Acute angle-closure glaucoma (most serious cause)
- Scleritis or episcleritis
- Subconjunctival hemorrhage

PEDIATRIC CONSIDERATIONS

- Gram stain and culture all cases of ophthalmia neonatorum
- Giemsa stain of conjunctival scrapings reveals diagnostic basophilic epithelial cytoplasmic inclusions in a significant number of infants with chlamydial disease
- Rapid enzyme immunoassay (EIA) test available for diagnosis of neonatal chlamydial conjunctivitis

Treatment

INITIAL STABILIZATION

- Initiate empiric antibiotic therapy with broad-spectrum topical agent
- Systemic therapy for gonococcal, chlamydial, and meningococcal conjunctivitis, ophthalmia neonatorum, and all severe infections regardless of cause
- Manage herpetic eye infections in consultation with an ophthalmologist

ED TREATMENT

- Remove discharge from the eye(s)
- Antibiotics—topical
  - —Instill drops every 2 hours with ointment at bedtime
  - —Continue therapy for 48 hours after clearing of symptoms
  - —Discontinue therapy and obtain cultures if no improvement in 48–72 hours (with good compliance)
- Antibiotics—systemic
  - —Parenteral therapy mandatory for gonococcal infection
  - —Chlamydia requires systemic treatment of sexual partners and parents of neonates
- Eye irrigation
  - —Indicated at least hourly in gonococcal ophthalmia
  - —Symptomatic relief in allergic or viral cases
  - —Use saline or buffered solutions, preferably without preservatives
- Personal hygiene—frequent handwashing and use of separate towels and washcloths
- Isolation—use precautions at work or school
- Allergic conjunctivitis (there may be a lag time of up to 2 weeks for improvement with these agents)
  - —Antihistamine drops (naphazoline [Naphcon-A])
  - —Cromolyn sodium ophthalmic solution
  - —Nedocromil (Alacril) drops
- Do not use steroids in the initial management

MEDICATIONS

General

- Bacitracin ophthalmologic ointment (no pseudomonal coverage)
- Ciprofloxacin: 0.35% 1 drop q1–6h (has antipseudomonal properties; may be used in children)
- Erythromycin: 0.5% ointment
- Gentamicin: 0.3% ointment q3–4h or drops q1–4h (has antipseudomonal coverage)
- Sulfacetamide: 10% 1 drop q1–6h (lacks pseudomonal coverage)
- Tobramycin: 0.3% ointment q3–4h or drops q1–6h

Chlamydia

- Doxycycline: 100 mg PO b.i.d. for 3 weeks
- Erythromycin: 500 mg PO q.i.d. for 3 weeks (peds: 50 mg/kg/d PO in 4 div doses for 14 days)
- Tetracycline: 250–500 mg PO q.i.d. for 3 weeks

Gonococcal

Adults

- Ceftriaxone: 1 g i.v. or i.m. daily for 3–5 days or as needed
- Erythromycin: 500 mg PO q.i.d. for 2–3 weeks or doxycycline 100 mg PO b.i.d. for 2–3 weeks
- *Plus* topical antibiotics as above

Neonates

- Penicillin G 100,000 IU/kg/d in 4 divided doses for 7 days or ceftriaxone 25–50 mg/kg IV daily for 7 days

Viral

- Artificial tears

HSV or HZV

- Trifluorothymidine: 1% 5 times per day, *or*
- Vidarabine: 3% ointment 5 times per day

Allergic

- Naphazoline (Naphcon-A): 1 drop b.i.d. to q.i.d.
- Nedocromil (Alacril): 1–2 drops b.i.d.
- Cromolyn sodium (Crolom): 1 drop q4–6h

Disposition

ADMISSION CRITERIA

- Known or suspected gonococcal infection (any age group)

DISCHARGE CRITERIA

- Close follow-up for all cases

Miscellaneous

ICD9: 372.30

ICD10: H10.9

SEE ALSO: RED EYE

SUGGESTED READINGS

Alteveer JG, McCans KM. The red eye, the swollen eye, and acute vision loss. Emerg Med Pract 2002;4(6):2–7.

Bertolini J, Pelucio M. The red eye. Emerg Med Clin North Am 1995;13(3):561–579.

Diamant JI, Hwang DG. Therapy for bacterial conjunctivitis. Ophthalmol Clin North Am 1999;12(1):15–20.

Rhee D, Pyfer M. The Wills eye manual: office and emergency room diagnosis and treatment of eye diseases, 3rd ed. Philadelphia: Lippincott Williams & Wilkins, 1999:119–128.

Author: Mary Stewart

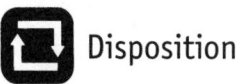

Conscious Sedation

Clinical Presentation

SIGNS AND SYMPTOMS

N/A

Pre-Hospital

N/A

Diagnosis

ESSENTIAL WORKUP

N/A

DIFFERENTIAL DIAGNOSIS

N/A

Treatment

INITIAL STABILIZATION

Preparation

- Have patient in area that has accessibility to resuscitation equipment
  - —Breathing masks, Ambu bag, oropharyngeal and nasal airways, laryngoscopes and endotracheal tubes appropriate for size of patient
  - —Defibrillator
  - —Emergency cart with all available medications to resuscitate the patient including flumazenil and naloxone
- Apply cardiorespiratory monitor, pulse oximeter, and BP monitor
- Gather medicines to use in procedure
- Oxygen supply
- Wall suction
- Acquire informed consent

Sedation Agents and Techniques

Sedative agents can be administered by various routes including IV, IM, PO, rectal, sublingual, transmucosal, and intranasal

- Benzodiazepines
  - —Provide anxiolysis and amnesia but *not* analgesia, so for painful procedure must not be the sole agent
  - —Benzodiazepines cause CNS and respiratory depression
  - —Midazolam is a negative inotrope and may induce hypotension
  - —Effects may be reversed with flumazenil
  - —Midazolam
    - -Dosage
      - *IV: 0.05–0.1 mg/kg (single max dose 2 mg) with subsequent incremental doses at 3-minute intervals to desired effect or to a total of 0.2 mg/kg
      - *IM: 0.3 mg/kg
      - *PO: 0.5–0.75 mg/kg (max dose of 15 mg)
      - *Nasal: 0.3–0.5 mg/kg (max dose of 5 mg)
    - -Duration of action: 30–45 minutes
  - —Diazepam (largely replaced by shorter acting midazolam)
    - -Dosage
      - *IV: 0.1–0.2 mg/kg (max 10 mg)
      - *PO: 0.2–0.3 mg/kg
      - *PR: 0.5 mg/kg
    - -Duration of action: 2–6 hours
- Sedative-hypnotics
  - —Chloral hydrate
    - -Dosage: PO/PR 50–75 mg/kg (max 2 g)
    - -Time of onset: 30–45 minutes
    - -Duration of action: 2–4 hours
    - -Cautions

*Nausea, vomiting, and paradoxic delirium/excitement
*Not reversible
*Serious effects of airway obstruction and death have been reported
*No analgesia
—Pentobarbital
-Dosage
*IV: 1–3 mg/kg
*IM: 2–6 mg/kg
-Onset: IV has actions within 30 seconds and appropriately sedated within 5 minutes
-Duration of action: 30–60 minutes, so better than chloral hydrate for procedures
-Cautions
*CNS and respiratory depression
*No analgesia
- Narcotics
—Can be administered with an anxiolytic for sedation for painful procedures
—Fentanyl
-Dosage
*IV: 1–3 μg/kg with onset in 1–3 minutes
*Transmucosal (oral lozenge [Oralet] allows patient to suck on drug and then can be removed by physician or patient when adequate sedation achieved): 10–15 μg/kg with onset in 15–20 minutes
-Duration of action: 30 minutes
-Cautions
*Respiratory depression
*Chest wall rigidity
*Use <⅓ dose in children younger than 6 months
*Emesis with transmucosal preparation
- Nitrous oxide
—Provides analgesia, anxiolysis, and sedation without the need for IV placement
—Administered in a 50% N_2O/O_2 concentration via inhalation
—Onset of action: 3–5 minutes
—Duration of action: 3–5 minutes after ceasing inhalation
—Cautions (side effects rare)
-Potent sedation if previous narcotic in past 4 hours
-Nausea and vomiting
-Pregnancy
-Pneumothorax or bowel obstruction
- Ketamine
—Produces analgesia, amnesia, and sedation due to its dissociative effect
—Spontaneous respirations and airway reflexes maintained
—Dosage
-IV: 1.0 mg/kg (use midazolam 0.05 mg/kg and atropine 0.01 mg/kg concurrently) with onset of action 5–10 minutes
-IM: 2.0–4.0 mg/kg (combine atropine and midazolam in same syringe) with onset of action 15–25 minutes
-PO: 10 mg/kg (use midazolam 0.5 mg/kg and atropine 0.02 mg/kg) with onset of 30–45 minutes
—Duration of action
-IV: 20–60 minutes
-IM: 30–90 minutes
-PO: 60–120 minutes
—Cautions
-Causes hypertension and tachycardia, so do not use if hypertension or cardiovascular disease
-Increases intracranial and intraocular pressure, so do not use with head injury or penetrating globe injury
-Stimulates salivary and tracheobronchial secretions, so must be administered with an anticholinergic such as atropine
-Emergence reactions with hallucinations reported but are less frequent in children younger than 10 years; the incidence can be reduced by premedicating the patient with midazolam
-Not for children younger than 3 months
- Propofol
—Produces amnesia and sedation but not analgesia
—Onset of action: seconds
—Dosage: 1.5–3.0 mg/kg bolus (usually given as 40-mg boluses every 10 seconds in adults until desired effect) followed by infusion of 0.1–0.2 mg/kg/min
—Duration of action: <2 minutes
—Cautions
-Dose-related respiratory depressant
-Deep sedation
-Hypotension
-Transient apnea
-Pain at injection site
-Used in children but studies are limited
- Reversal agents
—Naloxone
-Opioid antagonist
-For reversal of respiratory depression, apnea, and severe hypotension
-Dosage: 0.01–0.02 mg/kg i.v./i.m. in incremental doses (to total of 2 mg) every 1–2 minutes to the desired reversal effect
-Duration of action: 20–45 minutes
-Cautions
*Use smaller doses on patients who are dependent on opioids to prevent withdrawal reactions
—Flumazenil
-Benzodiazepine antagonist
-Reverses CNS depression and some degree of respiratory depression
-Dosage: 0.01 mg/kg/dose (max initial dose 0.2 mg) repeated at 1-minute intervals to desired effect or max of 0.05 mg/kg or 1.0 mg
-Duration of action: 20–45 minutes
-Cautions
*Not to be used in patients with chronic benzodiazepine therapy or TCA therapy because of seizures

ED TREATMENT

N/A

Disposition

ADMISSION CRITERIA

- Postprocedural sedation
- Inability to ambulate
- No responsible adult to accompany home
- Reason to undergo conscious sedation still present
- Complications of conscious sedation such as
  —Postprocedural sedation
  —Hemodynamic instability
  —Seizures
  —Respiratory complications such as aspiration or depression

DISCHARGE CRITERIA

- Stable hemodynamically
- Ambulatory 30 minutes before discharge
- Able to void
- Able to retain oral fluids
- Discharged with follow-up instructions both for the necessitating procedure and for conscious sedation
- Under observation of a responsible person and have transportation from the hospital

Miscellaneous

ICD9: N/A

ICD10: N/A

SUGGESTED READINGS

Fleisher G, Krauss B, Shannon M, et al. Guidelines for pediatric sedation. Dallas: American College of Emergency Physicians, 1998.

Marx JA, et al. Rosen's emergency medicine: clinical concepts and practice, 5th ed. St. Louis: Mosby, 2002.

Tintinalli J. Emergency medicine: a comprehensive study guide, 5th ed. New York: McGraw-Hill, 2000.

Author: Christopher Ross

Constipation

Clinical Presentation

SIGNS AND SYMPTOMS

- Constipation is a symptom, not a disease
- Passage of hard stool
- Straining/difficulty passing stool
- Infrequent bowel movements
- Abdominal distention/bloating
- Firm/hard stool on digital rectal exam
  - —May have empty rectal vault
- Diarrhea (liquid stool passes around firm feces)

MECHANISM/DESCRIPTION

- Less than two bowel movements per week

ETIOLOGY

- Metabolic and endocrine
  - —Diabetes
  - —Uremia
  - —Porphyria
  - —Hypothyroidism
  - —Hypercalcemia
  - —Pheochromocytoma
  - —Panhypopituitarism
  - —Pregnancy
- Functional and idiopathic
  - —Colonic irritable bowel syndrome
  - —Diverticular disease
  - —Colonic inertia
  - —Megacolon/rectum
  - —Pelvic intussusception
  - —Nonrelaxing puborectalis
  - —Rectocele/sigmoidocele
  - —Posthysterectomy syndrome
  - —Descending perineum
- Pharmacologic
  - —Analgesics
  - —Anesthetics
  - —Antacids
  - —Anticholinergics
  - —Anticonvulsants
  - —Antidepressants
  - —Antihypertensives
  - —Calcium channel blockers
  - —Diuretics
  - —Ferrous compounds
  - —Laxative abuse
  - —Monoamine oxidase inhibitors
  - —Opiates
  - —Paralytic agents
  - —Parasympatholytics
  - —Phenothiazines
  - —Psychotropics
- Neurologic
  - —Central Parkinson's disease
  - —Multiple sclerosis
  - —Cerebrovascular accidents
  - —Spinal cord lesions/injury
  - —Peripheral Hirschsprung's disease
  - —Chagas' disease
  - —Neurofibromatosis
  - —Autonomic neuropathy
- Mechanical obstruction
  - —Neoplasm
  - —Stricture
  - —Hernia
  - —Volvulus

PEDIATRIC CONSIDERATIONS

- 3% pediatric outpatient visits because of defecation disorders
- Cerebral palsy children often develop functional constipation
- Most common cause of fecal retention and soiling in children is functional fecal retention
  - —Caused by fears associated with defecation
  - —Associated with irritability, abdominal cramps, decreased appetite, early satiety

Pre-Hospital

N/A

Diagnosis

ESSENTIAL WORKUP

- Thorough history and physical exam
  - —Medical, surgical, and psychiatric investigation and date of onset
  - —Note abdominal distention, hernias, tenderness, or masses
  - —Complete anorectal exam for anal stenosis, fissure, neoplasm, sphincter tone, perineal descent, tenderness, spasm

LABORATORY

- Only necessary when considering metabolic/endocrine disorders
- CBC if inflammatory or neoplastic origin
- Electrolytes and calcium indicated if at risk of
  - —Hypokalemia
  - —Hypocalcemia
- Thyroid function test if patient appears to be hypothyroid

IMAGING/SPECIAL TESTS

- Rarely indicated unless an underlying process suspected
- Abdominal x-ray
  - —Large amount of feces in colon
  - —Dilated colon
- Barium enema study
  - —Diverticulosis
  - —Megarectum
  - —Megacolon
  - —Hirschsprung's disease
  - —Stricture

DIFFERENTIAL DIAGNOSIS

- See Etiology
- Bowel obstruction

PEDIATRIC CONSIDERATIONS

- Functional constipation in infants and preschool children
  - —Thorough history and physical to rule out neurologic, metabolic, or anatomic causes
  - —At least 2 weeks of
    - -Scybalous: pebble-like, hard stools
    - -Firm stools at least two times a week
    - -No evidence of structural, endocrine, or metabolic disease
- Functional fecal retention from infancy to 16 years old
  - —Physical exam: rectal fecal mass
  - —Neurologic exam: excludes occult spinal dysraphism
  - —At least 12 weeks of
    - -Passage of large-diameter stools fewer than two times per week
    - -Retentive posturing, avoiding defecation by contracting pelvic floor; as these muscles fatigue, the child uses gluteal muscles

Treatment

INITIAL STABILIZATION

N/A

ED TREATMENT

- Clean out colon
  - —Enemas, suppositories
  - —Manual disimpaction of hard stool
  - —Laxatives
- Maintain bowel regimen
  - —Increase noncaffeinated fluids (8–10 cups/d)
  - —Increase dietary fiber intake (20 g/d)
  - —Stool softeners
  - —Exercise
  - —Change medications causing constipation

MEDICATIONS

- Enemas
  - —Fleet: 120 mL (peds: 60–120 mL) p.r.
  - —Mineral oil: 60–150 mL (peds: 5–11 years old, 30–60 mL; older than 12 years, 60–150 mL) PR q.d.
  - —Tap water: 100–500 mL PR
- Fiber supplements
  - —Methylcellulose: 1 tbs in cup water PO q.d. to t.i.d.
  - —Psyllium: 1–2 tsp in cup of water/juice (peds: younger than 6 years, ¼–½ tsp in 2 oz water or juice; 6–11 years, ½–1 tsp in 4 oz water or juice; older than 12 years, 1–2 tsp in cup water or juice) PO q.d. to t.i.d.
- Laxatives (osmotic)
  - —Lactulose: 15–30 mL (peds: 1 mL/kg) PO q.d. to b.i.d.
  - —Polyethylene glycol: 17 g (peds: 0.8 g/kg/d dissolve in 4–8 oz of liquid) PO q.d. dissolved in liquid
- Laxatives (stimulant)
  - —Bisacodyl: 10–15 mg PO q.d. (peds: younger than 3 years, 5 mg PR q.d.; 3–12 years, 5–10 mg PO/PR q.d.; older than 12 years, 5–15 mg PO q.d. or 10 mg PR q.d.)
  - —Cascara sagrada: 5 mL (peds: infants, 1.25 mL; 2–12 years, 2.5 mL; older than 12 years, 5 mL) PO q.h.s. on an empty stomach
  - —Castor oil: 15–60 mL (peds: 2–12 years, 5–15 mL) PO q.d., do not take at bedtime
  - —Senna: 2–4 tabs PO q.d. to t.i.d. (peds: 2–6 years, ½–1 tab PO q.d. to b.i.d.; 6–12 years, 1–2 tabs PO q.d. to b.i.d.; older than 12 years, 2–4 tabs PO q.d. to b.i.d.)
- Stool softeners
  - —Docusate sodium: 100 mg (peds: 3–5 mg/kg/d in divided doses) PO q.d. to b.i.d.
  - —Mineral oil: 15–45 mL (peds: 5–15 mL) PO q.d.
- Suppositories
  - —Glycerin: 1 adult (peds: infant, 1 infant suppository) PR p.r.n.

PEDIATRIC CONSIDERATIONS

- Functional constipation
  - —In infants, increase stool water by fruit juices containing fructose and sorbitol (prune and pear); barley, corn syrup, lactulose, and sorbitol
  - —Adequate liquid and fiber ingestion: age (in years) + 5 = number of grams of dietary fiber per day
- Functional fecal retention
  - —Evacuate fecal mass with daily oral mineral oil or enemas and stimulant laxatives

Disposition

ADMISSION CRITERIA

- Patients with severe abdominal pain, nausea, and emesis
- Neurologically impaired, elderly, morbidly obese who cannot be cleaned out in the ED or home
- Bowel obstruction/peritonitis

DISCHARGE CRITERIA

- No comorbid illness requiring admission
- Pain free
- Adequately cleaned out

Miscellaneous

ICD9: 564.0

ICD10: K59.0

SUGGESTED READINGS

Prather C, Ortiz-Camacho C. Evaluation and treatment of constipation and fecal impaction in adults. Mayo Clin Proc 1998;73(9):881–887.

Rasquin-Weber A, Hyman PE, Cucchiara S, et al. Childhood functional gastrointestinal disorders. Gut 1999;45[Suppl II]:II60–II68.

Author: Julia Sone

Contact Dermatitis

Clinical Presentation

SIGNS AND SYMPTOMS

- *Acute lesions:* skin erythema and pruritus
  - —May see edema, papules, vesicles, bullae, serous discharge, or crusting
- *Subacute:* vesiculation less pronounced
- *Chronic lesions:* may see scaling, lichenification, pigmentation, or fissuring with little to no vesiculation; may have a characteristic distribution pattern

MECHANISM/DESCRIPTION

- Irritant
  - —An *eczematous eruption* (superficial inflammatory process primarily in the epidermis)
  - —Direct injury to the skin resulting in nonimmunologic inflammatory reaction with erythema, dryness, cracking, or fissuring; may see vesicles
  - —Lesions itch or burn
  - —Usually gradual onset with indistinct borders
  - —Most often seen on the hands
- Allergic
  - —Delayed hypersensitivity reaction (requires prior sensitization)
  - —Local edema, vesicles, erythema, pruritus, and/or burning
  - —Usually rapid onset (12–48 hours); may correspond to exact distribution of contact (e.g., watchband)

ETIOLOGY

- Irritant (80% of contact dermatitis)
  - —Strong soaps, solvents, chemicals, certain foods, urine, feces, continuous or repeated exposure to moisture (diaper rash), and others
- Allergic
  - —Common allergens include plants, cement (prolonged exposure may result in severe alkali burn), metals (especially nickel), solvents, epoxy, chemicals in rubber (e.g., elastic waistbands) or leather, lotions, cosmetics, topical medications (e.g., neomycin, benzocaine, paraben), some foods, and others
  - —Poison ivy, oak, sumac (rhus dermatitis)
    - -Common form of allergic contact dermatitis
    - -Direct: reaction to oleoresin from plant
    - -Indirect: contact with pet or clothes with oleoresin on surface or fur or in smoke from burning leaves
    - -Lesions may appear up to 3 days after exposure and may persist up to 3 weeks
    - -Fluid from vesicles is not contagious and does not produce new lesions
- Shoe dermatitis
  - —Common; identify by lesions limited to distal dorsal surface of foot usually sparing the interdigital spaces
- Photodermatitis
  - —Inflammatory reaction from exposure to an irritant (frequently plant sap) and sunlight

PEDIATRIC CONSIDERATIONS

- Allergic contact dermatitis is less frequent in children, especially infants, than adults
- Major sources of pediatric contact allergy
  - —Metals, shoes, preservatives or fragrances in cosmetics and topical medications, and plants
- Circumoral dermatitis: seen in infants and small children; may result from certain foods (irritant or allergic reaction)

Pre-Hospital

N/A

Diagnosis

ESSENTIAL WORKUP

- Medical history
  - —Include date of onset, time course, pattern of lesions, relationship to work, exposures (home and at work), new products (e.g., lotions and cosmetics), medications, and jewelry
- Physical exam
  - —Special attention to character and distribution of the rash

LABORATORY

- No specific tests in the ED are helpful

IMAGING/SPECIAL TESTS

- Patch testing
  - —Generally not done in the ED, refer to subspecialist
- When tinea is suspected, may use Wood's lamp for fluorescence

DIFFERENTIAL DIAGNOSIS

- Atopic dermatitis: associated with family history of atopy
- Seborrheic dermatitis: scaly or crusting "greasy" lesions
- Nummular dermatitis: "coin-like" lesions
- Intertrigo: dermatitis in which skin is in apposition
- Infectious eczematous dermatitis: dermatitis with secondary bacterial infection, usually *Staphylococcus aureus*
- Cellulitis: warm, blanching, painful lesion
- Impetigo: yellow crusting
- Scabies: intensely pruritic, frequently interdigital with "tracks"
- Psoriasis: silvery adherent, scaling, lesions well delineated, affecting extensor surfaces, scalp, and genital region
- Herpes simplex: groups of vesicles, painful, burning
- Herpes zoster: painful, follows dermatomal pattern
- Bullous pemphigoid: diffuse bullous lesions
- Tinea: maximal involvement at margins, fluoresces under Wood's lamp
- Pityriasis alba: discrete, asymptomatic, hypopigmented lesions
- Urticaria: pruritic raised lesions (wheal) frequently with surrounding erythema (flare)
- Acrodermatitis enteropathica: vesiculobullous lesion of hands and feet, associated with failure to thrive, diarrhea, and alopecia
- Letterer-Siwe tumor (Langerhans cell histiocytosis)
  - —Associated with hepatosplenomegaly and adenopathy

Treatment

INITIAL STABILIZATION

- Rarely required in absence of concomitant pathology

ED TREATMENT

General

- Primarily symptomatic
- Wash area with mild soap and water
- Remove or avoid offending agent (including washing clothes)
- Cool, wet compresses, especially effective during acute blistering phase
- Antipruritic agents
  - —Topical: calamine lotion, corticosteroids (does not penetrate blisters); avoid benzocaine-containing products, which may further sensitize skin
  - —Systemic: antihistamines, corticosteroids
- Aluminum acetate (Burrows) solution: weeping surfaces

Irritant Dermatitis

- Decrease wet/dry cycles (hand washing)
- Bland emollient
- Topical steroids for severe cases (ointment preferred) medium to high potency (hands) b.i.d. for several weeks

Allergic Dermatitis

- Topical steroids (ointment preferred) b.i.d. 2–3 weeks
  - —Face: low potency
  - —Arms, legs, trunk: medium potency
  - —Hands and feet: high potency
- Oral steroids for severe cases

Rhus Dermatitis

- Follow general measures plus
  - —Aseptic aspiration of bullae may relieve discomfort
  - —Severe reaction: systemic corticosteroids for 2–3 weeks with gradual taper; premature termination of corticosteroid therapy may result in rapid rebound of symptoms

Shoe Dermatitis

- Follow general measures plus
  - —Wear open-toe, canvas, or vinyl shoes
  - —Control perspiration: change socks, absorbent powder

MEDICATIONS

Systemic

- Antihistamine (H_1-receptor antagonist, first and second generation)
  - —Diphenhydramine hydrochloride (Benadryl): 25–50 mg i.v./i.m./PO q6h p.r.n. (peds: 5 mg/kg/24 h divided q6h p.r.n.)
  - —Hydroxyzine hydrochloride (Atarax): 25–50 mg PO i.m. up to q.i.d. p.r.n. (peds: 2 mg/kg/24 h PO divided q.i.d. or 0.5 mg/kg i.m. q4–6h p.r.n.
  - —Loratadine (Claritin): 10 mg PO b.i.d.
  - —Cetirizine (Zyrtec): adult and children 6 years or older, 5–10 mg PO q.d. (peds: 2–6 years, 2.5 mg PO q.d. to b.i.d.
  - —Or refractory pruritus, doxepin 75 mg q.d. may be effective
- Corticosteroid
  - —Prednisone: 40–60 mg PO q.d. (peds: 1–2 mg/kg/24 h, max 80 mg/24 h) divided q.d./b.i.d.

Topical

- Aluminum acetate (Burrows) solution: apply topically for 20 minutes t.i.d. until skin is dry
- Calamine lotion: q.i.d. p.r.n.
- Topical corticosteroid
  - —Hydrocortisone: cream 1%; ointment 0.5% or 1%; lotion 0.25%, 0.5%, or 1%; gel 0.5%; aerosol 0.5% t.i.d. q.i.d.
- Triamcinolone: ointment 0.025, 0.1%; cream 0.025, 0.1%; lotion 0.025, 0.1% t.i.d. q.i.d.

Disposition

ADMISSION CRITERIA

- Rarely indicated unless severe systemic reaction or significant secondary infection

DISCHARGE CRITERIA

- Symptomatic relief
- Adequate follow-up with PCP or dermatologic specialist

Miscellaneous

ICD9: 692.9

ICD10: L25.9

SUGGESTED READINGS

Habif TP. Skin disease diagnosis and treatment. St Louis: CV Mosby, 2001: 30–35.

Habif TP. Clinical dermatology. St Louis: CV Mosby, 1996:81–99.

Hurwitz S. Clinical pediatric dermatology. Philadelphia: WB Saunders, 1993:68–82.

Juckett G. Plant dermatitis. Postgrad Med 1996;100(3):159–171.

White IR. Occupational dermatitis. BMJ 1996;313:487–489.

Wolf R, Wolf D. Contact dermatitis. Clin Dermatol 2000;18(6):661–666.

Author: Jeffrey Horton

Cor Pulmonale

Clinical Presentation

SIGNS AND SYMPTOMS

- *Exertional dyspnea*
- *Easy fatigability*
- Weakness
- Syncope
- Cough
- Hemoptysis
- Wheezing
- Hoarseness
- Weight gain
- Jugular venous distention
  —Prominent a and v waves
- Hepatomegaly
- Ascites
- Hepatojugular reflex
- Peripheral edema
- Left parasternal heave on cardiac palpation
- Pulmonic component of the second heart sound increases in intensity

MECHANISM/DESCRIPTION

- Ventricular failure confined to the right ventricle
  —Right ventricular hypertrophy or dilation is an adaptive response to pulmonary hypertension
- The pulmonary circulation is a low-resistance, low-pressure system
  —The pulmonary arteries are thin walled and distensible
  —Mean pulmonary arterial pressure is usually 12–15 mm Hg
  —Normal left arterial pressure is 6–10 mm Hg
  —The resulting pressure difference driving the pulmonary circulation is only 6–9 mm Hg
- Three factors affect pulmonary arterial pressure
  —Cardiac output
  —Pulmonary venous pressure
  —Pulmonary vascular resistance
- Pulmonary hypertension can arise by a number of mechanisms
  —A marked increase in cardiac output
  —Left-to-right shunt secondary to congenital heart disease
  —Hypoxia
    -Most commonly causes pulmonary vascular resistance to increase
    -The resulting hypercapnia and acidosis induce vasoconstriction
    -Pulmonary venous pressure increase
    -A compensatory rise is seen in the pulmonary arterial system so flow is maintained across the pulmonary vascular bed
  —Pulmonary embolus causes such a change by increasing resistance to pulmonary blood flow
  —Left ventricular failure achieves the same result by directly influencing pulmonary venous pressure
  —Dramatic rises in blood viscosity or intrathoracic pressure impede blood flow

Incidence

- Approximately 86,000 patients die from COPD each year
  —Associated right ventricular failure is a significant factor in many of these cases
- In those older than 50 years with COPD, 50% develop pulmonary hypertension and are at risk of developing cor pulmonale
- The course of cor pulmonale is generally related to the progression of the underlying disease process
- Once biventricular failure is noted, life expectancy is usually <5 years

ETIOLOGY

- Chronic hypoxia
  —COPD
  —Chronic hypoxia at high altitude
  —Sleep apnea
    -Primary pulmonary hypertension
- Cystic fibrosis
- Congenital heart disease
  —Left-to-right shunts
- Severe anemia
- Pulmonary embolism
- Collagen vascular diseases
- Thoracic deformities
  —Kyphoscoliosis
- Obesity
- Mitral stenosis
- Pulmonary venoocclusive disease
- Increased blood viscosity
  —Polycythemia vera
  —Leukemia
- Increased intrathoracic pressure
  —COPD
  —Mechanical ventilation with positive end-expiratory pressure

Pre-Hospital

- Supportive therapy
  —Supplemental oxygen
- To an endpoint of 90% arterial saturation
  —IV access
  —Cardiac monitoring
  —Pulse oximetry
- Treat bronchospasm from associated respiratory disease
  —β-Agonist nebulizers

CAUTIONS

- Vasodilators and diuretics do not have a role in the field
- Severely hypoxic patients may require ETT intubation

Diagnosis

ESSENTIAL WORKUP

N/A

LABORATORY

- Pulse oximetry or arterial blood gas
  - —Resting PO_2 40–60 mm Hg
  - —Resting PCO_2 often 40–70 mm Hg
- Hematocrit
  - —Frequently elevated
- B-natriuretic peptide
  - —Often useful in distinguishing biventricular failure from respiratory disease
- Other laboratory tests are not generally useful

IMAGING/SPECIAL TESTS

- CXR
  - —Signs of pulmonary hypertension
    - -Large pulmonary arteries (>16–18 mm)
    - -An enlarged right ventricular silhouette
    - -98% sensitive for detection of cor pulmonale, but does not indicate the severity of disease
    - -Pleural effusions do not occur in the setting of cor pulmonale alone
- EKG
  - —Right-axis deviation
  - —Tall, peaked P waves (P pulmonale)
  - —Right ventricular hypertrophy (specific not sensitive)
  - —Transient changes due to hypoxia
  - —Right precordial T-wave flattening
  - —ST-segment depression in segments II, III, and aVF
- Echocardiography
  - —Noninvasive
  - —Right ventricular dilation or hypertrophy in the setting of normal left ventricular dimensions
  - —Assessment of tricuspid regurgitation
  - —Doppler quantitation of pulmonary artery pressure, right ventricular ejection fraction
- Ventilation/perfusion scans or pulmonary angiography
  - —Useful in the setting of acute cor pulmonale
- CT or MRI
  - —Delineates size and shape of the ventricles and pulmonary arteries
  - —Detection of larger pulmonary emboli
- Right heart catheterization
  - —The most precise estimate of pulmonary vascular hemodynamics
  - —Gives accurate measurements of pulmonary arterial pressure and pulmonary capillary wedge pressure

DIFFERENTIAL DIAGNOSIS

- Primary disease of the left side of the heart
- Congenital heart disease
- Hypothyroidism
- Cirrhosis

Treatment

INITIAL STABILIZATION

- ED therapy is directed at the underlying disease process and reducing pulmonary hypertension

ED TREATMENT

- Supplemental oxygen sufficient to raise arterial saturation to 90%
  - —Improving oxygenation reduces pulmonary arterial vasoconstriction and right ventricular afterload
  - —The improved cardiac output enhances diuresis of excess body water
  - —Care must be taken to monitor the patient's ventilatory status and PCO_2 as hypercapnia may reduce respiratory drive and cause an acidosis
- Diuretics, such as furosemide, may be added cautiously to reduce pulmonary artery pressure by contributing to the reduction of circulating blood volume
- Patients should be maintained on salt and fluid restriction
- There is no role for digoxin in the treatment of cor pulmonale
- Bronchodilator therapy is particularly helpful for those patients with COPD
  - —Selective β-adrenergic agents such as subcutaneous terbutaline 0.25 mg s.c.
  - —Bronchodilator affects and reduces ventricular afterload
  - —Theophylline may play a role to improve diaphragmatic contractility and reduce muscle fatigue
- Acutely decompensated COPD patients
  - —Early steroid therapy
  - —Antibiotic administration
- In general, improvement in the underlying respiratory disease results in improved right ventricular function

MEDICATIONS

- Furosemide: 20–60 mg i.v. (peds: 1 mg/kg may increase by 1 mg/kg q2h not to exceed 6 mg/kg)
- Terbutaline: 0.25 mg s.c.

Disposition

ADMISSION CRITERIA

- New-onset hypoxia
- Anasarca
- Severe respiratory failure
- Admission criteria for the underlying disease process

DISCHARGE CRITERIA

- Patients without hypoxia or a stable oxygen requirement
- Close follow-up as long as the underlying etiology has responded to acute management

Miscellaneous

ICD9: 415.0, 415.1, 416, 416.0, 416.1, 416.8, 416.9

ICD10: I27.9, I26.0

SUGGESTED READINGS

Arroliga AC, Matthay MA, Matthay RA. Pulmonary thromboembolism and other pulmonary vascular diseases. In: George RB, et al, eds. Chest medicine: essentials of pulmonary and critical care medicine, 3rd ed. Philadelphia: Lippincott Williams & Wilkins, 2000:251–255.

Braunwald E. Cor pulmonale. In: Braunwald E, et al, eds. Harrison's textbook of medicine, 15th ed. New York: McGraw-Hill, 2001:1355–1359.

McLaughlin VV, Rich S. Cor pulmonale. In: Braunwald E, et al, eds. Heart disease: a textbook of cardiovascular medicine, 6th ed. Philadelphia: WB Saunders, 2001:1936–1954.

Morrison LK, Harrison A, et al. Utility of a rapid B-natriuretic peptide assay in differentiating congestive heart failure from lung disease in patients presenting with dyspnea. J Am Coll Cardiol 2002;39(2):202–209.

Author: E. Jedd Roe

Corneal Abrasion

Clinical Presentation

SIGNS AND SYMPTOMS

- Severe ocular pain
- Tearing/ocular discharge
- Blepharospasm
- Foreign body sensation
- Photophobia
- Conjunctival injection
- Blurred vision
- Headache

MECHANISM/DESCRIPTION

- Traumatic desquamation of portions of the corneal epithelium
- Focal epithelial loss secondary to removal of corneal foreign body
- Previous corneal transplant, corneal surgery, or radial keratotomy
    - —Predispose patient to a more severe injury after minor trauma to eye

ETIOLOGY

- Contusive force
- Direct contact injury
    - —Human fingernail
    - —Branches
    - —Fingers/toes
    - —Hairbrushes/combs
    - —Sand/stones
    - —Metallic object
    - —Snow
    - —Pens/pencils
    - —Toys
    - —Activated charcoal
    - —Airbag deployment
- Mechanical action of eyelid
    - —Blinking or rubbing eye with loose foreign body
- Projectiles at high speeds (metal workers)
    - —Carefully examine for globe perforation
- Poorly fitting contact lens or prolonged use
    - —Extended-wear soft contact lenses increase infection rate 10–15% over daily-wear contact lenses

PEDIATRIC CONSIDERATIONS

- Signs and symptoms may differ
    - —Excessive crying
    - —Conjunctival erythema
    - —Tearing
    - —Eye rubbing
    - —Lid edema
    - —Grunting respiration
- Younger than 12 months
    - —Frequently no history of eye trauma
    - —Often no eye signs
- Older than 12 months
    - —More often will have history of minor eye trauma
    - —Positive eye signs
    - —No excessive crying
- Compression injuries to cornea associated with birth
    - —Localized edema
    - —Corneal clouding
    - —Clear within hours

Pre-Hospital

N/A

Diagnosis

ESSENTIAL WORKUP

- History
    - —Past ocular trauma
    - —Ocular/periocular surgery
    - —Preexisting visual impairment
    - —Glasses
    - —Contact lens use (extended wear has increased risk of corneal ulcer)
    - —Time of onset
    - —Associated symptoms
    - —Treatment before visit
    - —Use of safety glasses
    - —Systemic disease
- Complete eye exam
    - —Visual acuity
    - —Evert upper lids to check for retained foreign body
    - —Bright white light for visual inspection of cornea to rule out infiltrate/edema/loss of corneal luster
    - —Slit-lamp to evaluate anterior segment and depth of abrasion
    - —Fluorescein to identify area of damaged corneal epithelium

DIFFERENTIAL DIAGNOSIS

- Herpes simplex virus keratitis
- Recurrent corneal erosion syndrome
- Ultraviolet keratitis (snow blindness)
- Corneal ulcer
- Corneal dystrophy (inherited)
- More extensive injury than corneal abrasion
    - —Laceration of cornea
    - —Perforation of cornea
    - —Hyphema
    - —Iris prolapse
    - —Lens disruption

PEDIATRIC CONSIDERATIONS

- Hand-held slit-lamp and Wood's lamp: helpful in examination of pediatric eye

Treatment

INITIAL STABILIZATION

- Instill topical anesthetic (proparacaine/tetracaine)

ED TREATMENT

- Examination
- Removal of superficial foreign body
- Pain control (topical/oral)
  - —Diclofenac (topical)
  - —Ketorolac (topical)
  - —Oral narcotics
  - —Cool compresses
- Cycloplegic (optional)
  - —Cyclopentolate (mydriasis 1–2 days)
  - —Tropicamide (mydriasis 6 hours)
- Antibiotic ointment/drop options
  - —Ciprofloxacin
  - —Erythromycin
  - —Gentamicin
  - —Sulfacetamide
  - —Tobramycin
  - —Contact lens wearers must be covered for *Pseudomonas*
    - -Use aminoglycoside or quinolone
- Eye patch
  - —Controversial regarding efficacy
  - —No patch required for small abrasions
  - —Never patch contact lens–related injury
  - —Never patch infection prone injury
    - -Fingernail
    - -Vegetable matter
    - -Removal of wood particles
  - —Patch non–contact lens–related abrasions >10-mm^2 or recurrent corneal erosions
  - —Collagen shields/soft bandage contact lenses (currently under investigation)
- Disadvantages of patching
  - —Removes binocular vision/reduces visual field
  - —Uncomfortable
  - —Increases corneal temperature
  - —Decreases corneal oxygenation
  - —Slows reepithelialization
  - —Decrease tear exchange
  - —Prolongs healing
- Tetanus prophylaxis
  - —When contaminants include dirt, fecal material, or saliva
  - —Routine tetanus not necessary

MEDICATIONS

- Ciprofloxacin: 0.35% 1 gt q.i.d.
- Cyclopentolate: 0.5%, 1.0%, or 2.0% drops (mydriasis 1–2 gtt t.i.d.)
- Diclofenac: 0.1% drops 1 gt q.i.d.
- Erythromycin: 0.5% ointment q.i.d.
- Gentamicin: 0.3% ointment q.i.d.
- Gentamicin: 0.3% drops q6h
- Ketorolac: 0.5% drops 1 gt q.i.d.
- Proparacaine: 0.5% 1 gt
- Sulfacetamide: drops 10% q.i.d.
- Sulfacetamide: ointment 10% qid
- Tobramycin: 0.3% drops q6h
- Tobramycin: 0.3% ointment q6h
- Tropicamide: 0.5%, 1.0% drops (mydriasis 6 hours) 1 gt

PEDIATRIC CONSIDERATIONS

- Patching poorly tolerated

Disposition

ADMISSION CRITERIA

- Associated injuries requiring admission

DISCHARGE CRITERIA

- All simple corneal abrasions
- Follow-up in 24–48 hours with ophthalmologist for reexamination and ongoing care
- Follow-up with ED when access to specialist is limited

Miscellaneous

ICD9: 918.1

ICD10: S05.0

SEE ALSO: RED EYE

SUGGESTED READINGS

Aaron R, John C, eds. Office management of trauma. Clin Family Pract 2000;2(3).

Alteveer JG, McCans KM, eds. The red eye, the swollen eye, and acute visual loss. Emerg Med Pract 2002;4(6).

Arbour JD, Brunette I, Boisjoly HM, et al. Should we patch corneal erosions? Arch Ophthalmol 1997;115:313–317.

Brown MD, Cordell WH, Gee AS. Do ophthalmic nonsteroidal anti-inflammatory drugs reduce the pain associated with simple corneal abrasions without delayed healing? Ann Emerg Med 1999;34:526–534.

Donald TH, ed. Eye trauma: corneal abrasions. Pediatr Rev 1999;20(9).

Flynn CH, D'Amico F, Smith G. Should we patch corneal abrasions? A meta-analysis. J Family Pract 1998;47:264–270.

Kaiser PK, Pineda R. Corneal Abrasion Patching Study Group. A study of topical nonsteroidal anti-inflammatory drops and no pressure patching in the treatment of corneal abrasions. Ophthalmology 1997;104:1353–1359.

Le Sage N, Verreault R, Rochette LM. Efficacy of eye patching for traumatic corneal abrasions. Ann Emerg Med 2001;38:129–134.

Author: Kevin Kern

Corneal Burn

Clinical Presentation

SIGNS AND SYMPTOMS

- Severe ocular pain
- Photophobia
- Lacrimation
- Foreign body sensation
- Conjunctival injection
- Corneal edema
- Corneal opacification
- Impaired visual acuity
- Limbal blanching
- Lens opacification
- Vesicles clear fluid (hypothermal injury)
- Vesicles hemorrhagic fluid
- Necrosis of iris, ciliary body

MECHANISM/DESCRIPTION

- Inappropriate exposure of cornea to chemicals, heat, cold, electrical, or radiant energy causing damage to the cornea and often extending to adjacent structures
- Severity of injury related to duration of exposure, type of agent, anion concentration, pH level of solution
- Alkalis
  —Cause immediate rise in pH level
  —Highly soluble in lipid, so rapidly penetrate the eye causing severe corneal injury and continue to penetrate with time if no intervention
  —Penetration can occur in <1 minute
  —Exception: calcium alkalis penetrate relatively poorly secondary to SOAP formation; can cause corneal opacification, so may appear worse but actually have better prognosis than other alkali burns
- Acids
  —Immediately coagulate proteins of the corneal epithelium
  —Cause opacification
  —Coagulation produces a barrier to deeper penetration
  —Exception: the lipophilicity of HF acid causes it to act similar to a base with more rapid penetration
- Thermal burns
  —Cause direct injury to cornea
  —Damage primarily dependent on duration and intensity of heat
  —Globe often spared secondary to
    -Blinking
    -Bell's phenomenon (eyes roll up and outward)
    -Tears
    -Protective bony structure of the orbit
- Electrical injury
  —Occurs with current flow through the head, with input at or near the eye

ETIOLOGY

- Alkalis
  —Ammonia
    -Fertilizer, refrigerant, household ammonia, cleansing agents
  —Potassium hydroxide
    -Caustic potash
  —Magnesium hydroxide
    -Sparklers, flares, fireworks
  —Lye—NaOH
    -Caustic soda, drain cleaners
  —Lime—$CaOH_2$
    -Fresh lime, quicklime, calcium hydrate, slaked lime, hydrated lime, plaster, mortar, cement, whitewash
  —Nonspecific alkali
    -Motor vehicle airbag upon inflation releases alkali
- Acids
  —Sulfuric acid: H_2SO_4
    -Car battery acid
  —Sulfurous acid: H_2SO_3
    -Preservatives (fruit and vegetable), bleach, refrigerants
  —Hydrofluoric acid: HF
    -Used in etching silicon/glass, cleaning brick, electropolishing metals, control of fermentation in breweries, commercial/household rust removal
- Thermal
  —Hot liquids, molten metal
  —Flames
  —Hot smoke/gases
  —Flash burn
  —Steam
  —Cigarette burns

PEDIATRIC CONSIDERATIONS

- Consider child neglect or abuse

Pre-Hospital

CAUTIONS

- Irrigate at scene 15–30 minutes, unless other coexisting life-threatening conditions require immediate transfer
- Continuous irrigation en route to hospital with NS

Diagnosis

ESSENTIAL WORKUP

- History
  —Type of exposure
  —Duration of exposure
  —Time of onset
  —Time irrigation initiated
  —Preexisting visual impairment
  —Protective eyewear
  —Contact lens use
  —Treatment before arrival
- Complete eye exam (after irrigation)
  —Visual acuity
  —Bright white light for visual inspection of cornea/conjunctivae/limbus
  —Slit-lamp to evaluate anterior segment inflammation
  —Fluorescein to identify damaged corneal epithelium
  —Check for lenticular clarity
  —Fundus exam
  —Measure intraocular pressure (especially in delayed presentation)
  —Lid/eyelash exam
  —Check pH with acid/alkali burns with litmus paper or pH indicator on urine dipstick

DIFFERENTIAL DIAGNOSIS

- Infection
  —Viral keratitis
  —Corneal ulcer
- Corneal erosion syndrome
  —Corneal foreign body
  —Corneal abrasion
  —Hypothermal injury

PEDIATRIC CONSIDERATIONS

- Hand-held slit-lamp and Wood's lamp helpful in examination of pediatric eye

Treatment

INITIAL STABILIZATION

- Chemical exposure
  - —Irrigate with any available diluting substance but preferably water or NS
- Thermal exposure
  - —Cool moist dressing with overlying ice packs

ED TREATMENT

Chemical Exposure: Alkalis/Acids/Mace

- Continuous irrigation to achieve pH 7.3–7.5 (1–2 L via a Morgan lens over 30–60 minutes)
- pH should be evaluated at 5 and 30 minutes after irrigation to ensure normalization of pH
- Evaluate fornices in detail and eye in full range of motion to ensure removal of all particulate chemical substance
- Topical anesthetic (proparacaine)
- Examination
- Antibiotic prophylaxis for *Staphylococcus/Pseudomonas* until epithelialization is complete
  - —Gentamicin ointment plus erythromycin or
  - —Bacitracin
- Cycloplegics to minimize posterior synechiae formation
  - —Cyclopentolate 1%
  - —Atropine 1%
- Oral analgesics
- If increased intraocular pressure
  - —Immediate ophthalmologic consultation
  - —Administer acetazolamide 125 mg po q.i.d. and timolol 0.5% drops b.i.d.
- Topical steroids to control anterior uveitis (consult ophthalmology)
- Eye patch (consult ophthalmology)
- May require surgical intervention if frank corneal penetration
- Ophthalmologic consultation by phone in mild injuries
- Immediate ophthalmologic consultation in all moderate to severe injuries; if unavailable at your hospital, arrange transfer to closest eye center
- Hydrofluoric acid
  - —Treat as above, plus 1% calcium gluconate eyedrops
  - —Systemic analgesia × 24 hours

Thermal Exposure

- Frequent moist dressing changes
- Antibiotics drops q.i.d.
- Generous lubricant application
- Moisture chamber when extensive injury to eyelid
- Steroids (consult ophthalmologist; do not use for >1 week)

Electrical Injury

- Irrigation
- Wound care
- Antibiotic ointment
- Cycloplegic (if anterior uveitis)
- Analgesia

MEDICATIONS

- Artificial tears
- Atropine: 0.5%, 1.0%, 2.0% drops (cycloplegia 5–10 days, mydriasis 7–14 days) 1 gt t.i.d.
- Bacitracin ointment: q.i.d.
- Ciprofloxacin: 0.35% 1 gt q.i.d.
- Cyclopentolate: 0.5%, 1.0%, 2.0% drops (cycloplegia 1–2 days, mydriasis 1–2 days) 1 gt t.i.d.
- Erythromycin: 0.5% ointment q.i.d.
- Gentamicin: 0.3% ointment q.i.d.
- Gentamicin: 0.3% drops 1 gt q6h
- Proparacaine: 0.5% drops 1 gt
- Sulfacetamide: 10% ointment q.i.d.
- Sulfacetamide: 10% drops q.i.d.
- Tobramycin: 0.3% ointment q6h
- Tobramycin: 0.3% drops q6h
- Tropicamide: 0.5%, 1.0% drops (cycloplegia none; mydriasis 6 hours) 1 gt

PEDIATRIC CONSIDERATIONS

- Patching poorly tolerated
- May require systemic analgesia for complete examination

Disposition

ADMISSION CRITERIA

- Intractable pain
- Increased intraocular pressure
- Corneal penetration requiring immediate surgical intervention
- Hydrofluoric acid burn, admit for 24 hours of systemic analgesia
- Suspected child abuse

DISCHARGE CRITERIA

- All mild corneal burns
- Mandatory follow-up with ophthalmologist in 12–24 hours; arrange before patient discharge

Miscellaneous

ICD9: 940.4, 940.3, 940.2

ICD10: T26.1

SEE ALSO: CORNEAL ABRASION; RED EYE

SUGGESTED READINGS

Bouchard CS, Morno K, Perkins J, et al. Ocular complications of thermal injury. J Trauma 2001;50:79–82.

Hooper M. Prompt treatment for chemical eye injuries. Nursing Standard 1997;11:40–43.

Lipshy KA, Wheeler WE, Denning DE. Ophthalmic thermal injuries. Am Surg 1996;62(6):481–483.

Markoff DD, Chacko D, eds. Ophthalmologic emergencies. In: Emergency medicine reports textbook of adult and pediatric emergency medicine. Atlanta: American Health Consultants, 2000:1011–1021.

Michel FK, Sulewski ME. Focused assessment of the patient with eye trauma: the essentials. Topics Emerg Med 2000;22:1–8.

Watts DD, Kokiko J. Air bags and eye injuries: assessment and treatment. J Emerg Nursing 1999;25:572–574.

Author: Kevin Kern

Corneal Foreign Body

Clinical Presentation

SIGNS AND SYMPTOMS

- Foreign body sensation
- Eye pain
- Conjunctiva and sclera injection
- Tearing
- Blurred or decreased vision
- Photophobia
- Visible foreign body or rust ring
- Iritis

MECHANISM/DESCRIPTION

- Common complaint: something fell, flew, or otherwise landed in my eye
- Hot, high-speed projectiles may not produce pain initially
- Corneal epithelium disrupted
  —Abrasion if only epithelium disrupted
  —Scar if deeper layers of cornea involved

ETIOLOGY

- Poorly tolerated
  —Organic material (plant material, insect parts)
  —Inorganic material that oxidizes (iron, copper)
- Well tolerated
  —Inert objects (paint, glass, plastic, fiberglass, nonoxidizing metals)

Pre-Hospital

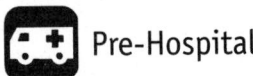

- Place a Fox shield and position the patient upright

Diagnosis

ESSENTIAL WORKUP

- Injury history to determine type of foreign body and likelihood of perforation
- Complete eye exam
  —Visual acuity
  —Visual fields
  —Extraocular movements
  —Lids and lashes
  —Pupils
  —Sclera
  —Conjunctiva
  —Fundi
  —Slit-lamp
  —Fluorescein exam
  —Intraocular pressure if no evidence of perforation

IMAGING/SPECIAL TESTS

- Ocular CT or B-mode US when suspect intraocular foreign body

DIFFERENTIAL DIAGNOSIS

- Conjunctival foreign body
- Corneal abrasion
- Corneal perforation with or without intraocular foreign body
- Corneal ulcer
- Keratitis

PEDIATRIC CONSIDERATIONS

- May require sedation to facilitate exam and foreign body removal

Treatment

INITIAL STABILIZATION

- Apply topical anesthetic to stop eye discomfort and assist in examination

ED TREATMENT

- Deep foreign bodies
  —Refer those penetrating Bowman's membrane (next layer under epithelium) to an ophthalmologist, because permanent scarring may occur
- Superficial foreign bodies
  —Irrigation removal technique
    -Apply topical anesthetic
    -Try to wash foreign body off cornea by directing a stream of 0.9% NS at an oblique angle to cornea
  —25-gauge needle or FB Spud removal technique
    -Using slit-lamp to immobilize patient's head and allow good visualization
    -Hold needle (bevel up) with thumb and forefinger allowing other fingers to be stabilized on the patient's cheek
    -Lift foreign body off cornea keeping needle parallel to corneal surface
- Rust rings removal
  —Within 3 hours, iron-containing foreign bodies oxidize, leaving a rust stain on adjacent epithelial cells
  —Removal recommended as rust rings delay healing and act as an irritant focus
  —Remove with needle or pothook burr either at same time as foreign body or delayed 24 hours

- Postremoval therapy
  - —Treat resultant corneal abrasion with antibiotic drops
  - —Initiate cycloplegic agent when suspect presence of keratitis
  - —Update tetanus
  - —Initiate analgesia (NSAID or acetaminophen with codeine)

MEDICATIONS

- Cyclopentolate 1–2%: 1 drop t.i.d. (lasts up to 2 days)
- Gentamicin ophthalmic: 2 drops q6h
- Homatropine 2% or 5%: 1 drop q.d. (lasts up to 3 days)
- Sulfacetamide 10%: 1 drop q6h
- Tobramycin ophthalmic: 2 drops q6h

Disposition

ADMISSION CRITERIA

- Globe penetration

DISCHARGE CRITERIA

- All corneal foreign bodies
- Ophthalmologist follow-up in 24 hours for
  - —Rust ring removal
  - —Vegetative material removal due to risk of ulceration

Miscellaneous

ICD9: 930.9

ICD10: T15.0

SUGGESTED READINGS

Kaiser P. A comparison of pressure patching versus no patching for corneal abrasions due to trauma or foreign body removal. Ophthalmology 1995;102(12): 1936–1942.

Newel F. Ophthalmology principles and concepts, 8th ed. St. Louis: Mosby-Year Book, 1996:184–185.

Rhee D, Pyfer M. The Wills eye manual: office and emergency room diagnosis and treatment of eye disease, 3rd ed. Philadelphia: Lippincott Williams & Wilkins, 1999:24–26.

Santen S, Scott J. Ophthalmologic procedures. Emerg Med Clin North Am 1995;13(3):681–694.

Author: David A. Harter

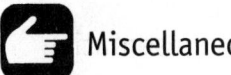

Cough

Clinical Presentation

SIGNS AND SYMPTOMS

- Sputum production
  - —Frothy (pulmonary edema)
  - —Mucopurulent
    - -Suggestive of bacterial pneumonia or bronchitis but also seen with viral infections
  - —Rust colored (pneumococcal pneumonia)
  - —"Currant jelly" (*Klebsiella* pneumonia)
  - —Hemoptysis
- Posttussive syncope or emesis (suggests pertussis)
- Shortness of breath
- Chest pain
- Chills/fever
- Night sweats
- Wheezing
- GERD
  - —Heartburn
  - —Dysphagia
  - —Regurgitation
  - —Belching
  - —Early satiety
- Malignancy
  - —Weight loss
  - —Poor appetite
  - —Fatigue

MECHANISM/DESCRIPTION

- Deep inspiration, glottis closes, expiratory muscles contract, intrapulmonary pressures increase, glottis opens, air expiration at high pressure, secretion and foreign material excretion, vocal cord vibration with tracheobronchial walls, lung parenchyma and secretions
- Defense mechanism to clear the airway of foreign material and secretions
  - —Voluntary or involuntary
  - —Reflex involves respiratory tissue receptor activation of afferent neurons to the central cough center followed by efferent output to the respiratory muscles
  - —Mechanical receptors in larynx, trachea, and carina sense touch and displacement
  - —Chemical receptors in larynx and bronchi are sensitive to gases and fumes
  - —Activated by irritants, mucus, edema, pus, thermal stimuli

ETIOLOGY

- Acute: <3 weeks
  - —Common cold
  - —Bacterial sinusitis
  - —Allergic rhinitis
  - —Environmental irritant rhinitis
  - —Pertussis
  - —Exacerbation of COPD
  - —Pneumonia
  - —Left ventricular failure
  - —Asthma
- Subacute: 3–8 weeks
  - —Postinfectious cough
  - —Bacterial sinusitis
  - —Asthma
- Chronic: >8 weeks
  - —Postnasal drip
  - —Asthma
  - —GERD
  - —Chronic bronchitis
  - —Bronchiectasis
  - —Eosinophilic bronchitis
  - —ACE inhibitor use
  - —Bronchogenic carcinoma
  - —Carcinomatosis
  - —Sarcoidosis
  - —Left ventricular failure
  - —Aspiration syndrome
  - —Psychogenic/habit

Pre-Hospital

CAUTIONS

- Oxygen
- Airway management if massive hemoptysis
- Respiratory precautions if suspect tuberculosis
- Bronchodilators if suspect asthma/reactive airway disease

Diagnosis

ESSENTIAL WORKUP

- Complete medical history
  - —Duration
  - —Associated symptoms
  - —Smoking exposure
  - —ACE inhibitor use
  - —HIV/immunocompromised state
  - —Potential exposure to tuberculosis
- Physical exam
  - —Vital signs
  - —Evidence of respiratory distress
    - -Use of accessory muscles
    - -Abdominal breathing

LABORATORY

- Order according to presenting signs and symptoms
  - —WBC count with differential
  - —Sputum Gram stain, cultures, and sensitivities
  - —AFB culture
  - —CD4 count
  - —Pertussis titers

IMAGING/SPECIAL TESTS

- CXR
  - —For immunosuppressed patient
  - —Abnormal lung sounds on exam
  - —Ill appearing
  - —Change in chronic cough
  - —Continued cough after discontinuation of ACE inhibitor
- EKG
  - —History of cardiac disease
  - —Associated chest pain or abnormal vital signs
  - —Lack of infectious symptoms
- Bronchoscopy
  - —For unknown mass on CXR
  - —Hemoptysis
  - —Suspected cancer
- Peak flow

DIFFERENTIAL DIAGNOSIS

See Etiology

PEDIATRIC CONSIDERATIONS

- Most frequent causes
  - —Asthma
  - —Sinusitis
  - —GERD
- Less common causes
  - —Tracheobronchomalacia
  - —Mediastinal tumor
  - —Acyanotic congenital heart disease
  - —Ventricular septal defect
  - —PDA
  - —Pulmonary stenosis
  - —Tetralogy of Fallot
  - —Lodged foreign body
  - —Chronic aspiration of milk
  - —Environmental exposure

- Consider
  - —Neonatal history
  - —Feeding history
  - —Growth and developmental history
  - —Allergies
  - —Eczema
  - —Sleep disorders
- Indications for CXR
  - —Suspicion of foreign body ingestion
  - —Suspect aspiration

Treatment

INITIAL STABILIZATION

- Assess airway, breathing, and circulation

ED TREATMENT

- Specific treatment related to cause
  - —Respiratory infection: consider antibiotics, decongestants, and antitussives
  - —Asthma: inhaled β_2-agonist and steroid
  - —GERD: H_2-blockers, proton pump inhibitors, and antacids
  - —Malignancy: supportive care

MEDICATIONS

- Antitussives
  - —Benzonatate (Tessalon Perles): 100–200 mg PO q6h
  - —Codeine: 10–20 mg (peds: 1–1.5 mg/kg/d) PO q4–6h
  - —Dextromethorphan: 10–20 mg (peds: 1 mg/kg/d) PO q6–8h
  - —Hydrocodone: 5–10 mg (peds: 0.6 mg/kg/d q6–8 h) PO q6–8h
- Bronchodilators
  - —Albuterol: 2.5 mg in 2.5 NS (peds: 0.1–0.15 mg/kg/dose every 20 minutes) every 20 minutes inhaled
  - —Ipratropium: 0.5 mg in 3 mL NS (peds: nebulizer 250–500 μg/dose q6h) q.h. $\times$ 3
- Decongestants
  - —Chlorpheniramine: 4–12 mg (peds: 2 mg PO q4–6h) PO q4–12h
  - —Phenylpropanolamine: 25–50 mg (peds: 6.25–12.5 mg PO q4h) PO q4–8h
- Mucolytics
  - —Guaifenesin: 5–20 mL (peds: 5–10 mL/dose if older than 6 years; 2.5–5 mL/dose if younger than 6 years) PO q4h
- Steroids
  - —Dexamethasone: 2 sprays/nostril b.i.d.
  - —Methylprednisolone: 60–125 mg i.v. (peds: 1–2 mg/kg/dose i.v./PO q6h)
  - —Prednisone: 40–60 mg (peds: 1–2 mg/kg/d q6–12h) PO

Disposition

ADMISSION CRITERIA

- Hypoxemia or critical illness
- Suspected tuberculosis with positive CXR result
- Immunocompromised with fever
- Risk of bacteremia or sepsis

DISCHARGE CRITERIA

- Oxygenation at baseline for patient
- Oral medications
- Safe environment at home

Miscellaneous

ICD9: 786.2

ICD10: R05

SUGGESTED READINGS

Irwin RS. Managing cough as a defense mechanism and as a symptom. Chest 1998;114(2):133S–181S.

Irwin RS. Primary care: the diagnosis and treatment of cough. N Engl J Med 2000;343(23):1715–1721.

Author: Alison Sisitsky

Croup

Clinical Presentation

SIGNS AND SYMPTOMS

- Nonspecific upper respiratory prodrome with or without fever
- Barking cough
- Hoarse voice
- Inspiratory stridor
- Accessory muscle use
- May progress to respiratory distress/failure

MECHANISM/DESCRIPTION

- Viral infection of the upper and lower respiratory tract
  - —Laryngotracheitis/laryngotracheobronchitis
  - —Inspiratory stridor due to extrathoracic airway obstruction
  - —Expiratory wheeze suggests lower airway involvement
  - —Inflammatory edema of subglottic region
  - —Narrowest part of pediatric airway
- Most commonly presents in children 6 months to 3 years
- Spasmodic croup
  - —Sudden onset at night without viral prodrome
  - —Consistent response to mist or cool night air
  - —Often recurrent
  - —May represent allergic reaction to viral antigen

ETIOLOGY

- Parainfluenza types 1, 2, and 3
- Influenza A and B
- Adenoviruses
- Respiratory syncytial virus
- Measles
- *Mycoplasma pneumoniae*
- Herpes simplex

Pre-Hospital

- Allow child to assume position of comfort
- Blow-by humidified oxygen
- Nebulized epinephrine after consulting medical control for severe distress

CAUTIONS

- Do not remove parent from child
- Avoid scary or painful procedures
  - —IV access
  - —Mask oxygen

Diagnosis

ESSENTIAL WORKUP

- History
  - —Prior intubation, duration of illness, previous episodes, immunization status
- Physical exam
  - —Mental status, stridor at rest, work of breathing, preferred position, hydration status, toxicity, drooling
- Westley Croup Score (maximum total points: 17)
  - —Stridor
    - -0 = None
    - -1 = Audible with stethoscope at rest
    - -2 = Audible without stethoscope at rest
  - —Retractions
    - -0 = None
    - -1 = Mild
    - -2 = Moderate
    - -3 = Severe
  - —Air entry
    - -0 = Normal
    - -1 = Decreased
    - -2 = Severely decreased
  - —Cyanosis
    - -0 = None
    - -4 = With agitation
    - -5 = At rest
  - —Level of consciousness
    - -0 = Normal
    - -5 = Altered

LABORATORY

- Pulse oximetry
- Other tests are not routinely indicated

IMAGING/SPECIAL TESTS

- AP and lateral neck radiographs
  - —"Steeple sign" indicates narrowing of subglottic trachea
  - —Not routinely indicated, unless atypical presentation or clinical course
  - —Subject to misinterpretation
  - —Should not delay definitive visualization and intubation in OR in child with concern for epiglottitis

DIFFERENTIAL DIAGNOSIS

- Infection
  - —Epiglottitis
  - —Bacterial tracheitis
  - —Peritonsillar abscess
  - —Retropharyngeal abscess
  - —Diphtheria
- Congenital airway anomaly
  - —Laryngomalacia
- Angioedema
- Vocal cord paralysis
- Acquired subglottic stenosis
- Foreign body (airway or esophageal)
- Thermal injury to upper airway
- Hemangioma
- Laryngeal papillomatosis

Treatment

INITIAL STABILIZATION

- Allow child to maintain position of comfort
- Defer interventions that distress child
  - —IV access
  - —IM injections
  - —Radiographs
- If severe distress
  - —Immediate nebulized epinephrine with humidified oxygen

ED TREATMENT

- Humidified O_2 (mist) (limited evidence of efficacy)
- Dexamethasone
  - —Decreases severity of disease
  - —Indicated in patients with stridor at rest and those receiving epinephrine
- Nebulized racemic epinephrine or L-epinephrine if any distress or stridor at rest
  - —L-epinephrine containing only the active isomer; has been shown to be therapeutically equivalent to racemic epinephrine
- If poor response to nebulized racemic epinephrine or L-epinephrine
  - —Consider trial of heliox
- Heliox, when available, has been used to decrease the work of breathing in patients with an incomplete response to epinephrine
- If impending or existing respiratory failure despite aforementioned therapy
  - —Tracheal intubation by most experienced person available
  - —Use uncuffed ETT 0.5 to 1.0 mm smaller than usual size
- Suspected epiglottitis
  - —To OR for inhalational anesthesia
  - —Direct laryngoscopy and intubation
  - —Surgeon standing by for emergent tracheostomy

MEDICATIONS

- Antibiotics: not indicated
- Dexamethasone: single dose of 0.6 mg/kg (max 10 mg) PO (use crushed tablet with flavored syrup) i.v. or i.m.; doses as low as 0.15 mg/kg may be effective
- Heliox (70% helium: 30% oxygen mixture administered via face mask or tent house)
- L-epinephrine 1:1,000: 5 mL (5 mg) nebulized
- Racemic epinephrine 2.25%: 0.25–0.5 mL nebulized in 2.5 mL NS

Disposition

ADMISSION CRITERIA

- Very young infants, preexisting upper airway obstruction
- Persistent stridor at rest unresponsive to nebulized epinephrine *or*
- Recurrent stridor 3–4 hours after initial treatment with epinephrine and dexamethasone
- PICU
  - —Persistent severe obstruction
  - —Need for frequent epinephrine treatments and/or heliox
  - —Tracheal intubation with assisted ventilation

DISCHARGE CRITERIA

- Normal oxygenation in room air
- No stridor at rest after brief observation *or*
- No recurrent stridor 3–4 hours after nebulized epinephrine
- Reliable caretaker, communication, transport

Miscellaneous

ICD9: 464.4

ICD10: J05.0

SUGGESTED READINGS

Ausejo M, et al. The effectiveness of glucocorticoids in treating croup: meta-analysis. BMJ 1999:595–600.

Ledwith CA, Shea LM, Mauro RD. Safety and efficacy of nebulized racemic epinephrine in conjunction with oral dexamethasone and mist in the outpatient treatment of croup. Ann Emerg Med 1995;25: 331–337.

Rittichier KK, Ledwith CA. Outpatient treatment of moderate croup with dexamethasone: intramuscular versus oral dosing. Pediatrics 2000;106:1344–1348.

Waisman Y, Klein BL, Boenning DA, et al. Prospective randomized double-blind study comparing L-epinephrine and racemic epinephrine aerosols in the treatment of laryngotracheitis (croup). Pediatrics 1992;89:302–306.

Weber JE, Chudnofsky CR, Younger JG, et al. A randomized comparison of helium-oxygen mixture (heliox) and racemic epinephrine for the treatment of moderate to severe croup. Pediatrics 2001;107:e96.

Author: Dale Steele

Cushing's Syndrome

Clinical Presentation

SIGNS AND SYMPTOMS

- Diagnosis suggested by
  - —*Abnormal fat deposition* with Moon facies
  - —Buffalo hump
  - —Central obesity with thin extremities
  - —Supraclavicular fat deposition: these findings raise suspicion in a stressed patient of potentially developing *Addisonian crisis*
- Hypokalemia while not on diuretic therapy
- Cardiovascular
  - —Uncontrolled hypertension
  - —Myocardial infarction
- Neurologic
  - —Atherosclerotic or embolic stroke
  - —Pseudotumor cerebri (primarily with exogenous glucocorticoid administration)
  - —Spinal lipomatosis with cord or nerve-root compression
- Gastroenterologic
  - —Peptic ulcers
  - —GI hemorrhage
  - —Pancreatitis (primarily with exogenous glucocorticoid administration)
  - —Fatty liver
- Psychiatric
  - —*Toxic psychosis*
  - —Mood disorders (40%)
  - —Depression
  - —Memory impairment
  - —Euphoria
- Musculoskeletal
  - —Myopathy (proximal weakness)
  - —Pathologic fractures
  - —Osteoporosis
  - —Aseptic necrosis humeral or femoral heads (primarily with exogenous glucocorticoid administration)
  - —Delayed bone age
- Endocrine
  - —Glucose intolerance
  - —Hyperlipidemia
  - —Amenorrhea, female with male pattern balding, or hirsutism
- Hematologic
  - —Increased neutrophils
  - —Decreased lymphocytes and eosinophils
  - —Opportunistic infections
- Ophthalmologic
  - —Cataracts (primarily with exogenous glucocorticoid administration)
  - —Glaucoma (primarily with exogenous glucocorticoid administration)
- Dermatologic
  - —Purple striae >1 cm in diameter
  - —Hyperpigmentation (if excess ACTH production)
  - —Facial plethora
  - —Thin skin
  - —Impaired wound healing
  - —Ecchymoses
  - —Acne
  - —Hyperhidrosis

MECHANISM/DESCRIPTION

- Cushing's disease: pituitary adenoma producing excess ACTH
- Cushing's syndrome: excessive glucocorticoid effects

ETIOLOGY

- Most commonly exogenous administration of glucocorticoids either therapeutically or surreptitiously
- Pituitary adenoma secreting ACTH
- Adrenal production of cortisol from adenoma, carcinoma, or micronodular disease
- Tumor-producing ectopic ACTH
  - —Small cell lung carcinoma (most common)
  - —Uterine cervical carcinoma
  - —Islet cell tumor of pancreas (MEA I-type syndrome)
  - —Medullary thyroid cancer
  - —Pheochromocytoma
  - —Ganglioneuroma
  - —Melanoma prostate carcinoma
  - —Carcinoid tumor (lung, pancreas, GI tract, thymus, or ovary)

PEDIATRIC CONSIDERATIONS

- Suspect if increasing in obesity while falling off in height on the growth chart

Pre-Hospital

CAUTIONS

- Acute addisonian crisis under stress may develop with iatrogenic Cushing's syndrome
- Patients may have extremely labile behavior
- Cause of death in untreated Cushing's syndrome is
  - —Infection
  - —Stroke
  - —Myocardial infarction
  - —Suicide

Diagnosis

ESSENTIAL WORKUP

- Cannot confirm diagnosis in ED
- Anticipate impending addisonian crisis
  - —Most frequent and common problem with Cushing's syndrome is its recognition in patient with intercurrent illness to prevent acute *addisonian crisis*
- Search for life-threatening conditions
  - —Myocardial infarction
  - —Stroke
  - —Sepsis
  - —Pathologic fracture
  - —Uncontrolled DM
  - —Psychiatric emergency necessitating admission

LABORATORY

- Electrolytes, BUN, Cr, glucose
  - —Hypokalemia
  - —10% with metabolic alkalosis
  - —Diminished glucose tolerance (75%)
    - -50% have glycosuria
    - -20% overt DM
- CBC
  - —Increased WBCs
  - —Decreased eosinophils

IMAGING/SPECIAL TESTS

- EKG for myocardial ischemia
- CXR for tumor-causing ectopic ACTH
- Plain films if suspect possible pathologic fractures

Nonemergent Testing

- MRI for pituitary tumor
- CT for adrenal carcinoma, adenoma, or hyperplasia
- Dexamethasone-suppression test (follow-up study with primary physician)
  - —If suspicion of endogenous Cushing's syndrome exists
  - —Screening test: 1 mg at 11:00 p.m. with an 8 a.m. cortisol level drawn
    - -Low specificity
    - -Decrease false-positive results by stopping alcohol, estrogens, spironolactone, phenytoin, and barbiturates
  - —High-dose dexamethasone-suppression test needed to confirm the diagnosis
    - -2 mg q.i.d. of dexamethasone with cortisol level 6 hours later
    - -Compare day 2 urine-free cortisol and 17-hydroxyketosteroids with baseline levels

DIFFERENTIAL DIAGNOSIS

- Alcohol-induced pseudo-Cushing's syndrome
- Obesity
- Psychiatric states
  - —Depression
  - —Obsessive-compulsive disorder
  - —Panic disorder
- Physiologic states
  - —Chronic stress
  - —Third-trimester pregnancy
  - —Chronic strenuous exercise
- Malnutrition

Treatment

INITIAL STABILIZATION

- Initiate treatment for associated complications
  - —Myocardial infarction
  - —Stroke
  - —Psychiatric stabilization

ED TREATMENT

- IV rehydration/glucose-lowering agents for hyperglycemia
- Appropriate cultures and antibiotics for suspected infection
- Antihypertensive agents for uncontrolled BP
- Administer steroids (hydrocortisone) with iatrogenic Cushing's if patient under stress to prevent addisonian crisis
- Medications to lower cortisol levels (bromocriptine, ketoconazole, aminoglutamide, metapyrone)
  - —Used rarely with severe symptoms in patients awaiting surgery
  - —Institute under the direction of an endocrinologist

Definitive Therapy

- Iatrogenic
  - —Taper steroids as rapidly as possible
  - —Calcium, vitamin D, and estrogen supplementation if possible
- Pituitary Cushing's
  - —Transsphenoidal surgery
  - —Radiation for surgical failures and a few select patients
- Adrenal adenoma/carcinoma
  - —Adrenal resection with medical therapy for metastatic lesions not resectable
- Ectopic ACTH
  - —Tumor resection (if possible) with medical therapy for metastatic lesions not resectable

MEDICATIONS

- Hydrocortisone: 100–200 mg (peds: 1–2 mg/kg) IVP

Disposition

ADMISSION CRITERIA

- Complications that require admission such as
  - —Myocardial infarction
  - —Stroke
  - —Sepsis
  - —Pathologic fracture
  - —Uncontrolled DM
  - —Psychiatric emergency
- Impending addisonian crisis

DISCHARGE CRITERIA

- Well-appearing, stable patient without admission criteria

Miscellaneous

ICD9: 255.0

ICD10: E24.9

SEE ALSO: ADRENAL INSUFFICIENCY

SUGGESTED READINGS

Goldman L, Bennett JC, eds. Cecil's textbook of medicine, 21st ed. Philadelphia: WB Saunders, 2000.

Marx JA, Hockenberger RS, Walls RM, et al, eds. Rosen's emergency medicine, 5th ed. Philadelphia: Mosby, 2002.

Wallach J, ed. Interpretation of diagnostic tests, 7th ed. Boston: Little, Brown and Company, 2000.

Author: Hugh Schuckman

Clinical Presentation

SIGNS AND SYMPTOMS

- Dermal exposure: standard decontamination
- Oral exposure: can be caustic, 50 mg has caused death
- Inhalational exposure
  - —50 parts/min causes anxiety, palpitations, dyspnea, headache
  - —100 parts/min results in death after 30 minutes
- Heart and brain—most sensitive organs—first to show manifestation of toxicity

CNS

- Headache
- Confusion
- Syncope
- Seizures
- Coma

Cardiovascular

- Dyspnea
- Chest pain
- Cardiorespiratory collapse and death

Other

- Nausea/vomiting

MECHANISM/DESCRIPTION

- Toxicity through inhalation, dermal, or GI tract absorption
- Intracellular toxin that inhibits aerobic metabolism through interruption of oxidative phosphorylation
  - —Leads to decreased O_2 utilization and ATP production
- Inhibits antioxidant defense enzymes; contributes to oxidative damage
- Stimulates neurotransmitter release in CNS/PNS

Cyanide Detoxification

- Rhodanese: a hepatic mitochondrial enzyme responsible for the metabolism
  - —Combines cyanide (CN) with sulfur (rate-limiting step) covalently (irreversible) to form a less toxic and water-soluble thiocyanate (T-CN)
  - —Forms less toxic reversible cyanhemoglobin when combined with hemoglobin (Fe^{2+})
  - —Forms nontoxic cyanocobalamin (B_{12}) when combined with hydroxocobalamin (B_{12a})
  - —Rate of CN removal requires adequate bioavailability of sulfur compounds (thiosulfate [TS])

ETIOLOGY

- Fires
  - —Combustion by product of natural and synthetic products
- Vehicle exhaust
- Industry
  - —Metal plating
  - —Chemical synthesis
  - —Plastic manufacturing
  - —Pesticides
- Solvents
  - —Artificial nail remover
  - —Metal polishes
- Byproduct of nitroprusside metabolism (nonenzymatic)
- Byproduct of *Pseudomonas aeruginosa* and pyocyaneus infections
- Amygdalin (converted by intestinal flora to CN)-containing plants (apricot and peach pits, apple and pear seeds, and cassava)

Pre-Hospital

CAUTIONS

- Remove the source of CN
- Prevent others from becoming contaminated
- Remove and bag all contaminated clothing and wash affected areas copiously with soap and water

Diagnosis

ESSENTIAL WORKUP

- History of exposure (not routinely available)
- Clinical clues (frequently absent)
  - —Peculiar odor of bitter almonds
  - —Bright red (arterialization) retinal vessels
  - —Abrupt onset and/or deteriorating toxic effects
  - —Lactic acidosis
  - —High venous O_2 saturation (due to blocked O_2 consumption); arterialization of venous blood gases

LABORATORY

- CBC
- Electrolytes, BUN, Cr, glucose
  - —Anion gap acidosis
- Liver profile
- CPK
- Carboxyhemoglobin (CO) level
- Methemoglobin (MH) level
- CN level
  - —Support the clinical diagnosis if performed in a timely fashion
  - —Analyze sample immediately after venipuncture because CN *in vitro* production and transformation are both time and temperature dependent
  - —Levels >0.5–1 mg/L: toxic
  - —Levels 2.5–3.0 mg/L: fatal
- Thiocyanate level
- Blood gas determinations
  - —Increased arterial saturation gap (calculated direct [measure] O_2 saturation [cooximeter])
  - —Elevated mixed venous O_2: MvO_2 (normal about 35–40)
  - —Elevated mixed venous O_2 saturation (cooximeter): $SmvO_2$ (normal about 75%)
  - —Decreased arteriovenous O_2 difference: AVO_2D (normal about 3–4.8 mL/dL)
- Elevated lactate level >8 mmol/L

IMAGING/SPECIAL TESTS

- Cyanomethemoglobin level
- Acetoacetate level
- β-Hydroxybutyrate level (normal about −0.3 μmol/L)
- Pyruvate level

DIFFERENTIAL DIAGNOSIS

- Carbon monoxide
- Hydrogen sulfide
- Methemoglobinemia (MH)
- Sulfhemoglobinemia
- Inert gases "asphyxiants"
- Causes of high anion gap metabolic acidosis

Treatment

Initial Stabilization

- ABCs
- Administer 100% oxygen
  - —Even in presence of normal PaO_2
  - —Acts synergistically with antidotes
- Gastric decontamination for oral ingestions if within 1 hour
  - —Perform gastric lavage and administer activated charcoal (AC) if ingestion of CN or CN-containing products and no contraindications
  - —Do not induce emesis

ED TREATMENT

Cyanide Antidote Kit

- Administer if manifesting significant CN toxicity with persistent high anion gap metabolic acidosis and a narrow arteriovenous O_2 difference
- Administration often instituted empirically; CN levels not immediately available
- Contents: amyl nitrite pearls, sodium nitrite, and TS
- Nitrite action
  - —Induce a CN-scavenging MH by oxidizing hemoglobin (Fe^{2+} to Fe^{3+}), which attracts extracellular CN away from the mitochondria-forming CN-MH, which is less toxic
  - —Do not administer empirically or prophylactically
- TS action
  - —Substrate for the enzyme rhodanase
  - —Combines with CN to form a less toxic T-CN
  - —May administer empirically
- Use clinical response and not methemoglobin levels to guide nitrite administration
- Side effects of nitrites
  - —Hypotension (nitrite-induced vasodilation)
  - —MH
    - -Does not function as O_2 transporter
    - -Impairs oxygen delivery
    - -Elevated level leads to further tissue hypoxia

Hydroxocobalamin (B_{12a})

- Alternate safe antidote
- Binds to CN
  - —Forms nontoxic cyanocobalamin (B_{12}); renally excreted
- Advantages
  - —No methemoglobin induction
  - —Does not cause hypotension
- Limitations
  - —Large amount needed to successfully treat poisoned patients (50 g B_{12a}:1 g CN)
  - —Use of TS combined with B_{12a} may reduce the amount of B_{12a} required

Combined TS and B_{12a} Therapy

- Victims of smoke inhalation may have combination of
  - —CN toxicity
  - —MH
  - —CO toxicity
- Avoid further reduction in oxygen transport; initially treat with TS and/or B_{12a} until the CO and MH levels are known

Hyperbaric Oxygen Therapy

- Maximizes tissue oxygenation despite toxic MH level
- Employ as adjunct to aforementioned antidotes in severe cases or when antidotes have failed

Antidote Alternatives

- Not yet FDA approved
- Do not institute empirically due to toxicity
- Dicobalt edetate
  - —Inactivates CN by chelation
  - —Associated with hypertension, dysrhythmias, and metabolic acidosis
- Dimethylaminophenol
  - —Induces a much faster scavenging MH
  - —Nephrotoxic

MEDICATIONS

- AC: 1–2 g/kg PO
- Hydroxocobalamin (B_{12a})
  - —Dose equivalent to 50 times the amount of CN exposure infused in 30 minutes
  - —Empiric single dose, 4–5 g (50 mg/kg) i.v. in D5W
  - —Prophylactic i.v. infusion at 25 mg/h in Nipride usage

Cyanide Antidote Kit (Eli Lilly Antidote Kit)

- Amyl nitrite pearls
  - —Crush 1–2 ampules in gauze and hold close to the nose, in the lip of the face mask, or within the Ambu bag
  - —Inhale for 30 sec/min until IV access obtained
- N-nitrite ($NaNO_2$): 10 mL (300 mg) (peds: 0.19–0.33 mL/kg) i.v. as 3% solution over 5–20 minutes
  - —May repeat once at one-half dose within 30–60 minutes
  - —Keep MH level $<30\%$
  - —Dilute; infuse slowly if hypotensive
- N-thiosulfate: 50 mL (12.5 g) (peds: 0.95–1.95 mL/kg) i.v. over 10–15 minutes of a 25% solution
  - —Half the initial dose may be given after 30–60 minutes

Disposition

ADMISSION CRITERIA

- ICU admission

DISCHARGE CRITERIA

- Asymptomatic patients after at least 4 hours of observation
- Survival after 4 hours of an acute exposure usually associated with complete recovery

Miscellaneous

ICD9: 989.0

ICD10: T65.0

SUGGESTED READINGS

Baud F, Borron S, Megarbane B, et al. Lactic acidosis in cyanide poisoning: pathophysiology and clinical considerations. J Toxicol Clin Toxicol 2001;39:244.

Eyer P. Therapeutic implications of the toxicokinetics and toxicodynamics in cyanide poisoning. J Toxicol Clin Toxicol 2000;38(2):212–214.

Ford M, Delaney K, Ling L, et al. Clinical toxicology, 1st ed. Philadelphia: WB Saunders, 2001:705–711.

Leikin J, Paloucek F. Leikin and Paloucek's poisoning and toxicology handbook, 3rd ed. Lexi-Corp Inc, 2002:424–426, 665.

Author: Kirk Cumpston

Cyanosis

Clinical Presentation

SIGNS AND SYMPTOMS

- A bluish color of the skin and mucous membranes
  - —Chocolate color
    - -Methemoglobinemia
  - —Slate gray color
    - -Methemoglobinemia or sulfhemoglobin
  - —Varies based on skin thickness or pigment
- Central or generalized
  - —Visible in lips, nailbeds, ears, or malar regions
- Peripheral or local cyanosis
  - —Limited to extremities
- Differential cyanosis
  - —Lower extremities involved but upper extremities spared
- Clubbing
- Dyspnea
- Fatigue
- Headache
- Occupational exposure or use of certain chemicals or drugs
- Asymptomatic
  - —Suggests methemoglobinemia

MECHANISM/DESCRIPTION

- Caused by abnormal elevations of hemoglobin or hemoglobin derivatives
  - —Reduced hemoglobin >5 g/dL
  - —Methemoglobin >1.5 g/dL
  - —Sulfhemoglobin >0.5 g/dL
- The amount of oxyhemoglobin does not affect the color
- Cyanosis is more common in polycythemia
- Cyanosis is less common in those with anemia
- Methemoglobinemia cyanosis with normal PO_2 and chocolate-colored blood

ETIOLOGY

Central Cyanosis/Decreased Saturation

- Impaired pulmonary function
  - —Hypoventilation
    - -Pneumonia
    - -COPD
    - -Pulmonary edema
  - —Ventilation/perfusion mismatch
    - -Asthma
    - -Pulmonary embolus
  - —Diffusion problems
    - -Interstitial lung disease
- Anatomic shunts
  - —Congenital cardiac causes
    - -Transposition
    - -Tetralogy
  - —Pulmonary a-v fistula
    - -Hereditary hemorrhagic telangiectasia
- High altitude decreased atmospheric pressure at 16,000 feet
- Low oxygen affinity hemoglobin mutants
  - —Hb Kansas
  - —Beth Israel
  - —St. Mande

Central Cyanosis/Hemoglobin Abnormalities

- Methemoglobinemia
  - —Congenital
    - -Cytochrome *b*5 reductase deficiency
    - -Hemoglobin M disease
  - —Most cases are acquired
    - -Aniline dyes
    - -Chloroquine, primaquine
    - -Dapsone
    - -Local anesthetic agents lidocaine
    - -High doses of methylene blue
    - -Naphthalene
    - -Nitrites, nitroglycerine
    - -Sulfonamides
- Sulfhemoglobin
  - —Generally benign
  - —Irreversible alteration of hemoglobin
  - —Caused by many medications
    - -Dimethyl sulfoxide (DMSO)
    - -Paint
    - -Phenacetin
    - -Phenazopyridine
    - -Phenylenediamine
    - -Phenylhydroxylamine
    - -Sulfanilamide
    - -Sulfapyridine
    - -Sulfathiazole
    - -Sulfur compounds

Peripheral Cyanosis

- Vasoconstriction to cold air or water
- Arterial obstruction seen in emboli or Raynaud's
- Venous obstruction thrombophlebitis
- Decreased cardiac output compensatory vasoconstriction

Differential Cyanosis

- Lower extremities involved but upper extremities spared
- Patent truncus arteriosus or pulmonary hypertension

Pediatric Cyanosis

- Cardiac
  - —Cyanotic congenital defects
    - -Tetralogy of Fallot
    - -Transposition of great vessels
    - -Truncus arteriosus
    - -Pulmonary and tricuspid atresia
    - -Ebstein's anomaly
  - —Total anomalous pulmonary venous return
  - —Pulmonary stenosis
  - —Any right-to-left shunting
- Respiratory
  - —Upper airway disorders
    - -Croup
    - -Bacterial tracheitis
    - -Epiglottitis
    - -Retropharyngeal abscess
    - -Foreign body
    - -Trauma
  - —Lower airway disorders
    - -Asthma
    - -Bronchiolitis
    - -Pneumonia
    - -Cystic fibrosis
    - -Pulmonary edema/CHF
    - -Pulmonary embolism
    - -Chest wall injury
    - -Pleural disorders pneumothorax or diaphragmatic hernia
- Neurologic
  - —CNS injury/lesions
  - —Infection
  - —Seizure
  - —Toxins
  - —Breath-holding
- Hemoglobinopathy

Pre-Hospital

- Assess and establish patent airway
- Correct any airway obstruction
- Recognize an incorrectly placed airway
- 100% O_2 via non-rebreather
- Ensure adequate ventilation
- Recognize need to establish definitive airway
- Protect c-spine if trauma suspected
- IV, monitor, pulse oximetry
- Albuterol nebulizer for bronchospasm
- Racemic epinephrine nebulizer for severe croup
- Management of pulmonary edema per protocol

Diagnosis

ESSENTIAL WORKUP

- Assess airway and ventilation as first priority
  - —Stabilize airway provide adequate ventilation
- Investigate hypoxemia causes
  - —Cardiac and respiratory most common
- Consider methemoglobinemia

LABORATORY

- Pulse oximetry
  - —Does not assess ventilation
  - —Results inaccurate with
    - -abnormal hemoglobins
    - -nail polish
    - -pigmented skin
    - -hypoperfusion
    - -when used with vital dyes
- Arterial blood gas
  - —Oxygen tension
  - —Measured hemoglobin saturation
  - —Cyanosis in face of normal PO_2, think methemoglobinemia
  - —Blood in methemoglobinemia chocolate color
- Methemoglobin level
- CBC
  - —Check hemoglobin
- Hyperoxia test for congenital cyanosis of newborn
  - —If PO_2 fails to increase to 100 mm Hg after 100% O_2, suspect congenital heart disease

IMAGING/SPECIAL TESTS

- CXR to investigate respiratory or cardiac pathology
  - —Inspiratory/expiratory views if foreign body
  - —Expiratory view if occult pneumothorax suspected
- X-ray of neck for upper airway disorders
  - —Foreign body
  - —Steeple sign (croup)
  - —Prevertebral swelling (retropharyngeal abscess)
  - —Epiglottic swelling
- EKG
  - —Arrhythmia, injury, or ischemia
- Echocardiography
  - —Bubble study if septal defect/shunt suspected
  - —Wall motion/valvular abnormalities
  - —Pericardial fluid

DIFFERENTIAL DIAGNOSIS

- Hyperpigmentation
  - —Drugs or metals
  - —Chronic high-dose chlorpromazine
  - —Minocycline
  - —Argyria (silver deposits)
  - —Tattoos
- Polycythemia

Treatment

INITIAL STABILIZATION

- Oxygen via 100% non-rebreather
- Immediately assess and address airway issues

ED TREATMENT

- Recognize and manage cardiopulmonary disorders
- Methylene blue for methemoglobinemia >30%
  - —Do not use if G6PD deficiency

MEDICATIONS

- Albuterol nebulized: 0.03 mL/kg (5 mg/mL)
- Dexamethasone: (croup) 0.6 mg/kg i.v./i.m.
- Furosemide: 1.0 mg/kg i.v. q6h
- Magnesium: 2.0 g i.v. over 10 minutes (40 mg/kg i.v. over 20 minutes)
- Methylene blue: 1–2 mg/kg of 1% solution over 5 minutes
- Methylprednisolone: 1–2 mg/kg i.v. q6h
- Morphine: 2–4 mg i.v. (0.05–0.1 mg/kg i.v. q2h p.r.n.)
- Nitroglycerine: 0.4 mg s.l. or i.v. (0.5–5 μg/kg/min i.v.)
- Prostaglandin E_1: 0.05–0.1 μg/kg/min i.v.; maximum 0.4 μg/kg/min)
- Racemic epinephrine nebulized: 0.05 mL/kg

Disposition

ADMISSION CRITERIA

- Most patients should be admitted
  - —ICU admission for any instability or cyanosis

DISCHARGE CRITERIA

- Reversible causes of hypoxia
  - —Reactive airway disease responsive to β-agonists
  - —Pulmonary edema in patient with known CHF no suspicion of myocardial injury and diuresis

Miscellaneous

ICD9: 782.5

ICD10: R23.0

SUGGESTED READINGS

Braunwald E. Hypoxia, polycythemia, and cyanosis. In: Harrison's principles of internal medicine, 13th ed. New York: McGraw-Hill, 1994:178–183.

Mansouri A, Lurie A. Concise review: methemoglobinemia. Am J Hematol 1993;42:7.

Stack A. Cyanosis. In: Fleisher GR, ed. Synopsis of pediatric emergency medicine, 4th ed. Philadelphia: Lippincott Williams & Wilkins, 2002:64–67.

Wright RO, Lewander WJ, Woolf AD. Methemoglobinemia: etiology, pharmacology, and clinical management. Ann Emerg Med 1999;34:646.

Author: Michael S. Murphy

Cystic Fibrosis

Clinical Presentation

SIGNS AND SYMPTOMS

- General
  —Failure to thrive
  —Recurrent respiratory tract infections
  —Anasarca in infancy
  —Salty taste of skin
- HEENT
  —Nasal polyps
  —Severe headaches due to sinusitis
- Pulmonary
  —Persistent, dry hacking paroxysmal cough
  —Recurrent pneumonitis or bronchiolitis in the first year of life
  —Wheezing
  —Hemoptysis
  —Pneumonia
  —Respiratory distress
  —Pneumothorax
  —Most common cause of hospitalization
- Cardiac
  —CHF
  —Cor pulmonale
  —Pulmonary hypertension
- GI
  —Abdominal pain
  —Distal ileal obstructive syndrome or "meconium ileus equivalent"
  —Cholelithiasis
  —Pancreatitis
  —Ileocecal intussusception
  —Foul smelling, fatty stools
  —Jaundice
  —Cirrhosis or cholelithiasis
  —Rectal prolapse
  —Hematemesis
- Extremities
  —Bone pain
  —Edema
  —Joint effusions
- Cardiorespiratory failure is most common cause of death

MECHANISM/DESCRIPTION

- Defect of the cystic fibrosis transmembrane conductance regulator (CFTR)
- CFTR functions as an ATP-regulated chloride channel that regulates the activity of chloride and sodium channels on the cell surface
  —Abnormal electrolyte transport in exocrine glands and secretory epithelia
  —Decreased exocrine pancreatic function with malabsorption
  —Thickened mucus, recurrent pulmonary infections, and progressive obstructive damage to the lungs
- Epidemiology
  —Affects 1/2,500 whites
  —More prevalent in white populations
  —Diagnosed in the first decade of life in about 70% of cases
- Median life expectancy in the U.S. is about 30 years

ETIOLOGY

- Recessively inherited genetic disease, involving the CFTR gene on the long arm of chromosome 7
  —Different mutations produce variable phenotypes
  —Classic disease is homozygous for the DF508 mutation
- Common organisms in patients with pneumonia; often multiple drug resistance
  —*Pseudomonas aeruginosa*
    -Prevalence increases with age; 70% of adults are chronically infected
  —*Haemophilus influenzae*
  —*Staphylococcus aureus*
  —*Burkholderia cepacia*
    -Prevalence 5%
    -Associated with rapid clinical deterioration
  —*Aspergillus*

Pre-Hospital

CAUTIONS

- Supportive measures
- Determine DNR status

Diagnosis

ESSENTIAL WORKUP

- Test patients with chronic or unusual respiratory and GI complaints
- Prior culture results may be helpful in patients with known CF

LABORATORY

- Sweat chloride test
  —Chloride concentration >80 mEq/L
  —With classic signs and symptoms, a positive test result confirms the diagnosis
- Stool sample
  —Trypsin or chymotrypsin absent or diminished
  —Increased fat in 72-hour fecal fat excretion
- Cytogenetic analysis
  —Indicated if symptoms are highly suggestive, but sweat test result is negative
  —Positive if two abnormal genes present
  —Genotyping, however, cannot establish the diagnosis
  —Detects 70 of 500 CTFR mutations
  —Ameliorating or neutralizing second mutation may be present
- ABG
  —Hypoxemia
  —Metabolic alkalosis
- Serum electrolytes
  —Hyponatremic, hypochloremic alkalosis
- Serum glucose
  —Hyperglycemia and new-onset diabetes occurs primarily in adolescents and adults; ketoacidosis is rare
- Sputum culture
  —Determine whether pseudomonal colonization is present
- CBC
  —Thrombocytopenia
- Liver function tests and PT
  —Indicated when CF is complicated by hematemesis or signs of liver failure

IMAGING/SPECIAL TESTS

- CXR
  —Hyperaeration
  —Peribronchial thickening
  —Atelectasis
  —Hilar lymphadenopathy
  —Possible pneumothorax
  —Bronchiectasis
  —Blebs
  —Compare with previous CXR for acute pulmonary deterioration
- Abdominal radiographs
  —Indicated if abdominal pain, vomiting, or abdominal distention
  —Distal ileal obstruction syndrome
  —Intussusception

- Barium enema
  - —Indicated if suspicion of intussusception
- Sinus films
  - —Limited use because routine sinus films are always cloudy
  - —CT scan is needed to assess sinuses
- Bronchoalveolar lavage
  - —High percentage of neutrophils and absolute neutrophil count
  - —Unnecessary in patients with obvious pulmonary symptoms
- Studies indicated in patients at high risk with a difficult diagnosis
  - —Semen analysis
  - —Azoospermia
  - —Nasal potential-difference measurements
  - —Complex and time-consuming study

DIFFERENTIAL DIAGNOSIS

- Respiratory
  - —Asthma
  - —Recurrent pneumonia
  - —Bronchiectasis
  - —Pertussis
  - —Immunodeficiency
- GI
  - —Chronic diarrhea
  - —Gastroenteritis
  - —Milk allergy
- Elevated electrolyte levels in sweat
  - —Fucosidosis
  - —Glycogen storage disease type I
  - —Mucopolysaccharidosis
  - —Hypothyroidism
  - —Vasopressin-resistant diabetes insipidus
  - —Adrenal insufficiency
  - —Familial cholestasis
  - —Familial hypoparathyroidism
  - —Malnutrition
  - —Ectodermal dysplasia
  - —Atopic dermatitis
  - —Infusion of prostaglandin E_1

Treatment

INITIAL STABILIZATION

- Oxygen if hypoxemia with PaO_2 <50 mm Hg
- Clarification of DNR status

ED TREATMENT

- Stabilize ABCs
  - —Correct fluid, respiratory, electrolyte, and glucose abnormalities
- Pneumothorax
  - —Observe if <5–10%
  - —Thoracostomy
- Consultation with the primary CF physician or pulmonary specialist
- Right heart failure
  - —Diuretics
- Hemoptysis
  - —Blood products
  - —Ventilatory support
- Distal ileal obstructive syndrome
  - —Usually requires surgery
  - —Blood products are used for the correction of coagulation abnormalities and red cells may be required for replacement in hematemesis
  - —Early consultation with an endoscopist to find the cause and help with therapy of hematemesis is useful
  - —Intussusception can be corrected with barium enema but at times requires surgery
  - —Manual reduction of rectal prolapse; surgical consult for difficult case or for recurrence
- Antibiotics
  - —Based on culture and sensitivity
  - —Pneumonia
  - —*S. aureus*
    - ∗Cephalothin
    - ∗Nafcillin
  - —*H. influenzae*
    - ∗Ticarcillin and clavulanate
  - —*P. aeruginosa*
    - ∗Tobramycin and ticarcillin
    - ∗Inhaled tobramycin (adults: 300 mg b.i.d.) has been shown to improve pulmonary function and decrease risk of hospitalization
  - —*S. aureus* and *P. aeruginosa*
    - ∗Ticarcillin and tobramycin
  - —*P. aeruginosa* and *Burkholderia cepacia*
    - ∗Ceftazidime and ciprofloxacin
  - —*B. cepacia*
    - ∗Chloramphenicol
    - ∗Trimethoprim-sulfamethoxazole
  - —Sinusitis
  - —Antibiotics based on cultures and sensitivities

MEDICATIONS

- Ceftazidime: 50–75 mg/kg q8h
- Cephalothin: 25–50 mg/kg q6h
- Chloramphenicol: 15–20 mg/kg q6h
- Gentamicin: 3 mg/kg q8h
- Nafcillin: 25-50 mg/kg q6h
- Ticarcillin: 100 mg/kg q6h
- Trimethoprim-sulfamethoxazole: 5/25 mg/kg q12h

Note: Because many patients are undernourished, pharmacokinetics of antibiotics (especially amino glycosides, penicillins, and cephalosporins) may be altered, requiring careful monitoring

Disposition

ADMISSION CRITERIA

- Pulmonary exacerbation with significant deterioration from baseline, resistant bacteria, failure of outpatient therapy
- Hemoptysis
- Hematemesis
- Intussusception or unexplained abdominal pain
- Hyperglycemia

DISCHARGE CRITERIA

- Close follow-up to verify the sensitivities of culture results and change therapy as needed
- Avoid hot weather
- Oral salt supplements during times of profuse sweating
- Chloride sweat test of newly diagnosed child with CF

Miscellaneous

ICD9: 277.0

ICD10: E84.9

SUGGESTED READINGS

Farrell DM, Kosorok MR, Rock MT, et al. Early diagnosis of cystic fibrosis through neonatal screening prevents severe malnutrition and improves long term growth. Pediatrics 2001;107:1–13.

Nishioka GJ, Cook PR. Paranasal sinus disease in patients with cystic fibrosis. Otolaryngol Clin North Am 1996;29(1): 193–205.

Ramsey BW. Management of pulmonary disease in patients with cystic fibrosis. N Engl J Med 1996;335(3):179–188.

Ramsey BW, Pepe MS, Quan TJ. Intermittent administration of inhaled tobramycin in patients with cystic fibrosis. N Engl J Med 1999;340:24–30.

Schindlow DV, Taussig LM, Knowles MR. Cystic Fibrosis Foundation consensus conference report on pulmonary complications of cystic fibrosis. Pediatr Pulmonol 1993;15(3):187–198.

Stern RC. The diagnosis of cystic fibrosis. N Engl J Med 1997;336(7):487–491.

Author: Roger M. Barkin

Dacryoadenitis

Clinical Presentation

SIGNS AND SYMPTOMS

- May present as sudden-onset unilateral eyelid erythema or as indolent swelling
  - —Bilateral uncommon
- Swelling and tenderness greatest in the temporal aspect of the upper lid under the orbital rim
  - —May be able to palpate mass
  - —May be associated with
    - -Extensive cellulitis
    - -Conjunctival discharge
    - -Increase or decrease in tear production
    - -Ipsilateral conjunctival injection and chemosis
    - -Ipsilateral preauricular adenopathy
- Normal visual acuity, slit-lamp, and funduscopic exam

MECHANISM/DESCRIPTION

- Inflammation of lacrimal gland
- Primary infection of lacrimal gland
  - —May occur secondary to contiguous spread from bacterial conjunctivitis or periorbital cellulitis

ETIOLOGY

- Most diseases causing inflammation of the lacrimal gland are not infectious
  - —Autoimmune diseases
  - —Sjögren's syndrome
  - —Sarcoidosis
  - —Tumor
    - ->25% of all lacrimal gland swelling
- Uncommon infection, usually seen in children and young adults
- Acute suppurative dacryoadenitis
  - —In adults, bacteria most common cause
    - -*Staphylococcus aureus*
    - -Streptococci
    - -*Chlamydia trachomatis*
    - -*Neisseria gonorrhea*
- Chronic dacryoadenitis
  - —Slowly progressive, painless swelling without systemic symptoms
  - —Viruses most common cause
    - -Mumps, measles (particularly in children)
    - -Epstein-Barr virus (EBV)
    - -Cytomegalovirus (CMV)
    - -Coxsackievirus
    - -Varicella-zoster virus

PEDIATRIC CONSIDERATIONS

- Viral—most common cause in children
  - —Mumps the most common
- Slowly enlarging mass may be a dermoid

Pre-Hospital

N/A

Diagnosis

ESSENTIAL WORKUP

- Complete eye exam, including visual acuity, slit-lamp, and funduscopic exam normal
- Determine the likelihood of gonorrhea as the etiology
  - —High-risk systemic illness and visual loss

LABORATORY

- Gram stain and culture of drainage
  - —May identify the pathogen and guide therapy
- CBC

IMAGING/SPECIAL TESTS

- Radiographic studies generally unnecessary
  - —Orbital CT (if diagnosis unclear) to rule out orbital cellulitis, tumor, or other etiology

DIFFERENTIAL DIAGNOSIS

- Autoimmune disease
- Lacrimal gland tumor
- Hordeolum
- Periorbital (preseptal) cellulitis
- Severe blepharitis
- Orbital cellulitis
- Acute conjunctivitis
- Acute dacryocystitis
- Insect bite
- Traumatic injury

Treatment

INITIAL STABILIZATION

- Exclude orbital cellulitis

ED TREATMENT

- Apply cool compresses to decrease inflammation and pain
- Antibiotics
  —Oral (cephalexin, amoxicillin/clavulanate) for mild infection
  —IV (cefazolin, ticarcillin/clavulanate) for severe infection
- Analgesics
- Tetanus toxoid if necessary
- Incision and drainage rarely necessary except in very severe cases
  —Perform with consultation to facial surgery service or ophthalmology

MEDICATIONS

- Amoxicillin/clavulanate (Augmentin): 250–500 mg (peds: 20–40 mg of amoxicillin/kg/24 h) PO q8h
- Cefazolin: 500–1000 mg (peds: 50–100 mg/kg/24 h) i.v. q6–8h
- Cephalexin: 250–500 mg (peds: 25–100 g/kg/24 h) PO q.i.d.
- Ticarcillin/clavulanate: 3.2 g (peds: 200–300 mg of ticarcillin/kg/24 h) i.v. q4–6h

PEDIATRIC CONSIDERATIONS

- Viral most commonly etiology
  —Treat with cold compresses and analgesics
- If etiology is unclear, treat with antibiotics as with adults

Disposition

ADMISSION CRITERIA

- Acutely ill, toxic appearing
- Immunocompromised

DISCHARGE CRITERIA

- Well-appearing who can tolerate oral antibiotics

Miscellaneous

ICD9: 375.00

ICD10: H04.0

SEE ALSO: DACROCYSTITIS

SUGGESTED READINGS

Boruchoff SA, Boruchoff SE. Infections of the lacrimal system. Infect Dis Clin North Am 1992;6(4):925–933.

Brook I, Frazier EH. Aerobic and anaerobic microbiology of dacryoadenitis. Am J Ophthalmol 1998;125(4):552–554.

Kanski JJ. Clinical ophthalmology. Oxford: Butterworth-Heinemann, 1994:66–69.

Rhee DJ, Pyfer MF, Rhee DM. The Wills eye manual: office and emergency room diagnosis and treatment of eye disease. Philadelphia: Lippincott Williams & Wilkins, 1999.

Rubin S, Hallagan L. Lids, lacrimals and lids. Emerg Med Clin North Am 1995;13(3): 631–647.

Author: Shari Schabowski

Dacryocystitis

Clinical Presentation

SIGNS AND SYMPTOMS

- Unilateral, red, painful, swollen mass extending inferior and medial from the inner canthus
- Excessive tearing
- Discharge
- Cellulitis extending to the lower lid in some cases
- Low-grade fever may be present, but patient rarely appears toxic

MECHANISM/DESCRIPTION

- Suppurative infection of the lacrimal sac, which is located adjacent to the lacrimal duct near the inner canthus of the eye
- Under normal conditions, tears drain via pumping action at the lacrimal duct, moving tears to the lacrimal sac and then to the middle turbinate into the sinuses
- Symptoms begin when the duct to the lacrimal sac becomes partially or completely obstructed
  —Stasis in this conduit results in overgrowth of bacteria and infection
- May also occur secondary to trauma or a dacryolith or after nasal surgery or sinus surgery
- Infection may be recurrent and may become chronic
- Complications include mucocele, fistula formation, conjunctivitis with or without corneal involvement, and facial, periorbital, or orbital cellulitis

ETIOLOGY

- Most common bacteria are ocular and sinus flora
- *Staphylococcus aureus*—most common organism in acquired acute dacryocystitis
- Most commonly occurs in infants and postmenopausal women

PEDIATRIC CONSIDERATIONS

- Congenital nasolacrimal obstruction due to stenosis occurs in about 2–4% of full-term newborns and presents as acute dacryocystitis
- *Streptococcus pneumoniae*—most common organism in congenital dacryocystitis

Pre-Hospital

N/A

Diagnosis

ESSENTIAL WORKUP

- Expression of purulent material from the punctum when pressure is applied to the mass confirms the diagnosis
- Visual acuity, complete eye exam, including slit-lamp and funduscopic exam
- Examination of nasal passages

LABORATORY

- Gram stain, culture and sensitivity, and chocolate agar plating of the expressed material
  —Helps direct specific antibiotic treatment

IMAGING/SPECIAL TESTS

- CT of orbit/sinus to evaluate deep tissue extension and particularly with recurrent cases

DIFFERENTIAL DIAGNOSIS

- Insect bite
- Traumatic injury
- Acute ethmoid sinusitis
- Acute maxillary sinusitis
- Periorbital (preseptal) cellulitis
- Orbital cellulitis
- Acute conjunctivitis
- Acute blepharitis

Treatment

INITIAL STABILIZATION

Initial Approach and Immediate Concerns

- Confirm diagnosis by expressing purulent material
- Begin treatment to avoid extension of infection to adjacent structures
- Determine whether symptoms are recurrent

ED TREATMENT

- Drainage of the infected sac is essential
  - —Warm compresses and gentle massage to relieve the obstruction
  - —Facilitate outflow from the obstructed tract with nasal packing with local anesthetic and strong vasoconstrictor
- Incision and drainage in severe cases
  - —Avoid if possible—may result in fistula formation
- Duct instrumentation to facilitate drainage not indicated in acute setting (controversial)
  - —Reserve instrumentation of the duct for the nonacute setting if necessary at all
  - —Only 50% of adults show improvement after manipulation
  - —Manipulation while the duct is inflamed may result in injury to the duct and permanent obstruction owing to scarring and stenosis
- Topical ophthalmic antibiotic drops to prevent secondary conjunctivitis
- Systemic antibiotics to resolve infection and prevent spread to adjacent structures
  - —Oral for mild infection
  - —IV when febrile or severe infection
- Analgesics

MEDICATIONS

- Amoxicillin/clavulanate (Augmentin): 250–500 mg (peds: 20–40 mg of amoxicillin/kg/24 h) PO q8h
- Cefaclor: 20–40 mg/kg/24 h PO q8h
- Cefazolin: 500–1000 mg (peds: 50–100 mg/kg/24 h) i.v. q6–8h
- Cefuroxime: 50–100 mg/kg/24 h i.v. q8h
- Cephalexin: 250–500 mg (peds: 25–100 g/kg/24 h) PO q.i.d.
- Cocaine hydrochloride: 4% topical solution single-dose nasal spray
- Erythromycin ophthalmic ointment: 2 drops q.i.d. to affected eye
- Tetracaine and phenylephrine topical solution single-dose nasal spray
- Trimethoprim-polymyxin ointment: 2 drops q.i.d. to affected eye

PEDIATRIC CONSIDERATION

- Newborns respond well to massage and topical antibiotics in about 95% of cases
- If no resolution in the first year of life, may require probing of the duct by an ophthalmologist
- Children <4 years of age (particularly 6 months–2 years) who develop dacryocystitis
  - —At increased risk for *Haemophilus influenzae* infection (those who have not completed two HiB vaccinations)
  - —*Haemophilus influenzae* type B carries a high risk for bacteremia, septicemia, and meningitis
  - —Treat afebrile, well-appearing patient with a responsible parent with oral cefaclor or amoxicillin/clavulanate
  - —Administer cefuroxime IV in acutely ill patient

Disposition

ADMISSION CRITERIA

- Adult
  - —Febrile toxic appearing
  - —Concomitant medical problems including diabetes or immunosuppression
  - —Extensive cellulitis
  - —Suspicion of adjacent spread with deep tissue involvement or meningitis
- Children
  - —Acutely ill appearance
  - —Concomitant medical problems
  - —Extensive cellulitis
  - —High risk for *Haemophilus influenzae*
  - —If reliable follow-up within 24 hours cannot be arranged

DISCHARGE CRITERIA

- Well-appearing, healthy individual

Miscellaneous

ICD9: 375.30

ICD10: H04.3

SEE ALSO: DACRYOADENITIS

SUGGESTED READINGS

Boruchoff SA, Boruchoff SE. Infections of the lacrimal system. Infect Dis Clin North Am 1992;6(4):925–933.

Kanski JJ. Clinical ophthalmology. Oxford: Butterworth-Heinemann, 1994:66–69.

Lueder GT. Neonatal dacryocystitis associated with nasolacrimal duct cysts. J Pediatr Ophthalmol Strabismus 1995; 32(2):102–106.

Rhee DJ, Pyfer MF, Rhee DM. The Wills eye manual: office and emergency room diagnosis and treatment of eye disease. Philadelphia: Lippincott Williams & Wilkins, 1999.

Rubin S, Hallagan L. Lids, lacrimals and lids. Emerg Med Clin North Am 1995;13(3): 631–647.

Thompson CJ. Review of the diagnosis and management of acquired nasolacrimal duct obstruction. Optometry 2001;72(2): 103–111.

Author: Shari Schabowski

Decompression Sickness

Clinical Presentation

SIGNS AND SYMPTOMS

Cutaneous

- Scarlatiniform, erysipeloid, or mottled rash
  - —Cutis marmorata
- Peau d'orange appearance owing to lymphatic obstruction

Musculoskeletal

- Pain
  - —"The bends"
  - —Dull, deep muscular aching
  - —Often in a joint (elbow and shoulder most common)
  - —Typically not exacerbated by movement or reproduced with palpation
- No external physical signs of trauma

GI

- Nausea and vomiting
- Abdominal pain

Pulmonary

- Shortness of breath
- "The chokes" triad of
  - —Substernal pressure
  - —Cough
  - —Dyspnea
  - —Thought due to bubbles in the pulmonary vascular tree

CNS

- Weakness and fatigue
- Numbness and paresthesia
- Agitation
- Headache
- Dizziness
- Vertigo
- Convulsion
- Bowel and bladder incontinence
- Lethargy
- Visual disturbance
- "The staggers"
  - —Vestibular system and the posterior column involvement

MECHANISM/DESCRIPTION

Henry's Law

- Amount of gas that will dissolve in a solution is directly proportional to the partial pressure of that gas
- Increases in partial pressure result in larger amount of gas dissolved in tissue
- Decreases in partial pressure result in gas coming out of solution

Dalton's Law

- Total pressure exerted by a mixture of gases is equal to the sum of the partial pressure of each of the component gases

Sequence

- Increases in ambient pressure cause an increase in partial pressure of nitrogen inspired (per Henry's law, above)
- Nitrogen accumulates in the tissues in increasing concentrations the longer ambient pressures remain elevated
- Decompression sickness (DCS) results when ambient pressure keeping nitrogen in solution decreases too rapidly (on ascent), preventing gradual removal of the excess body burden of nitrogen
- As the nitrogen removal gradient is overwhelmed, tissues become supersaturated, and bubble formation occurs

ETIOLOGY

- Bubble location determines clinical effects
  - —Blood flow obstruction and tissue ischemia from intravascular bubbles
  - —Tissue distention and compression from interstitial bubbles
  - —Compression of arterioles, nerves, and lymphatics
  - —Endothelial damage leading to stimulation of coagulation and clotting cascades
  - —Bubbles sensed as foreign by host defenses leading to the release of chemotactic and other factors
- Risk factors for DCS
  - —Greater depth (increased ambient pressures), longer bottom time, and quicker rate of ascent
  - —Proper use of dive tables and computers does *not* eliminate risk for DCS
  - —Increased incidence with age and weight (higher body fat), hypothermia, dehydration, exercise, multiple dives in a day
- Airplane flight following diving can precipitate DCS owing to lower cabin pressure

Pre-Hospital

CONTROVERSIES

- "In water" recompression
  - —Return injured diver/patient to a depth where symptoms are ameliorated
  - —Extremely difficult
  - —Need large amount of surface support
  - —Consider as last resort only

CAUTIONS

- Recognize DCS
  - —Postdive extremity pain often attributed to a muscle strain
  - —Serious neurologic complaints often minimized because the diver does not consider DCS
- Time after surfacing to presentation of DCS
  - —50%—symptoms within 1 hour
  - —95%—symptoms within 12 hours
  - —60% of neurologic DCS within 10 minutes

Diagnosis

ESSENTIAL WORKUP

- Clinical diagnosis: recognize risk factors and various clinical presentation
- Careful neurologic exam to document possible waning symptoms
- "Trial of pressure"
  —Rapid relief of symptoms upon recompression in a hyperbaric chamber may be the only way to diagnose DCS conclusively

LABORATORY

- CBC
  —Increased hematocrit owing to hemoconcentration
- Electrolytes, BUN, creatinine, glucose
- Urinalysis
- Arterial blood gas (ABG) and pulse oximetry
  —Monitor oxygenation

IMAGING

- Chest x-ray
  —Concomitant pulmonary barotrauma
  —Aspiration pneumonia
- Head CT when altered mental status or neurologic deficit

DIFFERENTIAL DIAGNOSIS

- Musculoskeletal injury unrelated to bubble formation
- Inner or middle ear barotrauma
- Arterial gas embolism
- Cerebrovascular accident (CVA)

Treatment

INITIAL STABILIZATION

- ABCs
- Provide normobaric (100%) oxygen via mask or endotracheal tube (ETT)
  —Increases inert gas (nitrogen) elimination from the tissues, reducing gas bubble size
  —Increases oxygen delivery to the injured tissue
- Early recompression in hyperbaric chamber

ED TREATMENT

- IV rehydration with 0.9% NS
  —Diver usually dehydrated owing to diuretic effect of pressure, exercise, breathing dry compressed air
  —Increased fluid assists with gas removal and dissolution of nitrogen
- Hyperbaric oxygen recompression therapy (see Hyperbaric Oxygen Therapy)
  —For all DCS except for cutaneous
  —Arrange transportation to nearest hyperbaric facility
  —Aircraft capable of full pressurization maintaining barometric pressure below 1,000 feet best suited for transfers
  —Prophylactic chest tube for simple pneumothorax to prevent conversion to tension pneumothorax
  —Fill endotracheal and Foley catheter balloons with water or saline to avoid shrinkage/damage during recompression
- Divers Alert Network (DAN)
  —Based at Duke University Medical Center
  —Provides a 24-hour emergency hotline for medical consultation on the treatment of dive-related injuries and for referrals to hyperbaric chambers (1-919-684-8111)

Disposition

ADMISSION CRITERIA

- Refer all patients with suspected or diagnosis DCS for hyperbaric therapy

DISCHARGE CRITERIA

- Patients not requiring hyperbaric treatment
- Stable patients with mild symptoms may be discharged post-hyperbaric oxygen treatment
- Air travel may exacerbate symptoms as ambient pressure decreases

Miscellaneous

ICD9: 993.3

ICD10: T70.3

SEE ALSO: ARTERIAL GAS EMBOLISM; BAROTRAUMA; HYPERBARIC OXYGEN THERAPY

SUGGESTED READINGS

Bartlett RB. Diving emergencies. In: Critical decisions in emergency medicine, Vol. 10, No. 10, Lesson 20. Dallas: American College of Emergency Physicians, 1997.

Kizer KW. Scuba diving and dysbarism. In: Auerbach PA, ed. Wilderness medicine, 3rd ed. St. Louis: CV Mosby, 1995: 1176–1208.

Madsen J, Hink J, Hyldegaard O. Diving physiology and pathophysiology. Clin Physiol 1994;14:597–626.

Moon RE, Vann RD, Bennett PB. The physiology of decompression illness. Sci Am 1995;(Aug):70–77.

Newton HB. Neurologic complications of scuba diving. Am Fam Physician 2001;63(11):2211–2218.

Author: Jeffrey Gordon

Deep Vein Thrombosis

Clinical Presentation

SIGNS AND SYMPTOMS

- Leg swelling
  - —Greater than 1 cm difference is usually significant
- Leg warmth and redness
- Leg pain and tenderness
- Palpable cord
- In superficial thrombophlebitis, a red pipe cleaner-like cord may be visible and palpable
- Arm swelling, warmth, or tenderness
  - —Upper extremity or subclavian vein involved
- Phlegmasia cerulea dolens
  - —Cold, tender, swollen and blue leg (secondary arterial insufficiency)
- In phlegmasia alba dolens
  - —Cold, tender and white leg (secondary arterial insufficiency)

MECHANISM/DESCRIPTION

- A constant balance exists between intravascular clot-promoting and clot-dissolving forces
  - —When the former overpowers the latter, clot results
- Subdivisions of thrombophlebitis
  - —Superficial (to the fascia)
  - —Deep
  - —Septic
  - —Bland
  - —Distal to the popliteal vein
  - —Proximal to the popliteal vein
  - —Pelvic
  - —Upper extremity

EPIDEMIOLOGY

- About 600,000 to 2,000,000 new cases present annually
- Prevalence increases with advancing age in the general population
- Diagnosis is more common using active surveillance rather than clinical suspicion
- Common in both medical and surgical hospitalized patients
- Other manifestation of thromboembolism
  - —Pulmonary embolism

ETIOLOGY

- Three generic factors promote clotting
- Hypercoagulable states
  - —Cancer
  - —Nephrotic syndrome
  - —Sepsis
  - —Inflammatory conditions
    - -Ulcerative colitis
  - —Increased estrogen
    - -Pregnancy
    - -Oral contraceptives
  - —Antiphospholipid syndrome
  - —Protein deficiencies
    - -Protein S
    - -Protein C
    - -Antithrombin III
  - —Newer hypercoagulable states continue to be identified
    - -Factor V
    - -Leiden
    - -Prothrombin gene mutations
- Stasis
  - —Prolonged bed rest
  - —Immobility from a cast
  - —Long plane or train ride
  - —Neurologic disorders with paralysis
  - —Congestive heart failure
  - —Obesity
- Vascular damage
  - —Trauma
  - —Surgery
  - —Central lines
    - -Especially in the case of upper extremity thrombophlebitis
- Multifactorial issues
  - —Advancing age
  - —Prior thromboembolism

CAUTIONS

- The initial ultrasound study may be falsely negative
  - —For patients who have a strong clinical (pretest) probability, consider a contrast venogram, or at least a repeat ultrasound, in 3–5 days
- Because deep vein thrombosis (DVT) and pulmonary embolism are two manifestations of the same disease, carefully question and examine the patients for symptoms and signs of clot in the lungs
- The complication of postphlebitic syndrome occurs in 20%–30% of cases of DVT
  - —The mechanism is thought to be loss of valve function within the veins
  - —Often mimics recurrent thrombophlebitis and can be difficult to distinguish by imaging studies unless the old and current studies are being compared

Diagnosis

ESSENTIAL WORKUP

- Determination of a patient's clinical (pretest) risk is a key step in a workup for venous thromboembolism
- A careful history and physical exam, interpreted in the context of the risk factor profile, is the most important driver of subsequent diagnostic evaluation

LABORATORY

- D-Dimer testing
  - —A byproduct of endogenous clot formation, becoming increasingly used in evaluation of patients for DVT
  - —Only useful when the result is negative (to exclude DVT)
  - —Methods of measuring D-dimer levels
    - -Latex agglutination (standard) testing not sufficiently sensitive
    - -Microlatex agglutination tests shows some promise but remain insufficiently tested as compared with other methods
    - -Whole-blood latex agglutination (SimpliRed) is valuable if negative in low probability patients (using Well's criteria)
    - -Enzyme-linked immunosorbent assay (ELISA) testing gives a quantitative result and has been validated in large clinical studies in ED patients

IMAGING/SPECIAL TESTS

- Contrast venography
  - —Once the imaging test of choice; now rarely performed because it is invasive, is expensive, and has complications
  - —Involves injection of contrast medium into a leg vein, the inflammation from which can cause thrombophlebitis in several percent of patients undergoing the procedure
  - —Reactions to the contrast dye may also cause reaction
- Radionuclide venography
  - —Radionuclide venous imaging is under investigation
  - —This test is not commonly used in routine clinical practice
- Impedance plethysmography
  - —Another uncommonly used test, which can miss smaller distal clots
- Compression ultrasound
  - —Standard first-line diagnostic test
  - —It looks for compression (which is normal) of the vein
  - —Color Doppler can be useful for identifying the vein but does not add substantially to accuracy

—Duplex scanning refers to the combination of compression B-mode ultrasound and color Doppler
—Has a sensitivity in the high 90% range
—Should be repeated (or followed up with a venogram) in high-risk patients with negative ultrasounds

DIFFERENTIAL DIAGNOSIS

- Superficial thrombophlebitis
- Cellulitis
- Torn muscle and/or ligaments (including plantaris and gastrocnemius tears)
- Ruptured Baker's cyst
- (Bilateral) edema secondary to heart, liver, or kidney disease
- (Unilateral) edema from abdominal mass (gravid uterus or tumor) or lymphedema
- Postphlebitic syndrome (from prior thrombophlebitis)

Treatment

INITIAL STABILIZATION

In cases of phlegmasia cerulea (or alba) dolens
- Intravenous access
- Supplemental oxygen
- Surgical or vascular consultation

ED TREATMENT

- Parenteral anticoagulation
  —In patients without contraindication
  —Use either unfractionated or low-molecular-weight heparin
  —Carefully selected patients can be primarily with treated with low-molecular-weight heparin as outpatients
- Warfarin
  —Started shortly after a heparin has been administered
  —Not before heparin because of the theoretic risk for inducing a transient hypercoagulable state
- Vena cava filters
  —Indications
  -Contraindications to systemic anticoagulation
  -New thromboembolic event while on adequate anticoagulation
  —Vena cava filters (or umbrellas) can be placed transcutaneously, usually by a vascular surgeon or radiologist
  —Empiric filter placement may be useful in certain settings
  -Ongoing risk such as cancer
  -Risk for a recurrent pulmonary embolism could be fatal because of poor cardiopulmonary reserve or a recent pulmonary embolism
  —Randomized data suggest that filter placement is no more effective than anticoagulation
  —Filters can also be deployed in the superior vena cava in the setting of upper extremity DVT
- Thrombolysis
  —Rarely indicated
  —Roughly a threefold increase in bleeding complications
  —Catheter-administered lytic therapy is used more commonly in upper extremity thrombophlebitis
- Thrombectomy
  —Occasionally recommended for patients with extensive disease
  —Coordinate with a vascular surgeon
- Septic thrombophlebitis
  —Surgical excision of the vein or intravenous antibiotics

MEDICATIONS

- Enoxaparin: 1 mg/kg SQ b.i.d. for outpatients (or inpatients); a dose of 1.5 mg/kg SQ qd is FDA-approved for inpatients
- Heparin (unfractionated): 80 units/kg bolus followed by an 18 U/kg/h drip, with the activated partial thromboplastin time (aPTT) titrated to 2–2.5 times normal
- Tinzaparin: 175 IU/kg SQ qd
- Warfarin: 5 mg/d with a prothrombin time being checked on the third day

Disposition

ADMISSION CRITERIA

- Patients with thrombophlebitis unable to receive low-molecular-weight heparin as an outpatient
- Patients with concomitant pulmonary embolism or other serious diseases

DISCHARGE CRITERIA

- Outpatient treatment with a low-molecular-weight heparin
  —No serious concomitant disease that requires hospitalization
  —Patient has means of communication and transportation to return to the hospital if needed
  —Patient (or family member) is willing and able to inject the medication
  —Patient needs hematocrit, platelet count, and INR checked in 2–3 days
  —aPTT does not need to be checked
  —Heparin-induced thrombocytopenia is less common with the low-molecular-weight heparins but still occurs
  —INR needs to be checked at about day 3
- Patients with superficial or distal thrombophlebitis can be discharged with close follow-up

Miscellaneous

ICD9: 451.9

ICD10: I80.2

SUGGESTED READINGS

Brown DFM. Treatment options for DVT. Emerg Med Clin North Am 2001;19:913–923.

Decoussis MN, et al. A clinical trial of vena cava filters in the prevention of pulmonary embolism in patients with proximal deep-vein thrombosis. N Engl J Med 1998;333:409–415.

Hirsh J, Hoak J. Management of DVT and PE. Circulation 1996;93:2212–2245.

Kelly J, Hunt BJ. Role of D-dimers in diagnosis of venous thromboembolism. Lancet 2002;359(9305):456–458.

Levine M, et al. A comparison of LMWH administered primarily at home with unfractionated heparin administered in the hospital for proximal DVT. N Engl J Med 1996;334:677–681.

Pearson SP, et al. A critical pathway to evaluate suspected DVT. Arch Intern Med 1995;155:1773–1778.

Rosen CL, Tracy JA. The diagnosis of lower extremity DVT. Emerg Med Clin North Am 2001;19:895–912.

Author: Jonathan Edlow

Defibrillators, Implantable

Clinical Presentation

SIGNS AND SYMPTOMS

Implantable Cardiac Defibrillators (ICDs) Fires

- How many shocks
- Were they sleeping at the time (phantom shocks)
- Determine symptoms before and after shock
  - —Asymptomatic
  - —Symptomatic
    - -Syncope or near syncope
    - -Lightheadedness or dizziness
    - -Shortness of breath
    - -Palpitations
    - -Chest discomfort or pain
    - -Diaphoresis
- Cardiac arrest

Implantation Site Related

- 2–6 weeks after implantation
  - —Warmth
  - —Erythema
  - —Pain
  - —Fluctuance
  - —Skin erosion
  - —Fever

Vascular

- Unilateral upper extremity edema
- Superior vena cava (SVC) syndrome rare
- Tachypnea, tachycardia, or pleuritic chest pain if pulmonary emboli

Psychiatric

- Adjustment disorders and panic attacks
- Major depression
- Phantom shocks
  - —Patient awakened from sleep by a perceived shock

MECHANISM/DESCRIPTION

- More than 10,000 ICDs have been implanted
  - —Ability to prevent death due to life-threatening arrhythmias
- Newer generations of ICDs incorporate advanced pacemaker technologies and may combine single-chamber pacing, dual-chamber pacing, and even biventricular pacing
- Pulse generator located in an anterior chest wall pocket

ETIOLOGY

ICD Fires

- Felt *well* before shock, feels *well* after
  - —Erroneous sensing of supraventricular tachyarrhythmias as ventricular (atrial fibrillation most common)
  - —Lead fractures can result in body motion artifact being sensed as ventricular arrhythmias
  - —Erroneous sensing of pacemaker spikes in patients with permanent pacemakers, diaphragmatic contractions, and T waves (being double counted as the QRS complex)
  - —Electrode migration may lead to inappropriate delivery of shocks resulting in ventricular fibrillation
  - —Phantom shock possible if patient was awoken from sleep by a perceived shock
- Felt *poor* before shock, feels *well* after
  - —Likely appropriate therapy for dysrhythmia
  - —Postinfarction (remote) V-tach is more likely
  - —Antiarrhythmic drugs and electrolyte abnormalities can be proarrhythmic
- Felt *poor* before shock, feels *poor* after
  - —Acute cardiac ischemic syndromes may present with unstable angina, myocardial infarction (MI), or congestive heart failure (CHF)

Infection

- *Staphylococcus aureus* (most aggressive and seen early)
- *Staphylococcus epidermidis* (more indolent and later)
- *Escherichia coli, Pseudomonas* species, and *Streptococcal* species (less common)

Vascular Related

- Venous thrombosis/embolism secondary to impedance of venous flow as a result of the ICD lead(s)

Pre-Hospital

CAUTIONS

- Follow standard advanced cardiac life support (ACLS) protocols during cardiac arrest situations
  - —External defibrillation may be necessary
  - —Avoid shocking directly over the device
- Deactivation of ICD
  - —Averts inappropriate firing of the unit
  - —All units may be temporarily inhibited from firing while a magnet is positioned on the skin over the pulse generator
- Avoid strong magnetic fields because they can deactivate ICDs
- Search for medical alert tags

Diagnosis

ESSENTIAL WORKUP

ICD Fires

- EKG
  - —Transient ST-segment changes and elevations of the cardiac enzymes may be seen after shock delivery and do not necessarily indicate myocardial damage
- Chest x-ray
  - —Lead fracture
  - —CHF
- Electrolytes
- Cardiac enzymes if ischemia suspected
- Interrogation of the unit by a cardiologist or electrophysiologist

Implantation Site Related

- CBC
- Erythrocyte sedimentation rate (ESR)
- Blood culture
- Chest x-ray
- Do not aspirate ICD pockets

Vascular Related

- Venous duplex of the upper extremity
  - —Demonstrates presence of venous thrombosis
- Ventilation/perfusion (V/Q) scan or chest CT angiogram
  - —Indicated if pulmonary embolus suspected

DIFFERENTIAL DIAGNOSIS

- Inappropriate shock versus
- Phantom shock
- Seroma
- Hematoma

INITIAL STABILIZATION

- ABCs
- Institute ACLS protocol for life-threatening dysrhythmia
- Place on monitor even with defibrillator
- IV access
- During cardiac arrest, defibrillation does not harm the device
  - —Avoid placing the paddles directly over the unit
  - —May deactivate with a ring magnet

ED TREATMENT

ICD Fires

- Consult with a cardiac electrophysiologist
- Patients with nonfunctioning ICDs need external defibrillator pads and close monitoring at all times
- Repeated firing necessitates prompt interrogation of the unit
- Appropriate ICD shock delivery
  - —Treatment of ischemia
  - —Institution of antiarrhythmic therapy
  - —Correction of electrolyte disturbances
- Inappropriate ICD shock delivery
  - —May warrant temporary deactivation with a ring magnet and close monitoring, until the unit can be reprogrammed
  - —Deactivation can usually be accomplished by placing the magnet directly over the unit

Implantation Site Inflammation

- Obtain blood cultures
  - —Do not aspirate material from ICD pocket
- Administer parenteral antibiotics
- Consult with a cardiologist regarding unit removal
- Prophylactic antibiotics are controversial if a seroma or hematoma is suspected

Vascular Related

- Venous thrombosis, unilateral upper extremity swelling
  - —Rarely embolic, but does require anticoagulation
  - —Conservative therapy with warm packs usually sufficient

Other

- MRI absolutely contraindicated
  - —Magnetic field may damage ICDs
- Electrocautery should generally be avoided

MEDICATIONS

- Cefazolin: 1 g i.v. q8h
- Vancomycin: 1 g i.v. q12h
- Cefalexin: 500 mg PO q.i.d.

Disposition

ADMISSION CRITERIA

- Felt poor before shock, feels poor after
- Signs of systemic infection
- Infected implantation site
- Expanding pocket hematoma with skin tension
- Upper extremity thrombosis

DISCHARGE CRITERIA

- Asymptomatic before and after shock with a negative workup in concert with the patient's cardiologist
- Symptomatic before shock but feels well after
  - —Usually indicates VT/VF and is the appropriate action of the device
  - —Discharge to home with appropriate follow-up after consultation with the patient's cardiologist
- Swelling at implantation site with absence of signs of systemic or local infection
  - —May be treated with oral antibiotics
  - —Frequent inspection as an outpatient to differentiate between seratoma/hematoma and early infection

Miscellaneous

ICD9: N/A

ICD10: N/A

SUGGESTED READINGS

Munter D. Assessment of implanted pacemaker/AICD devices. In: Roberts J, Hedges G, eds. Clinical procedures in emergency medicine, 3rd ed. Philadelphia: WB Saunders, 1998.

Peters R, Gold M. Cardiac arrhythmias: implantable cardiac defibrillators. Med Clin North Am 2001;85(2):343–367.

Pfeiffer D, Jung W, Fehske W, et al. Complications of pacemaker-defibrillator devices: diagnosis and management. Am Heart J 1994;127(42):1073–1080.

Pinski S. Scientific reviews: emergencies related to implantable cardioverter-defibrillators. Crit Care Med 2000;28(10): N174–180.

Pinski S, Troman R. Implantable cardioverter-defibrillators: implications for the non-electrophysiologist. Ann Intern Med 1995;122(10):770–777.

Author: Robert Sidman

Delirium

Clinical Presentation

SIGNS AND SYMPTOMS

- Disturbed consciousness
  - —Hyperalert
  - —Lethargic
  - —Stupor
  - —Coma
- Cognitive changes
  - —Disorientation
  - —Impaired memory
  - —Disorganized thinking and speech
  - —Misperceptions, illusions, delusions, and hallucinations
- Time course
  - —Hours to days
  - —Fluctuating course
- Reduced awareness of the environment
- Inattention
  - —Difficulties in focusing, shifting, and maintaining attention
  - —Restlessness
  - —Distractibility
  - —Lability

MECHANISM/DESCRIPTION

- Syndrome caused by multiple medical disorders
- Delirium is caused by an underlying medical condition
- Pathophysiology unknown
  - —Diffuse derangements of cerebral acetylcholine
  - —CNS dopamine, γ-aminobutyric acid, and serotonin may be involved

ETIOLOGY

- Life threats
  - —Withdrawal from barbiturates
  - —Wernicke's encephalopathy
  - —Hypoxia and hypoperfusion of the brain
  - —Hypertensive crisis
  - —Hypoglycemia
  - —Hyperthermia or hypothermia
  - —Intracranial bleed or mass
  - —Acute coronary syndromes
  - —Meningitis or encephalitis
  - —Poisoning or medications
  - —Status epilepticus
  - —Sepsis
- General categories of disorders causing delirium
  - —Medications
  - —Drug abuse
  - —Intoxication
  - —Withdrawal
  - —Metabolic abnormalities
  - —CNS pathology
  - —Hypoperfusion from cardiovascular disease
  - —Hypoxemia
  - —Vitamin deficiencies
  - —Endocrinopathies
  - —Infections
  - —Toxins
  - —Collagen vascular illnesses

Pre-Hospital

CAUTIONS

- Intravenous access
- Glucose measurement or empiric dextrose administration
- Naloxone (Narcan) if associated respiratory insufficiency
- Monitor patient
- Look for signs of an underlying cause
  - —Medications
  - —Medical alert bracelets
- Document a basic neurologic examination
  - —Glasgow Coma Scale score
  - —Pupils
  - —Extremity movements

Diagnosis

ESSENTIAL WORKUP

- Awareness of delirium as a syndrome is key
- Confusion assessment method
  - —Acute onset or fluctuating course
  - —Inattention
  - —Disorganized thinking
  - —Altered level of consciousness
- Vital signs and physical examination
- Neurologic examination with careful attention to the changes in mental status
- Ancillary studies to determine the underlying cause

LABORATORY

- Electrolytes, calcium
- BUN and creatinine
- Glucose
- CBC
- Toxicology screens
- Further studies based on signs and symptoms
  - —Arterial blood gases
  - —Liver functions tests
  - —Thyroid tests, thyroid-stimulating hormone measurement
  - —Cardiac enzymes

IMAGING/SPECIAL TESTS

- EKG
- Head CT scan
- Lumbar puncture
- Chest radiograph

DIFFERENTIAL DIAGNOSIS

- Cardiovascular diseases producing hypoperfusion
- Pulmonary diseases causing hypoxia
- Metabolic abnormalities
- Infections
- Environmental illness
- Adverse drug event
- Drug or alcohol withdrawal
- Psychiatric illness
- Dementia
- CNS disorders

Treatment

INITIAL STABILIZATION

- Most patients with delirium do not need medications acutely
- Treatment is based on etiology of delirium
- Chemical sedation in severely agitated patients
  —Benzodiazepines
  —Neuroleptics
  —If withdrawal is likely, consider lorazepam

ED TREATMENT

- Diagnosis and treatment of the underlying medical condition
- Thiamine is administered to alcoholic and malnourished patients
- For patients who are significantly agitated, treatment of the agitation may help facilitate the ED workup
  —Benzodiazepines
  —Neuroleptics

MEDICATIONS

- Alprazolam: 0.25–0.5 mg PO
- Diazepam: 2.5–5 mg PO or i.v.
- Haloperidol: 5–10 mg i.v. or i.m.
- Lorazepam: 0.5–2 mg i.v., i.m., or PO
- Thiamine: 100 mg i.v., i.m., or PO

Disposition

ADMISSION CRITERIA

- When the etiology is unclear, the patient is admitted
- If the delirium has not resolved, the patient is admitted

DISCHARGE CRITERIA

- Treatable cause of the delirium is found and treated
- The patient's mental status clears while in the ED

Miscellaneous

ICD9: 780.09

ICD10: F05.9

SUGGESTED READINGS

American College of Emergency Physicians. Clinical policy for the initial approach to patients presenting with altered mental status. Ann Emerg Med 1999;33: 251–280.

Inouye SK, van Dyck CH, Alessi CA, et al. Clarifying confusion: the confusion assessment method—a new method for detection of delirium. Ann Intern Med 1990;113:941–948.

Kalbfleisch N. Altered mental status. In: Emergency care of the elder person. St. Louis: Beverly Cracom Publications, 1996:119–142.

Lewis LM, Miller DK, Morley JE, et al. Unrecognized delirium in ED geriatric patients. Am J Emerg Med 1995;13(2): 142–145.

Murphy BA. Delirium. Emerg Med Clin North Am 2000;18:243–252.

Author: Arthur Sanders

Delivery, Uncomplicated

Clinical Presentation

SIGNS AND SYMPTOMS

- True labor presents as uterine contractions occurring at least every 5 minutes, and lasting 30–60 seconds
- Signs and symptoms of impending delivery include ruptured membranes (amniotic sac), bloody show (loss of mucous plug), urge to push or to have a bowel movement
- Signs of imminent delivery include a fully effaced and dilated cervix (about 10 cm in a term infant), palpable fetal parts, bulging of perineum, and widening of the vulvovaginal area
- Significant vaginal bleeding with labor demands immediate assessment for placenta previa or abruption

ETIOLOGY

- In general, delivery in the ED is rare
  - —The actual incidence of ED deliveries in the United States is not known
  - —Hospitals in which patients have little prenatal care tend to have a greater incidence of ED deliveries
- ED deliveries usually occur in one of the following three scenarios:
  - —The multiparous patient with a history of prior rapid labor
  - —The nulliparous patient who does not recognize the symptoms of labor
  - —Patients with lack of prenatal care, lack of transportation, or premature labor

Pre-Hospital

- Place patients in the left lateral recumbent position
- EMS personnel should be adequately trained and have proper equipment available for delivery
- EMS transportation of high-risk obstetric patients *before* delivery results in lower neonatal morbidity and mortality and is faster and less expensive when compared with transportation of the neonate *after* delivery
- The use of air transport for obstetric patients has been shown to be safe and effective
  - —If altitude during the flight can result in hypoxia for the compromised fetus, pregnant patients should be placed on supplemental oxygen

Diagnosis

ESSENTIAL WORKUP

- The bimanual pelvic exam is the most useful tool to assess the presence of labor and the possibility of imminent delivery
  - —Assess dilation, station, and effacement of the cervix
  - —Bimanual exam should *not* be done with vaginal bleeding until ultrasound can rule out placenta previa
- Fetal heart tones (FHTs) should be obtained by Doppler

LABORATORY

- If patient is in active labor, CBC, blood typing, and Rh screen should be sent
  - —Kleihauer-Betke testing should be ordered after delivery if an Rh-negative mother gives birth to an Rh-positive child
  - —Rh immunoglobulin can be administered to the mother within 72 hours of delivery
- Urinalysis if there is concern about urinary tract infection or preeclampsia

IMAGING/SPECIAL TESTS

- Imaging studies are not needed for uncomplicated vaginal deliveries
- Third-trimester vaginal bleeding should have emergent ultrasound to evaluate for placental abruption or placenta previa

DIFFERENTIAL DIAGNOSIS

- Braxton Hicks contractions
  - —Irregular uterine contractions that do not result in cervical dilation or effacement
- Muscular low back pain
- Round uterine ligament pain
- Other causes of abdominal pain, such as torsed ovary, appendicitis, nephrolithiasis

Treatment

INITIAL STABILIZATION

- Immediate pelvic examination to assess for cervical dilation, effacement, station, or presenting parts
- Patients in active labor should be transferred to Labor and Delivery immediately unless delivery is imminent
- If the patient is completely dilated and fetal parts are on the perineal verge, prepare for ED delivery

ED TREATMENT

- The obstetrician should be notified that delivery will be occurring in the ED
- If the patient is high risk or less than 36 weeks' gestational age, the pediatrician or neonatologist and NICU should be notified
- Begin IV saline and supplemental oxygen, and place patient in lithotomy position
- Assemble bulb syringe, two sterile Kelly clamps, sterile Mayo scissors, and an umbilical clamp (usually part of an "OB pack")
  - —Neonatal resuscitative equipment should also be available
- If time permits, sterilize vaginal area with povidone-iodine (Betadine)
- Uncomplicated vaginal delivery should occur as follows
  - —As crowning occurs, deliver the head in a controlled fashion, guiding it through the introitus with each contraction
  - —Routine episiotomy is not necessary; however, if the perineum is tearing, perform a midline episiotomy by placing two fingers behind the perineum and make a straight incision toward (but not including) the rectum with sterile Mayo scissors
  - —After the fetal head is delivered, quickly suction the nasopharynx, then feel around the neck for a nuchal cord
    - -If present, manually reduce over the head
    - -If the nuchal cord is too tight, double clamp, cut the cord, and deliver the infant immediately
  - —Apply gentle downward pressure on the fetal head with uterine contractions, and after delivery of the anterior shoulder, the posterior shoulder and remainder of the infant will rapidly deliver
  - —After delivery, the infant should be held at the level of the uterus and the oropharynx suctioned again
  - —Double clamp the cord with sterile Kelly clamps and cut between them
  - —The infant should be stimulated, warmed, and dried; if cyanosis is present, the infant should be given oxygen and resuscitated

—The placenta will spontaneously deliver in 20–30 minutes, and the mother should be observed closely because this is a potentially dangerous time because of postpartum hemorrhage
—Uterine massage can aid in the separation of the placenta from the uterus and limit uterine atony; avoid placing traction on the umbilical cord because this can lead to inversion of the uterus or rupture the cord
—If the patient has severe bleeding and the placenta is not passing spontaneously, the patient should be taken immediately to the operating room
—After delivery of the placenta, it should be examined for any irregular or torn areas suggestive of retained placental products
—If bleeding persists after delivery of the placenta, continue uterine massage; examine for lacerations, and if necessary, give oxytocin IV
—If uterine atony seems to be the cause of bleeding, administer methylergonovine maleate (Methergine) IM
—If bleeding is still not controlled, IM carboprost tromethamine (Hemabate) can be repeated every 15–60 minutes
—The obstetrician and operating room should be notified of continuous bleeding and the need for possible surgical intervention

- In an uncomplicated delivery, the utilization of drugs is not necessary.
  —Massage of the uterus is all that is needed to facilitate the cessation of bleeding after the placenta has been delivered
- However, uterine bleeding is a common postpartum complication, and initially, the uterus, vagina, and perineum should be inspected for a laceration
  —If no laceration is found, it can be assumed that the postpartum bleeding is caused by uterine atony
  —If the uterus does not contract in response to uterine massage, then administer oxytocin IV
  —Continued massage of the uterus may be helpful if the bleeding still persists, then give methylergonovine maleate (Methergine) IM
  —If the bleeding is not responding to these measures, then carboprost tromethamine (Hemabate) can be administered IM

MEDICATIONS

- Carboprost tromethamine (Hemabate): 0.25 mg i.m. every 15–60 minutes (up to two doses)
- Methylergonovine maleate (Methergine): 0.2 mg i.m.
- Oxytocin: 20–20 IU in 1 L of crystalloid infused at 250–500 mL/h i.v.

Disposition

ADMISSION CRITERIA

- All women with uncomplicated deliveries and no significant postpartum bleeding should be admitted to Labor and Delivery or the postpartum unit for care and monitoring
- All infants with respiratory distress, gestational age less than 36 weeks, weight less than 5 pounds, or low Apgar should have immediate pediatric or neonatal consultation and be admitted to a neonatal intensive care unit
- Term infants with none of the above complications may be admitted to the nursery or with the mother to a combined maternal-fetal unit

DISCHARGE CRITERIA

- Adequate recovery from delivery

Miscellaneous

ICD9: 650.0

ICD10: 080.9

SUGGESTED READINGS

Doan-Wiggins L. Emergency childbirth. In: Roberts J, Hedges J, eds. Clinical procedures in emergency medicine, 3rd ed. Philadelphia: WB Saunders, 1998:988–1015.

Druelinger L. Postpartum emergencies. Emerg Med Clin North Am 1994;12: 219–225.

Gianooulod JG. Emergency complications of labor and delivery. Emerg Med Clin North Am 1994;12:201–217.

Zlatnik FJ. Normal labor and delivery and its conduct. In: Scott J, et al., eds. Danforth's obstetrics and gynecology, 7th ed. Philadelphia: WB Saunders, 1998.

Author: James S. Walker

Dementia

Clinical Presentation

SIGNS AND SYMPTOMS

- Acquired loss of cognitive function leading to impairment of daily functioning, may be associated with the following:
  - —Loss of memory—short followed by long term
  - —Impairment of abstract thinking
  - —Impaired judgment and impulse control
  - —Agnosia—inability to recognize objects
  - —Aphasia—language disorder
  - —Apraxia—inability to perform motor functions
  - —Agitation
  - —Apathy
  - —Depression
  - —Inappropriate behavior
  - —Declining personal hygiene and appearance
  - —Urinary or fecal incontinence
- Physical examination
  - —Generally no focal neurologic findings
  - —May be associated with signs of Parkinson's disease tremor, masked facies, bradykinesia
  - —Level of alertness usually normal

MECHANISM/DESCRIPTION

- Progressive degenerative process of the CNS
- Prevalence 1% at age 60 years to 30–50% by age 85 years
- Pathophysiology varies, dependent on etiology
- Primary dementia
  - —Neurofibrillary tangles—Alzheimer's
  - —Gliosis—Pick's
- Secondary dementia
  - —Ischemic—multiinfarct dementia
  - —Subcortical degeneration—Parkinson's, Wilson's
  - —Toxic, metabolic, nutritional derangements—vitamin B_{12}
  - —Prions—Creutzfeldt-Jakob
  - —Virus—HIV dementia
  - —Bacterial—syphilis
  - —Vasculitis—systemic lupus erythematosus (SLE), thrombotic thrombocytopenic purpura (TTP)
- Characterized by gradual decline in cognitive functioning
  - —Generally evolves over a period of years
  - —Course is highly variable, months to years in duration

ETIOLOGY

- Primary dementia
  - —Alzheimer's disease
  - —Lewy's body variant
  - —Pick's
  - —Binswanger's
- Secondary dementia—see Differential Diagnosis

PEDIATRIC CONSIDERATIONS

- Congenital or inborn errors of metabolism
- Secondary etiologies in most nonneonatal presentations more likely to be reversible with early diagnosis and intervention

Pre-Hospital

- Obtain history from friends, family
- Provide for patient and staff safety
- Manage agitation
- Attentiveness to comorbid conditions
- Treat acute toxic and metabolic disorders
  - —Hypoglycemia
  - —Hypothermia
  - —Hyperthermia

Diagnosis

ESSENTIAL WORKUP

- Full and complete history
  - —Must include input from family and friends
  - —Complete list of medications
  - —Comorbid diseases
  - —Full and complete physical examination
  - —Head-to-toe evaluation, all organ systems
  - —Meticulous neurologic examination to include mental status evaluation
- Must eliminate acute reversible or exacerbating factors
- Extent of workup is related to history and course of illness
  - —Extensive evaluation for new diagnosis
  - —Directed evaluation for sudden change of dementia
  - —Limited evaluation for stable disease previously assessed

LABORATORY

- Extent of evaluation dependent on circumstances
- New diagnosis or sudden deterioration
  - —CBC
  - —Erythrocyte sedimentation rate (ESR)
  - —Glucose
  - —Electrolytes
  - —BUN, creatinine
  - —Liver enzymes
  - —Urinalysis
  - —Toxicology screen
  - —Thyroid-stimulating hormone
  - —Vitamin B_{12} level
  - —Syphilis serology (RPR)
  - —HIV
  - —Blood cultures if fever present
  - —Antinuclear antibody if SLE suspected
- Established diagnosis with stable disease, no tests may be required

IMAGING/SPECIAL TESTS

- New diagnosis or sudden deterioration in established dementia
  - —Chest x-ray if infection considered
  - —Head CT, without and with contrast
  - —Lumbar puncture and CSF analysis, syphilis serology
  - —Electroencephalogram if suspicion of seizure disorder
  - —Head MRI in selected cases
- Established diagnosis with stable disease, studies may not be required

DIFFERENTIAL DIAGNOSIS

- Toxic, metabolic, nutritional
  - —Narcotics, sedatives, hypnotics
  - —Alcohol
  - —Heavy metals
  - —Dehydration
  - —Hypothermia, hyperthermia
  - —Hypoglycemia, hyperglycemia
  - —Hyponatremia, hypernatremia
  - —Hypercalcemia
  - —Thiamine deficiency
  - —Vitamin B_{12} deficiency
  - —Niacin deficiency
- Infections
  - —Urinary tract infection (UTI)
  - —Pneumonia
  - —Sepsis
  - —Meningitis, encephalitis
- Seizures—frontal lobe status
- Head trauma
  - —Bilateral chronic subdural hematomas
  - —Pugilistic dementia
- Normal pressure hydrocephalus
- Stroke
- Tumor
- Vasculitis
  - —SLE
  - —TTP
- Depression

Treatment

INITIAL STABILIZATION

- Ensure adequate airway
- Administer O_2 if hypoxic
- Ensure normal vital signs
- Establish intravenous access if required
- In agitated patients provide for patient and staff safety

ED TREATMENT

- Evaluate for reversible causes of altered mental status
- Consider the full differential diagnosis—evaluate and treat appropriately
  - —Treat hypoglycemia with oral or IV dextrose
  - —Treat narcotic overdose or excess with naloxone
  - —Rewarm if hypothermic
  - —Antipyretic for hyperthermia
  - —Intravenous fluids for dehydration
  - —Correct electrolyte abnormalities
  - —Administer antibiotics for infection—UTI and pneumonia most common occult infections
  - —Treat seizures—lorazepam for status, phenytoin for long-term management
- Sedation for agitation—start with low doses and increase as necessary to achieve clinical result
  - —Neuroleptics—haloperidol, risperidone
  - —Benzodiazepines—lorazepam, midazolam
- Soft restraints if chemical sedation not effective
- Attempt to limit number of medications
  - —Reduced likelihood of toxicity
  - —Reduced likelihood of drug-drug interaction
  - —If agitation not an issue, eliminate all sedative-hypnotics
- Treat depression

MEDICATIONS

- Alzheimer's agents—always start at the lowest dose
  - —Donepezil: 5 to 10 mg PO qhs
  - —Tacrine: 10 to 40 mg PO q.i.d.
  - —Rivastigmine: 1.5 to 6 mg PO b.i.d.
  - —Galantamine: 2–12 mg PO b.i.d.
- Amitriptyline: 10–50 mg PO b.i.d., start with lowest dose, oversedation a problem, may worsen dementia useful in patients that cannot sleep
- Dextrose: 25 g slow i.v. push
- Droperidol: 0.625–2.5 mg i.v.—advantage rapid onset, disadvantage risk for QT prolongation, requires prolonged EKG monitoring
- Fluoxetine: 20–60 mg PO q.d., start with the lowest dose
- Haloperidol: 0.5–2 mg PO b.i.d., start with lowest dose 0.5–2.5 mg i.m. or i.v. if rapid onset required
- Lorazepam: 0.5–1 mg i.v., 0.5–2 mg PO
- Midazolam: 0.5–2 mg i.v. slow push
- Naloxone: 0.4–2 mg i.v. push
- Risperidone: 0.5–2 mg PO b.i.d., start with lowest dose

EXPECTED COURSE AND PROGNOSIS

- Primary dementia is characterized by slow steady progression; the course is generally 5 to 10 years from diagnosis to death
- The disease, although inexorable, can fluctuate as a consequence of intervening illness and comorbid conditions
- Cholinesterase medications can improve functional status in patients with Alzheimer's disease
- Careful attention to medications, secondary illnesses, and prompt intervention for infections can improve quality of life and longevity
- Death is generally a consequence of infection, cardiovascular disease, or injury

Disposition

ADMISSION CRITERIA

- Unstable vital signs
- Significant comorbid condition requiring parenteral medications
  - —Pneumonia
  - —UTI
  - —Fluid and electrolyte disorder
- Uncertain diagnosis requiring evaluation of an extent and in a time frame not suitable for outpatient management
- Inadequate home support coupled with an inability to arrange suitable placement from the ED

DISCHARGE CRITERIA

- Stable vital signs
- No significant comorbid conditions
- Secure diagnosis
- Adequate home support
- Reliable access to follow-up care

Miscellaneous

ICD9: 290.0, 294.1, 331.0

ICD10: F03

SUGGESTED READINGS

Conn DK. Cholinesterase inhibitors, comparing the options for mild to moderate dementia. Geriatrics 2001;56:56–57.

Geldmacher DA, Whitehouse PJ. Evaluation of dementia. N Engl J Med 1996;335: 330–336.

Rossor M. Dementia. In: Bradley WG, ed. Neurology in clinical practice, 3rd ed. Boston: Butterworth-Heinemann, 2000:1703–1743.

Smith J, Seirafi J. Organic brain syndrome. In: Marx JA, ed. Rosen's emergency medicine, 5th ed. St. Louis: Mosby, 2002:1468–1485.

Tune LE. Risperidone for the treatment of behavioral and psychological symptoms of dementia. J Clin Psychiatry 2001:62(Suppl 21):29–32.

Dengue Fever

Clinical Presentation

SIGNS AND SYMPTOMS

- Fever:
  - —Abrupt in onset rising to 39°C or higher
  - —2–7 days duration
  - —Biphasic, returning to almost normal after 2–7 days
  - —Associated with frontal or retroorbital headache
- Rash:
  - —Generalized maculopapular rash occurs with onset of fever
  - —After 3–4 days, rash becomes diffusely erythematous
  - —Faded areas appear
  - —Areas of desquamation may appear
  - —After defervescence of fever, scattered petechiae may develop over trunk, extensor surfaces of limbs, and axillae
  - —Palms and soles spared
- Musculoskeletal
  - —Arthralgias and myalgias after onset of fever
  - —Severe lumbar back pain
- GI
  - —Anorexia
  - —Nausea and vomiting
  - —Abdominal pain (sometimes severe)
  - —Altered taste
  - —Hepatomegaly
  - —GI bleeding
- Miscellaneous:
  - —Epistaxis
  - —Gingival bleeding
  - —Hemoptysis
  - —Hypotension
  - —Narrowed pulse pressure (<20 mm Hg)

MECHANISM

- Dengue fever occurs secondary to viral infection
- Poorly understood immunopathologic response causes Dengue hemorrhagic fever (DHF) and Dengue shock syndrome (DSS)
- DHF and DSS usually occur in patients with previous exposure to Dengue virus
- Hemorrhagic manifestations occur after defervescence of fever
- Vascular permeability increases
- Plasma extravasates into extravascular space, including pleural and abdominal cavities
- Shock may ensue
- Disseminated intravascular coagulation (DIC) may develop
- Dengue fever, DHF, and DSS are all self-limited

ETIOLOGY

- Occurs in tropical regions: Asia, Africa, Central and South America, and the Caribbean
- Caused by Dengue virus serotypes 1–4
- Transmitted by mosquitoes: *Aedes aegypti* and *Aedes albopictus*
- Incubation period of 4–7 days

PEDIATRIC CONSIDERATIONS

- Neonatal dengue can occur by vertical transmission if mother infected 0–8 days before delivery
- Infants may develop DHF or DSS because of passive maternal immunity
- DHF and DSS most common in children 7–12 years of age

Pre-Hospital

CAUTIONS

- Intravenous fluid for hypotension

Diagnosis

ESSENTIAL WORKUP

- Primarily a clinical diagnosis
- Suspect in endemic areas
- Suspect in patients with history of travel

LABORATORY

- CBC
  - —Thrombocytopenia
  - —Elevated hematocrit
- Chemistry panel
  - —Elevated BUN
- Liver function tests:
  - —Elevated aspartate transaminase (AST; or serum glutamic-oxaloacetic transaminase [SGOT])
- Coagulation profiles
  - —Prolonged prothrombin time (PT) and partial thromboplastin time (PTT)
  - —Low fibrinogen
  - —D-Dimer
- Virus isolation or detection of dengue virus-specific antibodies (available in only a few laboratories)

IMAGING/SPECIAL TESTS

- Chest x-ray
  - —Pleural effusions
- Tourniquet test:
  - —Inflate BP cuff to median BP in patient's extremity
  - —Test is positive when three or more petechiae appear per square centimeter
- World Health Organization–required criteria for diagnosis of DHF
  - —Fever
  - —Positive tourniquet test or bleeding phenomenon
  - —Hepatomegaly
  - —Shock
  - —Thrombocytopenia (<100,000/mm^3)
  - —Elevated hematocrit (>20%)

DIFFERENTIAL DIAGNOSIS

- Viral illness
- Influenza
- Rubella
- Measles
- Hepatitis
- Appendicitis
- Meningitis
- Malaria
- Rocky Mountain spotted fever
- Typhoid

Treatment

INITIAL STABILIZATION

- IV access
- IV crystalloids for hypotension
- O_2 and monitor for unstable patients

ED TREATMENT

- Treatment is supportive
- Intravenous fluids
- Acetaminophen (Tylenol) for fever
- Analgesics for pain
- Platelet transfusion for severe thrombocytopenia
- DIC therapy, if necessary
- Aspirin and NSAIDS are contraindicated

Disposition

ADMISSION CRITERIA

- ICU admission for the following:
  —Hypotension
  —DIC
  —Thrombocytopenia
  —Hemoconcentration
- Regular admission for the following
  —15 years of age or younger
  —All patients with previous Dengue exposure
  —Any patient where close follow-up is not available

DISCHARGE CRITERIA

- Close follow-up guaranteed
- Tolerating PO
- Pain controlled

Miscellaneous

ICD9: 061

ICD10: A90

SUGGESTED READINGS

Isturiz RE, Gubler DJ, del Castillo JB. Dengue and dengue hemorrhagic fever in Latin America and the Caribbean. Infect Dis Clin North Am 2000;14(1):121–140.

Kautner I, Robinson MJ, Kuhnle U. Dengue virus infection: epidemiology, pathogenesis, clinical presentation, diagnosis and prevention. J Pediatr 1997;131(4):516–524.

Mandell GL, Bennett JE, Douglas RG, eds. Principles and practice of infectious diseases, 5th ed. New York: Churchill Livingstone, 2000:1724–1731.

Author: Jessica Freedman

Dental Trauma

Clinical Presentation

SIGNS AND SYMPTOMS

- History of oral or facial trauma
- Facial edema
- Oral or facial laceration
- Oral or facial pain
  - —Tooth pain (may indicate pulp exposure or inflammation)
  - —Tooth looseness, mobility, or avulsion
  - —Jaw
  - —Ear
  - —Throat
- Exacerbating factors (may indicate pulp exposure or inflammation)
  - —Chewing
  - —Drinking
  - —Extremes of temperature
  - —Pain on palpation
- Bite malocclusion (suggests displaced teeth or maxillary or mandibular fracture)

MECHANISM/DESCRIPTION

- Tooth fractures classified according to the depth of penetration using the Ellis classification system
  - —Class I fracture
    - -Involves only minor chipping of the superficial enamel
    - -Fracture line has uniform chalky white surface
    - -Painless to percussion
  - —Class II fracture
    - -Involves the enamel and dentin
    - -Fracture line will have ivory or pale-yellow appearance
    - -Sensitive to temperature, air, percussion
  - —Class III fracture (*true dental emergency*)
    - -Involves enamel, dentin, and pulp
    - -May be either exquisitely painful or desensitized
    - -Pulp has pinkish, red, fleshy hue within surrounding dentin
    - -Blush of blood after wiping tooth surface indicates pulp violation
- Alveolar bone fractures
  - —Fractures of tooth-bearing portions of mandible, maxilla
  - —Bite malocclusion, painful bite, tooth mobility en bloc

ETIOLOGY

- Age periods of greatest predilection:
  - —Toddlers (falls and child abuse)
  - —School-aged children and preteens (bicycle and playground accidents)
  - —Adolescents (athletic events and altercations, motor vehicle crashes)
  - —Sporting dental injury greatly reduced with mouth guard use
- Assault
- Laryngoscopy
- Domestic violence
- Multiple trauma
- Motor vehicle crashes, motorcycle, bicycle
- Certain predisposing anatomic factors increase risk
  - —Anterior overbite >4 mm increases risk for fracture two to three times
  - —Short upper lip, mouth breathing, after normal occlusion, incompetent upper lip, physical disabilities

Pre-Hospital

- Maintain a patent airway
- Account for all teeth
- Immediate reimplantation of tooth if possible
  - —*Time is tooth:* each minute tooth is out of socket reduces tooth viability by 1%; best chance of success if done in <30 minutes; poor tooth viability if more than 2 hours
- Otherwise, place tooth in a transport solution (listed from most to least desirable, i.e., likelihood of preservation of tooth viability)
  - —Hanks balanced salt solution (HBSS)
    - -Available commercially in the Save-a-Tooth kit
    - -Works well even after 30 minutes avulsion or with dry tooth
  - —Cold milk
  - —Saline
  - —Saliva (patient or parent's mouth)
  - —Never use tap water or dry transport (will cause cell damage)

Diagnosis

ESSENTIAL WORKUP

- Mechanism
  - —Sufficient mechanism necessitates complete evaluation for multiple trauma
- Exact time of injury
- Mechanism
- Assess for changes in occlusion and midface stability
- Account for all missing teeth, tooth fragments, and prostheses (may have been swallowed, aspirated, or impacted into alveolus)
- Careful inspection of the oral cavity
  - —Adjacent soft tissue injuries
    - -Fractures to alveolar bone, mandible, maxilla, condylar injury
  - —Embedded fragments
  - —Associated injuries
    - -Salivary glands
    - -Ducts
    - -Nerves (test tooth sensitivity by tapping with tongue blade in addition to testing mental and infraorbital nerve function)
    - -Blood vessels

LABORATORY

N/A

IMAGING/SPECIAL TESTS

- Plain dental radiograph
  - —Ellis class III fractures
  - —Assess for associated root or alveolar fracture
- Panorex
  - —Indicated if there is a suspicion of associated mandibular fracture
    - -Foreign bodies
    - -Displacement of teeth
    - -Alveolar or jaw fractures
- Chest radiograph
  - —Indicated if a tooth or tooth fragment is unaccounted for
- CT
  - —Indicated for suspected condyle fractures (may be missed by plain film)
- Bronchoscopy
  - —Indicated for removal in cases of dental aspiration

DIFFERENTIAL DIAGNOSIS

- Rule out other significant concurrent facial or systemic injuries

Treatment

INITIAL STABILIZATION

- Ensure patent airway
- Control bleeding by having the patient bite on gauze
- Account for all teeth and tooth fragments
- Immediate reimplantation of avulsed tooth
- Consider early pain control, especially in children

ED TREATMENT

- Ellis class I
  - —File/smooth all sharp edges with an emery board (preventing further injury to soft tissue)
  - —Dental referral for cosmetic repair (nonemergent)
- Ellis class II
  - —Dressing of calcium hydroxide paste (Dycal)
  - —Cover with dry foil, a metal band, or enamel-bonded plastic
  - —Dental referral within 24 hours
  - —In children <12 years of age
    - -Protective dentin layer is thinner, placing pulp at risk for infection
    - -Dress in calcium hydroxide paste and cover in foil
    - -Treat like Ellis class III if pulp blush is visualized below thin dentin layer
    - -Urgent dental referral
- Ellis class III
  - —Immediate dental/oral surgeon referral
    - -Children with primary teeth
- Nerve block, pulpotomy by dentist
  - -Adults and older children
- Nerve block
- Dentist to provide root canal to avoid abscess formation
  - —If dental/oral surgeon is not immediately available
    - -Place a piece of moist cotton over the exposed pulp
    - -Cover with dry dental foil or seal with temporary root canal sealant
  - —Avoid topical anesthetics (may lead to sterile abscess)
- Subluxed tooth
  - —Analgesia, and reduce to normal position
  - —Soft diet if minimally mobile
  - —Mobile teeth require 10–14D of stabilization by dentist
- Tooth avulsion
  - —Gently rinse (do not scrub or sterilize) in saline
  - —Administer local anesthesia
  - —Irrigate socket to remove clots
  - —Reinsert holding the tooth only by the crown
  - —If tooth dry for >30 minutes outside mouth, soak in HBSS for 30 minutes before reimplanting
  - —Proper temporary stabilization with a splint or periodontal pack such as a Coe-Pak
    - -Mix resin and catalyst in even amounts to a firm consistency
    - -Apply to anterior and posterior surface of the avulsed tooth and adjacent two teeth
  - —Prophylactic antibiotic coverage for 5–7 days
  - —Liquid diet for 72 hours, then advance to soft mechanical
  - —Definitive stabilization by a dentist
  - —Primary teeth are never replaced because of potential for ankylosing facial deformity and damage to root bed
- Concussed teeth
  - —Soft diet and follow-up with dentist
- Displaced teeth
  - —Reposition to normal anatomic position by hand with anesthesia and splint
  - —Soft diet, no straws, warm rinses t.i.d., dentist in <24 hours
- Alveolar ridge fracture
  - —Pain control
  - —Oral surgery consult for stabilization
  - —Prophylactic antibiotic coverage
  - —Liquid diet, advance to soft mechanical, no straws, warm rinses t.i.d.
- Significant deep intraoral and through-and-through lacerations require prophylactic antibiotics, saline rinses six times a day, triple antibiotic ointment over skin, and wound check in 48–72 hours

MEDICATIONS

- Acetaminophen with codeine (Tylenol No. 3): 2 tablets PO q4–6h PRN; peds: codeine: 2.5–5.0 mg/kg/24 h (max, 30 mg) PO q4–6h for children 2–6 years old
- Acetaminophen with oxycodone (Tylox): 2 tablets PO q4–6h PRN; peds: oxycodone: 0.05–0.15 mg/kg/dose (max, 10 mg/dose)
- Clindamycin (use if penicillin allergic): 300 mg PO q6h; peds: 10–20 mg/kg/24 h PO q6h
- Erythromycin: adult: 500 mg PO q6h; peds: 30–50 mg/kg/24 h (max, 2 g) PO q6h
- Penicillin V: 500 mg PO q6h; peds: 25–50 mg/kg/24 h (max, 3 g) PO q6h
- Tetanus prophylaxis for dirty wounds, avulsed/intruded teeth and for deep lacerations

Disposition

ADMISSION CRITERIA

- Admission for other associated injuries
- Suspected child or elder abuse and no safe available environment

DISCHARGE CRITERIA

- Isolated dental fractures, Ellis class I
  - —Follow-up with a dentist (necessary not urgent)
- Avulsions, Ellis class II
  - —Dental follow-up within 24 hours
- Ellis class III fractures
  - —Require immediate dental referral owing to the risk for tooth loss and abscess formation
- Advise all patients that involved teeth may die and require future root canal therapy

Miscellaneous

ICD9: 525

ICD10: S09.9

SUGGESTED READINGS

Amsterdam JT. Traumatic dental emergencies. In: Rosen P, et al., eds. Emergency medicine: concepts and clinical practice, 5th ed. St. Louis: CV Mosby, 2002:902–905.

Baumann BM, Thomas LB. Dental injuries. In: Harwood-Nuss A, et al., eds. The clinical practice of emergency medicine, 3rd ed. Philadelphia: Lippincott Williams & Wilkins, 2001:475–480.

Medford HM, Curtis JW. Acute care of severe tooth fractures. Ann Emerg Med 1983;12:364–365.

Powers MP. Diagnosis and management of dentoalveolar injuries. In: Fonseca RJ, Walker RV, eds. Oral and maxillofacial trauma. Philadelphia: WB Saunders, 1991:323–358.

Author: Brian Corwell

Depression

Clinical Presentation

SIGNS AND SYMPTOMS

- Wide variety of presentations
  - —Dramatically in suicidal crisis
  - —Quietly with somatic complaints, panic attacks, or psychosocial distress
- Vague somatic complaints
  - —Weakness, malaise
  - —Weight loss
  - —Headache
  - —Back pain
- Diminished sense of self-esteem
- Loss of interest in or lack of enjoyment of pleasurable activities
- Loss of energy
- Poor appetite
- Sleep disturbance
- Decreased attention span
- Irritability

MECHANISM/DESCRIPTION

- Major depression
  - —Psychiatric illness with depressed mood and neurovegetative signs and symptoms lasting 2 weeks or more
  - —Significant associated morbidity and mortality
  - —Clinician should try to recognize this disorder in the medically ill

ETIOLOGY

- Major depression with suicidal ideations
  - —Biologic illness associated with derangements in several neurotransmitter systems of the brain, including serotonin
- Causes of neurobiologic derangement include
  - —Genetic predisposition
  - —Medical illness
  - —Effects of medications
  - —Chronic unremitting stressors in a predisposed individual
- Women are twice as likely to have major depression than men
  - —Men are more likely to complete suicide successfully

PEDIATRIC CONSIDERATIONS

- Depressed children and adolescents are difficult to diagnose because the criteria are not as easily recognized
- Indicators of major depression in children
  - —Irritability
  - —Changes in school, home, and social functioning
  - —Social withdrawal
  - —Substance abuse
- Consultation with a child psychiatrist is crucial in further assessment and disposition

Pre-Hospital

CAUTIONS

- Patients often seek nonpsychiatric medical care shortly before committing suicide
- Search potentially suicidal patients for weapons
- Obtain additional help for potentially suicidal or dangerous patients

Diagnosis

ESSENTIAL WORKUP

- Eliciting the signs and symptoms of major depression is key to making the diagnosis
- DSM-IV diagnostic criteria include
  - —The presence of *depressed mood or loss of interest or pleasure* for 2 weeks or longer accompanied by at least five of the following criteria
    - -Weight loss or gain
    - -Insomnia or hypersomnia
    - -Psychomotor agitation or retardation
    - -Fatigue or loss of energy
    - -Feelings of excessive guilt or worthlessness
    - -Diminished thinking or concentration or indecisiveness
    - -Suicidal ideation or preoccupation with death

LABORATORY

- Focus is on establishing the diagnosis as a psychiatric illness rather than due to a medical condition
- CBC
- Electrolytes, BUN, creatinine, glucose
- Liver function tests
- Thyroid screen

DIFFERENTIAL DIAGNOSIS

Depressive-like Psychiatric Illnesses

Dysthymia

- Adjustment reactions
- Bereavement
- Acute reactions to stress

Medical Causes of Depression

- Drug induced
  - —Antihypertensives
  - —Oral contraceptives
  - —Steroids
  - —Cimetidine and ranitidine
  - —Sedative-hypnotics
  - —Cocaine and amphetamine
  - —Beta-blockers
  - —Metoclopramide
- Endocrine disorders
  - —Thyroid
  - —Adrenal
  - —Diabetes mellitus
  - —Hyperparathyroid
- Tumors
  - —Pancreatic
  - —Lung
  - —Brain
- Neurologic disorders
  - —Dementia (early phase)
  - —Epilepsy
  - —Huntington's disease
  - —Multiple sclerosis
  - —Parkinson's disease
  - —Stroke
  - —Subdural hematoma
  - —Syphilis
- Infections
  - —Hepatitis
  - —Influenza
  - —Mononucleosis
- Nutritional disorders
  - —Folate deficiency
  - —Pellagra
  - —Vitamin B_{12} deficiency
- Electrolyte disturbances
- End-stage renal pulmonary and cardiovascular disease
- Chronic pain syndromes

Treatment

INITIAL STABILIZATION

- One-to-one nursing, or restrain any potentially suicidal patient for patient safety

ED TREATMENT

Psychological Management

- Empathetic listening to understand the stressors involved in the depression helps focus and encourage patients
- Emphasizing that depression is a treatable condition is reassuring as well as helpful in developing a treatment alliance

Drug Therapy

- For diagnosed neurovegetative, major depression
- Decision to initiate antidepressant medication should be for patients with established follow-up and only with enough medication given until the next appointment
- Low-dose benzodiazepines or neuroleptics maybe used for associated agitation, insomnia, or psychosis
- Usually takes weeks for antidepressant medications to resolve major depression
- Choice of drug for the initiation of antidepressant therapy depends on
  - —Efficacy
  - —Side-effect profile of the agent
  - —Potential lethality if used to overdose
  - —Compliance factors
- Selective serotonin reuptake inhibitors (fluoxetine, sertraline, paroxetine)
  - —Well tolerated
  - —Side effects include
    - -Mild nausea
    - -Decreased appetite
    - -Agitation
    - -Somnolence
    - -Sexual dysfunction
    - -Minimal overdose potential
  - —Starting dose is often final dose
  - —Sertraline better tolerated in the medically ill but may be titrated to 150–200 mg
- Tricyclic antidepressants (amitriptyline, imipramine, nortriptyline)
  - —Side effects include
    - -Anticholinergic effects
    - -Postural hypotension
    - -Sedation
    - -Decreased seizure threshold
    - -Overdoses of as little as 1 g of tricyclic antidepressant can be fatal
  - —Nortriptyline is best tolerated and effective
- Monoamine oxidase inhibitors (phenelzine, tranylcypromine)
  - —Dietary restrictions to avoid hypertensive crisis
  - —Best prescribed by psychiatrist

MEDICATIONS

- Amitriptyline: 25 mg PO t.i.d.
- Fluoxetine: 20 mg PO qd
- Imipramine: initial 25 mg PO t.i.d.
- Nortriptyline: 60 mg PO qd
- Paroxetine: 20 mg PO qd
- Phenelzine: 15 mg PO t.i.d.
- Sertraline: 50 mg PO qd
- Tranylcypromine: 10 mg PO t.i.d.

Disposition

ADMISSION CRITERIA

- Patient is suicidal or at high risk for suicide
- Minimal or unreliable social supports
- Previous history of suicide or poor treatment response
- Symptoms so severe that continual observation or nursing supportive care is required
- Psychotic features
- *Civil commitment* for psychiatric hospitalization is necessary if the patient is refusing treatment and is suicidal or otherwise judged to be at-risk to harm self or others

DISCHARGE CRITERIA

- Low suicide risk
- Adequate social support
- Close follow-up available

Miscellaneous

ICD9: 311

ICD10: F32.9

SUGGESTED READINGS

Arana GW, Rosenbaum JF. Antidepressant drugs. In: Arana GW, Rosenbaum JF, eds. Handbook of psychiatric drug therapy, 4th ed. Philadelphia: Lippincott Williams & Wilkins, 2000:53–113.

APA practice guidelines for the treatment of patients with major depressive disorder, 2nd ed. Washington DC: APPI, 2000.

Cassem NH. Depression. In: Cassem NH, ed. Handbook of general hospital psychiatry, 4th ed. St. Louis: Mosby–Year Book, 1997.

Gliatto MG, Caroff SN, Kaiser R, eds. Concise guide to psychiatry for the primary care practitioner. Washington, DC: APPI, 1999.

Author: Kathy Sanders

Dermatomyositis/Polymyositis

Clinical Presentation

SIGNS AND SYMPTOMS

- Polymyositis (PM) is distinguished from dermatomyositis (DM) by the absence of rash
- Patients with PM present with muscle pain and proximal muscle weakness
- DM presents with skin rash, muscle pain, and weakness
- Constitutional symptoms include weight loss, fever, anorexia, morning stiffness, myalgias, and arthralgias
- Often note fatigue doing customary tasks such as brushing hair, climbing stairs, reaching above the head, or rising from a chair
  - —May also complain of dysphagia, dyspnea, and cough
- Progressive weakness of the proximal limb and girdle muscles is seen early; distal muscle weakness can occur late in the disease
- Skin findings of DM
  - —Skin rash occurs with or precedes muscle weakness
  - —Heliotrope rash (lilac discoloration) on the upper eyelids associated with edema
  - —Gottron's sign: violaceous or erythematous papules over the extensor surfaces of the joints, particularly knuckles, knees, and elbows
  - —Shawl sign: a V-shaped erythematous rash occurring on the back and shoulders
  - —Periungual telangiectasias: nail-bed capillary changes that include thickened irregular and distorted cuticles
  - —"Machinist hands": darkened horizontal lines across the lateral and palmar aspects of the fingers

MECHANISM/DESCRIPTION

- DM/PM is a systemic inflammatory myopathy
  - —Progression of muscle weakness over weeks to months
  - —Respiratory insufficiency from respiratory muscle weakness
  - —Aspiration pneumonia due to a weak cough mechanism, pharyngeal muscle dysfunction, and esophageal dysmotility
  - —Cardiac manifestations include myocarditis and congestive heart failure (CHF)
  - —Arthralgias of the hands, wrists, knees, and shoulders
  - —Ocular muscles are not involved, and facial muscle weakness may be seen in advanced cases

ETIOLOGY

- Exact cause is unknown, although an autoimmune etiology is theorized
- Incidence about 1:100,000 with a female preponderance
- Association with HLA-B8 and HLA-DR3
- There may be an association between PM and viral, bacterial, and parasitic infections
- DM/PM occurs with collagen vascular disease about 20% of the time
- Deposition of complement is the earliest and most specific lesion, followed by inflammation, ischemia, microinfarcts, necrosis, and destruction of the muscle fibers

PEDIATRIC CONSIDERATIONS

- Although DM is seen in both children and adults, PM is rare in children
- Juvenile form may include vasculitis, ectopic calcifications (calcinosis cutis), and lipodystrophy
- The juvenile form may be associated with coxsackievirus

Pre-Hospital

N/A

Diagnosis

ESSENTIAL WORKUP

- Serum muscle enzymes: creatine phosphokinase (CPK), lactate dehydrogenase (LDH), aldolase, aspartate transaminase (AST), and serum glutamic-oxaloacetic transaminase (SGOT)
- EKG and urinalysis
- Diagnostic criteria established in 1975 by Bohan and Peter
  - —Symmetric proximal muscle weakness with dysphagia and respiratory muscle weakness
  - —Elevation of serum muscle enzymes
  - —Electromyographic features of myopathy
  - —Muscle biopsy showing features of inflammatory myopathy
- Confidence limits for diagnosis (typical rash must be seen for diagnosis of DM)
  - —Definite diagnosis: 3–4 criteria
  - —Probable diagnosis: 2 criteria
  - —Possible diagnosis: 1 criterion

LABORATORY

- Elevation of CPK is sensitive for muscle injury but not specific for dermatomyositis
- CPK may be normal in juvenile form
- Levels of aldolase, myoglobulin, creatinine, serum glutamate pyruvate transaminase (SGPT), SGOT, and LDH may be elevated
- Proteinuria, RBC casts, and sediment may be found on urinalysis
- CBC will generally be normal unless occult bleeding from vasculitis or other cause is present
- EKG may show nonspecific ST-T wave changes in up to 30% of patients

IMAGING/SPECIAL TESTS

- Chest x-ray may show interstitial lung disease, evidence of aspiration pneumonia, CHF, or cardiomyopathy
- Electromyogram (EMG) studies show myopathic potentials that are not specific for DM/PM
- Pulmonary function tests are useful in following the progression of interstitial lung disease
- Renal biopsies of patients may show focal proliferative glomerulonephritis
- *Muscle biopsy is the definitive test*
  —In PM, inflammatory infiltrates are often endomysial, although they may be perivascular
  —In DM, inflammatory infiltrates are mostly perivascular and include a high percentage of B cells

DIFFERENTIAL DIAGNOSIS

- Collagen vascular diseases
- Muscular dystrophies, spinal muscular atrophy, myasthenia gravis, amyotrophic lateral sclerosis, poliomyelitis, Guillain-Barré syndrome
- Hypothyroidism, hyperthyroidism, Cushing's syndrome
- Drug-induced: colchicine, zidovudine (AZT), penicillamine, ipecac, ethanol, chloroquine, corticosteroids
- Toxoplasmosis, trichinosis, coxsackievirus, HIV, influenza, Epstein-Barr virus
- Hypokalemia, hypercalcemia, hypomagnesemia, vasculitis, paraneoplastic neuromyopathy, hypereosinophilic myalgia syndrome

Treatment

INITIAL STABILIZATION

- Intubation and mechanical ventilation as required
- NG suction to prevent aspiration
- Pneumothorax has been described as a rare occurrence in childhood DM

ED TREATMENT

- Elevate head of the bed to prevent aspiration
- Begin *high-dose corticosteroids* to suppress inflammation and improve muscle weakness
- Avoid triamcinolone and dexamethasone because there is an associated myopathy
- Efficacy of prednisone determined by objective increase in muscle strength
- Immunosuppressive medications
  —Azathioprine is limited by GI intolerance and bone marrow suppression
  —Cyclosporine has been used but with limited success
  —Methotrexate
- Do not treat CPK level

OUTCOME

- Mortality rate of patient with DM four times that of the general population
- Death is due to pulmonary, renal, or cardiac complications
- Black females have a poorer prognosis
- 5-year survival rate greater than 75% with steroids

MEDICATIONS

- Azathioprine: 3 mg/kg/day for 4–6 months
- Methotrexate: 15–25 mg per week; peds: 0.5–1 mg/kg per week (not to exceed adult dose)
- Prednisone: 60 mg/d; peds: 1–2 mg/kg/d

Disposition

ADMISSION CRITERIA

- Respiratory insufficiency, aspiration pneumonia, muscle weakness, weakened cough mechanisms, and pharyngeal dysfunction, CHF

DISCHARGE CRITERIA

- Well-appearing patients with no respiratory dysfunction and no risk for aspiration
- Patients who can take oral corticosteroids and immunosuppressive agents as outpatients

Miscellaneous

ICD9: 710.4, 710.3

ICD10: M33.1, M33.2

SUGGESTED READINGS

Bohan A, Peter JB. Polymyositis and dermatomyositis. N Engl J Med 1975;292:344–347.

Caro I. Dermatomyositis as a systemic disease: collagen vascular diseases. Med Clin North Am 1989;73(5):1181–1191.

Dalakas MC. Polymyositis, dermatomyositis and inclusion-body myositis [Review]. N Engl J Med 1991;325:1487–1496.

Pachman L. Juvenile dermatomyositis: immunogenetics, pathophysiology, and disease expression. Rheum Dis Clin North Am 2002;28(3):579.

Shearer P, Jagoda A. Dermatomyositis. In: Marx JA, ed. Rosen's emergency medicine: concepts and clinical practice, 5th ed. St. Louis: Mosby, 2002:1525–1526.

Author: Stephen R. Hayden

Diabetes Insipidus

Clinical Presentation

SIGNS AND SYMPTOMS

- Polyuria (up to 16–24 L/d of urine)
- Polydipsia (often crave cold fluids)
- Headache
- Visual disturbance
- Hypernatremia (mild to severe)
- Dehydration
- Signs and symptoms of hypothalamic tumors
  - —Growth disturbances
  - —Cachexia
  - —Obesity
  - —Hyperpyrexia
  - —Sleep disturbances
  - —Sexual precocity
  - —Emotional disturbances

PEDIATRIC CONSIDERATIONS

- Polyuria and polydipsia may not be recognized by caregivers until symptoms of dehydration develop
- Neonatal diabetes insipidus (DI)
  - —Often present at birth
  - —If not recognized, the dehydration and hypernatremia may cause permanent CNS damage.
- In infants:
  - —Irritability
  - —Poor feeding
  - —Growth failure
  - —Intermittent high fever
  - —Abnormal behavior (hyperactivity, restlessness)
- Children
  - —Enuresis

MECHANISM/DESCRIPTION

- Failure of arginine vasopressin (AVP) release (central DI) or renal response to AVP (nephrogenic DI) resulting in passage of large amounts of dilute fluid through body
- Central DI: deficiency of vasopressin release; four types are
  - —No AVP to release (loss or malfunction of posterior pituitary neurons)
  - —Defective osmoreceptors—release AVP only in response to severe dehydration
  - —Elevated threshold for AVP release
  - —Subnormal amount of AVP released
- Genetics
  - —Central DI: familial cases have been reported (autosomal dominant)
  - —Nephrogenic DI: usually X-linked recessive in males

ETIOLOGY

Central DI

- Any condition that disrupts the osmoreceptor-hypothalamus-hypophyseal axis:
  - —Trauma (skull fractures, hemorrhage)
  - —CNS neoplasm—DI can be considered a tumor marker
    - -Pituitary adenomas
    - -Craniopharyngiomas
    - -Germinomas
    - -Pinealomas
    - -Metastatic tumors
    - -Leukemia
    - -Histiocytosis X
    - -Sarcoidosis
- Congenital CNS defects
- Pituitary or hypothalamic surgery
- CNS infections (e.g., meningitis, encephalitis)
- Pregnancy (Sheehan's syndrome, release of placental vasopressinase)
- Idiopathic (autoantibodies, occult tumor)
- Wolfram's syndrome (DI, diabetes mellitus, deafness)

Nephrogenic DI

- Congenital renal disorders
- Obstructive uropathy
- Renal dysplasia
- Polycystic disease
- Systemic disease with renal involvement
- Sickle cell disease
- Sarcoidosis
- Amyloidosis
- Drugs
  - —Amphotericin
  - —Phenytoin
  - —Lithium (persisting past discontinuation of drug)
  - —Aminoglycosides
  - —Methoxyflurane
  - —Demeclocycline
- Electrolyte disturbances
  - —Hypercalcemia
  - —Hypokalemia
  - —Osmotic diuresis

Pediatric Causes

- Newborn:
  - —Asphyxia
  - —Intraventricular hemorrhage
  - —Intravascular coagulopathy
  - —*Listeria monocytogenes* sepsis
  - —Group B streptococcal meningitis

Pre-Hospital

CAUTIONS

- IV access and fluids if signs of dehydration exist

Diagnosis

ESSENTIAL WORKUP

- History
  - —Amount of PO fluid intake per day
  - —Voiding frequency
  - —Drug intake
- Physical exam
  - —Signs of dehydration
  - —Signs of trauma

LABORATORY

- Serum and urine osmolality
  - —High serum osmolality
  - —Low urine osmolality
- Electrolytes, BUN, creatinine, glucose
  - —Hypernatremia
- Calcium
- CBC
  - —For anemia, which may be a sign of neoplasm
- Serum and urine AVP tests are expensive and unnecessary

IMAGING/SPECIAL TESTS

- Chest x-ray to search for neoplasm
- MRI of the pituitary axis

Dehydration Test

- Method
  - —No PO fluids for 3 hours or until urine osmolality stabilize
    - -Caution with fluid deprivation in small children
  - —Determine plasma osmolality (should be above 288 mmol/kg)
  - —AVP: 5 units given (or desmopressin 1 μg SQ or 10 μg intranasally)
  - —Urine osmolality at 0 minutes, 30 minutes and 60 minutes afterward
- In normal patients, osmolality will not change more than 9%
  - —Endogenous AVP will increase osmolality to maximum
  - —Extra AVP has no effect
- In central DI, osmolality rises more than 9%
  - —No or little endogenous AVP
  - —Extra AVP has significant concentrating effect
- In nephrogenic DI, there should be no response to AVP
  - —Renal tubules are insensitive to AVP

DIFFERENTIAL DIAGNOSIS

- Primary sodium excess
- Improperly mixed formula or rehydration solution
- Accidental substitution of NaCl for glucose in infant formulas
- Excessive sodium bicarbonate during resuscitation
- Hypernatremic enemas
- Ingestion of seawater
- Hypertonic saline intravenous administration
- NaCl used to induce vomiting
- Intentional salt poisoning
- High breast milk sodium
- Primary water deficit
- Diabetes mellitus or other solute diuresis
- Gastroenteritis (i.e., water loss greater than solute loss)
- Inadequate breast feeding
- Intentional withholding of water intake
- Increased insensible water loss (e.g., premature infant)
- Inadequate access to free water

Treatment

INITIAL STABILIZATION

- Be suspicious for head trauma and treat accordingly

ED TREATMENT

- Control fluid balance and prevent dehydration
  - —Avoid rapid correction of longstanding hypernatremia
- Central (vasopressin-deficient) DI
  - —Desmopressin
    - -Drug of choice to control symptoms
    - -Administer intranasally two times daily in dosage necessary to control polyuria or polydipsia
    - -Caution in postoperative patients because cerebral edema may develop
  - —Chlorpropamide enhances effect of vasopressin at renal tubule
  - —Clofibrate stimulates the release of endogenous vasopressin
- Nephrogenic DI
  - —Thiazide diuretics enhances sodium excretion
  - —Restrict solutes and avoid excessive drinking to prevent water intoxication
  - —Avoid alcohol (especially beer) intake
- Check weight daily
- Provide good skin and mouth care

MEDICATIONS

- Aqueous arginine vasopressin: 5–10 units SQ in the unconscious patient from head trauma or postop
- Chlorpropamide (Diabinese): 200–500 mg PO qd
- Clofibrate (Atromid-S): 500 mg q6h
- Desmopressin: 10–20 μg intranasally; 2–4 μ SQ or i.v.; 0.1 mg PO
- Hydrochlorothiazide (HCTZ): 50 mg PO qd
- Lypressin nasal spray: 1–2 nasal spray t.i.d. to q.i.d. as needed

Disposition

ADMISSION CRITERIA

- Patients requiring DDAVP testing or a trial of water restriction
- Severe dehydration
- Electrolyte abnormalities
- Associated trauma

DISCHARGE CRITERIA

- Known diagnosis of DI
- Stable electrolytes
- Adequately hydrated

Miscellaneous

ICD9: 253.5

ICD10: E23.2

SEE ALSO: HYPERNATREMIA

SUGGESTED READINGS

Behrman RE, ed. Nelson textbook of pediatrics, 16th ed. Philadelphia: WB Saunders, 2000.

Braunwald E, et al. Diabetes insipidus. In: Braunwald E, ed. Harrison's principles of internal medicine. New York: McGraw-Hill, 2002.

Goroll AH, ed. Primary care medicine, 4th ed. Philadelphia: Lippincott Williams & Wilkins, 2000.

Lee CC. Emergency department presentation of pituitary apoplexy. Am J Emerg Med 2000;18(3):328–331.

Zink BJ. Traumatic brain injury outcome: concepts for emergency care. Ann Emerg Med 2001;37(3):318–332.

Author: Rahul Patwari

Diabetes Mellitus, Juvenile

Clinical Presentation

SIGNS AND SYMPTOMS

- Polydipsia
- Polyuria
- Polyphagia
- Weight loss, unexplained
- Diabetic ketoacidosis (DKA)
  - —Initial presentation in 20–40% of patients
  - —Nausea
  - —Vomiting
  - —Abdominal pain, often resolving with reduction in ketosis
  - —Altered mental status, potentially from cerebral edema
  - —Hyperpnea
  - —Ketotic breath
  - —Dehydration
  - —Shock

MECHANISM/DESCRIPTION

- Insulin deficiency
- Counterregulatory hormones increased
- Hyperglycemia from decreased peripheral glucose utilization and increased hepatic gluconeogenesis
- Osmotic diuresis
- Ketoacidosis produced by increased free fatty acid metabolism
- Potassium deficit
  - —Intracellular shifts into extracellular space due to hydrogen ion exchange
  - —Loss from osmotic diuresis

ETIOLOGY

- Immune-mediated pancreatic islet β-cell destruction
- Precipitating events leading to DKA
  - —Infection
  - —Stress
  - —Pregnancy
  - —Hypoglycemic rebound
  - —Medication noncompliance

Pre-Hospital

- For DKA
  - —Monitor ABCs
  - —Airway protection
  - —Establish intravenous access and initiate fluid bolus

Diagnosis

ESSENTIAL WORKUP

- For DKA
  - —Hourly vital signs and neurologic checks
  - —Frequent blood chemistries

LABORATORY

- For DKA
  - —Glucose, serum and bedside
    - -Hyperglycemia
  - —Urinalysis
    - -Glycosuria
    - -Ketonuria
    - -Exclude urinary tract infection
  - —Blood chemistries every 2–4 hours until acidosis has resolved
  - —Electrolytes and venous pH
    - -Anion gap metabolic acidosis
    - -Potassium—high or normal (artifactual due to extracellular shift)
    - -Sodium—low or normal (may be artifactual due to hyperglycemia)
    - -Bicarbonate—low
  - —Serum ketones—elevated
  - —Serum osmolality
  - —CBC
    - -White blood cell count often elevated owing to stress or infection
  - —Calcium
  - —Phosphate
  - —Cultures as indicated

DIFFERENTIAL DIAGNOSIS

- Infection
  - —Urinary tract infection
  - —Gastroenteritis
  - —Appendicitis
  - —Sepsis
- Ingestion (salicylates, alcohols, glycols)
- Diabetes insipidus

Treatment

INITIAL STABLIZATION

- For DKA
  —Oxygen
  —Cardiac monitor
  —Intravenous access and volume resuscitation

ED TREATMENT

- For DKA
  —Fluid replacement
  -Assume fluid deficit of 10% of body weight
  -Initial volume expansion with 10–20 mL/kg of 0.9% NaCl; may repeat to achieve hemodynamic stability
  -Correct 50% of fluid deficit over first 8 hours, remainder over 24–48 hours
  -Do not give more than 3 L/m^2 over first 24 hours
  —Begin intravenous insulin infusion after ketoacidosis confirmed
  -Initial rate of continuous infusion (regular insulin) 0.1 U/kg/h
  -Adjust rate to drop serum glucose *maximum* of 100 mg/dL/h
  -Add dextrose when serum glucose <300 mg/dL
  -Change to subcutaneous insulin when no longer significantly acidotic and able to eat
  —Replace potassium and phosphate losses
  -Verify adequate urine output
  -Add to fluids as KCl and K_3PO_4 in equal amounts
  -Large doses of K^+ may be necessary; guide therapy by frequent monitoring of K^+
  —Monitor serum sodium
  -Risk for cerebral edema if Na^+ fails to rise as glucose falls
  —Bicarbonate therapy not recommended in most cases
  -Generally does not alter outcome
  -Increased risk for cerebral edema with its use
  —Treat cerebral edema as needed
  -Recognize early, if present
  -Usually occurs 8–12 hours after onset of treatment
  -Mortality rate, 90%
  -Risk factors include fluid rate >4 L/m^2/d, low arterial PCO_2 and high BUN at presentation, and bicarbonate use
  -Decrease fluid administration
  -Endotracheal intubation and hyperventilation
  -Mannitol

MEDICATIONS

- Insulin drip: start 0.1 U/kg/h i.v.
- Mannitol: 0.25–1 g/kg i.v.

Disposition

ADMISSION CRITERIA

- For DKA
  —Intensive care unit (ICU)
  -Altered mental status
  -Shock or cardiac dysrhythmia
  -Initial glucose >1000 mg/dL
  -Initial pH <7.0
  —Inpatient unit
  -Stable new-onset diabetic patients requiring intensive education
  -Patients with ketoacidosis not meeting requirements for ICU care
  -Compliance concerns or other social issues

DISCHARGE CRITERIA

- Known diabetic patients who respond well to therapy with normalization of glucose, pH, and ketosis
- Tolerating oral fluids
- Reliable parents
- Reliable follow-up within 24 hours

Miscellaneous

ICD9: 250.1

ICD10: E10

SUGGESTED READINGS

Finberg L. Why do patients with diabetic ketoacidosis have cerebral swelling and why does treatment sometimes make it worse. Arch Pediatr Adolesc Med 1996;150:785.

Glaser N, Barnett P, McCaslin I, et al. Risk factors for cerebral edema in children with diabetic ketoacidosis. N Engl J Med 2001;344:264–269.

Green SM, Rothrock SG, Ho JD, et al. Failure of adjunctive bicarbonate to improve outcome in severe pediatric diabetic ketoacidosis. Ann Emerg Med 1998;31:41–48.

Klekamp J, Churchwell KB. Diabetic ketoacidosis in children: initial clinical assessment and treatment. Pediatr Ann 1996;25:387–393.

Rosenbloom AL, Hamas R. Diabetic ketoacidosis (DKA): treatment guidelines. Clin Pediatr 1996;35:261–266.

Author: Stephanie Zimmerman

Diabetic Ketoacidosis

Clinical Presentation

SIGNS AND SYMPTOMS

- Dehydration
  - —Hypotension
  - —Tachycardia
  - —Sunken eyes
  - —Tenting of skin
  - —Dry mucous membranes
  - —Longitudinally furrowed tongue
- Metabolic acidosis
  - —Tachypnea
  - —Kussmaul's respiration (rapid, deep, sighing respiration)
  - —Myocardial depression
  - —Vasodilation
  - —Fruity odor on breath
- Nausea and vomiting
- Abdominal pain and tenderness

MECHANISM/DESCRIPTION

- Relative insulin deficiency and excess of counterregulatory hormones (glucagon, growth hormone, catecholamines and cortisol) resulting in a triad of
  - —Ketonemia—primary cause of metabolic acidosis
  - —Hyperglycemia—results in osmotic diuresis
  - —Metabolic acidosis
- Potassium exchanges with hydrogen as an intracellular buffer
- GI symptoms due to acidosis and hypokalemia-induced paralytic ileus

ETIOLOGY

- Infectious process
- Noncompliance with insulin/oral hypoglycemic agent
- New-onset diabetes mellitus (DM) (25%)
- Myocardial infarction (MI)
- Cerebrovascular accident (CVA)
- Pregnancy
- GI bleed

PEDIATRIC CONSIDERATIONS

- Overwhelming majority of children with diabetes have type I disease and are ketosis prone
- Diabetic ketoacidosis (DKA) is initial presentation of diabetes in 10% of children

Pre-Hospital

N/A

Diagnosis

ESSENTIAL WORKUP

- Diagnostic criteria
  - —Glucose >300 mg/dL
  - —HCO_3^- <15 mEq/L
  - —pH <7.3 with ketonemia and ketonuria
- Bedside glucose measurement (Accu-Chek)
- Arterial blood gas (ABG)
- Urine dip for ketones
- Search for precipitating factor

LABORATORY

- Serum glucose
  - —Essential to confirm results of reagent strips
- Electrolytes
  - —Increased anion gap metabolic acidosis
  - —Sodium
    - -Measured serum sodium often spuriously lowered by hyperglycemia
    - -Pseudohyponatremia correction factor: 1.6 mEq/L is added to measured value for every 100 mg/dL of blood glucose >100 mg/dL
    - -Sodium deficit with DKA
  - —Potassium
    - -Initial level usually normal to high owing to extracellular shift as compensation for acidosis
    - -Level decreases precipitously with fluid and insulin
    - -For every 0.1 increase in pH, potassium decreases by 0.6 mEq/L
    - -Deficit of total-body potassium common
- BUN, creatinine
  - —Elevated due to dehydration/renal damage
- Urinalysis
  - —Ketonuria glycosuria, proteinuria
  - —Check for urinary tract infection (UTI) as precipitant
- CBC
  - —WBC often increased to 15–20,000 mm^3 in absence of infection
  - —Suspect infection if left shift of differential present
- Serum human chorionic gonadotropin (hCG)
- Ketones
  - —May be spuriously low or absent because only acetone and acetoacetate measured
  - —β-Hydroxybutyrate not measured by nitroprusside reaction
- Serum osmolality—measured and calculated
  - —Calculated: $2(Na^+)$ + glucose/18 + BUN/2.8
  - —Normal range: 285–300
  - —Significant hyperosmolarity >320 mOsm/L
- Lab tests of secondary importance
  - —Mg^{2+}—decreased (changes follow serum potassium)
  - —Calcium—hypocalcemia may result from phosphate administration
  - —Phosphate—decreased (changes follow serum potassium)
  - —Amylase
  - —Lactate

IMAGING/SPECIAL TESTS

- Chest x-ray for pneumonia
  - —Common precipitant
  - —Aspiration if decreased level of consciousness
- EKG to rule out MI as a precipitant of DKA
- CT head—if altered mental status possibly due to primary CNS condition

DIFFERENTIAL DIAGNOSIS

- Nonketotic hyperosmolar coma
- Alcoholic ketoacidosis
- Methanol
- Uremia
- Paraldehyde
- Isoniazid
- Lactic acidosis
- Ethylene glycol
- Sepsis
- Alcohol or drug intoxication
- Starvation ketoacidosis

PEDIATRIC CONSIDERATIONS

- DKA may mimic bacterial sepsis as well as occur concomitantly with it
  - —If etiology of DKA uncertain, consider septic workup (including CBC, blood cultures, urinalysis, LP) and antibiotics

Treatment

INITIAL STABILIZATION

- ABCs with intubation if comatose
- Naloxone, thiamine, Accucheck (or dextrose) for coma of unknown etiology
- Aggressive 0.9% NS fluid resuscitation if hypovolemic

ED TREATMENT

- Rehydration
  —Average fluid deficit in DKA: 5-10 L
  —Administer first liter bolus over 30-60 minutes
  —Initial 2 L use 0.9% NS to replace intravascular deficit, then switch to 0.45% NS
  —Avoid volume overload in patients with congestive heart failure
  —Speed of rehydration may be related to risk for cerebral edema; many recommend slower rehydration
- Cardiac monitor until electrolyte disorder corrected
- Insulin
  —Stops ketosis and replenishes cellular glucose
  —Goal is to decrease glucose by 100 mg/dL/h
  —Initiate infusion 5-10 IU/h (0.1 IU/kg)
  —Increase insulin drip if glucose fails to respond within 1 hour
  —Switch to glucose-containing IV when blood glucose falls to 250 mg/dL
  —Continue glucose and insulin until pH >7.3
- Potassium
  —Depletion and imminent hypokalemia may only become apparent as
    -Rehydration is instituted
    -Potassium shifts back into cells
    -Renal excretion returns to normal
  —Add 10 mEq to each liter of IV fluid once renal function adequate, EKG is normal, and serum K <5.5 mEq/L
  —Add 40-80 mEq/h when K <3.5 mEq/L or if bicarb is given
  —Monitor electrolytes hourly until pH >7.3 and potassium repleted to K >4.0 mEq/L
- Phosphorus
  —Supplement if phosphorus level <1 mg/dL
  —Use potassium phosphate 20 mEq/L IV fluid with concomitant potassium depletion
- Sodium bicarbonate
  —Administer only for pH <7.0
  —Complications include cerebral edema, alkalosis, paradoxical cerebrospinal fluid acidosis
  —Administer 44 mEq if pH <7.0 but >6.9
  —Administer 88 mEq if pH <6.9
- Magnesium repletion if low level
  —0.35 mEq/kg magnesium in fluids for first 3-4 hours
  —2.5-3.0 g $MgSO_4$ in 70-kg patient

MEDICATIONS

- D50W: 1 amp (25 g) of 50% dextrose (peds: 2-4 mL/kg D25W) intravenous push (IVP)
- Insulin (regular, short acting)
- Naloxone: 2 mg (peds: 0.1 mg/kg) IVP
- Potassium phosphate: phosphates 3 μmol/mL and potassium 4.4 mEq/mL
- Sodium bicarbonate (1 amp = 50 mL = 44 mEq): 1-2 mEq/kg i.v.
- Thiamine: 100 mg (peds: 10-25 mg) IVP

PEDIATRIC CONSIDERATIONS

- Average fluid deficit is 100-150 mL/kg
- Initial volume replacement should be 20 mL/kg NS bolus over 1 hour
  —Repeat as necessary if in shock
- Replace deficit at 1.5 times maintenance needs over next 24-36 hours
- Switch to D5 0.45% NS when blood glucose <250 mg/dL

Disposition

ADMISSION CRITERIA

- ICU admission for pH <7.0, serious concurrent illness, mental obtundation or coma, age <2 years or >60 years
- Telemetry admission if patient has history of congestive heart failure or coronary artery disease
- Regular admission for moderate DKA
- Observation (12-24 hours) admission if bicarbonates >12 mEq/L with no serious precipitating event

DISCHARGE CRITERIA

- Resolution of anion gap acidosis
- Able to tolerate oral fluids
- No evidence of concurrent illness (infection) which may precipitate DKA

Miscellaneous

ICD9: 250.1

ICD10: E14.1; E10.1; E11.1

SEE ALSO: HYPEROSMOLAR SYNDROME

SUGGESTED READINGS

Carroll MF, Schade DS. Ten pivotal questions about diabetic ketoacidosis: answers that clarify new concepts in treatment. Postgrad Med 2001;110(5):89–92, 95.

Fleckman AM. Diabetic ketoacidoses. Endocrinol Metab Clin North Am 1993;22(2):181–207.

Kitabchi AE, Wall BM. Diabetic ketoacidosis. Med Clin North Am 1995;79(1):9–33.

Magee MF, Bhatt BA. Management of decompensated diabetes: diabetic ketoacidosis and hyperglycemic hyperosmolar syndrome. Crit Care Clin 2001;17(1):75–106.

Author: Steven Friedman

Dialysis Complications

Clinical Presentation

SIGNS AND SYMPTOMS

Vascular Access Related

- Bleeding from puncture sites
- Loss of bruit in the graft
- Local infection, cellulitis, fever
- Decreased sensation, strength distal to access

Non–Vascular Access Related

- Hypotension before, during, or after the procedure
- Dysrhythmias
- Chest pain (ischemic, pleuritic)
- Hemorrhage (GI, pleural, retroperitoneal)
- Shortness of breath
- Neurologic (disequilibrium syndrome)
  - —Headache
  - —Malaise
  - —Seizures
  - —Coma

Peritoneal

- Abdominal pain
- Cloudy dialysis effluent
- Vomiting
- Exudates or inflammation at insertion site of Tenckhoff catheter

MECHANISM/DESCRIPTION

Vascular Access Related

- Infections
  - —Due to *Staphylococcus aureus*
  - —Bacteremia may be present without local signs of infection

Non–Vascular Access Related

- Hypotension
  - —After dialysis: due to acute decrease in circulating blood volume
  - —During dialysis: hypovolemia or onset of cardiac tamponade due to compensated effusion suddenly becoming symptomatic after correction of volume overload
  - —Myocardial infarction (MI), sepsis, dysrhythmias
  - —Hemorrhage secondary to anticoagulation, platelet dysfunction of renal failure
- Shortness of breath
  - —Volume overload
  - —Development of dyspnea *during* dialysis (tamponade, pericardial effusion, hemorrhage, anaphylaxis, pulmonary emboli, or air emboli)
- Chest pain
  - —Ischemic: dialysis creates acute physiologic stressor with transient hypotension and hypoxemia and increased myocardial oxygen demand
  - —Pericarditis if pleuritic
- Neurologic dysfunction: disequilibrium syndrome
  - —Rapid decrease in serum osmolality during dialysis leaving the brain in a comparatively hyperosmolal state

Peritoneal

- Peritonitis
  - —Due to contamination of the peritoneal dialysate or tubing during an exchange
  - —*S. aureus* or *Staphylococcus epidermidis* (70%)
- Perforated viscus with severe abdominal pain, fever, brown or fecal material in the effluent, or localized tenderness
- Fibrinous blockage of the catheter resulting from infection or inflammation

Pre-Hospital

CAUTIONS

- Do not perform IV access and BP measurement in an extremity with a functioning access
- Run IV fluids slowly and keep to a minimum if possible
- Administer furosemide in pulmonary edema (use high doses up to 200 mg in anuric patients)

Diagnosis

ESSENTIAL WORKUP

- Infection
  - —Blood and wound cultures
  - —Cell count, Gram stain, and culture of peritoneal fluid
  - —Careful physical exam for occult sources of infection (odontogenic, perirectal abscess)
- Bleeding
  - —CBC to evaluate anemia and platelet count
  - —Coagulation studies
  - —Stool for guaiac
- Chest pain and shortness of breath
  - —EKG
  - —Chest x-ray
  - —Arterial blood gas (ABG)
  - —Cardiac enzymes
- Neurologic dysfunction
  - —CT of brain for intracranial hemorrhage

LABORATORY

- Electrolytes, BUN, creatinine, glucose
- CBC

IMAGING/SPECIAL TESTS

- Echocardiogram for suspected pericarditis, effusion, or tamponade
- Ultrasonography of access for possible clotted graft or fistula
- Peritoneal catheterogram for catheter blockages

DIFFERENTIAL DIAGNOSIS

- Hypotension
  - —Hypovolemia
  - —Cardiogenic shock, acute MI, tamponade, dysrhythmias
  - —Hyperkalemia or hypokalemia
  - —Hypercalcemia or hypocalcemia
  - —Hypermagnesemia
  - —Embolism: air or pulmonary
  - —Vascular instability: autonomic neuropathy, drug related, dialysate related
- Neurologic complications
  - —Cerebrovascular accident (CVA)
  - —Intracranial bleed
  - —Meningitis or abscess
  - —Disequilibrium syndrome
  - —Uremia
  - —Hypernatremia or hyponatremia
  - —Hyperglycemia or hypoglycemia
  - —Hypoxemia
- Peritoneal
  - —Peritonitis
  - —Hernia incarceration
  - —Perforated viscus
  - —Acute abdominal process: appendicitis, cholecystitis

Treatment

INITIAL STABILIZATION

- ABCs

Vascular Access Related

- Bleeding
  - —Firm pressure to site(s)
    - -Do not totally occlude the graft—may cause clotting
    - -Document presence of trill postpressure
  - —Apply Gelfoam

Non–Vascular Access Related

- Hypotension
  - —Search for underlying cause
  - —Vasopressors, fluid, saline
- Shortness of breath
  - —Attempt diuresis if fluid overloaded and arrange dialysis
- Hyperkalemia
  - —Administer IV calcium, bicarbonate, insulin, and glucose
  - —Monitor cardiac rhythm
  - —Administer ion exchange resin (Kayexalate)
  - —Arrange for dialysis
- Neurologic complications
  - —Narcan, thiamine, dextrose (or Accucheck) for altered mental status
  - —Control seizures with benzodiazepines

ED TREATMENT

Vascular Access–Related Complications

- Infection
  - —Initiate antistaphylococcal IV antibiotics
- Clotted access
  - —Analgesia
  - —Warm compresses
  - —Vascular surgery consult
- Hemorrhage
  - —Control bleeding
  - —Correct coagulopathies
  - —Administer IV fluids and blood products

Non–Vascular Access–Related Complications

- Electrolyte imbalances
  - —Treat hypercalcemia or hypermagnesemia with
    - -Saline infusion if tolerated (dilution)
    - -Diuresis with furosemide
    - -Dialysis
- Volume overload
  - —Attempt diuresis
  - —Arrange dialysis
- Pericardial effusion or tamponade
  - —Emergent pericardiocentesis may be necessary
  - —Arrange dialysis
- Acute MI
  - —Thrombolytics or angioplasty if candidate
  - —Nitrates to decrease myocardial workload
- Disequilibrium syndrome
  - —Rule out other causes of altered mental status
  - —Resolves over time
  - —May respond to hyperosmolar infusions (mannitol, hypertonic saline)

Peritoneal Complications

- Peritonitis: IV antibiotics or intraperitoneal antibiotics
- Catheter or tunnel infection culture, visible exudates
  - —Oral antibiotics (antistaphylococcal)
  - —If recurrent or tunnel, may need to be unroofed
  - —Meticulous site care
- Perforated viscus
  - —IV antibiotics
  - —Surgical consultation

MEDICATIONS

- Calcium gluconate: 1 g slowly i.v. (cardioprotective in hyperkalemia)
- Cefazolin: 1 g i.v. or i.m. followed by 250 mg/2 L bag × 10 days (peritonitis)
- Dextrose: D50W 1 amp (50 mL or 25 g) (peds: D25W 2–4 mL/kg) i.v. (hyperkalemia or hypoglycemia)
- Dopamine: 2–20 μg/kg/min i.v.
- Furosemide: 20–100 mg i.v. (may require doses of 300 mg or more to effect diuresis in chronic renal failure)
- Insulin: 5–10 U regular insulin i.v. (with D-50 for hyperkalemia)
- Naloxone (Narcan): 2 mg (peds: 0.1 mg/kg) i.v. or i.m. initial dose
- Nitroglycerin: 0.4 mg SL; 5–20 μg/min i.v.
- Sodium bicarbonate: 1 mEq/kg up to 50–100 mEq i.v. PRN
- Sodium polystyrene sulfonate (Kayexalate): 1 g/kg up to 15–60 PO or 30–50 g retention enema q6h PRN hyperkalemia
- Thiamine (Vitamin B_1): 100 mg (peds: 50 mg) i.v. or i.m.
- Tobramycin: 1.7 mg/kg i.v. or i.m.; then 10 mg/2 L bag × 10 days (peritonitis)
- Vancomycin: 1 g i.v. or i.m.; then 50 mg/2 L bag × 10 days (peritonitis)

Disposition

ADMISSION CRITERIA

- ICU admission for severe hyperkalemia, pulmonary edema, volume overload, persistent hypotension, uncontrolled seizures, acute MI, CVA, pericarditis, and sepsis
- Regular admission for fever, vomiting, non–life-threatening electrolyte disturbances, or inability to provide self-care for continuous ambulatory peritoneal dialysis (CAPD) with antibiotics

DISCHARGE CRITERIA

- Mild infections of the access site or peritonitis without toxic, systemic symptoms
- Same-day surgery for some thrombectomy procedures
- Control of hemostasis control at puncture sites

Miscellaneous

ICD9: N/A

ICD10 CODE: N/A

SEE ALSO: RENAL FAILURE

SUGGESTED READINGS

Feldman HI, Held PJ, Hutchinson JT, et al. Hemodialysis vascular access morbidity in the United States. Kidney Int 1993; 43(Suppl 41):S1091–1096.

Khan IH, Catto GRD. Long-term complications of dialysis: infection. Kidney Int 1993;43(Suppl 41):S143–S148.

Marx JA, et al., eds. Rosen's emergency medicine: concepts and clinical practice, 5th ed. St. Louis: CV Mosby, 2002: 1380–1388.

Author: Mary Stewart

Diaper Rash

Clinical Presentation

SIGNS AND SYMPTOMS

- Shiny, glazed appearance of the skin
- Maceration and fissures
- Beefy-red confluent patches
  - —"Kissing maculopapules"
- Candidal rashes
  - —Sharply demarcated with satellite lesions
- Pruritus
  - —May be seen in pinworm or *Tricophyton* species infection
- Pustules
  - —Secondarily infected rash
- Jacquet's syndrome
  - —Chronic severe irritant dermatitis with atrophic skin changes

MECHANISM/DESCRIPTION

- Most common dermatologic disorder of infancy
- Prevalence in the first year of life estimated at 7–35% with peak incidence in the first 4 weeks and again at 9–12 months
- Incidence in adults unknown but most common among incontinent patients
- Prolonged presence of moisture
  - —Moist skin provides a good growth medium for bacteria and candida
  - —Bacterial overgrowth leads to loss of integrity of epidermal barrier
  - —Trapped moisture in the diaper area causes erythema
- Friction
  - —Diaper against skin causes irritation
  - —On moist skin, less friction is needed to cause irritation
  - —Tape cuts from plastic adhesive tabs
  - —Maceration of the intertriginous areas
- Chemical irritation
  - —Stool enzymes, urine, or artificial scents
- Infection
  - —*Candida albicans*
    - -Clusters of erythematous papules and pustules
    - -Coalesce into a beefy-red confluent rash with sharply demarcated borders
    - -Satellite papules and pustules outside the border of the main rash are pathognomonic
    - -40% of infants with diaper rash for >72 hours may be secondarily infected with candida; 80% if >96 hours
  - —Pinworms infestation
    - -Erythema, edema, and excoriations of perianal areas (pruritus ani)
    - -Female pinworm migrates from the bowel out onto the perianal skin and lays eggs
    - -Usually occurs at night; hence, the tape test is best performed first thing in the morning
- Atopic dermatitis
  - —Similar in appearance to irritant dermatitis
  - —Look for similar lesions on other body surfaces
  - —Rash often more confluent and textured (cobblestone) than irritant dermatitis
- Seborrheic dermatitis
  - —Lesions with an erythematous base and greasy yellow or gray scale
  - —Look for similar lesion on other body surfaces

ETIOLOGY

- Irritant—moisture, friction, chemical
- Infection—*C. albicans, Enterobius vermicularis* (pinworms)
- Atopic
- Seborrheic

Pre-Hospital

N/A

Diagnosis

ESSENTIAL WORKUP

- Inquire about diaper-changing habits and urinary and fecal habits
- Examine other body areas to identify associated rashes
- Consider child abuse or neglect
  - —Child's overall hygiene
  - —Burns or other trauma

LABORATORY

- Skin surface scrapings with KOH prep
  - —Look for budding yeast and/or pseudohyphae
  - —Diagnosis usually empiric based on the appearance of the rash
- Cellophane adhesive tape test to assess for pinworm
  - —Press tape onto the perianal skin
  - —Examine for pinworm eggs under direct microscopy
  - —Best performed first thing in the morning

IMAGING/SPECIAL TESTS

N/A

DIFFERENTIAL DIAGNOSIS

- Infection
  - —Bullous impetigo
  - —Scabies
  - —Herpes simplex
  - —Varicella
  - —Congenital syphilis
- Child abuse
- Psoriasis
- Bullous pemphigoid
- Papular urticaria

Treatment

ED TREATMENT

- Topical barrier preparation (e.g., zinc oxide)
  —Provides moisture-impermeable barrier
  —Reduces friction
- Topical anti-yeast agent (e.g., Nystatin, Clotrimazole, Miconazole) if one or more of the following are present
  —Obvious candidal infection
  —Spreading or painful rash
  —Rash >72 hours old
  —KOH prep positive for yeast
- Oral antiparasitic agent if indicated (e.g., Mebendazole)
  —Evidence of pinworm eggs by tape test
- *Avoid* mid- to high-potency halogenated steroid preparations because these may lead to systemic effects and skin changes

MEDICATIONS

- Clotrimazole: apply q.i.d. or with each diaper change
- Hydrocortisone (1% topical); for primary irritant dermatitis only, apply t.i.d. or q.i.d.
- Miconazole: apply q.i.d. or with each diaper change
- Mebendazole: for pinworm infestation, 100 mg PO single dose, repeat in 2 weeks
- Nystatin: apply q.i.d. or with each diaper change
- Zinc oxide: apply at earliest sign of diaper rash and b.i.d. or t.i.d. thereafter

Disposition

ADMISSION CRITERIA

- Evidence of child abuse or severe neglect
- Evidence of sepsis

DISCHARGE CRITERIA

- Instruct parents/caregivers:
  —Remove irritants
  —Diaper change every 2 hours
  —Leave baby without diaper as much as possible; naps are a good time
  —Gentle rinsing of affected area with warm water followed by air drying
  —Avoid soaps or alcohol wipes because these may irritate or degrade the protective epithelial layer
  —Cornstarch is contraindicated because it serves as a culture medium for candida
  —Ensure proper fit of diapers to minimize friction; superabsorbent diapers may be helpful

Miscellaneous

ICD9: 691.0

ICD10: L22

SUGGESTED READINGS

Daniel GL, Longo WE, Vernava AM 3rd. Pruritus ani: causes and concerns. Dis Colon Rectum 1994;37(3):670–674.

Sires UL, Mallory SB. Diaper dermatitis: how to treat and prevent. Postgrad Med 1995;98:79–84.

Ward DB, Fleischer AB Jr, Feldman SR, et al. Characterization of diaper dermatitis in the United States. Arch Pediatr Adolesc Med 2000;154(9):943–946.

Wolf R, Wolf D, Tuzun B, Tuzun Y. Diaper dermatitis. Clin Dermatol 2000;18(6):657–660.

Authors: Stephen C. Copps; Deepi G. Goyal

Diaphragmatic Trauma

Clinical Presentation

SIGNS AND SYMPTOMS

- Signs and symptoms vary depending on whether phase is acute, latent, or obstructive
- *Acute phase:* tachypnea, hypotension, absence of breath sounds, abdominal distention, or bowel sounds in the chest
- *Latent phase:* abdominal discomfort caused by intermittent herniation of abdominal contents into thorax
  —Nonspecific symptoms such as abdominal pain that is worse postprandially or exacerbated by lying supine
  —Pain may radiate to the left shoulder, be relieved by sitting or standing
  —Nausea, vomiting, or belching
- *Obstructive phase:* severe abdominal pain, obstipation, nausea, vomiting, and abdominal distention
- Abdominal organs, strangulated and necrotic, may perforate and spill abdominal contents into the chest
  —Respiratory compromise, sepsis, and death

MECHANISM/DESCRIPTION

- Penetrating injury: violation of the diaphragm by the penetrating object (knife and gunshot wounds)
  —May involve any portion of the diaphragm
  —The defect is usually less than 2 cm in length
- Blunt injury: increased intraabdominal or intrathoracic pressure is transmitted to the diaphragm, causing rupture
  —Injuries are typically in a radial orientation, in the posterolateral area of the left side of the diaphragm
  —Embryologic point of weakness; injuries are frequently between 5 and 15 cm in length
- Diaphragmatic defects do not heal spontaneously because of the pleuroperitoneal pressure gradient, which may exceed 100 cm H_2O during maximal respiratory effort
  —Promotes herniation of the abdominal contents through the rent in the diaphragm and into the chest

ETIOLOGY

- Incidence is estimated to be 1–6% in all patients sustaining multiple-system trauma
- Lateral torso impact is three times more likely to result in ipsilateral blunt diaphragmatic rupture than frontal impact
- Diaphragmatic injury should be suspected with penetrating trauma to the thoracoabdominal area, or injuries that cross the plane of the diaphragm

Pre-Hospital

CAUTIONS

- Herniation of abdominal contents into the chest wall may mimic hemothorax or tension pneumothorax
  —Bowel sounds in the chest may help distinguish
  —Be suspicious of diaphragmatic injury with lateral compression of the chest, and be cautious in placement of needle or tube thoracostomies

Diagnosis

- In the acute phase, there may be no abdominal visceral herniation
  —This injury may even be missed on initial laparotomy

ESSENTIAL WORKUP

- Chest x-ray is essential and may reveal herniated loops of bowel or other abdominal viscera in the thorax
  —Pathognomonic finding is the presence of a nasogastric tube above the diaphragm
  —Findings are often nonspecific: a unilaterally elevated diaphragm, mediastinal shift away from the affected side, unilateral pleural thickening, areas of atelectasis or consolidation at the bases, or small hemothorax or pneumothorax
  —50% of initial chest x-rays may be normal
- Diagnosis may be difficult in the latent phase because of the intermittent nature of herniation
  —Contrast studies of the gastrointestinal tract may be helpful

LABORATORY

- If diagnostic peritoneal lavage (DPL) is performed, a red blood cell count of 5000 RBC/mm^3 is the recommended level for interpretation as positive
- No laboratory studies confirm or rule out the presence of diaphragmatic injury

IMAGING/SPECIAL TESTS

- Gastrointestinal contrast studies are the most useful in diagnosing chronic herniation of abdominal contents through the diaphragm
- Ultrasound has been successfully used to diagnose traumatic diaphragmatic rupture, particularly on the right side with accompanying hepatic herniation
- CT has been used; it is rarely diagnostic and has poor sensitivity
- MRI may be useful
- Diagnostic pneumoperitoneography is a technique whereby air is injected through a DPL catheter, and pneumothorax on subsequent chest x-ray is diagnostic of diaphragmatic injury
  —Poorly tolerated by unstable patients and may require chest tube placement
- Thoracoscopy and laparoscopy are potentially valuable tools, both diagnostically and therapeutically

DIFFERENTIAL DIAGNOSIS

- Atelectasis, hemothorax, pneumothorax
- Gastric dilation, pulmonary contusion, intraabdominal fluid
- Traumatic pneumatocele, subdiaphragmatic abscess, intrathoracic cyst
- Empyema, congenital eventration of the diaphragm

Treatment

INITIAL STABILIZATION

- Follow advanced trauma life support (ATLS) protocols
- If respiratory distress is present, immediate placement of a nasogastric tube may decompress herniated abdominal contents

ED TREATMENT

- Palpate within the chest wall completely for visceral organs before placing chest tube
- Patients with visceral perforations are septic and need aggressive resuscitation and antibiotic therapy
- Early surgical intervention is paramount
- Thoracoscopy is useful in selected injuries
- Empiric broad-spectrum antibiotics are indicated in the case of perforated viscera

MEDICATIONS

- Gram-negative aerobes
  —Gentamicin: adults/peds: 2–5 mg/kg i.v.
- Gram-negative anaerobes
  —Clindamycin: 900 mg (peds: 20–40 mg/kg/24 h) i.v. q8h
  —Metronidazole: 1 g (peds: 15 mg/kg) i.v. load, then 500 mg (peds: 7.5 mg/kg) i.v. q6h
- Both aerobic and anaerobic
  —Ampicillin/sulbactam: 1.5–3 g (peds: 100–400 mg/kg/24 h) i.v. q6h
  —Cefotetan: 2 g (peds: 40–80 mg/kg/24 h) i.v. q12h
  —Cefoxitin: 2 g (peds: 80–160 mg/kg/24 h) i.v. q12h
  —Ticarcillin/clavulanate: 3.1 g (peds: 50 mg/kg/dose) i.v. q6h

Disposition

ADMISSION CRITERIA

- Patients with suspicion for diaphragmatic injury must be admitted to the care of a trauma surgeon
- Patients should be admitted to a monitored or intensive care unit setting

DISCHARGE CRITERIA

- Patients with diaphragmatic injury must not be discharged from the ED

Miscellaneous

ICD9: 862.0

ICD10: S27.8

SUGGESTED READINGS

Kanowitz A, Markovchick V. Esophageal and diaphragmatic trauma. In: Rosen P, et al., eds. Emergency medicine: concepts and clinical practice, 4th ed. St. Louis: CV Mosby, 1998:546–554.

Mansour KA. Trauma to the diaphragm. Chest Surg Clin North Am 1997;7(2):373–383.

Rosati C. Acute traumatic injury of the diaphragm. Chest Surg Clin North Am 1998;8(2):371–379.

Shah R, Sabanathan S, Mearns AJ, et al. Traumatic rupture of the diaphragm. Ann Thorac Surg 1995;60(5):1444–1449.

Sharma OP. Pericardio-diaphragmatic rupture: five new cases and literature review. J Emerg Med 1999;17(6):963–968.

Author: Robert S. Hamilton

Diarrhea, Adult

Clinical Presentation

SIGNS AND SYMPTOMS

- Loose, watery bowel movements
- Bloody stools with mucus
- Abdominal pain and cramps, tenesmus, flatulence
- Fever, headache, myalgias
- Nausea, vomiting
- Dehydration, lethargy and stupor
- Perianal inflammation, fissure, fistula

ETIOLOGY

Infectious

Viruses

- 50–70% of all cases

Invasive Bacteria

- *Campylobacter*
  —Contaminated food or water, wilderness water, birds and animals
  —Most common bacterial diarrhea
  —Gross or occult blood is found in 60–90%
- *Salmonella*
  —Contaminated water, eggs, poultry, or dairy products
  —Typhoid fever (*Salmonella typhi*) characterized by unremitting fever, abdominal pain, rose spots, splenomegaly, and bradycardia
- *Shigella*
  —Fecal or oral route
- *Vibrio parahaemolyticus*
  —Raw and undercooked seafood
- *Yersinia*
  —Contaminated food (pork), water, and milk
  —May present as mesenteric adenitis or mimic appendicitis

Bacterial Toxin

- *Escherichia coli*
- Major cause of traveler's diarrhea
- Ingestion of food or water contaminated by feces
- *Staphylococcal aureus*
  —Most common toxin-related disease
  —Symptoms 1–6 hours after ingesting food
- *Bacillus cereus*
  —Classic source—fried rice left on steam tables
  —Symptoms within 1–36 hours
- *Clostridium difficile*
  —Antibiotic-associated enteritis linked to pseudomembranous colitis
  —Incubation period within 10 days of exposure or initiation of antibiotics
- *Aeromonas hydrophila*
  —Aquatic sources primarily
  —Affects children younger than 3 years of age
  —Fecal leukocytes absent
- Cholera
  —Caused by an enterotoxin produced by *Vibrio cholerae*
  —Profuse watery stools with mucus (classic appearance of "rice-water" stools)

Protozoa

- *Giardia lamblia*
  —Most common cause of parasite gastroenteritis in North America
  —High-risk groups: travelers, children in day care centers, institutionalized people, homosexual men, and campers who drink untreated mountain water
- *Cryptosporidium parvum*
  —Commonly carried in patients with AIDS
- *Entamoeba histolytica* (entamebiasis)
  —5–10% extraintestinal manifestations (hepatic amebic abscess)

PEDIATRIC CONSIDERATIONS

- Most are viral in origin and self-limited
  —Rotavirus accounts for 50%
- *Shigella*: infections associated with seizures
- Focus evaluation on state of hydration

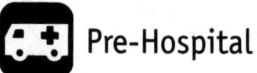

Pre-Hospital

CAUTIONS

- Difficult IV access with severe dehydration
- Avoid exposure to contaminated clothes or body substances

Diagnosis

ESSENTIAL WORKUP

- Digital rectal examination to determine the presence of gross or occult blood
- Fecal leukocyte determination
  - —Present with invasive bacteria
  - —Absent in protozoal infections, viral, toxin-induced food poisoning

LABORATORY

- CBC—indications
  - —Significant blood loss
  - —Systemic toxicity
- Electrolytes, glucose, BUN, creatinine—indications
  - —Lethargy, significant dehydration, toxicity, or altered mental status
  - —Diuretic use, persistent diarrhea, chronic liver or renal disease
- Stool culture—indications
  - —Presence of fecal leukocytes
  - —Historical markers: immunocompromised, travel, homosexual
  - —Public health: food handler, day care or health care worker, institutionalized
- Blood cultures—indications
  - —Suspected bacteremia or systemic infections
  - —Ill patients requiring admission
  - —Immunocompromised
  - —Elderly patients and infants

IMAGING/SPECIAL TESTS

- Abdominal x-rays
  - —No value unless an obstruction or a toxic megacolon suspected

DIFFERENTIAL DIAGNOSIS

- Ulcerative colitis
- Crohn's disease
- Mesenteric ischemia
- Diverticulitis, anal fissures, hemorrhoids
- Irritable bowel syndrome
- Milk and food allergies
- Malrotation with midgut volvulus
- Meckel's diverticulum
- Intussusception
- Drugs and toxins:
  - —Mannitol
  - —Sorbitol
  - —Phenolphthalein
  - —Magnesium-containing antacids
  - —Quinidine
  - —Colchicine
  - —Mushrooms
  - —Mercury poisoning

Treatment

INITIAL STABILIZATION

- ABCs
- IV fluid with 0.9% NS resuscitation for severely dehydrated

ED MANAGEMENT

- Oral fluids for mild dehydration (Gatorade/Pedialyte)
- IV fluids for
  - —Hypotension, nausea and vomiting, obtundation, metabolic acidosis, significant hypernatremia or hyponatremia
  - —0.9% NS bolus (500 mL-1 L adults, 20 mL/kg pediatrics) for resuscitation then 0.9% NS or D5W 0.45% NS (D5W 0.25% NS pediatrics) to maintain an adequate urine output
- Bismuth subsalicylate (Pepto-Bismol)
  - —Antisecretory agent
  - —Effective clinical relief without adverse effects
- Kaolin-pectin (Kaopectate)
  - —Reduces fluidity of stools
  - —Does not influence the course of the disease
- Antimotility drugs: diphenoxylate (Lomotil), loperamide (Imodium), paregoric, and codeine
  - —Appropriate in noninfectious diarrhea
  - —Initial use of sparse amounts to control symptoms in infectious diarrhea
  - —Avoid prolonged use in infectious diarrhea—may increase the duration of fever, diarrhea, and bacteremia and may precipitate a toxic megacolon

Antibiotics for Infectious Pathogens

- *Campylobacter*: quinolones or erythromycin
- *Salmonella*: quinolones or trimethoprim-sulfamethoxazole (TMP-SMX)
- Typhoid fever: ceftriaxone
- *Shigella*: quinolone, TMP-SMX, or ampicillin
- *Vibrio parahaemolyticus:* tetracycline or doxycycline
- *Clostridium difficile:* vancomycin
- *Escherichia coli:* quinolones or TMP-SMX
- *Giardia lamblia:* metronidazole or quinacrine
- *Entamoeba histolytica* (entamebiasis): iodoquinol or metronidazole

MEDICATIONS

- Ampicillin: 500 mg (peds: 20 mg/kg/24 h) PO or i.v. q6h
- Bactrim DS (TMP-SMX): 1 tab (peds: 8–10 mg TMP/40–50 mg SMX/kg/24 h) PO or 4–5 mg/kg TMP i.v. b.i.d.
- Ciprofloxacin (quinolone): 500 mg PO or 400 mg i.v. b.i.d.
- Doxycycline: 100 mg PO or 400 mg i.v. b.i.d.
- Erythromycin: 500 mg (peds: 40–50 mg/kg/24 h) PO q.i.d.
- Iodoquinol: 650 mg (peds: 30–40 mg/kg/24 h) PO t.i.d.
- Metronidazole: 250 mg (peds: 35 mg/kg/24 h) PO t.i.d.
- Quinacrine: 100 mg (peds: 6 mg/kg/24 h) PO t.i.d.
- Tetracycline: 500 mg PO or i.v. q6h
- Vancomycin: 500 mg (peds: 10–50 mg/kg/24 h) i.v. q.i.d.

Disposition

ADMISSION CRITERIA

- Hypotension, unresponsive to IV fluids
- Significant bleeding
- Signs of sepsis or toxicity
- Intractable vomiting or abdominal pain
- Severe electrolyte imbalance or metabolic acidosis
- Altered mental status
- Children with >10–15% dehydration

DISCHARGE CRITERIA

- Mild cases requiring oral hydration
- Dehydration responsive to IV fluids

Miscellaneous

ICD9: 787.91

ICD10: A09

SEE ALSO: GASTROENTERITIS

SUGGESTED READINGS

Bitterman RA. Acute gastroenteritides. In: Marx JA, Hockberger RS, Walls RM, et al., eds. Rosen's emergency medicine: concepts and clinical practice, 5th ed. St. Louis: Mosby-Year Book, 2002:1301–1325.

Gough JE, Clement PA. Diarrhea. In: Marx JA, Hockberger RS, Walls RM, et al., eds. Rosen's emergency medicine: concepts and clinical practice, 5th ed. St. Louis: Mosby-Year Book, 2002:200–208.

Hogan D. The emergency department approach to diarrhea. Emerg Med Clin North Am 1996;14(4):673–694.

Reisdorff E, Pflug V. Infectious diarrhea: beyond supportive care. Emerg Med Rep 1996;17(14):141–150.

Surawicz CM. Infectious diarrhea. Gastroenterol Clin North Am 2001;30(3).

Author: Isam Nasr

Diarrhea, Pediatric

Clinical Presentation

SIGNS AND SYMPTOMS

- Frequent, loose stools
  - —Watery
  - —Bloody
  - —Mucoid
- Signs of dehydration reflect loss of total-body water
- Categorization of degree of dehydration
  - —Mental status
    - -Mild (<5%): alert
    - -Moderate (5–10%): irritable
    - -Severe (≥15%): lethargic
  - —Mucous membrane
    - -Mild: variably dry
    - -Moderate: dry
    - -Severe: dry
  - —Skin turgor
    - -Mild: normal
    - -Moderate: variably reduced
    - -Severe: reduced
  - —Anterior fontanel
    - -Mild: normal
    - -Moderate: depressed
    - -Severe: depressed
  - —Blood pressure
    - -Mild: normal
    - -Moderate: variably orthostatic
    - -Severe: orthostatic or decreased
  - —Pulse
    - -Mild: normal
    - -Moderate: tachycardia
    - -Severe: markedly tachycardic
  - —Capillary refill
    - -Mild: <2 seconds
    - -Moderate: 2-3 seconds
    - -Severe: ≥4 seconds
  - —Urine output
    - -Mild: mild decreased
    - -Moderate: oliguria
    - -Severe: oliguria/anuria
- Fever
- Abdominal pain, distention
- Vomiting
- Tenesmus
- Impaired nutritional status or abnormal growth parameters

MECHANISM/DESCRIPTION

- One of the most common pediatric complaints; second only to respiratory infections in overall disease frequency
- Leading cause of illness and death in children worldwide
- Acute infectious enteritis (AIE)
  - —Vomiting and diarrhea
  - —Children <5 years in the United States typically have two episodes annually
  - —Responsible for about 10% of all pediatric ED visits and hospital admissions
- Acute change in the "normal" bowel pattern that leads to increased number or volume of stools and lasts less than 7 days
  - —Chronic if the diarrhea persists for more than 2 weeks

ETIOLOGY

Acute Enteritis

- Infectious
  - —Viruses: 70–80% of cases
    - -Rotavirus and Norwalk viruses in the winter months
    - -Enteroviruses in the summer and early autumn
    - -Bacteria: 10–20%
    - -*Escherichia coli*
    - -*Campylobacter*
    - -*Salmonella*
    - -*Shigella*
    - -*Yersinia enterocolitica*
    - -*Clostridium difficile*
  - —Parasites: 5%
- Food poisoning
- Postinfectious
- Milk allergy
- Associated with other infections
  - —Otitis media
  - —Urinary tract infection

Chronic Diarrhea

- Osmotic
  - —Lactose intolerance (increased sorbitol or fructose from fruit juices)
- Secretory
  - —Increased secretion due to secretagogues (bacterial toxins, failure reabsorption, hormone-producing tumors)
- Altered motility
  - —Increased gut transit (irritable bowel syndrome)
- Exudative diarrhea
  - —Inflammatory conditions where there is disruption of the mucosa of the intestines (inflammatory bowel disease, Henoch-Schönlein purpura, bacterial colitis)
- Malabsorption (cystic fibrosis)

Pre-Hospital

CAUTIONS

- Severely dehydrated (>10% dehydration) children in shock or near-shock must receive
  - —Immediate IV bolus with 0.9% NS 20 mL/kg; may repeat
  - —Blood glucose determination; treat if hypoglycemia
  - —100% O_2 via non-rebreather
  - —Cardiac monitoring; oximetry

Diagnosis

ESSENTIAL WORKUP

- Gross examination of stool
- Guaiac and Wright stain for fecal leucocytes
  - —Watery diarrhea without blood or mucus associated with viral enteritis or related to bacterial enterotoxins
  - —Diarrhea with blood or mucus suggests an enteroinvasive inflammatory or cytotoxin-mediated process (*Salmonella,* invasive *E. coli*)
  - —Microscopic examination of a Wright-stained smear of the mucoid part of stool revealing >5 fecal leucocytes per high-power field is suggestive of bacterial infection
    - -*Shigella*
    - -*Salmonella*
    - -*Campylobacter*
    - -*Yersinia*
    - -Invasive *E. coli*

LABORATORY

- Serum electrolytes, BUN, creatinine assist in the assessment of dehydration
- Urinalysis assists in the assessment of dehydration
- Stool pH <5.5 or positive stool reducing substances in viral infection

IMAGING/SPECIAL TESTS

- Stool culture
  - —Unnecessary in most cases unless there is a high likelihood of identifying bacterial pathogens where the clinical course and period of contagion may be altered by antibiotic therapy

DIFFERENTIAL DIAGNOSIS

- Infectious
  - —Bacterial gastroenteritis
  - —Temperature >39°C
  - —Toxic clinical appearance
  - —Crampy abdominal pain
  - —Bloody mucoid stools
  - —Viral gastroenteritis
  - —Seasonal epidemics
  - —Guaiac-negative stool
  - —Parasitic (*Giardia lamblia*)
  - —Chronic diarrhea
- Postinfectious
  - —Follows acute or bacterial or viral gastroenteritis; often associated with malabsorption, esp. lactose
  - —*C. difficile* may follow use of antibiotics
- Noninfectious
  - —Milk allergy
  - —Heme-positive stool
  - —Vomiting
  - —Malrotation with midgut volvulus
  - —Inflammatory bowel disease
  - —Intussusception
  - —"Currant jelly" stool
  - —Abdominal mass

Treatment

INITIAL STABILIZATION

- For severely dehydrated children in shock or near-shock, intravenous or intraosseous access with 20 mL/kg 0.9% NS, and 1 g/kg dextrose if hypoglycemic
- Pulse oximetry
- Endotracheal intubation may be required for children in shock

ED TREATMENT

- For mild to moderate dehydration, correct dehydration using oral rehydration therapy (ORT), 50 mL/kg and 100 mL/kg, respectively, over a 4-hour period
  —Replace ongoing losses with 10 mL/kg of ORT for each stool
- For moderate to severe dehydration correct dehydration using parenteral fluids combining maintenance and deficit requirements
- If diarrhea is not associated with dehydration, use 10 mL/kg of ORT for each stool alone
- Antibiotics only for defined acute enteritis
  —*Campylobacter jejuni*
    -Erythromycin
  —*Salmonella*—uncomplicated
    -No antibiotics
  —*Salmonella*—complicated (infant <6 months old, disseminated, bacteremia, immunocompromised host, enteric fever)
    -Ampicillin or trimethoprim-sulfamethoxazole (TMP-SMX) for 10 days
  —*Shigella*
    -TMP-SMX for 5 days
  —*Yersinia*
    -None or TMP-SMX for 5 days
  —*C. difficile*—carrier
    -None
  —*C. difficile*—severe and or prolonged enteritis
    -Metronidazole or vancomycin for 7 days
  —*E. coli*—enterotoxigenic, enteropathogenic
    -None
  —*E. coli*—enteroinvasive
    -TMP-SMX for 5 days
  —*E. coli*—enteroadherent
    -Neomycin for 5 days
  —*G. lamblia*
    -Furazolidone or metronidazole for 10 days
- Antidiarrheal agents *not* recommended, although some promising studies suggest that loperamide may be helpful
  —Alter intestinal motility (loperamide, opiates, opiate-atropine combinations)
  —Alter secretion (bismuth subsalicylate)
  —Adsorb fluid and toxins (kaolin-pectin, fiber, activated charcoal, attapulgite)
  —Alter intestinal microflora (*Lactobacillus*-containing compounds, probiotics)

POST-ED DIET

- On rehydration, feed children with diarrhea age-appropriate diets
- Well-tolerated foods
  —Rich in complex carbohydrates (rice, potatoes, bread)
  —Lean meats
  —Yogurt
  —Fruits
  —Vegetables
  —Full-strength milk and formula unless there is a strong suspicion of lactose intolerance
- Avoid fatty foods and foods high in simple sugars

MEDICATIONS

- Ampicillin: 50–200 mg/kg/24 h i.v. or PO q6h
- Erythromycin: 40 mg/kg/24 h PO q6h; 10–20 mg/kg/24 h i.v. q6h
- Furazolidone: 6 mg/kg/24 h q6h
- Metronidazole: 15–30 mg/kg/24 h
- Neomycin: 100 mg/kg/24 h PO q4h
- ORT (45–50 mmol/L of sodium): as described above
- TMP-SMX: 6–12 mg/kg/24 h as TMP q12h
- Vancomycin: 20–40 mg/kg/24 h PO q6h
- Loperamide (not for use in children <6 years old or in those with heme-positive stools): age 6–8 years, 2 mg PO b.i.d.; age 8–12 years, 2 mg PO t.i.d.

Disposition

ADMISSION CRITERIA

- Surgical abdomen
- Inability to tolerate oral fluids
- ≥10% dehydration
- Suspected complicated *Salmonella* enteritis
- Toxic-appearing child

DISCHARGE CRITERIA

- ORT tolerated
- Improvement in the patient's condition
- Caregivers of child can follow through with appropriate ORT and diet
- Caregivers able to report signs and symptoms of dehydration

Miscellaneous

ICD9: 787.91

ICD10: A09

SEE ALSO: VOMITING, PEDIATRIC

SUGGESTED READINGS

Bonadio WA. Acute infectious enteritis in children—emergency department diagnosis and management. Emerg Med Clin North Am 1995;13:457–472.

Kaplan MA, Prior MJ, McKonly KI, et al. A multicenter randomized controlled trial of a liquid loperamide product versus placebo in the treatment of acute diarrhea in children. Clin Pediatr 1999;38:579–591.

Merrick N, Davidson B, Fox S. Treatment of acute gastroenteritis: too much and too little care. Clin Pediatr 1996;9:429–436.

Provisional Committee on Quality Improvement, Subcommittee on Acute Gastroenteritis. Practice parameter: the management of acute gastroenteritis in young children. Pediatrics 1996;97: 424–436.

Salazar-Lindo E, Santisteban-Ponce J, Chea-Woo E, et al. Racecadotril in the treatment of acute watery diarrhea in children. N Engl J Med 2000;343:463–467.

Author: Richard Lichenstein

Digoxin, Poisoning

Clinical Presentation

SIGNS AND SYMPTOMS

Cardiovascular

- Dysrhythmias
  - —Paroxysmal atrial tachycardia (PAT) with atrioventricular (AV) block and bidirectional ventricular tachycardia
    - -Classic dysrhythmia
    - -Uncommon
  - —Premature ventricular contractions (PVCs) most common
  - —Nonparoxysmal accelerated junctional tachycardia
  - —Ventricular tachycardia (VT)
  - —Regularized atrial fibrillation (AFib)
  - —Bigeminy
  - —Bradycardia
  - —Nonparoxysmal atrial tachycardia
  - —AV blocks
  - —Sinus arrhythmia
  - —Premature atrial contraction
- Congestive heart failure (CHF) exacerbation
- Hypotension
- Shock
- Cardiovascular collapse
- Syncope

CNS

- Mental status changes
  - —Agitation
  - —Lethargy
  - —Psychosis
- Visual perception
  - —Blurred
  - —Scotoma
  - —Green to yellow halo
  - —Photophobia
  - —Hallucinations
  - —Color perception changes

GI

- Anorexia
- Nausea and vomiting
- Diarrhea
- Abdominal pain

General

- Headache
- Weakness
- Lightheadedness

MECHANISM/DESCRIPTION

Acute Digitalis Effects (Elevated Levels in Children and Intentional Overdose)

- Inhibits sodium-potassium ATPase pump in cell membranes
- Allows more calcium ions to enter the cell and cardiac cells to contract more strongly
- Increases K^+ extracellularly
- Increases vagal tone
- Slows AV node conduction
- Increases automaticity and conduction system refractory period
- Bradydysrhythmias

Chronic Digitalis Effects (Therapeutic to Toxic Levels in Elderly Patients)

- Inhibits sodium-potassium ATPase pump in cell membranes
- Increases intracellular calcium
- Increases vagal tone
- Increases automaticity
- Usually hypokalemic secondary to diuretic use
- Tachydysrhythmias

ETIOLOGY

- Onset: 2 hours after PO ingestion and 15 minutes following IV
- Toxicity
  - —Occurs with normal digoxin levels
  - —May be absent with elevated digoxin levels
- Plants and animals containing cardiac glycosides
  - —Foxglove
  - —Oleander
  - —Lily of the valley
  - —Dogbane
  - —Red squill
  - —Cane toad, Colorado River toad

Pre-Hospital

CAUTIONS

- If cardioversion is necessary for tachydysrhythmias, use low levels (50 J)
  - —May precipitate refractory tachydysrhythmias

Diagnosis

ESSENTIAL WORKUP

- EKG
  - —For dysrhythmia (see above)
- Digoxin level
  - —Normal range: 0.5–2.0 ng/mL
  - —Distribution after oral intake not complete until 6 hours; therefore, a 6-hour level is most accurate
  - —False elevations possible with spironolactone use, pregnancy, hyperbilirubinemia, chronic renal failure
  - —Will be falsely elevated after digoxin immune Fab antibodies given

LABORATORY

- Electrolytes, BUN, creatinine, glucose
  - —Hypokalemia contributes to digitalis toxicity
  - —Hyperkalemia seen in acute toxicity and correlates with acute digitalis mortality better than digoxin serum levels
  - —Follow K^+ serially
- Calcium, magnesium

DIFFERENTIAL DIAGNOSES

- Overdoses
  - —Calcium channel blockers
  - —Beta-blockers
  - —Quinidine, procainamide
  - —Clonidine
  - —Organophosphates
- Primary cardiac dysrhythmias
- Acute gastroenteritis

Treatment

INITIAL STABILIZATION

- ABCs
- IV, oxygen, monitor
  - —IV fluid bolus if hypovolemic
- Administer naloxone, thiamine, dextrose, for altered mental status

ED TREATMENT

Cardiac Arrest Resuscitation

- Defibrillate for ventricular fibrillation, pulseless VT
- Standard advanced cardiac life support (ACLS) protocol
- Administer digoxin-specific antibody Fab fragments (Digibind), up to 20 vials IV push (IVP)
- $MgSO_4$, 2 g IVP
- Continue resuscitation for 30 minutes after digoxin immune Fab antibodies

General Measures

- Gastric lavage if <1 hour after acute ingestion and history of significant ingestion, hemodynamically stable, and airway stabilization
  - —May cause bradycardia, asystole
  - —Use caution if bradycardia or AV block present
  - —Consider atropine pretreatment
- Avoid ipecac and induction of emesis
- Activated charcoal if acute ingestion
- Potassium replacement to achieve level above 4.0 mEq/L
  - —Use with caution if bradycardia or AV block
- Replete magnesium
- Treat hyperkalemia with insulin, dextrose, bicarbonate, sodium polystyrene sulfonate
  - —Calcium *contraindicated*

Dysrhythmia Management

- Initiate the following while waiting for digoxin specific immune fragments
  —Lidocaine
    -For ventricular dysrhythmias without AV block
    -Not harmful but not very effective
  —Phenytoin
    -Drug of choice for ventricular dysrhythmias
    -Suppresses automaticity without suppressing conduction
    -Action at AV node and beneficial response in supraventricular dysrhythmias (atrial tachycardia with AV block)
  —Amiodarone
  —For bradydysrhythmias
    -Atropine
    -Pacing for symptomatic bradydysrhythmia
  —Beta blockade (propranolol, esmolol) for supraventricular tachycardia
    -Avoid with AV block, bradycardia
  —$MgSO_4$ for ventricular dysrhythmias
  —Bretylium and catecholamines may exacerbate toxicity
  —Quinidine, procainamide contraindicated
- Cardioversion is a last resort for severe, life-threatening tachydysrhythmia
  —Start at low energy 10 to 50 J, then increase to high levels if ineffective
  —Safe if digoxin level <2.0 ng/mL
- Pacemaker

Digoxin-Specific Antibody Fab Fragments (Digibind)

- Indications
  —Serum digoxin concentration ≥15 ng/mL at any time or ≥10 ng/mL at steady state
  —Ingestion of >10 mg in adults or 0.2 mg/kg or 4 mg in children
  —Hyperkalemia >5.0–5.5 mEq/L
  —Hemodynamically unstable or life-threatening dysrhythmias
  —Ventricular tachycardia, ventricular fibrillation
  —Atrial tachycardia
  —Variable AV block
  —Bradycardia with no response to atropine
  —Hypotension
- Onset: 20–30 minutes
- Digoxin levels increase after therapy due to antibody complexes
- Renal clearance of the drug-antibody complexes
  —Too large to be removed by dialysis
- Second dose if rebound toxicity
- Complications
  —Exacerbation of CHF
  —Hypokalemia
  —AFib with rapid ventricular response

MEDICATIONS

- Activated charcoal slurry: 10:1 grams per gram PO if amount of digoxin ingested is known
  —1 mg/kg if amount of drug is unknown
- Amiodarone: 15 mg/min 150-mg load, 1 mg/min q6h, then 0.5 mg/min
- Atropine: 0.5 mg (peds: 0.02 mg/kg) i.v.; repeat 0.5–1.0 mg i.v. (peds: 0.04 mg/kg)
- Dextrose: D50W 1 amp (50 mL or 25 g) (peds: D25W 2–4 mL/kg) i.v.
- Digoxin-specific antibody Fab fragments
  —40 mg per vial neutralizes 0.6 mg of digoxin
  —If amount ingested known:
    -Number of vials needed equals amount ingested mg/0.6
  —If steady serum level known:
    -Number of vials needed equals serum digoxin level multiplied by patient's weight in kg/100
  —If neither amount ingested or serum level known:
    -Acute toxicity: 10–15 vials adults or children
    -Chronic toxicity: 2–3 vials adults
  —Bolus for cardiac arrest
  —Additional doses as needed
- Esmolol: 50–200 mg/kg/min
- Insulin and glucose: 10 U (peds: 0.25 U/kg) regular insulin plus 50 mL 50% (peds: 1 g/kg) dextrose i.v.
- Lidocaine: 1 mg/kg i.v., then 0.5 mg/kg every 10 minutes to max 3 mg/kg
- Magnesium sulfate: 2 g (peds: 25–50 mg/kg/dose) IVPB
- Naloxone: 2 mg (peds: 0.1 mg/kg) i.v. or i.m.
- Phenytoin: 15–18 mg/kg i.v.
- Propranolol: 1 mg (peds: 0.01–0.1 mg/kg) i.v.
- Sodium bicarbonate: 1–3 amp (44 mEq) i.v. over 20–30 minutes (peds: 1–2 mEq/kg/dose)
- Sodium polystyrene sulfonate (Kayexalate)
  —Oral: 15 g mixed with water or 50 mL of sorbitol
  —Rectal enema: 50 g in 200 mL of sorbitol
  —Peds: 1.0 g/kg PO or PR
- Sorbitol: 1–2 g/kg to a max of 100 g (peds: >1 year old: 1–1.5 g/kg as a 35% solution to a max of 50 g) PO
- Thiamine: 100 mg (peds: 50 mg) i.v. or i.m.

Disposition

ADMISSION CRITERIA

- ICU
  —Symptomatic toxicity or digoxin level >2 ng/mL with acute exposure
  —Postdigoxin immune Fab (for 24 hours) administration
  —Unstable acute or chronic toxicity
- Telemetry
  —Asymptomatic or mildly symptomatic dysrhythmia, especially following large doses
  —High risk for developing toxicity

DISCHARGE CRITERIA

- Acute ingestion
  —Digoxin level <2.0 ng/mL
  —Asymptomatic for 6 hours and no EKG abnormalities
- Chronic exposure
  —Digoxin level <2.5 ng/mL
  —Asymptomatic for 6 hours and no EKG abnormalities

Miscellaneous

ICD9: 972.1

ICD10: T46.0

SUGGESTED READINGS

Ford M, Delaney K, Ling L, et al. Clinical toxicology, 1st ed. Philadelphia: WB Saunders, 2001:379–389.

Goldfrank L, Flomenbaum N, Lewin N, et al. Goldfrank's toxicologic emergencies, 6th ed. Stamford, CT: Appleton & Lange, 1998:791–798.

Hickey A, Wenger T, Carpenter V, et al. Digoxin immune Fab therapy in the management of digitalis intoxication: safety and efficacy results of an observational surveillance study. J Am Coll Cardiol 1991;17:590–598.

Leikin J, Paloucek F. Leikin and Paloucek's poisoning and toxicology handbook, 3rd ed. Digoxin. Hudson, Ohio: Digibind Lexi-Comp, 2002:484–488.

Mauskopf J. Cost-effectiveness analysis of the use of digoxin immune Fab(ovine) for treatment of digoxin toxicity. Am J Cardiol 1991;68:1709–1714.

Author: Kirk Cumpston

Disseminated Intravascular Coagulation

Clinical Presentation

SIGNS AND SYMPTOMS

- Excessive bleeding
  - —Petechiae
  - —Purpura
  - —Hemorrhagic bullae
  - —Wound bleeding
  - —Epistaxis
  - —Hemoptysis
  - —Gastrointestinal bleeding
- Excessive thrombosis
  - —Large vessels
  - —Microvascular thrombosis and end-organ dysfunction
  - —Cardiac, pulmonary, renal, hepatic, CNS
  - —Thrombophlebitis
  - —Pulmonary embolus
  - —Nonbacterial thrombotic endocarditis
  - —Gangrene
  - —Ischemic infarcts of kidney, liver, CNS, bowel
- Acute DIC
  - —Hemorrhagic complications predominate
- Chronic DIC
  - —Thrombotic complications predominate

MECHANISM/DESCRIPTION

- Normal coagulation
  - —A series of *local* reactions among blood vessels, platelets, and clotting factors
- DIC is *systemic* activation of coagulation and fibrinolysis by some other primary disease process
- Coagulation system activation results in systemic circulation of thrombin and plasmin
  - —Role of thrombin in DIC
    - -Thrombin circulates and converts fibrinogen to fibrin monomer
    - -Fibrin monomer polymerizes into fibrin (clot) in the circulation
    - -Clots cause microvascular and macrovascular thrombosis with resultant peripheral ischemia and end-organ damage
    - -Platelets become trapped in clot with resultant thrombocytopenia
  - —Role of plasmin in DIC
    - -Plasmin circulates systemically converting fibrinogen into fibrin degradation products (FDPs)
    - -FDPs combine with fibrin monomers
    - -FDP-monomer complexes interfere with normal polymerization and impair hemostasis
    - -FDPs also interfere with platelet function
- Acute DIC—uncompensated form
  - —Clotting factors used more rapidly than the body can replace them
  - —Hemorrhage predominant clinical feature, which overshadows ongoing thrombosis
- Chronic DIC—compensated form
  - —Body able to keep up with pace of clotting factor consumption
  - —Thrombosis predominant clinical feature

ETIOLOGY

- Precipitated by many disease states
- Complications of pregnancy
  - —Retained fetus
  - —Amniotic fluid embolism
  - —Placental abruption
  - —Abortion
  - —Eclampsia
- Sepsis
  - —Gram-negative (endotoxin-mediated meningococcemia)
  - —Gram-positive (mucopolysaccharide mediated)
- Trauma
  - —Crush injury
  - —Severe burns
  - —Severe head injury
- Malignancy
  - —Metastatic disease
  - —Leukemia
- Intravascular hemolysis
  - —Transfusion reactions
  - —Massive transfusion
- Thrombocytopenia
  - —Thrombotic thrombocytopenic purpura
  - —Idiopathic thrombocytopenic purpura

Pre-Hospital

N/A

Diagnosis

ESSENTIAL WORKUP

- Depends on precipitating illness
- Diagnosis generally not made in the ED
- Platelet count
  - —Decreased
  - —<100,000/mm^3
  - —May be normal in chronic DIC
- Prothrombin time (PT)/partial thromboplastin time (PTT)
  - —Increased
  - —May be normal in chronic DIC
- Fibrinogen
  - —Decreased
  - —<150 mg/dL in 70%
  - —May be normal in chronic DIC
- FDPs
  - —Increased
  - —>40 μg/mL
- D-Dimer
  - —Increased

LABORATORY

- CBC/peripheral smear
  - —Red cell fragments
  - —Low platelets
  - —Peripheral smear confirms disease in chronic DIC
- Electrolytes, BUN, creatinine, glucose
  - —Elevated BUN, creatinine due to renal insufficiency
- Arterial blood gases (ABGs)
  - —Oxygen, acid base status

IMAGING/SPECIAL TESTS

- Chest x-ray for suspected pneumonia/sepsis
- Brain CT for altered mental status

DIFFERENTIAL DIAGNOSIS

- Inherited coagulation disorders
  - —Factor deficiencies
- Other acquired coagulation disorders
  - —Anticoagulant therapy
  - —Drugs
  - —Hepatic disease
- Platelet dysfunction

Treatment

INITIAL STABILIZATION

- ABCs
  - —Control bleeding
  - —Establish IV access
  - —Restore and maintain circulating blood volume
- Initiate therapy of precipitating disease
  - —Antibiotics in sepsis
  - —Evacuate uterus of retained dead fetus
  - —Chemotherapy in malignancy
  - —Débridement of devitalized tissue in trauma

ED TREATMENT

Overview

- Therapy of DIC is controversial and should be individualized based on
  - —Age
  - —Hemodynamic status
  - —Severity of hemorrhage
  - —Severity of thrombosis
- Involve admitting service before initiating specific DIC therapy
- DIC therapy
- Replace depleted blood components
  - —Fresh frozen plasma (FFP)
    - -For prolonged PT
    - -Provides clotting factors and volume replacement
    - -Dose: 2 U or 10–15 mL/kg
  - —Platelets
    - -If platelet count <20,000 or platelet count <50,000 with ongoing bleeding
    - -Dose: 1 U/10 kg body weight
  - —Cryoprecipitate
    - -Higher fibrinogen content than whole plasma
    - -For severe hypofibrinogenemia (<50 mg/dL) or for active bleeding with fibrinogen <100 mg/dL
    - -Dose: 8 U
  - —Washed packed cells
  - —Albumin
- —Nonclotting volume expanders
- Inhibition of intravascular clotting
  - —Heparin (use is controversial)
    - -May be effective in mild to moderate DIC
    - -Efficacy undetermined in severe DIC
    - -Possible indications
      - ∗Purpura fulminans (gangrene of digits, extremities)
      - ∗Acute promyelocytic leukemia
      - ∗"Dead fetus syndrome"—several weeks after intrauterine fetal death
      - ∗Thromboembolic complications of large vessels
      - ∗Before surgery with metastatic carcinoma
    - -Low-dose regimen: 5–10 U/kg/h i.v. for chronic DIC
    - -High-dose regimen: 10,000 U bolus followed by 1000 U/h; 20–30,000 U every 24 hours via constant infusion
  - —Antithrombin concentrates (controversial)
  - —Used alone or in combination with heparin
- Inhibition of fibrinolysis
  - —Block secondary compensatory fibrinolysis that accompanies DIC
  - —Use complicated by severe thrombosis
  - —Use only when DIC accompanied by primary fibrinolysis
    - -Promyelocytic leukemia
    - -Giant hemangioma
    - -Heat stroke
    - -Amniotic fluid embolism
    - -Metastatic carcinoma of prostate
  - —Initiate in extreme cases only
    - -Profuse bleeding not responding to replacement therapy
    - -Excessive fibrinolysis present (rapid whole blood lysis/short euglobulin lysis time)
    - -ϵ-Aminocaproic acid (EACA)

Disposition

ADMISSION CRITERIA

- Severe precipitating illness in combination with DIC requires ICU admission

DISCHARGE CRITERIA

- None

Miscellaneous

ICD9: 286.6

ICD10: D65

SUGGESTED READINGS

Bick RL. Disseminated intravascular coagulation: objective clinical and laboratory diagnosis, treatment and assessment of therapeutic response. Semin Thromb Hemost 1996;22(1):69.

Gusset A, et al. In: Lee G, et al., eds. Wintrobe's clinical hematology, 10th ed. Philadelphia: Lippincott Williams & Wilkins, 1999:1733–1780.

Seligsohn U. Disseminated intravascular coagulation. In: Beutler E, et al., eds. Williams hematology, 6th ed. New York: McGraw-Hill, 2001:1677–1659.

Author: Steven Bowman

Disulfiram Reaction

Clinical Presentation

SIGNS AND SYMPTOMS

Disulfiram Overdose

- Symptoms rare with less than 3 g ingested
- 10–30 g may be lethal
- Tachycardia, hypotension, tachypnea
- Abdominal pain, diarrhea, garlic or rotten-egg breath
- Agitation, irritability, ataxia
- Dysarthria, hallucinations
- Lethargy, coma, seizures, flaccidity
- Parkinson-like syndrome

Disulfiram-Ethanol Reaction

- Hypotension, tachycardia, tachypnea
- Flushing of face, neck, torso
- Pruritus, diaphoresis, sensation of warmth
- Nausea, vomiting, abdominal pain, diarrhea
- Headache, ataxia, confusion, anxiety, dizziness
- Dyspnea, pulmonary edema, chest pain, dysrhythmias, myocardial infarction

MECHANISM/DESCRIPTION

- Inhibits various enzymes, and its active metabolites exert additional effects
- Disulfiram—ethanol reaction
  - —Usually occurs 8–12 hours after taking the drug and should not be observed greater than 24 hours after dosing
  - —Competitively and irreversibly inactivates aldehyde dehydrogenase
  - —Ethanol metabolism is blocked, resulting in accumulation of acetaldehyde
  - —Acetaldehyde produces a release of histamine, causing vasodilation and hypotension
  - —Severe reactions may occur in ethanol drinkers with levels of 50–100 mg/dL
  - —Severity and duration of reaction is proportional to the amount of ethanol ingested
- Disulfiram blocks dopamine β-hydroxylase and limits the synthesis of norepinephrine from dopamine
  - —Relative excess of dopamine may contribute to altered behavior
  - —Relative depletion of norepinephrine may contribute to hypotension
- Disulfiram metabolite (carbon disulfide) interacts with pyridoxal 5-phosphate
  - —Diminishes concentration of pyridoxine available for the formation of γ-aminobutyric acid (GABA) in the CNS
  - —Potentially lowers the seizure threshold
  - —Carbon disulfide is also cardiotoxic, hepatotoxic, and inhibits cytochrome P-450
- Disulfiram metabolites can chelate important metals (copper, zinc, iron) essential in various enzyme systems
- Disulfiram metabolites can cause peripheral neuropathies that are dose and duration dependent

ETIOLOGY

- Used as a deterrent to ethanol consumption in the treatment of chronic ethanol abuse
- Many users of the medication wear a medical alert bracelet
- A major metabolite investigated as an inhibitor of HIV replication and as an immune stimulant

Other Agents Producing Disulfiram-like Reactions

- Antibiotics
  - —Cephalosporins
  - —Nitrofurantoin
  - —Metronidazole
- Oral hypoglycemics
  - —Sulfonylureas
- Industrial agents
  - —Carbon disulfide
  - —Hydrogen sulfide
- Mushrooms
  - —*Coprinus atramentarius*
  - —*Clitocybe clavipes*

Pre-Hospital

N/A

Diagnosis

ESSENTIAL WORKUP

- Suspect disulfiram-ethanol reaction with the following:
  - —Typical signs and symptoms are present
  - —Treatment for chronic ethanol abuse in conjunction with recent ethanol ingestion, or exposure to ethanol-containing foods or medications

LABORATORY

- Ethanol level
- Electrolytes, BUN, creatinine, and glucose
- Liver function tests if hepatitis is suspected
- Creatine phosphokinase (CPK) if considering rhabdomyolysis in light of seizures or agitation

IMAGING/SPECIAL TESTS

- EKG to assess cardiac ischemia
- CT scan or MRI
  - —Indicated with altered mental status/ seizure
  - —Basal ganglia ischemia and infarction have been reported
- Electroencephalogram (EEG)
  - —Diffuse slowing without focal abnormalities has been seen in cases of acute toxicity with coma

DIFFERENTIAL DIAGNOSIS

- Sepsis
- Meningitis, encephalitis
- Cardiogenic shock secondary to acute coronary syndrome
- Anaphylactoid/anaphylactic reaction
- Gastroenteritis/pancreatitis with dehydration
- Ethanol withdrawal

PEDIATRIC CONSIDERATIONS

- Acute poisonings yield mainly severe CNS toxicity
- Ataxia, weakness, lethargy, seizures
- A Reye's syndrome–like encephalopathy in severe cases
- Adult symptoms may also be present

Treatment

INITIAL STABILIZATION

- ABCs
  - —Airway protection if necessary
  - —Supplemental oxygen
  - —Mechanical ventilation as needed
  - —0.9% NS IV resuscitation for hypotension
  - —Pressor support with *norepinephrine* for refractory hypotension

ED TREATMENT

- Supportive care is key to management
- No specific antidote available
- GI decontamination
  - —Activated charcoal in cases of disulfiram overdose
  - —Syrup of ipecac and gastric lavage unnecessary
- Alleviation of flushing
  - —Antihistamines (H_1 and H_2 antagonists)
  - —Prostaglandin inhibitors (indomethacin, ketorolac)
- Antiemetics for intractable vomiting (ondansetron, metoclopramide)
- Seizures
  - —Benzodiazepines (diazepam, lorazepam)
  - —Pyridoxine (for disulfiram overdose)
- 4-Methylpyrazole
  - —Inhibits ethanol metabolism at the alcohol dehydrogenase enzyme
  - —Has no indication for disulfiram-ethanol reactions or disulfiram overdose
- Hemodialysis
  - —Consider after massive ingestion of disulfiram and ethanol with refractory hypotension
  - —No studies documenting beneficial effect

MEDICATIONS

- Diazepam: 5–10 mg (peds: 0.2–0.5 mg/kg) i.v.
- Diphenhydramine: 25–50 mg (peds: 1–2 mg/kg) i.v.
- Indomethacin: 50 mg PO (peds: 0.6 mg/kg PO for age >14 years)
- Lorazepam: 2–6 mg (peds: 0.03–0.05 mg/kg) i.v.
- Metoclopramide: 10 mg (peds: 1–2 mg/kg) i.v.
- Norepinephrine: 4 mL in 1000 mL of D5W, infused at 0.1–0.2 μg/kg/min
- Ondansetron: 4 mg (0.15 mg/kg) i.v.
- Pyridoxine: 1 g (peds: 500 mg) i.v., repeat PRN

Disposition

ADMISSION CRITERIA

- ICU admission for mechanical ventilation, coma, refractory hypotension requiring pressors, cardiac ischemia, refractory seizures, and severe agitation
- Persistent vomiting, abdominal pain, or flushing
- Elderly patients or those who have preexisting cardiac disease

DISCHARGE CRITERIA

- Mild reactions that resolve with supportive care after an observation period of 8–12 hours
  - —Symptoms may recur upon rechallenge with ethanol up to 7–10 days after the last dose of disulfiram or agents that cause disulfiram-like reactions
  - —Abstain from ethanol use until at least 2 weeks after last dose of such agents
- Appropriate follow-up needed to assess the development of any hepatic or neurologic sequelae as a result of disulfiram toxicity

Miscellaneous

ICD9: N/A

ICD10: N/A

SEE ALSO: ALCOHOL POISONING

SUGGESTED READINGS

Enghusen Poulsen H, Loft S, Anderson JR, et al. Disulfiram therapy—adverse drug reactions and interactions. Acta Psychiatr Scand 1992;86:59–66.

Goldfrank LR. Disulfiram and disulfiram-like reactions. In: Goldfrank LR, ed. Goldfrank's toxicologic emergencies. East Stamford, CT: Appleton & Lange, 1998.

Johansson B. A review of the pharmacokinetics and pharmacodynamics of disulfiram and its metabolites. Acta Psychiatr Scand 1992;86:15–26.

Leikin J, Paloucek F. Disulfiram. In: Poisoning and toxicology handbook. Hudson, OH: Lexi-Comp, 2002.

Park CW, Rissio S. Disulfiram-ethanol induced delirium. Ann Pharmacother 2001;35:32–35.

Petersen EN. The pharmacology and toxicology of disulfiram and its metabolites. Acta Psychiatr Scand 1992;86:7–13.

Watson WA. Disulfiram. In: Ford MD, Delaney KA, Ling LJ, et al., eds. Clinical toxicology. Philadelphia, PA: WB Saunders, 2001.

Author: Sean Bryant

Diverticulitis

Clinical Presentation

SIGNS AND SYMPTOMS

General

- Symptoms develop over hours to days
- Anorexia
- Nausea, vomiting
- Low-grade fever
- Malaise

GI

- Abdominal pain
  - —Persistent
  - —Initially vague
  - —Becomes localized to left lower abdomen
- Tenderness at left lower quadrant with occasional mass palpated (phlegmon)
  - —*Phlegmon*—inflamed bowel loops or abscess
- Abdominal distention
- Bowel sounds normal, increased, or decreased
- Rectal tenderness with heme-positive stool
  - —Massive gross rectal bleeding rare
- Diarrhea (colon irritation) or constipation (inflammatory obstruction)
- Flatulence, heartburn
- Peritoneal signs if
  - —Perforation has occurred
- Unremarkable examination if
  - —Elderly
  - —Immunocompromised
  - —Taking corticosteroids

Other

- Urinary frequency
  - —Due to contact of inflamed colon against the bladder
- Resultant complications
  - —Bowel obstruction
  - —Fistulas after recurrent attacks
    - -Colovesical fistula (most common) presents with dysuria, frequency, urgency, pneumaturia, and fecaluria

MECHANISM/DESCRIPTION

- Perforation of a diverticulum

ETIOLOGY

- Fecal material becomes lodged in a diverticulum and hardens, forming a fecalith
- Fecalith can either abrade the mucosa or compromise surrounding blood supply, causing inflammation
- Inflammation causes microperforation of the bowel wall
  - —Peridiverticulitis: inflammation of colonic wall not extending beyond serosa
  - —Pericolic abscess: perforation of serosal layer though inflammation remains localized
  - —Peritonitis: perforation of serosal layer with generalized spread of inflammation

Pre-Hospital

CAUTION

- Avoid analgesics in abdominal pain when the underlying etiology is uncertain

Diagnosis

ESSENTIAL WORKUP

- CBC
  - —Elevated WBC with a left shift
  - —Iron-deficiency anemia suggests underlying carcinoma etiology
- Abdominal (supine and upright) and chest radiographs
  - —Perforation indicated by free air
  - —Obstruction indicated by air-fluid levels
- CT of abdomen
  - —Preferred diagnostic modality
  - —Better than contrast studies at diagnosing extraluminal processes (e.g., diverticulitis)
  - —Diagnostic criteria include:
    - -Wall thickening >5 mm
    - -Inflammation of pericolic fat
    - -Pericolic abscess
  - —Nondiagnostic criteria include:
    - -Stricture
    - -Diverticula
    - -Fistula
  - —Ability to diagnose nondiverticular causes of abdominal pain
  - —CT-guided percutaneous needle aspiration of localized abscesses avoids further surgery

LABORATORY

- Urinalysis
  - —WBC/RBC common
  - —Colovesical fistula results in WBC, bacteria, or feces
- Blood cultures
  - —If hospitalized with peritonitis

IMAGING/SPECIAL TESTS

- Avoid endoscopic procedures and contrast studies in acute cases so as not to cause perforation
  - —In select cases, water-soluble contrast may be a safe alternative
- Barium enema
  - —Indicated after resolution of acute illness to rule out fistula or other colonic pathology (e.g., carcinoma)
- Endoscopy
  - —Not necessary to diagnose acute illness
  - —Rigid sigmoidoscopy aids in diagnosing nondiverticular causes of abdominal pain (spasm, stricture, edema, pus, or peridiverticular erythema)
- Ultrasonography
  - —For diagnosing colonic wall thickening, inflammation, mass, abscess, or fistula
  - —Greatly operator dependent
  - —Not reliable in the presence of intestinal gas

DIFFERENTIAL DIAGNOSIS

- Colon carcinoma with perforation
- Ischemic colitis
- Bacterial colitis
- Appendicitis
  —Left-sided pain if peritonitis from ruptured appendix
  —Right-sided diverticular pain with cecal diverticulum (rare) or redundant sigmoid colon
- Inflammatory bowel disease
- Irritable bowel syndrome
- Ruptured or torsed ovarian cyst
- Pelvic inflammatory disease
- Peptic ulcer disease
- Renal colic

Treatment

INITIAL STABILIZATION

- Rehydration with 0.9% NS to replace intravascular volume depletion
- Bowel rest
  —NPO
  —NG tube if persistent vomiting or bowel obstruction present

ED MANAGEMENT

Analgesia

- Anticholinergics (dicyclomine)
  —Reduces colonic spasm
  —Does not mask underlying pathology
- Opiates for more aggressive pain management (IV morphine or demerol though morphine can cause colonic spasm)
  —If hemodynamically stable
  —When not dependent on repeat abdominal examinations for diagnostic or therapeutic decisions

Antibiotics

- Mild, uncomplicated cases (without perforation)
  —Outpatient oral agents include:
    -Trimethoprim-sulfamethoxazole (TMP-SMX) DS
    -Ciprofloxacin plus metronidazole
    -Amoxicillin/clavulanate (alternative)
  —Duration of therapy is 7–10 days or until afebrile for 3–5 days
- Moderate cases (focal inflammatory process)
  —Inpatient parenteral therapy includes:
    -Ampicillin/sulbactam
    -Piperacillin/tazobactam
    -Ticarcillin/clavulanate
    -Cefoxitin (alternative)
    -Cefotetan (alternative)
    -Ciprofloxacin plus metronidazole (alternative)
- Complicated cases (with peritonitis from perforation)
  —Imipenem/cilastatin
  —Meropenem
  —Trovafloxacin (alternative)
  —Ampicillin plus metronidazole plus gentamicin (alternative)
  —Ampicillin plus metronidazole plus ciprofloxacin (alternative)

Surgery

- Emergent surgery
  —Indicated for generalized peritonitis from perforation
  —Two-stage procedure with resection of diseased segment of colon and a proximal colostomy followed later with a reanastomosis
- Elective surgery
  —Indicated for
    -Multiple recurrent attacks without generalized peritonitis
    -Fistula formation
    -Intractable pain
    -Unresolved obstruction
    -Failure of medical therapy
    -Single serious attack under 40 years of age (controversial)
  —One-stage procedure following initial medical therapy allowing resolution of inflammation
- Peridiverticular abscess drainage
  —Indicated if well circumscribed and easily accessible
  —Accomplished by CT- or ultrasound-guided percutaneous needle aspiration

Ongoing Therapy

- When acute condition has resolved
- High-fiber, low-fat diet to decrease recurrence of attacks

MEDICATIONS

- Amoxicillin/clavulanate: 500/125 mg PO t.i.d.
- Ampicillin 2.0 g i.v. q6h
- Ampicillin/sulbactam: 3.0 g i.v. q6h
- Cefotetan: 2.0 g i.v. q12h
- Cefoxitin: 2.0 g i.v. q8h
- Ciprofloxacin: 400 mg i.v. q12h or 500 mg PO b.i.d.
- Dicyclomine: 20 mg PO q.i.d. (up to 40 mg PO q.i.d.) or 20 mg i.m. q.i.d. (*not* for IV use)
- Gentamicin: multiple daily dose (MDD) regimen, 2.0 mg/kg load then 1.7 mg/kg i.v. q8h, or once-daily dose (OD) regimen, 5.1 (7.0 if critically ill) mg/kg i.v. q24h (assuming normal renal function)
- Imipenem/cilastatin: 500 mg i.v. q6h
- Meropenem: 1 g i.v. q8h
- Meperidine: 50–100 mg i.m. q3–4h PRN or 25–50 mg i.v. and titrate to clinical response
- Metronidazole: 500 mg i.v. q6h or 500 mg PO q6h
- Morphine sulfate: 2–10 mg/70 kg body weight i.v. push slowly
- Piperacillin/tazobactam: 3.375 g i.v. q6h or 4.5 g i.v. q8h
- Ticarcillin/clavulanate: 3.1 g i.v. q6h
- Trimethoprim-sulfamethoxazole DS: 1 tablet PO b.i.d.
- Trovafloxacin: 300 mg i.v. for first dose then 200 mg i.v./PO daily

Disposition

ADMISSION CRITERIA

- Intractable pain
- High fever
- Peritonitis
- Failure to respond to outpatient management
- Immunocompromised or steroid-dependent patients
- Extreme of age
- Uncertainty of diagnosis

DISCHARGE CRITERIA

- Mild cases (low-grade fever, mild discomfort) of known diverticular disease

Miscellaneous

ICD9 CODE: 562.11

ICD10: K57.9

SEE ALSO: DIVERTICULOSIS

SUGGESTED READINGS

Ambrosetti P, et al. Acute left colonic diverticulitis in young patients. J Am Coll Surg 1994;179:156–160.

Ferzoco LB, Raptopoulos V, Silen W. Acute diverticulitis. N Engl J Med 1998;338: 1521–1526.

Freeman SR, McNally PR. Gastrointestinal emergencies: diverticulitis. Med Clin North Am 1993;77(5):1149–1165.

Gilbert DN, Moellering RC, Sande MA, eds. The Sanford guide to antimicrobial therapy, 32nd ed. Vermont: Jeb C. Sanford, Publisher, 2002.

Kohler L, et al. Diagnosis and treatment of diverticular disease: results of a consensus development conference. The Scientific Committee of the European Association for Endoscopic Surgery. Surg Endosc 1999;13(4):430–436.

Vignati PV, et al. Long-term management of diverticulitis in young patients. Dis Colon Rectum 1995;38:627–629.

Author: Dino Rumoro

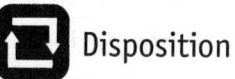

Diverticulosis

Clinical Presentation

SIGNS AND SYMPTOMS

Subdivisions

- Asymptomatic (90%)
- Symptomatic (painful)
- Hemorrhagic (3%)

GI

- Chronic or intermittent left lower quadrant pain
- Acute, painless bleeding with hematochezia or maroon stools
- Constipation (or diarrhea)
- Flatulence
  —Sometimes relieving the pain
- Dyspepsia
- Abdominal palpation
  —Tenderness in left lower quadrant
  —Firm sigmoid colon in the left lower quadrant
- Rectal exam
  —Predominantly reveals heme-negative stool
  —Bleeding typically mild
  —Most common cause of massive GI bleed

Other

- Fever: absent
- Diverticulitis and diverticular bleeding are separate entities and rarely coexist

MECHANISM/DESCRIPTION

- Single (diverticulum) or multiple (diverticula) colonic wall outpouchings as a result of colonic muscle dysfunction
- Sequence
  —Insufficient amounts of dietary fiber causes diminished stool bulk
  —Increased colonic contractions necessary to propel stool through colon, causing an increase in intraluminal pressure
  —Increased pressure forces mucosa and submucosa to herniate through the muscularis propria at its weakest point (site of nutrient artery penetration)

ETIOLOGY

- Occur anywhere in the GI tract, although diverticulosis generally refers to colonic disease
  —Sigmoid colon—most common site
- Pseudodiverticula
  —Most common form of colonic diverticula
- True diverticula (uncommon) contain all bowel wall layers
- Incidence directly related to increase in age
- Common in westernized society owing to refined diet and low fiber intake
- Massive bleeding usually from right colon
  —Fecalith (dry, hard stool) erodes through arterial branch

Pre-Hospital

CAUTIONS

- Avoid analgesics in abdominal pain when the underlying etiology is uncertain
- Establish two large-bore IVs with 0.9% NS if significant rectal bleeding/hemodynamic instability
- For hypotension
  —1–2 L (20 mL/kg) bolus 0.9% NS IV
  —Trendelenburg position

Diagnosis

ESSENTIAL WORKUP

- Thorough history and physical examination essential to avoid excessive workup

LABORATORY

- Asymptomatic diverticulosis
  —Requires no testing
- Uncomplicated painful disease (no peritoneal signs) with known history
  —Requires no workup
- Uncomplicated painful disease (no peritoneal signs) without previous history
  —Requires workup to rule out carcinoma (if weight loss, anorexia, heme-positive stool)
  —CBC for leukocytosis or anemia
  —Urinalysis to exclude hematuria or pyuria
- Hemorrhagic diverticulosis
  —CBC
  —Electrolytes, BUN, creatinine, glucose, calcium
  —Type and cross for 4 U of packed red blood cells (PRBCs)
  —Prothrombin time (PT), partial thromboplastin time (PTT), platelet count
  —EKG

IMAGING/SPECIAL TESTS

- Uncomplicated painful diverticulosis (as an outpatient)
  —Barium enema: search for classic diverticula and exclude carcinoma or polyps
  —Sigmoidoscopy: rule out carcinoma (done before barium studies so as not to have visualization hindered)
- Hemorrhagic diverticulosis
  —Anoscopy: if mild bleeding to rule out hemorrhoids
  —Proctosigmoidoscopy: if no blood in stool above rectum, assume rectal bleed
  —Colonoscopy: requires a clean colon, and bleeding cannot be excessive, otherwise difficult to visualize pathology
  —Radionuclide imaging
    -Safe
    -Localizes bleeding site
    -Ideal for detecting intermittent bleeding owing to the long half-life of the radioisotope (24–36 hours)
  —Angiography: identifies site of bleeding (more exact after radionuclide scanning)
  —Barium enema
    -Identifies diverticula but not bleeding
    -Can hinder visualization via other imaging techniques; therefore, rarely indicated

DIFFERENTIAL DIAGNOSIS

- Painful diverticulosis
  - —Irritable bowel syndrome (clinical presentation is almost identical)
  - —Diverticulitis
  - —Colon carcinoma
  - —Crohn's disease
  - —Urologic (renal colic)
  - —Gynecologic (ruptured or torsed ovarian cyst)
- Hemorrhagic diverticulosis
  - —Hemorrhoids
  - —Anal fissure
  - —Proctitis
  - —Colitis
  - —Carcinoma
  - —Polyps
  - —Ischemic enteritis
  - —Angiodysplasia
  - —Amyloidosis
  - —Vascular-enteric fistula
  - —Upper GI source

Treatment

INITIAL STABILIZATION

- Hemorrhagic diverticulosis (massive)
- Airway control (100% oxygen or intubate if unresponsive)
- Intravenous access with at least one large-bore catheter or two if unstable
- 0.9% NS bolus 1–2 L (20 mL/kg) for hypotension
- Central catheter placement if unstable following initial fluid resuscitation for more efficient delivery of fluids and monitoring of central venous pressure
- NG tube to rule out upper GI bleed
- Bladder catheter to monitor urine output
- Transfuse O-negative red blood cells immediately if impending arrest
- Most diverticular bleeding stops spontaneously

ED MANAGEMENT

- Uncomplicated symptomatic diverticulosis
  - —High-fiber diet and/or hydrophilic bulk laxative (e.g., psyllium)
  - —Antispasmodic (dicyclomine)
  - —Warm compresses to abdomen
  - —Reassurance
  - —Avoid cathartic laxatives
- Hemorrhagic diverticulosis (massive)
  - —Transfuse IV fluids and PRBCs (monitor electrolytes, calcium)
  - —Monitor fluid status (input/output)
  - —Consult surgeon
  - —Prepare for radionuclide scan followed by angiography if necessary
  - —Surgical intervention for segmental colectomy if bleeding on radionuclide scan
  - —Consider selective angiography with injection of vasopressin to control bleeding
  - —Embolization not recommended for colonic hemorrhage

MEDICATIONS

- Dicyclomine: 20 mg PO q.i.d. (up to 40 mg PO q.i.d.) or 20 mg i.m. q.i.d. (*not* for IV use)

Disposition

ADMISSION CRITERIA

- ICU admission if unstable with massive hemorrhagic diverticulosis
- Regular admission for mild or intermittent hemorrhagic diverticulosis that is otherwise stable to determine site of bleeding, and to evaluate need for definitive treatment

DISCHARGE CRITERIA

- Uncomplicated, symptomatic diverticulosis
- Stable with trace heme-positive stool, negative gastric aspirate, no anemia, and no other complaints

Miscellaneous

ICD9: 562.10

ICD10: K57.9

SEE ALSO: DIVERTICULITIS

SUGGESTED READINGS

Bono MJ. Gastrointestinal emergencies. Part I. Lower gastrointestinal tract bleeding. Emerg Med Clin North Am 1996;14(3):547–556.

Kim YI, et al. Injection therapy for colonic diverticular bleeding. J Clin Gastroenterol 1993;17(1):46–48.

Kohler L, et al. Diagnosis and treatment of diverticular disease: results of a consensus development conference. The Scientific Committee of the European Association for Endoscopic Surgery. Surg Endosc 1999;13(4):430–436.

McGuire HH. Bleeding colonic diverticula: a reappraisal of natural history and management. Ann Surg 1994;220(5): 653–656.

Author: Dino Rumoro

Dizziness

Clinical Presentation

SIGNS AND SYMPTOMS

- Dizziness is used to describe a wide range of symptoms
  —Abnormal sensation of motion
  —Feeling faint or fainting
  —Lightheadedness
  —Unsteadiness
- Classify dizziness into one of four categories by asking the patient to explain the sensation without using the word dizzy
  —Vertigo
    -Abnormal sensation of movement and position in space
    -Nystagmus
    -Nausea
    -Vomiting
    -Diaphoresis
  —Disequilibrium
    -Disorder of coordination and rhythm
    -Loss of equilibrium
    -May include sensory deficits such as peripheral neuropathy
  —Near syncope/syncope
    -Diaphoresis
    -Palpitations
    -Pallor during the episode
  —Other
    -Depression
    -Fatigue
    -Weakness
    -Hyperventilation

MECHANISM/DESCRIPTION

- Dizziness may be caused by a number of problems
  —Vertigo
    -Vestibular dysfunction
    -Cerebellar disease
  —Disequilibrium
    -Suggests a structural CNS disorder
    -Multiple sensory deficits
  —Near syncope/syncope
    -Cardiovascular insufficiency
    -Faintness that is postural or paroxysmal suggests a cardiovascular disorder
  —Other
    -Psychiatric illness
    -Constant ill-defined dizziness unrelated to posture suggests a psychogenic etiology
    -Metabolic derangement

ETIOLOGY

Vertigo

- Peripheral (85%)
  —Benign paroxysmal positional (most common)
  —Acute labyrinthitis
  —Ménière's disease
  —Vestibule neuritis
  —Acoustic neuroma
  —Ototoxic drugs
    -Aminoglycosides
    -Antimalarials
    -Erythromycin
    -Furosemide
  —Otitis media and serous otitis with effusion
  —Foreign body in ear canal

Central (15%)

—Cerebellar hemorrhage
—Vertebral basilar artery insufficiency
—Cerebellar trauma
—Cerebellopontine angle tumor
—Temporal lobe epilepsy
—Vertebral basilar migraines
—Multiple sclerosis
—Subclavian steal syndrome
—Drugs suppressing the reticular activating system
  -Sedative-hypnotics
  -Anticonvulsants

Disequilibrium

- Multiple sensory defects
- Frontal lobe disorder
  —Tumors
    -Meningioma
    -Glioma
    -Metastatic tumor
  —Anterior cerebral artery syndrome
  —Hydrocephalus
- Subcortical disorders
  —Multiple strokes
  —Ataxic hemiparesis
- Brainstem disorders
  —Stroke
  —Multiple sclerosis
- Cerebellar disorders
  —Cerebellar hemorrhage, infarct, tumor
  —Spinocerebellar degeneration
  —Alcoholism
  —Acute cerebellitis

Cardiac and Vascular Insufficiency

- Hypovolemia
- Orthostatic hypotension
- Anemia
- Myocardial ischemia
- Structural cardiac or valvular disease
- Cardiac dysrhythmias
  —Preexcitation
  —Prolonged QT syndrome
  —Hypokalemia
  —Supraventricular tachycardia
  —Ventricular dysrhythmia
- Pulmonary embolism
- Subarachnoid hemorrhage
- Hypoglycemia
- Hypoxia
- Hypercarbia
- Hyperventilation syndrome
- Vasovagal episode

Other

- Psychogenic
  —Anxiety
  —Hyperventilation syndrome
  —Depression
- Chronic fatigue syndrome
- Familial periodic paralysis
- Hypothyroidism

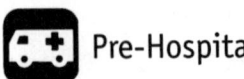

Pre-Hospital

CAUTIONS

- Acute onset of dizziness may be due to a transient ischemic attack, stroke, or hemorrhage
  —Monitor
  —Supplemental oxygen
- Observe mental status carefully as deterioration may warrant field endotracheal intubation

Diagnosis

ESSENTIAL WORKUP

N/A

LABORATORY

- Hematocrit
- Glucose
- Electrolytes
- Toxicologic screen

IMAGING/SPECIAL TESTS

- EKG to detect cardiac causes of near syncope and weakness
- CT scan if central vertigo or ataxia is present
- MR angiogram if vertebral basilar insufficiency is suspected

DIFFERENTIAL DIAGNOSIS

- See Etiology

Treatment

INITIAL STABILIZATION

- Supplemental oxygen
- Stabilization should be determined by more specific classification of dizziness based on the history, physical examination, and ancillary studies

ED TREATMENT

- Treatment should be determined by the underlying cause

MEDICATIONS

- Diazepam: 2.5–5 mg i.v. q8h *or* 2–10 mg PO q8h
- Diphenhydramine: 25–50 mg i.v., i.m., or PO q6h
- Meclizine: 25 mg PO q6h PRN
- Promethazine: 12.5 mg i.v. q6h *or* 25–50 mg PO, i.m., or PR q6h

Disposition

ADMISSION CRITERIA

- Admission of patients with dizziness should be based on the underlying etiology or associated symptoms

DISCHARGE CRITERIA

- Referral for completion of workup as an outpatient to a primary care physician or a neurologist

Miscellaneous

ICD9: 386,780.2

ICD10: R42

SEE ALSO: VERTIGO

SUGGESTED READINGS

Baloh RW. Approach to the dizzy patient. In: Baloh RW, ed. *Neurotology.* Baillieres Clin Neurol 1994;3:453.

Brown JJ. A systematic approach to the dizzy patient. Neurol Clin 1990;8:209–224.

Herr RD, Zun L, Mathews JJ. A directed approach to the dizzy patient. Ann Emerg Med 1989;18:664.

Pigott DC, Rosco CJ. The dizzy patient: an evidence-based diagnosis and treatment strategy. Emerg Med Pract 2001;3(3): 1–20.

Walker JS, Barnes SB. Dizziness. Emerg Med Clin North Am 1998;16(4):845–875.

Authors: Mitchell Adelstein; Jonathan Edlow

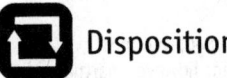

Domestic Violence

Clinical Presentation

SIGNS AND SYMPTOMS

- Traumatic injuries
  - —Small subset of presenting complaints
  - —Fractures
  - —Contusions
  - —Lacerations
  - —Penetrating and blunt trauma to the body
- Psychiatric
  - —Chronic pain syndromes
  - —Physical symptoms related to stress
  - —Anhedonia
  - —Insomnia
  - —Anorexia
  - —Somatic complaints
  - —Anxiety
  - —Depression and suicidal ideation
- Clinical clues of domestic violence
  - —History not compatible with exam
  - —Repeat visits for the same chief complaint
  - —Delay in seeking care
  - —Any injury during pregnancy
  - —Interaction between woman and partner that suggests interpersonal problems
  - —Evidence of trauma not attributable to a motor vehicle accident
  - —Multiple symptoms without obvious physical findings

MECHANISM/DESCRIPTION

- Intimate partner violence and abuse (IPVA) is the infliction or threat of physical harm against an intimate partner; it occurs in dating, married, cohabiting, or separated relationships
- IPVA is a pattern of assaultive and coercive behaviors that includes physical, sexual, and psychological attacks against the victims; these tactics are used to attain compliance and control over their partner
- Below are listed tactics used by perpetrators to gain power and control over their partner
  - —Pushing, shoving, slapping, punching, kicking, choking, holding, or tying down
  - —Verbal abuse
  - —Threats of harm (including children or pets), intimidation, or destruction of property
  - —Isolation of a victim physically or socially
  - —Degrading or humiliating behavior
  - —Attempting or forcing to perform sexual acts against a person's will or without protection against pregnancy
  - —Causing physical harm during sex or assaulting genitalia

ETIOLOGY

- Most victims are women, and most perpetrators are men; however, partners of same sex relationships and men may also be victims
- Most rapes and assaults of women are by known assailants

Diagnosis

- Diagnosis and recognition of IPVA in the ED, clinic, or office remains difficult and problematic

ESSENTIAL WORKUP

- Short screening questions of all female patients may be an effective means of identifying victims of domestic violence in the ED
- Screening should be direct, nonjudgmental, supportive, and private
- Patients who have sustained blunt trauma should have a thorough, focused exam of the affected areas

DIFFERENTIAL DIAGNOSIS

- Partner violence may be the acute precipitant of the patient's reason for presenting to the ED, or it may be part of the patient's past or present social history; there is no traumatic or nontraumatic presentation that is pathognomonic for intimate partner violence

Treatment

INITIAL STABILIZATION

- Provide timely and appropriate medical attention
- Maintain advocacy by expressing messages of support and validating the victim's dilemma

ED TREATMENT

- Document the victim's allegations in the chart in their own words
- Diagram or photograph injuries (after consent) and incorporate them into the clinical record
- Address the patient's safety in returning to the same home environment
  —Important determinants in predicting future danger include violence that is increasing in frequency and severity, threats of homicide or suicide by the partner, or the availability of a lethal weapon
- With the aid of social services or domestic violence advocates, review the patient's options: outpatient victim services, emergency shelter information, hot lines, restraining order information, and legal services
- Mandatory reporting requirements vary from state to state
  —Some states require a health care practitioner to make a report verbally and in writing if they suspect the wound or physical injury is the result of assaultive and abusive conduct
  —Determine how local authorities respond to reports of IPVA by health care practitioners
  —Recognize that mandatory reporting requirements may place the victim in more danger and create ethical dilemmas for physicians when the victim does not want the case reported to police or social service agencies

MEDICATIONS

- Acetaminophen: 650–975 mg PO
- Ibuprofen: 300–800 mg PO
- Meperidine: 1–1.8 mg/kg/dose i.v. or i.m.
- Morphine sulfate: 0.1 mg/kg/dose i.v. or i.m.

Disposition

ADMISSION CRITERIA

- A victim whose life is in imminent danger and has no place to be safely discharged (home, family, friends, or shelter) may need to be admitted to the hospital (under an assumed name)
- Use appropriate admission guidelines depending on the degree of trauma sustained

DISCHARGE CRITERIA

- A victim whose safety is assured and whose injuries can be managed as an outpatient may be discharged

Miscellaneous

ICD9: V15.49, V15.41

ICD10: R45.6

SUGGESTED READINGS

Abbott J. Injuries and illnesses of domestic violence. Ann Emerg Med 1997;29: 781–785.

Hayden SR, Barton ED, Hayden M. Domestic violence in the emergency department: how do women prefer to disclose and discuss the issues? J Emerg Med 1997;15(4):1–5.

Hyman A, Schillinger D, Lo B. Laws mandating reporting of domestic violence: do they promote well-being? JAMA 1995;273:1781–1787.

Salber PR, Taliaferro E. The physician's guide to domestic violence. Volcano, CA: Volcano Press, 1995.

Salber PR, Taliaferro E. Intimate partner violence and abuse. In: Marx J, Hockberger RS, Walls R, eds. Rosen's emergency medicine concepts and clinical practice, 5th ed. St. Louis: Mosby, 2002:863–875.

Author: Jim Comes

Duodenal Trauma

Clinical Presentation

SIGNS AND SYMPTOMS

- Complaints may be minimal with vague abdominal, flank, and back pain
- High gastrointestinal obstruction may be seen with duodenal hematomas

MECHANISM/DESCRIPTION

- The duodenum is 12 inches long, C shaped, divided into four sections (last three sections intraperitoneal), and lies mostly over the first three lumbar vertebrae
- The second section is the one most commonly injured
- Types of injury include duodenal wall hematoma, wall perforation, and hemorrhage
- Incidence of duodenal injury is about 5% of all intraabdominal injuries
- Penetrating trauma accounts for 85% of duodenal injuries
- Mortality ranges from 13–28%
  —Mostly from exsanguination
- Blunt duodenal injuries have a higher mortality
- Late mortality is usually from sepsis
- If blunt duodenal injury is diagnosed in less than 24 hours, the mortality rate is about 11%; if more than 24 hours, it approaches 40%

PEDIATRIC CONSIDERATIONS

- Intramural duodenal hematomas are commonly seen in child abuse, but most are secondary to recreational injuries (e.g., bicycle injuries)
- In children, the hematoma is most commonly seen in the first portion of the duodenum, and in adults, in the second and third portions

Pre-Hospital

CAUTIONS

- Follow trauma protocols
- Important to have pre-hospital personnel provide clear description of the mechanism of injury

Diagnosis

ESSENTIAL WORKUP

- Elicit tenderness or ecchymosis of upper abdomen or penetrating wounds to right upper quadrant or lower chest

LABORATORY

- Laboratory tests are of little value
  —50% of patients with duodenal injuries have elevated serum amylase

IMAGING/SPECIAL TESTS

Diagnostic Peritoneal Lavage

- Often *positive* for blood, bile, or bowel content
  —A *negative* lavage does not exclude injury!

Upright Chest and Abdominal Radiographs

- May show intraperitoneal air, retroperitoneal air, or air in the biliary tree
- Look for scoliosis to the right, loss of psoas shadow, and air around the right kidney
- Injecting air into the nasogastric tube may demonstrate retroperitoneal air more clearly
- Intramural hematomas without leakage may see a coiled spring appearance in plain radiographs of the affected portion

CT with Contrast

- Perhaps the best diagnostic test that shows small amounts of *retroperitoneal gas* and *extravasated contrast material*
- Also used to look for a *sausage-shaped mass* in the duodenal wall, which strongly suggests duodenal hematoma

DIFFERENTIAL DIAGNOSIS

- Injury to hollow organs (stomach, small and large intestines)
- Liver and biliary tree injuries
- Vascular injuries (aortic and mesenteric arteries as well as venous injuries)
  —Postoperative complications from prior duodenal injury repair such as infection and suture line dehiscence

Treatment

INITIAL STABILIZATION

- ABCs of multiple trauma care
- Aggressive fluid resuscitation with warmed normal saline or lactated Ringer's
- Central line for unstable patients
- Nasogastric decompression
- Early trauma surgical consultation

ED TREATMENT

- Tetanus prophylaxis for penetrating wounds and antibiotic prophylaxis
- Definitive treatment involves laparotomy in the OR with extensive exploration of the duodenum for injuries
- If unable to maintain perfusion in penetrating trauma may need to perform open thoracotomy to cross-clamp the aorta in order to survive to the operating room
- Broad-spectrum antibiotics to combat subsequent development of sepsis in patients with known perforation

MEDICATIONS

- Cefoxitin: 2 g i.v. in adults; 40 mg/kg i.v. in peds *plus*
- Gentamicin: 2 mg/kg i.v. loading dose (adult and peds) *or*
- Cefotetan: 2 g i.v. in adults; 20 mg/kg i.v. in peds *plus*
- Gentamicin: 2 mg/kg i.v. loading dose (adult and peds) *or*
- Clindamycin: 600 mg i.v. in adults; 20–40 mg/kg/d i.v. in 3–4 divided doses in peds *plus*
- Gentamicin: 2 mg/kg i.v. loading dose (adult and peds) *or*
- Ceftriaxone: 1–2 g i.v. in adults; 50–75 mg/kg/d in two divided doses not to exceed 2 g in peds *plus*
- Metronidazole: 15 mg/kg i.v.

Pediatric Considerations

- If nonaccidental trauma is suspected, then prompt referral to appropriate child protective agencies is required along with medical treatment

Disposition

ADMISSION CRITERIA

- Patients with duodenal injuries need admission to a trauma surgical service
- Minor duodenal hematomas that do not require immediate surgery may require nasogastric decompression for obstruction (up to 7 days) and observation for possible expansion or rupture of the hematoma
- Postoperative patients also require nasogastric decompression and need to be observed for possible fistula formation and other postoperative complications

DISCHARGE CRITERIA

- All patients with duodenal trauma require admission

Miscellaneous

ICD9: 863.21

ICD10: S36.4

SUGGESTED READINGS

Carrillo EH, Richardson JD, Miller FB, et al. Evolution in the management of duodenal injuries. J Trauma 1996;40(6):1037–1046.

Degiannis E, Boffard K. Duodenal injuries. Br J Surg 2000;87(11):1473–1479.

Ivatury RR, et al. Complex duodenal injuries. Surg Clin North Am 1996;76(4):797–812.

Tyburski JG, et al. Infectious complications following duodenal and/or pancreatic trauma. Am Surg 2001;67(3):227–230.

Weigelt JA. Duodenal injuries. Surg Clin North Am 1990;70(3):529–539.

Author: Hagop Isnar

Dysfunctional Uterine Bleeding

Clinical Presentation

SIGNS AND SYMPTOMS

- Excessive (>80 mL) or prolonged vaginal bleeding
- Vaginal bleeding that is significantly changed from a patient's normal pattern
- Pallor, tachycardia, hypotension, orthostasis in severe cases
- Bilateral ovarian enlargement if polycystic ovary disease is the etiology

MECHANISM/DESCRIPTION

- Abnormal uterine bleeding in the absence of systemic or structural disease
  —Includes bleeding between normal menstrual cycles, change in normal pattern of menstrual cycle, increased or decreased amount of menstrual bleeding
- Usually associated with anovulation (75%)
- Diagnosis of exclusion

ETIOLOGY

- Immature hypothalamic-pituitary-ovarian axis
- Perimenopause
- Obesity
- Polycystic ovary syndrome
- Very-low-calorie diets, intense exercise, rapid weight change, psychological stress

PEDIATRIC CONSIDERATIONS

- Common in adolescence due to immaturity of the hypothalamic-pituitary-ovarian axis

Pre-Hospital

- ABCs

CAUTIONS

- It is rare for women to be hemodynamically unstable simply from dysfunctional uterine bleeding; if such instability is present, concern is for ectopic pregnancy or other cause for hemorrhage

Diagnosis

ESSENTIAL WORKUP

- Exclude causes listed in differential diagnosis
- Thorough history and physical examination will suggest the etiology of bleeding in most cases
- Pregnancy test

LABORATORY

- CBC, prothrombin time (PT), partial thromboplastin time (PTT), type and screen, cross-match
- Iron studies, thyroid-stimulating hormone, luteinizing hormone, follicle-stimulating hormone, prolactin level, cervical cultures may be sent for routine follow-up by gynecologist

IMAGING/SPECIAL TESTS

- Endometrial biopsy if over 35 years of age
- Pelvic ultrasound may be necessary to evaluate for structural uterine, tubal, or ovarian abnormality

DIFFERENTIAL DIAGNOSIS

- Pregnancy complication: threatened, incomplete, or spontaneous abortion, ectopic or molar pregnancy
- Infectious: vaginitis, cervicitis, pelvic inflammatory disease (PID)
- Coagulopathies: von Willebrand's, idiopathic thrombocytopenic purpura, platelet defects, thalassemia major
- Medications: warfarin, aspirin, oral contraceptives, tricyclic antidepressants, major tranquilizers
- Systemic illness: adrenal, hepatic, renal, thyroid dysfunction, diabetes mellitus, or other endocrinopathies
- Anatomic lesions: fibroids, endometriosis, polyps, endometrial hyperplasia, neoplasms
- Intrauterine devices, trauma

Treatment

INITIAL STABILIZATION

- ABCs
  - —Packed RBCs for significant bleeding unresponsive to crystalloids

ED TREATMENT

- Rule out pregnancy
- Gynecology consultation if bleeding is severe and requires crystalloid resuscitation or blood products
- Dilation and curettage (D&C) may be necessary in the ED for hemodynamic instability
- Hysteroscopy or hysterectomy when symptoms unresponsive to estrogen treatment

MEDICATIONS

- Conjugated estrogen: 25 mg i.v. over 15 minutes for hemodynamically unstable patients, repeat every 2–4 hours until bleeding controlled, then oral estrogen 25 mg PO q.i.d.
- Multiple hormonal treatments available for outpatient therapy
  - —Combination oral contraceptive: 4 pills q.d. for 7 days or slow taper 4 pills × 2 days, then 3 pills × 2 days, then 2 pills × 2 days, then 1 pill × 3 days
  - —Medroxyprogesterone: 10 mg q.d. for 10–12 days every month
  - —Depot medroxyprogesterone acetate: 150 mg i.m.
  - —In hemodynamically stable, older patients, defer hormonal therapy until endometrial biopsy can be performed

PEDIATRIC CONSIDERATIONS

- Observation may be adequate if no instability
- Oral contraceptives often effective

Disposition

ADMISSION CRITERIA

- Significant blood loss
- Continued bleeding, hematocrit <20
- Unresponsive hemodynamic instability for possible D&C or operative treatment

DISCHARGE CRITERIA

- Most patients can be discharged with gynecology referral once bleeding is controlled and hemodynamically stable

Miscellaneous

ICD9: 626.8

ICD10: N93.8

SUGGESTED READINGS

Bradford JC, Kyriakedes CG. Vaginal bleeding. In: Marx JA, et al., eds. Rosen's emergency medicine: concepts and clinical practice. 5th ed. St. Louis: Mosby-Year Book, 2002:226–233.

Chuong CJ, Brenner JF. Management of abnormal uterine bleeding. Am J Obstet Gynecol 1996;175(3):787–791.

Morrison L, Spence J. Obstetrics and gynecology: vaginal bleeding and pelvic pain in the non pregnant patient. In: Tintinalli JE, ed. Emergency medicine: a comprehensive study guide, 5th ed. New York: McGraw-Hill, 2000:669–680.

Munro MG. Dysfunctional uterine bleeding: advances in diagnosis and treatment. Curr Opin Obstet Gynecol 2001;13:475–489.

Author: Christy Mohler

Dysphagia

Clinical Presentation

SIGNS AND SYMPTOMS

Oropharyngeal (Transfer) Dysphagia

- Difficulty initiating a swallow
  - —Immediate, within seconds of swallowing
- Sensation of the bolus not passing below the cervical esophagus
- Nasal or oral regurgitation
- Coughing or choking
  - —Indicating aspiration
- Gurgling noise after swallowing
  - —Suggests Zenker's diverticulum
- Vocal quality changes
  - —Results from bulbar muscle weakness

Esophageal (Transport) Dysphagia

- Retrosternal sticking sensation 10–15 seconds after swallowing
- Nocturnal regurgitation
- Drooling or regurgitation of undigested food and liquid
  - —Characteristic of esophageal obstruction

MECHANISM/DESCRIPTION

- Dysphagia
  - —Impaired swallowing
  - —Can be neuromuscular or mechanical
  - —Frequency and severity increase with advancing age
- Classification
  - —Oropharyngeal
    - -Difficulty transferring from the oropharynx to the proximal esophagus
    - -Usually a neuromuscular disorder resulting in bulbar muscle weakness or impaired coordination
  - —Esophageal
    - -Failure of normal transit through the esophagus
    - -Usually obstructive but consider motility disorders
- Odynophagia
  - —*Pain* with swallowing
  - —Separate, but often related, entity
- Pain pattern
  - —Voluntary striated muscle in the upper one third transitions to involuntary nonstriated muscle in the lower two thirds
  - —Somatic nerve fibers in the upper esophagus—excellent pain localization
  - —Afferents, from the vagus nerve along with the cervical and thoracic sympathetic ganglia, innervate the lower esophagus—poor pain localization
  - —Visceral pain from the lower esophagus may be difficult to distinguish from that of acute coronary syndrome

Pre-Hospital

CAUTIONS

- Vigilant airway attention
- Position of comfort with suction available

Diagnosis

ESSENTIAL WORKUP

- Three important questions
  - —What causes symptoms?
    - -Solids *and* liquids suggests a neuromuscular disorder
    - -Solids *only* or progression from solids to liquids suggests a structural abnormality
  - —Are symptoms intermittent or progressive?
    - -Intermittent symptoms suggest rings or webs
    - -Progressive symptoms suggest peptic or malignant strictures
    - -Motility disorders can be intermittent or progressive
  - —Are there concomitant symptoms?
    - -Odynophagia or chest pains
    - -Chronic cough or nocturnal wheezing
- Physical examination
  - —Often unremarkable
  - —Oropharyngeal inspection
  - —Pulmonary auscultation
  - —Neurologic exam with emphasis on cranial nerves
- EKG
  - —Consider cardiac etiology for chest discomfort
  - —Heart and esophagus share a common neural pathway

LABORATORY

- CBC and chemistries may be appropriate

IMAGING/SPECIAL TESTS

- Chest x-ray
  - —Food dilating the esophagus
  - —Aspiration pneumonitis
  - —Extrinsic compressing mass
- Soft tissue lateral neck radiograph
- Fluoroscopic barium swallow
  - —Defines esophageal anatomy
  - —Assesses function
  - —Do not perform if endoscopy anticipated
- Esophagoscopy
  - —Indicated to relieve obstruction and inspect the esophageal anatomy
- CT of the head
  - —Indicated for new-onset neuromuscular dysphagia

DIFFERENTIAL DIAGNOSIS

- Oropharyngeal
  - —Neuromuscular
    - -Cerebrovascular accident (CVA)
    - -Multiple sclerosis
    - -Amyotrophic lateral sclerosis (ALS)
    - -Parkinson's disease
    - -Huntington's chorea
    - -Myasthenia gravis
  - —Inflammatory
    - -Dermatomyositis
    - -Infectious pharyngitis
- Esophageal
  - —Mechanical
    - -Foreign body
    - -Peptic esophageal stricture
    - -Neoplasm
    - -Schatzki's ring
    - -Diverticula
  - —Motor
    - -Scleroderma
    - -Achalasia
    - -Diffuse esophageal spasm
    - -Nutcracker esophagus
    - -Nonspecific motor disorders

Treatment

INITIAL STABILIZATION

- Vigilant airway attention
- Position of comfort with suction available
- NPO
  - —Due to risk for aspiration
- 0.9% NS 500 mL bolus (peds: 20 mL/kg) i.v. fluid bolus for significant dehydration

ED TREATMENT

- Nitroglycerin for esophageal spasm
- Glucagon for impacted foreign body
- Treat complications
  - —Airway obstruction
  - —Aspiration, pneumonia, lung abscess
  - —Dehydration, malnutrition

MEDICATIONS

- Glucagon: 0.5 mg i.v. followed by second dose of 1 mg after 5 minutes if there is no improvement in symptoms
- Nitroglycerin: 0.4 mg SL every 5 minutes repeated up to 3 times

Disposition

ADMISSION CRITERIA

- Esophageal obstruction
- Compromised fluid or nutrition status

DISCHARGE CRITERIA

- Well-hydrated patient
- Urgent neurology, otolaryngology, or gastroenterology referral arranged for further evaluation and treatment

Miscellaneous

ICD9: 787.2

ICD10: R13

SUGGESTED READINGS

Baker BM. Symptoms, diagnosis, and management of dysphagia. J Ky Med Assoc 1998;96(9):362–367.

Cefalu CA. Diagnosing and treating dysphagia. Provider 1999;25(11): 71–72,74–75.

Rothstein RD. A systematic approach to the patient with dysphagia. Hosp Pract 1997;32(3):169–175.

Swann LA, Munter DW. Esophageal emergencies. Emerg Med Clin North Am 1996;14(3):557–570.

Authors: Timothy J. Mader; J. Brian Liddy

Dyspnea

Clinical Presentation

SIGNS AND SYMPTOMS

- Difficult, labored, or uncomfortable breathing
- Upper airway
  - —Stridor
  - —Upper airway obstruction
- Pulmonary
  - —Tachypnea
  - —Accessory muscle use
  - —Wheezing
  - —Rales
  - —Asymmetric breath sounds
  - —Poor air movement
- Cardiovascular
  - —S3 gallop
  - —Murmur
  - —Jugular venous distention
- CNS
  - —Altered levels of consciousness
- General
  - —Diaphoretic/cool versus hot/dry skin
  - —Pallor
  - —Upright patient position
  - —Clubbing
  - —Cyanosis
  - —Edema
  - —Ketotic breath odor

MECHANISM/DESCRIPTION

- Dyspnea comes from the Greek word for "hard breathing"
- Often described as "shortness of breath"
- Usually an unconscious activity, dyspnea is the subjective sensation of breathing, from mild discomfort to feelings of suffocation

ETIOLOGY

- Dyspnea usually reflects an impairment in ventilation, perfusion, metabolic function, or CNS drive
- Mechanisms that control breathing
  - —Control centers
    - -Brainstem and cerebral cortex affect both automatic and voluntary control of breathing
  - —Chemo, stretch, and irritant sensors
    - -CO_2 receptors located centrally and PO_2 receptors located peripherally
    - -Mechanoreceptors lie in respiratory muscles and respond to stretch
    - -Intrapulmonary mechanoreceptors respond to chemical irritation, engorgement, and stretch
  - —Effectors of respiratory center output are in the respiratory muscles and respond to central stimulation to move air in and out of the thoracic cavity
  - —Motor-sensory control of the diaphragm and muscles of respiration are controlled by C-3 to C-8 nerves and T-1 to T-12 nerves
- Derangements of any of these neurosensory pathways produces dyspnea
  - —Many etiologies for the sensation of dyspnea are due to complex nature of mechanisms that control breathing

Pre-Hospital

CAUTIONS

- Place all patients on supplemental oxygen, pulse oximetry, and cardiac monitor
- Initiate therapy for suspected cause of dyspnea when indicated
  - —Asthma
  - —Chronic obstructive pulmonary disease (COPD)
  - —Congestive heart failure (CHF)
- Intubate patients in the face of impending respiratory failure

Diagnosis

ESSENTIAL WORKUP

- Pulse oximetry
  - —May be falsely elevated due to increased ventilation or carbon monoxide
- Chest x-ray
  - —For diagnosis of pulmonary conditions
  - —Assess heart size and evidence of CHF
- Arterial blood gas
  - —Oxygenation
  - —Calculate arterial-alveolar gradient
    - -A-a (at sea level) $= 150 - (PO_2 - PCO_2)/0.8$
    - -Normal $= 5\text{–}20$
  - —Assess degree of acidosis

LABORATORY

- CBC
  - —Evaluation of anemia
  - —Neutrophil count helpful in evaluation of infectious processes
- Electrolyte, BUN, creatinine, glucose
  - —Consider when specific metabolic derangements are suspected
- Toxicology screen
- Methemoglobin/carboxyhemoglobin level
- Thyroid function tests

IMAGING/SPECIAL TESTS

- EKG for suspected myocardial ischemia, CHF
- Ventilation-perfusion scan or CT pulmonary angiogram for suspected pulmonary embolism
- Soft tissue neck radiograph or fiberoptic visualization for suspected upper airway obstruction
- Echocardiography for suspected pericardial effusion/tamponade
- Peak expiratory flow/spirometry to assess for reactive airway disease
- Tensilon test for suspected myasthenia gravis

DIFFERENTIAL DIAGNOSIS

- Upper airway
  - —Epiglottitis
  - —Laryngeal obstruction
  - —Tracheitis or tracheobronchitis
  - —Angioedema
- Pulmonary
  - —Airway mass
  - —Asthma
  - —Bronchitis
  - —Chest wall trauma
  - —CHF
  - —Drug-induced conditions (e.g., crack lung, aspirin overdose)
  - —Effusion
  - —Emphysema
  - —Metastatic disease
  - —Pneumonia
  - —Pneumothorax
  - —Pulmonary embolism
  - —Pulmonary hypertension
  - —Restrictive lung disease
- Cardiovascular
  - —Arrhythmia
  - —Coronary artery disease
  - —Intracardiac shunt
  - —LV failure
  - —Myxoma
  - —Pericardial disease
  - —Valvular disease
- Neuromuscular
  - —CNS disorders
  - —Myopathy and neuropathy
  - —Phrenic nerve and diaphragmatic disorders
  - —Spinal cord disorders
  - —Systemic neuromuscular disorders
- Other
  - —Acidosis
  - —Altitude
  - —Anaphylaxis
  - —Anemia
  - —Thyroid disorders
  - —Psychogenic
  - —Sepsis

PEDIATRIC CONSIDERATIONS

- Unique conditions in differential diagnosis for age <2 years
  - —Croup
  - —Congenital anomalies of the airway
  - —Congenital heart disease
  - —Foreign-body aspiration
  - —Nasopharyngeal obstruction
  - —Shock

Treatment

INITIAL STABILIZATION

- ABCs
- Immediate intubation for impending respiratory distress

ED TREATMENT

- Supplemental oxygen for hypoxia or to increase A-a gradient
- Initiate therapy for underlying condition

Disposition

ADMISSION CRITERIA

- Assisted ventilation
- Hypoxia
- A-a gradient >40
- Medical condition requiring hospital therapy

DISCHARGE CRITERIA

- Adequate oxygenation
- Stable medical illness that can be managed as outpatient

Miscellaneous

ICD9: 786.09

ICD10: R06.0

SEE ALSO: RESPIRATORY DISTRESS

SUGGESTED READINGS

Michelson E, Hollrah S. Evaluation of the patient with shortness of breath: an evidence based approach. Emerg Med Clin North Am 1999;17(1):221–237.

Schwartzstein RM, Manning HL. Pathophysiology of dyspnea. N Engl J Med 1995;12(3):1547–1552.

Tobin MJ. Dyspnea: pathophysiologic basis, clinical presentation, and management. Arch Intern Med 1990;8:1604–1612.

Weisman IM, Zeballos RJ. Clinical evaluation of unexplained dyspnea. Cardiologia 1996;41(7):621–634.

Author: Elizabeth Mitchell

Dystonic Reaction

Clinical Presentation

SIGNS AND SYMPTOMS

General

- Usually occur within 5 hours of ingestion and almost always within the first 4 days after exposure to the offending drug
- Age
  - —Twice as common in males
  - —More common in cocaine abusers
  - —Uncommon in older patients
  - —Children are more susceptible
- Difficulty with vocalization
- Completely alert and able to answer questions

Characteristic Motor Spasms

- Oculogyric crisis
  - —Involves the eye and periorbital muscles
  - —Starts as blepharospasm
  - —Evolves into a painful upward or lateral deviation of the eyes
- Buccolingual crisis
  - —Involves the facial muscles and tongue
  - —Bizarre grimacing
  - —Trismus
  - —Tongue protrusion
  - —Dysarthria
  - —Rarely causes spasm of the pharynx and larynx that can be severe enough to cause choking and respiratory distress
- Torticollic crisis
  - —Twisting of the neck
- Tortipelvic crisis
  - —Abdominal wall muscle spasm
- Opisthotonos
  - —Involves the muscles of the trunk and back
  - —Twisting and arching of the spine

MECHANISM/DESCRIPTION

- Normal pattern of CNS neurotransmission maintained by a balance between dopaminergic and cholinergic receptors
  - —Certain drugs disrupt this balance by blocking dopaminergic D_2 receptors, leading to involuntary muscle spasms
- Although the spasms are uncomfortable, they are not life threatening

ETIOLOGY

- Usually occur after the patient has taken an antipsychotic, antiemetic, or antidepressant drug either for therapeutic or recreational purposes
- Incidence of dystonic reactions in patients taking neuroleptics is 2–25%, depending on the agent
- Neuroleptic agents
  - —Phenothiazine (Thorazine, Mellaril, Prolixin, Compazine, Stelazine, Phenergan)
  - —Thioxanthenes (Navane)
  - —Butyrophenones (Haldol, Droperidol)
  - —Indole (Moban)
  - —Dibenzoxipine (Loxitane)
- Dystonic reactions caused by other agents
  - —Metoclopramide (Reglan)
  - —Trimethobenzamide (Tigan)
- Can last for prolonged periods and can be difficult to treat
  - —Cyclic antidepressants
  - —Antihistamines
  - —Doxepin
  - —Cimetidine
  - —Prozac

PEDIATRIC CONSIDERATIONS

- Children are particularly vulnerable to dystonic reactions when dehydrated or febrile

Pre-Hospital

CAUTIONS

- Rarely life threatening
- Direct attention toward spasm of larynx and tongue to be sure dystonic reaction is not causing respiratory compromise
- Ask family and friends about ingestions of antipsychotic medications, antiemetics, and recreational drugs
- Transport pill bottles

Diagnosis

ESSENTIAL WORKUP

- Clinical diagnosis is based on characteristic signs and symptoms with history of possible drug exposure
- Diagnosis is confirmed by response to treatment

DIFFERENTIAL DIAGNOSIS

- Seizure
  - —History of prior seizures
  - —Not responsive to verbal stimuli
  - —Tonic-clonic-type motor movements rather than spasm
- Hysteria or pseudoseizure
  - —History of a precipitating emotional event
  - —Tonic-clonic motor activity rather than a sustained spasm
- Tetanus
- Strychnine poisoning
- Chronic dystonias
  - —Cerebral palsy, familial choreas
  - —Usually the history of dystonia is associated with a chronic neurologic process
- Scorpion envenomation
  - —Oculogyric crisis and opisthotonos are common manifestations of scorpion envenomation
  - —Patient lacks a history of drug exposure

PEDIATRIC CONSIDERATIONS

- Meningitis and encephalitis may present with atypical seizures that mimic dystonic reaction

Treatment

INITIAL STABILIZATION

- Stabilize airway to prevent spasm of the larynx or tongue from causing respiratory compromise

ED TREATMENT

- Administer diphenhydramine (Benadryl) or benztropine mesylate (Cogentin)
  —Rapid resolution of the muscular spasm by restoring cholinergic-dopaminergic balance in the CNS
  —IV administration is preferred route of treatment
  —Onset of relief in 2–5 minutes
  —Complete resolution of symptoms in 15 minutes
  —IM administration is alternate route of treatment
  —Begins to work in 15–30 minutes
  —Continue oral administration for 3 days to prevent redevelopment of symptoms
- Diazepam (Valium)
  —Administer in cases of dystonia unresponsive to adequate doses of anticholinergic medications
  —A failure to respond to standard treatment should lead the physician to consider other diagnoses

MEDICATIONS

- Benztropine mesylate (Cogentin): 1–2 mg either i.v. (over 2 minutes) or i.m. followed by 1–2 mg PO b.i.d. for 3 days
  —Not to be used in children <3 years old
  —For children >3 years old: 0.02 mg/kg i.v. (over 2 minutes) or i.m. followed by 0.02 mg/kg PO b.i.d. for 3 days
- Diphenhydramine (Benadryl): 1–2 mg/kg up to 100 mg either i.v. (over 2 minutes) or i.m. followed by 25–50 mg (peds: 1–2 mg/kg) PO t.i.d. for 3 days, *or*
- Diazepam: 5–10 mg i.v. followed by 5 mg PO q4–6h as necessary for 3 days

Disposition

ADMISSION CRITERIA

- None

DISCHARGE CRITERIA

- Discharge after resolution of symptoms
- Patient should not drive or perform tasks that require full alertness while taking sedating medications

Miscellaneous

ICD9: N/A

ICD10: G24.0

SUGGESTED READINGS

Diederich NJ, Goetz CG. Drug-induced movement disorders. Neurol Clin 1998;16:125–139.

Ellenhorn MJ, Schonwald S, Ordog G, et al. Neuroleptic drugs. In: Ellenhorn MJ, ed. Ellenhorn's medical toxicology: diagnosis and treatment of human poisoning. Baltimore: Williams & Wilkins, 1997:662–670.

McCormick MA, Manognerra AS. Dystonic reactions. In: Harwood-Nuss A, ed. The clinical practice of emergency medicine. Philadelphia: Lippincott Williams & Wilkins, 2001:1496–1498.

Van Harten PN, Hoek HW, Kahn RS. Acute dystonia induced by drug treatment. BMJ 1999;319:623–626.

Author: Kenneth Jackimczyk

Eating Disorders

Clinical Presentation

SIGNS AND SYMPTOMS

- Prevalence of partial syndrome eating disorders is 5–10% of the population
- A range of disordered eating attitudes and behaviors should be considered

Anorexia Nervosa (AN)

- Refusal to maintain body weight at or above a minimally normal weight for age and height
  —Failure to make expected weight gain during a period of growth
- Intense fear of gaining weight or becoming fat, even though underweight
- Disturbance in the way body weight or shape is experienced
- Undue influence of body weight and shape on self-evaluation
- Denial of seriousness of low body weight
- In postmenarchal females, amenorrhea for three consecutive cycles

Bulimia Nervosa (BN)

- Recurrent episodes of binge eating characterized by
  —Eating a larger than usual amount of food in a discrete period of time
  —A sense of loss of control over eating during the episode
- Recurrent inappropriate compensatory behaviors used to prevent weight gain
  —Self-induced vomiting
  —Misuse of laxatives
  —Diuretics
  —Enemas or other medications
  —Fasting
  —Excessive exercise

Binge-Eating Disorder (BED)

- Recurrent episodes of binge eating characterized by
  —Eating a larger than usual amount of food in a discrete period of time
  —A sense of loss of control over eating during the episode
- Binge-eating episodes associated with three or more of the following
  —Eating much more rapidly than normal
  —Eating until feeling uncomfortably full
  —Eating large amounts of food when not feeling physically hungry
  —Eating alone because of being embarrassed by how much one is eating
  —Feeling disgusted with oneself, depressed, or very guilty after overeating
  —Marked distress regarding binge eating

Medical Complications

- Endocrine, metabolic
  —Electrolyte imbalances
- Growth retardation
- Nutritionally based osteoporosis
- Cardiovascular problems
  —Arrhythmias
  —Bradycardia
  —Ipecac cardiomyopathy
- Renal complications
  —Hypokalemia
  —Edema
- Hematologic complications
  —Hematologic changes
  —Anemia
  —Leukopenia
  —Thrombocytopenia
- Potentially irreversible structural brain changes

MECHANISM/DESCRIPTION

- Prevalence
  —AN: 0.5% of the U.S. female population
  —BN: 2%
  —BED: 2%
- 5–10% of AN and BN cases, and 40% of BED cases occur in boys and men

ETIOLOGY

- Typical age of onset for AN is bimodal at 13–14 years and 17–18 years
- Typical anorexic is a teenager whose dieting behavior escalates into an obsessive preoccupation with weight and thinness
- BN and BED typically onset in late adolescence or early adulthood
- Typical bulimic
  —Has attempted many diets and failed
  —May have learned purging behaviors from a friend or family member
- BED associated with a history of obesity, weight cycling, and dieting

Pre-Hospital

N/A

Diagnosis

ESSENTIAL WORKUP

- Clinical diagnosis
- Medical evaluation
- Nutritional assessment
- Psychiatric interview
- Family evaluation when patient lives with her/his family

LABORATORY

- CBC
- Electrolytes, BUN, creatinine, glucose
- Liver function tests for serum albumin

DIFFERENTIAL DIAGNOSIS

- Mood disorders
- Anxiety disorders (especially obsessive-compulsive disorder)
- Substance abuse
- Kleptomania
- Variety of personality disorders (especially borderline personality disorder) warrant assessment
- Medical conditions
  —Crohn's disease
  —Diabetes mellitus

Treatment

INITIAL STABILIZATION

- ABCs
- IV 0.9% NS 1 L bolus (peds: 20 mL/kg) for severe dehydration
- Accucheck, correct hypoglycemia with dextrose

ED TREATMENT

- Outpatient treatment
  - —Requires a multimodal, multidisciplinary team approach comprised of
    - -Psychotherapy
    - -Nutritional guidance
    - -Medical monitoring
    - -Pharmacotherapy
    - -Family therapy
    - -Group therapy
  - —Establish modest goals and clear parameters
    - -Expected weight gain for anorexic patients
  - —Cognitive behavioral therapy and interpersonal psychotherapy
    - -Most effective forms of psychotherapy for eating disorders
- Medical therapy
  - —Pharmacotherapy
    - -Often indicated within the context of psychotherapy
    - -When other psychopathology requires treatment
  - —Antidepressant medications shown to reduce binging and purging behaviors significantly
    - -Selective serotonin reuptake inhibitors (SSRIs; fluoxetine)
    - -Tricyclic antidepressants (amitriptyline, imipramine)
    - -Appetite suppressants in the treatment of BED (sibutramine)
    - -No accepted pharmacologic treatment of AN
- Prognosis
  - —Anorexics
    - -20% of anorexics continue on a chronic course
    - -30% improve
    - -50% recover
    - -Mortality rate 5.6% per decade

MEDICATIONS

- Amitriptyline: 25 mg PO t.i.d.
- Fluoxetine: 20 mg PO q.d.
- Imipramine: initial 25 mg PO t.i.d.
- Sibutramine: 10 mg PO q.d.

Disposition

ADMISSION CRITERIA

- Medical risk
  - —Extremely low weight
  - —Rapid weight loss
  - —Serum electrolyte imbalance
- Psychiatric risk
  - —Severe depression
  - —Suicidality
  - —Severe denial
  - —Severe impairment in functioning
  - —Toxic family environment

DISCHARGE CRITERIA

- In AN patients, safe weight and a decrease in unhealthy eating behaviors
- In BN patients, significant decrease in the frequency, severity, and paralyzing nature of binging and purging behaviors is necessary

Miscellaneous

ICD9: 307.50

ICD10: F50

SUGGESTED READINGS

Anonymous. Practice guideline for the treatment of patients with eating disorders (revision). American Psychiatric Association. Practice guideline for eating disorders. Am J Psychiatry 2000;157:1–39.

Becker AE, Grinspoon SK, Klibanski A, et al. Eating disorders. N Engl J Med 1999;340: 1092–1098.

Herzog DB, Becker AE. Eating disorders. In: Nicholi A, ed. The new Harvard guide to psychiatry. Cambridge, MA: Belknap Press, 1999;400–411.

Herzog DB, Beresin EV, Charat VE. Anorexia nervosa. In: Weiner JM, ed. Textbook of child and adolescent psychiatry, 3rd ed. Washington, DC: American Psychiatric Publishing (in press).

Kreipe RE, Birndorf SA. Eating disorders in adolescents and young adults. Psychiatr Clin North Am 2000;84:1027–1049.

Rigotti NA. Approach to eating disorders. In: Goroll AH, May LA, Mulley JB, eds. Primary care medicine: office evaluation and management of the adult patient, 3rd ed. Philadelphia: JB Lippincott, 1995.

Rigotti NA. Eating disorders. In: Carlson KJ, Eisenstat SA, Frigoletto FD, Schiff IS, eds. Primary care of women. St. Louis: Mosby-Year Book, 1995.

Authors: David Herzog; Valerie Charat; Ana Richards

Ectopic Pregnancy

Clinical Presentation

SIGNS AND SYMPTOMS

- The classic triad of amenorrhea, vaginal bleeding, and abdominal pain are present in only 15% of women with ectopic pregnancies
- Amenorrhea (75–95%)
- Abdominal pain (80–100%), frequently unilateral
- Abnormal vaginal bleeding (50–80%)
- Symptoms of pregnancy (10–25%)
- Orthostatic hypotension, dizziness, and syncope (5–35%)
- Abdominal tenderness (55–95%)
- Adnexal tenderness (75–90%)
- Adnexal mass (35–50%)
- Cervical motion tenderness (43%)

MECHANISM/DESCRIPTION

- Implantation of a fertilized ovum outside of the uterus, most commonly the fallopian tube
  —Abdominal and peritoneal implantations associated with higher morbidities because of the difficulty in diagnosis and their tendency to bleed
  —Incidence is 16.8 cases per 1000 pregnancies
- Risk factors include
  —Woman >35 years old
  —African American
  —Any factor that prevents or delays the fertilized egg from reaching the uterus
  —Previous fallopian tube damage from infections, such as pelvic inflammatory disease (PID)
  —Previous tubal surgery, such as history of tubal ligation
  —History of previous ectopic pregnancy
  —History of intrauterine device (IUD) use
  —DES exposure
  —In vitro fertilizations
  —43% of women with ectopic pregnancies have no risk factors

Pre-Hospital

CAUTIONS

- Female patients of childbearing age presenting in shock may have an unrecognized ruptured ectopic pregnancy

Diagnosis

ESSENTIAL WORKUP

- Pregnancy testing
  —Women presenting with vaginal bleeding or abdominal pain *must* have a urine or serum pregnancy test and be ruled out for an ectopic pregnancy
  —Do not forget to include patients with history of recent elective or spontaneous abortion, tubal ligations or IUD use

Vital Signs Unstable

- Type and cross-match, hematocrit (HCT)
- Bedside ultrasound (US), if immediately available, simultaneous with resuscitation
- Although rarely performed, culdocentesis can be performed quickly and the presence of blood in the cul-de-sac suggests bleeding ectopic pregnancy
- Consult gynecology and prepare for immediate surgical intervention

Vital Signs Stable

- Rapid hemoglobin determination
- Type and Rh
- Pelvic exam: note uterine size, adnexal size, and tenderness
- Ultrasonography

LABORATORY

- Urine pregnancy (ICON) can detect β-human chorionic gonadotropin (β-hCG) levels of 50 mIU/L
- β-hCG levels of 25 mIU/L can be detected with serum tests
- For pregnant patients with no demonstrable IUP
  —Quantitative serum β-hCG; for diagnosis and follow-up
  -Doubles every 2 days in a normal early pregnancy (early pregnancy <10,000 β-hCG mIU/L)
  —Serum progesterone; adjunct for diagnosing normal pregnancy
  ->25 ng/mL 97% of normal pregnancy
  -<5 ng/mL almost 100% prediction of abnormal pregnancy
  -10–20 ng/mL not helpful in predicting

ULTRASOUND IN CONJUNCTION WITH QUANTITATIVE β-HCG

- Patients with β-hCG levels >6,500 mIU/L and no intrauterine gestational sac seen on ultrasound have a 100% chance of having an ectopic pregnancy
- Patients with β-hCG levels >6,500 mIU/L with intrauterine gestational sacs present have a 94% chance of having a normal pregnancy
- Patients with β-hCG <2,000 mIU/L are too early to have a gestational sac seen by abdominal ultrasound and thus cannot be ruled out for an ectopic pregnancy
- Patients with β-hCG >2,000 and <6,500 mIU/L should have an IUP visualized on transvaginal US; suspect ectopic pregnancy if IUP is absent

IMAGING

- Ultrasonographic evidence of an IUP makes ectopic pregnancy very unlikely
  —Positive IUP is indicated by a double-ringed gestational sac and yolk sac, fetal pole, and heartbeat seen in the uterus
  —The use of transvaginal ultrasound allows for the visualization of these structures 1 week earlier
  —Transvaginal ultrasound; gestational sac at 5 weeks, cardiac activity at 6.5 weeks
  —Transabdominal ultrasound; gestational sac at 6 weeks, cardiac activity at 8 weeks
  —Complex adnexal mass and fluid in the cul-de-sac seen in 22% of ectopics and has a 94% positive predictive value when present
  —Positive pregnancy test with no confirmed IUP and fluid in the pelvis; high risk for bleeding ectopic pregnancy

DIFFERENTIAL DIAGNOSIS

- Positive pregnancy test with vaginal bleeding
  —Spontaneous abortion, cervicitis, trauma
- Positive pregnancy test with no evidence of an IUP
  —Completed spontaneous abortion
  —Early threatened abortion
- Positive pregnancy test with evidence of an IUP, abdominal pain, or adnexal tenderness
  —Septic abortion, threatened abortion, corpus luteal cyst, ovarian torsion, urinary tract infection (UTI), nephrolithiasis, gastroenteritis, appendicitis

Treatment

INITIAL STABILIZATION

Vital Signs Unstable

- ABCs
- Fluid resuscitation with two large-bore IVs, oxygen and monitor
- Type specific, or O-negative blood if hypotensive after initial fluid bolus
- Consult gynecology and then transport to the OR immediately for surgery

Vital Signs Stable

- Evidence of ectopic pregnancy on ultrasound–obstetric-gynecologic evaluation for surgery versus outpatient methotrexate treatment
- No evidence of ectopic pregnancy (early IUP or early ectopic)
  - —*Desired pregnancy:* β-hCG levels in a normal IUP should double every 2 days; stable, reliable patients may be followed for serial β-hCG tests in conjunction with obstetrician-gynecologist
  - —*Undesired pregnancy:* dilation and curettage (D&C) to evacuate the uterus and confirm the presence of intrauterine products of conception

MEDICATIONS

- RhoGAM in Rh-negative women: 50 μg i.m. in women $\leq$12 weeks pregnant; 300 μg i.m. in women >12 weeks pregnant
- Methotrexate: initiated in conjunction with obstetric consultant
  - —Reliable patients with unruptured ectopic pregnancies <3.5 cm
  - —Contraindications are renal or hepatic dysfunction, active peptic ulcer disease, and blood dyscrasias
  - —Most common dosing, single dose (50 mg/m^2); serial β-hCG on days 2, 4, and 7. If <15% decline in β-hCG between days 4 and 7, a second dose is given
  - —Most common side effects are worsening abdominal pain, nausea, vomiting, and diarrhea
  - —Most common complication, tubal rupture in 4%

Disposition

ADMISSION CRITERIA

- Any patient with a confirmed ectopic pregnancy that is hemodynamically unstable
- Unreliable patients with increased risk factors, no available ultrasound, β-hCG >6,500 with no evidence of an IUP should be admitted for observation and serial β-hCG tests

DISCHARGE CRITERIA

- Decision for outpatient management should be made in conjunction with obstetrician-gynecologist
- Hemodynamically stable and reliable patients with workup that cannot rule out ectopic pregnancy
  - —Strict follow-up for serial β-hCG tests every 2 days
  - —Patients should be recorded in a logbook with phone numbers to ensure follow-up
  - —*Ectopic precautions:* patients should return to the emergency room immediately for increasing abdominal pain, vaginal bleeding, syncope, or dizziness; patients should not be left alone until the diagnosis of ectopic pregnancy can be safely ruled out; family and friends should also be instructed on the warning signs and symptoms of ruptured/bleeding ectopic pregnancies

Miscellaneous

ICD9: 633.9

ICD10: 000.9

SUGGESTED READINGS

Abbott J. Complications related to pregnancy. In: Rosen P, et al., eds. Emergency medicine: concepts and clinical practice, 3rd ed. St. Louis: CV Mosby, 1992.

Cartwright PS. Diagnosis of ectopic pregnancy. Obstet Gynecol Clin North Am 1991;18:19.

Hockberger RS. Ectopic pregnancy. Emerg Med Clin North Am 1987;5:481.

Kaplan BC, et al. Ectopic pregnancy: prospective study with improved diagnostic accuracy. Ann Emerg Med 1996;28:10.

Lipscomb GH, Stovall TG, Ling FW. Nonsurgical treatment of ectopic pregnancy. N Engl J Med 2000;343(18): 1325–1329.

Stovall TG, Ling FW. Single dose methotrexate: an expanded clinical trial. Obstet Gynecol 1993;168:1759–1765.

Turner LM. Vaginal bleeding during pregnancy. Emerg Med Clin North Am 1994;12:45.

Author: Aviva Zigman

Eczema/Atopic Dermatitis

Clinical Presentation

SIGNS AND SYMPTOMS

- Chronic disease: hyperpigmentation, hypopigmentation, lichenification, and scaling
- Acute flares:
  - —Mild/moderate: erythematous, scaly patches with crusting and excoriation
  - —Severe: diffuse, exfoliative erythroderma
- Distribution varies with age:
  - —Infancy: tends to be more widespread with prominent facial and scalp involvement; from 8–12 months, extensor surface involvement prominent
  - —Childhood: wrists, ankles, antecubital and popliteal fossae
  - —Adolescents/adults: flexural areas, hands, feet, face, and neck
- Other exam findings commonly associated with atopic dermatitis (AD) include:
  - —Dennie-Morgan folds (infraorbital grooves)
  - —"Allergic shiners" (infraorbital darkening)
  - —Exaggerated linear nasal crease
  - —Geographic tongue
  - —Pityriasis alba (dry, white patches to the face and upper body)
  - —Facial pallor
  - —Hyperlinear palms
  - —Follicular accentuation
  - —Keratosis pilaris (flesh-colored, keratotic papules on upper arms, thighs, buttocks)
  - —Dermatographism

MECHANISM/DESCRIPTION

- Chronic disease with acute flares
- Superinfection with bacteria (especially *Staphylococcus aureus*) common
- Altered cell-mediated immunity predisposes to increased infection with herpes simplex virus (HSV; eczema herpeticum), moluscum contagiosum, common warts, and fungi

ETIOLOGY

- Unknown although likely multifactorial
  - —Genetic: AD patients have family members with "atopy" (asthma, allergic rhinitis) 30–70% of the time; if both parents are "atopic" individuals, the incidence of AD in their child is 79%
  - —Immunologic: decreased capacity of circulating mononuclear cells to produce interferon-γ (IFN-γ), increased synthesis of granulocyte-macrophage colony-stimulating factor (GM-CSF) by monocytes leading to decreased apoptosis, *elevated levels of serum immunoglobulin E (IgE)* and circulating eosinophils

PEDIATRIC CONSIDERATIONS

- Occurs in 10–15% of children <5 years of age
- Onset <6 months of age in 48–75% of patients

Pre-Hospital

N/A

Diagnosis

ESSENTIAL WORKUP

- None

LABORATORY

- Serum IgE levels and eosinophils are often elevated
- CBC with differential and blood cultures if febrile or toxic appearing
- Tzanck smear, viral culture and HSV direct fluorescent antibody (DFA) test if eczema herpeticum suspected

IMAGING/SPECIAL TESTS

- Generally reserved for settings outside of the ED but can include
  - —Patch testing can help distinguish AD from contact dermatitis
  - —Radioallergosorbent test (RAST) can sometimes help identify allergic triggers
  - —Skin biopsy may help rule out other disorders

DIFFERENTIAL DIAGNOSIS

- Seborrheic dermatitis
- Allergic contact dermatitis
- Irritant dermatitis
- Psoriasis
- Scabies
- Histiocytosis X
- Acrodermatitis enteropathica
- Wiskott-Aldrich syndrome
- Hyperimmunoglobulin E syndrome
- Phenylketonuria

Treatment

INITIAL STABILIZATION

N/A

ED TREATMENT

- Treatment is two-fold: chronic maintenance and control of acute flares
- Chronic maintenance
  - —Avoidance of excessive bathing
  - —Use of tepid water and mild soaps
  - —Frequent use of appropriate emollients (Eucerin cream, Aquaphor ointment)
  - —Avoidance of irritants: tobacco smoke, wool or other harsh fabrics, feather/down bed products, stuffed animals, dust mites and pets
  - —Reduction of perspiration
- Control of acute flares
  - —Emollients
  - —Mild disease/face: hydrocortisone 2.5% ointment (low potency)
  - —Moderate disease: triamcinolone 0.1% ointment (moderate potency)
  - —Severe disease: fluocinonide 0.05% ointment (high potency)
  - —Systemic corticosteroids are rarely used owing to the chronicity of AD and the high likelihood of relapse upon discontinuation
  - —New topical immunomodulator medications: topical pimecrolimus and tacrolimus (second-line agents at this point)
- Antihistamines: diphenhydramine, hydroxyzine, Zyrtec, Claritin, or Allegra to help reduce itching
- Bacterial superinfection: cephalexin, cefazolin
- Eczema herpeticum
  - —Acyclovir
  - —Hold topic steroids

MEDICATIONS

- Acyclovir: 400 mg (peds: 80 mg/kg/24 h) PO q8h
- Acyclovir: 750 mg/m^2/24 h (peds: same dosage but if CNS infection suspected then 60 mg/kg/24 h) i.v. divided q8h
- Aquaphor ointment: apply to affected areas b.i.d.
- Cefazolin: 1–2 g (peds >1 month 50–100 mg/kg/24 h, <1 month, see PDR) i.v. q8h
- Cephalexin: 250 mg–1 g (peds: 25–100 mg/kg/24 h) PO q6h
- Cetirizine: 5–10 mg (peds: 2.5–5 mg) PO q.d.
- Diphenhydramine: 25–50 mg (peds: 5 mg/kg/24 h) PO or i.v. q6h
- Eucerin cream: apply to affected areas b.i.d.
- Fexofenadine: 60 mg (peds >12 years) PO q.d. to b.i.d.
- Fluocinonide 0.05% ointment: apply to affected areas of body b.i.d. (high potency)
- Hydrocortisone 2.5% ointment: apply to affected areas of body/face b.i.d. (low potency)
- Hydroxyzine: 25–100 mg (peds: 2 mg/kg/24 h) PO q4–6h
- Loratadine: 10 mg (peds <30 kg: 5 mg) PO q.d.
- Pimecrolimus 1% cream: apply to affected areas b.i.d. (peds >2 years of age)
- Tacrolimus ointment: 0.1% (peds >2 years of age: 0.03%) apply to affected areas b.i.d.
- Triamcinolone 0.1% ointment: apply to affected areas of body b.i.d. (mid potency)

PEDIATRIC CONSIDERATIONS

- Young infants with eczema herpeticum are at risk for CNS involvement (HSV encephalitis) and should have a lumbar puncture with HSV polymerase chain reaction (PCR) if signs of CNS infection are present, such as lethargy, irritability, or seizure; if CSF pleocytosis is found, IV acyclovir is the treatment of choice

Disposition

ADMISSION CRITERIA

- Severe eczema herpeticum in a patient who is toxic appearing, is immunocompromised, or will not tolerate PO acyclovir
- Severe bacterial superinfection where there is concern of systemic involvement (e.g., toxic shock-like picture) or inability to take PO meds

DISCHARGE CRITERIA

- Those that do not meet the above admission criteria
- Primary care provider or dermatologist follow-up assured

PEDIATRIC CONSIDERATIONS

- Consider lowering admission threshold for any child with unreliable caregiver

Miscellaneous

ICD9: 619.8

ICD10: L30.9, L20.9

SUGGESTED READINGS

Boguniewicz M. Advances in the understanding and treatment of atopic dermatitis. Curr Opin Pediatr 1997;9(6):577–581.

Hanifin J, Ling M, Langley R, et al. Tacrolimus ointment for the treatment of atopic dermatitis in adult patients: part I, efficacy. J Am Acad Dermatol 2001; 44(1 Suppl):S28–38.

Odom RB, James WD, Berger TG, eds. Andrews' diseases of the skin, 9th ed. Philadelphia: WB Saunders, 2000:69–95.

Paller A, McCalister R, Doyle J, et al. Atopic dermatitis in pediatric patients: perceptions of physicians and parents. Presented at the American Academy of Dermatology Annual Meeting, March 2000, San Francisco.

Sieberry G, Iannone R, eds. The Harriet-Lane handbook, 15th ed. St. Louis: Mosby, 2000:908–909.

Soter NA, Fleischer AB Jr, Webster GF, et al. Tacrolimus ointment for the treatment of atopic dermatitis in adult patients. Part II: safety. J Am Acad Dermatol 2001; 44(1 Suppl):S39–46.

Author: Jon Ludwig

Edema

Clinical Presentation

SIGNS AND SYMPTOMS

- Weight gain of several kilograms
- Discomfort in the affected areas
- Swelling
- Tenderness
- Pitting edema
  - —Increased venous hydrostatic pressure or decreased oncotic pressure
- Nonpitting edema
  - —Protein-rich extravasated fluid

Generalized Edema (Anasarca)

- Edema is most prominent in dependent areas
  - —Feet
  - —Sacrum
  - —Bilateral lower extremities
- Cardiac
  - —Dyspnea
  - —Orthopnea
  - —Paroxysmal nocturnal dyspnea
  - —Increased jugular venous pressure (JVP)
  - —Rales
  - —S3 gallop
- Renal
  - —Anorexia
  - —Puffy eyelids
  - —Frothy urine
  - —Oliguria
  - —Dark urine
  - —Hematuria
  - —Hypertension
- Hepatic
  - —Jaundice
  - —Spider angiomas
  - —Palmar erythema
  - —Gynecomastia
  - —Testicular atrophy

Localized

- Ascites
- Hydrothorax
- Associated signs and symptoms by type of disorder
  - —History of trauma
    - -Mechanical, thermal, radiation
  - —Infectious
    - -Chills
    - -Fever
    - -Erythema
    - -Increased warmth
  - —Allergic
    - -Pruritus
    - -Hives
    - -Involvement of the lips and the oral mucosa
  - —Myxedema
    - -Pretibial nonpitting edema
    - -Periorbital edema
    - -Fatigue
    - -Cold intolerance
    - -Weight gain
    - -Constipation
    - -Slowed deep-tendon reflex relaxation
  - —Idiopathic
    - -Diurnal weight gain/loss

MECHANISM/DESCRIPTION

- Clinically apparent accumulation of extravascular fluid due to a derangement in the balance of oncotic and hydrostatic forces
  - —Increase in venous hydrostatic pressure
    - -Systemically as with congestive heart failure
    - -Locally as with deep vein thrombosis
  - —Increase in lymphatic hydrostatic pressure
  - —Decrease in oncotic pressure
    - -Systemically from hypoalbuminemia
    - -Locally from increased capillary permeability
  - —Increased venous hydrostatic pressure or decreased oncotic pressure results in pitting edema
  - —Protein-rich extravasated fluid results in nonpitting edema
    - -Lymphedema
    - -Increased capillary permeability
- In certain disorders, there is no clear relation to Starling forces
  - —Myxedema
  - —Idiopathic (cyclic) edema
    - -Worsened with heat
    - -More common in women
    - -Not necessarily related to menses

ETIOLOGY

Generalized

- Right heart failure
- Constrictive pericarditis
- Acute glomerulonephritis
- Renal failure
- Salt retention
  - —Steroids/estrogen therapy
  - —NSAIDs
  - —Antihypertensives (especially vasodilators)
  - —Lithium
  - —Cyclosporine
  - —Acute withdrawal of diuretics
- Idiopathic (cyclic) edema
- Cirrhosis
- Nephrotic syndrome
- Protein-losing enteropathy
- Starvation

Localized

- Thrombophlebitis
- Cellulitis
- Baker's cyst
- Vasculitis
- Angioedema
  - —Allergic
  - —Acquired
- Mechanical trauma
- Thermal injuries
- Radiation injuries
- Chemical burns
- Hemiplegia
- Compressive or invasive tumor
- Postsurgical resection of lymphatics
- Postirradiation
- Filariasis

Pre-Hospital

N/A

Diagnosis

ESSENTIAL WORKUP

- Diagnostic studies should be directed by the underlying etiology suggested by the history and physical examination

LABORATORY

- Renal etiology suspected
  - —Electrolytes
  - —BUN and creatinine
  - —Urinalysis
  - —Urine electrolytes and protein
- Hepatic etiology suspected
  - —Serum albumin
  - —Liver function tests
  - —Prothrombin time (PT) and partial thromboplastin time (PTT)
- Myxedema suspected
  - —Thyroid function tests

IMAGING/SPECIAL TESTS

- Cardiac etiology suspected
  - —EKG
  - —Chest radiograph
  - —Echocardiography
- Localized edema to an extremity
  - —Ultrasound (duplex scanning) or contrast venography

DIFFERENTIAL DIAGNOSIS

- Cellulitis
- Contact dermatitis
- Diffuse subcutaneous infiltrative process
- Lymphedema
- Obesity

Treatment

INITIAL STABILIZATION

See ED Treatment

ED TREATMENT

- Treatment should be directed toward the underlying cause
- Diuretics are indicated in cases of generalized edema but are not required emergently

MEDICATIONS

- Amiloride: 5–20 mg PO q.d.
- Captopril: 12.5–50 mg PO t.i.d.
- Furosemide: 20–40 mg i.v.; 20–80 mg PO q.d.
- Hydrochlorothiazide: 25–100 mg PO q.d.
- Spironolactone: 25–100 mg PO q.d.

Disposition

ADMISSION CRITERIA

- Base the decision to admit the patient on the underlying etiology
- Inability to ambulate without adequate home support
- Hypoxia

DISCHARGE CRITERIA

- Patient should be advised to decrease salt intake
- Elastic support stockings

Miscellaneous

ICD9: 782.3

ICD10: R60.9

SUGGESTED READINGS

Brater DC. Diuretic therapy. N Engl J Med 1998;339:387–395.

Braunwald E. Edema. In: Braunwald E., et al., eds. Harrison's principles of internal medicine, 15th ed., New York: McGraw-Hill, 2001.

Kay A, Davis DL. Idiopathic edema. Am J Kidney Dis 1999;34:405–423.

Author: Laura Macnow

Elbow Injuries

Clinical Presentation

SIGNS AND SYMPTOMS

Bony Injuries

- How patient carries the arm may give clues to diagnosis
- *Supracondylar fracture*
  —Flexion type: patient supports injured forearm with other arm and elbow in 90-degree flexion, loss of olecranon prominence
  —Extension type: patient holds arm at side in S-type configuration

Soft Tissue Injuries

- Elbow dislocations
  —Posterior: abnormal prominence of olecranon
  —Anterior: loss of olecranon prominence
- Radial head subluxation
  —Elbow slightly flexed and forearm pronated, resists moving arm at the elbow
- Medial/lateral epicondylitis
  —Gradual onset of dull ache over inner/outer aspect of the elbow referred to the forearm
  —Pain increases with grasping and twisting motions

MECHANISM/DESCRIPTION

Bony Injuries

- Supracondylar fracture
  —Most common in children
  —Peak ages 5–10 years, rarely occurs after age 15 years
  —Extension type (98%): FOOSH (*F*all *O*n an *O*ut *S*tretched *H*and) with fully extended or hyperextended arm
  -Type 1: minimal or no displacement
  -Type 2: slightly displaced fracture; posterior cortex intact
  -Type 3: totally displaced fracture; posterior cortex broken
  —Flexion type: a blow directly to a flexed elbow
  -Type 1: minimal or no displacement
  -Type 2: slightly displaced fracture; anterior cortex intact
  -Type 3: totally displaced fracture; anterior cortex broken
- Radial head fracture
  —Usually indirect mechanism, i.e., FOOSH
  —Radial head driven into the capitellum

Soft Tissue Injuries

- Elbow dislocation
  —Second only to shoulder as most dislocated joint
  —Most are posterior
- Medial/lateral epicondylitis
  —Overuse injuries usually related to rotary motion at the elbow involving the attachment points of the hand and wrist flexor/extensor muscular groups to the elbow
  —Plumbers, carpenters, tennis players, golfers
  —Pain made worse by resisted contraction of the particular muscle groups

ETIOLOGY

- Mechanism aids in determining the expected injury
- Trauma predominates
- Most elbow injuries caused by indirect trauma transmitted through the bones of the forearm (FOOSH)
- Direct blows account for very few fractures or dislocations

PEDIATRIC CONSIDERATIONS

- Subluxed radial head (nursemaid's elbow)
  —20% of all upper extremity injuries in children
  —Peak age 1–4 years; occurs more frequently in females than males
  —Sudden longitudinal pull on forearm with forearm pronated

Pre-Hospital

CAUTIONS

- Injuries to the ipsilateral upper limb, particularly fractures to the midshaft humerus and distal forearm are common
- Evaluate for associated neurovascular injuries (up to 20%)

Diagnosis

ESSENTIAL WORKUP

- Radiographs
- Assess wrist and shoulder for associated injury
- Evaluate neurovascular status of limb
- Assess skin integrity
- Examine for compartment syndrome, which is more common in supracondylar fractures

LABORATORY

- None specific for elbow injuries

IMAGING/SPECIAL TESTS

Radiographs

- Not usually necessary if overuse injury suspected
- Routine AP and lateral; add oblique for assessment of subtle injuries to radial head/distal humerus
- Fat pad sign
  —Seen with intraarticular injuries
  —Normally the anterior fat pad is a narrow radiolucent strip anterior to humerus, posterior fat pad is normally *not* visible
  —*Anterior fat pad sign* indicates joint effusion/injury when raised and becomes more perpendicular to the anterior humeral cortex (sail sign)
  —*Posterior fat pad sign* indicates effusion/injury
  -In adults, posterior fat pad sign implies radial head fracture; in children, it implies supracondylar fracture

DIFFERENTIAL DIAGNOSIS

- Sprain/strain
- Effusion
- Contusion
- Bursitis

PEDIATRIC CONSIDERATIONS

- Fractures in children often occur through unossified cartilage, making radiographic interpretation confusing
- A line drawn down the anterior surface of the humerus should always bisect the capitellum in lateral view
- If any bony relationships appear questionable on radiographs, obtain a comparison view of the uninvolved elbow
- Suspect nonaccidental trauma if history does not fit injury

COMPLICATIONS

- Neurovascular injuries to the numerous structures that pass about the elbow, including the anterior interosseus nerve, ulnar and radial nerve, brachial artery
- Volkmann's ischemic contracture is compartment syndrome of the forearm

Treatment

INITIAL STABILIZATION

- Immobilization to prevent further injury before taking radiographs is essential

ED TREATMENT

- Orthopedic consultation is recommended for all but nondisplaced, stable fractures that can generally be splinted with 24- to 48-hour orthopedic follow-up
- Fractures generally requiring orthopedic consultation
  —Transcondylar, intercondylar, condylar, epicondylar fractures
  —Fractures involving articular surfaces such as capitellum or trochlea
- Supracondylar fractures
  —Type 1 can be handled by ED physician with 24- to 48-hour orthopedic follow-up
  —Elbow may be flexed and splinted with posterior splint
  —Types 2 and 3 require immediate orthopedic consult
  —Reduce these in ED when fracture is associated with vascular compromise
- Anterior dislocation
  —Reduce immediately if vascular structures compromised
  —Then flex to 90 degrees and place posterior splint
- Posterior dislocation
  —Reduce immediately if vascular structures compromised
  —Then flex to 90 degrees and place posterior splint
- Radial head fracture
  —Minimally displaced fractures may be aspirated to remove hemarthrosis, instill bupivacaine (Marcaine), and immobilize
  —Other types should have orthopedic consult
- Radial head subluxation
  —In one continuous motion, supinate and flex the elbow while placing slight pressure on the radial head
  —Often will feel a click with reduction
  —If exam suggests fracture but x-ray is negative, splint and have patient follow-up in 24–48 hours for reevaluation
- Medial/lateral epicondylitis
  —Severe cases can be splinted
  —Rest, heat, antiinflammatory agents

MEDICATIONS

- Conscious sedation is often required to achieve reductions; see Conscious Sedation

PEDIATRIC CONSIDERATIONS

- Ossification centers: first appears
  —Capitellum: 3–6 months
  —Radial head: 3–5 years
  —Medial epicondyle: 5–7 years
  —Trochlea: 9–10 years
  —Olecranon: 9–10 years
  —Lateral epicondyle: 9–13 years

Disposition

ADMISSION CRITERIA

- Vascular injuries, open fractures
- Fractures requiring operative reduction or internal fixation
- Admit all patients with extensive swelling or ecchymosis for overnight observation and elevation to decrease the risk for compartment syndrome

DISCHARGE CRITERIA

- Stable fractures or reduced dislocations with none of above features
- Splint and arrange orthopedic follow-up in 24–48 hours
- Uncomplicated soft tissue injuries

Miscellaneous

ICD9: 959.3

ICD10: S59.9

SUGGESTED READINGS

Minkowitz B, et al. Supracondylar humerus fractures: current trends and controversies. Orthop Clin North Am 1994;25:4.

Nicholson DA, et al. ABC of emergency radiology: the elbow. BMJ 1993;307:23.

Simon R, Koenigsknecht S. Emergency orthopedics: the extremities, 4th ed. E. Norwalk, CT: Appleton & Lange, 1996.

Author: Christian Sloane

Electrical Injury

Clinical Presentation

SIGNS AND SYMPTOMS

General

- Severity ranges from minor cutaneous burns to crush-type trauma involving deep tissues
- Minor skin burns may mask major deep injury
- Effect of electricity
  - —0.2–2 mA at 60 Hz: tingling sensation
  - —1–4 mA at 60 Hz: pain
  - —6–22 mA at 60 Hz: inability to let go/tetanic contractions
  - —30–50 mA at 60 Hz: diaphragm/intercostals tetany
  - —100 mA at 60 Hz: ventricular fibrillation
  - —1,000 mA at 60 Hz: ventricular standstill

Cardiac

- Cardiac standstill is the leading cause of death from electrical injuries
- Sinus tach, A-fib, and premature ventricular contractions (PVCs) are most common
  - —Usually resolve spontaneously
- Ventricular fibrillation
  - —Most common lethal dysrhythmia
  - —Induced by alternating current at levels of 50–60 Hz (household current)
- Asystole results from direct current and high-voltage alternating current
- Myocardial damage occurs rarely
  - —Generally epicardial, not transmural
  - —Patch-like damage does not follow distribution of coronary arteries
  - —EKG will not show standard injury patterns

Respiratory

- Respiratory arrest may occur from
  - —Brain injury causing respiratory center inhibition
  - —Tetanic contraction of chest wall/diaphragm muscles
  - —Prolonged paralysis of respiratory muscles
  - —Postcardiac arrest respiratory arrest

Neurologic

- Acute
  - —Respiratory arrest
  - —Amnesia
  - —Altered mental status
  - —Seizures
  - —Coma
  - —Quadriplegia
  - —Localized paresis
- Delayed
  - —Ascending paralysis
  - —Transverse myelitis
  - —Amyotrophic lateral sclerosis
  - —Reflex sympathetic dystrophy

Vascular

- Venous thrombosis
- Compartment syndromes secondary to edema

Renal

- Renal failure secondary to myoglobinuria

Musculoskeletal

- Orthopedic injuries result from
  - —Forceful muscle contraction from electrostimulation
  - —Secondary injury from falls (most common cause)
- Common injuries
  - —Vertebral column fracture
  - —Posterior shoulder dislocation
  - —Femoral neck fracture

Ophthalmologic

- Cataracts (onset 4–6 months postinjury)
- Corneal burns
- Intraocular hemorrhage
- Uveitis
- Retinal injuries
- Optic nerve atrophy

Dermatologic

- Thermal burns from current arcing or clothes burning
- Kissing burns from flexor surface arcing as current exits and reenters skin
- Entry/exit wounds

MECHANISM/DESCRIPTION

- Ohm's law: voltage (V) = current (I) × resistance (R)
  - —Amperage (electron flow or current) is proportional to voltage (potential difference) and indirectly proportional to resistance
- Alternating current (AC)
  - —Has periodic reversal of direction (60 Hz in United States)
  - —Found in residential power supply
  - —Can produce tetanic muscle contraction prolonging contact
  - —More likely to result in V-fib at household current level
- Direct current (DC)
  - —Continuous in one direction
  - —Defibrillators and pacemakers
  - —Tends to throw patient from source
  - —More likely to result in asystole
- Factors that *increase* severity of injury
  - —*Higher* voltage (>600 V considered "high voltage")
  - —*Higher* current
  - —*Lower* tissue resistance (wet skin worse than dry skin)
  - —Longer time of contact with source (AC >DC)
  - —Current pathway through torso (hand-to-foot worse than hand-to-hand or foot-to-foot)
  - —Immersion in water

Levels of Electrical Exposure in Voltage

- Telephone lines: 65 V
- Household circuits: 110 V
- Electrical range or dryer: 220 V
- House power lines: 220 V
- Subway third rail: 600 V
- Residential trunk line: 7,620 V

PEDIATRIC CONSIDERATIONS

- Fetus much less resistant to electrical shock than mother
  - —All pregnant patients must undergo a period of fetal monitoring
- Oral commissure burn
  - —Results from child biting an electrical cord
  - —Associated with bleeding from the labial artery 3–5 days after injury
  - —May heal with significant contractures
- Trimodal distribution of electrical injuries
  - —Toddlers (household outlets and cords)
  - —Teenagers (risk-taking behavior)
  - —Adults (work-related injuries)

Pre-Hospital

CAUTIONS

- Care must be exercised in removing patients to ensure that rescuers do not contact live electrical sources
- Spinal precautions for transport
- Standard basic life support (BLS)/advanced cardiac life support (ACLS) care
- Remove smoldering clothes

Diagnosis

ESSENTIAL WORKUP
- EKG
- Urinalysis for myoglobin
- Cardiac monitor
  - —Controversy abounds on the need for 24-hour monitoring
  - —Prolonged monitoring is *not* necessary in asymptomatic patients with a normal EKG, no arrhythmias, and an exposure to <240 V
- Head CT if altered mentation, high voltage, head trauma
- C-spine, skeletal x-rays in high-voltage injury when pain present or in unconscious patient

LABORATORY
- Determined by the nature of the injury
- For most exposures to household current, no testing indicated
- Creatinine kinase (CK) indications
  - —Positive urine myoglobin
  - —High-voltage exposures
- Troponin, CK-MB indications
  - —Abnormal EKG or dysrhythmia
- Electrolytes, BUN, creatinine
  - —For high-voltage exposures
  - —Provides baseline renal function
  - —Hyperkalemia occurs due to cell death
  - —Metabolic acidosis with significant injury

DIFFERENTIAL DIAGNOSIS
- Thermal burns from electrical arcing flash injuries

Treatment

INITIAL STABILIZATION
- ABCs
- Standard ACLS measures for arrhythmias
- Spine immobilization when indicated

ED TREATMENT
- IV fluid resuscitation
  - —Larger fluid volumes required owing to extensive third spacing in injured muscle
  - —Rapid administration to reach urine output of 1 mL/kg/h
  - —Titrate to urine output and central venous pressure (CVP) measurement
- Foley catheter
- Prevent renal failure from myoglobinuria
  - —Maintain good urine output
  - —IV bicarbonate increases solubility of myoglobin in urine
  - —Furosemide/mannitol
  - —Monitor renal function
- Immobilize/reduce fractures and dislocations
- Local wound care for thermal burns
- Tetanus prophylaxis

MEDICATIONS
- Bicarbonate: 1 ampule i.v., then 2 ampules added to 1 L of D5W to maintain urine pH >7.45
- Furosemide: 0.5 mg/kg i.v.
- Mannitol: 25 g (peds: 0.25–0.5 mg/kg) i.v. bolus, then 12.5 mg/kg/h i.v. titrated to urine flow >1 mL/kg/h

Disposition

ADMISSION CRITERIA
- Documented loss of consciousness (LOC)
- Dysrhythmias, abnormal EKG or evidence of myocardial damage
- Suspicion of deep tissue burns
- Myoglobinuria
- Acidosis
- Significant skin burns/associated injury

DISCHARGE CRITERIA
- Minor, low voltage injury (<240 W) with no associated injuries and normal EKG

PEDIATRIC CONSIDERATIONS
- Advise parents of children with oral commissure burns of risk for delayed labial artery bleeding and contractures
  - —24-hour wound check and plastic surgery follow-up

Miscellaneous

ICD9: 994.8

ICD10: T75.4

SEE ALSO: LIGHTNING INJURY

SUGGESTED READINGS

Bailey B, Gaudreault P, Thivierge R, et al. Cardiac monitoring of children with household electrical injuries. Ann Emerg Med 1995;25(5):612–617.

Chinnis A, Williams J, Treat K. Electrical Injuries. In: Tintinalli JE, ed. Emergency medicine: a comprehensive study guide, 5th ed. New York: McGraw-Hill, 2000:1292–1297.

Fish R. Electrical injuries, parts I, II, III. J Emerg Med 1999;17:977–983, 2000;18:27–34, 2000;18:181–187.

Rai J, Jeschke M, Barrow R, et al. Electrical injuries: a 30-year review. J Trauma 1999;46:933–936.

Subin J, Venkata B. Electrical and lightning injuries. Crit Care Clin 1999;15:319–331.

Author: Marc Doucette

Encephalitis

Clinical Presentation

SIGNS AND SYMPTOMS

- Often begins with a preceding flulike illness over a few days
  - —Mild headache, fever, sore throat, reduced appetite, myalgias
- Altered level of consciousness, drowsiness, coma
- Impaired cognitive ability and personality change, hallucinations, psychosis
- Restlessness, agitation, irritability, delirium
- Rash (Lyme disease, Rocky Mountain spotted fever, varicella, herpes simplex virus [HSV])
- Seizures
- Fever, headache, vomiting, possible meningismus
- Focal neurologic deficits, tremor, ataxia, cranial nerve palsies (more common than meningitis)
- Papilledema on fundoscopy
- Clinical picture varies from mild headache and mild cognitive/emotional lability to severe agitation, seizures, coma, permanent neurologic sequelae, and death
- Clinical course of symptoms may be slow-moving or rapidly progressive

MECHANISM/DESCRIPTION

- Acute infectious inflammation of the brain
- 20,000 cases in United States annually
- Mortality 10%
- Inflammatory reaction occurs within brain parenchyma with destruction of neurons, parenchymal edema, and petechial hemorrhages
- Route of CNS infection usually hematogenous; search for another site
- Neural migration occurs with rabies, HSV, and varicella-zoster encephalitis

ETIOLOGY

- Viral is most common
- 50% of cases have no identifiable cause

Specific Viruses

- HSV
  - —10–20% of all encephalitides
  - —Primary or reactivation
  - —Early treatment improves prognosis
- Arbovirus
  - —10–15% of all encephalitides
  - —Zoonotic transmission (mosquitoes, ticks) in warm months
  - —Eastern equine causes fulminant encephalitis
    - -Tropism for the hippocampus
    - -Abrupt onset of headache, fever, vomiting
  - —Western equine occurs mostly in the western two thirds of the United States
    - -Often preceded by nonspecific upper respiratory/GI tract symptoms
  - —Japanese—most prevalent arboviral encephalitis worldwide
    - -Indolent course of fever, headache, myalgias, and fatigue followed by confusion, delirium, masklike facies, and parkinsonisms, seizures, brainstem dysfunction, coma, and death
- Flavivirus
  - —West Nile virus—increased incidence in North America
    - -Found in mosquitos and birds
    - -Febrile illness, often with rash
    - -Headache
    - -Lymphadenopathy
    - -Polyarthropathy
    - -Increased morbidity/mortality in elderly patients
- Enteroviral
  - —Occurs mainly in children <10 years old
  - —Relatively benign course with little or no long-term sequelae
- Measles encephalitis
  - —Occurs several days to 2–3 weeks after primary infection and rash, or after years of latent infection
  - —Abrupt onset and rapid progression to coma
  - —Seizures common (50–60%)
  - —Postimmunization incidence of 1 per 1 million vaccinated
- HIV encephalitis
  - —Lower CD4 counts predispose to encephalitis
  - —Typical features include motor spasticity and dementia
  - —Involvement of white matter with extensive neural degeneration
- Rhabdovirus: rabies

Nonviral

- *Mycoplasma pneumoniae*
- *Toxoplasma gondii*
- *Rickettsia rickettsii*
- *Mycobacterium tuberculosis*
- *Borrelia burgdorferi*
- *Coccidioides immitis*
- Leptospirosis

Immunocompromised/HIV Patients

- Histoplasma
- *Cryptococcus neoformans*
- Varicella-zoster
- *Listeria monocytogenes*
- Cytomegalovirus
- *Toxoplasma gondii*
- Human herpesvirus type 6 (HHV-6)

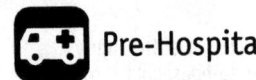

Pre-Hospital

N/A

Diagnosis

ESSENTIAL WORKUP

- Lumbar puncture—CSF analysis for
  - —Cell count/chemistry
    - -Elevated WBC, predominantly lymphocytes
    - -Elevated protein
    - -Glucose (normal in viral disease)
    - -Gram stain with or without India ink for suspected/confirmed HIV
  - —Viral and bacterial cultures (fungi if indicated by history)
  - —Antigen assays for
    - -HSV
    - -Cryptococcus
    - -Toxoplasmosis
    - -Other viral antigen and antibody assays if available (enterovirus, adenovirus, cytomegalovirus, mumps, and varicella-zoster)

LABORATORY

- CBC
  - —WBC usually elevated; however, a normal WBC does not rule out infection
- Electrolytes, glucose, BUN, creatinine
- Bacterial and viral blood cultures
- Liver function tests if hepatic failure suspected
- Carboxyhemoglobin level if CO poisoning suspected
- Toxicology screen if ingestion suspected in differential
- Polymerase chain reaction (PCR)
  - —Confirm viral nucleic acids in CSF
  - —HSV, varicella, enteroviruses, others

IMAGING/SPECIAL TESTS

- CT scan
  - —To rule out trauma, hemorrhagic conditions, and mass lesions
  - —Cerebral edema may be the only finding consistent with encephalitis
  - —HSV may show parenchymal hemorrhagic areas of the frontal and temporal lobes, along with edema
- MRI
  - —Hypodense temporal lobes in HSV

DIFFERENTIAL DIAGNOSIS

- Meningitis
- Brain abscess
- Sepsis
- Stroke (hemorrhagic or ischemic)
- Head injury
- Subarachnoid hemorrhage
- Encephalopathy (hepatic, uremic)
- Metabolic
  - —Electrolyte abnormalities (Na^{2+}, K^+, Cl^-, Ca^{2+}, Mg^{2+}, phosphate)
  - —Hypoglycemia
  - —Hyperglycemic nonketotic coma
- Neoplastic
- Drugs/toxins
- CO inhalation

Treatment

INITIAL STABILIZATION

- ABCs
  - —Intubate obtunded/comatose/absent gag reflex
- Naloxone, thiamine, glucose (or Accucheck) for altered mental status
- For signs of raised intracranial pressure on fundoscopy or CT
  - —Hyperventilate to PCO_2 of 25–30 mm Hg
  - —Administer mannitol
  - —Neurosurgical consult for suspected hydrocephalus
- Run IV saline at TKO or half-maintenance to avoid cerebral edema

ED TREATMENT

- Seizure control
  - —Abort with diazepam
  - —Initiate antiseizure medication (dilantin or phenobarbital) if more than one seizure has occurred
- No specific treatment for most viral encephalitides
  - —Steroid use controversial
- Treat HSV encephalitis with acyclovir IV
  - —Initiate if considered likely based on clinical grounds, CT, and CSF findings
- Initiate ganciclovir for suspected immunocompromised related infections (CMV, HHV-6)
- Administer antibiotic to cover for meningitis if diagnosis uncertain, especially when rash present (e.g., meningococcemia, rickettsia)

MEDICATIONS

- Acyclovir: 5–10 mg/kg i.v. q8h, maximum 15 mg/kg/d (peds: 250 mg/m^2 i.v. q8h, maximum 750 mg/m^2/d)
- Diazepam: 5 mg i.v. (peds: 0.1–0.2 mg/kg i.v. or PR) per dose
- Dilantin: loading dose 15 mg/kg i.v. to a maximum of 1 g
- Ganciclovir: 5 mg/kg i.v. q12h
- Mannitol: 0.5–1 g/kg of a 20% solution to run i.v. over 20–30 minutes
- Phenobarbital: load 15–20 mg/kg to 300–800 mg i.v. at 25–50 mg/min

Disposition

ADMISSION CRITERIA

- All patients

DISCHARGE CRITERIA

- None

Miscellaneous

ICD9: 323.9

ICD10: G04.9

SEE ALSO: MENINGITIS

SUGGESTED READINGS

Kimberlin DW, Whitley RJ. Viral encephalitis. Pediatr Rev 1999;20: 192–198.

Mandell GL, ed. Principles and practice of infectious disease. 5th ed. New York: Churchill Livingstone, 2000.

Mortgenstern LB, ed. Encephalitis. In: Neurologic clinics, Vol. 17, No. 4. Philadelphia: WB Saunders, 1999.

Rakel RE, ed. Conn's current therapy 2002, 5th ed. Philadelphia: WB Saunders, 2002.

Author: Neil Troost

Endocarditis

Clinical Presentation

SIGNS AND SYMPTOMS

General

- Fever
  - —Most common symptom
  - —Often absent in certain settings
    - -Elderly
    - -Congestive heart failure
    - -Severe debility
    - -Chronic renal failure
- Flulike illness
- Chills
- Sweats
- Rigors
- Malaise

HEENT

- Retinal hemorrhages or Roth's spots

Respiratory

- Dyspnea
- Cough

Cardiac

- A new or changing murmur in 80–85% of patients

Abdominal

- Abdominal or back pain
- Splenomegaly (15–50%)

Extremities

- Myalgias
- Arthralgias
- Digital clubbing

Neurologic

- Septic embolization (stroke or mycotic aneurysm)

Skin

- Cutaneous vasculitic lesions
  - —Mucosal and conjunctival petechiae
  - —Splinter hemorrhages
  - —Osler's nodes
    - -Erythematous, painful tender nodules
  - —Janeway's lesions
    - -Erythematous or hemorrhagic, macular or nodular lesions, a few millimeters in diameter on the hands and feet

MECHANISM/DESCRIPTION

- A microbial infection of the endothelial surface of the heart
- Characterized by the vegetation (a thrombus with superimposed microorganisms)
- Older population
- Frequently male
- Fewer patients demonstrating the classic signs once noted by Osler
- Risk factors
  - —Poor dental hygiene
  - —Intravenous drug abuse
    - -Greater risk than rheumatic heart disease or prosthetic valves
    - -IV drug abuse has a predilection for right-sided heart valves
    - -Risk factor for recurrent endocarditis
  - —Structural heart disease serves as common vegetative sites due to altered intracardiac flow
    - -Mitral valve prolapse
    - -Aortic valve dysfunction
  - —Congenital heart disorders in the pediatric populations
    - -Tetralogy of Fallot
    - -Aortic stenosis
    - -Patent ductus arteriosus
    - -Ventricular septal defects
    - -Aortic coarctation
  - —Prosthetic valves
  - —Indwelling catheters
  - —Any mechanical devices may serve as a portal of entry or attachment for microorganisms

ETIOLOGY

- Major categories
  - —Bacterial endocarditis
  - —Prosthetic valve endocarditis
  - —Nonbacterial thrombotic endocarditis
    - -Malignancy
    - -Uremia
    - -Burns
    - -Systemic lupus erythematosus
- Common organisms
  - —*Streptococcus viridans*
    - -Found in oropharynx, common agent in native valve endocarditis
  - —*Streptococcus bovis*
    - -Common association with colonic polyps or GI malignancy
  - —*Streptococcus pneumoniae*
    - -Causes rapid valvular destruction, abscess, and congestive heart failure (CHF)
    - -Risk factor alcoholism
  - —*Staphylococcus epidermidis*
  - —*Staphylococcus aureus*
    - -Seen in all populations, especially intravenous drug abuse (IVDA) and toxic illness
    - -Sometimes metastatic
  - —Enterococci
    - -Seen in young women and old men following instrumentation or infection
  - —*Candida* and *Aspergillus*
    - -Found in IVDA, prosthetic valves, or immunocompromised patients
  - —HACEK (*Haemophilus* species)
  - —Cause of culture-negative endocarditis

Pre-Hospital

N/A

Diagnosis

ESSENTIAL WORKUP

- Identify risk factors for endocarditis in patients with fever of unknown etiology
- Blood cultures
- Echocardiography is needed to confirm the diagnostic

LABORATORY

- CBC
  - —Anemia (sometimes hemolytic)
  - —Leukocytosis (with granulocytosis and bandemia)
- Blood cultures
  - —Multiple sets (three sets over a time period) should be obtained before antibiotic administration
- Elevated sedimentation rate and C-reactive protein (lacks specificity)
- Urinalysis
  - —Microscopic hematuria

IMAGING/SPECIAL TESTS

- Chest radiography
  - —CHF
  - —Septic pulmonic emboli, which may be seen in right-sided endocarditis
- EKG
  - —Arrhythmia, new heart block
- Echocardiography
  - —Acute valvular pathology
  - —Abscess
  - —Vegetations
  - —Transesophageal echocardiography provides greater sensitivity

DIFFERENTIAL DIAGNOSIS

- Rheumatic fever
- Atrial myxoma
- Acute pericarditis
- Myocardial infarction
- Aortic dissection with regurgitant valve
- Thrombotic thrombocytopenic purpura
- Systemic lupus erythematosus
- Occult neoplasm with metastasis
- Septicemia

Treatment

INITIAL STABILIZATION

- Monitor for signs of heart failure
- Operative repair if
  —Severe valvular dysfunction causing failure
  —Unstable prosthesis
  —Perivalvular extension with intracardiac abscess
  —Antimicrobial therapy failure
  —Large or fungal vegetations
- Antibiotic therapy
  —Intravenous, bactericidal, and empiric, pending culture results
  —Native valve or congenital abnormality
    -Penicillin G + nafcillin + gentamicin
    -Vancomycin + gentamicin
  —Prosthetic valve or history of IVDA
    -Vancomycin + gentamicin + rifampin
    -Nafcillin + gentamicin (if methicillin-resistant *S. aureus* [MRSA] is not suspected)
  —Fungal
    -Amphotericin B
  —HACEK
    -Ceftriaxone

MEDICATIONS

- Amphotericin B
  —Test dose 0.1 mg/kg up to 1 mg slow i.v.
  —Wait 2–4 hours
  —If tolerated then begin 0.25 mg/kg i.v. and advance to 0.6 mg/kg i.v. q.d.
- Ceftriaxone: 2 g i.v. q.d.
- Gentamicin: 1 mg/kg i.v. q8h
- Nafcillin: 2 g i.v. q4h
- Penicillin G: 20 million IU i.v. q.d.
- Rifampin: 600 mg PO q.d.
- Vancomycin: 15 mg/kg i.v. q12h

Disposition

ADMISSION CRITERIA

- Patients with risk factors who exhibit pathologic criteria or clinical findings
- All intravenous drug users with fever
- Admit patients with cardiovascular instability to an ICU/monitored setting

DISCHARGE CRITERIA

- None

EXPECTED COURSE

- Most patients will defervesce within 1 week

COMPLICATIONS

- Cardiac—CHF, valve abscess, pericarditis, fistula
- Neurologic—embolic stroke, abscess, hemorrhage
- Embolization—CNS, pulmonary, ischemic extremities
- Mycotic aneurysms—cerebral or systemic
- Renal—infarction, nephritis, abscess
- Metastatic abscess—kidney, spleen, tissue

Miscellaneous

ICD9: 421

ICD10: I38

SUGGESTED READINGS

Berbari E, Cockerill F, et al. Infective endocarditis due to unusual or fastidious microorganisms. Mayo Clin Proc 1997;72: 532–542.

Hogevik H, Alestig K. Fungal endocarditis: a report on seven cases and a brief review. Infection 1996;24(1):17–21.

Karchmer A. Infective endocarditis. In: Braunwald E, ed. Heart disease: a textbook of cardiovascular medicine, 5th ed. Philadelphia: WB Saunders, 1997: 1077–1104.

Mylonakis E, Calderwood S. Infective endocarditis in adults. N Engl J Med 2001;345(18):1318–1330.

Salman L, Prince A, et al. Pediatric infective endocarditis in the modern era. J Pediatr 1993;122:847–853.

Author: Michael S. Murphy

Endometriosis

Clinical Presentation

SIGNS AND SYMPTOMS
- Pelvic or back pain, usually cyclic
- Dysmenorrhea, often severe
- Dyspareunia
- Infertility
- Pelvic exam nonspecific; rarely tender, nodular masses are present
- Abdominal exam typically benign unless ruptured endometrioma produces peritoneal signs

ETIOLOGY
- Ectopic endometrial tissue with cyclic hormonal responsiveness
- Invades tissues, spreads locally and hematogenously
- Theories include retrograde menstruation, immunologic factors, and metaplastic transformation

PEDIATRIC CONSIDERATIONS
- Not seen before menarche

Pre-Hospital

- No specific pre-hospital considerations

Diagnosis

ESSENTIAL WORKUP
- Must rule out other, life-threatening diagnoses, as directed by history and physical exam (e.g., ectopic pregnancy, appendicitis)
- Pregnancy test

IMAGING/SPECIAL TESTS
- Ultrasound, CT, and MRI may show ovarian endometriomas, but rarely reveal implants
- Surgery, usually laparoscopy, required for definitive diagnosis

DIFFERENTIAL DIAGNOSIS
- Appendicitis
- Ovarian cysts
- Ovarian torsion
- Pelvic inflammatory disease
- Menstrual cramps/mittelschmerz
- Inflammatory bowel disease
- Irritable bowel disease
- Diverticulosis
- Gastroenteritis

Treatment

INITIAL STABILIZATION

- ABCs
- May require IV crystalloid if pain is severe and patient is unable to tolerate oral fluids/medications

ED TREATMENT

- Once other diagnoses ruled out, adequate analgesia is necessary
  —Analgesic of choice
- Oral contraceptives, gonadotropin-releasing hormone agonists (e.g., leoprolide [Lupron]), or other hormonal manipulation may be started in consultation with primary care physician or gynecologist

MEDICATIONS

- Acetaminophen: 650–1000 mg PO q.i.d.
- Ketorolac: 15–30 mg i.v. or i.m. q6h
- Morphine: 2–10 mg i.v., repeat as necessary
- NSAIDs (ibuprofen): 600 mg PO q.i.d.

Disposition

ADMISSION CRITERIA

- Refractory pain
- Unclear diagnosis for exploratory surgery or to follow serial exams
- Ruptured ovarian endometrioma with peritoneal signs

DISCHARGE CRITERIA

- Most patients with a clear exacerbation of endometriosis can be discharged with gynecology follow-up once pain is controlled

Miscellaneous

ICD9: 617.9

ICD10: N80.9

SUGGESTED READINGS

Dart R. Acute Pelvic Pain. In: Marx JA, et al., eds. Rosen's emergency medicine: concepts and clinical practice, 5th ed. St. Louis: Mosby–Year Book, 2002: 219–226.

Morrison L, Spence J. Gynecology and obstetrics: vaginal bleeding and pelvic pain in the non pregnant patient. In: Tintinalli JE, ed. Emergency medicine: a comprehensive study guide, 5th ed. New York: McGraw-Hill, 2000:678.

Olive DL, Pritts EA. Treatment of endometriosis. N Engl J Med 2001;345(4): 266–275.

Prentice A. Endometriosis. BMJ 2001; 323:93–95.

Author: Christy Mohler

Epididymitis and Orchitis

Clinical Presentation

SIGNS AND SYMPTOMS

- Pain: gradual onset of mild to moderate testicular or scrotal pain; may be bilateral
- Progressive scrotal swelling
- Dysuria (30%)
  - —Recent urinary tract infection (24% will have positive urine bacterial cultures)
  - —History of abnormal bladder function
- Urethral discharge
  - —Of patients with gonococcal epididymitis, 21–30% did not complain of urethral discharge and did not have demonstrable urethral discharge 50% of time
- Fever (14–28%)
- Recent urinary instrumentation
- Tenderness in groin, lower abdomen, or scrotum
- Scrotal skin commonly erythematous and warm (60%)
- Early: may feel swollen, indurated epididymis; later: may not be able to distinguish epididymis from testis
- Spermatic cord may be edematous
- Coexistent prostatitis is rare (8%)
- If pyogenic bacterial orchitis, patients usually are acutely ill with fever, intense discomfort, swelling of testicle, and often reactive hydrocele

MECHANISM/DESCRIPTION

Epididymitis

- Definition: inflammation or infection of the epididymis
- Rare in prepubertal boys
- Pathogenesis
  - —Initial stages: cellular inflammation begins in vas deferens and descends to lower pole of epididymis (flank and groin pain)
  - —Acute phase: epididymis is swollen and indurated in upper and lower poles; spermatic cord thickened
  - —Testis may become edematous owing to passive congestion or inflammation
  - —Resolution: may be complete without sequelae; although often peritubular fibrosis develops, occluding ductules
- Complications
  - —Two thirds of men have atrophy because of partial vascular thrombosis of testicular artery
  - —Abscess and infarction rare (5%)
  - —Incidence of infertility with unilateral epididymitis unknown; 50% with bilateral epididymitis

Orchitis

- Definition: inflammation or acute infection of the testicle
  - —Usually from direct extension of the same process within the epididymis
  - —Isolated testicular infection is rare; can result from hematogenous spread of bacteria or following mumps infection
- Categories
  - —Pyogenic bacterial orchitis: secondary to bacterial involvement of epididymis
  - —Viral orchitis: most commonly due to mumps
    - -Rare in prepubertal boys; occurs in 20–30% of postpubertal boys with mumps
    - -Occurs 4–6 days after parotitis but can occur without parotitis
    - -Unilateral in 70% of patients
    - -Usually resolution in 4–5 days
    - ->50% of testes involved have residual atrophy; rarely affects fertility
  - —Granulomatous orchitis: syphilis and mycobacterium and fungal diseases; usually occurs in immunocompromised host

ETIOLOGY

Epididymitis

- Children
  - —Coliform or pseudomonal urinary tract infections
  - —Sexually transmitted diseases rare in prepubertal males
  - —Associated with predisposing structural, neurologic, or functional abnormalities of lower urinary tract
- Young men, age <35 years
  - —Usually sexually transmitted
  - —*Chlamydia trachomatis* (28–88%): severe inflammation with minimal destruction
  - —*Neisseria gonorrhoeae* (3–28%)
  - —Coliform bacteria (7–24%): highly destructive with tendency for abscess
    - -Coliform bacteria more common in insertive partners in anal intercourse
  - —*Ureaplasma urealyticum* (sole organism in only 6% of cases)
- Older men, age >35 years
  - —Commonly associated with underlying urologic pathology (benign prostatic hypertrophy [BPH], prostate cancer, strictures)
  - —May have acute or chronic bacterial prostatitis
  - —Coliform bacteria more common (23–67%), especially after instrumentation
  - —*Chlamydia trachomatis* (8–80%)
  - —*Klebsiella* and *Pseudomonas* species
  - —*Neisseria gonorrhoeae* (15%)
  - —Gram-positive cocci
- Drug related
  - —Amiodarone-induced epididymitis: usually with amiodarone levels higher than therapeutic levels
- Granulomatous: syphilis or mycobacterial and fungal causes; may be presenting feature of *Mycobacterium tuberculosis* in high prevalence regions; urine cultures often negative for *M. tuberculosis*
- Vasculitis: polyarteritis nodosa, Behçet's disease, Henoch-Schönlein purpura

Orchitis

- Pyogenic bacterial orchitis
  - —*Escherichia coli*
  - —*Klebsiella pneumoniae*
  - —*Pseudomonas aeruginosa*
  - —Staphylococci
  - —Streptococci
- Viral orchitis
  - —Mumps
    - -20% of patients with mumps may develop epididymoorchitis
    - -Rarely associated with live-attenuated mumps vaccine
  - —Coxsackie A and lymphocytic choriomeningitis virus
- Granulomatous orchitis: syphilis and mycobacterial and fungal diseases
- Fungal orchitis
  - —Blastomycosis in endemic regions
  - —Invasive candidal infections in immunosuppressed hosts
- Posttraumatic orchitis: inflammation

Pre-Hospital

- ABCs
- IV access
- Crystalloid fluid boluses if patient appears systemically ill or septic

Diagnosis

ESSENTIAL WORKUP

- *Must differentiate from testicular torsion*
- Ultrasonography: color Doppler imaging
  - 82–100% sensitivity, 100% specificity in detecting testicular torsion; decreased blood flow
  - Epididymoorchitis: hyperemia, increased vascularity and blood flow
  - Advantages: if torsion not present, can evaluate for epididymitis or other causes of scrotal pain
  - Disadvantages: highly examiner dependent, difficult in infants or children
- Testicular scintigraphy: radionuclide study to analyze testicular perfusion
  - 90–100% sensitivity, 89–97% specificity in detecting testicular torsion
  - Inflammatory processes have increased flow and uptake
  - False-positive scans in large fluid collections in scrotum: abscess, hydrocele, hematocele, bowel herniation
  - False-negative scans in early torsion, spontaneous detorsion, small children or infants
- Early consultation with urologist

LABORATORY

- CBC; often leukocytosis in range of 10,000–30,000/mm^3
- Urinalysis and culture
  - 24% of patients with epididymoorchitis have pyuria
  - May or may not reveal bacterial source of infection
  - Urine chlamydial enzyme immunoassay (EIA) low sensitivity (50–70%)
- Urethral swab (50–73% have demonstrable urethritis despite minority of symptoms)
  - Gram stain and culture
  - Chlamydia testing
  - Avoid bladder emptying within 2 hours of tests (lowers sensitivity)
  - Especially for postpubertal and sexually active males
- Blood culture if systemically ill

IMAGING/SPECIAL TESTS

- Color Doppler ultrasound
- Technetium scan

DIFFERENTIAL DIAGNOSIS

- Testicular torsion
- Testicular tumor
- Torsion of testicular appendages
- Trauma to scrotum
- Acute hernia
- Acute hydrocele

Treatment

INITIAL STABILIZATION

- ABCs
- IV access
- IV fluids, especially if systemically ill

ED TREATMENT

- Imaging and laboratory as above
- Antibiotics:
  - Cover for chlamydial and gonococcal etiologies if adult or presumed sexually transmitted
  - Cover for coliform etiology if child, adult >35 years of age, or presumed nonsexually transmitted
  - Adjust according to culture and sensitivity results
  - Treat sexual partners
- Bed rest and scrotal support with elevation and ice packs
- Analgesics and antiinflammatories
- Urologic consultation and follow-up
  - Children need workup for urologic abnormalities: voiding cystourethrography and renal ultrasound
  - If bacteriuria present, examination of lower tract with cystoscopy after treatment completed
  - Surgical indications
    - Scrotal abscess
    - If another scrotal problem, such as torsion, cannot be excluded
    - Suspected or proved ischemia caused by severe epididymitis
    - Patient with solitary testicle
    - Scrotal fixation: indicates severe inflammation and potential suppuration

MEDICATIONS

Age <35 Years

- Primary: ceftriaxone 250 mg i.m. × 1, *plus* doxycycline 100 mg PO b.i.d. × 10 days *or* ofloxacin 300 mg PO b.i.d. × 10 days
- Alternative: ciprofloxacin 500 mg PO *or* ofloxacin 400 mg PO *plus* tetracycline 500 mg PO q.i.d. × 10 days

Age >35 Years or Insertive Partners in Anal Intercourse

- Primary: ciprofloxacin 500 mg PO b.i.d. or 400 mg i.v. b.i.d. (*or* ofloxacin 200 mg PO b.i.d.) × 10–14 days
- Alternative: amoxicillin (Augmentin)/ sulbactam 3 g i.v. q6h *or* cefotaxime 2 g i.v. q.d. *or* ceftriaxone 2 g i.v. q.d.

Disposition

ADMISSION CRITERIA

- Surgical indications present
- Older age group if it is the only way to ensure appropriate workup
  - Many will have underlying urologic pathology
- Systemically ill: fever, nausea, vomiting
- Scrotal abscess

DISCHARGE CRITERIA

- Fails to meet admission criteria
- Patient with good follow-up
- Able to take oral antibiotics

Miscellaneous

ICD9: 604.90

ICD10: N45.9

SUGGESTED READINGS

Berger RE. Acute epididymitis: etiology and therapy. Semin Urol 1991;9:28–31.

Herberner TE. Ultrasound in the assessment of the acute scrotum. J Clin Ultrasound 1996;24:405–421.

Kass EJ, Lundak B. The acute scrotum. Pediatr Urol 1997;44:1251–1266.

Luzzi GA, O'Brien TS. Acute epididymitis. Br J Urol Int 2001;87:747–754.

Marcozzi D, Suner S. The nontraumatic acute scrotum. Emerg Med Clin North Am 2001;19:547–568.

Schul MW, Keating MA. The acute pediatric scrotum. J Emerg Med 1993;11:565–577.

Vordermark JS, Deshon GE, Jones TA. Role of surgery in management of acute bacterial epididymitis. Urology 1990;4:283–287.

Author: Tami Gash-Kim

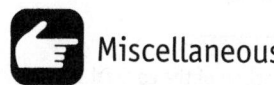

Epidural Abscess

Clinical Presentation

SIGNS AND SYMPTOMS

- *Classic presentation:* severe, progressive back and radicular pain with fever and eventual neurologic deficit (weakness or paralysis, sensory level, sphincter disturbance)
- May present with signs and symptoms of sepsis without prominent back pain
- Occurs at all ages including infants; peak is at ages 60–70 years of age
- Most patients have predisposing condition (diabetes, malignancy, IV drug abuse, chronic steroids, chronic alcoholism, instrumentation [s/p discogram] or spinal surgery)
- May occur in the absence of identifiable predisposing factors

MECHANISM/DESCRIPTION

- A pyogenic infection of the epidural space
- Most common in the thoracic spine, followed by the lumbar and cervical areas

ETIOLOGY

- Focus of infection present followed by either hematogenous spread (~50%) or direct extension
- The most common sources are skin structure infections, but any pyogenic infection may be a source
- *Staphylococcus aureus* accounts for more than 50% of cases, with streptococcus the second most common organism
- *Haemophilus influenzae,* Gram-negative bacilli, mycobacteria, anaerobic and mixed infections also occur
- May occur after lumbar puncture (usually follows multiple attempts)

PEDIATRIC CONSIDERATIONS

- Children present similar to adults with back pain, fever, and neurologic signs as well as nonspecific systemic symptoms
- Infants may exhibit only fever, irritability, and associated meningitis
- Sphincter disturbance is frequently seen
- Most cases are secondary to hematogenous spread
- Location and bacteriology similar to adults

Pre-Hospital

N/A

Diagnosis

- Fever and severe back pain represent a potentially serious combination
  - —If the pain is radicular or there is a neurologic disturbance, the likelihood of epidural abscess is increased

ESSENTIAL WORKUP

- History should include predisposing conditions when this diagnosis is suspected
- Physical exam for a source of infection, localized spinal tenderness, and neurologic findings, especially *decreased sphincter tone,* saddle anesthesia, and lower extremity weakness
- Voided urine followed by postvoid catheterization
  - —Younger adults should have less than 50 mL postvoid residual urine
  - —Older adults may normally have higher residuals up to 100 mL
- MRI is the diagnostic test of choice; when not available, obtain CT myelogram
  - —Suspected epidural abscess is a true neurosurgical emergency and requires emergent imaging

LABORATORY

- Erythrocyte sedimentation rate (ESR) is almost always elevated (~100%) but is nonspecific
  - —A normal ESR makes the diagnosis much less likely
- Blood cultures are often positive (~60%)
- Leukocytosis with a left shift is common (~70%)
- CSF often abnormal but is nondiagnostic; routine lumbar puncture should be avoided when epidural abscess is suspected (may cause meningitis)

IMAGING/SPECIAL TESTS

- MRI is at least 90% sensitive; shows high-intensity lesion on T2 imaging
- Myelography and CT myelography are also sensitive but risk dissemination
- Plain films are usually abnormal but nonspecific
  - —May demonstrate occult traumatic injury

DIFFERENTIAL DIAGNOSIS

- Diagnosis is difficult owing to rarity of the condition and nonspecific symptoms; multiple physician encounters commonly precede the diagnosis; most common initial diagnosis is benign musculoskeletal pathology
- *Early presentation:* muscular or ligamentous pain, degenerative arthritis, compression fracture, discogenic pain
- *Back pain with fever, systemic signs and symptoms:* vertebral osteomyelitis, spinal tumor, meningitis, spinal subdural abscess, discitis, pyelonephritis
- *Back pain with neurologic signs and symptoms:* cord compression, cord ischemia, disc herniation

PEDIATRIC CONSIDERATIONS

- Fever and back pain should be urgently investigated with MRI when epidural abscess is suspected

Treatment

INITIAL STABILIZATION

- Broad-spectrum parenteral antibiotics early for signs of sepsis, must include coverage for *S. aureus* and streptococci
- Ceftriaxone and clindamycin are appropriate initial coverage

ED TREATMENT

- Urgent imaging is essential when diagnosis is considered; delay in definitive treatment is associated with a poor outcome
- Urgent neurosurgical consultation or transfer for definitive therapy (surgical decompression) after diagnosis and antibiotic Rx

MEDICATIONS

- Ceftriaxone: 1–2 g i.v. q12h
- Clindamycin: 600–900 mg i.v. q8h

Disposition

ADMISSION CRITERIA

- Suspected epidural abscess should be admitted; an MRI is needed emergently, transfer the patient if necessary
- Patients with spinal epidural abscess require admission to a facility with neurosurgical capability

DISCHARGE CRITERIA

- Patients with epidural abscess should not be discharged

Miscellaneous

ICD9: 324.9

ICD10: G06.2

SUGGESTED READINGS

Martin MJ, Yuan HA. Neurosurgical care of spinal epidural, subdural, and intramedullary abscesses and arachnoiditis. Orthop Clin North Am 1996;27(1):125–136.

Maslin DR, et al. Spinal epidural abscess. Arch Intern Med 1993;153(14):1713–1721.

Redekop GJ, Del Maestro RF. Diagnosis and management of spinal epidural abscess. Can J Neurol Sci 1992;19(2):180–187.

Rubin G, et al. Spinal epidural abscess in the pediatric age group: case report and review of the literature. Pediatr Infect Dis J 1993;12(12):1007–1011.

Vilke VM Honingford EA. Cervical spine epidural abscess in a patient with no predisposing risk factors. Ann Emerg Med 1996;27(6):777–780.

Wheeler D, et al. Medical management of spinal epidural abscesses: case report and review. Clin Infect Dis 1992;15(1):22–27.

Author: Richard Krause

Epidural Hematoma

Clinical Presentation

SIGNS AND SYMPTOMS

- Altered or deteriorating level of consciousness (LOC)
- LOC: 85% will have at some point in course
  - —Only 11–30% will have a "lucid" interval
- Nausea and vomiting: 40%
- Pupillary dilation: 20–40%
  - —Usually on same side as lesion (90%)
- Hemiparesis more than one third
  - —Usually contralateral (80%)

MECHANISM/DESCRIPTION

- Direct skull trauma
- Inward bending of calvarium causes bleeding when dura separates from skull
  - —Middle meningeal artery is involved in bleed >50% of time
  - —Meningeal vein is involved in one third
  - —Diploic venous sinus bleed is seen in <10%
- Skull fracture is associated in 75% of cases, less commonly in children
- Greater than 50% have epidural hematoma (EDH) as isolated head injury
  - —Most commonly associated with subdural hematoma (SDH) and cerebral contusion
- Classic CT finding is lenticular, unilateral convexity, usually in temporal region
- It usually does not cross suture lines, but may cross midline

ETIOLOGY

- Accounts for 1.5% of traumatic brain injury (TBI)
- Male/female incidence is 3:1
- Peak incidence is second to third decade of life
- Motor vehicle accidents (MVAs), assault, and falls are most common causes
  - —Of all blunt mechanisms, assault has the highest association with intracranial injury requiring neurosurgical intervention
- Uncommon in very young (younger than 5 years) or elderly patients
- Mortality is 12% and is related to preoperative condition

PEDIATRIC CONSIDERATIONS

- Head injury is the most common cause of death and acquired disability in childhood
- Falls, pedestrian struck bicycle accidents are most common causes
  - —Most severe head injuries in children are from MVA
  - —Always consider the possibility of nonaccidental trauma
- Less than 50% have LOC
  - —If EDH in DD, CT should be obtained
- Bleeding is more likely to be venous
- Good outcome in 95% of children younger than 5 years

Pre-Hospital

CAUTIONS

- Head-injured patients have improved outcome when triaged to regional trauma centers
- Spinal immobilization is essential
- Ensure adequate oxygenation throughout transport
  - —Intubation and airway protection may be necessary

Diagnosis

ESSENTIAL WORKUP

- Noncontrast CT of head
- Spine series
- Further workup of trauma as indicated

LABORATORY

- ABG, CBC, chemistry, PT/PTT
- Blood ETOH/drug screen

IMAGING/SPECIAL TESTS

- All patients need a noncontrast CT promptly
  - —Lenticular, biconvex hematoma with smooth borders may be seen
  - —Most commonly seen in temporal parietal region
- Plain films may show skull fractures

DIFFERENTIAL DIAGNOSIS

- History of recent head trauma lends itself to the diagnosis
  - —Trauma may be minor in infants/toddlers
- Consider other diagnosis
  - —SDH
  - —Cerebral concussion/contusion
  - —Intracerebral bleed
  - —Diffuse axonal injury
  - —Subdural hygroma
  - —Shaken baby syndrome
  - —Toxic, metabolic, or infectious causes

PEDIATRIC CONSIDERATIONS

- US may be used for diagnosis in infants with open fontanels
- Many times the only clinical sign is a drop in HCT of 40% in infants
- Bulging fontanel with vomiting, seizures, or lethargy also suggest EDH
- Posterior fossa lesions are seen more commonly in children

Treatment

INITIAL STABILIZATION

- ABCs: prevent hypoxia and hypotension
  - —Rapid-sequence intubation for signs of deterioration or increased ICP
  - —Avoid induction agents, which may increase ICP (e.g., ketamine)
- Stabilize spine
- Elevate head of bed 15–20% after adequate fluid resuscitation
- Perform rapid neurologic assessment
  - —Glasgow coma scale (GCS) score
    - -14–15; minor head injury
    - -9–13; moderate head injury
    - -<8; severe
  - —Reflexes; pupils, corneal, gag, brain stem reflexes
- Secondary survey will reveal coexisting injury in >50%

ED TREATMENT

- Early surgical intervention (<4 hours) in comatose patients with EDH improves meaningful survival
  - —Burr hole is placed at fracture site or side with ipsilateral pupillary dilation
  - —Rapid craniectomy is occasionally performed if bleeding is not controlled at site of burr hole
- Nonsurgical intervention in asymptomatic patients is associated with high rate of deterioration; >30% requiring surgical intervention
- Maintain euvolic status with isotonic fluids
  - —Arterial line placement will affect close monitoring of MAP, PO_2, PCO_2
  - —Foley catheter to monitor I/O status
- Control ICP
  - —Prevent pain, posturing, and increased respiratory effort
    - -Sedation with benzodiazepines
    - -Neuromuscular blockade with vecuronium or pancuronium in intubated patients; etomidate is a good induction agent
    - -Barbiturate coma should be executed for refractory increased ICP in the neurosurgical ICU
  - —Mannitol may be used once euvolemic
    - -Shown to increase MAP < CPP and CBF, as well as decrease ICP
    - -Keep osmolality between 295–310
    - -Use furosemide (Lasix) as an adjunct only if no risk of hypovolemia
  - —Treat hypertension
    - -Labetalol or hydralazine

- Treat hyperglycemia if present; it is associated with increased lactic acidosis and mortality in patients with TBI
- Treat and prevent seizures
  - —Diazepam and dilantin
- Not considered helpful
  - —Steroids
  - —Antibiotic prophylaxis
  - —Hyperventilation
  - —Fluid restriction
  - —Calcium channel blockers
- Factors associated with poor outcome
  - —Age older than 40 years
  - —Large hematoma with rapid expansion
  - —Increased midline shift
  - —Lower admission GCS score or unconsciousness at presentation
  - —Postoperative ICP >3
  - —Prolonged anisocoria
  - —Associated brain injuries or concomitant trauma injuries

MEDICATIONS

- Diazepam: 5–10 mg i.v. (0.1–0.2 mg/kg i.v.)
- Dilantin: adult/peds, load 18 mg/kg at 25,050 mg/min
- Etomidate: 3 mg/kg i.v.
- Furosemide (Lasix): adults/peds, 0.5 mg/kg i.v.
- Hydralazine: 10/mg/h i.v. (peds: safety not established)
- Labetalol: 15–30 mg/h i.v. (peds: safety not established)
- Lidocaine: as preinduction agent, 1.5 mg/kg i.v.
- Mannitol: adults/peds, 0.25–1 g/kg i.v. q4h
- Pentobarbital: 1–5 mg i.v. q6h
- Thiopental: as induction agent, 20 mg/kg i.v.
- Versed: 2–4 mg/h i.v. p.r.n. (peds: safety not established)

PEDIATRIC CONSIDERATIONS

- Hemodynamically significant blood loss can result from scalp lacerations and subgaleal hematomas; direct pressure and control of bleeding is indicated

Disposition

ADMISSION CRITERIA

- All patients with CT abnormality or altered LOC should be admitted to an ICU setting with frequent neurologic assessment
  - —Patients should have repeated CT examination in 12–24 hours
  - —Patients at increased risk of deterioration include those with rapid bleeds, associated skull fracture, or lower GCS scores or neurologic deficits

DISCHARGE CRITERIA

- Admission is necessary in all patients with EDH
- If CT scan is normal, there are no neurologic deficits, and GCS is 15, patients may be safely discharged with head injury precautions and acetaminophen as needed for headaches
  - —Follow-up is necessary within 48 hours

Miscellaneous

ICD9: 852.40

ICD10: S06.4

SUGGESTED READINGS

Cooper PR, Golfinos JG. Head injury. New York: McGraw-Hill, 2000:1–348.

Marion DW. Head and spinal cord injury: traumatic brain injuries. Neurol Clin 1998;16(2):485–494.

Ono JI, et al. Outcome prediction in severe head injury: analyses of clinical prognostic factors. J Clin Neurosci 2001;8(2): 120–123.

Stieg PE, Kase CS. Neurologic emergencies: intracranial hemorrhage: diagnosis and emergency management. Neurol Clin 1998;16(2):373–390.

Zink BJ. Traumatic brain injury outcome: concepts for emergency care. Ann Emerg Med 2001;37(3):318–332.

Author: Colleen Campbell

Epiglottitis, Adult

Clinical Presentation

SIGNS AND SYMPTOMS

- General
  - —Fever
  - —Upper respiratory tract infection (URTI) symptoms
    - -Prodrome
    - -Absent in significant number of cases
  - —Toxic appearance
  - —Drooling
- HEENT
  - —Dysphagia
  - —Muffled voice
  - —Voice change
    - -"Hot potato voice"
    - -Hoarseness
  - —Foreign body sensation in throat
  - —Associated tonsillar, peritonsillar, uvula findings
  - —"Cherry red" epiglottis is classic, may be pale and edematous in up to 50%
  - —Hyoid/thyroid cartilage tender to gentle palpation
  - —Lymphadenopathy
- Respiratory
  - —Respiratory compromise
  - —Subjective sense of obstructed airway
  - —Stridor
  - —Sudden loss of airway
  - —May be more indolent in adults than pediatrics; rapid progression to total airway occlusion still seen in adults

MECHANISM/DESCRIPTION

- Inflammation of supraglottic structures
  - —Epiglottis
    - -Involvement of this is of primary airway concern
    - -May be primary or secondary from adjacent structures
  - —Valleculae
  - —Arytenoids
- Uncommon
  - —Incidence is rising
  - —Unclear true incidence versus improved diagnosis
  - —1/100,000 adults
  - —2.5 times more common in adults
- Adult mortality
  - —5–7% versus pediatric 1%
  - —Likely due to underrecognition, comorbidities, or more conservative management
- Male/female ratio is 3:1
- Average age 40–50 years
- Immune compromised patients may be particularly fulminant, with minimally associated symptoms and unusual pathogens, such as candida
- Complications
  - —Total airway obstruction
  - —Retropharyngeal abscess
  - —ARDS
  - —Pneumonia
  - —Empyema
- 35–50% patients have been evaluated in the previous 48 hours without visualization of the epiglottitis

ETIOLOGY

- Infectious
  - —*Haemophilus influenzae* B
  - —*Streptococcus pneumoniae*
  - —Group A strep
  - —Herpes simplex
  - —*Neisseria meningitis*
  - —Cytomegalovirus
  - —Numerous other uncommon agents
- Physical agents
  - —Chemical burns
  - —Thermal burns
  - —Toxic or illicit drug inhalation
  - —Trauma, instrumentation

Pre-Hospital

- Transport patients in position of comfort
- Supplemental oxygen as tolerated, avoid increasing anxiety
- Intubation indicated only if patient in severe respiratory distress
  - —Likely difficult airway and significant chance of exacerbating compromise with laryngoscopy attempts
- Inhaled agents, racemic epinephrine, and β-agonists have no demonstrated value

Diagnosis

ESSENTIAL WORKUP

- If significant respiratory distress
  - —No invasive diagnostic procedures
  - —Manage empirically with antibiotics and control of airway
- Portable lateral soft-tissue x-ray

LABORATORY

- CBC with differential
- Blood cultures
- Cultures of pharynx
  - —Only if no signs of respiratory distress

IMAGING/SPECIAL TESTS

- Nasopharyngoscopy (mini-fiberoptic scope)
- Indirect laryngoscopy
- Portable lateral soft-tissue x-ray
  - —If patient not in distress
  - —Epiglottic "thumb" sign
  - —"Vallecula" sign
  - —Significant false negative with imaging
  - —If suspected with negative film results rule out with indirect visualization

DIFFERENTIAL DIAGNOSIS

- Airway foreign body
- Anaphylaxis
- Paradoxic vocal cord dysfunction
- Angioedema
- Laryngitis
- Pharyngitis
- Oropharyngeal abscess

Treatment

INITIAL STABILIZATION

- Be prepared with all equipment on hand for definitive airway management, including a surgical airway, from presentation until diagnosis ruled out or transport to ICU setting
- Orotracheal intubation in patients with signs of obstruction or significant respiratory distress
  - —Respiratory distress/airway failure may develop precipitously
  - —Consider ENT/surgical consult if patient's condition permits for possible difficult/surgical airway
- Needle jet insufflation may be life-saving temporizing measure if surgical airway not immediately attainable with failed intubation

ED TREATMENT

- Humidified oxygen support
- IV access, hydration as indicated
- Begin antibiotic coverage empirically
- Corticosteroids controversial

MEDICATIONS

- First line
  - —Cefotaxime: 1–2 g i.v. initially, then 180 mg/kg/d in four divided doses
  - —Ceftriaxone: 1–2 g i.v. initially, then 100 mg/kg/d in two doses
- Second line
  - —Ampicillin/sulbactam: 3 g i.v. initially, then 200–300 mg/kg/d in four divided doses
  - —Trimethoprim-sulfamethoxazole: 320 mg i.v. initially, then 4–5 mg/kg i.v. q12h

Disposition

ADMISSION CRITERIA

- Any patient with a suspected or confirmed diagnosis of epiglottitis should be admitted to an ICU setting for IV antibiotics and airway management

DISCHARGE CRITERIA

- Patients should not be discharged unless the diagnosis has been ruled out by visualization of the supraglottic structures by a physician familiar with physical appearance of the disease
- Close contacts should receive prophylactic treatment with rifampin

Miscellaneous

ICD9: 464.3, 464.30, 464.31

ICD10: J05.1

SUGGESTED READINGS

Burns JE, Hendley JO. Epiglottitis. In: Mandell GL, Bennett JE, Dolin R, eds. Mandell: principles and practice of infectious diseases, 5th ed. Philadelphia: Churchill Livingstone, 2000.

Carey MJ. Epiglottitis in adults. Am J Emerg Med 1996;14:421–424.

Ducic Y, Herbert PC, MacLachlan L, et al. Description and evaluation of the vallecula sign: a new radiologic sign in the diagnosis of adult epiglottitis. Ann Emerg Med 1997;30:1–6.

Mayo-Smith MF, Spinale JW, Donskey CJ, et al. Acute epiglottitis. An 18 year experience in Rhode Island. Chest 1995;108:1640–1647.

Melio FR. Upper respiratory tract infections. In: Marx JA, et al, eds. Marx: Rosen's emergency medicine: concepts and clinical practice, 5th ed. Philadelphia: Mosby, 2001.

Nakamura H, Tanaka H, Matsuda A, et al. Acute epiglottitis: a review of 80 patients. J Laryngol Otolaryngol 2001;115:31–34.

Author: Owen M. Lander

Epiglottitis, Pediatric

Clinical Presentation

SIGNS AND SYMPTOMS

- Usually fulminant presentation without prodromal illness
- General
  - —Initial irritability with progressive lethargy
  - —*Toxic* appearing
  - —High fever is typical (>38.4°C)
- HEENT
  - —Sore throat
  - —Drooling
  - —Odynophagia
  - —Muffled voice
- Respiratory
  - —Rapidly progressive respiratory distress (dyspnea in only one third of adults)
  - —Children usually prefer to sit upright, leaning forward with open mouth ("sniffing position") to maximize air entry
  - —*Subtle stridor* that may progress to severe stridor (stridor in only 10% of adults)
- Complications
  - —Pulmonary edema
  - —Epiglottic abscess
  - —Pulmonary atelectasis

MECHANISM/DESCRIPTION

- Inflammation of the epiglottis and surrounding supraglottic region
- Children are at greatest risk of upper airway obstruction because of small caliber airways due to
  - —Decreased cross-sectional area of the upper airway (Resistance inversely changes as the radius to the fourth power)
  - —Cricoid ring is the narrowest part of the airway
  - —Loose attachment of mucosal surface and increased vascularity of mucosa allows for edema
  - —Dynamic collapse of the airway
- A precipitous decline in the incidence of childhood epiglottitis since the introduction of the *Haemophilus influenzae* vaccination
- Typically occurs in children from 7 months to 16 years of age with peak incidence between 2 and 6 years
- Epiglottitis predominates in the winter and spring but may occur throughout the year

ETIOLOGY

- Infection
  - —*H. influenzae*
  - —β-hemolytic streptococci
  - —Herpes simplex virus (rare)
  - —Anaerobes (rare)
  - —*Klebsiella*
  - —*Aspergillus* (usually seen only in patients with underlying disease)
- Caustic
- Thermal
- Traumatic

Pre-Hospital

- Notification to receiving ED to prepare OR for visualization and possible airway management in a controlled setting
- Do nothing that agitates any patient, particularly a child with stridor and respiratory distress
- Most children will be most calm when held by or sitting with a parent
- If the patient allows, administer 100% O_2 by mask or by cannula
- Generally, do not attempt IV access prior to securing airway
- Bag-valve-mask ventilation with 100% O_2 followed by emergency airway procedures if acute obstruction

Diagnosis

ESSENTIAL WORKUP

- Epiglottitis is a clinical diagnosis
- Indirect laryngoscopy or any attempts to directly visualize the epiglottis are not indicated in children with suspected epiglottis unless performed in a controlled environment (controversial in adults)
- If infection is suspected, obtain cultures of the epiglottis during laryngoscopy

LABORATORY

- Avoid laboratory tests until airway is controlled
- Throat cultures
- Blood cultures
  - —Often positive if *H. influenzae* is the pathogen

IMAGING/SPECIAL TESTS

- X-rays of the soft tissue lateral neck
  - —Usually not necessary to make the diagnosis
  - —Creates additional risk by delaying stabilization of the airway, promoting airway obstruction by agitating the patient, and often removing the child from the ED to an uncontrolled environment
  - —Variable findings
    - -Normal
    - -Swelling of the epiglottis and often supraglottic region
    - -"Thumbprint" sign from thickened aryepiglottic folds and normal subglottis
    - -An EW/C3W (epiglottic width to third cervical vertebral body width) ratio of >0.5
- Laryngoscopy
  - —In a controlled environment whenever possible
  - —Cultures of the epiglottis during laryngoscopy to clarify pathogens and direct treatment

DIFFERENTIAL DIAGNOSIS

- Other infectious processes
  - —Bacterial tracheitis
  - —Mononucleosis
  - —Diphtheria
  - —Pertussis
  - —Croup (primarily in younger children, but there is a significant overlap in the ages of presentation)
  - —Ludwig's angina
  - —Peritonsillar infection
  - —Retropharyngeal abscess
- Allergic reactions
- Angioneurotic edema
- Airway foreign bodies
- Laryngeal trauma
- Laryngospasm
- Inhalation or aspiration of toxins (e.g., hydrocarbons)

- Airway burns (have been related to crack cocaine)
- Systemic diseases: amyloid, sarcoid, pemphigus, pemphigoid, Wegner's granulomatosis
- Hyperventilation
- CNS disorders

Treatment

INITIAL STABILIZATION

- Airway management in patients in extremis
  - —Bag-valve-mask ventilation with 100% O_2 with cricoid pressure often provides adequate ventilation and time to move the patient to the OR
  - —Oral intubation
    - -Use an ETT size 1 mm smaller than indicated by age
    - -Direct compression of the anterior neck in the glottic region may help visualize air bubbles at the opening of the swollen glottis
  - —When oral intubation fails
    - -Emergency cricothyrotomy if age older than 10–12 years
    - -Needle cricothyrotomy if age younger than 10–12 years

ED TREATMENT

- 100% O_2 as tolerated by patient
- Racemic epinephrine may temporize symptoms but must be done with extreme caution avoiding agitating child
- Avoid procedures that agitate the patient
- Empiric invasive airway management may be indicated
  - —Patients with rapidly progressive respiratory difficulty, tachypnea, worsening throat pain, tachycardia, or hypoxemia
  - —Patients at high risk of acute obstruction (e.g., children with immunocompetency disorders)
- Intubate in OR or controlled environment by most skilled person
- Inhalational anesthesia is used before intubation
- Have appropriate various diameters of ETT available to accommodate the inflamed supraglottic region
- Surgical backup required in case intubation not possible, then emergency tracheotomy or cricothyrotomy can be performed
- Administer IV antibiotics: second- or third-generation cephalosporin is active against β-lactamase-producing *H. influenzae*
- Equipment for intubation and for a surgical airway or needle cricothyrotomy must be available at the bedside
- Steroids are controversial but frequently administered, particularly in patients with chemical or thermal epiglottitis

MEDICATIONS

- Ampicillin: 100–200 mg/kg/24 h q4h i.v.
- Cefotaxime: 50–150 mg/kg/24 h q6h i.v.
- Ceftriaxone: 50–75 mg/kg/24 h q12h i.v.
- Chloramphenicol: 75–100 mg/kg/24 h q6h i.v.
- Epinephrine, racemic: 0.05 mL/kg (max, 0.5 mL) every 30 minutes in 2.5 mL NS via nebulizer
- Rifampin: 20 mg/kg (max, 600 mg) q.d. × 4 days

Disposition

ADMISSION CRITERIA

- All patients with suspected epiglottitis

DISCHARGE CRITERIA

- Close contacts should be treated with rifampin prophylaxis

Miscellaneous

ICD9: 464.3, 464.30, 464.31

ICD10: J05.1

SEE ALSO: BACTERIAL TRACHEITIS

SUGGESTED READINGS

Bank D, Krug S. New approaches to upper airway disease. Emerg Med Clin North Am 1995;13(2):473–487.

Damm M, Eckel HE, Jungehulsing M, et al. Management of acute inflammatory childhood stridor. Otolaryngol Head Neck Surg 1999;121(5):633–638.

Frantz T, Ragson B, Quesenberry C. Acute epiglottitis in adults: analysis of 129 cases. JAMA 1994;272(17):1358–1360.

Lai SH, Wong KS, Liao SL, et al. Non-infectious epiglottitis in children: two case reports. Int J Pediatr Otorhinolaryngol 2000;55(1):57–60.

Rothrock S, et al. Radiologic diagnosis of epiglottitis: objective criteria for all ages. Ann Emerg Med 1990;9:978–982.

Stroud RH, Friedman NR. An update on inflammatory disorders of the pediatric airway: epiglottitis, croup and tracheitis. Am J Otolaryngol 2001;22(4):268–275.

Author: Susan J. Duffy

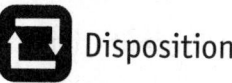

Epiphyseal Injuries

Clinical Presentation

SIGNS AND SYMPTOMS

- Pain and localized tenderness
- Limited mobility of affected joint
- Swelling
- Ecchymosis
- Bony deformities

MECHANISM/DESCRIPTION

- More common than sprains in children
  —Relative weakness of the physis compared with ligaments or metaphyseal bone
  —Ligaments often insert into the epiphyses
- Common mechanisms
  —Shearing
  —Tension
  —Compression
- Most common during peak growth
- Salter-Harris classification
  —Type I
    -Fracture line is confined to physis
    -Epiphyseal separation from metaphysis
    -No growth disturbance
  —Type II
    -Fracture propagates along physis and a fragment from metaphysis accompanies displaced epiphysis
    -Periosteum torn opposite metaphyseal fragment
    -Most common epiphyseal fracture
    -No growth disturbance
  —Type III
    -Fracture through a portion of physis extending through epiphysis and articular surface
    -Phalanges and distal tibia most commonly affected
    -Require anatomic alignment due to displacement of both physis and articular surface
    -Growth disturbance may occur despite anatomic reduction
  —Type IV
    -Fracture originates at articular surface
    -Extends through physis and into metaphysis
    -Distal humerus and distal tibia most commonly affected
    -Anatomic reduction is essential and frequently requires surgical intervention
    -Growth arrest is common
  —Type V
    -Result from crush injuries to physis
    -No immediately visible radiographic alteration
    -Often found in retrospect with premature physeal closure
    -Usually involve knee or ankle
    -Growth arrest is common
  —Type VI
    -Not described in original Salter-Harris classification
    -Involves periosteum surrounding physis
    -Reactive formation of bone external to growth plate causing tethering of the epiphysis to the metaphysis and restricting further expansion at the physis
    -May result from ligamentous avulsion or thermal injuries
  —Type VII
    -Not described in original Salter-Harris classification
    -Fracture involves epiphysis only
- Long-term complications
  —Overreduction
  —Bone growth disturbances
  —Reduced joint mobility

ETIOLOGY

- Traumatic injury, often without specific history in young children
- Occur most frequently in distal radius, phalanges, and distal tibia

Pre-Hospital

- Immobilize limb in the position found
- Apply ice or cold packs to injury
- Assess injured extremity for neurologic and vascular function
- Consider concomitant injuries

Diagnosis

ESSENTIAL WORKUP

- Assess pulses and capillary filling distal to injury
- Evaluate distal motor and sensory function
- Verify integrity of the skin overlying injury
- Address and manage coexisting injuries

IMAGING/SPECIAL TESTS

- Plain radiography of the injured extremity
  —Type I fractures
    -May appreciate a slightly separated physis or an associated joint effusion; usually unremarkable film
    -Consider comparison views of the contralateral joint to detect small defects
    -Callus may be present on subsequent follow-up films
  —Types II through IV
    -Films diagnostic of fracture
  —Types V and VI
    -Initial film often normal
    -Subsequent radiographs may reveal premature bone arrest
- Radionuclide bone scan
  —Rarely necessary
  —Fractures must be at least 24–48 hours old
  —Valuable adjunct if child abuse is suspected
- CT scan
  —Helpful in assessing integrity of articular surfaces in type III and IV fractures
- MRI
  —If diagnosis remains equivocal and identification of a fracture would alter management
  —Allows for early detection of growth arrest

DIFFERENTIAL DIAGNOSIS

- Sprain
- Strain
- Contusion

Treatment

INITIAL STABILIZATION

- Control hemorrhage
- Apply sterile dressings to open wounds
- Analgesia

ED TREATMENT

- Reduction/alignment
  —Displacement requires anatomic alignment
  —Vascular or neurologic compromise distal to injury
- Immobilization
  —A splint must immobilize joints proximal and distal to injury in anatomic alignment
  —Elevate injured limb
- Open fractures
  —IV antibiotics with staphylococcal and streptococcal coverage
  —Copious irrigation with saline
  —Sterile dressing
  —Orthopedic consultation

MEDICATIONS

- Cefazolin: 25–50 mg/kg/d i.v./i.m. q6–8h
- Clindamycin: 20–40 mg/kg/d i.v. q6–8h
- Fentanyl: 2-3 μg/kg i.v.; transmucosal lollipops, 5–15 μg/kg, max 400 mg, contraindicated if $<$10 kg
- Morphine: 0.1 mg/kg i.v./i.m.

Disposition

ADMISSION CRITERIA

- Open fractures
- Open surgical reduction required
- Type III and IV fractures

DISCHARGE CRITERIA

- Type I, II, V, VI, and VII epiphyseal injuries
- Orthopedic follow-up within 1 week
- Splint for comfort
- Analgesics
- Ice packs
- Elevation of affected limb

Miscellaneous

ICD9: N/A

ICD10: N/A

SUGGESTED READINGS

England SP, Sundberg S. Management of common pediatric fractures. Pediatr Clin North Am 1996;43(5):991–1012.

Morrissy RT, Weinstein SL, eds. Lovell and Winter's pediatric orthopaedics, 5th ed. Philadelphia: Lippincott Williams & Wilkins, 2001.

Ozonoff MB. Pediatric orthopedic radiology, 2nd ed. Philadelphia: WB Saunders, 1992.

Rogers LF, Poznanski AK. Imaging of epiphyseal injuries. Radiology 1994; 91:297.

Salter R, Harris W. Injuries involving the epiphyseal plate. J Bone Joint Surg 1963;45A:587.

Authors: Steven F. Fisher; Daniel L. Savitt

Epistaxis

Clinical Presentation

SIGNS AND SYMPTOMS

- Bleeding from nare(s)
- Complaints of vomiting or coughing blood
- Hemorrhage
- Tachycardia
- Hypotension
- Airway compromise
- Anxiety

MECHANISM/DESCRIPTION

- Anterior epistaxis (90% of cases)
  —Source: Kiesselbach's plexus of anterior inferior septum
  —Generally unilateral
- Posterior epistaxis (10% of cases)
  —Source: posterior branch of sphenopalatine artery

ETIOLOGY

- Local factors
  —Trauma (including postoperative)
  —Nose picking
  —Dry nasal mucosa (low humidity)
  —Environmental irritants (ammonia, gasoline, sulfuric acid, glutaraldehyde)
  —Inflammation from infections or allergens
  —Neoplasia (e.g., papilloma and polyp)
- Systemic factors
  —Atherosclerosis of nasal vasculature
  —Barotrauma
  —Hypertension (controversial whether this is cause or effect)
  —Coagulopathy (familial): hemophilia A or B, von Willebrand's disease
  —Coagulopathy (acquired): thrombocytopenia, liver disease, renal failure/uremia
  —Drug induced: salicylates, NSAIDs, heparin, coumadin
  —Diabetes mellitus
  —Alcoholism
  —Hereditary hemorrhagic telangiectasia (Osler-Weber-Rendu disease)

Pre-Hospital

- Stable patients: patient should bend forward at the waist, pinch nares closed, and spit out blood rather than swallow it
- Unstable patients
  —Intubation if airway compromise
  —IV access
  —Crystalloid resuscitation if signs of hypovolemia

Diagnosis

ESSENTIAL WORKUP

- Assess stability: airway compromise, hemorrhage
- Determine source (anterior vs. posterior)
- Consider underlying coagulopathy

LABORATORY

- Consider for severe bleeding or suspected coagulopathy
  —Type and cross-match, hematocrit, PT, PTT, BUN

IMAGING/SPECIAL TESTS

- Direct visualization of nasal mucosa with nasal speculum
  —Pretreat with topical vasoconstricting agent and anesthetic
  —Ensure adequate lighting (i.e., headlamp) and suction

DIFFERENTIAL DIAGNOSIS

- Hematemesis
- Hemoptysis

PEDIATRIC CONSIDERATIONS

- Posterior epistaxis is rare in children; consider further workup for bleeding diatheses
- Consider nasal foreign bodies or neoplasms such as juvenile angiofibroma or papilloma

Treatment

INITIAL STABILIZATION

- Secure the airway in patients who are unconscious, have major facial trauma, or are otherwise at risk of obstruction or aspiration
- Treat hypotension with crystalloids and blood products if necessary, and ensure adequate IV access

ED TREATMENT

- Universal precautions against blood/fluid contamination
- Anterior source:
  —Instruct patient to bend forward at waist, pinch nares closed for 15 minutes, and spit out blood rather than swallow it
  —If bleeding persists, use bayonet forceps to place cotton pledgets soaked in vasoconstricting and anesthetic agents (cocaine, lidocaine and epinephrine, oxymetolazone, or phenylephrine) into affected nares
  —Visualize source of bleeding, and cauterize limited area with silver nitrate
  —Consider Gelfoam or Surgicel
  —Consider anterior packing with Vaseline ribbon gauze if cautery unsuccessful, ensuring that both ends protrude from nares, that the strip is removed by 48 hours, and that antibiotics (cephalexin, amoxicillin-clavulanate, or others) are prescribed for toxic shock/sinusitis prophylaxis
  —Merocel synthetic sponge tampon is an alternative to ribbon gauze packing
  —After anterior packing, persistent new bleeding may be a sign of inadequate packing or posterior source
- Posterior source:
  —Posterior packing with balloon device such as Nasostat, Epistat; these are left in for 2–5 days, with antibiotic prophylaxis as for anterior packing
  —If commercial packs unavailable, a Foley catheter may be directed into posterior nares, inflated with water until uncomfortable, held in place by umbilical clamp, with Vaseline gauze then placed for anterior packing
  —Endoscopic cautery by otolaryngology is also useful and may obviate need for admission
- Complications of posterior packing
  —Nasal trauma
  —Vagal response
  —Aspiration
  —Infection
  —Hypoxia

MEDICATIONS

- Vasoactive solutions
  —4% cocaine
  —1:1 mixture of 2% tetracaine and epinephrine (1:1,000)
  —1:1 mixture of oxymetazoline 0.05% (Afrin) and lidocaine solution 4%
  —Phenylephrine (Neo-Synephrine)
- Amoxicillin-clavulanate potassium: 250 mg PO q8h
- Cephalexin: 250 mg PO q6h
- Clindamycin: 150 mg PO q6h
- Trimethoprim-sulfamethoxazole: 160/800 mg PO q12h

Disposition

ADMISSION CRITERIA

- Severe blood loss, requiring transfusion
- Severe coagulopathy that places patient at risk of further blood loss
- Posterior nasal packing: otolaryngology consult, and admission for supplemental oxygen, sedation, and observation, possible further surgical intervention (e.g., arterial ligation or embolization)

DISCHARGE CRITERIA

- Stable patients
  —Use Afrin nasal spray for 2 days
  —Lubricate nares with an antibiotic ointment
  —Humidify air
  —Avoid nose picking
- Return to ED for bleeding not controlled by pressure, fever, difficulty breathing, vomiting

Miscellaneous

ICD9: 784.7

ICD10: R04.0

SUGGESTED READINGS

Frazee TA, Hauser MS. Nonsurgical management of epistaxis. J Oral Maxillofac Surg 2000;58:419–424.

Pfaff JA, Moore GP. Otolaryngology. In: Marx J, Hockberger R, Walls R, eds. Emergency medicine: concepts and clinical practice, 5th ed. St. Louis: Mosby, 2002: 933–935.

Tan LS, Calhoun KH. Epistaxis. Med Clin North Am 1999;83:43–56.

Author: Bret P. Nelson

Erysipelas

Clinical Presentation

SIGNS AND SYMPTOMS

- Most common site of involvement is the face, lower legs, and ears
- Skin has an intense "fiery red" color, earning the nickname "St. Anthony's fire"
- The involved skin is an edematous, indurated (peau d'orange), painful, well-circumscribed plaque with a sharp, clearly demarcated edge
- Vesicles and bullae may be present in more serious infection
- Predilection for infants, children, and the elderly
- Systemic symptoms may include malaise, fever, chills, nausea, and vomiting
- Traumatic portal of entry on skin is not always apparent
- Rarely there may be an associated periorbital cellulitis or cavernous sinus involvement

MECHANISM/DESCRIPTION

- Superficial cellulitis of the skin with prominent lymphatic involvement
- Group A β-hemolytic streptococcus is the causative organism (uncommonly, group C or G)
- Portals of entry are commonly skin ulcers, local trauma, or abrasions; psoriatic or eczematous lesions; or fungal infections

PEDIATRIC CONSIDERATIONS

- *Haemophilus influenzae* type b causes facial cellulitis in children that may appear similar to erysipelas
- Group B streptococci can cause erysipelas in the newborn
- Can develop from infection of umbilical stump

Pre-Hospital

N/A

Diagnosis

ESSENTIAL WORKUP

- The diagnosis is clinical based on the characteristic skin findings and the clinical setting
  - —Classical "butterfly" rash on cheeks and across nose when affecting face
- Needle aspirate wound cultures are seldom positive and not indicated
- Positive blood cultures in only 3%; leukocytosis is common; when complicating infected ulcers, cultures are positive in 30%

DIFFERENT DIAGNOSIS

- Allergic inflammation
- Cellulitis
- Contact dermatitis
- Familial Mediterranean fever
- Herpes zoster
- Impetigo
- Viral exanthem
- Diffuse inflammatory carcinoma of the breast

Treatment

INITIAL STABILIZATION

- Patients with periorbital cellulitis or cavernous sinus thrombosis may be toxic and in need of IV fluid resuscitation or pressure support

ED TREATMENT

- Appropriate antibiotic therapy
  - —Patients with extensive involvement may benefit from a parenteral antibiotic dose in the ED
  - —Penicillin is the drug of choice when clearly the symptoms are consistent with erysipelas
  - —If there is difficulty in distinguishing from cellulitis, staphylococcal coverage should be added
  - —Facial cellulitis in children may be caused by *H. influenzae* in patients who have not been immunized; many will be bacteremic and require admission

MEDICATIONS

- Cefuroxime: peds, 50–100 mg/kg/d PO divided q8h
- Cephalexin: 500 mg PO q6h (peds: 40 mg/kg/d PO divided q8h)
- Dicloxacillin: 500 mg PO q6h (peds: 30–50 mg/kg/d PO divided q6h)
- Erythromycin ethylsuccinate: 250–500 mg PO q6h (peds: 40 mg/kg/d PO in divided doses q6h)
- Penicillin G: 2 million units q4h i.v. (peds: 25,000 U/kg i.v. q6h)
- Penicillin V: 500 mg PO q6h (peds: 25–50 mg/kg/d divided q6–8h)

Disposition

ADMISSION CRITERIA

- Patients with extensive involvement, fever, toxic appearance
- Children more often require admission; blood cultures, IV antibiotics, including coverage for *H. influenzae,* should be initiated for patients who have not been immunized

DISCHARGE CRITERIA

- Most patients can be discharged on oral therapy if nontoxic appearing, good compliance, and close follow-up can be ensured
- Minimal facial involvement
- Nontoxic appearing
- Not immunosuppressed
- Able to tolerate and comply with oral therapy
- Adequate follow-up

Miscellaneous

ICD9: 035

ICD10: A46

SUGGESTED READINGS

Bisno AI, Stevens DL. Streptococcal infections of skin and soft tissues. N Engl J Med 1996;334:240–244.

Kahn RM, Goldstein EJ. Common bacterial skin infections. Postgrad Med 1993;93(6): 175–182.

Author: Irving "Jake" Jacoby

Erythema Infectiosum

Clinical Presentation

SIGNS AND SYMPTOMS

- Following the incubation period mild constitutional symptoms
  - —Low-grade fever
  - —Headache
  - —During this time, the child is contagious

Rash

- Begins 1 week after initial onset of symptoms
- Three stages
  - —First stage
    - -"Slapped cheek" appearance occurs in 75%
    - -Erythematous
    - -Warm
    - -Nontender
  - —Second stage
    - -Occurs 1–4 days after facial rash
    - -Pink to dull red, lacy macular eruption
    - -Occurs on the extremities and trunk
    - -May be pruritic
    - -Usually spares the palms and soles
  - —Third stage
    - -Rash may recur secondary to cutaneous vasodilation, especially during periods of stress, exercise, sun exposure, and bathing
    - -Resolves in 1–3 weeks but can recur over a period of months

Possible Complications

- Arthritis
  - —Common complication in adults
- Transient aplastic crisis in patients with hemolytic anemias
  - —Fever
  - —Pallor
  - —Weakness
  - —Lethargy
  - —Hepatosplenomegaly
  - —Evidence of heart failure

MECHANISM/DESCRIPTION

- Infectious exanthem also known as *fifth disease*
  - —Derived from the historical numbering of infectious exanthems
    - -1 Measles
    - -2 Scarlet fever
    - -3 Rubella
    - -4 Filatov-Dukes disease (this was a variant of scarlet fever, which is no longer recognized)
    - -5 Erythema infectiosum
    - -6 Roseola

ETIOLOGY

- Caused by human parvovirus B19
- Incubation period typically is 4–14 days
- Seasonal predilection for late winter and spring
- Spreads via respiratory transmission
- School-aged children typically infected
- Adults infrequently affected

Pre-Hospital

N/A

Diagnosis

ESSENTIAL WORKUP

- Clinical diagnosis based on typical signs and symptoms

LABORATORY

- No workup necessary unless concerns for an aplastic crisis or arthritis are present
- CBC

IMAGING/SPECIAL TESTS

- IgM antibody assay
  - —Diagnostic testing is available only at a few sites
  - —Confirms acute infection

DIFFERENTIAL DIAGNOSIS

- Scarlet fever
- Rubella
- Roseola
- Infectious mononucleosis
- Echovirus
- Coxsackie virus
- Drug eruptions

Treatment

INITIAL STABILIZATION

- ABCs for septic or ill-appearing patient

ED TREATMENT

- No specific antiviral treatment or vaccine is available
- Symptomatic treatment with fluids and acetaminophen
- Hospitalization and respiratory isolation for aplastic crisis

Expected Course

- Rash usually resolves in 1–3 weeks but can recur over a period of months; most children do very well
- Exposed pregnant women have an increased incidence of nonimmune hydrops fetalis
- Once the rash is present, the patient is no longer contagious
  —May return to school or daycare

Disposition

ADMISSION CRITERIA

- Aplastic crisis
- Significant arthritis
- Overall ill appearance

DISCHARGE CRITERIA

- Almost all patients
- Well appearing with rash and no signs of aplastic crisis or arthritis

Miscellaneous

ICD9: 057.0

ICD10: B08.3

SUGGESTED READINGS

Adams DM, Ware RE. Parvovirus B19: how much should you worry? Contemp Pediatr 1996;13:85–96.

Anderson MJ, Higgins PG, Davis LR, et al. Experimental parvoviral infection in humans. Infect Dis 1985;152:257–265.

Ussery X, Demmler G. Human parvovirus B19. Semin Pediatr Infect Dis 1996;7(2): 89–96.

Author: Kathlene Bassett

Erythema Multiforme

Clinical Presentation

SIGNS AND SYMPTOMS

- Prodrome: infrequent systemic symptoms (mild fever/malaise), antecedent (within 3 weeks) herpes simplex virus (HSV) in most cases
- Rash: characteristic "target" lesions spread from the extremities toward the trunk, may be mildly pruritic

MECHANISM/DESCRIPTION

- Divided into major and minor types
- Erythema multiforme major: separate disease pattern that includes more severe disorders (see Toxic Epidermal Necrolysis and Stevens-Johnson syndrome)
- Erythema multiforme minor is characterized by a benign, self-limited rash, generally not associated with acute, serious illness; simply referred to as *erythema multiforme;* it features
  - —Lesions: symmetric dull red macules and papules, evolving into round, well-demarcated "target" lesions with central clearing; "multiforme" refers to the evolution of the rash through various stages at different times
  - —Distribution: extremities, dorsal hands and feet, palms and soles, extensor surfaces, especially elbows and knees
  - —Spread: from extremities toward trunk
  - —Mucosal involvement: occasional erosions in the mouth
  - —Duration: usually 1–4 weeks, but may become chronic or recurrent
  - —Population: children and young adults (>50% younger than 20 years); males are affected more often than females

ETIOLOGY

- Hypersensitivity reaction, probably a transient autoimmune defect
- Initial and recurrent HSV is the most common precipitant (>70%)
- Other causes include idiopathic, medications (antibiotics: penicillin, sulfur-based, phenytoin, and others), malignancy, and *Mycoplasma* infections

Pre-Hospital

- Not contagious and does not require isolation or postexposure prophylaxis for exposed personnel

Diagnosis

ESSENTIAL WORKUP

- Complete history and physical exam, with special attention to the skin, genitourinary system, and recent infectious symptoms

LABORATORY

- No specific laboratory tests needed
- History and physical examination dictate workup for underlying illnesses

IMAGING/SPECIAL TESTS

- *Skin biopsy* reveals mononuclear cell infiltrate around upper dermal blood vessels, without leukocytoclastic vasculitis; also, necrosis of epidermal keratinocytes

DIFFERENTIAL DIAGNOSIS

- Systemic lupus erythematosus
- Fixed drug eruption
- Pityriasis rosea
- Secondary syphilis
- Erythema migrans
- Urticaria

Treatment

INITIAL STABILIZATION

- Generally benign and self-limited, requiring no initial stabilization

ED TREATMENT

- Attempt to identify, treat, or remove underlying cause or precipitant
- Symptomatic: cool compresses, antipruritics

MEDICATIONS

- Antipruritic agents
  - —Cetirizine (Zyrtec): 10 mg PO q.d.
  - —Diphenhydramine: 25–50 mg (peds: 5 mg/kg/24 h) PO q6–8h
  - —Hydroxyzine: 25 mg PO q6–8h
- Antiviral therapy
  - —If HSV infection is present, see Herpes for specific treatment options

Disposition

ADMISSION CRITERIA

- None, unless required for other concurrent disorders

DISCHARGE CRITERIA

- Erythema multiforme is a benign disorder that does not require admission

Miscellaneous

ICD9: 695.1

ICD10: L51.9

SUGGESTED READINGS

Assier H, Bastuji-Garin S, Revuz J, et al. Erythema multiforme with mucous membrane involvement and Stevens-Johnson syndrome are clinically different disorders with distinct causes. Arch Dermatol 1995;131:539–543.

Kerob D, Assier-Bonnet H. Recurrent erythema multiforme unresponsive to acyclovir prophylaxis and responsive to valacyclovir continuous therapy. Arch Dermatol 1998;134:877–878.

Leaute-Labreze C, Lamireau T, Chawki D, et al. Diagnosis, classification, and management of erythema multiforme and Stevens-Johnson syndrome. Arch Dis Child 2000;83:347–352.

Weston WL. What is erythema multiforme? Pediatr Ann 1996;25(2):106–109.

Authors: Gregory W. Hendey; Thomas A. Utecht

Erythema Nodosum

Clinical Presentation

SIGNS AND SYMPTOMS

- Tender SC erythematous nodules symmetrically distributed on extensor surface of lower legs
- Lesions occasionally occur on fingers, hands, arms, calves, and thighs
- In bedridden patients, dependent areas may be involved
- Patients may have fever, malaise, leukocytosis, arthralgias, arthritis, and unilateral or bilateral hilar adenopathy with any form of the disease

MECHANISM/DESCRIPTION

- Erythema nodosum is characterized by multiple symmetric, nonulcerative tender nodules on the extensor surface of the lower extremities typically in young adults
- Peak incidence in third decade, more common in women (4:1)
- Nodules are round with poorly demarcated edges and vary in size from 1–10 cm
- Skin lesions are initially red, become progressively "ecchymotic appearing" as they resolve over 3–6 weeks
- Lesions are caused by inflammation of the septa between SC fat nodules (septal panniculitis)
- Natural history of idiopathic form or with treatment of underlying disease is spontaneous regression of lesions within 3–6 weeks
- Major disease variants include erythema nodosum migrans (usually mild unilateral disease with little or no systemic symptoms) and chronic erythema nodosum (lesions spread via extension, and though associated systemic symptoms occur as with traditional acute form, they tend to be milder)

ETIOLOGY

- A common dermatologic disease generally considered an immune-mediated response; 30–50% of the time the etiology is idiopathic
- Often a marker for underlying disease; specific etiologies include
  - —Drug reactions (oral contraceptives, sulfonamides, penicillins)
  - —Infections including streptococcal, mycobacterium TB, atypical mycobacteria, and coccidioidomycosis, hepatitis, syphilis, chlamydia, rickettsia, salmonella, *Campylobacter*, yersinia, parasites, and leprosy
  - —Systemic diseases such as sarcoidosis, inflammatory bowel disease, Behçet's, and connective tissue disorders
  - —Malignancies such as lymphoma and leukemia
  - —HIV infection
  - —Rarely can be caused by vaccines for hepatitis and TB (BCG)
- Incidence of the different etiologies vary according to the time of year and the geographic location and ethnicity of the population being studied
- Typically erythema nodosum begins 2–3 weeks after the onset of pharyngitis in children

Pre-Hospital

N/A

Diagnosis

ESSENTIAL WORKUP

- Careful history and physical exam directed at detecting precipitating etiology

LABORATORY

- CBC, ESR, appropriate chemistry tests; TB and coccidioidomycosis skin tests may be useful initial screening tests for lymphoma, leukemia, TB, and cocci

IMAGING/SPECIAL TEST

- CXR can serve as initial screen for sarcoidosis
- Definitive diagnosis made by deep elliptical biopsy and histopathologic evaluation (punch biopsy may be inadequate as SC fat sample must be obtained)

DIFFERENTIAL DIAGNOSIS

- Erythema nodosum migrans and chronic erythema nodosum
- Any type of panniculitis can resemble erythema nodosum
- Differences can be determined histopathologically
- Other disorders include periarteritis nodosum, migratory thrombophlebitis, superficial varicose thrombophlebitis, scleroderma, systemic lupus erythematosus, α_1-antitrypsin deficiency, Behçet's syndrome, lipodystrophies, leukemic infiltration of fat, and panniculitis associated with steroid use, cold, and infection

PEDIATRIC CONSIDERATIONS

- In children, streptococcal pharyngitis is the most likely etiology

Treatment

INITIAL STABILIZATION

- ABCs, IV, oxygen, monitoring as appropriate

ED TREATMENT

- Treatment should be directed at the underlying disease
- Typically only supportive therapies, such as analgesics, are necessary for dermatologic lesions
- Treatment of the underlying pathology usually ensures disappearance of the lesions within 1–2 months
- Specific therapies such as potassium iodide and systemic corticosteroids are used only when the underlying process is known
- Systemic corticosteroids are contraindicated in presence of certain underlying infections such as TB or coccidioidomycosis, which may disseminate with their use

MEDICATIONS

- Aspirin: 650 mg PO q4–6h p.r.n. (peds: contraindicated)
- NSAIDs
  —Ibuprofen: 300–800 mg PO q8h (peds: 5–10 mg/kg PO q6h)
  —Indomethacin: 25–50 mg PO q8h
- Potassium iodide/SSKI (used for resistant disease; contraindicated in hyperthyroidism): 900 mg PO q.d. × 3–4 weeks
- Systemic corticosteroids

Disposition

ADMISSION CRITERIA

- Dictated by the severity of symptoms and the etiologic agent

DISCHARGE CRITERIA

- Nontoxic patients, able to take oral fluids without difficulty
- Scheduled follow-up should be arranged

Miscellaneous

ICD9: 695.2

ICD10: L52

SUGGESTED READINGS

Gonzalez-Gay MA. Erythema nodosum: a clinical approach. Clin Exp Rheumatol 2001;19:365–368.

Myerson MS. Erythema nodosum leprosum. Int J Dermatol 1996;35(6):389–392.

Psychos DN, Voulgari PV. Erythema nodosum: the underlying conditions. Clin Rheumatol 2000;19:212–216.

Authors: Herbert G. Bivins; Theresa Schwab

Esophageal Trauma

Clinical Presentation

SIGNS AND SYMPTOMS

General

- Dysphagia: difficulty swallowing
- Odynophagia: pain with swallowing
- Chest pain: angina-like, often pleuritic, severe and unrelenting
- Hoarseness
- Dyspnea

Tears or Perforations

- Bleeding
- Hematemesis
- SC air at the base of the neck
- Hamman's crunch: systolic crunching sound due to air in the mediastinum
- Shock
- Septicemia
- Peritonitis
- Associated neck, chest, or abdominal injury with trauma; most commonly trachea, associated with penetrating/blunt trauma

Ingestions/Foreign Bodies

- Drooling or excessive salivation
- Choking, gagging, vomiting, stridor, or wheezing
- Inability of food or liquid to pass

MECHANISM/DESCRIPTION

Foreign Bodies/Food Impactions (See Foreign Body, Esophageal)

- Adults often associated with prisoners, psychiatric patients, intoxication, or edentulous
- Sites of esophageal narrowing: cricopharyngeal muscle (upper esophageal sphincter); crossover of left mainstem bronchus and aortic arch; gastroesophageal junction (lower esophageal sphincter); and areas of disease (cancer, webs, or Schatzki's ring)

Partial- and Full-thickness Tears

- Foreign bodies via direct penetration, pressure necrosis, or chemical necrosis
- Caustic ingestions: accidental or intentional
  - —Alkali: liquefaction necrosis causing burns, airway edema or compromise, perforation, chronic stricture, and cancer, more likely to perforate than acids
  - —Acid: coagulation necrosis, thermal injury, and dehydration causing perforation, ulceration, and infection
- Large pressure differences between thorax and intraabdominal cavity may lead to lacerations or perforation
- Perforation: penetrating trauma, foreign bodies, instrumentation, may lead to mediastinitis, sepsis, shock, and death
- Mallory-Weiss syndrome: longitudinal tears in distal esophagus with bleeding (see Mallory-Weiss Syndrome)
- Boerhaave's syndrome: rupture of distal esophagus, classically after alcohol or large meals and vomiting (see Boerhaave's Syndrome)

ETIOLOGY

External Forces or Agents (30%)

- Penetrating: stab wounds, missile wounds
- Blunt: motor vehicle accident
- Caustic ingestions/burns: acid pH <2, alkali pH >12
- Swallowed foreign bodies: coins, bones, buttons, marbles, pins, button batteries
- Food bolus impaction: meat most common

Iatrogenic (55%)

- Perforation secondary to instrumentation
- Endoscopy: most common
- Nasotracheal intubation/nasogastric tube: most common in ED

Increased Gastric Pressure (15%)

- Mallory-Weiss syndrome
- Boerhaave's syndrome (spontaneous esophageal rupture)

PEDIATRIC CONSIDERATIONS

- Account for 75–80% of swallowed foreign bodies, typically 18–48 months
- Entrapment usually at upper esophageal sphincter

Pre-Hospital

CAUTIONS

- Chest pain should be presumed cardiac until proven otherwise
- Airway protection, frequent suctioning
- IV crystalloid if patient hypotensive, vomiting, or if hematemesis present

Diagnosis

ESSENTIAL WORKUP

- High level of suspicion and early diagnosis are the keys
  - —Mortality <5% for perforation if repaired within 24 hours; 75% if delayed
- History of ingestions (type, time, amount)
- EKG in patients with chest pain

LABORATORY

- CBC in cases of GI bleeding
- Coagulation studies
- Electrolytes for protracted vomiting or prolonged foreign body retention

IMAGING/SPECIAL TESTS

- CXR for foreign body or perforation (pneumomediastinum, widened mediastinum, pneumothorax, or pleural effusion)
- Lateral C-spine films, for foreign body or perforation (retropharyngeal air or fluid, cervical emphysema)
- Fiberoptic nasopharyngoscopy for foreign body removal
- Esophagram for foreign bodies or suspected perforation (10–25% false-negative rate), current recommendations for water soluble first if perforation likely
  - —Barium may limit visibility for later endoscopy, more irritating if extravasates into mediastinum
  - —Water-soluble contrast provides better visibility, less reaction if extravasates into mediastinum, may cause chemical pneumonitis if aspirated
  - —Nonionic contrast may be safest, but more expensive
- Endoscopy for suspected perforation: operator dependent

DIFFERENTIAL DIAGNOSIS

Pulmonary

- Tracheal injury
- Pneumothorax

Cardiovascular

- Myocardial infarction
- Aortic dissection
- Spontaneous pneumomediastinum

Other Esophageal Emergencies

- Peptic stricture
- Esophageal neoplasm
- Schatzki's ring
- Diverticula
- Achalasia
- Diffuse esophageal spasm
- Nutcracker esophagus
- Gastroesophageal reflux
- Esophagitis

Treatment

INITIAL STABILIZATION

- ABCs, IV access, monitoring
- Airway protection
- Early intubation for penetrating neck and chest wounds
- Frequent suctioning of copious secretions
- Fluid replacement

ED TREATMENT

Foreign Bodies/Food Impaction

- 80% pass, 20% need endoscopy, 1% need surgery
- Glucagon may be tried
- Nitroglycerin or nifedipine may be tried
- Carbonated beverages may be tried
- Valium may be of benefit for foreign bodies in the upper (striated muscle) esophagus
- GI consultation and endoscopic extraction

Ingestions

- Emesis/lavage *contraindicated*
- Immediate decontamination with water or milk
- GI consultation

Tears/Perforations

- Partial-thickness tears usually heal spontaneously
- GI consultation may be needed for diagnosis (endoscopy)
- Perforation requires surgical consultation for thoracotomy and primary repair
- Broad-spectrum parenteral antibiotics for perforation

MEDICATIONS

Foreign Bodies/Food Impactions

- Glucagon: 1–2 mg (peds: 0.02–0.03 mg/kg) i.v.; may repeat once in 20 minutes
- Nifedipine: 10 mg s.l.
- Nitroglycerin: 0.4 mg s.l.
- Valium: 5–10 mg (peds: 1–2 mg) i.v.

Ingestions

- Antibiotics if perforated

Perforation

- Cefoxitin: 1–2 g (peds: 100–160 mg/kg/24 h) i.v. q6–8h
- Gentamicin: 1–1.7 mg/kg (peds: 1.5–2.5 mg/kg/24 h) i.v. q8h

PEDIATRIC CONSIDERATIONS

- Certain swallowed foreign bodies require GI consultation and endoscopic removal
  —Sharp objects: fish bones, straight pins, and razor blades
  —Caustic objects: button batteries
- Other objects may pass on their own if below the lower esophageal sphincter and require follow-up only
  —Coins, buttons, marbles, etc.
  —Open safety pins may pass spontaneously if blunt end forward; consult pediatric GI specialist

Disposition

ADMISSION CRITERIA

- Caustic ingestion
- Sharp foreign bodies
- Airway compromise
- Penetrating neck or chest trauma
- Evidence of sepsis, mediastinitis, or esophageal perforation
- Significant bleeding
- Inability to tolerate oral fluids

DISCHARGE CRITERIA

- Self-limited bleeding from partial-thickness tear
- Foreign body or food impaction that has passed the lower esophageal sphincter

Miscellaneous

ESOPHAGUS INJURY SCALE

I	Contusion/hematoma; partial thickness
II	Laceration $\leq$50% circumference
III	Laceration $>$50% circumference
IV	Segmental loss or devascularization $<$2 cm
V	Segmental loss or devascularization $>$2 cm

ICD9: 862.22; 862.32

ICD10: S27.8, S19.8, S11.2

SEE ALSO: FOREIGN BODY, ESOPHAGEAL; MALLORY-WEISS SYNDROME; BOERHAAVE'S SYNDROME

SUGGESTED READINGS

Richardson JD, et al. Complex thoracic injuries. Surg Clin North Am 1996;76(4):725–748.

Shanmuganathan K. Imaging diagnosis of nonaortic thoracic injury. Radiol Clin North Am 1999;37(3):533–551.

Stack L, Munter D. Foreign bodies in the gastrointestinal tract. Emerg Med Clin North Am 1996;14(3):557–570.

Swann L, Munter D. Esophageal emergencies. Emerg Med Clin North Am 1996;14(3):557–570.

Authors: Adam Thomas; Susan Dufel

Ethylene Glycol, Poisoning

Clinical Presentation

SIGNS AND SYMPTOMS

Cardiovascular

- Tachycardia/bradycardia/other dysrhythmias
- Hypertension/hypotension

Central Nervous System

- Inebriation/irritability
- Ataxia
- Obtundation
- Coma
- Cerebral edema
- Convulsions

GI

- Nausea/vomiting
- Abdominal pain

Pulmonary

- Hyperventilation/tachypnea/Kussmaul's breathing
- Pulmonary edema

Renal

- Acute renal failure
- Costal-vertebral angle tenderness
- Crystalluria

MECHANISM/DESCRIPTION

- Peak levels in 1–4 hours
- Half-life, 2.5–4.5 hours
- $<$20% excreted unmetabolized by the kidneys
- *Three stages* (may be overlap)
  - —First stage
    - -1–12 hours after ingestion
    - -CNS depression
    - -GI symptoms
    - -Worsening acidosis
    - -Coma, convulsions, cerebral edema
    - -Tetany and myoclonus secondary to hypocalcemia
  - —Second stage
    - -12–36 hours after ingestion
    - -Cardiopulmonary symptoms
    - -Most deaths occur
  - —Third stage
    - -36–72 hours after ingestion
    - -Oliguria, flank pain, acute renal failure
    - -Bone marrow suppression and pancytopenia

Pathophysiology

- Metabolized by hepatic alcohol dehydrogenase and aldehyde dehydrogenase ultimately to oxalic acid
  - —Results in aldehyde and acid metabolites
  - —Directly toxic to the CNS, lungs, and kidney
  - —Metabolites inhibit metabolic pathways, including oxidative phosphorylation

ETIOLOGY

- Ethylene glycol-containing products
  - —Antifreeze
  - —Solvents
- Minimum reported lethal dose is 30 mL of 100% ethylene glycol

Pre-Hospital

- Bring containers of all possible ingestants

Diagnosis

ESSENTIAL WORKUP

- History of all substances ingested
- Drawn *simultaneously*
  - —ABGs
  - —Serum ethylene glycol, methanol, isopropyl alcohol, and ethanol levels
  - —Electrolytes, BUN/Cr, glucose
  - —Measured serum osmolality (by freezing point depression)
  - —Serum calcium, phosphorus, magnesium

LABORATORY

- Determine the anion gap
  - —Anion gap = $(Na^+) - (Cl^- + HCO_3^-)$
  - —Normal anion gap is 8–12
- Determine osmol gap
  - —Osmol gap = measured osmolality − calculated osmolarity
  - —Calculated osmolarity = $2\,(Na^+)$ + glucose/18 + BUN/2.8 + ethanol (in mg/dL)/4.6
  - —Calculated to screen for ethylene glycol ingestion because toxic alcohol levels are not commonly available in a timely manner from most clinical laboratories
  - —Most useful early in the course of ethylene glycol poisoning or with concurrent ethanol ingestion
  - —With concurrent ethanol ingestion, osmol gap tends to be larger and acidosis tends to be less severe because relatively less ethylene glycol has been converted to acid-producing metabolites
  - —Increased osmol gap: $>$10
  - —Normal osmol gap does not rule out ethylene glycol ingestion
- Ethylene glycol level
- Ethanol level
  - —Measured to determine the amount of ethanol bolus necessary to attain a therapeutic level
- Urinalysis
  - —Envelope-shaped oxalate crystals: an insensitive but specific finding
  - —Ketones may be due to isopropyl alcohol ingestion, starvation, or DKA

IMAGING/SPECIAL TESTS

- Wood's lamp inspection of urine or gastric contents
  - —Detects the presence of fluorescein, a common antifreeze additive
  - —Insensitive but specific marker of antifreeze ingestion

DIFFERENTIAL DIAGNOSIS

- Increased osmol gap: *ME DIE A*
  - —*M*ethanol
  - —*E*thanol
  - —*D*iuretics (mannitol, glycerin, sorbitol)
  - —*I*sopropyl alcohol
  - —*E*thylene glycol
  - —*A*cetone, ammonia
- Elevated anion gap metabolic acidosis: *ACAT MUDPILES*
  - —*A*lcoholic ketoacidosis
  - —*C*yanide, CO, H_2S, others
  - —*A*SA, other salicylates
  - —*T*oluene
  - —*M*ethanol, metformin
  - —*U*remia
  - —*D*iabetic ketoacidosis
  - —*P*araldehyde, phenformin
  - —*I*ron, INH
  - —*L*actic acidosis from other causes
  - —*E*thylene glycol
  - —*S*tarvation ketosis

Treatment

INITIAL STABILIZATION

- ABCs
- Supplemental oxygen, cardiac monitor, secured IV with 0.9% NS
- D50W (or Accucheck), naloxone, and thiamine for altered mental status

ED TREATMENT

Prevent Further Ethylene Glycol Absorption

- Gastric lavage with NGT
  - —If $<$1 hour since ingestion, if the patient is in a coma, or if history of a large ingestion
- Ipecac contraindicated
- Initial dose of activated charcoal for potential co-ingestants, but unlikely to help if only ethylene glycol
  - —Activated charcoal poorly adsorbs ethylene glycol

Prevent Ethylene Glycol Conversion to Toxic Metabolites

- 4-Methylpyrazole (4-MP, Antizol)
  - —Initiate before the ethylene glycol level returns if
    - -Accidental ingestion greater than a sip or intentional ingestion
    - -Altered mental status associated with an unexplained osmol gap or elevated anion gap acidosis
  - —Competitive inhibitor of alcohol dehydrogenase
  - —Disadvantages over ethanol
    - -More expensive
  - —Advantages over ethanol
    - -Easy dosing
    - -No need for continuous infusion
    - -No inebriation/CNS depression
    - -No hypoglycemia, no hyponatremia, no hyperosmolality
    - -Not necessary to check ethanol levels
    - -Reduction in degree of nursing care and monitoring
- Ethanol therapy
  - —Initiate before the ethylene glycol level returns if a potentially toxic ingestion suspected
  - —Ethanol: greater affinity than ethylene glycol for alcohol dehydrogenase
  - —Slows conversion to toxic metabolites
  - —Indications
    - -History of accidental ethylene glycol ingestion of greater than a sip or intentional ethylene glycol ingestion
    - -Altered mental status associated with an unexplained osmol gap or elevated anion gap metabolic acidosis
  - —Goal: serum ethanol level of 100–150 mg/dL
  - —Continue ethanol therapy until the ethylene glycol level is zero

Enhance Elimination

- Hemodialysis
  - —Decreases the elimination half-life of ethylene glycol and removes toxic metabolites
  - —Indications
    - -Severe acidosis or osmol gap, no ethylene glycol levels, and clinical suspicion of a significant ingestion
    - -Persistent electrolyte or fluid disturbance
    - -Renal insufficiency
    - -Pulmonary edema
    - -Cerebral edema
    - -Serum ethylene glycol level >25–50 mg/dL
  - —Continue hemodialysis until ethylene glycol level approaches zero
- Administer thiamine, pyridoxine, and magnesium
  - —Thiamine, pyridoxine, and magnesium are cofactors in the metabolism of ethylene glycol that may promote the conversion to nontoxic metabolites
  - —No human data supporting this theory

Correct Secondary Disorders

- Ensure adequate urine output via IV fluids
- Sodium bicarbonate therapy for acidemia with pH <7.1
- Monitor/replace calcium
  - —Deposition of calcium into tissues can result in hypocalcemia

MEDICATIONS

- Activated charcoal: 1 g/kg PO
- Dextrose: D50W 1 ampule (50 mL or 25 g) (peds: D25W 2–4 mL/kg) i.v.
- Ethanol
  - —Oral: 50% ethanol solution (100 proof liquor) via NGT
    - -Loading dose: 1.5 mL/kg
    - -Maintenance dose: 0.2–0.4 mL/kg/h
    - -Maintenance dose during hemodialysis: 0.4–0.7 mL/kg/h
  - —IV: 10% ethanol in D5W
    - -Loading dose: 7.5 mL/kg over 30–60 minutes
    - -Maintenance infusion: 1–2 mL/kg/h
    - -Maintenance infusion during hemodialysis: 2–3.5 mL/kg/h
- 4-MP
  - —Loading dose: 15 mg/kg slow infusion over 30 minutes
  - —Maintenance dose: 10 mg/kg q12h for four doses, then 15 mg/kg q12h until ethylene glycol levels reduced to <20 mg/dL
  - —Dosing related to hemodialysis
    - -Do not administer a dose at the beginning of dialysis if the last dose was <6 hours previously
    - -Administer the next dose if the last dose was >6 hours previously
    - -Dose every 4 hours during dialysis
    - -If the time between the last dose and the end of dialysis was <1 hour from last dose, do not administer a new dose
    - -If the time between the last dose and the end of dialysis was 1–3 hours from last dose, administer one half of next scheduled dose
    - -If the time between the last dose and the end of dialysis was >3 hours from last dose, administer next scheduled dose
- Naloxone: 2 mg (peds: 0.1 mg/kg) i.v. or i.m. initial dose
- Pyridoxine: 100 mg/d × 2 days
- Sodium bicarbonate: 1–2 mEq/kg in D5 i.v.
- Thiamine: 100 mg (peds: 50 mg) i.v. or i.m. per day × 2 days

PEDIATRIC CONSIDERATIONS

- Measure fingerstick glucose hourly to monitor for ethanol-induced hypoglycemia
- Monitor serum chemistry for hyponatremia if on ethanol drip

Disposition

ADMISSION CRITERIA

- All patients with significant ethylene glycol ingestion even if initially asymptomatic
- ICU admission for seriously ill patients
- Transfer to another facility if hemodialysis or MP is indicated but not readily available

DISCHARGE CRITERIA

- Asymptomatic patient with isolated ethylene glycol ingestion if the serum ethylene glycol level is undetectable

Miscellaneous

ICD9: 982.8

ICD10: T52.8

SUGGESTED READINGS

Barceloux D, Krenzelok E, Olson K, et al. American academy of clinical toxicology, practice, guidelines on the treatment of ethylene glycol poisoning. J Toxicol Clin Toxicol 1999;37(5):537–560.

Brent J, McMartin K, Phillips S, et al. Fomepizole for the treatment of ethylene glycol poisoning. N Engl J Med 1999;340:832–838.

Ford M, McMartin K. Ethylene glycol and methanol. In: Ford M, Delaney K, Ling I, et al, eds. Clinical toxicology, 1st ed. Philadelphia: WB Saunders, 2001: 757–767.

Leikin J, Paloucek F. Ethylene glycol. Alcohol. Fomepizole. In: Leikin and Paloucek's poisoning and toxicology handbook, 3rd ed. Lexicomp, Inc, 2002:556–557, 201–202, 599–600.

Author: Kirk Cumpston

External Ear Chondritis/Abscess

Clinical Presentation

SIGNS AND SYMPTOMS

- Initially a dull pain that increases in severity
- Pinna
  —Painful
  —Exquisite tenderness
  —Erythematous
  —Warmth
  —Loss of contours caused by edema often with sparing of the lobule
- Increase of the auriculocephalic angle
- Fluctuant areas develop with eventual breakdown and suppuration
- Entire ear involvement if untreated
  —Disfigurement can occur
- Fever
- Chills

MECHANISM/DESCRIPTION

- Inflammation and infection of the pinna
- Cartilage of the external ear is easily damaged due to
  —Lack of overlying SC tissue
  —Relative avascularity
  —Exposed position
- Chondritis
  —Most commonly a secondary complication of otic trauma and burns
  —Onset often insidious and may be delayed until apparent healing has occurred
- Disfiguration of the pinna occurs without proper treatment
  —Ranges from being shriveled, cauliflower-like ear to complete loss of the external ear and possible stenosis of the auditory meatus

ETIOLOGY

- Common causes of chondritis include
  —Chemical or thermal burns
  —Frostbite
  —Hematoma formation
  —Mastoid surgery
  —Human bites
  —Deep abrasions
  —External otitis
  —High piercing of the ear lobe
- Bacteria involved
  —*Pseudomonas aeruginosa*
  —Staphylococcus
  —Proteus

Pre-Hospital

N/A

Diagnosis

ESSENTIAL WORKUP

- Clinical diagnosis
  —Typical physical findings in combination with aforementioned causes

LABORATORY

- Blood culture if systemic signs of infection

DIFFERENTIAL DIAGNOSIS

N/A

Treatment

INITIAL STABILIZATION

N/A

ED TREATMENT

Antibiotics

- Oral antibiotics for minor cases of early ear lobe inflammation
  - —Ciprofloxacin preferred (older than 18 years)
  - —First-generation cephalosporin or dicloxacillin
- IV antibiotics for severe infection
- Apply topical antibiotics when break in skin barrier

ENT Consult

- For chondritis, abscess, and necrosis of the involved cartilage
- Early surgical drainage for chondritis
- Aggressive early management may prevent gross ear deformity

General Postinjury Preventive Measures

- Prevention of chondritis is of the utmost importance
  - —Difficult management and disfiguring potential
- Avoid pressure to the injured ear
- Minimize active débridement of eschars and crusts
- Gentle washing twice daily with antibacterial soap and water followed by complete drying and application of topical antibiotics
- Keep hair away from the ear

MEDICATIONS

- Cephalexin: 500 mg (peds: 50 mg/kg/d) PO q.i.d.
- Ciprofloxacin: 500 mg PO b.i.d. (adult)
- Dicloxacillin: 500 mg (peds: 25 mg/kg/d) PO q.i.d.

Disposition

ADMISSION CRITERIA

- Parenteral antibiotics and early surgical drainage for patients with chondritis
- Edema, erythema, and significant ear tenderness
- Toxic patient with fever and chills
- Immunocompromised patient
- Unreliable patient or caretaker

DISCHARGE CRITERIA

- Stable patient without systemic signs with close ENT follow-up

Miscellaneous

ICD9: 733.99

ICD10: H60.0, M94.8

SUGGESTED READINGS

Bentrem DJ, Bill TJ, Himel HN, et al. Chondritis of the ear: a late sequela of deep partial thickness burns of the face. J Emerg Med 1996;14:469–471.

More DR, Seidel JS, Bryan PA. Ear-piercing techniques as a cause of auricular chondritis. Pediatr Emerg Care 1999;15(3): 189–192.

Staley R, Fitzgibbon JJ, Anderson C. Auricular infections caused by high ear piercing in adolescents. Pediatrics 1997;99:610–611.

Author: Assaad J. Sayah

Extremity Trauma, Penetrating

Clinical Presentation

SIGNS AND SYMPTOMS

- Entry and exit wound (if present), lacerations
- High muzzle-velocity gunshot wounds produce a shockwave that results in significant tissue injury
  - —Often exit wound demonstrates more tissue damage than entrance wound
- Vascular injury
  - —Arterial injury is indicated by decreased or absent distal pulse, distal ischemic changes, expanding hematoma, bruit, or thrill over the injury
  - —The presence of a distal pulse does not exclude a proximal vascular injury
- Neurologic injury
  - —Paresthesias, decreased or absent motor function, or sensation distal to the injury
- Musculoskeletal injury
  - —Visible deformity
  - —Ligamentous laxity in joints adjacent to the injury suggests tendon injury
  - —An effusion in an adjacent joint indicates fracture or ligamentous injury
- Compartment syndrome
  - —Suggested by severe and constant pain over the involved compartment
  - —Pain on active and passive extension or flexion of the distal extremity
  - —Weakness, pain on palpation of the compartment, and hypesthesia of the nerves in the compartment
  - —Pulselessness and pallor are late findings

Pre-Hospital

CAUTIONS

- Control hemorrhage with direct digital pressure over site
- Elevate extremity
- Evaluate neurovascular status
- Leave impaled objects in place and stabilize in current position

Diagnosis

ESSENTIAL WORKUP

History

- Mechanism of injury (stab, puncture, gunshot, laceration, bite, high-pressure injection injury)
- Age of wound
- Circumstances of wounding (assault, self-inflicted wound, domestic abuse)
- Comorbid conditions (immunosuppression, diabetes, valvular heart disease, asplenia, peripheral vascular disease)

Physical Examination

- Note location, length, depth, and shape of the primary wound and the exit wound, if present
- Vascular injury
  - —Compare distal pulses by palpation and with Doppler study
  - —Assess capillary refill: abnormal if >2 seconds
  - —Ankle-brachial index (ABI): take BP in calf and arm (involved extremity); a systolic pressure difference of >10 mm Hg suggests vascular injury
  - —Expanding hematoma, bruit, or thrill over the injury also indicates vascular injury
- Neurologic injury
  - —Assess distal motor function and sensory function (two-point discrimination, light touch, proprioception)
- Musculoskeletal injury
  - —Note associated crush, tendon, or ligamentous injury and bony deformity
  - —Examine adjacent joints for range of motion
  - —Assess for compartment syndrome
- Explore the wound for *foreign body*

LABORATORY

- Culture of acute wounds is not indicated
- Wounds with signs of infection may be cultured to guide antibiotic choice

IMAGING/SPECIAL TESTS

- X-ray to evaluate for radiopaque foreign body or underlying fracture; at minimum AP and lateral views
- Radiolucent foreign bodies may be located by fluoroscopy, US, or CT
- Arteriogram is indicated when vascular injury is suspected and immediate vascular surgery is not required

DIFFERENTIAL DIAGNOSIS

N/A

Treatment

INITIAL STABILIZATION

- ABCs of trauma care
- Expose the wound completely and remove constricting clothing or jewelry
- Control hemorrhage with direct pressure
- Blind clamping within the wound and prolonged tourniquet use are not recommended

ED TREATMENT

- Pain control
- Complete neurologic assessment before local anesthesia
- Prolonged soaking of wounds, particularly with cytotoxic agents, is *not* recommended
- Remove any visible debris and débride devitalized tissue
- Most important is copious high-pressure irrigation with saline
- Tetanus prophylaxis
- Stab wounds and gunshot wounds should receive a single dose of cefazolin in the ED
- Immobilize the extremity if there is suspicion of significant vascular injury, tendon injury, fracture, or joint violation
- Loss of pulse or distal ischemia requires emergent surgery
  - —Do not delay surgical management for arteriogram
- Lacerations may be closed if they have been adequately cleaned, have minimal tissue loss, and are seen within 6–8 hours of injury
  - —Delayed primary closure is an alternative for older or contaminated wounds
- Puncture or gunshot wounds should *not* be closed primarily

Special Considerations

- Plantar puncture wounds
  - —Examine the wound carefully under bright light, remove any foreign material, and clean the wound carefully; coring the wound is controversial and should be reserved for removal of devitalized tissue or imbedded debris
  - —Probing or high-pressure irrigation of a puncture wound will only force particulate matter further into the wound
  - —Prophylactic antibiotics are not recommended (unless the patient is diabetic or immunocompromised)
  - —Close follow-up is necessary to assess for smoldering infection from an unseen foreign body that if not treated with aggressive débridement can lead to osteomyelitis
- High-pressure injuries of the hand
  - —Orthopedic evaluation in the ED is essential because wounds that appear trivial on the surface may have the product that was being sprayed track up the tendon sheaths into more proximal aspects of the hand

MEDICATIONS

- Tetanus prophylaxis: TD 0.5 mL i.m.
- Wounds more than 12 hours old, especially of the hands and lower extremities, crush wounds with devitalized tissue, contaminated wounds
  - —Cefazolin: 1 g i.v./i.m. (peds: 20–40 mg/kg i.m./i.v. single dose in the ED)
  - —Cephalexin: 500 mg PO q.i.d. (peds: 25–50 mg/kg/d q.i.d. × 7 days *or*
  - -Amoxicillin/clavulanate: 875/125 mg PO b.i.d. (peds: 25 mg/kg/d b.i.d. × 7 days
  - —Erythromycin: 333 mg PO t.i.d. (peds: 40 mg/kg/d q6h × 7 days)
- Contaminated wounds in patients with preexisting valvular heart disease
  - —Cefazolin: 1 g i.m./i.v., then cephalexin, 500 mg PO q.i.d. × 7 days
  - —If penicillin allergic
  - —EES: 800 mg PO, then 400 mg PO q6h × 7 days *or*
  - -Clindamycin: 300 mg PO q6h × 7 days

Disposition

ADMISSION CRITERIA

- Emergent surgical consultation and admission are required for any penetrating wounds with potential for vascular compromise, with associated compartment syndrome, and with joint penetration
- High muzzle-velocity penetrating gunshot wounds
- Diabetic or immunocompromised patients with contaminated wounds

DISCHARGE CRITERIA

- Penetrating extremity injuries not requiring surgical intervention may be discharged after appropriate wound care with instructions to elevate the extremity, keep the wound clean, and to return for recheck in 24–48 hours or for any signs of infection

Miscellaneous

ICD9: 959.8

SUGGESTED READINGS

American College of Emergency Physicians. Clinical policy for the initial approach to patients presenting with penetrating extremity trauma. Ann Emerg Med 1994;23:1147–1156.

Haverstock BD, Grossman JP. Puncture wounds of the foot. Evaluation and treatment. Clin Podiatr Med Surg 1999;16(4):583–596.

Schnall SB, Mirzayan R. High pressure injuries to the hand. Hand Clin 1999; 15(2):245–248.

Author: Gary M. Vilke

Facial Fractures

Clinical Presentation

SIGNS AND SYMPTOMS

- Most posttraumatic deformities of the face represent underlying fractures
- Pain, swelling, ecchymosis and deformity
- CSF rhinorrhea, facial hemorrhage, epistaxis, raccoon eyes
- Facial anesthesia represents nerve entrapment or injury
- Associated injuries are common, including teeth, mandible, eye, tear duct, skull, and neck
- A bluish fluid-filled sac overlying the nasal septum is a septal hematoma and is critical to detect

MECHANISM/DESCRIPTION

- Typically blunt trauma from motor vehicle accidents (MVAs), direct blows, or falls
- Physical assault and domestic violence
- Open fractures are common
- Le Fort fractures involve the maxilla and are classified as
  —Le Fort I: transverse fracture of the maxilla below the nose but above the teeth through the lateral wall of the maxillary sinus to the lateral pterygoid plate
  —Le Fort II: pyramidal fracture from the nasal and ethmoid bones through the zygomaticomaxillary suture and the maxilla, often involving the maxillary sinuses and the infraorbital rims
  —Le Fort III: craniofacial disjunction with elongated, flattened face, due to fractures through the frontozygomatic suture, orbit, base of the nose, and ethmoid bone
  —Le Fort IV: includes the frontal bone in addition to Le Fort III

ETIOLOGY

- Zygomatic arch fractures often occur in two to three places and can involve the orbit and maxilla (tripod fracture)
- Inner plate frontal sinus fractures are associated with CSF leaks and ocular injuries

PEDIATRIC CONSIDERATIONS

- Maxillofacial fractures are rarely seen in children younger than 6 years, suspect nonaccidental trauma
- Falls and MVAs account for most cases
- There is a higher incidence of associated head injury

Pre-Hospital

CAUTIONS

- Airway control takes precedence
  —Severe facial fractures may preclude the use of oral intubation
    -Nasotracheal intubation is contraindicated in massive facial or nasal trauma
    -Cricothyrotomy is the airway of choice if intubation using RSI cannot be performed
- If associated injuries are present, protect the C spine

Diagnosis

ESSENTIAL WORKUP

- Immediately assess the airway
- The physical exam is the most important aspect
  —Palpate the entire face, looking for tenderness, step-offs, depressions, and crepitance; check for mandibular injuries or malocclusion
  —Perform a nasal speculum exam looking for blood, septal hematoma, or CSF leak
  —Assess for areas of facial anesthesia
  —Careful eye exam including funduscopic exam, obtain a visual acuity
    -Look for telecanthus (intercanthal width >30–35 mm), which can indicate a nasofrontoethmoid fracture
- Le Fort fractures are assessed by placing the thumb of index finger of one hand on the bridge of the nose and pulling the upper teeth with the other hand
  —Le Fort I: movement of the hard palate and maxillary dentition only (your hand on the nose will not feel movement)
  —Le Fort II: movement of the hard palate, maxillary dentition, and nose (your hand on the nose will feel movement)
  —Le Fort III: movement of the entire midface

IMAGING/SPECIAL TESTS

- CT scanning is the imaging modality of choice for complex facial injuries
- Obtain x-rays of any area of tenderness, crepitance, depression, or deformity, with the exception of isolated nasal injuries
- A Water's view is a good screening exam; Caldwell and lateral facial films are less helpful
  —These views may show fractures, asymmetry, or blood in the sinuses
- Jug-handle views (submental vertex) may be needed to view zygomatic arch fractures

DIFFERENTIAL DIAGNOSIS

- Nasal fracture
- Zygoma fractures (arch or tripod fracture)
- Le Fort fracture
- Skull fractures including frontal sinus fractures and cribriform plate fractures
- Nasofrontoethmoid complex fractures
- Mandibular fractures
- Associated injuries to teeth, neck, brain
- Contusions or lacerations without underlying fractures

PEDIATRIC CONSIDERATIONS

- Sedation with diazepam or midazolam may be needed to perform an adequate exam (sedate with caution if there is a head injury)

Treatment

INITIAL STABILIZATION

- *Aggressively manage the airway:* RSI is the initial airway management of choice in massive facial injuries; use etomidate or midazolam (or ketamine in children) and vecuronium or succinylcholine for RSI
- Surgical airway (cricothyroidotomy or needle cricothyroidotomy) may be required if RSI is unsuccessful
- Nasotracheal intubation is contraindicated in most facial fractures
- Protect the C spine until clinically or radiographically cleared
- Once the airway is secure, other major injuries take precedence over facial injuries
- Bleeding may be difficult to control and may require posterior packing if direct pressure does not work

ED TREATMENT

- Consult ENT, plastic surgery, or oral surgery for operative repair of complex fractures including all Le Fort fractures and frontal sinus fractures involving the posterior table
- Antibiotics (cefazolin or clindamycin in penicillin allergic patients) are indicated for open fractures and CSF leak
- Tetanus prophylaxis
- Parenteral pain medication (morphine, meperidine, or fentanyl)
- A septal hematoma must be drained in the ED
  —Anesthetize, aspirate with an 18–20-gauge needle, and pack both nares with Vaseline gauze to prevent reaccumulation
  —Discharge on amoxicillin or erythromycin with recheck in 3–5 days by ENT
- Nondisplaced zygomatic fractures can be discharged with analgesics (acetaminophen or ibuprofen); refer displaced zygoma and tripod fractures that are otherwise stable for outpatient reduction in 2–3 days after swelling is reduced
- Overlying lacerations with simple fractures can be sutured in the ED, if discharged, treat with amoxicillin or erythromycin

MEDICATIONS

- Acetaminophen: 650 mg (peds: 10–15 mg/kg) PO q4h
- Amoxicillin: 250 mg (peds: 30–50 mg/kg/24 h) PO q8h
- Cefazolin: 1 g (peds: 50–100 mg/kg/24 h) i.v. or i.m.
- Clindamycin: 600–900 mg (peds: 25–40 mg/kg/24 h) PO q8h
- Diazepam: 5–10 mg (peds: 0.1–0.2 mg/kg) i.v.
- Erythromycin: 500 mg (peds: 30–50 mg/kg/24 h) PO q.i.d.
- Etomidate: 0.2–0.3 mg/kg (peds: 0.2–0.3 mg/kg) i.v.
- Fentanyl: 2–10 μg/kg (peds: 2–3 μg/kg) i.v.
- Ibuprofen: 600–800 mg (peds: 20–40 mg/kg/24 h) PO t.i.d. to q.i.d.
- Ketamine: 2 mg/kg (peds: 1–2 mg/kg) i.v.
- Meperidine: 1–2 mg/kg (peds: 1–2 mg/kg) i.v. q1–4h titrated
- Midazolam: 2–5 mg (peds: safety not established but 0.02–0.05 mg/kg/dose has been used) i.v.
- Morphine sulfate: 0.1–0.2 mg/kg (peds: 0.1–0.2 mg/kg) i.v. q1–4h titrated
- Succinylcholine: 1–1.5 mg/kg (peds: 1–2 mg/kg) i.v.
- Vecuronium: 0.1–0.3 mg/kg (peds: 0.1–0.3 mg/kg) i.v.

PEDIATRIC CONSIDERATIONS

- Surgical cricothyroidotomy should not be performed in children younger than 8 years
  —Needle cricothyroidotomy with jet ventilation may be performed
- Children are at high risk of associated injuries
- Definitive repair of facial fractures should not be delayed more than 3–4 days because of the rapid healing of facial fractures and the risk of malunion and cosmetic deformity

Disposition

ADMISSION CRITERIA

- Significant associated trauma
- Airway compromise
- Le Fort II and III fractures
- CSF leak
- Posterior table frontal sinus fractures
- Most open fractures excluding simple nasal fractures with lacerations

DISCHARGE CRITERIA

- No evidence of significant head, neck, or other injuries
- Closed fractures of the zygoma or anterior table of the frontal sinus with appropriate follow-up in 24–36 hours
- Septal hematomas that have been drained in the ED require follow-up in 24 hours

PEDIATRIC CONSIDERATIONS

- Consult child protective services for any suspicion of nonaccidental trauma
- Fibrous union begins in only 3–4 days; early referral for repair is indicated

Miscellaneous

ICD9: 801.1, 802.4

ICD10: S02.9

SUGGESTED READINGS

Druelinger L, Guenther M, Marchand EG. Radiographic evaluation of the facial complex. Emerg Med Clin North Am 2000;18:393–410.

Ellis E, Scott K. Assessment of patients with facial fractures. Emerg Med Clin North Am 2000;18:411–447.

Hunter JG. Pediatric maxillofacial trauma. Pediatr Clin North Am 1992;39:1127–1143.

Iiada S, Koso M, Sugivia T, et al. Retrospective analysis of 1502 patients with facial fractures. Int J Oral Maxillofac Surg 2001;30:286–290.

Olucciello SA, Sternbach G, Walker SB. The treacherous and complex spectrum of maxillofacial trauma: etiologies, evaluation, and emergency stabilization. Emerg Med Rep 1995;16:59–69.

Author: David W. Munter

Failure to Thrive

Clinical Presentation

SIGNS AND SYMPTOMS

- Failure to achieve or maintain a growth rate appropriate for age
  - —Fall off in growth across two major growth percentile lines in a short time (e.g., from seventy-fifth to twenty-fifth percentile), reflecting a change in the velocity of growth
- Calorie or protein deprivation initially results in weight loss, followed by impaired linear and head circumference growth
- Muscle wasting of extremities with redundant hanging skin
- Temporal wasting
- Alopecia
- Edema
- Developmental delays common in infants, particularly if failure to thrive (FTT) occurs in first few months of life

MECHANISM/DESCRIPTION

- Inadequate nourishment
  - —Poor GI function
  - —Most common cause
- Acute or chronic disease
- Psychosocial issues
  - —May be contributory

ETIOLOGY

- Multifactorial

See Differential Diagnosis

Pre-Hospital

N/A

Diagnosis

ESSENTIAL WORKUP

- Complete history and physical
  - —Birth history including perinatal illnesses, drug exposures, prenatal care, and hereditary illnesses in family
  - —Growth records and plotted growth curves for height, weight, head circumference
  - —History of feeding behavior, patterns, and developmental milestones
  - —Observation of family–child interactivity
  - —Examination for any congenital abnormalities
  - —Evidence of poor hygiene or inappropriate childhood socialization

LABORATORY

- CBC and ESR
  - —Infections
  - —Anemia
  - —Lead poisoning
  - —Malignancy
- Chemistry panel (electrolytes, BUN, creatinine, glucose, liver function, protein, albumin, calcium, phosphate, magnesium)
  - —Hydration and acidosis
  - —Metabolic disorders
  - —Diabetes mellitus
- Urinalysis with culture
  - —Renal disease
  - —Infection

IMAGING/SPECIAL TESTS

- Reducing substances for inborn metabolic errors
- Lead level
- Tuberculin test
- EKG
- HIV test
- Skeletal survey for nonaccidental trauma
- Bone radiographs for infection, metabolic, and hereditary or acquired bone disease; bone age of wrist

DIFFERENTIAL DIAGNOSIS

Organic Causes

- Congenital
  - —Congenital syndromes
  - —Chromosomal abnormalities
  - —Congenital heart disease
  - —Inborn errors of metabolism
- GI
  - —Malabsorption syndromes (celiac disease, lactose intolerance, cystic fibrosis)
  - —Inflammatory bowel disease
  - —Hepatobiliary disease (hepatitis, cirrhosis)
  - —Obstructive disease (pyloric stenosis, Hirschsprung's disease)
  - —Gastroesophageal reflux
  - —Pancreatic insufficiency

- Hematologic
  - —Sickle cell anemia
  - —Iron deficiency anemia
  - —Thalassemia
- Cardiopulmonary
  - —Acquired heart disease
  - —Chronic lung disease (asthma, bronchopulmonary dysplasia)
- Renal
  - —Chronic renal insufficiency
  - —Renal tubular acidosis
  - —Renal failure
- Immunologic
  - —Severe combined immunodeficiency
  - —AIDS
  - —DiGeorge syndrome
  - —Food allergies
- Endocrine
  - —Diabetes mellitus
  - —Thyroid/parathyroid disease
  - —Adrenal disease
  - —Growth hormone deficiency
  - —Hypopituitarism
- Neurologic
  - —Degenerative disorders
  - —Cerebral palsy
  - —Oral-motor dysfunction
  - —Mental retardation
  - —Brain tumors
- Infections
  - —Tuberculosis
  - —Parasite
  - —Chronic urinary tract infection
  - —Chronic sinusitis
  - —Recurrent tonsillitis/adenoiditis
- Orthopedic
  - —Rickets
  - —Osteogenesis imperfecta
  - —Chondrodystrophies
- Toxic
  - —Fetal exposure to alcohol/drugs
  - —Hypervitaminosis
  - —Lead or mercury poisoning

Nonorganic Causes

- Parent-child dysfunction
  - —Mother-infant bonding problems
  - —Maternal mental illness/substance abuse
  - —Inexperienced mother
  - —Absent caretaker
  - —Breast-feeding difficulties
  - —Improper formula preparation
  - —Chaotic family environment
  - —Developmental delay
  - —Child abuse or neglect
  - —Munchausen syndrome by proxy

Treatment

INITIAL STABILIZATION

- Check for hypoglycemia
- Fluid resuscitation when dehydrated
- Begin gradual correction of electrolyte abnormalities
- Supportive environment

ED TREATMENT

- Recognize/identify child with FTT
- Rule out organic abnormalities
- Social services consult
- Admission to hospital for multidisciplinary team evaluation and teaching and nourishment

Disposition

ADMISSION CRITERIA

- Any child who has fallen across two major growth percentiles unless already under treatment for identified cause
- Child abuse/neglect
- Child younger than 1 year old with severe FTT
- Severe dehydration, malnutrition, or electrolyte imbalance are at risk of refeeding syndrome and should be hospitalized
- Hyperalimentation need

DISCHARGE CRITERIA

- Outpatient care for mild FTT when good extended follow-up with involved primary care practitioner available and supportive family
- Physiologically stable with satisfactory evaluation by physician and social or child services
- When alternative custody arrangement available in cases of severe abuse or neglect or where danger is still present in home environment
- Referral to appropriate subspecialist when medical cause discovered

Miscellaneous

ICD9: 783.4

ICD10: R62.8

SUGGESTED READINGS

Bithoney WG, Dubowitz H, Egan H. Failure to thrive/growth deficiency. Pediatr Rev 1992;13:453–460.

Gahagan S, Holmes R. A stepwise approach to evaluation of undernutrition and failure to thrive. Pediatr Clin North Am 1998;45(1):169–187.

Maggioni A, Lifshitz F. Nutritional management of failure to thrive. Pediatr Clin North Am 1995;42:791–810.

Author: Jeffrey Proudfoot

Fatigue

Clinical Presentation

SIGNS AND SYMPTOMS

- Perception of being physically, intellectually, or emotionally exhausted
- Occurs with or without objective findings on physical exam
- Focal or generalized motor weakness may accompany fatigue
- Typically persists even after resting
- May present as subjective weakness, tiredness, exhaustion, or decreased energy level
- May be associated with multiple nonspecific symptoms

MECHANISM/DESCRIPTION

Localized Motor Fatigue

- Deconditioning of nerves or muscle results in loss of function
- Localized muscular fatigue occurs after overuse or trauma to a muscle group

Generalized Fatigue

- Infection and immunologic mechanisms
  - —Increase cytokines, inflammation, and immunoglobulin complexes
- Endocrine disorders
  - —Alter metabolic status hydration, and electrolyte balance
- Neoplastic disease
  - —Alter chemical and cellular mediators
- Drugs
  - —Cause electrolyte disturbances
  - —Decreased sympathetic tone or energy uncoupling
- Nutritional deficiency
  - —Produces catabolism
- Psychiatric disorders
  - —Produce imbalances in neurotransmitters
- Chronic fatigue syndrome (CFS)
  - —Associated with abnormalities in the reticular activating system

Pre-Hospital

CAUTIONS

- Apply cardiac monitor
- Insert IV catheter
- Administer oxygen for patient with or suspected to have low oxygen saturation
- Perform Accu-Chek and administer glucose for hypoglycemia

Diagnosis

ESSENTIAL WORKUP

- Thorough history to include
  - —Timing, duration, pattern
  - —Exacerbating or mitigating factors
  - —Sleep patterns
  - —Presence of myalgias or arthralgias
  - —Medications
  - —Mood and psychiatric history
  - —Activity patterns
  - —Major life events or changes
  - —Diet, appetite, weight loss/gain
  - —Alcohol, tobacco, caffeine use
  - —Medications
  - —Full review of systems
- CFS is clinical diagnosis
  - —Persistent or relapsing fatigue >6 months
  - —>50% reduction in daily activity
  - —Minor symptoms such as
    - -Headaches
    - -Migratory arthralgia
    - -Sleep disturbances
    - -Mild fever or chills
    - -Myalgia
    - -Exercise intolerance
    - -Painful lymphadenopathy
  - —Exclusion of other diseases or psychiatric illness
- Fatigue may be a symptom of many other disorders

LABORATORY

- Electrolytes, BUN/Cr
  - —Hyperkalemia
  - —Hypokalemia
  - —Renal failure
  - —Adrenal insufficiency
- Magnesium, calcium, phosphorous
- Glucose
  - —Hyperglycemia or hypoglycemia
- CBC
  - —Leukemia
  - —Infection
  - —Anemia
- Additional laboratory tests may be indicated based on the presentation
  - —Pregnancy test
  - —Liver function tests
  - —ESR
  - —Monospot and/or EBV test
  - —ANA
  - —HIV
  - —ABG or pulse oximetry for oxygen saturation

IMAGING/SPECIAL TESTS

- EKG
  - —Silent ischemia
  - —Arrhythmias
- CXR
  - —Pneumonia
  - —CHF
  - —Tumors
- Head CT
- Tests for specific diseases include
  - —Cosyntropin test
  - —Thyroid studies
  - —Lyme titers
  - —PPD

DIFFERENTIAL DIAGNOSIS

- Infection
  - —Bacteremia
  - —Urosepsis
  - —Pneumonia
  - —Viral syndromes
  - —Abscess
  - —EBV
  - —CMV
  - —HIV
  - —HHV-6
- Immunologic/connective tissue
  - —Rheumatologic (rheumatoid arthritis, systemic lupus erythematosus, JRA)
  - —Osteoarthritis
  - —Fibromyalgia
  - —Myasthenia gravis
  - —Lambert-Eaton syndrome
- Neoplastic
  - —Solid or hematologic cancers
- Metabolic
  - —Electrolyte abnormalities
  - —Mitochondrial diseases
  - —Bromism
- Hematologic
  - —Anemia
  - —Hypovolemia
  - —Hemoglobinopathy
- Endocrine
  - —Hyperthyroid or hypothyroid
  - —Adrenal insufficiency
  - —Diabetes
  - —Hypoglycemia
- Neurologic
  - —MS
  - —Cerebrovascular accident
  - —Amyotrophic lateral sclerosis
- Cardiovascular
  - —Myocardial infarction
  - —Cardiomyopathy
  - —CHF
- Pulmonary
  - —Pneumonia
  - —COPD
  - —Asthma
  - —Sleep apnea
- GI
  - —Reflux
  - —Peptic ulcer disease
  - —Liver disease
- Autonomic dysfunction
- Lifestyle
  - —Excessive or insufficient exercise
  - —Obesity
- Psychiatric
  - —Major depression
  - —Anxiety
  - —Grief
  - —Stress
- Medication related
  - —Drug interactions
  - —Commonly caused by BP, cardiovascular, psychiatric, and narcotic medications
- Dehydration

Treatment

INITIAL STABILIZATION

- ABCs
- Administer supplemental oxygen for hypoxia
- IV fluid bolus for signs of dehydration

ED TREATMENT

- Exclude serious infection or treat if present
- Correct metabolic and hematologic disturbances
- Diagnose progressive neurologic disease and acute psychiatric crisis
- Initiate workup for endocrine and neoplastic disease
- Decrease or eliminate alcohol or caffeine consumption
- Recommend appropriate diet or exercise regimen
- CFS treatment options
  - —IV IgG
  - —Magnesium
  - —Monoamine oxidase inhibitors (moclobemide)
  - —Cognitive-behavioral therapy

Disposition

ADMISSION CRITERIA

- Underlying disease requiring IV medication or monitoring
- Failure to thrive as outpatient
- Unable to provide for self

DISCHARGE CRITERIA

- Able to care for self
- Serious disturbances have been excluded
- Adequate follow-up is arranged

Miscellaneous

ICD9: 780.7

ICD10: R53

SUGGESTED READINGS

Buchwald D, Wener MH, Pearlman T, et al. Markers of inflammation and immune activation in chronic fatigue and chronic fatigue syndrome. J Rheumatol 1997; 24(2):372–376.

Dickinson CJ. Chronic fatigue syndrome—etiological aspects. Eur J Clin Invest 1997;27(4):257–267.

Fukuda K. The chronic fatigue syndrome: a comprehensive approach to its definition and study. International Chronic Fatigue Syndrome Study Group. Ann Intern Med 1994;121(12):953–959.

Maul AC. Chronic fatigue syndrome. Immunol Invest 1997;26(1-2):269–273.

Morrison RE, Keating HJ. Fatigue in primary care. Obstet Gynecol Clin 2001;28(2).

Authors: Christopher Lipinski; John Matheson

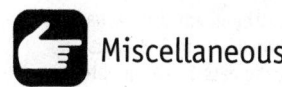

Feeding Problems, Pediatric

Clinical Presentation

SIGNS AND SYMPTOMS

Symptoms

- Define nature of problems
  - —Frequency, duration, and quantity of feeding
  - —Onset, duration, and severity
  - —Findings during feeding
    - -Cough, dyspnea, color change
    - -Vomiting, spitting
- Variability in feeding patterns is typical; parental impression of normal feeding is best guide
  - —Full-term healthy infant usually has 2–3 ounces of formula every 2–3 hours
  - —Breast-fed baby eats 10–20 minutes on each breast every 2–3 hours
  - —1-month-old normally eats 4 ounces every 4 hours
- Poor weight gain
- Irritability

Signs

- Vital signs variable
- Hydration variable
- Growth (especially weight) velocity slow; impaired nutritional status
- Cough, tachypnea, color change
- Oropharyngeal inflammation, infection, or anatomic abnormality
- Chest: evidence of aspiration
- Neurologic status: muscle tone, reflexes, mental status

Complication

- Poor nutrition may lead to abnormal brain development, immunocompromise, and other long-term adverse outcomes

MECHANISM/DESCRIPTION

- Feeding requires a coordinated series of actions involving several components
- Getting food into the oral cavity: appetite, food-seeking behavior, ingestion
- Swallowing good: oral and pharyngeal phases
- Ingestion and absorption: esophageal swallowing, GI phase
- Infant requires a minimum of 100–120 calories/kg/d
  - —Formula and human breast milk provide 20 calories/oz

ETIOLOGY

- Structural abnormalities
  - —Retrognathic jaw
  - —Cleft palate
  - —Posterior tongue placement
  - —Macroglossia
  - —Tracheotomy
  - —Esophageal strictures or stenosis
- Neurologic conditions
  - —Cerebral palsy
  - —Muscular dystrophies
  - —Cranial nerve dysfunction
  - —Mental retardation/developmental disabilities
  - —Brainstem injury
  - —Pervasive developmental disorder
- Behavioral issues
  - —Poor environmental stimulation
  - —Dysfunctional feeder-child interaction
  - —Selective food refusal
  - —Rumination
  - —Phobias
  - —Conditioned emotional reactions
  - —Depression
- Cardiorespiratory problems: tachypnea
- Metabolic dysfunction
  - —Hereditary fructose intolerance
  - —Dumping syndrome

Pre-Hospital

- Assess vital signs and hydration, and resuscitate as necessary

Diagnosis

ESSENTIAL WORKUP

- Medical and dietary history
- Observation of caretaker feeding the child and parent-child interactions

LABORATORY

- Initial assessment if child failing to thrive or dehydrated
  - —CBC, urinalysis, electrolytes, BUN, glucose; consider ESR and thyroid functions
- CXR, oximetry, and ABG if suspected cardiopulmonary concerns
- Cultures of blood, urine, and cerebrospinal fluid (CSF) if evidence of infection

IMAGING/SPECIAL TESTS

- Fluoroscopy, contrast radiographs, endoscopy, and US may be needed on an individual basis to define nature of swallowing, reflux, and associated conditions

DIFFERENTIAL DIAGNOSIS

- Family dysfunction, stress leading to potential neglect
- Difficulty getting food into the oral cavity
  - —Depression or other behavioral issues
  - —Deprivation
  - —Infection of oropharynx: herpes, aphthous ulcers, etc
  - —CNS or endocrine disease (thyroid or adrenal dysfunction)
  - —Sensory deficit
  - —Neuromuscular disease
  - —Continued dysphagia and fatigue due to overwhelming infection (sepsis, meningitis, UTI)
  - —Anemia
  - —Cardiopulmonary disease (CHF, congenital heart disease, bronchopulmonary dysplasia, bronchiolitis, pneumonia)
- Difficulty swallowing
  - —Anatomic abnormalities of oropharynx or esophagus: congenital or acquired
  - —Cardiopulmonary disease
  - —Neuromuscular disorder
  - —Disorder of esophagus: peristalsis, mucosal inflammation, esophagitis, reflux

Treatment

INITIAL STABILIZATION
- Resuscitation as required

ED TREATMENT
- Observe feeding session with primary caretaker; note gagging, coughing, emesis, noisy airway sounds, ability to handle secretions

Disposition

ADMISSION CRITERIA
- Suspected system infection
- Moderate to severe dehydration
- Significant failure to thrive
- Decompensated cardiopulmonary disease
- Severe esophagitis or reflux
- Symptomatic anemia or endocrine dysfunction
- Negligent caretaker

DISCHARGE CRITERIA
- Demonstrated ability to tolerate oral feedings
- Weight gain if failure to thrive
- Reliable caretaker and follow-up
- Behavioral therapy may be needed

Miscellaneous

ICD9: 783.3

ICD10: R63.3, P92.9

SUGGESTED READINGS

Burklow KA, Phelps AN, Schultz JR, et al. Classifying complex pediatric feeding disorders. J Pediatr Gastroenterol Nutr 1998;27(2):143–147.

Rudolph CD. Feeding disorders in infants and children. J Pediatr 1994;125: S116–S124.

Authors: Niels Rathlev; Hanan Sedik

Feeding Tube Complications

Clinical Presentation

SIGNS AND SYMPTOMS

Extubation

- Tube removed from source

Occlusion

- Unable to pass liquid through tube

Tube Migration

- Distal displacement of percutaneous endoscopic gastrostomy (PEG) tube
- Obstruction at or distal to the pylorus
- Dumping syndrome
- Ischemia
- Intussusception
- Evidence of distal prolapse on external tube (if marked)

Peristomal Wound Infections

- Cellulitis
- Necrotizing fasciitis
- Abscess formation

Stoma Leak

- Leakage of feedings/GI tract contents around stoma
- Usually mild and short lived

Aspiration Pneumonia

- Cough
- Dyspnea
- Hypoxia
- Food coloring in pulmonary secretions
- Fever
- Misplacement of nasoenteric tube (NET) in the pulmonary tree
  - —Pneumothorax
  - —Hydrothorax
  - —Pleural effusion
  - —Bronchopleural fistula

Diarrhea

- Frequent loose stools
- Dehydration

Esophageal Bezoars

- Formula and sucralfate

Intolerance to Enteral Nutrition

- High residuals
- Associated with increased risk of aspiration

MECHANISM/DESCRIPTION

Extubation

- Accidental or intentional
- More common with NET compared with PEG tubes, gastrostomy (G tube), or jejunostomy (J tube) tubes

Occlusion

- Due to small diameter
  - —Most common with NET
  - —Polyurethane tubes and solution with high pH level less likely to occlude
- Due to pill fragments (especially if enteric coated or sustained release)
- Physical incompatibilities between formula and medications
  - —Adherence of formula residue to the inner wall
- Essential to R/O malposition, fracture, and dislodgment

Peristomal Wound Infections

- Risk factors
  - —Malnutrition
  - —Poor wound healing
  - —Stomal leak
  - —Local irritation
  - —Poor wound care
  - —Immunosuppression
  - —Diabetes mellitus (DM)
  - —Obesity
  - —Excessive traction on the tube
- Leads to delayed maturation of gastrocutaneous tract

Stoma Leak

- Problematic with distal obstruction (mechanical or dysmotility); more common with high gastric residual

Aspiration Pneumonia

- At risk
  - —Impaired cough/gag reflex
  - —Delayed gastric emptying due to ileus
  - —Obstruction
  - —Gastroparesis (in DM or head trauma)
  - —Gastroesophageal reflux (frequent with large NET)

Diarrhea

- Medication induced
  - —Antibiotics
  - —Sorbitol or magnesium-containing medications
  - —Overgrowth of *Clostridium difficile,* other bacteria, or candida

Formula Intolerance

- 150–200 mL residual suggests GI motility dysfunction
  - —Too rapid delivery
  - —High osmolarity
  - —Lactose or fat intolerance
  - —Low serum albumin

Pre-Hospital

CAUTIONS

- If extubation of tube has occurred, transport tube with patient to facilitate easier replacement

Diagnosis

ESSENTIAL WORKUP

- Careful examination of feeding tube site and position of feeding tube within wound

LABORATORY

Peristomal Wound Infections

- CBC for significant infections

Aspiration Pneumonia

- ABG or pulse oximeter
- CBC
- Electrolytes, BUN/Cr, glucose
- U/A
- Blood and sputum culture

Diarrhea

- Stool for WBC/culture/*C. difficile* toxin

IMAGING/SPECIAL TESTS

- CXR
  - —For NET position
  - —Aspiration pneumonia

Tube Migration

- Endoscopy or upper GI barium study to confirm migration of tube into GI tract

DIFFERENTIAL DIAGNOSIS

N/A

Treatment

INITIAL STABILIZATION

- ABCs
- IV fluid resuscitation for dehydration/sepsis

ED TREATMENT

Extubation

- NET
  - —Replaced in the ED
  - —Confirm position by x-ray before use
- PEG tube
  - —Takes up to 6 weeks for the gastrocutaneous tract/fistula to mature
    - -Improper or aggressive attempt at tube replacement could lead to disruption of the gastrocutaneous tract and subsequent peritonitis
  - —PEG tube in place >1 week before extubation
    - -Replace in ED
    - -May use a Foley catheter
    - -Confirm by Gastrografin study if there is doubt about placement
    - -Secure the catheter to the abdominal wall to prevent distal migration
  - —PEG tube in place <1 week before extubation
    - -Fistula may not close promptly
    - -Do not replace the tube in the ED
    - -Watch for signs of peritonitis due to intraperitoneal leak of gastric contents
    - -May need hospital admission and endoscopic tube replacement
- Surgical gastrostomy (G tube) or jejunostomy (J tube)
  - —Management similar to that for PEG tube
  - —Early dislodgment within first 3 days requires emergency surgical consult and antibiotic coverage for peritonitis

Occlusion

- Attempt gentle irrigation with NS, water, or carbonated soda
- If irrigation fails, replace the tube
- Do not use meat tenderizer or pancreatic enzymes

Tube Migration

- If retraction of the tube is possible and well tolerated
  - —Secure the tube externally
  - —Discharge home after brief trial of tube feeding
- If the feeding is not tolerated, or if there are signs of persistent obstruction or peritonitis
  - —Admit with consult to the appropriate service (surgical/GI)
- If the external tube is cut (accidental or intentional)
  - —The inner bumper usually passes through the GI tract
  - —Cases of obstruction, subsequent perforation, and peritonitis have been reported, especially in children

Peristomal Wound Infections

- Local wound care with hydrogen peroxide
- Antibiotics
  - —First-generation cephalosporin (cefazolin or cephalexin)
  - —Ampicillin/sulbactam
  - —Amoxicillin/clavulanic acid
- Outpatient management for milder cases
- More severe cases require surgical consult for possible drainage/débridement and inpatient care
- Prophylactic use of antibiotic (cefazolin) before tube placement decreases wound infection

Stoma Leak

- Change from intermittent to continuous delivery
- Decrease the rate of infusion
- Administer prokinetic agents (e.g., metoclopramide, cisapride, or erythromycin)
- Local care
  - —Keep the site clean and dry
  - —Use sucralfate powder or stoma adhesive powder

Aspiration Pneumonia

- Stop enteral feeding
- Administer oxygen and broad-spectrum antibiotics
- Endotracheal intubation with mechanical ventilation for respiratory failure and airway protection when indicated
- Prevent by
  - —Elevation of head of bed
  - —Monitoring gastric residual
  - —Use of continuous infusion at graduated rate
  - —Use of prokinetic agent

Diarrhea

- Manage etiology
- Correct fluid and electrolyte imbalance
- Try isotonic, hypotonic, or fat- or lactose-free formulas
- High-fiber formula if aforementioned measures fail
- Antimotility agents
  - —Loperamide
  - —Kaopectate
  - —Cholestyramine

Formula Intolerance

- Prokinetic agents promote gastric emptying

MEDICATIONS

- Amoxicillin/clavulanic acid (Augmentin): 250–500 mg (peds: 40 mg/kg/24 h) PO t.i.d.
- Ampicillin/sulbactam: 1.5–3 g i.v. q6h
- Cefazolin (Ancef, Kefzol): 500 mg–1 g (peds: 25–100 mg/kg/24 h) i.v. q6h
- Cephalexin (Keflex): 250–500 mg (peds: 25–50 mg/kg/24 h) PO q.i.d.
- Cholestyramine: 4 g PO 1–6 times/d
- Kaopectate: 30 mL (peds: 3–6 years old, 7.5 mg; 6–12 years old, 15 mL) PO after each loose bowel movement up to 7 times/d
- Loperamide (Imodium): 4 mg initially then 2 mg (peds: 1 mg t.i.d. if 13–20 kg; 2 mg b.i.d. if 20–30 kg; 2 mg t.i.d. if >30 kg) PO up to 16 mg/d
- Metoclopramide: 10 mg PO/i.v./i.m. q.i.d. (30 minutes before feeds and q.h.s.)

Disposition

ADMISSION CRITERIA

- PEG tube extubation within 1 week of placement
- Surgical gastrostomy (G-tube) or jejunostomy (J-tube) extubation within 3 days of placement
- Significant peristomal wound infection with fever/leukocytosis
- Aspiration pneumonia
- Diarrhea associated with dehydration
- Peritonitis

DISCHARGE CRITERIA

- Successful replacement of extubated feeding tube

Miscellaneous

ICD9: N/A

ICD10: N/A

SUGGESTED READINGS

Fleming CR. Enteral nutrition. Gastrointest Dis Today 1996;5(2):1–9.

Kirby DF, Delegg MH, Fleming CR. American Gastroenterological Association technical review on tube feeding for enteral nutrition. Gastroenterology 1995;108: 1282–1301.

MacLaren R. Intolerance to intragastric enteral nutrition in critically ill patients: complications and management. Pharm 2000;20(12):1486–1498.

Rassias AF, Ball PA, Corwin HL. A prospective study of tracheopulmonary complications associated with the placement of narrow-bore enteral feeding tubes. Crit Care 1998;2(1):25–28.

Schapira GD, Edmundowicz SA. Complications of percutaneous endoscopic gastrostomy. Gastrointest Endosc Clin North Am 1996;6:409–422.

Author: Craig Houston

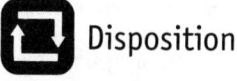

Femur Fracture

Clinical Presentation

SIGNS AND SYMPTOMS

- Thigh pain, deformity, swelling, shortening
- Patient unable to move hip or knee
- Commonly presents with multitrauma: chest, abdominal, pelvic, hip, knee injury, including dislocation
- Rarely open fracture unless injury is result of penetrating trauma
- Patient may be hypotensive as a result of hemorrhage into the thigh
- Patient may have impaired circulation in the foot because of vascular compromise, compartment syndrome

MECHANISM/DESCRIPTION

- Usually requires major, high-energy trauma
- Patients are mostly young adults with high-energy injuries (motor vehicle accidents, GSWs, falls)
  —Spiral fractures with falls from height
- Consider pathologic fracture if minor mechanism
- Can occasionally be caused by stress fracture from repetitive activity
- Complications include compartment syndrome, fat embolism, ARDS, hemorrhage

Fractures classified according to

- Location
  —Proximal third (subtrochanteric region)
  —For fractures of the femoral head, neck, and intertrochanteric regions, see Hip Injury
  —Middle third
  —Distal third (distal metaphyseal-diaphyseal junction)
  -Geometry (spiral, transverse, oblique, segmental)
  -Extent of soft tissue injury
  -Degree of comminution: Winquist and Hansen classification
  *Grade I: fracture with small fragment <25% width of femoral shaft; stable lengthwise and rotationally
  *Grade II: fracture with 25–50% width of femoral shaft; stable lengthwise; may or may not have rotational stability
  *Grade III: fracture with >50% width of femoral shaft; unstable lengthwise and rotationally
  *Grade IV: circumferential loss of cortex; unstable lengthwise and rotationally

PEDIATRIC CONSIDERATIONS

- 70% of femoral fractures in children younger than 3 years are the result of nonaccidental trauma (NAT)
- Spiral fractures of the femur strongly suggest NAT

Pre-Hospital

- Immobilization of the extremity and application of a traction splint can be important for tamponade of further blood loss into the thigh
  —Also, backboard immobilization, rigid splinting, support of extremity for position of comfort
  —Pneumatic antishock garment (PASG) can be used for immobilization
- Contraindications to external traction
  —Fractures close to the knee
  —Fracture or dislocation of the ipsilateral hip
  —Fractures of the pelvis
  —Fractures of the lower leg
  —May need skeletal traction (Steinmann pin)

CAUTIONS

- Do not attempt to reduce open fractures in the field; cover open wounds with sterile dressings
- Monitor closely for development of hemorrhagic shock because thigh can contain 4–6 units of blood

Diagnosis

ESSENTIAL WORKUP

- Radiographs (see later discussion)
- Assess distal pulses, palpate compartments, evaluate sensation and motor function
- If pulses are not equal or palpable, bedside Doppler or angiography may be necessary
- Search for associated injuries with multisystem trauma
- In suspected child abuse, obtain skeletal survey or bone scan

LABORATORY

- CBC, type, and cross-match

IMAGING/SPECIAL TESTS

- AP pelvis; true lateral of the hip; AP and lateral views of the femur; and complete knee series
- Baseline CXR; other films as indicated by trauma protocols

DIFFERENTIAL DIAGNOSIS

- Hip fracture or dislocation
- Knee fracture or dislocation
- Thigh contusion or hematoma

PEDIATRIC CONSIDERATIONS

- Cartilaginous components of the proximal and distal ends of the developing femur alter the fracture patterns seen in hip and knee injuries in children

Treatment

INITIAL STABILIZATION

- ABCs of trauma care
- Monitor BP continuously for signs of hemorrhagic shock

ED TREATMENT

- Maintain lower extremity stability
- Remove splint and clothing
- Pain control
  —Isolated femur injuries: parenteral analgesia
  —Multitrauma or pediatric patients: femoral nerve block
- Orthopedic consultation necessary for all femur fractures
  —Emergent if neurovascular compromise
  —Open fractures must go directly to the OR for irrigation and débridement
- Antibiotics
  —Fractures requiring surgery: cefazolin
  —If open fracture with laceration, extensive soft tissue damage, contamination: add gentamicin/tobramycin, tetanus
  —If highly contaminated wound: add penicillin G to cover clostridial species
- Femur fractures with diminished or absent distal pulses, an expanding hematoma, or a palpable pulsatile mass require immediate angiography or femoral artery exploration
- Skeletal traction should be applied if the patient will not go to the OR immediately

MEDICATIONS

- Cefazolin: 2 g (peds: 20 mg/kg) i.m./i.v.
- Gentamicin/tobramycin: 1.5 mg/kg i.v.
- Penicillin G: 2 million IU i.v. (peds: 25,000 IU/kg/d i.v. q8h)

PEDIATRIC CONSIDERATIONS

- Assess markers for NAT
  —Delay in presentation
  —History of mechanism inconsistent with the injury
  —Isolated trauma to the thigh, associated burns, bruises, or linear abrasions
- Assess for dislocation of the femoral capital epiphysis
- Depending on the age of the patient and the fracture type, pediatric femoral fractures may not require operative treatment

Disposition

ADMISSION CRITERIA

- All femur fractures must be admitted except as noted under Discharge Criteria
- Any suspicion of NAT in children

DISCHARGE CRITERIA

- In certain rare circumstances of pathologic fracture or femur fractures in patients who are not ambulatory and would not undergo operative fixation, discharge can be considered in consultation with orthopedics if adequate pain control can be achieved and proper follow-up ensured

Miscellaneous

ICD9: 821.00

ICD10: S72.9

SEE ALSO: HIP INJURY

SUGGESTED READINGS

Abarbanell N. Prehospital midthigh trauma and traction splint use: recommendations for treatment protocols. Am J Emerg Med 2001;19:137–140.

Brien W, et al. Management of gunshot wounds to the femur. Orthop Clin North Am 1995;26(1):133–138.

Buckley S. Current trends in the treatment of femoral shaft fractures in children and adolescents. Clin Orthop 1997;338:60–73.

Rockwood C, et al. Fractures of the femoral shaft. In: Rockwood and Green's fractures in adults and children. Philadelphia: Lippincott Williams & Wilkins 2001.

Rudman N, McIlmail D. Emergency department evaluation and treatment of hip and thigh injuries. Emerg Med Clin North Am 2000;18:29–66.

Ward K, Yealy D. Systemic analgesia and sedation in managing orthopedic emergencies. Emerg Med Clin North Am 2000;18:141–166.

Author: Colleen Buono

Fever, Adult

Clinical Presentation

SIGNS AND SYMPTOMS

- Elevated core temperature
  - —Temperature >38°C (100.4°F) rectally or 37.5°C (99.5°F) orally
  - —Lower thresholds in patients older than 65 years, as the febrile response is not as strong
- Anorexia
- Changes in mental status
  - —Can range from irritability to frank delirium and obtundation
- Chills, shivering, and rigors
  - —Mechanisms to raise body core temperature
- Fatigue
- Malaise
- Myalgias
- Night sweats
  - —Suggestive of lymphoma, solid tumor, chronic inflammatory disease, or tuberculosis (TB)
- Rash
  - —Type of lesions and distribution can offer important clues to diagnosis
  - —Petechial rashes concerning for meningococcemia and Rocky Mountain spotted fever
- Specific fever patterns
  - —Relapsing fevers; febrile episode with alternating afebrile intervals
    - -Seen in malaria, *Borrelia* infections, rat-bite fever, and lymphoma (Pel Ebstein fevers)
  - —Remittent fever; temperature falls daily but does not return to normal
    - -Seen in TB and viral diseases
  - —Intermittent fevers; exaggerated circadian rhythm
    - -Seen in systemic infections, malignancy, and drug fever
  - —Reversal of normal circadian patterns
    - -Sometimes seen in typhoid fever and disseminated TB
- Changes in heart rate
  - —Tachycardia commonly seen
  - —Temperature pulse dissociation (relative bradycardia) seen in typhoid, brucellosis, psittacosis, leptospirosis, Legionnaire's disease, Lyme disease, and factitious fevers

MECHANISM/DESCRIPTION

- Fever represents an elevation in the body's set thermoregulatory point
- Core temperature is regulated by the anterior hypothalamus at 37°C ± 2°C
- Fever caused by increased prostaglandin E_2 (PGE_2) synthesis in the hypothalamus
- Autonomic discharge from hypothalamus raises core temperature through shivering and dermal vasoconstriction
- Normal circadian variation in core temperature occurs with nadir in early morning and peak in late afternoon
- Both exogenous and endogenous factors can raise the body's set thermoregulatory point
  - —Endogenous factors include IL-1 and IL-6, tumor necrosis factor, and IFN-γ
  - —Exogenous factors include endotoxin (lipopolysaccharide) and other toxins and metabolites produced by infectious organisms

ETIOLOGY

- Any infectious process may present with fever
  - —Cardiac (endocarditis, pericarditis)
  - —Respiratory (pneumonia, upper respiratory tract infection, sinusitis)
  - —Genitourinary (urinary tract infection, pyelonephritis, prostatitis)
  - —GI (infectious diarrhea, gastroenteritis, hepatitis, pancreatitis, appendicitis)
  - —CNS (meningitis, encephalitis)
  - —Skin and connective tissue (cellulitis, abscess, osteomyelitis)
  - —Gynecologic (pelvic inflammatory disease)
  - —Systemic (Epstein-Barr virus, cytomegalovirus, HIV, sepsis)
  - —Iatrogenic (indwelling catheters, prostheses)
- Drugs: nearly all drugs may cause fever
  - —Antibiotics (penicillins, sulfonamides)
  - —NSAIDs
  - —Antihypertensives (nifedipine, hydralazine, methyldopa)
  - —Antiarrhythmics (procainamide, quinidine)
  - —Anticonvulsants (barbiturates, carbamazepine, phenytoin)
  - —Antidepressants (TCAs, monoamine oxidase inhibitors)
  - —Drugs of abuse (cocaine, amphetamines)
- Systemic inflammatory
  - —Collagen vascular diseases
  - —Rheumatic fever
  - —Rheumatoid arthritis
  - —Systemic lupus erythematosus
  - —Vasculitis
  - —Polymyalgia rheumatica
  - —Temporal arteritis
  - —Granulomatous diseases
  - —Sarcoidosis
  - —Inflammatory bowel disease
  - —Sickle cell disease
  - —Hemolytic anemia
- Neoplastic disease
  - —Lymphomas and leukemias
  - —Hepatoma
  - —Metastatic carcinomas
  - —Atrial myxomas
- Endocrine
  - —Hyperthyroidism or thyrotoxicosis
  - —Pheochromocytoma
- Pulmonary embolus
- Familial Mediterranean fever
- CNS lesions
- Fever of unknown origin
  - —Defined as fever >38.3°C for at least 3 weeks as an outpatient *or* 1 week after inpatient workup
  - —A diagnosis of exclusion rarely made in the ED

Pre-Hospital

CAUTIONS

- No specific field interventions required
- Monitoring and IV access should be obtained in the field for unstable patients or patients with altered mental status

Diagnosis

ESSENTIAL WORKUP

- Core temperature is most acutely measured rectally
- Careful history and physical exam (PE) necessary to determine need for further diagnostic testing
  - —History should elicit any sick contacts, previous infections, recent travel, medications, and immunization status

LABORATORY

- CBC
  - —Commonly performed, but rarely helpful in management of fever in the ED
  - —Important in determining neutropenia in patients with risk factors
  - —Differential WBC count is unreliable but may give clues to certain etiologies
  - —Neutrophilia and bandemia suggestive of bacterial infection
  - —Lymphocytosis suggestive of typhoid, TB, brucellosis, and viral disease
  - —Atypical lymphocytosis seen in mononucleosis, cytomegalovirus, HIV, rubella, varicella, measles, and viral hepatitis
  - —Monocytosis suggestive of TB, brucellosis, viral illness, and lymphoma
  - —Platelet count <150,000 may be predictor of sepsis
- ESR is generally not useful in ED diagnosis of fever
  - —Very high values suggestive of endocarditis, temporal arteritis, TB, and polymyalgia rheumatica
- C-reactive protein is nonspecific and minimally useful in ED workup
- Urinalysis and urine culture
  - —Helpful if fever etiology is uncertain after PE
- Blood cultures
  - —Obtain for patients with signs of sepsis or altered mental status and ill-appearing patients
  - —Ideally should be attained before antimicrobial therapy, but antibiotics should be started immediately in unstable patients or patients with altered mental status

IMAGING/SPECIAL TESTS

- Lumbar puncture for patients with headache, meningeal signs, and change in mental status
- CXR
  - —In patients with PE finding of cardiopulmonary disease and patients with unclear fever source
- CT scanning or US may be indicated based on history and PE findings

DIFFERENTIAL DIAGNOSIS

- Failure of thermoregulatory systems
  - —Core temperatures >41°C more common in these states
  - —Neuroleptic malignant syndrome
  - —Malignant hyperthermia
  - —Serotonin syndrome
  - —Heat stroke
- Factitious fever

Treatment

INITIAL STABILIZATION

- Immediate treatment rarely required
- Airway control, breathing and circulatory support for unstable patients
- Initiate broad-spectrum antibiotic treatment immediately for immunocompromised patients and patients with unstable vital signs or profound mental status changes

ED TREATMENT

- Antipyretics
  - —Acetaminophen, NSAIDs, or salicylates
  - —Inhibit the cyclooxygenase enzyme, thereby blocking synthesis of prostaglandins
  - —Most febrile patients do not require antipyretic medication other than for comfort
  - —Selected patients require more aggressive antipyretic interventions
  - —Pregnant women
  - —Patients with history of seizure disorders
  - —Patients with significant cardiac disease
  - —Hemodynamically unstable patients
  - —Patients with altered mental status
- Glucocorticoids
  - —Inhibit phospholipase A_2 blocking prostaglandin synthesis
  - —Indicated only in chronic inflammatory conditions; contraindicated in infectious etiologies
- Empiric antibiotics for unstable or immunocompromised patients
- External cooling mechanism rarely indicated

MEDICATIONS

- Acetaminophen: 650–1,000 mg PO/p.r. q4–6h
- Aspirin: 650 mg PO q4h
- Empiric antibiotics for unstable patients with unidentified source of fever
  - —Gentamicin: 2 mg/kg i.v. loading dose then 1 mg/kg q8h plus piperacillin/tazobactam (3.375 g i.v. q6h) or ticarcillin/clavulanate (3.1 g i.v. q6h)
  - —Imipenem 500–1,000 mg i.v. q8h
  - —Meropenem: 1 g i.v. q8h
- Ibuprofen: 800 mg PO q6h

Disposition

ADMISSION CRITERIA

- Patients with unstable vital signs require ICU admission
- Certain high-risk groups require admission for fever
  - —Neutropenic patients or patients with known malignancy
  - —Immunosuppressed or immunocompromised patients
  - —Asplenic patients
  - —IV drug abusers (high risk of endocarditis)
- Lower thresholds for admission in patients older than 60 years and diabetics

DISCHARGE CRITERIA

- Immunocompetent patients with stable vital signs and an identified source of fever with appropriate outpatient treatment and follow-up may be safely discharged

Miscellaneous

ICD9: 780.6

ICD10: R50.9

SUGGESTED READINGS

Gelfand JA, Dinarello CA. Fever and hyperthermia. In: Fauci AS, Braunwald E, Isselbacher KJ, et al. eds. Harrison's principles of internal medicine, 14th ed. New York: McGraw-Hill, 1998:84–90.

Mackowiak PA. Concepts of fever. Arch Intern Med 1998;158:1870–1881.

McKinnon HD Jr, Howard T. Evaluating the febrile patient with a rash. Am Fam Phys 2000;62(4):804–815.

Mendelson M. Fever in the immunocompromised host. Emerg Med Clin North Am 1998;16(4):761–778.

Plaisance KI, Mackowiak PA. Antipyretic therapy. Arch Intern Med 2000;160: 449–456.

Author: Teriggi J. Ciccone

Fever, Pediatric

Clinical Presentation

SIGNS AND SYMPTOMS

- Clinical appearance must be evaluated
- Toxicity associated with lethargy, poor perfusion, hypoventilation/hyperventilation, weak cry, decreased PO intake; purpuric or petechial rash
- Altered mental status
  - —Lethargy presenting with decreased level of consciousness
  - —Irritability
  - —Impaired interaction with environment, parents, physician, toys
- Physical exam (PE) to search for underlying condition
- Febrile seizures
- Temperatures >42°C often have a noninfectious etiology
- Serious infection may occur in the absence of fever
- Antipyretics may change findings without impacting underlying disease
- Approximately 20% of children will have fever without source after history and PE

MECHANISM/DESCRIPTION

- Fever is defined as a temperature of 38°C (100.4°F) rectally
  - —Oral and tympanic temperatures are generally 0.6–1.0°C lower
- Tympanic temperatures are not accurate in children younger than 6 months
- Axillary temperatures are generally unreliable
- After 3 months of age, significant fever is defined as a temperature of 39°C
- Children who are afebrile but have a reliable history of documented fever should be considered to be febrile to the degree reported

ETIOLOGY

- Bacteremia (*Haemophilus influenzae* type B and *Streptococcus pneumoniae* vaccines have decreased incidence of invasive *Haemophilus* and pneumococcal disease), viral exanthem (varicella, roseola, rubella), coxsackievirus (hand-foot-mouth disease), abscess
- CNS: meningitis, encephalitis
- HEENT: otitis media, facial cellulitis, orbital/periorbital cellulitis, pharyngitis (group A β-hemolytic streptococcus, herpangina, adenovirus pharyngoconjunctival fever), viral gingivostomatitis (herpes and coxsackievirus), cervical adenitis, sinusitis, mastoiditis, conjunctivitis, peritonsillar/retropharyngeal abscess
- Respiratory: croup (paramyxovirus), epiglottitis, bronchiolitis (RSV), pneumonia, empyema
- Cardiovascular: purulent pericarditis, endocarditis, myocarditis
- GU: cystitis, pyelonephritis
- GI: bacterial diarrhea, intussusception, appendicitis, hepatitis
- Extremity: osteomyelitis, septic arthritis, cellulitis
- Miscellaneous: Kawasaki disease, vaccine (DPT) reaction, heat exhaustion/stroke, factitious, familial dysautonomia, thyrotoxicosis, collagen vascular disease, vasculitis, rheumatic fever, malignancy, drug induced, overbundling (recheck 15 minutes after unbundling)

Pre-Hospital

- Resuscitate as appropriate
- Begin cooling with antipyretics or tepid towels

Diagnosis

ESSENTIAL WORKUP

- Oxygen saturation as mandatory fifth vital sign
- Resuscitate as appropriate
- Determine duration of illness, degree and level of fever, use of antipyretics, past medical history, drug allergies, vaccination status, recent medications/antibiotics, birth history if younger than 6 months of age, exposures, feeding, activity, urine/bowel habits, travel history, and relevant review of systems
- Search for underlying condition
- Initiate antipyretic therapy

LABORATORY

- CBC with differential
- Urinalysis and culture in all male infants younger than 6 months, uncircumcised infants younger than 12 months, and girls younger than 2 years
- Blood culture
  - —The development of automated blood culture systems has led to more rapid detection of bacterial pathogens
- CSF for cell counts/culture for children toxic or 0–28 days of age; consider for non-toxic-appearing children 28–90 days of age as well as older
- Stool for WBCs and culture when diarrhea present

IMAGING/SPECIAL TESTS

- CXR to exclude pneumonia if patient tachypneic or hypoxic
- Lumbar puncture as indicated
- Other studies as indicated to evaluate for underlying infection

DIFFERENTIAL DIAGNOSIS

See Etiology

Treatment

INITIAL STABILIZATION

- Treat any life-threatening conditions
- Antipyretic therapy
- Evaporative cooling techniques such as sponge bath

ED TREATMENT

- Focal infections require evaluation and treatment
- Toxic children require prompt septic workup and appropriate antibiotics
- All potential life-threatening conditions must be excluded before treating a minor acute illness, which is more common
- Infants 0–28 days old need a full septic workup: CBC, UA, cultures (blood, urine, CSF), lumbar puncture, CXR
  —Antibiotics: cefotaxime and ampicillin
  —Admit
- Nontoxic infants 28–90 days old need workup, selective antibiotic use (ceftriaxone), and reevaluation within 24 hours of admission
  —*H. influenzae* type B and *S. pneumoniae* incidence has declined significantly with widespread vaccination
  —It is currently reasonable to perform blood culture and urine culture with selective lumbar puncture, coupled with ceftriaxone IM in low-risk patients (see definition under Disposition) if reevaluation in 24 hours is ensured
  —Lumbar puncture is optional in this setting but should be done if empiric antibiotics (ceftriaxone) are given to ensure that subsequent reevaluation is not compromised
- Children 3 months–3 years of age are evaluated selectively; antibiotic use is individualized for specific identifiable infections and pending appropriate cultures
  —Nontoxic children with temperatures >39°C receive urinalysis/culture as indicated, CXR as indicated, CBC/blood culture, and selective empiric antibiotics
  —Children with WBC >15,000/mm^3 may benefit from empiric antibiotics pending culture results, especially if not vaccinated with *H. influenzae* type B and pneumococcal vaccines
- Immunocompromised children need aggressive evaluation, as do children with fever and petechiae/purpura

MEDICATIONS

- Acetaminophen: 15 mg/kg/dose PO/p.r. q6h
- Amoxicillin: 50 mg/kg/d PO t.i.d.
- Ampicillin: 150 mg/kg/d i.v. q4–6h
- Cefotaxime: 100 mg/kg/d i.v. q6–8h
- Ceftriaxone: 50–100 mg/kg/d i.v./i.v. q12h
- Ibuprofen: 10 mg/kg/dose PO q6h
- Penicillin V: 25–50 mg/kg/d PO b.i.d. to q.i.d.

Disposition

ADMISSION CRITERIA

- All toxic patients
- Infants 0–28 days of age with temperature >38°C
- Nontoxic infants 28–90 days of age with temperature >38°C who do not meet low-risk criteria (see definition under Discharge Criteria)
- Poor compliance or followup

DISCHARGE CRITERIA

- Infants 28–90 days of age meeting low-risk criteria
  —No prior hospitalizations, chronic illness, antibiotic therapy, prematurity
  —Reliable, mature parents with home phone, available transport, thermometer, and living in relative proximity to ED
  —No evidence of focal infection (except otitis media), non-toxic appearing, normal activity, perfusion and hydration with age-appropriate vital signs
  —Normal WBC (5–15,000/mm^3), urine (negative Gram stain of unspun urine or leukocyte esterase or <5 WBC/HPF), stool (<5 WBC/HPF) if performed, and CSF (<8 WBC/mm^3 and negative Gram stain) if performed
- Infants 3 to 36 months of age who are nontoxic and previously healthy with good follow-up
  —Antipyretics
  —Consider ceftriaxone and close follow-up
- Follow-up by phone in 12–24 hours and reevaluate in 24–48 hours with parental instructions to return if concerns develop or patient worsens

Miscellaneous

ICD9: 780.6

ICD10: P81.9

SUGGESTED READINGS

Abramson JS, Baker CJ, Fisher MC. American Academy of Pediatrics. Committee on Infectious Diseases. Technical report: prevention of pneumococcal infections, including the use of pneumococcal conjugate and polysaccharide vaccines and antibiotic prophylaxis. Pediatrics 2000;106:367–376.

Baraff LJ. Management of fever without source in infants and children. Ann Emerg Med 2000;36:602–614.

Bulloch B, Craig WR, Klassen TP. The use of antibiotics to prevent serious sequelae in children at risk for occult bacteremia: a meta-analysis. Acad Emerg Med 1997;4:679–683.

Lee GM, Harper MB. Risk of bacteremia for febrile young children in the post-*Haemophilus influenzae* type b era. Arch Pediatr Adolesc Med 1998;152:624–628.

Authors: Nathan Mick; David A. Peak; Andrew S. Ulrich

Fibrocystic Breast Disease

Clinical Presentation

SIGNS AND SYMPTOMS

- Pain (mastodynia) and tenderness
- Usually bilateral, can be unilateral
  —Especially premenstrual phase of normal menstrual cycle
- Lumpiness, nodularity: may be localized or generalized, unilateral or bilateral
- Excessive nodularity
- Increased engorgement and breast density; breasts described as being dull and heavy with fluctuations in the size of the cystic areas
- Occasional spontaneous nipple discharge

MECHANISM/DESCRIPTION

- *Fibrocystic change* (FCC) is a term that has no specificity and is usually physiologic nodularity and is more descriptive of the symptoms and clinical findings
- Can be defined as palpable thickening or lumpiness in the breast, associated with pain and tenderness that fluctuates with the menstrual cycle; often become progressively worse until menopause; many feel these symptoms are exaggerated physiologic phenomena
- Synonyms: fibrocystic breast, cystic mastitis, symptomatic chronic cystic mastopathy, Schimmelbusch's disease, Reclus disease, mammary dysplasia
- FCCs are found histologically in 50% of women with normal breasts
- *Three clinical stages of fibrocystic changes*
  —*Mazoplasia:* intense proliferation of the breast stroma; pain usually in upper outer breast quadrant with most tender area in axillary tail; generally affects women in their 20s
  —*Adenosis:* marked proliferation and hyperplasia of ducts, ductless, and alveolar cells; multiple breast nodules: 2-10 mm; premenstrual pain and tenderness; generally affects women in their 20s and 30s
  —*Cystic:* solitary (Cooper's disease) or multiple (Reclus disease); lumps are cystic when palpated and tender, slightly mobile, and well delineated; vary in size from microscopic to 5 cm in diameter; deeply imbedded or clustered; usually not painful, unless rapid increases in cyst size and lump appears; fluid aspirated is straw colored or dark brown to green

ETIOLOGY

- Enhanced or exaggerated reaction by breast tissue to cyclic levels of ovarian hormones; therefore, most common in reproductive, premenopausal years
- Risk factors: nulliparity, late age at natural menopause, high social status; age, genetic makeup, and lactational history may affect development of FCC as well

Pre-Hospital

N/A

Diagnosis

ESSENTIAL WORKUP

- Clinical examination: ideally 7–9 days after onset of menstrual flow when breasts are least congested
- Ultrasonography
  —Can differentiate cystic from solid breast masses
  —Useful in palpable masses and nonpalpable masses that appear on screening mammography
  —Benign cystic masses typically have uniform outer margin without asymmetry or irregular thickness of the cyst wall; there are no echoes centrally, and posterior wall enhancement is noted
  —Can assist in aspiration of deep cysts or those not palpated
  —Can conservatively follow size of cysts

IMAGING/SPECIAL TESTS

- Mammography
  —Sensitivity of approximately 85% in detecting malignancies
  —However, mammographic findings of benign processes of the breast can appear as malignant and vice versa
  —Should be done either before aspiration or 7–10 days after aspiration to avoid artifacts
- Needle aspiration
  —Should completely evacuate cyst
  —Can be done for symptomatic or large masses
- Excisional biopsy
  —Gold standard diagnostic test for patients with abnormal results of mammogram, a breast mass, or normal results of mammogram and a palpable mass that has not been proved cystic

DIFFERENTIAL DIAGNOSIS

- Benign breast masses
- Malignant breast masses
- Chest wall pain
- Physiologic symptoms associated with menses

Treatment

INITIAL STABILIZATION

N/A

ED TREATMENT

- Referral to PCP
- Reassurance if only minimal symptoms
- Conservative therapy
  - —Support bra: reduces tension on supporting ligaments of breast and can reduce inflammatory response and edema
  - —Mild diuretic for 2–3 days before onset of menses
  - —Dietary changes: reduction in dietary methylxanthines reduces level of cAMP and cGMP and has been found by some authors to reduce symptoms and changes of FCC
  - —NSAIDs
- Hormonal therapy
  - —Oral contraceptives: can decrease the symptoms of FCC, particularly after 1 year of treatment
- Sex hormone inhibitors: should be prescribed by PCP to enable follow-up during course of treatment
  - —Danazol: a synthetic androgen with greater anabolic than androgenic activity; variable results in reduction of breast nodularity
  - —Tamoxifen; a partial estrogen antagonist; response rate of 65–75%; fewer side effects than danazol
  - —Bromocriptine: inhibits prolactin production; most patients (75%) have relief from mastalgia and reduced nodularity
- Surgical intervention: if a nodule in a breast remains, excision is recommended regardless of mammographic or US findings; if a large cyst recurs after aspiration on two occasions, it should be excised and studied histologically; referral to general surgeon

MEDICATIONS

- Danazol: 100–400 mg/d in two divided doses for 6 months
- Oral contraceptives: for example, combination with 0.02 mg of ethinyl estradiol and 1 mg norethindrone acetate: 1 tablet/d

Disposition

ADMISSION CRITERIA

N/A

DISCHARGE CRITERIA

- All patients may be discharged if the diagnosis is fibrocystic changes
- It is important for patient satisfaction, as well as patient health and disease prevention, to ensure follow-up for all patients with breast masses
- Referral to a PCP or even a general surgeon should be provided

Miscellaneous

ICD9: 610.1

ICD10: N60.1

SUGGESTED READINGS

Drukker BH. Fibrocystic change of the breast. Clin Obstet Gynecol 1994;37:903.

Fiorica JV. Fibrocystic changes. Obstet Gynecol Clin North Am 1994;21:445.

Hutter RVP. Consensus meetings. Is "fibrocystic disease" of the breast precancerous? Arch Pathol Lab Med 1986;110:171.

Marchant DJ. Benign breast disease. Obstet Gynecol Clin North Am 2002;29:1.

Scanlon EF. The early diagnosis of breast cancer. Cancer 1981;48:523.

Author: Tami Gash-Kim

Fibromyalgia

Clinical Presentation

SIGNS AND SYMPTOMS

- Generalized musculoskeletal pain and morning stiffness
- Weakness and fatigue
- Sleep disturbance
- Tension headaches
- GI complaints (e.g., irritable bowel syndrome)
- Paresthesias
- Sensation of swollen hands
- Skinfold tenderness
- Postexertional pain
- Cold intolerance
- Dermatographism

MECHANISM/DESCRIPTION

- Nonarticular, noninflammatory form of muscular rheumatism
  —*Widespread* pain, tender points, fatigue, sleep disturbance with limited physical findings
- Not a diagnosis of exclusion, may occur with other rheumatic diseases
- Painful symptoms believed to be muscular in origin
- Abnormalities identified as possible mechanism
  —Decreased ATP/phosphocreatine level
  —Prolonged muscle ischemia/tension
  —Low blood flow in exercise muscles of patients with fibromyalgia
- Muscle biopsies from tender points have shown no reproducible abnormalities
- Other mechanisms may involve the neuroendocrine system or a combination of peripheral and central mechanisms; see Etiology

ETIOLOGY

- Unknown
- Genetic predisposition may play a role when symptoms triggered by exposure to environmental stressors
- Other factors such as
  —Physiologic imbalance in the hypothalamic-pituitary-adrenal axis with decreased free cortisol production
  —Low serum levels of insulin growth factor
  —Elevated levels of substance P (enhances pain perception) in CSF
  —Reduced serotonin levels
  —Sleep disturbance of normal stage 3 and 4 phases (non-REM), resulting in nonrestorative sleep and immunologic dysfunction
- Psychologic distress

Pre-Hospital

N/A

Diagnosis

ESSENTIAL WORKUP

- History and characteristic physical findings are key to making the diagnosis
- Use the classification criteria established by the American College of Rheumatology (ACR) for fibromyalgia
  —Absence or less than the number of required *tender points* do not exclude the syndrome
  —*Widespread* pain present for at least 3 months on both the left and the right side of the body, with pain above and below the waist, axial skeletal pain must be present (cervical or anterior chest or thoracic spine or low back pain)
  —11 of 18 specific tender points on digital palpation with a force of 4 kg (the amount of pressure required to blanch a thumbnail); the nine *paired* (bilateral) tender points are located at the
    -Occiput: suboccipital muscle insertions
    -Low cervical: anterior aspects of the C-5, C-7 intertransverse spaces
    -Trapezius: midpoint of the upper border
    -Supraspinatus: above the medial border of the scapular spine
    -Second rib: second costochondral junction about 3 cm lateral to the sternal border
    -Lateral epicondyle: about 2 cm below the bony prominence
    -Gluteal: upper outer quadrant of the buttocks
    -Greater trochanter: posterior to the trochanteric prominence
    -Knee: medial fat pad proximal to the joint line

LABORATORY

- CBC, blood chemistries, ESR, and thyroid function tests may help rule out alternative diagnoses
- No specific laboratory abnormalities are characteristic of fibromyalgia

IMAGING/SPECIAL TESTS

- No specific radiographic abnormalities are characteristic

DIFFERENTIAL DIAGNOSIS

- Myofascial pain syndrome (*trigger points* present not *tender points*)
- Polymyalgia rheumatica
- Axial arthritis
- Hypothyroidism
- Electrolyte imbalance
- Myopathies (metabolic and drug induced)
- Early collagen disease
- Osteomalacia
- Psychogenic rheumatism
- Chronic fatigue syndrome
- Eosinophilia-myalgia syndrome

Treatment

INITIAL STABILIZATION
- None required

ED TREATMENT
- Patient education and reassurance
  - —Emphasize that fibromyalgia is not life threatening and does not reduce life expectancy
  - —The disorder is chronic but not crippling or deforming
  - —Goal is to manage pain and improve functional disability
- *Psyche:* patients with poor coping skills will require psychiatric intervention

Pharmacologic Therapy
- Medications alone or in combination (e.g., amitriptyline and fluoxetine or amitriptyline and cyclobenzaprine) are beneficial in improving sleep quality and relaxing painful muscles
- TCAs (amitriptyline, nortriptyline)
- Selective serotonin reuptake inhibitors (fluoxetine, paroxetine)
- Muscle relaxants (cyclobenzaprine)
- Benzodiazepines (alprazolam, temazepam) given at bedtime
- NSAIDs and corticosteroids have not been shown to be effective
- Steroids or local anesthetic (lidocaine) injection into tender points is controversial; no studies available to prove efficacy
- Opioids: no data showing benefit in long term

MEDICATIONS
- Alprazolam: 0.5–1 mg/d PO h.s.
- Amitriptyline: 10–50 mg/d PO h.s.
- Cyclobenzaprine: 10–30 mg/d PO in q.d. to t.i.d.
- Fluoxetine: 20 mg/d PO
- Paroxetine: 10 mg/d PO
- Temazepam: 15 mg/d PO h.s.
- Zolpidem: 10 mg/d PO h.s.

Lifestyle Modifications
- Physical exercise should be encouraged
  - —Exercise program should be gradual to avoid overexertion and discouragement
  - —Aerobic exercise may be more beneficial than simple stretching
- Good sleep pattern should also be discussed
  - —Establishing a nightly ritual in preparation for sleep
  - —Avoiding caffeine-containing beverages or foods in the afternoon or evenings
- Encourage stress management and coping strategies
- Participation in educational programs (e.g., cognitive-behavioral therapy)

Disposition

ADMISSION CRITERIA
- Patients with serious underlying disease, intractable pain, or immunocompromised
- Patients with suicidal ideation

DISCHARGE CRITERIA
- Patients with uncomplicated fibromyalgia can be managed as outpatients

Miscellaneous

ICD9: 729.1

ICD10: M79.0

SUGGESTED READINGS

Arthritis Foundation. Primer on the rheumatic diseases, 12th ed. 2001: 188–193.

Goldenberg D, et al. A randomized, double-blind crossover trial of fluoxetine and amitriptyline in the treatment of fibromyalgia. Arthr Rheum 1996;39(11): 1852–1859.

Leventhal, Lawrence J. Management of fibromyalgia. Ann Intern Med 1999;131: 850–858.

Wolfe F, and the Vancouver Fibromyalgia Consensus Group. Special report. The fibromyalgia syndrome: a consensus report on fibromyalgia and disability. J Rheumatol 1996;23:534–539.

Wolfe F. The fibromyalgia problem [Editorial]. J Rheumatol 1997;24: 1247–1249.

Author: Karlene Chin

Flail Chest

Clinical Presentation

SIGNS AND SYMPTOMS

- *Flail chest* paradoxically moves inward during inspiration and outward during expiration
  - —Initially this may not be seen because of muscle splinting
- Localized chest wall pain increases with deep inspiration or coughing
- Ecchymosis, bony crepitus, and tenderness associated with multiple rib fractures
- Splinting respirations
- Intercostal muscle spasm
- Dyspnea, tachypnea; onset may be insidious, increasing over time
- Hemoptysis
- Cyanosis, tachycardia, hypotension
- Auscultation: initially normal breath sounds progressing to wet rales or absent breath sounds
- Flail chest is most commonly associated with *pulmonary contusion*

MECHANISM/DESCRIPTION

- Direct chest wall trauma, fall from height, motor vehicle accident (MVA)
- Flail chest is a free-floating segment of chest wall, resulting when three or more adjacent ribs are fractured in two or more places or from rib fractures in conjunction with sternal fractures or costochondral separations
- Ribs usually break at the point of impact or the posterior angle, which is the structurally weakest region
- Direct injury from the transfer of kinetic energy to the lung parenchyma causes disruption of the alveolocapillary membrane and development of pulmonary contusion
- Arteriovenous shunting, ventilation/perfusion mismatch, hypoxemia, and potential respiratory failure result
- The main problem with flail chest is the resultant pulmonary contusion, not alteration in ventilatory mechanics due to the free-floating segment

PEDIATRIC CONSIDERATIONS

- Relatively elastic chest wall make rib fractures less common in children

Pre-Hospital

CAUTIONS

- In the field, positioning the patient injured side down can stabilize the involved chest wall and improve ventilation in the noninjured hemithorax
- Patients with thoracic trauma associated with a MVA, significant fall, or preexisting lung disease should be routed to the nearest available trauma facility

Diagnosis

ESSENTIAL WORKUP

- Diagnosis is based on clinical exam
  - —Inspection under tangential light may magnify the paradoxic motion of the chest wall segment
  - —The thorax should be palpated in search of tenderness and crepitus
- CXR aids diagnosis, revealing multiple rib fractures
  - —Associated intrathoracic pathology such as pneumothorax, hemothorax, and widened mediastinum
  - —*Pulmonary contusion* appears within 6–12 hours after injury and ranges from patchy alveolar infiltrates to frank consolidation

LABORATORY

- ABG analysis may reveal hypoxemia and an elevated A-a gradient

IMAGING/SPECIAL TESTS

- Thoracic CT may be a useful adjunct in defining associated thoracic injuries not identified on CXR

DIFFERENTIAL DIAGNOSIS

- Rib contusion or intercostal muscle strain
- Costochondral separation
- Sternal fracture and dislocation
- Radiographic differential diagnosis includes
  - —ARDS
  - —Pulmonary laceration
  - —CHF
  - —Pneumonia or other infectious process
  - —Noncardiogenic causes of pulmonary edema

Treatment

INITIAL STABILIZATION

- ABCs, IV, O_2, continuous cardiac and pulse oximetry monitoring
- Control airway
  - —Endotracheal intubation is indicated for patients with severe hypoxemia (PaO_2 <60 mm Hg on room air, <80 mm Hg on 100% O_2), significant underlying lung disease or impending respiratory failure

ED TREATMENT

- Maintain adequate oxygenation, monitor O_2 saturation and respiratory rate
- In the conscious and alert patient, O_2 administration via face mask is first-line therapy
  - —If the patient cannot maintain a PaO_2 >80 mm Hg on high-flow oxygen, then CPAP via mask or nasal BiPAP can be attempted
- If adequate oxygenation cannot be maintained with mask/CPAP/BiPAP, early endotracheal intubation and mechanical ventilation should be instituted with PEEP
  - —This results in a physiologic internal fixation of the flail segment
- External fixation or stabilization of the flail segment is not indicated
- Adequate pain control is key to maintaining adequate pulmonary function and avoiding splinting, atelectasis, and subsequent pneumonia
- Search for associated injuries, treat exacerbation of underlying lung disease
- *Intercostal nerve blocks with 0.5% bupivacaine are safe and effective when performed properly, providing 6–12 hours of pain relief*
  - —The intercostal nerve can be blocked posteriorly 2–3 finger breadths from the midline
  - —The neurovascular bundle runs just along the undersurface of the rib; aspirate first to be sure the intercostal vessels have not been punctured
- *Avoid overhydration:* in the setting of pulmonary contusion, the need for IV crystalloid resuscitation must be weighed against the risk of increasing interstitial pulmonary edema
- Prophylactic antibiotics are not indicated

MEDICATIONS

- Acetaminophen: 325 mg/oxycodone 5 mg (Percocet) 1–2 tabs PO q6h
- Bupivacaine 0.5% for intercostal nerve blocks
- Hydromorphone (Dilaudid): 1–2 mg i.v./i.m./s.c. q4–6h
- Meperidine (Demerol): 50–150 mg (peds: 0.75–2.0 mg/kg) i.v./i.m. q3–4h
- Morphine sulfate: 2–10 mg (peds: 0.05–0.1 mg/kg) i.v./i.m./s.c. q4–6h
- For the admitted patient, thoracic epidural block or patient-controlled analgesia (PCA) is an effective alternative to traditional parenteral narcotics
  - —Consider these for patients with refractory pain, oversedation, or hypoventilation secondary to narcotic analgesics

Disposition

ADMISSION CRITERIA

- All patients with flail chest are admitted to a critical care setting for close monitoring and pain control

DISCHARGE CRITERIA

- Patients found to have flail chest, with or without pulmonary contusion, should not be discharged

Miscellaneous

ICD9: 807.4

ICD10: S22.5

SUGGESTED READINGS

Committee on Trauma, American College of Surgeons. Advanced trauma life support instructor manual, 5th ed. Chicago: American College of Surgeons, 1993.

Scott Bjerke H. Flail chest. eMedicine Journal 2002;3(1). Available at www.emedicine.com.

Vukich D, Markovchick V. Thoracic trauma. In: Rosen P, et al. eds. Emergency medicine: concepts and clinical practice, 4th ed. St. Louis: Mosby, 1998:514.

Wilson R. Thoracic trauma. In: Tintinalli J, et al. eds. Emergency medicine: a comprehensive study guide, 4th ed. New York: McGraw-Hill, 1996:1156.

Author: Gregory Lampe

Foot Fractures

Clinical Presentation

SIGNS AND SYMPTOMS

- Ecchymosis, pain, swelling, or deformity of foot
- Pain with weight bearing
- Joint instability

MECHANISM/DESCRIPTION

- The most common foot injuries are the metatarsals (MTs) and phalanges
- The calcaneus is the most commonly fractured among the tarsal bones
- Calcaneus fractures: compression injury from sudden high-velocity impact to heel
  - —75% are intraarticular; 50% have associated injuries
    - -10% spine fractures
    - -25% with associated lower extremity trauma
    - -5% bilateral, 5% open
- MT fractures: divided into stress fractures, twisting injuries, or direct trauma
  - —First MT: direct applied force
  - —Second and third MTs are most often involved in stress fractures and twisting injuries
  - —Fifth MT: avulsion fracture (dancer's fracture) of proximal apophysis is the most common injury
  - —Jones fracture: transverse fracture of the metaphyseal-diaphyseal junction of fifth MT
    - -Results from twisting while foot inverted
- Talus: caused by dorsiflexion with axial load, common snow-boarder's injury
- Tarsal-MT (TMT) injuries "Lisfranc": these are high-energy injuries
  - —Axial load on plantar-flexed foot, or hindfoot fixed with forced foot eversion
  - —Unstable forefoot on hindfoot
  - —20% go undiagnosed on initial visit
- Navicular: results from axial compression or stress fractures
- Cuboid and cuneiform fractures are rare and occur in conjunction with other injuries, often with TMT injuries

Pre-Hospital

- **Patients should have ice bag placed on affected foot and immobilization of foot and ankle**
- **All patients suspected of calcaneus fracture should have spinal immobilization; often the mechanism is fall from height >6 feet**

Diagnosis

ESSENTIAL WORKUP

- Physical exam of extremity is necessary to assess neurovascular status, skin integrity, gross swelling, deformity, or loss of function
- Examination of the spine is also essential in suspected calcaneus fractures, as there is a 10% incidence of coexistent injury
- AP/lateral and oblique views are necessary for all foot fractures

IMAGING AND SPECIAL TESTS

- Special views may be needed for some fractures
  - —Lisfranc fractures may require stress views with weight bearing
  - —Calcaneus fractures require an axial view and may require CT
  - —Boehler angle <20 degrees suggests a compression fracture of calcaneus
  - —LS spine films are necessary in all patients with calcaneus fractures
- Stress fractures may require 2 weeks to appear on plain films; bone scan or CT may be used to elucidate suspected fractures

Complications

- Compartment syndrome most commonly presents as severe pain in a swollen foot
  - —Pressures >35 mm Hg require opening of all major foot compartments
- Nonunion and avascular necrosis are common complications with talar neck fractures due to distal blood supply
- Calcaneus fractures may be accompanied by sural nerve injury; test sensation along lateral aspect of foot

DIFFERENTIAL DIAGNOSIS

N/A

PEDIATRIC CONSIDERATIONS

- MT fractures account for 90% of foot fractures in children
  - —Avulsion fractures of the fifth MT are most common
  - —Physeal injury may occur with proximal first MT fractures
- Other common injuries include phalangeal fractures (17%) and navicular fractures (5%)

Treatment

INITIAL STABILIZATION

- ABCs of trauma first
- Assess for neurovascular compromise distal to fracture site
- Dislocations must be reduced as quickly as possible with assessment of neurovascular status before and after procedure
  - —Conscious sedation is usually required (see Conscious Sedation)
- Immobilize, ice, and elevate in a bulky splint; application of cast should be delayed until swelling subsides
- Pain management
  - —If there is a large amount of swelling and pain with toe movement, suspect compartment syndrome
- Orthopedic consult is indicated early for displaced fractures
  - —Many injuries require repair within 6 hours of injury to prevent delay of ORIF for 6–10 days due to swelling

ED TREATMENT

- Almost all fractures that are displaced >2 mm or have loss of height or instability require anatomic reduction
  - —Calcaneus fractures: most commonly undergo ORIF with "H" plate and screws
  - —Lisfranc fractures; ORIF is treatment of choice
  - —MT-head fracture may respond to closed reduction and pinning; closed reduction may be attempted using digital block
  - —Talus: ORIF with screws or 3.5-mm cortical screw/Kirschner wires
  - —Navicular, cuneiform, and cuboid fractures will need ORIF if displaced
- Assume all fractures are non-weight bearing and place in bulky splint unless instructed otherwise by involved orthopedic surgeon
- Open fractures have a high incidence of infection
  - —High-pressure irrigation of wound is necessary in the ED if there is a delay to OR
  - —Antistaphylococcal and streptococcal antibiotics should be given

MEDICATIONS

- Cefazolin: 1 g i.v./i.m. (peds: 25 mg/kg i.v./i.m.)
- Fentanyl: 50–250 μg i.v. titrated (peds: 2 μg/kg i.v.)
- Ibuprofen: 800 mg p.o. (peds: 10 mg/kg PO)
- Meperidine: 25–100 mg i.v./i.m. titrated (peds: 1–1.75 mg/kg i.v./i.m.)
- Morphine: 2–10 mg i.v./i.m. titrated (peds: 0.1 mg/kg i.v.)

Disposition

ADMISSION CRITERIA

- Open fracture
- Evidence of compartment syndrome or neurovascular injury
- Open reduction internal fixation required immediately

DISCHARGE CRITERIA

- Most MT fractures can be discharged with orthopedic follow-up

Miscellaneous

ICD9: 825

ICD10: S92.9

SUGGESTED READINGS

Crawford Adams J, Hamblen D. Outline of fractures; the foot, 11th ed. London: Churchill Livingstone, 1999:278–285.

Hansen ST Jr. Skeletal trauma: foot injuries, 2nd ed. Philadelphia: WB Saunders, 1998:2405–2433.

Heckman JD, et al. Rockwood and Greens fractures in adults, 5th ed. Philadelphia: 2001:2091–2245.

Swiontkowski MF. Skeletal trauma in children: fractures and dislocations of the foot and ankle, 2nd ed. Philadelphia: WB Saunders, 1998:530–555.

Author: Colleen J. Campbell

Forearm Fractures Shaft/Distal

Clinical Presentation

SIGNS AND SYMPTOMS

- Forearm pain, crepitus, tenderness to palpation, deformity, shortening of the forearm
- Forearm edema, ecchymosis, elbow or wrist joint effusions
- Abnormal mobility or loss of function at elbow/wrist/hand
- Neurologic abnormalities, vascular compromise

MECHANISM/DESCRIPTION

- Direct blow to forearm
- Longitudinal compression load, fall on outstretched hand (FOOSH), horizontal force
- Excessive pronation, supination, hyperextension, or hyperflexion
- Shaft fractures (single and paired) are often displaced by contraction of the muscles of the arm and are sometimes associated with dislocations
  - —*Galeazzi* fracture is a distal radius fracture, associated with distal radioulnar dislocation
  - —*Monteggia* fracture is a proximal ulnar fracture, associated with dislocation of the radial head
- Distal fractures include extension, flexion, and intraarticular classifications
  - —*Colles* fracture is a hyperextension fracture of the distal radius (distal fragment displaced dorsally with radial deviation) that may also involve the ulnar styloid and the distal radioulnar joint
  - —*Smith* fracture is a hyperflexion fracture of the distal radius (distal fragment displaced volarly)
  - —*Barton* fracture is an intraarticular fracture of the dorsal rim of the distal radius, often associated with dislocation of the carpal bones
  - —*Hutchinson* fracture is an intraarticular fracture of the radial styloid

PEDIATRIC CONSIDERATIONS

- Shaft fractures
  - —*Torus* fracture involves compression (buckling) of the cortex on one or both sides
  - —*Greenstick* fracture involves distraction of one side of the cortex with the opposite side intact
  - —*Plastic deformity* results in bowing of the radius or ulna without apparent disruption of the cortex (multiple microfractures)
- Distal fractures
  - —*Salter-Harris*-type fractures (see chapter on Salter-Harris classification)

Pre-Hospital

CAUTIONS

- All suspected forearm fractures should be elevated, splinted, and immobilized, including the elbow and wrist joints
- All open fractures should be wrapped with a sterile dressing before splinting/ immobilization
  - —Do not reduce open fractures back under the skin in the field
- In patients without altered mental status or complicated abdominal trauma, analgesia may be administered in the pre-hospital setting

Diagnosis

ESSENTIAL WORKUP

- History should include occupation and hand dominance
- Physical exam with special attention to skin integrity, deformity, and neurovascular status
- All suspected forearm fractures require AP and lateral radiographs, including wrist and elbow

IMAGING/SPECIAL TESTS

- Compartment pressures should be measured for suspected compartment syndrome
- Some intraarticular fractures may require CT imaging

DIFFERENTIAL DIAGNOSIS

- Upper extremity muscle, ligamentous injury
- Elbow or wrist dislocations, including the pediatric nursemaid's elbow
- Forearm contusions, hematomas, cellulitis, abscesses, soft tissue masses
- Forearm osteogenic tumors, osteomyelitis
- Upper extremity vascular or neurologic injuries
- Elbow or wrist arthritis, joint effusions
- Pediatric growth plates, nutrient vessels may be mistaken for fractures

Treatment

INITIAL STABILIZATION

- All suspected forearm fractures should be immobilized, elevated, and have a cold compress applied
- Appropriate pain medication
- Open fractures need early systemic antibiotics and tetanus prophylaxis as indicated

ED TREATMENT

- Shaft fractures, nondisplaced
  - —Long-arm splint
  - —Orthopedic referral
- Shaft fractures, displaced
  - —Orthopedic consultation (often require open reduction, internal fixation)
- Distal fractures, nondisplaced
  - —Forearm sugar-tong or AP splint; orthopedic referral
- Distal fractures: *Colles/Smith*
  - —Simple, noncomminuted, extraarticular Colles and Smith fractures may be reduced, splinted (long-arm sugar-tong splint), placed in a sling, and referred to orthopedics
  - —Complicated Colles and Smith fractures require orthopedic consultation
- Distal fractures: *Barton/Hutchinson*
  - —Uncomplicated Barton and Hutchinson fractures can be splinted (AP or sugar-tong splint), placed in a sling, and referred to orthopedics
  - —Complicated fractures require orthopedic consultation
- Open fractures
  - —Open fractures should be covered with sterile dressings, given IM/IV antibiotics tetanus immunization (if indicated), splinted, and require immediate orthopedic consultation
  - —Forearm fractures associated with compartment syndrome or neurovascular compromise require immediate orthopedic consultation
- Special pediatric considerations
  - —*Torus* and *Greenstick* fractures with <10 degrees of angulation may be treated with a long-arm splint, sling, and orthopedic referral
  - —*Plastic deformities* require orthopedic consultation; some minimally displaced plastic deformities may be placed in a long-arm splint and sling
  - —*Salter-Harris*-type fractures require orthopedic consultation

MEDICATIONS

- Acetaminophen: 325–1,000 mg PO q4h (peds: 10–15 mg/kg q4h PO)
- Antibiotics
  - —Cefazolin: 1–2 g i.m./i.v. or equivalent first-generation cephalosporin; if contaminated, add an aminoglycoside
  - —Open fractures require IM/IV antibiotics
- Codeine: 15–60 mg PO/i.m. q4h (peds: older than 2 years, 0.5–1.0 mg/kg q4h PO/i.m.)
- Hydrocodone: 5–10 mg PO q4h
- Ibuprofen: 200–800 mg q4–8h (peds: older than 6 months, 5–10 mg/kg/dose q6h)
- Morphine sulfate: 2–10 mg i.v./i.m. titrate to pain (peds: 0.01 mg/kg/dose i.v./i.m.)
- Tetanus (Td): 0.5 mL i.m. q10yr

Disposition

ADMISSION CRITERIA

- Open fractures
- Fractures with compartment syndrome or neurovascular compromise
- Fractures needing immediate operative management or general anesthesia for reduction
- Suspected child abuse

DISCHARGE CRITERIA

- Appropriate reduction and immobilization
- Arranged orthopedic follow-up
- Adequate pain control measures
- Cast/splint care discharge instructions provided and understood by patient
- Documentation of intact neurovascular function after ED treatment

Miscellaneous

ICD9: 813.20, 813.40

ICD10: S52.9

SUGGESTED READINGS

Dicke TE, Nunley JA. Distal forearm fractures in children: complications and surgical indications. Orthop Clin North Am 1993;24(2):333.

Patzakis MJ, Wilkens J. Factors influencing infection rate in open fracture wounds. Clin Orthop 1988;243:36.

Price CT. Injuries to the shafts of the radius and ulna. In: Rockwood CA, Wilkins KE, Beaty JH, eds. Fractures in children, 4th ed, vol 3. Philadelphia: JB Lippincott Co, 1996:449–586.

Richards RR, Corley FG. Fractures of the shafts of the radius and ulna. In: Rockwood CA, Green DP, Bucholz RW, et al. eds. Fractures in adults, 4th ed, vol 1. Philadelphia: JB Lippincott Co, 1996:869–929.

Szabo RM. Extra-articular fractures of the distal radius. Orthop Clin North Am 1993;24(2):229.

Wilkins KE, O'Brien E. Fractures of the distal radius and ulna. In: Rockwood CA, Wilkins KE, Beaty JH, eds. Fractures in children, 4th ed, vol 3. Philadelphia: JB Lippincott Co, 1996:586–653.

Authors: Trevor J. Mills; Peter M. C. DeBlieux

Foreign Body, Ear

Clinical Presentation

SIGNS AND SYMPTOMS

- Decreased hearing
- Unilateral ear pain
- Fullness
- Loud noises
- Buzzing sound (with live insects)
- Nausea
- Dizziness
- Ipsilateral tearing
- Purulent discharge from the external ear
- Itching
- Bleeding

MECHANISM/DESCRIPTION

- Foreign bodies lodged in the external auditory canal (EAC)
- Types of foreign bodies with children
  - —Stones
  - —Small beads
  - —Paper
  - —Toys
  - —Seeds and popcorn kernels
  - —Beans and other food and organic materials
- Types of foreign bodies with competent adults
  - —Cotton-swab tips
  - —Earplugs
  - —Insects
- Inanimate objects are often associated with delayed presentations
- Most objects tend to become trapped in the outer two thirds of the EAC
- Children and psychiatric patients may place anything sufficiently small to enter the EAC
- Ear foreign bodies are most common in children younger than 8 years
- Complications
  - —Canal laceration
  - —Perforation of the tympanic membrane
  - —More likely to result from the removal procedure
  - —Otitis externa
- Symptoms usually resolve within a few days after foreign body removal

Pre-Hospital

CAUTIONS

- Severe ear pain, sensation of movement, and a loud buzzing sound
  - —Typical signs of a live insect in the external auditory canal
  - —Instill warm lidocaine or mineral oil in the affected ear to kill the insect

CONTROVERSIES

- Attempts at removal in the field are not indicated
  - —Lack of appropriate equipment
  - —Prior failed attempts may make future attempts more difficult

Diagnosis

ESSENTIAL WORKUP

- Always seek to identify the nature of the foreign body before trying to remove it
  - —Live insect
  - —Vegetable
  - —Inanimate object
- Careful otoscopic examination
  - —Minimize pain
  - —Gain the patient's trust
  - —Achieve optimal visualization by having an assistant exert gentle, steady traction on the patient's lobule
  - —Perform a bilateral examination
  - —Especially important in children and psychiatric patients
  - —Prevents overlooking a quiescent foreign body in the contralateral ear
  - —Repeat exam after removal to assess possible trauma of external canal or tympanic membrane

IMAGING/SPECIAL TESTS

- Operating microscope
  - —Use if ED removal fails
- Radiographs are not indicated

DIFFERENTIAL DIAGNOSIS

- Cerumen impaction
- Granuloma
- Hematoma
- Injury
- Otitis externa
- Perforated tympanic membrane
- Residual otitis externa after self-extraction of the foreign body
- Tumor

Treatment

INITIAL STABILIZATION

- For a patient in distress because of a live insect
  - —Drown or immobilize insect before any removal attempts
  - —Instill warm solution into the EAC
    - -Mineral oil
    - -Viscous lidocaine
    - -Ether
    - -2% lidocaine
    - -Microscope immersion oil
    - -Cold fluids should not be used so as to avoid a caloric response

ED TREATMENT

- Appropriate instruments
  - —Otoscope
  - —Alligator forceps
  - —Cupped forceps
  - —Number 3, 5, and 7 suction tips, preferably with Frazier suction cups
  - —A wire loop
  - —Ear curettes
  - —A right-angled blunt hook
- Achieve proper head immobilization
- Vegetable matter removal
  - —Visualize
  - —Attempt removal with forceps
  - —Be certain to delineate clearly between foreign body and inflamed EAC tissue
  - —Do not irrigate the EAC if the foreign body is of such a nature that it might swell
- Nonvegetable inanimate foreign body removal
  - —Visualize
  - —If easily grasped, attempt removal with forceps
  - —If not accessible, attempt removal with irrigation
  - —Perform careful visualization
  - —Place an Angiocath catheter adjacent to, or preferably distal to, the foreign body
  - —Inject warm water or sterile saline through catheter via a syringe
  - —Backwash the foreign body out
  - —Never attempt removal by irrigation when the foreign body is a button battery
- Polished or smooth object extraction
  - —Visualize
  - —Direct suction
  - —Blunt right-angled probe: pass beyond the foreign body; rotate 90 degrees; remove it with the foreign body
  - —Fogarty catheter: carefully pass beyond the foreign body and inflate and withdraw; this approach puts the tympanic membrane at particular risk of inadvertent injury
  - —Cyanoacrylate glue (Super-Glue): place on the tip of a blunt probe; place on the foreign body for 10 seconds and then pull; quick bonding may allow foreign body removal with the probe
- Insect removal
  - —Once killed, remove with forceps or by irrigation
  - —Reexamine to ensure all insect parts are removed
- Sharp objects
  - —Remove with operating microscope
  - —Consider otolaryngologic referral if evidence of trauma or if patient uncooperative
- Anesthesia or analgesia
  - —None needed in adults for simple foreign body removal
  - —Four-quadrant local anesthetic block
  - —1% or 2% lidocaine, with or without epinephrine
  - —Infiltrate around the EAC
  - —Conscious sedation
  - —Indicated for children and uncooperative adults
  - —Use before attempts, as unsuccessful efforts may produce bleeding, edema, or injury to the tympanic membrane
  - —Ketamine for children
  - —Benzodiazepines for older patients

MEDICATIONS

- Fentanyl: 1 μg/kg
- Ketamine: 1–2 mg/kg i.v. or 4 mg/kg i.m.
- Midazolam: 1 mg i.v. slowly q2–3min up to 5 mg (peds: 6 months–5 years, 0.05–0.1 mg/kg, titrate to maximum of 0.6 mg/kg; 6–12 years, 0.025–0.05 mg/kg, titrate to maximum of 0.4 mg/kg)

Disposition

ADMISSION CRITERIA

- Hospital admission is usually not necessary

DISCHARGE CRITERIA

- The patient should be instructed not to place any objects in the ear
- A short course of analgesics after traumatic foreign body removal
- Otitis externa
  - —Topical antimicrobial such as Cortisporin suspension
- Immunocompromised patients may require oral antibiotics
- Perforated tympanic membrane
  - —Prophylaxis with antibiotics
  - —ENT follow-up
- Avoid submersion in water until follow-up if trauma or infection present

Miscellaneous

ICD9: 931

ICD10: T16

SUGGESTED READINGS

Ansley JF, Cunningham MJ. Treatment of aural foreign bodies in children. Pediatrics 1998;101:638–641.

Balbani AP, Sanchez TG, Butugan O, et al. Ear and nose foreign body removal in children. Int J Pediatr Otorhinolaryngol 1998;46:37–42.

Bressler K, Shelton C. Ear foreign body removal: a review of 98 consecutive cases. Laryngoscope 1993;103:367–370.

Davies PH, Benger JR. Foreign bodies in the nose and ear: a review of techniques for removal in the emergency department. J Accid Emerg Med 2000;17:91–94.

Authors: Kathleen Nasci; Charles Pollack

Foreign Body, Esophageal

Clinical Presentation

SIGNS AND SYMPTOMS

Acute Ingestion

- Dysphagia
- Odynophagia
- Drooling
- Vomiting
- Choking
- Gagging
- Blood-stained saliva

Chronically Retained Foreign Body

- Respiratory symptoms predominate (paraesophageal tissue swelling compromises adjacent trachea)
  - —Cough
  - —Stridor
  - —Hoarseness
- Chest pain
- Site of foreign body (FB) sensation usually corresponds to esophageal level of FB
- Esophageal perforation
  - —Redness
  - —Swelling
  - —Crepitus in the neck
- <20% asymptomatic

MECHANISM/DESCRIPTION

- Esophageal FBs typically lodge at three sites of physiologic constriction
  - —Cricopharyngeal muscle (C-6) (most common)
  - —Aortic arch (T-4)
  - —Gastroesophageal junction (T-11)
- 90% of ingested FB pass spontaneously

ETIOLOGY

- Most common adult and adolescent FBs are food boluses and bones
  - —Esophageal pathology almost always underlies food impactions
- Increased risk
  - —Edentulous adults
  - —Intoxicated patients
  - —Patients with underlying esophageal disease

PEDIATRIC CONSIDERATIONS

- 80% of FB ingestions occur in the pediatric age-group, particularly younger than 2 years
- Coins
  - —Most common
  - —80% of esophageal FB
- Infants: signs/symptoms
  - —Refusal to eat
  - —Stridor
  - —Upper respiratory tract infection
  - —Neck/throat pain
- Predisposing factor: esophageal strictures

Pre-Hospital

CAUTIONS

- Airway maintenance and prevention of aspiration paramount
- Oxygen for patients in distress
- Place patient in whatever position gives the most comfort
- Ipecac and cathartics are contraindicated

Diagnosis

ESSENTIAL WORKUP

- History about the object ingested: type, when, and how
- Physical exam focused by the degree of distress exhibited
  - —Esophagus for
    - -Obstruction
    - -Perforation
    - -Hemorrhage
  - —Oropharynx for
    - -Red, irritated throat
    - -Palatal abrasions
  - —Lung for
    - -Stridor and wheezing
  - —Abdomen for
    - -Peritonitis or bowel obstruction
- Direct or indirect laryngoscopy can be useful

IMAGING/SPECIAL TESTS

- CXR includes all of neck for FB localization
  - —Need for additional radiographs is dictated by the clinical situation
  - —Those with food bolus need no radiographs usually
  - —Esophageal FBs usually align themselves in the coronal plane
  - —Esophageal perforation is noted by air in the retropharyngeal space, in the soft tissues of the neck, or by pneumomediastinum
- Esophageal contrast studies for nonradiopaque FBs
  - —Changes in the contour of the barium column localize FB
  - —Passage of the contrast solution into the stomach: partial versus complete obstruction
  - —*Caution*
    - -Oral contrast in high-grade esophageal obstructions can increase the risk of aspiration, and barium may coat the mucosa, limiting subsequent endoscopy
    - -Traditional water-soluble contrast can cause severe tissue reaction in perforations because of its hyperosmolality
- Metal detectors have been used in localizing ingested metal, particularly coins
- Endoscopy
  - —Method of choice for localizing and managing most esophageal FBs
  - —Ability to inspect the surrounding esophageal mucosa for pathology
- CT can often detect FBs not identified by other means

DIFFERENTIAL DIAGNOSIS

- Globus phenomenon
- Esophagitis
- Croup
- Epiglottitis
- Upper respiratory tract infection
- Retropharyngeal abscess

Treatment

INITIAL STABILIZATION

- ABCs first priority
- Prevent aspiration

ED TREATMENT

- FBs lodged in the upper or mid-esophagus
  - —Extraction required
- Asymptomatic patients with coins or smooth objects in the distal esophagus
  - —Observe up to 24 hours after ingestion to see whether it will pass into the stomach
- Impacted food bolus obstructing the esophagus
  - —Emergent removal indicated
  - —Digestion with proteolytic enzymes (papain) not recommended because of serious morbidity including esophageal perforation and aspiration
- Extricate sharp or pointed esophageal FBs regardless of their location
- Button batteries
  - —Extract emergently wherever they lodge in the esophagus
  - —Batteries frequently leak: potassium hydroxide and mercury are the most toxic constituents
  - —Mucosal burns can occur within 4–6 hours

Removal Techniques

- Fluoroscopically guided Foley catheter extraction
  - —Successful and safe in experienced hands
  - —Foley catheter (10–16 French) placed nasally, passed into esophagus, tip and balloon pushed beyond the FB under fluoroscopic control
  - —Foley balloon inflated with contrast and the catheter slowly withdrawn
  - —Contraindicated in chronic ingestions, uncooperative patients, sharp-pointed objects
- Foley catheters may also be used to push a distal FB into the stomach
- Endoscopy
  - —Preferred method to remove acute or chronic FBs
  - —Always used with impactions of long duration (>2–4 days) because of associated esophageal irritation/edema
  - —General endotracheal anesthesia needed in difficult cases
    - -Infants
    - -Psychiatric patients
    - -Difficult FB
- Bougienage: using dilator to push FB into stomach
- IV glucagon
  - —Decreases LES tone without interfering with esophageal contractions
  - —Often permits distal food boluses to pass into the stomach
  - —For impactions <24 hours' duration
- Gas forming agents
  - —Useful in patients with esophageal food impactions <24 hours
  - —Combining IV glucagon followed by oral gas-forming agents has also been successful
- Surgical intervention
  - —Reserved for patients in whom the FB cannot be removed by other methods
  - —Approximately 2% of all patients
  - —Toothpicks and bones common objects

MEDICATIONS

- E-Z Gas: 30 mL solution ($NaHCO_3$, citric acid and simethicone) orally
- Glucagon: 1–2 mg i.v. push after test dose to determine hypersensitivity

Disposition

ADMISSION CRITERIA

- Seriously ill patients and those with complications such as esophageal perforation, migration of FB through esophageal wall, significant bleeding
- Airway compromise
- Symptomatic patients in whom attempts to remove the FB are unsuccessful

DISCHARGE CRITERIA

- Asymptomatic patients in whom the FB has been removed or passed distal to the esophagus
- Asymptomatic patients with distal esophageal smooth FBs need reexamination within 12–24 hours to ascertain whether spontaneous passage into the stomach has occurred

Miscellaneous

ICD9: 935.1

ICD10: T18.1

SUGGESTED READINGS

Calkins CM, Christians KK, Sell LL. Cost analysis in the management of esophageal coins: endoscopy vs. bougienage. J Pediatr Surg 1999;34:412–414.

MacPherson RI, Hill JG, Othersen HB, et al. Esophageal foreign bodies in children: diagnosis, treatment and complications. AJR Am J Roentgenol 1996;166:911–924.

Mosca S, Manes G, Martion R, et al. Endoscopic management of foreign bodies in the upper gastrointestinal tract: report on a series of 414 adult patients. Endoscopy 2001;33:692–696.

Soprano JV, Mandl KD. Four strategies for the management of esophageal coins in children. Pediatrics 2000;105:1497–1501.

Weinstock LB, Shatz BA, Thyssen ED. Esophageal food bolun obstruction: evaluation of extraction and modified push techniques in 75 cases. Endoscopy 1999;31:421–425.

Author: Thomas W. Lukens

Foreign Body, Nasal

Clinical Presentation

SIGNS AND SYMPTOMS

- Most nasal foreign bodies (FBs) asymptomatic
- Someone witnesses child putting object into nare
- FB noticed by parent or caretaker
- Nasal discharge
  - —Acute or chronic
  - —Unilateral
  - —Foul smelling
  - —Halitosis
- Sinus discomfort
- Epistaxis
- Local inflammation
- Septal perforation
- Ingestion or aspiration of FB

MECHANISM/DESCRIPTION

- Types of FBs
  - —Limited only by nostril size and imagination, activity of the child
  - —Most innocuous; sinusitis the principal risk
    - -Food
    - -Paper
    - -Pieces of toys
    - -Beads
    - -Rocks
    - -Button batteries high risk of complications compared with other FBs: tissue necrosis; septal perforation; require rapid removal
- Average patient age 2–4 years
- Age not associated with particular type of FB

Pre-Hospital

CAUTIONS

- Transport in sitting position
  - -Avoid posterior displacement, possible aspiration of FB
- Avoid interventions that upset the child

Diagnosis

ESSENTIAL WORKUP

- Visualization of the FB in the nostril
  - —Always check both nostrils

IMAGING/SPECIAL TESTS

- Fiberoptic visualization if FB cannot be visualized on rhinoscopy
- Sinus films if present for extended period
  - —Symptom persistence despite removal of the FB and antibiotics

DIFFERENTIAL DIAGNOSIS

- Sinusitis
- Epistaxis
- Intranasal mass

Treatment

INITIAL STABILIZATION

N/A

ED TREATMENT

- Topical vasoconstrictors
  - —Presence of mucosal edema or bleeding secondary to removal attempts
    - -Nebulized epinephrine
    - -Cocaine 4%
    - -Oxymetazoline 0.05%
    - -Phenylephrine 0.125–0.5%
- Positive pressure
  - —Occlude contralateral nostril
  - —Positive pressure applied to mouth only
  - —Deliver brisk puff as child begins to inhale
  - —Parent may tell the child they will be given a "big kiss"
  - —Placement of 4-by-4-inch gauze pads on caregiver's cheek
  - —FB dislodges onto cheek of the provider or into room
  - —Repeated as necessary
  - —Alternatively deliver puff with a bag-mask over the mouth and O_2 at 10–15 L/min
  - —Alternatively into contralateral nostril male–male adapter on oxygen tubing, deliver wall oxygen at 10–15 L/min
  - —Nasal wash with 7 mL saline via bulb syringe contralateral nostril described; controversial; aspiration risk
- Hooked probe, alligator forceps
  - —Anterior FBs that are easily grasped
  - —Headlamp, nasal speculum facilitate use
  - —Risk of further posterior displacement
- Balloon catheters
  - —Used primarily when instrumentation fails
  - —5-French or 6-French Foley or Fogarty balloon catheter lubricated with 2% lidocaine jelly
  - —Advance catheter past object
  - —After inflation with 2–3 mL of air, catheter gently withdrawn
- Suction catheter
  - —Best for round, smooth objects
  - —Optimal retrieval with Schunkt-neck suction catheter
    - -Metal with plastic umbrella at the tip
  - —Suction tip placed against the object
  - —Suction turned up to 100–140 mm Hg
  - —Catheter and object withdrawn
- Cyanoacrylate tissue glue
  - —Film of glue applied to cut end of hollow plastic swab handle
  - —Apply against object for 60 seconds, then withdraw
  - —Caution with nontissue cyanoacrylate glues; tissue irritation
- Magnet for removal of metal FB described; limited experience

MEDICATIONS

- Cocaine: 4% solution, 2 drops affected nares
- Lidocaine: 4% solution, 2 drops affected nares
- Oxymetazoline 0.05%: 2–3 drops or sprays affected nares
- Phenylephrine 0.125–0.5%: 2–3 sprays affected nares

Disposition

ADMISSION CRITERIA

- Referral for ambulatory surgical removal
  - —FB cannot be recovered in ED
  - —Removal under general anesthesia required

DISCHARGE CRITERIA

- Ensure all FBs removed, both nares
- Return if bleeding, infection (nasal discharge)
- If a button battery was removed
  - —Mandatory follow-up with ENT specialist
  - —Monitor for delayed sequelae
    - -Ischemic mucosa
    - -Turbinate or septal damage
    - -Saddle-nose deformity

Miscellaneous

ICD9: 933.0

ICD10: T17.1

SUGGESTED READINGS

Backlin SA. Positive-pressure technique for nasal foreign body removal in children. Ann Emerg Med 1995;25(4):554–555.

Douglas SA, Mirza S, Stafford FW. Magnetic removal of a nasal foreign body. Int J Pediatr Otorhinolaryngol 2002;62(2):165–167.

Kadish HA, Corneli HM. Removal of nasal foreign bodies in the pediatric population. Am J Emerg Med 1997;15(1):54–56.

Lichenstein R, Guidice EL. Nasal wash technique for nasal foreign body removal. Pediatr Emerg Care 2000;16(1):59–60.

Navitsky RC, Beamsley A, McLaughlin S. Nasal positive-pressure technique for nasal foreign body removal in children. Am J Emerg Med 2002;20(2):103–104.

Palmer O, Natarajan B, Johnstone A, et al. Button battery in the nose—an unusual foreign body. J Laryngol Otol 1994;108:871–872.

Author: Paul Blackburn

Foreign Body, Rectal

Clinical Presentation

SIGNS AND SYMPTOMS

- Complaint of rectal foreign body (FB)
- Rectal fullness
- Rectal pain
- Perirectal abscess (with imbedded bones/toothpick)
- FB on rectal examination

MECHANISM/DESCRIPTION

- Self-insertion (autoeroticism)
  - —Phallic substitutes inserted by patient or partner
  - —FBs used to aid in removal of feces
- Ingested
  - —Chicken bones
  - —Fish bones
  - —Toothpick
- Iatrogenic
  - —Thermometer
  - —Enema tips
- Assault
  - —Knife or pipe forcibly inserted
  - —Incidence of perforation is very high

Pre-Hospital

CAUTIONS

- Patient has usually tried to remove the FB and failed
- Further attempts at extraction will not work and could cause a perforation

Diagnosis

ESSENTIAL WORKUP

- Identify the number, type, and duration of FBs and mechanism of insertion
- Physical exam with emphasis on abdominal and rectal exam
- Biplane x-ray films to confirm number and size of FBs
- For assaulted patients, workup as for blunt trauma to abdomen

LABORATORY

- CBC
  - —For bleeding or peritonitis
- Urinalysis
  - —For urethral/bladder injuries

DIFFERENTIAL DIAGNOSIS

- Pseudo-FB
  - —Patients insist there is a FB when x-ray, rectal exams, and proctoscopy results are normal
- Perirectal abscess
- Hemorrhoid

Treatment

INITIAL STABILIZATION

- Perforation with peritonitis and sepsis
  - —0.9% NS i.v. fluid 500-mL bolus
  - —Broad-spectrum antibiotics
  - —Gentamicin, clindamycin, ampicillin
  - —Urgent surgical consult
- ATLS with multiple trauma victims

ED TREATMENT

Foreign Body Removal

- Small objects that are not fragile or sharp
  - —Can be removed if the object can be firmly held
  - —Remove with gentle but firm continuous traction to overcome the anal sphincter
  - —Colonic mucosa tightly adherent to distal end of FB creates vacuum and impedes withdrawal of object
  - —Passage of a Foley catheter beyond the object with insufflation of air breaks vacuum and permits retrieval
- Removal with some direct visualization and a large operating anoscope (after blockage of sphincter and pudendal nerve with local anesthesia) for
  - —Larger objects
  - —Objects that have remained >24 hours with resulting edema
  - —Objects with sharp edges
- Proctoscopy/sigmoidoscopy after extraction to examine the colonic mucosa

MEDICATIONS

- Ampicillin: 1–2 g (peds: 50–200 mg/kg/24 h) i.v. q4–6h
- Clindamycin: 600–900 mg (peds: 20–40 mg/kg/24 h) i.v. q8h
- Gentamicin: 1 mg/kg (peds: 2–2.5 mg/kg) i.v. q8h

PEDIATRIC CONSIDERATIONS

- Removal under general anesthesia for children who are too young to cooperate
- It is probably child abuse if a FB other than enema tips or thermometer is present

Disposition

ADMISSION CRITERIA

- Failed extraction in ED requires surgical removal in OR
- Evidence of mucosal tear on proctoscopy should be observed for 24 hours (no antibiotic indicated)
- Symptoms of rectal pain associated with removal of a sharp FB indicates the possibility of a small perforation with developing abscess and requires examination under anesthesia

DISCHARGE CRITERIA

- Reliable patient with an atraumatic insertion and removal of a rectal FB
  - —Instruct to return for rectal pain, abdominal pain, fever, or massive rectal bleeding

Miscellaneous

ICD9: 937

ICD10: T18.5

SUGGESTED READINGS

Abcarian H. Colorectal foreign bodies. In: Mazier PW, et al. eds. Surgery of the colon, rectum, and anus. Philadelphia: WB Saunders, 1995.

Eftaiha M, Hambrick E, Abcarian H. Principles of management of colorectal foreign bodies. Dis Colon Rectum 1977;112: 691–695.

Janicke DM, Pundt MR. Anorectal disorders. Emerg Med Clinic North Am 1996;14: 757–788.

Nehme-Kingsley A, Abcarian H. Colorectal foreign bodies management update. Dis Colon Rectum 1985;28:941–944.

Author: Charles Orsay

Fournier's Gangrene

Clinical Presentation

SIGNS AND SYMPTOMS

- A *rapidly progressive* necrotizing infection of the *perineum* involving the subcutaneous and fascial tissues and often muscle layers; usually seen in diabetics or immunocompromised patients
- Patients are often *toxic* in appearance with nausea, vomiting, fever, chills, and complaints of pain
- Sources of infection may be flora from *genitourinary, rectal,* or *penile/scrotal* regions
- Skin findings include bronze or violaceous discoloration of the skin, a thin brown watery discharge, ulceration, bullous vesicles, crepitance, subcutaneous air, frank necrosis, and eschar formation
- Early on, pain is out of proportion to the examination, but eventually the dead tissue becomes *insensate*
- Lethargy and an inappropriate indifference to the illness are common

MECHANISM/DESCRIPTION

- Inadequate hygiene leads to *skin maceration* and *excoriation,* providing bacteria access to the subcutaneous tissue
- Once the skin barrier is broken, polymicrobial flora spread along the *fascial planes* of the perineum
- Colles fascia fuses with the urogenital diaphragm, slowing propagation posteriorly and laterally
- Anteriorly, Buck and Scarpa fascia are continuous, allowing rapid extension to anterior abdominal wall and laterally along the fascia lata
- *The testes and urethra are usually spared*
- Three anatomic origins account for most cases
  —40% lower urinary tract: urethral strictures, indwelling catheters
  —30% penile or scrotal: condom catheters, hydradenitis, and balanitis
  —30% anorectal: fistulas, perirectal infections, and hemorrhoids
- Rarely, intraabdominal sources such as perforating appendicitis, diverticulitis, or pancreatitis has produced Fournier's gangrene by dependent contiguous spread

ETIOLOGY

- An infection by *polymicrobial flora* (mixed aerobic and anaerobic organisms)
- The mixed bacteria exert a synergistic tissue-destructive effect
- End arterial thrombosis in the subcutaneous tissues produces an anaerobic environment, promoting extension of the infection
- Bacterial toxins and tissue necrosis factors may contribute to the clinical presentation
- Risk factors include trauma, diabetes, alcoholism, other immunocompromised states, morbid obesity, and abdominal surgery

PEDIATRIC CONSIDERATIONS

- Though unusual in children, >50 cases in children have been described
- Most often are complications of burns, circumcision, balanitis, severe diaper rashes, or insect bites
- Organisms are more frequently *Staphylococcus* or *Streptococcus*
- Pediatric patients have more local disease and are less toxic

Pre-Hospital

CAUTIONS

- Patients may be hypotensive from septic shock and require fluid resuscitation and pressor support

Diagnosis

ESSENTIAL WORKUP

- Fournier's gangrene is a clinical diagnosis
- History and physical exam with special attention to the perineum, and evaluating for signs of sepsis
- *Early surgical consultation* for emergent débridement is essential
- Other workup directed toward the relevant comorbid factors such as diabetes or immunocompromised status

LABORATORY

- Other than Gram stain of tissue and the associated drainage, there are *no specific laboratory tests* that are diagnostic of Fournier's gangrene
- Urinalysis should be performed
- Leukocytosis, anemia, electrolyte imbalances, acidosis, and renal failure are common
- Disseminated intravascular coagulation (DIC) may be present; PT, PTT, fibrin-split products, and fibrinogen levels help identify
- If patient is suspected of or known to have diabetes, glucose, electrolytes, and serum ketones to evaluate for diabetes and DKA
- Culture of blood, urine, and tissue (when available)

IMAGING/SPECIAL TESTS

- Plain films of the pelvis may reveal *subcutaneous emphysema* and an ileus
- CT scanning helps if an intraabdominal or ischiorectal source is suspected
- US may be useful in differentiating from other causes of acute scrotum
- Retrograde urethrography, anoscopy, proctosigmoidoscopy, and barium enemas may be helpful to localize anatomic sources of infection

DIFFERENTIAL DIAGNOSIS

- Testicular torsion
- Scrotal cellulitis
- Epididymitis/orchitis
- Tinea cruris
- Scrotal abscess/inguinal abscess
- Perirectal infections
- Insect and human bites

PEDIATRIC CONSIDERATIONS

- Early pediatric consultation to assist with medical management and guide a *more conservative* surgical approach

Treatment

INITIAL STABILIZATION
- ABCs
- Central venous access, fluid resuscitation, and pressure support as indicated
- Avoid femoral access, femoral venipuncture, and lower extremity venous access
- Foley catheter placement or suprapubic access if indicated

ED TREATMENT
- Empiric *broad-spectrum antibiotics*
- Early *emergent aggressive surgical débridement*
- Adjunctive *hyperbaric oxygen therapy* coordinated with surgical care
- Treat dehydration and correct electrolytes
- Blood products as needed for DIC or anemia; oxygen debt can be minimized by keeping the hematocrit >30%
- Tetanus prophylaxis as indicated

MEDICATIONS
- Antibiotic regimens
  - —Multidrug regimen
    - -Ampicillin: 2 g i.v. q6h (peds: 50 mg/kg) *and*
    - -Clindamycin: 900 mg i.v. q8h (peds: 10 mg/kg) *and*
    - -Gentamicin: 5 mg/kg daily load i.v. q8h
  - —Single-drug regimens (peds: safety not established)
    - -Ampicillin/sulbactam: 3 g i.v. initial ED dose
    - -Imipenem: 1 g i.v. initial ED dose
    - -Piperacillin/tazobactam: 3.375 g i.v. initial ED dose
    - -Ticarcillin/clavulanate: 3.1 g i.v. initial ED dose *or*
- Blood products as indicated
- Dopamine or dobutamine IV drips starting at 5 μg/kg/min titrating to effect if hypotensive after aggressive hydration
- Insulin adjusted to control glucose and acidosis

PEDIATRIC CONSIDERATIONS
- More conservative surgical approach
- Adequate staphylococcal coverage

Disposition

ADMISSION CRITERIA
- *All* patients with Fournier's gangrene require admission and surgical ICU admission
- Mortality estimates of up to 67% emphasize the need for early aggressive care

DISCHARGE CRITERIA
- No patients with Fournier's gangrene should be discharged

Miscellaneous

ICD9: 608.83

ICD10: N49.8

SUGGESTED READINGS

Adams JR, Mata JA, Venable DD, et al. Fournier's gangrene in children. Urology 1990;35(5):439–441.

Corman JM, Moody JA, Aronson WJ. Fournier's gangrene in a modern surgical setting: improved survival with aggressive management. Br J Urol 1999;84:85–88.

Eke N. Fourier's gangrene: a review of 1726 cases. Br J Surg 2000;87:718–728.

Norton KS, Johnson LW, Perry T, et al. Management of Fournier's gangrene: and eleven year retrospective analysis of early recognition, diagnosis and treatment. Am Surg 2002;68:709–713.

Author: Gary M. Vilke

Fracture, Open

Clinical Presentation

SIGNS AND SYMPTOMS

- Deformity with nearby violation in skin integrity
- Neurovascular compromise may be present

MECHANISM/DESCRIPTION

- Continuity between skin violation and fracture site, ranging from a puncture wound to grossly exposed bone
- Predisposition to complications
  - —Massive soft tissue damage
  - —Severe wound contamination
  - —Compromised vascularity
  - —Fracture instability
  - —Compromised host (diabetes, vascular disease, etc)

Pre-Hospital

- Sterile dressings over open wound
- Immobilize the joints above and below the fracture
- Do not reduce long-bone fractures unless severely angulated or neurovascularly compromised
- Military antishock trousers (MAST) can be used to immobilize the hip in femur fractures if a traction device is not available

Diagnosis

ESSENTIAL WORKUP

- Complete neurologic and vascular examination
- Plain radiographs including joints above and below the affected area
- Perform saline arthrogram by intraarticular injection of saline or methylene blue if joint involvement suspected
  - —Positive test result is saline or methylene blue visible in nearby wound

LABORATORY

- CBC, coagulation studies for large-bone (femur, pelvis) fractures
- Type and screen or type and cross-match for significant blood loss

IMAGING/SPECIAL TESTS

- Angiography to assess vascular damage with the following indications
  - —Ischemic extremity
  - —Knee dislocation
  - —High-energy fracture patterns
  - —Massive soft tissue injury in high-risk areas
- Measurement of compartment pressures if compartment syndrome suspected

DIFFERENTIAL DIAGNOSIS

- Noncontinuous laceration/abrasion

Treatment

INITIAL STABILIZATION

- ABCs of trauma care
  - —30% of patients with open lower extremity fractures are multiple-trauma victims
- Reduction of fracture with steady, longitudinal traction
- Immobilization with nonradiopaque device

ED TREATMENT

- IV access
- Administer tetanus, if needed, and parenteral antibiotics
- Early orthopedic consultation for formal irrigation, débridement, and operative fixation, if needed, within 6 hours to reduce likelihood of infection
- Minimize the number of times dressing is removed to avoid secondary contamination
- Examine regularly for compartment syndrome and neurovascular status

MEDICATIONS

- Cefazolin: 1–2 g (peds: 20 mg/kg i.m./i.v. within 3 hours of injury)
- Gentamicin: 2–5 mg/kg i.m./i.v.
- Morphine sulfate: 2–10 mg (peds: 0.1 mg/kg/dose i.v. or equivalent analgesic)
- Penicillin: 4–5 million units i.v./i.m. in farmyard injuries or wounds at risk of contamination with *Clostridium*
- Tetanus booster: 0.5 mL i.m.
- Tetanus immunoglobulin (TIG): 250 IU i.m. if not previously immunized against tetanus

PEDIATRIC CONSIDERATIONS

- Diphtheria-pertussis-tetanus booster for children younger than 7 years

Disposition

ADMISSION CRITERIA

- Most patients will be admitted for washout and possibly débridement or operative fixation and IV antibiotics

DISCHARGE CRITERIA

- Simple open fractures may be washed out and immobilized in the ED after consultation with an orthopaedic surgeon and discharged with oral antibiotics and very close follow-up in 24 hours

Miscellaneous

ICD9: 829.1

SUGGESTED READINGS

Alonso JE, Lee J, Burgess AR, et al. The management of complex orthopedic injuries. Surg Clin North Am 1996;76(4): 879–901.

Chapman MW. Open fractures. In: Chapman MW, ed. Chapman's orthopaedic surgery, 3rd ed. Philadelphia: Lippincott Williams & Wilkins, 2001:381–392.

Geiderman JM. General principles of orthopaedic injuries. In: Marx JA, et al. eds. Rosen's emergency medicine: concepts and clinical practice, 5th ed. St. Louis: Mosby–Year Book, 2002:467–492.

Menkes JS. Injuries to bones, joints & soft tissues: initial evaluation and management of orthopaedic injuries. In: Tintinalli JE, ed. Emergency medicine: a comprehensive study guide, 5th ed. New York: McGraw-Hill, 2000:1739–1753.

Author: Christy Rosa Mohler

Fractures, Pediatric

Clinical Presentation

SIGNS AND SYMPTOMS

- Decreased limb movement, "pseudoparalysis"
- Swelling
- Tenderness
- Deformity
- Ecchymoses
- Crepitus
- Limp
- Abnormal neurovascular status of extremity
  —Severe pain in forearm or calf, pain with passive stretching of fingers or toes, or sensory deficit in the distal extremity more sensitive indicators of ischemia
- Open fracture may be obvious or subtle (collection of blood with fat globules under skin)
- Complications (long term)
  —Nonunion of capitulum fracture
  —Avascular necrosis of femoral head after femoral neck fracture
  —Neurovascular compromise
  —Posttraumatic ossification of elbow after displaced fracture or dislocation
  —Growth arrest if growth plate crushed
  —Angulation or rotational deformity from initial injury or subsequent differential growth
  —Reflex sympathetic dystrophy

MECHANISM/DESCRIPTION

- Anatomy
  —Diaphysis: physis to physis; bone shaft
  —Epiphysis: cartilaginous center at or near end of bone that is site of bone growth
  —Physis (equals epiphyseal or metaphyseal growth plate): radiolucent line between epiphysis and metaphysis; cartilaginous
  —Metaphysis: region of rapidly growing trabecular bone underlying base of cartilaginous growth plate; between diaphysis and epiphysis
- Bones are highly resilient, elastic, and "springy"
- Cartilaginous growth plates are potential areas of injury
- Ligaments more resistant to injury than growth plates
  —Fractures often accompany dislocations
- Nonaccidental trauma (NAT) if history inconsistent with findings

Salter-Harris Classification

- Risk of growth disturbance increases from type I to type V
- Type I
  —Separation of epiphysis from metaphysis without displacement or injury to the growth plate
  —Tenderness and pain at point of growth plate
  —X-ray normal initially, repeat in 7–10 days to look for calcification and new bone formation
  —Growth disturbance is rare
- Type II
  —Epiphyseal plate slip with fracture through the metaphysis
  —Most common
  —Growth disturbance is rare
- Type III
  —Epiphyseal plate slip with an intraarticular fracture involving the epiphysis
  —Most common site is distal tibial epiphysis
  —Growth disturbance possible
- Type IV
  —Intraarticular fracture extending through the epiphysis, epiphyseal plate, and metaphysis; lateral condyle of humerus is most common site
  —Growth disturbance highly likely
- Type V
  —Crush injury to epiphyseal plate, producing growth arrest
  —Usually occurs in joints that move in only one plane such as knee or ankle

ETIOLOGY

- Mechanism is useful in defining the potential and type of injury
  —Falls, motor vehicle accidents, blunt trauma, NAT
- Obesity and rapid growth spurts are risk factors
- Common fractures include lower forearm, clavicle, tibia or fibula, supracondylar fracture of humerus
- NAT: consider in specific fractures
  —Fractures of the radius/ulna, tibia/fibula, or femur in children younger than 1 year
  —Midshaft or metaphyseal fractures of the humerus in children younger than 3 years
  —Epiphyseal lesions (especially chip fractures)
  —Rib fractures
  —Skull fractures, especially in children younger than 1 year
  —Unexplained, inconsistent, or multiple fractures (especially at different stages of healing)
  —Subperiosteal ossification without previous known fracture
  —Unusual behavior in child or parent

Pre-Hospital

CAUTIONS

- Immobilize/splint involved extremity
- Assess neurovascular status

Diagnosis

ESSENTIAL WORKUP

- Assess neurovascular status
- Exclude concurrent injuries
- Ensure that history consistent with injury
- AP, lateral, and oblique radiographs as necessary, including the joint above and below the fracture
  —Comparison views may be useful if growth plates involved

LABORATORY

- Required only if concomitant injuries, surgery anticipated, or multiple/major bone involvement
- CBC, ESR if infection suspected

IMAGING/SPECIAL TESTS

- Follow-up radiographs at 7–10 days may be required to exclude Salter I fracture
- Bone scan/CT/MRI may be useful to exclude fractures if plain radiographs are unhelpful or to evaluate for infection

DIFFERENTIAL DIAGNOSIS

- Infection
- Tumor
- Neurologic deficits
- Subtle dislocations such as radial head subluxation (nursemaid's elbow)
- NAT

Treatment

INITIAL STABILIZATION

- Resuscitation for concurrent injuries

ED TREATMENT

- Management of life-threatening concurrent injuries
- Dislocations require immediate assessment and attention to neurovascular compromise
- Mechanism helps in understanding the direction of the force required to relocate
- Alignment is essential, particularly when it involves a joint surface
- Angulation of metaphyseal fractures is tolerated; remodeling often with up to 30 degrees
- Open fractures: need to convert an open wound to a clean closed wound
- Appropriate reporting of NAT

Salter-Harris Fractures

- Type I and type II fractures require 3 weeks of immobilization for upper extremity and 6 weeks for lower extremities
- Type II distal femur fractures, type III, and type IV require referral for anatomic reduction
- Type V fractures require immobilization and consultation
- Anatomic reduction does not eliminate possibility of growth disturbance in type III fractures and higher

Clavicle Fracture

- Figure-of-eight splint and sling as tolerated for comfort
- Distal third clavicle fractures should be referred with initial sling and swathe or shoulder immobilizer

Supracondylar Humerus Fracture

- Orthopedic consultation because of potential complications
  —Brachial artery injury, median nerve injury
  —Volar compartment syndrome of forearm
  —Epiphyseal injury with long-term growth abnormalities

Distal Radius and Ulnar Fractures

- Rotational deformities must be eliminated
- Reduce angulated fractures >15 degrees
- Immobilize for 4–6 weeks
- *Torus fracture* (incomplete fracture; buckling or angulation on the compression side of the bone only)
  —Age 5–11 years
  —Occurs at junction of metaphysis and diaphysis
  —Immobilize in short-arm splint for 3–4 weeks or until nontender at fracture site
- *Greenstick fracture* (incomplete fracture of diaphysis of long bone with fracture on tension side of cortex)
  —Immobilize in long-arm splint for 4–6 weeks
  —Reduction if angulation >30 degrees in infants, >15 degrees in children
- Colles fracture
  —Reduce by traction in the line of deformity to disimpact the fragments, followed by pressure on the dorsal aspect of the distal fragment and volar aspect of the proximal fragment
  —Correct radial deviation
  —Immobilize the hand in ulnar deviation, wrist in neutral, and forearm in full pronation
  —Orthopedic consultation

Tibial or Fibular Fracture

- Isolated fibular fractures: short-leg walking cast
- Nondisplaced tibial fracture: long-leg posterior splint, non-weight bearing
- Displaced tibial fracture and complex fractures require consultation

MEDICATIONS

- For sedation/analgesia during reduction
  —Fentanyl (Sublimaze): 1-5 μg/kg i.v. (20-minute half-life)
  —Hematoma block: 1% lidocaine without epi (maximum, 3-5 mg/kg)
  —Ketamine: 1-5 mg/kg i.m., to maximum of 50 mg/dose, with atropine 0.01 mg/kg
  -Most useful in children aged 3 months to 7 years because of side effects
  —Midazolam (Versed): 0.05–0.10 mg/kg/dose i.v. over 1–2 minutes to maximum of 4 mg/dose
  -Often used with fentanyl
  —Nitrous oxide: 50% nitrous oxide in oxygen in children older than 4 years; 3-minute prereduction, maximum 30 minutes; best with hematoma block

Disposition

ADMISSION CRITERIA

- NAT (or per social services)
- Potential neurovascular compromise
  —Condylar or supracondylar humerus fracture
  —Femoral shaft
  —Complete patella

DISCHARGE CRITERIA

- Uncomplicated fracture: no concurrent injury or neurovascular/compartment compromise
- Follow-up arranged and parents understand injury and management

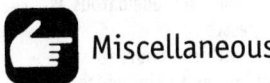

Miscellaneous

ICD9: 829.0

SUGGESTED READINGS

Adams J, Hamblen D. Outline of fractures, 10th ed. New York: Churchill Livingstone, 1992.

Gall O, et al. Adverse events of premixed nitrous oxide and oxygen for procedural sedation in children. Lancet 2001;358: 1514–1515.

Hennrikus WL, et al. Self-administered nitrous oxide and a hematoma block for analgesia in the outpatient reduction of fracture in children. J Bone Joint Surg 1995;77-A(3):335–338.

Leventhal J, et al. Fractures in young children. Distinguishing child abuse from unintentional injuries. Am J Dis Child 1993;147:87–92.

Marx JA. Rosen's emergency medicine concepts and clinical practice, 5th ed. St. Louis: Mosby, 2002.

Wheeless CR. Wheeless textbook of orthopedics. 1996. Available at: *www.medmedia.com/med.htm*.

Authors: Leslie Milne; Adam Barkin

Frostbite

Clinical Presentation

SIGNS AND SYMPTOMS

- Extremities (fingers, toes) and head (ears, nose) most commonly affected
- Initial appearance of an injury often fails to predict eventual depth or outcome

Superficial Frostbite

- Skin structures only involved
  —No tissue loss
- Frozen skin loses touch, pain, or temperature sensation
- Stinging, numbness, burning
- Appearance
  —Initially white/waxy/mottled
  —Becomes hyperemic and edematous as warming progresses
- Rewarming leads within 3 hours to hyperemia, swelling, and pain, which resolve within 2–3 days

Deep Frostbite

- Subcutaneous, muscle, nerve, or bone involved
  —Tissue loss inevitable
- Initially insensate, injuries develop severe pain/burning upon rewarming
- Tissue feels hard, woody to the touch
- Post-rewarming appearance
  —Edema within 3 hours and lasts 5 days
  —Large clear blebs within 6–24 hours
  —Small, hemorrhagic blebs form after 24 hours
  —Eschar forms in 9–15 days
  —Mummification in 3–6 weeks
- Reduced mobility, persistent mottling, anesthesia despite edema after rewarming are unfavorable prognostic indicators
- Devitalized tissue demarcates as the injury evolves over weeks to months

MECHANISM/DESCRIPTION

- Tissue damage results from
  —*Direct cell damage:* due to intracellular ice crystal formation
  —*Indirect cell damage:* extracellular ice crystal formation leads to intracellular dehydration through osmosis
  —*Microvascular stasis and thrombosis:* erythrocyte sludging leads to hypoxia then vasospasm, ischemia, tissue necrosis
  —*Progressive dermal ischemia:* mediated by thromboxane and prostaglandins in blisters
  —*Reperfusion injury:* after thawing, caused by edema then thrombosis, inflammatory leukocyte infiltration, and necrosis
  —*Thermal shock:* direct cell death due to the extreme cold
- Devitalized tissue demarcates as the injury evolves over weeks to months, hence the expectant management of severe frostbite

ETIOLOGY

- Cold exposure with increased vulnerability due to
  —Extremes of age
  —Poor self-care
    -Intoxication
    -Altered mental status
    -Immobility
  —Poor circulatory status

Pre-Hospital

CAUTIONS

- Protect and immobilize frostbitten area during transport
- Remove restrictive or wet garments
- Avoid dry rewarming of the frostbitten limb if a likelihood of refreezing of the injury
  —If evacuation will be delayed and suitable facilities are available, field rewarming in warm (40–42°C) water can be attempted
- Rubbing, manipulating the limb, or applying snow while it is still frozen is contraindicated
- Hypothermia
  —Common in frostbite victims
  —Avoid rough handling to minimize possibility of cardiac dysrhythmias in the seriously hypothermic patient
- Evaluate for underlying etiology
  —Intoxication
  —Head injury
  —Trauma
  —Hypoglycemia
  —Cardiac or neurologic problems

Diagnosis

ESSENTIAL WORKUP

- Diagnosis is based on the clinical presentation

LABORATORY

- None indicated in most cases
- For severe frostbite
  —CBC
  —Electrolytes, BUN/Cr, glucose
  —Urinalysis for evidence for myoglobinuria
- Cultures and Gram stains from open areas when infection suspected
- Technetium-99 scintigraphy
  —Helpful in early identification of unsalvageable bone
  —Permits earlier decision about amputation
  —Perform 2–7 days after cold injury

DIFFERENTIAL DIAGNOSIS

- Frostnip
  —Superficial, reversible ice crystal formation without tissue destruction
  —Transient numbness and paresthesia resolve after rewarming
- Trench foot
  —Exposure to wet cold for prolonged periods
  —Neurovascular damage without ice crystal formation
  —Pallor, mottling, paresthesias, pulselessness, paralysis, and numbness
  —Hyperemia with rewarming lasting up to 6 weeks
- Chilblains
  —Chronic repeated exposure to dry cold
  —Localized erythema, cyanosis, plaques, and vesicles

Treatment

INITIAL STABILIZATION

- ABCs
- Identify and correct hypothermia
- IV fluid volume expansion with 0.9% NS for severe frostbite
- Protect frostbitten areas from excessive handling or dry warming during resuscitation

ED TREATMENT

- If the injury is <24 hours' old and has not yet been rewarmed
  —Initiate rapid thawing of the injured extremity for 10–30 minutes in 40–42°C water
  —Stop treatment when the limb is warm, red, and pliable
  —Monitor water temperature closely to prevent thermal injury
- Analgesia
- NSAIDs (e.g., ibuprofen) to combat the effects of prostaglandins on skin necrosis
- Aloe Vera topical cream
  —Combats the arachidonic cascade
  —Recommended for all intact blisters
  —Avoid preparations containing alcohol, scent, salicylates, which interfere with its effectiveness
- Blister débridement or aspiration
  —Indicated for clear blebs
    -Removes thromboxane and prostaglandins
  —Contraindicated for hemorrhagic blebs
    -Exposes deeper structures to dehydration and infection)
- Tetanus prophylaxis
- Antibacterial prophylaxis
  —Consider during the hyperemic recovery phase (at least 2–3 days) in severely frostbitten areas
  —Against streptococci, staphylococci, and pseudomonads species (cephalosporin, penicillinase-resistant penicillin, quinolone)
  —Topical antibacterial agents interfere with the use of Aloe Vera cream and should be considered a second-line approach
- Elevation and splinting of frostbitten area
- Change dressing two to four times daily
- Avoid vasoconstrictive agents (including tobacco)

MEDICATIONS

- Aloe Vera: topical cream 70% concentration q6h
- Cephalexin (cephalosporin): 500 mg (peds: 25–50 mg/kg/24 h q6h) PO q.i.d.
- Ciprofloxacin (quinolone): 500 mg PO b.i.d.
- Dicloxacillin (penicillinase-resistant penicillin): 500 mg (peds: 25–100 mg/kg/ 24 h q6h) PO q.i.d.
- Ibuprofen (NSAID): 800 mg (peds: 40 mg/kg/ 24 h q6–8h) PO t.i.d.
- Morphine sulfate: 0.1–0.2 mg/kg (peds: 0.1 mg/kg) i.v. or i.m. p.r.n. (titrate to patient response)

Disposition

ADMISSION CRITERIA

- All but the most superficial and painless cases should be admitted for at least 24–48 hours after rewarming
- Lower admission threshold where risk of refreezing exists

DISCHARGE CRITERIA

- Rewarmed injury with evidence of only superficial injury and close follow-up availability

Miscellaneous

ICD9: 991.3

ICD10: T35.7

SEE ALSO: HYPOTHERMIA

SUGGESTED READINGS

Hayes DW Jr, et al. Pentoxifylline. Adjunctive therapy in the treatment of pedal frostbite [Review]. Clin Podiatr Med Surg 2000;17(4):715–722.

Marx JA, Hockenberger RS, Walls RM, et al, eds. Rosen's emergency medicine, 5th ed. Philadelphia: Mosby, 2002.

McCauley RL, et al. Frostbite: methods to minimize tissue loss. Postgrad Med 1990;88(8):67–77.

McCauley RL, et al. Frostbite and other cold-induced injuries. In: Auerbach PS, ed. Wilderness medicine. St. Louis: Mosby, 1995:129–145.

Author: Paul Arnold

Gallstone Ileus

Clinical Presentation

SIGNS AND SYMPTOMS

- Abdominal cramping
  —Pain, episodic
- Nausea
- Vomiting
  —Can be feculent
- Obstipation
- Abdominal distention
- Abdominal tenderness
  —Peritoneal findings late
- Abnormal bowel sounds
- Jaundice in 10%
- Initial pain may be suggestive of biliary colic

MECHANISM/DESCRIPTION

- Mechanical intestinal obstruction secondary to the impaction of a gallstone in the bowel lumen
- Gallstone ileus
  —1–4% of all intestinal obstructions
  —25% of bowel obstruction in patients older than 65 years

ETIOLOGY

- Chronic gallbladder inflammation causes adhesions between the gallbladder and adjacent bowel wall
- Cholecystenteric fistula develops permitting stone passage into the intestine
  —Most fistulas occur between the gallbladder and duodenum
- Stones usually lodge in the terminal ileum (narrowest portion of the small intestine), causing complete or partial obstruction of the bowel
  —Gallstone obstruction of large bowel is rare
- Cholecystocolic fistulas in 15% of patients
- Stones spilled intraperitoneally during cholecystectomy—open or laparoscopic—may also lead to bowel obstruction
- Recurrent obstruction in 2–10%: additional stones present in the bowel
  —Migration of common duct stones

PEDIATRIC CONSIDERATION

- Very uncommon in children but case report of a 13-year-old

Pre-Hospital

CAUTIONS

- Initiate fluid replacement for dehydrated or hypotensive patients

Diagnosis

ESSENTIAL WORKUP

- Evaluation for intestinal obstruction

LABORATORY

- Electrolytes, BUN/Cr, glucose; vomiting leads to
  —Hypochloremia
  —Hypokalemia
  —Hyponatremia
  —Alkalosis
- Amylase
  —Elevated in late obstructions
- CBC/hematocrit
  —Hemoconcentration secondary to dehydration

IMAGING/SPECIAL TESTS

- Flat and upright abdominal radiographs
  —Multiple air fluid levels and distended bowel consistent with bowel obstruction
- CXR
  —Pneumoperitoneum
- Criteria for radiographic diagnosis of gallstone ileus: Rigler triad (two of three needed)
  —Air in the biliary tree (pneumobilia)
  —Partial or complete bowel obstruction
  —Aberrant gallstone visualized or indirect visualization via contrast medium in the bowel.
- Abdominal CT scan
  —Effective in delineating causes of bowel obstruction including gallstone ileus
- Abdominal US

DIFFERENTIAL DIAGNOSIS

- Paralytic ileus
- Extrinsic bowel obstruction: adhesions, volvulus, hernia, intussusception
- GI malignancy
- Diverticulitis
- Bezoar
- Inflammatory bowel disease
- Pseudoobstruction

Treatment

INITIAL STABILIZATION
- Fluid resuscitation

ED TREATMENT
- Nasogastric suction to decompress the stomach and intestine
- NPO
- Electrolyte replacement
- Monitor urine output
- Analgesics
- Observation
- Surgical consultation

Disposition

ADMISSION CRITERIA
- Admit all patients with bowel obstruction

DISCHARGE CRITERIA
- None

Miscellaneous

ICD9: 560.31

ICD10: K56.3

SEE ALSO: BOWEL OBSTRUCTION

SUGGESTED READINGS

Aricite A, Czeiger D, Gortzak Y, et al. Gastric outlet obstruction by gallstone: Bouveret syndrome. Can J Gastroenterol 2000;35:781–783.

Draganil BD, Reece-Smith H. Gallstone ileus without a gallbladder. Ann R Coll Surg Engl 1997;79:231–232.

Resiner RM, Cohen JR. Gallstone ileus: a review of 1,001 reported cases. Am Surg 1994;60:441–446.

Ripolles T, Mighel-Dasit A, Errando J, et al. Gallstone ileus: increased diagnostic sensitivity by combining plain film with ultrasound. Abdom Imaging 2001;26: 401–405.

Swift SE, Spencer JA. Gallstone ileus: CT findings. Clin Radiol 1998;53:451–454.

Author: Thomas W. Lukens

Gangrene

Clinical Presentation

SIGNS AND SYMPTOMS

- Sudden severe pain of extremity or involved area
- Low-grade fever
- Tachycardia out of proportion to fever
- Bronzing of the skin over involved area
- Crepitus
- Formation of blebs and bullae
- Thin, serosanguineous exudate with a sweet odor
- Rapid local extension
- Obtunded sensorium
- Systemic toxicity

MECHANISM/DESCRIPTION

- Gas gangrene or clostridial myonecrosis is an acute, rapidly progressive, gas-forming necrotizing infection of muscle and subcutaneous tissue that can be seen in posttraumatic or postoperative situations

ETIOLOGY

- Clostridial organisms, a facultative anaerobic, spore-forming, gram-positive bacillus, produce a number of toxins; the most prevalent and lethal is α-toxin
- *Clostridium perfringens* is the most common bacteria; found in 80–90% of wounds
- Other clostridial bacteria isolated include *Clostridium novyi, Clostridium septicum, Clostridium histolyticum, Clostridium bifermentans* and *Clostridium fallux*
- Two distinct mechanisms for introduction of clostridial organisms
  —Traumatic and postoperative
  —Nontraumatic (associated with diabetes mellitus, peripheral vascular disease, alcoholism, IVDA, and malignancies)

PEDIATRIC CONSIDERATIONS

- Similar presentation as adults

Pre-Hospital

N/A

Diagnosis

ESSENTIAL WORKUP

- History and physical exam with special attention to clinical evidence of crepitus in soft tissue
- Soft tissue x-rays of involved area to detect gas dissecting along fascial planes (however, the absence of gas does not rule out significant disease)
- Stat Gram stain of wound exudate for gram-positive bacillus with paucity of leukocytes

LABORATORY

- CBC with differential, electrolytes, BUN, and creatinine
- Coagulation studies
- Evaluate for hemolysis
- Stat Gram stain of wound exudate
- Anaerobic cultures of wound or tissue biopsy

IMAGING/SPECIAL TESTS

- X-rays may reveal soft tissue gas
- CT if area involves abdomen or flank

DIFFERENTIAL DIAGNOSIS

- Cellulitis
- Necrotizing fasciitis
- Nonclostridial myositis and myonecrosis
- Other causes of gas in tissues, as from dissection from respiratory or GI tracts

Treatment

INITIAL STABILIZATION

- ABCs
  - —Control airway as needed
  - —Supplemental oxygen; cardiac and oxygen saturation monitors should be placed
  - —IV access; consider CVP monitoring
  - —Aggressive volume expansion including crystalloid, plasma, packed RBCs, and albumin

ED TREATMENT

- Parenteral antibiotic therapy
  - —Primary: penicillin G plus clindamycin
  - —Alternative: ceftriaxone or erythromycin
  - —If mixed infection: penicillin plus clindamycin, metronidazole, or vancomycin and gram-negative coverage with gentamicin
- Surgical consultation
  - —Débridement, amputation, or fasciotomy are *required*
- Hyperbaric oxygen as adjunctive therapy
  - —Early transfer to hyperbaric facility may be life saving
- Tetanus prophylaxis
- Observe for major complications including ARDS, renal failure, myocardial irritability, and DIC
- Polyvalent antitoxin is not made in the U.S. and studies have not demonstrated efficacy; because of the unacceptable hypersensitivity reactions, it is not routinely recommended

MEDICATIONS

- Ceftriaxone: 2.0 g (peds: 100 mg/kg/24 h; maximum 4 g) i.v. q24h
- Clindamycin: 900 mg (peds: 40 mg/kg/d q6h) i.v. q8h i.v.
- Gentamicin: 2.0 mg/kg (peds: 2.0 mg/kg i.v. q8h) i.v. q8h
- Metronidazole: 500 mg (peds: safety not established) i.v. q8h
- Penicillin G: 24 million IU/24 h (peds: 250,000 IU/kg/24 h) i.v. q4–6h
- Tetanus immune globulin: 500 IU i.m.
- Tetanus toxoid: 0.5 mg i.m.

Disposition

ADMISSION CRITERIA

- All patients with gas gangrene and evidence of myonecrosis *must be admitted* for surgical débridement and IV antibiotics
- Use of hyperbaric oxygen therapy is an important adjunct

DISCHARGE CRITERIA

- No patient with acute gangrene should be discharged

Miscellaneous

ICD9: 040.0

ICD10: R02

SUGGESTED READINGS

Chapnick EK, Abter EI. Necrotizing soft-tissue infections. Infect Dis Clin North Am 1996;10(4):835–855.

Clark LA, Moon RE. Hyperbaric oxygen in the treatment of life-threatening soft-tissue infection. Respir Care Clin North Am 1999;5(2):203–219.

Gonzalez MH. Necrotizing fasciitis and gangrene of the upper extremity. Hand Clin 1998;14(4):635–645.

Sasaki T, Nanjo H, Takahashi M, et al. Non-traumatic gas gangrene in the abdomen: report of six autopsy cases. J Gastroenterol 2000;35(5):382–390.

Author: Karen Van Hoesen

Gastric Outlet Obstruction

Clinical Presentation

SIGNS AND SYMPTOMS

- Early satiety
- Postprandial fullness
- Epigastric discomfort relieved with emesis
- Vomiting
  - —Occurs approximately 20–30 minutes after eating
  - —With blood if bleeding ulcer/Mallory-Weiss tear
- Vital signs
  - —Usually normal
  - —Tachycardia, hypotension with significant volume depletion
- Abdominal examination
  - —Minimal epigastric distention
  - —Tympany
  - —Succussion splash >4 hours after eating

MECHANISM/DESCRIPTION

- Edema, scarring, stricture, or hyperplasia at pylorus or duodenum
- Intrinsic or extrinsic mass, causing compression at pylorus or proximal duodenum

ETIOLOGY

- Peptic ulcer disease
- Pyloric stenosis
- Neoplasms
- Inflammation
- Strictures postcaustic ingestion
- Tuberculosis

PEDIATRIC CONSIDERATIONS

- Pyloric stenosis
  - —Most common cause in pediatric population
  - —May present as early as first week after birth and up to age 3 months
  - —Presentation
    - -Initially occasional nonprojectile postprandial vomiting
    - -Progress to nonbilious projectile vomiting
  - —Midepigastric peristaltic wave may be seen before vomiting
  - —Epigastric rounded mass "olive" palpable in 80–90% of patients

Pre-Hospital

N/A

Diagnosis

ESSENTIAL WORKUP

- Careful history and physical exam reveals diagnosis
- Abdominal US in pediatric patients
  - —Reveals elongated hypertrophic pyloric sphincter

LABORATORY

- CBC
  - —Anemia if blood loss from ulcer
  - —High hematocrit indicates hemoconcentration
- Electrolytes, BUN/Cr, glucose
  - —Hypokalemia
  - —Hypochloremic metabolic alkalosis
  - —Hypoglycemia
  - —Prerenal azotemia
- Urinalysis
- Amylase/lipase

IMAGING/SPECIAL TESTS

- Plain abdominal radiographs
  - —Dilated stomach
  - —Absence of air distally in bowel
- Abdominal CT for detecting neoplastic cause of obstruction
- EKG in elderly/at risk of coronary artery disease
- Upper GI/endoscopy to define and diagnose etiology

DIFFERENTIAL DIAGNOSIS

- Proximal bowel obstruction
- Exacerbation of peptic ulcer disease
- Gastroenteritis
- Cholecystitis
- Acute pancreatitis
- Cholelithiasis
- Diabetic gastroparesis
- Psychogenic vomiting

Treatment

INITIAL STABILIZATION

- 0.9% NS IV fluid resuscitation for prolonged obstruction and significant volume depletion
  - —1-L bolus in adult
  - —20-mL/kg bolus in children
- Correct electrolyte abnormalities, especially hypokalemia

ED TREATMENT

- NGT
- Foley catheter to monitor urine output
- Surgical consultation

Disposition

ADMISSION CRITERIA

- All patients with gastric outlet obstruction will require admission for fluid resuscitation and possible surgical intervention

DISCHARGE CRITERIA

- None

Miscellaneous

ICD9: 537.0

ICD10: K31.1

SEE ALSO: PYLORIC STENOSIS

SUGGESTED READINGS

Feldman. Sleisenger & Fordtran's gastrointestinal and liver disease, 6th ed. Philadelphia: WB Saunders, 1998:666–668.

Holder W. Intestinal obstruction. Gastroenterol Clin North Am 1988;17(2): 317.

Marx. Rosen's emergency medicine: concepts and clinical practice, 5th ed. St. Louis: Mosby, 2002:1243.

Shaffer H. Perforation and obstruction of the gastrointestinal tract. Radiol Clin North Am 1992;30(2):405.

Sivit C. Gastrointestinal emergencies in older infants and children. Radiol Clin North Am 1997;35(4):865.

Author: Julio Silva

Gastritis

Clinical Presentation

SIGNS AND SYMPTOMS

- Dyspepsia
- Epigastric pain or discomfort (episodic and chronic)
- Bloating, indigestion, eructation, flatulence, and heartburn
- Anorexia, nausea/vomiting
- Dehydration, tachycardia, and electrolyte disturbances (with vomiting)
- Hematemesis, melena, pallor, and signs of volume depletion (hemorrhagic gastritis)

MECHANISM/DESCRIPTION

- Inflammatory response of the gastric mucosa to injury
- Three lines of defense of the gastric mucosa
  —Mucous layer that forms a protective pH gradient
  —Surface epithelial cells that can repair small defects
  —Postepithelial barrier that neutralizes the acid that has traversed the first two layers
- No definite link between histologic gastritis and dyspeptic symptoms

ETIOLOGY

Acute Gastritis

- Caused by
  —Aspirin
  —Steroids
  —Alcohol
  —NSAIDs
  —Burns
  —Sepsis
  —Trauma
- Stress (sepsis, burns, trauma)
  —Decrease in splanchnic blood flow leading to decreased mucus production, bicarbonate secretion, and prostaglandin synthesis
  —Results in mucosal erosions and hemorrhage
- Alcohol
  —Induces production of leukotrienes that cause microvascular stasis, engorgement, and increased vascular permeability
  —Leads to hemorrhage
- NSAIDs
  —Interfere with prostaglandin synthesis, leading to a similar cascade as induced by alcohol
  —Results in mucosal erosions

Chronic Gastritis

- Produced by *Helicobacter pylori*
- Mechanism of *H. pylori* unclear
  —Gram-negative spiral bacteria found in the gastric mucous layer
  —Contains an enzyme urease that allows it to change the pH level (alkaline) of its microenvironment

Pre-Hospital

CAUTIONS

- ABCs with significant blood loss producing tachycardia and hypotension
  —Two large-bore IV lines infusing lactated Ringer's solution or 0.9% NS for fluid resuscitation
- Do not underestimate the degree of blood loss in a patient with a history of hypertension with a normal BP

Diagnosis

ESSENTIAL WORKUP

- Careful physical exam including stool Hemoccult testing and vital signs with orthostatics
- NGT when history of hematemesis or unstable vital signs
- Hematocrit determination

LABORATORY

- Normal laboratory values in uncomplicated gastritis
- CBC
  —Anemia with acute hemorrhagic gastritis
  —Leukocytosis: infection
- Amylase/lipase for pancreatitis in differential
- Urinalysis
  —Assess dehydration/ketosis (starvation)
  —Bilirubin present with hepatitis

IMAGING/SPECIAL TESTS

- EKG
  —For elderly patients
  —Myocardial ischemia in differential
- Endoscopy
  —Outpatient unless significant hemorrhage
  —Allows for visualization of the bleeding sites, histologic confirmation of mucosal inflammation, and detection of *H. pylori*
- Noninvasive *H. pylori* testing
  —^{13}C and ^{14}C urea breath tests
  —Stool antigen test
  —Serology to detect antibodies to *H. pylori*

DIFFERENTIAL DIAGNOSIS

- Peptic ulcer disease (PUD)
- "Nonulcer dyspepsia" (symptoms and no ulcer on endoscopy)
- Gastroesophageal reflux
- Biliary colic
- Cholecystitis
- Pancreatitis
- Hepatitis
- Abdominal aortic aneurysm
- Aortic dissection
- Myocardial infarction

Treatment

INITIAL STABILIZATION

- ABCs with acute erosive or hemorrhagic gastritis that presents with hemodynamic instability
- IV fluid resuscitation with lactated Ringer's solution or 0.9% NS via two large-bore catheters
- NGT for gastric decompression and lavage
- Foley catheterization to assess volume replacement

ED TREATMENT

- Pain control with
  - —Antacids
  - —GI cocktail
    - -30 mL antacids plus 10–20 mL viscous lidocaine
  - —H_2 antagonists
  - —Sucralfate
  - —Avoid narcotics because may mask serious illness

Acute Hemorrhagic Gastritis

- IV fluid resuscitation
- Blood transfusion if low hematocrit
- Reverse causes (alcohol, sepsis, NSAIDs, or trauma)
- Prevent *acute* or *erosive* gastritis in critically ill
  - —Antacids hourly or IV H_2 antagonists
  - —Goal is to keep pH level at more than 4

Chronic Gastritis

- Treatment of *H. pylori* infection
  - —Invasive or noninvasive testing to confirm infection
  - —Oral (PO) eradication antibiotic therapy options
    - -The most common regimen consists of omeprazole 20 mg or lansoprazole 30 mg plus clarithromycin 500 mg and amoxicillin 1 g all taken b.i.d. for 2 weeks.
    - -For penicillin allergic patients: proton pump inhibitor plus clarithromycin 500 mg b.i.d. plus metronidazole 500 mg b.i.d. for 14 days
    - -H_2 blocker, bismuth subsalicylate (Pepto-Bismol) plus either amoxicillin 1,000 mg b.i.d. or tetracycline 500 mg q.i.d. in combination with either metronidazole 250 mg q.i.d. or clarithromycin 500 mg b.i.d. for 14 days
  - —Resistance
    - -Increasing antibiotic resistance to metronidazole 30–48% and clarithromycin is now more than 10%
    - -Uncommon resistance to amoxicillin and tetracycline
    - -No resistance to bismuth
  - —Treatment controversial for asymptomatic or nonulcer dyspepsia gastritis
- Vitamin B_{12} supplementation for *atrophic gastritis*

MEDICATIONS

- Bismuth subsalicylate: 525-mg tabs 2 PO q.i.d.
- Cimetidine (H_2-blocker): 800 mg PO q.h.s. × 6–8 weeks
- Famotidine (H_2-blocker): 40 mg PO q.h.s. × 6–8 weeks
- Misoprostol: 100–200 μg PO q.i.d.
- Maalox plus: 2–4 tablets PO q.i.d.
- Mylanta II: 2–4 tablets PO q.i.d.
- Nizatidine (H_2-blocker): 300 mg PO q.h.s. × 6–8 weeks
- Omeprazole (20 mg) or lansoprazole (30 mg): PO b.i.d. × 2 weeks
- Ranitidine (H_2-blocker): 300 mg PO q.h.s. × 6–8 weeks
- Sucralfate: 1 g PO q.i.d. × 6–8 weeks

Disposition

ADMISSION CRITERIA

- Acute hemorrhagic or erosive gastritis that presents with upper GI tract bleeding, tachycardia and hypotension
- Uncontrolled pain or vomiting
- Coagulopathy from medication or liver disease

DISCHARGE CRITERIA

- Unremarkable physical exam with normal CBC and heme-negative stools
- If heme-positive stools, discharge if stable vital signs, normal hematocrit, and negative NGT aspiration for upper GI tract hemorrhage
- Outpatient evaluation for endoscopy

Miscellaneous

ICD9: 535.5

ICD10: K29.7

SEE ALSO: GASTROINTESTINAL BLEEDING; PEPTIC ULCER DISEASE

SUGGESTED READINGS

Heatley RV, et al. Gastritis and duodenitis. In: Bockus, ed. Gastroenterology, vol 1, 5th ed. 1995:635–643.

Leung WK, et al. Ulcer and gastritis. Prim Care 2001;28(3):487–503.

McGuirk TD, et al. Upper gastrointestinal tract bleeding. Emerg Med Clin North Am 1996;14(3):530–533.

Smoot DT, Go MF, Cryes B. Peptic ulcer disease. Prim Care 2001;33(1):8–15.

Soll AH, Isenberg JI, Graham DY. Gastritis, peptic ulcer disease, medical therapy. In: Bennett JC, Plum F, eds. Cecil's textbook of medicine. Philadelphia: WB Saunders, 1996:659–669.

Sung JJ, Chung SC, et al. Antibacterial treatment of gastric ulcers associated with *Helicobacter pylori*. N Engl J Med 1995;332: 139–142.

Author: Marco Cordero

Gastroenteritis

Clinical Presentation

SIGNS AND SYMPTOMS

- Nausea, vomiting, diarrhea
- Bloody/mucous diarrhea
- Abdominal cramps or pain
- Fever
- Malaise, myalgias, headache, anorexia
- Tachycardia, hypotension, lethargy, and dehydration (severe cases)

ETIOLOGY

Infections

Viruses

- 50–70% of all cases

Invasive Bacteria

- *Campylobacter:* contaminated food/water, wilderness water, birds, and other animals
  —Most common cause
  —Gross or occult blood is found in 60–90%
- Salmonella: contaminated water, eggs, poultry or dairy products
  —*Typhoid fever (Salmonella typhi)* characterized by unremitting fever, abdominal pain, rose spots, splenomegaly, and bradycardia
  —Immunocompromised susceptible
- *Shigella:* fecal-oral route
- *Vibrio parahaemolyticus:* raw and undercooked seafood
- *Yersinia:* contaminated food (pork), water, and milk
  —May present as mesenteric adenitis or mimic appendicitis

Specific Food-borne Disease (Food Poisoning)

- *Staphylococcus aureus*
  —Most common toxin-related disease
  —Symptoms 1–6 hours after ingesting food
- *Bacillus cereus*
  —Classic source is fried rice left on steam tables
  —Symptoms within 1–36 hours
- Cholera: profuse watery stools with mucous ("rice-water" stools)
- Ciguatera
  —Fish intoxication
  —Onset 5 minutes to 30 hours (average 6 hours) after ingestion
  —Paresthesias, hypotension, peripheral muscle weakness
  —Amitriptyline may be therapeutic
- Scombroid
  —Caused by "blood fish": tuna, albacore, mackerel, and mahi mahi
  —Flushing, headache, erythema, dizziness, blurred vision, and generalized burning sensation
  —Symptoms last <6 hours
  —Treatment includes antihistamines

Protozoa

- *Giardia lamblia*
  —High-risk groups: travelers, day care children, homosexual men, and campers who drink untreated mountain water

Noninfectious Causes

- Toxins
  —Zinc, copper, cadmium
  —Organic chemicals: polyvinyl chlorides
  —Pesticides: organophosphates
  —Radioactive substances
  —Alkyl mercury
- Altered host response to a food substance (tyramine, monosodium glutamate, tryptamine)

PEDIATRIC CONSIDERATIONS

- Focus evaluation on state of hydration
- Majority of viral origin and self-limited
- Rotavirus accounts for up to 50%
- *Shigella* infections associated with seizures

Pre-Hospital

CAUTIONS

- Difficult IV access in severe dehydration
- Avoid exposure to contaminated clothes or body substances

Diagnosis

ESSENTIAL WORKUP

- Digital rectal examination to determine the presence of gross or occult blood
- Fecal leukocyte determination
  —Present with invasive bacteria
  —Absent in protozoal infections, viral, toxin-induced food poisoning

LABORATORY

- CBC indications
  —Significant blood loss
  —Systemic toxicity
- Electrolytes, glucose, BUN/Cr indications
  —Lethargy, significant dehydration, toxicity, or altered mental status
  —Diuretic use, persistent diarrhea, chronic liver or renal disease
- Stool culture indications
  —Presence of fecal leukocytes
  —Historical markers (immunocompromised, travel, homosexual)
  —Public health (food handler, day/health care worker)
- Blood cultures indications
  —Suspected bacteremia/systemic infections
  —Ill patients requiring admission

IMAGING/SPECIAL TESTS

- Abdominal x-ray films have no value unless an obstruction or a toxic megacolon suspected

DIFFERENTIAL DIAGNOSIS

- Gastritis/peptic ulcer disease
- Milk and food allergies
- Appendicitis
- Irritable bowel syndrome
- Ulcerative colitis/Crohn disease
- Malrotation with midget volvulus
- Meckel's diverticulum
- Drugs and toxins
  —Mannitol
  —Sorbitol
  —Phenolphthalein
  —Magnesium-containing antacids
  —Quinidine
  —Colchicine
  —Mushrooms
  —Mercury poisoning

PEDIATRIC CONSIDERATIONS

- Laboratory studies not required in most cases
- Rotazyme assay detects rotavirus
  —Rarely indicated in managing outpatients
  —Helpful to cohort and avoid cross-contamination among inpatients
- Stool cultures indication
  —Fecal leukocytes
  —Toxic
  —Infants
  —Immunocompromised

Treatment

INITIAL STABILIZATION

- IV fluid with 0.9% NS resuscitation for severely dehydrated

ED TREATMENT

- Oral fluids for mild dehydration (Gatorade/Pedialyte)
- IV fluids for
  - —Hypotension, nausea/vomiting, obtundation, metabolic acidosis, significant hypernatremia or hyponatremia
  - —0.9% NS 500-mL to 1-L bolus (peds: 20 mL/kg) for resuscitation then 0.9% NS or D5 0.45% NS (peds: D5 0.25% NS) to maintain an adequate urine output
- Bismuth subsalicylate (Pepto-Bismol)
  - —Antisecretory agent
  - —Effective clinical relief without adverse effects
- Kaolin-pectin (Kaopectate)
  - —Reduces fluidity of stools
  - —Does not influence the course of the disease
- Antimotility drugs (diphenoxylate (Lomotil), loperamide (Imodium), paregoric, and codeine)
  - —Appropriate in noninfectious diarrhea
  - —Initial use of sparse amounts to control symptoms in infectious diarrhea
  - —Avoid prolonged use in infectious diarrhea—may increase the duration of fever, diarrhea, and bacteremia, and may precipitate a toxic megacolon
- Antiemetics: prochlorperazine (Compazine) and promethazine (Phenergan) for nausea/vomiting

Antibiotics for Infectious Pathogens

- Campylobacter: quinolone or erythromycin
- Salmonella: quinolone or trimethoprim-sulfamethoxazole (TMP/SMX)
- Ceftriaxone for typhoid fever
- Shigella: quinolone, TMP/SMX, or ampicillin
- *Vibrio parahaemolyticus:* tetracycline or doxycycline
- *Clostridium difficile:* vancomycin
- *Escherichia coli:* quinolone or TMP/SMX
- *G. lamblia:* metronidazole

MEDICATIONS

- Ampicillin: 500 mg (peds: 20 mg/kg/24 h) PO/i.v. q6h
- Bactrim DS (TMP/SMX): 1 tab (peds: 8–10 mg TMP/40–50 mg SMX/kg/24 h) PO or 4–5 mg/kg TMP i.v. b.i.d.
- Ciprofloxacin (quinolone): 500 mg PO or 400 mg i.v. b.i.d. (older than 18 years)
- Doxycycline: 100 mg PO/i.v. b.i.d.
- Erythromycin: 500 mg (peds: 40–50 mg/kg/24 h) PO q.i.d.
- Metronidazole: 250 mg (peds: 35 mg/kg/24 h) PO t.i.d. (older than 8 years)
- Tetracycline: 500 mg PO/i.v. q6h
- Prochlorperazine (Compazine): 5–10 mg IVP q3–4h; 10 mg PO q8h; 25 mg PR; q12h p.r.n.
- Promethazine (Phenergan): 25 mg i.m./i.v. q4h; 25 mg PO/PR q12h p.r.n. (peds: 0.25–1 mg/kg PO/PR/i.m. q4–6h)

Disposition

ADMISSION CRITERIA

- Hypotension unresponsive to IV fluids
- Significant bleeding
- Signs of sepsis/toxicity
- Intractable vomiting or abdominal pain
- Severe electrolyte imbalance
- Metabolic acidosis
- Altered mental status
- Children with >10–15% dehydration

DISCHARGE CRITERIA

- Mild cases requiring oral hydration
- Dehydration responsive to IV fluids

Miscellaneous

ICD9: 558.9

ICD10: A06

SEE ALSO: DIARRHEA, ADULT; DIARRHEA, PEDIATRIC

SUGGESTED READINGS

Bitterman R. Acute gastroenteritides. In: Marx JA, Hockberger RS, Walls RM, et al. eds. Rosen's emergency medicine: concepts and clinical practice, 5th ed. St. Louis: Mosby-Year Book, 2002:1301–1325.

Blacklow NR, Greenberg HB. Viral gastroenteritis. N Engl J Med 1991; 325:252.

DuPont H, Miranda A. Small intestine: infections with common bacterial and viral pathogens. In: Yamada T, et al. eds. Textbook of gastroenterology, 2d ed. Philadelphia: JB Lippincott Co, 1995:1605–1629.

Fleisher GR. Gastrointestinal infections. In: Fleisher G, Ludwig S, eds. Pediatric emergency medicine, 3rd ed. Baltimore: Williams & Wilkins, 1993:628–633.

Author: Isam Nasr

Gastroesophageal Reflux Disease

Clinical Presentation

SIGNS AND SYMPTOMS

- Heartburn (pyrosis)
  - —Retrosternal burning pain
  - —Radiates from epigastrium through the chest to the neck and throat
- Dysphagia
  - —Dysphagia suggests esophageal spasm or stricture
- Odynophagia
  - —Odynophagia suggests ulcerative esophagitis
- Regurgitation
- Water brash
- Belching
- Esophageal structures, bleeding
- Barrett esophagus (esophageal carcinoma)
- Early satiety, nausea, anorexia, weight loss
- Symptoms worse with recumbency or bending over
- Symptoms usually relieved with antacids, though temporarily

Atypical Signs

- Noncardiac chest pain
- Asthma
- Persistent cough, hiccups
- Hoarseness
- Globus sensation
- Pharyngeal/laryngeal ulcers and carcinoma
- Frequent throat clearing
- Recurrent pneumonitis
- Nocturnal choking
- Upper GI tract bleeding

DESCRIPTION

- Spectrum of pathology in which gastric reflux causes symptoms and damage to the esophageal mucosa
- Approximately 40% of the general population experience symptoms monthly

ETIOLOGY

- Incompetent reflux barrier allowing an increase in the frequency and duration of gastric contents into the esophagus
  - —The exposed esophageal mucosa becomes acidified and with time necrosed
- Main antireflux barrier
  - —Lower esophageal sphincter (LES)
  - —Crural diaphragm attachment (diaphragmatic sphincter)
  - —Both contribute to the pressure barrier at the gastroesophageal junction
  - —Esophageal acid clearance via peristalsis and esophageal mucosal resistance are additional barriers
- Most healthy individuals have brief episodes of reflux without symptoms
- Decreased LES tone
  - —Smoking
  - —Foods: alcohol, chocolate, onion
  - —Drugs: calcium channel blockers, morphine, meperidine, barbiturates, theophylline
- Delayed gastric emptying gastric distention contribute to reflux
- Hiatal hernias associated with GERD
  - —Significance varies in any given individual
  - —Most persons with hiatal hernias do not have clinically evident reflux disease
- Acid secretion is the same in those with or without GERD

PEDIATRIC CONSIDERATIONS

- Regurgitation is common in infants
  - —Incidence decreases from twice daily in 50% of those age 2 months to 1% of 1-year-olds
- Signs
  - —Frequent vomiting, irritability, cough, crying, and malaise
  - —Arching the body (hyperextension) at feeding and refusals of feedings

Pre-Hospital

CAUTIONS

- Esophageal pain may mimic angina
- Airway control needs maintaining secondary to vomiting

Diagnosis

ESSENTIAL WORKUP

- Differentiated GERD from more emergent conditions such as ischemic heart pain or esophageal perforation
- History: typical
- Physical exam is nonspecific

LABORATORY

- CBC
  - —Chronic anemia from esophagitis
- Stool testing for occult bleeding

IMAGING/SPECIAL TESTS

- No imaging routine
  - —CXR: evidence of esophageal perforation, hiatal hernia
- Diagnostic trial of antacid
  - —Those with persistent symptoms should be referred for endoscopy
- Barium esophagram for prominent dysphagia
- Esophageal pH monitoring
  - —Best test for evaluation of GERD

DIFFERENTIAL DIAGNOSIS

- Ischemic heart disease
- Asthma
- Peptic ulcer disease
- Gastritis
- Esophageal perforation
- Esophageal foreign body
- Esophageal infection
- Cholecystitis
- Mesenteric ischemia

PEDIATRIC CONSIDERATIONS

- Failure to thrive
- Formula intolerance
- Sepsis

Treatment

INITIAL STABILIZATION

- ABCs need to be evaluated
- IV fluid resuscitation for blood loss or shock

ED TREATMENT

- Symptomatic relief
  - —Antacids
  - —Antacids with viscous lidocaine
  - —Sublingual nitroglycerine for esophageal spasm
  - —Analgesics
- Lifestyle modifications
  - —Avoid late-night meals
  - —Minimize time in the supine position after eating
  - —Elevation of the head of the bed
  - —Weight loss
- Avoid direct esophageal irritants such as citric juices and coffee
- Avoid foods that decrease LES pressures such as fatty foods, chocolate, coffee
- Avoid drugs that lower LES tone
- Antacids
  - —Treatment of mild and infrequent reflux symptoms
  - —Not effective for healing esophagitis
  - —Alginic acid slurry floats on surface of gastric contents providing a mechanical barrier
- Sucralfate
  - —Binds pepsin, bile salts, and exposed submucosa, thereby limiting inflammation
- Metoclopramide
  - —Prokinetic drug
    - -Improves peristalsis
    - -Accelerates gastric emptying
    - -Increases LES pressure
  - —Bethanechol has a considerable incidence of side effects and is of questionable value
- H_2-blockers
  - —Effective for mild to moderate disease
  - —Severe disease requires greater dosage than that used for peptic ulcer disease
- Proton pump inhibitors
  - —More potent long acting inhibitors of gastric acid secretion
  - —Faster healing than other drug therapies
  - —More efficacious in severe GERD and frank esophagitis
- Antireflux surgery
  - —Chronic reflux, younger patients, nonhealing ulceration, severe bleeding
  - —Fundoplication can be more effective than medical therapy in selected cases

MEDICATIONS

- Antacids: 30 mL plus viscous lidocaine, 10 mL, PO
- Cimetidine: 400–800 mg b.i.d.
- Esomeprazole: 20–40 mg q.d.
- Famotidine: 20 mg b.i.d.
- Lansoprazole: 15–30 mg q.d.
- Metoclopramide: 10–15 mg q.i.d. before meals and qh5
- Nizatidine: 150 mg b.i.d.
- Omeprazole: 20–40 mg q.d.
- Pantoprazole: 40 mg q.d.
- Rabeprazole: 20 mg q.d.
- Ranitidine: 150 mg b.i.d. or 300 mg qh5
- Sucralfate: 1 g q.i.d.

Disposition

ADMISSION CRITERIA

- Seriously ill patients
- Significant esophageal bleeding
- Uncontrolled reactive asthma
- Dehydration
- Starvation and failure to thrive

DISCHARGE CRITERIA

- Uncomplicated GERD: refer to patient's PCP or a gastroenterologist for further evaluation

Miscellaneous

ICD9: 530.81

ICD10: K21.9

SUGGESTED READINGS

DeVault KR, Castell DV. Updated guidelines for the diagnosis and treatment of gastroesophageal reflux disease. Am J Gastroenterol 1999;94:1434–1442.

Klinkenberg-Knol EC, Nelis F, Dent J, et al. Long term omeprazole treatment in resistant gastroesophageal reflux disease: efficacy, safety and influence on gastric mucosa. Gastroenterology 2000;118: 661–669.

Lundell L, Miettinen P, Myrvold HE, et al. Long term management of gastro-esophageal reflux disease with omeprazole or open antireflux surgery: results of a prospective, randomized clinical trial. Eur J Gastroenterol Hepatol 2000;12: 879–887.

Richter JE. Typical and atypical presentations of gastroesophageal reflux disease. Gastroenterol Clinics North Am 1996;25:75–103.

Spechler SJ, Lee E, Ahnen D, et al. Long term outcome of medical and surgical therapies for gastroesophageal reflux disease. JAMA 2001;205:2331–2338.

Author: Thomas W. Lukens

Gastrointestinal Bleeding

Clinical Presentation

SIGNS AND SYMPTOMS

- Fatigue
- Weakness
- Dyspnea on exertion
- Anxiety
- Altered level of consciousness
- Tachycardia
- Orthostasis
- Pale appearance
- Pale conjunctiva, mucous membranes
- Pale nail beds

Upper GI Tract Bleeding

- Hematemesis
- Abdominal pain
  —Sharp, burning
  —Epigastric, sometimes to back
- Coffee ground emesis
- Black stools

Lower GI Tract Bleeding

- Bright red blood per rectum
- Melena
- Black stools
- Blood in toilet bowl

MECHANISM/DESCRIPTION

- Black melanotic stool requires rapid loss of at least 100 mL of blood above the ligament of Treitz
- Mortality rate for GI tract bleeding
  —Increases as age increases
  —Ranges from <5% in children to as high as 25% in adults older than 70 years
- Two categories
  —Upper—proximal to the ligament of Treitz
  —Lower—distal to the ligament of Treitz
- Range
  —Occult—a heme-positive stool or new anemia
  —Massive

ETIOLOGY

- Most common causes of upper GI tract bleeding include
  —Peptic ulcer disease
  —Gastritis
  —Esophageal varices
  —Mallory-Weiss tear
  —Caustic ingestions
- Most common causes of lower GI tract bleeding include
  —Diverticular disease
  —Angiodysplasia
  —GI tract polyps
  —Hemorrhoids
  —Anal fissures

PEDIATRIC CONSIDERATIONS

- Common causes of lower GI tract bleeding
  —Meckel diverticulum
  —Intussusception

Pre-Hospital

CAUTIONS

- Stabilize the airway
  —Place the patient on 100% oxygen via mask
  —Intubation for massive upper GI tract bleeding
- Insert at least one large-bore IV line (14–16 g) and administer crystalloids to attempt to maintain a BP >90 mm Hg systolic
  —Attempt second IV while transport is undertaken
  —Do not remain at the scene for a second IV line

Diagnosis

ESSENTIAL WORKUP

- Hematocrit
- Nasogastric aspiration for suspected upper GI tract bleeding
  —Most useful test for determining current upper GI tract bleeding
  —Follow by room-temperature saline lavage to demonstrate any active bleeding
  —25% falsely negative if bleeding source duodenal
    -Lower false-negative rate if aspirate contains bile
  —Iced lavage is not useful
    -Causes hypothermia and does not stop bleeding
- Rectal examination with stool for melena and Hemoccult testing
  —False-positive Hemoccult result
    -Raw meat
    -Some iron preparations
  —Agents causing black stools aside from GI tract bleeding
    -Iron
    -Charcoal
    -Bismuth
    -Food dyes
    -Beets

LABORATORY

- CBC
  —For anemia
  —Low MCV associated with chronic blood loss
  —For thrombocytopenia
- Electrolytes, BUN/Cr, glucose
- PT/PTT/INR
- Type and cross for active bleeding or unstable patient

IMAGING/SPECIAL TESTS

- Panendoscopy
  —Reveals the location of GI tract bleeding in up to 90% of cases
  —May be therapeutic
- Upright CXR/abdominal series
  —If signs of acute peritonitis
  —For perforation or obstruction
- Angiography
  —Diagnostic and therapeutic
- Radionuclide scans for slow bleeding in attempt to locate source
- EKG for cardiac ischemia

DIFFERENTIAL DIAGNOSIS

- Acute abdomen
- Aortoenteric fistula
- Visceral trauma

Treatment

INITIAL STABILIZATION

- Control airway in massive GI tract bleed with unstable vital signs and altered mental status
- Administer oxygen
- Place cardiac, pulse oximetry, and noninvasive BP monitors
- Initiate two large-bore IV access with 0.9% NS
  - —Administer 1-L bolus (peds: 20 mL/kg)
  - —Administer blood if no response to 2-L 0.9% NS bolus
  - —Administer fresh frozen plasma (FFP) if coagulopathic and bleeding

ED TREATMENT

- Consult gastroenterology or surgery for emergent endoscopy if significant ongoing bleeding
- Follow serial hematocrit
  - —May take several hours for level to reflect blood loss
- Place Foley catheter to follow urine output
  - —Good indicator of response to volume resuscitation
- Blood transfusion
  - —For patients with ongoing chest pain or ischemic changes on EKG
  - —For continued hypotension unresponsive to crystalloid infusion with ongoing bleeding regardless of hematocrit

Upper GI Tract Bleeding

- Place NGT
  - —Aspirate for blood
  - —Place on suction
  - —Lavage with water to determine whether continued bleeding
  - —May not detect duodenal bleed with competent pyloric sphincter
- Initiate H_2-blockers (cimetidine, famotidine, ranitidine)
  - —May help prevent rebleeding in gastritis
- Consider IV proton pump inhibitor (pantoprazole)
  - —May help prevent rebleeding in gastritis
- Emergent endoscopy
  - —Indications
    - -Active bleeding that does not clear with lavage
    - -Hemodynamic instability in setting of liver disease
  - —Therapeutic options
    - -Cauterization of bleeding ulcers or vessels
    - -Injection sclerosis of visible vessels
- Variceal bleeding treatment
  - —Endoscopic sclerotherapy
    - -Most effective
  - —Vasopressin
    - -Potent vasoconstrictor
    - -May be used concurrently with sclerotherapy
    - -Administered concurrently with IV nitroglycerin to prevent tissue necrosis/myocardial ischemia
  - —Balloon tamponade
    - -Sengstaken-Blakemore tube
    - -For confirmed variceal bleeding unresponsive to aforementioned measures
- Spontaneous resolution
  - —60% from variceal bleeding
  - —80% from other upper GI tract sources

Lower GI Tract Bleeding

- Anoscopy for suspected hemorrhoidal bleeding
- Flexible fiberoptic colonoscopy
  - —Best if done after adequate bowel preparation
- Angiography for massive or continuous bleeding
  - —Diagnostic and therapeutic
- Spontaneous resolution
  - —80% of the time
  - —25% rate of rebleeding

MEDICATIONS

- Cimetidine: 300 mg i.v. q6h; 400 mg PO b.i.d.
- Famotidine: 20 mg i.v. q12h; 40 mg PO q.h.s.
- Nitroglycerin: 5–20 μg/min i.v.
- IV pantoprazole (Protonix): 40–80 mg i.v.
- Ranitidine: 50 mg i.v. q8h; 300 mg PO q.h.s.
- Vasopressin: 0.2–0.4 IU/min (peds: 0.1–0.3 IU/min) initial dose then titrate up i.v.

Disposition

ADMISSION CRITERIA

- Unstable vital signs at any time
- Decreased hematocrit with recent GI tract bleed
- Coagulopathy
- Advanced age/comorbid conditions
- Active upper GI tract bleeding
- Lower GI tract bleeding
  - —Significant initial blood loss
  - —Continued bleeding

DISCHARGE CRITERIA

- Resolution of upper GI tract bleeding with negative NGT aspirate and endoscopy
- Minor, resolved lower GI tract bleed
- Stable vital signs
- Stable hematocrit >30%
- Normal coagulation function

Miscellaneous

ICD9: 578.9

ICD10: K92.2

SUGGESTED READINGS

Bono MJ. Lower gastrointestinal tract bleeding. Emerg Med Clin North Am 1996;14(3):547–555.

Jensen DM, Machicado GA, Jutabha R, et al. Urgent colonoscopy for the diagnosis and treatment of severe diverticular hemorrhage. N Engl J Med 2000;342(2): 78–82.

McGuirck TD, Coyle WJ. Upper gastrointestinal tract bleeding. Emerg Med Clin North Am 1996;14(3):523–539.

Sharara AI, Rockey DC. Medical progress: gastroesophageal variceal hemorrhage. N Engl J Med 2001;345(9):669–681.

Spiegel BM, Vakil NB, Ofman JJ. Endoscopy for acute nonvariceal upper gastrointestinal tract hemorrhage: is sooner better? A systematic review. Arch Intern Med 2001;161(11):1393–1404.

Van Dam J, Brugge WR. Medical progress: endoscopy of the upper gastrointestinal tract. N Engl J Med 1999;341(23): 1738–1748.

Author: Dean E. Johnson

γ-Hydroxybutyrate (GHB), Poisoning

Clinical Presentation

SIGNS AND SYMPTOMS

CNS
- CNS depression
- Ataxia/dizziness
- Impaired judgment
- Aggressive behavior
- Clonic movements of the extremities
- Coma
- Seizures

Pulmonary
- Respiratory depression
- Apnea
- Laryngospasm (rare)

Gastrointestinal
- Nausea
- Vomiting

Cardiovascular
- Bradycardia
- AV block
- Hypotension

Other
- Nystagmus
- Hypothermia

Withdrawal
- Hypertension
- Tachycardia
- Agitation
- Diaphoresis
- Tremors
- Nausea/vomiting/abdominal cramping
- Hallucinations/delusions/psychosis

MECHANISM/DESCRIPTION
- Naturally occurring analog of GABA
- Used medically for narcolepsy
- Nonmedical uses
  - —Body-building agent
  - —Euphoric agent
  - —Date-rape agent
- Onset of activity: 15–30 minutes after ingestion
- Duration of effect: 2–6 hours

Pre-Hospital

CAUTIONS
- Transport all pills/bottles/drug paraphernalia involved in overdose for identification in ED
- GHB precursors (GBL and 1,4-BD) have same effects as GHB
- Do not induce emesis due to risk of CNS depression and aspiration
- Provide respiratory support

CONTROVERSIES
- Physostigmine administration has not been demonstrated to reliably reverse GHB intoxication

Diagnosis

ESSENTIAL WORKUP
- Diagnosis based on clinical presentation and an accurate history
- Exclude co-ingestants if signs and symptoms inconsistent with GHB intoxication

LABORATORY
- Urine or plasma toxicology screen will confirm GHB ingestion, but levels do not guide management
- Urine toxicology screen to exclude co-ingestants
- Serum alcohol level
- Urinalysis and creatine kinase if suspected rhabdomyolysis from prolonged immobilization

IMAGING/SPECIAL TESTS
- EKG
  - —Sinus bradycardia
  - —AV block
- CXR
  - —Aspiration pneumonia
- Head CT if suspected occult head trauma

DIFFERENTIAL DIAGNOSIS
- Alcohol intoxication
- Barbiturate overdose
- Benzodiazepine overdose
- Neuroleptic overdose
- Opiate overdose
- Withdrawal
  - —Alcohol withdrawal
  - —Sedative-hypnotic withdrawal

Treatment

INITIAL STABILIZATION

- ABCs
  - —Airway control essential
  - —Administer supplemental oxygen
  - —Intubate if indicated
- Administer thiamine, dextrose (or Accu-Chek), and naloxone for depressed mental status

ED TREATMENT

- Supportive care
- Decontamination
  - —Consider activated charcoal for recent ingestion
- Bradycardia
  - —Atropine
  - —Temporary pacing
- Hypotension
  - —0.9% NS i.v. fluid bolus
  - —Trendelenburg
  - —Dopamine titrated to pressure
- Seizures
  - —Treat initially with benzodiazepine
  - —Treat refractory seizures with phenobarbital
- Withdrawal
  - —Treat aggressively with benzodiazepine
  - —Treat with phenobarbital if large doses of benzodiazepines unsuccessful

MEDICATIONS

- Activated charcoal: 1–2 g/kg PO
- Dextrose: 50–100 mL D50 (peds: 2 mL/kg of D25 over 1 min) i.v.; repeat if necessary
- Diazepam: 5–10 mg (peds: 0.2–0.5 mg/kg) i.v. q10–15 min
- Dopamine: 2–20 μg/kg/min with titration to effect
- Lorazepam: 2–4 mg (peds: 0.03–0.05 mg/kg) i.v. q10–15 min
- Naloxone: 0.4–2 mg (peds: 0.1 mg/kg; neonatal: 10–30 μg/kg) i.v. or i.m.
- Phenobarbital: 10–20 mg/kg i.v. (loading dose)
- Thiamine (vitamin B_1): 100 mg (peds: 50 mg) i.v. or i.m.

Disposition

ADMISSION CRITERIA

- Intubated patient
- Patient with hypothermia or other hemodynamic instability
- Co-ingestion prolonging the duration of intoxication

DISCHARGE CRITERIA

- Asymptomatic after 6 hours of observation
- No clinical evidence of withdrawal syndrome

Miscellaneous

ICD9: 967.8

SUGGESTED READINGS

Dyer JE, Roth B, Hyma BA. Gamma-hydroxybutyrate withdrawal syndrome. Ann Emerg Med 2001;37(2):147–153.

Li J, Stokes SA, Wockener A. A tale of novel intoxication: a review of the effects of γ-hydroxybutyric acid with recommendations for management. Ann Emerg Med 1998;31(6):729–736.

Shannon M, Quang LS. Gamma-hydroxybutyrate, gamma-butyrolactone, and 1,4-butanediol: a case report and review of the literature. Pediatr Emerg Care 2000;16(6):435–440.

Authors: Daniel Belmont; Mark B. Mycyk

Giardia

Clinical Presentation

SIGNS AND SYMPTOMS

- Onset 1 to 2 weeks postexposure
- Infection may be asymptomatic (most common)
- Diarrhea of acute onset (90% of symptomatic patients)
  - —Foul-smelling stools
  - —Steatorrhea
  - —Nonbloody
  - —Self-limiting within 2 to 4 weeks
- Flatulence and bloating (70–75%)
- Abdominal cramping (70%)
- Nausea (70%)
- Vomiting (30%)
- Malaise (86%)
- Anorexia (66%)
- Weight loss (60–70%)
- Fever is rare (15%)
- Abdominal exam is benign
- Extraintestinal manifestations (10% of patients):
  - —Polyarthritis
  - —Urticaria
  - —Aphthous ulcers
  - —Maculopapular rash
  - —Biliary tract disease
- 30–50% of acute cases progress to chronic giardiasis (>4 weeks)
  - —Fat malabsorption
  - —Severe macrocytic anemia secondary to folate deficiency
  - —Secondary lactase deficiency (in 40% of patients)

MECHANISM/DESCRIPTION

- Found worldwide
- Most common intestinal parasite in the U.S.
- Fecal-oral transmission
  - —Humans are major reservoir
  - —Zoonotic reservoir in domestic (dogs, cats, sheep, cattle) and wild animals (beavers, deer, rodents)
  - —Reservoir in contaminated surface water
- Populations at risk:
  - —Travelers to endemic areas (developing countries, wilderness areas of U.S.)
  - —Children in day care centers
  - —Institutionalized persons
  - —Practitioners of anal sexual activity
- Biphasic life cycle of *Giardia:*
  - —Ingested as cysts
  - —As few as 10 cysts shown to produce infection
  - —Cysts become trophozoites in the duodenum and attach to intestinal villi
  - —Trophozoites re-encyst in the ileum and cysts are shed in the feces
- Noninvasive diarrhea
- No toxin produced

ETIOLOGY

- *Giardia lamblia*
  - —A protozoan flagellate
- Also called *Giardia intestinalis* or *Giardia duodenalis*

PEDIATRIC CONSIDERATIONS

- With acute infection:
  - —Severe dehydration
- With chronic infection:
  - —Failure to thrive
  - —Growth retardation due to nutrient malabsorption

Pre-Hospital

CAUTIONS

- Universal precautions
  - —Avoid contact with fecal matter and/or contaminated items
  - —Wear gloves
  - —Strict hand washing
- For severely dehydrated children (>10% dehydration)
  - —IV bolus with 0.9% NS at 20 cc/kg
  - —Cardiac monitor
  - —Blood glucose determination

Diagnosis

ESSENTIAL WORKUP

- History
  - —Possible sources of exposure
  - —Membership in high-risk group
- Physical exam
  - —If gross or occult blood on digital rectal exam, unlikely to be *Giardia*
- Stool sample for microscopy (ova and parasites)
  - —50–70% sensitive if one sample
  - —85–90% sensitive if three samples taken at 2-day intervals (ideal)
  - —100% specific
  - —Ability to detect other parasites

LABORATORY

- Electrolytes, BUN/Cr, glucose
  - —If prolonged diarrhea or evidence of dehydration
- CBC
  - —Macrocytic anemia in chronic giardiasis
  - —Nondiagnostic in acute giardiasis

IMAGING/SPECIAL TESTS

- Stool ELISA for *Giardia* antigen
  - —95% sensitive, 95–100% specific
  - —Unlike microscopy, cannot rule out other parasites
- Duodenal sampling
  - —Entero-Test (patient swallows a weighted string, which is later retrieved and examined for *Giardia*)
  - —Duodenal aspiration
  - —Endoscopic biopsy
- Fecal leukocytes and stool culture unnecessary unless enteroinvasive organisms suspected (fever, bloody stool)
- Abdominal x-rays of no value

DIFFERENTIAL DIAGNOSIS

- Viral gastroenteritis
  - —Norwalk virus
  - —Rotavirus
  - —Hepatitis A
- Bacterial infections
  - —*Staphylococcus*
  - —*E. coli*
  - —*Shigella*
  - —*Salmonella*
  - —*Yersinia*
  - —*Campylobacter*
  - —*Clostridium difficile*
  - —*Vibrio cholera*
- Other protozoa
  - —*Cryptosporidium*
  - —*Microsporidium*
  - —*Cyclospora*
  - —*Isospora*
  - —*Entamoeba*
- Inflammatory bowel disease
- Irritable bowel syndrome
- Lactase deficiency
- Tropical sprue
- Drugs and toxins
  - —Antibiotics
  - —Calcium channel blockers
  - —Magnesium antacids
  - —Caffeine
  - —Alcohol
  - —Sorbitol
  - —Laxative abuse
  - —Quinidine
  - —Colchicine
  - —Mercury poisoning
- Endocrine
  - —Addison's disease
  - —Thyroid disorders
- Malignancy
  - —Colorectal carcinoma
  - —Medullary carcinoma of the thyroid

Treatment

INITIAL STABILIZATION

- ABCs
- IV 0.9 NS if signs of significant dehydration

ED MANAGEMENT

- Oral fluids for mild dehydration
- Correct any serum electrolyte imbalances
- Stool sample for microscopy
- If stool sample is positive for *Giardia:*
  - —Metronidazole is first-line anti-parasitic drug in U.S.
    - -80–95% cure rate
    - -Contraindicated in children and first-trimester pregnancy
  - —Albendazole if metronidazole unsuccessful
  - —Furazolidone in children
  - —Paromomycin or furazolidone in first-trimester pregnancy
  - —Quinacrine and tinidazole highly effective but not available in U.S.
- If stool sample negative for *Giardia:*
  - —Refer to gastroenterologist for further specialized testing
  - —Consider empiric course of metronidazole if high suspicion for *Giardia*

MEDICATIONS

- Albendazole: 400 mg (peds: 15 mg/kg/24 hours) PO qd × 3 days
- Furazolidone: 100 mg (peds: 6–8 mg/kg/24 hours) PO q6h × 7 days
- Metronidazole: 250 mg PO q8h × 5 days
- Paromomycin: (25–30 mg/kg/24 hours) PO q8h × 7 days
- Quinacrine: 100 mg (peds: 6 mg/kg/24 hours) PO q8h × 5 days
- Tinidazole: 2,000 mg (peds: 50–75 mg/kg) PO × 1

Disposition

ADMISSION CRITERIA

- Hypotension or tachycardia unresponsive to IV fluids
- Severe electrolyte imbalance
- Children with >10% dehydration
- Signs of sepsis/toxicity (rare in isolated giardiasis)
- Patients unable to maintain adequate oral hydration
  - —Extremes of age, cognitive impairment, significant comorbid illness

DISCHARGE CRITERIA

- Able to maintain adequate oral hydration
- Dehydration responsive to IV fluids

Miscellaneous

ICD9: 007.1

ICD10: A07.1

SEE ALSO: DIARRHEA, ADULT

SUGGESTED READINGS

Adachi JA, Backer HD, DuPont HL. Infectious diarrhea from wilderness and foreign travel. In: Auerbach PS, ed. Wilderness medicine, 4th ed. St. Louis: Mosby, 2001:1237–1270.

Farthing MJG. Giardiasis. Gastroenterol Clin North Am 1996;25:493–515.

Okhuysen PC. Traveler's diarrhea due to intestinal protozoa. Travel Med 2001;33: 110–114.

Ortega YR, Adam RD. Giardia: overview and update. Clin Infect Dis 1997;25: 545–550.

Vesy CJ, Peterson WL. Review article: the management of giardiasis. Aliment Pharmacol Ther 1999;13:843–850.

Author: Ann Nguyen

Glaucoma

Clinical Presentation

SIGNS AND SYMPTOMS

Acute Closed-Angle

- Severe eye or forehead pain
- Blurred vision
- Halos around lights
- Injected sclera
- Hazy cornea
- Shallow anterior chamber angle
- Mid-dilated pupils
- Decreased visual acuity
- Firm eyes with digital ballottement
- Nausea and vomiting
- Abdominal pain (nonspecific)

Open-Angle

- Painless, gradual loss of vision
- Disc pallor and cupping
- Visual field defects

MECHANISM/DESCRIPTION

- Increased intraocular pressure due to overproduction of aqueous humor or decreased aqueous humor outflow leads to
  —Corneal edema
  —Pupillary sphincter paralysis
  —Optic nerve degeneration
  —Eventual blindness

ETIOLOGY

- Glaucoma classifications
  —*Primary* (unknown cause)—open-angle, closed-angle, or congenital
  —*Developmental*—developmental abnormality in the aqueous outflow tract
  —*Secondary*—a condition that leads to a secondary rise in intraocular pressure
    -Inflammation (uveitis, scleritis, keratitis)
    -Trauma (blunt or penetrating)
    -Intraocular blood
    -Systemic diseases (amyloidosis, diabetes mellitus, thyroid disease)

Closed-Angle

- Most common type presenting to ED because of the rapid onset and painful nature
- Abnormally narrow anterior chamber angles allow for occlusion of aqueous humor outflow
- Inciting agents
  —Trauma
  —Stress
  —Entering a darkened room
  —Sneezing
  —Pharmacologic dilation of the eye
    -Intentional with an ophthalmologic examination
    -Unintentional as with inhaled β-agonists or atropine, or intranasal use of cocaine that accidentally enters the eye
- Both eyes are at risk, abnormality usually bilateral

Open-Angle

- Normal anterior chamber angle
- Risk factors
  —Age >35 years old
  —Diabetics (three times more likely)

PEDIATRIC CONSIDERATIONS

- Tearing, photophobia, blepharospasm, and irritability
  —Often the first signs
  —Secondary to corneal irritation from corneal edema
- Cornea appearance
  —Hazy due to edema
  —Haab's striae (breaks in Descemet's membrane, which causes linear ridging)
  —Enlarged due to the elasticity of a child's eye
- Entire eye may be enlarged (buphthalmos, "ox eye")
- Older children have progressive myopia due to the eye's change in shape from continued intraocular pressure

Pre-Hospital

N/A

Diagnosis

ESSENTIAL WORKUP

- Detailed history and ocular examination
- Visual acuity
- Tonometry (normal intraocular pressure = 10–21 mm Hg)
  —Pressures >21 mm Hg are suspicious
  —Pressures >24 mm Hg are abnormal

DIFFERENTIAL DIAGNOSIS

- Broad differential depending on whether the chief symptom is a painful red eye, headache, gastrointestinal complaint, or chronic loss of vision
  —Diagnosis of glaucoma made with increased intraocular pressure
- Headache
  —Migraine
  —Cluster
  —Tension
- Red eye
  —Conjunctivitis
  —Iritis
  —Allergic/toxic
  —Corneal abrasion
  —Trauma

PEDIATRIC CONSIDERATIONS

- Consider developmental glaucoma (relatively rare: 1:10,000 live births) in an irritable photophobic child or when "big eyes" noted
- Children (<5 years) may need general anesthesia for a good ophthalmologic examination

Treatment

INITIAL STABILIZATION

- Initiate steps to lower intraocular pressure in acute closed-angle glaucoma

ED TREATMENT

Acute Closed-Angle

- Goals of treatment
  - —Decreasing intraocular pressure in the affected eye
  - —Preventing an episode in the other eye
- Decrease aqueous humor production
  - —*Carbonic anhydrase inhibitors* (acetazolamide)
    - -Inhibits the generation of carbonic acid needed in the production of aqueous humor
    - -Results in less aqueous humor formation
    - -Do not administer acetazolamide in sickle cell patients secondary to a hyphema—may induce sickling and worsen the prognosis
  - —β-blockers (timolol, betaxolol) decrease aqueous production and increase outflow
- Decrease intraocular volume
  - —Hyperosmotic drugs (mannitol, glycerol) raise blood osmolality rapidly, thereby inducing an osmotic gradient between the blood and ocular fluids
    - -Water moves from the eye to the plasma to decrease the intraocular volume
- Decrease pupil size
  - —Cholinergic drugs (pilocarpine)—miotics that cause pupillary constriction
    - -Allows for angle widening and increased aqueous outflow
    - -Cholinergic drugs may worsen the condition in cases of pupillary ischemia due to pupillary block as the pupil will not constrict but the lens will move forward
- Move lens posteriorly
  - —Supine position uses gravity to allow the lens to move posteriorly
  - —May relieve some degree of pupillary block

Open-Angle

- Not generally treated in the ED
- Symptoms occur gradually and the patients do not come to ED for this complaint
- If increased intraocular pressure found, refer to an ophthalmologist

PEDIATRIC CONSIDERATIONS

- Complications of β-adrenergic antagonists (asthma, bradycardia, drowsiness, and hyperactivity) more common in children

MEDICATIONS

- Acetazolamide
  - —IV: 500 mg (peds: 20–40 mg/kg/24 hours q6h) initially followed by 250 mg every 4 hours
  - —PO: 500 mg sustained-release (peds: 8–30 mg/kg/24 hours q6–8h) PO b.i.d.
- Betaxolol: 0.5% 1 drop b.i.d.
- Glycerol: 1–1.5 ml/kg PO
- Mannitol: 1.5–2 g/kg i.v.
- Pilocarpine 2%
  - —Affected eye: 1 drop q 15 min for 5 times, then 1 drop q2–3h
  - —Unaffected eye: 1 drop q6h
- Timolol: 0.25–0.5% 1 drop b.i.d.

Disposition

ADMISSION CRITERIA

- Acute closed-angle glaucoma with immediate ophthalmologic consultation

DISCHARGE CRITERIA

- Primary open-angle glaucoma with ophthalmologic follow-up as this is a chronic progressive disease

Miscellaneous

ICD9: 365.9

ICD10: H40.9

SEE ALSO: RED EYE

SUGGESTED READINGS

Bertolini J, Pelucio M. The red eye. Emerg Med Clin North Am 1995;13(3):561–580.

Hartwick AT. Beyond intraocular pressure: neuroprotective strategies for future glaucoma therapy. Optom Vis Sci 2001;78(2):85–94.

Migdal C. Glaucoma medical treatment: philosophy, principles and practice. Eye 2002;14(pt 3B):515–518.

Patel KH, Javitt JC, Tielsch JM, et al. Incidence of acute angle-closure glaucoma after pharmacologic mydriasis. Am J Ophthalmol 1995;120(6):709–717.

Schuman JS. Antiglaucoma medications: a review of safety and tolerability issues related to their use. Clin Ther 2000;22(2):167–208.

Author: Eric Reichman

Globe Rupture

Clinical Presentation

SIGNS AND SYMPTOMS

- Markedly decreased visual acuity
- Severe subconjunctival hemorrhage and edema
- Abnormally deep anterior chamber
- Hyphema (sometimes with clotted blood)
- Limited extraocular motion
- Extrusion of intraocular contents
- Full-thickness scleral or corneal laceration (indicates penetrating injury)
- Low intraocular pressure (occasionally can be normal or high)
- Irregular pupil
- Iridodialysis/cyclodialysis
- Subluxed lens
- Commotio retinae
  - —Gray-white discoloration of the retina
- Choroidal rupture
- Traumatic optic neuropathy

MECHANISM/DESCRIPTION

- Blunt trauma to the eye
  - —Causes an abrupt rise in intraocular pressure
  - —Subsequent rupture of the eye at the weakest points
    - -Extraocular muscle insertion
    - -Corneoscleral junction
- Penetrating injuries
  - —Occur with sharp or pointed objects or projectiles injuring the scleral or anterior eye directly
  - —Most common anteriorly, the bony orbit protects laterally and posteriorly
  - —Posterior injury can occur with fracture of the bony orbit or with penetrating injuries of the eyelid or eyebrow
- Hemorrhage within the eye portends a poor prognosis
  - —Blood is both a source of fibrosis and an aggravating influence on fibrosis in the posterior portion of the eye

ETIOLOGY

- Falls, impact injuries
- Sport-related injuries (e.g., elbow impacts, ball impacts, etc.)
- Indirect concussive injuries (explosions)
- Sharp instrument/stabbing injuries, accidental or intentional
- Projectile injuries (industrial, firearms, etc.)

Pre-Hospital

CAUTIONS

- Do not manipulate the eye if a ruptured globe is suspected
- Place a shield (not patch) over eye with no pressure on the globe

Diagnosis

ESSENTIAL WORKUP

- Penlight or slit-lamp examination observing for signs of globe rupture
- Defer complete ocular examination until the time of surgical repair in the operating room once the diagnosis of ruptured globe is made
  - —Prevents placing any undue pressure onto the eye and risking extrusion of the intraocular contents
- If no evidence of globe rupture on initial survey, proceed with thorough ophthalmologic examination
  - —Visual acuity
  - —Slit-lamp examination
    - -Corneal
    - -Anterior chamber
    - -Iris
    - -Sclera
    - -Posterior chamber
  - —Fluorescein
    - -Observe if fluorescein moves away as contents leak out of globe (Seidel test: positive indicates rupture)
  - —Visualize fundus/retina
  - —Measure intraocular pressure
    - -Only perform if globe rupture is *not* present

LABORATORY

- Preoperative labs as indicated
  - —CBC
  - —Electrolytes, BUN/Cr, glucose

IMAGING/SPECIAL TESTS

- Orbital radiograph (AP/lat) for metallic intraocular foreign body with penetrating injuries
- CT scan of the orbits (axial and coronal views)
- MRI scan of the orbits after retained metallic foreign body is ruled out
- B-scan ultrasound of the eye

DIFFERENTIAL DIAGNOSIS

- Intraocular foreign body
- Hypemia
- Severe subconjunctival hemorrhage and chemosis
- Partial corneal laceration
- Partial scleral laceration

PEDIATRIC CONSIDERATIONS

- Childhood injuries are generally much more devastating secondary to more marked and more rapid fibrosis
- Early aggressive therapy indicated to establish best visual stimulus as quickly as possible to prevent amblyopia

Treatment

INITIAL STABILIZATION

- Protect eye with shield

ED TREATMENT

- Emergent ophthalmologic consultation
- Bed rest
- No food or drink (NPO)
- Administer antiemetic for nausea/vomiting
  —Prochlorperazine (Compazine)
  —Promethazine
- Administer tetanus prophylaxis
- Administer prophylactic antibiotics
  —First-generation cephalosporin (Ancef) with an aminoglycoside (gentamicin)
- Avoid succinylcholine if rapid sequence intubation required (increase intraocular pressure)

MEDICATIONS

- Cefazolin (Ancef): 1 g (peds: 25–50 mg/kg/24 hours) i.v. q6–8h
- Gentamicin: 1 mg/kg (peds: 2–2.5 mg/kg) i.v. q8h
- Prochlorperazine (Compazine): 5–10 mg i.v./i.m. (peds: 0.13 mg/kg/dose i.m.)
- Promethazine: 12.5–25 mg (peds: 0.25–1 mg/kg) PO/i.m./i.v. q4–6h

Disposition

ADMISSION CRITERIA

- All patients with globe-rupture/penetrating eye injuries
- Early enucleation for devastating eye injury in which there is no hope of salvageable vision

DISCHARGE CRITERIA

- Globe penetration excluded

Miscellaneous

ICD9: 871.0

ICD10: S05.3

SEE ALSO: CORNEAL ABRASION, RED EYE

SUGGESTED READINGS

DeJuan E Jr, Sternberg P Jr, Michels RG. Penetrating ocular injury: types of injuries and visual results. Ophthalmology 1983; 90(11):1313–1322.

Dunya IM, Rubin PAD, Shore JW. Penetrating orbital trauma. Int Ophthalmol Clin 1994;34:25–36.

Klystra JA, Lamkin JC, Runyan DR. Clinical predictors of scleral rupture after blunt ocular trauma. Am J Ophthalmol 1993; 115(4):530–535.

Linden JA, Renner GS. Trauma to the globe. Emerg Med Clin North Am 1995;13(3): 581–605.

Navon SE. Management of the ruptured globe. Int Ophthalmol Clin 1994;34:71–91.

Author: Eric Reichman

Glomerulonephritis

Clinical Presentation

SIGNS AND SYMPTOMS

- Cardinal signs
  - —Proteinuria
  - —Hematuria
- Edema
  - —Periorbital
  - —Ascites
  - —Pleural effusion
  - —Due to renal salt and water retention
- Hypertension (diastolic)
  - —Mild in 50%
  - —+/— Oliguria
- Azotemia—commonly in older patients
- Congestive heart failure—older patients with associated hypertension
- Renal failure
- Autoimmune disorders
  - —Arthralgias
  - —Arthritis
  - —Rash
  - —Fever
- Nonspecific manifestations:
  - —Fatigue
  - —Weight loss
  - —Abdominal pain
  - —Nausea/vomiting

MECHANISM/DESCRIPTION

- Third most common cause of end-stage renal disease (ESRD) in developing countries
- Group of conditions affecting the glomerulus resulting in
  - —Proteinuria (typically <3.5 g/d)
  - —Edema
  - —Hypertension
  - —Azotemia
  - —Abnormal urine sediment (dysmorphic red blood cells (RBC), RBC casts, leukocytes, etc.)
- Immunologic mechanism
  - —Due to individual host response to specific antigen, reticuloendothelial system function, and genetic makeup of host, resulting in diffuse inflammatory changes in renal glomeruli
  - —Autoimmune response to stimuli results in immune-complex deposits or cell-mediated immune response to antigen in glomeruli

ETIOLOGY

- Grouped according to presentation
  - —Acute nephritic syndrome (see Nephritic Syndrome)
  - —Rapidly progressive glomerulonephritis (RPGN)
  - —Idiopathic renal hematuric syndrome
  - —Nephrotic syndrome (see Nephrotic Syndrome)
  - —Chronic nephritic syndrome
- Causative agent unknown in most cases
  - —Infectious: poststreptococcal GN (PSGN) most common
  - —Systemic diseases: vasculitis, Henoch-Schönlein purpura, Goodpasture's disease, SLE
  - —Primary glomerular diseases: membranoproliferative GN (MPGN), IgA nephropathy (Berger's disease)
  - —Drugs (penicillamine, hydralazine, rifampin)
  - —Rarer causes: hemolytic uremic syndrome, acute hypersensitivity interstitial nephritis, serum sickness

Rapidly Progressive Glomerulonephritis (RPGN)

- Clinical syndrome of GN and rapid decrease of renal function—rare condition
- Development of *acute renal failure* within days to weeks
- Medical emergency; need early aggressive treatment to prevent ESRD
- Can occur with any form of GN
- Onset insidious, nonspecific symptoms
- *Edema* in 50%
- Hypertension uncommon
- >50% require dialysis within 6 months of onset

Idiopathic Renal Hematuric Syndrome

- Asymptomatic minimal urinary abnormalities
  - —Gross hematuria (episodic)
  - —Proteinuria (minimal)
  - —*Without* edema, azotemia, and hypertension
- Most common: MPGN, e.g., IgA nephropathy, "orthostatic" proteinuria, focal and segmental glomerulosclerosis, diabetes, amyloidosis
- IgA nephropathy most common form of GN worldwide; occurs most commonly in 20–40 age group, with male/female occurrence rate of 2:1
- Frequently associated within 1–2 days after URI or GI infection; ESRD develops in 20–40% of patients over lifetime

Chronic Glomerulonephritis

- *Persistent abnormal proteinuria* (*nonnephrotic*) with associated hypertension, reduced GFR, and abnormal urinary sediment
- Irreversible end-stage renal failure occurs over a number of years

Pre-Hospital

N/A

Diagnosis

ESSENTIAL WORKUP

- Urinalysis for
  - —Hematuria, proteinuria, and RBC casts

LABORATORY

- Electrolytes, BUN, Cr, glucose
  - —Baseline renal function
  - —Hyperkalemia
  - —For diabetes
- Albumin, total protein
  - —Varying degrees of hypoalbuminemia depending on clinical process
- CBC
  - —Anemia secondary to chronic renal disease, neoplasm, Goodpasture's disease
  - —+/— elevated WBC in infections
- PT, PTT, platelets (abnormal in neoplasms, nephrotic syndromes)
- ABG if renal failure

IMAGING/SPECIAL TESTS

- Renal ultrasound
  - —Kidney size predictor of potential reversibility of disease, alternative diagnosis (neoplasm, stone)
- CXR: heart size, pulmonary edema, or hemorrhage
- Renal biopsy: discern primary glomerulopathies versus other causes

Diagnostic Tests

- Cultures—throat, skin, blood (if infection suspected)
- Calcium—hypocalcemia (nephrotic patients)
- 24-hour urine collection—protein, urine electrolytes
- Streptozyme or antistreptolysin O titer
- Complement levels (C1, C3, C4, CH_{50})—reduced in PSGN, MPGN, SLE
- ANA, rheumatoid factor—connective tissue diseases
- Anti-glomerular basement membrane (GBM)—Goodpasture's
- ANCA, PR3—Wegner's
- Serum and urine protein electrophoresis—multiple myeloma, amyloidosis
- Viral studies—hepatitis B + C, Epstein-Barr, CMV
- Cryoglobulins and immune complexes—vasculitis, various acute GN
- Endocrine—glucose tolerance test, TSH (hypothyroidism; nephrotic syndrome)

DIFFERENTIAL DIAGNOSIS

- *Hematologic*—sickle cell disease, coagulopathy
- *Renal*—infectious, malformation, neoplasm, ischemic, trauma, vasculitis
- *Postrenal*
  —Mechanical (stones, reflux, obstruction, catheterization)
  —Inflammatory (cystitis, prostatitis, epididymitis, endometriosis, periurethritis)
  —Neoplasm
- *Factitious*—food, drugs, pigmenturia (myoglobin, porphyria, hemoglobinemia), vaginal bleeding

Treatment

INITIAL STABILIZATION

- ABCs

ED TREATMENT

- Treatment mainly supportive care
- Fluid and sodium restriction
- Loop diuretics
  —Furosemide
  —May precipitate acute renal failure with intrinsic renal disease
- Blood pressure stabilization to decrease proteinuria, retard progression of GN
  —ACE inhibitor
  —Hypertensive emergency: nitroprusside, diazoxide
- Dialysis for
  —Severe hyperkalemia
  —Fluid overload
  —Uremia

Specific Medical Treatments

- Antibiotics
  —If suspected bacterial infection
  —Penicillin for PSGN
  —Trimethoprim-sulfamethoxazole (cotrimoxazole) for Wegner's (decreases relapse)
- Albumin—not recommended
- Plasmapheresis—may be beneficial, e.g., RPGN
- Erythropoietin—for anemia due to chronic renal disease

RPGN Treatment

- Combination of steroids and cytotoxic drugs maximize improvement in renal function by decreasing antibody formation
- Steroid pulse therapy—methylprednisolone, followed by daily prednisone (decreases pulmonary hemorrhage risk)
- Cytotoxic agents—azathioprine, cyclosporine
- Plasma exchange—commonly used to remove circulating anti-GBM antibody
- Dialysis

MEDICATIONS

- Azathioprine: 2 mg/kg/d
- Benazepril: 10–80 mg PO qd
- Cyclophosphamide: 2 mg/kg/d
- Diazoxide: 1–3 mg/kg i.v., max 150 mg, repeat q 15 min
- Dopamine: 1–3 μg/kg/min i.v.
- Erythromycin: 250 mg (peds: 30–50 mg/kg/24 hours) PO q6h for 7–10 days
- Furosemide: 20–100 mg (peds: 1 mg/kg/dose max 6 mg/kg) i.v.; max 2 mg/kg/d
- Methylprednisolone: 30 mg/kg i.v. on alternative days × 3 doses, followed by oral prednisone
- Morphine sulfate: 2–4 mg (peds: 0.1 mg/kg/dose; max 15 mg/dose) i.v. q 5 min
- Nitroprusside: 0.5–10 mg/kg/min i.v.
- Penicillin
  —Benzathine penicillin: 1.2 million units (peds: 0.6 million units for <30 kg) i.m.
  —Penicillin: 2 million units PO q6h for 7–10 days
- Prednisone: 0.5–1 mg/kg/d

Disposition

ADMISSION CRITERIA

- Unstable vital signs
- Oliguria, anuria
- Uremia
- Acute renal failure
- Electrolyte abnormality
- Malignant hypertension
- Congestive heart failure
- Infectious cause of GN

DISCHARGE CRITERIA

- Healthy patients with no comorbid illness who present with mild proteinuria and hematuria with
  —Stable vital signs
  —No signs of infection
  —Otherwise normal lab work
  —Close follow-up recommended

Miscellaneous

ICD9: 583.9

ICD10: N05

SEE ALSO: NEPHRITIC SYNDROME, NEPHROTIC SYNDROME, AND RENAL FAILURE

SUGGESTED READINGS

Couser WG. Glomerulonephritis. Lancet 1999;353(9163):1509–1515.

Glassock RJ. Management of rapidly progressive glomerulonephritis. Hosp Pract (Office Ed) 2000;35(2):59–62, 65–66, 69–70.

Hricik DE, Chung-Park M, Sedor JR. Glomerulonephritis. N Engl J Med 1998;339(13):888–899.

Madaio MP, Harrington JT. The diagnosis of glomerular diseases: acute glomerulonephritis and the nephrotic syndrome. Arch Intern Med 2001;161(1):25–34.

Author: Shirley Lee

Gonococcal Disease

Clinical Presentation

SIGNS AND SYMPTOMS

Female

- Cervicitis
  - —Many asymptomatic for prolonged periods
  - —Yellow or white thick mucopurulent endocervical discharge
  - —Cervical edema, congestion, and friability
  - —Abnormal vaginal bleeding
- Pelvic inflammatory disease (10–20% infected females)
  - —Abdominal pain/tenderness
  - —Fever
  - —Cervical motion tenderness
  - —Bilateral adnexal tenderness
  - —Nausea/vomiting
- Fitz-Hugh-Curtis syndrome
  - —Right upper quadrant pain/tenderness
- Vaginal itching
- Dysuria
- 30–40% asymptomatic carriers
- Proctitis
  - —May self-inoculate

Male

- Incubation period 3–7 days and symptoms usually within 10–14 days
- Urethritis with yellow-white thick discharge
  - —Cannot be reliably differentiated from chlamydia clinically
- Urinary tract infection symptoms
  - —Dysuria
- Prostatitis
- Epididymitis
- Proctitis
  - —Often asymptomatic
  - —May have tenesmus, pruritus ani rectal bleeding (1–2% infected individuals)

Disseminated (1–2% Infected Individuals)

- Females more common, 1 week postmenses
- Fever
- Chills
- Migratory tenosynovitis
  - —Involve flexor tendon sheaths of wrist/Achilles tendon
- Rash
  - —Two thirds accompanies tenosynovitis
  - —Hemorrhagic, necrotic pustules on erythematous base
  - —Begin distally
  - —Resembles meningococcus
  - —Healing crust in 4 days
- Arthralgia (usually less than three joints)
- Arthritis
  - —Especially of knees, ankle, and wrist
  - —Swollen, warm joint with effusion
- Endocarditis

Other

- Pharyngitis
- Conjunctivitis
  - —Severe purulent discharge
  - —Conjunctival injection/irritation

MECHANISM/DESCRIPTION

- Common sexually transmitted disease—600,000 new cases/year
- Often seen with *Chlamydia*
- Humans only known host for *Neisseria gonorrhea*
- 60–80% of females in contact with males with urethral gonorrhea develop infection
- 20–30% of males in contact with females with gonorrhea develop infection

ETIOLOGY

- *N. gonorrhea*
  - —Gram-negative aerobic, diplococcus bacteria
  - —Die rapidly when outside normal environment

PEDIATRIC CONSIDERATIONS

- Ophthalmia neonatorum
  - —Bilateral conjunctivitis 2–5 days postbirth
  - —Untreated leads to perforation of globe and blindness

Pre-Hospital

N/A

Diagnosis

ESSENTIAL WORKUP

- Clinical diagnosis in male gonorrhea
  - —Gram stain of urethral exudate with 95% sensitivity and 97% specificity
- Cervical culture in female gonorrhea
  - —Gram stain cervical discharge with 65% sensitivity and 90% specificity

LABORATORY

- Culture on Thayer-Martin media is gold standard
- Antigen detection techniques (ELISA, DFA), DNA probes, nucleic acid complication tests (PCR, LLR)
  - —From simple cervical or urethral swabs
  - —LCR can be performed on urine but lower sensitivity
  - —Accurate
- Blood cultures for disseminated GC
- Joint arthrocentesis/analysis
  - —Neutrophilic leukocytosis (usually >50,000 leukocytes/mm^3)
  - —Positive culture when >80,000 leukocytes/mm^3
- Pharyngeal/rectal cultures for local symptoms in high-risk individuals
- CBC for suspected PID
- Urinalysis for suspected PID/lower abdominal pain in females
- Pregnancy test for lower abdominal pain

DIFFERENTIAL DIAGNOSIS

- Urethritis
  - —Chlamydia
  - —Trichomonas
  - —Urinary tract infection
  - —Syphilis
- Disseminated GC
  - —Meningococcus (rash)
  - —Reiter's syndrome
  - —Rheumatic fever
  - —Systemic lupus
  - —Hepatitis

Treatment

INITIAL STABILIZATION

- 0.9% NS 500 cc i.v. fluid bolus for dehydration due to nausea/vomiting

ED TREATMENT

Genital Infection

- Treat all patients for gonorrhea and *Chlamydia*
- Uncomplicated male genital or female/male pharyngeal/rectal infection
  - —1 dose of the following plus 7-day course of doxycycline or 1 dose of azithromycin
    - -Ceftriaxone 250 mg i.m.
    - -Cefixime 400 mg PO
    - -Ofloxacin 400 mg PO
    - -Ciprofloxin 500 mg PO
    - -Avoid quinolones in pregnant or nursing women or patients less than 18 years old
    - -Quinolone resistance has been noted
- Salpingitis/pelvic inflammatory disease
  - —Outpatient options
    - -1 dose cefixime/ceftriaxone/ spectinomycin plus 14-day course of doxycycline
    - -Ofloxacin 400 mg b.i.d. plus clindamycin 450 mg t.i.d. or metronidazole 500 mg b.i.d. for 14 days
  - —Inpatient options
    - -Cefoxitin i.v. plus doxycycline i.v.
- Gonorrhea in pregnancy
  - —1 dose ceftriaxone or spectinomycin plus 7-day course of erythromycin
- Treat sexual partners within 60 days
- Recommend syphilis (RPR) and HIV testing

Nongenital Infections

- Disseminated GC
  - —Open drainage of septic joints rarely indicated
  - —Inpatient antibiotics for moderate to severe infection
  - —Oral outpatient antibiotics to conclude 7-day course once improvement
  - —Outpatient antibiotics for mild infection not involving weight-bearing joints
  - —Initial antibiotic options
    - -Ceftriaxone 1 g i.m. q24h
    - -Ceftizoxime 1 g i.v. q8h
    - -Cefotaxime 1 g i.v. q8h
    - -Spectinomycin 2 mg i.m. q12h
  - —After 24–48 hours of above and improvement for 7 days of therapy
    - -Cefixime 400 mg PO b.i.d.
    - -Ciprofloxacin 500 mg PO b.i.d.
    - -Ofloxacin 400 mg PO b.i.d.
- Conjunctivitis
  - —Adults—ceftriaxone 1 g i.m. × 1 dose
  - —Ophthalmia neonatorum options
    - -Penicillin G 100,000 IU/kg/24 hours q6h
    - -Ceftriaxone 25–50 mg/kg/24 hours qd
    - -Ceftriaxone 125 mg i.m./i.v.
- Pharyngitis—one of the following plus azithromycin 1 g or doxycycline 100 mg b.i.d. × 7 days
  - —Ceftriaxone 125 mg i.m. × 1 dose
  - —Ciprofloxin 500 mg PO × 1 dose
  - —Ofloxacin 400 mg PO × 1 dose
- Meningitis and endocarditis
  - —Ceftriaxone 1–2 g i.v. q12h
  - —Treat meningitis for 10–14 days
  - —Treat endocarditis for 4 weeks

MEDICATIONS

- Azithromycin: 1 g PO
- Cefixime: 400 mg PO
- Cefotaxime: 1 g i.v. q8h
- Cefoxitin: 2 g i.v. q6h
- Ceftizoxime: 1 g i.v. q8h
- Ceftriaxone: 125–250 mg i.m.; 1 g (peds: 25–50 mg/kg/24 hours) i.v. q24h
- Ciprofloxin: 500 mg PO
- Clindamycin: 450 mg PO t.i.d.
- Doxycycline: 100 mg IV/PO q12h
- Erythromycin: 500 mg PO q6h
- Metronidazole: 500 mg PO b.i.d.
- Ofloxacin: 400 mg PO
- Penicillin G: 100,000 IU/kg/24 hours q6h
- Spectinomycin: 2 g i.m. q12h

Disposition

ADMISSION CRITERIA

- Moderate to severe disseminated GC with arthritis involving weight-bearing joints
- PID with
  - —Peritoneal signs
  - —WBC >15,000/mm^3
  - —Vomiting
  - —Conjunctivitis requiring IV antibiotics

DISCHARGE CRITERIA

- Uncomplicated genital, pharyngeal, or conjunctival infection
- Mild disseminated GC in nontoxic patient without arthritis in weight-bearing joints
- Encourage treatment of sexual partners

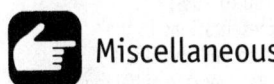

Miscellaneous

ICD9: 98.0

ICD10: A54.9

SEE ALSO: URETHRITIS

SUGGESTED READINGS

Berger RE. Sexually transmitted diseases. Adv Urol 1997;2:97.

Drugs for Sexually Transmitted Infections. Med Lett Drugs Ther 1999;41:85–90.

Kreipe RE. Sexually transmitted diseases in adolescents. Pediatr Infect Dis J 1998;17: 921–922.

McKinzie J. Sexually transmitted disease. Emerg Med Clin North Am 2001;19(3): 723–743.

Author: David Levine

Gout/Pseudogout

Clinical Presentation

SIGNS AND SYMPTOMS

- Gout and pseudogout both present as acute monoarticular or polyarticular arthritis
- Increased warmth, erythema, and joint swelling are present
- Early attacks subside spontaneously within 3–21 days, even without treatment
- Later attacks may last longer, cluster, be more severe, and be polyarticular

Gout

- The most common of the crystalline diseases
- Symptoms present maximally within 12–24 hours
- Tophi and joint desquamation may be present
- Women predominantly present after menopause and have polyarticular predominance (up to 70%)
- Less dramatic presentations in the immunosuppressed and the elderly
- Most common: 1st metatarsophalangeal joint (75%) > ankle; tarsal area; knee > hand; wrist

Pseudogout

- Typically involves larger joints than gout
- Most common: knee > wrist > metacarpals; shoulder; elbow; ankle > hip; tarsal joints
- Monoarticular (25%)
- Asymptomatic (25%)
- Pseudo-osteoarthritis (45%): progressive degeneration, often symmetric
- Pseudorheumatoid arthritis (in the elderly): a polyarticular variant with fever and confusion

MECHANISM/DESCRIPTION

- Gout affects mainly middle-aged men and postmenopausal women
- Urologic deposition of uric acid calculi may cause renal dysfunction
- Risk factors
  —Age >40
  —Male/female ratio 2:1 to 6:1 <65 years old; 1:1 ≥65 years old
  —Renal disease; myeloproliferative disorder; ethanol intake; diabetes; hyperlipidemia; hypertension; vascular disease; psoriasis; obesity

Four Phases

- Asymptomatic hyperuricemia (serum urate >7 mg/dL)
- Acute gout
- Intercritical gout: quiet intervening periods
- Tophaceous gout (up to 45% of cases)
  —Chalky deposits of sodium urate on x-ray (tophi)
  —Usually evident 10 years after first attack but early in postmenopausal women
  —Associated with avascular necrosis and deforming arthritis
  —Most frequent in previously damaged joints; synovium; subchondral bone, bursae (olecranon; infrapatellar; prepatellar); Achilles tendon; extensor surface of the forearms; toes; fingers; ear; rarely CNS or cardiac (valves)

Pseudogout (Chondrocalcinosis)

- The most common cause of acute monarthritis after age 60
- Risk factors
  —Hypercalcemia (e.g., hyperparathyroidism, familial); hemochromatosis; hemosiderosis
  —Hypo- and hyperthyroidism, hypophosphatemia, hypomagnesemia, amyloidosis, or gout

ETIOLOGY

- Gout is caused by deposition of *monosodium urate crystals* in tissues from supersaturated extracellular fluid, due to:
  —Underexcretion (most commonly) or excessive production of uric acid
  —Any rapid change in uric acid levels (e.g., the initiation or cessation of diuretics, alcohol, salicylates, cyclosporine, lead acetate poisoning, and uricosurics or allopurinol)
- Pseudogout occurs secondary to excess synovial accumulation of *calcium pyrophosphate* crystals
- Precipitants for both gout and pseudogout include minor trauma and acute illnesses (e.g., surgery, ischemic heart disease)

Pre-Hospital

N/A

Diagnosis

ESSENTIAL WORKUP

- Arthrocentesis and aspiration of tophi
  —Examine aspirant for crystals, Gram stain, cultures, leukocyte count, and differential
  —Fluid is typically thick pasty white
  —*Gout:* 20,000–100,000 WBC/mm^3; poor string and mucin clot; no bacteria
  —*Pseudogout:* up to 50,000 WBC/mm^3; no bacteria
- Microscopic examination of crystals under polarized light
  —*Gout:* needle-shaped; strong birefringence; negative elongation
  —*Pseudogout:* rhomboid; weak birefringence; positive elongation

LABORATORY

- CBC often shows a leukocytosis
- Chemistry panel to assess for renal impairment
- Magnesium and calcium, TSH, and serum iron
- Uric acid level has limited value
- If infectious arthritis is suspected
  —Blood and urine cultures
  —Urethral, cervical, rectal, or pharyngeal gonococcal cultures

IMAGING/SPECIAL TESTS

- Plain radiographs to assess the presence of:
  —Effusion
  —Joint space narrowing
  —The baseline status of the joint
  —Contiguous osteomyelitis
  —Fractures or foreign body
  —*Acute gout:* soft tissue swelling; normal mineralization; joint space preservation
  —*Chronic gout:* calcified tophi; asymmetric bony erosions; overhanging edges; bony shaft tapering
  —*Pseudogout:* chondrocalcinosis; subchondral sclerosis or cysts (wrist); radiopaque calcification of cartilage, tendons, and ligaments; radiopaque osteophytes

DIFFERENTIAL DIAGNOSIS

- Infectious arthritis
- Trauma
- Osteoarthritis
- Reactive arthritis
- Miscellaneous crystalline arthritis
- Aseptic necrosis
- Rheumatoid arthritis
- Systemic lupus erythematosus
- Sickle cell
- Osteomyelitis

Treatment

INITIAL STABILIZATION

- Relieve pain
- Rule out infectious etiology

ED TREATMENT

- NSAIDs are first-line treatment
- If NSAIDS ineffective or contraindicated:
  - —Steroids (oral, intravascular, intramuscular, intraarticular)
  - —Colchicine (limited by toxicity)
- Joint aspiration
- Avoid aspirin
- Reduction of hyperuricemia and the long-term management of gout and pseudogout are not within the usual scope of ED care; strategies include:
  - —Careful withdrawal of gout-producing agent
  - —Uricosurics (e.g., probenecid, sulfinpyrazone) to increase uric acid excretion
  - —Allopurinol to reduce uric acid synthesis, especially for overproducers, renal disease, those undergoing cytotoxic therapy, uricosuric failure, frequent attacks, and tophaceous disease
  - —Increased fluid intake and urine alkalization to prevent renal stones
  - —Long-term colchicine or NSAIDs prophylactically for pseudogout and gout

MEDICATIONS

- Allopurinol: 50–100 mg PO qd, max 200–300 mg qd
- NSAIDs in maximal doses initially × 3 days, then taper over 4 days
  - —Ibuprofen: 800 mg PO q.i.d.
  - —Indomethacin: 25–50 mg PO t.i.d.–q.i.d.
  - —Ketorolac: 15–30 mg i.m./i.v. in ED, may repeat × 1 dose
  - —Naproxen: 500 mg PO t.i.d.
  - —Sulindac: 200 mg PO t.i.d.
- Colchicine: 0.5 mg/h PO up to pain relief, 8 mg total, or GI toxicity
- Corticosteroids
  - —Methylprednisolone: 40 mg i.m. or i.v. qd × 3–4 days
  - —Prednisone: 40 mg PO qd × 3–4 days; taper over 7–14 days
  - —Triamcinolone: 10–40 mg plus dexamethasone 2–10 mg intraarticularly
- Probenecid: 250–500 mg PO b.i.d., max 3 g qd
- Sulfinpyrazone: 50 mg t.i.d., max 800 mg qd

Disposition

ADMISSION CRITERIA

- Suspected infectious arthritis
- Acute renal failure
- Intractable pain

DISCHARGE CRITERIA

- No evidence of infection
- Adequate pain relief

Miscellaneous

ICD9: 274.9, 275.49

ICD10: M10.9

SUGGESTED READINGS

Agudelo CA, Wise CM. Crystal-associated arthritis in the elderly. Rheum Dis Clin North Am 2000;26(3):527–546.

Buckley TJ. Radiologic features of gout. Am Fam Physician 1996;54(4):1232–1238.

Harris MD, Siegel LB, Alloway JA. Gout and hyperuricemia. Am Fam Physician 1999;59(4):925–934.

Joseph J, McGrath H. Gout or "pseudogout": how to differentiate crystal-induced arthropathies. Geriatrics 1995;50(4):33–39.

McGill NW. Gout and other crystal arthropathies. Med J Aust 1997;66:33–38.

Authors: Delaram Ghadishah; A. Antoine Kazzi

Granulocytopenia

Clinical Presentation

SIGNS AND SYMPTOMS

- Fever
- Localized erythema or fluctuance
- Signs of lung consolidation
  - —Rales
  - —Rhonchi
  - —Dullness
- Dysuria
- Urinary retention, urgency, or frequency
- Change in bowel habits
- Mucosal lesions

MECHANISM/DESCRIPTION

- Less than normal number of polymorphonuclear (PMN) leukocytes
- Number of PMN + bands $<500/mm^3$
  - —Patients with a count below 1,000 that has recently or rapidly fallen are at greater risk for infection than those with a count below 500 but rising
  - —Patients with myelodysplastic syndromes should be considered granulocytopenic with higher counts because of defective neutrophils

ETIOLOGY

- Most commonly seen in patients undergoing myelosuppressive drug therapy or radiation treatment for neoplasms
- Chemicals
- Immune-related
  - —Bone marrow infiltration
- Infection
  - —Bacterial primarily staphylococcal and gram-negative
  - —Fungal
- Vitamin deficiency (B_{12}/folate)

Pre-Hospital

N/A

Diagnosis

ESSENTIAL WORKUP

- Complete physical examination
  - —Detailed examination of oral mucosa and perianal area
  - —Palpation of skin
  - —Location of fluctuances or tenderness
  - —Careful lung examination
  - —Rectal examination if symptoms suggest perirectal abscess

LABORATORY

- CBC with differential
- Blood culture from two different sites, with one from IV catheter site if present
- Urinalysis and urine culture
  - —Urinalysis may be normal

IMAGING/SPECIAL TESTS

- Chest radiography even in absence of lung findings
- CSF analysis for altered mental status/signs of meningitis

DIFFERENTIAL DIAGNOSIS

- Infection
  - —Bacterial
  - —Fungal
  - —Viral
  - —Protozoal/parasitic
- Immune suppression
  - —Cell-mediated
  - —Antineoplastic agents

Treatment

INITIAL STABILIZATION

- ABCs
- Initiate IV, O_2, monitor
- For hypotension
  —Administer 1 L 0.9% NS IV fluid bolus (peds: 20 cc/kg)
  —Initiate pressors as needed to stabilize blood pressure if no response to IV fluids

ED TREATMENT

- Strict isolation
- Administer broad-spectrum combination antibiotics after cultures for suspected or documented infection
  —Imipenem-cilastatin or fluoroquinolone
  —Ceftazidime alone or with aminoglycoside (amikacin, tobramycin, gentamicin)
- Cefepime alone
  —Aminoglycoside plus antipseudomonal β-lactam (mezlocillin, piperacillin, or ticarcillin)
  —Vancomycin if patient is at risk to be carrier of *Staphylococcus aureus* or has a history of previous staphylococcal infections

MEDICATIONS

- Amikacin: 15 mg/kg/24 hours (peds: 15–30 mg/kg/24 hours) divided q8–24h i.v.
- Cefepime: 0.5–2 g q12h i.v.
- Ceftazidime: 1–2 g (peds: 30–50 mg/kg q8h) q8–12h i.v.
- Gentamicin: 1 mg/kg (peds 2–2.5 mg/kg) q8h or 5 mg/kg q24h
- Imipenem-cilastatin: 250 mg–1000 mg q6–8h
- Levofloxacin: 500 mg i.v. qd
- Mezlocillin: 3 g q4h over 30 min
- Piperacillin: 3 g q4h over 30 min
- Ticarcillin: 3 g (peds: 200–300 mg/kg/ 24 hours) q4h over 30 min
- Tobramycin: 1 mg/kg/ q8h i.v. (peds: 2–2.5 mg/kg q8h i.v.)
- Vancomycin: 1–2 mg/kg q8–12h i.v.

Disposition

ADMISSION CRITERIA

- Signs of infection
- Unreliable patient
- Close follow-up unavailable

DISCHARGE CRITERIA

- Previously diagnosed granulocytopenia
- Completely asymptomatic
- Close follow-up assured
- Reliable patient

Miscellaneous

ICD9: 288.0

ICD10: D70

SUGGESTED READINGS

Avery RK, Longworth DL. Evolving concepts in the management of patients with neutropenia and fever. Cleve Clin J Med 1999;66(3):173–180.

Bagby GC. Disorders of neutrophil production. In: Bennett JC, et al. Cecil's textbook of medicine. Philadelphia: WB Saunders, 1996:908–915.

Calandra T. Spectrum and treatment of bacterial infections in cancer patients with granulocytopenia. Recent Results Cancer Res 1991;121:329–336.

Schimpff SC. Infections in the cancer patient—diagnosis, prevention, and treatment. In: Mandel G, et al., eds. Mandel, Douglas and Bennet's principles and practice of infectious disease. New York: Churchill Livingstone, 1995: 2666–2684.

Vogelzang NJ, Flaherty JP. Fever and granulocytopenia: a viewpoint from an academic setting. Recent Results Cancer Res 1993;132:79–88.

Author: Elicia Sinor Kennedy

Guillain-Barré Syndrome

Clinical Presentation

SIGNS AND SYMPTOMS

- Rapidly evolving, symmetric, ascending paralysis
- Loss of deep tendon reflexes
- Absent or mild sensory symptoms
  - —Paresthesias of fingertips or toes
- Pain, commonly of pelvis and shoulder girdles
- Preceding bacterial or viral infection
- Acute or subacute onset of weakness, reaching a peak in 2–4 weeks
- Spontaneous resolution of symptoms over weeks to months
- Autonomic dysfunction
  - —Hypertension
  - —Orthostatic hypotension
  - —Ileus
  - —Dysrhythmias
  - —Urinary retention
- Miller Fisher syndrome (MFS)
  - —Ophthalmoplegia
  - —Ataxia
  - —Areflexia
- Features that suggest alternative diagnoses
  - —Fever
  - —Normal reflexes
  - —Upper motor neuron signs
  - —Asymmetric neurologic deficits
  - —Sharply demarcated sensory level

MECHANISM/DESCRIPTION

- Leading cause of acute flaccid paralysis in Western countries
- All ages, rare in infancy
- Annual incidence 1–2 per 100,000
- Reactive, self-limited autoimmune disease triggered by preceding infection
- Peripheral nerves only, central nerves unaffected
- Acute inflammatory demyelinating polyradiculoneuropathy (AIDP)
  - —Most prevalent form of GBS (90%)
  - —Usually complete recovery
  - —Formerly synonymous with GBS
- Uncommon forms of GBS
  - —Acute motor-sensory axonal neuropathy (AMSAN): affects motor and sensory nerves, fulminant course
  - —Acute motor axonal neuropathy (AMAN): affects motor nerves, clinically identical to AIDP
  - —Miller Fisher syndrome
- Outcome favorable with 70% with complete recovery in 1 year
- Mortality 5–8%
- Common causes of death: ARDS, sepsis, dysautonomia

ETIOLOGY

- Postinfectious
  - —Two thirds with antecedent illness, usually respiratory or gastrointestinal
  - —1–3 weeks between prodromal illness and neurologic symptoms
  - —*Campylobacter jejuni* most common antecedent infection
  - —Cytomegalovirus most common viral infection
- Postvaccination
  - —Rabies vaccine prepared from infected brain of adult animals
  - —Relationship to oral polio vaccine questionable

PEDIATRIC CONSIDERATIONS

- Pain may be initial symptom
- Cranial nerve palsies
- Occasionally, evolving ataxia
- Older child may present with distal paresthesias

Pre-Hospital

- May need ventilatory support

ESSENTIAL WORKUP

- Clinical diagnosis
- Electrolytes
- Lumbar puncture

LABORATORY

- CSF
  - —Albuminocytologic dissociation may be present only after 7–10 days
  - —Normal opening pressure
  - —Few or no WBCs
  - —Increased protein (55–250)

IMAGING/SPECIAL TESTS

- Abnormal electrophysiologic studies
- CT or MRI to rule out cord compression

DIFFERENTIAL DIAGNOSIS

- Cord compression
- Lyme disease
- Tick paralysis
- Transverse myelitis
- Botulism
- Myasthenia gravis
- Neoplastic meningitis
- Tetrodotoxin poisoning
- Chronic heavy metal poisoning
- Acute periodic paralysis
- Acute intermittent porphyria
- Eaton-Lambert syndrome
- Poliomyelitis
- Diphtheria
- Psychogenic, malingering

Treatment

INITIAL STABILIZATION

- Airway
  - Progression to respiratory failure can be rapid

ED TREATMENT

- Focus is on airway management
  - 33% need ventilatory support
  - May need intubation within 24–48 hours from time of onset
- Forced vital capacity (FVC)
  - Assists in guiding need for airway intervention
  - ICU admission is recommended when FVC is less than 20 mL/kg
  - Intubation is recommended in most cases when FVC is less than 15 mL/kg
- Watch for autonomic dysfunction
- Supportive therapy
- Early neurology consult
- Steroids not beneficial

MEDICATIONS

- Plasmapheresis
- Intravenous immunoglobulin
- Administered in consultation with neurology

Disposition

ADMISSION CRITERIA

- All patients with diagnosis of GBS need admission for close observation
- ICU admission for those with respiratory compromise or autonomic dysfunction, FVC <20 mL/kg
- Evolution and severity of neurologic deficits is variable

DISCHARGE CRITERIA

- Patients should be considered for discharge only in consultation with a neurologist

Miscellaneous

ICD9: 357.0

ICD10: G61.0

SUGGESTED READINGS

Brody AJ, Sternbach G. Octave Landry: Guillain-Barré syndrome. J Emerg Med 1994;12(6):833–837.

Hahn A. Guillain-Barré syndrome. Lancet 1998;352(9128):635–641.

Jones HR. Childhood Guillain-Barré syndrome: clinical presentation, diagnosis, and therapy. J Child Neurol 1996;11(1): 4–12.

Lindenbaum Y, Kissel JT, Mendell JR. Treatment approaches for Guillain-Barré syndrome and chronic inflammatory demyelinating polyradiculoneuropathy. Neurol Clin 2001;19(1):187–204.

Author: Angela Loh

Hallucinogen, Poisoning

Clinical Presentation

SIGNS AND SYMPTOMS

- Considerable individual variation
- Usually oriented and able to give a history of exposure, even while having delusions
- Initial symptoms
  - —Nausea
  - —Flushing
  - —Chills
  - —Tachycardia
  - —Hypertension
  - —Piloerection
  - —Tremor

NEUROLOGIC SYMPTOMS

- Restlessness and dizziness early after ingestion
- Affective lability
- Desire to laugh (especially with *Psilocybe* mushrooms)
- Anxiety, despair, helplessness, incipient dread
- Exaggeration of preexisting mood (medical personnel are more likely to see patients anxious moods, or "bad trips")
- Intensified perceptions
- Visual distortions/intensification
- Auditory distortions/intensification
- Tactile distortions (especially with mescaline)
- Synesthesia: blending of sensory modalities (e.g., seeing sounds)
- Distortions of reality
- Time-space distortions
- Distortions of body image
- Sensation of rapid aging
- Loss of ego boundaries and feeling of unity with the universe
- Religious or mystical experiences
- Sleep disruption

NEUROLOGIC SIGNS

- Unusual behavior
- Speech disruption
- Markedly dilated pupils, especially with lysergic acid diethylamide (LSD)
- Piloerection
- Hyperreflexia
- Coma, with massive exposures
- Convulsions
  - —Paramethoxyamphetamine (PMA) and methylenedioxymethamphetamine (MDMA; ecstasy)
  - —Children who become hyperpyrexic after *Psilocybe* mushroom ingestion

PULMONARY

- Mild tachypnea
- Respiratory arrest with massive exposures

CARDIOVASCULAR

- Tachycardia
- Hypertension (with hallucinogenic amphetamines)
- Dysrhythmias (with hallucinogenic amphetamines)
- Intracerebral hemorrhage (with hallucinogenic amphetamines)

GASTROINTESTINAL

- Nausea/vomiting (especially with mescaline)

METABOLIC

- Hyperpyrexia
  - —Especially with MDMA and PMA use at "Rave" clubs
  - —Hepatic failure, renal failure, and disseminated intravascular coagulopathy may follow
  - —May be lethal
- Hyponatremia
  - —With MDMA use

HEMOPOIETIC

- Coagulopathies and hemorrhage at high doses
  - —Due to disruption of platelet serotonin function

MECHANISM/DESCRIPTION

- Characteristics
  - —Predominantly alters perception, cognition, and mood
  - —Minimal memory loss, intellectual deficits, stupor, autonomic nervous system dysfunction
- Symptoms characterized by sympathetic arousal
- Structurally similar to neurotransmitters
  - —Serotonin (5-hydroxytryptamine, 5-HT)
    - -Hallucinogens act as agonists at some 5-HT receptor subtypes and as antagonists at other 5-HT receptor subtypes
    - -Possible long-term damage to serotonin system with MDMA use
  - —Norepinephrine (NE)
  - —Epinephrine (Epi)
  - —Dopamine (DA)

ETIOLOGY

- Most exposures are intentional
- Common hallucinogens include:
  - —LSD (duration 6–12 hours)
  - —Hallucinogenic amphetamines
    - -Methylenedioxyamphetamine (MDA) (duration 8–12 hours)
    - -Methylenedioxyethamphetamine (MDEA)
    - -MDMA—Ecstasy (duration 4–6 hours)
    - -PMA
    - -Dimethoxyamphetamine (DOM or STP)
  - —Mescaline (peyote cactus) (duration 6–12 hours)
  - —Psilocybin (*Psilocybe* mushrooms)
- LSD
  - —Prototypical hallucinogen
  - —Street-marketed peyote cactus "buttons" and *Psilocybe* mushrooms are often adulterated with LSD
  - —Focus on signs and symptoms described above
  - —Other hallucinogens present similarly

Pre-Hospital

CONTROVERSIES

- Sedation with benzodiazepines versus haloperidol versus physical restraints
  - —Benzodiazepines are generally preferred
  - —Sedation masks symptoms and may limit history

CAUTIONS

- Sedate or restrain patient to ensure safe transport
- For the hyperthermic patient:
  - —Employ sedation rather than physical restraint
  - —Begin cooling measures

Diagnosis

ESSENTIAL WORKUP
- Measure core temperature
- Determine risk of rhabdomyolysis
  —Urine dip or myoglobin level
  —CPK level

LABORATORY
- Electrolytes, BUN/Cr, glucose
- Urine toxicology screen
  —Rarely indicated
  —Distinguishing between hallucinogens is of little value
  —The clinical syndromes and treatments are similar
  —Most do not detect LSD

IMAGING/SPECIAL TESTS
- Generally not indicated

DIFFERENTIAL DIAGNOSIS
- Meningitis
- Intracranial bleeds or lesions
- Psychiatric illnesses
  —LSD associated with prolonged psychoses, resembling schizoaffective disorders
  —Patients with true psychosis are usually not oriented or able to give their own history
- Exposure to other hallucinogenic substances
  —Anticholinergic drugs (e.g., diphenhydramine)
  —Plants (e.g., jimsonweed, morning glory, and marijuana)
  —Phencyclidine (PCP)
  —Chronic amphetamine abuse
  —Chronic cocaine abuse
  —Steroids
- Infectious/febrile seizures in the hyperpyretic child

PEDIATRIC CONSIDERATIONS
- Assess parent-child relationships for possibility of neglect or abuse

Treatment

INITIAL STABILIZATION
- ABCs
- Aggressive cooling if hyperthermic
- IV access/rehydration with isotonic fluids if significant fluid loss
- Naloxone, Accucheck, dextrose, and thiamine if altered mental status

ED TREATMENT
- Cooling measures
  —Cool mist and fans
  —Benzodiazepines if agitated
  —Paralytics if needed (generally not succinylcholine)
- Sedate if agitated
  —Benzodiazepines
  —Rarely neuroleptics
    -May intensify hallucinogenic experience
    -May lower seizure threshold
- Activated charcoal if oral ingestion
- Place in a quiet, calm environment
- Hydration and urine alkalinization for treatment of rhabdomyolysis

MEDICATIONS
- Dextrose: D50W 1 amp (25 g/50 mL) (peds D25W 0.5–1 g/kg or 2–4 mL/kg) i.v.
- Diazepam (benzodiazepine): 5–10 mg (peds 0.2–0.5 mg/kg) i.v.
- Haloperidol (Haldol): 2.5–10 mg i.v./i.m. (not recommended for peds)
- Mannitol: 1 g/kg i.v. over 30 min
- Naloxone (Narcan): 2 mg (peds 0.01–0.1 mg/kg) i.v. or i.m. initial dose
- Sodium bicarbonate drip: 2 amp in 1 L of D5W to run at 1.5–2 times maintenance rates and to keep urine alkalinized
- Thiamine (vitamin B_1): 100 mg (peds 25 mg) i.v. or i.m.

PEDIATRIC CONSIDERATIONS
- Avoid haloperidol in children

Disposition

ADMISSION CRITERIA
- Severely intoxicated
- Atypical presentations
- Prolonged symptoms (>12 hours postexposure)
- Prolonged periods of agitation and hyperthermia
  —Risk of rhabdomyolysis or organ damage

DISCHARGE CRITERIA
- Most patients, after receiving supportive therapy and observation, can be discharged once asymptomatic

PEDIATRIC CONSIDERATIONS
- Suspected cases of child abuse or neglect require referral to child protection agencies

Miscellaneous

ICD9: 969.6

ICD10: T40.9

SUGGESTED READINGS

Abraham HD, Aldridge AM, Gogia P. The psychopharmacology of hallucinogens. Neuropsychopharmacology 1996;14:285–298.

Acute reactions to drugs of abuse. Med Lett 2002;44(1125):21–24.

Golub A, Johnson BD, Sifaneck SJ, et al. Is the U.S. experiencing an incipient epidemic of hallucinogen use? Substance Use Misuse 2001;36:1699–1729.

Kalant H. The pharmacology and toxicology of "ecstasy" (MDMA) and related drugs. Can Med Assoc J 2001;165:917–928.

O'Shea B, Fagan J. Lysergic acid diethylamide. Ir Med J 2001;94:217.

Author: Kimberlie A. Graeme

Hand Infection

Clinical Presentation

SIGNS AND SYMPTOMS

Paronychia

- Localized edema, erythema, and pain in proximal portion of lateral nail fold
- Fluctuance may be present and may extend beneath the nail margin to the nail bed
- Systemic signs and symptoms are usually not present

Felon

- Erythema and tense swelling of the distal pulp space that does *not* extend proximal to the PIP
- Aching pain early, severe throbbing pain late
- Systemic signs and symptoms are usually not present

Herpetic Whitlow

- Distal pulp space is swollen, but remains soft
- Lateral nail folds may be affected
- Throbbing pain of the distal pulp space
- Vesicles containing nonpurulent fluid are present and may form bullae
- Systemic symptoms may be present, as fever, lymphadenopathy, and constitutional symptoms

Flexor Tenosynovitis

- Severe pain and symmetric edema of the digit, usually the thumb, index finger, or middle finger
- Severe tenderness over the course of the tendon sheath
- Flexed position of the finger at rest
- Pain on passive extension of the finger—may be the only finding in early infection

Clenched Fist Injury

- Laceration over the MCP from striking an object with a clenched fist
- Any laceration over the MCP must be assumed to be a *human bite wound* until proven otherwise

Web Space Abscess

- Pain and edema of the affected web space and adjacent palm
- Fingers are held abducted

Palmar Space Infections

- Thenar space infection
  - —Pain, tenderness, tense edema of thenar eminence
  - —Dorsal edema without tenderness
  - —Thumb is held abducted and flexed, and passive adduction is painful
- Midpalmar space infection
  - —Pain, edema, and tenderness of the midpalmar space
  - —Dorsal edema without tenderness
  - —Motion of middle and ring fingers is painful
- Hypothenar space infection
  - —Pain and fullness over hypothenar eminence
  - —No limitation of finger movement

ETIOLOGY

- Bacterial infection of the hand is associated with skin pathogens, *Staphylococcus* or *Streptococcus* species, and history of a puncture wound
- Anaerobes are identified in 75% of paronychia in children due to thumb sucking and nail biting
- Chronic paronychia may be caused by *Candida albicans*
- Herpetic whitlow is caused by type 1 or 2 herpes simplex virus
- Clenched fist injuries involve a variety of pathogens, including anaerobic *Streptococcus* and *Eikenella* sp.

Pre-Hospital

- Elevation of extremity
- Pain relief may be necessary

Diagnosis

ESSENTIAL WORKUP

- Most hand infections are diagnosed by history and physical examination with special attention to neurovascular status

LABORATORY

- Although usually not necessary, herpetic whitlow may be confirmed by Tzank test
- Gram stain and culture may guide antibiotic choice in felons
- Blood cultures are not routinely indicated

IMAGING/SPECIAL TESTS

- Radiographs are usually not helpful in paronychia unless there has been trauma or a suspected foreign body
- With felon, flexor tenosynovitis, and palmar space infection, radiograph may identify osteomyelitis or foreign body
- Radiographs in clenched fist injury may reveal a fracture

DIFFERENTIAL DIAGNOSIS

- Paronychia should be differentiated from herpetic whitlow and felon
- The differential for palmar space infection includes flexor tenosynovitis, cellulitis, and web space infection

Treatment

INITIAL STABILIZATION

- ABCs if patient is toxic or above conditions occur in the setting of sepsis or other injury

ED TREATMENT

Paronychia

- Early paronychia/simple cellulitis without purulence present may be managed with oral antibiotics, and rest
  —Cephalexin, dicloxacillin
  —Clindamycin or erythromycin if associated with nail biting or oral contact
- Superficial infections are drained by inserting a No. 11 blade between nail and eponychium and lifting the eponychium from the nail
- If necessary, the lateral nail fold may be incised tangential to the curvature of the nail
- When pus is present under the adjacent nail, one fourth of the nail should be removed
- When pus is present under the dorsal roof of the proximal nail, remove one third of the proximal nail

Felon

- A lateral incision avoiding the neurovascular bundle is preferred to drain most distal pulp infections
- More extensive felons are drained through a unilateral longitudinal incision that does not cross the DIP flexor crease
- Disruption of fibrous septa is no longer recommended because it results in an unstable fingertip; however, loculations may need to be broken
- Give oral antibiotics to cover skin pathogens, place a drain, and recheck in 48 hours
  —Cephalexin, dicloxacillin

Herpetic Whitlow

- Usually self-limited; do not incise and drain
- Oral acyclovir may be given to patients with systemic involvement

Flexor Tenosynovitis, Web Space Abscess, Palmar Space Infection

- Elevation, IV antibiotics, and pain control in the ED
  —Ampicillin/sulbactam, cefoxitin, ticarcillin/clavulanate
- All of these infections require immediate consultation with a hand surgeon for admission and drainage

Clenched Fist Injury

- Elevation, IV antibiotics, tetanus prophylaxis, and pain control in the ED
  —Ampicillin/sulbactam, cefoxitin, ticarcillin/clavulanate
- All bite wounds with evidence of infection or joint involvement require emergent consultation with a hand surgeon as tendon involvement almost universal
- If there are no signs of infection and no joint penetration, patients may be considered for outpatient treatment with oral antibiotics after appropriate irrigation and wound care
  —Ampicillin/clavulanate or penicillin V plus cephalexin or dicloxacillin
  —Do *not* primarily close lacerations associated with a human bite; delayed primary closure or healing by secondary intention is appropriate

MEDICATIONS

- Acyclovir: adult: 400 mg PO t.i.d. for 10 days; peds: not recommended for herpetic whitlow
- Ampicillin/clavulanate: adult: 875/125 mg PO b.i.d.; peds: 40 mg/kg/d PO div q6h
- Ampicillin/sulbactam: adult: 1.5 to 3.0 g i.v. q6h; peds: safety not established
- Cefoxitin: adult: 2 g i.v. q8h; peds: 80–160 mg/kg/d i.v. or i.m. div q6h
- Cephalexin: adult: 500 g PO q.i.d. for 7 days; peds: 40 mg/kg/d PO div q6h
- Clindamycin: adult: 300 mg PO q.i.d. for 7 days; peds: 20–40 mg/kg/d div q6h PO i.v., i.m.
- Dicloxacillin: adult: 500 mg PO q.i.d. for 7 days; peds: 12.5–50 mg/kg/d PO div q6h
- Erythromycin: adult: 500 mg PO q.i.d. for 7 days; peds: 40 mg/kg/d div q6h PO
- Penicillin V: adult: 250 mg PO q.i.d.; peds: 40 mg/kg/d PO div q6h
- Ticarcillin/clavulanate: adult: 3.1 g i.v. q4–6h; peds: safety not established

Disposition

ADMISSION CRITERIA

Flexor Tenosynovitis, Web Space Abscess, Palmar Space Infections

- All these infections require admission for IV antibiotics and drainage

Clenched Fist Injury with Signs of Infection

- Requires admission for surgical débridement and IV antimicrobials

DISCHARGE CRITERIA

Paronychia and Felons

- Patients with uncomplicated paronychia or felon may be discharged from the ED with a recheck and drain removal in 48 hours

Herpetic Whitlow

- Patients with herpetic whitlow may be discharged from the ED with appropriate follow-up

Clenched Fist Injury Without Infection

- May be discharged on oral antibiotics with follow-up in 24 hours

Miscellaneous

ICD9: 136.9

ICD10: L08.9, L70.8, M70.1

SUGGESTED READINGS

Antosia RE, Lyn E. The hand. In: Rosen P, et al., eds. Emergency medicine: concepts and clinical practice, 4th ed. St. Louis: CV Mosby, 1998:625–668.

Hausman MR, Lisser SP. Hand infections. Orthop Clin North Am 1992;23(1): 171–185.

Tintinalli JE, Kelen GD, Stapcynski JS, eds. Emergency medicine: a comprehensive study guide. Hand Infect 1999;277–280.

Author: Chet Shermer

Hazmat

Clinical Presentation

SIGNS AND SYMPTOMS

Skin

- Chemical burns, may appear deceptively mild at first
- Visible liquid or powder on skin
- Absorption through skin may cause systemic toxicity

Mucous Membranes (Eyes, Nasopharynx)

- Ranges from subjective irritation to serious mucosal burns
- Potential airway compromise
- See Corneal Burn

Pulmonary

- Cough
- Pleuritic chest pain
- Bronchospasm
- Dyspnea
- Pulmonary edema (immediate or delayed)

Systemic (After Skin or Pulmonary Absorption)

- Altered mental status
- Seizures
- Tachy/brady dysrhythmias
- Hypo/hypertension
- GI symptoms
- Electrolyte disturbances
- Carboxy/met hemoglobinemias
- Cholinergic syndrome, see Chemical Weapons Poisoning (Nerve Agents)

MECHANISM

- Acids cause coagulation necrosis with eschar usually limiting penetration to deeper tissue
- Alkalis cause liquefaction necrosis and soluble complexes that penetrate into deep tissues
- Damage also occurs through oxidation, protein denaturation, cellular dehydration, local ischemia, and by metabolic competition/inhibition

ETIOLOGY

- Hazardous materials are encountered in the household, industry, agriculture, transportation accidents, and in criminal/terrorist activities

Pre-Hospital

CAUTIONS

Recognize a HAZMAT Incident

- Accident at industrial/agricultural site
- Accident involving transport of hazardous materials
- Suspected terrorist mass casualty incident
- Cholinergic syndrome
- Irritant mucous membrane symptoms
- Chemical burns

Protect Yourself

- Approach from upwind
- Do not enter scene until safety of material is determined
- Level A protective gear if safety not established
- Personal chemical protective equipment
  - —Level A: positive pressure self-contained breathing apparatus (SCBA), fully encapsulated chemical resistant suit, double chemical resistant gloves, chemical resistant boots, airtight seals between suit, gloves, boots
  - —Level B: SCBA, nonencapsulated chemical suit, double gloves, boots
  - —Level C: air purification device, suit, gloves, boots
  - —Level D: common work clothes

Identify Substance

- Department of Transportation (DOT) placard, Material Safety Data Sheet (MSDS), shipping papers, hazard labels
- If unsuccessful, call Chemical Transportation Emergency Center (CHEMTREC) at 1-800-424-9300 to determine substance and toxicity
- HAZMAT teams can do chemical testing

Determine Toxicity and Need for Decontamination

- Poison control
- CHEMTREC

Decontaminate

- HAZMAT team

Treat

- Provide BLS and ALS care as indicated
- Generally BLS only in a hot zone
- Irrigate skin and ocular burns immediately and continue until arrival at hospital

Diagnosis

ESSENTIAL WORKUP

- Attempt to identify substance using pre-hospital providers, MSDS, and CHEMTREC
- MSDS is useful for identifying chemicals, vapor vs skin hazard, and need for decontamination but has limited treatment data
- Determine route and duration of exposure
  - —Inhalation injury more likely in an enclosed space
- Determine toxicity using poison control, computerized databases such as POISINDEX or TOXNET, or standard toxicology text
- Observe as needed for systemic toxicity

LABORATORY

- Depends on substance
- Electrolytes, BUN, Cr, glucose
- Liver function tests
- Ca, Mg, phosphorus
- ABG for
  - —Metabolic acidosis
  - —Carboxy/methemoglobinemias
  - —Respiratory failure

IMAGING/SPECIAL TESTS

- CXR for pulmonary edema

DIFFERENTIAL DIAGNOSIS

- Skin
  - —Hypersensitivity reaction
  - —Thermal burns
- Pulmonary
  - —Pneumonia
  - —Pulmonary embolism
  - —Anaphylaxis
- Systemic
  - —Status epilepticus
  - —Overdose
  - —Psychiatric illness
  - —Myocardial infarction

Treatment

INITIAL STABILIZATION

- Protect ED personnel
  - —Secondary contamination can occur from dermal contact or through inhalation of volatile gases/particles
- Keep patients outside in designated hot zones until decontaminated
- When in doubt decontaminate
- Expect contaminated patients to arrive via EMS or private vehicle
- If treatment is required before/during decontamination
  - —Use minimum necessary staff in appropriate personal protection gear
  - —Focus on life/limb saving care only
- Decontamination
  - —Security to enforce hot zone
  - —Remove and double bag clothing
  - —Copious irrigation with soap and water for 10–15 minutes with special attention to obviously contaminated areas, wounds, and exposed eyes
  - —If possible, recapture water to prevent contamination of the sewer and downstream areas
    - -In an emergency or mass casualty situation, it is acceptable to let water drain into the sewer
  - —Hydrotherapy is the mainstay of therapy for chemical burns and is contraindicated only for elemental metals (sodium and potassium)
  - —If possible, allow the patient to decontaminate himself, or use a trained decontamination team
  - —If necessary, gloves, masks, goggles, and disposable gowns provide some protection
  - —Remove/replace bandages, tourniquets, airway adjuncts, IV sets
  - —Re-triage after decontamination

ED TREATMENT

- Provide supportive care as needed
- Determine if antidotal treatment would be effective and available
- HAZMAT incidents provoke extreme fear
  - —Expect casualties suffering from collective hysteria
  - —Knowledge of toxicologic profile can exclude contamination in these patients
- ED staff may become symptomatic even if chemical concentrations in the air are below toxic levels, and may need to be escorted to fresh air
- Chemical burns
  - —Irrigation should be started as soon as possible and if due to a strong alkali may need to be continued for hours
  - —Aggressive fluid resuscitation 2–4 cc/kg LR per total burn surface area (TBSA) percent over 24 hours with one half given over the first 8 hours
  - —Pain control
- Pulmonary symptoms
  - —Bronchodilators, oxygen, intubation, and mechanical ventilation
- Selected special treatments
  - —Hydrofluoric acid burns:
    - -Calcium gluconate via topical cutaneous gel, subcutaneous or intraarterial
    - -For systemic toxicity: IV calcium and magnesium
  - —Phenol burns:
    - -Remove phenol from skin with polyethylene glycol (PEG) 300 or 400 or with isopropyl alcohol
  - —Nitrates:
    - -Ingested or extensive burns may cause methemoglobinemia
    - -Treat levels greater than 30% with high-flow oxygen and IV methylene blue
  - —Elemental metals (sodium/potassium):
    - -Water lavage is contraindicated and dangerous
    - -Cover with oil until substance can be débrided from skin
  - —Organophosphates/carbamate insecticides:
    - -See Chemical Weapons Poisoning (Nerve Agent)

MEDICATIONS

- Albuterol 2.5–5.0 mg nebulized
- Methylene blue 1–2 mg/kg slow i.v.

Disposition

ADMISSION CRITERIA

- Airway compromise, respiratory difficulty (hypoxia)
- Any significant systemic symptoms
- Admit chemical burns to a burn center

DISCHARGE CRITERIA

- Patients who are well after a period of observation and consultation with poison control
- Superficial chemical burns due to a toxin without potential for systemic toxicity (weak acid/alkali)

Miscellaneous

ICD9: N/A

ICD10: N/A

SEE ALSO: CHEMICAL WEAPONS POISONING, AND RADIATION INJURY

SUGGESTED READINGS

Burgess JL, Kirk M, Borron SW, et al. Emergency department hazardous materials protocol for contaminated patients. Ann Emerg Med 1999;34:205–212.

Goldfrank LR, Flomenbaum NE, Lewin NE. Goldrank's toxicologic emergencies, 6th ed. New York: McGraw-Hill, 1998.

Greenberg MI, Cone DC, Roberts JR. Material Safety Data Sheet: a useful resource for the emergency physician. Ann Emerg Med 1996;27:347–352.

Author: Dan Huhn

Head Trauma, Blunt

Clinical Presentation

SIGNS AND SYMPTOMS

- Evidence of trauma to head includes:
  - —Scalp laceration, cephalohematoma, or ecchymosis
  - —Raccoon's eyes: bilateral ecchymosis of orbits associated with basilar skull fractures
  - —Battle's sign: ecchymosis behind the ear at mastoid process associated with basilar skull fracture
  - —Hemotympanum
  - —Cerebral spinal fluid rhinorrhea or otorrhea
- Evidence of increasing intracranial pressure (ICP) includes:
  - —Decreasing level of consciousness, falling Glasgow Coma Scale (GCS) score
  - —Cushing's response; bradycardia, hypertension, and diminished respiratory rate
  - —Dilated pupils associated with decorticate or decerebrate posturing

ETIOLOGY

- Blunt trauma to head may cause several types of closed head injuries
  - —*Concussion:* head trauma associated with transient loss of consciousness or amnesia with no evidence of intracranial pathology on CT
  - —*Subdural hematoma:* tearing of subdural bridging veins and bleeding into the subdural space
  - —*Epidural hematoma:* dural arterial injury, especially the middle meningeal artery often associated with a skull fracture
    - -Classically, transient loss of consciousness followed by a *lucid interval,* then rapid demise
  - —*Subarachnoid hemorrhage:* bleeding into the subarachnoid space following trauma
  - —*Cerebral contusion:* focal injuries to the brain characterized as coup (beneath area of impact) or contrecoup (area remote from impact)
  - —*Intracerebral hemorrhage:* mass intracranial lesion with bleeding into the brain parenchyma
  - —*Diffuse axonal injury:* microscopic injuries scattered throughout the brain in a patient in deep coma

Pre-Hospital

- Blunt head trauma patients with risk for intracranial lesion must go to a trauma center.
  - —*High-risk* patients include depressed consciousness, focal neurologic signs, multiple trauma, or palpable depressed skull fractures
- Moderate risk patients should go to a hospital with availability of prompt neurosurgical consultation
  - —*Moderate risk* patients include progressive headache, alcohol or drug intoxication, unreliable history, posttraumatic seizure, repeated vomiting, posttraumatic amnesia, signs of basilar skull fracture
- Protect and manage the airway including intubation
  - —Routine hyperventilation without signs of cerebral herniation should be avoided
- If evidence of cerebral herniation (extensor posturing, pupillary asymmetry, or nonreactivity in a comatose patient) or progressive neurologic deterioration, then initiate measures to decrease ICP including:
  - —*Mild* hyperventilation: 16–20 breaths per minute (bpm) in adults, 20–24 bpm in children, and 24–26 bpm in infants
  - —Elevating head of bed 20–30 degrees
- C-spine precautions must be maintained in all patients

CAUTIONS

- Hypotension [systolic blood pressure (SBP) <90 mm Hg] should be avoided; utilize crystalloid solutions intravenously to maintain BP
- Hypoxia (O_2 sat $<90\%$) should be avoided; administer 100% O_2
- Check blood glucose

Diagnosis

ESSENTIAL WORKUP

- *Head CT* should be performed in patients with any of the following:
  - —Loss of consciousness or amnesia of events
  - —Progressive headache, alcohol or drug intoxication, unreliable history, posttraumatic seizure, repeated vomiting, signs of basilar skull fracture, possible skull penetration or depressed skull fracture, GCS score <15, or focal neurologic findings
  - —Patients on Coumadin, heparin, or with history of bleeding dyscrasias must be imaged
  - —Elderly patients and alcoholics are at higher risk for intracranial hemorrhage, so have low threshold to scan

LABORATORY

- Rapid check of blood glucose
- CBC, platelet count, coagulation parameters
- Type and cross-match for surgical candidates
- Baseline electrolytes, BUN, and creatinine levels
- Alcohol levels if indicated

IMAGING/SPECIAL TESTS

- Head CT as above
- Cervical spine x-ray, including AP, lateral, and odontoid, should be obtained when indicated

DIFFERENTIAL DIAGNOSIS

- Penetrating head trauma
- Any condition that alters mental status that may have produced a fall and caused external evidence of head trauma (e.g., hypoglycemic episode, seizure)

Treatment

INITIAL STABILIZATION

- ABCs of trauma care
  - —Control airway as needed; RSI intubation if GCS score <8, unable to protect airway, or evidence of hypoxia
  - —Treatment with etomidate or fentanyl as induction agent, succinylcholine (pretreat with mini-dose paralytic), rocuronium or vecuronium; morphine for ongoing sedation
  - —Caution with fentanyl in a patient who is hemodynamically labile
  - —IV catheter placement with crystalloid solution as needed to avoid hypotension (keep SBP >90 mm Hg)
  - —Cervical spine precautions

ED TREATMENT

- Early neurosurgical consultation
- If patient has evidence of cerebral herniation (see above), then initiate measures to decrease ICP including:
  - —*Mild* hyperventilation: 16–20 bpm in adults, 20–24 bpm in children, and 24–26 bpm in infants to keep $PaCO_2$ about 35, which correlates to an end-tidal CO_2 of 32–35
  - —Elevating head of bed 20–30 degrees
  - —Mannitol boluses IV; do not administer mannitol unless SBP >100 mm Hg and patient is adequately fluid resuscitated
- Phenytoin to prevent *early* posttraumatic seizures
- The use of glucocorticoids is *not* recommended to lower ICP in head trauma patients
- Barbiturates are *not* recommended in the initial ED treatment of head-injured patients
- If definitive neurosurgical care is not immediately available, a single burr hole may preserve life until neurosurgical intervention can be obtained
  - —This should only be done in comatose patients with decerebrate or decorticate posturing on the side of a known mass lesion who have not responded to hyperventilation and mannitol
- Transfuse as needed to keep hematocrit above 30%
- Avoid hypothermia, as this will increase risks of coagulopathy during surgery

MEDICATIONS

- Etomidate: 0.2–0.3 mg/kg i.v.
- Fentanyl: 3–5 μg/kg i.v. if SBP >100 mm Hg
- Mannitol: 0.25–1 g/kg i.v. boluses
- Morphine sulfate: adult: 2–20 mg i.v.; peds: 0.1 mg/kg up to adult doses
- Phenytoin: 15–20 mg/kg i.v. up to 1,000 mg
- Rocuronium: 0.6 mg/kg i.v.
- Succinylcholine: 1–2 mg/kg i.v.
- Vecuronium bromide: 0.1 mg/kg i.v., mini-dose pretreatment: 0.01 mg/kg i.v.

Disposition

ADMISSION CRITERIA

- Patients with mass lesion associated with head trauma must be admitted to the ICU or OR
- Patients with subarachnoid hemorrhage and diffuse axonal injury should be initially admitted to the ICU
- Patients with ongoing symptoms including repetitive questioning, anterograde amnesia, or disorientation should be admitted to a monitored unit for neurologic evaluation

DISCHARGE CRITERIA

- Patients with resolved symptoms, negative head CT, and no other comorbid factors (e.g., intoxication, additional trauma needing treatment) may be discharged
- Patients with minor head trauma, no loss of consciousness or amnesia, and normal neurologic exam can be discharged home with a friend or family member and head injury instructions

Miscellaneous

ICD9: 959.01

ICD10: S09.9

SUGGESTED READINGS

Brain Trauma Foundation. Management and prognosis of severe traumatic brain injury. New York: Brain Trauma Foundation, 2000.

Brain Trauma Foundation. Guidelines for prehospital management of traumatic brain injury. New York: Brain Trauma Foundation, 1999.

Chestnut RM, Marshall LF, Klauber MR, et al. The role of secondary brain injury in determining outcome from severe head injury. J Trauma 1993;34:216–222.

Cold GE. Cerebral blood flow in acute head injury. Acta Neurochir 1990;[suppl 49]: 3–64.

Committee on Trauma. Head trauma. In: Advanced trauma life support. Chicago: American College of Surgeons, 1997.

Gennarelli TA. Emergency department management of head injuries. Emerg Med Clin North Am 1984;2:749–760.

Author: Gary M. Vilke

Head Trauma, Penetrating

Clinical Presentation

SIGNS AND SYMPTOMS

- Alteration in level of consciousness and neurologic exam varies based on object and location
- Evidence of increasing intracranial pressure (ICP) include
  - —Decreasing level of consciousness, falling Glasgow Coma Scale (GCS) score
  - —Cushing's response: bradycardia, hypertension, and diminished respiratory rate
  - —Blown pupil associated with decorticate or decerebrate posturing
- Evidence of penetrating injury to head or basilar skull fracture, or object still remaining in head
  - —Raccoon's eyes: bilateral ecchymosis of orbits associated with basilar skull fractures
  - —Battle's sign: ecchymosis behind the ear at mastoid process associated with basilar skull fracture
  - —Hemotympanum
  - —Cerebral spinal fluid rhinorrhea or otorrhea

MECHANISM/DESCRIPTION

- Penetrating injury to the intracranial contents
  - —*High-velocity penetration:* usually bullets, which cause trauma directly to brain tissue, but also have a "shock wave" injury to local surrounding brain tissue along the bullet's path
  - —*Low-velocity penetration:* usually knives, picks, or other sharp objects, with direct local trauma to brain tissue

ETIOLOGY

- Direct penetration of the skull into the intracranial cavity by foreign objects
- The object itself may cause direct or local damage to brain tissue
- The trauma can cause intracranial hemorrhage, including subdural, epidural, and intraparenchymal bleeds
- A bullet that hits the skull, ricochets off, and does not fracture the skull can still cause significant trauma to the underlying brain tissue

Pre-Hospital

CAUTIONS

- If the foreign object is still in the patient's head (e.g., a knife), stabilize it, but *do not* remove
- Determine the weapon type or caliber of weapon at scene
- Protect and manage the airway as needed to avoid hypoxemia, but routine hyperventilation without signs of cerebral herniation should be avoided
- If evidence of cerebral herniation (extensor posturing, pupillary asymmetry or nonreactivity in a comatose patient, or progressive neurologic deterioration with a decrease in GCS of 2 or more points in a patient with an initial GCS less than 9), initiate measures to decrease ICP, including:
  - —*Mild* hyperventilation: 16–20 breaths per minute (bpm) in adults, 20–24 bpm in children, and 24–26 bpm in infants
  - —Elevating head of bed 20–30 degrees
- Maintain C-spine precautions
- Patient must go to a trauma center
- Hypotension [systolic blood pressure (SBP) <90 mm Hg], should be avoided; use crystalloid solutions intravenously as needed to maintain BP
- Hypoxia (O_2 sat <90%) should be avoided; administer 100% O_2

Diagnosis

ESSENTIAL WORKUP

- *Head CT:* location of the lesion and extent of damage can be best evaluated with this study; side-to-side injuries and those lower in the brain tend to be more ominous

LABORATORY

- CBC, platelet count, coagulation perimeters
- Type and crossmatch
- Electrolytes, BUN, and creatinine baseline levels

IMAGING/SPECIAL TESTS

- Head CT as discussed above
- Occasionally, skull radiographs can assess depth of impalement, location of bone fragments, and whether multiple fragments are within the cranium
- Cervical spine evaluation, including AP, lateral, and odontoid, should be obtained when indicated

DIFFERENTIAL DIAGNOSIS

- Blunt head trauma
- Basilar skull fracture
- Any condition that alters mental status that may have induced a fall and caused secondary penetrating trauma

Treatment

INITIAL STABILIZATION

- ABCs
  - —Control airway as needed; RSI intubation if GCS <8, unable to protect airway, or evidence of hypoxia or cerebral herniation
  - —Medications for RSI should include etomidate or fentanyl as induction agent, succinylcholine (pretreat with mini-dose paralytic), rocuronium, or vecuronium; caution with fentanyl in the hemodynamically labile patient; morphine sulfate for ongoing sedation
  - —Intravenous catheter placement, crystalloid solution as needed to keep SBP >90 mm Hg
  - —Address other sources of associated trauma
  - —Cervical spine precautions should be maintained

ED TREATMENT

- Early neurosurgical consultation is necessary
- If patient demonstrates signs of cerebral herniation (see above), initiate measures to decrease ICP including:
  - —*Mild* hyperventilation: 16–20 bpm in adults, 20–24 bpm in children, and 24–26 bpm in infants to keep $PaCO_2$ about 35, which correlates to an end-tidal CO_2 of 32–35
  - —Elevating head of bed 20–30 degrees
  - —Mannitol boluses IV; do not administer mannitol unless SBP >100 mm Hg and patient is adequately fluid resuscitated
- Phenytoin IV to prevent *early* posttraumatic seizures
- The use of glucocorticoids is *not* recommended to lower ICP in head trauma patients
- Barbiturates are *not* recommended in the initial ED treatment of penetrating head-injured patients
- Transfuse as needed to keep hematocrit above 30%
- If definitive neurosurgical care is not immediately available, a single burr hole may preserve life until neurosurgical intervention can be attained; this should only be done in comatose patients with decerebrate or decorticate posturing on the side of a known mass lesion/hematoma who have not responded to hyperventilation and mannitol
- Avoid hypothermia, as this will increase risks of coagulopathy during surgery

MEDICATIONS

- Etomidate: 0.2–0.3 mg/kg i.v.
- Fentanyl: 3–5 μg/kg i.v. if SBP >100 mm Hg
- Mannitol: 0.25–1 g/kg i.v. boluses
- Morphine sulfate: adult: 2–20 mg i.v.; peds: 0.1 mg/kg up to adult doses
- Phenytoin: 15–20 mg/kg i.v. up to 1,000 mg
- Rocuronium: 0.6 mg/kg i.v.
- Succinylcholine: 1–2 mg/kg i.v.
- Vecuronium bromide: 0.1 mg/kg i.v., pretreatment mini-dose: 0.01 mg/kg i.v.

Disposition

ADMISSION CRITERIA

- All patients with penetrating head trauma must be admitted to the ICU, if not directly to the operating room

DISCHARGE CRITERIA

- Patients with penetrating head injury should not be discharged

Miscellaneous

ICD9: 959.01

ICD10: S01.9

SUGGESTED READINGS

Brain Trauma Foundation. Management and prognosis of severe traumatic brain injury. New York: Brain Trauma Foundation, 2000.

Brain Trauma Foundation. Guidelines for prehospital management of traumatic brain injury. New York: Brain Trauma Foundation, 1999.

Chestnut RM, Marshall LF, Klauber MR, et al. The role of secondary brain injury in determining outcome from severe head injury. J Trauma 1993;34:216–222.

Cold GE. Cerebral blood flow in acute head injury. Acta Neurochir 1990;[suppl 49]: 3–64.

Committee on Trauma. Head trauma. In: Advanced trauma life support. Chicago: American College of Surgeons, 1997.

Author: Gary M. Vilke

Headache

Clinical Presentation

SIGNS AND SYMPTOMS

- Migraine
  - —Fully reversible aura (usually visual)
  - —Recurring, variable frequency
  - —Gradual onset
  - —Pulsating
  - —Moderate to severe intensity
  - —4–72-hour duration
  - —Nausea and vomiting
  - —Photophobia
  - —Phonophobia
- Tension
  - —Most common recurrent pain syndrome
  - —Recurring
  - —Bilateral
  - —Nonpulsatile
  - —Bandlike
  - —Mild to moderate intensity
  - —4–13-hour duration
- Cluster
  - —Recurring clusters (many over 24 hours)
  - —Unilateral
  - —Penetrating (pt holding or rubbing eye)
  - —Severe intensity
  - —Sudden onset
  - —45–60-minute duration
  - —Lacrimation
  - —Conjunctival injection
  - —Rhinorrhea
  - —Ptosis
  - —No aura
- Potentially life-threatening headaches
  - —New onset
  - —Severe headache or "worst headache of my life"
  - —Abnormal vital signs
    - -Diastolic BP >130 mm Hg
    - -Fever
  - —Altered level of consciousness
  - —Altered mental status
  - —Abnormal neurologic findings or meningismus

MECHANISM/DESCRIPTION

- Vascular
  - —Severe, throbbing headache
  - —Divided into migraine (the majority) and vascular nonmigrainous
  - —Triggered by stress, hormone fluctuations, lack of sleep, certain foods
- Tension (muscle contraction headache)
  - —Most common type of chronic recurring headache
  - —Secondary to sustained contraction of head and neck muscles
  - —Triggered by poor posture, stress, anxiety, depression, cervical osteoarthritis
- Cluster headaches
  - —Triggered by alcohol, certain foods, altered sleep habits, strong emotions
- Intracranial (traction)
  - —Mass lesions inside the calvarium stretching arteries and other pain sensitive structures
- Extracranial (nontension)
  - —Pathology from an extracranial site causing pain in a peripheral nerve of the head and neck

ETIOLOGY

- Vascular
  - —Intra/extracranial vasodilatation and constriction of pain-sensitive blood vessels
- Tension
  - —Unknown (possibly serotonin imbalance, decreased endorphins)
- Other headaches
  - —Multiple etiologies depending on cause (see differential diagnosis)
  - —Generally through traction, tension, or inflammation of the pain-sensitive structures; the vasculature, meninges, and cranial nerves V, IX, and X

PEDIATRIC CONSIDERATIONS

- Migraine
  - —Most common headache in children
  - —70–90% have positive family history
  - —May manifest only as cyclic vomiting or vertigo

Pre-Hospital

N/A

Diagnosis

ESSENTIAL WORKUP

- Detailed history and CNS examination
- Workup is strongly dependent on the clinical differential diagnosis

LABORATORY

- ESR
  - —If temporal arteritis or other inflammatory disorders suspected
- Tests appropriate for patient's underlying medical condition (e.g., ABG, glucose)
- Tests appropriate for physical examination abnormalities

IMAGING/SPECIAL TESTS

- Head CT scan
  - —Indications
    - -Unclear diagnosis based on history and physical examination
    - -Signs of increased ICP
    - -Worst or first headache
    - -Acute onset
    - -Focal neurologic abnormalities
    - -Papilledema
    - -Recurrent morning headache
    - -Persistent vomiting
    - -Headache associated with fever, rash, and nausea without systemic illness
    - -Head trauma with loss of consciousness (LOC), focal neurologic findings, or lethargy
    - -Altered mental status, meningismus
  - —90% sensitive for subarachnoid hemorrhage (SAH) <24 hours old
    - -Must do lumbar puncture (LP) if SAH suspected and CT is negative
- Lumbar puncture
  - —Intracranial infections
  - —Detect blood not evident on CT scan
- Sinus imaging
  - —Suspect sinusitis
- Vascular assessment with angiogram or MR angiography
  - —May be indicated if nonmigrainous vascular cause suspected
- MRI
  - —Suspected posterior fossa lesion (not imaged well on CT)

DIFFERENTIAL DIAGNOSIS

- Vascular
  - —Migraine: classic (with aura), common (without aura), cluster, ophthalmoplegic, hemiplegic, migraine equivalents
  - —Hypertensive headache: throbbing, occipital, SBP >130 mm Hg
  - —Anoxic: carbon monoxide toxicity, sleep apnea, anemia
- Tension
  - —Muscular contraction
  - —Conversion reaction
  - —Chronic anxiety states
- Intracranial (traction)
  - —Subarachnoid hemorrhage: "first or worst," sudden onset, vomiting, meningismus
  - —Aneurysm/AVM: sudden onset, unilateral, severe, decreased vision
  - —Meningitis/encephalitis: fever, nonfocal, meningismus
  - —Acute subdural hematoma: mental status, depression, or focal findings
  - —Chronic subdural hematoma: hemiparesis, focal seizures
  - —Epidural hematoma: trauma, brief LOC, rapid progression of neurologic symptoms
  - —Brain tumor: pain on awakening, progressively worsens, worse with Valsalva, ataxia
  - —Brain abscess: fever, nausea/vomiting, seizures
  - —Pseudotumor cerebri: young obese female, irregular menses, papilledema
- Extracranial
  - —Trigeminal neuralgia: transient, shocklike facial pain
  - —Temporal arteritis: elderly, severe, scalp artery tenderness/swelling
  - —Sinusitis: stabbing/aching, worse with bending or coughing
  - —Metabolic: fever, hypoglycemia, high altitude, acute anemia
  - —Acute glaucoma: nausea/vomiting, eye pain, conjunctival injection, increased IOP
  - —Cervical: spondylosis, trauma, arthritis
  - —Temporomandibular joint syndrome

Treatment

INITIAL STABILIZATION

- ABCs
- IV fluids, oxygen, and monitoring if necessary

ED TREATMENT

- Migraine
  - —Abortive therapy
    - -NSAID
    - -Ergotamine
    - -Phenothiazine
    - -5-Hydroxytryptamine (5-HT) receptor agonists (triptan class)
  - —Analgesia/comfort
    - -Narcotics (most common but suboptimal)
    - -Dark quiet room
    - -Prophylactic measures (beta-blockers, calcium blockers)
    - -Not recommended for ED use
- Tension
  - —Aspirin
  - —Acetaminophen
  - —NSAID
  - —Nonpharmacologic (meditation, massage, biofeedback)
- Cluster
  - —Oxygen
  - —Sumatriptan, DHE
  - —Prednisone
- Temporal arteritis
  - —Steroids
- Intracranial infection: see Meningitis
- Intracranial hemorrhage: see Subarachnoid Hemorrhage

MEDICATIONS

- Chlorpromazine: 25–50 mg i.m./i.v. (peds: 0.5–1 mg/kg/dose i.m./i.v./PO) q4–6h
- Dihydroergotamine: 1 mg i.m./i.v., repeat q1h; max dose 3 mg
- Ergotamine: 2 mg PO/SL at onset, then 1 mg PO q 30 min; max dose 10 mg/wk
- Ketorolac: 30–60 mg i.m.; 15–30 mg i.v. once, then 15–30 mg q6h (peds 1 mg/kg i.v. q6h)
- Lidocaine 4%: 1 mL intranasal on same side as symptoms
- Metoclopramide: 5–10 mg PO/i.v./i.m. q6–8h
- Morphine: 2.5–20 mg (peds: 0.1–0.2 mg/kg/dose) i.m./i.v./s.c. q2–6h
- Prochlorperazine: 5–10 mg i.v./PO/i.m. t.i.d.–q.i.d.; max 40 mg/day
- Sumatriptan: 6 mg s.c., repeat in 1 hour, up to 12 mg/24 hours

Disposition

ADMISSION CRITERIA

- Headache secondary to suspected organic disease
- Chronic daily headache, pain refractory to outpatient management
- Persistent migraine with intractable vomiting and dehydration
- Headache complicated by significant surgical or medical history
- Intracranial infection
- Intracranial hemorrhage
- Consider ICU admission
  - —Suspected aneurysm
  - —Acute subdural hematoma
  - —Subarachnoid hemorrhage
  - —Stroke
  - —Increased ICP
  - —Severe headache following trauma
  - —Intracranial infection

DISCHARGE CRITERIA

- Most migraine, cluster, and tension headaches after pain relief
- Local or minor systemic infections

Miscellaneous

ICD9: 784.0

ICD10: R51

SUGGESTED READINGS

American College of Emergency Physicians. Clinical policy: critical issues in the evaluation and management of patients presenting to the emergency department with acute headache. Ann Emerg Med 2002;39:108–122.

American College of Emergency Physicians. Clinical policy for the initial approach to adolescents and adults presenting to the emergency department with a chief complaint of headache. Ann Emerg Med 1996;27:821–844.

Henry GL. Headache. In: Marx, ed. Rosen's emergency medicine: concepts and clinical practice, 5th ed. St. Louis: CV Mosby, 2002:149–155.

Kwiatkowski T, Alagappan K. Headache. In: Marx, ed. Rosen's emergency medicine: concepts and clinical practice, 5th ed. St. Louis: CV Mosby, 2002:1456–1467.

Perkins AT, Ondo W. When to worry about headache: head pain as a clue to intracranial disease. Postgrad Med 1995;98(2):197–208.

Author: Abhishek Mehrotra

Headache, Cluster

Clinical Presentation

SIGNS AND SYMPTOMS

- Unilateral, excruciating, nonthrobbing, incapacitating headache
- Pain is ocular or retrobulbar
- Rarely lasts longer than 2 hours; often lasts a few minutes
- Associated with nasal congestion, lacrimation, rhinorrhea, conjunctival injection, or facial flushing on the same side
- Horner's syndrome may be seen
- Headaches occur in clusters; several times per day for weeks or months at a time
- Occurs predominantly in middle-aged men
- Attacks are more likely after ingestion of alcohol, nitroglycerine, or histamine-containing compounds
- Episodes are often nocturnal, and are more common in spring and fall
- More likely in times of stress, prolonged strain, overwork, and upsetting emotional experiences
- No prodrome or aura

MECHANISM/DESCRIPTION

- Not clearly understood, but may be the result of vasoactive substances released from mast cells

ETIOLOGY

- Etiology is unclear at present
- Affects 0.1% of the population

Pre-Hospital

CAUTIONS

- Recognize more severe life-threatening causes of headache
- Administration of oxygen by face mask may alleviate symptoms

Diagnosis

ESSENTIAL WORKUP

- An accurate history and physical examination should confirm the diagnosis

LABORATORY

- Lumbar puncture (if meningitis or subarachnoid hemorrhage is suspected)
- ESR (if temporal arteritis is suspected)

IMAGING/SPECIAL TESTS

- CT scan/MRI (to rule out hemorrhage, tumor)

DIFFERENTIAL DIAGNOSIS

- Migraine headache
- Trigeminal neuralgia
- Meningitis
- Temporal arteritis
- Intracerebral mass lesion
- Herpes zoster
- Intracerebral bleed
- Dental causes
- Orbital/ocular disease (acute glaucoma)
- Temporal mandibular joint syndrome

Treatment

INITIAL STABILIZATION

- ABCs
- Rule out life-threatening causes of headache
- Administration of supplemental oxygen

ED TREATMENT

- Pain management

MEDICATIONS

- Ergots: DHE 1 cc i.m. or i.v.; repeat in 1 hour if necessary
- Fentanyl: 2–3 mcg/kg i.v.
- NSAIDs: ketorolac 15–30 mg i.m. or i.v.
- Meperidine: 50–75 mg i.m. or i.v.
- Morphine: 2–4 mg i.v. or i.m., may repeat q 10 min
- Oxygen: 100% via face mask
- Prochlorperazine: 10 mg i.m. or i.v.
- Sumatriptan: 6 mg s.c., may repeat in 1 hour (max of 2 doses in 24 hours)

Disposition

ADMISSION CRITERIA

- Persistent headache unresponsive to usual measures
- Unclear headache diagnosis

DISCHARGE CRITERIA

- Patients with moderate to complete pain relief, a normal neurologic exam and with a confident diagnosis of cluster headache
- Follow-up with a neurologist should be arranged

Miscellaneous

ICD9: 346.20

ICD10: G44.0

SUGGESTED READINGS

Diamond S. The management of migraine and cluster headaches. Compr Ther 1995; 21(9):492–498.

Kumar KL. Recent advances in the acute management of migraine and cluster headaches. J Gen Intern Med 1994;9(6):339–348.

Author: Gary Johnson

Headache, Migraine

Clinical Presentation

SIGNS AND SYMPTOMS

- *Common migraine*
  - —Headache that is recurrent, throbbing, and frequently unilateral
  - —Usually associated with photophobia, phonophobia, nausea, anorexia, and vomiting
- *Classic migraine:* very similar to common migraine except it is preceded by a prodrome; usually visual symptoms such as bright lights or jagged lines
- *Complex migraine:* migraine headache with associated focal neurologic symptoms such as numbness, weakness, paralysis, or aphasia

MECHANISM/DESCRIPTION

- Migraine may begin with intracranial artery vasoconstriction, which results in reduced cerebral blood flow; this produces the *aura,* the type of which is dependent on the area of reduced flow
  - —This is followed by a rebound vasodilation of the arteries during which the headache occurs
  - —The arterial dilation and plasma leak may give rise to pain

ETIOLOGY

- Idiopathic
- May be precipitated by chocolate, cheese, nuts, alcohol, sulfites, MSG, stress, tension, or puberty
- There is a family history of migraines in 60%
- Affects 5–15% of the population (women three times more than men)

PEDIATRIC CONSIDERATIONS

- Migraines do present in the pediatric age group, but are less common
- The typical pediatric patient is a prepubertal girl with a strong family history of migraine

Pre-Hospital

CAUTIONS

- It is important to recognize life-threatening causes of headache and transport rapidly
  - —Sudden onset of symptoms, altered mental status, neck stiffness, fever, or neurologic deficit is a useful sign that suggests a more serious cause of headache
  - —Prior history of similar headache, absence of above symptoms, or strong family history is more suggestive of migraine
- Allow patients with migraine headache to be in a calm, dark environment

Diagnosis

ESSENTIAL WORKUP

- An accurate history and physical exam should confirm the diagnosis
- Patients with new onset of headache syndrome need an objective evaluation to rule out more serious causes of severe headaches
  - —Complete neurologic examination
  - —CT or MRI of the head
  - —Lumbar puncture (LP)
  - —If the patient can be provided close follow-up, imaging studies and LP can be done as an outpatient if the clinical presentation does not suggest a life-threatening cause of headache

LABORATORY

- Not needed for classic migraine or established migraines with typical symptoms
- LP if meningitis, intracranial hemorrhage, or pseudotumor cerebri is suspected
- ESR if temporal arteritis is suspected
- Carbon monoxide (CO) level if there is history or suspicion of CO exposure

IMAGING/SPECIAL TESTS

- CT scan or MRI to rule out intracranial hemorrhage or tumor

DIFFERENTIAL DIAGNOSIS

- Meningitis/encephalitis
- Subarachnoid/intracranial hemorrhage
- Cerebral ischemia (if complex migraine)
- Hypertension
- Brain tumor
- Carbon monoxide intoxication
- Temporal mandibular joint (TMJ) syndrome
- Glaucoma
- Pseudotumor cerebri
- Temporal arteritis

Treatment

INITIAL STABILIZATION

- ABCs
- Patients with evidence of increased intracranial pressure may need rapid sequence intubation and controlled ventilation

ED TREATMENT

- Abortive therapy and pain management are the primary issues for patients in which life-threatening causes of headache have been ruled out
- Generally, abortive therapy options such as sumatriptan should be attempted first
- Narcotic pain medications may be administered as rescue therapy
- Intravenous saline hydration is often a helpful adjunct for migraine headaches

MEDICATIONS

- Abortive therapy in ED
  —Droperidol: 0.625–2.5 mg i.m. or i.v.
  —Ergot alkaloids: DHE 1 mg i.m. or i.v., then repeat in 1 hour if necessary
  —Metoclopramide: 10 mg i.v.
  —NSAIDs: ketorolac 15–30 mg i.m./i.v.
  —Prochlorperazine: 10 mg i.v.
  —Sumatriptan: 6 mg s.c., may repeat in 1 hour (max of 2 doses per 24 hours)
- Rescue pain medication
  —Meperidine: 25–100 mg i.m./i.v. per dose
  —Morphine: 2–10 mg i.m./i.v. per dose
- Prophylactic therapy
  —Beta-blockers: propranolol 40 mg PO b.i.d.
  —Ca^{2+} channel blockers: verapamil 40 mg PO t.i.d.
  —Cyclic antidepressants: amitriptyline 25 mg PO t.i.d.

Disposition

ADMISSION CRITERIA

- Severe intractable headache pain
- Intractable vomiting, electrolyte imbalance, or inability to take oral food or fluid
- Suicidal ideation secondary to unremitting headache

DISCHARGE CRITERIA

- Patients with moderate to complete pain relief, a normal neurologic exam, and a confident diagnosis of migraine

Miscellaneous

ICD9: 346.90

ICD10: G43.9

SUGGESTED READINGS

Goadsby PJ, Olesen J. Diagnosis and management of migraine. Br Med J 1996;312(7041):1279–1283.

Lipton R, Stewart W, Stone A, et al. Stratified care vs step care strategies for migraine: The Disability in Strategies of Care (DISC) Study: a randomized trial. JAMA 2000;284(20):2599–2605.

Noack H, Rothrock JF. Migraine: Definitions, mechanisms, and treatment. South Med J 1996;89(8):762–769.

Author: Gary Johnson

Heart Murmur

Clinical Presentation

SIGNS AND SYMPTOMS

- Aortic stenosis
  - —Systolic crescendo decrescendo murmur radiating to carotids
  - —Carotid pulse is described as parvus and tardus (diminished intensity and late upstroke)
  - —Angina
  - —Dyspnea on exertion
  - —Exertional syncope
- Aortic regurgitation
  - —Diastolic blowing murmur at left sternal border
  - —Austin Flint murmur is a diastolic rumble from exposure of the mitral valve to the aortic regurgitant flow
  - —Pulmonary edema
  - —Dyspnea
  - —Tachycardia
  - —Chest pain
  - —Pulse pressure may be widened
  - —Corrigan's pulse or water hammer pulse, a rapid upstroke and downstroke of the carotid pulse
  - —Quincke's pulse, pulsations seen at the nailbeds
  - —Musset's sign, bobbing with carotid pulse
- Idiopathic hypertrophic subaortic stenosis
  - —Systolic, harsh, crescendo decrescendo murmur heard at left sternal border
  - —Increases in volume of the left ventricle at end diastole will decrease the intensity of the murmur
  - —Dyspnea
  - —Chest pain
  - —Exertional syncope
  - —Sudden death
- Mitral stenosis
  - —Diastolic, rumbling murmur heard at the apex
  - —Loud S_1 with an opening snap
  - —Dyspnea
  - —Orthopnea
  - —Hemoptysis
  - —Pulmonary edema
  - —Emboli to systemic circulation
  - —Atrial fibrillation
- Mitral regurgitation, acute
  - —Systolic, harsh, crescendo decrescendo murmur heard at the base
  - —Pulmonary edema
- Mitral regurgitation, chronic
  - —Holosystolic murmur heard at the apex radiating to the axilla
  - —Dyspnea on exertion
  - —Fatigue
  - —Atrial fibrillation is common
- Mitral valve prolapse
  - —Early to midsystolic click often followed by systolic murmur
  - —Palpitations
  - —Chest pain
- Tricuspid stenosis
  - —Diastolic, high-pitched murmur
  - —Peripheral edema
  - —Hepatosplenomegaly
  - —Ascites
  - —Fatigue
  - —Atrial fibrillation is common
  - —Large a wave in the jugular venous pulse
- Tricuspid regurgitation
  - —Holosystolic, blowing murmur best heard along the left sternal margin
  - —Peripheral edema
  - —Hepatosplenomegaly
  - —Ascites
  - —Atrial fibrillation is common
  - —Large v wave in the jugular venous pulse
- Patent ductus arteriosus
  - —Continuous machinery murmur
  - —Congestive heart failure
- Pericardial friction rub
  - —Intermittent murmur
  - —May have systolic and/or diastolic component
  - —Symptoms due to pericarditis or pericardial effusion

MECHANISM/DESCRIPTION

- Stenotic lesions lead to pressure overload in the chamber preceding the valve
- Pressure overload leads to hypertrophy of the chamber in an attempt to overcome the increased resistance
- Regurgitant lesions lead to volume overload of the chamber preceding the valve
- Volume overload leads to chamber dilatation in an attempt to accommodate the regurgitant blood volume

ETIOLOGY

- Aortic stenosis
  - —Rheumatic heart disease
  - —Congenital bicuspid valve
  - —Calcification of valve from aging
  - —Prosthetic valve
- Aortic regurgitation
  - —Rheumatic heart disease
  - —Endocarditis
  - —Aortic dissection
  - —Prosthetic valve
- Idiopathic hypertrophic subaortic stenosis
  - —Congenital
- Mitral stenosis
  - —Rheumatic heart disease
  - —Rheumatologic disorders (SLE)
  - —Calcification
  - —Cardiac tumors (atrial myxoma)
  - —Congenital
  - —Prosthetic valve
- Mitral regurgitation, acute
  - —Endocarditis
  - —Papillary muscle dysfunction
  - —Rupture of papillary muscle
  - —Rupture of chordae tendineae
  - —Prosthetic valve
- Mitral regurgitation, chronic
  - —Rheumatic heart disease
  - —Mitral valve prolapse
  - —Connective tissue disease (Marfan's)
- Mitral valve prolapse
  - —Congenital
  - —Connective tissue disease
- Tricuspid stenosis
  - —Rheumatic heart disease
- Tricuspid regurgitation
  - —Rheumatic heart disease
  - —Endocarditis
  - —Pulmonary hypertension
- Patent ductus arteriosus
  - —Congenital
- Pericardial friction rub
  - —Pericarditis
  - —Pericardial effusion

Pre-Hospital

- Patients with critical aortic stenosis are very sensitive to fluid shifts; care should be exercised when giving fluids or preload reducers
- Intravenous access, oxygen as appropriate

Diagnosis

ESSENTIAL WORKUP

- See Valvular Heart Disease, Mitral Valve Prolapse, Congenital Heart Disease, Patent Ductus Arteriosus, Pericarditis, and Pericardial Effusion/Tamponade for more details
- EKG
- Chest x-ray
- Echocardiogram may be useful in evaluation of valves, chambers, and flow
- CT when aortic dissection is considered
- Consider cardiac catheterization in acute regurgitant lesions

DIFFERENTIAL DIAGNOSIS

- See etiology

Treatment

INITIAL STABILIZATION

- Oxygen
- IV access
- Cardiac monitor
- Treat symptoms (CHF, dysrhythmias)
- Exercise care with fluids and medications in aortic stenosis

ED TREATMENT

- See Valvular Heart Disease, Mitral Valve Prolapse, Congenital Heart Disease, Patent Ductus Arteriosus, Pericarditis, and Pericardial Effusion/Tamponade for more details
- Acute mitral and aortic regurgitation may necessitate emergency surgery
- Intraaortic balloon pump may be a useful temporizing measure
- Antibiotics for endocarditis
- Treat pulmonary edema and dysrhythmias as appropriate
- Avoid diuretics and ionotropes in IHSS
- Critical aortic stenosis necessitates surgery to improve mortality
- Anticoagulation as necessary for atrial fibrillation

MEDICATIONS

- Digoxin: 0.5 mg i.v., then 0.25 mg i.v. × 2 q6h
- Diltiazem (Cardizem): 0.25 mg/kg (17.5 mg for 70-kg person) i.v. over 2 minutes, may rebolus after 15 minutes with 0.35 mg/kg; start drip at 5 to 15 mg/h
- Furosemide (Lasix): 20–80 mg i.v. may increase dose if necessary, max dose of 600 mg in 24 hours
- Heparin: 80 units/kg bolus, then drip at 18 units/kg/h monitor PTT
- Metoprolol (Lopressor): 5 mg i.v. q 5–15 min ×3 as tolerated
- Nitroglycerin: 10–20 μg/min i.v. titrate to effect, max of 300 μg/min
- Nitroprusside: 0.3 μg/kg/min titrate to effect, max 10 μg/kg/min; protect bag from light, thiocyanate toxicity from prolonged use
- Propranolol (Inderal): 1 mg i.v. every 2 minutes

Disposition

ADMISSION CRITERIA

- Signs of cardiac ischemia
- Syncope or near syncope
- Pulmonary edema
- Hemodynamic instability
- Endocarditis
- Arrhythmia

DISCHARGE CRITERIA

- Asymptomatic
- Hemodynamically stable

Miscellaneous

ICD9: 785.2

ICD10: R01.1

SEE ALSO: VALVULAR HEART DISEASE

SUGGESTED READINGS

Carabello BA, Crawford FA. Valvular heart disease. N Engl J Med 1997;337:32–41

Dunmire SM. Infective endocarditis and acquired valvular heart disease. In: Rosen P, et al., eds. Emergency medicine: concepts and clinical practice, 4th ed. St Louis: CV Mosby, 1998:1745–1754.

Author: Leon D. Sanchez

HELLP Syndrome

(*H*emolysis, *E*levated *L*iver *E*nzymes, and *L*ow *P*latelets)

Clinical Presentation

SIGNS AND SYMPTOMS

- Frequently white, multiparous, older pregnant women
  - —Usually develops in second trimester
- Symptoms: nausea, vomiting, moderate to severe epigastric or right upper quadrant pain, headache, and perhaps visual changes
  - —Epigastric pain and nausea increase as the severity of HELLP worsens
- May present with flu-like symptoms such as fatigue or malaise
- Continuum with severe preeclampsia; most patients will be hypertensive
  - —Patients with HELLP may not have systolic or diastolic hypertension
- Symptoms of significant morbidity include cardiogenic/noncardiogenic pulmonary edema, cardiac or pulmonary arrest, pulmonary embolus, chest pain with myocardial ischemia, hypertensive encephalopathy, cerebral edema with change in mental status, seizures, blindness, peripheral edema, ascites, hematuria, and renal failure

MECHANISM/DESCRIPTION

- Signs/symptoms of hemolysis, abnormal LFTs, and thrombocytopenia were recognized 100 years ago; the term *HELLP syndrome* coined by Weinstein in 1982
- HELLP considered a complication of preeclampsia/eclampsia
  - —20% of women with preeclampsia/eclampsia will develop HELLP
  - —Estimated HELLP occurs in 0.3% of all pregnancies
- Liver involvement is hallmark of the disease; other organs may also be involved such as the brain and kidneys
- HELLP syndrome recently divided into three groups, representing severity of the disease; *severity is directly related to the platelet count*
  - —Class 1: most severe form; platelet nadir less than 50,000 cells/μL
  - —Class 2: less severe; platelet nadir between 50,000 and 100,000 cells/μL
  - —Class 3: least severe; platelet nadir between 100,000 and 150,000 cells/μL
- Most maternal deaths occur with class 1
- Increased mortality rate is associated with hemorrhage in the hepatic or central nervous systems, or vascular insult to the cardiopulmonary or renal systems
- Perinatal mortality is greater in infants of women with HELLP

ETIOLOGY

- Etiology remains unclear
- Vasospasm is the basis of the problem
  - —Vascular constriction causes resistance to blood flow and hypertension
  - —Vasospasm probably damages vessels directly
  - —Angiotensin II causes endothelial cells to contract
  - —Endothelial cell damage and interendothelial cell leaks are the result
- Leaks develop in small vessels
  - —Platelets and fibrinogen get deposited subendothelially
  - —Fibrin deposition develops in severe cases
- Vascular changes and local tissue hypoxia lead to hemorrhage, necrosis, and end-organ damage

Pre-Hospital

CAUTIONS

- Transport patient in left lateral decubitus position to prevent IVC syndrome
- Venous access advisable for anticipated seizure activity
- Routine seizure management (preferably with $MgSO_4$, if available pre-hospital) if the patient seizes
- *Transport to a facility capable of providing high-risk obstetric care*

Diagnosis

ESSENTIAL WORKUP

- History and physical exam with attention to symptoms of abdominal pain, nausea, vomiting, and headache
- Vital signs with attention to blood pressure (anything greater than 140/90 is abnormal)
- Stat blood for CBC with platelet count and smear, BUN, creatinine, LFTs, coagulation profile, and magnesium level
- Urinalysis for protein; screen for UTI
- Weigh patient to determine recent weight gain

LABORATORY

- CBC will reveal anemia and thrombocytopenia
  - —Peripheral smear demonstrates microangiopathic hemolytic anemia (burr cells or schistocytes)
  - —Other hemolysis markers are elevated LDH levels, increased reticulocyte count, and elevated bilirubin and urobilinogen levels
  - —Platelet counts less than 100,000 cells/μL
- Hepatic dysfunction will show an increased aspartate aminotransferase (AST) level >40 IU/L, increased alanine aminotransferase (ALT) level >40 IU/L, or both, with increased lactate dehydrogenase (LDH) >600 IU/L
- PT/PTT to evaluate coagulation
- DIC screen if patient is bleeding or DIC suspected
- BUN/Cr to evaluate renal function

IMAGING/SPECIAL TESTS

- CXR if suspect pulmonary edema
- CT of head if any mental status changes (cerebral edema)
- Ultrasound of the pelvis (transabdominal or transvaginal) to image fetus and placenta
  - —*Determination of gestational age and fetal viability is critical in HELLP*

DIFFERENTIAL DIAGNOSIS

- Gastrointestinal: cholecystitis, cholelithiasis, biliary colic, pancreatitis, hepatitis, ulcer disease, acute fatty liver of pregnancy, acute gastritis, hiatal hernia, severe gastroesophageal reflux
- Hematologic: preeclampsia-associated thrombocytopenia, gestational thrombocytopenia, ITP, TTP, HUS
- Neurologic: epilepsy, encephalitis, meningitis, encephalopathy, brain tumor, intracranial hemorrhage
- Other: Drug abuse, pyelonephritis, sepsis

Treatment

INITIAL STABILIZATION

- ABCs
- Left lateral decubitus position to prevent IVC syndrome
- 100% O_2 via face mask
- Maternal cardiac, pulse oximetry, and tocographic monitoring
- Fetal monitoring

ED TREATMENT

- Control hypertension with antihypertensives (see Medications, below)
- Avoid ACE inhibitors because of fetal side effects
- Treat preeclampsia or eclampsia if present with IV $MgSO_4$
  - —$MgSO_4$ is not given to treat hypertension
- Order type and screen for possible transfusion
- Call for emergent OB consult, consider neonatology consult
- Discuss administration of glucocorticoid with consultant
  - —Helps fetal lung maturity
  - —IV dexamethasone more effective than IM betamethasone
  - —Depends on gestational age of fetus
- Limit IV fluid administration unless clinical evidence of dehydration
  - —Excess fluids promote further capillary leak
  - —Ringer's lactate at 60 mL/h (no more than 125 mL/h)
  - —Monitor urine output with Foley catheter
- Discuss emergent delivery with OB consultant

Blood Products

- Correct thrombocytopenia by platelet transfusion in women with platelet counts of less than 20,000 cells/μL, even without active bleeding, as risk of postpartum bleeding is significantly increased
  - —Platelet counts above 40,000/μL are generally considered safe for vaginal delivery
- Correct thrombocytopenia to platelet counts >50,000/μL if delivery by cesarean section is planned
- If coagulation dysfunction is present, transfusion with FFP and PRBC in consultation with OB
- Transfusion with PRBC is recommended for hemoglobin less than 10 g/dL

MEDICATIONS

- Hydralazine: 2.5 mg i.v., then 5–10 mg every 15–20 min, up to 40 mg total dose, to keep diastolic BP <110; i.v. drip 5–10 mg/h titrated
- Labetalol: 10 mg i.v., then 40–80 mg i.v. every 10 min, up to 300 mg total dose; i.v. drip 1–2 mg/min titrated
- Nifedipine: 10 mg PO, repeated every 30 min PO
- Nitroprusside: 0.25 μg/kg/min as a drip, increase 0.25 μg/kg/min every 5 min; use only if no response to hydralazine, labetalol, or nifedipine
- Avoid ACE inhibitors
- Magnesium sulfate: 4–6 g in 100 mL i.v. over 15–20 min loading dose, then maintenance drip starting at 2 g/h and titrate to clinical effect
  - —Watch for toxicity (antidote is calcium gluconate 10%, 10 mL i.v. over 3 min)
  - —Measure $MgSO_4$ level at 4–6 hours, adjust drip to achieve levels between 4 and 7 mEq/L

Disposition

ADMISSION CRITERIA

- All women with HELLP should be admitted to the OB service for close continuous monitoring of both mother and fetus
- After stabilization in the ED, transfer to facility capable of managing high-risk obstetric conditions is warranted, unless delivery is imminent
- Patients with pulmonary edema/respiratory failure, cerebral edema, or GI bleeding with hemodynamic instability should be admitted to an ICU setting

Miscellaneous

ICD9: 642.50

ICD10: 014.0

SUGGESTED READINGS

Audibert F, Friedman SA, Frangieh AY, et al. Clinical utility of strict diagnostic criteria for the HELLP (hemolysis, elevated liver enzymes, and low platelets) syndrome. Am J Obstet Gynecol 1996;175(2):460–464.

Isler CM. A prospective, randomized trial comparing the efficacy of dexamethasone and betamethasone for the treatment of antepartum HELLP (hemolysis, elevated liver enzymes, and low platelet count) syndrome. Am J Obstet Gynecol 2001;184(7):1332–1137.

Houry D, Abbott J. Acute complications of pregnancy. In: Rosen P, et al., eds. Emergency medicine: concepts and clinical practice, 5th ed. St. Louis: CV Mosby, 2002:2413–2433.

Martin JN, Rinehart BK, May WL, et al. The spectrum of severe preeclampsia: comparative analysis by HELLP (hemolysis, elevated liver enzymes, and low platelet count) syndrome classification. Am J Obstet Gynecol 1999;180(6 pt 1): 1373–1384.

Hypertensive disorders in pregnancy. In: Cunningham FG, et al., eds. Williams' obstetrics, 21st ed. New York: McGraw-Hill, 2001:567–618.

Author: Michael J. Bono

Hematuria and Proteinuria

Clinical Presentation

SIGNS AND SYMPTOMS

- Dysuria
- Blood in urine
- Fever
- Flank pain
- Flank ecchymosis
- Initial hematuria (anterior urethral lesion)
- Terminal hematuria (posterior urethra, bladder, neck, trigone)
- Cyclic hematuria (endometriosis or urinary tract)
- Previous upper respiratory tract infection (10–21 days prior)
- Previous skin infection (10–21 days prior)
- Deafness (Alport's syndrome)
- Peripheral edema
- Hemoptysis (Goodpasture's disease)
- Concurrent menstruation
- Testicular, epididymal, and prostatic tenderness or trauma
- Terminal urethral lesion
- Enlarged prostate
- Penile/scrotal hematoma
- Atrial fibrillation (renal artery embolus or thrombus)
- Organomegaly, flank mass
- Risk factors for more significant disease in asymptomatic hematuria
  —Tobacco use
  —Occupational exposure to benzenes, aromatic amines, dyes
  —History of gross hematuria
  —Age greater than 40 years old
  —History of urologic disorder or disease
  —History of irritative voiding symptoms
  —History of urinary tract infections
  —Analgesic abuse
  —History of pelvic irradiation

MECHANISM/DESCRIPTION

- Microscopic hematuria: three or more red blood cells per high power field in two of three properly collected urine specimens
- Gross hematuria: visible blood to the naked eye in properly collected urine specimen
- Proteinuria: urinary protein excretion of greater than 150 mg/d

Pre-Hospital

- Airway, breathing, circulation (ABCs)
- Control other trauma, if present

Diagnosis

ESSENTIAL WORKUP

- Urine dipstick
- Urinalysis with microscopic analysis
- Blood urea nitrogen
- Serum creatinine
- Complete blood count

LABORATORY

- Urine culture
- Urine cytology
- Coagulation studies
- Serum and urine protein electrophoresis
- 24-hour urine protein, creatinine
- Spot ratio of urine protein to creatinine
- Spot ratio of urine protein to osmolality

IMAGING/SPECIAL TESTS

- Intravenous pyelogram
- Helical CT
- Renal ultrasound
- Cystourethroscopy
- Urethrogram
- Cystogram
- Retrograde pyelography

DIFFERENTIAL DIAGNOSIS

- Glomerular hematuria
  —IgA nephropathy (Berger's disease)
  —Postinfectious glomerulonephritis
  —Membranoproliferative glomerulonephritis
  —Focal glomerular sclerosis
  —Lupus nephritis
  —Wegener's granulomatosis
  —Polyarteritis nodosa
  —Henoch-Schönlein syndrome
  —Thrombotic thrombocytopenic purpura
  —Hemolytic uremic syndrome
  —Alport's syndrome
  —Goodpasture's disease
- Nonglomerular hematuria
  —Infection (pyelonephritis, tuberculosis, schistosomiasis)
  —Inflammation (drug induced, radiation induced)
  —Renal and extrarenal tumor
  —Interstitial nephritis
  —Papillary necrosis
  —Polycystic kidney disease
  —Medullary sponge disease
  —Renal artery embolism/thrombosis
  —Renal vein thrombosis
  —Sickle cell disease
  —Malignant hypertension
  —Hypercalcuria
  —Hyperuricosuria
  —Urolithiasis
  —Strictures
  —Endometriosis
  —Foreign bodies
  —Benign prostatic hypertrophy
  —Coagulopathy/bleeding disorders
  —Trauma (renal pedicle injuries, urethral disruptions, bladder rupture)
  —Recent instrumentation
  —Frequent or interrupted coitus
  —Factitious
- Glomerular proteinuria (>2.0 g/d)
  —Minimal change disease
  —Membranous glomerulonephritis
  —Focal segmental glomerulonephritis
  —Membranoproliferative glomerulonephritis
  —Diabetes mellitus
  —Collagen vascular diseases
  —Amyloidosis
  —Preeclampsia
  —Infection (HIV, hepatitis B, hepatitis C, poststreptococcal infection, syphilis)
  —Lymphoma
  —Chronic renal transplant rejection
  —Heroin
  —Penicillamine
- Tubular proteinuria
  —Hypertensive nephrosclerosis
  —Uric acid nephropathy
  —Acute hypersensitivity interstitial nephritis
  —Fanconi syndrome
  —Sickle cell disease
- Overflow proteinuria
  —Monoclonal gammopathy
  —Leukemia
- Proteinuria, other
  —Dehydration
  —Stress
  —Fever
  —Heat injury
  —Inflammatory process
  —Orthostatic proteinuria

Treatment

INITIAL STABILIZATION

- ABCs
- Treat hemodynamically unstable injuries first, if present
- Obtain initial labs (urinalysis with microscopic analysis, blood urea nitrogen, serum creatinine)

ED TREATMENT

- Uncomplicated urinary tract infections
  - —Only 3-day treatment required
  - —TMP/SMX is first-line therapy
  - —Ciprofloxacin or levofloxacin when the patient is allergic to sulfa or after failure of TMP/SMX
- Pyelonephritis
  - —Outpatient treatment with 7 days of ciprofloxacin or levofloxacin or 14 days of amoxicillin/clavulanate
  - —Analgesics for stone disease and pain
- Steroid therapy for rapidly progressing glomerulonephropathies (consultation with specialists needed)
- Hemodialysis for acute renal failure (consultation with specialists needed)
- Gross hematuria: placement of three-way Foley catheter with bladder irrigation to clear blood clots that may cause urinary retention from bladder obstruction

MEDICATIONS

- Uncomplicated urinary tract infection
  - —Ciprofloxacin 250 mg PO b.i.d. for 3 days
  - —Levofloxacin 250 mg PO qd for 3 days
  - —Nitrofurantoin 2 mg/kg PO qd
  - —TMP/SMX DS PO b.i.d. × 3 days (peds: 2 mg TMP/10 mg SMX/kg PO qd)
- Outpatient pyelonephritis
  - —Amoxicillin/clavulanate 500/125 mg PO t.i.d. for 14 days
  - —Ciprofloxacin 500 mg PO b.i.d. for 7 days
  - —Levofloxacin 250 mg PO qd for 7 days
  - —TMP/SMX DS PO b.i.d. for 14 days

Disposition

ADMISSION CRITERIA

- Intractable pain
- Intolerance of oral fluids and medications
- Hemodynamic instability
- Hematuria with traumatic injuries
- Obstructing ureteral stones with infection or renal failure
- Hypertensive emergency
- Acute renal failure: azotemia/uremia/hyperkalemia
- Oliguria/anuria
- Pregnant with preeclampsia, pyelonephritis, obstructing nephrolithiasis

DISCHARGE CRITERIA

- Hemodynamically stable without life-threatening issues

Miscellaneous

ICD9: 599.7, 791.0

ICD10: R31, R80

SUGGESTED READINGS

Ahmed Z, Lee J. Asymptomatic urinary abnormalities. Med Clin North Am 1997;81(3):641–652.

Grossfeld GD, Wolf JS, Litwin MS, et al. Asymptomatic microscopic hematuria in adults: summary of the AUA best practice policy recommendations. Am Fam Physician 2001;63(6):1145–1154.

Sokolosky MC. Hematuria. Emerg Med Clin North Am 2001;19(3):621–632.

Tintinalli JE, Kelen GD, Stapczynski JS, eds. Emergency medicine: a comprehensive study guide, 5th ed. New York: McGraw-Hill, 2000.

Author: David Wang

Hemophilia

Clinical Presentation

SIGNS AND SYMPTOMS

- Bleeding
  - —Hemarthrosis (most common)
    - -Knee (most common) > elbow > ankle > shoulder > wrist (least common)
  - —Muscle hemorrhage
  - —Postextraction or oral mucosal bleeding
  - —Epistaxis (only in severe disease)
  - —Hematuria
  - —Sustained from minor trauma
  - —Intracranial hemorrhage
  - —Gastrointestinal bleeding
  - —Pseudotumors (blood cysts)

MECHANISM/DESCRIPTION

- Caused by deficiency of factor VIII or factor IX
- Absence of factors causes partial inactivation of coagulation cascade and impaired hemostasis
- Two types
  - —Hemophilia A: factor VIII deficiency
  - —Hemophilia B (Christmas disease): factor IX deficiency
- Severity varies among different individuals reflecting available natural factor activity
  - —70% of type A hemophiliacs are severe
- Symptomatology dependent on factor availability
  - —5–30% factor activity (mild hemophilia)
    - -Bleeding almost exclusively with trauma
  - —1–5% factor activity
    - -Occasional spontaneous hemorrhages
  - —<1%
    - -Frequent spontaneous hemorrhages

ETIOLOGY

- Genetic transmission; sex-linked recessive occurring in males
- Rare disease
  - —Hemophilia A occurs in approximately 1 in 10,000 males
  - —Hemophilia B occurs in approximately 1 in 30,000 males

Pre-Hospital

CAUTIONS

- Control bleeding with direct pressure

Diagnosis

- Generally not made in ED
- Consider in undiagnosed patients if:
  - —Positive family history
  - —Recurrent prior episodes of bleeding

ESSENTIAL WORKUP

- Thorough physical examination
- Factor-specific assays (see below)

LABORATORY

- CBC
- Platelet count: normal
- PT/PTT
  - —PT: normal
  - —PTT: increased
- Bleeding time: normal
- Urinalysis
  - —Asymptomatic hematuria is a common finding

IMAGING/SPECIAL TESTS

- Specific factor assays
  - —Factor VIII:Ag (measures factor VIII quantity): decreased
  - —Factor VIII:c (measures factor VIII activity): decreased
  - —vWF (measures von Willebrand factor activity): normal
  - —vWF:Ag (measures von Willebrand factor quantity): normal
- Radiographic studies may be required in certain circumstances
  - —Head CT to evaluate or exclude intracranial bleed
  - —Renal US/IVP to evaluate excessive hematuria or renal trauma
  - —Abdominal CT to evaluate or exclude retroperitoneal bleeding

DIFFERENTIAL DIAGNOSIS

- Von Willebrand's disease
- Anticoagulant drugs
- Antiplatelet agents
- Thrombocytopenia
- Hepatic dysfunction

Treatment

INITIAL STABILIZATION

- ABCs
  - —Control bleeding
  - —Establish IV access

ED TREATMENT

General

- Goals of ED therapy
  - —Abort current bleeding episode by raising factor level
  - —Prevent additional morbidity
  - —Coordinate ED care with primary provider (hematologist)
- Approach to therapy
  - —Patients generally have excellent understanding of their disease
  - —Determine desired factor level based on risk of bleeding and location/system
  - —Factor VIII required (in units) = wt (kg) × 0.5 × (% factor activity desired)
    - -1 IU factor VIII/kg raises activity approximately 2%
  - —Factor IX required (in units) = wt (kg) × 1.0 × (% factor activity desired)
    - -1 IU factor IX/kg raises activity approximately 1%
  - —May need to increase dose if inhibitors (antibodies to factor) are present or use special factor replacement
    - -Patient/primary care provider usually has this information
  - —Avoid all IM injections
  - —Avoid aspirin and aspirin-containing products

Approach to Factor Replacement

- Low to moderate risk of bleeding
  - —Examples
    - -Soft tissue injury
    - -Joint or muscle bleeding
  - —Desired hemostatic factor level
    - -30–50%
  - —Empirical factor VIII therapy
    - -25–50 IU/kg
- Moderate to severe risk of bleeding
  - —Examples
    - -GI or GU bleeding
  - —Desired hemostatic factor level
    - -50–100%
  - —Empirical factor VIII therapy
    - -25–50 IU/kg
- Severe risk of bleeding
  - —Examples
    - -CNS injury
    - -Major trauma
  - —Desired hemostatic factor level
    - -100%
  - —Empirical factor VIII therapy
    - -50 IU/kg

Factor Replacement Options

- Cryoprecipitates
  - —Obtained from FFP after thawing at 4°C
  - —Contains multiple proteins but high in VIII, vWF, and fibrinogen
  - —Only use if purified factor not available
  - —Not useful in hemophilia B; does not contain factor IX
- Factor VIII concentrates
  - —Mainstay of modern hemophilia therapy
  - —Choice based on patient's profile, prior agents, cost
  - —Intermediate-purity products
    - -Low factor VIII specific activity
    - -Contain fibronectin, fibrinogen, other proteins
    - -Viruses killed by solvent detergent extraction or pasteurization
    - -Indicated for older hemophiliacs, patients with prior exposure to blood products
    - -Examples: Humate-P, Profilate
  - —High-purity products
    - -High factor VIII specific activity
    - -Contain fewer plasma proteins
    - -Examples: Alphanate
  - —Very high purity products
    - -Highest factor VIII specific activity
    - -Contains no plasma proteins
    - -Either plasma derived and monoclonal antibody purified or produced using recombinant DNA technology
    - -Indications: pediatric patients; those with limited prior exposure to blood products
    - -Very expensive
    - -Examples: Monoclate-P
- Factor IX concentrates
  - —Fewer options
  - —Low-purity products also known as prothrombin complex concentrates (PCCs)
    - -Plasma derived; contain factors VII, X, and prothrombin
    - -May be activated, i.e., able to initiate coagulation cascade (APCCs)
    - -If administered at frequent or prolonged intervals, may cause DIC or thrombosis
    - -Examples: Profilnine (PCC); Autoplex (APCC)
  - —High-purity concentrates
    - -Plasma derived; purified either using chromatography or immunoaffinity
    - -Expensive
    - -Example: Alphanine
- Adjuncts
  - —DDAVP
    - -Synthetic analogue of the antidiuretic hormone L-arginine vasopressin
    - -Raises factor VIII level 2–4 times in patients with activity >5%
    - -Not useful in patients with hemophilia B
    - -Maximal effect occurs 15–30 minutes after infusion
    - -Side effects: mild flushing, headache, tachycardia, hypotension, hyponatremia
    - -Dose 0.3 μg/kg of DDVAP diluted in 50 mL 0.9% NS given over 15–30 minutes
  - —Amicar
    - -Only for mucosal bleeding
    - -Do not use in children
    - -Do not use in hemarthrosis or hematuria

Specific Management Considerations

- Hemarthrosis
  - —Replace factor promptly
  - —Splint
  - —Ace, ice
  - —Avoid aspirin
  - —Arthrocentesis rarely indicated
- Muscle hemorrhage
  - —Replace factor promptly
  - —Forearm/calf—consider compartment syndrome
  - —Avoid cylindrical casts
  - —Psoas hematoma—groin pain, femoral nerve paresthesias
- Postextraction or oral mucosal bleeding
  - —Treat locally with Avitene or microfibrillar collagen
  - —Replace factor if severe
  - —Amicar may be useful
- Hematuria
  - —Generally mild
  - —Replace factor if symptoms >2 days (50–100%)
  - —Hydrate
  - —Avoid Amicar and cryoprecipitate
- Intracranial hemorrhage
  - —All head injuries should be considered significant, especially in children
  - —Don't delay therapy for diagnostic testing
  - —Replace factor to 100%
  - —CT scan aggressively
- Gastrointestinal bleeding
  - —Secondary to ulcers, polyps, hemorrhoids
  - —Replace factor promptly (50–100%)
  - —Replace factor prior to endoscopy

Disposition

ADMISSION CRITERIA

- Low threshold for admission
- Generally observe 23 hours for resolution of bleeding
- Bleeding episodes may require multiple infusions
- Severe complications
- Head trauma

DISCHARGE CRITERIA

- Minor bleeding with resolution
- If subjective symptoms only

Miscellaneous

ICD9: 286.0

ICD10: D66

SEE ALSO: VON WILLEBRAND DISEASE

SUGGESTED READINGS

Cohen AJ, Kessler CM. Treatment of inherited coagulation disorders. Am J Med 1995;99:675.

DiMichele D. Hemophilia 1996: new approach to an old disease. Pediatr Clin North Am 1996;43:709.

Furie B, Limentani SA, Rosenfield C. A practical guide to the evaluation and treatment of hemophilia. Blood 1994;84–3.

Roberts HR, et al. Hemophilia. In: Beutler E, et al., eds. Williams' hematology, 6th ed. New York: McGraw-Hill, 2001:1639–1657.

Rodgers G, et al. Inherited coagulation disorders. In: Lee G, et al., eds. Wintrobe's clinical hematology, 10th ed. Philadelphia: Lippincott Williams & Wilkins, 1999: 1682–1732.

Author: Steven Bowman

Hemoptysis

Clinical Presentation

SIGNS AND SYMPTOMS

- Expectoration of blood
- Presence of blood in sputum

General

- Acute infectious symptoms
  - —Cough
  - —Fever
  - —Chest pain
  - —Upper respiratory symptoms—congestion/rhinorrhea/sore throat
  - —Sinusitis
  - —General malaise
- Chronic constitutional symptoms (malignancy or tuberculosis)
  - —Weight loss
  - —Night sweats
  - —Development of adenopathy
- Chest pain
  - —Dyspnea
- Coagulopathy/bleeding diathesis
- Symptoms of congestive heart failure (CHF)—orthopnea, pedal edema, dyspnea
- Hematuria
- Gingival bleeding
- Epistaxis
- Petechiae
- Nasal and sinus pain or bleeding

MECHANISM/DESCRIPTION

- Expectoration of blood or the presence of blood in sputum
- May be the manifestation of a wide variety of disease processes or entities in patients of any age
- More common in adults (children under age 6 usually swallow their sputum and rarely present with hemoptysis unless they have substantial bleeding)
- Massive hemoptysis
  - —100–600 mL over 24 hours (>8 mL/kg per 24 hours in child) or 1,000 mL over several days
  - —Rare (<5%)
  - —Potential life-threatening event

ETIOLOGY

- Most common—bronchitis, bronchogenic carcinoma, bronchiectasis

Infection

- Both URI and LRI
  - —Acute or chronic bronchitis
  - —Sinusitis
  - —Pneumonia (especially *Staphylococcus, Klebsiella, Legionella, Pneumococcus*)
  - —Lung abscess
  - —Tuberculosis
  - —Mycetoma
- Fungal
- Viral
- Parasitic

Neoplastic

- Lung cancer (squamous cell, small cell, carcinoid)
- Bronchial adenoma
- Metastasis

Cardiac

- Mitral stenosis
- CHF
- Any left-sided obstructive lesion

Pulmonary

- Bronchiectasis
- Cystic fibrosis
- Pulmonary thromboembolism/infarction
- Bullous emphysema

Systemic Disease

- Goodpasture's syndrome
- Systemic lupus erythematosus
- Vasculitis (e.g., Wegener's granulomatosis, Henoch-Schönlein purpura)

Hematologic

- Coagulopathy
- Thrombocytopenia
- Platelet dysfunction
- DIC

Vascular

- Pulmonary hypertension
- Arteriovenous malformation
- Aortic aneurysm
- Aortobronchial fistula

Drugs/Toxins

- Aspirin
- Anticoagulants
- Penicillamine
- Solvents
- Cocaine

Trauma

- Fat embolism
- Tracheobronchial rupture

Iatrogenic

- Bronchoscopy
- Lung biopsy
- Transtracheal aspirate
- Central venous line placement

Miscellaneous

- Foreign body
- Endometriosis—catamenial hemoptysis
- Amyloidosis
- Bronchopleural fistula
- Factitious or Munchausen syndrome
- Idiopathic
  - —As high as 30% of cases

Pre-Hospital

- Airway management
  - —Oxygen
  - —Endotracheal intubation for respiratory distress
- IV access
- Cardiac monitoring

ESSENTIAL WORKUP

- Careful history
- *Essential to differentiate between hemoptysis and hematemesis*
  - —Blood originating in the airway
  - —Bright red and frothy
  - —Alkaline
  - —Often mixed with sputum
  - —Accompanied by coughing or preceded by a gurgling noise
- Gastrointestinal blood
  - —Usually has a dark red, brown, or "coffee grounds" color
  - —Acidic
  - —May contain food particles
  - —Usually accompanied by nausea, retching, or emesis
  - —Gastric lavage and stool testing for occult blood may be necessary to distinguish the source
- Duration of hemoptysis
- Smoking or chronic lung disease
- Chronic alcohol abuse (increased risk of lung abscess or tuberculosis)
- Recent travel abroad (parasitic disease or tuberculosis)

PEDIATRIC CONSIDERATIONS

- Chronic productive cough or wheezing
- Congenital or rheumatic heart disease
- Foreign body aspiration (majority of cases in children <4 years old)
- Physical examination
  - —Inspect oropharynx and nose to exclude an oral lesion or epistaxis
  - —Poor dentition may predispose to lung abscess
  - —Wheezing over one lung segment may suggest a focal obstruction or foreign body
  - —Crackles may point to pneumonia, CHF, or alveolar hemorrhage
  - —Digital clubbing suggests chronic lung disease, cancer, or congenital heart disease
  - —Diffuse petechiae or purpura points to a possible coagulopathy
  - —Telangiectasias or hemangiomas may indicate the presence of arteriovenous malformations

LABORATORY

- CBC with differential
- PT, PTT
- Massive hemoptysis
  - —Type and cross
  - —Electrolytes, renal function, liver function tests
  - —Arterial blood gas
- If infectious etiology, sputum Gram and acid-fast stains with cultures and cytology
- If considering pulmonary-renal syndrome
  - —Urinalysis for hematuria
  - —Electrolytes, BUN/Cr
- Pregnancy testing in women of child-bearing potential
- Consider arterial blood gas

IMAGING/SPECIAL TESTS

- Chest radiography
  - —Foreign body, mass, infection, nodule, heart failure, cavitary lesions
- Ventilation-perfusion scan and/or pulmonary arteriography or CT angiography for pulmonary embolism
- Bronchoscopy
  - —Initial invasive procedure of choice for life-threatening, massive hemoptysis
- CT
  - —Before bronchoscopy unless life-threatening hemoptysis
- *Controversy* exists over bronchoscopy vs CT as next line test in evaluation of hemoptysis

PEDIATRIC CONSIDERATIONS

- Sweat chloride test if cystic fibrosis suspected
- CT of chest more useful in children, as part of the initial evaluation of stable patients, particularly if the CXR reveals a mass, foreign body, or other abnormality

INITIAL STABILIZATION

- Airway and breathing
  - —Asphyxia most immediate threat to life
  - —Endotracheal intubation for impending respiratory failure
  - —Large-diameter tube (>8 French)
  - —Careful suctioning once intubated to prevent further airway trauma
  - —Supplemental oxygen
- Massive hemoptysis
  - —Large-bore IV access with volume resuscitation
  - —Oxygen
  - —Place patient in upright position
  - —Cardiac monitor
  - —Pulse oximetry

ED TREATMENT

- Volume resuscitation as needed with IV fluid and blood
- If *massive* hemoptysis:
  - —Consider airway control
  - —Correct coagulation abnormalities as indicated by lab and coagulation studies
  - —Consult with pulmonologist and thoracic surgeon
  - —Essential to find etiology and site of hemoptysis
- Place patient in lateral decubitus position with involved side down
  - —If bleeding can be localized to one lung, attempt mainstem intubation of nonbleeding lung
  - —Treat underlying pathology
- Ensure respiratory isolation measures until proven that the patient does not have active pulmonary tuberculosis

ADMISSION CRITERIA

- ICU
  - —Massive hemoptysis
  - —Hemodynamic instability
  - —Hypovolemic shock
  - —Severe hypoxemia
  - —Threatened airway
  - —Intubation/mechanical ventilation
  - —Suspected pulmonary embolism
- General
  - —Cavitary lung disease
  - —Lung abscess
  - —Suspected active pulmonary tuberculosis
  - —Foreign bodies for bronchoscopy or surgical removal

DISCHARGE CRITERIA

- Minor hemoptysis due to tracheobronchitis
- Pneumonia amenable to outpatient treatment
- Bronchogenic carcinoma
- Discharge with cough suppressants (codeine, etc.) and appropriate oral antibiotic
- Close follow-up

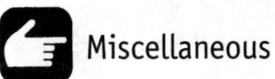

Miscellaneous

ICD9: 786.3

ICD10: R04.2

SUGGESTED READINGS

Cahill B, Ingbar D. Massive hemoptysis: assessment and management. Clin Chest Med 1994;15(1):147–167.

Goldman J. Hemoptysis: emergency assessment and management. Emerg Med Clin North Am 1989;7(2):325–338.

Jean-Baptiste E. Clinical assessment and management of massive hemoptysis. Crit Care Med 2000;28:1642–1647.

Pianosi P, Al-Sadoon H. Hemoptysis in children. Pediatr Rev 1996;17(10): 344–348.

Weinbergeer S. Etiology and evaluation of hemoptysis. *WWW.UpToDate.Com*, 1999.

Author: Peter S. Pang

Hemorrhagic Fevers

Clinical Presentation

SIGNS AND SYMPTOMS

- Most common (>50%)
  —Acute febrile illness
  —Malaise
  —Headache
  —Nausea/vomiting
  —Flushing
  —Diarrhea (nonbloody)
  —Abdominal pain
  —Myalgias
- Less common (<30%)
  —Gingival hemorrhage
  —Conjunctival injection/hemorrhage
  —Petechia
  —Hematemesis
  —Melena
  —Epistaxis
- Delayed presentations (>3 days into the disease)
  —As above with hemorrhagic symptoms becoming more prominent
- Bleeding from the gums, nose, lungs, GI tract, or uterus
  —Exanthems
- Marburg and Ebola—nonpruritic centripetal, papular, erythematous eruption appearing between days 5 and 7, which then coalesce into well-demarcated macules that may be hemorrhagic
- Yellow fever—jaundice
- Dengue—bright maculopapular truncal erythroderma that blanches dramatically under light pressure
  —Shock
  —Seizures
  —Coma

ETIOLOGY

- Infection with RNA viruses that have zoonotic life cycles in specific geographic areas
- Short incubation period of <10 days but may extend out to 21 days
- Examples of viral hemorrhagic fevers (VHF):
  —Filoviruses—unknown reservoir and vector
    -Ebola
    -Marburg
  —Arenaviruses—rodent reservoir, transmitted via inhalation of aerosolized virus in rodent excreta
    -Lassa
    -South American hemorrhagic fevers (SAHF)
  —Flaviviruses—human reservoir, transmitted via mosquito
    -Dengue hemorrhagic fever (DHF)
    -Yellow fever
  —Bunyaviridae—small mammal reservoir, transmitted via mosquitoes or ticks
    -Rift valley fever (RVF)
    -Crimean-Congo hemorrhagic fever (CCHF)
  —Hantavirus—rodent reservoir, transmitted via inhalation of aerosolized virus in rodent excreta.
    -Hemorrhagic fever with renal syndrome (HFRS)

PATHOGENESIS

- VHF cause endothelial damage and increase vascular permeability, hemorrhage, and hypovolemic shock
- DIC appears to be a regular feature of Marburg and CCHF but is less frequent with Arenavirus infections
- DHF is thought to be immune mediated and is usually the result of a second infection

BIOWARFARE THREAT

- These viruses are highly infectious by aerosol (with the exception of dengue)
- Associated with high morbidity and in some cases high mortality
- Replicate well in cell culture, which permits weaponization

Pre-Hospital

CAUTIONS

- Any place in the world can now be reached within a period of time significantly shorter than the incubation period of almost all infectious diseases
- Early detection of VHF, natural or biologic attack, is the key to control an outbreak
- Most cases will derive from patients who traveled to or had contact with persons from parts of the world where the viruses are endemic

Diagnosis

ESSENTIAL WORKUP

- Workup focuses on differentiating from other acute febrile illnesses especially in the returned traveler
- Recognize a possible biologic attack when an unusual number of patients present with similar and/or unusual findings

LABORATORY

- CBC
  —May see leukocytosis or leukopenia, thrombocytopenia
- Electrolytes, BUN/Cr, glucose
  —Look for renal failure
- LFTs
  —Hepatic involvement is common but jaundice occurs mainly with yellow fever
- PT/PTT, d-dimer
  —Look for a coagulopathy and DIC (seen in CCHF, Ebola, and Marburg)

SPECIAL TESTS

- In specialized laboratories (biohazard level 4), definitive diagnosis can be made by viral isolation, PCR, and immunohistochemistry
  —Coordinated with the CDC
- Thick and thin smears to help differentiate from malaria

DIFFERENTIAL DIAGNOSIS

- Malaria
  —Real concern in the returned traveler with fever
- Dengue fever
  —Common source of fever in the returned traveler
- Rickettsial
  —Rocky Mountain spotted fever
  —Typhus
- Bacterial
  —Meningococcemia
  —Sepsis
- Systemic disease
  —Leukemia
  —TTP
- Pit viper envenomation

Treatment

INITIAL STABILIZATION

- Protection of health care workers
  - —Universal blood and body precautions
  - —Isolation of the patient
  - —Use of protective clothing plus HEPA-filtered respirators to minimize exposure to aerosols for those involved in procedures such as suctioning, catheter placement and wound dressing
  - —Notify the CDC at 404-639-2888 for all suspected cases

ED TREATMENT

- Mainly supportive
- Empiric therapy with antimalarial regimens until a definitive diagnosis is obtained
- Aggressively treat secondary infections
- Bleeding is usually mild, and life-threatening loss of blood is rare
  - —If indicated, hemorrhage can be managed by replacement of blood, platelets, and clotting factors
- Pulmonary artery catheter to manage shock
  - —Patients are often hypovolemic because of third spacing and hemorrhage but may readily develop pulmonary edema with crystalloid infusion
- Ribavirin—a synthetic nucleoside
  - —Useful for Lassa, SAHF, CCHF, and HFRS; ineffective against filoviruses
  - —Causes a reversible hemolytic anemia
- Transfusion of immune plasma (convalescent plasma therapy) for SAHF within the first week of symptoms

MEDICATIONS

- Ribavirin
  - —IV loading dose of 33 mg/kg followed by 16 mg/kg every 6 hours for 4 days, then 8 mg/kg every 8 hours for 3 days
  - —Prophylactic—500 mg by mouth every 6 hours for 7 days
- Vaccines
  - —Yellow fever is widely available
  - —SAHF, RVF, and Hantavirus are under development
- Other medications under investigation
  - —Nucleoside analogue inhibitors of S-adenosylhomocysteine hydrolase inhibit Ebola replication in mice

Disposition

ADMISSION CRITERIA

- Admit all suspected cases of VHF to isolation rooms
  - —ICU bed if signs of shock or multiorgan system failure

DISCHARGE CRITERIA

N/A

Miscellaneous

ICD9: 065

ICD10: A94

SUGGESTED READINGS

Anonymous. Update: Management of patients with suspected viral hemorrhagic fever—United States. MMWR 1995;44: 475–479.

Anonymous. Management of patients with suspected viral hemorrhagic fever. MMWR 1988;37(S3):1–16.

Boyle TJ, Bryan RT, Peters CJ. Emerging infectious diseases: viral hemorrhagic fevers and Hantavirus infections in the Americas. Infect Dis Clin North Am 1998;12:95–110.

Franz DR, Jarling PB, Friedlander AM, et al. Clinical recognition and management of patients exposed to biological warfare agents. JAMA 1997;278:399–411.

Mayers DL. Advances in military dermatology: exotic virus infections of military significance. Dermatol Clin 1999;17:29–39.

Author: David Tanen

Hemorrhagic Shock

Clinical Presentation

SIGNS AND SYMPTOMS

- *Class I hemorrhage:* loss of up to 15% of blood volume (up to 750 cc in 70-kg adult)
  —Minimal tachycardia
  —Increase in pulse pressure
  —Slight anxiety
- *Class II hemorrhage:* loss of 15–30% of blood volume (750–1,500 cc)
  —Tachycardia
  —Tachypnea
  —Decreased pulse pressure
  —Elevated diastolic BP
  —Mild anxiety
  —Small decrease in urine output
- *Class III hemorrhage:* loss of 30–40% of blood volume (1,500–2,000 cc)
  —Marked tachycardia
  —Tachypnea
  —Decreased pulse pressure
  —Fall in systolic BP
  —Significant change in mental status
  -Anxiety
  -Confusion
  —Marked decrease in urine output
- *Class IV hemorrhage:* loss of greater than 40% of blood volume (greater than 2,000 cc)
  —Marked tachycardia
  —Tachypnea
  —Very narrow pulse pressure
  —Significant fall in systolic BP
  —Depressed mental status
  -Confusion
  -Lethargy
  -Loss of consciousness
  —Negligible urine output
  —Cold and pale skin

MECHANISM/DESCRIPTION

- Shock occurs when loss of effective circulating blood volume results in inadequate organ perfusion
- At the tissue level, hypoperfusion leads to inadequate oxygenation, anaerobic metabolism, cellular injury, and death
- Compensated shock occurs when the patient's physiologic reserve prevents significant alteration in vital signs
- Decompensated shock occurs when there is a loss of circulating volume that overcomes the patient's physiologic reserve, resulting in signification alteration in vital signs
- Blood loss can be estimated by multiplying 70 mL/kg (adult blood volume) times body weight (kg) times percentage loss as determined by class of hemorrhage

PEDIATRIC CONSIDERATIONS

- Children often have greater physiologic reserve and can preserve normal vital signs longer
- Systemic responses to blood loss in the pediatric patient include:
  —<25% volume loss: weak, thready pulse and tachycardia; lethargy, irritability, confusion; cool, clammy skin; decreased urine output (UO) with increased urine specific gravity
  —25–40% volume loss: tachycardia; marked change in consciousness, dulled response to pain; cyanotic, cold extremities with decreased capillary refill; minimal UO
  —>40% volume loss: hypotension, tachycardia, or bradycardia; comatose; pale, cold skin; no UO

Pre-Hospital

CONTROVERSIES

- The current standard of care calls for IV crystalloid resuscitation in trauma patients; follow local protocols

ETIOLOGIES

- Abdominal trauma, blunt or penetrating
- Abortion—complete, partial, or inevitable
- Aneurysms
  —Abdominal aortic aneurysm most common
  —Mycotic aneurysm secondary to endocarditis
  —May lead to thoracic, retroperitoneal, or intraperitoneal bleeding
- Aortogastric fistula
- Arteriovenous malformations
  —May lead to thoracic, retroperitoneal, or intraperitoneal bleeding
- Blunt trauma
  —Splenic injury (40% of abdominal hemorrhage)
  —Liver injury (20% of abdominal hemorrhage)
- Ectopic pregnancy
- Epistaxis
- Fractures (especially long bones)
- Hemoptysis
- Lower GI bleed
- Malignancies
- Mallory-Weiss tear
- Penetrating trauma
- Placenta previa
- Postpartum hemorrhage
- Retroperitoneal bleeds
- Splenic rupture
- Upper GI bleed
- Vascular injuries

Diagnosis

ESSENTIAL WORKUP

- Rectal examination and nasogastric tube
  —Indicated in undifferentiated hypovolemic shock to rule out GI hemorrhage
- Blood type and cross-match
- Hemoglobin/hematocrit

LABORATORY

- Coagulation studies (PT/PTT, INR, and platelet count) may be useful
- Other measures of shock and tissue hypoperfusion include arterial blood gas, base deficit, and serum lactate level to determine acid–base status
- Serum electrolytes to assess renal function and intravascular volume status

IMAGING/SPECIAL TESTS

- Chest x-ray
  —Hemothorax
  -Blunt chest injuries
  -Thoracic AV malformation
- Pelvic x-ray
  —Pelvic fracture
- Abdominal ultrasound (FAST exam)
  —Indicated following abdominal trauma, for possible abdominal aortic aneurysm, or when nontraumatic intraperitoneal hemorrhage is suspected
  —Fluid in Morison's pouch implies significant hemorrhage or ascites
  —A negative study does not rule out intraperitoneal hemorrhage
  —Bedside evaluation for an abdominal aortic aneurysm
- Endovaginal ultrasound
  —Indicated in women with a positive pregnancy test
  —Fluid in the cul-de-sac
  —Ectopic pregnancy
- Diagnostic peritoneal lavage
  —Indicated in unstable trauma patients when the ultrasound fails to show intraperitoneal hemorrhage
  —Detects intraperitoneal bleeding only
  —Aspiration of 10 cc of blood defines the need for emergent laparotomy in unstable patients
- Abdominal CT scan
  —Detects both intraperitoneal and retroperitoneal hemorrhage
  —Should only be performed once the patient has been stabilized
  —Abdominal aortic aneurysm
- Endoscopy
  —In the setting of upper and lower GI bleeding

- Angiography
  - —Indications
    - -Pelvic fracture
    - -Retroperitoneal hemorrhage
    - -Lower GI bleeding
    - -Embolization therapy for bleeding from arterial sources can be performed

DIFFERENTIAL DIAGNOSIS

See Shock

Treatment

INITIAL STABILIZATION

- Airway and breathing
  - —Intubation as indicated by patient's respiratory and mental status
  - —100% oxygen via face mask should be administered
- Circulation
  - —Two large-bore peripheral IV lines should be established (16-gauge or larger)
  - —Venous cutdown (saphenous) may be necessary
  - —Aggressive crystalloid resuscitation should be initiated early in the course in the ED
  - —3:1 rule: for one unit volume of blood loss, give three volumes of crystalloid
- With evidence of class III or IV hemorrhage, initiate blood transfusion early
  - —Type-specific and cross-matched blood is preferred when time permits, often 1 hour
  - —Type-specific blood is usually available within 10–15 minutes
  - —Type O blood can be used in immediate, life-threatening situations (type O Rh negative blood only for women of child-bearing age)

ED TREATMENT

- If possible, obtain control of hemorrhage (direct pressure, pelvic fixation/stabilization, etc.)
- Place patient on continuous monitor; insert Foley catheter to monitor urine output
- Central venous access may be indicated for CVP monitoring, but placement of such lines should not interfere with resuscitation measures
- Continually reassess patient for clinical response or deterioration
  - —Monitor vital signs, mental status, urine output
  - —Follow serial blood gas, lactate level, hemoglobin/hematocrit measurements
  - —Maintain urine output at 50 cc/hr
- The response to initial fluid resuscitation is the key to determining subsequent therapy
  - —Rapid response to fluid administration indicates minimal (<20%) blood loss
  - —Transient response to volume resuscitation indicates ongoing hemorrhage or inadequate resuscitation; continue fluid and blood administration and rapidly obtain necessary studies and consultations
  - —Minimal or no response to volume resuscitation indicates ongoing severe blood loss; immediate angiography or surgical intervention is warranted
- Use fluids warmed (approximately 39°C) by means of microwave ovens, warm water baths, or blood warmers
- Transfuse platelets and coagulation factors as indicated
- Consider autotransfusion devices with tube thoracostomy treatment and decompression of large hemothoraces

MEDICATIONS

- Crystalloids: normal saline or lactated ringers IV: adults: 1–2 L bolus, reassess for perfusion; peds: 20 mL/kg bolus
- Blood products: cross-matched, type-specific, or O-negative: adult: initiate with 4–6 units PRBC; peds: 10 mL/kg of PRBC
- Other blood products: platelets, coagulation factors such as fresh frozen plasma (large transfusions of packed RBCs as opposed to whole blood may lead to significant dilution of platelet and coagulation factors)
- Hemoglobin substitutes currently under study, but of no proven benefit

PEDIATRIC CONSIDERATIONS

- Access may be obtained by intraosseous route after one or two unsuccessful attempts at peripheral access
- Maintain urine output at 1 cc/kg/h for children and 2 cc/kg/h for infants

Disposition

ADMISSION CRITERIA

- All patients with hemorrhage should be admitted to the appropriate service

DISCHARGE CRITERIA

- No patients with acute hemorrhagic shock in the ED should be discharged home

Miscellaneous

ICD9: 958.4, 785.59

ICD10: R57.1

SEE ALSO: SHOCK

SUGGESTED READINGS

American College of Surgeons, Committee on Trauma. Advanced trauma life support program. Chicago: American College of Surgeons, 1997.

Baron BJ, Scalea TM. Acute blood loss. Emerg Med Clin North Am 1996;14(1):35.

Kline JA. Shock. In: Marx J, et al., eds. Rosen's emergency medicine: concepts and clinical practice, 5th ed. St. Louis: CV Mosby, 2001:33–47.

Stainsby D, MacLennan S, Hamilton PJ. Management of massive blood loss: a template guideline. Br J Anaesth 2000;85(3):487–491.

Author: Theodore C. Chan

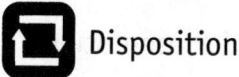

Hemorrhoid

Clinical Presentation

SIGNS AND SYMPTOMS

- Painless, rectal bleeding with defecation
- Blood on stool or toilet paper
- Blood drips into toilet bowel
- Severe pain if:
  —Internal hemorrhoids prolapse and strangulate
  —External hemorrhoids thrombose
- Pruritus ani
- May also have fissure

MECHANISM/DESCRIPTION

- No precise definition exists
- Abnormal vascular cushions of anal canal
- Do not cause pain unless thrombosed/ strangulated
- Discrete masses of thick submucosa contain:
  —Blood vessels
  —Smooth muscle
  —Elastic and connective tissue
- Sliding down of part of anal canal lining
- External hemorrhoids:
  —Vessels situated below dentate line
  —Covered by skin/anoderm
  —Drain to internal iliac veins
- Internal hemorrhoids:
  —Submucosal vessels above dentate line
  —Drain to portal system
  —Usually at left lateral, right posterolateral, and right anterolateral positions
  —Grade 1 = painless, bleeding
  —Grade 2 = prolapse with BM, spontaneously reduce
  —Grade 3 = prolapse with BM, require manual reduction
  —Grade 4 = chronically prolapsed, not reducible

ETIOLOGY

- Exact etiology unknown
- Associated with straining and irregular bowel habits
  —Hard, bulky stools or diarrhea cause tenesmus/straining
  —Push anal cushions out of anal canal
  —Weakens submucosal tissue
- Higher resting anal pressures
- Erect posture
- Heredity
  —Absence of valves in veins
- Increased intraabdominal pressure
  —Ascites
  —Pregnancy
- Portal hypertension

Pre-Hospital

N/A

Diagnosis

ESSENTIAL WORKUP

- History
  —Length of bleeding
    -Pain?
    -Duration?
  —Any new lumps or masses by rectum?
- Examination of perianal area
  —Gently spread buttocks
  —Discrete, dark blue, tender mass covered with skin = thrombosed external hemorrhoid
    -Can have internal component
  —Purplish, tender mucosal covered mass = prolapsed, strangulated internal hemorrhoid
    -Usually associated with enlarged, thrombosed external hemorrhoid
  —Have patient bear down to check for prolapsing hemorrhoids
  —Digital rectal exam mandatory to r/o cancer

LABORATORY

- Hct if history of significant blood loss
- Plt and PT/PTT if pt on anticoagulants or severe comorbid condition

IMAGING/SPECIAL TESTS

- Anoscopy to visualize anal canal
  —Identify bleeding internal hemorrhoids

DIFFERENTIAL DIAGNOSIS

- Rectal prolapse
- Anal fissure
- Perirectal abscess

Treatment

INITIAL STABILIZATION

- Direct digital pressure to control bleeding

ED TREATMENT

- Conservative therapy for all
  - —Hot sitz baths for 15 minutes three times a day and after each bowel movement
  - —High-fiber diet = 30 g/d
    - -Eat more fresh fruits and vegetables
    - -Increase "bran" intake
  - —10–12 glasses of water per day
  - —Stool softeners
  - —Bulk-forming laxatives
- Excise thrombosed external hemorrhoid if severe pain and if the hemorrhoid is less than 5 days old
  - —Follow with conservative therapy
  - —Place patient in prone jack-knife position or left lateral decubitus
  - —Infiltrate surrounding skin and underneath clot using 27-gauge needle with lidocaine containing epinephrine
  - —Make an elliptical incision to excise clot/skin
  - —Place a small piece of Gelfoam and/or gauze onto the wound and tape
  - —Remove dressing at time of first sitz bath in about 6 hours
  - —Give analgesics
    - -NSAIDs
    - -Acetaminophen
    - -0.2% topical nitroglycerin ointment to anus
      - *Decreases pain by inhibiting sphincter spasm
- Manually reduce nonthrombosed, prolapsed internal hemorrhoids
  - —Follow with conservative therapy
  - —May need topical anesthetic or anal sphincter block with local
  - —Can sclerose bleeding internal hemorrhoids
  - —Can rubber band ligate 1–2 internal hemorrhoids
- Nonreducible internal hemorrhoids
  - —Nonstrangulated = conservative management and surgical referral
  - —Strangulated = immediate surgical referral for excision

MEDICATIONS

- Acetaminophen: 325–650 mg (peds: 15 mg/kg) with codeine 15–30 mg (peds 0.5 mg/kg) PO q4h PRN
- Bran/fiber: 20 g PO qd
- Docusate sodium (Colace): 50–200 mg (peds: <3 years = 10–40 mg/d; 3–6 years = 20–60 mg/d; >6–12 years = 40–150 mg/day) PO q12h
- ELA-Max 5 (5% lidocaine anorectal cream): apply to perianal area q4h PRN pain (peds: not for <12 years of age)
- Ibuprofen (Motrin): 400–600 mg (peds: 40 mg/kg/d) PO q6h
- Psyllium seeds: 1–2 tsp (peds: 0.25–1 tsp/day) PO q24h

Disposition

ADMISSION CRITERIA

- Strangulated grade 4 hemorrhoids
  - —Surgical consult for prolapsed, thrombosed internal hemorrhoids
- Severe anemia with bleeding hemorrhoids

DISCHARGE CRITERIA

- Majority of patients will go home
- Surgical referral for:
  - —Grade 3 or 4 internal hemorrhoids
  - —Suspected anorectal or colonic tumors, inflammatory bowel disease, coagulopathy, pregnancy, or immunocompromised

Miscellaneous

ICD9: 455.6

ICD10: I84.9

SUGGESTED READINGS

Janicke DM, Pundt MR. Anorectal disorders. Emerg Med Clin North Am 1994;14:757–788.

Pfenninger JL, Surrell J. Nonsurgical treatment options for internal hemorrhoids. Am Fam Physician 1995;52:821–834.

Author: Julia Sone

Hemothorax

Clinical Presentation

SIGNS AND SYMPTOMS

- Small amount of blood in thorax (less than 400 cc): little or no change in patient's appearance, vital signs, or physical findings
- Large amount of blood (more than 1,000 cc): restlessness, anxiety, pallor, pleuritic pain, hemoptysis, dyspnea, or air hunger
- Tachycardia, tachypnea, hypotension
- Chest inspection: asymmetric expansion, paradoxical wall movement, abrasion, contusion
- Chest wall palpation: tenderness or crepitus over ribs, clavicles, scapulae, or the sternum; subcutaneous emphysema, dullness to percussion
- Auscultation: ipsilateral decreased breath sounds

MECHANISM/DESCRIPTION

- Accumulation of blood in the intrapleural space after blunt or penetrating chest trauma causing lung compression
  - —Results in decreased vital capacity, hypoxia, and respiratory compromise
  - —Commonly associated with pneumothorax (25% of cases) as well as extrathoracic injuries (73% of cases)
- Hemothorax can cause increased intrathoracic pressure resulting in compromised venous return and decreased cardiac output
- Loss of large intravascular volume results in hemodynamic instability
- Large hemothoraces cause the release of substances that can act as anticoagulants and contribute to continued intrathoracic bleeding

ETIOLOGY

- Traumatic injuries to major vessels: laceration of major blood vessels, including pulmonary artery, pulmonary vein, intercostal artery, internal mammary artery, aorta, vena cava, and heart are associated with hemorrhage into the thoracic cavity
- Traumatic lung parenchymal injuries: often stops spontaneously by nature of the low pulmonary pressures and high concentrations of tissue thromboplastin in the lung
- Nontraumatic spontaneous hemothoraces: very rare; coagulation disorder, malignancy, primary vascular event (such as aortic dissection), infection, and complication of spontaneous pneumothoraces

Pre-Hospital

CAUTIONS

- Difficult to differentiate hemothoraces from pneumothoraces clinically
  - —All may present with dyspnea, pleuritic chest pain, decreased breath sounds, and hemodynamic instability
  - —Certain clues aid in making the diagnosis such as subcutaneous emphysema for pneumothorax, and dullness to percussion for hemothorax
- Perform needle thoracostomy for potential tension pneumothorax if the patient hemodynamically unstable

Diagnosis

ESSENTIAL WORKUP

- Chest radiography is the single best diagnostic tool; fluid collections >200–300 cc can usually be seen on good upright to decubitus radiograph of the chest
  - —In the supine position, which is often the initial view available, up to 1,000 cc of blood may not be readily apparent
  - —Hemothorax appears as a slight haziness over the involved hemithorax on the AP radiograph
  - —In the hemodynamically stable patient, the optimal technique is an upright PA projection at full inspiration
- Pulse-oximetry, arterial blood gas

LABORATORY

- Hematocrit may be helpful if it shows a drop or changes on serial evaluations
- Type and cross-match

IMAGING/SPECIAL TESTS

- Ultrasound diagnostic imaging is a valuable tool in the evaluation of intrapleural fluid collection.
- CT is useful in detecting small amounts of intrapleural fluid not visible on the chest radiograph

DIFFERENTIAL DIAGNOSIS

- Hemopneumothorax
- Pneumothorax
- Pulmonary contusion

Treatment

INITIAL STABILIZATION

- ABCs
  - —Control airway as needed; endotracheal intubation for patients with impending respiratory failure
  - —Supplemental oxygen: 100% non-rebreather mask
  - —Intravenous access: two large-bore intravenous catheters to restore circulating blood volume
  - —Needle thoracostomy should be performed in patients with hemodynamic instability unless chest tube kit is immediately available

ED TREATMENT

- Hemothorax is treated by evacuating accumulated blood in the intrapleural space
- Tube thoracostomy evacuates blood; allows for reexpansion of the lung as well as constant monitoring of blood loss
- Tube thoracostomy: use a large-bore chest tube (36–40 French) inserted in the fourth or fifth intercostal space at the midaxillary line aiming posteriorly and superiorly; the tube is then connected to underwater-seal drainage and suction (20–30 mL H_2O)
- Autotransfusion should be used if available to replace blood loss
- Indications for *thoracotomy*
  - —Initial tube drainage greater than 20 cc/kg of blood (or 1,000 mL of blood for adults from the pleural cavity)
  - —Persistent bleeding at a rate greater than 7 cc/kg/h (or 200 mL/h for 4 hours)
  - —Increasing hemothorax seen on chest radiography
  - —Patient remains hypotensive despite adequate blood replacement and other sites of blood loss have been ruled out
  - —Patient decompensates after initial response to resuscitation
- Indications for ED thoracotomy
  - —Penetrating trauma: traumatic arrest at any point with initial signs of life in the field; blood pressure <50 mm Hg systolic after fluid resuscitation; severe shock with clinical signs of cardiac tamponade
  - —Blunt trauma: traumatic arrest in the ED

MEDICATIONS

- Local anesthetics for cutaneous anesthesia prior to tube thoracostomy in awake, conscious patients
- Conscious sedation (midazolam) and analgesia (fentanyl) should be used for stable, awake patients prior to tube thoracostomy
  - —Fentanyl: adult/peds: 2–5 μg/kg/dose
  - —Midazolam: adult/peds: 0.02–0.04 mg/kg/dose

Disposition

ADMISSION CRITERIA

- Hemothoraces large enough to require tube thoracostomies should be admitted for monitoring and thoracostomy tube management

DISCHARGE CRITERIA

- Isolated small hemothoraces (detected incidentally on ultrasound or CT imaging) may be considered for discharge after 4–6 hours of observation if there is no evidence of continued bleeding and the patient is not hypoxic

Miscellaneous

ICD9: 511.8

ICD10: J94.2

SUGGESTED READINGS

Eddy CA, Carrico CJ, Rusch VW. Injury to the lung and pleura. In: Moore EE, Mattox KL, Feliciano DV, eds. Trauma, 2nd ed. East Norwalk, CT: Appleton & Lange, 1991.

Meredith JW. Chest wall injury. In: Trunkey D, Lewis FR Jr, eds. Current therapy of trauma, 3rd ed. Philadelphia: BC Decker, 1991:216–219.

Parry GW, Morgan WE, Salama FD. Management of haemothorax. Ann R Coll Surg Engl 1996;78(4):325–326.

Vukich DJ, Markovchick V. Thoracic trauma. In: Rosen P, et al., eds. Emergency medicine: concept and clinical practice, 5th ed. St. Louis: CV Mosby, 2001:391–392.

Author: Thomas C. Lee

Henoch Schönlein Purpura

Clinical Presentation

SIGNS AND SYMPTOMS

General

- Well-appearing child, despite nature and extent of rash
- Recent or current upper respiratory tract infection
- Malaise
- Low-grade fever
- Hypertension, if associated renal failure
- Children <3 months may have only skin manifestations

Skin

- Purpuric rash
  - —Presenting sign in 50% of patients
  - —100% of patients develop purpura
  - —First appears as pink rounded papules that blanch
  - —Progresses to 2–3 cm circular palpable purpura within 24 hours; may be discrete, confluent, or confluent
  - —Rash begins in gravity dependent areas of legs and buttocks
  - —Symmetric distribution
  - —May involve lower back
  - —Rarely involves the face
  - —Rash recurs in up to 40% of patients (within 6 weeks)

Abdominal

- Abdominal pain
  - —70–80% of cases
  - —Colicky to severe
  - —Abdominal findings may precede the rash by 4 weeks
- GI bleeding
  - —75% of cases
  - —Occult to severe blood loss
  - —Intussusception (ileo-ileal or ileocolic)

Renal-Genitourinary

- Asymptomatic hematuria
  - —Occurs in 80% of cases
- Scrotal pain
- Testicular swelling
- Renal failure

Extremities

- Arthritis
  - —70–80% of cases
  - —Migratory periarticular pain
  - —Most frequent in knees and ankles
  - —Angioedema

Neurologic

- Headache
- Seizure
- Focal deficits

MECHANISM/DESCRIPTION

- Vasculitis
- Increased serum IgA
  - —Circulating IgA complexes
  - —Glomerular mesangial deposition of IgA
- Peak incidence school-aged children and young adults
- More common in Caucasians
- Males > females
- Occurs more often in winter/spring
- Multisystem involvement can lead to life-threatening or long-term complications
  - —Intussusception
  - —Proliferative glomerulonephritis
  - —Chronic renal failure
    - -More common in older children and adults (13–14%)
  - —Intracranial hemorrhage

ETIOLOGY

- Although etiology is undefined, there are many associated conditions
  - —Infections
  - —Group A strep
  - —Mycoplasma
  - —Viral: varicella, Epstein-Barr (EB)
  - —Drugs: penicillin, tetracycline, aspirin, sulfonamides, erythromycin
  - —Allergens: insect bites, chocolate, milk, wheat

Pre-Hospital

N/A

Diagnosis

ESSENTIAL WORKUP

- Exclude life-threatening causes of purpura, severe abdominal pain, hematuria, and CNS findings, if appropriate

LABORATORY

- CBC
  - —Platelet count normal
  - —WBC often elevated
- PT, PTT (if bleeding or in shock; or if unsure of diagnosis and concerned about possibility of coagulopathy)
- Electrolytes (if hypertension or urinalysis abnormal)
- BUN, creatinine (if hypertension or urinalysis abnormal)
  - —May be elevated in cases with serious renal complications
- Urinalysis
  - —Hematuria is common
  - —Proteinuria is suggestive of glomerulonephritis
- Cultures to exclude common infections

IMAGING/SPECIAL TESTS

- Abdominal imaging studies
  - —Indicated if abdominal pain or GI bleeding
  - —Flat and upright abdominal films of limited utility
  - —Abdominal ultrasound, barium enema, or CT scan may be necessary to rule out intussusception
- Testicular ultrasound
  - —Indicated in patients with testicular pain and swelling
- Head CT
  - —Indicated if CNS findings to exclude bleed

DIFFERENTIAL DIAGNOSIS

- Abdominal pain
  - —Gastroenteritis
  - —Appendicitis
  - —Inflammatory bowel disease
  - —Intussusception
  - —Meckel's diverticulum
- Arthralgias
  - —Acute rheumatic fever
  - —Polyarthritis nodosa
  - —Juvenile rheumatoid arthritis
  - —Systemic lupus erythematosus

- Rash
  - —Infection
    - -Meningococcemia
    - -Bacterial sepsis: streptococcal or staphylococcal
    - -Rocky Mountain spotted fever
    - -Infectious mononucleosis
    - -Bacterial endocarditis
    - -Viral exanthem
  - —Trauma/child abuse
  - —Functional platelet disorders
  - —Thrombocytopenia
  - —Vasculitis
  - —Erythema nodosum
  - —Drugs/toxins
- Renal disease
  - —Acute glomerulonephritis
- Testicular swelling
  - —Incarcerated hernia
  - —Orchitis
  - —Testicular torsion

Treatment

INITIAL STABILIZATION

- Intravenous fluids for shock
- Packed red blood cells for massive GI hemorrhage

ED TREATMENT

- Emergent intervention for life-threatening conditions, if any
- NSAIDs (ibuprofen)
  - —Arthralgias
- Prednisone
  - —Severe abdominal pain once life-threatening pathology excluded
  - —Painful subcutaneous edema or arthritis
  - —Renal disease (high-dose pulse therapy required)
  - —Central nervous system involvement
- Polyclonal immunoglobulin therapy
  - —Severe, life-threatening disease (controversial)

MEDICATIONS

- Ibuprofen: 600 mg (5–10 mg/kg/dose) PO q6h
- Prednisone: 60 mg (1–2 mg/kg/24 hours) PO qd for 5–7 days

Disposition

ADMISSION CRITERIA

- Severe abdominal pain
- CNS findings
- Gastrointestinal bleeding
- Intussusception
- Evidence of renal failure

DISCHARGE CRITERIA

- Normal platelet count
- Normal renal function
- Minimal or no abdominal pain
- If steroids started, follow up within 24 hours

Miscellaneous

ICD9: 287.0

ICD10: D69.0

SEE ALSO: RASH, PEDIATRIC

SUGGESTED READINGS

Causey AL, Woodall BN, Wahl NG, et al. Henoch-Schönlein purpura: four cases and a review. J Emerg Med 1994;12(3): 331–341.

Durbin DR, Liacouras CA. Gastrointestinal emergencies. In: Fleisher GR, Ludwig S, ed. Textbook of pediatric emergency medicine, 4th ed. Philadelphia: Lippincott Williams & Wilkins, 2000:1017–1041.

Hurwitz S. Clinical pediatric dermatology, 2nd ed. Philadelphia: WB Saunders, 1993:539–541.

Robson W, Leung A. Henoch-Schonlein purpura. Adv Pediatr 1994;41:163.

Rostoker G. Schonlein-Henoch purpura in children and adults. Diagnosis, pathophysiology and management. Biodrugs 2001;15(2):99–138.

Rostoker G, et al. High dose immunoglobulin therapy for severe IGA nephropathy and Henoch-Schonlein purpura. Ann Intern Med 1994;120:476.

Szer IS. Henoch-Schönlein purpura: when and how to treat. J Rheumatol 1996; 23(9):1661–1665.

Author: Mark Hostetler

Hepatic Encephalopathy

Clinical Presentation

SIGNS AND SYMPTOMS

- Wide range of mental status changes affecting behavioral, intellectual, neuromuscular function, and level of consciousness
- Symptoms and signs of associated chronic liver disease, portal hypertension, or fulminant hepatic failure (FHF)
  - —Ascites
  - —Spider angiomata
  - —Testicular atrophy
  - —Muscle wasting
  - —Easy bruising
  - —Palmar erythema
  - —Gynecomastia
- Asterixis with mild to moderate encephalopathy
- Fetor hepaticus—peculiar sweet odor

Grading (West Haven Criteria)

- Stage 0
  - —No apparent clinical changes
  - —Abnormal neurophysiologic and neuropsychological tests
- Stage I
  - —Euphoria or depression
  - —Reversal of normal sleep pattern
  - —Impairment of writing, drawing, addition, subtraction
- Stage II
  - —Lethargy
  - —Slow responses
  - —Inappropriate behavior
  - —Asterixis
  - —Slurred speech
  - —Ataxia
- Stage III
  - —Disorientation to time and place
  - —Amnesia
  - —Paranoia
  - —Nystagmus
  - —Hyperactive reflexes
  - —Positive Babinski reflex
  - —Semistupor to stupor
- Stage IV
  - —Dilated pupils
  - —Opisthion
  - —Stupor or coma

MECHANISM/DESCRIPTION

- Changes in behavior and consciousness due to collection of nitrogenous substances from hepatic insufficiency
  - —Accumulation of ammonia from
    - -Protein degradation by colonic bacteria
    - -Deamination of glutamine in small bowel
  - —Other neurotoxins
    - -Short-chain fatty acids
    - -Phenols
    - -Mercaptans
    - -Amino acids such as tryptophan
- Increased levels of inhibitory neurotransmitters:
  - —Benzodiazepines
  - —GABA
  - —Serotonin
- Decreased levels of excitatory neurotransmitters:
  - —Glutamate
  - —Dopamine
  - —Aspartate
  - —Catecholamine
- Other contributing factors to hepatic encephalopathy (HE)
  - —Decreased cerebral blood flow and oxygen
  - —Glucose consumption
  - —Zinc deficiency

ETIOLOGY

- Advanced cirrhosis or FHF with hepatocellular dysfunction often in association with portal hypertension
- Postsurgical or transjugular intrahepatic portosystemic stent/shunt (TIPS)
- Precipitating events
  - —GI bleeding (more common in elderly)
  - —Hypokalemia
  - —Alkalosis
  - —Sepsis (e.g., spontaneous bacterial peritonitis)
  - —Constipation
  - —Noncompliance with lactulose
  - —High-protein diet
  - —Hypoglycemia
  - —Hypovolemia (e.g., post-large-volume paracentesis)
  - —Azotemia (e.g., diuretic-induced)
  - —Narcotics or sedatives, including alcohol
  - —Zinc deficiency
  - —Zinc needed for normal nitrogen metabolism
  - —Hepatocellular injury
  - —Viral- or drug-induced hepatitis
  - —Recurrent encephalopathy can occur without precipitating factor

Pre-Hospital

CAUTIONS

- With advanced grades HE or associated active GI bleeding
  - —Maintain airway
  - —Aspiration precautions
  - —Provide adequate ventilation
  - —Treat hypoglycemia

Diagnosis

ESSENTIAL WORKUP

- Elicit history of liver disease and prior episodes of HE
- Clinical diagnosis—altered mental status with evidence of liver failure or portal hypertension
- Search for precipitating cause (particularly GI bleeding and sepsis)

LABORATORY

- Arterial ammonia level
  - —Increased in HE
  - —Ammonia levels $>200\ \mu g/dL$ associated with cerebral edema and herniation
  - —Level correlates poorly with the degree of HE
  - —Helpful in detecting HE in cases of altered mental status of unknown cause
  - —Normal ammonia level with suspected HE warrants search for other causes of altered mental status
  - —Serial measurements helpful in monitoring individual patients
  - —Level affected by
    - -Azotemia
    - -Infusion of amino acid solution
    - -Massive tissue breakdown
- Hemoccult testing and nasogastric lavage to rule out GI bleeding
- CBC
  - —Anemia
  - —Leukocytosis suggests infection
  - —Cultures of blood, urine, and ascitic fluid
- Electrolytes, BUN, Cr, glucose
- PT, PTT
- Liver profile/liver enzymes
- ABG
- Toxicology screen
  - —Acetaminophen and alcohol level
- TSH
- Urinalysis
- Magnesium
- Zinc level
- Viral serology

IMAGING/SPECIAL TESTS

- CXR for pneumonia and signs of CHF
- EKG for arrhythmia and electrolyte imbalance
- Head CT scan
  - —New-onset altered mental status
  - —Focal neurologic deficit
  - —Suspected trauma
  - —Cerebral edema and atrophy associated with HE
- CSF examination
  - —For new onset or unexplained worsening of HE
  - —CSF glutamine level correlates with severity of HE

DIFFERENTIAL DIAGNOSIS

- Alcohol withdrawal syndromes including delirium tremens
  - —Signs of sympathetic hyperactivity
  - —Hallucinations
  - —Anxiety
  - —Tremors
  - —Seizures
- *Asterixis* seen in other metabolic encephalopathies
  - —Uremia
  - —CO_2 narcosis
  - —CHF
  - —Sedative overdose
- Uremia
- Hypoglycemia
- Sedative use including alcohol intoxication
- Medications or drug-induced toxic confusional states
- Head trauma
- Cerebrovascular accident and neuropsychiatric disorders
- Meningitis or encephalitis

PEDIATRIC CONSIDERATIONS

- Consider Reye's syndrome early (most common cause of FHF in children) even if PT is only mildly prolonged
- Consider fatty acid β-oxidation disorder
  - —Freeze serum and urine sample for subsequent testing

Treatment

INITIAL STABILIZATION

- Advanced stages of HE
  - —Oxygen and airway protection
  - —Cardiac monitor
  - —Fluid resuscitation
  - —Naloxone, D50W (or Accucheck) and thiamine for altered mental status

ED TREATMENT

- Identification and removal of precipitating factors is key
- Treatment of complicating conditions:
  - —Acute GI bleeding
  - —Sepsis
  - —Coagulopathy
  - —Renal and electrolytes disturbances
- Avoid sedative/narcotics
  - —Use agents not metabolized by the liver
  - —Oxazepam 10–30 mg carefully titrated
- Increase nitrogen elimination
  - —Bowel cleansing with laxatives and nonabsorbable disaccharides
    - -Lactulose
  - —Ileorectal anastomosis with surgical excision of colon—rarely performed
- Decrease ammonia producing intestinal flora
  - —Neomycin (nephrotoxic and ototoxic)
  - —Metronidazole
  - —Combine with lactulose treatment
- Clean bowel with Fleet's, sorbitol, or lactulose enema
- Correct zinc deficiency with zinc acetate or sulfate
- Short-term restriction of protein intake in diet
- Flumazenil or bromocriptine in patients who have received benzodiazepines
- Occlusion of large portal-systemic shunts via ultrasound or angiography
- Precautions to prevent bodily harm to the confused patient with HE
- *Liver transplantation provides cure* for severe, spontaneous, or recurrent HE

MEDICATIONS

- Bromocriptine: 30 mg PO b.i.d. for chronic encephalopathy not responsive to other treatment
- Dextrose: D50W 1 amp (50 mL or 25 g) (peds: D25W 2–4 mL/kg) i.v.
- Flumazenil (Romazicon)
  - —Initial: 0.2 mg i.v. over 30 sec
  - —If no response: 0.3 mg i.v. after 30 sec
  - —If still no response: 0.5 mg i.v. and repeat q 30–60 sec if needed up to maximum dose of 3–5 mg
- Lactulose: 15–45 mL (peds: 0.3 mL/kg) PO or via NG tube every hour titrated to produce 2–3 soft stools per day and stool pH <5 (can also be given as enema)
- Metronidazole: 250 mg (peds: 10–30 mg/kg/d) b.i.d.—t.i.d. for 2 weeks
- Naloxone (Narcan): 0.4–2 mg (peds: 0.1 mg/kg) i.v. or i.m.
- Neomycin: 0.5 g q4–6h up to 3–6 g per day (peds: 50–100 mg/kg/24 hours) PO for 1–2 weeks
- Thiamine (vitamin B_1): 100 mg (peds: 50 mg) i.v. or i.m.
- Zinc acetate or sulfate: 220 mg PO b.i.d.

Disposition

ADMISSION CRITERIA

- HE stage II, III, or IV, or inadequate social support
- Advanced stages of HE to ICU with urgent GI consult
- Associated complicating condition (GI bleeding and sepsis)
- Uncertainty about the cause of altered mental status

DISCHARGE CRITERIA

- Known chronic or intermittent HE
- Grades 0 or I with remediable cause
- Adequate supervision at home
- Close follow-up

Miscellaneous

ICD9: 572.2

ICD10: K72.9

SEE ALSO: HEPATITIS

SUGGESTED READINGS

Blei AT, Cordoba J. Hepatic encephalopathy. Am J Gastroenterol 2001;96(7):1968–1976.

Bosch J, Bruix J, Mas A, et al. The treatment of major complications of cirrhosis. Aliment Pharmacol Ther 1994;8:639.

Jalan R, Seery JP, Taylor-Robinson SD. Pathogenesis and treatment of chronic hepatic encephalopathy. Aliment Pharmacol Ther 1996;10:681.

Marsano L, McClain C. How to manage both acute and chronic hepatic encephalopathy. J Crit Illness 1993;8:579.

Ong JP, Mullen KD. Hepatic encephalopathy. Eur J Gastroenterol Hepatol 2001;13(4):325–334.

Riordan SM, Williams R. Treatment of hepatic encephalopathy. N Engl J Med 1997;337:473–479.

Author: Anita Kulkarni

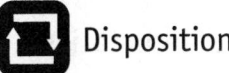

Hepatic Injury

Clinical Presentation

SIGNS AND SYMPTOMS

- Systemic signs due to acute blood loss
  - —May present with dizziness and weakness
  - —Profound hypotension or clinical shock
- Local signs include right upper quadrant tenderness, guarding, abdominal distention, rigidity, or rebound
- Contusions, abrasions, or penetrating wounds to the right chest, flank, or abdomen may be indicative of underlying hepatic injury
- Fractures of lower right ribs are commonly seen in association with hepatic injuries
- Physical exam is neither sensitive nor specific for hepatic injury

MECHANISM/DESCRIPTION

- The size of the liver alone, occupying most of the right upper quadrant, places it at significant risk for any penetrating injury
- The liver is the most frequently injured solid organ in penetrating trauma
- The position of the liver, under the lower rib cage, makes it highly susceptible to blunt injuries, either by direct blow or deceleration forces
- Mechanism of injury and kinematic forces are important factors in evaluating patients for possible hepatic injury
  - —For blunt trauma, obtain information about the forces and direction (horizontal or vertical) of any deceleration or compressive forces
  - —In penetrating trauma, the type and caliber of the weapon, distance from the weapon, and variety and length of knife or impaling object are important
- Hepatic injuries are graded by severity, ranging from subcapsular hematoma and lacerations to severe hepatic fragmentation

PEDIATRIC CONSIDERATIONS

- Poorly developed musculature and relatively smaller anterior-posterior diameter increase the vulnerability of abdominal contents to compressive forces in children
- Nonoperative management of isolated blunt hepatic trauma is widely utilized in pediatric trauma

Pre-Hospital

CAUTIONS

- Obtain details of mechanism of injury from the pre-hospital providers
- Initiate IV access as hemorrhage is major threat to life
- Penetrating wounds or evisceration should be covered with moist saline dressings
- Direct pressure should be used to control active bleeding

Diagnosis

ESSENTIAL WORKUP

- Physical exam is neither specific nor sensitive for hepatic injury
- Objective evaluation for intraperitoneal bleeding and liver injury is mandatory for significant abdominal injuries

LABORATORY

- No hematologic laboratory studies are specific for diagnosis of injury to the liver
- Obtain baseline hemoglobin
- Liver function tests are not helpful in the acute setting

IMAGING/SPECIAL TESTS

- Plain abdominal x-rays are of little value
- Bedside ultrasound is rapidly becoming the initial procedure of choice as it may detect intraabdominal fluid in the hepatorenal (Morison's) pouch as well as other findings suggestive of hepatic injury
- Diagnostic peritoneal lavage is extremely sensitive for the presence of hemoperitoneum, although nonspecific for source of bleeding
- CT scan best depicts the presence and extent of hepatic injury as well as injuries to adjacent organs
  - —Patient must be stable enough to go to the CT scanner
  - —IV contrast may demonstrate extravasation during the arterial phase of injection indicative of a vascular or high-grade liver injury requiring operative management

DIFFERENTIAL DIAGNOSIS

- Other causes of intraperitoneal injury
- Retroperitoneal injury
- Thoracic injury
- Diaphragmatic injury

Treatment

INITIAL STABILIZATION

- ABCs (including C-spine immobilization)
  - —Control airway as needed; may have associated injuries including closed head injury
  - —Supplemental oxygen, cardiac monitor, pulse oximetry
  - —Adequate IV access, including central lines and cutdowns as dictated by the patient's hemodynamic status
  - —Fluid resuscitation, initially with 2 L of crystalloid (NS or LR), followed by blood products as needed

ED TREATMENT

- Immediate laparotomy may be appropriate in the acutely injured patient who is hemodynamically unstable with presumed hemoperitoneum and hepatic injury
- Bedside US or diagnostic peritoneal lavage (DPL) may be helpful in confirming clinically suspected intraabdominal hemorrhage in the patient with blunt multiple trauma
- Gunshot wounds to the anterior abdomen are routinely explored in the OR
- Stab wounds can be managed by local wound exploration followed by US or DPL when intraperitoneal penetration is demonstrated or equivocal
- Operative versus nonoperative management
  - —Patients with frank signs of intraperitoneal hemorrhage, those with indications based on diagnostic procedures, and those who fail nonoperative management should undergo laparotomy
  - —Nonoperative management may be considered for those who are hemodynamically stable, no evidence of other intraabdominal injury, and isolated low-grade (grades 1–3) hepatic injury confirmed by imaging study, most commonly CT scan
  - —High-grade liver injuries (grades 4–5) have less successful nonoperative rates
  - —Selective use of angiography with embolization in patients with persistent bleeding may decrease the need for operative management
  - —All patients with suspected hepatic injury should remain NPO with strict bed rest

Disposition

ADMISSION CRITERIA

- All patients with hepatic injury require hospitalization for definitive laparotomy or observation with serial exams and hematocrit determinations
- ICU admission is usually indicated in the first 48 hours after injury

DISCHARGE CRITERIA

- Patients with hepatic injuries should not be discharged

Miscellaneous

ICD9: 864.00

ICD10: S36.1

SUGGESTED READINGS

Croce MA, et al. Nonoperative management of blunt hepatic trauma is the treatment of choice for hemodynamically stable patients. Ann Surg 1995;221(6): 744–755.

Jacobs IA. Nonoperative management of blunt splenic and hepatic trauma in the pediatric population. Am Surg 2001;67(2): 149–154.

Leone RT Jr. Nonoperative management of pediatric blunt hepatic trauma. Am Surg 2001;67(2):138–142.

Marx J. Abdominal trauma. In: Rosen P, et al., eds. Emergency medicine: concepts and clinical practice, 5th ed. St. Louis: CV Mosby, 2002:415–436.

Ochsner MG, Jaffin JH, Golocovsky M, et al. Major hepatic trauma. Surg Clin North Am 1993;73(2):337–352.

Pachter HL, Liang HG, Hofstetter SR. Liver and biliary tract trauma. In: Felicano D, et al., eds. Trauma, 3rd ed. Stamford, CT: Appleton and Lange, 1996:487–524.

Townsend CM. Abdominal trauma. In: Towsend CM, Beauchamp DR, Evers MB, Mattox KL, eds. Sabiston textbook of surgery, 16th ed. Philadelphia: WB Saunders, 2001:336–338.

Author: Sean Deitch

Hepatitis

Clinical Presentation

SIGNS AND SYMPTOMS

- Often asymptomatic and subclinical
- Preicteric phase
  —Flu-like illness with fever, chills, malaise
  —Nausea, vomiting, anorexia
  —Aversion to smoking or certain foods
  —60% remain anicteric
- Icteric phase
  —Tender hepatomegaly
  —Jaundice
  —Pruritus
  —Dark urine
- May present in fulminant hepatic failure (FHF), with ascites or hepatic encephalopathy (HE)
- FHF in:
  —2% of hepatitis B (HBV)
  —3% of hepatitis D (HDV) co-infection with HBV
  —30% of HDV superinfection or chronic HBV
  —0.2% of hepatitis A (HAV)
  —1% of hepatitis E (HEV)
  —Up to 20% of pregnant women with HEV
- Chronic viral hepatitis
  —Often asymptomatic or nonspecific symptom
  —Abnormal liver tests
  —With hepatitis C/C-GB and B (with or without HDV)
  —May first present as cirrhosis or hepatocellular carcinoma
- Extrahepatic manifestation of HCV or HBV
  —Urticaria/angioedema
  —Porphyria
  —Polyarteritis nodosa
  —Synovitis
  —Glomerulonephritis

MECHANISM/DESCRIPTION

- A (HAV)
  —Incubation 2–6 weeks
  —Blood product transmission rarely occurs
  —Enteric transmission occurs
  —No sexual transmission
  —Body fluid transmission very rarely occurs
- B (HBV)
  —Incubation 12–26 weeks
  —Blood product transmission occurs
  —Enteric transmission occurs
  —Sexual transmission occurs
  —Body fluid transmission occurs
- C (HCV/C-GB)
  —Incubation 6–7 weeks
  —Blood product transmission occurs
  —No enteric transmission
  —Sexual transmission rarely occurs
  —No body fluid transmission
- E (HEV)
  —Incubation 2–6 weeks
  —Blood product transmission rarely occurs
  —Enteric transmission occurs
  —No sexual transmission
  —No body fluid transmission
- D (HDV)
  —Incubation 4–7 weeks
  —Blood product transmission occurs as co-infection/superinfection with HBV
  —Enteric transmission occurs
  —No sexual transmission
  —No body fluid transmission
- Primary hepatitis viruses (A, B, C/C-GB, D, and E)
  —Account for 95% of cases
  —Attack primarily the liver
- Secondary hepatitis viruses
  —Involve the liver in the course of infection of other organs
- In acute hepatitis, liver biopsy shows hepatocellular necrosis and mononuclear infiltrate
- Toxins and drugs cause hepatocellular necrosis

ETIOLOGY

- Hepatitis A
  —Fecal/oral transmission
- Hepatitis C/C-GB
  —Unknown mode of transmission in one fourth of patients
- Secondary hepatitis viruses
  —Epstein-Barr, cytomegalovirus, herpes viruses, HIV, adenovirus, Coxsackie
  —Seen mostly in immune-compromised host
- Toxin induced
  —Drugs
    -Ethanol
    -Acetaminophen
    -Isoniazid
    -Azathioprine
    -Chemotherapeutics
  —Chemicals
    -Industrial solvents
    -Cleaning solutions

PEDIATRIC CONSIDERATIONS

- Majority of cases are hepatitis A
- Usually subclinical
- Up to 90% of newborns of HB_sAg-positive mothers (especially if HB_eAg is positive) develop chronic HBV

Pre-Hospital

N/A

Diagnosis

ESSENTIAL WORKUP

- Detailed history for *risk factors* for hepatitis, including possible toxic exposure and drug overdose
- Clinical picture consistent with hepatitis

LABORATORY

- Electrolytes, BUN, Cr, glucose
  —Azotemia with hepatorenal syndrome
  —Hypoglycemia with severe liver damage
- Urinalysis
  —Dark-tea colored
  —+ Bilirubin
- CBC for:
  —Leukopenia
  —Thrombocytopenia
  —Aplastic anemia is a rare complication of HBV and HCV

Liver Function Tests

- Liver enzymes
  —Elevation reflects injury
  —AST and ALT increased 10–1,000 times
  —Degree of elevation does not correlate with severity
  —Lower enzyme elevation in chronic hepatitis
- Alkaline phosphatase
  —Mild to moderate elevation except in the less common cholestatic form (seen with HAV)
- Conjugated bilirubin
  —Mild to moderate elevation
- Prolongation of INR/PT reflects more severe diseases
- Serum albumin, globulin

Viral Serology

- Hepatitis A
  —IgM anti-HAV—excellent marker for acute infection
  —IgG anti-HAV—previous exposure and immunity
- Hepatitis B
  —Acute hepatitis B
    -HB_sAg may or may not be positive
    -IgM anti-HB_c—almost always positive
  —Chronic hepatitis
    -HB_sAg-positive
    -Positive HB_eAg indicates active viral replication and high infectivity
    -Negative HB_eAg indicates low viral replication or a carrier state if liver enzymes and histology are normal
  —HB_s antibody (titer of >10 mIU/mL)—reflects immunity
  —Isolated presence of IgG anti-HB_c (with all other serologic markers negative) reflects remote infection with hepatitis B or rarely false-positive test

- Hepatitis C
  - —ELISA II is negative in the acute stage but viral RNA (by PCR) is usually positive
  - —ELISA III, RIBA II, or viral RNA (tested by PCR) may be used to confirm the diagnosis
  - —Only a few laboratories can test for HC-GB viral RNA
- Hepatitis D
  - —Hepatitis D antibody (IgM or IgG) or viral RNA
- Hepatitis E
  - —Hepatitis E antibody (IgM or IgG) or viral RNA

Additional Testing

- α-Fetoprotein—every 12 months for surveillance for hepatocellular carcinoma in long-standing hepatitis B or C/C-GB
- Monospot—for Epstein-Barr virus

IMAGING/SPECIAL TESTS

- Head CT scan in cases of hepatic encephalopathy
- RUQ US for biliary obstruction

DIFFERENTIAL DIAGNOSIS

- Drug- or toxin-induced hepatitis: isoniazid, acetaminophen, α-methyldopa, amiodarone, valproate, phenytoin, halothane, cocaine
- Ischemic or hypoxic hepatitis: hypotension, hypoxemia, or CHF
- Alcoholic hepatitis
  - —Elevation of AST is 2–3 times more than ALT
  - —Elevation is usually less than 300 units
  - —Encephalopathy, high bilirubin, and prolonged PT indicate poor prognosis
- Autoimmune hepatitis
- Wilson's disease (adolescents)
- Pregnancy-associated hepatitis
  - —HELLP syndrome
  - —Acute fatty liver of pregnancy
- Reye's syndrome
- Infectious mononucleosis

Treatment

INITIAL STABILIZATION

- ABCs for fulminant hepatic failure
- Naloxone, thiamine, glucose (or Accucheck) for altered mental status

ED TREATMENT

- Treat hypovolemia with IV 0.9% NS
- Correct electrolyte imbalance
- Control vomiting with metoclopramide or trimethobenzamide
- Avoid hepatotoxic agents, or those metabolized in the liver (phenothiazines, alcohol, and acetaminophen)
- Vitamin K 10 mg s.c. (give daily for 3 days) if PT is prolonged
- Ursodeoxycholic acid or cholestyramine for cholestasis-induced itching

Contact Immunoprophylaxis

- Hepatitis A
  - —Immune globulin 0.02 mL/kg i.m. (within 2 weeks of exposure)
  - —For household, day care, or institutional contacts
    - -HAV vaccine 1 mL (peds: 2–17 years: 0.5 mL) i.m., repeated in 6 months
    - -Complete 2 weeks before expected exposure (e.g., travel)
- Hepatitis B
  - —Hepatitis B immune globulin 0.06 mL/kg i.m.
    - -Within 10 days of HBV exposure
    - -Sexual contact, percutaneous, transmucosal exposure
  - —HBV vaccine 1 mL (peds: 0.5 mL) i.m. given at 0, 1, and 6 months
    - -For infants and children; particularly newborns of HB_sAg-positive mothers
    - -Post-HBV exposure
- Hepatitis C: no vaccine or effective immune prophylaxis
- Hepatitis D: prevent HBV
- Hepatitis E: no vaccine or effective immune prophylaxis
  - —Interferon s.c. 3 times a week
    - -For chronic hepatitis B: 10 million units (6 million units/m^2) for 4–6 months
    - -For chronic hepatitis C: 3 million units (3 million units/m^2) for 12 months

MEDICATIONS

- Cholestyramine: 4 g PO 1–6 times/day
- Dextrose: D50W 1 amp (50 mL or 25 g) (peds: D25W 2–4 mL/kg) i.v.
- Metoclopramide (Reglan): 10 mg i.v./i.m. q6–8h PRN; 10–30 mg PO q.i.d.
- Naloxone (Narcan): 2 mg (peds: 0.1 mg/kg) i.v. or i.m. initial dose
- Thiamine (vitamin B_1): 100 mg (peds: 50 mg) i.v. or i.m.
- Trimethobenzamide (Tigan): 250 mg PO t.i.d.–q.i.d.; 200 mg i.m./PR q6–8h (peds: 100–200 mg/dose if >15 kg)
- Ursodeoxycholic acid: 8–10 mg/kg/24 hours t.i.d.

Disposition

ADMISSION CRITERIA

- Intractable vomiting, dehydration, or electrolyte imbalance not responding to ED treatment
- Acute hepatitis with evidence of liver dysfunction
  - —INR >1.5 or PT >3 seconds above control
  - —Bilirubin >20 mg/dL
  - —Hypoglycemia
  - —Albumin <2.5 g/dL
- ICU admission for fulminant hepatic failure
- Hepatic encephalopathy
- Pregnancy, immunocompromised host, or possible toxic hepatitis

DISCHARGE CRITERIA

- Outpatient management usual
- Food handlers with enteric pathogens should not return to work as long as they are infectious

Miscellaneous

ICD9: 573.3

ICD10: K75.9

SEE ALSO: HEPATIC ENCEPHALOPATHY

SUGGESTED READINGS

Bondesson JD, Saperston AR. Hepatitis. Emerg Med Clin North Am 1996;14: 695–718.

Lemon SM, Thomas DL. Vaccines to prevent viral hepatitis. N Engl J Med 1997;336:196.

Sjogren M. Serologic diagnosis of viral hepatitis. Med Clin North Am 1996; 80:929.

Wolf JL. Liver disease in pregnancy. Med Clin North Am 1996;80:1167.

Author: Stuart Feldman

Hepatorenal Syndrome

Clinical Presentation

SIGNS AND SYMPTOMS

- Signs of acute or chronic liver disease
- Signs of portal hypertension
- Ascites, often tense
- Progressive oliguria
- Jaundice or hepatic encephalopathy
- Coagulopathy
- Tachycardia
- Hypotension

MECHANISM/DESCRIPTION

- Renal failure (RF) in patients with acute or chronic liver disease with no other identifiable cause of renal pathology
  —Type I hepatorenal syndrome (HRS)
    -Acute form with spontaneous RF in patients with liver disease
    -Rapidly progressive
    -80% mortality within 2 weeks
    -Seen with acute liver failure or alcoholic hepatitis
  —Type II HRS
    -Slow course of RF
    -Seen in patients with diuretic resistant ascites
    -Lower mortality rate than type I HRS
- Hallmarks of HRS
  —Reversible renal vasoconstriction and mild systemic hypotension
  —Kidneys have normal histology and structure
- Liver disease causes systemic vasodilation with decrease in arterial blood volume:
  —Reflex activation of sympathetic nervous system
  —Activation of renin-angiotensin-aldosterone system (RAAS)
  —Stimulation of numerous vasoactive substances
    -Nitric oxide
    -Prostacyclin
    -Atrial natriuretic peptide (ANP)
    -Arachidonic acid metabolites
    -Platelet-activating factor
    -Endothelins
    -Catecholamines
    -Angiotensin II
    -Thromboxane
- Action of vasoconstrictors prevails over vasodilator effects
  —Renal hypoperfusion ensues due to renal cortical vasoconstriction
  —Decrease in renal blood flow and glomerular filtration rates

ETIOLOGY

- Chronic liver disease, especially alcoholic
- Fulminant hepatic failure
- Precipitating factors
  —Decreased effective blood volume
    -GI bleeding
    -Vigorous diuresis
    -Large-volume paracentesis
  —Use of nephrotoxic agent
    -NSAIDs
    -Aminoglycoside
  —Sepsis

Pre-Hospital

CAUTIONS

- Attention to hypotension, active GI bleeding, respiratory distress

Diagnosis

ESSENTIAL WORKUP

- Azotemia in setting of liver disease
- Identify any precipitating factors

LABORATORY

- CBC
  —Anemia due to GI bleed
- Electrolytes
  —Hyperkalemia
  —Acidosis
- Elevated BUN, Cr
  —Normal Cr found with low GFR in association with muscle wasting, poor nutrition, and ascites
  —Cr increased by some medications (cimetidine, trimethoprim, and spironolactone) due to inhibition of tubular secretion of creatinine
  —Hyperbilirubinemia can artifactually lower serum creatinine
- Glucose
- PT, PTT
- Urinalysis
  —Absence of casts from acute tubular necrosis (ATN)
  —Check for UTI
- Spot urine sodium and creatinine, and serum and urine osmolality
  —Spot urine Na^+ <10 mEq/L
  —Fractional excretion of Na^+ <1%
  —Urine/plasma creatinine >30:1
  —Hyperosmolar urine
- Blood, ascitic fluid, and urine culture as indicated
- Urinary excretion of β_2-microglobulin—useful marker of acute tubular damage

IMAGING/SPECIAL TESTS

- CXR for signs of CHF or fluid overload
- EKG for dysrhythmia or signs of hyperkalemia
- Renal ultrasound: for obstruction as etiology
- Central venous pressure (CVP) measurements
  —Differentiates prerenal (low) from HRS (elevated)

DIFFERENTIAL DIAGNOSIS

- ATN
  —Urine sodium >30 mEq/L
  —Urine osmolality equals plasma osmolality
  —Urine casts and cellular debris
- Prerenal azotemia
  —Urine output improves following correction of hypovolemia
- Obstruction
- Interstitial nephritis
- Post-liver transplant renal dysfunction due to:
  —HRS due to failure of transplanted liver
  —Medications, e.g., cyclosporine
  —Preexisting renal disease
  —Perioperative hypovolemia

Treatment

INITIAL STABILIZATION

- ABCs
- Aggressive correction of hypovolemia with
  - —0.9% NS IV fluid
  - —Colloid volume expanders: 100 g albumin in 500 mL of normal saline
  - —Closely monitor clinical status including use of CVP
  - —Urine output should improve with prerenal azotemia
- Manage life-threatening emergencies of renal failure
  - —Hyperkalemia
  - —Severe acidosis

ED TREATMENT

- Exclude reversible or treatable causes of HRS
- Supportive care until hepatic function recovers
- *Do no harm*—discontinue potentially nephrotoxic agents
  - —NSAIDs
  - —Aminoglycosides
  - —Demeclocycline
- Search for and treat coexisting renal disease
- Correct electrolyte imbalances
- Treat any associated cardiopulmonary disorder and hypoxia
- Initiate broad-spectrum antibiotics if sepsis suspected
- Correct liver associated complications
  - —Obstructive jaundice
  - —Hepatic encephalopathy
  - —Hypoglycemia
- Large-volume paracentesis with IV albumin replacement (to relieve tense ascites)
  - —Increases renal blood flow
  - —May briefly improve HRS
- Dialysis
  - —Useful in correcting fluid, electrolytes, acid-base imbalances, pulmonary edema
  - —Indicated for patients who have a likelihood of hepatic regeneration, hepatic recovery, or liver transplantation
- Liver transplant
  - —Only available cure

MEDICATIONS

- Dopamine (renal dose): 2–5 μg/kg/min
  - —May improve renal function
  - —Not curative
- Midodrine and octreotide
  - —Octreotide is analogue of somatostatin
  - —Midodrine is a sympathomimetic drug
- Misoprostol: 0.4 mg PO q.i.d.
  - —Synthetic analogue of prostaglandin E_1
- Ornipressin: 2-hour infusion at 6 IU/h
  - —Vasopressin analogue
  - —Increases renal perfusion pressure and function
- Terlipressin: 2 mg/day for 2 days
  - —Synthetic analogue of vasopressin
  - —Intrinsic vasoconstrictor activity

Disposition

ADMISSION CRITERIA

- All suspected HRS with GI and nephrology consults
- ICU admission for associated cardiopulmonary disease, hepatic encephalopathy, marked electrolyte imbalances

DISCHARGE CRITERIA

- None

Miscellaneous

ICD9: 572.4

ICD10: K76.7

SEE ALSO: HEPATIC ENCEPHALOPATHY AND HEPATITIS

SUGGESTED READINGS

Badalamenti S, Graziani G, Salerno F, et al. Hepatorenal syndrome. Arch Intern Med 1993;153:1957.

Dagher L, Moore K. The hepatorenal syndrome. Gut 2001;49(5):729–737.

Forrest EH, Jalan R, Hayes PC. Renal and circulatory changes in cirrhosis—pathogenesis and therapeutic perspective. Aliment Pharmacol Ther 1996;10:219.

Gentilini P, Vizzutti F, et al. Ascites and hepatorenal syndrome. Eur J Gastroenterol Hepatol 2001;13:313–316.

Roberts LR, Kamath PS. Ascites and hepatorenal syndrome: Pathophysiology and management. Mayo Clin Proc 1996;71:874.

Author: Anita Kulkarni

Hernia

Clinical Presentation

SIGNS AND SYMPTOMS

General

- Pain/swelling
  - —Localized to region of hernia
- Constant pain, vomiting, fever may indicate
  - —Incarceration
  - —Strangulation
  - —Obstruction

Inguinal Hernia

- Pain
  - —Localized to inguinal region
  - —Exacerbated by straining/positional changes
  - —Relieved by rest
- Swelling
  - —Males: intermittent bulge in scrotum
  - —Females: bulge immediately inferior to inguinal ligament or in labia
- Swelling of spermatic cord, scrotum, or testes
- Valsalva maneuver done while finger directed toward internal ring—may allow hernia sac to descend against finger

Femoral Hernia

- Pain/swelling
  - —Localized to femoral orifice inferior to inguinal ligament

Incisional Hernia

- Pain/swelling
  - —Localized to previous incision/scar

Obturator Hernia

- Nonspecific abdominal pain
- Intermittent intestinal obstruction
- Weight loss
- Pain
  - —Due to pressure on obturator nerve from hernia (Howship-Romberg sign)
  - —Along medial thigh
  - —Radiating to hip
  - —Relieved with thigh flexion
  - —Exacerbated by hip extension, adduction, or external rotation

Spigelian Hernia

- Abdominal pain/mass along anterior abdominal wall
- Increased pain with maneuvers increasing intraabdominal pressure
- Intermittent bowel obstruction
- Palpable mass along spigelian line
  - —Convex line extending from costal arch to pubic tubercle along lateral edge of rectus muscle

MECHANISM/DESCRIPTION

- Abnormal protrusion of peritoneal contents through a defect in the abdominal wall
- Incarceration
  - —When contents in hernia sac cannot be manipulated back into abdomen
- Strangulation
  - —Compromise of vascular supply to bowel contained in hernia leading to ischemia and gangrene
  - —Tender irreducible hernia with nausea/vomiting, fever, leukocytosis

ETIOLOGY

- Indirect inguinal hernia
  - —Results from persistent process vaginalis
  - —Herniation of peritoneal contents through internal ring
  - —Right side more common than left
- Direct inguinal hernia
  - —Due to defect or weakness in transversalis area in Hesselbach's triangle
    - -Inguinal ligament inferiorly
    - -Inferior epigastric vessels laterally
    - -Lateral border of rectus abdominus medially
  - —Herniation through Hesselbach's triangle
- Incisional hernia
  - —Resultant breakdown of surgical fascial closure
  - —Herniation through surgical fascia
- Femoral hernia
  - —Peritoneum herniates into the femoral canal beneath the inguinal ligament
- Obturator hernia
  - —Passes through obturator membrane and exits beneath pectineal muscle
- Umbilical hernia
  - —Failure of umbilical ring closure
  - —Herniation through umbilical ring/umbilicus

PEDIATRIC CONSIDERATIONS

- Diagnosis difficult
  - —Parents complain of a bulge in inguinal area often no longer present at time of exam
  - —Incarcerated hernias may present with irritability, abdominal pain, or intermittent vomiting
- Incidence of incarceration/strangulation is 10–20%
  - —Greater than 50% occurring in patients less than 6 months of age
- Incidence of incarceration higher in girls than boys
- Umbilical hernias
  - —Strangulation and incarceration rare
  - —Majority close spontaneously
  - —Most surgeons will delay closure until age 4

Pre-Hospital

N/A

Diagnosis

ESSENTIAL WORKUP

- Diagnosis based on history and careful clinical exam
  - —Palpate inguinal/femoral area for tenderness/masses
  - —Repeat examination while standing/straining

LABORATORY

- CBC
  - —Leukocytosis with strangulation
- Electrolytes, BUN/Cr, glucose
  - —If vomiting/dehydration
- Urinalysis
  - —For identifying GU causes of groin pain

IMAGING/SPECIAL TESTS

- Plain abdominal radiographs
  - —Bowel obstructive pattern with incarceration or strangulation
- Ultrasound
  - —For identifying testicular source of scrotal swelling

DIFFERENTIAL DIAGNOSIS

- Hydrocele
- Varicocele
- Lymphadenitis
- Testicular torsion
- Testicular tumor
- Undescended testis
- Lymphogranuloma venereum

Treatment

INITIAL STABILIZATION

- 0.9% NS IV fluid resuscitation when bowel strangulation, obstruction, or sepsis
  - —Adults: 1 L bolus
  - —Children: 20 cc/kg

ED TREATMENT

Incarceration Irreducible/Strangulation

- IVF
- Nasogastric tube
- Immediate surgical consultation
- Preoperative antibiotics for strangulated hernia

Hernia Reduction Method

- Intravenous sedation (benzodiazepine) and analgesia (opiate)
- Place in Trendelenburg position
- Allow 20–30 minutes for spontaneous reduction of hernia
- Manual reduction
  - —Place constant, gentle pressure on hernia
  - —For inguinal hernias, achieve reduction by putting fingers of one hand on internal ring while gently pulling then pressing on hernia distal to external ring
- Obtain surgical consultation if reduction is unsuccessful after one or two attempts
- Contraindications to reduction include:
  - —Fever
  - —Leukocytosis
- Complications
  - —Reduction of strangulated bowel into abdomen
    - -Further ischemia/necrosis occurs with no clinical improvement

MEDICATIONS

- Cefoxitin: 1–2 g q6–8h (peds: 0–7 d, 40 mg/kg/24 hours q12h; >7 d, 80–160 mg/kg/24 hours q6h) i.v. PB
- Fentanyl: 1–4 μg/kg IVP
- Meperidine (Demerol): 25-mg increments (peds: 1 mg/kg) i.v. PRN
- Midazolam (Versed): 2.5–5 mg (peds: 0.07 mg/kg) i.v.
- Morphine sulfate: 2–4 mg increments (peds: 0.1 mg/kg) i.v. PRN

PEDIATRIC CONSIDERATIONS

- Reduction in girls is harder since ovary may be wrapped in hernia

Disposition

ADMISSION CRITERIA

- Strangulated hernias require immediate surgical intervention
- Incarcerated hernias require admission for urgent surgical intervention
- Intestinal obstruction
- Peritonitis
- Vomiting
- Severe pain

DISCHARGE CRITERIA

- After successful reduction has been achieved
- Scheduled reevaluation in 24 hours and referral to surgery

Miscellaneous

ICD9: 553.9

ICD10: K46.9

SUGGESTED READINGS

Mensching JJ, Musielewicz AJ. Abdominal wall hernias. Emerg Med Clin North Am 1996;14(4):739–756.

Miller PA, Mezwa DG, Feczko PJ, et al. Imaging of abdominal hernias. Radiographics 1995;15(2):333–347.

Townsend. Sabiston textbook of surgery, 16th ed. Philadelphia: WB Saunders, 2001:783–800.

Author: Julio Silva

Herpes Simplex

Clinical Presentation

SIGNS AND SYMPTOMS

- HSV causes six common syndromes (orofacial, genital, CNS, neonatal, skin, and ophthalmic) presenting as either primary or recurrent disease
- Each syndrome has unique presentations, although some common signs and symptoms
  —Classically presents with grouped 1–3 mm vesicles on an erythematous base
  —Vesicles may be filled with clear or cloudy fluid, or may appear as frank pustules

Orofacial Infection

- Primary infection
  —Fever, malaise, irritability, and myalgias
  —Cervical adenopathy
  —Gingivostomatitis or pharyngitis
  —Inability to eat due to pain
- Recurrent infection
  —Usually involves lips, specifically the vermilion border
  —Commonly incited by sunlight, heat, stress, trauma, or immunosuppression
  —Prodrome of itching, tingling, throbbing, or burning

Genital Infection

See Herpes, Genital

CNS/Encephalitis

- Acute onset of fever, altered mental status, and focal neurologic deficits
- Patient may have olfactory hallucinations (noxious smell) secondary to temporal lobe involvement
- Complication of either primary or recurrent disease
- Ages 5–30 and age >50 most commonly affected

Neonatal Infections—Three Syndromes

- Skin, eye, mouth disease
  —Vesicular lesions appear on presenting birth part (usually face, eyes, mouth), or areas such as scalp monitor sites
- CNS disease
  —Cranial nerve abnormalities; focal and generalized seizures
  —Apnea and bradycardia
  —May or may not develop skin lesions
  —Presents in second to third week of life
- Disseminated disease
  —Any organ system may be involved
  —Presents in first week of life

Skin

- Includes herpetic whitlow and herpes gladiatorum, eczema herpeticum, Darier's and Sézary's syndromes, and erythema multiforme
- History of exposure to HSV-1 or HSV-2
- Abrupt-onset fever, edema, erythema, and localized tenderness

Eye

- Caused by extension of facial lesions or direct inoculation
- Acute onset of pain and photophobia, blurring of vision, chemosis, and conjunctivitis; may be unilateral or bilateral
- Dendritic lesions of cornea noted on fluorescein exam
- Different from herpes varicella-zoster as dermatome not involved

MECHANISM/DESCRIPTION

- Viral disease characterized by recurrent painful vesicular lesions of mucocutaneous areas
- Lips, genitalia, rectum, hands, and eyes most commonly involved
- Characterized by latency and reactivation
- Incubation period is approximately 4 days from exposure
- Viral shedding occurs from 7–10 days (up to 23 days) in primary infection
- 70% of untreated patients die and only 2.5% return to normal neurologic function with CNS involvement
- Neonatal infections can occur in utero, intrapartum, or postnatal; occurs in 1 in 2,000–5,000 births/year in U.S.

ETIOLOGY

- Herpes simplex type I (HSV-1) or type 2 (HSV-2), both DNA viruses of the Herpesviridae family
- Virus transmission occurs through mucosa or abraded skin
- Both viruses infect oral or genital mucosa, predilection of HSV-1 with orofacial infection and HSV-2 with genital infection

PEDIATRIC CONSIDERATIONS

- See Neonatal Infections—Three Syndromes, above
- Primary maternal HSV infection will result in CNS or disseminated disease in 70% of exposed neonates
- Vesicular skin lesions may or may not be present on initial exam
- Orofacial disease is most likely to present as gingivostomatitis in children less than 5 years
- Whitlow may be caused by thumb-sucking children with oral herpes

Pre-Hospital

CAUTIONS

- Maintain universal precautions

Diagnosis

ESSENTIAL WORKUP

- Orofacial
  —Presumptive diagnosis made by history and exam
  —If definitive diagnosis is necessary (e.g., systemic disease, child abuse)
    -Viral culture of vesicles
    -Fluorescent antibody detection of antigen; serum antibody studies
    -Scrapings for Tzanck smear or Papanicolaou stain
- Encephalitis
  —CT or MRI
  —Lumbar puncture with CSF pleocytosis and negative bacterial antigens
  —CSF polymerase chain reaction (PCR)
  —EEG diagnostic if spike and slow waves in temporal region
- Neonatal
  —*All* neonatal disease mandates complete workup because progression to systemic disease is likely
  —CT or MRI, EEG, and lumbar puncture
  —Liver function studies and chest x-ray
- Eye
  —Dendritic corneal lesions by fluorescein exam
  —Swab of affected area for viral culture or fluorescent antibody detection

LABORATORY

- Lesion scrapings
  —Virus isolation by tissue culture or fluorescent antibody provides isolate that can be typed
  —Tzanck smear demonstrating *multinucleated giant cells*, atypical keratinocytes, and large nuclei
- Serum testing has limited ED utility
  —ELISA testing may demonstrate HSV antibodies, determining past exposure only
  —Require from 2 weeks to >3 months to detect seroconversion
  —New tests distinguishing HSV-1 from HSV-2 are now available
- CSF
  —Polymerase chain reaction (PCR) is preferred diagnostic method; 100% specific, 75–98% sensitive
  —CSF will remain PCR positive up to 1 week in infected patients

DIFFERENTIAL DIAGNOSIS

- Orofacial and skin
  - —Bacterial pharyngitis
  - —Mycoplasma pneumoniae pharyngitis
  - —Stevens-Johnson syndrome
  - —Herpes zoster
  - —Varicella
  - —Pemphigus
  - —Contact or chemical dermatitis
  - —Impetigo
- Encephalitis/meningitis
  - —Bacterial, viral, fungal, tuberculous, parasitic, or vasculitic
  - —Cerebrovascular accident
  - —Brain tumor
- Neonatal
  - —Sepsis of any etiology
- Eye
  - —Conjunctivitis: viral, bacterial, or allergic
  - —Herpes zoster ophthalmicus
  - —Scleritis/episcleritis
  - —Angle-closure glaucoma

Treatment

INITIAL STABILIZATION

- Protect airway in comatose or obtunded patients with suspected CNS disease
- Parenteral antiviral is indicated for neonatal HSV, encephalitis, and severe infections in immunocompromised patients

ED TREATMENT

- Orofacial/gingivostomatitis
  - —Primary disease in children: oral acyclovir
  - —Primary disease in normal host with mild disease:
    - -Supportive treatment with hydration and topical anesthetics (viscous lidocaine, diphenhydramine elixir)
    - -Recommendations exist for penciclovir, or famciclovir with or without fluocinonide
  - —Severe disease or immunocompromised patients: IV or oral acyclovir, valacyclovir, or famciclovir
- Encephalitis
  - —Acyclovir IV is the drug of choice
- Neonatal
  - —All syndromes treated with intravenous acyclovir
- Skin (other than orofacial or genital)
  - —May be treated with oral acyclovir
  - —Antibiotics if secondary bacterial infection occurs
  - —*Do not incise and drain,* may lead to spread of infection
- Eye
  - —Topical antiviral therapy with trifluridine
  - —Vidarabine ointment for children
  - —*Do not treat with steroids,* may cause increased viral replication
  - —Suppressive therapy with oral acyclovir
  - —Consult with ophthalmology

MEDICATIONS

- Acyclovir
  - —Orofacial: adults: 400 mg PO t.i.d. for 10–14 days or 5 mg/kg i.v. (infused over 1 hour) q8h for 7–14 days; peds (primary infection): 15 mg/kg PO 5×/d for 7 days
  - —Encephalitis: adults: 10–15 mg/kg i.v. (infused over 1 hour) q8h for 14–21 days; peds (3 mo–12 y/o): 10–20 mg/kg i.v. q8h for 14–21 days; neonatal (0–3 months): 10 mg/kg i.v. q8h
  - —Skin (not orofacial or genital): adults: 400 mg PO t.i.d. for 10 days; peds: 20 mg/kg PO t.i.d. for 10 days
  - —Eyes: For suppression therapy 400 mg PO b.i.d.
- Famciclovir: for orofacial/ immunocompromised host 250–500 mg PO t.i.d. for 5 days
- Fluocinonides: adults: topical 0.05% gel q8h for 5 days
- Penciclovir: adults: topical 1% cream applied q2h while awake for 4 days
- Trifluridine: adults and peds: 1 drop of 1% ophthalmic solution to eye q2h while awake (max. 9 drops per day) for 14–21 days
- Valacyclovir: adults: 500–1,000 mg PO b.i.d. for 7 days (not FDA approved)
- Vidarabine: adults or peds: topical 0.5-inch ribbon of 3% ophthalmic ointment to eye 5 times per day

Disposition

ADMISSION CRITERIA

- Encephalitis, disseminated disease, dehydration
- Severe local or disseminated disease in immunocompromised host
- Neonatal HSV
  - —ICU vs. ward based on toxicity and need for airway support

DISCHARGE CRITERIA

- Uncomplicated local disease

Miscellaneous

ICD9: 054.9

ICD10: B00.9

SEE ALSO: HERPES, GENITAL

SUGGESTED READINGS

Annunziato PW, Gershon A. Herpes simplex virus infections. Pediatr Rev 1996;17: 415–423.

Barequest IS, O'Brien TP. Ocular infections: update on therapy. Ophthalmol Clin North Am 1999;12:63–69.

Miller CS, Redding SW. Diagnosis and management of orofacial herpes simplex virus infections. Dent Clin North Am 1992;36:879–895.

Whitley RJ, Lakeman FL. Herpes simplex virus infections of the central nervous system: therapeutic and diagnostic considerations. Clin Infect Dis 1995;20: 414–420.

Whitley RJ, Roizman B. Herpes simplex virus infections. Lancet 2001;357: 1513–1518.

Authors: Susan C. Zapalac; Mark G. Richmond

Herpes Zoster

Clinical Presentation

SIGNS AND SYMPTOMS

- Prodrome of pain and paresthesias in a dermatomal distribution
  —Character of pain may be sharp, dull, tingling, burning, or intense pruritus
  —Pain precedes rash by 1–10 days
  —Young patients are less likely to have a prodrome
- Classical rash is grouped vesicles on an erythematous base
  —The lesions begin as patches of erythema
  —Vesicles rapidly follow erythema
  —Initially appear clear, become cloudy, progress to scab and crust formation over 10–12 days
  —Crusts fall off in 2–3 weeks
  —Lesions evolve synchronously, as opposed to primary varicella, in which lesions of varying stages of development are pathognomonic
  —One dermatome typically affected, rarely crosses midline
  —Most common nerve distributions are the second thoracic to second lumbar, followed by trigeminal and cervical
- Ocular involvement occurs in half of cases involving the ophthalmic division of the trigeminal nerve
  —Closely associated with disease occurring at the tip of the nose or the eyelid
  —Corneal involvement is most common, beginning as a punctate keratitis, which may coalesce to form a pseudodendritic or stellate pattern
- Disseminated disease may cause signs and symptoms of meningoencephalitis, myelitis, peripheral neuropathy, and hepatic disease
- Immunosuppressed patients generally have similar signs and symptoms, but of greater severity

MECHANISM/DESCRIPTION

- Commonly known as "shingles," may be referred to as "dermatomal zoster" or "zona"
- Most common in 50- to 80-year-old patients
- Disease disseminates in 1–2% of normal hosts and frequently in immunocompromised hosts
- *Ramsay Hunt syndrome* is characterized by zoster oticus, peripheral facial palsy, regional adenopathy, vertigo, and anesthesia of the anterior two thirds of the hemitongue
  —Secondary to seventh and eighth cranial nerve involvement
- Postherpetic neuralgia (PHN) is a complication of zoster
  —Described as pain that persists at the site of zoster lesions for more than 1 month after the cutaneous disease has healed
  —10–70% of patients will have pain after resolution of lesions
  —Incidence increases with age
- Syndrome of identical signs and symptoms as herpes zoster occurring without rash is called *zoster sine herpete*

ETIOLOGY

- Caused by varicella zoster virus (VZV), a DNA virus in the Herpesviridae family
- Occurs exclusively in individuals with a prior history of chickenpox
- Is a reactivation disease from virus that lies dormant in the dorsal root ganglia

PEDIATRIC CONSIDERATIONS

- Herpes zoster during pregnancy is associated with an extremely low rate of fetal complications; there is no need to consider termination
- Childhood zoster is most common when varicella occurred in utero or within the first 6 months of life

Pre-Hospital

CAUTIONS

- Zoster is potentially contagious and may cause varicella in nonimmune health care workers; lesions should be covered to minimize viral transmission
- Maintain universal precautions

Diagnosis

ESSENTIAL WORKUP

- The patient should be isolated and considered contagious until crusts are present on every vesicle
- Clinical presentation is sufficient for diagnosis in most patients
- If definitive diagnosis is necessary, tissue culture is recommended
- Herpes zoster ophthalmicus (HZO) is diagnosed by slit-lamp exam
  —The pseudodendrites of HZO are broader, more opaque, and stain less brightly with fluorescein than the lesions of herpes simplex

LABORATORY

- Cell yields are highest if the base of vesicular lesions are scraped
- Numerous rapid immunofluorescence assays exist to detect VZV in vesicular fluid
- Tzanck smear demonstrates giant cells and intranuclear inclusions
- IgM and IgG is most commonly measured by ELISA; antibody titers rise 2 weeks after acute infection
- Polymerase chain reaction (PCR) may be useful in CSF analysis or verrucous lesions in which cultures are otherwise negative

DIFFERENTIAL DIAGNOSIS

- Zosteriform herpes simplex
- Varicella
- Herpes simplex
- Nonherpetic conjunctivitis
- Enteroviral infections (e.g., hand-foot-and-mouth disease)
- Insect bites
- Bullous impetigo
- *Molluscum contagiosum*

PEDIATRIC CONSIDERATIONS

- Zoster may be the first manifestation of VZV infection after primary infection in utero

Treatment

INITIAL STABILIZATION

- Rarely necessary
- IV access to administer fluids and antiviral therapy
- Disseminated disease to CNS or lungs may require airway support

ED TREATMENT

- Goal of treatment is to treat the acute viral infection, decrease pain, and prevent postherpetic neuralgia
- Acyclovir, valacyclovir, or famciclovir is recommended in patients with moderate to severe pain at rash onset, patients >50 years old, and those who are immunocompromised
  —Should be instituted within 72 hours of rash formation
- Foscarnet recommended for acyclovir-resistant VZV in immunocompromised patients
- Ocular involvement
  —Necessitates ophthalmologic consultation
  —Oral (normal host) or intravenous (immunocompromised host) acyclovir is best started within 72 hours, may be beneficial up to 1 week after symptom onset
- Oral corticosteroids in acute zoster is controversial
  —May reduce the pain associated with zoster
  —May or may not help prevent PHN
  —If not contraindicated, recommended in patients >50 years old, severe disease (>21 lesions), or severe pain
- Long-acting narcotics and topical lidocaine patches are recommended for moderate to severe pain, over-the-counter analgesia for mild pain
- Postherpetic neuralgia (PHN) is difficult to manage
  —Early use of antiviral drugs in acute zoster may prevent it
  —Lidocaine patch or lidocaine and prilocaine cream provides short-term relief
  —Topical capsaicin is controversial and should not be initiated in the ED
  —Sustained release oxycodone useful for analgesia
  —Tricyclic antidepressants recommended; nortriptyline and desipramine as beneficial but with fewer side effects than amitriptyline
  —Gabapentin safe and effective for PHN
  —A list of pain clinics can be obtained from the American Pain Society, telephone 708-966-5595

MEDICATIONS

- Acyclovir: adults: 800 mg PO 5 times/d for 7–10 days; immunocompromised with severe disease 10–12 mg/kg i.v. infused over 1 hour q8h; peds: 20 mg/kg PO q.i.d. × 5 days, 10 mg/kg i.v. q8h
- Famciclovir: adults: 500 mg PO t.i.d. × 7 days; peds: not approved
- Foscarnet: 40 mg/kg i.v. q8h for 14–26 days
- Gabapentin: 100–300 mg qhs increasing 100–300 mg q3d until adequate response or maximum dose of 3,600 mg/d divided t.i.d.
- Lidocaine patch 5%: apply <3 patches for <12 hours within a 24-hour period
- Nortriptyline: 10–25 mg PO qhs, increase dosage by 25 mg q 2–4 weeks until response adequate, maximum dose 125 mg per day
- Prednisone: 30 mg PO b.i.d. days 1–7, 15 mg PO b.i.d. days 8–14, and 7.5 mg b.i.d. days 15–21
- Valacyclovir: 1,000 mg PO t.i.d. × 7 days; peds: not approved
- Varicella-Zoster immune globulin (VZIG) adults: specialized dosing; peds: specialized dosing

PEDIATRIC CONSIDERATIONS

- Aspirin should be avoided as in varicella because of the potential risk of Reye's syndrome

Disposition

ADMISSION CRITERIA

- Disseminated disease
- Immunocompromised patients with any of the following:
  —Involvement of trigeminal nerve
  —Herpes zoster ophthalmicus
  —Ramsay Hunt syndrome
  —Involvement of more than two dermatomes
- Intractable pain
- ICU versus ward depends on severity of disease

DISCHARGE CRITERIA

- Most patients are managed as outpatients with referral to primary care or specialist as needed
- Postherpetic neuralgia may require long-term follow-up and management, referral to pain specialist may be required
- Patients should be instructed that lesions may heal with scarring or may leave depigmented areas
- Isolation from steroid-dependent, pregnant, or immunocompromised persons is recommended prior to onset of vesicles if zoster prodrome is suspected and until lesions are crusted
  —VZIG recommended within 72 hours for exposed immunocompromised contacts

PEDIATRIC CONSIDERATIONS

- Zoster in the neonate (<28 days old) requires admission and treatment with IV acyclovir; ward versus ICU depends on severity of disease
- Neonates born to seronegative mothers that are exposed to zoster should receive VZIG within 24 hours

Miscellaneous

ICD9: 053.9

ICD10: B02.9

SUGGESTED READINGS

Cohen JI, Brunnell PA, Straus SE, et al. Recent advances in varicella-Zoster virus infection. Ann Intern Med 1999;130(11): 922–932.

Kanzai GE, Johnson RW, Dworkin RH. Treatment of postherpetic neuralgia: an update. Drugs 2000;59(5):1113–1126.

Karlin JD. Herpes zoster ophthalmicus: the virus strikes back. Ann Ophthalmol 1993;25:208–215.

Kost RG, Straus SE, Wood AJ. Postherpetic neuralgia—pathogenesis, treatment, and prevention. N Engl J Med 1996;335: 32–42.

Rowbotham M, Harden N, Stacey B. Gabapentin for the treatment of postherpetic neuralgia. JAMA 1998;280: 1837–1842.

Authors: Susan C. Zapalac; Mark G. Richmond

Herpes, Genital

Clinical Presentation

SIGNS AND SYMPTOMS

- Local pain and itching
- Grouped vesicles on an erythematous base
- Lesions ulcerate, crust over, and then heal
- Lesions on vulva, vagina, cervix, perineum, buttocks; penile shaft or glans
- Vesicles may not be apparent on moist mucosal surfaces; ulcers may predominate
- Herpetic cervicitis, vaginitis, or urethritis may present with dysuria, urinary hesitancy or retention, vaginal discharge, or pelvic pain
- Systemic symptoms like fever, headache, malaise, photophobia, anorexia, myalgias, and lymphadenopathy are more common with primary infection
- Atypical features may include localized edema, erythema, crusts, or fissures

MECHANISM/DISEASE

First Episode/Primary HSV Infection

- Primary infection may have more prominent clinical syndrome and complications (e.g., encephalitis, meningitis)
- Primary infection may also go unnoticed; greater than 50% of first recognized signs and symptoms are not primary infection
- 2–12 day incubation; symptoms peak 8–10 days after onset; lesions heal in 3 weeks

Recurrent HSV Infection

- Average patient has 3–4 recurrences per year
- Virus reactivated from dorsal root ganglia
- Triggered by local trauma, emotional stress, fever, sunlight, cold or heat, menstruation, infection, etc.
- 1–2 day prodrome of local tingling, burning, itching, or pain prior to eruption (can mimic sciatica)
- Milder clinical syndrome; fewer lesions that usually heal within 10 days

Asymptomatic HSV Infection

- Positive cultures without lesions or symptoms can occur
- Virus is shed intermittently and often transmitted by persons who are asymptomatic

ETIOLOGY

- 70–90% of cases caused by a DNA virus herpes simplex virus, type 2 (HSV-2)
- 5–30% of cases caused by herpes simplex virus, type 1 (HSV-1), which usually causes herpes labialis (cold sores); tends to be milder than HSV-2; increasing in prevalence
- 22% of Americans seropositive for HSV-2 but most are asymptomatic
- High association with HIV and other STDs

PEDIATRIC CONSIDERATIONS

- Neonatal infections are often disseminated or involve the CNS
- Congenital HSV in the neonate without vesicles may mimic rubella, CMV, or toxoplasmosis

Pre-Hospital

CAUTIONS

- Contact isolation should be maintained in the form of gloves to protect health care workers

Diagnosis

ESSENTIAL WORKUP

- Diagnosis usually based on typical history and physical examination

LABORATORY

- Tzanck prep (Wright's or Giemsa stain of vesicle fluid from ulcer base) revealing multinucleated giant cells positive in half of cases
- Viral culture of vesicle fluid or ulcer base positive in 80–95% of cases
- Serologic tests not helpful in acute disease
  - —Require from 2 weeks to >3 months to detect seroconversion
  - —Cannot distinguish acute from chronic disease
  - —Tests to distinguish HSV-1 from HSV-2 are now available

DIFFERENTIAL DIAGNOSIS

- Syphilis
- Chancroid
- Lymphogranuloma venereum (LGV)
- Granuloma inguinale
- Candidiasis
- Behçet's syndrome

Treatment

INITIAL STABILIZATION

- Rarely required unless associated with systemic symptoms

ED TREATMENT

- Treatment not curative, aimed at preventing expression of disease
- Acyclovir interferes with viral DNA polymerase; equally effective medications with less frequent dosing regimens are famciclovir and valacyclovir
- Severe disease requiring hospitalization such as disseminated infection, hepatitis, pneumonitis, or CNS involvement: acyclovir 5–10 mg/kg i.v. q8h × 5–7 days
- Resistance to acyclovir in immunocompromised individuals is 5–10%; intravenous foscarnet may be effective
- Episodic treatment of recurrences may shorten the duration of lesions or ameliorate recurrences
- Daily suppressive therapy in patients with frequent recurrences (six or more per year) reduces the frequency of recurrences by 75%
- Women with primary HSV infection during pregnancy should receive antiviral therapy; therapy should also be considered for first episode and recurrent infections after 36 weeks
- Analgesics and antipruritics as needed
- Dysuria and urinary retention may be relieved with sitz baths or pouring warm water over lesions during urination
- Avoid any sexual contact from prodrome until healing
- Practice safe sex techniques even if there are no lesions
- Consider testing for concomitant STDs

MEDICATIONS

Acyclovir (Zovirax)

- First episode
  - —Adult: 400 mg PO t.i.d. or 200 mg 5 times/day; treat for 10 days
  - —Peds: 20 mg/kg PO q8h × 7–10 days *or* 5 mg/kg i.v. q8h over 1 hour
- Recurrent infection
  - —Adult: 400 mg PO t.i.d. or 200 mg PO 5 times/day or 800 mg PO b.i.d. for 5 days
- Suppressive therapy
  - —Adult: 400 mg PO b.i.d.

Famciclovir (Famvir)

- Not approved for pediatric dosing
- First episode
  - —250 mg PO t.i.d. for 10 days
- Recurrent infection
  - —125 mg PO b.i.d. for 5 days
- Suppressive therapy
  - —250 mg PO b.i.d.

Valacyclovir (Valtrex)

- Not approved for pediatric dosing
- First episode
  - —1 g PO b.i.d. for 10 days
- Recurrent infection
  - —500 mg PO b.i.d. for 5 days
- Suppressive therapy
  - —500–1,000 mg PO qd

PEDIATRIC CONSIDERATIONS

- Consider sexual abuse in children with genital HSV; culture lesions and test for other STDs in all suspected cases

Disposition

ADMISSION CRITERIA

- Systemic involvement (encephalitis, meningitis), significant dissemination
- Severe local symptoms (pain, urinary retention)
- Severely immunocompromised patient

DISCHARGE CRITERIA

- Immunocompetent patient without systemic involvement

Miscellaneous

ICD9: 054.10

ICD10: A60.0

SUGGESTED READINGS

Brown TJ. An overview of sexually transmitted diseases. Part I. J Am Acad Dermatol 1999;41(4):511–532.

Drake S, Taylor S, Brown D, et al. Improving the care of patients with genital herpes. Br Med J 2000;321:619–623.

Leung DT, Sacks SL. Current recommendations for the treatment of genital herpes. Drugs 2000;60(6): 1329–1352.

1998 guidelines for treatment of sexually transmitted diseases. Centers for Disease Control and Prevention. MMWR 1998;47: 1–111.

Preboth M. ACOG practice bulletin on management of herpes in pregnancy. American College of Obstetricians and Gynecologists. Am Fam Physician 2000;61(2):556–561.

Authors: Torrey Laack; Mark Richmond

Hiccups

Clinical Presentation

SIGNS AND SYMPTOMS

- Characteristic sound abruptly ending an inspiratory effort
- Attacks usually occur at brief intervals and last only a few seconds or minutes
- Attacks lasting more than 48 hours or persisting during sleep suggest an underlying disorder
- Described as *persistent* if duration longer than 48 hours; *intractable* if greater than 1 month

MECHANISM/DESCRIPTION

- Sudden, involuntary, contraction of the diaphragm (usually unilateral) and other inspiratory muscles terminated by abrupt closure of the glottis
- Usually occur with a frequency of 4–60 per minute
- Results from stimulation of one or more limbs of the hiccup reflex arc
  —Involves irritation of the vagus and phrenic nerves
  —"Hiccup center" is located in the upper spinal cord
- Male/female ratio 4:1
  —In men, greater than 90% have an organic basis
  —In women, a psychogenic cause is more likely

ETIOLOGY

- Idiopathic
- Gastrointestinal
  —Gastric distention
  —Esophageal lesions
  —Reflux esophagitis
  —Achalasia
  —Candida esophagitis
  —Carcinoma
  —Obstruction
  —Gastric lesions
  —Ulcer
  —Cancer
  —Hepatic lesions
  —Hepatitis
  —Hepatoma
  —Pancreatic lesions
  —Pancreatitis
  —Pseudocysts
  —Inflammatory bowel disease
  —Cholelithiasis
  —Cholecystitis
  —Appendicitis
  —Abdominal aortic aneurysm
  —Postoperative, abdominal procedure
- Diaphragmatic irritation
  —Hiatal hernia
  —Tumors
  —Pericarditis
  —Eventration
  —Splenomegaly
  —Hepatomegaly
  —Peritonitis
- CNS lesions
  —Encephalitis
  —Ventriculoperitoneal shunt
  —Stroke
  —Subarachnoid hemorrhage
  —Arteriovenous malformations
  —Parkinson's disease
  —Multiple sclerosis
- Mediastinal and other thoracic lesions
  —Pneumonia
  —Aortic aneurysm
  —Tuberculosis
  —Myocardial infarction
  —Lung cancer
  —Mediastinal adenopathy
- Metabolic causes
  —Uremia
  —Hyponatremia
  —Gout
  —Hypocalcemia
  —Diabetes
- Toxic/drug induced
  —α-Methyldopa
  —Benzodiazepines
  —Steroids
  —Barbiturates
  —General anesthesia
- Psychogenic causes
  —Stress/excitement
  —Grief
  —Malingering
  —Conversion disorder
- Head and neck
  —Otic foreign body irritating the tympanic membrane
  —Pharyngitis
  —Laryngitis
  —Goiter
  —Retropharyngeal/peritonsillar abscess

Pre-Hospital

N/A

Diagnosis

ESSENTIAL WORKUP

- Targeted history and review of systems to determine likelihood of potential underlying etiology
  —Severity and duration of current episode
  —History of previous episodes and treatment attempts
- Careful physical examination in search of an underlying cause
- Consider further diagnostic testing, dictated by history and physical, if hiccups are persistent or chronic

LABORATORY

- CBC with differential
- Electrolytes, BUN, creatinine

IMAGING/SPECIAL TESTS

- Chest radiography
- Further imaging may be indicated depending on clinical suspicion of a particular etiology; often can be performed on an outpatient basis

DIFFERENTIAL DIAGNOSIS

- Eructation

Treatment

INITIAL STABILIZATION

N/A

ED TREATMENT

- Treat specific causes when identified
  - —Remove foreign bodies from the ear
  - —Relieve gastric distention with a nasogastric tube
- Nonpharmacologic maneuvers
  - —Catheter stimulation of the posterior pharynx
  - —Direct stimulation of the uvula with a cotton swab
  - —Supraorbital pressure
  - —Carotid sinus massage
  - —Digital rectal massage
- Pharmacologic treatment
  - —Chlorpromazine
  - —Haloperidol
  - —Baclofen
  - —Nebulized lidocaine
  - —Amitriptyline
  - —Phenytoin
  - —Metoclopramide

MEDICATIONS

- Amitriptyline: 10 mg PO t.i.d.
- Baclofen: 10 mg PO t.i.d.
- Chlorpromazine: 25–50 mg i.v./i.m., 25–50 mg PO t.i.d.
- Haloperidol: 2–5 mg i.m.
- Lidocaine (4%): 3 mL nebulized, repeat if necessary
- Metoclopramide: 10 mg i.v./i.m., 10–20 mg PO q.i.d.
- Phenytoin: 200 mg i.v.

Disposition

ADMISSION CRITERIA

- Admission is not indicated for uncomplicated cases of hiccups

DISCHARGE CRITERIA

- Remedies that can be tried at home in case of recurrence:
  - —Swallowing a spoonful of sugar
  - —Sucking on a hard candy or swallowing peanut butter
  - —Breath holding/Valsalva maneuver
  - —Tongue traction
  - —Lifting the uvula with a cold spoon
  - —Drinking from the far side of a glass
  - —Inducing fright
  - —Smelling salts
  - —Rebreathing into a paper bag
- Referral in cases of intractable hiccups for investigation into underlying cause and more definitive therapeutic measures
  - —Phrenic nerve block of dominant diaphragm
  - —Phrenic nerve crush or transection
  - —Psychiatric interventions
  - —Hypnosis
  - —Behavioral modification

Miscellaneous

ICD9: 786.8

ICD10: R06.6

SUGGESTED READINGS

Kolodzik PW, Eilers MA. Hiccups (singultus): review and approach to management. Ann Emerg Med 1991;20: 565–573.

Lewis JH. Hiccups: reasons and remedies. In: Lewis JH, ed. A pharmacologic approach to gastrointestinal disorders. Baltimore: Williams & Wilkins, 1994:1–16.

Rosseau P. Hiccups. South Med J 1995; 88(2):175–181.

Author: Carrie Tibbles

High Altitude Illness

Clinical Presentation

SIGNS AND SYMPTOMS

Acute Mountain Sickness (AMS)

- Generally benign and self-limited
- Symptoms may become debilitating
- Onset 4–12 hours after ascent
- Headache plus at least one of the following:
  —Nausea/vomiting
  —Fatigue/lassitude
  —Dizziness
  —Difficulty sleeping

High Altitude Pulmonary Edema (HAPE)

- Onset 2–4 days after ascent, most commonly second night
- Cough early (dry at first, then productive)
- Dyspnea at rest
- Tachypnea
- Rales
- Cyanosis
- Fever may be present
- Severe respiratory distress and death may occur

High Altitude Cerebral Edema (HACE)

- Life-threatening
- Occurs in presence of HAPE and/or AMS
  —Seen rarely as an isolated entity
- Onset
  —May occur 12 hours after the onset of AMS
  —Usually requires 2–4 days for development
- Ataxia
- Severe headache
- Altered mental status/global encephalopathy
  —Focal neurologic deficit less common
- Nausea/vomiting
- Coma
- Seizure (rare)

MECHANISM/DESCRIPTION

- Incidence dependent on:
  —Rate of ascent
  —Final altitude
  —Sleeping altitude
  —Duration at altitude
- AMS incidence
  —Up to 67% incidence with rapid ascent (1–2 days) to >14,000 feet
  —22% incidence for skiers visiting resorts and sleeping at 7,000–9,000 feet, 40% at 10,000 feet
- AMS risk factors
  —Previous history of high altitude illness
  —Exertion
  —Younger persons (<50)
  —Physical fitness not protective
- HAPE incidence
  —<1–2%
  —Varies with rate of ascent
- HACE incidence <1%

PEDIATRIC CONSIDERATIONS

- AMS in infants and young children manifested by:
  —Increased fussiness
  —Decreased playfulness
  —Decreased appetite
  —Vomiting
  —Sleep disturbances
- Incidence of HAPE greater in younger individuals (<20 years) than adults
- No cases of HAPE or HACE reported in children <4 years old

Pre-Hospital

CAUTIONS

- Severe cases require immediate evacuation to a lower altitude
- Do not proceed to higher altitude in the presence of symptoms
- Oxygen delivery or simulated descent in a portable hyperbaric chamber (Gamow bag) can be a life-saving temporary measure making self-rescue possible

Diagnosis

ESSENTIAL WORKUP

- Clinical diagnosis in setting of recent altitude gain

AMS

- Diagnosis made with a history of a headache plus at least one of the following:
  —Nausea/vomiting
  —Lassitude/fatigue
  —Dizziness
  —Insomnia
- No diagnostic laboratory or imaging studies

HAPE

- Dyspnea on exertion—universal finding at altitude
- Dyspnea at rest—symptom of HAPE, worse at night
- Rales, cyanosis, or cough support the diagnosis
- Tachycardia, tachypnea correlate with severity

HACE

- Cerebellar ataxia with or without other symptoms of AMS
- Papilledema, retinal hemorrhages are associated findings

LABORATORY

- ABG for HAPE
  —Reveals hypoxemia (pO_2 30–50) and respiratory alkalosis, *not* acidosis

IMAGING/SPECIAL TESTS

- CXR in HAPE
  —Reveals patchy alveolar infiltrates with areas of clearing between the patches
  —Unilateral or bilateral infiltrates (right mid-lung field being most common)
  —Cardiomegaly, "batwing" distribution of infiltrates, and Kerley B lines (typical of cardiogenic pulmonary edema)—absent in HAPE
- Swan Ganz monitoring in HAPE
  —Increased pulmonary vascular resistance
  —Elevated pulmonary artery pressures
  —Normal pulmonary wedge pressures
- EKG in HAPE
  —Tachycardia
  —Evidence of right-heart strain
- CT and MRI scans in HACE
  —Vasogenic edema of the white matter

DIFFERENTIAL DIAGNOSIS

AMS

- Viral syndrome
- Exhaustion
- Alcohol hangover
- Carbon monoxide poisoning

HAPE

- Pneumonia
- High altitude bronchitis and pharyngitis
- Pulmonary embolism
  - —More rapid onset
  - —Pleuritic chest pain

HACE

- Cerebrovascular accidents/transient ischemic attacks
  - —Focal neurologic signs suggest a vascular lesion

Treatment

INITIAL STABILIZATION

HAPE and HACE

- ABCs
  - —Endotracheal intubation for impending respiratory failure, hyperventilation, or airway protection
- Establish IV access
- Supplemental oxygen and monitoring
- Continuous positive airway pressure (CPAP) for HAPE

ED MANAGEMENT

AMS

- Mild cases usually self-limited
  - —Symptomatic treatment
  - —Halt ascent until symptoms resolve
- Acetazolamide for moderate to severe symptoms
- Ibuprofen or acetaminophen for headache
- Promethazine for nausea
- Supplemental oxygen in severe cases
- Descent for severe or persistent symptoms
- Acetazolamide for AMS prophylaxis
  - —In high-risk individual with planned rapid ascent

HAPE

- Immediate descent for moderate/severe symptoms
- Mild cases may be managed without descent if:
  - —Adequate oxygen supplies available
  - —Serial medical examinations possible
  - —Immediate descent for any deterioration in clinical status
- Bed rest to avoid exercise-induced pulmonary hypertension
- Supplemental oxygen
  - —High flow rates (6–8 L/min) until improvement, then continue with lower flow rates
- Nifedipine when other interventions are unavailable
- β-agonist inhalers may be helpful

HACE

- *Immediate evacuation to lower altitude*
- Oxygen
- Dexamethasone
- Bed rest with elevation of head at 30 degrees and in severe cases the aggressive management of elevated intracranial pressure

MEDICATIONS

- Acetazolamide:
  - —AMS treatment: 250–500 mg (peds: 5 mg/kg) PO b.i.d. for AMS treatment
  - —AMS prophylaxis: 250 mg PO b.i.d. (peds: 5 mg/kg) PO b.i.d. start 24 hours before ascent
- Dexamethasone: 8 mg i.v., then 4 mg PO/i.v. q.i.d.
- Ibuprofen 800 mg (peds: 5–10 mg/kg) PO t.i.d.
- Nifedipine: 10 mg PO, then 30 mg SR PO b.i.d.
- Promethazine: 12.5–25 mg (peds: 0.25–1 mg/kg) PO/PR/i.m. q4–6h

Disposition

ADMISSION CRITERIA

- Descent to a lower facility mandatory in severe cases
- Persistent symptoms after observation in the lower altitude ED require admission

DISCHARGE CRITERIA

- Once clinical improvement seen and oxygen saturation >95% on room air
- Offer prophylactic therapy for future ascents in patients with recurrent AMS (acetazolamide) or HAPE (nifedipine)

Miscellaneous

ICD9: 993.2

ICD10: T70.2

SUGGESTED READINGS

Grissom CK, Roach RC, Sarnquist FH, et al. Acetazolamide in the treatment of acute mountain sickness: clinical efficacy and effect on gas exchange. Ann Intern Med 1992;116(6):461–465.

Hacket PH, Roach RC. High altitude illness. N Engl J Med 2001;345(2):107–114.

Hacket PH, Roach RC. High altitude medicine. In: Auerbach PS, ed. Wilderness medicine, 4th ed. St. Louis: Mosby, 2001:2–43.

Honigman B, Theis MK, McLain J, et al. Acute mountain sickness in a general tourist population at moderate altitudes. Ann Intern Med 1993;118(8):587–592.

Yaron M, Waldman N, Niermeyer S, et al. The diagnosis of acute mountain sickness in preverbal children. Arch Pediatr Adolesc Med 1998;152:683–687.

Author: Marc Doucette

Hip Injury

Clinical Presentation

SIGNS AND SYMPTOMS

- Groin, hip, thigh, medial knee pain, pain with ambulation/weight bearing
- Minor trauma in the elderly due to osteoporosis, high-impact trauma in young adults
- Obvious signs of trauma
  —Deformity or angulation, swelling, open fracture, or missile entrance wound
- Lower extremity held in position of comfort
  —Hip fracture: flexion, abduction, external rotation
  —Posterior hip dislocation: flexion, *adduction, internal rotation* of hip, flexion of knee
  —Anterior hip dislocation: flexion, *abduction, external rotation* of hip, thigh shortening

MECHANISM/DESCRIPTION

- Hip fracture = fracture of proximal femur
  —Classified by location, displacement/angulation, open/closed, comminution, fracture lines, neurovascular state
- Femoral head/neck fracture (intracapsular)
  —Minor mechanism in elderly, high-energy mechanism in young
  —Patient may or may not be ambulatory
  —Associated with hip dislocations (anterior > posterior)
  —Nondisplaced head/neck fractures difficult to visualize; increased morbidity when fracture goes from nondisplaced to displaced
  —Femoral neck is occasional site of stress fracture in runners and military recruits (repetitive activity)
- Intertrochanteric fracture (extracapsular)
  —Often due to fall in elderly patients
  —Nonambulatory with significant pain
  —Extremity often shortened, externally rotated
  —Significant blood loss
- Subtrochanteric fracture
  —Direct trauma in young patients, lesser trauma in elderly
  —Common site for pathologic fracture
  —Extremity shortened, displacement of proximal fragment
  —Can be site of significant blood loss
  -Greater/lesser trochanter fractures
  —In young patients; usually avulsion
- Hip dislocation = disarticulation of femoral head
- Posterior dislocation (most common)
  —Often from MVA, where knees strike dashboard
  —10% associated with sciatic nerve injury
- Anterior dislocation
  —Often due to trauma with sudden abduction of thigh
  —Associated femoral head fractures, femoral nerve injury
  -Central dislocation with acetabular fracture
  —Usually from direct impact to greater trochanter
  —Associated significant blood loss, sciatic nerve injury

PEDIATRIC CONSIDERATIONS

- Usually posterior hip dislocation
- Fracture usually requires high-impact trauma
- Suspect nonaccidental trauma (NAT)

Pre-Hospital

- Neurovascular exam is essential
- Immobilize extremity in position of comfort

CAUTIONS

- DO NOT apply traction
- Monitor closely for development of hemorrhagic shock as thigh can contain 4–6 units of blood

Diagnosis

ESSENTIAL WORKUP

- Assess distal pulses, palpate compartments, evaluate sensation and motor function
- If pulses are not equal or palpable, bedside Doppler or angiography may be necessary
- Search for associated injuries
- Radiographs as outlined below
  —Remove splints and clothing when taking films
  —Positive exam and negative X-ray = hip fracture until proven otherwise
- In suspected child abuse, obtain skeletal survey or bone scan

LABORATORY

- CBC, type and cross-match

IMAGING/SPECIAL TESTS

- Standard films: AP pelvis and true lateral of hip
- Femoral neck: AP pelvis with hip internally rotated 15–20 degrees
- Pubic rami and acetabular fractures: pelvic inlet and outlet views
- Acetabular fractures: Judet views (oblique views of hip)
- High suspicion with negative plain films: CT, MRI, or bone scan
- Joint aspiration with or without arthrogram under fluoroscope if suspect a septic joint, foreign body, or hemarthrosis, especially in gunshot wound to hip

DIFFERENTIAL DIAGNOSIS

- Pubic ramus fracture
- Acetabular fracture
- Septic joint
- Thigh, knee, ankle, or foot injury
- Trochanteric bursitis
- Iliotibial band tendinitis
- Hip contusion

PEDIATRIC CONSIDERATIONS

- Pediatric fracture patterns different due to developing cartilaginous components
- Suspect NAT without obvious mechanism of injury
- Consider hip pain due to a separate process (limb-length discrepancy, neuromuscular disorders, neoplastic invasion of bone)

Treatment

INITIAL STABILIZATION

- ABCs of trauma care
- Monitor blood pressure continuously

ED TREATMENT

- Maintain pelvis and hip stability
- Remove splint and clothing
- Pain control
  - —Isolated hip injuries: parenteral analgesia
  - —Multitrauma or pediatric patients: femoral nerve block
- Orthopedic consultation necessary for all hip fractures and dislocations
  - —Emergent if neurovascular compromise
  - —Open fractures must go directly to the OR for irrigation and débridement
  - -Antibiotics
  - —Fractures requiring surgery: cefazolin
  - —If open fracture with laceration, extensive soft tissue damage, contamination: add gentamicin/tobramycin, tetanus
  - —If highly contaminated wound: add penicillin G to cover clostridial species
- Gunshot wounds: culture missile track, sterile dressing

Hip Dislocation

- True orthopedic emergency
  - —Incidence of avascular necrosis and degenerative joint disease increases linearly with time to reduction
- Perform reduction in ED, ideally <6 hours from onset
  - —Allis or Stimson maneuvers
  - —Also described: lateral decubitus, move hip from flexed and adducted position to full external rotation with tibia perpendicular to floor
- Moderate sedation with etomidate, ketamine or methohexital + midazolam, propofol + fentanyl
- Look for fractures on postreduction imaging (plain film, CT)
- Patients with prior hip arthroplasty may be reduced in the ED with moderate sedation and appropriate monitoring

MEDICATIONS

Antibiotics

- Cefazolin: adults: 2 g i.m./i.v.; peds: 20 mg/kg i.m./i.v.
- Gentamicin/tobramycin: 1.5 mg/kg i.v.
- Penicillin G: adults: 2 million IU i.v.; peds: 25,000 IU/kg/d i.v. divided q8h

Moderate Sedation

- Etomidate: adults: 0.1–0.3 mg/kg i.v.; peds: not recommended for under 12 years of age
- Fentanyl: adults and peds (>6 mos): 1–5 μg/kg i.v.
- Ketamine: adults: 0.5–1.0 mg/kg i.v., 2–4 mg/kg i.m.; peds: 1.0–1.5 mg/kg i.v., 2–5 mg/kg i.m.
- Methohexital: adults: 1–3 mg/kg i.v.; peds: not recommended
- Midazolam: adults: 0.03–0.01 mg/kg i.v.; peds: 0.05–0.15 mg/kg i.v./i.m., 0.5–0.7 mg/kg PO, 0.2–0.5 mg/kg nasally
- Propofol: adults/peds: 50–70 μg/kg/min i.v. continuous infusion

PEDIATRIC CONSIDERATIONS

- Assess for NAT
  - —Delay in presentation; mechanism inconsistent with injury
  - —Isolated trauma to the thigh, associated burns, bruises, linear abrasions
  - —Assess for dislocation of the femoral capital epiphysis
- Trivial force required for posterior hip locations in children <6 years old

Disposition

ADMISSION CRITERIA

- All hip fractures or dislocations
- Suspicion of occult fracture
- Suspicion of NAT in children

DISCHARGE CRITERIA

- Hip pain attributable to other cause
- Fracture ruled out (negative radiographs plus negative clinical exam)
- Patient with successful reduction of dislocated hip arthroplasty may be considered for discharge in consultation with orthopedics and with appropriate follow-up

Miscellaneous

ICD9: 959.6

ICD10: S79.9

SUGGESTED READINGS

Dursteler B, Wightman J. Etomidate-facilitated hip reduction in the emergency department. Am J Emerg Med 2000;18:204–208.

Hughes L, Beaty J. Fractures of the head and neck of the femur in children. J Bone Joint Surg 1994;76A(2):283–292.

Kutty S, et al. Traumatic posterior hip location of hip in children. Pediatr Emerg Care 2001;17:32–35.

Long W, et al. Management of civilian gunshot injuries to the hip. Orthop Clin North Am 1995;26(1):123–131.

Lyons R. Clinical outcomes and treatment of hip fractures. Am J Med 1997;103(2A):51S–64S.

McMurty A, Quaile A. Closed reduction of the traumatically dislocated hip: a new technique. Injury 2001;32:162–164.

Rudman N, McIlmail D. Emergency department evaluation and treatment of hip and thigh injuries. Emerg Med Clin North Am 2000;18:29–66.

Ward K, Yealy D. Systemic analgesia and sedation in managing orthopedic emergencies. Emerg Med Clin North Am 2000;18:141–166.

Zuckerman J. Hip fracture. N Engl J Med 1996;334(23):1519–1525.

Author: Colleen Buono

Hirschsprung's Disease

Clinical Presentation

SIGNS AND SYMPTOMS

- Also known as congenital aganglionosis megacolon
- Three presentations
  —Neonatal
    -Abdominal distention
    -Delayed passage of meconium in first 48 hours
    -Vomiting
    -Neonatal enterocolitis
  —Infancy
    -Severe constipation
    -Chronic abdominal distention
    -Vomiting
    -Failure to thrive
  —Later childhood and adulthood
    -Chronic constipation with obstruction
    -Enterocolitis at any age
- Bowel movements frequently require rectal stimulation or enemas
- Narrow caliber stools
- Encopresis and diarrhea are uncommon
- Absence of inciting factors associated with functional constipation (i.e., fissures, toilet training, diet)
- Possible palpable colon on the left
- Occult blood possibly due to enterocolitis or anal fissures (constipation)
- Complications
  —Enterocolitis
    -Fever
    -Lethargic or toxic-appearing child
    -Abdominal distention
    -Bloody, foul-smelling diarrhea
  —Malnutrition
  —Reversible urinary tract infection (hydronephrosis, hydroureter, recurrent UTIs)
  —Acute appendicitis
  —Septicemia

MECHANISM/DESCRIPTION

- Absence of enteric ganglia in the distal bowel
  —Creates functional obstruction to passage of stool
  —Mutations of the *ret* proto-oncogene found in both familial and sporadic forms
- Failure of neural crest cells to migrate into parasympathetic Meissner's (submucosal) and Auerbach's (myenteric) ganglions
- Begins at the internal anal sphincter and involves the rectosigmoid colon (75% of cases)
- May extend entire length of gastrointestinal tract—(often fatal)
- Aganglionic segment chronically contracts, forming an obstruction to the passage of stool
  —Proximal colon distends to hold stool that has not passed
  —Stimulation of the anus allows passage of stool
  —Toxic megacolon may develop

EPIDEMIOLOGY

- 1:5,000 live births
- Male to female ratio—4:1
- 8% have positive family history; 5–12% of siblings
- Chromosomal abnormality (12%) most commonly Down syndrome
- Other congenital anomalies (GI, cardiac, craniofacial, cleft palate) (18%)

Pre-Hospital

- Infants may be dehydrated, acidotic, and hypoglycemic

Diagnosis

ESSENTIAL WORKUP

- Abdominal x-rays
  —Distended small bowel and proximal colon with an empty rectum are common findings
  —Transition zone into a narrowed rectosigmoid segment
  —In neonates, films will commonly show a distal obstructive pattern
  —In children, with chronic constipation films may show only large amounts of stool
  —In children with enterocolitis, bowel wall edema or *pneumatosis intestinales* may be present

LABORATORY

- CBC, electrolytes, glucose, urinalysis, blood culture if toxic

IMAGING/SPECIAL TESTS

- Barium enema
  —Obtain after stabilization
  —Dilated colon proximal to the contracted aganglionic colon with uncoordinated peristalsis
  —Delayed barium evacuation
- Rectal manometry may assist in diagnosis but is often abnormal in long-standing constipation
- Full-thickness rectal biopsy confirms diagnosis by the lack of ganglion cells

DIFFERENTIAL DIAGNOSIS

Infants

- Meconium ileus or meconium plug from cystic fibrosis
- Congenital disorder
  —Intestinal or anal atresia or hypoplasia
- Malrotation or duplication with volvulus
- Necrotizing enterocolitis
- Functional constipation
- Sepsis

Children

- Functional constipation
- Toxic
  —Opiates, anticholinergics
- Infectious
  —Botulism, *Trypanosoma cruzi* acquired aganglionic colon
- Metabolic or endocrine
  —Hypothyroid/parathyroid, adrenal insufficiency, electrolyte abnormality
- Structural
  —Spinal cord defects, abdominal masses

Treatment

INITIAL STABILIZATION

- Ill-appearing children
  - —ABCs with monitoring
  - —Initial bolus 0.9% fluids (20 mL/kg) for shock, dehydration, sepsis

ED TREATMENT

- Infants should be managed for bowel obstruction
- Consultation with a pediatric surgeon and pediatric gastroenterology
  - —Unstable patient may require decompression by loop colostomy; stoma must contain normal bowel
- Stable children
  - —Workup may be done as an outpatient
  - —Definitive treatment is resection of the aganglionic section of bowel; staging unnecessary in relatively well child
  - —Return to normal bowel function is the usual result
  - —Enterocolitis may occur at any time
- Ultimate surgical goal is to place normal ganglion containing bowel within 1 cm of the anal opening

MEDICATIONS

- When the child is toxic or has enterocolitis, then use triple IV antibiotic coverage
  - —Ampicillin: 50 mg/kg q8–12h
  - —Flagyl: 7.5 mg/kg q12–48h
  - —Gentamicin: 2.5 mg/kg q6–12h

Disposition

ADMISSION CRITERIA

- Infants and neonates presenting with bowel obstruction
- Enterocolitis
- Ill-appearing infants should be admitted to the PICU/NICU
- If pediatric surgery is not available, transfer to a pediatric tertiary care center

DISCHARGE CRITERIA

- Older children with constipation
- Well hydrated and taking oral fluid
- Responsible parents

Miscellaneous

ICD9: 751.31

ICD10: Q43.1

SUGGESTED READINGS

Amiel J, Lyonnet S. Hirschsprung disease, associated syndromes, and genetics: a review. J Med Genet 2001;38:729–739.

Kays DW. Surgical conditions of the neonatal intestinal tract. Clin Perinatol 1996;23:353–375.

Rudolph C, Benaroch L. Hirschsprung disease. Pediatr Rev 1995;16:5–11.

Skinner MA. Hirschsprung disease. Curr Prob Surg 1996;399–460.

Sullivan PB. Hirschsprung's disease. Arch Dis Child 1996;74:5.

Authors: Sally Santen; Andrea Bracikowski

HIV/AIDS

Clinical Presentation

SIGNS AND SYMPTOMS

- Primary HIV infection
  - —Fever
  - —Malaise
  - —Rash on face and trunk
  - —Headache
  - —Photophobia
  - —Meningismus
  - —Flu-like syndrome with lymphadenopathy and hepatosplenomegaly
    - -Commonly described as "mono-like"
  - —Asymptomatic period averaging 8 or more years after initial infection
- Advanced disease (CD4 <200)
  - —Fatigue
  - —Fevers
  - —Night sweats
  - —Weight loss/wasting
  - —Alopecia
  - —Chronic diarrhea with severe dehydration and electrolyte abnormalities
  - —Cough
  - —Dyspnea
  - —Hemoptysis
  - —Chronic low-grade headache
  - —Altered mental status
  - —Seizures
  - —Dementia
  - —Neuropathy
  - —Painless visual loss
  - —Skin lesions
    - -Kaposi's sarcoma
    - -Chronic dermatologic conditions

ETIOLOGY

- The HIV retrovirus impedes the immune system by destroying the CD4 lymphocytes
- Risk factors
  - —Prostitution
  - —Intravenous drug abuse
  - —Homosexuality
  - —Blood transfusions prior to 1985
  - —Unprotected sex with partners at-risk
  - —Children of women who engage in high-risk behavior

MECHANISMS/DESCRIPTION

- Opportunistic diseases occur with decreasing CD4 counts
  - —CD <500 cells/mm^3
    - -Oral candidiasis
    - -Pneumococcal infection
    - -Hairy leukoplakia
    - -Immune thrombocytopenic purpura
  - —CD4 <200 cells/mm^3
    - -*Pneumocystis carinii* pneumonia
    - -Cryptococcal infection, tuberculosis
    - -Cryptosporidiosis
    - -Isosporiasis
    - -Toxoplasmosis
    - -Histoplasmosis
  - —CD4 <50 cells/mm^3
    - -CNS lymphoma
    - -*Mycobacterium avium* complex (MAC)
    - -Cytomegalovirus (CMV)
    - -Cholangiopathy
- Common medication complications
  - —Both dideoxyinosine (DDI) and dideoxycytidine (DDC) can cause pancreatitis
  - —DDC and stavudine (D4T) can cause peripheral neuropathy
  - —Indinavir can cause kidney stones
  - —Dapsone (used for treatment of TB) can cause hemolytic anemia
  - —Pentamidine can cause hypoglycemia
  - —Many of the antiretroviral medications can cause some hematologic effects (anemia or bone marrow suppression), gastrointestinal upset, and rash

PEDIATRIC CONSIDERATIONS

- Infants infected with HIV may present with failure to thrive, recurrent bacterial infections, unexplained organomegaly or lymphadenopathy, and unexplained developmental delay

Pre-Hospital

CAUTIONS

- Universal precautions

Diagnosis

ESSENTIAL WORKUP

- HIV serologic tests as noted below
  - —There is a "window" of 6 months between primary infection and seroconversion, during which tests may be negative
- Respiratory symptoms
  - —Chest x-ray, ABG, and induced sputum for Gram stain, silver stain, acid-fast bacillus (AFB), and culture
- Neurologic symptoms
  - —Head CT and lumbar puncture
  - —CSF for glucose, protein, Gram stain and culture, cell count with differential, AFB smear, India ink stain, cryptococcus titer, and VDRL
- Gastrointestinal symptoms
  - —Stool for ova and parasites, Gram stain, culture, and *Clostridium difficile* assay
- Fever workup
  - —Include aerobic/anaerobic, fungal, AFB, and MAC blood cultures

LABORATORY

- ELISA immunoassay
  - —Detects IgG antibody against HIV
  - —Sensitivity and specificity are approximately 99%
  - —Can be negative during the window period
- Western blot
  - —Detects IgG antibody against HIV proteins p24, gp120, gp 41
  - —More specific than ELISA
  - —Used to confirm a positive ELISA
- The p24 antigen assay and PCR and viral cultures for HIV
  - —Able to detect HIV during the window period
- PCP pneumonia
  - —Increased A-a gradient on arterial blood gas analysis
  - —Elevated serum LDH
  - —*Pneumocystis* identified on silver stain
- Cryptococcal meningitis
  - —Positive CSF India ink
  - —Cryptococcal antigen assay
    - -More sensitive than India ink test

IMAGING/SPECIAL TESTS

- Chest x-ray
  - —Bilateral interstitial infiltrates or pneumothorax
    - -PCP
  - —Reticulonodular infiltrates
    - -TB, KS, or fungal pneumonia
  - —Hilar lymphadenopathy with infiltrate
    - -TB
  - —Lobar consolidation
    - -Bacterial pneumonia
  - —Cavitation
    - -TB, necrotizing bacterial pneumonia, coccidioidomycosis
  - —Normal
    - -Does not rule out PCP or TB
- Head CT
  - —IV contrast
  - —Multiple ring-enhancing lesions with edema in basal ganglia or cortex
    - -Toxoplasmosis
  - —Weakly enhancing periventricular lesions with edema
    - -CNS lymphoma
  - —Multiple subcortical nonenhancing lesions
    - -Progressive multifocal leukoencephalopathy

DIFFERENTIAL DIAGNOSIS

- Mononucleosis
- Hepatitis
- Syphilis
- Rubella
- Disseminated gonococcal infection
- Pulmonary emboli
- TB
- Pneumonia
- Pulmonary malignancies
- Lymphocytic interstitial pneumonitis
- Neurosyphilis
- CMV encephalitis
- CNS lymphoma
- Coccidioidal meningitis
- Subarachnoid hemorrhage
- Cerebral infarction
- Cerebral edema

Treatment

INITIAL STABILIZATION

- ABCs
  - —Supplemental oxygen or intubation as necessary
  - —Identify code status prior to intubation

ED TREATMENT

- Patients who appear to have bacterial infections, appear toxic, or have rapidly progressive symptoms should receive their first dose of antibiotics in the ED
- Primary HIV infection and maintenance
  - —HIV treatment strategies use three antiretroviral medications: two nucleoside analogues plus either a protease inhibitor or a nonnucleoside reverse transcriptase inhibitor
- Cryptococcal meningitis
  - —Amphotericin B with or without flucytosine
- Esophageal candidiasis
  - —Ketoconazole or fluconazole
- MAC
  - —Rifabutin
- PCP
  - —Trimethoprim (TMP)/sulfamethoxazole (SMX)
  - —Pentamidine for sulfa-allergic patients
  - —If PaO_2 <70 mm Hg or A-a gradient >35 mm Hg, add prednisone 80 mg PO once per day for 5 days, then taper

MEDICATIONS

- Nucleoside analogues
  - —Abacavir (ABC): 300 mg PO twice per day
  - —Didanosine (DDI): <60 kg: 250 mg PO per day; ≥60 kg: 400 mg PO per day
  - —Lamivudine (3TC): 150 mg PO b.i.d.
  - —Stavudine (D4T): 40 mg PO b.i.d.
  - —Zalcitabine (DDC): 0.75 mg PO t.i.d.
  - —Zidovudine (AZT): 100 mg PO 5 times per day
- Protease inhibitors
  - —Amprenavir: 20 mg/kg PO b.i.d.
  - —Indinavir: 800 mg PO t.i.d.
  - —Lopinavir/ritonavir: 400 mg/100 mg PO b.i.d.
  - —Nelfinavir: 750 mg PO t.i.d.
  - —Ritonavir: 600 mg PO b.i.d.
  - —Saquinavir: 1,200 mg PO t.i.d.
- Nonnucleoside reverse transcriptase inhibitors
  - —Delavirdine: 400 mg PO t.i.d.
  - —Efavirenz: 600 mg PO qd
  - —Nevirapine: 200 mg PO b.i.d.
- Amphotericin B: 0.3–0.6 mg/kg/d i.v.
- Fluconazole: 100–200 mg/d PO
- Flucytosine: 25–37.5 mg/kg PO q.i.d.
- Ketoconazole: 400 mg/d PO
- Pentamidine: 4 mg/kg i.v.
- Rifabutin: 300 mg PO qd
- Trimethoprim (TMP)/sulfamethoxazole (SMX): 20 mg/kg/d as i.v./PO divided into four times per day dosing

PEDIATRIC CONSIDERATIONS

- The oral polio vaccine is contraindicated in HIV-positive patients
- Immunization with the pneumococcal vaccine and tetanus booster is recommended

Disposition

ADMISSION CRITERIA

- Unexplained fever with CNS involvement or suspected endocarditis
- Severe hypoxemia (PaO_2 <70 mm Hg)
- Suspected bacterial pneumonia or TB
- A change in neurologic status
- New-onset seizures
- Inability to ambulate
- Inability to tolerate oral intake
- Intractable diarrhea with dehydration

DISCHARGE CRITERIA

- The patient can maintain adequate oral intake, provide self-care, and ambulate

Miscellaneous

ICD9: 042

ICD10: B24

SUGGESTED READINGS

Barbaro G, Fisher SD, Giancaspro G, et al. HIV-associated cardiovascular complications: a new challenge for emergency physicians. Am J Emerg Med 2001;19(7):566–574.

Fein JA, Friedland LR, Rutstein R, et al. Children with unrecognized human immunodeficiency virus infection. An emergency department perspective. Am J Dis Child 1993;147(10):1104–1108.

Guss DA. The acquired immune deficiency syndrome: an overview for the emergency physician, part I. J Emerg Med 1994;12(3): 375–384.

Guss DA. The acquired immune deficiency syndrome: An overview for the emergency physician, Part II. J Emerg Med 1994;12(4): 491–497.

Hovanessian HC. New developments in the treatment of HIV disease: an overview. Ann Emerg Med 1999;33(5):546–555.

Moran GJ, House HR. HIV-related illnesses: the challenge of ED management. Emerg Med Pract 2002;4(1):1-28.

Authors: Amal Mattu; Sejal G. Mattu

Hordeolum and Chalazion

Clinical Presentation

- Result from inflammatory processes involving the glands within the eyelid
  - —Hordeolum—acute glandular obstruction resulting in inflammation
  - —Chalazion—end result of a chronic granulomatous inflammation

SIGNS AND SYMPTOMS

Hordeolum

- Develops acutely when glandular outflow is obstructed
- Red, tender, painful, swollen mass on the eyelid
- Typically solitary but may be multiple
- Nontoxic-appearing patient
- Presentation depends on which gland is affected
  - —External hordeolum
    - -Originates from obstruction of the superficial sebaceous or sweat glands whose ducts are located between the eye lashes
    - -Exquisitely tender small mass that points anteriorly
  - —Internal hordeolum
    - -Originates from obstruction of the sebaceous glands whose ducts are located on the inner aspect of the lid margin
    - -Painful small mass that is palpable through the eyelid
    - -May cause a foreign body sensation in the eye
    - -Typically more inflamed, larger, and more painful
    - -Most commonly drains through the conjunctival surface but may drain through the skin
- Associated with localized inflammation in the surrounding tissue
  - —May lead to preseptal cellulitis
- Tender preauricular lymph nodes may be present

Chalazion

- Firm, circumscribed, nontender, or minimally tender nodule
- Noninflamed
- Typically long-standing
- Symptoms most commonly due to physical properties
  - —Disrupts natural contour of eye
  - —Obstructs visual field/peripheral vision
  - —Pressure on globe

MECHANISM/DESCRIPTION

Hordeolum

- Develops due to outflow obstruction in one or more of the glands of the eyelid
- The eyelid has many secretory glands
  - —External hordeolum
    - -Glands of Zeis—superficial sebaceous glands
    - -Glands of Moll—superficial sweat glands
  - —Internal hordeolum
    - -Meibomian glands—deeper modified sebaceous glands
- Obstructed glands may become secondarily infected
- May progress to localized abscess formation

Chalazion

- Chronic granulomatous inflammation in the meibomian gland
  - —Originates from inspissated secretions
  - —May evolve from incompletely drained internal hordeolum

ETIOLOGY

Hordeolum

- Secondarily infected with *Staphylococcal aureus*

Pre-Hospital

N/A

Diagnosis

ESSENTIAL WORKUP

- Complete ophthalmologic examination

Hordeolum

- Identify the origin of the abscess
- Determine extent of surrounding inflammation/cellulitis

Chalazion

- Determine whether physical properties of chalazion result in corneal exposure and injury

DIFFERENTIAL DIAGNOSIS

- Hordeolum
- Chalazion
- Blepharitis
- Dacryocystitis
- Dacryoadenitis
- Preseptal cellulitis
- Pyogenic granuloma
- Sebaceous cell carcinoma

Treatment

INITIAL STABILIZATION

N/A

ED TREATMENT

Hordeolum

- Relieve obstruction and prevent abscess formation
  - —Warm compresses for 15 minutes 4 to 6 times per day
  - —Gently massage the nodule to express obstructed material
  - —Rarely, in severe cases, incision and drainage of internal hordeolum may be necessary
    - -Typically done by ophthalmologist
    - -If pointed toward the conjunctiva, vertical incision is made to avoid injury to the meibomian glands
  - —Prophylactic topical antistaphylococcal antibiotic ointment is applied in the cul-de-sac and massaged along the lid margin to stimulate duct and prevent secondary conjunctivitis

Chalazion

- For chalazion, complaints typically reflect nonemergent aesthetic and cumbersome physical properties of the mass
  - —Referral to ophthalmology for incision and curettage or steroid injection
  - —Lubricating eye drops may provide symptomatic relief

MEDICATIONS

- Lacri-Lube ophthalmologic drops as needed for comfort
- Sulfacetamide ophthalmologic ointment applied every 2–4 hours until 24 hours after symptoms resolve completely
- Gentamicin ophthalmologic ointment applied every 2–4 hours until 24 hours after symptoms resolve completely

Disposition

ADMISSION CRITERIA

- Secondary cellulitis or deep tissue infection develop

DISCHARGE CRITERIA

- All uncomplicated cases may be discharged
- If incision and drainage is necessary, follow-up with ophthalmology within 1 to 2 days
- Symptoms are expected to resolve completely within 3–4 weeks, more typically complete resolution is seen within 7–10 days

Miscellaneous

ICD9: 373.2; 373.11

ICD10: H00.1; H00.0

SUGGESTED READINGS

Cullom R. The Will's eye manual: office and emergency room diagnosis and treatment of eye disease. Philadelphia: Lippincott-Raven, 1994:133–134.

Kanski JJ. Clinical ophthalmology. London: Butterworth-Heinemann, 1994:2–4.

Lavrich JB, Nelson LB. Disorders of the lacrimal system apparatus. Pediatr Clin North Am 1993;40:767–804.

Lederman C, Miller M. Disorders of the lacrimal system apparatus. Hordeola and chalazia. Pediatr Rev 1999;20(8):283–284.

Rubin S, Hallagan L. Lids, lacrimals and lashes. Emerg Clin North Am 1995;13(3):631–647.

Author: Shari Schabowski

Horner's Syndrome

Clinical Presentation

SIGNS AND SYMPTOMS

- Horner's syndrome is characterized by:
  - —*Ptosis:* drooping of the eyelid on the affected side, usually slight
  - —*Miosis:* a decrease in pupillary size on the involved side (pupillary asymmetry = 1 mm)
  - —*Anhidrosis:* lack of sweating on the involved side of the face
- The importance of Horner's syndrome is its association with certain disease states

MECHANISM/DESCRIPTION

- Unilateral sympathetic denervation produces the signs of Horner's syndrome
  - —Relaxation of the retracting muscles in the upper and lower lids—ptosis
  - —Loss of pupillary dilator innervation—miosis (unopposed pupillary constriction)
  - —Loss of sympathetic stimulation of the sweat glands—anhidrosis

ETIOLOGY

- Tumors of the lung or metastases to the cervical nodes: may interrupt the preganglionic sympathetic fibers (between the thoracic sympathetic trunk and superior cervical ganglion)
- Trauma: penetrating neck wounds
- Pneumothorax: tension pneumothorax may cause traction on the sympathetic fibers due to shift of mediastinal structures
- Infiltration or infection of cervical nodes: sarcoidosis, tuberculosis
- Vascular disorders: migraine or cluster headaches, carotid artery dissection

PEDIATRIC CONSIDERATIONS

- Hereditary Horner's syndrome: associated with a blue iris (or irregular coloration) on the affected side and brown on the unaffected side (heterochromia iridis)
- Birth trauma: may cause damage to the sympathetic chain

Pre-Hospital

CAUTIONS

- The importance of Horner's syndrome is its association with more serious underlying conditions; patients with increased ICP or tension pneumothorax must be recognized immediately

Diagnosis

ESSENTIAL WORKUP

- History and physical exam focused on neurologic findings
- Chest x-ray to screen for tumor or pneumothorax

IMAGING/SPECIAL TESTS

- Pharmacologic (cocaine) testing confirms the diagnosis of a sympathetic ocular lesion
  - —One drop of 5% ocular cocaine solution is instilled into each eye.
  - —Failure of pupil on the involved side to dilate as much as the other pupil (an increase in the amount of anisocoria) in 1 hour is confirmatory (positive test)
- CT or MRI of the head, neck, or chest may be indicated depending on the signs and symptoms
- Ocular tonometry for suspected glaucoma
- Carotid Doppler US may be indicated to evaluate for carotid dissection

DIFFERENTIAL DIAGNOSIS

- Increased ICP: almost always associated with altered LOC, headache
- *Simple anisocoria (pseudo-Horner's syndrome):* 15–20% of the population has anisocoria and 3–4% also have miosis and ptosis
  - —The cocaine test is negative (both pupils dilate equally)
  - —Inspect photo ID for preexisting anisocoria
- Topical medications or exposures
- Migraine or cluster headache
- Glaucoma, inflammatory ocular diseases, or ocular trauma

PEDIATRIC CONSIDERATIONS

- Birth trauma in newborns
- Hereditary Horner's syndrome

Treatment

INITIAL STABILIZATION

- If increased ICP is suspected: measures to control ICP (intubation, osmotic diuretics)
- Tension pneumothorax: needle thoracostomy followed by chest tube

ED TREATMENT

- Horner's syndrome per se requires no ED treatment

MEDICATIONS

- Cocaine: 5% (adult), 2.5% (pediatric) ophthalmic solution: 1 drop in each eye is diagnostic

Disposition

ADMISSION CRITERIA

- Admission for isolated Horner's syndrome is not needed
  —Admission may be needed for the underlying condition

DISCHARGE CRITERIA

- Patients with Horner's syndrome may be discharged with appropriate follow-up arranged for continued workup as an outpatient

Miscellaneous

ICD9: 337.9

ICD10: G90.2

SUGGESTED READINGS

Cook T, Kietzman L, Leibold R. "Pneumo-ptosis" in the emergency department. Am J Emerg Med 1992;10:431–434.

Corbett J, Thompson H. Pupillary function and dysfunction. In: Asbury A, McKhann G, MacDonald W, eds. Diseases of the nervous system: clinical neurobiology. Philadelphia: WB Saunders, 1992:495–500.

Fields C, Barker F. Review of Horner's syndrome and a case report. Optom Vis Sci 1992;69(6):481–485.

Wilheim H, et al. Horner's syndrome: a retrospective analysis of 90 cases and recommendations for clinical handling. Ger J Ophthalmol 1992;1(2):96–102.

Author: Richard S. Krause

Humerus Fractures

Clinical Presentation

SIGNS AND SYMPTOMS

- Pain, swelling, and tenderness
- Difficulty in initiating active motion
- Arm often closely held against the chest
- Crepitus may be present
- Ecchymoses within 24–48 hours at area of fracture
- Diminished peripheral pulses
  —Decreased sensation over the deltoid muscle (axillary nerve), or forearm/first web space (radial nerve)

MECHANISM/DESCRIPTION

- Fall onto an outstretched hand
- High-energy direct trauma
- Excessive rotation of the arm in the abducted position
- Electrical shock or seizure
- Pathologic fracture from metastatic disease
- Ball throwing
- Proximal humeral fractures involve the humeral head, lesser tuberosity, greater tuberosity, bicipital groove, and proximal humeral shaft
- Typically seen in adults over the age of 45 years and the elderly
- Proximal humeral fractures account for 5% of all fractures
- Humeral shaft fractures are of three types: nondisplaced, displaced or angulated, or severely displaced or associated with neurovascular compromise
- Humeral shaft fractures account for 3% of all fractures

Pre-Hospital

CAUTIONS

- Excessive movement of the arm may produce further neurovascular injury
- Immobilization with sling and swath and transport
- Rapid transport in presence of neurologic or vascular deficits

Diagnosis

ESSENTIAL WORKUP

- Assessment of neurovascular status
  —Assess function of radial, median, ulnar, axillary (sensation to the lateral aspect of the shoulder), and musculocutaneous nerve (sensation to the extensor aspect of the forearm)
  —Presence of radial, ulnar, and brachial pulses, and good capillary refill in all digits
- Diagnosis is confirmed by x-ray

IMAGING/SPECIAL TESTS

Proximal Humerus Fractures

- Anteroposterior, lateral and axillary views or transthoracic or "y" view
  —The axillary view to assess tuberosity displacement, the glenoid articular surface, and the relationship of the humeral head to the glenoid
  —CT scan can be useful in evaluating articular surfaces of glenoid and humeral head

Humeral Shaft Fractures

- AP and lateral views of the entire humerus are mandatory
  —Include shoulder and elbow views to exclude associated joint involvement

DIFFERENTIAL DIAGNOSIS

- Acute hemorrhagic bursitis
- Traumatic rotator cuff tear
- Dislocation
- Acromioclavicular separation
- Calcific tendinitis
- Contusion
- Tendon rupture
- Neuropraxia
- Pathologic fracture

PEDIATRIC CONSIDERATIONS

- Children <5 years: Salter-Harris I fractures are seen
  —Neonatal fractures occur from obstetric trauma and pseudoparalysis are often seen
  —Physeal separation in the infant may also be the result of physical abuse
- Children 5–10 years: metaphyseal fractures due to rapid growth and thinning of the metaphyseal cortex; most fractures are transverse or short oblique
- Children ≥ 11 years: Salter-Harris II fractures
- Always consider child abuse especially with spiral fractures of the humerus, which implies a rotational component to the injury

Treatment

INITIAL STABILIZATION

- ABCs and secondary survey for associated injuries
- Immediate immobilization to prevent further fracture displacement or neurovascular injury
  —Sling with arm supported at the side or in the Velpeau position
  —Axillary pad may also be used for comfort
  —After immobilization perform another neurovascular exam
- Pain control with NSAIDs or narcotic analgesics
- Application of ice to limit swelling
- Open humerus fractures require covering with a sterile dressing, tetanus prophylaxis, and parenteral prophylactic antibiotics

ED TREATMENT

- Immobilization
  —Orthopedic consultation
  —Pain management
- *Operative versus nonoperative treatment* is decided in conjunction with orthopedics

Proximal Humerus Fractures

- *Neer classification:* this system identifies the number of fragments and their location
  —The fractures consist of 2-part to 4-part fractures, and the locations include the anatomic neck, the surgical neck, the greater tuberosity, and the lesser tuberosity
  —Fracture-dislocation and humeral head splitting are also part of the Neer classification
  —In general, the higher the number of fragments in the fracture and the greater the degree of displacement, the more difficult it is to manage the patient with a closed reduction
- *Nonoperative treatment*
  —Initial immobilization and early motion: succeeds in many cases as most proximal humeral fractures are minimally displaced
  —Use a sling, swath, and axillary pad to immobilize
  —Closed reduction with consultation of orthopedics
  —Conscious sedation for all closed reductions
  —1-part and 2-part fractures are often successfully treated with closed reduction, but 3-part and 4-part fractures are unstable and may need ORIF

Humeral Shaft Fractures

- Usually don't require elaborate reduction or immobilization
- Nondisplaced fractures can be treated with a sugar-tong splint of the upper extremity
- Grossly displaced or comminuted fractures require immobilization with a light hanging cast
- Open fractures or fractures associated with neurovascular compromise require immediate orthopedic consultation

MEDICATIONS

- Pain medications
- Conscious sedation with closed reductions (see Conscious Sedation)

PEDIATRIC CONSIDERATIONS

- In children nearing skeletal maturity, determining the degree of displacement or separation of the proximal humeral epiphysis is essential as exact reduction is important to prevent later growth disturbance

Disposition

ADMISSION CRITERIA

- Open fractures for operative management and parenteral antibiotic therapy
- Fractures associated with neurovascular compromise
- Displaced fracture that cannot be treated through closed reduction
- Significant associated injuries that require admission and observation

DISCHARGE CRITERIA

- Nondisplaced fracture or a fracture that is successfully treated with closed reduction and no associated injuries

PEDIATRIC CONSIDERATIONS

- Pediatric patients are often less compliant with immobilization and less able to verbalize complaints and may benefit from admission

Miscellaneous

ICD9: 812.09, 812.21

ICD10: S42.3

SUGGESTED READINGS

Bucholz RW, Heckman JD. Rockwood and Green's fractures in adults, 5th ed. Philadelphia: Lippincott Williams & Wilkins, 2002.

Gregory PR. Fractures of the shaft of the humerus. In: Bucholz RW, Heckman JD, eds. Rockwood and Green's fractures in adults, 5th ed. Philadelphia: Lippincott Williams & Wilkins, 2002.

Hawkins RJ, Angelo RL. Displaced proximal humeral fractures: selecting treatment, avoiding pitfalls. Orthop Clin North Am 1987;18(3):421–431.

Morrissy RT, Weinstein SL. Lovell and Winter's pediatric orthopaedics, vol 2, 5th ed. Philadelphia: Lippincott Williams & Wilkins, 2001.

Neer CS. Displaced proximal humeral fractures: I. Classification and evaluation. J Bone Joint Surg 1970;52A:1077–1089.

Rasmussen S, Hvass I, Dalsgaard J, et al. Displaced proximal humeral fractures: results of conservative treatment. Injury 1992;23(1):41–42.

Simon R, Koenigskhecht S. Emergency orthopedics, the extremities, 3rd ed. Norwalk, CT: Appleton & Lange, 1993.

Authors: William Goldberg; Nancy Kwon; Wallace Carter

Hydatidiform Mole

Clinical Presentation

SIGNS AND SYMPTOMS

- Findings consistent with pregnancy, usually exaggerated subjective symptoms
- Hyperemesis gravidarum
- Vaginal bleeding is most common symptom (97%)
  - —Usually late first trimester or early second trimester
  - —Usually painless bleeding
  - —May have passage of tissue; edematous trophoblasts passed through dilated cervical os
- Uterine dates/size discrepancy (50–66%)
  - —Usually larger than date would indicate; due to marked trophoblastic growth
  - —Can be smaller than date would indicate, especially partial mole
- Adnexal masses
  - —Prominent ovarian theca lutein cysts, due to high levels of circulating human chorionic gonadotrophin (hCG)

Complete Mole

- Toxemia (27%): visual changes, hypertension, proteinuria, hyperreflexia, rarely convulsions
- Hyperthyroidism (7%): marked tachycardia, tremor
- Acute respiratory distress (2%): tachypnea, tachycardia, mental status changes (agitation, confusion)
  - —Cause is multifactorial: trophoblastic pulmonary embolism or cardiopulmonary changes from toxemia, hyperthyroidism, and vigorous fluid replacement
  - —Diffuse rales
- Absent fetal heart tones

Partial Mole

- Usually do not exhibit the dramatic clinical features of complete mole
- Usually presents with symptoms similar to patients with threatened abortion (AB) or spontaneous AB
- Usually presents at more advanced gestational age
- Typically uterine growth is less than expected for gestational age
- May have fetal heart tones

MECHANISM/DESCRIPTION

- Complete mole
  - —Diffuse chorionic villi swelling
  - —Diffuse trophoblastic hyperplasia
  - —Fetal or embryonic tissue absent
  - —Karyotype: 46,XX (90%); 46,XY (10%)
  - —Paternal nuclear DNA
  - —Mechanism: 1 or 2 sperm "fertilize" empty egg
  - —Risk of persistent gestational trophoblastic tumor (GTT): 20%
- Partial mole
  - —Focal chorionic villi swelling
  - —Focal trophoblastic hyperplasia
  - —Fetal or embryonic tissue present
  - —Karyotype: triploid (90%); diploid (10%)
  - —Paternal and maternal nuclear DNA
  - —Mechanism: 2 sperm fertilize normal egg
  - —Risk of persistent GTT: 2–4%
- Risk factors for gestational trophoblastic tumor (GTT): marked trophoblastic proliferation (elevated hCG, excessive uterine enlargement, prominent theca lutein ovarian cysts), older patients, and repetitive molar pregnancies
- When compared to low-risk patients, high-risk patients have a higher incidence of local invasion (31% vs. 3.4%) and metastatic disease (8.8% vs. 0.6%)

ETIOLOGY

- Largely unknown
- Frequency more common in Asian countries, 1 per 125 live births, and less common in Western Europe and U.S., 1 per 1,500 live births
- Socioeconomic and nutritional factors; vitamin A deficiency
- Advanced maternal age; women older than 40 have a 5- to 10-fold greater risk

Pre-Hospital

- Ensure patent airway, provide oxygen, and establish IV access
  - —If convulsions are present, treat with diazepam
  - —Save any passed tissue for histologic evaluation

Diagnosis

ESSENTIAL WORKUP

- Ultrasonography
  - —Complete molar pregnancy produces characteristic vesicular sonographic pattern from swelling of chorionic villi ("snowstorm" appearance)
  - —Partial molar pregnancy may have cystic changes in placenta and changes in the shape of gestational sac (transverse to anteroposterior dimension ratio of 1.5); also scalloping of villi
  - —Theca lutein ovarian cysts, associated with high hCG levels
- hCG and free subunits
  - —Complete mole: often β-hCG $>$100,000 mIU/mL; mean ratio of β-hCG to α-hCG is 20.9; higher serum level of percent free β-hCG
  - —Partial mole: mean ratio of β-hCG to α-hCG is 2.4; higher serum level of percent free α-hCG
  - —Prognostic indicator: pretreatment hCG $>$40,000 mIU/mL is poor prognosis
  - —Can be followed as indication of persistent disease

LABORATORY

- Hemoglobin and hematocrit
- Blood type and Rh (RhoGAM should be given as in normal pregnancy when indicated)
- CBC, electrolytes, liver function tests, urinalysis if toxemia suspected
- TSH, thyroxine (free T_4) if hyperthyroidism suspected
- Pathologic evaluation of products of conception; partial moles may only be diagnosed via pathology

IMAGING

- Chest x-ray if suspect acute respiratory distress or for baseline to check for metastatic disease

DIFFERENTIAL DIAGNOSIS

- Threatened abortion
- Missed abortion
- Incomplete abortion
- Ectopic pregnancy

Treatment

INITIAL STABILIZATION

- ABCs
- IV access
- Type and cross-match for blood, especially if patient needs uterine extraction

ED TREATMENT

Acute Respiratory Distress

- CXR: may show bilateral pulmonary infiltrates
- Intubation and mechanical ventilation

Hyperthyroidism

- β-adrenergic blockers
  —Administer before molar evacuation
  —Stress of anesthesia or surgery may precipitate thyroid storm with tachyarrhythmia, high-output failure, hyperthermia and convulsions

Preeclampsia

- Benzodiazepine if convulsions
- Magnesium sulfate

Suction Curettage

- Done by obstetrician, possibly in ED
- Method of choice in women wishing to preserve fertility
- Oxytocin infusion after anesthesia started to induce myometrial tone
- Cervix carefully dilated
- 12-mm cannula to permit rapid evacuation and involution of the uterus to control bleeding
- Sharp curettage to remove residual chorionic tissue
- Submit suction and curettage specimen separately

Chemoprophylaxis

- Should be prescribed by obstetrician for patients with follow-up
- Use of chemoprophylaxis at time of evacuation remains controversial
- Kim et al. showed chemoprophylaxis reduced the incidence of postmolar tumor from 47% to 14% in patients with high-risk complete mole.
- Berkowitz et al. showed that actinomycin D reduces risk of persistent GTT in patients with high-risk complete mole
- Chemoprophylaxis may be useful in high-risk complete mole or if hormonal follow-up is unavailable or unreliable

MEDICATIONS

- Actinomycin D: 12 μg/kg/d i.v. for 5 days every 2 weeks, or 1.5 mg i.v. every 14 days
- Methotrexate: 0.4 μg/kg/d, 5 days i.m. every 2 weeks
- Oxytocin: Postpartum bleeding: 10 units i.m. or 10–40 units in 1000 mL NS i.v.
- Propranolol: 1 mg i.v. increments every 2 min
- RhoGAM: 1 vial within 72 hours if mother Rh−
- Diazepam: 0.2–0.4 mg/kg up to 5–10 mg i.v., or 0.3–0.5 mg/kg PR

Disposition

ADMISSION CRITERIA

- Enlargement of uterus beyond 16 weeks gestational size; the larger the uterus, the greater the risk for uterine perforation during suction curettage, hemorrhage, and pulmonary complications
- Clinical evidence of preeclampsia, hyperthyroidism, respiratory distress
- Indications for hysterectomy: patient in older age group or patient who does not want to preserve fertility; should be considered in patient with high-risk disease; hysterectomy ensures removal of entire primary neoplasm but does not prevent metastases
- Partial molar pregnancies: often need larger grasping instruments to remove abnormal fetus
- Hemodynamic instability

DISCHARGE CRITERIA

- Uncomplicated dilation and curettage of low-risk and small size mole (less than 16 weeks) in reliable patient with good follow-up
- Meticulous follow-up is mandatory due to the risk of persistent trophoblastic neoplasia
- Weekly β-hCG testing until three consecutive normal levels are achieved; then monthly β-hCG levels for 6 months; contraception for the entire follow-up period

Miscellaneous

ICD9: 630

ICD10: 001.9

SUGGESTED READINGS

Berkowitz RS, Goldstein DP. Management of molar pregnancy and gestational trophoblastic tumors. In: Knapp RC, Berkowitz RS, eds. Gynecologic oncology, 2nd ed. New York: McGraw-Hill, 1993: 328–338.

Goldstein DP, Berkowitz RS. Current management of complete and partial molar pregnancy. J Reprod Med 1994;39: 139–146.

Hancock BW, Tidy JA. Current management of molar pregnancy. J Reprod Med 2002;47:347–353.

Homesley HD. Development of single-agent chemotherapy regimens for gestational trophoblastic disease. J Reprod Med 1994;39:185–192.

Kim DS, et al. Effects of prophylactic chemotherapy on persistent trophoblastic disease in patients with complete hydatidiform mole. Obstet Gynecol 1986;67:690–694.

Shapter AP, McLellan R. Gestational trophoblastic disease. Obstet Gynecol Clin North Am 2001;28:805–817.

Soper JT. Surgical therapy for gestational trophoblastic disease. J Reprod Med 1994;39:168–174.

Author: Tami Gash-Kim

Hydrocarbon, Poisoning

Clinical Presentation

SIGNS AND SYMPTOMS

- Often asymptomatic at presentation
- Odor of hydrocarbons on breath
- Pulmonary
  —Mild to severe respiratory distress
  —Cyanosis
  —Aspiration (primary complication)
- CNS
  —Intoxication
  —Euphoria
  —Slurred speech
  —Lethargy
  —Coma
- GI
  —Local mucosal irritation
  —Gastritis
  —Diarrhea
- Cardiac
  —Tachycardia
  —Dysrhythmias (volatile substance abuse)
- Dermal
  —Local erythema
  —Maculopapular or vesicular eruptions
  —Defatting dermatitis from chronic skin exposure
  —Huffer's rash of the face seen in chronic abusers

ETIOLOGY

- Accidental exposures—typical in young children
- Inhalation abuse of volatile hydrocarbons
- Suicide attempts in adolescents and adults

Major Classes of Hydrocarbons

- Aliphatics, or straight-chain compounds
  —Include kerosene, mineral oil, seal oil, gasoline, solvents, and paint thinners
  —Pulmonary toxicity via aspiration
  —Asphyxiation from gaseous methane and butane by displacement of alveolar oxygen
- Halogenated hydrocarbons
  —Carbon tetrachloride, and trichloroethane
  —Found in industrial settings as solvents
  —Well absorbed by the lungs and the gut
  —High toxicity
  —Liver and renal failure are associated with ingestion
- Cyclics or aromatic compounds
  —Toluene and xylene highly volatile and well absorbed from the gut
  —Death from benzene reported with 15-mL ingestion
- Terpenes or wood distillates (turpentine and pine oil)
  —Significant GI absorption
  —Great degree of CNS depression

MECHANISM/DESCRIPTION

- Physical properties that determine the type and extent of toxicity
  —Viscosity (resistance to flow): aspiration risk
  —Volatility (ability of a substance to vaporize): hypoxia from aromatic hydrocarbons displacing alveolar air
  —Surface tension (the ability to adhere to itself at the liquid's surface): low surface tension allows easy spread from the oropharynx to the trachea, promoting aspiration, e.g., mineral oil, seal oil
- Volatile substance abuse
  —Common solvents abused: typewriter correction fluid, adhesive, or other halogenated hydrocarbons such as gasoline or cigarette-lighter fluid
  —*Huffing:* product inhaled through a soaked rag held to face
  —*Bagging:* product poured into a bag and multiple inhalations taken from bag
  —Symptoms:
  -Early: euphoria, disinhibition
  -Late: dysphoria, ataxia, confusion, and hallucination
  -Sudden sniffing death: cardiac arrest in volatile substance abusers secondary to hypersensitization of the myocardium leading to malignant dysrhythmias upon adrenergic stimulation

Pre-Hospital

CAUTIONS

- Do not induce emesis
- Avoid gastric lavage when possible
- Ipecac contraindicated due to increased risk of aspiration
- Keep volatile-substance abusers calm and avoid interventions that cause anxiety or distress

CONTROVERSIES

- Management of *accidental* hydrocarbon exposures at home
  —<1% required physician intervention
  —For asymptomatic or quickly asymptomatic after ingestion with reliable observer available
  —Only applies when the exact product and its components are known and there is no indication for gastric decontamination or possibility for delayed organ toxicity

Diagnosis

ESSENTIAL WORKUP

- Obtain
  - —Product: exact name on label, manufacturer, and ingredients
  - —Nature of ingestion or exposure: accidental or intentional
  - —Estimated amount ingested
  - —In industrial settings, the manufacturer safety data sheets (MSDS)

LABORATORY

- Pulse oximetry
  - —If abnormal follow with ABG
- Electrolytes, BUN, Cr, glucose, liver function tests
  - —For halogenated and aromatic hydrocarbon exposure
  - —Metabolic acidosis
  - —Hypokalemia
- Carboxyhemoglobin levels for methylene chloride exposure
  - —Methylene chloride metabolized to carbon monoxide in vivo

IMAGING/SPECIAL TESTS

- EKG for intoxicated volatile substance abusers
- CXR
  - —Abnormalities as early as 20 minutes or as late as 24 hours
  - —Increased bronchovascular marking and bibasilar and perihilar infiltrates (typical)
  - —Lobar consolidation (uncommon)
  - —Pneumothorax, pneumomediastinum, and pleural effusion (rare)
  - —Pneumatoceles—resolve over weeks
- Abdominal radiograph
  - —Radiopaque halogenated hydrocarbons may be visible

DIFFERENTIAL DIAGNOSIS

- Caustic, pesticide, or toxic alcohol ingestions
- Accidental vs. intentional: psychiatric evaluation for all intentional ingestions
- Child neglect—poor supervision or unsafe home environment

Treatment

INITIAL STABILIZATION

- ABCs
- Naloxone, thiamine, glucose for altered mental status
- IV access and fluid resuscitation if hypotensive or ongoing fluid losses
- Cardiac monitoring for halogenated hydrocarbons (*baggers* and *huffers*)

ED TREATMENT

- Supportive care
- Respiratory symptoms
  - —Oxygen
  - —Nebulized β_2-agonist for bronchospasm (albuterol)
  - —Endotracheal intubation and mechanical ventilation for respiratory failure
  - —Steroids not indicated for bronchospasm
- Gastric evacuation generally not indicated
  - —Aspiration risk higher than the risk of systemic absorption for aliphatic hydrocarbon mixtures that account for most ingestions
  - —Contraindicated if spontaneous emesis has occurred
  - —Evacuation indicated for CHAMP containing hydrocarbon ingestions
    - -CHAMP: camphor, halogenated hydrocarbons, aromatic hydrocarbons, metals (e.g., lead, mercury), pesticides
    - -Use small-bore lavage tube (petroleum distillates are liquids)
    - -Consider endotracheal intubation with a cuffed tube for airway protection during lavage if no gag reflex or altered mental status
- Activated charcoal not indicated except for significant co-ingestants
- Cathartics not indicated—diarrhea from the hydrocarbon common

MEDICATIONS

- Dextrose: D50W 1 amp (50 mL or 25 g) (peds: D25W 2–4 mL/kg) i.v.
- Naloxone (Narcan): 2 mg (peds: 0.1 mg/kg) i.v. or i.m. initial dose
- Thiamine (vitamin B_1): 100 mg (peds: 50 mg) i.v. or i.m.

Disposition

ADMISSION CRITERIA

- All symptomatic patients
- Potential delayed organ toxicity (carbon tetrachloride or other toxic additives)

DISCHARGE CRITERIA

- Observe for 6 hours, then discharge
  - —Asymptomatic patients with a normal chest x-ray and pulse oximetry
  - —Asymptomatic patients with abnormal chest x-ray and normal oxygenation and respiratory rate may be discharged if reliable follow-up ensured
  - —Symptomatic patients on presentation who quickly become asymptomatic may be evaluated as above
- Observe volatile substance abusers until mental status clears

Miscellaneous

ICD9: 987.1

SUGGESTED READINGS

Anas N, Namasonthi V, Ginsburg C. Criteria for hospitalizing children who have ingested products containing hydrocarbons. JAMA 1981;246:840–843.

Dice WH, Ward G, Kelly J, et al. Pulmonary toxicity following gastrointestinal ingestion of kerosene. Ann Emerg Med 1982;11:138–142.

Esmail A, Meyer L, Pottier A, et al. Deaths from volatile substance abuse in those under 18 years: results from a national epidemiological study. Arch Dis Child 1993;69:356.

Machado B, Cross K, Snodgrass WR. Accidental hydrocarbon ingestion cases telephoned to a regional poison center. Ann Emerg Med 1988;17:804–807.

Author: Bonnie McManus

Hydrocele

Clinical Presentation

SIGNS AND SYMPTOMS

- Progressive painless swelling on the involved side of the scrotum
- May be unilateral or bilateral
- Symptoms may include sensation of heaviness

MECHANISM/DESCRIPTION

- *Communicating hydrocele* occurs in those patients with patent processus vaginalis and the scrotum fills and empties with peritoneal fluid depending on body position
- *Noncommunicating hydrocele* is due to the production of serous fluid by a disease process

ETIOLOGY

- Hydrocele results from an imbalance between the production and resorption of fluid within the space between the tunica vaginalis and the tunica albuginea
- Disease processes causing adult noncommunicating hydrocele include:
  - —Epididymitis
  - —Hypoalbuminemia
  - —Tuberculosis
  - —Trauma
  - —Mumps
  - —Spermatic vein ligation
  - —In the Third World, hydrocele is primarily caused by infections such as *Wuchereria bancrofti* or *Loa Loa*
  - —Rarely malignancy (first-degree testicular neoplasm or lymphoma)
- Rare etiology is the "abdominoscrotal hydrocele" that may cause hydroureter or unilateral limb edema due to compression
  - —Ultrasound reveals single sac extending from scrotum into the abdominal cavity via the deep inguinal ring

PEDIATRIC CONSIDERATIONS

- Congenital in 6% of newborn boys
- Usually diagnosed in the newborn nursery
- Caused by a patent processus vaginalis, a structure that remains patent in 85% of newborns
- As it communicates with the abdominal cavity, it may vary in size due to position or crying; patients may present with a history of a scrotal mass that has resolved

Pre-Hospital

N/A

Diagnosis

ESSENTIAL WORKUP

- History and examination with special attention to identifying torsion of the testicle
- Initial diagnostic test is transillumination of the affected side
- Due to the possibility in adults that a hydrocele may be due to a primary neoplasm, the testicle must be palpated in its entirety
- In cases of massive hydrocele, or if the testicle can not be palpated, direct visualization with ultrasound is indicated

LABORATORY

- No specific laboratory testing is indicated unless underlying etiology demands it

IMAGING/SPECIAL TESTS

- Ultrasound is diagnostic and allows visualization of testicular anatomy
  - —Appears as a large fluid-filled space surrounding the testicle

Treatment

INITIAL STABILIZATION

- Stabilization should focus on the underlying cause (e.g., trauma)

ED MANAGEMENT

- Appropriate examination of testicle to exclude primary neoplasm and referral

MEDICATIONS

- Treat underlying etiology

PEDIATRIC CONSIDERATIONS

See Disposition, below

Disposition

ADMISSION CRITERIA

- Patients with secondary hydrocele may need admission for further evaluation of underlying pathology (e.g., neoplasm, trauma)

DISCHARGE CRITERIA

- Otherwise healthy patients without comorbid illness may be referred for further evaluation to a urologist
- Hydrocele is usually repaired if cosmesis is a factor or in cases where it causes discomfort
- Repair can be:
  —Surgical
  —Medical—with aspiration of hydrocele contents and sclerotherapy to prevent recurrence

PEDIATRIC CONSIDERATIONS

- Most hydroceles in the infant population will spontaneously resolve by 12 months of age; referral and observation are appropriate once the diagnosis is made
- After the age of 12–18 months refer for surgical repair as communicating hydroceles usually have a hernia that needs repair

Miscellaneous

ICD9: 603.9

ICD10: N43.3

SUGGESTED READINGS

Kaplan GW. Scrotal swelling in children. Pediatr Rev 2000;21:311–314.

Lau MW, Taylor PM, Payne SR. The indications for scrotal ultrasound. Br J Radiol 1999;72:833–837.

Rabinowitz R, Hulbert WC. Acute scrotal swelling. Urol Clin North Am 1995;22: 101–105.

Schul MW, Keating MA. The acute pediatric scrotum. J Emerg Med 1993;11:565–577.

Author: Sean O. Henderson

Hydrocephalus

Clinical Presentation

SIGNS AND SYMPTOMS

Obstructive (Noncommunicating) Hydrocephalus

- Headache, with nausea and vomiting, decreased level of consciousness (LOC), urinary incontinence
- Ocular palsies, papilledema, decreased vision
- Pupillary dilation and the Cushing's response (raised systolic pressure and bradycardia)
- *Pediatric patients:* full fontanelle, irritability, and lethargy
- May present like nonobstructive hydrocephalus if obstruction develops slowly

Nonobstructing (Communicating) Hydrocephalus

- Progressive dementia, somnolence
- Gait disturbance, urinary incontinence, impaired upward gaze, generalized weakness, and lethargy
- Dementia is often insidious with subacute onset of progressive intellectual deterioration
- No headache or papilledema
- Pediatric patients increase CSF volume slowly resulting in craniomegaly, retardation, prominent scalp veins, and impaired upward gaze ("setting sun" sign)

MECHANISM/DESCRIPTION

- The signs and symptoms of hydrocephalus result from increased fluid in the cranium
- *Obstructive hydrocephalus* is the most common form
  - —The obstruction is within the ventricular system or in the subarachnoid space
- Acute obstructive hydrocephalus may cause acute rises in ICP, rapidly leading to death or permanent cerebral damage
- *Nonobstructive hydrocephalus* causes subacute symptoms and is a potentially treatable form of dementia

ETIOLOGY

- *Obstructive hydrocephalus*
  - —Obstruction of the foramen of Monro, third ventricle, fourth ventricle, aqueduct of Sylvius, or foramina of Luschka and Magendie (tumor or other masses) or the subarachnoid space around the brainstem (postinfectious or post-SAH)
  - —Acute presentations usually secondary to CSF shunt blockage, SAH, or severe head trauma
- *Nonobstructive hydrocephalus*
  - —Normal pressure hydrocephalus: increased intracranial volume without intracranial hypertension
  - —Increased ventricular size on CT
- *Pediatric hydrocephalus*
  - —Congenital hydrocephalus due to neonatal hemorrhages, congenital malformations, or acquired postmeningitis secondary to subarachnoid scarring around the brain stem

Pre-Hospital

CAUTIONS

- Elevated ICP cannot be definitively diagnosed in the field
- When it is suspected, supplemental O_2 and aggressive airway management are indicated
- If not contraindicated, patients should be transported with head elevated at 30 degrees

Diagnosis

ESSENTIAL WORKUP

- CT scan of the head will allow assessment of ventricular size and symmetry and aid in the diagnosis of cerebral edema, mass lesions, and hemorrhage

LABORATORY

- Lumbar puncture is typically performed after head CT
  - —The opening pressure on LP will reflect increased ICP in nonobstructive hydrocephalus
  - —CSF should be sent for routine tests (Gram stain, culture, protein, and glucose) if an infectious or inflammatory process is suspected

IMAGING/SPECIAL TESTS

- MRI of brain reveals ventricular size and symmetry and may allow for better visualization of masses than CT

DIFFERENTIAL DIAGNOSIS

- Acute cerebral infarction or hemorrhage
- Intracranial infection
- Mass effect from fast-growing tumor or hematoma
- Dementia or delirium of other cause
- Toxic or metabolic encephalopathies

PEDIATRIC CONSIDERATIONS

- Suspect hydrocephalus in an infant whose head circumference is increasing excessively
- Congenital anomalies, e.g., constitutional macrocrania, megalencephaly, Dandy-Walker malformation, Arnold-Chiari malformation, meningomyelocele, choroid plexus papilloma, hypoplasia/dysfunction of arachnoid villi
- Infections, e.g., rubella, CMV, toxoplasmosis, syphilis, bacterial meningitis, Reye's syndrome
- Tumors, especially posterior fossa tumors, e.g., medulloblastoma, astrocytoma, ependymoma
- Hemorrhage, e.g., intraventricular bleed and fibrosis, subarachnoid bleed

Treatment

INITIAL STABILIZATION

- Signs of impending herniation
  - —Rapid sequence intubation (RSI); thiopental or etomidate for induction; paralytic choice is controversial
  - —Depolarizing agents (succinylcholine) may increase ICP, though this effect may not be clinically significant
  - —Nondepolarizing agents (rocuronium, vecuronium) may be preferable
  - —Controlled ventilation to maintain $PaCO_2$ ~35 mm Hg
  - —Maintain systolic bp >100 mm Hg (adult) with fluids or pressors
  - —Mannitol
- If a CSF shunt is present and there are signs of impending herniation
  - —Forced pumping of shunt chamber: flush the device with 1 cc saline to remove distal obstruction; slow drainage of CSF from the reservoir to achieve pressure <20 cm H_2O; IV mannitol to lower ICP

ED TREATMENT

- When signs of impending herniation or acute shunt malfunction are absent, hydrocephalus does not require ED treatment
- Definitive treatment involves either placement (or revision) of a shunting device or treatment of the underlying cause (e.g., tumor)
- Increased ICP refractory to other treatments may respond to controlled lumbar drainage
- Neurologic symptoms (gait disturbance) or severe headache associated with normal pressure hydrocephalus may respond to removal of 25–30 cc of CSF

MEDICATIONS

- Atropine: 0.02 mg/kg i.v. (max 0.1 mg)
- Etomidate: 0.2–0.3 mg/kg
- Lidocaine: 1 mg/kg i.v.
- Mannitol: 0.5–1 mg/kg
- Rocuronium: 0.6 mg/kg i.v.
- Succinylcholine: 1–1.5 mg/kg i.v.
- Vecuronium: 0.1 mg/kg

Disposition

ADMISSION CRITERIA

- Evidence of increased ICP or shunt malfunction requires admission

DISCHARGE CRITERIA

- Patients with presumed normal pressure hydrocephalus may be discharged for follow-up

Miscellaneous

ICD9: 331.4

ICD10: G91.9

SUGGESTED READINGS

Adams RD, Victor M, Ropper AH. Principles of neurology, 6th ed. New York: McGraw-Hill, 1997:539–553.

Del Bigio MR. Neuropathological changes caused by hydrocephalus. Acta Neuropathol 1993;85(6):573–585.

Ledin T, Bynke O, Odkvist LM. Influence of cerebrospinal fluid tapping on dynamic equilibrium in suspected hydrocephalus. Acta Otolaryngol 1995;520[pt 2 suppl]: 317–319.

Marmarou A, Foda M, Bandoh K, et al. Posttraumatic ventriculomegaly: hydrocephalus or atrophy? A new approach for diagnosis using CSF dynamics. J Neurosurg 1996;85:1026–1035.

Mori K. Current concept of hydrocephalus: evolution of new classifications. Childs Nerv Syst 1995;11(9):523–531.

Rowland LP. Merritt's textbook of neurology, 9th ed. Baltimore: Williams & Wilkins, 1995:294–309.

Vanaclocha V, Saiz-Sapena N, Leiva J. Shunt malfunction as related to shunt infection. Acta Neurochir 1996;138(7):829–834.

Author: Richard S. Krause

Hyperbaric Oxygen Therapy

Clinical Presentation

SIGNS AND SYMPTOMS

Indications for Hyperbaric Oxygen (HBO)

- Arterial gas embolism
- Decompression sickness
- Toxic inhalations
  —Carbon monoxide
  —Cyanide
  —Hydrogen sulfide
- Wound care (requires multiple treatments)
  —Gas gangrene (*Clostridium*)
  —Osteomyelitis
  —Postradiation tissue injury
  —Burns
  —Crush injuries and acute peripheral extremity ischemic injuries
  —Increased tissue oxygen level improves function of neutrophils and allows more effective antimicrobial function
- Indications continuously evolving

MECHANISM/DESCRIPTION

- Definition: administration of 100% oxygen at pressure greater than sea level (1 atm)
- Two effects of HBO
  —Mechanical effect—compression of formed gas bubbles
  —Chemical effect—increase in the amount of oxygen available at the cellular level due to increased oxygen dissolved in plasma
    -At 3 atm pressure and breathing 100% oxygen—enough oxygen is dissolved in plasma to supply baseline tissue requirements, and hemoglobin is not necessary for oxygen transport
- Types of HBO chambers
  —Monoplace
    -Accommodates a single supine patient monitored by a technician outside the clear tube
    -Compressed with 100% oxygen
  —Multiplace
    -Holds multiple patients as well as tenders who "dive" with the patients
    -Air locks allow for transfer of medication and equipment in and out of the chamber
    -Compressed with air: patients breathe oxygen by mask, face tent, or endotracheal tube
- Due to the risk of oxygen toxicity and seizures, most hyperbaric protocols limit depth to 2–2.8 atm (60 feet) for no more that 90–120 minutes

Pre-Hospital

CAUTIONS

- Administer 100% oxygen for all patients being transported to HBO facility
- Establish IV access

CONTROVERSIES

- A recent study questions the presumed efficacy of HBO in the treatment of carbon monoxide poisoning; more investigation is needed

Diagnosis

ESSENTIAL WORKUP

- Determine need for HBO treatment by above diagnosis
- Document a comprehensive neurologic exam to establish baseline for subsequent posttreatment examinations

LABORATORY

- ABG
  —Baseline measure useful for hypoxic patients
  —Serial measurements of the suspected inhaled toxin (CO, CN, HS) may be necessary

IMAGING/SPECIAL TESTS

- CXR to rule out any untreated pneumothorax

Treatment

INITIAL STABILIZATION

- Only absolute contraindication to HBO therapy
  - —Untreated pneumothorax
    - -Increased pressure converts a simple pneumothorax into a tension pneumothorax
- Cardiovascular stability required for treatment in monoplace chambers
- Multiplace chambers allow for nursing and other personnel to provide ongoing care

ED TREATMENT

- Patient equipment/devices with balloons (i.e., Foley catheters, endotracheal tubes) must be filled with fluid to avoid rupture
- Pretreatment with decongestants if sinus congestion present
- Tympanostomy tubes for patients who experience middle ear discomfort (squeeze) during compression and who cannot equalize the ear pressures
- Multiplace chambers can accommodate IVs, ventilators, and most medical therapies
- No smoking or any potentially flammable devices
- Divers Alert Network (DAN)
  - —Based at Duke University Medical Center in North Carolina
  - —Provides a 24-hour emergency hotline for medical consultation on the treatment of dive-related injuries and for referrals to hyperbaric chambers
  - —Telephone: 919-684-8111

MEDICATIONS

- Pseudoephedrine (Sudafed): 60 mg (peds: 6–12 years old, 30 mg; 2–5 years old, 15 mg/dose) PO q4–6h

Disposition

ADMISSION CRITERIA

- Arterial gas embolism/decompression sickness should be admitted for repeat neurologic exam
- Severe inhalational injury with CO or CN

DISCHARGE CRITERIA

- Mild toxic inhalations may be discharged post-HBO therapy if their oxygenation status is acceptable and there are no other injuries

Miscellaneous

ICD9: N/A

ICD10: N/A

SEE ALSO: ARTERIAL GAS EMBOLISM, DECOMPRESSION SICKNESS, AND BAROTRAUMA

SUGGESTED READINGS

Scheinkestel CD, et al. Hyperbaric or normobaric oxygen for acute carbon monoxide poisoning: a randomized controlled clinical trial. Med J Aust 1999;170(5):203–210.

Tibbles PM, Edelsberg JS. Hyperbaric oxygen therapy. N Engl J Med 1996; 334(25):1642–1648.

Author: Jeffrey Gordon

Hypercalcemia

Clinical Presentation

SIGNS AND SYMPTOMS

General

- Severity depends on level of serum calcium and rate of its rise
- Hypercalcemic crisis, usually above 14 mg/dL, associated with serious signs and symptoms

Neurologic

- Headache
- Fatigue
- Weakness
- Difficulty concentrating
- Confusion
- Irritable
- Lethargy
- Stupor
- Coma
- Hyporeflexia

Cardiovascular

- Hypotension, if severely volume depleted or hypertension
- EKG
  - —Shortening of QT interval
  - —Prolongation of PR interval
  - —QRS widening
- Accentuates side effects of digoxin
- Sinus bradycardia, bundle branch block, AV block, cardiac arrest with severe hypercalcemia (rare)

Renal

- Dehydration
- Polyuria, polydipsia
- Oliguric renal failure
- Chronically: renal calculi, nephrocalcinosis, interstitial nephritis

Gastrointestinal

- Anorexia
- Nausea
- Vomiting
- Abdominal pain
- Constipation
- Intestinal ileus
- Chronically: increased risk of peptic ulcer disease and pancreatitis

Dermatologic

- Pruritus
- Band keratopathy
- Ectopic calcification

MECHANISM/DESCRIPTION

- 0.1–1% of patients on routine laboratory screening
- Most cases mild (<12 mg/dL) and asymptomatic
- Calcium in bloodstream in three forms
  - —Ionized: 45%
  - —Bound to protein (primarily albumin): 40%
  - —Bound to other anions: 15%
- Ionized calcium—only physiologically active form

ETIOLOGY

- Primary hyperparathyroidism
- Malignancy
- Miscellaneous

PEDIATRIC CONSIDERATIONS

Infantile Hypercalcemia

- Characteristic facies: pug nose, fat nasal bridge, "cupid's bow" upper lip
- Failure to thrive
- Slow development
- Hypotonia
- Associated with pulmonic and supravalvular aortic stenosis
- Mental retardation may ensue

Pre-Hospital

N/A

Diagnosis

ESSENTIAL WORKUP

- Ionized and total serum calcium levels, albumin levels
  - —Normal total calcium level is <10.5 mg/dL
  - —Must correct for calcium that is protein-bound, primarily to albumin
  - —Corrected total calcium (mg/dL) = measured total calcium (mg/dL) + 0.8 × [4.0 − albumin concentration (g/dL)]
- Electrolytes, BUN/Cr, glucose
- EKG

LABORATORY

- Phosphate
- Protein
- Urinalysis
- Parathyroid hormone level
- Vitamin D level, if suspected
- Digoxin level, if taking
- Thyroid function tests

IMAGING/SPECIAL TESTS

- CT head, if altered mental status
- Workup for occult malignancy, if no other cause

DIFFERENTIAL DIAGNOSIS

Primary Hyperparathyroidism

- Most common cause in outpatients
- Usually mild, less than 11.2 mg/dL
- Increased bone resorption, relative decrease in calcium excretion, increased intestinal calcium absorption

Malignancy

- Most common cause in hospitalized patients
- Most common paraneoplastic complication of cancer
- Most commonly from production of parathyroid hormone-related protein with similar actions
- May result from production of other bone-resorbing substances by tumor
- May result from local effects of osteolytic skeletal metastasis

MISCELLANEOUS

- Excessive calcium supplements
- Thiazide diuretics increase renal reabsorption
- Granulomatous disorders may lead to activation of vitamin D
- Acute vitamin A intoxication
- Increased exogenous vitamin D intake
- Milk-alkali syndrome from excessive ingestion of calcium and nonabsorbable antacids such as milk or calcium carbonate
- Long-term lithium therapy
- Renal transplantation
- Hyperthyroidism
- Acute tubular necrosis

PEDIATRIC CONSIDERATIONS

- Differential diagnosis: differences from adults
  - —Primary hyperparathyroidism
    - -Less common than in adults
  - —Infantile hypercalcemia
    - -Uncertain etiology
    - -Possibly hypersensitivity and in utero excessive exposure to vitamin D
  - —Immobilization hypercalcemia
    - -Typically adolescent who is growing rapidly
    - -Prolonged immobilization, especially in traction, leads to hypercalciuria and then hypercalcemia
    - -Presumably from increased bone resorption with decreased or arrested bone mineralization

Treatment

INITIAL STABILIZATION

- ABCs, intravenous access, oxygen, cardiac monitor
- 0.9% NS 1 L bolus (20 mL/kg) for hypotension or severe dehydration
- Naloxone, thiamine, D50W (or Accucheck) for altered mental status

ED TREATMENT

General

- Immediate therapy for severe hypercalcemia (corrected total >14 mg/dL) regardless of symptoms, and for symptomatic hypercalcemia
- Asymptomatic, mild hypercalcemia does not require emergency treatment

Fluid Administration

- Isotonic saline for restoration of intravascular volume
- Often need 2–5 L per day
- Correct other electrolyte abnormalities
- Cardiovascular status of patient may necessitate central venous pressure monitoring to adjust fluid administration rates

Renal Elimination

- After volume expansion and if needed to avoid overload, administer loop diuretics like furosemide
- Avoid thiazide diuretics
- May need peritoneal or hemodialysis against a low calcium dialysate in renal failure

Inhibition of Osteoclastic Activity

- Reduce mobilization of calcium from bone
- Administer drug therapy when corrected calcium level >14 mg/dL or signs or symptoms
- First-line drug therapy
  - —Bisphosphonates: pamidronate (more potent and possibly less toxic), etidronate
  - —Calcitonin: rapid onset but modest decrease in levels
- Other potential drug therapy
  - —Plicamycin: efficacious but numerous side effects
  - —Hydrocortisone: especially useful with malignancies, granulomatous disorders, or vitamin D intoxication
- Encourage ambulation in appropriate patients

Underlying Disorder

- Prepare to treat underlying cause
- Parathyroidectomy for primary hyperparathyroidism resulting in symptomatic or severe hypercalcemia
- Treat tumor for malignancy
- Discontinue medication if cause

MEDICATIONS

- Calcitonin: 4 IU/kg q12h i.v.
- Etidronate: 7.5 mg/kg over 4 hours daily for 3–7 days i.v.
- Furosemide: 10–40 mg q6–8h (peds: 1–2 mg/kg) i.v.
- Gallium nitrate: continuous infusion of 200 mg/m^2/d for 5 days i.v.
- Hydrocortisone: 200–300 mg/day i.v. (peds: consult pediatrician)
- Pamidronate: single 24-hr infusion of 60–90 mg i.v. (peds: consult pediatrician)
- Plicamycin: 25 μg/kg over 4 hours i.v.

PEDIATRIC CONSIDERATIONS

- Fluid at 2–3 times daily maintenance in otherwise normal patients

Disposition

ADMISSION CRITERIA

- Corrected total calcium level above 13.0 mg/dL
- Signs or symptoms attributed to hypercalcemia
- Monitored bed or ICU for corrected level >14 or serious signs and symptoms

DISCHARGE CRITERIA

- Corrected calcium level below 13.0 mg/dL and no signs or symptoms of hypercalcemia
- Rapid follow-up arranged to determine cause and long-term therapy

Miscellaneous

ICD9: 275.4

ICD10: E83.5

SUGGESTED READINGS

Edelson GW, Kleerekoper M. Hypercalcemic crisis. In: Ober KP, ed. Med Clin North Am 1995;79(1):79–92.

Kaye TB. Hypercalcemia. How to pinpoint the cause and customize treatment. Postgrad Med 1995;97(1):153–155, 159–160.

Kirmsky WS, Behrens RJ, Kerkvliet GJ. Oncologic emergencies for the internist. Cleve Clin J Med 2002;69(3):209–210, 213–214, 216–217, 221–222.

Marx J, et al., eds. Rosen's emergency medicine: concepts and clinical practice, 5th ed. St. Louis: CV Mosby, 2002:1732–1736.

Author: Jeffrey King

Hyperemesis Gravidarum

Clinical Presentation

SIGNS AND SYMPTOMS

- Nausea and vomiting during pregnancy is common, affecting between 50% and 90%
- Onset of symptoms by the 4th to 10th week of pregnancy with resolution by the 20th
  - —Symptoms after the 20th week should raise one's suspicion of another process
- Hyperemesis gravidarum is a clinical diagnosis
- Hyperemesis is defined by the following:
  - —Persistent, severe nausea and vomiting
  - —Dehydration
  - —Weight loss of >5% of total body weight
  - —Laboratory findings: increased urine specific gravity, ketonuria, electrolyte disturbances, ketonemia

MECHANISM/DESCRIPTION

- Hyperemesis gravidarum, also known as pernicious vomiting of pregnancy, is the most severe form along the continuum of nausea and vomiting of pregnancy

ETIOLOGY

- The exact etiology is unknown; however, possible etiologies include the following:
  - —Elevated gestational associated hormone levels
  - —Thyrotoxicosis
  - —Upper GI motility dysfunction
  - —Hepatic abnormalities
  - —Autonomic nervous system dysfunction
  - —Psychological factors
  - —*Helicobacter pylori* infection

Pre-Hospital

N/A

Diagnosis

ESSENTIAL WORKUP

- History and physical examination with special attention to state of hydration and abdominal exam for other diagnoses associated with vomiting (appendicitis, cholecystitis, etc.)
- The only mandated test is an uncontaminated urinalysis
- If patient has unremitting vomiting for greater than 24 hours, obtain a CBC, electrolytes, renal function, liver enzymes, bilirubin, and amylase or lipase

LABORATORY

- Urinalysis
  - —Increased specific gravity and ketonuria
  - —Presence of glucose mandates checking serum glucose to rule out diabetes
  - —Presence of bilirubin mandates a search to rule out hepatobiliary cause for the vomiting
- CBC
  - —May have an elevated hematocrit due to dehydration
  - —White blood cell count is usually normal
- Electrolytes
  - —Elevated blood urea nitrogen indicating volume depletion
  - —Hyponatremia, hypokalemia, hypochloremia, and metabolic alkalosis from loss of HCl in emesis
- Liver function tests
  - —Mild increases in bilirubin may occur but should be below 4 mg/dL
  - —AST and ALT may also be mildly elevated, but not over 100 IU/L
- Amylase/lipase
  - —In one study amylase was elevated in 24% of patients with hyperemesis gravidarum; however, the amylase was not pancreatic in origin; thus, use lipase rather than amylase to evaluate for pancreatitis

DIFFERENTIAL DIAGNOSIS

- Pyelonephritis; most commonly missed
- Gastroenteritis
- Hepatobiliary disease; hepatitis, cholecystitis, fatty liver of pregnancy
- Pancreatitis
- Appendicitis
- Diabetic ketoacidosis
- Hyperthyroidism
- Uremia; persistent nausea and vomiting are seen with severe renal dysfunction

Treatment

INITIAL STABILIZATION

- IV hydration using a crystalloid with dextrose (D5LR or D5NS)

ED TREATMENT

- IV hydration using up to 3 L of D5LR or D5NS
- The dextrose is added to help break the cycle of the ketosis
- Treat until the patient is no longer symptomatic from hypovolemia
- Antiemetics administered IV are given to break the vomiting cycle
- The most commonly used medications are the phenothiazines (promethazine and chlorpromazine both FDA category C), metoclopramide (FDA category B), or droperidol (FDA category C)
  - —These medications have been used extensively in pregnancy and there is little or no evidence that these antiemetics are associated with an increased risk of congenital anomalies
  - —Parenteral antiemetics are clearly preferable to the risk of prolonged ketosis and the associated hypovolemia
- Oral rehydration in the ED after the initial fluid resuscitation and antiemetics are given
- Thiamine 100 mg IV or IM in the patient who has a protracted course of symptoms
  - —There are case reports of patients developing Wernicke's encephalopathy due to hyperemesis gravidarum
- Methylprednisolone may be effective for patients with hyperemesis gravidarum
  - —Two studies demonstrated relief in symptoms and decreased need for admission for hyperemesis

MEDICATIONS

- Droperidol (pregnancy category C): 0.625–1.25 mg i.v.
- Methylprednisolone (category C): 48 mg i.v. or PO
- Metoclopramide (category B): 10–20 mg i.v.
- Prochlorperazine (category C): 5–10 mg i.v. not to exceed 40 mg/d
- Promethazine (category C): 12.5–25 mg i.v.

DISCHARGE MEDICATIONS

- Use first-line medications and elevate to the second-line agents for repeated visits
- Meclizine (category B): 25 mg PO q6h PRN, first line
- Metoclopramide (category B): 10 mg PO q6–8h PRN, second line
- Prochlorperazine (category C): 5–10 mg PO q6h or 25 mg PR b.i.d. PRN, second line
- Promethazine (category C): 12.5–25 mg PO or PR q4–6h PRN, second line
- Pyridoxine (vitamin B_6) (category A): 25 mg PO t.i.d. first line (over-the-counter)

Disposition

ADMISSION CRITERIA

- Inability to tolerate oral intake after treatment
- Inability to control the emesis despite treatment
- Severe electrolyte or metabolic disturbances

DISCHARGE CRITERIA

- The majority of patients can be discharged as long as they are able to tolerate oral intake and have adequate follow-up
- Correction of the dehydration and associated symptoms
- Decreased ketonuria
- Patients should be reassured that their symptoms are common and almost always self-limited
- Patients should be counseled to eat frequent, small meals, stopping short of satiety; their meals should contain simple carbohydrates and be low in fats; they should avoid all irritant or spicy foods
- Home IV therapy can be arranged if indicated

Miscellaneous

ICD9: 643.00

ICD10: 021

SUGGESTED READINGS

Broussard C, Richter J. Nausea and vomiting of pregnancy. Gastroenterol Clin North Am 1998;27:123–151.

Eliakim R, Abulafia O, Sherer D. Hyperemesis gravidarum: a current review. Am J Perinatol 2000;17(4):207–218.

Goodwin T: Hyperemesis gravidarum. Clin Obstet Gynecol 1998;41(3):597–605.

Safari H, Alsulyman O, Gherman R, et al. Experience with oral methylprednisolone in the treatment of refractory hyperemesis gravidarum. Am J Obstet Gynecol 1998;178(5):1054–1058.

Author: David Della-Giustina

Hyperkalemia

Clinical Presentation

SIGNS AND SYMPTOMS

- Cardiac dysrhythmias—initial manifestation
  - —See EKG changes in diagnosis section
- Muscular weakness (rare except in severe cases)
  - —Generalized weakness—may progress to flaccid paralysis
  - —Dyspnea due to respiratory muscle weakness

MECHANISM/DESCRIPTION

- Potassium distribution
  - —Extracellular space: 2%
  - —Intracellular space: 98%
- Potassium excretion
  - —90% renal
  - —10% GI
- Renal and extrarenal mechanisms maintain a normal plasma concentration between 3.5 and 5.0 mmol/L
- Renal excretion of potassium affected by:
  - —Dietary intake
  - —Distal renal tubular function
  - —Acid–base balance
  - —Mineralocorticoids
- Regulation between intracellular and extracellular potassium balance affected by:
  - —Acid–base balance
  - —Insulin
  - —Mineralocorticoids
  - —Catecholamines
  - —Osmolarity
  - —Drugs

ETIOLOGY

Decreased Potassium Excretion

- Most common cause: renal failure (acute or chronic)
- Distal tubular diseases
  - —Acute interstitial nephritis
  - —Renal transplant rejection
  - —Sickle cell nephropathy
- Mineralocorticoid deficiency
  - —Addison's disease
  - —Hypoaldosteronism
- Drugs
  - —ACE inhibitors/angiotensin receptor blockers
  - —Beta-blockers
  - —Potassium-sparing diuretics
  - —NSAIDs
  - —Cyclosporine
  - —High-dose trimethoprim
  - —Lithium toxicity

Intracellular to Extracellular Potassium Shifts

- Metabolic acidosis
  - —Serum K^+ rises 0.2–1.7 mmol/L for each 0.1 unit fall in arterial pH
- Hyperosmolar states
- Insulin deficiency
- Cell necrosis
- Rhabdomyolysis
- Hemolysis
- Chemotherapy
- Drugs
  - —Digitalis toxicity
  - —Depolarizing muscle relaxants (e.g., succinylcholine)
  - —Beta-blockers
  - —α-Agonists
- Hyperkalemic periodic paralysis

Excess Exogenous Potassium Load

- Salt substitutes
- Oral potassium
- Potassium penicillin G
- Rapid transfusions of banked blood

Pseudohyperkalemia

- Traumatic venipuncture with hemolysis
- Postvenipuncture release of potassium can occur in the setting of:
  - —Thrombocytosis (platelets $>800{,}000/mm^3$)
  - —Extreme leukocytosis (WBC $>100{,}000/mm^3$)

Pre-Hospital

CAUTIONS

- Treatment of hyperkalemic-induced dysrhythmias/cardiac arrest involves different drugs from the usual ACLS measures (see Treatment, below)
- Diagnosis suggested by the pre-hospital rhythm strip or in at-risk populations (renal failure)

Diagnosis

ESSENTIAL WORKUP

- Serum potassium >5.0 mmol/L
- Collect in heparinized tube if pseudohyperkalemia suspected

LABORATORY

- Electrolytes, BUN, Cr, glucose
  - —Elevated BUN, Cr in renal failure
  - —Hyponatremia with mineralocorticoid deficiency
  - —Mild metabolic acidosis with type IV renal tubular acidosis
- Arterial blood gases
  - —Assesses acid–base status
- Creatinine kinase
- Ca^{2+}
- For hyperkalemia in the face of normal renal function, calculate transtubular potassium gradient (TTKG)
  - —TTKG = Urine K × Posm/Plasma K × Uosm
  - —Posm = plasma osmolality; Uosm = urine osmolality
  - —TTKG >8 suggests an extrarenal cause; TTKG <6 indicates a renal excretory defect

IMAGING/SPECIAL TESTS

- EKG: Changes correlate with the degree of hyperkalemia
  - —>5.0–6.5: Peaking of T waves; shortening of QT_c interval
  - —>6.5–8.0: PR prolongation; loss of P waves; widening of QRS complexes
  - —>8.0: Intraventricular blocks; bundle branch blocks; QRS axis shifts; sine wave complex

DIFFERENTIAL DIAGNOSIS

- Pseudohyperkalemia

Treatment

INITIAL STABILIZATION

- ABCs
- IV access
- Cardiac monitor

ED TREATMENT

Hyperkalemia with EKG Changes (Widened QRS Complexes/Dysrhythmia): Antagonize Potassium-Mediated Cardiotoxicity

- Administer calcium gluconate or calcium chloride
  —Onset 1–3 minutes
  —30- to 60-minute duration
  —No effect on serum potassium levels

Severe (>7.0) or Moderate (6.0–7.0) with EKG Changes: Shift Potassium Intracellularly

- Administer combination of insulin and glucose
  —Onset 20–30 minutes
  —2- to 4-hour duration
- IV sodium bicarbonate
  —Onset 20 minutes
  —2-hour duration
  —Caution in patients at risk for volume overload
  —Worsens concomitant hypocalcemia
- Inhaled albuterol
  —Onset within 30 minutes
  —2- to 4-hour duration

Enhanced Excretion for K^+ >6.0

- Administer cation exchange resin
  —Calcium or sodium polystyrene sulfonate PO or PR
  —Avoid in patients with suspected ileus or bowel obstruction

All Patients

- Limit exogenous potassium and potassium-sparing drugs
- Treat the underlying cause

Special Situations

- Renal failure
  —Arrange for dialysis
  —Hemodialysis immediately effective at removing potassium
- Furosemide
  —Effective in the absence of oliguric renal failure
  —Causes a potassium-losing diuresis
- Cardiac arrest
  —Administer $CaCl_2$ and $NaHCO_3$ with known or suspected hyperkalemia
- Digoxin toxicity
  —Avoid calcium
  -When necessary, administer small doses extremely slowly
  —Consider Digibind for K^+ >5.5 mmol/L
- Mineralocorticoid deficiency
  —Hydrocortisone

MEDICATIONS

- Albuterol: 10–20 mg (peds: 2.5 mg if <25 kg; 5.0 mg if ≥25 kg) nebulized over 10 min
- Calcium chloride 10%: 10-mL amp (peds: 0.2–0.3 mL/kg/dose) i.v. over 2–5 min
- Calcium gluconate 10%: 20-mL amp (peds: 0.1 mL/kg) i.v. over 2–5 min
- Furosemide: 40–80 mg (peds: 1.0 mg/kg) i.v.—modify dose to achieve appropriate diuresis
- Hydrocortisone: 100 mg (peds: 1–2 mg/kg) i.v.
- Insulin and glucose: 10 IU (peds: 0.1 IU/kg) regular insulin plus 50 mL 50% (peds: 0.5–1 g/kg) dextrose i.v.
- Sodium bicarbonate: 1–3 amp (44 mEq per amp) i.v. over 20–30 min (peds: 1.0–2.0 mEq/kg/dose)
- Sodium polystyrene sulfonate (Kayexalate) or calcium polystyrene sulfonate (preferred with volume overload)
  —Oral: 15 g mixed with water or 50 mL of sorbitol q2h to a total of 5 doses
  —Rectal enema: 50 g in 200 mL of sorbitol q4–6h
  —Peds: 1.0 g/kg orally or rectally

Disposition

ADMISSION CRITERIA

- Admit most cases
  —Process of potassium removal relatively slow
  —Levels may continue to rise

DISCHARGE CRITERIA

- Mild hyperkalemia (<6.0 mmol/L) provided that:
  —Response to treatment has been demonstrated
  —Known correctable cause
  —Further rises in serum potassium not anticipated
  —Early follow-up possible

Miscellaneous

ICD9: 276.7

ICD10: E87.5

SUGGESTED READINGS

Halperin M, Kamel K. Potassium. Lancet 1998;352:135–140.

Mattu A, Brady W, Robinson D. Electrocardiographic manifestations of hyperkalemia. Am J Emerg Med 2000; 18(6):721–728.

Rastegar A, Soleimani M. Hypokalaemia and hyperkalaemia. Postgrad Med J 2001; 77:759–764.

Rodríguez-Soriano J. Potassium homeostasis and its disturbances in children. Pediatr Nephrol 1995;9(3): 364–374.

Author: Paul Byskosh

Hypernatremia

Clinical Presentation

SIGNS AND SYMPTOMS

General

- Most symptoms attributed to the underlying cause (dehydration)
- More marked with acute changes
- Death likely to occur with sodium of ≥185 mEq/L
- May see the following symptoms, usually at levels ≥160 mEq/L:

Neurologic

- Tremulous
- Irritability
- Ataxia
- Mental confusion
- Delirium
- Seizures
- Coma
- Hyperreflexia
- Subarachnoid, intracerebral, and subdural hemorrhages

Musculoskeletal

- Spasticity
- Muscle weakness

Other

- Venous sinus thrombosis

Hypovolemic Hypernatremia

- Tachycardia
- Orthostasis
- Dry mucous membranes
- Oliguria
- Azotemia

Hypervolemic Hypernatremia

- Pulmonary edema
- Peripheral edema

MECHANISM/DESCRIPTION

- Hypernatremia definition: sodium >145 mEq/L
  —Mild hypernatremia serum sodium 146–155 mEq/L
  —Severe hypernatremia serum sodium >155 mEq/L

ETIOLOGY

- Divided into three categories:

Hypovolemic Hypernatremia

- Most common
- Loss or deficiency of water and sodium with water losses being greater than sodium losses
- Examples
  —Diuretics
  —Glucosuria
  —Mannitol
  —Renal failure
  —High-protein feedings
  —Lactulose
  —Excess sweating
  —Respiratory loss
  —Defective thirst mechanism
  —Lack of access to water
  —Diarrhea/vomiting

Isovolemic Hypernatremia

- Water deficiency without sodium loss
- Examples
  —Fever
  —Hypothalamic diabetes insipidus
    -Head trauma
    -Tumor
    -Infection (TB, syphilis, mycoses, toxoplasmosis, encephalitis)
    -Granulomatous disease (sarcoid, Wegner's)
    -Cerebrovascular accident
    -Aneurysm
  —Nephrogenic diabetes insipidus
    -Congenital
    -Drugs (lithium, amphotericin B, foscarnet, demeclocycline)
    -Obstructive uropathy
    -Chronic tubulointerstitial disease (sickle cell nephropathy, multiple myeloma, amyloidosis, sarcoidosis, systemic lupus erythematosus, polycystic kidney)
    -Electrolyte disorders (hypercalcemia, potassium depletion)

Hypervolemic Hypernatremia

- Gain of water and sodium, with sodium gain greater than water gain
- Examples
  —Iatrogenic—most common cause
    -Sodium bicarbonate administration
    -NaCl tablets
    -Hypertonic IVF
    -Hypertonic dialysis
  —Cushing's disease
  —Adrenal hyperplasia
  —Primary aldosteronism

PEDIATRIC CONSIDERATIONS

- More prone to iatrogenic causes
- More likely to die or to have permanent neurologic sequela
- Morbidity ranges from 25–50%
- May present with high pitched cry, lethargy, irritable, muscle weakness

Pre-Hospital

N/A

Diagnosis

ESSENTIAL WORKUP

- Serum Na^+ level

LABORATORY

- Electrolytes, BUN/Cr, glucose
- CBC
- Urinalysis
  - —Specific gravity

IMAGING/SPECIAL TESTS

- CXR
  - —For infection/aspiration
  - —Pulmonary edema with hypervolemic hypernatremia
- CT brain
  - —For altered mental status
  - —Urine/serum osmolality
  - —Urine Na^+

DIFFERENTIAL DIAGNOSIS

- Diabetic ketoacidosis
- Hyperosmolar coma
- Primary CNS lesions

Treatment

INITIAL STABILIZATION

- ABCs
- 0.9% NS IV bolus for severe hypotension
- Naloxone, thiamine, D50W (or Accucheck) for altered mental status

ED TREATMENT

General

- Calculate water deficit
  - —Water deficit $= 0.6$ (weight in kg) $\times$ (actual Na^+ $-$ desired Na^+)/(actual Na^+)
- Do not rapidly correct hypertonicity to a normal serum osmolality
  - —Rapid correction may cause seizures
  - —Reduce serum sodium level by <0.5–0.7 mEq/L/h

Hypovolemic Hypernatremia

- Replace volume contraction with 0.9% NS IV bolus
- Change to D5W or hypotonic saline once volume repleted and hemodynamically stable

Isovolemic Hypernatremia

- Calculate water deficit
- Correct water deficit with D5W or hypotonic saline
  - —Replace half of deficit in first 24 hours, then remainder over 1–2 days

Hypervolemic Hypernatremia

- Remove excess water with diuretics or dialysis
- When euvolemic, replace water deficit with D5W
- Avoid hypotonic saline solutions because already have an excess of total body sodium

Diabetes Insipidus (DI) Hypernatremia

- Sodium restriction
- Desmopressin
  - —Aqueous vasopressin (DDAVP) 1–2 μg i.v./s.c. q12h or 5–20 μg intranasally
  - —Best therapeutic agent
- Chlorpropamide (Diabinese) 100–500 mg/day enhances effect of vasopressin at renal tubule
- Carbamazepine causes release of vasopressin
- Hydrochlorothiazide enhances sodium excretion
- Discontinue DI-inducing drugs

MEDICATIONS

- Chlorpropamide (Diabinese) 100–500 mg/d
- Vasopressin (DDAVP) 1–2 μg i.v./s.c. q12h or 5–20 μg intranasally

Disposition

ADMISSION CRITERIA

- Newly diagnosed sodium >150 mEq/L for monitoring and treatment
- Admit sodium >160 mEq/L or symptomatic patients to ICU

DISCHARGE CRITERIA

- Sodium <150 mEq/L in asymptomatic patient
- Sodium >150 mEq/L in patients with history of chronically elevated sodium who are at their baseline and asymptomatic

Miscellaneous

ICD9: 276.0

ICD10: E87.0

SUGGESTED READINGS

Adrogue HS, Madias NE. Hypernatremia. N Engl J Med 2000;342(20):1493–1499.

Fall P. Hyponatremia and hypernatremia—a systematic approach to causes and their correction. Postgrad Med 2000;107(5): 75–82.

Fried LF, Palevsky PM. Hyponatremia and hypernatremia. Med Clin North Am 1997; 81(3):585–609.

Kugler JP, Hustead T. Hyponatremia and hypernatremia in the elderly. Am Fam Physician 2000;61(12):3623–3630.

Author: Linda Mueller

Hyperosmolar Syndrome

Clinical Presentation

SIGNS AND SYMPTOMS

- Polyuria/polydipsia/weight loss
- Dizziness/weakness
- Marked dehydration
- Decreased sweating, dry mucous membranes
- Orthostasis
- Hypotension
- Tachycardia
- Collapsed neck veins
- Decreased skin turgor
- Urinary output maintained until late
- Lethargy/drowsiness
- Seizures/focal neurologic deficits/coma

MECHANISM/DESCRIPTION

- Results from a relative insulin deficiency in the undiagnosed or undertreated diabetic
- Sustained hyperglycemia creates an osmotic diuresis and dehydration
  - —Extracellular space maintained by the osmotic gradient at the expense of the intracellular space
  - —Eventually profound intracellular dehydration occurs
- Total body deficits of H_2O, Na^+, K^+, PO_4^-, and Mg^+
- In contrast to diabetic ketoacidosis (DKA), significant ketoacidosis does not occur:
  - —Circulating insulin levels are higher
  - —The elevation of insulin counterregulatory hormones is less marked
  - —The hyperosmolar state itself inhibits lipolysis (the release of free fatty acids) and subsequent generation of ketoacids
- Most commonly occurs in mild type 2 elderly diabetic with renal insufficiency who experiences some stressful illness that precipitates worsening hyperglycemia and reduced renal function
- Less common than DKA but with a greater mortality

ETIOLOGY

- Factors that may contribute to the hyperosmolar state include:
  - —Increase in endogenous glucose: in the undertreated diabetic
  - —Increase in exogenous glucose: with dietary indiscretion or improperly managed parenteral hyperalimentation
  - —Decreased insulin or impaired insulin action: caused by excess catecholamines during periods of physiologic stress, such as serious infections, burns, trauma, pancreatitis, myocardial ischemia, pulmonary emboli, CVA, GI bleeding, or as side effect of common medications such as beta-blockers, Dilantin, diazoxide, and diuretics
  - —Impaired peripheral action of insulin as with type 2 diabetes
  - —Decrease in patient's ability to keep up with fluid loss: particularly in older debilitated patients, altered mental status, and those with impaired thirst
  - —Increased renal glucose threshold with renal insufficiency
  - —Impaired renal elimination of glucose—use of thiazide diuretics

PEDIATRIC CONSIDERATIONS

- Rare in childhood

Pre-Hospital

CAUTIONS

- Avoid routine use of D50W in all cases of altered mental state without first performing a fingerstick glucose check
  - —Exacerbates the hyperosmolar state

Diagnosis

ESSENTIAL WORKUP

- Diagnostic criteria
  - —Serum glucose $\geq$ 600 mg/dL (usually >1,000 mg/dL)
  - —Absence of ketosis—Acetest $\leq$ 2+, pH $\geq$ 7.30, $HCO_3 \geq$ 15 mEq/L
  - —Increased serum osmolarity
  - —>350 Osm/L or
  - —$\geq$ 320 Osm/L with at least mild disturbance in mentation

LABORATORY

- Electrolytes
  - —Initially elevated levels of K^+ found even in presence of total body deficit due to shift from intracellular space to extracellular space
  - —Mild anion gap metabolic acidosis due to lactic acid, β-hydroxybutyric acid or renal insufficiency
  - —Increased sodium—must correct for hyperglycemia (raise Na^+ by 1.6 for each 100 mg/dL of glucose over 100)
- BUN, Cr
  - —Azotemia with elevated BUN/Cr ratio due to prerenal and renal causes
- ABG to rapidly determine pH
- Serum osmolarity = $2 \times Na^+ + \text{glucose}/18 + \text{BUN}/2.8$
- CBC
  - —Leukocytosis
  - —Increased Hct due to hemoconcentration
- Amylase
  - —Pancreatitis common
- Urinalysis
  - —Check for ketones/glucose
  - —Assess renal function
  - —Investigate for UTI
- Magnesium, phosphate
- Blood cultures if febrile

IMAGING/SPECIAL TESTS

- EKG for ischemia or infarction
- CXR to check for pneumonia, the most common precipitant
- Head CT (non-contrast-enhanced) indicated if comatose or with a focal neurologic deficit

DIFFERENTIAL DIAGNOSIS

- Differentiate from DKA
  - —If acidosis present, determine if from ketosis (DKA) or from lactate (hypoperfusion, sepsis, or postictal)

Treatment

INITIAL STABILIZATION

- ABCs
  - —Secure airway in comatose patients
  - —Place on cardiac monitor
  - —Naloxane, thiamine, and blood glucose for coma of unknown etiology
- Restore hemodynamic stability with IV fluids
  - —0.9% NS 1–2 L over the first hour
  - —Larger volumes of fluid may be needed to normalize the vital signs and establish urine output
  - —If serum osmolarity $\geq$320, consider 0.45% saline as alternative

ED TREATMENT

General Strategy

- Frequent reassessment of volume status and mental status
- Electrolyte assessment difficult
  - —Serum levels of Na^+, K^+, PO_4^- do not accurately reflect the total body solute deficits or the intracellular environment
  - —Repeat $Na^+$and K^+ levels to determine replacement therapy
- Search for a precipitating illness

Fluids

- Once hemodynamic stability is restored, the fluid should be switched to 0.45% saline
- Replace 50% of the predicted volume deficit within the first 12 hours
  - —Average deficit is 9 L
- Lower the serum glucose no faster than 100–200 mg/dL each hour

Potassium

- Anticipate hypokalemia
  - —Total body deficit of approximately 5–10 mEq/kg body weight (replace over 3 days)
- Begin potassium repletion as soon as urine output is established
  - —If the initial K^+ is normal (3.5–5.5 mEq/L) give 20–30 mEq KCl in the first liter of fluids, then give 20 mEq/h
  - —If the initial K^+ is low (<3.5 mEq/L), begin 40 mEq KCl/h and avoid insulin
- Follow repeat serum K^+ levels every 1–2 hours and adjust treatment accordingly

Insulin

- Some patients will not require insulin
- Begin insulin only after restoring hemodynamic stability and after instituting K^+ replacement
- Earlier use of insulin may cause rapid correction of hyperglycemia with collapse of the intravascular space, hypotension, and shock; overzealous use of insulin can contribute to unnecessary morbidity
- If insulin is used, begin at 0.05 U/kg/h

Other Electrolyte Replacement

- Phosphate
  - —Supplement if phosphorus level <1 mg/dL
  - —Potassium phosphate 20 mEq/L IV fluid with concomitant potassium depletion
- Magnesium
  - —0.35 mEq/kg magnesium in fluids for first 3–4 hours (= 2.5–3.0 g $MgSO_4$ in 70-kg patient)
  - —Caution with acute renal failure

Anticoagulation

- Arterial thrombosis may complicate hyperosmolar state; low-dose heparin may be given as prophylaxis
- Clinician should remain vigilant to detect thrombotic complications, e.g., myocardial infarction, pulmonary embolus, mesenteric ischemia

Pitfalls to Avoid

- Too rapid correction of glucose—may lead to hypotension
- Continuing isotonic fluids after volume resuscitation—may lead to hypernatremia
- Continuing hypotonic fluids without frequent electrolytes—may lead to cellular edema, cerebral edema
- Failure to prevent hypokalemia: respiratory depression, dysrhythmias
- Avoid Dilantin in the event of seizure activity
  - —Inhibits the endogenous release of insulin

MEDICATIONS

- Insulin: begin with 0.05–0.1 U/kg/h, modify after assessing clinical response
- $MgSO_4$ (magnesium sulfate): 50% (5 g/10 mL; dilute to at least 20% before IV use)
- Naloxone: 2 mg (peds: 0.1 mg/kg) IVP
- Potassium phosphate: phosphates 3 mmol/mL and potassium 4.4 mEq/ml
- Thiamine: 100 mg (peds: 10–25 mg) IVP

Disposition

ADMISSION CRITERIA

- All but the mildest cases should be admitted to ICU
  - —Frequent serial labs for the first 24 hours
  - —Rapid shifts in fluids and electrolytes and the potential for deterioration in mental status and arrhythmias mandate close monitoring
- Mild cases may be managed in an observation unit over 12–24 hours

DISCHARGE CRITERIA

- Patients meeting the diagnostic criteria for hyperosmolar syndrome should not be discharged
- Mild hyperglycemia patients with mild volume deficits and normal serum osmolarity can be discharged after hydration and correction of hyperglycemia

Miscellaneous

ICD9: 276.0

SEE ALSO: DIABETIC KETOACIDOSIS

SUGGESTED READINGS

Lorber D. Nonketotic hypertonicity in diabetes mellitus. Med Clin North Am 1995;79(1):39–52.

Magee MF, Bhatt BA. Management of decompensated diabetes. Diabetic ketoacidosis and hyperglycemia hyperosmolar syndrome. Crit Care Clin 2001;17(1):75–106.

Matz R. Management of the hyperosmolar hyperglycemic syndrome. Am Fam Physician 1999;60(5):1468–1476.

Umpierrez GE, et al. Review: diabetic ketoacidosis and hyperglycemia hyperosmolar nonketotic syndrome. Am J Med Sci 1996;311(5):225–233.

Author: Karen Cosby

Hyperparathyroidism

Clinical Presentation

SIGNS AND SYMPTOMS
- Dehydration
- Depend on the severity and rapidity of hypercalcemia
- Cardiac
  - —Hypertension (even in the face of dehydration)
  - —Cardiac conduction abnormalities (*not* proportional to degree of hypercalcemia)
  - —Bradydysrhythmia
  - —Bundle branch blocks
  - —Complete heart block
  - —Asystole
  - —Short QT interval
  - —Potentiation of digitalis effects
- Neurologic
  - —Headaches
  - —Decreased reflexes
  - —Proximal muscle weakness
  - —Dementia
  - —Lethargy
  - —Coma
- Psychiatric
  - —Personality changes
  - —Depression
  - —Inability to concentrate
  - —Anxiety
  - —Psychosis
- GI
  - —Anorexia, nausea, vomiting
  - —Constipation
  - —Peptic ulcer disease
  - —Pancreatitis
- General
  - —Fatigue
  - —Weight loss
  - —Polyuria and polydipsia
- Musculoskeletal
  - —Gout/pseudogout
  - —Bone pain, bone cysts (osteitis cystica)
  - —Arthralgias
  - —Chondrocalcinosis
- Renal
  - —Kidney stones
  - —Nephrocalcinosis
  - —Decreased renal concentrating ability

Hypercalcemic Crisis
- Anorexia
- Nausea, vomiting
- Mental obtundation

MECHANISM/DESCRIPTION
- Parathyroid hormone (PTH) actions
  - —Decreases urinary Ca^{2+} loss
  - —Increases urinary PO_4^{-2} loss
  - —Stimulates vitamin D conversion from 25(OH)-D to 1,25$(OH)_2$-D in kidney
  - —Liberates Ca^{2+} and PO_4^{-2} from bone
- Magnesium
  - —Cofactor in production of PTH
  - —Essential for action of PTH in target tissues
  - —Hypercalcuria produces increased magnesium losses in urine

ETIOLOGY
- Excess secretion of PTH due to:
  - —Primary hyperparathyroidism (adenoma 85%, hyperplasia 14%, carcinoma <1%)
  - —Secondary hyperparathyroidism (response to vitamin D deficiency or chronic renal failure with hyperphosphatemia)

PEDIATRIC CONSIDERATIONS
- Hypotonia, weakness, and listlessness
- May present as critically ill infant with calcium as high as 25 mg/dL
- Mid-teens presentation with nonspecific symptoms of hypercalcemia
- Associated with multiple endocrine neoplasia syndromes I and II
- Newborns following delivery to hypoparathyroid mothers
- Hypercalcemic infants present with:
  - —Broad forehead
  - —Epicanthal folds
  - —Underdeveloped nasal bridge
  - —Prominent upper lip
  - —Mental retardation

Pre-Hospital

CAUTIONS
- May present as a primarily psychiatric disorder

Diagnosis

ESSENTIAL WORKUP
- Calcium level
- Albumin
  - —Elevated albumin—falsely elevated calcium level
  - —Low albumin—falsely lowered calcium level
- Evaluate for symptoms of hypercalcemia especially impending parathyroid storm
- Review history for medication ingestion (see Differential Diagnosis, below)
- No further ED workup if:
  - —Asymptomatic
  - —Normal EKG
  - —Calcium level <14 mg/dL when corrected for albumin
- If symptomatic with Ca^{2+} <14 mg/dL or any patient with $Ca^{2+} \geq 14$ mg/dL check:
  - —CXR
  - —Phosphorus
  - —Electrolytes, BUN, creatinine
  - —Sed rate
  - —Alkaline phosphatase
  - —Magnesium
  - —TSH
  - —CBC

LABORATORY
- Calcium correction for albumin
  - —Corrected Ca^{2+} (mg/dL) = measured Ca^{2+} (mg/dL) + 0.8 [4.0 − albumin (g/dL)]
  - —Acidosis
  - —Shifts binding to albumin—increases ionized (metabolically active) Ca^{2+}
  - —Decrease of 0.1 pH unit increases the ionized Ca^{2+} by 3–8%
- Phosphorus
  - —Low in primary hyperparathyroidism
  - —Variable in secondary hyperparathyroidism
  - —Normal or high in malignancy-related hypercalcemia
- Chloride/PO_4^{-2} ratio
  - —>33—hyperparathyroidism
  - —<30—malignancy
- Alkaline phosphatase
  - —Increased in 50% of patients with hyperparathyroidism
  - —Normal with vitamin D excess

- ESR
  - —Normal in hyperparathyroidism
  - —Elevated in malignancy or granulomatous diseases
- Anemia
  - —Present with malignancy or granulomatous disease
  - —Absent in hyperparathyroidism
- Magnesium
  - —Low or low normal
- Parathyroid hormone (PTH)
  - —Elevated in primary and secondary hyperparathyroidism
- PTH-related peptide
  - —Secreted by squamous cell carcinomas of lung, head, neck; renal carcinomas, bladder carcinomas, adenocarcinomas, and lymphomas

IMAGING/SPECIAL TESTS

- CXR for:
  - —CHF risk during IV hydration
  - —Granulomatous disease or malignancy if cause of hypercalcemia is uncertain

DIFFERENTIAL DIAGNOSIS

Causes of Hypercalcemia

- PTH related
  - —Primary or secondary hyperparathyroidism
  - —Familial hypocalciuric hypercalcemia
- Malignancy related
  - —PTH-related peptide or Ca^{2+} release from osteolytic tumor
- Vitamin D related
  - —Excess vitamin D intake or vitamin D production by granulomas
- Immobilization—associated with Paget's disease
- Drug induced
  - —Thiazide diuretics
  - —Lithium
  - —Aluminum-containing antacids
  - —Tamoxifen
  - —Estrogens
  - —Androgens
  - —Vitamin A

Treatment

INITIAL STABILIZATION

- Cardiac monitor if:
  - —Symptomatic hypercalcemia
  - —Ca^{2+} level >14 mg/dL
- Hydration with IV 0.9% NS

ED TREATMENT

- Treat hypercalcemia
  - —Vigorous hydration with 0.9% NS at minimum of 250 mL/h unless CHF
    - -Lowers calcium 1.5–2.0 mg/dL in 24 hours
    - -Achieve urine output 100 mL/h
  - —Administer furosemide or other loop diuretic (calciuric) after adequate volume replacement or in presence of CHF
    - -Common error: administration of furosemide before adequate hydration; if urinary sodium losses exceed replacement sodium, then renal conservation measures retard calcium excretion
  - —Avoid thiazide diuretics (retard calcium excretion)
  - —Consider glucocorticoid administration (decreases gut absorption and increases renal excretion of Ca^{2+}) most effective with vitamin D intoxication or granulomatous diseases
  - —Administer calcitonin if poor response to saline diuresis
  - —Start bisphosphonates (pamidronate or etidronate) in conjunction with primary physician (inhibits calcium mobilization from bone)
- Treat cardiac dysrhythmias
- Determine the etiology of the hypercalcemia
- Stop all medications that may contribute to hypercalcemia
- Use extreme caution in use of digoxin
- Anticipate CHF and electrolyte imbalance with frequent reassessment of patient and monitoring of serum electrolytes and magnesium levels
- Emergent dialysis with renal failure

MEDICATIONS

- Calcitonin: 4–8 IU/kg s.c. q6h
- Etidronate: 7.5 mg/kg over 2 hours
- Furosemide: 40 mg i.v. q6h after assurance of adequate hydration
- Hydrocortisone: 100 mg (peds: 1–2 mg/kg) i.v.
- Pamidronate: 30 mg i.v. over 4 hours or 90 mg i.v. over 24 hours
- Prednisone: 40–80 mg PO

Disposition

ADMISSION CRITERIA

- Calcium >14 mg/dl
- Symptomatic hypercalcemia
- Evidence of abnormal cardiac rhythm or conduction

DISCHARGE CRITERIA

- Able to maintain adequate hydration

Miscellaneous

ICD9: 252.0, 259.3, 588.8

ICD10: E21.3

SEE ALSO: HYPERCALCEMIA

SUGGESTED READINGS

Goldman L, Bennett JC, eds. Cecil's textbook of medicine, 21st ed. Philadelphia: WB Saunders, 2000.

Marx JA, Hockenberger RS, Walls RM, et al., eds. Rosen's emergency medicine, 5th ed. Philadelphia: Mosby, 2002.

Wallach J, ed. Interpretation of diagnostic tests, 7th ed. Boston: Little, Brown, 2000.

Author: Hugh Schuckman

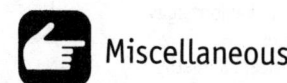

Hypertensive Emergencies

Clinical Presentation

SIGNS AND SYMPTOMS

- Malignant hypertension
  - —Headache
  - —Visual changes
  - —Nocturia
  - —Weakness
  - —Chest pain
  - —Dyspnea
  - —Funduscopic abnormalities
    - -Papilledema (most common finding)
    - -Retinal flame hemorrhages
    - -Soft exudates
- Hypertensive encephalopathy
  - —Headaches
  - —Nausea
  - —Vomiting
  - —Visual changes
  - —Confusion
  - —Weakness
  - —Disorientation
  - —Altered mental status
  - —Papilledema
  - —Focal weakness
  - —Seizures

MECHANISM/DESCRIPTION

- A severe elevation in blood pressure
  - —Diastolic pressure of greater than 140 mm Hg
    - -Acute progressive end-organ damage
- Abrupt increase in systemic vascular resistance
  - —Increase in circulating vasoconstrictors
    - -Norepinephrine
    - -Angiotensin II
  - —Arteriolar fibrinoid necrosis
  - —Endothelial damage
  - —Platelet and fibrin deposition
  - —Loss of autoregulation of blood flow
  - —End-organ ischemia
    - -Prompts the renewed release of vasoconstrictors
    - -Triggers a vicious cycle
  - —2% of hypertensive patients will have a hypertensive emergency
  - —Malignant hypertension
    - -Young black men
    - -Underlying renal disease

ETIOLOGY

- Central nervous system abnormalities
  - —Subarachnoid hemorrhage
  - —Intracranial hemorrhage
  - —Thrombotic infarction
  - —Encephalopathy
  - —Head trauma
  - —Transient ischemic attacks
- Cardiovascular abnormalities
  - —Acute coronary insufficiency
  - —Acute aortic dissection
  - —Accelerated hypertension
  - —Acute heart failure
  - —Myocardial infarction
  - —Unstable angina
- Renal system abnormalities
  - —Acute renal insufficiency
  - —Acute glomerulonephritis
- Excessive catecholamine states
  - —Pheochromocytoma
  - —Adrenocortical tumors
  - —Monoamine oxidase inhibitor interactions
- Antihypertensive medication withdrawal
- Pregnancy-induced hypertension
- Preeclampsia
- Drugs
  - —Cocaine
  - —Amphetamines
  - —Oral contraceptives
  - —Corticosteroids
  - —Toxins
  - —Heavy metals

Pre-Hospital

CAUTIONS

- Intravenous access
- Cardiac monitoring
- Pulse oximetry
- Oxygen administration
- Twelve-lead EKG when available
- Follow standard pre-hospital protocols
  - —Chest pain
  - —Congestive heart failure

Diagnosis

ESSENTIAL WORKUP

- Exclusion of other causes of severe symptomatic hypertension

LABORATORY

- BUN, creatinine
  - —Acute elevation if renal damage
- Serum electrolytes
- Urinalysis
  - —Proteinuria and casts

IMAGING/SPECIAL TESTS

- EKG
  - —Assess for myocardial ischemia
- Intraarterial line
  - —Continuous blood pressure monitoring during initial treatment
- Head CT
  - —Exclude subarachnoid and intracerebral hemorrhage
- Lumbar puncture
  - —Exclude subarachnoid hemorrhage
  - —When CT is negative

DIFFERENTIAL DIAGNOSIS

- Subarachnoid hemorrhage
- Intracerebral hemorrhage
- Cerebral infarction
- Acute myocardial ischemia
- Acute myocardial infarction
- Acute pulmonary edema
- Aortic dissection
- Preeclampsia/eclampsia
- Withdrawal syndromes
  - —Beta-blockers
  - —Central acting antihypertensive agents (e.g., clonidine)
- States of catecholamine excess
  - —Pheochromocytoma
  - —Cocaine/sympathomimetic drug intoxication
  - —Tyramine ingestion in patients on monoamine oxidase inhibitors

Treatment

INITIAL STABILIZATION

- Cardiac monitoring
- Pulse oximetry
- Oxygen administration
- Intravenous access
- Antiischemic therapy
  - —With signs of acute myocardial ischemia or infarction

ED TREATMENT

Goals of Parenteral Antihypertensive Therapy

- Reduce the mean arterial pressure by no more than 30%
- Decrease the diastolic blood pressure to 100–110 mm Hg
  - —The reduction should occur over several minutes to hours
  - —More gradual reduction in certain settings
    - -Long history of poorly controlled hypertension
    - -Acute ongoing injury to the central nervous system
    - -Cardiac involvement
  - —Further blood pressure reduction should be avoided in the ED

Nitroprusside

- Potent vasodilator
- Immediate onset
- Brief (2–3 minutes) duration of action
- Indications
  - —First-line agent
  - —Malignant hypertension
  - —Hypertensive encephalopathy
  - —Aortic dissection
    - -Administer concomitantly with beta-blockers to reduce aortic wall stress and eliminate reflex tachycardia caused by nitroprusside
- Complications
  - —Hypotension
  - —Nausea and vomiting
  - —Reflex tachycardia
  - —Thiocyanate toxicity
  - —Degraded by light
- Contraindications
  - —Pregnancy

Fenoldopam

- Selective postsynaptic dopaminergic receptor (DA1) agonist
- Onset of action 3–4 minutes
- Duration of action 8–10 minutes
- Does not appear to cause reflex tachycardia
- Indications
  - —In clinical trials very promising for treatment of HTN emergencies, but not yet FDA approved for this use
- Complications (most mild and diminish after 24 hours)
  - —Flushing
  - —Headache
  - —Dizziness
  - —Tachy- or bradycardia
  - —EKG changes (not related to cardiac ischemia)
  - —Increased intraocular pressure
- Contraindication
  - —Glaucoma (relative)

Labetalol

- A combined alpha- and beta-blocker
- Onset of action of 5–10 minutes
- 3- to 6-hour duration of action
- Does not cause reflex tachycardia
- Easily converted to oral therapy
- Indications
  - —Acceptable alternative to nitroprusside
  - —All hypertensive emergencies
- Contraindications
  - —To beta-blockers

Diazoxide

- A smooth-muscle relaxant
- Indications
  - —Hypertensive encephalopathy
  - —Malignant hypertension
  - —Pregnancy-induced hypertension
  - —Preeclampsia/eclampsia
- Complications
  - —Reflex sympathetic stimulation
- Contraindications
  - —Aortic dissection
  - —Acute myocardial ischemia

Phentolamine

- Alpha-blocker
- Agent of choice in states of catecholamine excess
- Indications
  - —Pheochromocytoma
  - —MAO inhibitor reactions
  - —Stimulant abuse
  - —Antihypertensive drug withdrawal states
- Caution
  - —Beta-blockers should be avoided in states of catecholamine excess
  - —Only after alpha-blockade
  - —Only for tachydysrhythmias

Second-Line Agents

- Trimethaphan camsylate
  - —A ganglionic blocker
  - —Lowers aortic wall stress
  - —Indicated in aortic dissection
- Nicardipine
  - —Intravenous calcium channel blocker
- Enalapril
  - —An intravenous angiotensin-converting enzyme inhibitor
  - —Useful in patients with high renin states
  - —Congestive heart failure
- Hydralazine
  - —Eclampsia
- Nitroglycerin
  - —Myocardial ischemia
  - —Heart failure

MEDICATIONS

- Diazoxide: 50–100 mg i.v. q 5–10 min or 10–30 mg/min i.v. infusion
- Enalapril: 1.25–5 mg q6h
- Fenoldopam: 0.05 to 0.1 μg/kg/min, increased by 0.1 mg/kg/min to max 1.6 mg/kg/min or DBP $<$110 mm Hg
- Hydralazine: 5–10 mg i.v. or i.m. q 20 min up to 20 mg
- Labetalol: 20–80 mg i.v. q 5–10 min or 0.5–2.0 mg/kg i.v. infusion
- Nicardipine: 5–15 mg/h i.v. infusion
- Nitroglycerin: 5–200 μg/min i.v. infusion
- Nitroprusside: 0.2–0.5 μg/kg/min initial i.v.; infusion up to 8–10 μg/kg/min
- Phentolamine: 5–10 mg i.v. q 5–15 min
- Trimethaphan: 1–15 mg/min i.v. infusion

Disposition

ADMISSION CRITERIA

- All patients hypertensive emergencies
  - —Signs of end-organ damage
  - —ICU for cardiac and blood pressure monitoring

DISCHARGE CRITERIA

- Hypertensive urgencies
  - —Absence of ocular, cardiac, or renal damage
- Instruct to return with chest pain or headache

Miscellaneous

ICD9: 401.0, 401.1, 401.9

SUGGESTED READINGS

Abdelwahab W, Frishman W, Landau A. Management of hypertensive urgencies and emergencies. J Clin Pharmacol 1995;35: 747–762.

Calhoun DA, Oparil S. Treatment of hypertensive crisis. N Engl J Med 1990; 323:1177–1183.

Houston M. Hypertensive emergencies and urgencies: pathophysiology and clinical aspects. Am Heart J 1986;111:205–210.

Murphy M, Murray C, Shorten GD. Fenoldopam: a selective peripheral dopamine-receptor agonist for the treatment of severe hypertension. N Engl J Med 2001;345:1548–1557.

Rubenstein EB, Escalante C. Hypertensive crisis. Crit Care Clin 1989;5:477–495.

Authors: David F. M. Brown; Christo Courban

Hyperthermia

Clinical Presentation

SIGNS AND SYMPTOMS

Heat Stroke

- Classic triad: hyperthermia, CNS dysfunction, anhydrosis
  —Perspiration is often present in early stages
- Core temp: >105°F (40.5°C)
- CNS:
  —Severe confusion
  —Lethargy
  —Coma
  —Seizure
  —Ataxia
- CV:
  —Tachycardia
  —Hypotension
- Pulmonary: tachypnea
- GI:
  —Nausea
  —Vomiting
  —Diarrhea
- Skin:
  —Dry and hot if severe dehydration
  —Sweating may be present if not dehydrated
- Acute oliguric renal failure due to rhabdomyolysis, dehydration
- Hepatic failure

Heat Exhaustion

- Core temp: <104°F (40°C)
- CNS:
  —Headache
  —Fatigue
  —Malaise
  —Confusion
  —Agitation
- CV:
  —Mild tachycardia
  —Dehydration
- Pulmonary: tachypnea
- GI:
  —Nausea
  —Vomiting
- Skin: perspiration present, often profuse

Heat Cramps

- Cramps in heavily exercised muscles
- During or after exercise
- Primarily in lower extremities

Heat Tetany

- Carpal-pedal spasm—secondary to hyperventilation

Heat Edema

- Swelling of dependent areas of body
- Resolves after acclimatization

Prickly Heat

- Pruritic maculopapular rash over clothed areas

MECHANISM/DESCRIPTION

- Continuum of increasingly severe illnesses secondary to overwhelming heat stress
- Begins with dehydration and electrolyte abnormalities and progresses to thermoregulatory dysfunction and multisystem organ failure

Heat Stroke

- Loss of thermoregulatory function, severe CNS dysfunction, and multisystem organ failure
- Classic heat stroke
  —Occurs in those with compromised homeostatic mechanisms (elderly, debilitated)
  —Develops over days to weeks
  —Severe dehydration, skin warm and dry
- Exertional heat stroke
  —Occurs in younger, athletic individuals with a combined environmental and exertional heat stress
  —Develops over hours
  —Internal heat production overwhelms dissipating mechanisms
  —May be sweating

Heat Exhaustion

- Fluid and electrolyte depletion
- Thermoregulatory function is maintained
- CNS function is preserved

Heat Cramps

- Secondary to excessive sweating and sodium loss

Prickly Heat

- Blockage of sweat glands leading to rash

ETIOLOGY

- Preexisting conditions that hinder the body's ability to dissipate heat
  —Age extremes
  —Dehydration
  —Cardiovascular disease
  —Obesity
  —Hyperthyroidism
  —Febrile illness
  —Skin diseases that hinder sweating (psoriasis, eczema)
- Pharmacologic contributors
  —Sympathomimetics
  —LSD/PCP
  —MAO inhibitors
  —Anticholinergics
  —Antihistamines
  —Beta-blockers
  —Diuretics
  —Laxatives
  —Drug or alcohol withdrawal
- Physical/environmental factors
  —Prolonged exertion
  —Lack of mobility
  —Lack of air conditioning
  —Excessive humidity
  —Lack of acclimatization

PEDIATRIC CONSIDERATIONS

- Children are at increased risk of heat illness due to increased body surface area to mass ratio

Pre-Hospital

CAUTIONS

- Institute cooling measures for severe heat illness
  —Remove from heat stress
  —Disrobe patient
  —Ice packs to axilla, groin, and neck
  —Cover body with wet sheet
- IV 0.9% NS 500 cc fluid bolus if hypotensive
- If altered mental status administer glucose (or Accucheck), thiamine, naloxone

Diagnosis

ESSENTIAL WORKUP

- Accurate core temperature
- History of heat exposure
- Heat exhaustion—diagnosis of exclusion
- Core temperature >105°F (40.5°C) and CNS dysfunction required to make diagnosis of heat stroke

LABORATORY

For Heat Stroke and Heat Exhaustion

- CBC
  - —Leukocytosis, hemoconcentration often present
- Electrolytes, BUN, Cr, glucose
  - —Hypernatremia with severe dehydration
  - —Hyponatremia can occur if drinking copious free water
  - —Acute renal failure
- UA
  - —Myoglobin present in rhabdomyolysis

For Heat Stroke

- Liver function tests
  - —Hepatic necrosis presents with elevated transaminases
- PT/PTT/DIC panel
  - —Clotting abnormalities, DIC

IMAGING/SPECIAL TESTS

- EKG indicated in elderly or at cardiac risk
- CT head for altered mental status
- CXR for ARDS, aspiration pneumonia

DIFFERENTIAL DIAGNOSIS

- Febrile illness/sepsis
- Thyroid storm
- Pheochromocytoma
- Malignant hyperthermia
- Cocaine
- PCP
- Anticholinergics
- MAO inhibitors
- Meningitis
- Encephalitis
- Cerebral falciparum malaria
- Delirium tremens

Treatment

INITIAL STABILIZATION

- ABCs
- Immediate/rapid cooling if temperature >104°F (40°C)

ED MANAGEMENT

Cooling Measures

- Initiate for body temperature >104°F (40°C)
- Evaporative cooling
  - —Extremely effective (0.05–0.3°C/min)
  - —Spray disrobed patient with fine mist of warm water (prevents shivering)
  - —Airflow with fans blowing over patient
- Conductive cooling
  - —Ice packs to groin/axilla—combine with evaporative cooling treatment above
  - —Iced or cold water immersion—effective but impractical
- Iced peritoneal lavage and cardiopulmonary bypass for refractory cases
- To avoid hypothermia stop cooling therapy at 102°F (39°C)

Supportive Measures

- Rehydration for heat stroke/heat exhaustion
  - —Initial rehydration with 0.5–1.0 L 0.9% NS
  - —Avoid overhydration may contribute to development of ARDS
  - —Peds: 20-cc/kg bolus
  - —Place Foley catheter to monitor urine output for heat stroke victims
- Glucose/naloxone/thiamine for altered mental status
- Benzodiazepines for seizure, or to stop shivering
- Analgesics and oral or IV hydration with electrolyte-containing fluid for heat cramps
- Reassurance/calming measures/rebreathing in closed system (bag or nonrebreather without oxygen) for hyperventilation heat tetany
- Lower extremity elevation/removal from heat stress for heat edema

MEDICATIONS

- Dextrose: 50–100 cc D50 (peds: 2 cc/kg of D25W over 1 min) i.v.
- Diazepam (benzodiazepine): 5–10 mg (peds: 0.2–0.4 mg/kg) i.v. push
- Lorazepam: 1–2 mg (peds 0.05–0.1 mg/kg) i.v. push
- Naloxone (Narcan): 2 mg (peds: 0.1 mg/kg) i.v.

Disposition

ADMISSION CRITERIA

- Heat stroke to the ICU
- Heat exhaustion
  - —Severe electrolyte abnormalities
  - —Renal failure/evidence of rhabdomyolysis
  - —Elderly

DISCHARGE CRITERIA

- All patients except those with heat stroke or severe heat exhaustion may be discharged

Miscellaneous

ICD9: 780.6

ICD10: R50.9

SUGGESTED READINGS

Khosla R, Guntupalli K. Heat-related illness. Crit Care Clin 1999;15:251–263.

Lee-Chiong TL, Stitt JT. Heat stroke and other heat-related illnesses. Postgrad Med 1995;98(1):26–36.

Simon HB. Hyperthermia. N Engl J Med 1993;329(7):483–487.

Walker JS, Barnes SB. Heat emergencies. In: Tintinalli JE, ed. Emergency medicine: a comprehensive study guide, 5th ed. New York: McGraw-Hill, 2000:1237–1242.

Author: Marc Doucette

Hyperthyroidism

Clinical Presentation

SIGNS AND SYMPTOMS

- Reflect end-organ responsiveness to thyroid hormone

Symptoms

- Weight loss
- Palpitations
- Dyspnea
- Chest pain
- Weakness
- Diarrhea
- Abdominal pain
- Myalgia
- Nervousness
- Heat intolerance

Signs

- Fever
- Tachycardia disproportional to fever
- CHF
- Wide pulse pressure
- Thyromegaly
- Shock
- Jaundice
- Tremor
- Disorientation
- Psychosis
- Coma
- Tender liver
- Thyrotoxic stare

Apathetic Hyperthyroidism

- Seen in the elderly
- Due to multinodular goiter
- Subtle clinical findings
  - —Often reflecting single-organ dysfunction (CHF)
  - —Weight loss
  - —Depressed mentation
  - —Tremor
  - —Hyperactivity

MECHANISM/DESCRIPTION

- Excessive thyroid function results in continuum of disease
  - —Mild hyperthyroidism
  - —Thyrotoxicosis
  - —Thyroid storm or thyrotoxic crisis with life-threatening manifestations
- 1–2% of patients with hyperthyroidism progress to thyroid storm

ETIOLOGY

- Toxic diffuse goiter (Graves' disease)
- Toxic multinodular or uninodular goiter
- Factitious thyrotoxicosis
- T_3 toxicosis
- Hashimoto's thyroiditis
- Malignancy
- Hypothalamic hyperthyroidism
- TSH-producing pituitary tumor

Pre-Hospital

N/A

Diagnosis

ESSENTIAL WORKUP

- Plasma thyroid-stimulating hormone (TSH) assay is the initial test of choice in the ED
  - —Normal level usually excludes hyperthyroidism
  - —If TSH levels are not available, strong clinical picture should prompt initiation of therapy
- Thyroid storm—exaggerated signs and symptoms of thyrotoxicosis
  - —Goiter
  - —Extreme tachycardia
  - —Hyperpyrexia
- Disorientation and mental status changes common

LABORATORY

- Thyroid function tests for:
  - —Elderly patient with new-onset CHF
  - —New AFib/SVT
- TSH
- Free T_4
  - —If free T_4 is unavailable, total T_4 and resin T_3 uptake
- EKG
  - —Tachydysrhythmias
  - —Atrial fibrillation
- CBC
  - —Anemia
- Electrolytes, BUN, Cr, glucose
  - —BUN, creatinine, 2° dehydration
  - —Hypokalemia
- Calcium
- Liver function tests
- Arterial blood gases for hypoxemia
- Search for the underlying etiology

DIFFERENTIAL DIAGNOSIS

- Pheochromocytoma
- Sepsis
- Sympathomimetic ingestion
- Psychosis

Treatment

INITIAL STABILIZATION

- ABCs
- Cardiac monitor
- Supplemental oxygen to meet metabolic needs
- Initiate cooling measures
  - —Avoid aspirin

ED TREATMENT

- Inhibit hormone synthesis using thioamides
  - —Propylthiouracil (PTU)
- Block hormone release
  - —Potassium iodide, or
  - —Oral Lugol's solutions, or
  - —Sodium iodide
  - —Administer iodine therapy at least 1 hour after thioamides to prevent organification of the iodine
- Prevent peripheral conversion of T_4 to T_3
  - —PTU or
  - —Dexamethasone
- Block the peripheral effects of thyroid hormone
  - —Beta-blockade
    - -Propranolol
    - -Esmolol
    - -Contraindicated/caution advised with CHF, diabetes mellitus, and reactive airway disease
  - —When beta-blockers contraindicated, use:
    - -Reserpine
    - -Guanethidine
- Treatment of thyrotoxicosis, 2° thyroiditis consists of:
  - —Beta-blockade
  - —Antiinflammatory medications
- General support
  - —Acetaminophen for hyperpyrexia (aspirin contraindicated; displaces thyroid hormone from thyroglobulin)
  - —Control congestive heart failure
  - —Manage dehydration
- Identify and treat the precipitating event

MEDICATIONS

- Dexamethasone: 2 mg (peds: 0.15 mg/kg) i.v. q6h
- Esmolol: 500 μg/kg i.v. over 1 min followed by maintenance dose of 50 μg/kg min i.v. titrate to effect
- Guanethidine: 10 mg/day initially, then increased to 25–50 mg/day in three divided doses
- Lugol's solutions: 30 drops q12h
- Potassium iodide: 5–10 drops SSKI
- Propranolol: 1–2 mg IV repeated every 10–15 min
- Propylthiouracil (PTU): 300 mg (peds: 5–7 mg/kg/24 hours) q6h PO or per NGT
- Reserpine: 1–5 mg IM every 4–6 hours up to 15 mg/24 hours
- Sodium iodide: 1 g q8–12h

Disposition

ADMISSION CRITERIA

- Thyroid storm
- Requiring IV medications to control HR
- Symptomatic patients (tachycardia, fever)

DISCHARGE CRITERIA

- Minimally symptomatic individuals that respond well to oral therapy

Miscellaneous

ICD9: 242.9

ICD10: E05.9

SUGGESTED READINGS

Larson R, Davies TF, Hay ID. The thyroid. In: Wilson JD, ed. Williams' textbook of endocrinology, 9th ed. St. Louis: WB Saunders, 2001:389–516.

Tietgens ST, Leinung MC. Thyroid storm. Med Clin North Am 1995;79:169–184.

Wogan JM. Endocrine disorders. In: Marx J, et al., eds. Rosen's emergency medicine: concepts and clinical practice, 5th ed. St. Louis: CV Mosby, 2001:1770–1784.

Author: Rita Cydulka

Hyperventilation

Clinical Presentation

SIGNS AND SYMPTOMS

- Cardiac
  - —Chest pain
  - —Dyspnea
  - —"Air hunger"
  - —Palpitations
- Neurologic
  - —Dizziness
  - —Light-headedness
  - —Syncope
  - —Paresthesias
  - —Headache
  - —Carpopedal spasm
  - —Tetany
- Psychiatric
  - —Intense fear, anxiety
  - —Giddiness
  - —Feeling of unreality
- General
  - —Fatigue
  - —Weakness
  - —Malaise
- Clinical signs are rare and varied
  - —Tachypnea may not be present
    - -Patient may increase tidal volume rather than respiratory rate
- Carpopedal spasm
  - —May be dramatic
  - —Chvostek's sign may be present

MECHANISM/DESCRIPTION

- Constellation of symptoms produced by a *nonphysiologic* increase in minute ventilation; minute ventilation may be increased by increasing respiratory rate or tidal volume (sighs)
  - —Etiology of symptoms is unclear; symptoms may be related to hypocapnia, hypophosphatemia, or hypocalcemia, but significant controversy exists in the literature
- More common in females (may be related to progesterone)
- Incidence is approximately 10–15% in the general population

ETIOLOGY

- Usually a response to psychological stressors
- Therapy directed at alleviating those stressors

Pre-Hospital

CAUTIONS

- IV access and pulse oximetry with abnormal vital signs
- Supplemental oxygen if hypoxic

Diagnosis

ESSENTIAL WORKUP

- Diagnosis of exclusion
  - —Primary pathologic causes of hyperventilation must be investigated and excluded
- Clinical diagnosis based on the history and physical exam
- All patients with abnormal vital signs at presentation need further investigation
- Pulse oximetry

LABORATORY

- Arterial blood gas in any hypoxic patient
- Electrolytes, BUN/Cr, glucose for suspected acidosis/diabetic ketoacidosis

IMAGING/SPECIAL TESTS

- Chest x-ray study in any patient with hypoxia or focal findings on lung exam
- Electrocardiogram if chest pain present
- Hyperventilation provocation test
  - —Once symptoms have resolved
  - —Forced overbreathing for 3 minutes may be attempted to reproduce the symptoms
  - —Diagnostic accuracy is controversial
  - —Reproducibility of the symptoms may help the patient understand the role of overbreathing and help manage future attacks

DIFFERENTIAL DIAGNOSIS

- Hypoxia
  - —Asthma
  - —CHF
  - —Pulmonary embolus
  - —Pneumonia
- Severe pain
- CNS lesions
- Acidosis
- Pulmonary hypertension
- Hypoglycemia
- Mild asthma
- Pregnancy
- Pyrexia
- Altitude
- Drugs
  - —Aspirin intoxication
  - —Withdrawal syndrome (e.g., alcohol, benzodiazepines)

Treatment

INITIAL STABILIZATION

- IV access and pulse oximetry for patients with abnormal vital signs
- Initiate therapy for primary cause of hyperventilation

ED TREATMENT

- Initiate the treatment below if:
  - —Initial workup does not support a physiologic cause
  - —History and physical suggest the diagnosis of hyperventilation syndrome
- Reassurance, calming, and explanation of the voluntary component of the patient's symptoms often have immediate dramatic results
  - —Do not use paper bag rebreathing
- Benzodiazepine if symptoms persist
  - —Used to break the cycle of anxiety and hyperventilation
- Clarification of the psychological stressors help the patient avoid further attacks
  - —Assess for need of psychiatric evaluation
    - -Suicidal ideation
- Anxiolytics
  - —Short course of anxiolytics may benefit certain patients with definable temporary stressors

MEDICATIONS

- Buspirone: 5 mg PO t.i.d. for outpatient treatment
- Lorazepam: 1–2 mg PO or i.v. for ED treatment
- Valium: 2–5 mg PO or i.v. for ED or outpatient treatment

Disposition

ADMISSION CRITERIA

- Hyperventilation syndrome does not require admission

DISCHARGE CRITERIA

- Exclusion or successful treatment of primary pathologic causes of hyperventilation
- No acute psychiatric issues
- Adequate follow-up with a primary care physician

Miscellaneous

ICD9: 306.1

ICD10: R06.4

SUGGESTED READINGS

Block M, Szidon P. Hyperventilation syndromes. Compr Ther 1994;20(5): 306–311.

Gardner W. The pathophysiology of hyperventilation disorders. Chest 1996; 109:516–534.

Gardner WN, Bass C. Hyperventilation in clinical practice. Br J Hosp Med 1989; 41(1):73–81.

Hanashiro PK. Hyperventilation. Benign symptom or harbinger of catastrophe? Postgrad Med 1990;88(1):191–193.

Jozefowicz RF. Neurological manifestations of pulmonary disease. Neurol Clin 1989; 7(3):605–616.

Tobin MJ. Dyspnea. Pathologic basis, clinical presentation, and management. Arch Intern Med 1990;150(8):1604–1613.

Author: Robert F. McCormack

Hyperviscosity Syndrome

Clinical Presentation

SIGNS AND SYMPTOMS

- Signs and symptoms reflect end-organ dysfunction from hypoperfusion
- Hematologic
  - —Bleeding is the most common manifestation
  - —Epistaxis
  - —Gingival, rectal, uterine bleeding
  - —Prolonged postprocedural bleeding
  - —Blood dyscrasias
  - —Pruritus due to red cell breakdown products
  - —Splenic enlargement (extramedullary hematopoiesis)
- Ocular
  - —Change in visual acuity (blurring, diplopia, visual loss)
    - -Characteristic "link-sausage effect" on funduscopy
    - -Alternating bulges and constrictions within the retinal veins
  - —Retinal hemorrhage, detachment,
  - —Exudate, microaneurysm formation
  - —Papilledema
- Renal
  - —Nephritic or nephrotic syndrome
  - —Hematuria
  - —Sterile pyuria
- Neurologic
  - —Headache
  - —Ataxia
  - —Mental status changes/coma
  - —Dizziness/vertigo
  - —Nystagmus
  - —Tinnitus, hearing loss
  - —Paresthesia, peripheral neuropathy
  - —Seizure
- Cardiovascular
  - —Angina or myocardial infarction
  - —Dysrhythmias
  - —Congestive heart failure
- Dermatologic
  - —Raynaud's phenomenon
  - —Livedo reticularis
  - —Palpable purpura
  - —Eruptive spider nevus-like lesions
  - —Digital infarcts
  - —Peripheral gangrene

MECHANISM/DESCRIPTION

- Oxygen delivery proportional to blood flow
  - —Increased viscosity due to increase in plasma proteins or cell number
- Hyperviscosity syndrome (HVS) includes the disorders of blood viscosity such as:
  - —Erythrocytosis (polycythemia rubra vera)
  - —Leukocytosis (acute leukemia, chronic myelocytic leukemia)
  - —Sickle cell disease
  - —Paraproteinemia (Waldenström macroglobulinemia, multiple myeloma, heavy chain disease, primary amyloidosis)
- Primary HVS
  - —Conditions in which a primary blood abnormality causes impairment in blood flow such as in polycythemia or leukemia
- Secondary HVS
  - —Conditions in which vascular obstruction or stenosis causes a reduction of blood flow provoking tissue ischemia such as in myocardial infarction or stroke
- Syndromes associated with blood hyperviscosity include:
  - —Diabetes
  - —Shock
  - —Surgery
  - —Rheumatologic diseases

ETIOLOGY

- Increased concentration of circulating cells and blood volume
- Viscosity rises quickly with hematocrit (usually greater than 50%)
- Decreased deformability of erythrocytes or increased amounts of rigid leukemic cells
- Waldenström's macroglobulinemia
  - —Most common cause of HVS accounting for 85–90% of cases
  - —HVS is the presenting feature in 10–30% of cases
- Multiple myeloma
  - —Second most common cause of HVS
- Blastic phase of leukemias
  - —WBC $>$100,000
- Polycythemia vera

Pre-Hospital

CAUTIONS

- IV fluid resuscitation with hemorrhage

Diagnosis

ESSENTIAL WORKUP

- Evaluation of end-organ ischemia and bleeding
- Direct measurement of the serum or whole blood viscosity
- Suspect diagnosis if the laboratory evaluation is hampered by serum stasis and increased viscosity causing analyzer blockage

LABORATORY

- CBC with WBC differential
  - —Anemia or erythrocytosis can be seen in HVS
    - -Anemia usually normocytic and normochromic
  - —Rouleaux of erythrocytes on the peripheral smear—important diagnostic clue
  - —WBC for leukemia
- Electrolyte, BUN/Cr, glucose
  - —Renal dysfunction is commonly noted in HVS
  - —Hypercalcemia and pseudohyponatremia in multiple myeloma
- Coagulation profile
- Serum and urine protein electrophoresis
- Measurement of serum viscosity
  - —By an Ostwald viscosimeter
  - —Normal range for the serum viscosity relative to water is 1.4 to 1.8
  - —Minimal viscosity at which symptoms develop is 4.0 centipoise (cp)
- Elevated leukocyte alkaline phosphatase, LDH, and serum B_{12}

DIFFERENTIAL DIAGNOSIS

- Bleeding and clotting disorders
  - —Platelet disorders (qualitative and quantitative)
  - —Hereditary factor deficiencies
  - —Acquired disorders (vitamin K deficiency, liver disease)
  - —Disseminated intravascular coagulation

Treatment

INITIAL STABILIZATION

- Rehydrate with 0.9% NS IV fluid
- Bleeding or end-organ ischemia may not be controlled by any treatment except plasmapheresis
- In patients with anemia and a leukemic picture, avoid blood transfusion until pheresis is performed as an exacerbation of HVS may occur

ED TREATMENT

- Plasmapheresis/leukapheresis
  —Recommended exchange
    -40 mL/kg of body weight in stable patients
    -60 mL/kg of body weight in critical patients
  —Many patients require more than one plasmapheresis
  —Side effects
    -Hypocalcemia with use of a citrate-containing anticoagulant
    -Dysrhythmias (rare)
- Phlebotomy
  —Useful in acute severe cases if plasmapheresis not readily available
  —100–200 mL of blood can be withdrawn and volume replaced with isotonic saline

Disposition

ADMISSION CRITERIA

- Evidence of end-organ ischemia or hemorrhage
- ICU admission for:
  —Hemorrhage
  —Altered mental status
  —Acute myocardial infarction
- Regular admission for less severe presentations

DISCHARGE CRITERIA

- Definitive treatment of the underlying disorder

Miscellaneous

ICD9: 273.3

SUGGESTED READINGS

Forconi S, Pieragalli D, Guerrini M, et al. Primary and secondary blood hyperviscosity syndromes and syndromes associated with blood hyperviscosity. Drug 1987;33[suppl 2]:19–26.

Geraci JM, Hansen RM, Kueck BD. Plasma cell leukemia and hyperviscosity syndrome. South Med J 1990;83(7):800–805.

Pimentel L. Medical complications of oncologic disease. Emerg Med Clin North Am 1993;22(2):407–419.

Somer T, Meiselman HJ. Disorders of blood viscosity. Ann Med 1993;25:31–39.

Stolz JF, Donner M, Larcan A. Introduction to hemorheology: theoretical aspects and hyperviscosity syndromes. Int Angiol 1987;6:119–132.

Author: Christopher A. Lipinski

Hyphema

Clinical Presentation

SIGNS AND SYMPTOMS

- Photophobia
- Blurring of vision/decreased visual acuity
- Ocular pain
- Blood in the anterior chamber
  - —Noted on slit-lamp examination
  - —Red-pigmented substance settling to the bottom of the anterior chamber in an individual whose head is elevated
- Evidence of blunt periorbital or orbital eye trauma including:
  - —Ecchymosis
  - —Corneal abrasion
  - —Subconjunctival hemorrhage
- Penetrating corneal injuries

MECHANISM/DESCRIPTION

- Defined as blood in the anterior chamber of the eye
- Four grades (classifications) depending on the percentage of the anterior chamber occluded by blood
  - —Grade I: <1/3 of the anterior chamber
  - —Grade II: 1/3 to 1/2 of the anterior chamber
  - —Grade III: >1/2 of the anterior chamber
  - —Grade IV: total (also called "eight-ball" hyphema)
- Higher grade hyphemas:
  - —More likely to rebleed (25% of grade I rebleed compared to 67% of grade III)
  - —More likely to experience glaucoma
  - —More likely to experience corneal staining
  - —Less likely to recover visual acuity
- Blunt trauma
  - —An orbital blow deforms the cornea inward causing an acute elevation of intraocular pressure and an anterior chamber fluid wave
  - —Limbal tissue stretches and blood vessels tear at the angle
- Penetrating trauma—stromal vessels directly injured or ruptured by sudden decrease in intraocular pressure
- Spontaneous—any vessel in the anterior chamber begins to bleed without trauma

ETIOLOGY

- Traumatic (blunt or penetrating), surgical, or spontaneous
- Most traumatic hyphemas result from blunt ocular trauma (71–94%)
- Spontaneous causes include:
  - —Tumors
    - -Melanoma
    - -Retinoblastoma
    - -Metastatic tumors
    - -Xanthogranulomas
  - —Blood dyscrasias
    - -Hemophilia
    - -Leukemia
    - -Coagulopathies
  - —Drugs
    - -Aspirin
    - -Alcohol
    - -Anticoagulants
  - —Vascular anomalies: neovascularization
  - —Sudden lowering of an inflamed eyes intraocular pressure

Pre-Hospital

CAUTIONS

- Place an eye shield in case of corneal perforation
- Keep head upright to allow the blood to settle to bottom of anterior chamber

Diagnosis

ESSENTIAL WORKUP

- Thorough history including:
  - —Previous visual acuity
  - —Prior eye surgery
  - —Medications
  - —Sickle cell disease
  - —Other injuries
  - —Concurrent medical problems
- Visual acuity (mandatory)
- Inspection of the cornea and anterior chamber for perforation
- Slit-lamp examination
- Fluorescein evaluation
- Tonometry
  - —Exclude global perforation prior to pressure measurement

LABORATORY TEST

- Laboratory tests should be individualized depending on etiology
- Sickle cell screen
- PT/PTT/bleeding time if bleeding disorder suspected
- Platelet count for those at risk for thrombocytopenia
- BUN and Cr if aminocaproic acid to be used

IMAGING/SPECIAL TESTS

- Orbital radiographs, CT, ultrasound, or MRI if the retina and vitreous chamber cannot be visualized or an intraocular foreign body is suspected

Treatment

INITIAL STABILIZATION

- Hard metal shield

ED TREATMENT

- Restrict activity that increases eye movements (e.g., reading)
- Avoid bending, straining, or exertion
- Elevate the head of the bed to 45 degrees
- Antiemetics for nausea/vomiting (increases IOP)
- Analgesics
  - —Avoid NSAID- or aspirin-containing products
- Treat elevated intraocular pressure if present (>21–24 mm Hg) as in glaucoma
  - —Carbonic anhydrase inhibitors (acetazolamide)
  - —Beta-blockers (timolol, betaxolol)
  - —Hyperosmotic drugs (mannitol, glycerol)
  - —Cholinergic drugs (pilocarpine)
  - —In sickle cell patients avoid acetazolamide, pilocarpine, epinephrine, or hyperosmotics, which can increase sickling and lead to increased intraocular pressure
- Stop anticoagulants and aspirin if possible
- Topical steroids may decrease inflammation from iritis but do not decrease rebleeds
- Cycloplegics may help decrease the pain from iritis
- Oral steroids and antifibrinolytics (aminocaproic acid)
  - —Extremely controversial
  - —Best left to the discretion of the consulting ophthalmologist
- Oral stool softeners and bulking agents to prevent constipation and straining (which increases intraocular pressure)

MEDICATIONS

- Acetazolamide
  - —i.v.: 500 mg (peds: 20–40 mg/kg/24 hours q6h) initially, followed by 250 mg q4h
  - —PO: 500 mg sustained-release (peds: 8–30 mg/kg/24 hours q6–8h) PO b.i.d.
- Aminocaproic acid: 50 mg/kg q4h for 5 days orally (30 g/day max)
- Betaxolol 0.5%: 1 drop b.i.d.
- Docusate sodium: 100 mg (peds: 10–20 mg) PO b.i.d.
- Glycerol: 1–1.5 ml/kg PO
- Mannitol: 1.5–2 g/kg i.v.
- Pilocarpine 2%: affected eye—1 drop q 15 min for 5 times, then q2–3h
- Psyllium: 1 tsp in liquid PO qd or b.i.d.
- Timolol 0.25–0.5%: 1 drop b.i.d.

Disposition

ADMISSION CRITERIA

- Unreliable patient
- Disease that increases the risk of rebleeding or increases the risk of increased intraocular pressure (sickle cell disease)
- Ongoing bleeding
- Ruptured globe
- Visibility of the vitreous chamber is obscured by blood

DISCHARGE CRITERIA

- No patient should be discharged before consultation with an ophthalmologist
- Treat small hyphemas on an outpatient basis with daily follow-up to assess the complications of corneal staining, rebleeding, increased intraocular pressure, and synechiae

Miscellaneous

ICD9: 364.41

ICD10: H21.0

SEE ALSO: GLOBE RUPTURE

SUGGESTED READINGS

Berrios RR, Dreyer EB. Traumatic hyphema. Int Ophthalmol Clin 1995;35:93–103.

Crouch ER Jr, Crouch ER. Management of traumatic hyphema: therapeutic options. J Pediatr Ophthalmol Strabismus 1999; 35(5):238–250.

Endo EG, Mead MD. The management of traumatic hyphema. Int Ophthalmol Clin 1994;34:1–7.

Hamill MB. Current concepts in the treatment of traumatic injury to the anterior segment. Ophthalmol Clin North Am 1999;12(3):457–464.

Hemphill RR, Doe EA. Right eye pain and redness. Acad Emerg Med 1997;4(2): 142–143, 147–149.

Author: Eric Reichman

Hypocalcemia

Clinical Presentation

SIGNS AND SYMPTOMS

- Occur when ionized calcium falls below 3.2 mg/dL
- Reflect both the absolute and the rate of fall in calcium concentration

Neuromuscular

- Paresthesias
- Hyperreflexia
- Muscle spasm
- Latent tetany (Chvostek's and Trousseau's sign)
- Tetany
- Laryngeal stridor
- Seizures

Cardiovascular

- Dysrhythmias
- Hypotension
- Impaired contractility (CHF)
- QT and ST prolongation
- T-wave abnormalities

Psychiatric

- Irritability
- Mental status changes
- Psychosis
- Depression
- Confusion
- Delusions
- Chorea
- Parkinsonisms

Ocular

- Papilledema
- Cataracts

MECHANISM/DESCRIPTION

- Intravascular calcium circulates in three forms
  - —Bound to proteins (mainly albumin): 45–50%
  - —Bound to complexing ions (citrate, phosphate, carbonate): 5–10%
  - —Ionized (free) calcium (physiologically active form): 45–50%
- Normal total serum calcium concentrations = 8.7–10.5 mg/dL
  - —Under normal conditions the ionized calcium level is approximately half of the total calcium level
  - —In critically ill patients, the total calcium level is a poor indicator of ionized calcium levels
- Hypocalcemia = total plasma calcium levels below 8.7 mg/dL
  - —Ionized calcium may be normal and therefore have no clinical manifestations occurring
- Incidence in the general population is 0.6%

ETIOLOGY

- Serum levels of calcium controlled primarily by the activity of three hormones
  - —Parathyroid hormone (PTH)
    - -Decrease in calcium levels leads to an increase in PTH secretion (increasing bone resorption, renal absorption, intestinal absorption, and urinary phosphate excretion)
  - —Vitamin D (1,25-dihydroxyvitamin D)
    - -Decrease in calcium levels activates vitamin D (increasing bone resorption and intestinal absorption)
  - —Calcitonin
    - -Causes a direct inhibition of bone resorption with increased calcium levels
- Hypoalbuminemia is most common cause of hypocalcemia
  - —Each g/dL decrease in serum albumin decreases protein-bound serum calcium by 0.8 mg/dL
    - -Will not change ionized (free) calcium
- Hypomagnesemia
  - —Decreased secretion of PTH
  - —End-organ resistance to PTH
  - —Chronic illnesses/critical illnesses

PEDIATRIC CONSIDERATIONS

- Children have higher values of normal calcium (9.2–11 mg/dL)
- Neonatal hypocalcemia = total serum calcium concentrations <7.0 mg/dL or serum-ionized calcium levels <4.4 mg/dL
- Frequent symptoms of hypocalcemia in infancy
  - —Hyperactivity, jitteriness
  - —Tachypnea
  - —Apneic spells with cyanosis
  - —Vomiting

Pre-Hospital

N/A

Diagnosis

ESSENTIAL WORKUP

- Serum-ionized calcium level confirms the diagnosis

LABORATORY

- Arterial blood gas
  - —Change from normal pH of 0.1 units equals a reciprocal change in ionized calcium of approximately 1.7 mg/dL
- Serum albumin
  - —Total serum calcium reduced by approximately 0.8 mg/dL for every g/dL by which the albumin is below the normal value
- Electrolytes, BUN/Cr, glucose
- Magnesium
  - —Hypomagnesemia can cause hypocalcemia
- Phosphate
  - —Differentiates hypoparathyroidism from vitamin D deficiency
  - —Increase in phosphate associated with hypoparathyroidism
  - —Decrease in phosphate associated with vitamin D deficiency
- PTH
  - —Very high levels of PTH associated with pseudohypoparathyroidism
  - —High levels of PTH associated with vitamin D deficiency
  - —Low levels of PTH associated with hypoparathyroidism

IMAGING/SPECIAL TESTS

- EKG
  - —Prolonged QT interval
  - —Heart block

DIFFERENTIAL DIAGNOSIS

- Impaired PTH action or secretion
  - —Autoimmune congenital neck surgery or irradiation
  - —Neonatal secondary to maternal hyperparathyroidism
  - —Magnesium disorder
  - —Pseudohypoparathyroidism
  - —Infiltrative (amyloidosis, sarcoidosis)
- Impaired vitamin D synthesis or action
  - —Nutritional malabsorption
  - —Renal or liver disease
  - —Sepsis
  - —Rickets disease
- Calcium complex formation or sequestration
  - —Hyperphosphatemia
  - —Ethylene glycol, ethylenediaminetetraacetic acid (EDTA), citrate (from transfusion)
  - —Pancreatitis, rhabdomyolysis
  - —Alkalosis (i.e., hyperventilation)
- Medications
  - —Mithramycin, plicamycin, phosphate, calcitonin, bisphosphonates
  - —Phenobarbital, Dilantin
  - —Cisplatin
  - —Cadmium, colchicine
  - —Fluoride, citrate
- Malignancies
  - —Prostate cancer
  - —Breast cancer
  - —Lung cancer
  - —Chondrosarcoma
- "Hungry bone syndrome"
  - —After parathyroid removal
  - —Rapid accretion of calcium as bone is remineralized

Treatment

INITIAL STABILIZATION

- ABCs
  - —Control airway and provide supplemental oxygen as needed
  - —Establish intravenous catheter access
  - —Cardiac monitor

ED TREATMENT

Acute Management

- Treat symptomatic hypocalcemia as a medical emergency with parenteral calcium administration
- Calcium
  - —Administer 100–300 mg of elemental calcium for an adult
    - -10-mL ampules of 10% calcium chloride contains 360 mg of elemental calcium
    - -10-mL ampules of 10% calcium gluconate contains 93 mg of elemental calcium
  - —Faster IV rates
    - -Can cause cardiac dysrhythmias
    - -Calcium salts are irritating to veins
  - —Intramuscular calcium gluceptate or calcium gluconate if IV access not available
  - —Bolus calcium doses increase ionized calcium for only 1–2 hours
  - —Must follow by an infusion
- Calcium infusion
  - —Calcium infusion rate = 0.5–2 mg/kg/h
  - —Do not mix calcium with bicarbonate or phosphate
    - -Precipitates of calcium salts may form
  - —Administer cautiously in digitalis patients
    - -Can initiate and exacerbate digitalis toxicity
- Response to therapy
  - —Individual responses vary
  - —Monitor calcium concentrations q1–4h during therapy
  - —Titrate treatment to symptoms or EKG changes
  - —Consider hypomagnesemia if the patient fails to respond to calcium therapy
    - -Correct hypomagnesemia with magnesium 2 g IVPB
  - —In setting of acidosis, correct calcium first, alkalosis will further reduce ionized calcium
  - —Side effects of IV calcium
    - -Nausea, vomiting
    - -Hypotension
    - -Dysrhythmias

Chronic Management

- Oral calcium supplementation
- 1–4 g/d of elemental calcium in divided doses
- Vitamin D
  - —Enhances intestinal absorption
  - —Initiate when calcium supplementation alone not sufficient to restore calcium levels
  - —Dose:
    - -200 IU for ages 19–50
    - -400 IU for ages 51–70
    - -600–800 for ages >70
  - —Multivitamin contains 400 IU of vitamin D
- Vitamin D preparations
  - —Ergocalciferol: 125 μg/d
  - —Dihydrotachysterol: 100–400 μg/d
  - —Calcifediol: 50–200 μg/d
  - —Calcitriol 0.25–1.0 μg/d

MEDICATIONS

- Calcium (i.v.)
  - —Chloride: 1 g in 10 mL [1 g = 360 mg (13.6 mEq) elemental calcium]
  - —Gluceptate (i.v./i.m.): 1 g in 5 mL [1 g = 90 mg (4.5 mEq) elemental calcium]
  - —Gluconate: 1 g in 10 mL [1 g = 90 mg (4.5 mEq) elemental calcium]
- Oral calcium
  - —Glubionate: 18 g/5 mL of syrup (1 g = 65 mg elemental calcium)
  - —Carbonate: 350- to 1,500-mg tablets (1 g = 400 mg)
  - —Citrate: 950-mg tablets (1 g = 211 mg elemental calcium)
  - —Gluconate: 500- to 1,000-mg tablets (1 g = 90 mg elemental calcium)
  - —Lactate: 350- to 1,000-mg tablets (1 g = 130 mg elemental calcium)

PEDIATRIC CONSIDERATIONS

- Initial calcium bolus with 10% calcium gluconate should be 9–18 mg of elemental calcium/kg or 1–2 mL/kg not to exceed 5 mL in premature infants or 10 mL in term infants
- Calcitriol dose in children ranges from 0.1–3 μg/day

Miscellaneous

- Calcium content of common foods
  - —Milk or yogurt, 8 oz = 300 mg
  - —Cheddar cheese, 1 oz = 200 mg
  - —Calcium-fortified cereal, 1 cup = 300 mg
  - —Calcium-fortified orange juice, 1 cup = 270 mg
  - —Shrimp, 3 oz = 50 mg
  - —Peanuts = 130 mg
  - —Oranges = 50 mg

Disposition

ADMISSION CRITERIA

- Symptomatic or severe ionized hypocalcemia (<3.2 mg/dL)
- Continuous IV calcium preparations necessary to maintain calcium levels

DISCHARGE CRITERIA

- Asymptomatic hypocalcemia
- Ionized calcium >3.2 mg/dL in healthy patients with no comorbid illness

Miscellaneous

ICD9: 275.4

ICD10: E83.5

SUGGESTED READINGS

Anagnos A, Ruff RL, Kaminski HJ. Endocrine neuromyopathies. Neurol Clin 1997;15(3):673–696.

Fulop M. Algorithms for diagnosing some electrolyte disorders. Am J Emerg Med 1998;16(1):76–84.

Horak HA, Poumand R. Endocrine myopathies. Neurol Clin 2000;18(1): 203–213.

Kapoor M, Chan Z. Fluid and electrolyte abnormalities. Crit Care Clin 2001;17(3): 503–529.

Riggs JE. Neurologic manifestations of electrolyte disturbances. Neurol Clin 2002;20(1):227–239, vii.

Thomas MK, Demay MB. Vitamin D deficiency and disorders of vitamin D metabolism. Endocrinol Metab Clin North Am 2000;29(3):611–627, viii.

Author: Christopher Ervin

Hypoglycemia

Clinical Presentation

SIGNS AND SYMPTOMS

- Adrenergic
  - —Diaphoresis
  - —Anxiety
  - —Tachycardia
  - —Hunger
- Neuroglycopenic
  - —Dizziness
  - —Confusion
  - —Hyperactive or psychotic behavior
  - —Slurred speech
  - —Cranial-nerve palsies
  - —Seizures
  - —Hemiplegia
  - —Decerebrate posturing
- Neonatal presentation
  - —Asymptomatic
  - —Limp
  - —Bradycardia
  - —Irritable
  - —Tremulous
  - —Seizures

MECHANISM/DESCRIPTION

- Deficiency in counterregulatory hormones (glucagon, epinephrine, cortisol, growth hormone) or excessive insulin response
- Fall in serum glucose (<40 mg/dL) stimulates sympathetic catecholamine release

ETIOLOGY

- Increased insulin levels
  - —Overdose of oral hypoglycemic agent or insulin
  - —Sepsis
  - —Insulinoma
- Underproduction of glucose
  - —Alcohol (inhibitory effect on glycogen storage and gluconeogenesis)
  - —Salicylates
  - —Beta-blockers
  - —Adrenal insufficiency
  - —Liver disease
  - —Malnutrition
  - —Dehydration
  - —Cerebral edema

PEDIATRIC CONSIDERATIONS

- Infants at greatest risk of hypoglycemia
  - —Mothers with DM
  - —Premature/postmature
  - —Small for gestational age
  - —Intrapartum hypoxia
- Common in critically ill children
- Definitions
  - —<20 mg/dL in preterm infant during first 24 hours of life
  - —<30 mg/dL in newborn
  - —40 mg/dL in infants

Pre-Hospital

CAUTIONS

- Diagnosis with finger stick glucose (Accucheck)
- Oral glucose-containing fluids or IV dextrose for hypoglycemia
- Administer thiamine along with dextrose IV to prevent precipitation of Wernicke's encephalopathy

Diagnosis

ESSENTIAL WORKUP

- Diagnosis requires:
  - —Demonstration of neuroglycopenic signs and symptoms as defined above
  - —Lab evidence of hypoglycemia (Accucheck/Dextrostix)
  - —Clearing of symptoms following glucose administration

LABORATORY

- Blood glucose
  - —Initial and posttreatment, monitor
- Electrolytes, BUN, Cr
  - —Order if mental status does not improve post-glucose administration
- CBC
  - —Order if sepsis present
- Urinalysis

IMAGING/SPECIAL TESTS

- EKG if suspect MI/ischemia due to hypoglycemia
- CXR for
  - —Possible aspiration
  - —Pneumonia as source of sepsis

DIFFERENTIAL DIAGNOSIS

- Neurologic
  - —CVA/TIA
  - —Seizure disorder
- Drug or alcohol intoxication
- Psychosis or depression
- Pediatric considerations
  - —Salicylate ingestion
  - —Reye's syndrome
  - —Growth hormone deficiency
  - —Ketotic hypoglycemia
  - —Inborn errors of metabolism

Treatment

INITIAL STABILIZATION

- Glucose
  - —Dextrose IVP
  - —Oral glucose in awake patient (with no IV) without risk of aspiration
  - —Glucagon IM if unable to establish IV access
- ABCs with aspiration and seizure precautions

ED TREATMENT

- Administer 50 cc D50W for decreased level of consciousness
  - —Second or third ampule may be necessary
  - —Complications include volume overload and hypokalemia
- Initiate continuous IV infusion of 5–20% glucose solution for persistent mild hypoglycemia or if patient cannot eat
- Administer glucagon
  - —If hypoglycemia refractory to glucose
  - —If IV access delayed
  - —Effective in 10–20 minutes
  - —Ineffective in alcohol-induced hypoglycemia
  - —May repeat twice
- Monitor blood glucose every 2–3 hours and prior to discharge
- Adrenal insufficiency: administer hydrocortisone 100 mg and glucagon 1 mg
- For cases of resistant hypoglycemia due to sulfonylureas administer diazoxide 300 mg IV over 30 minutes every 4 hours PRN
  - —Beware of potent hypotensive effect

MEDICATIONS

- D50W: 1 amp (= 25 g) of 50% dextrose, 1–2 cc/kg (peds: 1–2 mL/kg D25W) IVP
- Diazoxide: 1–3 mg/kg IVP, max 150 mg
- Glucagon: 1–2 mg (peds: <6 years: 0.5 mg; ≥6 years: 1.0 mg) i.v./i.m./s.c.
- Hydrocortisone: 100 mg (peds: 1–2 mg/kg) i.v.
- Oral glucose: 20 g orally equals ~12 oz nondiet fruit juice, 14 oz nondiet cola, 2.5 oz chocolate

PEDIATRIC CONSIDERATIONS

- Children: use D25W 1–2 cc/kg i.v. or glucagon if unable to achieve i.v. access
- Infants: D10W i.v./intraosseous as needed

Disposition

ADMISSION CRITERIA

- Overdoses of oral hypoglycemic agent or long-acting insulin mandate observation for at least 24 hours
- Failure of neuroglycopenic symptoms to improve after 1 hour suggests neurologic injury, preexisting neurologic condition, or another cause for these symptoms
- Recurrent hypoglycemic state in ED
- Older patients may require several days for complete recovery from severe or prolonged hypoglycemia

DISCHARGE CRITERIA

- Discharge mild unintentional insulin over usage if blood glucose normal, symptoms resolved, tolerating oral intake, and can be observed

Miscellaneous

ICD9: 251.2

ICD10: E16.2

SUGGESTED READINGS

Comi RJ. Approach to acute hypoglycemia. Endocrinol Metab Clin North Am 1993; 22(2):247–262.

Service FJ. Hypoglycemia. Med Clin North Am 1995;79(1):1–6.

Service FJ. Hypoglycemia disorders. N Engl J Med 1995;27:1144–1150.

Authors: Michelle Ervin; Steven Friedman

Hypoglycemic Agent, Poisoning

Clinical Presentation

SIGNS AND SYMPTOMS

Insulin or Sulfonylureas

- Overdose causes hypoglycemia
  - —Symptoms most often occur when glucose <40–60 mg/dL (may occur at higher levels in diabetics)
  - —Symptoms blunted by β-antagonists
- Facial flushing, diaphoresis, pallor, piloerection
- Hunger, nausea, abdominal cramping
- Labored respirations, apnea
- Headache, blurred vision
- Paresthesias, weakness, incoordination, tremor
- Anxiety, irritability, bizarre behavior, confusion, stupor, coma, seizures
- Palpitations, tachycardia, bradycardia (late)
- Hypertension
- Hypothermia

Biguanides

- Toxicity primarily due to lactic acid accumulation
- Nausea, vomiting, abdominal pain
- Agitation, confusion, lethargy, coma
- Kussmaul respirations
- Hypotension, tachycardia

MECHANISM/DESCRIPTION

- Insulin
  - —Enhances glucose uptake into cells
  - —Limits glucose availability to the brain (most sensitive to hypoglycemia)
  - —Influences potassium redistribution
- Sulfonylurea agents
  - —Enhance insulin release from β cells, reduce hepatic glucose production, and increase peripheral insulin sensitivity
  - —Hypoglycemic effect enhanced by polypharmacy, alcohol use, hepatic dysfunction, and renal insufficiency
- Biguanide agents (metformin)
  - —Antihyperglycemic agents
  - —Decrease elevated serum glucose concentrations, but generally do not cause hypoglycemia on their own
  - —In the presence of insulin, biguanides do the following:
    - -Increase glucose uptake into cells
    - -Decrease gastrointestinal glucose absorption
    - -Decrease hepatic gluconeogenesis
  - —Metabolize glucose to lactate in intestinal cells, which may accumulate and lead to lactic acidosis
- Thiazolidinediones
  - —In the presence of insulin, thiazolidinediones increase glucose uptake and utilization and decrease gluconeogenesis
- α-Glucosidase inhibitors
  - —Lower systemic glucose by decreasing gastrointestinal absorption of carbohydrates

PEDIATRIC CONSIDERATIONS

- Neonatal hypoglycemia may occur after maternal use of sulfonylureas during labor
- Ingestion of one sulfonylurea tablet may cause hypoglycemia in a child
- Onset of symptomatic hypoglycemia may be delayed up to 8 hours

Pre-Hospital

CAUTIONS

- Symptomatic hypoglycemia is a true emergency
  - —Sequelae of hypoglycemia dependent on duration of neuroglycopenia
  - —Administer glucose immediately when hypoglycemia suspected or confirmed
  - —Administer glucagon IM if IV access impossible (action delayed and transient)
  - —Obtain all pills/pill bottles from the scene for identification in the ED

Diagnosis

ESSENTIAL WORKUP

- Monitor serum glucose concentration
- Monitor vital signs and neurologic status
- Obtain serum electrolytes and lactate for biguanide ingestion
- Obtain liver function tests for thiazolidinedione ingestion

LABORATORY

- Serum glucose, before and after treatment
- Electrolytes
  - —Check for hypokalemia
  - —Anion gap acidosis
- BUN, Cr
  - —May reveal renal insufficiency, causing drug accumulation
- CBC
- Ethanol level
- Lactate level
- Liver function tests
- Arterial blood gas
- Assays for immunoreactive insulin and C-peptide levels
  - —Do not correlate with severity of clinical symptoms
  - —Confirm surreptitious self-administration of exogenous insulin if insulin level is high and C-peptide is low in the setting of hypoglycemia
- Assays for sulfonylureas
  - —Do not correlate with severity of clinical symptoms
  - —Confirm surreptitious drug ingestions when suspected

IMAGING/SPECIAL TESTS

- EKG: sinus tachycardia, PVCs, atrial dysrhythmias
- EEG: diffuse slowing without focal abnormalities
- CT scan: cerebral edema if prolonged hypoglycemia
- CXR: aspiration pneumonia or pulmonary edema

DIFFERENTIAL DIAGNOSIS

- Addison's disease
- Panhypopituitarism
- Sepsis
- Insulinoma
- Neuroendocrine tumors
- Cirrhosis
- Chronic ethanol abuse
- Ethanol ingestion
- Salicylate ingestion
- β-antagonist ingestion
- Ackee fruit poisoning

Treatment

INITIAL STABILIZATION

- ABCs
- Administer 50% dextrose IV

ED TREATMENT

- Supportive care
- Hypotension
  - —0.9% NS IV fluid bolus
  - —Trendelenburg position
  - —Dopamine titrated to pressure
  - —Pressors may increase lactate production; use cautiously with biguanide induced lactic acidosis
- Neuroglycopenia
  - —May persist shortly after serum glucose corrected
  - —Persistent symptoms requires further dextrose administration
- Hypoglycemia
  - —IV infusion D5W or D10W to maintain euglycemia or mild hyperglycemia
  - —Food
- Administer activated charcoal for recent or large ingestion of oral agent (sulfonylurea or biguanide)
- Administer sodium bicarbonate for biguanide-induced lactic acidosis if pH <7.0
- Administer benzodiazepines for seizures
- Inhibit insulin secretion for sulfonylurea overdose with recurrent hypoglycemia, with:
  - —Octreotide
  - —Diazoxide (watch for hypotension)
- Early hemodialysis beneficial in cases of biguanide-induced lactic acidosis
  - —Corrects acid/base abnormalities
  - —Enhances elimination of the drug

MEDICATIONS

- Activated charcoal: 1 g/kg PO
- Dextrose: 50–100 cc D50 (peds: 2 cc/kg of D25 over 1 min) i.v.; repeat if necessary
- Diazepam (benzodiazepine): 5–10 mg (peds: 0.2–0.5 mg/kg) i.v.; repeat if necessary
- Diazoxide: 200 mg PO or 1–3 mg/kg i.v. (infant: 8–15 mg/kg/24 hours q8–12h PO/i.v.; child: 3–8 mg/kg/24 hours q8h PO/i.v.)
- Glucagon: 1–2 mg (peds: 0.03–0.1 mg/kg) i.m./s.c./i.v.
- Lorazepam (benzodiazepine): 2–6 mg (peds: 0.03–0.05 mg/kg) i.v.; repeat if necessary
- Octreotide: 50–100 μg q8–12h s.c./i.v.
- Sodium bicarbonate: 1–2 mEq/kg i.v.

Disposition

ADMISSION CRITERIA

- Hypoglycemia due to sulfonylurea agents (may require several days of monitoring) or long-acting insulin preparations
- Intentional overdose or self-injection of insulin warrants admission for 24 hours glucose monitoring
- All children with accidental ingestion of sulfonylureas
- Metabolic alterations due to biguanide ingestion or accumulation

DISCHARGE CRITERIA

- Accidental hypoglycemia due to short-acting insulin injection in the setting of dietary insufficiency
- Discharge after glucose correction and a 4-hour period of observation

Miscellaneous

ICD9: 977.9

ICD10: T50.8; T38.3

SUGGESTED READINGS

Kruse JA. Metformin associated lactic acidosis. J Emerg Med 2001;20(3): 267–272.

McLaughlin SA, Crandall CS, McKinney PE. Octreotide: an antidote for sulfonylurea-induced hypoglycemia. Ann Emerg Med 2000;36(2):133–138.

Spiller HA. Management of antidiabetic medications in overdose. Drug Safety 1998;19(5):411–424.

Wolf LR, Smeeks F, Policastro M. Oral hypoglycemic agents. In: Ford MD, Delaney KA, Ling LJ, et al., eds. Clinical toxicology. Philadelphia: WB Saunders, 2001:423–432.

Author: Mark B. Mycyk

Hypokalemia

Clinical Presentation

SIGNS AND SYMPTOMS

Cardiovascular

- Ventricular dysrhythmias (especially in the setting of heart disease)
- Potentiation of digoxin toxicity

Neuromuscular

- Weakness
  —Severe weakness (K^+ <2.5)
  —May progress to paralysis
- Cramps
- Constipation, ileus
- Increased risk of rhabdomyolysis
- Endocrine
  —Hypokalemia inhibits insulin release
  —Glucose levels may rise

Renal

- Polyuria (inhibits kidneys' ability to concentrate urine)
- Metabolic alkalosis

MECHANISM/DESCRIPTION

- Increase in the normal intracellular to extracellular potassium gradient
  —Alters the depolarization threshold for muscles and nerves
  —Inhibits the termination of action potentials
- Alterations in intracellular potassium directly affect cellular function

ETIOLOGY

Intracellular Shift of Potassium

- Alkalosis
- Insulin
- Adrenergic excess
  —Severe stress (trauma, myocardial infarction, sepsis)
  —Treatment of asthma
- Hypokalemic periodic paralysis
  —Familial
  —Thyrotoxic
  —Barium poisoning

Potassium Losses

- Renal losses
  —Diuretics (thiazides, loop diuretics, carbonic anhydrase inhibitors)
    -Usually associated with loss of other cations (Mg^{2+}, Ca^{2+}, P^{3+}, Na^+)
  —Vomiting causes volume depletion and metabolic alkalosis, which increases renal losses of potassium
  —Renal tubular damage
  —Primary renal tubular disorders
  —Hyperaldosteronism
    -Primary
    -Pseudohyperaldosteronism (licorice ingestion)
  —Hypomagnesemia
  —DKA
- GI losses
  —Diarrhea
  —Vomiting, nasogastric suction
  —Ureterosigmoidostomy
  —Villous adenomas
  —Laxative abuse
  —Intestinal fistulae, ileostomy
  —Cystic fibrosis

Poor Intake (Rare as a Sole Etiology)

- Nutritional
- Eating disorders

Pre-Hospital

N/A

Diagnosis

ESSENTIAL WORKUP

- Serum potassium <3.5 mEq/L

LABORATORY

- Electrolytes, BUN, Cr, glucose
- Calcium
- Urinalysis
  - —Check for myoglobin
  - —Hypokalemia may cause rhabdomyolysis
- Magnesium
  - —Hypomagnesemia may lead to inability to correct hypokalemia
- ABG
  - —Acid-base status

IMAGING/SPECIAL TESTS

- EKG shows
  - —Low-voltage T waves
  - —Sagging of the ST segments
  - —U waves
  - —Atrial and ventricular dysrhythmias, especially in patients on digoxin

Parameter for Etiology of Hypokalemia

- Normotensive
  - —Urine K^+ <25 mEq/L and serum bicarbonate low or normal: lower GI losses, poor intake
  - —Urine K^+ <25 mEq/L and serum bicarbonate high: prior diuretic use
  - —Urine K^+ >25 mEq/L and serum bicarbonate low: renal tubular acidosis, DKA
  - —Urine K^+ >25 mEq/L and serum bicarbonate high: vomiting, current diuretic use, Bartter's syndrome
- Hypertensive
  - —Measure plasma renin
    - -High renin: primary aldosteronism vs renal artery stenosis
    - -Low renin: measure aldosterone

DIFFERENTIAL DIAGNOSIS

- Intrinsic cardiac disease with arrhythmias

Causes of Muscular Weakness

- Neuromuscular junction disease
  - —Myasthenia gravis
  - —Organophosphate poisoning
  - —Botulism
- Spinal cord disease
- Polyneuropathies
- Primary acute myopathies

Treatment

INITIAL STABILIZATION

- ABCs
- Cardiac monitor
- IV access

ED TREATMENT

- Treat predisposing condition
- Correct volume deficit and acid-base disorder

Potassium Replacement

- Because potassium is an intracellular ion, a low serum potassium may reflect a much greater total potassium deficit
  - —At levels above 2.0 mEq/L
    - -Estimate a total potassium deficit of 100–200 mEq for every 1 mEq/L reduction in serum potassium (based on a normal serum pH)
  - —At levels below 2.0 mEq/L
    - -Deficit much higher since a significant portion of exogenous potassium excreted by the kidneys
    - -Total replacement dose required greater than the estimated deficit
- Oral potassium
  - —Preferable to IV therapy whenever possible
  - —Gradual oral repletion effective
  - —Potassium chloride
    - -Oral forms associated with GI upset
    - -Enteric-coated forms associated with small bowel ulceration
  - —Use potassium gluconate or citrate in acidotic patients
- IV potassium (KCl)
  - —For serious dysrhythmias or severe weakness
  - —Emergent situations: rates up to 40 mEq/h (peds: 0.3 mEq/kg/h)
  - —Less urgent situations: 10–20 mEq/h
  - —Use central lines for concentrations in excess of 40 mEq/L
  - —Frequent monitoring of potassium levels when large amounts of K^+ are infused
- Increase dietary potassium

Correct Other Electrolyte Abnormalities

- Magnesium
- Chloride
- Calcium

MEDICATIONS

- IV potassium chloride
  - —Emergent situations
    - -Max rate: 40 mEq/h (peds: 0.3 mEq/kg/h)
    - -Max concentration via peripheral line: 40 mEq/L
  - —Nonemergent situations
    - -Max rate: 10–20 mEq/h
- Magnesium sulfate: 1–2 g i.v. (over minutes when required, or as an infusion)
- Oral potassium
  - —Potassium chloride/potassium citrate/potassium gluconate
  - —Available in elixir, soluble preparations, and tablets
  - —Unit doses contain from 10–40 mEq K^+
  - —Replacement dose: adult: 40–100 mEq/d; peds: 3–5 mEq/kg/d

Disposition

ADMISSION CRITERIA

- Need of IV potassium repletion
- Dysrhythmias
- Serum potassium level <2.5 mEq/L

DISCHARGE CRITERIA

- Asymptomatic
- Able to replete deficiency with oral potassium
- Early follow up available

Miscellaneous

ICD9: 276.8

ICD10: E87.6

SUGGESTED READINGS

Halperin M, Kamel K. Potassium. Lancet 1998;352:135–140.

Rastegar A, Soleimani M. Hypokalaemia and hyperkalaemia. Postgrad Med J 2001;77:759–764.

Rodríguez-Soriano J. Potassium homeostasis and its disturbances in children. Pediatr Nephrol 1995;9(3):364–374.

Author: Paul Byskosh

Hyponatremia

Clinical Presentation

SIGNS AND SYMPTOMS

Mild: $Na^+ > 120$ mEq/L

- Headache
- Nausea
- Vomiting
- Weakness
- Anorexia
- Muscle cramps
- Rhabdomyolysis

Moderate: Na^+ Between 110 and 120 mEq/L

- Impaired response to verbal stimuli
- Decreased response to painful stimuli
- Visual/auditory hallucinations
- Bizarre behavior
- Incontinence
- Hyperventilation
- Gait disturbance

Severe: $Na^+ < 110$ mEq/L

- Signs of herniation
  —Decorticate/decerebrate posturing
- Bradycardia
- Hypertension
- Altered temperature regulation
- Dilated pupils
- Seizure activity
- Respiratory arrest
- Coma/unresponsive

Chronic

- May be asymptomatic

MECHANISM/DESCRIPTION

- Sodium <130 mEq/L
- Most common electrolyte disturbance (1–4% of hospitalized patients)

ETIOLOGY

Pseudohyponatremia

- Low-measured serum sodium but normal measured serum osmolarity
- Occurs secondary to the displacement of sodium to aqueous phase of serum
- Seen with elevated lipids or proteins
- Disease examples include:
  —Multiple myeloma
  —Hyperlipidemia

Hyponatremia with Normal Osmolarity and Fluid Overload

- Inappropriate retention of water
- Disease examples include:
  —CHF
  —Cirrhosis
  —Renal failure
  —Nephrotic syndrome

Hyponatremia with Normal Osmolarity and Euvolemia

- Tend to have increased total body water without marked edema
- Purest form of dilutional hyponatremia
- Disease examples include:
  —Endocrine abnormalities
    -Hypothyroid
    -Stress
    -SIADH
  —Diseases that cause SIADH:
    -Pulmonary disease
    -CNS disorders (bleeding, malignancy, trauma)
    -Cancer (small cell lung, pancreas, duodenum)
    -HIV infection
  —Water intoxication (3–7% of institutionalized psychotic patients)
  —Mineralocorticoid abnormalities
  —Postoperative hyponatremia (particularly after TURP)

Hyponatremia with Normal Osmolarity and Hypovolemia

- Deficits in total body water and total body sodium
- Sodium deficits exceed water deficits
- Possible etiologies include:
  —GI losses
  —Sweating
  —Burns
  —Cystic fibrosis
  —Salt-wasting nephropathies
  —Diuretics

Drug-induced

- Drugs may stimulate ADH and cause hyponatremia
  —Clofibrate
  —Cyclophosphamide
  —Carbamazepine
  —Vincristine, vinblastine
  —Oxytocin
  —Bromocriptine
  —Barbiturates
  —Opiates
- Drugs may increase sensitivity to ADH and cause hyponatremia
  —Chlorpropamide
  —NSAIDs
- Drugs may stimulate thirst and cause hyponatremia
  —Thiothixene
  —Amitriptyline
  —Fluphenazine
  —Ecstasy
  —Fluoxetine
  —Sertraline
  —Haloperidol

Hyponatremia with Hyperosmolarity

- Due to excessive osmotically active substances
- Possible etiologies include:
  —Elevated glucose (most common cause of hyponatremia)
  —Corrected $Na^+ = 0.016\times$ (measured glucose $-$ 100) $+$ measured sodium
  —Mannitol infusion
  —Maltose and glycine

PEDIATRIC CONSIDERATIONS

- More prone to water intoxication
- High incidence of iatrogenic hyponatremia

Pre-Hospital

N/A

Diagnosis

ESSENTIAL WORKUP

- Serum sodium level
  —Recheck sodium to verify
- Review patient medication list
- Obtain good medical history for possible etiologies

LABORATORY

- Electrolytes, BUN/Cr
- Glucose
  —Correct sodium value accordingly if severe hyperglycemia

IMAGING/SPECIAL TESTS

- Urine sodium

DIFFERENTIAL DIAGNOSIS

- Pseudohyponatremia due to:
  —Hyperglycemia
  —Hyperlipidemia
  —Hyperproteinemia

Treatment

INITIAL STABILIZATION

- ABCs
- Initiate IV fluid with 0.9% NS
- Naloxone, thiamine, D50W (or Accucheck) for altered mental status

ED TREATMENT

- Depends on severity and chronicity of hyponatremia and underlying etiology

Acute Hyponatremia with Severe CNS Symptoms

- Goal
  - —Raise serum sodium by 10 mEq/L or to level >120–125 mEq/L over 6 hours with administration of hypertonic saline
- Calculate sodium deficit
  - —Na^+ deficit = 0.6(weight in kg)(140 − Na^+)
- 250 mL of 3% or 5% saline solution in adult over 4–6 hours will raise serum sodium by 10–15 mEq/L
  - —*OR* may dose 1–2 mL/kg/h of 3% saline solution
- Sodium contents:
  - —1 L 0.9% NS = 154 mEq of sodium
  - —1 L 3% saline = 513 mEq of sodium

Hypovolemic Hyponatremia

- Correct underlying cause
- Replete volume with 0.9% NS IV
- Primary goals to restore
  - —Extracellular fluid
  - —Cardiac output
  - —Organ perfusion

Treatment for Hypervolemic/Euvolemic Hyponatremia

- Water restriction to less than 1 L per day with high dietary salt intake
- For faster correction of sodium
  - —Administer IV 0.9% NS with loop diuretic (furosemide)
- Maximum rate of correction = 0.5 mEq/L/h

MEDICATIONS

- Calculate Na^+ deficit
- Replace no more than half of requirement over 8–12 h
- Furosemide: 20–40 mg IVP

Disposition

ADMISSION CRITERIA

- Symptomatic hyponatremia
- Sodium <120 mEq/L
- Asymptomatic, mild hyponatremia (Na^+ 120–127 mEq/L), with comorbid factors

DISCHARGE CRITERIA

- Sodium greater than 130 mEq/L and asymptomatic
- Known chronic history of hyponatremia with no acute changes
- Asymptomatic, mild hyponatremia (Na^+ 120–127 mEq/L) with no comorbid factors; however, must have close outpatient follow-up

Miscellaneous

ICD9: 276.1

ICD10: E87.1

SUGGESTED READINGS

Fall PJ. Hyponatremia and hypernatremia: a systematic approach to causes and their correction. Postgrad Med 2000;107(5):75–82.

Fried LF, Palevsky PM. Hyponatremia and hypernatremia. Med Clin North Am 1997;81(3):585–609.

Kugler JP, Hustead T. Hyponatremia and hypernatremia in the elderly. Am Fam Physician 2000;61(12):3623–3630.

Kumar S, Berl T. Sodium. Lancet 1998;352:220–228.

Mulloy AL, Caruana RJ. Hyponatremic emergencies. Med Clin North Am 1995;79:155–167.

Author: Linda Mueller

Hypoparathyroidism

Clinical Presentation

SIGNS AND SYMPTOMS

- Related to severity, rapidity of onset, and duration of hypocalcemia
- General
  —Weakness
  —Malaise
- Neuromuscular
  —Paresthesias (especially circumoral and extremities)
  —Carpal pedal spasm
  —Latent spasm elicited by:
  -Chvostek's sign (twitching of circumoral muscles after tapping facial nerve in front of the tragus)
  -Trousseau's sign (spasm after inflating blood pressure cuff 20 mm above patient's systolic BP for 3 minutes)
  —Laryngospasm/bronchospasm
  —Blepharospasm
  —Muscle cramps
  —Tetany
  —Seizures (presenting symptom of one third with hypoparathyroidism)
  —Increased ICP with papilledema
  —Parkinson's syndrome and other extrapyramidal disorders
  —Myelopathy
- Cardiovascular
  —Prolonged QT interval (due to ST segment prolongation)
  —Heart block
  —CHF
  —VFib
  —Vasoconstriction
- Psychiatric
  —Impaired memory
  —Confusion
  —Hallucinations
  —Dementia
- Dermatologic
  —Brittle hair and nails
  —Psoriasis
  —Hyperpigmentation
- Lenticular cataracts

MECHANISM/DESCRIPTION

- Parathyroid hormone (PTH)
  —Decreases urinary Ca^{2+} loss
  —Increases urinary PO_4 loss
  —Stimulates vitamin D conversion from 25(OH)-D to $1,25(OH)_2$-D in kidney,
  —Liberates Ca^{2+} and PO_4 from bone
- Calcitonin
  —Promotes deposition of Ca^{2+} and PO_4 into bone (produced primarily in C cells in thyroid)
- Magnesium
  —Cofactor in production of PTH
  —Essential for action of PTH in target tissues
- Hypoparathyroidism
  —Primary failure of the parathyroid gland (may have associated Addison's disease)
- Pseudohypoparathyroidism
  —Tissue unresponsiveness with elevated PTH levels
  —Associated with hypothyroidism and hypogonadism

ETIOLOGY

- Failure of parathyroid gland
  —Congenital absence
  —Autoimmune destruction
  —Surgical interruption of blood supply or gland removal
  —Radiation damage
  —Hypomagnesemia as PTH cofactor
- End-organ unresponsiveness to PTH
- DiGeorge's syndrome
  —Hypoparathyroidism
  —Thymic dysplasia
  —Severe immunodeficiency
- Wilson's disease
  —Destruction of gland due to copper deposition
- Autoimmune polyglandular syndrome type I
  —Hypoparathyroidism
  —Adrenal insufficiency
  —Mucocutaneous candidiasis
- Albright's syndrome (hereditary osteodystrophy)
  —Short stature
  —Obesity
  —Round face
  —Short neck
  —Short 4th and 5th metacarpals and metatarsals (type I pseudohypoparathyroidism)

PEDIATRIC CONSIDERATIONS

- Neonates/infants
  —Transient hypoparathyroidism in first year of life
  —Subnormal intelligence proportional to duration of hypocalcemia
  —Dental hypoplasia

Pre-Hospital

CAUTIONS

- Administer calcium in refractory VFib or status epilepticus in addition to usual medications if known hypoparathyroidism
- Stridor may herald laryngospasm

Diagnosis

ESSENTIAL WORKUP

- If asymptomatic with hypocalcemia, check albumin level
  —In hypoalbuminemia ionized Ca^{2+} normal
- If symptomatic with normal total Ca^{2+}, check pH
  —Ionized Ca^{2+}—active form
  —Metabolic or respiratory alkalosis increases the binding to albumin reducing the ionized Ca^{2+}
- If symptomatic with low Ca^{2+}, check a PTH level
  —Low in primary hypoparathyroidism and in vitamin D deficiency
  —Elevated in pseudohypoparathyroidism and hypocalcemia from renal failure

LABORATORY

- Calcium: correct for albumin using formula
  —Corrected Ca^{2+} (mg/dL) = measured Ca^{2+} (mg/dL) + 0.8[4.0 − albumin (g/dL)]
- Ionized Ca^{2+} if symptomatic with low total calcium
- Electrolytes, BUN, Cr, glucose
- Magnesium
- ABG if symptomatic with normal total Ca^{2+}
  —Elevation of 0.1 pH unit decreases the ionized Ca^{2+} by 3–8%
- Phosphorus
  —Elevated except when hypocalcemia due to vitamin D deficiency

IMAGING/SPECIAL TESTS

- EKG
  - —Prolonged QT interval

DIFFERENTIAL DIAGNOSIS

- Causes of hypocalcemia
- Lab artifact
  - —Low total calcium that is normal when corrected for albumin level with no symptoms of hypocalcemia
- Symptomatic hypocalcemia with a normal total calcium—alkalosis
- Low ionized calcium
- Hypoparathyroidism
  - —Gland failure
  - —Hypomagnesemia (needed for PTH secretion)
  - —PTH resistance (congenital)
  - —PTH suppression by ethanol, chemotherapeutics, or cimetidine
- Vitamin D deficiency (low Ca^{2+} + low PO_4)
  - —Anticonvulsant use
  - —Liver disease
  - —Resistance to vitamin D
  - —Malabsorption or dietary deficiency
- Gram-negative sepsis
- Renal failure or nephrotic syndrome
- Chelation
  - —Pancreatitis (fatty acids chelate calcium)
  - —Ammonium bifluoride (tire cleaner spray)
  - —Hydrofluoric acid
  - —Citrated blood
  - —Acute hyperphosphatemia
    - -Fleet enemas
    - -Rhabdomyolysis
    - -Acute renal failure

PEDIATRIC CONSIDERATIONS

- Suspect hypocalcemia [due to exposure to phosphates or ammonium bifluoride (tire cleaner spray)] in pediatric cardiac arrest of unclear etiology

Treatment

INITIAL STABILIZATION

- ABCs
  - —Manage airway if laryngospasm
- Administer IV calcium bolus (chloride or gluconate) if unstable cardiac rhythm or tetany
  - —Slow infusion much safer unless patient markedly symptomatic
- Prepare for ventricular dysrhythmias including ventricular fibrillation
- Seizure precautions

ED TREATMENT

- Calcium replacement
  - —10% calcium chloride (27.2 mg elemental Ca^{2+}/mL)
    - -For life-threatening conditions: 1 amp (10 mL) over 3–5 min IV or 10%
  - —Calcium gluconate (9 mg elemental Ca^{2+}/mL):
    - -For life-threatening conditions: 1–3 amp (10 mL/amp) over 5–10 min/amp
  - —For non-life-threatening conditions administer calcium via slow infusion of 500–1000 mg elemental Ca^{2+} over 6–24 hours with frequent checks of serum Ca^{2+} levels (peds: 100 mg elemental Ca^{2+}/kg/24 hours)
  - —Stop infusion if bradycardia develops
  - —Calcium administration may precipitate digitalis toxicity
  - —Supplement to lowest possible Ca^{2+} level keeping the patient asymptomatic since soft tissue calcification may occur with elevated phosphorus levels
- Replace magnesium if low
- Bind phosphorus with
  - —Aluminum hydroxide containing antacids (Maalox, Mylanta, or Gelusil) if creatinine <2
  - —Calcium acetate (Phos-lo) or calcium carbonate when concurrent renal failure if creatinine ≥ 2
- Begin vitamin D supplementation
- Avoid carbonated beverages (high in phosphorus)
- Assess for associated endocrinopathies

MEDICATIONS

- Calcium chloride 10% (27.2 mg elemental Ca^{2+}/ml): 1 amp over 3–5 min i.v. if life-threatening condition; otherwise, slow infusion—see ED Treatment, above
- Calcium gluconate 10% (9 mg elemental Ca^{2+}/mL): 1–3 amp over 5–10 min/amp if life-threatening condition; otherwise, slow infusion—see ED Treatment, above
- Vitamin D: 400 IU/day

Disposition

ADMISSION CRITERIA

- Symptomatic hypocalcemia
- Abnormal EKG
- Inability to take vitamin D or calcium orally
- Corrected calcium <5 mg/dL

DISCHARGE CRITERIA

- Asymptomatic hypocalcemia

Miscellaneous

ICD9: 252.1

ICD10: E20.9

SEE ALSO: HYPOCALCEMIA

SUGGESTED READINGS

Goldman L, Bennett JC, eds. Cecil's textbook of medicine, 21st ed. Philadelphia: WB Saunders, 2000.

Marx JA, Hockenberger RS, Walls RM, et al., eds. Rosen's emergency medicine, 5th ed. Philadelphia: Mosby, 2002.

Wallach J, ed. Interpretation of diagnostic tests, 7th ed. Boston: Little, Brown, 2000.

Author: Hugh Schuckman

Hypothermia

Clinical Presentation

SIGNS AND SYMPTOMS

Signs and Symptoms Based on Temperature (°C)

- 35: Maximum shivering
- 34: Amnesia/dysarthria
- 33: Ataxia/apathy
- 32: Stuporous
- 31: Shivering ceases
- 30: AFib
- 28: VFib
- 27: Reflexes/voluntary motion cease
- 24: Significant hypotension
- 19: EEG flat
- 18: Asystole
- 14.2: Lowest accidental hypothermia survival (infant)
- 13.7: Lowest accidental hypothermia survival (adult)

Cardiovascular

- Early tachycardia followed by bradycardia
  - —Caused by decreased spontaneous depolarization of pacemaker cells
  - —Refractory to atropine
- Cardiac cycle lengthens resulting in increased intervals
- Osborn J wave = hypothermic hump
  - —Repolarization abnormality seen at the junction of the QRS and ST segments at temperatures less than 32°C
- Core temperature after drop
  - —Decline in a temperature after removal from the cold
  - —Most common during active external rewarming where peripheral vasoconstriction and AV shunting are reversed

Respiratory System

- Progressive respiratory depression with CO_2 retention

Renal System

- Paradoxical large initial diuresis due to:
  - —Relative central hypovolemia
  - —Cold-induced defects in distal tubular reabsorption of sodium and water
  - —Renal blood flow depressed 50% at 27–30°C

MECHANISM/DESCRIPTION

- Definition = body temperature <35°C

ETIOLOGY

- Decreased heat production
  - —At age extremes
  - —With endocrine failure and malnutrition
- Impaired thermoregulation
  - —Central CNS conditions affecting the hypothalamus
  - —Spinal cord transection
- Medications/toxins decrease the body's ability to respond to cold stress
- Immersion in cold water and wet clothes increase heat loss
- Shivering increases the metabolic rate

PEDIATRIC CONSIDERATIONS

- Infants have a large body surface to mass ratio and are at greater risk for hypothermia

Pre-Hospital

CONTROVERSIES

- CPR not recommended if:
  - —Electrical rhythm present without palpable pulse or blood pressure with short transport time

CAUTIONS

- Prolonged palpation/auscultation for cardiac activity
  - —Apparent cardiovascular collapse may be depressed cardiac output, often sufficient to meet metabolic demands

Diagnosis

ESSENTIAL WORKUP

- Accurate core temperature confirms diagnosis

LABORATORY

- ABG
  - —Temperature correction not needed
- CBC
  - —Hematocrit rises due to decreased plasma volume
  - —Leukopenia does not imply absence of infection
- Electrolytes, BUN, Cr
  - —Vary during rewarming; recheck frequently
- PT, PTT, and platelets
  - —Prolonged clotting times with thrombocytopenia common
- Toxicology screen
- Alcohol/drug ingestions—common risk factors

IMAGING/SPECIAL TESTS

- CXR—pneumonia common complication

DIFFERENTIAL DIAGNOSIS

- Environmental
- Sepsis
- Primary CNS disorder

Treatment

INITIAL STABILIZATION

- ABCs
  - —Supplemental oxygen
  - —Oral and nasotracheal intubation are safe
    - -Place NG tube postintubation
  - —Cardiac monitor
  - —Warmed D5.9 NS preferred over lactated Ringer's
- Remove wet clothing and begin passive external rewarming
- Administer Narcan, D50W (or Accucheck), and thiamine with an altered mental status
- Obtain accurate core temperatures using rectal temperature

ED TREATMENT

Cardiac Arrest Resuscitation

- VFib induction occurs with rough handling, chest compressions, hypoxia, and acid–base changes
- CPR is less effective due to decreased chest wall elasticity
- Defibrillation is rarely successful at temperatures <28–30°C
  - —Defibrillate 1–3 times and then again post-rewarming
  - —Direct current results in myocardial damage

Arrhythmia Management

- Atrial fibrillation
  - —Common below 32°C
  - —Usually converts spontaneously with rewarming
- Malignant ventricular arrhythmias
  - —Bretylium—drug of choice
  - —Avoid lidocaine and procainamide—may increase ventricular fibrillation

Rewarming Techniques

- Faster rewarming rates (1–2°C/h) generally have better prognosis than slower rewarming rates (<0.5°C/h)
- Active rewarming is necessary at core temperatures below 32°C
  - —Internal thermogenesis (shivering extinguished) insufficient to increase the body temperature
- *Passive external rewarming*
  - —Ideal technique for the majority of healthy patients with mild hypothermia
  - —Cover the patient with dry insulating material
  - —Endogenous thermogenesis must generate an acceptable rate of rewarming
- *Active external rewarming* delivers heat directly to the skin
  - —Cover trunk preferential
  - —Bair Hugger device provides forced warm air
  - —Associated with core temperature after drop
  - —Safe in previously healthy young acutely hypothermic victims

Active Core Rewarming Techniques

- *Airway rewarming* (complete humidification at 40–45°C)
  - —Administer to all patients
- *Heated IV* (40–42°C)
  - —Administer to all patients
  - —High flow rates must be maintained to deliver warmed fluid
  - —Heat 1 L of crystalloid in a microwave set at high in 2 minutes
- *Heated gastric irrigation* via nasogastric or orogastric tubes
  - —Not recommended
  - —Low amount of surface area
  - —Aspiration risk if the airway not been secured
- *Pleural irrigation* (0.9% NS at 30–42°C)
  - —Use in severe hypothermia without cardiac activity
  - —One or two chest tubes
  - —Contraindicated in patients with a cardiac rhythm because the chest tube may induce VFib
- *Heated peritoneal lavage* (0.9% NS at 40–45°C)
  - —Use in unstable hypothermic patients or stable patients with severe hypothermia whose rewarming rates are <1°C/h
  - —One or two catheters
  - —Advantageous in patients with an overdose or rhabdomyolysis
- *Hemodialysis*
  - —Initiate for patients with drug overdoses or severe electrolyte disturbances
- *Continuous arteriovenous rewarming*
  - —Blood pressure must be >60 mm Hg
  - —Blood circulated through warmer from percutaneously inserted femoral arterial and contralateral femoral venous catheters
- *Extracorporeal venovenous rewarming*
  - —Blood is removed a central venous catheter, heated to 40°C, and returned via a second central or large peripheral venous catheter
- *Cardiopulmonary bypass*
  - —Treatment of choice in severe hypothermia especially for those patients in cardiac arrest
  - —Complications include:
    - -Hemolysis
    - -Arterial injury
    - -Air embolism
    - -Those associated with systemic heparinization

Additional Therapy

- Administer methylprednisolone or hydrocortisone for suspicion of adrenocortical insufficiency or steroid dependence
- Empiric treatment with levothyroxine only for myxedematous patients

MEDICATIONS

- Bretylium: 5–10 mg/kg IVP
- Dextrose: D50W 1 amp (50 mL or 25 g) (peds: D25W 2–4 ml/kg) i.v.
- Hydrocortisone 250 mg IVP
- Levothyroxine 50 to 500 μg i.v. over several minutes
- Methylprednisolone 30 mg/kg IVP
- Naloxone (Narcan): 2 mg (peds: 0.1 mg/kg) i.v. or i.m. initial dose
- Thiamine (vitamin B_1): 100 mg (peds: 50 mg) i.v. or i.m.

Disposition

ADMISSION CRITERIA

- Moderate to severe hypothermia (<32°C)
- Young, healthy patients with no comorbid illness who have mild accidental hypothermia (>32°C) that responds well to warming
  - —Admit to an observation area
  - —Discharge if asymptomatic after 8–12 hours and they remain asymptomatic

DISCHARGE CRITERIA

- Young, healthy patients with no comorbid illness
- Very mild accidental hypothermia (>35°C) that responds well to warming
- Safe, warm environment to go to after discharge

Miscellaneous

ICD9: 991.6

ICD10: T68

SUGGESTED READINGS

Cheng D. The EKG of hypothermia. J Emerg Med 2002;22(1):87–91.

Daniel F, Danzl DF. Accidental hypothermia. In: Marx JA, ed. Rosen's emergency medicine: concepts and clinical practice, 5th ed. St. Louis: Mosby, 2002: 1979–1996.

Hanania NA, Zimmerman JL. Accidental hypothermia. Crit Care Clin 1999;15(2): 235–249.

Walpoth BH, Walpoth-Aslan BN, Mattle HP, et al. Outcome of survivors of accidental deep hypothermia and circulatory arrest treated with extracorporeal blood warming. N Engl J Med 1997;337(21):1500–1505.

Author: Jeffrey Schaider

Hypothyroidism

Clinical Presentation

SIGNS AND SYMPTOMS

Symptoms

- Weakness/fatigue/drowsiness
- Cold intolerance
- Headaches
- Mental status changes
- Myalgias
- Menorrhagia
- Constipation
- Weight gain
- Emotional lability

SIGNS

- Puffy eyelids
- Sparse pubic, axillary hair
- Absent lateral one-third eyebrows
- Prolonged relaxation phase DTRs
- Yellow tinged/dry skin
- Pallor
- Goiter
- Myxedema—dry, waxy swelling of skin/subcutaneous tissues
- Swelling of hands/feet
- Huskiness of voice
- Galactorrhea

Myxedema Coma

- Extreme form of hypothyroidism (see above)
- Hypothermia
- Bradycardia
- Hypotension
- Coma/altered mental status

MECHANISM/DESCRIPTION

- Results from a deficiency of thyroid hormone
- Primarily due to thyroid disease caused by:
  - —Autoimmune process
  - —Iatrogenic failure
- Pituitary disease or secondary failure accounts for less than 4% of cases
- Usually follows an indolent course with decompensation after specific stress factors
- *Myedema coma* caused by:
  - —Hypothyroidism with hypoxia
  - —Hypothermia
  - —Hypotension
  - —Hypoglycemia
  - —Hyponatremia
  - —Adrenal insufficiency
  - —Sedative hypnotic drugs

ETIOLOGY

Primary

- Congenital
- Autoimmune
  - —Hypothyroidism
  - —Thyroiditis
  - —Hashimoto's disease
- Idiopathic
- Iatrogenic
  - —Postsurgical
  - —External radiation
  - —Radioiodine therapy
  - —Antithyroid drugs (iodides, lithium)
- Inherited defect:
  - —Aplasia
  - —Hypoplasia
  - —Enzymatic defect
  - —Ingestion of drugs or goitrogens during pregnancy
- Neoplasm: primary (carcinoma) or secondary infiltration
- Infection: viral (rarely aerobic or anaerobic bacteria)
- Trauma: neck injury

Secondary

- Pituitary tumor
- Infiltrative disease (sarcoid) or tumor
- Trauma

Pre-Hospital

N/A

Diagnosis

ESSENTIAL WORKUP

- Laboratory confirmation of the diagnosis of hypothyroidism/myxedema coma is usually not possible in the ED
- Myxedema coma—life-threatening condition
  - —Initiate therapy if a high index of suspicion
- Thyroid function studies
  - —Free T_4 (low)
  - —High-sensitivity TSH (increased)
  - —If free T_4 unavailable—total T_4 (decreased) and resin T_3 uptake (increased)
- EKG
  - —Profound bradycardia

LABORATORY

- CBC
  - —Anemia
- Electrolytes, BUN, Cr, glucose
  - —Hyponatremia
  - —Hypoglycemia
- AST, LDH, CPK
- Arterial blood gases
  - —Hypoxemia/hypercapnia
  - —Acidosis
- Search for the underlying etiology

IMAGING/SPECIAL TESTS

- CXR
  - —Enlarged heart/CHF
  - —Pericardial/pleural effusion
- Echocardiogram for suspected pericardial effusion

DIFFERENTIAL DIAGNOSIS

- Nephrotic syndrome
- Chronic nephritis
- Hypoalbuminemia
- Chronic renal disease
- Sepsis
- Depression
- CHF

Treatment

INITIAL STABILIZATION

- ABCs
  - —Intubation and ventilation may be necessary
- Cardiac monitor
- Blood pressure support
- Supplemental oxygen to meet metabolic needs
- Correct hypothermia
  - —Initiate passive warming measures

ED TREATMENT

- Mild hypothyroidism—oral thyroid replacement as an outpatient

Myxedema Coma

- Thyroid hormone replacement
  - —Prompt IV replacement improves survival
  - —L-thyroxine or liothyronine
    - -Reassess 4 hours after initial dose
  - —Use smaller doses of thyroid hormone in the elderly or patients with cardiac disease
- Hydrocortisone to prevent addisonian crisis
- Dextrose for hypoglycemia
- IV fluid bolus for hypotension
  - —Avoid pressors, if possible, as they may precipitate arrhythmias
  - —Response to pressors is poor until thyroid replacement initiated
  - —Thyroid hormone augments action of pressors
- Correct the underlying precipitant

MEDICATIONS

- Dextrose: 50–100 cc D50 (peds: 2 cc/kg of D10 over 1 min) i.v.
- Hydrocortisone: 100 mg (peds: 4 mg/kg) i.v.
- L-thyroxine: 300–500 μg load i.v. followed by 50–100 μg i.v. daily
- Liothyronine: 25–50 μg load i.v.

Disposition

ADMISSION CRITERIA

- Myxedema coma (admit to ICU)

DISCHARGE CRITERIA

- Hypothyroid patients should be referred to a primary care taker for initiation of oral thyroid hormone replacement therapy

Miscellaneous

ICD9: 244.9

ICD10: E03.9

SUGGESTED READINGS

Holmes L, Lakshmanan M. The patient with chronic endocrine disease. In: Herr RD, Cydulka RK, eds. Emergency care of the compromised patient. Philadelphia: Lippincott-Raven, 1994:123–133.

Jordan RM. Myxedema coma. Pathophysiology, therapy, and factors affecting prognosis. Med Clin North Am 1995;79:185–194.

Larson R, Davies TF, Hay ID. The thyroid. In: Wilson JD, ed. Williams' textbook of endocrinology, 9th ed. St. Louis: WB Saunders, 2001:389–516.

Tsitouras PD. Myxedema coma. Clin Geriatr Med 1995;11:251–258.

Wogan JM. Endocrine disorders. In: Marx JA, Hockenberger RS, Walls RM, et al., eds. Rosen's emergency medicine, 5th ed. Philadelphia: Mosby, 2002.

Author: Rita Cydulka

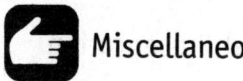

Idiopathic Thrombocytopenic Purpura

Clinical Presentation

SIGNS AND SYMPTOMS

- Bleeding into superficial sites
  - —Skin and mucous membranes = purpura
  - —Genitourinary tract = hematuria
  - —Gastrointestinal = hematemesis, hematochezia, or melena
- Neurologic deficits secondary to intracranial hemorrhage
- Bleeding begins immediately after trauma

MECHANISM/DEFINITION

- Thrombocytopenia without abnormalities in other cell lines or apparent cause for low platelets
- Immune-mediated destruction of circulating platelets primarily in the spleen

Acute Idiopathic Thrombocytopenia Purpura (ITP)

- Severe thrombocytopenia following recovery from viral exanthem or upper respiratory illness
- 90% of ITP are pediatric cases
- 90% recover within 3–6 months

Chronic Idiopathic Thrombocytopenia Purpura

- Chronic form of ITP is primarily an adult disease
- Women aged 20–40 most commonly afflicted
- Caused by autoimmune disorder
- More indolent than acute ITP

Pre-Hospital

N/A

Diagnosis

ESSENTIAL WORKUP

- Diagnosis based on excluding other causes of thrombocytopenia
- Complete history
  - —Assess type of bleeding to differentiate platelet-related mucocutaneous bleeding from coagulation disorder, which usually causes delayed visceral hematomas
  - —Rule out drug-induced thrombocytopenias
  - —Exclude systemic illnesses as cause of thrombocytopenia
- Directed physical exam excluding other causes of thrombocytopenia
  - —Type of bleeding (mucocutaneous vs visceral)
  - —Evidence of liver dysfunction, autoimmune disorders
  - —Evaluate for signs of thrombosis
  - —Evidence of infection (bacteremia or HIV)
  - —Neurologic exam to exclude intracranial hemorrhage

LABORATORY

- CBC/peripheral smear
  - —Results consistent with diagnosis of ITP
    - -Thrombocytopenia
    - -Normal platelet size
    - -Normal red blood cell morphology
    - -Normal white blood cell morphology
- Antigen-specific assays to detect glycoprotein (GP) IIb/IIIa antibodies
- HIV antibody

IMAGING/SPECIAL TESTS

- Abdominal CT scan or ultrasound for patients with splenomegaly on exam
- Head CT scan for neurologic findings consistent with intracranial bleeding
- Bone marrow aspiration
  - —Not routinely indicated
  - —Indications
    - -Children with persistent thrombocytopenia >6–12 months
    - -Children unresponsive to intravenous immunoglobulin (IV IG)
    - -Adults >60
    - -Patients considering splenectomy

DIFFERENTIAL DIAGNOSIS (OF THROMBOCYTOPENIA)

- Impaired bone marrow production
  - —Bone marrow fibrosis
  - —Bone marrow infiltration with malignant cells
  - —Cytotoxic drugs used in chemotherapy
  - —Congenital bone marrow abnormalities
- Splenic sequestration
  - —As spleen enlarges, the fraction of platelets sequestered increases
  - —Common causes
    - -Portal hypertension
    - -Splenic infiltration with tumor
- Accelerated destruction of platelets
  - —Nonimmunologic thrombocytopenia
    - -Vasculitis
    - -Hemolytic uremic syndrome
    - -Thrombotic thrombocytopenic purpura (TTP)
    - -Disseminated intravascular coagulation (DIC)
    - -Cardiac valve abnormalities
  - —Immunologic thrombocytopenia
    - -Immune (idiopathic) thrombocytopenic purpura
    - -Autoantibodies against platelet GP IIb/IIIa
    - -Platelets and megakaryocytes coated with antibodies, immune complex, or complement rapidly cleared in spleen
    - -Results in platelet destruction and inhibition thrombopoiesis
- Drug-induced thrombocytopenia
  - —Suppress platelet production
    - -Chemotherapeutics
    - -Thiazide diuretics
    - -Ethanol
    - -Estrogen
  - —Cause immunologic platelet destruction
    - -Aspirin
    - -Chlorpropamide
    - -Chloroquine
    - -Gold salts
    - -Insecticides
    - -Sulfa drugs

Treatment

INITIAL STABILIZATION

- ABCs
- Stabilize severe life-threatening bleeding
  - —Intracranial hemorrhage
    - -Airway control
    - -Hyperventilation
    - -Neurosurgery consult
  - —Hemorrhagic shock
    - -Large-bore IV lines
    - -Control bleeding with direct pressure if possible
    - -Blood and platelet transfusion
    - -IV glucocorticoids
    - -IV immune globulin (pooled vs monoclonal)
- Mucous membrane bleeding
  - —Apply topical collagen sponge

ED TREATMENT

- Initial treatment options for ITP are based on:
  - —Degree of thrombocytopenia
  - —Severity of illness
  - —Type of ITP (acute vs chronic)
  - —Age
  - —Risk factors for bleeding (hypertension, peptic ulcer disease, vigorous lifestyle)
- Efficacy of specific treatment options demonstrated in terms of platelet recovery time and not in terms of morbidity and mortality

Specific Treatment Options

- Acute ITP
  - —Children without bleeding complications or profound thrombocytopenia (platelet count <30,000)
    - -Observation recommended
  - —90% of children will have spontaneous resolution within 6 months
- Chronic or profound ITP (platelet count <30,000)
  - —High-dose oral corticosteroids (suppresses immune response)
  - —Intravenous immune globulin (IVIG)
    - -Causes temporary phagocytic blockade
    - -Combined with glucocorticoids considered first-line treatment in children
  - —Splenectomy
    - -Second-line treatment
    - -Inadequate data to make evidence-based recommendations on appropriate indications and timing for emergency and elective splenectomy
    - -Adverse risks: operative, fatal bacterial infection
    - -Indications:
      - *Glucocorticoid therapy unsuccessful
      - *Children with ITP for 1 year, bleeding symptoms, platelet count <x10,000
      - *Adults with ITP for 6 weeks, platelet count <10,000
      - *Adults with ITP for 3 months, platelet count <30,000

MEDICATION

- Anti-D immune globulin (anti-D): 45-50 μg/kg i.v. one time
- Collagen absorbable hemostat sponges: apply directly to bleeding surface with pressure 1- × 2-inch, 3- × 4-inch sponges
- IVIG (pooled): 1–2 g/kg i.v. one time
- Methylprednisolone: 1 g (peds: 30 mg/kg/24 hours) i.v. q8h
- Prednisone: 1–2 mg/kg/d (peds: 4 mg/kg/d) PO

Disposition

ADMISSION CRITERIA

- Life-threatening bleeding regardless of platelet count
- Mucous membrane bleeding and platelet count <20,000
- Asymptomatic patient with platelet count <20,000 who may become inaccessible or noncompliant

DISCHARGE CRITERIA

- Asymptomatic patients
- Patients with only minor purpura and platelet count >30,000/mm^3

Miscellaneous

ICD9: 287.2

ICD10: D69.3

SEE ALSO: THROMBOTIC THROMBOCYTOPENIC PURPURA

SUGGESTED READINGS

Cines DB. Immune thrombocytopenic purpura. N Engl J Med 2002;346(13): 995–1008.

George JN. Management of patients with chronic, refractory idiopathic thrombocytopenic purpura. Semin Hematol 2000;37(3):290–298.

George JN, et al. Idiopathic thrombocytopenic purpura: a practice guideline developed by explicit methods for the American Society of Hematology. Blood 1996;88(1):3–40.

McMillan R. The pathogenesis of chronic immune (idiopathic) thrombocytopenic purpura. Semin Hematol 2000;37[1 suppl 1]:5–9

Nugent DJ. Immune thrombocytopenic purpura: why treat? J Pediatr 1999; 134:3–4.

Reid MM. Chronic idiopathic thrombocytopenic purpura: incidence, treatment, and outcome. Arch Dis Child 1995;72(2):125–128.

Tarantino MD. Treatment of childhood acute immune thrombocytopenic purpura with anti-D immune globulin or pooled immune globulin. J Pediatr 1999;134:21–26.

Author: John McCourt

Immunosuppression

Clinical Presentation

SIGNS AND SYMPTOMS

- The principal concern is for occult infection
- Fever
- Altered mental status
- Abdominal pain without peritoneal signs
- Generalized weakness
- Malaise
- Meningitis without meningeal signs
- Fever in the neutropenic patient
  —Single temperature $\geq$ 38.3°C or sustained temperature $\geq$38.0°C over 1–2 hours

MECHANISM/DESCRIPTION

- At least half of neutropenic patients with fever have an established or occult infection
- Greater than 20% of patients with neutrophil counts $<100/mm^3$ are bacteremic
- Most common sites of infection in neutropenia:
  —Lung (25%)
  —Mouth and pharynx (25%)
  —Skin, soft tissue, and intravascular catheters (15%)
  —Perineum and anorectal area (10%)
  —Urinary tract (5%)
  —Nose and sinuses (5%)
  —Gastrointestinal tract (5%)
- Gram-positive cocci responsible for 60–70% of documented infections:
  —*Escherichia coli*
  —*Klebsiella* species
  —*Pseudomonas aeruginosa*
  —*Staphylococcus epidermidis*
  —α-Hemolytic streptococcal species
  —*Enterococcus faecalis*
  —*Staphylococcus aureus*
- Fungal infections
  —Seen in patients on broad-spectrum antibiotics
  —Persistent fever and neutropenia for >7 days
  —*Aspergillus flavus*
  —*Aspergillus fumigatus*
  —*Candida albicans*
  —*Candida tropicalis*

DEFINITION

- Deficiency in ability to fight infection
  —Congenital (incidence 1:10,000 patients)
    -Antibody (B cell)
    -Cellular (T cell)
    -Combined
    -Phagocytic dysfunction
  —Acquired

ETIOLOGY

- Old age (>75)
  —Decreased antibody and cellular immunity
  —Decreased cough reflex
  —Poor circulation and wound healing
  —Communal living (nosocomial infections)
  —Physiologic responses to infection are blunted
  —Blunted leukocytosis
  —Lack of classic peritoneal signs despite perforated viscus
- Organ transplant recipients
  —Immunosuppressive medications
- Intravenous drug abuse (IVDA)
  —Opiates suppress phagocytosis and bactericidal activity
  —Depressed cellular immunity with methadone and morphine
  —Risk factor for AIDS
- HIV infection (see HIV/AIDS)
- Diabetes
  —Hyperglycemia causes defective immune function while euglycemia improves it
  —Vascular insufficiency (small and large vessel)
  —Peripheral neuropathy leads to wound neglect
- Malnutrition
  —Homelessness
  —Alcoholism
- Cancer and chemoradiotherapy
  —Neutropenia from chemotherapy or native disease process
    -Defined as absolute neutrophil count (ANC) $<500/mm^3$ or $<1,000/mm^3$ with predicted decrease to <500
    -Risk of infection increases as ANC drops, and as neutropenia persists over several days
  —Impairment in T-cell and B-cell function

Pre-Hospital

CAUTIONS

- Observe universal precautions for patient and provider protection
- Patients in septic shock require aggressive fluid resuscitation
- Obtain bedside glucose test
  —Hypoglycemia can occur with sepsis

Diagnosis

ESSENTIAL WORKUP

- Workup must be tailored to the specific presenting complaint
- Focus on site of pain, even in the absence of physical findings
- CBC, differential, urinalysis, CXR
- Pitfalls in identifying infection with neutropenia
  —Overt signs of inflammation (redness, drainage, swelling) may not be present
  —Peritonitis may not manifest
  —Pyuria can be absent with urinary tract infection
  —Meningitis may be present without CSF pleocytosis (especially cryptococcal meningitis)
  —Lung infection may be present without pulmonary infiltrates

LABORATORY

- Obtain cultures
  —Two sets bacterial
  —One fungal culture
  —At least one bacterial culture from an indwelling central line
  —Gram stain of overt pus or drainage from indwelling catheters; fungal culture of drainage from line as well
  —Urine culture
  —Lumbar puncture if there is suspicion of meningitis (low-grade headache, confusion)
  —Send CSF for cryptococcal antigen, even if no CSF pleocytosis.
  —D-dimer (ELISA method) if cancer and abrupt-onset shortness of breath or hypotension

IMAGING/SPECIAL TESTS

- Chest x-ray should be obtained in all patients with fever and immunosuppression
- Sinus CT should be performed if facial pain or swelling is present
- CT, MRI, or radionuclide studies may be indicated to localize site of infection
- Spiral chest CT if pulmonary embolism suspected (abrupt onset, tachypnea, dyspnea, hypotension with or without fever)

Treatment

INITIAL STABILIZATION

- Hypotension
  - —Fluid resuscitation; may need 1–4 L NS or more for sepsis with hypotension
  - —Consider CVP catheter to monitor fluid balance
  - —Bedside cardiac ultrasound to rule-out malignant pericardial effusion/tamponade
  - —Pressors if hypotension unresponsive to fluids
    - -Systolic blood pressure ≥70: Dopamine 5–20 μg/kg/min
    - -Systolic blood pressure <70: Norepinephrine 0.5–30 μg/kg/min; usual adult dose 2–12 μg/kg/min
- Airway management for ventilatory failure, hypoxia unresponsive to high-flow face-mask oxygen
- Cardiac monitor and pulse oximetry

ED TREATMENT

- Start broad-spectrum antimicrobial therapy in the ED after appropriate cultures obtained

High-Risk Patients

- Risk factors
  - —ANC <100/mm^3, pulmonary infiltrates
  - —Abnormal renal or hepatic function tests
  - —IV catheter site infection
  - —Active malignancy
  - —Peak temperature >39.0°C
  - —Mental status changes
  - —Ill appearance
  - —Abdominal pain or comorbid conditions
- Use one of the following combination therapies
  - —Aminoglycoside (gentamicin) *plus* extended spectrum penicillin (mezlocillin) or ticarcillin with clavulanate or piperacillin with tazobactam
  - —Aminoglycoside (gentamicin) *plus* an antipseudomonal cephalosporin (ceftazidime or cefepime), or a carbapenem (imipenem-cilastin or meropenem)
  - —Extended spectrum penicillin (mezlocillin) or ticarcillin with clavulanate, or piperacillin with tazobactam *plus* antipseudomonal third-generation cephalosporin (ceftazidime)
- Add vancomycin to the regimen if suspicion of serious catheter-related infection, known colonization with penicillin-resistant pneumococci or methicillin-resistant *S. aureus*, or hypotension upon presentation

Low-Risk Patients

- Use one of the following:
  - —IV monotherapy (cefepime, ceftazidime, or a carbapenem) or oral combination therapy (ciprofloxacin plus amoxicillin-clavulanate) is acceptable
  - —For penicillin allergic patients aztreonam *plus* vancomycin
- If anaerobes are suspected (i.e., oral, abdominal, or perianal infection), add clindamycin

MEDICATIONS

- Aztreonam: adult: 2 g i.v.; peds: 120 mg/kg/d i.v. div q6h
- Cefepime: adult: 2 g i.v.; peds: 150 mg/kg/d i.v. div q8h
- Ceftazidime: adult: 2 g i.v.; peds: 150 mg/kg/day i.v. div q8h
- Clindamycin: adult: 900 mg i.v.; peds: 25–40 mg/kg/d i.v., i.m. div q6h
- Gentamicin: adult: 2–5 mg/kg i.v.; peds: 5 mg/kg/d i.v., i.m. div q12h
- Imipenem: adult: 0.5 g i.v.; peds: safety not established
- Mezlocillin: adult: 3 g i.v.; peds: safety not established
- Piperacillin/tazobactam: adult: 3.375 g i.v.; peds: safety not established
- Ticarcillin/clavulanate: adult: 3.1 g i.v.: peds: safety not established
- Vancomycin: adult: 1 g i.v.; peds: 40–60 mg/kg/d i.v. div q6h

Disposition

ADMISSION CRITERIA

- All febrile patients with neutropenia or organ transplant
- Admit to intensive care if signs of hemodynamic instability
- Admit elderly patients and diabetics with fever and signs of infection
- Admit intravenous drug users with fever, as approximately 20% have serious bacterial infection (pneumonia, endocarditis, bacteremia)

DISCHARGE CRITERIA

- If ED workup is negative, patient has ANC >100, and has no localized infection, and is reliable, well appearing, tolerating PO liquids, and close follow-up is assured, a trial of outpatient therapy is warranted
- If discharging patient, parenteral antibiotic therapy should be given in ED and oral antibiotics as an outpatient; patient must follow up in 1 day for reevaluation and to check culture results

Miscellaneous

ICD9: 279.3

SUGGESTED READINGS

Hughes WT, Armstrong D, Bodey GP, et al. 2002 Guidelines for the use of antimicrobial agents in neutropenic patients with cancer. Clin Infect Dis 2002;34:730–751.

Rosenberg AS, Brown AE. Infection in the cancer patient. Dis Mon 1993;39: 507–569.

Rubin JT, Lotze T. Immune function and dysfunction: A primer for the radiologist. Radiol Clin North Am 1992;30:507.

Schimpff SC. Infections in the cancer patient—diagnosis, prevention and treatment. In: Mandell GL, Bennett JE, Dolin R, eds. Principles and practice of infectious diseases, 4th ed. New York: Churchill Livingstone, 1995:2666–2675.

Sternbach GL. Infections in alcoholic patients. Emerg Med Clin North Am 1990;8:793.

Swenson KK, Rose MA, Ritz L, et al. Recognition and evaluation of oncology-related symptoms in the emergency department. Ann Emerg Med 1995;26:12.

Author: Mark I. Langdorf

Impetigo

Clinical Presentation

SIGNS AND SYMPTOMS

Classical (Nonbullous) Impetigo

- Begins as a single 2- to 4-mm erythematous macule or papule that may evolve into a vesicle or pustule, on a red base
- Rupture of the vesicle, usually within 24 hours, leaves a honey-colored, dark brown, or reddish black exudative crust
- Highly contagious
- Often pruritic, may be spread from the original site of infection by scratching
- Mild lymphadenopathy may be seen, usually not lymphadenitis
- Systemic manifestations are rare

Bullous Impetigo

- Occurs most commonly in the neonate, but can occur at any age
- Large, fragile bullae may have ruptured leaving only a shiny, erythematous base with peeling edges
- Weakness, fever, and diarrhea are common systemic manifestations

MECHANISM/DESCRIPTION

Classic Impetigo

- The result of bacteria entering through traumatic skin portal from scratch, abrasion, or insect bite
- Caused by either *Staphylococcus aureus,* group A β-hemolytic streptococci, or both
- More prevalent in warm climates and warm seasons

Bullous Impetigo

- Caused by *S. aureus* alone
- Epidermal cleavage is caused by a staphylococcal exotoxin called exfoliatin or exfoliative toxin

Pre-Hospital

CAUTIONS

- Maintain universal precautions

Diagnosis

ESSENTIAL WORKUP

- The diagnosis is made based on observation of the classic exam findings
  - —Cultures of bullous fluid may be considered in those cases refractory to traditional therapy

DIFFERENTIAL DIAGNOSIS

- Herpes simplex
- Varicella
- Atopic dermatitis
- Contact dermatitis
- Dermatophytosis
- Erysipelas
- Candidiasis
- Scabies
- Pediculosis
- Pemphigus vulgaris
- Bullous pemphigoid
- Thermal burns
- Stevens-Johnson syndrome
- Bullous erythema multiforme
- Staphylococcal scalded skin syndrome (caused by systemic spread of exfoliation in susceptible individuals)

Treatment

INITIAL STABILIZATION

- In healthy children or adults, classic or bullous impetigo is not a life-threatening condition and does not require resuscitative measures

ED TREATMENT

- Small lesions may be treated with topical therapy alone using mupirocin or in conjunction with systemic therapy
- Larger, widespread lesions with systemic therapy
- Treatment should employ a β-lactamase-resistant penicillin, cephalosporin, or macrolide antimicrobial for 7 days
- Systemic antibiotic advisable during epidemics of acute poststreptococcal glomerulonephritis
- Local care should include cleansing, removal of crusts, and application of wet dressings to the affected areas

MEDICATIONS

- All treatment regimens are 7 to 10 days
- Avoid use of erythromycin if high incidence of erythromycin resistance in the community

Oral

- Ampicillin/clavulanate: adult: 250 mg PO q8h; peds: 20 mg/kg/d PO in divided doses q8h
- Azithromycin: adult: 500 mg PO on day 1; 250 mg PO days 2–5; peds: 10 mg/kg PO on day 1; 5 mg/kg PO days 2–5
- Cephalexin: adult: 500 mg PO q12h; peds: 40 mg/kg/day PO in divided doses q8h
- Clarithromycin: adult: 250 mg PO q12h; peds: 15 mg/kg
- Clindamycin: adult: 150 mg PO t.i.d.; peds: 5 mg/kg t.i.d.
- Dicloxacillin: adult: 250 mg PO q6h; peds: 30 mg/kg/d PO in divided doses q6h
- Erythromycin ethylsuccinate: adult: 250 mg PO q6h; peds: 40 mg/kg/d PO in divided doses q6h
- Linezolid: adult: 600 mg PO b.i.d. (extremely expensive, used only for multiallergic patients or MRSA); peds: not approved for children

Topical

- Mupirocin (2% ointment): adult and peds: apply topically to affected area t.i.d.

Disposition

ADMISSION CRITERIA

- Admission for impetigo alone is rarely necessary
- Patients with disease that is widespread, esp. widespread bullae, or refractory to outpatient therapy
- Toxic, ill-appearing, or immunocompromised patients require admission
- Nephritis may already be present at time patients present for care, if presentation delayed more than 4–5 days

DISCHARGE CRITERIA

- Patients should not be toxic appearing
- Patients should be able to comply with the recommended treatment regimen
- Follow-up for reevaluation

Miscellaneous

- Siblings of affected children in same household should be checked for lesions

ICD9: 684

ICD10: L01.0

SUGGESTED READING

Hirschmann JV. Impetigo: etiology and therapy. In: Remington JS, Swartz M, eds. Current clinical topics in infectious diseases, vol 22. Malden, MA: Blackwell, 2002:42–51.

Author: Irving "Jake" Jacoby

Inborn Errors of Metabolism

Clinical Presentation

SIGNS AND SYMPTOMS

- Rapid decompensation may occur
- Neonates, initial presentation
  - —Hypothermia
  - —Hypo/hypertonia
  - —Apnea
  - —Seizures
  - —Coma
  - —Vomiting
  - —Poor feeding, growth
  - —Jaundice
  - —Hypoglycemia
- Older children, untreated
  - —General
    - -Failure to thrive
    - -Dehydration
  - —GI
    - -Vomiting
    - -Diarrhea
    - -Food intolerance
  - —Neurologic
    - -Lethargy
    - -Ataxia
    - -Seizures
    - -Mental retardation
- Physical examination
  - —Abnormal odor
  - —Altered mental status
  - —Tachypnea
  - —Abnormal facies
  - —Cataract
  - —Cardiomyopathy
  - —Hepatomegaly
  - —Splenomegaly
  - —Dermatitis

MECHANISM/DESCRIPTION

- Manifestations related to the defect and amount and toxicity of metabolites that accumulate
- Common inherited metabolic diseases
  - —Urea cycle defects
  - —Organic acidemias
  - —Disorders of amino acid metabolism
  - —Defects in fatty acid oxidation
  - —Mitochondrial disorders
  - —Carbohydrate disorders
  - —Mucopolysaccharidoses
  - —Sphingolipidoses
  - —Peroxisomal disorders

ETIOLOGY

- Diverse group of disorders involving a genetic deficiency of an enzyme of an intermediary metabolite or a membrane transport system
- Rare, occurring in 1:100,000–200,000 births
- Over 300 human diseases due to inborn errors of metabolism are now recognized

Pre-Hospital

CAUTIONS

- Careful assessment of the ABCs
- IV glucose infusion takes precedence over fluid boluses unless the patient is in shock
- Avoid lactated Ringer's solution

Diagnosis

ESSENTIAL WORKUP

- Key is to consider in differential diagnosis
  - —Deteriorating neurologic status
  - —Unexplained failure to thrive with dehydration, persistent vomiting, or acidosis

LABORATORY

- Bedside glucose determination
- Electrolytes, BUN/Cr, glucose
- CBC with differential
- Calcium
- Liver function tests, fractionated bilirubin, prothrombin time
- Arterial or venous blood gases
- Uric acid
- Urinalysis

IMAGING/SPECIAL TESTS

- Chemistries
  - —Ammonia level
  - —Quantitative serum amino acids
  - —Urine organic and amino acids
  - —Lactate and pyruvate levels
- CT scan for altered mental status
- Cultures: blood and CSF
- CXR

DIFFERENTIAL DIAGNOSIS

- Often misdiagnosed as sepsis, dehydration, failure to thrive, ingestion or nonaccidental trauma
- Infection
  - —Sepsis
  - —Meningitis
  - —Encephalitis
- Metabolic
  - —Reye's syndrome
  - —Hepatic encephalopathy
  - —Hyperinsulinemia
  - —Hormonal abnormality
- Renal
  - —Renal failure
  - —Renal tubular acidosis
- Toxic ingestion
- CNS mass lesions
- Nonaccidental trauma

Treatment

INITIAL STABILIZATION

- ABCs
- For altered mental status, administer Narcan, glucose (or Accucheck), and thiamine

ED TREATMENT

- Initiate IV glucose at a rate of 8–10 mg/kg/min to prevent catabolism
  - —Corresponds to D10 at 1.5 times maintenance
  - —Do not delay glucose infusion to give a "bolus" of isotonic saline; may be given concurrently in a child in shock
  - —If a patient is severely hypoglycemic, give IV glucose bolus of D25
- Rehydrate if hypovolemic
  - —Restore normal acid-base balance
- Administer bicarbonate if the pH is <7.0
  - —Initiate dialysis if severe acidosis does not improve quickly
- Increase urine output to help in removal of some toxins
- Stop all oral intake
  - —Amino acid metabolites may be neurotoxic
- Treat severe hyperammonemia with dialysis or with ammonia-trapping drugs such as arginine hydrochloride, sodium benzoate, sodium phenylacetate, or sodium phenylbutyrate
  - —Dosages vary with disease, and a metabolic physician should be consulted before their use
- Identify and treat intercurrent or precipitating infection/illness
- Consult a metabolic physician when any child presents with a suspected inherited metabolic disease

MEDICATIONS

- D25: 2–4 cc/kg i.v.
- Sodium bicarbonate: 1–2 mEq/kg i.v.

Disposition

ADMISSION CRITERIA

- Infants and children presenting with a new onset of a suspected inherited metabolic disease
- Significant urinary ketones or not tolerating oral intake
- ICU admission for significant altered mental status, severe or persistent acidosis, unresponsive hypoglycemia, or hyperammonemia
  - —Transfer of these patients to a specialized pediatric center may also be indicated

DISCHARGE CRITERIA

- Normal mental status
- Normal hydration with unremarkable labs
- No evidence of significant intercurrent illness
- Close follow-up arranged with primary care physician

Miscellaneous

ICD9: 277.9

SUGGESTED READINGS

D'Agata ID, Balistreri WF. Evaluation of liver disease in the pediatric patient. Pediatr Rev 1999;20(11):376–390.

Goodman SI, Green CL. Metabolic disorders of the newborn. Pediatr Rev 1994;15(9): 359–365.

Korson MS. Advances in newborn screening for metabolic disorders: what the pediatrician needs to know. Pediatr Ann 2000;29(5):294–301.

Leonard JV. Inborn errors of metabolism around time of birth. Lancet 2000; 356(9229):583–587.

Thoene JG. Treatment of urea cycle disorders. J Pediatr 1999;134(3): 255–256.

Wolf AD, Lavine JE. Hepatomegaly in neonates and children. Pediatr Rev 2000; 21(9):303–310.

Author: David A. Perlstein

Inflammatory Bowel Disease

Clinical Presentation

SIGNS AND SYMPTOMS

- Crohn's disease can present with any of the clinical correlates of a chronic inflammatory, fibrostenotic, or fistulizing process
- Ulcerative colitis (UC) may begin subtly or as a catastrophic illness
- Constitutional, gastrointestinal, and extraintestinal manifestations are common with both Crohn's and UC

Constitutional

- Crohn's disease
  - —Low-grade fever
  - —Night sweats
  - —Weight loss
  - —Fatigue
- Ulcerative colitis
  - —Fever usually only in fulminant disease
  - —Weight loss
  - —Fatigue

Gastrointestinal

- Abdominal pain/tenderness
  - —Crohn's disease
    - -Episodic
    - -Periumbilical—may localize to RLQ with ileal disease
    - -Generalized with more diffuse intestinal involvement
    - -Can localize to area of intraabdominal abscess or fistulous involvement
    - -Tenderness and distention suggest obstruction or toxic megacolon
  - —Ulcerative colitis
    - -More generalized than Crohn's disease
    - -Often limited to peri-defecatory period
    - -Tenderness and distension implies toxic dilation
- Stool
  - —Crohn's disease
    - -Mild loose stool
    - -Rarely more than 4-5/d
    - -~50% bloody
  - —Ulcerative colitis
    - -Diarrhea variable, can be severe
    - -Vast majority bloody, sometimes with severe hemorrhage
    - -Mucus
    - -Tenesmus and urgency common
- Nausea/vomiting
  - —Crohn's disease
    - -Obstruction common with ileocolonic disease
  - —Ulcerative colitis
    - -Obstruction rare
    - -Diminished bowel sounds with toxic dilation
- Perianal
  - —Crohn's disease
    - -Perianal abscess
    - -Fissure—characteristically painless
    - -Fistula
    - -Half of patients with colonic disease
    - -May present prior to other manifestations of illness
  - —Ulcerative colitis
    - -No perianal involvement

Extraintestinal—Occur in 25–35%

- Eye
  - —Uveitis
  - —Episcleritis
  - —Keratitis
- Oral—aphthous stomatitis
- Liver
  - —Sclerosing cholangitis
  - —Cholelithiasis in 35-60% of Crohn's patients
- Renal
  - —Nephrolithiasis
  - —Obstructive hydronephrosis
- Musculoskeletal
  - —Peripheral arthritis/arthralgias—follows intestinal disease activity
  - —Axial arthritis (ankylosing spondylitis, sacroiliitis)—course not related to underlying disease activity
- Skin
  - —Erythema nodosum
  - —Pyoderma gangrenosum

MECHANISM/DESCRIPTION

- Idiopathic, chronic, inflammatory disease of the intestines
- Differences between Crohn's and UC
  - —Rectum almost always involved in UC with continuous inflammation proximally in colon
  - —Small intestine not involved in UC
  - —Crohn's occurs anywhere from mouth to anus, often with normal GI tract segments between affected areas
  - —Crohn's involves transmural inflammation, whereas UC is confined to submucosa
- Similarities between Crohn's and UC
  - —Higher rate of colon cancer with disease >10 years
  - —Pattern of exacerbation/remission
  - —Bimodal age distribution with early peak between teens and early 30s and second peak about age 60
- Crohn's disease clinical pattern
  - —Ileocecal: ~40%
  - —Small bowel: ~30%
  - —Colon: ~25%
  - —Other: ~5%
- UC clinical pattern on presentation
  - —Pancolitis: 30%
    - -Most severe clinical course
  - —Proctitis or proctosigmoiditis: 30%
    - -Relatively mild clinical course
  - —Left-sided colitis (up to splenic flexure): 40%
    - -Between the two in severity

ETIOLOGY

- Unknown
- Two diseases—separate conditions with a common genetic predisposition
- Multifactorial origin involving interplay among the following factors:
  - —Genetic
  - —Environmental
  - —Immune
- Pathogenesis
  - —Gut wall becomes unable to downregulate its immune responses, ultimately resulting in inflammation
- No definitive evidence for etiologic role of infectious agent
- Psychogenic factors play a role in some symptomatic exacerbations

PEDIATRIC CONSIDERATIONS

- Can occur in the first few years of life
- Extraintestinal manifestations predominate
  - —May be confused with:
    - -Juvenile rheumatoid arthritis
    - -Idiopathic growth failure
    - -Anorexia nervosa

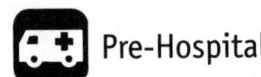

Pre-Hospital

N/A

Diagnosis

ESSENTIAL WORKUP

- May present as initial onset of disease or exacerbation of existing disease
- Maintain high index of suspicion due to subtle presentation of Crohn's disease

LABORATORY

- Nothing diagnostic
- CBC
  —Anemia secondary to chronic or acute blood loss
- Electrolytes, BUN/Cr, glucose
- Stool examination
  —Occult blood
  —Fecal leukocytes may be present
  —Culture to exclude infectious cause of enteritis
- ESR
  —Elevated

IMAGING/SPECIAL TESTS

- Plain abdominal films for
  —Toxic megacolon (>6 cm dilation)
  —Obstruction
  —Air in wall of colon (may indicate impending perforation)
  —Perforation—subdiaphragmatic air or free air outlining liver or gallbladder
- CT abdomen
  —To distinguish abscess from localized inflammatory mass in Crohn's
- Colonoscopy with biopsy confirms diagnosis of UC
  —Do not perform with severe symptoms due to perforation risk
- Lower endoscopy with biopsy and radiographic imaging of small bowel (especially terminal ileum) confirms diagnosis of Crohn's

DIFFERENTIAL DIAGNOSIS

- Infectious enteritis
- Pseudomembranous colitis (*Clostridium difficile*)
- Appendicitis
- Diverticulitis
- Diverticulosis
- Functional bowel disease
- Lymphoma involving bowel
- Ischemic colitis
- Gonococcal or chlamydial proctitis
- Vasculitis
- Amyloidosis

Treatment

INITIAL STABILIZATION

- IV 0.9% NS volume replacement if dehydrated
- Transfusion if significant blood loss
- NG suction if obstruction or toxic dilation suspected
- Broad-spectrum antibiotics for fulminant UC or suspected perforation

ED MANAGEMENT

Indications for Surgical Evaluation

- Free perforation
- Intestinal obstruction
- Massive, unresponsive hemorrhage
- Toxic dilation
  —Not an absolute indication for surgical intervention
  —Intensive medical management with small bowel suction and close radiographic monitoring and surgical consultation
- Walled-off perforation with abscess
  —Usually not an indication for emergent surgery
  —Careful observation for peritonitis

Medical Therapy

- Treatment usually not initiated unless already established diagnosis
- Refill or restart medications in a patient with known disease
- ED prescribed medical regime should be individualized
  —Aminosalicylate (sulfasalazine, mesalamine) for mild to moderate disease
  —Antidiarrheal agent (Lomotil/Imodium)
    -Not with severe disease if suspect toxic dilation
  —Steroid (prednisone, budesonide, or hydrocortisone enema, ACTH) for moderate to severe disease
  —Antibiotics (metronidazole and/or ciprofloxacin) aid in treatment of Crohn's with colon/perineum involvement
  —Immunosuppressive agents (azathioprine, cyclosporin A, methotrexate, 6-mercaptopurine) for refractory disease
  —Monoclonal antibody therapy targeting tumor necrosis factor-α (infliximab, CDP571) used in severe Crohn's disease

MEDICATIONS

- ACTH: 80–120 IU/24 hours i.m. or i.v.
- Ciprofloxacin: 500 mg PO q12h
- Hydrocortisone enema: 60 mg
- Mesalamine enemas: 1–4 g retention enema—retain overnight
- Mesalamine suppositories: 500 mg PR b.i.d.
- Mesalamine tablets: (Asacol sustained-release 400 mg; Pentasa 250 mg) 800 mg PO t.i.d.; 1,000 mg PO q.i.d.
- Metronidazole: 250–500 mg (peds: 30 mg/kg/24 hours) PO t.i.d.
- Prednisone: 40–60 mg PO qd
- Sulfasalazine (Azulfidine): 500 mg PO q.i.d.

Disposition

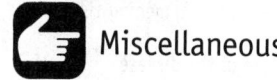

ADMISSION CRITERIA

- Surgical indication
  —Massive, unresponsive hemorrhage
  —Perforation
  —Toxic dilation
  —Obstruction
- Severe flare-up
  —Electrolyte imbalance
  —Severe dehydration
  —Severe pain
  —High fever
  —Significant bleeding

DISCHARGE CRITERIA

- Initial presentation of diarrhea, mild pain, without toxicity, with close follow-up
- Mild to moderate exacerbation of known disease without obstruction, severe bleeding, severe pain, dehydration, with close follow-up, on renewed therapy or with addition of steroid

Miscellaneous

ICD9: 555.9, 556.9

ICD10: K50.9; K51.9

SEE ALSO: DIARRHEA AND GASTROENTERITIS

SUGGESTED READINGS

Chutkan RK. Inflammatory bowel disease. Prim Care Clin Office Pract 2001;28(3):539–556, vi.

Hyams JS. Inflammatory bowel disease. Pediatr Rev 2000;21(9):291–295.

Stotland BR, Stein RB, Lichenstein GR. Advances in inflammatory bowel disease. Med Clin North Am 2000;84(5):1107–1124.

Author: Michael P. Jones

Influenza

Clinical Presentation

SIGNS AND SYMPTOMS

- Abrupt onset of high fever: 38–40°C (100–104°F)
- Chills, shivering
- Myalgias
- Headache
- Malaise
- Anorexia
- Nasal discharge
- Conjunctivitis
- Pharyngitis
- Dry cough
- Elderly may present with high fever, lassitude, and confusion without pulmonary complications

MECHANISM/DESCRIPTION

- Acute, usually self-limited, viral infection
- Transmission: by dispersion in small-particle aerosols created by sneezing, cough, and talking
- Virus deposited on respiratory tract epithelium and absorbed
- Incubation period: 1–2 days
- Duration: 3 days
  - —Severity of symptoms in proportion to height of the fever
- Outbreaks usually occur during winter months
- Common complications
  - —Primary influenza viral pneumonia
  - —Secondary bacterial pneumonia
  - —Exacerbations of COPD
  - —Rare complications: myositis, myocarditis, pericarditis, and aseptic meningitis
- Key features
  - —Epidemic nature of the disease
  - —Mortality results largely from pulmonary complications

ETIOLOGY

- Majority caused by three genera of the Orthomyxoviridae family: influenza virus type A, B, and C
- Epidemics
  - —Every 1–3 years
  - —Caused by *antigenic drift*—new variants from minor changes in surface protein
  - —Majority of cases occur in 2–3 weeks
  - —Duration of the epidemic <6 weeks
- Pandemics
  - —Every 10 years
  - —Caused by new strains created by *antigenic shift*—major changes in virus structure
- Waterfowl reservoir of influenza virus

PEDIATRIC CONSIDERATIONS

- Children exhibit more lower-respiratory involvement (croup, bronchitis, bronchiolitis, pneumonitis) and higher temperatures than adults
- Myalgias in the calf muscle
- Febrile convulsions occur in approximately 10% of children under 5 with influenza infection
- Reye's syndrome
  - —Influenza may be predisposing factor
  - —Rare and severe complication
  - —Characterized by fatty degeneration of the liver and cerebral edema
  - —Symptoms:
    - -Nausea
    - -Vomiting
    - -Stupor
  - —Strong correlation with salicylates: avoid aspirin products in children with influenza

Pre-Hospital

N/A

Diagnosis

ESSENTIAL WORKUP

- Clinical diagnosis based on the signs and symptoms of influenza during the winter months in the setting of an known outbreak

LABORATORY

- CBC
  - —WBC: normal to mildly decreased
- Culture of nasopharyngeal swab or aspirate
- Pulse oximetry/ABG for significant pulmonary symptoms

IMAGING/SPECIAL TESTS

- CXR for prominent lower respiratory symptoms
  - —Normal (50–90%)
  - —Bilateral interstitial infiltration
- Rapid ELISA antigen test
  - —Can distinguish types A and B
  - —Sensitivity about 75%, specificity 90%, within 2 days of symptom onset
  - —Nasal swab better than throat

DIFFERENTIAL DIAGNOSIS

- Indistinguishable from most viral infections (URI)
- Bronchitis
- Atypical pneumonia
- Epstein-Barr infection (infectious mononucleosis)
- Distinguishing features from anthrax
  - —Influenza is much more likely to include a sore throat and rhinorrhea
  - —Anthrax much more likely to include dyspnea and nausea

Treatment

INITIAL STABILIZATION

- Aggressive fluid resuscitation, supplemental oxygen, and positive-pressure ventilation as clinical circumstances dictate

ED TREATMENT

- Supportive and symptomatic
  - —Antipyretics (acetaminophen or NSAIDs)—avoid aspirin
  - —Cough suppressants
  - —Rehydration
- Antivirals effective if given within 48 hours of symptom onset
  - —Amantadine and rimantadine effective against influenza A
  - —Zanamivir and oseltamivir have activity against types A and B
  - —Reduce symptom duration of 1 day
  - —Costly, except for amantadine
  - —Accelerates functional recovery
  - —Recommended for:
    - -Pneumonia
    - -Patient with severe disease
    - -Immunocompromised
    - -Patients at high risk for complications

PREVENTION

- Polyvalent influenza vaccine recommended annually for
  - —Adults >65 years
  - —High-risk individuals (COPD, cardiovascular disease, immunocompromised, diabetics)
  - —Health care workers
- Chemoprophylaxis in the following settings
  - —Short-term prophylaxis during outbreak of influenza A in high-risk patients who did not receive vaccine
  - —In conjunction with vaccine in high-risk patients expected to respond poorly to vaccine, including HIV infections
  - —In lieu of vaccine when vaccine is contraindicated in high-risk individuals
  - —In individuals providing care for high-risk persons
  - —Zanamivir not approved for prophylaxis

MEDICATIONS

- Amantadine: 200 mg PO initially, then 100 mg PO b.i.d. for 3–5 d
- Oseltamivir: 75 mg PO b.i.d. for 3–4 d
- Rimantadine: 200 mg PO initially, then 100 mg PO b.i.d. for 3–5 d
- Zanamivir: 10 mg nasal insufflation b.i.d. for 3–5 d

Disposition

ADMISSION CRITERIA

- Hypoxia, pneumonia, severe dehydration

DISCHARGE CRITERIA

- Most patients will have a short, self-limited course provided they are able to tolerate fluids and antipyretics

Miscellaneous

ICD9: 487

ICD10: J11.1

SEE ALSO: ANTHRAX

SUGGESTED READINGS

Arruda E, Hayden FG. Update on therapy of influenza and rhinovirus infections. Adv Exp Med Biol 1996;394:174–187.

Betts RF. Influenza virus. In: Mandell Gl, Bennett JE, Dolin R, eds. Mandell, Douglas, and Bennett's principles and practice of infectious diseases, 4th ed. New York: Churchill Livingstone 1995.

CDC, National Center for Infectious Disease, *http://www.cdc.gov/ncidod/diseases/submenus/sub_flu.htm.*

CDC. Notice to readers: considerations for distinguishing influenza-like illness from inhalational anthrax. MMWR 2001;50(44): 984–986.

Fleming DM. Managing influenza: amantadine, rimantadine and beyond. Int J Clin Pract 2001;55(3):189–195.

Mossad SB. Prophylactic and symptomatic treatment of influenza. Current and developing options. Postgrad Med 2001;109(1):97–105.

Nicholson KG. Clinical features of influenza. Semin Respir Infect 1992;7(1):26–37.

Ryan-Poirier K. Influenza virus infection in children. Adv Pediatr Infect Dis 1995;10: 125–156.

Author: Philip Shayne

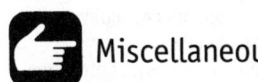

Intracerebral Hemorrhage

Clinical Presentation

SIGNS AND SYMPTOMS

- Severe headache, typically sudden in onset
- Hypertension
- Seizures
- Evidence of head injury
- Meningismus; vomiting
- Altered level of consciousness (may be comatose); altered mental status may occur as late as 24–48 hours after head injury
- Variable neurologic deficits depending on the site of intracerebral hemorrhage
  —Putamen hemorrhage (35%): contralateral hemiparesis and hemisensory loss, with occasional dysphagia or neglect
  —Lobar hemorrhage (30%): variable signs depending on involved area
  —Cerebellar hemorrhage (15%): vomiting, ataxia, and nystagmus
  —Thalamic hemorrhage (10%): similar to putamen, but may also have eye movement abnormalities
  —Caudate hemorrhage (5%): confusion, memory loss, hemiparesis, gaze paresis
  —Pontine hemorrhage (5%): quadriplegia, pin-point pupils, ataxia, sensorimotor loss

MECHANISM/DESCRIPTION

- Injury occurs primarily from hemorrhage into brain parenchyma leading to compression of brain tissues. Secondary injury results from cerebral edema leading to increased intracranial pressure and the possibility of brain herniation

ETIOLOGY

- Intracerebral hemorrhage can occur spontaneously or secondary to traumatic head injury
  —Uncontrolled or acute hypertension (most common)
  —Vascular malformations (arteriovenous malformation, venous angiomas, and ruptured aneurysms)
  —Neoplasm (particularly melanoma and glioma)
  —Anticoagulant therapy (Coumadin, heparin)
  —Thrombolytic agents
  —Illicit drugs (cocaine, amphetamines)
  —Bleeding disorders (hemophilia)
  —Cerebral amyloid angiopathy
  —Traumatic hemorrhage secondary to blunt or penetrating injury

Pre-Hospital

CAUTIONS

- C-spine precautions if head or neck injury is suspected
- Elevation of head with C-spine control
- Initial pre-hospital responder must ascertain the neurologic defect to be able to note progression of symptoms

Diagnosis

ESSENTIAL WORKUP

- Immediate noncontrast head CT (acute hemorrhage appears as a high-density lesion)

LABORATORY

- Check coagulation studies (PT/PTT, INR, platelets)

IMAGING/SPECIAL TESTS

- CT as above
- MRI not indicated because of long scan time, and it is difficult or impossible to manage unstable patients in the scanner

DIFFERENTIAL DIAGNOSIS

- Differential diagnosis based on mental status change, neurologic deficit, headache, etc., is vast and includes:
  —Seizure
  —CNS infection
  —CNS mass
  —Electrolyte or acid-base abnormality
  —Intoxication/Wernicke's encephalitis
  —Migraine headache
  —Transient ischemic attack (TIA)
  —Todd's paralysis
  —Air embolism
- Differential diagnosis once bleed is seen on CT:
  —Spontaneous hemorrhage (hypertensive, AVM, neoplasm, etc.)
  —Traumatic hemorrhage
  —Subarachnoid hemorrhage
  —Subdural hematoma
  —Epidural hematoma

PEDIATRIC CONSIDERATIONS

- Additional differential diagnoses include:
  —Moyamoya disease
  —Acute infantile hemiplegia

Treatment

INITIAL STABILIZATION

- ABCs
  - —Patients with depressed level of consciousness should be intubated immediately and administered controlled ventilation
- Early neurosurgical consultation

ED MANAGEMENT

- Blood pressure management
  - —Must use caution in blood pressure control because acute lowering of BP to normal in the setting of increased intracranial pressure (ICP) could reduce cerebral perfusion to ischemic levels
  - —Only correct hypertension if systolic blood pressure is >200 mm Hg or if diastolic blood pressure is >120 mm Hg
  - —Use nitroprusside, esmolol, or labetalol to slowly lower diastolic blood pressure initially by 10%
  - —Normotensive levels should be achieved over 12–24 hours
  - —May use hydralazine as an alternative
- Treatment of elevated intracranial pressure
  - —Controlled ventilation to $PaCO_2$ of 35 torr
  - —Fluid restriction; elevate head of bed 30 degrees
  - —Mannitol—osmotic diuresis
  - —Use furosemide as an alternative
  - —Correct coagulopathies if present
  - —Consider anticonvulsants: phenytoin

MEDICATIONS

- Esmolol: 0.5–1 mg/kg initial bolus i.v., followed by 50–150 μg/kg/min infusion
- Furosemide: 20–40 mg i.v.; may repeat as necessary (peds: 0.5–1.0 mg/kg/dose)
- Hydralazine: 10–40 mg i.v.; may repeat as necessary (peds: 0.1–0.2 mg/kg/dose)
- Labetalol: 20 mg i.v.; may give additional 40–80 mg i.v. q 10 min to max 300 mg (peds: 0.3–1.0 mg/kg/dose)
- Mannitol: 1 g/kg i.v.
- Nitroprusside: 0.5 μg/kg/min i.v. initially and titrate to effect
- Phenytoin: 15–20 mg/kg/dose at rate of 40–50 mg/h (peds: 0.5–1.0 mg/kg/min)

Disposition

ADMISSION CRITERIA

- To the OR if surgical intervention is indicated
- To the ICU if intubated; altered level of consciousness; or on IV infusion for blood pressure control
- Admit to neurologic observation unit if normal neurologic exam without evidence of progression of bleed, and hemodynamically stable

DISCHARGE CRITERIA

- All patients with intracerebral hemorrhage should be admitted

Miscellaneous

ICD9: 431

ICD10: I61.9

SUGGESTED READINGS

Broderick JP, Adams HP Jr, Barsan W. Guidelines for the management of spontaneous intracerebral hemorrhage: a statement for healthcare professionals from a special writing group of the stroke council, American Heart Association. Stroke 1999;30(4):905–915.

Diringer MH. Intracerebral hemorrhage: pathophysiology and management. Crit Care Med 1993;21(10):1591–1603.

Heiskanen O. Treatment of spontaneous intracerebral and intracerebellar hemorrhage. Stroke 1993;24(12): I-94–I-95.

MacKenzie JM. Intracerebral hemorrhage. J Clin Pathol 1996;49(5):360–364.

Ojemann RG, Heros RC. Spontaneous brain hemorrhage. Stroke 1983;14(4):468–475.

Authors: Atul Gupta; Rebecca Smith-Coggins

Intussusception

Clinical Presentation

SIGNS AND SYMPTOMS

- Classic triad (present in <50% of patients)
  - —Abdominal pain
  - —Vomiting, often bilious
  - —Stools have blood and mucus ("currant jelly" stools)
- Recurrent painful episodes accompanied by pallor and drawing up of the legs; intermittent fits of sudden intense pain with screaming and flexion of legs
  - —Occur in 5- to 20-minute intervals
- Mental status changes
  - —Irritability
  - —Lethargy or listlessness; child can be limp or have a "rag doll" appearance
  - —May preceded abdominal findings
- Stool variable
  - —Heme-positive (occult), bloody or "currant jelly"
- Fever
- Preceding illness several days or weeks prior to the onset of abdominal pain
  - —Diarrhea
  - —Viral syndrome
  - —Henoch-Schönlein purpura
- Abdomen distended and swollen
  - —A "sausage" mass may be palpated in the right upper quadrant
  - —May have absent cecum in right iliac fossa
  - —Peristaltic wave may be present
  - —Rectal examination may reveal bloody stool and palpable mass
- Dependent on the time from onset to diagnosis, perforation with peritonitis and sepsis may be present
- Recurrent intussusception occurs in less than 10% of patients

MECHANISM/DESCRIPTION

- The proximal bowel invaginates into the distal bowel, producing infarction and gangrene of the inner bowel
  - —Greater than 80% involve the ileocecal region
- Often occurs with a pathologic lead point in children >2 years
  - —Hypertrophied lymphoid patches may be present in infants
  - —Children >2 years, one third of patients have pathologic lead point
  - —Children >6 years, lymphoma is the most common lead point
  - —Adults usually have a pathologic lead point
- The most common cause of intestinal obstruction within the first 2 years of life
  - —Most frequently between 5 and 9 months of age
- Epidemiology in the U.S.
  - —The incidence is 2.4 cases per 1,000 live births
  - —Male to female predominance of 2:1
  - —Mortality is less than 1%
- Morbidity increases with delayed diagnosis

ETIOLOGY

- Most cases (85%) have no apparent underlying pathology
- Predisposing conditions that create a lead point for invagination
  - —Masses/tumors
    - -Lymphoma
    - -Lipoma
    - -Polyp
    - -Hypertrophied lymphoid patches
    - -Meckel's diverticulum
  - —Infection
    - -Adenovirus or rotavirus infection
    - -Parasites
  - —Foreign body
  - —Henoch-Schönlein purpura
  - —Celiac disease and cystic fibrosis (small intestine intussusception)

Pre-Hospital

- Intravenous access
- IV bolus of 20 cc/kg of 0.9% NS if evidence of hypovolemia, abdominal distention, peritonitis, sepsis
- Diagnosis rarely confirmed in pre-hospital setting

Diagnosis

ESSENTIAL WORKUP

- The diagnosis is suggested by the history and is proven radiographically
- A heme-positive stool may aid in the diagnosis, particularly in the presence of lethargy or listlessness

LABORATORY

- CBC
- Serum electrolytes, BUN
- Type and cross-match

IMAGING/SPECIAL TESTS

- Abdominal radiograph
  - —Abnormal in 35–40% of patients
  - —Decreased bowel gas and fecal material in the right colon
  - —Abdominal mass
  - —Apex of intussusceptum outlined by gas
  - —Small bowel distention and air-fluid levels secondary to mechanical obstruction
  - —May aid in excluding intestinal perforation
- Enema
  - —Often both diagnostic and therapeutic
    - -74% successful if intussusception present ≤24 hours
    - -32% effective when present >24 hours
    - -More distal the intussusception, the lower the ability to reduce it radiographically
    - -Recurrent disease has similar success to initial episode
  - —Complications include bowel perforation, reduction of necrotic bowel, incomplete reduction with delay in surgery and overlooking pathologic lead point
  - —Barium
    - -Standard for diagnosis of intussusception
    - -Characteristic "coiled spring" appearance
  - —Air
    - -Fluoroscopic guidance
    - -Avoids peritoneal contamination of perforation
  - —Contraindications
    - -Peritonitis
    - -Perforation
    - -Unstable patients secondary to sepsis or shock
- Ultrasound is highly accurate and may be useful as a screening technique; operator dependent
  - —Typical appearance is a "donut" structure, with hyperechoic core surrounded by hypoechoic rim of homogeneous thickness

DIFFERENTIAL DIAGNOSIS

- Infection/inflammation
- Acute gastroenteritis
- Appendicitis
- Inflammatory bowel disease
- Infectious mononucleosis
- Pneumonia
- Pharyngitis/group A streptococcal
- Pyelonephritis
- Colic
- Intestinal obstruction/peritonitis
- Strangulated hernia
- Malrotation/volvulus
- Hirschsprung's disease
- Trauma
- Intestinal vascular/hemorrhagic disorder
- Anal fissure/hemorrhoids
- Ulcer disease
- Vascular malformations
- Protein-sensitive enterocolitis
- Diabetes mellitus
- Coagulopathy

Treatment

INITIAL STABILIZATION

- Intravenous access and initiation of 0.9% NS at 20 cc/kg bolus
- Nasogastric tube

ED TREATMENT

- Stabilize patient hemodynamically
- Surgical consultation
- Abdominal x-ray film series
- Interventional radiography for reduction if no contraindications
  - —Barium enemas are 75–80% successful at reduction, reflecting duration of condition
  - —Recurrences may also be reduced radiographically
- Antibiotics
  - —Initiate if evidence of peritonitis, perforation, or sepsis
  - —Ampicillin, clindamycin, and gentamicin
- Laparotomy
  - —Indications
    - -Enema is unsuccessful
    - -Enema contraindicated
    - -Pathologic lead point
    - -Multiple recurrences
  - —Procedure
    - -Gentle milking of the intussusceptum
    - -Resection of any nonviable bowel as well as any lead points that are identified

MEDICATIONS

- Ampicillin: 100–200 mg/kg q4h i.v.
- Clindamycin: 30–40 mg/kg q6h i.v.
- Gentamicin: 5.0–7.5 mg/kg q8h i.v.

Disposition

ADMISSION CRITERIA

- Patients undergoing successful enema reduction should be observed for 24–48 hours for complications or reoccurrence
- Patients undergoing surgery

DISCHARGE CRITERIA

- May be considered after a prolonged period of observation following successful enema reduction
  - —Stable patient
  - —Symptomatic relief of abdominal pain during the postreduction period

Miscellaneous

ICD9: 560.0

ICD10: K56.1

SUGGESTED READINGS

Champoux AN, Del Becarro MA, Nazar-Stewart V. Recurrent intussusception: risks and features. Arch Pediatr Adolesc Med 1994;148:474–478.

Fecteau A, Flageole H, Nguyen LT, et al. Recurrent intussusception: safe use of hydrostatic enema. J Pediatr Surg 1996;31(6):859–861.

McCabe JB, et al. Intussusception. A supplement to the mnemonic for coma. Pediatr Emerg Care 1987;3:118.

Stein M, Alton DJ, Daneman A. Pneumatic reduction of intussusception: 5-year experience. Radiology 1992;183:681.

Stringer MD, Pablot SM, Brererton RJ. Paediatric intussusception. Br J Surg 1992;79:867–876.

Winslow BT, Westfall JM, Nicholas RA. Intussusception. Am Fam Physician 1996;54(1):213–217.

Author: Roger M. Barkin

Clinical Presentation

SIGNS AND SYMPTOMS

- Ocular pain, red eye
- Photophobia (consensual)
- Lacrimation
- Decreased visual acuity (usually mild)
- Cells and flare in anterior chamber; hypopyon
- Posterior synechiae (adhesions of iris to the lens)
- Miosis
- Low intraocular pressure (occasionally may be high)
- Injection of perilimbal vessels (ciliary flush)

MECHANISM/DESCRIPTION

- An inflammation of the anterior segment of the uvea—anterior uveitis

ETIOLOGY

- Most cases are idiopathic but may be traumatic or associated with numerous infectious and noninfectious systemic diseases

Noninfectious Systemic Diseases

- Ankylosing spondylitis
- Reiter's syndrome
- Sarcoidosis
- Behçet's disease
- Inflammatory bowel disease
- Juvenile rheumatoid arthritis
- Kawasaki syndrome
- Interstitial nephritis
- IgA nephropathy
- Drug reactions
- Sjögren's syndrome
- Psoriatic arthritis

Infectious

- Viral:
  - —Rubella
  - —Measles
  - —Adenovirus
  - —Herpes simplex virus
  - —Herpes zoster virus
  - —HIV
  - —Mumps
  - —Varicella
  - —Cytomegalovirus
- Bacterial:
  - —TB
  - —Syphilis
  - —Pertussis
  - —Brucellosis
  - —Lyme disease
  - —Chlamydia
  - —Rickettsia
  - —Gonorrhea
  - —Leprosy
- Fungal

Malignancies

- Leukemia
- Lymphoma
- Malignant melanoma

Other

- Cocaine use
- Exposure to pesticides
- Corneal foreign body
- Blunt trauma

Pre-Hospital

N/A

Diagnosis

ESSENTIAL WORKUP

- History and review of systems—up to 50% may be associated with systemic disease
- Slit-lamp exam (SLE)—flare and inflammatory cells in the anterior chamber are diagnostic
  - —Flare is a homogeneous fog secondary to protein leakage into aqueous humor
  - —Use short, wide beam to best appreciate cells and flare
  - —Cellular deposits with more severe inflammation
- Intraocular pressure
- If topical anesthesia relieves pain, probably *not* iritis

LABORATORY

- None usually indicated
- Tailored outpatient workup if history, signs, and symptoms point strongly to a certain etiology (with referral to ophthalmology, rheumatology, or internal medicine)
  - —Ankylosing spondylitis: sacroiliac spine x-rays, ESR, HLA-B27
  - —Inflammatory bowel disease: HLA-B27, GI consult
  - —Reiter's syndrome: cultures of conjunctiva, urethra, HLA-B27, rheumatology consult
  - —Psoriatic arthritis: HLA-B27, rheumatology consult
  - —Lyme disease: immunoassays
  - —JRA: ANA, rheumatoid factor, rheumatology consult
  - —Sarcoidosis: ACE, serum lysozyme, PPD, chest x-ray
  - —Sexually transmitted diseases: RPR or VDRL, FTA-ABS, appropriate cultures
  - —TB: PPD, chest x-ray

DIFFERENTIAL DIAGNOSIS

- Conjunctivitis
- Keratitis
- Acute angle-closure glaucoma
- Episcleritis
- Corneal abrasion
- Corneal foreign body

Treatment

INITIAL STABILIZATION

- Goal: reduce inflammation and prevent complications
- Cycloplegic agent (short acting)
  - —Decreases pain, photophobia
  - —Prevents development of posterior synechiae

ED MANAGEMENT

- Cycloplegia
- Topical steroids—if indicated
  - —Use with caution, in consultation with ophthalmologist
  - —May cause significant complications, i.e., progression of HSV keratitis
- Treat secondary glaucoma
- Supportive measures
  - —Warm compresses
  - —Dark glasses
  - —Analgesia
- If specific etiology identified, initiate appropriate management
- Ankylosing spondylitis: systemic antiinflammatory agents, physical therapy
- Inflammatory bowel disease: systemic steroids, sulfadiazine, vitamin A
- Reiter's syndrome: treat urethritis (and sexual contacts)
- Behçet's disease: systemic steroids or immunosuppressive agents
- Infectious causes: appropriate management of underlying infection

MEDICATIONS

- Acetaminophen with codeine: 1 or 2 tabs q4–6h
- Atropine 1%: 1 gt t.i.d. for moderate to severe inflammation (lasts 7–14 days)
- Cyclopentolate 1–2%: 1 gt t.i.d. for mild to moderate inflammation (lasts up to 2 days)
- Homatropine 2% or 5%: 1 gt qd t.i.d. (lasts up to 3 days)
- Hydrocodone 5–10 mg q4–6h
- Prednisolone acetate 1%: 1 gt q1–6h, depending on severity

PEDIATRIC CONSIDERATIONS

- Cycloplegics not recommended in children <6 years
  - —May cause systemic anticholinergic toxicity with blurred vision, flushing, tachycardia, hypotension, and hallucinations

Disposition

ADMISSION CRITERIA

- Not indicated unless significant systemic illness

DISCHARGE CRITERIA

- Refer to an ophthalmologist within 24 hours for follow-up care and possible steroid therapy

Miscellaneous

ICD9: 364.3

ICD10: H20.9

SEE ALSO: RED EYE, CORNEAL ABRASION, GLAUCOMA

SUGGESTED READINGS

Bertolini J, Pelucio M. The red eye. Emerg Med Clin North Am 1995;13(3):561–579.

Rhee DJ, ed. The Will's eye manual: office and emergency room diagnosis and treatment of eye diseases, 3rd ed. Philadelphia: Lippincott Williams & Wilkins, 1999:393–400.

Rothenhaus TC, Polis MA. Ocular manifestations of systemic disease. Emerg Med Clin North Am 1995;13(3):607–630.

Weinberg RS. Uveitis. Ophthalmology Clin North Am 1999;12(1):71–79.

Author: Mary Stewart

Iron, Poisoning

Clinical Presentation

SIGNS AND SYMPTOMS

- Classically divided into 5 stages
  —Stage 1: gastrointestinal (0.5–6 hours)
    -Abdominal pain
    -Vomiting
    -Diarrhea
    -Hematemesis
    -Hematochezia
  —Stage 2: latent/quiescent (6–24 hours)
    -Resolution of GI symptoms
    -Deceptive phase
    -Possible hypotension and acidosis
  —Stage 3: shock and organ failure (6–72 hours)
    -Hypoperfusion
    -Metabolic acidosis
    -Coma
    -Coagulopathy
  —Stage 4: hepatic failure (2–3 days)
    -Coagulopathy
    -Hypoglycemia
    -Jaundice
    -Elevated LFTs and bilirubin
  —Stage 5: obstruction (2–4 weeks)
    -Gastric outlet and small bowel obstruction
    -Abdominal pain, vomiting
- Patient may present in or skip any of the five stages
- If onset of stage 1 does not occur within 6 hours, likely not a significant ingestion

MECHANISM

- Peak concentrations are 2–4 hours postingestion
- Serum concentrations obtained more than 4–6 hours not reliable
  —Enteric coated or sustained release—erratic and may warrant serial levels
- Postabsorption: iron redistributes into the tissues and a *fall* in serum iron occurs as the free iron then causes damage at the cellular level
- Injury patterns
  —Corrosive to the intestinal mucosa, causing damage, profound fluid loss (shock), hemorrhage, and perforations
  —Liver receives the largest load of iron because of portal venous circulation—has the highest injury (hemorrhagic periportal necrosis)
- Free iron
  —Concentrates in the mitochondria, disrupting oxidative-phosphorylation, catalyzes lipid peroxidation, and free radical formation, resulting in cell death and increases anaerobic metabolism and acidosis
  —Causes myocardial depression, venodilation, and cerebral edema
- Hydration of the ferric form yields three protons, resulting in acidosis

ETIOLOGY

- Elemental iron ingestion
  —Nontoxic <20 mg/kg
  —Moderate to severe >40 mg/kg
  —Lethality possible >60 mg/kg
  —Elemental iron equivalents
    -Ferrous sulfate = 20% (325 mg = 65 mg Fe)
    -Ferrous gluconate = 12%
    -Ferrous fumarate = 33%
    -Prenatal vitamins vary from 60–90 mg elemental iron/tablet
    -Children's vitamins may contain 5–18 mg elemental iron/tablet

PEDIATRIC CONSIDERATIONS

- Highest mortality rate among pediatric accidental exposures (adult iron products)
- Children's chewable iron products have been shown to be safe

Pre-Hospital

CAUTION

- Early recognition of iron exposure essential
- Obtain empty bottles to calculate the actual elemental iron exposure dose
- IV fluid resuscitation with 0.9% NS 20 cc/kg bolus for hypotension/shock

Diagnosis

ESSENTIAL WORKUP

- Acute iron poisoning is a clinical diagnosis, regardless of laboratory results

LABORATORY

- Serum iron levels (μg/dL)
  —Peak absorption between 2–6 hours
  —4 hours most common time for peak level
  —Delayed peak with enteric coated/ sustained release
- Electrolytes, BUN/Cr, glucose
  —Anion gap metabolic acidosis
  —Hyperglycemia early
  —Hypoglycemia late
- ABG
  —Metabolic acidosis
- CBC
  —Anemia with significant hemorrhage
  —Leukocytosis
- Liver function
- Coagulation profile
- Lactic acid levels
- Type and screen if hemorrhage
- TIBC is not useful

IMAGING

- Abdominal radiograph check for:
  —Tablets (children's chewables rarely visible)
  —Absence of pill fragment interpretation
    -Patient did not ingest iron
    -Iron was in solution or has already dissolved
    -Patient ingested a pediatric multivitamin product
    -Absence of radiopacities does not rule out a significant or lethal ingestion
  —Perforation

DIFFERENTIAL DIAGNOSIS

- Sepsis
- Acetaminophen toxicity
- Toxic ingestions causing an anion gap acidosis
  —Salicylate
  —Cyanide
  —Methanol
  —Ethylene glycol
- Mushrooms
- Other metals
- Theophylline toxicity
- GI bleed from other causes (alcoholic liver disease)

Treatment

INITIAL STABILIZATION

- ABCs
  - —Airway if needed
  - —Venous access and fluids for hypotension
  - —Cardiac monitor and pulse oximeter
- Narcan, thiamine, dextrose (or Accu-Chek) as needed for altered mental status

ED TREATMENT

Decontamination

- Iron is poorly adsorbed to activated charcoal
- Ipecac and gastric lavage have not been shown to be effective
- $NaHCO_3$, phospho soda, and oral deferoxamine not recommended
- If pill fragments are visualized or history of significant ingestion:
  - —Administer whole bowel irrigation (WBI) with administration of Go-Lytely (peds: 10–15 cc/kg/h; adult: 1–2 L/h) while monitoring progression with KUBs
  - —Caution with GI bleed
- Endoscopy or gastrotomy can remove bezoar formation after massive ingestions (>240 mg/kg)

Chelation with Deferoxamine (DFO)

- DFO is a highly specific chelator of parenteral iron
- IV infusion results in more constant DFO levels and is route of choice
  - —Must be given as soon as possible (<24 hours)
- Administration techniques
  - —Increase IV infusion rate to 15 mg/kg/h over 20 minutes, monitoring for hypotension
  - —Slow the rate if hypotension occurs
  - —Infusion rates as high as 45 mg/kg/h have been used and tolerated
  - —Disregard the manufacturer's recommendation of maximum daily doses of 6 g in serious iron exposures
- IM DFO challenge test is not advocated
- Indication for administration
  - —Sustained GI symptoms
  - —Altered mental status
  - —Hypotension, lethargy, metabolic acidosis, or shock
  - —Serum iron >500 μg/dL
  - —Serum iron >350 μg/dL *and* pills seen on KUB
  - —Rising serum iron levels
  - —Interpret serum levels cautiously—time since ingestion must be considered
    - -Treatment may be indicated in a patient who presents late, after the distribution stage (>8 hours postingestion) with a serum iron level <350 μg/dL
  - —If serum iron levels not readily available, base treatment decisions on clinical course
- Length of infusion (controversial)
  - —DFO-iron complex causes urine to turn *vin rose* color—suggest continuing the infusion until the urine returns to normal
  - —Resolution of signs and symptoms of significant toxicity is criteria for discontinuing DFO
  - —Prolonged DFO therapy longer than 24–48 hours may precipitate ARDS
  - —In severe cases with continued signs and symptoms, the infusion may be continued cautiously at a lower dose
- Controversies
  - —Safety of DFO infusions given for >24 hours
  - —Maximal infusion rates and total amount of DFO given
  - —Serum iron level at which to treat
  - —End point of treatment
  - —Role of extracorporeal elimination
- Contact regional poison centers for moderate to severe iron exposures

Disposition

- Accidental ingestions or ingestions of <20 mg/kg may be monitored at home if brief or no GI symptoms
- Evaluation in the ED warranted in intentional overdoses, or ≥20 mg/kg ingested

ADMISSION CRITERIA

- GI symptoms and/or dehydration
- Any patient who warrants treatment with deferoxamine
- ICU admission for coma, shock, metabolic acidosis, or iron levels >1,000 μg/dL

DISCHARGE CRITERIA

- Asymptomatic with negative radiograph
- Minimal to no symptoms after 6-hour observation
- Mild GI symptoms that have resolved without evidence of metabolic acidosis and serum iron <350 μg/dL

Miscellaneous

ICD9: 964.0

ICD10: T45.4

SUGGESTED READINGS

Anderson BD, Turchen SG, Manoguerra AS, et al. Prospective analysis of ingestions of iron containing products in the United States: are there differences between chewable vitamins and adult preparations? J Emerg Med 2000;19:255–258.

Leikin J, Paloucek F. Iron. In: Poisoning and toxicology handbook. Hudson, OH: Lexi-comp, 2002.

Mills KD, Curry SC. Acute iron poisoning. Emerg Med Clin North Am 1994;12(2): 397–413.

Perrone J. Iron. In: Goldfrank LR, ed. Goldfrank's toxicologic emergencies. East Stamford, CT: Appleton & Lange, 1998.

Tenenbein M. Benefits of parenteral deferoxamine for acute iron poisoning. J Toxicol Clin Toxicol 1996;34(5):485–489.

Tenenbein M. Iron. In: Ford MD, Delaney KA, Ling LJ, et al., eds. Clinical toxicology. Philadelphia: WB Saunders, 2001.

Author: Sean Bryant

Irritable Bowel

Clinical Presentation

SIGNS AND SYMPTOMS

- At least 3 months of continuous or recurrent symptoms (Rome criteria)
  - —Abdominal pain or discomfort that is:
    - -Relieved by defecation or
    - -Associated with change in stool frequency or consistency
  - —Two or more of the following at least 25% of days:
    - -Altered stool frequency (>3 stools/day or <3 stools/week)
    - -Altered stool form (lumpy/hard or loose/watery)
    - -Altered stool passage (straining, urgency, or feeling of incomplete evacuation)
    - -Passage of mucus
    - -Bloating or feeling of abdominal distention
- Other symptoms
  - —Postprandial upper abdominal discomfort (dyspepsia)
  - —Gastroesophageal reflux
  - —Nausea, vomiting
  - —Flatulence
  - —Dysmenorrhea
  - —Dyspareunia
  - —Symptoms tend to be worse around the time of menses
  - —Most patients are women under age 40
  - —Examination usually unremarkable

MECHANISMS/DESCRIPTION

- Dysfunction of the sensory/perception pathways leading to disordered motility to various stimuli, such as meal or rectal distention
- Altered gut sensation due to lower pain threshold (*visceral hyperalgesia*) for pathophysiologic events and increased awareness of normal GI events
- Altered CNS processing of end-organ motor and sensory activity
- Gut irritants such as malabsorbed sugars, food allergen, bile acids, and short-chain fatty acids
- High association with functional dyspepsia
- The mean duration of postprandial motor activity is shorter in patients with irritable bowel syndrome (IBS)
- Patients may have general hyperresponsiveness of smooth muscle not limited to the GI tract (50% of IBS patients have bladder dysfunction or bronchospasm)

ETIOLOGY

- Main cause of ED visits with nonspecific abdominal pain
- Dietary factors
  - —Some vegetables (e.g., broccoli, cabbage, and legumes), lactose, sorbitol, fructose, aspartame, or tyramine rich products
  - —Large meals, fatty, or spicy food causes enhanced gastrocolic reflex
- Bereavement, physical, or sexual abuse in women or during childhood
- Patients adopt the "sick role"; seeking medical attention more than control for non-GI symptoms such as headaches, myalgia, backache, palpitation, and fatigue
- Patients score high on tests of psychoneurotic behavior, and reactions to psychological stress

PEDIATRIC CONSIDERATIONS

- Recurrent abdominal pain, missing many days from school, or chronic nausea

Pre-Hospital

N/A

Diagnosis

ESSENTIAL WORKUP

- Location of abdominal pain, duration, severity, exacerbating factors, associated symptoms, and results of previous workup and treatments
- Detailed history searching for dietary factors or medications
- Sudden onset of symptoms, peritoneal signs, blood or fat in stool, fever, weight loss, or other systemic symptoms should alert to different etiology
- Avoid excessive investigation, especially for patients under age 40

LABORATORY

- To rule out other disorders
- CBC, ESR, C-reactive protein, serum albumin, U/A, LFTs
  - —Normal
- Stool studies for leukocytes, ova, and parasites
  - —Negative
- Serum calcium, TSH, and *Giardia* antibody

IMAGING/SPECIAL TESTS

- KUB: distention of either of the flexures
- Flexible sigmoidoscopy/biopsy for:
  - —Rectal bleeding
  - —New onset of symptoms
  - —Atypical features
- Upper GI endoscopy and ultrasound if upper GI symptoms are most bothersome
- Colonoscopy—rarely helpful especially in patients under age 40
- Screen stool for laxative abuse
- Hydrogen breath test if lactose intolerance suspected

DIFFERENTIAL DIAGNOSIS

- Cholelithiasis/cholecystitis
- Acute diverticulitis
- Small bowel obstruction
- Inflammatory bowel disease (IBD)
  —Family history, tenesmus, rectal bleeding, systemic symptoms, and abnormal lab tests
- Microscopic colitis: watery diarrhea in older patient, and NSAID use
- Endometriosis and PID
  —Abnormal pelvic examination, or ultrasound
- Infectious diarrhea
  —Symptoms after recent exposure or travel to endemic area; particularly giardiasis, amebiasis, *Campylobacter*, and *Yersinia*
- Nonulcer dyspepsia
- Colorectal adenoma or carcinoma: family history or Hemoccult positive stool
- Diverticular disease or diverticulitis
  —Acute onset in older patient with localized tenderness and high WBC
- Intestinal vascular insufficiency in older patients with cardiovascular disease
- Lactose intolerance and laxative abuse
- Chronic pancreatitis
- Diabetes
- Hypo- or hyperthyroidism
- Psychiatric conditions such as depression, anxiety, panic attacks, hypochondriasis, and somatization

PEDIATRIC CONSIDERATIONS

- Other family members, especially mothers, of children with IBS often have a bowel disease, especially IBS

Treatment

INITIAL STABILIZATION

- 0.9% NS IV 500 cc IV fluid bolus for dehydration with vomiting

ED TREATMENT

- Empathetic approach, and therapeutic physician-patient relationship
- Avoidance of dietary factors, and medications that trigger the symptoms
- Counseling abused patients
- Constipation predominant
  —Psyllium seeds, polycarbophil, or methylcellulose, and bowel training
  —If laxative is needed, use warm water enema or oral lactulose, mineral oil, Go-Lytely, or cisapride
- Diarrhea predominant
  —Loperamide
  —Cholestyramine—a bile acid binder, anticholinergic agent
- Pain predominant
  —For postprandial pain use anticholinergic with or without sedative (dicyclomine and hyoscyamine)
  —For chronic pain use tricyclic antidepressant starting with a small dose
- Flatulence
  —Activated charcoal may reduce the odor
  —Simethicone has no effect on abdominal gas
- Selective serotonin reuptake inhibitors (SSRIs)
  —May improve or worsen IBS—use selectively
- For the difficult to manage case
  —Benzodiazepine (clonazepam), in small dose, followed by antihistamine (cyproheptadine)
- Lactose intolerance
  —Lactase capsules: 1–2 PO prior to ingesting milk (if unable to avoid dairy products)

MEDICATIONS

- Cisapride: 10–30 mg PO t.i.d.
- Clonazepam: 0.5 mg PO t.i.d.
- Cholestyramine: 4 g PO t.i.d.
- Cyproheptadine: 4 mg PO t.i.d.
- Dicyclomine: 10–20 mg PO q.i.d.
- Hyoscyamine: 0.125–0.25 mg PO/SL
- Loperamide: 2 mg PO q 4 PRN

PEDIATRIC CONSIDERATIONS

- The need for psychological counseling is more frequent in children than in adults

Disposition

ADMISSION CRITERIA

- Suspicion of an emergent abdominal condition
- Severe symptoms with associated psychiatric disorder
- Uncertainty about the diagnosis

DISCHARGE CRITERIA

- Almost all patients managed as outpatients

Miscellaneous

ICD9: 564.1

ICD10: K58.9

SUGGESTED READINGS

Almounajed G, Drossman DA. Newer aspects of the irritable bowel syndrome. Prim Care Clin North Am 1996;23:477.

Berstad A. Today's therapy of functional gastrointestinal disorders–Does it help? Eur J Surg 1998;suppl 583:92–97.

Camilleri M, Prather CM. Irritable bowel syndrome: mechanisms and practical approach to management. Ann Intern Med 1992;116:1001.

Dromman DA, Whitehead WE, Camilleri M. Irritable bowel syndrome. A review of practice guidelines developed. Gastroenterology 1997;112:2120.

Farthing MSG. Irritable bowel, irritable body or irritable brain? Br Med J 1995; 310:171.

Maxwell R, Mendall MA, Kumar D. Irritable bowel syndrome. Lancet 1997;350: 1691–1695.

Mertz HR. New concepts of irritable bowel syndrome. Curr Gastroenterol Rep 1999; 1(5):433–440.

Authors: Abbas Zagnoon; Craig Huston

Irritable Infant

Clinical Presentation

SIGNS AND SYMPTOMS

General (may be helpful in defining cause)

- Behavior
  - —Degree of irritability
  - —Lethargy
  - —Mental status change
- Vital signs
  - —Fever, oximetry, pulse, respirations, blood pressure
- Hypoxia, cyanosis
- Skin
  - —Purpura
  - —Petechiae
  - —Rashes
- Change in feeding or voiding pattern
  - —Diarrhea
  - —Vomiting
  - —Constipation
- Toxidrome

Nature of Crying

- Onset of crying—sudden, sporadic, or progressive
- Duration
- Intensity
- Type
  - —Screaming
  - —Grunting
  - —Whining
  - —High pitched
- Exacerbating/alleviating factors
  - —Rocking or holding
  - —Feeding or flatulence

MECHANISM/DESCRIPTION

- Most children have some period of the day when they are most irritable, usually toward the evening
  - —Normal infant crying ranges from 1 to 4 hours by 6 weeks of age
- Irritability based on a comparison with the child's normal pattern
- Colic is the most common cause of inconsolable crying in infants, occurring in as many as 25% of healthy children
  - —Episodes of screaming accompanied by drawing up knees and passage of flatus
  - —Usually begins at 2–3 weeks and may continue through 12 weeks
  - —Diagnosis of exclusion

ETIOLOGY

- Infection/inflammation
  - —Minor acute infections (upper respiratory infection, otitis media, thrush, gingivostomatitis)
  - —Urinary tract infection
  - —Meningitis
  - —Osteomyelitis
  - —Pneumonia
  - —Gastroenteritis
  - —Gastroesophageal reflux, esophagitis
- Colic
- Teething
- Constipation
- Parental anxiety
- Trauma
  - —Foreign body, fracture, tourniquet (hair around digit or penis)
  - —Hematoma—subdural, epidural
  - —Corneal abrasion
  - —Child abuse
  - —Diaper pin
  - —Splinter
  - —Anal fissure
- Sickle cell crisis
- Incarcerated hernia, testicular torsion
- Intussusception
- Medications
  - —DPT vaccine reaction
  - —New prescription
  - —Home remedy
  - —Vitamin use/overdose
- Deficiency
  - —Malnutrition
  - —Iron deficiency/anemia
- Hypoxia—cardiopulmonary disorder
  - —Supraventricular tachycardia
  - —Congestive heart failure
- Endocrine/metabolic
  - —Hypoglycemia
- Vascular

Pre-Hospital

- Resuscitate ABCs as necessary

Diagnosis

ESSENTIAL WORKUP

- Manage underlying conditions
- Support child and family
- Obtain complete history including routine feeding, crying, and sleeping patterns as well as birth history
- Perform a thorough physical exam with infant completely undressed

LABORATORY

- CBC, urinalysis, chemistries, and cultures as indicated

IMAGING/SPECIAL TESTS (TO BE PERFORMED AS INDICATED)

- Fluorescein eye exam
- Chest x-ray to exclude cardiopulmonary disease
- ECG
- Skeletal survey
- CT scan of the head
- Stool Hemoccult test
- Contrast x-ray studies such as barium enema for specific indications
- Stat blood glucose at bedside

DIFFERENTIAL DIAGNOSIS

See Etiology, above

Treatment

INITIAL STABILIZATION

- Manage underlying conditions; stabilize ABCs
- Immediate removal of hair tourniquets, splinters, etc.

ED TREATMENT

- Initial evaluation of the child focusing on parent–child interaction and then on potential underlying conditions
- Colic responds to soothing, rhythmic activities, avoiding stimulants (coffee, cola), minimizing daytime sleep
  - —Soy or hydrolyzed casein formula may be transiently beneficial
  - —Parents must reduce stress
  - —No proven pharmacologic therapy
- Support, empathy, close follow-up
- Prolonged observation of the child is usually appropriate

Disposition

ADMISSION CRITERIA

- Life-threatening underlying condition
- Significant parental stress secondary to crying infant

DISCHARGE CRITERIA

- No serious condition
- Functional and supportive family
- Excellent follow-up is essential; parents must feel that their observations and concerns are not being ignored; close follow-up and ongoing observation will occur

Miscellaneous

ICD9: 799.2

ICD10: R68.1

SUGGESTED READINGS

Barnett RM. Psychiatric and behavioral disorders. In: Barkin RM, ed. Pediatric emergency medicine, 2nd ed. St. Louis: CV Mosby, 1997:1042–1055.

Barr RG. Colic and crying syndromes in infants. Pediatrics 1998;102(5 suppl E): 1282–1286.

Garrison MM, Christakis DA. A systematic review of treatments for infant colic. Pediatrics 2000;106(1 pt 2):184–190.

Ruiz-Contreras J, Urquia L, Bastero R. Persistent crying as predominant manifestation of sepsis in infants and newborns. Pediatr Emerg Care 1999;15(2):113–115.

Trocinski DR, Pearigen PD. The crying infant. Emerg Med Clin North Am 1998;16(4):895–910.

Authors: Stacey A. Suecoff; David H. Rubin

Irritant Gas Exposure

Clinical Presentation

SIGNS AND SYMPTOMS

- Depends on water solubility

Highly Water-Soluble Gases

- Eye, nose, throat burning
- Shortness of breath
- Wheezing
- Cough
- Hoarseness
- Stridor
- Obstruction

Intermediate Water Solubility

- Upper and lower tract involvement
- Mucosal irritation
- Bronchospasm
- Dyspnea
- Wheezing
- Cough
- Rales
- Possible delayed pulmonary edema

Other

- Dermal irritation
- Headache
- Nausea
- Vomiting
- Confusion
- Seizures
- Syncope

MECHANISM/DESCRIPTION

- Definition
  —Irritant: any noncorrosive substance that on immediate, prolonged, or repeated contact with respiratory mucosa will induce a local inflammatory reaction
- Respiratory irritants are inhaled as gases, fumes, particles, or liquid aerosols
- Inhaled irritants
  —Pulmonary toxicity determined primarily by its water solubility
  —Cause cellular injury through interaction with respiratory mucosal water with the subsequent formation of acids, alkalis, and free radicals
- Inhalation accidents frequently involve a mixture of irritant gases as well as chemical asphyxiants (carbon monoxide, hydrogen cyanide, hydrogen sulfide, and oxides of nitrogen)

ETIOLOGY

- Settings
  —Industrial: chemical manufacturing, mining, plastics, and petroleum industries
  —Improper use or storage of cleaning chemicals in the home
  —Fires: combustion yields toxic gases
- *Immediate onset of upper airway inflammation* with highly water soluble irritant gases, or with aerodynamic diameter of $>5\ \mu m$
  —Ammonia (fertilizers, refrigerants, dyes, plastics, synthetic fibers, cleaning agents)
    -Immediate symptoms ranging from mild edema and erythema to full-thickness burns and airway obstruction
  —Sulfur dioxide (fumigation of produce, bleaching, tanning, brewing, and wine making; combustion of coal and smelting of sulfide containing ores)
    -Combines with water forming sulfuric acid
  —Hydrogen chloride (formed during combustion of chlorinated hydrocarbons such as polyvinyl chloride)
    -Combines with water forming hydrochloric acid
  —Chloramine (generated when ammonia and bleach are mixed)
    -When exposed to moist surfaces, releases hydrochlorous acid
  —Acrolein (production of plastics, pharmaceuticals, synthetic fibers; formed during combustion of petroleum products, cellulose, wood, paper)
    -May cause protein damage via free radical production and sulfhydryl binding
  —Formaldehyde (production of plywood, particle board, insulation; combustion product of gas stoves and heaters)
    -Combines with water to form sulfuric acid and formic acid
  —Hydrogen fluoride (combustion of fluorinated hydrocarbons)
    -Depletes calcium stores, resulting in cell death
- Latent period of minutes to hours before onset of symptoms with irritant gases of intermediate water solubility or aerodynamic diameter of 1–5 μm
  —Chlorine (product of chlorinated chemicals; a bleaching agent)
    -Upper and lower airway damage after reacting with water to form hydrochloric and hydrochlorous acids
- Delayed onset of symptoms up to 24 hours after inhalation with irritant gases of poor water solubility or aerodynamic diameter of $<1\ \mu m$ (with little or no warning of exposure)
  —Oxides of nitrogen/nitrogen dioxide [produced in the manufacture of dyes, fertilizers, celluloid; acetylene/electric arc welding and gas blowing; fermentation of nitrogen-rich silage ("Silo-fillers disease"); combustion of nitrocellulose and polyamides]
  —Phosgene/carbonyl chloride (arc welding and pesticide production: combustion of chlorinated hydrocarbons, and solvents)
  —Ozone (produced during arc welding)
  —Cadmium oxide (oxyacetylene welding and electroplating)

Pre-Hospital

CAUTIONS

- Rescuers may need to wear appropriate self-contained breathing apparatus and protective clothing to prevent self-contamination

Diagnosis

ESSENTIAL WORKUP

- History of exposure to irritant gases in addition to noted symptoms confirms the diagnosis

LABORATORY

- Arterial blood gas
  - —To assess oxygenation, ventilation, and evidence of acidosis
  - —Pulse oximetry unreliable
- Carbon monoxide level
  - —If smoke inhalation with concomitant irritant gas inhalation (see Carbon Monoxide, Poisoning)
- Methemoglobin level
  - —If oxides of nitrogen are suspected
- Serum calcium level
  - —If hydrogen fluoride is suspected
- Lactate
  - —Elevation may indicate cellular poisoning from carbon monoxide or cyanide
- Pregnancy test in all females of childbearing age
- Rapid dextrose

IMAGING/SPECIAL TESTS

- Spirometry: assess clinical evidence of airway narrowing and bronchoconstriction
- CXR
  - —Initially frequently normal
  - —May take up to 24 hours to reveal pulmonary edema or evidence of diffuse injury
- Direct laryngoscopy to assess evidence of upper airway edema
- Corneal fluorescein for corneal burns
- EKG in elderly, those with cardiac history, or evidence of significant pulmonary symptoms
- Cardiac enzymes if acute coronary syndrome suspected

DIFFERENTIAL DIAGNOSIS

- Asthma exacerbation
- Allergic stimuli (pollen)
- Physical stimuli (cold air)
- Bronchitis
- Pneumonia
- Occupational asthma
- Hypersensitivity pneumonitis
- Congestive heart failure

Treatment

INITIAL STABILIZATION

- ABCs
  - —100% oxygen through a tight fitting non-rebreathing face mask to prevent hypoxia
  - —Early intubation if necessary to protect airway prior to edema
  - —Mechanical ventilation
  - —CPAP or PEEP to enhance oxygenation
- Decontaminate by removing clothes and irrigating skin and ocular tissues

ED TREATMENT

- Inhaled nebulized β_2-adrenergic agonists (albuterol) for bronchoconstriction
- Inhaled/IV/PO corticosteroids: beclomethasone, methylprednisolone, prednisone
  - —Controversial
  - —No controlled trials that document the benefit of acute corticosteroids after irritant gas inhalation
- Nebulized sodium bicarbonate (3.75% solution) after chlorine gas exposure
  - —Reported to improve oxygenation in several case reports/series
- Nebulized calcium gluconate after acute hydrogen fluoride inhalation
  - —Reported, but without proven benefit
- Cyanide antidote kit if hydrogen cyanide is suspected. (see Cyanide, Poisoning)
- Oxygen or hyperbaric oxygen therapy if carbon monoxide poisoning documented

MEDICATIONS

- Albuterol: 0.5 cc (peds: 0.03 cc or 0.15 mg/kg/dose) of 0.5% sol diluted in NS to 3 cc aerosolized
- Calcium gluconate: nebulized (2.5–3% solution) prepared by adding 0.15 g of calcium gluconate to 6 cc of NS
- Metaproterenol: 0.3 cc (peds: 0.1–0.3 cc) of 5% sol diluted in NS to 3 cc aerosolized
- Sodium bicarbonate: nebulized (3 cc of 8.4% sodium bicarbonate mixed with 2 cc of NS to prepare 5 cc of a 5% solution) repeat as needed

Disposition

ADMISSION CRITERIA

- ICU admission for intubated patients, or those with significant respiratory difficulty with potential upper airway obstruction or respiratory insufficiency
- Persistently symptomatic with bronchospasm or oxygen requirement
- Exposure to irritant gases that affect peripheral airways
  - —Delayed pulmonary edema and respiratory failure may occur
- Lower criteria for children, pregnant females, elderly patients, or those with preexisting COPD or coronary disease

DISCHARGE CRITERIA

- Mild exposures that respond well to supportive care, and have no oxygen requirement or bronchospasm after a 4- to 6-hour observation period

Miscellaneous

ICD9: 987.9

SEE ALSO: CYANIDE, POISONING AND CARBON MONOXIDE, POISONING

SUGGESTED READINGS

Bosse GM. Nebulized sodium bicarbonate in the treatment of chlorine gas inhalation. J Toxicol Clin Toxicol 1994;32:233–241.

Newman-Taylor AJ. Respiratory irritants encountered at work. Thorax 1996;51: 541–545.

Rorison DG, McPherson SJ. Acute toxic inhalations. Emerg Med Clin North Am 1992;10(2):409–435.

Vinsel PJ. Treatment of acute chlorine gas inhalation with nebulized sodium bicarbonate. J Emerg Med 1990;8:327–329.

Weiner AL, Bayer MJ. Inhalation: gases with immediate toxicity. In: Ford MD, Delaney KA, Ling LJ, et al., eds. Clinical toxicology. Philadelphia: WB Saunders, 2001.

Weiss SM, Lakshminarayan S. Acute inhalation injury. Clin Chest Med 1994;15(1):103–116.

Author: Sean Bryant

Isoniazid, Poisoning

Clinical Presentation

SIGNS AND SYMPTOMS

Acute Toxicity

- Neurologic
  —Altered mental status
  —Seizures refractory to traditional methods of control
  —Agitation
  —Coma
  —Dizziness
  —Ataxia
  —Hyperreflexia
  —Slurred speech
  —Hallucinations
  —Psychosis
- Gastrointestinal
  —Nausea
  —Vomiting
- Renal
  —Anuria
  —Oliguria
- Cardiovascular
  —Hypotension
  —Tachycardia
  —Shock
  —Cyanosis
- Metabolic
  —Profound anion gag metabolic acidosis
  —Hyperthermia

Chronic Toxicity

- Neurologic
  —Peripheral neuropathy
  —Optic neuritis, optic atrophy
  —Psychosis
  —Insomnia
  —Vertigo
  —Pellagra
- Gastrointestinal hepatitis
  —Liver failure, hepatitis
  —Nausea, vomiting, constipation
  —Anorexia

MECHANISM/DESCRIPTION

- Complexes with and inactivates pyridoxal-5 phosphate, the active form of pyridoxine (vitamin B_6)
- Complexes with pyridoxine, which is then renally eliminated
- Inhibits pyridoxine phosphokinase, hindering the conversion of pyridoxine to its active form
- Interfering with pyridoxine levels yields a net decrease in GABA production
- Depressed GABA causes cerebral excitability and seizures
- Inhibits lactate dehydrogenase, decreasing the conversion of lactate to pyruvate
  —Contributes to the profound anion gap acidosis
- Chronic toxicity
  —Interferes with synthesis of nicotinic acid (niacin)
  —Causes syndrome indistinguishable from pellagra after months of therapy (niacin deficiency)
- Action similar to the MAO inhibitors
  —Reports of a tyramine-like reaction to INH
  —Rare cases of mania, diaphoresis, depression, obsessive-compulsive disorder, and psychosis

Pharmacokinetics

- Rapidly absorbed reaching peak levels within 1–2 hours
- Volume of distribution 0.6 L/kg and 10% protein binding
- Renally excreted within 24 hours after acetylation in the liver
- Half life <1 hour in fast acetylators, and 2–4 hours in slow-acetylating individuals

ETIOLOGY

- High risk includes immigrants, homeless, HIV infected, alcoholics, and lower socioeconomic status populations
- Slow acetylators (60% of African Americans and Caucasians compared to 20% of Asians) are more prone to chronic effects/toxicity
- LD50 in humans estimated to be 80–150 mg/kg
- Ingestions less than 1.5 g lead to mild toxicity, and those of 10 g or more often result in fatality

Pre-Hospital

CAUTIONS

- Induction of emesis contraindicated in light of lowered seizure threshold

Diagnosis

ESSENTIAL WORKUP

- Without specific history of ingestion, initiate general workup for:
  - —Altered mental status
  - —Seizures
  - —Metabolic acidosis

LABORATORY

- ABG
  - —Profound metabolic acidosis
- Electrolytes, BUN/Cr, glucose
  - —Elevated anion gap acidosis
  - —Hyperglycemia
- CBC
  - —Acute toxicity:
    - -Leukocytosis
    - -Eosinophilia
  - —Chronic toxicity:
    - -Agranulocytosis
    - -Eosinophilia
    - -Hemolysis
    - -Anemia

IMAGING/SPECIAL TESTS

- CXR
  - —Presence of tuberculous disease increases suspicion for toxicity
  - —For aspiration pneumonia
- CT/LP if indicated and questionable history

DIFFERENTIAL DIAGNOSIS

- Toxins
  - —Tricyclic antidepressants (TCAs)
  - —ASA
  - —Theophylline
  - —Methanol/ethylene glycol
  - —Paraldehyde
  - —Lithium
  - —Carbon monoxide
  - —Cocaine
  - —Agents that cause metabolic acidosis
- CNS
  - —CVA
  - —Intracranial hemorrhage/mass/trauma/abscess
- Hypoglycemia
- Uremia
- Thyrotoxicosis

Treatment

INITIAL STABILIZATION

- ABCs
  - —Supplemental oxygen
  - —Intubate if necessary for airway protection
  - —Cardiac monitor
  - —0.9% NS access
- Narcan, thiamine, D50W (Accu-Chek) if altered mental status

ED TREATMENT

- Vitamin B_6 (pyridoxine)
  - —Antidote for INH toxicity
  - —Administer 1 g of pyridoxine for each gram of INH ingested (1 g every 2–3 minutes)
  - —Administer 5 g for unknown amount ingested
  - —May repeat in 20 minutes for refractory seizures or persistent coma
  - —If insufficient quantity of pyridoxine available, contact other hospital pharmacies and your regional poison control center to obtain more
  - —If no parenteral pyridoxine available, crush tablets and administer as a slurry in same dose
- Seizure control
  - —Pyridoxine restores deficiency in GABA
  - —Benzodiazepines are synergistic with pyridoxine
  - —Phenytoin has no role
- Gastric decontamination after stabilization
  - —Gastric lavage only in life-threatening ingestions presenting within 1 hour with protected airway
  - —Activated charcoal dosed at 10:1 ratio
  - —Avoid syrup of ipecac
- Dialysis
  - —Persistent symptoms despite adequate therapy
  - —Renal insufficiency in symptomatic patients
- Sodium bicarbonate
  - —For severe metabolic acidosis
  - —Acidosis usually resolves spontaneously after elimination of seizures

MEDICATIONS

- Dextrose: D50W 1 amp (50 mL or 25 g) (peds: D25W 2–4 mL/kg) i.v.
- Diazepam (benzodiazepine): 5–10 mg (peds: 0.2–0.5 mg/kg) i.v.
- Lorazepam (benzodiazepine): 2–6 mg (peds: 0.03–0.05 mg/kg) i.v.
- Naloxone (Narcan): 2 mg (peds: 0.1 mg/kg) i.v. or i.m. initial dose
- Pyridoxine (vitamin B_6): 1 g i.v. for each gram of INH ingested (see above)
- Thiamine (vitamin B_1): 100 mg (peds: 50 mg) i.v. or i.m.

Disposition

ADMISSION CRITERIA

- ICU admission for refractory seizures, severe acidosis, coma, altered mental status
- Uncontrolled nausea/vomiting, unclear history of ingestion, or suicidal

DISCHARGE CRITERIA

- Symptoms are usually observed within 45 minutes of an acute overdose but may be delayed for 2 hours or longer
- Discharge if asymptomatic after 6 hours

Miscellaneous

ICD9: 961.8

ICD10: T37.1

SUGGESTED READINGS

Brent J, Vo N, Kulig K, et al. Reversal of prolonged isoniazid-induced coma by pyridoxine. Arch Intern Med 1990;150: 1751–1753.

Henry GC, Haynes S. Isoniazid and other antituberculous drugs. In: Ford MD, Delaney KA, Ling LJ, et al., eds. Clinical toxicology. Philadelphia: WB Saunders, 2001.

Leikin J, Paloucek F. Isoniazid. In: Poisoning and toxicology handbook. Hudson, OH: Lexi-comp, 2002.

Mcfee RB, Mofenson HC, Carracio TR. Isoniazid poisoning. Emerg Med 2000;32:57–58.

Osborn H. Antituberculous agents. In: Goldfrank LR, ed. Goldfrank's toxicologic emergencies. East Stamford, CT: Appleton & Lange, 1998.

Author: Sean Bryant

Isopropanol, Poisoning

Clinical Presentation

SIGNS AND SYMPTOMS

- Usually occur within 30–60 minutes of ingestion

Neurologic

- Lethargy
- Weakness
- Headache
- Inebriation
- Vertigo
- Ataxia
- Apnea
- Coma
- Initial excitation phase seen with ethanol ingestion is absent

Gastrointestinal

- Nausea/vomiting
- Abdominal pain
- Gastritis
- Hematemesis

Cardiovascular

- Hypotension
- Tachycardia
- Myocardial depression
- Peripheral vascular dilatation

Pulmonary

- Respiratory depression
- Hemorrhagic tracheobronchitis

Dermatologic

- Skin irritation
- Burns

Ocular

- Irritation
- Lacrimation

MECHANISM/DESCRIPTION

- CNS depressant effect of isopropanol is 2–3 times as potent as ethanol
- Many products that contain isopropanol also contain methanol, ethylene glycol, and ethanol
- Rapidly absorbed following oral ingestion
- Ketogenic but does not cause significant acidosis
- Metabolized by alcohol dehydrogenase to acetone (a CNS depressant)
- Acetone eliminated by lung and kidney
- $T_{1/2}$
  —Isopropanol: 3–16 hours
  —Acetone: 7.5–26 hours
- Concomitant ethanol ingestion doubles the half-life of isopropanol but not acetone

ETIOLOGY

- Isopropanol (isopropyl alcohol): clear, colorless, volatile liquid with a faint odor of acetone and a bitter taste
- Available as a 70% rubbing alcohol solution
  —May contain a blue dye that was added to inhibit its abuse ("Blue Heaven")
- Found in:
  —Various toiletries
  —Disinfectants
  —Window cleaning solutions
  —Paint remover
  —Solvents
  —Jewelry cleaners
  —Detergents
  —Antifreeze
- Typical adult patient: a chronic alcoholic who has been on a drinking binge and recently depleted his ethanol supply
- Rectal administration can cause systemic toxicity

PEDIATRIC CONSIDERATIONS

- Accidental ingestions common <6 years old
- Rubbing alcohol sponge baths may cause inhalational toxicity (rare)

Diagnosis

ESSENTIAL WORKUP

- History of ingestion
- Odor of isopropanol or acetone on patient's breath

LABORATORY

- Electrolytes, BUN/Cr, glucose
  —Hypoglycemia occurs
  —Does *not* produce significant acidosis unless accompanied by end-organ hypoperfusion
  —Acetone can produce a false elevation of serum Cr
    -When acetone levels exceeds 40 mg/dL, Cr values rise at approximately 1 mg Cr per 100 mg/dL acetone
    -Cr returns to baseline following acetone metabolism
- CBC
  —Decreased Hct with significant hemorrhagic gastritis
- ABG
  —Acidosis rare unless due to hypoperfusion or co-ingestant
- Urinalysis
  —Ketones present
- Serum osmolality
  —Osmolar gap—difference between measured and calculated osmolality
  —Calculated osmolality $= 2\ Na^{+}\ BUN/2.8 +$ glucose/18 + ethanol/4.3
  —Osmolar gap present if measured minus calculated osmolality >10
  —Gap increases by 1 mOsm/kg for each 5.9 mg/dL of isopropanol and 5.5 mg/dL of acetone
- Serum ketones present
- Isopropanol level
  —Coma with level >150 mg/dL

IMAGING/SPECIAL TESTS

- CXR: for aspiration pneumonia with AMS and vomiting
- CT head: concomitant head injury occurs

DIFFERENTIAL DIAGNOSIS

- For CNS depression and an elevated osmolar gap includes
  —Ethanol
  —Ethylene glycol
  —Methanol
  —Glycerol
  —Mannitol

PEDIATRIC CONSIDERATIONS

- Prone to hypoglycemia following exposure

Treatment

INITIAL STABILIZATION

- ABCs
  - —Maintain the airway and assist in ventilation if necessary
- Hypotension
  - —Treat initially with 0.9% NS IV fluid bolus
  - —Initiate dopamine or norepinephrine infusion if hypotension persists
  - —PRBC with significant hemorrhagic gastritis
- Narcan, thiamine, dextrose (or Accu-Chek) if altered mental status

ED TREATMENT

- Primarily supportive therapy—no specific antidote
- Irrigate skin/eyes for dermal or ocular exposure
- Activated charcoal
  - —For co-ingestants
  - —Large doses can absorb significant amounts of isopropanol
- Do *not* treat with an ethanol infusion or 4-methylpyrazole
- Hemodialysis
  - —Effectively removes isopropanol and acetone
  - —Most managed with supportive care alone
  - —Indications
    - -Hemodynamically instability despite fluid replacement and the use of pressors
    - -Levels >400 mg/dL (associated with severe hypotension and prolonged coma)

MEDICATIONS

- Activated charcoal slurry: 1–2 g/kg up to 90 g PO
- Sorbitol: 1–2 g/kg to a max of 150 g (peds >1 year old: 1–1.5 g/kg as a 35% sol to a max of 50 g) PO mixed in the activated charcoal slurry
- Dextrose: D50W 1 amp (50 mL or 25 g) (peds: D25W 2–4 mL/kg) i.v.
- Naloxone (Narcan): 2 mg (peds: 0.1 mg/kg) i.v. or i.m. initial dose
- Thiamine (vitamin B_1): 100 mg (peds: 50 mg) i.v. or i.m.
- Dopamine: 2–20 μg/kg/min i.v.

Disposition

ADMISSION CRITERIA

- Moderate to severe isopropanol toxicity (altered mental status, hypotension)

DISCHARGE CRITERIA

- Observe asymptomatic patients following ingestion for 2–4 hours before discharge
- Mild intoxication that resolves over 4–6 hours

Miscellaneous

ICD9: 980.2

ICD10: T55.2

SUGGESTED READINGS

Burkhart KK, Kulig K. The other alcohols methanol, ethylene glycol, and isopropanol. Emerg Med Clin North Am 1990;8(4):913–928.

Ellenhorn MJ, Schoonwald S, Ordog G, et al. Isopropyl alcohol. In: Ellenhorn MJ, ed. Ellenhorn's medical toxicology, 2nd ed. Baltimore: Williams & Wilkins, 1997: 1148–1149.

Goldfrank LR, Flomenbaum NE. Toxic alcohols. In: Goldfrank LR, Flomenbaum NE, Lewin NA, et al., eds. Goldfrank's toxicologic emergencies, 6th ed. Stamford, CT: Appleton & Lange, 1998:1049–1060.

Author: Paul Kolecki

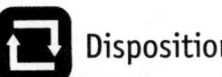

Jaundice

Clinical Presentation

SIGNS AND SYMPTOMS

- Cholestasis
  - —Pruritus
  - —Pale stools
  - —Dark urine
- Malignancy
  - —Anorexia
  - —Weight loss
  - —Malaise
- Abdominal pain
- Right upper quadrant tenderness
  - —Courvoisier's rule
  - —Painless jaundice and a palpable, nontender gallbladder represent malignant common duct obstruction
- Stigmata of cirrhosis
  - —Spider telangiectasis
  - —Palmar erythema
  - —Dupuytren's contractures
  - —Abdominal collateral circulation including caput medusae, hepatosplenomegaly, or hepatic atrophy
  - —Ascites
- Palpable gallbladder
- Hepatomegaly
- Splenomegaly
- Abdominal mass
- Evidence of cachexia
- Kayser-Fleischer rings
  - —Wilson's disease

MECHANISM/DESCRIPTION

- Yellow pigmentation of tissues and body fluids due to elevated serum bilirubin
- *Un*conjugated hyperbilirubinemia: unconjugated bilirubin is the direct breakdown product of heme, is water *in*soluble, and is measured as *in*direct bilirubin
- Causes include
  - —Hemolytic (excessive production of unconjugated bilirubin)
  - —Hepatic (decreased conjugation of bilirubin, Gilbert's syndrome)
  - —Decreased uptake (i.e., physiologic jaundice)
- Conjugated hyperbilirubinemia
  - —Conjugated bilirubin is water soluble and is measured as direct bilirubin
  - —In conjugated hyperbilirubinemia, bilirubin is returned to the bloodstream after conjugation in the liver, instead of draining into the bile ducts
  - —Causes include
    - -Hepatocellular dysfunction (i.e., hepatitis, cirrhosis, tumor invasion, toxic injury)
    - -Intrahepatic (nonobstructive) cholestasis
    - -Extrahepatic (obstructive) cholestasis

PEDIATRIC CONSIDERATIONS

- Physiologic jaundice
  - —Full-term infant: bilirubin peaks on the third or fourth day (about 5.5 mg/dL in white and black infants, and up to 10 mg/dL in Asian infants), then steadily decreases by 1–2 weeks
  - —Premature newborns: peak occurs at day 5 to 7 and returns to normal over several weeks
  - —Pathologic jaundice appears within the first 24 hours
  - -Characterized by rapidly rising bilirubin, prolonged jaundice, or an elevated direct bilirubin (>2 mg/dL or >20% of total serum bilirubin)
  - -Conjugated hyperbilirubinemia in the newborn never has a physiologic cause and must always be investigated
- Breast milk jaundice
  - —Normal prolongation of increased enterohepatic circulation of bilirubin caused by a factor in human milk that promotes intestinal absorption
  - —Elevated bilirubin levels persist in more than two thirds into the third week of life (half of these are clinically jaundiced)
  - —In most breast-fed infants, clinical jaundice resolves by the beginning of the second month of life

Pre-Hospital

N/A

Diagnosis

ESSENTIAL WORKUP

- History and physical examination, together with routine laboratory tests, will suggest the diagnosis in about 80% of patients with jaundice
- Bilirubin level: unconjugated versus conjugated
  - —Severity may suggest cause of obstruction
    - -Malignancy causes highest levels (10–30 mg/dL)
    - -Choledocholithiasis rarely exceeds 15 mg/dL

LABORATORY

- Alkaline phosphatase
  - —If no bone disease or pregnancy, then elevation suggests impaired biliary tract function
  - —2×: hepatitis and cirrhosis
  - —3×: extrahepatic biliary obstruction (i.e., choledocholithiasis) and intrahepatic cholestasis (i.e., drug-induced and biliary cirrhosis)
- Aminotransferases: provide evidence of hepatocellular damage
- Alanine aminotransferase (ALT, SGPT): primarily in the liver
- Aspartate aminotransferase (AST, SGOT): liver, heart, kidney, skeletal muscle, and brain
- GGTP (γ-glutamyl transpeptidase): throughout hepatobiliary system, pancreas, heart, kidneys, and lungs
  - —May be the most sensitive indicator of biliary tract disease
- 5′-Nucleotidase: widespread tissue distribution
  - —Confirms hepatic origin of an elevated alkaline phosphatase level
- Albumin: decreased level associated with severe liver disease
- Prothrombin time: prolonged level is an important prognostic indicator in patients with acute hepatitis

IMAGING/SPECIAL TESTS

- Ultrasound: most effective initial imaging technique
  - —Ductal dilation is a reliable indicator of extrahepatic obstruction
  - —A dilated common bile duct (CBD) and gallbladder suggest distal obstruction, whereas dilation of the intrahepatic ducts (without CBD dilation) suggests proximal obstruction
    - -More than 90% effective in identifying cholelithiasis
  - —Tumors of the liver and head of pancreas usually well visualized
  - —Distinguishes solid liver tumors from cystic structures
- Plain radiographs
  - —May show evidence of hepatic and splenic enlargement or biliary calcifications
- Hepatic nuclear scan (HIDA)
  - —Accurate method of diagnosing acute cholecystitis or cystic duct obstruction because the gallbladder cannot be visualized with these agents
- CT
  - —Superior to ultrasound in detecting pancreatic and intraabdominal tumors
  - —Can help differentiate fluid-containing structures
- Endoscopic retrograde cholangiopancreatography (ERCP)
  - —Diagnostic: stones seen as filling defects within bile duct lumen
  - —Malignancies seen as strictures
- Therapeutic
  - —Extraction of common bile duct stones by insertion of stents to bypass malignant obstructions
  - —Biopsies under direct vision
- Neonatal jaundice workup
  - —Serum bilirubin
- Full-term healthy newborn
  - —Blood group typing of infant and mother, direct Coombs' test, serum bilirubin

- Premature, ill, or significant jaundice (>15 mg/dL): CBC, reticulocyte count, blood smear, direct bilirubin
- Asian or Greek ethnicity (African Americans after oxidative agent exposure): glucose-6-phosphate dehydrogenase (G6PD)

DIFFERENTIAL DIAGNOSIS

- Prehepatic
  —Hemolysis (sickle cell, other hemoglobinopathies)
  —Ineffective erythropoiesis
  —Drugs
  —Gilbert's syndrome
  —Crigler-Najjar syndrome
  —Prolonged fasting
- Hepatocellular
  —Hepatitis (infectious, alcoholic, autoimmune, toxin, drug induced)
  —Cirrhosis
  —Postischemia
  —Hemochromatosis
- Intrahepatic cholestasis
  —Pregnancy
  —Drugs
  —Dubin-Johnson syndrome
  —Rotor's syndrome
  —Benign recurrent cholestasia
  —Familial syndromes
  —Sepsis
  —Postoperative jaundice
  —Lymphoma
- Extrahepatic obstruction
  —Common duct stone
  —Biliary stricture
  —Bacterial cholangitis
  —Sclerosing cholangitis
  —Carcinoma (ampulla, gallbladder, pancreas), cholangiosarcoma
  —Pancreatitis, pancreatic pseudocyst
  —Hemobilia
  —Duodenal diverticula
  —Ascariasis
  —Post-laparoscopic cholecystectomy complications
  —Congenital biliary atresia
  —Congenital choledochal cyst

Pediatric

- Intrahepatic cholestasis
  —Cardiovascular (congenital heart disease, congestive heart failure, shock, asphyxia)
  —Metabolic or genetic (α_1-antitrypsin deficiency, trisomy 18 and 21, cystic fibrosis, Gaucher's disease, Niemann-Pick disease, glycogen storage disease type IV)
  —Infectious (bacterial sepsis, cytomegalovirus (CMV), enterovirus, herpes simplex virus (HSV), rubella, syphilis, tuberculosis, varicella, viral hepatitis)
  —Hematologic (severe isoimmune hemolytic disease)

Treatment

INITIAL STABILIZATION

- Isotonic intravenous fluid therapy if dehydrated
- Toxic-appearing patients
  —Supplemental oxygen, cardiac monitoring
  —Nasogastric suction and bladder catheterization

ED TREATMENT

- For bacterial cholangitis/sepsis, obtain blood cultures and administer parenteral antibiotics
  —Ampicillin, gentamicin, and metronidazole *or*
  —Ticarcillin, or piperacillin, and metronidazole *or*
  —Cefoxitin and tobramycin
- Obstructive extrahepatic jaundice
  —Surgical consult
- Choledocholithiasis
  —ERCP papillotomy, balloon or basket retrieval, or open surgery
- Obstructive intrahepatic or nonobstructive jaundice
  —Medical management
    -Withdraw causative drug, ethanol
    -Interferon for chronic hepatitis B and C
    -Penicillamine and phlebotomy for Wilson's disease and hemochromatosis
    -Corticosteroids for chronic hepatitis of autoimmune origin

PEDIATRIC CONSIDERATIONS

- Exchange transfusion
  —Emergent treatment of markedly elevated bilirubin (>20 mg/dL in full-term infants) and for correction of anemia caused by isoimmune hemolytic disease
- Phototherapy: for neonatal jaundice when bilirubin = 17 mg/dL
  —Measure bilirubin once to twice daily and stop when bilirubin has been reduced by about 4-5 mg/dL
- Phenobarbital: in sepsis and drug-induced causes; decreases conjugated bilirubin
- Metalloporphyrins: investigational inhibitors of heme oxygenase

MEDICATIONS

- Ampicillin: 2 g i.v. q6h (peds: 25 mg/kg i.v. q6–8h)
- Cefoxitin: 2 g i.v. q6h (peds: 40–160 mg/kg/d div. q6–12h)
- Gentamicin: 2–5 mg/kg i.v. q8h (peds: same)
- Metronidazole: 1 g i.v. q12h (peds: 30 mg/kg/d div. q12h)
- Piperacillin/TZ: 3 g i.v. q6h (peds: 300 mg/kg/d div. q6h [>2 months of age])
- Ticarcillin/CL: 3 g i.v. q6h (peds: 75–100 mg/kg/d div. q6h)
- Tobramycin: 2–5 mg/kg i.v. q6h (peds: same)

Disposition

ADMISSION CRITERIA

- Bacterial cholangitis
- Intractable pain
- Intractable emesis
- Associated pancreatitis
- Elevated prothrombin time

DISCHARGE CRITERIA

- No evidence of infection (evaluate as outpatient)

Miscellaneous

ICD9: 782.4

ICD10: R17

SUGGESTED READINGS

Dennery PA, Seidman DS, Stevenson DK. Neonatal hyperbilirubinemia. N Engl J Med 2001;344:581-590.

Frank BB. Clinical evaluation of jaundice: a guideline of the Patient Care Committee of the American Gastroenterological Association. JAMA 1989;262(21):3031-3034.

Gartner LM, Herschel M. Jaundice and breastfeeding. Pediatr Clin North Am 2001;48:389-399.

Lasker MR, Holzman IR. Neonatal jaundice. Postgrad Med 1996;99(3):187-198.

McKnight JT, Jones JE. Jaundice. Am Fam Phys 1992;45(3):1139-1148.

Rossi RL, Traverso LW, Pimentel F. Malignant obstructive jaundice. Surg Clin North Am 1996;76:63-70.

Author: Andrew Chang

Kaposi's Sarcoma

Clinical Presentation

SIGNS AND SYMPTOMS

- Cutaneous
  - —Defining characteristic of Kaposi's sarcoma (KS)
  - —Skin lesions occur most commonly on the lower extremities, face, nose, oral mucosa, and genitalia
  - —Lesions may be red, brown, pink, or purple, depending on vascularity, with occasional yellow perilesional halos
  - —Usually papular, ranging in size from several millimeters to several centimeters
  - —Lesions are painless and nonpruritic
  - —Often elliptical in shape and may be arranged in linear fashion along lines of skin tension; may also be symmetrically distributed
  - —Less commonly may be plaquelike or exophytic and fungating with breakdown of the overlying skin, especially on thighs and soles of feet
  - —Lymphedema of face, genitalia, and lower extremities can occur, often out of proportion to amount of skin lesions
  - —May look like cigarette burns
- Oral
  - —Seen in one third of patients with KS
  - —Most commonly on palate, followed by gingiva
  - —Easily traumatized by normal chewing, causing bleeding, ulceration, and secondary infection
- Gastrointestinal
  - —Involved in 40 percent of patients at initial diagnosis of KS
  - —Lesions can occur anywhere in GI tract, most often in stomach and large bowel
  - —Asymptomatic, or can have weight loss, abdominal pain, nausea and vomiting, upper or lower GI bleeding, malabsorption, diarrhea, or obstruction
- Respiratory
  - —Incidence 21–49% in AIDS patients with cutaneous KS and respiratory symptoms
  - —Rarely seen without cutaneous KS
  - —Lesions can be found in tracheobronchial tree, pulmonary parenchyma, and pleura
  - —Most common presentations are dyspnea and cough; fever and night sweats suggest concomitant infection
  - —Hemoptysis, wheezing, and pleuritic chest pain
  - —Stridor and hoarseness are infrequent and indicate laryngeal or tracheal involvement; life-threatening airway obstruction and hypoxia are rare
- Systemic involvement
  - —Lymphadenopathy even in the absence of cutaneous involvement
  - —Widespread dissemination to visceral solid organs, such as liver, pancreas, heart, testes, and bone marrow, can occur

MECHANISM/DESCRIPTION

- Low-grade vascular tumor associated with human herpesvirus type 8 (HHV-8), also known as KS-associated herpesvirus (KSHV)
- Endothelial cells lining ectatic vascular spaces surrounded by spindle cells admixed with mononuclear immune cells and extravasated red blood cells
- Four epidemiologic forms
  - —Classic: usually indolent, cutaneous proliferative disease affecting elderly men of Jewish and Mediterranean origin
  - —African: found in all parts of equatorial Africa, not typically associated with immune deficiency
  - —Iatrogenic/organ transplant associated: often by transmission of KSHV through solid organ transplant to immunosuppressed host; more severe with cyclosporine use
  - —Epidemic/AIDS related: most common tumor arising in HIV-infected persons
    - -AIDS-defining illness
    - -Male-to-female ratio greater than 20:1
    - -Incidence of new KS cases has declined rapidly since the mid-1990s following widespread use of highly active antiretroviral therapy (HAART)

Pre-Hospital

N/A

Diagnosis

ESSENTIAL WORKUP

- Cutaneous lesions are diagnosed with a simple skin biopsy, rarely done in ED
- Careful oral examination for palate or gingival lesions
- Gastrointestinal involvement best screened for with fecal occult blood; positive occult blood should be followed with endoscopy
- Respiratory involvement should be screened with chest x-ray

IMAGING/SPECIAL TESTS

- Chest x-ray may show nodular, interstitial, or alveolar infiltrates; pleural effusion; hilar or mediastinal adenopathy
- Bronchoscopy is procedure of choice for diagnosis if chest x-ray is abnormal, showing cherry-red nodules
- Thallium-gallium scan shows thallium avid and gallium negative, whereas infections are usually thallium negative and gallium positive
- Chest CT can be used to guide biopsy of extrabronchial lesions
- Endoscopy may show hemorrhagic nodules anywhere in GI tract

DIFFERENTIAL DIAGNOSIS

- Cutaneous lesions: most important is bacillary angiomatosis (BA), caused by *Bartonella* species infection of the skin and treated with antibiotics; BA can occur simultaneously with KS and is diagnosed with Warthin silver stain
- Other skin diagnoses include: purpura of various causes, hematoma, angioma, dermatofibroma, nevi
- Pulmonary KS may be mistaken for *Pneumocystis carinii* pneumonia

Treatment

INITIAL STABILIZATION

- Cutaneous lesions: no specific considerations
- Gastrointestinal: GI bleeding with anemia may require fluid resuscitation and blood transfusion
- Respiratory: airway assessment and possible protection, although acute upper airway compromise is rare

ED TREATMENT

- Usually done for palliation of symptoms
- Consultation with hematologist/oncologist
- Local lesions can be injected directly with vinblastine, usually repeated in 3–4 weeks; alitretinoin (Panretin) gel is approved for topical use of cutaneous lesions
- Radiation therapy can be done for symptomatic disease that is too large for local injection but not extensive enough for chemotherapy, such as large lesions on the sole of the foot
- Systemic chemotherapy can be given for palliation of extensive disease; current first-line agents are pegylated liposomal doxorubicin and liposomal daunorubicin; paclitaxel (Taxol) is a second-line agent; interferon-α has been used with some efficacy
- For AIDS-related KS, treatment with HAART has shown to reduce significantly the development of new KS

MEDICATIONS

- No specific medications commonly used in the ED

Disposition

ADMISSION CRITERIA

- Patients with KS do not require admission solely for KS lesions
- Severe complications of KS such as airway compromise, hypoxia, GI bleeding, bowel obstruction, or secondary infections with sepsis may require admission

DISCHARGE CRITERIA

- Patients with uncomplicated KS may be discharged with appropriate referral

Miscellaneous

ICD9: 176.9

ICD10: M9104/3

SUGGESTED READINGS

Aboulafia DM. The epidemiologic, pathologic, and clinical features of AIDS-associated pulmonary Kaposi's sarcoma. Chest 2000;117(4):1128–1145.

Dezube BJ, Groopman JE. AIDS-related Kaposi's sarcoma: clinical features and treatment [Online]. Available: *http://www.uptodate.com/topics/topics/4363Q5.htm.*

Gascon, P, Schwartz RA. Kaposi's sarcoma: new treatment modalities. Dermatol Clin 2000;18(1):169–175.

Miner JE, Egan TE. An AIDS-associated cause of the difficult airway: supraglottic Kaposi's sarcoma. Anesth Analg 2000;90(5):1223–1226.

O'Connor PG, Scadden DT. AIDS oncology. Infect Dis Clin North Am 2000;14(4):945–965.

Author: Adam Wos

Kawasaki Disease

Clinical Presentation

SIGNS AND SYMPTOMS

- Diagnostic criteria
  —Temperature higher than 38.5°C (often spiking) for at least 5 days
    -Begins abruptly and may last as long as 23 days (average, 11 days)
  —Bilateral conjunctival injection without exudates
    -Bulbar conjunctiva is more frequently involved than palpebral conjunctiva
    -Usually within 2 days of onset of fever and lasting 1–2 weeks
  —Changes in oral mucosa
    -Erythema, dry and fissured lips, strawberry tongue, pharyngeal erythema
  —Cervical lymphadenopathy (node diameter >1.5 cm)
  —Rash, primarily on the trunk
    -May be maculopapular, scarlatiniform, or erythema multiforme-like; erythroderma
  —Changes in the hands or feet—erythema, edema (acute phase); unwilling to bear weight
    -Desquamation (subacute phase) of the tips of fingers and toes 2–3 weeks after onset of illness
- Cardiac
  —Myocarditis
  —Congestive heart failure
  —Pericarditis
  —Myocardial infarction
- Arthralgia, arthritis
- Neurologic
  —Extreme irritability
  —Meningismus
  —CSF pleocytosis
  —Photophobia, uveitis, iritis
- Gastrointestinal
  —Diarrhea
  —Vomiting
  —Right upper quadrant pain
  —Hydrops of the gallbladder
- Cardiac
  —Myocarditis
  —Congestive heart failure
  —Pericarditis
  —Myocardial infarction
- Genitourinary
  —Urethritis
  —Pyuria, proteinuria
- Complications
  —Coronary artery disease caused by arteritis, aneurysm, or thrombosis
  —20% of patients; greatest risk in children <1 year old and >5 years old at onset of disease
  —Onset as long as 45 days after the first of fever

MECHANISM/DESCRIPTION

- Vasculitis most severe in medium-sized arteries, including coronary arteries
- Stages
  —Acute (lasts 1–2 weeks)
    -Fever, oral mucosal erythema, conjunctival injection, erythema and edema of hands and feet, cervical adenopathy, aseptic meningitis, hepatic dysfunction, diarrhea
    -Myocarditis, pericardial effusion, no aneurysms by echocardiography
  —Subacute (when fever, rash and lymphadenopathy resolve until about 4 weeks)
    -Anorexia, irritability, desquamation of hands and feet, thrombocytosis
    -Coronary artery aneurysms visible on echocardiography
    -Risk for sudden death is highest
  —Convalescent phase (about 6–8 weeks)
    -Clinical signs are absent
    -Erythrocyte sedimentation rate (ESR) normalizes
- Epidemiology
  —80% of cases occur in children <4 years old; peak at 1–2 years; rare in infants <3 months old
  —Adult cases have been reported
  —Asians are at highest risk
- Etiology
  —Unknown—thought to be infectious based upon manifestations of disease, epidemics, and increased numbers of cases in winter and early spring

Pre-Hospital

N/A

Diagnosis

ESSENTIAL WORKUP

- Diagnostic criteria
  —Fever for 5 days plus four of the five following criteria
    -Bilateral conjunctival injection
    -Changes in oral mucosa
    -Changes in hands or feet
    -Cervical lymphadenopathy >1.5 cm
    -Rash
- Atypical cases can be seen without meeting diagnostic criteria
- Experienced clinicians can make the diagnosis before 5 days of fever

LABORATORY

- CBC
  —WBC—normally elevated with shift to left in acute phase
  —Normocytic anemia
  —Thrombocytopenia if myocardial infarction or several coronary disease
  —Thrombocytosis usually in second to third week
- Urinalysis
  —Sterile pyuria
- ESR elevated from first week until 4–6 weeks
- Increased C-reactive protein
- Aseptic meningitis
- Cultures: negative blood, urine, CSF, throat
- Increased transaminases and bilirubin

IMAGING/SPECIAL TESTS

- Echocardiogram
  —Acute phase (baseline)
  —2–3 weeks
  —6–8 weeks
- ECG if concern about myocardial infarction or pericarditis
- Slit-lamp exam—uveitis

DIFFERENTIAL DIAGNOSIS

- Viral infections
  —Adenovirus
  —Enterovirus
  —Measles
  —Epstein-Barr virus
  —Rubella
  —Rubeola
  —Stevens-Johnson syndrome
- Bacterial infection
  —Scarlet fever (responds rapidly to penicillin)
  —Staphylococcal scalded skin syndrome
  —Rickettsial disease, including Rocky Mountain spotted fever and leptospirosis
- Drug reaction
  —Stevens-Johnson syndrome
  —Erythema multiforme

Treatment

INITIAL STABILIZATION

- ABCs with focus on cardiovascular system

ED TREATMENT

- Initiate intravenous gammaglobulin (IVIG) and aspirin therapy
  —Do not generally need to monitor salicylate levels because decreased absorption and increased clearance
- Treatment within the first 10 days of illness reduces cardiac sequelae from 20–25% to 2–4%
- Cardiology consultation
- Treatment of myocardial infarctions as in adults

MEDICATIONS

- IVIG: 2 g/kg i.v. over 10–12 hours; retreatment may be required for persistent (>48–72 hours) or recrudescent fever
- Aspirin: 80–100 mg/kg/d PO q6h until about day 14 when fever has resolved; then 3–5 mg/kg/day PO q.d. for 6–8 weeks

Disposition

ADMISSION CRITERIA

- Admit all patients who fulfill diagnostic criteria for Kawasaki disease
- Admit toxic-appearing patients who do not yet meet the criteria for Kawasaki disease

DISCHARGE CRITERIA

- Nontoxic children who do not fulfill diagnostic criteria
- Close follow-up is required

Miscellaneous

ICD9: 446.1

ICD10: M30.3

SUGGESTED READINGS

Burns JC. Kawasaki disease. Adv Pediatr 2001;48:157–177.

Newburger JW. Kawasaki disease. Curr Treat Options Cardiovasc Med 2000;2: 227–236.

Rowley AH, Shulman ST. Kawasaki syndrome. Pediatr Clin North Am 1999;2:313.

Williams RV, Minich LL, Tani LY. Pharmacological therapy for patients with Kawasaki disease. Paediatr Drugs 2001;3:649–660.

Author: Adam Z. Barkin

Knee Dislocation

Clinical Presentation

SIGNS AND SYMPTOMS

- Popliteal artery injury is primary concern
- Grossly deformed knee
- Grossly unstable knee in AP plane, or on varus/valgus stress
  —Anterior and posterior cruciate ligament, and collateral ligament injury
- Lack of distal pulses
- Signs of distal ischemia
  —Pallor, paresthesias, pain, paralysis
- Unequal temperature of lower extremities

ETIOLOGY

- High-energy injuries such as motor vehicle crash, auto versus pedestrian, and athletic injuries
  —Football most common

MECHANISM/DESCRIPTION

- Defined by the position of the tibia in relationship to the distal femur
- *Anterior dislocation*
  —Most common dislocation, accounts for 60%
  —Hyperextension of the knee
  —Rupture of the posterior capsule at 30 degrees
  —Rupture of the posterior cruciate ligament (PCL) and popliteal artery (PA) occurs at 50 degrees
- *Posterior dislocation*
  —Direct blow to the anterior tibia with the knee flexed at 90 degrees
  —Anterior cruciate ligament (ACL) is usually spared
- *Medial dislocation*
  —Varus stress causing tear to ACL, PCL, and lateral collateral ligament (LCL)
- *Lateral dislocation*
  —Valgus stress causing tear to ACL, PCL, and medial collateral ligament (MCL)
- *Popliteal artery injury*
  —PA injury occurs in 33% of dislocations
  —Failure to revascularize within 6–8 hours, amputation rate approaches 90%
  —Anterior dislocations place traction on the PA and cause contusion or intimal injury, which may result in delayed thrombosis
  —Posterior dislocations cause direct intimal fracture or transection of the artery with immediate thrombosis
- *Peroneal nerve injury*
  —Less common than PA injury
  —If present, must rule out concomitant arterial insult
  —Hypesthesia of first web space and inability to dorsiflex foot
  —Poor prognosis for recovery
  —Medial dislocations cause injury by traction to the nerve
  —Rotatory injuries have a high incidence of traction and transection

Pre-Hospital

CAUTIONS

- Documentation of pulses and motor response is essential
- Splint in slight flexion to prevent PA traction or compression

Diagnosis

ESSENTIAL WORKUP

- Complete and careful physical exam including
  —*Pulses*—by palpation, Doppler, ankle-brachial pressure indexes, and distal perfusion
  —*Neurologic*—sensation to the first web space and great toe, movement of the toes, dorsiflexion of the foot
- Knee x-rays
- Repeat examination if any closed reduction is attempted
- Arterial imaging if any signs of limb ischemia exist

IMAGING/SPECIAL TESTS

- AP and lateral plain x-rays
- Angiogram indicated for poor distal perfusion, pulse return after reduction, abnormal pulses, signs of peroneal nerve injury, and ischemic symptoms despite normal pulse

DIFFERENTIAL DIAGNOSIS

- Tibial plateau fracture
- Supracondylar femoral fracture

Treatment

INITIAL STABILIZATION

- ABCs especially when motor vehicle crash or auto versus pedestrian is mechanism
- Fluid resuscitation, hypotension may alter distal pulses and perfusion
- Closed reduction must be performed immediately for any limb ischemia
- Early surgical consultation in an open injury or a high suspicion of arterial injury

ED TREATMENT

- Closed reduction by longitudinal traction and lifting femur into normal alignment without placing pressure PA
- Posterior leg splint in 15 degrees of flexion at knee
- IV analgesia for patient comfort
- Surgical consultation for: open injury, evidence of PA, or unable to reduce dislocation

Disposition

ADMISSION CRITERIA

- All patients require admission for PA repair or to observe limb perfusion

Miscellaneous

ICD9: 836.50

ICD10: S83.1

SUGGESTED READINGS

Ghalambor N, Vangsness CT. Traumatic dislocation of the knee: a review of the literature. Bull Hosp J Dis 1995;54(1): 19–24.

Kendell RW, Taylor DC, Salvian AJ, et al. The role of arteriography in assessing vascular injuries associated with dislocations of the knee. J Trauma 1993;35(6):875–878.

Martinez D, Sweatman MS, Thompson EC. Popliteal artery injury associated with knee dislocations. Am Surg 2001;67(2): 165–167.

Simon RR, Koenigsknecht SJ, eds. Emergency orthopedics, the extremities, 3rd ed, Chap 28. Norwalk, CT: Appleton & Lange, 1995.

Stewart C. Knee injuries: diagnosis and repair. EM Med Rep 1997;18(1):1–12.

Author: Kelly Anne Foley

Labor

Clinical Presentation

SIGNS AND SYMPTOMS

- Symptoms of labor include intermittent low abdominal pain with or without low back pain occurring regularly at least every 5 minutes and lasting 30–60 seconds
- Preterm labor is labor of sufficient frequency and intensity to bring about changes in dilation or effacement of the cervix before 37 weeks' gestational age
- Labor is not associated with vaginal bleeding, and any patient with third-trimester abdominal pain or vaginal bleeding should raise suspicion of placenta previa or placental abruption
- The sudden release of clear fluid from the vagina or a feeling of constant perineal wetness can represent rupture of membranes
  - —This is not always associated with labor but often leads to onset of labor

MECHANISM/DESCRIPTION

- Labor brings about changes in the cervix to allow passage of the fetus through the birth canal
- Synchronous, coordinated contractions of the uterus
- Contractions progress in magnitude, duration, and frequency to produce dilation of the cervix and the ultimate delivery
- Labor is divided into three stages
  - —Stage 1: From the onset of uterine contractions to the full dilation of the cervix; stage 1 is further divided into a latent and active phase
    - -The *latent phase* is a time of uterine contraction with little change in cervical dilation or effacement; contractions are mild, short (<45 seconds), and irregular
    - -This is followed by the *active phase*, which generally begins around the time of cervical dilation of 3–4 cm; contractions are strong, regular (every 2–3 minutes), and last longer (>45 seconds)
  - —Stage 2: From the onset of complete cervical dilation to the time of delivery of the infant
  - —Stage 3: From the time of delivery of the baby to the time of placental delivery
- The total duration of labor varies with each woman
- Generally, the lengths of the first and second stages of labor are significantly longer for the nulliparous woman
  - —Nulliparous: the mean length for the first stage of labor is 14.4 hours and 1.0 hours for the second stage of labor
  - —Parous: The mean length of the first stage of labor is 7.7 hours and 0.2 hours for the second stage of labor
- The length of the second stage of labor is greatly influenced by the "three Ps":
  - —Passenger (infant size and presentation)
  - —Passageway (size of the bony pelvis and soft tissues)
  - —Powers (uterine contractions)
- Problems with any of these three Ps can cause an abnormal progression of labor (e.g., fetal malposition, uterine dysfunction, cephalopelvic disproportion)
- False labor (Braxton-Hicks contractions) is characterized by irregular, nonsynchronous contractions of the uterus several weeks to days before the onset of true labor and does not cause cervical dilation

ETIOLOGY

- Premature labor occurs in 8–10% of pregnancies
- About 30–40% of premature labor is due to uterine, cervical, or urinary tract infections
- Premature rupture of membranes is defined as the rupture of the amniotic/chorionic membranes at least 2 hours before the onset of labor in a patient before 37 weeks' gestation
  - —This occurs in only 3% of pregnancies but accounts for 30–40% of all premature births

Pre-Hospital

- EMS personnel should place patients in labor on oxygen and in the left lateral recumbent position to maximize delivery of oxygen to the uterus
- In cases of hospital transfer of high-risk obstetric patients, maternal transport before delivery has been shown to be quicker, easier, and more cost-effective and results in lower infant morbidity and mortality than the transfer of the neonate after delivery
- Air transport of high-risk obstetric patients has been shown to be beneficial and cost-effective
- Patients in labor who are transported by aircraft should have high-flow oxygen available in the event of cabin decompression at high altitudes

Diagnosis

ESSENTIAL WORKUP

- All patients presenting in possible labor should have an *immediate pelvic exam* to assess dilation, effacement of the cervix, and the possibility of imminent delivery
- A bimanual pelvic exam should not be done in the third-trimester patient with vaginal bleeding until ultrasound can be done to assess for placenta previa or placental abruption
- Patients with suspected rupture of membranes should have a sterile speculum exam with visual examination of the cervix and collection of fluid from the vaginal area
  - —The presence of *ferning* when the fluid is allowed to dry on a slide and examined under a microscope, the presence of *pooling* of fluid in the vagina, and the *change of color of litmus paper* from yellow to blue are suggestive of rupture of membranes
- Patients with preterm labor and with cervical changes should have urinalysis with culture and cervical cultures
- Fetal monitoring should be initiated

LABORATORY

- If patient is in labor, CBC, type, and screen should be sent; urinalysis for proteinuria
- In patients with no prenatal care, obtain Rh factor and antibody screen
- Cervical cultures and urine culture in patients with preterm labor

IMAGING/SPECIAL TESTS

- Not generally needed
- Third-trimester patients with abdominal pain and vaginal bleeding should have emergent ultrasound to evaluate for placenta previa or abruption

DIFFERENTIAL DIAGNOSIS

- Braxton-Hicks contractions are irregular uterine contractions without associated cervical changes
- Round uterine ligament pain, musculoskeletal back pain
- Other common causes of abdominal pain, such as appendicitis

Treatment

INITIAL STABILIZATION

- If delivery is imminent (presenting part visible), prepare for immediate vaginal delivery in the ED (see Delivery, Uncomplicated)

ED TREATMENT

- Unless delivery is imminent, patient should be sent directly to labor and delivery unit
- If transport to labor and delivery will be delayed, or if transfer to another facility is necessary, these steps should be taken
  —IV hydration with 1 L of normal saline or D-5-LR over 30–60 minutes
  —Maternal monitoring and, if available, fetal monitoring
  —If labor needs to be arrested (premature fetus), begin a tocolytic such as the β-agonist terbutaline or $MgSO_4$
    -Magnesium toxicity is suggested by loss of deep tendon reflexes
    -High doses of magnesium can cause cardiac arrhythmias and respiratory depression

MEDICATIONS

- Magnesium sulfate: 4–6 g i.v. over 30 minutes, followed by 2–6 g/h
- Terbutaline: 0.25 mg subcutaneously; may repeat same dose in 30 minutes

Disposition

ADMISSION CRITERIA

- All patients in labor who are not at risk for imminent delivery should be admitted to a labor and delivery department
- Preterm patients in labor demand immediate obstetric consultation and should be admitted to a labor and delivery department for further treatment

DISCHARGE CRITERIA

N/A

Miscellaneous

ICD9: 650.0

SUGGESTED READINGS

Elliott JP, O'Keefe DF, Freeman RK. Helicopter transportation of patients with obstetric emergencies in an urban area. Am J Obstet Gynecol 1982;143:157–162.

Gianopoulos JG. Emergency complications of labor and delivery. Emerg Med Clin North Am 1994;12:201–217.

Parer T. Effects of hypoxia on the mother and fetus with emphasis on maternal air transport. Am J Obstet Gynecol 1982;142:957–961.

Author: James S. Walker

Labyrinthitis

Clinical Presentation

SIGNS AND SYMPTOMS

- Acute onset of peripheral vertigo
  - —Horizontal or rotational
  - —Extinguishable
  - —Positional
  - —Attenuates with fixation
- Associated autonomic symptoms
  - —Nausea and vomiting
  - —Diaphoresis
- No auditory symptoms
- No focal neurological findings
- Labyrinthitis
  - —No consensus on definition
  - —Peripheral vertigo
  - —Single episode of prolonged vertigo lasting days to weeks
  - —Peak onset 30–60 years old
  - —Recent upper respiratory tract infection in 50% of patients
  - —Recovery phase gradual over weeks to months, symptoms predominantly with head movement
- Benign paroxysmal positional vertigo (BPPV)
  - —Positional peripheral vertigo
  - —Recurrent episodes usually last less than 60 seconds
  - —May take months to resolve completely
- The three most common causes of peripheral vertigo are
  - —BPPV
  - —Ménière's disease
  - —Labyrinthitis

MECHANISM/DESCRIPTION

- The labyrinth system
  - —Consists of three semicircular canals (SCCs) and the otolithic organs
  - —The role of the labyrinth is to maintain equilibrium and to direct visual tracking during head movements (vestibuloocular reflex)
- Labyrinthitis
  - —An inflammation that decreases afferent firing from the labyrinth
  - —The CNS interprets this decreased signal as head rotation away from the diseased labyrinth
  - —The resulting imbalance in firing from the labyrinth results in spontaneous nystagmus with the fast phase away from the pathologic side
- BPPV
  - —Otoconia debris dislodged from the utricle stimulates the SCC, causing an increase in afferent firing from the labyrinth
  - —The brain interprets the increased firing as head rotation toward the stimulated SCC
  - —The increased signal causes positional nystagmus with fast phase toward the pathologic side

ETIOLOGY

- Labyrinthitis
  - —Serous—viral or bacterial
  - —Suppurative—bacterial
  - —Chronic
- BPPV
  - —Idiopathic—49%
  - —Posttraumatic—18%
  - —Sequela of labyrinthitis—15%
  - —Sequela of ischemic insult

PEDIATRIC CONSIDERATIONS

- Suppurative and serous labyrinthitis
  - —Usually secondary to acute otitis media, mastoiditis, or meningitis
- BPPV
  - —Onset between 1 and 5 years of age
  - —Symptoms: abrupt onset of crying, nystagmus, diaphoresis, emesis, ataxia
  - —Recurrences for up to 3 years
  - —Migraine-BPPV complex is the most common etiology of pediatric vertigo
- Ménière's disease
  - —Rare before 10 years of age

Pre-Hospital

- Antiemetics for nausea and vomiting
- IV fluids for dehydration
- Fall precautions
- Assessment for acute stroke
- Telemetry for arrhythmia
- Finger-stick glucose to exclude hypoglycemia
- Blood pressure check for hypotension

Diagnosis

ESSENTIAL WORKUP

- Thorough neurologic exam
- Evaluation for peripheral nystagmus
  - —Acute onset
  - —Positional
  - —Fatigable
  - —Attenuation with fixation
- Evaluate for central nystagmus
  - —Acute or gradual onset
  - —Not positional
  - —Nonfatigable
  - —Minimal effect with fixation
- Evaluation for infections
  - —Acute otitis media
  - —Meningitis
  - —Ramsay Hunt syndrome (herpetic lesions on the tympanic membrane)
- Caloric testing
  - —Irrigate external ear canal with cold water for 20 seconds
  - —Normal response causes horizontal nystagmus with the fast phase away from the irrigated ear
  - —Labyrinthitis produces partial or complete loss of response
- Dix-Hallpike maneuver
  - —The patient's head is rotated 45 degrees, the patient is then brought from a sitting position to a supine position with the head extending 20 degrees below the exam table; the maneuver is then repeated with the head turned to the opposite side
  - —Test is positive for BPPV when the patient has latent nystagmus and vertigo that is fatigable with repeat testing
- Orthostatics

LABORATORY

- Finger-stick glucose
- Thyroid function tests
- Syphilis screening
- Rheumatoid factor

IMAGING/SPECIAL TESTS

- EKG and telemetry for arrhythmias
- Head CT with fine cuts through the cerebellum
  - —Patients with suspected central vertigo
  - —Patients over 45 years of age with cardiovascular risk factors
- MRI to evaluate the posterior fossa and the eighth cranial nerve

DIFFERENTIAL DIAGNOSIS

- Peripheral vertigo
  - —Acoustic neuroma
  - —Autoimmune inner ear disease
  - —Benign paroxysmal positional vertigo
  - —Cholesteatoma
  - —Ménière's disease (associated tinnitus)
  - —Otosyphilis
  - —Ototoxic drugs (loop diuretics, aminoglycosides, streptomycin, salicylates, ethanol)
  - —Perforated tympanic membrane
  - —Perilymph fistula
  - —Posttraumatic vestibular concussion
  - —Suppurative labyrinthitis (toxic appearance)
  - —Temporal bone fracture
- Central vertigo—often presents with symptoms indistinguishable from peripheral vertigo because the labyrinth has a monosynaptic connection to the brainstem
  - —Brainstem ischemia
  - —Cerebellar hemorrhage
  - —Inferior cerebellar ischemia
  - —Multiple sclerosis
  - —Partial seizures
  - —Vestibular-masseter syndrome (associated masseter muscle weakness)
  - —Vestibular migraine (30% have vertigo independent of headaches)
  - —Wallenberg's syndrome (associated Horner's syndrome, crossed sensory signs)
- Cardiac arrhythmia
- Hypoglycemia
- Hypotension
- Hypothyroidism

PEDIATRIC CONSIDERATIONS

- Laboratory workup should include evaluation for hypoglycemia and anemia
- EKG to assess for arrhythmia
- Lumbar puncture if any clinical suspicion of meningitis
- Consider toxicology screen, EEG for patients with a loss of consciousness, and MRI or CT to evaluated for posterior fossa pathology

Treatment

INITIAL STABILIZATION

- IV fluid hydration
- Medications to alleviate symptoms
- Medications similar therapy for both labyrinthitis and BPPV
  - —Vestibular suppressants: diazepam, meclizine, scopolamine
  - —Antiemetics: prochlorperazine, promethazine
  - —Corticosteroids
  - —Prednisone taper of questionable benefit for labyrinthitis
- By referral to otolaryngology:
  - —Debris repositioning therapy for BPPV
    - -Epley's maneuver
    - -Semont's maneuver
  - —Vestibular enhancement exercises
  - —Surgery for failed medical and physical therapy

MEDICATIONS

- Diazepam (benzodiazepine): 2–10 mg i.v.; 5–10 mg (0.1–0.3 mg/kg/24h) PO q6–12h
- Meclizine (antihistamine): 25 mg (50 mg/24 h over 12 years old) PO q6h
- Prochlorperazine: 5–10 mg (0.3 mg/kg/24 h i.m. or PO over 2 years old) i.v., i.m. or PO q6–8h
- Promethazine: 12.5–25 mg (1.5—2.0 mg/kg/24 h) i.v. or PO q4–6h
- Scopolamine (anticholinergic, not approved in pediatrics): 0.6 mg PO q4–6h; 1.5 mg transdermal patch q3d

PEDIATRIC CONSIDERATIONS

- Dimenhydrinate: 5 mg/kg/24 h PO, i.m., i.v., or PR
- Bacterial labyrinthitis
  - —Antibiotics IV
  - —Surgical débridement

Disposition

ADMISSION CRITERIA

- Intractable nausea and vomiting
- Severe dehydration
- Unsteady gait
- Symptoms concerning for an acute stroke or central etiology of vertigo

DISCHARGE CRITERIA

- Tolerate oral fluids
- Steady gait
- Normal neurologic exam
- Avoid driving, heights, and operating dangerous equipment
- Fall precautions
- Arrange neurology or otolaryngology follow-up

Miscellaneous

ICD9: 386.0; 386.1; 386.2; 386.30

ICD10: H83.0

SEE ALSO: DIZZINESS; VERTIGO

SUGGESTED READINGS

Cummings CW, Harker LA, et al., eds. Otolaryngology. Saint Louis: Mosby, 1998.

Goebel JA. Management options for acute versus chronic vertigo. Otolaryngol Clin North Am 2000;33(3):483–493.

Hotson JR, Baloh RW. Acute vestibular syndrome. N Engl J Med 1998;339(10): 680–685.

Teach SJ. Dizziness. In: Fleisher GR, Ludwig S, eds. Pediatric emergency medicine, 4th ed. Philadelphia: Lippincott Williams & Wilkins, 2000:217–222.

Tusa RJ. Vertigo. Neurol Clin 2001;19(1): 23–55.

Authors: Paul A. Andrulonis; Charles V. Pollack, Jr.

Laceration Management

Clinical Presentation

SIGNS AND SYMPTOMS

- Lacerations may be accompanied by
  - —Bleeding
  - —Tissue foreign bodies
  - —Hematoma
  - —Pain or numbness
  - —Loss of motor function
  - —Diminished pulses, delayed capillary refill

MECHANISM/DESCRIPTION

- A laceration is a disruption in skin integrity most often resulting from trauma
- May be single or multiple layered

Pre-Hospital

CAUTIONS

- Obtain hemostasis, or control of bleeding with direct pressure
- Unkink any flaps of skin whose blood supply may be strangulated
- Universal precautions

PEDIATRIC CONSIDERATIONS

- Assess for possible nonaccidental trauma

Diagnosis

ESSENTIAL WORKUP

- Mechanism and circumstances of injury
- Time of injury
- History of foreign body (glass, splinter, teeth)
  - —Avoid digital exploration if the object is believed to be sharp
- Tetanus immunization
- Comorbid condition that may impede wound healing
- Evaluate nerve and motor function
- Document associated neurovascular injury
- Assess presence of devitalized tissue, debris from foreign materials, bone or joint violation

LABORATORY

N/A

IMAGING/SPECIAL TESTS

- Evaluation for possible foreign bodies
- Plain radiography
  - —Soft tissue views may aid in visualization
  - —Objects with the same density as soft tissue may not be seen (wood, plants)
- Ultrasonography

DIFFERENTIAL DIAGNOSIS

- Skin avulsion
- Contusion
- Abrasion

Treatment

INITIAL STABILIZATION

- ABCs
- Control of hemostasis

ED TREATMENT

Time of Onset

- Lacerations may be closed primarily up to 8 hours old in areas of poorer circulation
- Lacerations may be closed up to 12 hours old in areas of normal circulation
- On face, lacerations may be closed up to 24 hours if clean and well irrigated
- If not closed, wound may heal by secondary intention or by delayed primary closure (DPC) in 3–5 days

Analgesia and Conscious Sedation

- Adequate analgesia is crucial for good wound management
- Conscious sedation may be required (see Conscious Sedation)

Local Anesthetics

- Topical
  - —TAC (tetracaine, adrenaline, cocaine)
  - —EMLA ("eutectic mixture," lidocaine, prilocaine)
- Local/regional
  - —Lidocaine, bupivacaine
  - —Epinephrine will cause vasoconstriction and improve duration of action
  - —Avoid epinephrine in the penis, digits, toes, ears, eyelids, skin flaps (necrosis), and severely contaminated wounds (impairs defense)
  - —For patient comfort, inject slowly with small-gauge needle; buffer every 9 mL of 1% lidocaine with 1 mL 8.4% sodium bicarbonate
  - —Consider a 1% diphenhydramine solution in the lidocaine allergic patient

Exploration and Removal of Foreign Body

- Indications for removal of a foreign body include
  - —Potential or actual injury to tendons, nerves, vasculature
  - —Toxic substance, or reactive agent
  - —Continued pain

Irrigation and Débridement

- Surrounding intact skin may be cleaned with an antiseptic solution (povidone-iodine)
  - —Do not use antiseptic solution within the wound itself because it may impair healing
- Scrub with a fine-pore sponge only if significant contamination or particulate matter
- Irrigation with 200 mL or more of NS
  - —Optimal pressure (5–8 psi) generated with 30-mL syringe through 18- to 20-gauge needle
  - —Débride devitalized tissue

Wound Repair

- Universal precautions
- Wounds that cannot be cleaned adequately should heal by secondary intention or DPC
- Reapproximate all anatomic borders carefully (e.g., skin-vermilion border of lip)
- Consider tissue adhesive for wounds with clean borders, low tension

Simple Layered Closure

- Simple interrupted sutures
  —Avoid in lacerations under tension
- Horizontal mattress sutures (running or interrupted)
  —Edematous finger and hand wounds
  —Ideal in skin flaps where edges at risk for necrosis
- Vertical mattress
  —For wounds under greater tension

Multiple-Layered Closure

- Closes deep tissue dead space
- Lessens tension at the epidermal level, improves cosmetic result
- Buried interrupted absorbable suture, simple or running nonabsorbable sutures for epidermis

Dressing

- Dress wound with antibiotic ointment and nonadherent semiporous dressing
- Inform patient about scarring and risk for infection, use of sunscreen

Antimicrobial Agents

- Uncomplicated lacerations do not need antibiotic prophylaxis
- Lacerations with high likelihood of infection
  —Human bite to hand (see Hand Infection)
  —Contaminated with dirt, bodily fluids, feces
  —Polymicrobial, enteric prophylaxis
- Tetanus immunization

MEDICATIONS

- See Conscious Sedation
- Tetanus (Td adults, DT peds): 0.5 mL i.m.

Local Anesthetics

- Topical, applied directly to wound with cotton, gauze
  —EMLA (eutectic mixture, 5% lidocaine and prilocaine): apply for 60 minutes
  —TAC (0.5% tetracaine, 1:2000 adrenaline, 11.8% cocaine): apply for 20–30 minutes
- Injected
  —Bupivacaine (maximum dose: 2 mg/kg; duration 3–10 hours)
  —Lidocaine (maximum dose: 4.5 mg/kg; duration 1.5–3.5 hours)

MATERIALS

Suture Materials

Absorbable

- For use in mucous membranes and buried muscle/fascial layer closures
  —Natural—dissolve < 1 week, poor tensile strength, local inflammation
  —Plain catgut
  —Chromic
  —Fast-absorbing gut for certain facial lacerations where cosmesis is important
  —Synthetic braided—tensile strength diminishing over 1 month, mild inflammation
  —Polyglycolic acid (Dexon)
  —Polyglactin 910 (Vicryl)
  —Synthetic monofilament—tensile strength 70% at 1 month, inflammation degree unknown
  —Polydioxanone (PDS)
  —Polyglyconate (Maxon)

Nonabsorbable

- Greatest tensile strength
  —Monofilament
  —Nylon (Ethilon, Dermalon)
  —Polypropylene (Prolene)
  —Polybutester (Novofil): can stretch with wound edema
  —Polyethylene, stainless steel
  —Multifilament
  —Cotton
  —Silk (local inflammation)

Needle Types

- Cutting (cuticular and plastic) types are most often used in outpatient wound repair

Staples

- For linear lacerations of scalp, torso, extremities
- Avoid in hands, face, and areas requiring CT or MRI

Adhesive Tapes (Steri-Strips)

- For lacerations that are clean, small, and under minimal tension
- Avoid in wounds that have potential to become very swollen
- Pretreat wound edges with tincture of benzoin to improve adhesion

Tissue Adhesives

- Good cosmetic results have been achieved in simple lacerations with low skin tension
- An alternative to sutures/staples especially in children

Disposition

ADMISSION CRITERIA

- Few lacerations by themselves necessitate admission unless they require significant débridement or ongoing intravenous antibiotics, or are complicated by extensive wound care issues or comorbid processes (head injury, abdominal trauma)

DISCHARGE CRITERIA

- Wounds at risk for infection or poor healing requiring a wound check within 48 hours
- Time of suture removal dependent on location and peripheral perfusion
  —Scalp: 7–10 days
  —Face: 3–5 days
  —Oral: 7 days
  —Neck: 4–6 days
  —Abdomen, back, chest, hands, feet: 7–10 days
  —Upper extremity: 7–10 days
  —Lower extremity: 10–14 days

PEDIATRIC CONSIDERATIONS

- If it is unsafe for a child to return home if nonaccidental trauma is suspected

Miscellaneous

ICD9: 998.2

SEE ALSO: HAND INFECTION

SUGGESTED READINGS

Chisolm C, Howell JM. Soft tissue emergencies. Emerg Med Clin North Am 1992;10(4):665–705.

Edich RF, Rodeheover GT, Thacker JG. Wound preparation. In: Tintinalli JE, Ruiz E, Krome RL, eds. Emergency medicine a comprehensive study guide, 4th ed. New York: McGraw-Hill, 1996:279–283.

Hollander JE, Singer AJ. Laceration management. Ann Emerg Med 1999;34(3):356–367.

Roberts PA, Lamacraft G. Techniques to reduce the discomfort of pediatric laceration repair. MJA 1996;164(1):32–35.

Author: Gordon Chew

Laryngitis

Clinical Presentation

SIGNS AND SYMPTOMS

- Hoarseness
- Abnormal sounding voice
- Throat tickling
- Feeling of throat rawness
- Constant urge to clear the throat
- Cough
- Fever
- Malaise
- Dysphagia
- Regional lymphadenopathy
- Stridor in infants

MECHANISM/DESCRIPTION

- Inflammation of the mucosa of the larynx
- Peaks parallel epidemics of individual viruses
- Most common during late fall, winter, early spring

ETIOLOGY

- Viral upper respiratory infections most common
  —Influenza A and B
  —Parainfluenza types 1 and 2
  —Adenovirus
  —Coronavirus
  —Coxsackievirus
  —Adenovirus
  —Respiratory syncytial virus
  —Measles
  —Rhinovirus
- Bacterial infections in 10% of cases
  —β-Hemolytic streptococcus
  —*Streptococcus pneumoniae*
  —*Haemophilus influenzae*
  —*Moraxella catarrhalis*
  —Diphtheria
  —Tuberculosis
  —Syphilis
  —Leprosy
- Fungal infections
  —Histoplasmosis
  —Blastomycosis
  —Candidiasis
  —Actinomycosis
- Allergic
- Voice abuse or misuse
- Inhalation of caustic substances or other airborne irritants
- Autoimmune
- Idiopathic

PEDIATRIC CONSIDERATIONS

- Acute spasmodic laryngitis (spasmodic croup)

Pre-Hospital

- Supportive care and ambulance transport are not generally indicated

CAUTIONS

- If there are signs of respiratory distress, epiglottitis should be suspected
  —Transport sitting up
  —Provide supplemental oxygen
  —Intubation may be difficult or impossible and should only be attempted in patients in extremis

Diagnosis

ESSENTIAL WORKUP

- Acute laryngitis
  —In most cases, the history and inspection of the throat suffice to distinguish between viral and bacterial laryngitis
- Chronic laryngitis (>3 weeks)
  —The workup should be directed toward chronic infections, gastroesophageal reflux, neurologic disorders, and tumors
  —Visualization of the larynx should be performed
  —The patient should be referred to ENT for biopsy
  —Visualization of nodules indicate the need to admit to rule out tuberculosis

LABORATORY

- Blood tests are not generally indicated
  —An elevated WBC is not a reliable way to distinguish between bacterial and viral illness
- Throat culture
  —Indicated when throat inspection suggests a bacterial infection

IMAGING/SPECIAL TESTS

- Soft tissue neck films
  —Rarely indicated because direct laryngoscopy provides a more comprehensive assessment
- Direct laryngoscopy
  —Red, inflamed vocal cords, with rounded edges
  —Occasionally hemorrhage or exudate
  —Demonstration of laryngeal pseudomembrane to distinguishing diphtheria from other infectious forms of laryngitis
  —This procedure is mainly used to rule out epiglottitis

DIFFERENTIAL DIAGNOSIS

- Epiglottitis
- Esophageal reflux
- Vocal nodules
- Laryngeal or thyroid malignancy
- Croup/laryngotracheobronchitis
- Foreign body inhalation or other trauma

Treatment

INITIAL STABILIZATION

- Stabilization is only required if the patient show signs of respiratory distress
  - —The patient should be managed for epiglottitis
  - —Supplemental oxygen via a non-rebreathing mask
  - —Orotracheal intubation when time permits in the OR
  - —The neck should be prepped and the equipment ready for a surgical airway

ED TREATMENT

- Antibiotics should be administered only for bacterial infection
  - —Oral penicillin for streptococcal infections
  - —Erythromycin for *M. catarrhalis*
- Steroids may aid in decreasing the time to resolution of symptoms

MEDICATIONS

- Penicillin V: 250 mg q.i.d. PO
- Erythromycin: 250 mg q.i.d. PO

Disposition

ADMISSION CRITERIA

- Tuberculous laryngitis
  - —Highly contagious requiring isolation
- Signs of epiglottitis, respiratory distress, neck trauma, or anaphylaxis

DISCHARGE CRITERIA

- Voice rest (whispering not recommended because it puts further strain on inflamed vocal cords)
- Steam inhalations or cool-mist humidifier
- Increase fluid intake
- Analgesics
- Avoid smoking
- Symptoms usually resolve in 10–14 days if viral cause
- Refer patients with chronic laryngitis to otolaryngologist

Miscellaneous

ICD9: 464.0; 476.0

ICD10: J04.0

SUGGESTED READINGS

Ballenger JI, Snow JB, eds. Otorhinolaryngology head and neck surgery, 15th ed. Philadelphia: Williams & Wilkins, 1996.

Behrman RE, Kliegman R, Jenson H, eds. Nelson textbook of pediatrics, 16th ed. Philadelphia: WB Saunders, 2002.

Lynch JS, Roberti CG. Acute laryngitis. Lippincott's Primary Care Practice: Ear, Nose, and Throat Problems 2000;4(5): 534–538.

Author: Yi-Mei Chng

Larynx Fracture

Clinical Presentation

SIGNS AND SYMPTOMS

- May be subtle or delayed for hours
- Neck tenderness
- Bruising or abrasions over the anterior neck
- Hoarseness or voice changes
- Hemoptysis
- Dysphonia
- Stridor
- Subcutaneous emphysema
- Dyspnea
- Loss of normal cartilaginous landmarks of neck

MECHANISM/DESCRIPTION

- Disruption of any of the cartilaginous structures between the pharynx and trachea
  —Epiglottis, thyroid, arytenoid, cricoid, corniculate, and cuneiform cartilages

ETIOLOGY

- Rare injury, accounts for less than 1% of all blunt trauma
- Blunt trauma to the anterior neck associated with motor vehicle/cycle crash, assault, or recreational activities
- The typical mechanism is hyperextension of neck with a direct blow to the exposed anterior neck
- "Clothesline" injury is a classic mechanism (victim struck in neck by cord, wire, branch, etc., hung across path of travel)

PEDIATRIC CONSIDERATIONS

- Bicycle handlebars—extended neck hits the bar, compressing structures between the bar and vertebral column

Pre-Hospital

CAUTIONS

- Aggressive airway management is necessary: oxygen, suction
- Cervical spine immobilization
- Injury may be overlooked if intubated pre-hospital for other injuries due to loss of subjective complaints

CONTROVERSIES

- Elective intubation not advocated

Diagnosis

ESSENTIAL WORKUP

Radiography

- Cervical spine radiographs—to examine for concomitant spinal injury as well as soft tissue swelling and subcutaneous emphysema
- Chest—to identify pneumothorax, pneumomediastinum, and subcutaneous emphysema
- CT scan of larynx—recommended unless the patient is going directly to the OR
  —Useful even in cases of apparently less severe symptoms and minor abnormalities on indirect laryngoscopy

Fiberoptic Laryngoscopy

- Allows visualization of injuries involving the airway, vocal cords

LABORATORY

- Pulse oximetry
- Arterial blood gas if the patient is having respiratory difficulty—identifies hypoxia, hypercarbia

IMAGING/SPECIAL TESTS

- Arteriography—only if there is a concern that there are associated vascular injuries
- Surgical exploration
- Fiberoptic bronchoscopy and esophagoscopy

DIFFERENTIAL DIAGNOSIS

- Associated injuries
  —Hyoid fracture
  —Thyroid cartilage disruption
  —Recurrent laryngeal nerve disruption
  —Carotid artery injury
  —Phrenic nerve injury
  —Cervical spine injury
  —Hypoxic cerebral injury
  —Airway edema
  —Aspiration pneumonitis
  —Air embolism

PEDIATRIC CONSIDERATIONS

- Pediatric larynx located higher in the neck, more cartilaginous and mobile than adults; thus, pediatric patients are more resistant to laryngeal fractures
- Loosely attached submucosal tissue allows for greater soft tissue trauma, massive edema, and hematoma formation
  —With smaller airway diameters, rapid airway compromise can occur
- Neck tenderness is a more common complaint than dysphagia or dyspnea

Treatment

INITIAL STABILIZATION

- Airway management is of primary concern
  - —Severe injuries of the larynx may require operative management
  - —Early intubation to preclude respiratory embarrassment
  - —Formal tracheostomy under local rather than endotracheal intubation, especially with more severe injuries
  - —*Avoid* repeated intubation attempts—proceed to surgical airway
  - —Cricothyrotomy may be necessary if severe maxillofacial injuries are present and injury is superior to cricothyroid cartilage
  - —*Avoid* cricothyrotomy if a hematoma is seen over the cricothyroid membrane or if there is evidence of cricotracheal disruption
  - —Emergent tracheostomy may be the only option to secure an airway

ED TREATMENT

- Supplemental humidified oxygen
- Elevate head of bed to decrease cerebral and neck soft tissue edema
- IV access
- Consult otolaryngologist for surgical evaluation
- Positive end-expiratory pressure and volume-controlled ventilation for severe pulmonary injury associated with acute respiratory distress syndrome (ARDS) or aspiration pneumonitis

MEDICATIONS

Laryngeal Injury With Subcutaneous Emphysema

- Assume that the mucosa of the upper airway has communicated with the deep tissue of the neck
  - —Ampicillin/sulbactam: 1.5–3.0 g (peds: 50 mg/kg) i.v. q6h
  - —Clindamycin: 600–900 mg (peds: 25–40 mg/kg/24 h) i.v. q8h
  - —H_2 blockers to prevent irritation to mucosal injuries

Laryngeal Edema

- Steroids
  - —Not routinely used, but may be used for massive edema
  - —Dexamethasone: adult: 4 mg i.v.; peds: 0.15–0.6 mg/kg/dose i.v.

PEDIATRIC CONSIDERATIONS

- Elective intubation is potentially dangerous
- Mandatory flexible fiberoptic laryngoscopy
- CT scan if management course in doubt

Disposition

ADMISSION CRITERIA

- Patients with true laryngeal injuries must be admitted to a monitored setting for observation and airway management.; prepare for emergent surgical correction of laryngeal defect
- Patients with suspected laryngeal injury or highly suspicious mechanism must be admitted to a monitored setting for observation and serial flexible fiberoptic laryngoscopic examinations

DISCHARGE CRITERIA

- Patients that have been ruled out for serious laryngeal injury by objective testing and who have no evidence of airway edema or compromise after an appropriate period of observation in the ED (usually 6 hours) can be considered for discharge
- Patients can appear deceptively normal for several hours after injury; if there is any doubt, admit to a monitored setting

PEDIATRIC CONSIDERATIONS

- Mandatory admission recommended in all patients for oximetry, oxygen, and serial fiberoptic laryngoscopy examinations

Miscellaneous

ICD9: 959.09

ICD10: S12.8

SUGGESTED READINGS

Francis S, Gaspard D, Rogers N, et al. Diagnosis and management of laryngotracheal trauma. J Natl Med Assoc 2002;94(1):21–24.

Gold SM, Gerber ME, Hott SR, et al. Blunt laryngotracheal trauma in children. Arch Otolaryngol Head Neck Surg 1997;123(1): 83–87.

Ikram M, Naviwala S. Case report: acute management of external laryngeal trauma. Ear Nose Throat J 2000;79(10):802–804.

Kleinsasser NH, Priemer FG, Schulze W, et al. External trauma to the larynx: classification, diagnosis, therapy. Eur Arch Otorhinolaryngol 2000;257(8):439–444.

O'Mara W, Herbert AF. External laryngeal trauma. J La State Med Soc 2000;152(5): 218–222.

Authors: Diane Devita; David Della-Guistina

Lead, Poisoning

Clinical Presentation

SIGNS AND SYMPTOMS

- Subacute or chronic intoxication is more common than acute intoxication

Constitutional

- Malaise
- Fatigue
- Metallic taste

Gastrointestinal

- Nausea/vomiting
- Anorexia
- Abdominal pain
- Milky emesis (due to lead chloride)
- Black stools (due to lead sulfite)
- Constipation
- Intestinal spasms (lead colic)
- Gingival pigmentation
  - —Dark blue-black discoloration of gingivae at the dental border

NEUROLOGIC

- Insomnia
- Irritability
- Vertigo
- Ataxia
- Headache
- Memory loss
- Peripheral neuropathy
  - —Wrist drop
  - —Paresthesias
- Visual disturbances
- Encephalopathy
  - —Confusion
  - —Delirium
  - —Convulsions
  - —Coma
  - —Papilledema
- Peds: changes in activity level

Renal

- Interstitial neuropathy
- Proteinuria
- Hematuria
- Cast cells
- Nuclear inclusion bodies (lead–protein complexes)

Hematologic

- Basophilic stippling
- Hypochromic/microcytic anemia
- Karyorrhexia (rupture of RBC nucleus)

Dermatologic

- Ashen color
- Retinal stippling
- Lead lines (deposition of lead sulfite along gingival border)

MECHANISM/DESCRIPTION

- Binds to sulfhydryl groups of proteins and enzymes, altering their structure and function
- Interferes with calcium transport, synthesis and release of neurotransmitters, and activity of protein kinase C
- Organic lead much more toxic than inorganic lead
- Intoxication after single oral ingestion rare
- Children absorb 50% of dietary load; adults 10%
- Half-life in bone is 30 years

ETIOLOGY

- Common sources of exposure include
  - —Lead storage batteries
  - —Pigments
  - —Ceramics
  - —Glass
  - —Moonshine whisky (up to 5 years after consumption)
  - —Soldier
  - —Paint (predominately house paint sold before the early 1970s)

PEDIATRIC CONSIDERATIONS

- Toxic neurologic effects more common than in adults
- 25% of affected children with CNS involvement die
  - —40% of survivors have permanent neurologic defects
- Chronic exposure results in decreased intelligence and impaired neurobehavioral development
- Greater level of deposition in bone

Pre-Hospital

CAUTIONS

- Secure ABCs
- Remove patient from exposure
- Treat seizures with benzodiazepines, barbiturates, or other appropriate anticonvulsants
- Treat coma with glucose, thiamine, naloxone, oxygen

Diagnosis

ESSENTIAL WORKUP
- Lead level

LABORATORY
- CBC
  - —Anemia (microcytic or normocytic)
  - —Basophilic stippling of erythrocytes
- Electrolytes, BUN, creatinine, glucose
  - —Increased BUN, creatinine
- Urinalysis
  - —Proteinuria
  - —Hematuria
  - —Cast cells
  - —Nuclear inclusion bodies (lead-protein complexes)

Lead Level
- Store whole blood lead sample in lead-free tubes or tubes containing heparin or EDTA
- Level <10 μg/dL
  - —Normal
- Level 10–25 μg/dL
  - —Decreased intelligence and impaired neurobehavioral development in young children
  - —No effect in adults
- Level 25–60 μg/dL
  - —Headache, irritability, neuropsychiatric effects
  - —Subclinical anemia
- Level 60–80 μg/dL
  - —Gastrointestinal symptoms
  - —Subclinical renal effects
- Level >80 μg/dL
  - —Abdominal pain
  - —Neuropathy
- Level >100 μg/dL
  - —Neuropathy and encephalopathy

IMAGING/SPECIAL TESTS
- Long bone x-rays: lead lines (level >40 μg/dL)
- Abdominal radiographs
  - —For acute ingestion
  - —Lead radiopaque
- Free erythrocyte protoporphyrin
  - —Elevation reflects lead-induced inhibition of heme synthesis
  - —Affects actively forming and not mature erythrocytes and therefore lags lead exposure by few weeks
  - —Nonspecific and may also occur with iron deficiency
- Urinary lead excretion
  - —Increases and decreases more rapidly than blood levels
- CT scan of the head/lumber puncture for altered mental status if indicated

DIFFERENTIAL DIAGNOSIS
- Encephalopathy (hepatic, toxic, infectious, metabolic)
- Arsenic and mercury toxicity
- Cyclic antidepressant poisoning
- Intracerebral hemorrhage
- Sickle cell crisis
- Hepatic porphyrias
- Pancreatitis
- Guillain-Barré
- Peptic ulcer disease
- Gastroenteritis

Treatment

INITIAL STABILIZATION
- Secure ABCs and monitoring
- Control seizures with benzodiazepines, phenytoin, or barbiturates
- D50W, thiamine, naloxone if altered mental status

ED TREATMENT

Decontamination
- Acute oral ingestion
  - —Gastric lavage if recent (<1–2 hours) ingestion
  - —Activated charcoal
  - —Whole-bowel irrigation (if lead-containing material visible on x-ray after initial treatment)
- Dermal exposure
  - —If stable, decontaminate in the ED decontamination room before further evaluation

MEDICATIONS

Chelation Therapy
- Adults with severe encephalopathy
  - —Dimercaprol (BAL): 4 mg/kg i.m., then 4 mg/kg i.m. q4h, *with*
  - —Calcium EDTA: 50 mg/kg i.v. or i.m. over 24 hours q4h to start after the first dose of BAL
  - —*Continue* BAL and EDTA for 48 hours, then check level; if level >90 μg/dL, continue for 5 days
- Adults with mild encephalopathy
  - —Dimercaprol (BAL): 4 mg/kg i.m.; if level >90 μg/dL, give 3 mg/kg q4h i.m. *with*
  - —Calcium EDTA: 75 mg/kg i.v. or i.m. over 24 hours q4h to start after the first dose of BAL
  - —*Continue* BAL and EDTA for 2–7 days until lead level <90 μg/dL
- Adults with mild symptomatic encephalopathy (level 45–70 μg/dL)
  - —Oral DMSA (succimer): 10 mg/kg q8h for 5 days, then q12h for 14 days, *or*
  - —Calcium EDTA: 25 mg/kg infused over 24 hours
- Asymptomatic adults
  - —Remove from exposure and observe
  - —If level is >80 μg/dL, administer oral DMSA (succimer), 10 mg/kg q8h for 5 days, then q12h for 14 days
- Children with acute encephalopathy
  - —Dimercaprol (BAL): 75 mg/m^2 i.m. q4h (max, 450 mg/m^2 in 24 hours), *with*
  - —Calcium EDTA: 1500 mg/m^2 i.v. or i.m. over 24 hours q4h
  - —*Continue* for 5 days and recheck level, repeat for 5 more days if level high
- Children with mild symptomatic encephalopathy
  - —Dimercaprol (BAL): 50 mg/m^2 i.m. (max, 450 mg/m^2 in 24 hours), *with*
  - —Calcium EDTA: 1000 mg/m^2 over 24 hours q4h
  - —*Continue* for 5 days and recheck level; repeat for 5 more days if level high
  - —Aggressive environmental intervention
  - —Follow-up lead level
  - —Oral chelation with DMSA or D-penicillamine (30 mg/kg/d) if levels remain elevated
- Asymptomatic children with levels <25 μg/dL
  - —Aggressive environmental intervention
  - —Follow-up lead level

Disposition

ADMISSION CRITERIA
- All symptomatic patients
- Lead level >60 μg/dL
- IV chelation therapy

DISCHARGE CRITERIA
- Level <60 μg/dL and minimal symptoms or asymptomatic

Miscellaneous

ICD9: 984.9

ICD10: T56.0

SUGGESTED READINGS

Caset R, et al. Longitudinal assessment for lead poisoning. Clin Pediatr 1996;35(2): 58–61.

Ellenhorn MJ, Schoonwald S, Ordog G, et al. Arsenic. In: Ellenhorn's medical toxicology, 2nd ed. Baltimore: Williams & Wilkins, 1997:1563–1578.

Nadig R. Lead. In: Goldfrank's toxicologic emergencies, 6th ed. Norwalk, CT: Appleton & Lange, 1998:1029–1050.

Authors: Meika Neblett; Lisandro Irizarry

Legg-Calvé-Perthes Disease

Clinical Presentation

SIGNS AND SYMPTOMS

- Insidious onset
- Limp
  - —Often presenting complaint
  - —Antalgic gait
- Pain
  - —May be mild
  - —Aching in hip, groin, anteromedial thigh or anteromedial knee
  - —Aggravated by activity
  - —Relieved by rest
- Tenderness over anterior aspect of hip joint
- Joint stiffness
  - —Limitation of internal rotation seen earliest
  - —Limited abduction
- Muscle spasm common complaint early in course of disease
- Muscle atrophy and shortening of leg on affected side late findings
- Otherwise well-appearing and afebrile
- May be asymptomatic

MECHANISM/DESCRIPTION

- Avascular necrosis of all or part of femoral head in children
- Multiple episodes of infarction causing characteristic findings
- Progression through four stages of disease:
  - —Synovitis: brief duration (weeks), reaction to ischemia
  - —Necrosis and collapse of femoral head
  - —Fragmentation: resorption of avascular bone
    - -Deformation of femoral head often occurs at this stage
  - —Reconstitution: formation of new bone
- More common in boys with male-to-female ratio of 4:1
- Most commonly occurs between ages of 3 and 9 years
  - —Range, 2–18 years of age
- Bilateral in 10–15% of cases
- Associated with short stature and delayed skeletal maturation

ETIOLOGY

- Disruption of vascular supply to femoral head with exact underlying cause unknown
- Growing evidence implicating hypercoagulable states
- May be multifactorial

Pre-Hospital

N/A

Diagnosis

ESSENTIAL WORKUP

- Radiographs of hip for evaluation of complaint of limp in children
- Consider and exclude septic arthritis (usually an acute febrile illness)
- If radiographs normal, patient should still be referred to orthopedist for evaluation of limp

LABORATORY

- CBC, erythrocyte sedimentation rate (ESR)
  - —If significantly elevated should raise suspicion for septic arthritis
- See Arthritis, Septic for further discussion

IMAGING/SPECIAL TESTS

- Hip radiographs
  - —Anteroposterior and frog-leg views of hip
  - —Early findings:
    - -Joint space widening from cartilaginous overgrowth
    - -Subchondral fracture (Caffey's sign): crescentic subchondral radiolucency
    - -Minimal lateral shift of femoral head in acetabulum from cartilaginous overgrowth
    - -Minimal joint effusion
    - -Prominence of soft tissues over capsule
  - —Over subsequent weeks:
    - -Increased opacity of femoral head
    - -Fragmentation of femoral head
    - -May see metaphyseal "cysts" (also known as physeal bridge): radiolucent areas in metaphysis representing ingrowth of cartilage from growth plate
    - -May see flattening of femoral head (coxa plana)
- Ultrasound
  - —Evaluate for effusion
  - —Evaluate articular cartilage for thickening and enlargement
  - —Evaluate deformity and containment of femoral head
- Technetium-99m bone scan
  - —Detects changes in femoral head earlier than plain radiographs
  - —Shows decreased uptake in femoral head on affected side
  - —Can help differentiate from transient synovitis
- Magnetic resonance imaging
  - —Shows low signal density in femoral head

DIFFERENTIAL DIAGNOSIS

- Unilateral involvement
  —Transient (or toxic) synovitis
  —Septic arthritis
  —Osteomyelitis
  —Juvenile rheumatoid arthritis
  —Rheumatic fever
  —Trauma
    -Femoral neck fracture
    -Hip dislocation
    -Slipped capital femoral epiphysis
  —Tuberculosis
  —Tumor
- Bilateral involvement
  —Hypothyroidism
  —Epiphyseal dysplasia
  —Gaucher's disease

Treatment

INITIAL STABILIZATION

N/A

ED TREATMENT

- Pain control main ED intervention
  —NSAIDs
  —Muscle relaxants
- May need crutches to avoid weight bearing
- Orthopedic consultation to determine management
  —Very young or minimal involvement usually does well without treatment
  —Restoration or maintenance of range of motion
    -Physical therapy, stretching exercises
    -Traction to relieve muscle spasm sometimes necessary
  —Traction: for a few days to several weeks
    -At home or in hospital
    -Maintains hip in abduction and slight internal rotation
  —Containment of femoral head
    -May be indicated for older children or more severe disease
    -Sphericity of femoral head can be regained if kept within acetabulum to allow molding during remodeling
    -Achieved through orthotic brace or surgical osteotomy
    -Orthotics often poorly tolerated by children

MEDICATIONS

- Diazepam: 0.1–0.2 mg/kg/dose (max, 5 mg) PO q6–8h PRN muscle spasm
- Ibuprofen: 10–15 mg/kg/dose PO q6–8h PRN pain

Disposition

ADMISSION CRITERIA

- Need for admission rare, indicated for:
  —Severe pain or muscle spasm not controlled by oral medications
  —Social considerations
    -Bedrest/care at home not possible

DISCHARGE CRITERIA

- Adequate pain control with oral medications
- Orthopedic follow-up arranged

Miscellaneous

ICD9: 732.1

ICD10: M91.1

SUGGESTED READINGS

Staheli L. Practice of pediatric orthopedics. Philadelphia: Lippincott Williams & Wilkins, 2001:146–151.

Tachdijan M. Clinical pediatric orthopedics. Stanford: Appleton & Lange, 1997: 210–223.

Wall E. Legg-Calvé-Perthes disease. Curr Opin Pediatr 1999;11(1):76–79.

Author: Brandon Backlund

Leukemia

Clinical Presentation

SIGNS AND SYMPTOMS

Chronic Myelogenous Leukemia (CML)

- Asymptomatic
- Fatigue
- Weight loss
- Left upper quadrant pain, tenderness
- Abdominal fullness
- Splenomegaly (most common)
- Later stage
  - —Headaches
  - —Bone pain
  - —Arthralgias
  - —Fever
  - —Leukotactic symptoms
    - -Dyspnea
    - -Drowsiness
    - -Confusion

Chronic Lymphocytic Leukemia (CLL)

- Asymptomatic
- Fatigue
- Lethargy
- Weight loss
- Lymphadenopathy
- Splenomegaly
- Hepatomegaly

Acute Lymphocytic Leukemia (ALL); Acute Myelogenous Leukemia (AML)

- Fever
- Fatigue
- Pallor
- Headache
- Angina
- Congestive heart failure, dyspnea on exertion
- Bone pain
- Granulocytic sarcoma (isolated mass of leukemic blasts)
- Easy bleeding (thrombocytopenia)
  - —Petechiae
  - —Ecchymosis
  - —Epistaxis
  - —Hemorrhage
- Infections (granulocytopenic)
- Organ involvement with advanced ALL
  - —Lymphadenopathy
  - —Hepatomegaly
  - —Splenomegaly
  - —Leukemic meningitis
    - -Headache
    - -Nausea
    - -Seizures

MECHANISM/DESCRIPTION

- Neoplasms of white blood cells that have undergone a malignant transformation
- Hyperleukocytosis
  - —Occurs with WBC $>100,000/mm^3$
  - —Leads to occlusions of small vessels primarily in brain or lungs
  - —Present with confusion, stupor, or shortness of breath

CML

- Overproduction of granulocytic WBCs (neutrophils)
  - —Neutrophil function preserved
- Thrombocytosis
- Basophilia
- Philadelphia chromosome present in bone marrow of >95%

CLL

- Most common leukemia in adults
- Overproduction of monoclonal lymphocytes
- Cells accumulate in lymph nodes, bone marrow, liver, spleen
- Particularly prone to herpes virus infections

Acute Leukemias

- Proliferation of undifferentiated immature cells
  - —AML—immature myeloid cells
  - —ALL—immature lymphoid cells (blasts)
- Rapidly fatal

ETIOLOGY

- Cause unknown
- Familial clustering in CLL
- Increased incidence of AML, ALL, and CML with ionizing radiation

PEDIATRIC CONSIDERATIONS

- Usually have ALL
  - —Most common pediatric cancer
- 60–80% remission in those who are standard risk
- Better overall prognosis, except if under 1 year of age
- May develop leukostasis at lower levels

Pre-Hospital

N/A

Diagnosis

ESSENTIAL WORKUP

- CBC/platelets
  - —CML
    - -WBC range, 10,000–1 million/mm^3
    - -Neutrophils predominate
    - -Thrombocytosis in 50%
  - —CLL
    - -Absolute lymphocytosis >5000
    - -WBC range, 40,000–150,000/mm^3
  - —Acute leukemia (AML/ALL)
    - -Anemia
    - -Thrombocytopenia
    - -Elevation/depression of WBC

LABORATORY

- Electrolytes, BUN, creatinine, glucose, calcium
- Uric acid level
  - —Frequently elevated especially in ALL
- Lactate dehydrogenase
  - —Increased in acute leukemias
- Coagulation profile
  - —Prothrombin time (PT), partial thromboplastin time (PTT), fibrinogen, fibrin-split products
  - —If disseminated, suspect intravascular coagulation
- Blood/urine cultures if fever
- Arterial blood gases/pulse oximetry for shortness of breath

IMAGING/SPECIAL TESTS

- Bone marrow biopsy
  - —Required to make diagnosis
  - —CML—hypercellular with myeloid hyperplasia
  - —CLL—lymphocytosis (30–100%)
  - —Acute leukemia—hypercellular with blast cells, which replace normal marrow
- Leukocyte alkaline phosphatase test
  - —Decreased in neutrophils in CML
- Ph1 chromosome present in CML
- Chest x-ray

DIFFERENTIAL DIAGNOSIS

CML

- Lymphoma
- Myeloproliferative syndromes
- Systemic lupus erythematosus
- Infection—bacterial, fungal, mycobacterial

CLL

- Pertussis
- Infectious lymphocytosis
- Cytomegalovirus
- Epstein-Barr virus/mononucleosis
- Hepatitis
- Rubella

Acute Leukemia

- Aplastic anemia
- Leukemoid reactions to infections

Treatment

INITIAL STABILIZATION

- 100% oxygen for hypoxia/shortness of breath
- IV access with 0.9% NS
- Initiate platelet transfusion for severe bleeding from thrombocytopenia
- Begin broad-spectrum antibiotics for fever and granulocytopenia
- Treat disseminated intravascular coagulation (see Disseminated Intravascular Coagulation)

ED TREATMENT

- Treat leukostasis
  - —Rehydrate with 500-mL bolus (20 mL/kg) i.v. 0.9% NS
  - —Administer acetazolamide to alkalinize urine
  - —Initiate allopurinol
  - —Arrange for leukapheresis
  - —Whole-brain radiation for CNS effects
  - —Administer hydroxyurea for CML: 20–30 mg/kg single dose daily
- Transfuse packed RBCs for symptomatic anemia
  - —May require irradiated, filtered, and HLA-type specific blood

POST-ED TREATMENT

- CLL
  - —Chemotherapy
  - —Prednisone for immune-mediated thrombocytopenia
  - —Radiation to localized nodular masses/enlarged spleen
- CML
  - —Interferon therapy
  - —Chemotherapy
  - —Bone marrow transplantation
- ALL
  - —Chemotherapy
  - —CNS prophylaxis with intrathecal methotrexate/cranial radiation
  - —Bone marrow transplantation
- AML
  - —Chemotherapy
  - —Bone marrow transplantation

Disposition

ADMISSION CRITERIA

- Newly diagnosed leukemia with
  - —Symptomatic anemia
  - —WBC >30,000
  - —Thrombocytopenia
- ICU admission for unstable patients with disseminated intravascular coagulation, blast crisis, or bleeding

DISCHARGE CRITERIA

- Asymptomatic patients without significant laboratory abnormalities

Miscellaneous

ICD9: 208.9

ICD10: C95.9

SUGGESTED READINGS

Abramson N. Leukocytosis: basics of clinical assessment. Am Fam Physician 2000;62(9):2053–2060.

Applebaum FR. The acute leukemias. In: Bennet JC, Plum F, et al., eds. Cecil's textbook of medicine, 20th ed. Philadelphia: WB Saunders, 1996: 936–940.

Keating MJ. The chronic leukemias. In: Bennet JC, Plum F, et al., eds. Cecil's textbook of medicine, 20th ed. Philadelphia: WB Saunders, 1996: 925–935.

Lowenberg B. Acute myeloid leukemia. N Engl J Med 1999;341(14):1051–1062.

Pui C. Acute lymphoblastic leukemia. N Engl J Med 1998;339(9):605–614.

Sawyers C. Chronic myeloid leukemia. N Engl J Med 1999;340(17):1330–1340.

Tsiodras S. Infection and immunity in chronic lymphocytic leukemia. Mayo Clin Proc 2000;75:1039–1054.

Author: Linda Mueller

Lightning Injuries

Clinical Presentation

SIGNS AND SYMPTOMS

Cardiorespiratory

- Cardiac asystole
  - —Due to direct current injury
  - —May resolve spontaneously as the heart's intrinsic automaticity resumes
- Respiratory arrest
  - —Due to paralysis of medullary respiratory center
  - —May persist longer than cardiac asystole and lead to hypoxia-induced ventricular fibrillation
- Rarely, acute myocardial infarction
- Shock
  - —Neurogenic (spinal injury)
  - —Hypovolemic (trauma)
- Mottled or cold extremities
  - —Due to autonomic vasomotor instability
  - —Usually resolves spontaneously in a few hours

Neurological Injuries

- Confusion, cognitive or memory defects
- Altered level of consciousness (>70% of cases)
- Flaccid motor paralysis
- Seizures
- Fixed dilated pupils due either to serious head injury or autonomic dysfunction

Traumatic Injuries

- Blunt trauma
  - —To the head or spine
  - —Fractures, dislocations, muscle tears, and compartment syndromes
- Ruptured tympanic membrane with ossicular disruption (up to 50%)
- Burns
  - —Discrete entrance and exit wounds uncommon
  - —Thermal burns can arise from evaporation of water on skin, ignited clothing, heated metal objects (buckles/jewelry)
    - -Direct thermal injury is uncommon due to the brevity of electrical currents
- Feathering (fernlike pattern) "burns"
  - —Cutaneous imprints from electron showers that track over skin
  - —Pathognomonic of lightning injury
  - —Resolve within 24 hours

Ophthalmologic Injuries

- Cataracts occur days to years after injury
- Corneal lesions
- Intraocular hemorrhages
- Retinal detachment

MECHANISM/DESCRIPTION

- Due to the brief duration (1–100 milliseconds) of lightning
  - —Current passes over the skin rather than through the body (flashover)
  - —Deep tissue injuries are rare
- Mechanisms of injury
  - —Direct strike
  - —Splash injury
    - -Current moves from another object to the victim
  - —Ground strike
    - -Current moves through ground surface and may injure multiple victims
  - —Blunt injury due to atmospheric shock wave, fall
  - —Thermal burning

Pre-Hospital

CONTROVERSIES

- Field triage should rapidly focus on providing ventilatory support to unconscious victims or those in cardiopulmonary arrest
  - —Prevents reversible asystolic cardiac arrest from degenerating into hypoxia-induced ventricular fibrillation
- Conscious victims are at lower risk for imminent demise

CAUTIONS

- Spine immobilization for
  - —Cardiopulmonary arrest (suspected trauma)
  - —Significant mechanical trauma
  - —Suspected loss of consciousness at any time
- Cover superficial burns with sterile saline dressings
- Immobilize injured extremities
- Rapid extrication to decrease risk for repeat lightning strikes

Diagnosis

ESSENTIAL WORKUP

- Confirmatory history from bystanders or rescuers of the circumstances of the injury

LABORATORY

- CBC for baseline hematocrit
- Urinalysis for myoglobin
- Electrolytes for acidosis
- BUN, creatinine for renal function
- Troponin, creatine kinase (CK), and cardiac enzymes for muscle/cardiac damage

IMAGING/SPECIAL TESTS

- X-rays
  - —Chest x-ray
  - —Cervical spine
  - —CT head for altered mental status or significant head trauma
  - —Relevant imaging for specific injuries
- EKG
  - —Nonspecific ST changes common
  - —Acute myocardial infarction rare

DIFFERENTIAL DIAGNOSIS

- Consider lightning strike in unwitnessed falls, cardiac arrests, or unexplained coma in an outdoor setting
- Lightning can strike indoor victims who are handling ungrounded electrical equipment or telephones
- Other causes of coma, cardiac dysrhythmia, or trauma:
  - —Hypoglycemia
  - —Intoxication
  - —Drug overdose
  - —Cardiovascular disease
  - —Cerebrovascular accident (CVA)

Treatment

INITIAL STABILIZATION

- ABCs
- Standard advanced cardiac life support (ACLS) measures for cardiac arrest
- Diligent primary and secondary survey for traumatic injuries and other causes of collapse/injury
  - —Maintain cervical spine precautions until cleared
- Treat altered mental status with glucose, naloxone, or thiamine as indicated
- Hypotension requires volume expansion and pressor agents

ED TREATMENT

- IV access for medication administration
- Clean and dress burns
- Tetanus prophylaxis
- Treat myoglobinuria if present
  - —Diuretics, such as furosemide or mannitol
  - —Alkalinize urine to a pH = 7.45
  - —Maintain urine output with IV fluid administration
- Volume expansion
  - —Do not follow burn treatment formulas because flashover burns are rarely the cause of fluid loss
  - —Occult deep burn injury is rare when compared with other types of electrical current injury
  - —Titrate volume administration to urine output
    - -Fluid loading may be dangerous with head injuries
- Compartment syndrome
  - —Must be distinguished from vasospasm, autonomic dysfunction, and paralysis, which are usually self-limited phenomena
  - —Delay fasciotomy if possible because it will rarely be necessary
- NSAIDs and high-dose steroids have been proposed to reduce long-term neurologic and corneal damage

MEDICATIONS

- Furosemide: 1 mg/kg i.v. slow bolus q6h
- Mannitol: 0.5 mg/kg i.v., repeat PRN
- Sodium bicarbonate: 1 amp i.v. push (peds: 1 mEq/kg) followed by 2–3 amps/L D5W i.v. fluid

Disposition

ADMISSION CRITERIA

- Seriously injured and postcardiac arrest victims
- History of change in mental status/altered level of consciousness
- Myoglobinuria
- Acidosis
- History dysrhythmias or EKG changes
  - —May not resolve spontaneously
  - —24- to 48-hour observation period to identify potentially unstable cases

DISCHARGE CRITERIA

- Asymptomatic patients with no injuries
- Close follow-up required owing to the risk for delayed sequelae
  - —Neurologic
  - —Psychological
  - —Ophthalmologic

Miscellaneous

ICD9: 994.0

ICD10: T75.0

SEE ALSO: ELECTRICAL INJURY

SUGGESTED READINGS

Browne BJ, Gaasch WR. Lightening. Emerg Med Clin North Am 1992;10:2:211–230.

Cooper MA. Lightning injuries. In: Marx JA, Hockenberger RS, Walls RM, et al. eds. Rosen's emergency medicine, 5th ed. Philadelphia: Mosby, 2002.

Cooper MA, Andrew CJ. Lightning injuries. In: Auerbach P, ed. Wilderness medicine. St. Louis: CV Mosby, 1995:261–290.

Lichtenberg R, et al. Cardiovascular effects of lightning strikes. J Am Coll Cardiol 1993;21(2):531–536.

Author: Paul Arnold

Lithium, Poisoning

Clinical Presentation

SIGNS AND SYMPTOMS

Acute Toxicity

- Generally less common and less serious

Neurologic

- Mild
  - —Weakness
  - —Fine tremor
  - —Lightheadedness
- Moderate
  - —Ataxia
  - —Slurred speech
  - —Blurred vision
  - —Tinnitus
  - —Profound weakness
  - —Coarse tremor
  - —Fasciculations
  - —Hyperreflexia
  - —Apathy
- Severe
  - —Confusion
  - —Coma
  - —Clonus
  - —Extrapyramidal symptoms
  - —Seizure

Gastrointestinal

- Very common
- Nausea/vomiting
- Diarrhea
- Abdominal pain

Cardiac

- Prolonged QT, ST depression
- T-wave flattening *most common* EKG abnormality
- U waves
- Serious arrhythmia (rare)

Chronic Toxicity

Neurologic

- Most common signs and symptoms
- Same symptoms as acute
- Severe toxicity:
  - —Parkinson's type symptoms
  - —Psychosis
  - —Memory deficits

Renal

- Nephrogenic diabetes insipidus
- Interstitial nephritis
- Distal tubular acidosis
- Direct cellular damage

Dermatologic

- Dermatitis
- Ulcers
- Localized edema

Endocrine

- Hypothyroidism

Hematologic

- Leukocytosis
- Aplastic anemia

MECHANISM/DESCRIPTION

- Oral absorption is rapid
  - —Regular release: peak serum levels 2–4 hours
  - —Sustained release: peak serum levels 4–12 hours
- Half-life of 24 hours
- Slow distribution
- Volume of distribution (V_d) 0.6–0.9 L/kg
- Elimination
  - —*Not* metabolized
  - —Excreted unchanged by the kidneys
  - —Reabsorbed in the *proximal* tubules by sodium transport mechanism
  - —Elimination half life (therapeutic) is 20–24 hours and prolonged in chronic users
- Therapeutic and toxic indices
  - —Therapeutic and toxic effects occur *only* when lithium is intracellular
  - —Narrow toxic-to-therapeutic ratio
  - —Therapeutic level 0.6–1.2 mEq/L (after intracellular/extracellular equilibration)
  - —Handled similarly to sodium, potassium, and magnesium

ETIOLOGY

- Acute conditions increasing risk for toxicity
  - —Dehydration (decreases renal filtration and increases reabsorption)
  - —Intentional overdose
- Chronic conditions increasing risk of toxicity
  - —Hypertension
  - —Diabetes mellitus
  - —Renal failure
  - —Congestive heart failure
  - —Advanced age
  - —Dose change
  - —Drug interactions
  - —Lithium therapy
  - —Low-salt diet
- Increase serum lithium levels due to decrease renal clearance
  - —NSAIDs
  - —Thiazides
  - —Angiotensin-converting enzyme (ACE) inhibitors
  - —Dilantin
  - —Potentiate lithium effects
  - —Tricyclic antidepressants
  - —Phenothiazines

Pre-Hospital

CAUTIONS

- Transport all appropriate pill bottles to hospital
- Support by stabilizing ABCs
- Initiate IV, O_2, monitor

Diagnosis

ESSENTIAL WORKUP

- Lithium level
  - —Repeat in 2 hours to detect any trend
  - —Prolonged observation/admission warrants every-4-hour levels
- Stratify patient into one of three categories to interpret lithium level and predict toxicity
  - —Acute toxicity
    - -Intentional overdose in a patient not previously taking lithium
    - -Poor correlation between lithium level and symptoms because intracellular distribution has not yet occurred
    - -Toxic levels may appear in asymptomatic patients
    - -Lithium level >4 mEq/L is toxic as clearance is slow and complications are possible
  - —Acute on chronic toxicity
    - -Intentional or accidental overdose in a patient on lithium therapy
    - -Lithium level >3 mEq/L usually associated with symptoms
  - —Chronic toxicity
    - -Patients on lithium therapy who progressively develop toxicity secondary to factors other than acute ingestion
    - -Stronger correlation between lithium level and symptoms
    - -Lithium level >1.5 mEq/L may be toxic

LABORATORY

- Electrolytes, BUN, creatinine, glucose for electrolyte disturbances/renal function
- Aspirin and acetaminophen (APAP) levels may be indicated
- Urinalysis
  - —Specific gravity

DIFFERENTIAL DIAGNOSIS

- Consider lithium toxicity with altered mental status and fasciculations
- Endocrine: hypoglycemia
- Toxicologic
  - —Organophosphates
  - —Cholinergic substances
  - —Heavy-metal poisoning
  - —Neuroleptic overdose
  - —Black widow/scorpion envenomation
  - —Strychnine poisoning

Treatment

INITIAL STABILIZATION

- ABCs
- Secure IV access with 0.9% NS
- Cardiac monitor
- Naloxone, thiamine, dextrose (or Accucheck) if altered mental status
- Administer diazepam for seizures

ED TREATMENT

Prevent Absorption

- Syrup of ipecac is of no use
- Gastric lavage only if patient presents within 1 hour of acute life threatening ingestion and has a protected airway
- Charcoal
  - —Lithium not absorbed by charcoal
  - —Consider one dose of activated charcoal with sorbitol if possibility of co-ingestion
- Whole-bowel irrigation
  - —Polyethylene glycol solution (PEG/GoLYTELY)
  - —Indicated with sustained-release products
  - —Flushes out toxin
  - —Administer until rectal effluent is clear
  - —Contraindications
    - -Bowel obstruction or perforation
    - -Ileus or hypotension
    - -Unprotected airway in obtunded or seizing patient

Enhance Elimination

- IV fluids
  - —Rapidly correct any preexisting fluid deficit with 0.9% NS at 150–300 mL/h
  - —Saline hydration improves glomerular filtration and decreases proximal tubule reabsorption of lithium
  - —Maintain urine output between 1–2 mL/kg/h
  - —Limited value once glomerular filtration rate (GFR) maximized
  - —Sodium bicarbonate offers no additional advantage
- Loop, thiazide, and osmotic diuretics not recommended
  - —Dehydration may result which worsens toxicity
  - —No direct effect on renal reabsorption because lithium is reabsorbed in proximal tubules
- Kayexalate (sodium polystyrene sulfonate)
  - —Animal studies indicate reduced lithium levels
  - —Only very large doses studied
  - —Complications include hypokalemia, hyperkalemia, fluid overload, and dysrhythmias

Dialysis

- Peritoneal dialysis not recommended
- Hemodialysis
  - —Best method for augmenting elimination
  - —For severe cases or acute ingestions with high levels indicating imminent toxicity
  - —Controversial indications
    - -Severe and progressive neurologic abnormalities
    - -Renal failure
    - -Altered mental status
    - -Ventricular arrhythmia/cardiogenic shock
    - -History of congestive heart failure or pulmonary edema
    - -Acute ingestions with levels >4 mEq/L
    - -Chronic ingestions with levels >2.5 mEq/L
    - -Standard end point is lithium level <1 mEq/L
    - -Obtain repeat lithium level 6 hours after dialysis
    - -May need to repeat dialysis due to rebound effect (redistribution of intracellular lithium)
    - -Reduces the potential for developing permanent neurologic sequelae with chronic toxicity

Supportive Care

- Correct electrolyte abnormalities
- Continuous cardiac monitoring
- Maintain well-hydrated state
- Observe for neurologic changes

MEDICATIONS

- Dextrose: D50 1 amp (25 g) (peds: D25W 4 mL/kg) i.v.
- Diazepam: 5 mg (peds: 0.2–0.4 mg/kg) i.v. every 5 minutes until seizures controlled
- Naloxone: 2 mg (peds: 0.1 mg/kg) i.v. or ET
- Polyethylene glycol: 2 L/h (peds: 2 mL/kg/h) NGT
- Thiamine: 100 mg i.v.

Disposition

ADMISSION CRITERIA

- Symptomatic
- Requiring hemodialysis
- Lithium level unchanged, increased, or greater than 2 mEq/L despite ED intervention
- Moderate to severe symptoms with chronic levels >4 mEq/L warrant ICU
- Psychiatric consultation for intentional ingestion

DISCHARGE CRITERIA

- Decreasing lithium levels q4h in an *asymptomatic* patient *and*
- Most recent serum lithium level <2 mEq/L

Miscellaneous

ICD9: 985.8

ICD10: T56.8

SUGGESTED READINGS

Bailey B, McGuigan M. Comparisons of patients hemodialyzed for lithium poisoning and those for whom dialysis was recommended by PCC but not done: what lesson can we learn? Clin Neurol 2000;54:388–392.

Belanger DR, Tierney MG, Dickinson G. Effect of sodium polystyrene sulfonate on lithium bioavailability. Ann Emerg Med 1992;21:1312–1315.

Bosse GM, Arnold TC. Overdose with sustained release lithium preparation. J Emerg Med 1992;10:719–721.

Henry GC. Lithium. In: Goldfrank LR, ed. Goldfrank's toxicologic emergencies. East Stamford, CT: Appleton & Lange, 1998.

Leikin J, Paloucek F. Lithium. In: Poisoning and toxicology handbook. Hudson, OH: Lexi-Comp, 2002.

Osborn HH, Malkevich D. Lithium. In: Ford MD, Delaney KA, Ling LJ, Erickson T, eds. Clinical toxicology. Philadelphia, PA: WB Saunders, 2001.

Scharman EJ. Methods used to decrease lithium absorption or enhance elimination. Clin Toxicol 1997;35:601–608.

Author: Sean Bryant

Ludwig's Angina

Clinical Presentation

SIGNS AND SYMPTOMS

- Submandibular pain
- Tongue elevation, protrusion
- Trismus
  —Difficult to examine mouth, pharynx
- Dysphonia
- Odynophagia
- Stridor
- Anxiety
- Salivary incontinence
- Fever
- Tachypneic, tachycardic
- Patient will prefer sitting/"sniffing" position
- Submandibular area hard, "woody," painful

MECHANISM/DESCRIPTION

- A life-threatening infection of the floor of the mouth
- Rapidly spreading gangrenous cellulitis, necrotizing fasciitis of submaxillary, sublingual, submandibular spaces
- First described by von Ludwig in 1836
- Mortality exceeded 50% in preantibiotic era
- Most deaths due to respiratory obstruction
- Improved dental care, antibiotics reduce incidence
- Four cardinal aspects
  —Bilateral involvement of more than one deep tissue space
  —Gangrene with serosanguineous, putrid infiltration; little or no frank pus
  —Involvement of connective tissue, fasciae, and muscles; not glandular structures
  —Spread by fascial space continuity, not lymphatics
- Brawny, painful induration of suprahyoid neck results in woody edema of the floor of the mouth; tongue, soft tissues forced superiorly, posteriorly
- Rapid respiratory obstruction (asphyxia) can occur

ETIOLOGY

- Odontogenic 50–90% of reported cases
  —Most commonly second, third mandibular molars
  —Children less likely to have odontogenic source
- Less commonly
  —IV drug injections into neck veins
  —Mandibular fractures
  —Oral lacerations
  —Sialadenitis
  —Peritonsillar abscess
  —Tongue piercing
- Invariably polymicrobial, oral flora
  —Most common pathogens *Streptococcus viridans, Staphylococcus aureus, Staphylococcus epidermidis*
  -Anaerobes: most commonly *Bacteroides* species

Pre-Hospital

- Transport in sitting position
  —Supplemental oxygen, suction secretions as needed
- Early, aggressive airway protection

Diagnosis

ESSENTIAL WORKUP

- Diagnosis apparent from the history, physical examination

LABORATORY

- Consider WBC count (systemic response), screening studies
- Consider blood cultures

IMAGING/SPECIAL TESTS

- Soft tissue films of neck
  —Edema, presence of gas
- CT, MRI detect severe cellulitis, abscesses, intrathoracic extension
- Panorex detects odontogenic abscesses
- Chest x-ray
  —Intrathoracic extension
- Ultrasound detects abscesses

DIFFERENTIAL DIAGNOSIS

- Cellulitis
- Peritonsillar abscess
- Salivary gland abscess
- Lymphadenitis
- Angioneurotic edema
- Lingual carcinoma
- Sublingual hematoma secondary to anticoagulation

Treatment

INITIAL STABILIZATION

- Airway compromise the primary concern
- *Expect difficulty: altered anatomy, swollen tissue, trismus*
- Rapid-sequence intubation may result in loss of supporting structures; loss of visualization, patent airway
- Sedation-assisted orotracheal intubation preferred
  —Ultrashort agents (etomidate, thiopental)
- Awake, fiberoptic intubation recommended first-line approach
- Avoid blind nasotracheal intubation
  —Distorted anatomy
  —Induce bleeding, perforate abscess
- Cricothyrotomy, jet ventilation may be difficult
- Tracheostomy the gold standard management
  —Risk for intrathoracic spread with procedure

ED TREATMENT

- Initiate broad-spectrum antibiotics
  —Aerobic/anaerobic/polymicrobial infection
  —Clindamycin or penicillin G plus metronidazole; also cefoxitin, ticarcillin/clavulanate, piperacillin/tazobactam, ampicillin/sulbactam
- Steroids of no proven benefit
- Hyperbaric oxygen if mediastinitis, necrotizing fasciitis of the chest wall

MEDICATIONS

- Antibiotics
  —Ampicillin/SB: 3 g i.v. q6h
  —Cefoxitin: 2 g i.v. q8h
  —Clindamycin: 900 mg i.v. q8h
  —Metronidazole: 500 mg i.v. q6h
  —Penicillin G: 4 million units i.v. q4–6h
  —Piperacillin/TZ: 3 g i.v. q6h
  —Ticarcillin/CL: 3 g i.v. q4–6h
- Sedatives
  —Etomidate: 0.2–0.3 mg/kg i.v.
  —Thiopental: 3–5 mg/kg i.v.

Disposition

ADMISSION CRITERIA

- All are admitted
- ICU or monitored setting; airway compromise can be precipitous

DISCHARGE CRITERIA

N/A

Miscellaneous

ICD9: 528.3

ICD10: K12.2

SUGGESTED READINGS

Barakate MS, Jensen MJ, Hemli JM, et al. Ludwig's angina: report of a case and review of management issues. Ann Otol Rhinol Laryngol 2001;110(5 Pt 1): 453–456.

Britt JC, Josephson GD, Gross CW. Ludwig's angina in the pediatric population: report of a case and review of the literature. Int J Pediatr Otorhinolaryngol 2000;52(1): 79–87.

Busch RF, Shah D. Ludwig's angina: improved treatment. Otolaryngol Head Neck Surg 1997;117(6):S172–175.

Neff SP, Merry AF, Anderson B. Airway management in Ludwig's angina. Anaesth Intensive Care 1999;27(6):659–661.

Spitalnic SJ, Sucov A. Ludwig's angina: case report and review. J Emerg Med 1995;13(4):499–503.

Author: Paul Blackburn

Lunate Dislocation

Clinical Presentation

SIGNS AND SYMPTOMS

- Pain and tenderness in the wrist
- Mass or swelling in the wrist, either dorsally or volarly depending on direction of dislocation
- May display signs of median nerve injury (paresthesias, diminished two-point discrimination)
- Easily missed injury; look carefully at lateral wrist x-ray

MECHANISM/DESCRIPTION

- Usually high-energy hyperextension with ulnar deviation of the wrist, such as fall from height or motor vehicle accident
- Dislocation of the lunate relative to the radius and distal row of metacarpals, either dorsally or volarly
- Implies disruption of all four perilunate ligaments, radiocarpal ligament
- In volar dislocations, median nerve injury occurs in the carpal tunnel
- Associated fractures of the radial styloid, scaphoid, capitate, and triquetrum are common and, if present, should raise suspicion of an occult perilunate ligamentous injury

Pre-Hospital

- Consider other injuries
- Dress open wounds
- Immobilize in neutral position
- Elevate; ice to reduce swelling

Diagnosis

ESSENTIAL WORKUP

- Clinical exam is frequently not diagnostic
- Assess skin integrity and neurovascular status, including two-point discrimination
- Radiographs as outlined below

IMAGING/SPECIAL TESTS

- Radiographic imaging to include three views of the wrist
- On a lateral radiograph (most useful view):
  - —Disruption of the normal imaginary longitudinal line through the centers of the radius, lunate, and capitate indicates dislocation or subluxation
  - —In volar dislocations, the lunate is frequently tilted with the opening of the "cup" toward the palm *(spilled teacup sign)*
- On a PA view:
  - —The dislocated lunate has a triangular (as opposed to the usual quadrangular) appearance
  - —Disruption of a smooth and continuous arc formed by the radiocarpal row suggests lunate dislocation

DIFFERENTIAL DIAGNOSIS

- Lunate fracture
- Perilunate dislocation
- Scapholunate dissociation
- Scaphoid fracture

PEDIATRIC CONSIDERATIONS

- X-ray can be difficult to interpret unless full ossification is present

Treatment

INITIAL STABILIZATION

- Immobilize in position of comfort with a volar or "sugar-tong" splint

ED TREATMENT

- Identify multiple trauma or other injuries
- Contact a hand surgeon for immediate reduction and possible operative intervention
- Closed reduction can be difficult or unstable and frequently open reduction and internal fixation is needed
- Even with optimal management, chronic carpal instability can result, leading to degenerative arthritis, chronic pain and disability

MEDICATIONS

- Pain control pending definitive management

PEDIATRIC CONSIDERATIONS

- Wrists are rarely sprained in children, and the x-ray is difficult to interpret
- Although serious injury is unusual, children with wrist pain should be splinted and referred for ongoing evaluation of possible occult fractures

Disposition

ADMISSION CRITERIA

- Dislocations should be reduced immediately; therefore, patients usually are admitted at the contact point for definitive orthopedic care
- Open fracture, presence of multiple trauma, or other more serious injuries mandates admission

DISCHARGE CRITERIA

- Closed dislocations or fractures that have been adequately reduced and immobilized in the ED may be discharged with orthopedic follow-up

Miscellaneous

ICD9: 833.00

SUGGESTED READINGS

American Society for Surgery of the Hand. The hand: primary care of common problems, 2nd ed. New York: Churchill Livingstone, 1990:637–649.

Eisenhauer MA. Forearm and wrist. In: Rosen P, et al., eds. Emergency medicine: concepts and clinical practice, 4th ed. St. Louis: Mosby–Year Book, 2002:535–542.

Perron AD. Orthopedic pitfalls in the ED: lunate and perilunate injuries. Am J Emerg Med 2001;19(2):157–162.

Simon RR, Koenigsknecht SJ, eds. Emergency orthopedics: the extremities, 4th ed. New York: McGraw-Hill, 2001:176–180.

Uehara DT. The hand in emergency medicine. Emerg Clin North Am 1993;11(3):781–796.

Author: Mary Anne Fuchs

Lyme Disease

Clinical Presentation

SIGNS AND SYMPTOMS

Stage I (Early)

- Onset a few days to a month after tick bite (arthropod transmission)
- 30–50% of patients recall tick bite
- Erythema chronicum migrans (ECM)
  - —Pathognomonic finding
    - -*"Bull's-eye"* rash
  - —Maculopapular, irregular expanding annular lesion
    - -Single or multiple
    - -Central clearing with red outer border
    - -Diameter >5 cm
- Regional adenopathy
- Low-grade, intermittent fever
- Headache
- Myalgia
- Arthralgias
- Fatigue
- Malaise

Stage II (Secondary, Disseminated)

- Days to weeks after tick bite
- Intermittent and fluctuating symptoms with eventual disappearance
- Triad of aseptic meningitis, cranial neuritis, and radiculoneuritis
  - —Facial (Bell's) palsy the most common cranial neuritis
  - —May present without rash
  - —Prognosis generally good
- Cardiac
  - —Tachycardia
  - —Bradycardia
  - —Atrioventricular block
  - —Myopericarditis

Stage III (Tertiary, Late)

- Onset greater than 1 year after disease onset
- Acrodermatitis chronica atrophicans
  - —Extensor surfaces of extremities, especially lower leg
  - —Initial edematous infiltration evolving to atrophic lesions
  - —Resembles scleroderma
- Arthritis
  - —Brief arthritis attacks
  - —Monoarthritis
  - —Oligoarthritis
  - —Occasionally migratory
  - —Most common joints (descending order)
    - -Knee
    - -Shoulder
    - -Elbow

Other

- Gastrointestinal
  - —Hepatitis
  - —Right upper quadrant pain
- Ocular
  - —Keratitis
  - —Uveitis
  - —Iritis
  - —Optic neuritis
- Jarisch-Herxheimer reaction
  - —Worsening of symptoms a few hours after treatment initiated
  - —More common in patients with multiple ECM lesions
- Babesiosis occurs simultaneously in endemic areas

Persistent Lyme Disease

- Articular and neurologic symptoms despite treatment
  - —Chronic axonal polyneuropathy or encephalopathy

Recurrent Lyme Disease

- Relapse despite treatment
- Second episodes less severe

ETIOLOGY

- Most common tick-borne illness in North America
- Endemic in northeastern, upper midwestern, and northwestern California
- Peak between April and November; 80–90% in the summer months
- Spirochete *Borrelia burgdorferi* introduced by *Ixodes* tick
  - —*Ixodes dammini* (deer tick) the most common
- <50% of patients recall tick bite
- Pathogenesis—combination of
  - —Organism induced local inflammation
  - —Cytokine release
  - —Autoimmunity
- No person-to-person transmission

PEDIATRIC CONSIDERATIONS

- More likely than adults to be febrile
- Only 50% of children with arthralgias have a history of ECM
- Facial palsy accompanied by aseptic meningitis in one third
- Asymptomatic cardiac involvement with abnormal EKGs
- Appropriately treated children have excellent prognosis for unimpaired cognitive functioning
- Untreated children may have keratitis, joint pain, or chronic encephalopathy

Pre-Hospital

N/A

Diagnosis

ESSENTIAL WORKUP

- Clinical diagnosis
  - —Presence of ECM obviates serologic tests
- Careful search for tick
- Lumbar puncture when meningeal signs
- Arthrocentesis for acute arthritis
- EKG

LABORATORY

- CBC
  - —Leukocytosis
  - —Anemia
  - —Thrombocytopenia
- Erythrocyte sedimentation rate (ESR)
  - —>30 mm/h
  - —Most common laboratory abnormality
- Electrolytes, BUN, creatinine, glucose
- Liver function tests
  - —Elevated liver enzymes (gamma-glutamyl transferase [GGT] most common)
- Culture
  - —Low yield
  - —Not indicated
- CSF
  - —Pleocytosis
  - —Elevated protein
  - —Obtain CSF spirochete antibodies

IMAGING/SPECIAL TESTS

- Serology
  - —Obtain enzyme-linked immunosorbent assay (ELISA), immunofluorescence assay (IFA), and Western blot when disease suggested without ECM lesion
  - —Antibodies may persist for months to years
  - —Positive serology or previous Lyme disease does not ensure protective immunity
- Polymerase chain reaction assay
  - —Highly specific and sensitive
  - —Not available for routine use
- Joint fluid
  - —Cryoglobulin increased five-fold compared with serum
- Joint films may show soft tissue, cartilaginous, osseous changes

DIFFERENTIAL DIAGNOSIS

- Other tick-borne illnesses
  - —Deer tick usually larger (1 cm) than ixodid ticks (1–2 mm)
  - —Rocky Mountain spotted fever
  - —Tularemia
  - —Relapsing fever
  - —Colorado tick fever
  - —Tick-bite paralysis
- Rheumatic fever
  - —Rash of erythema marginatum
  - —Temporomandibular joint arthritis more common than in Lyme disease
  - —Valvular involvement rather than heart block
  - —Chorea may be isolated finding
- Viral meningitis
- Syphilis
- Septic arthritis
- Parvovirus B19 infection—polyarticular arthritis
- Infectious endocarditis
- Juvenile rheumatoid arthritis
- Reiter's syndrome
- Brown recluse spider bite
- Fibromyalgia
- Chronic fatigue syndrome

Treatment

INITIAL STABILIZATION

- 500 mL (20 mL/kg) 0.9% NS IV fluid bolus fluids for dehydration
- IV access for neurologic and cardiac involvement
- Cardiac monitoring
- Temporary pacemaker for heart block

ED TREATMENT

- Remove tick
  - —Disinfect site
  - —With blunt instrument grasp tick close to skin and pull upward with gentle pressure
- Administer
  - —Aspirin as adjunctive therapy for cardiac involvement
  - —NSAIDs for arthritis and arthralgias

Stage I

- Amoxicillin, doxycycline, or cefuroxime (21 days)
- Azithromycin (14–21 days)
- Parenteral therapy in pregnant patients

Stage II

- Oral therapy for isolated Bell's palsy and mild involvement
  - —Amoxicillin with probenecid (30 days) or doxycycline (avoid if pregnant or <9 years old) (10–21 days)
- Parenteral therapy for more severe involvement (meningitis, carditis, severe arthritis)
  - —Ceftriaxone, cefotaxime (14–21 days), or penicillin G (14–28 days)

Stage III

- Parenteral therapy
  - —Penicillin G, cefotaxime (14–21 days), or ceftriaxone (14–28 days)

MEDICATIONS

- Amoxicillin: 500 mg (peds: 40 mg/kg/24 h) PO t.i.d.
- Aspirin: 80–100 mg/kg/d (peds: 50–100 mg/kg/d in 6 divided doses) PO
- Azithromycin: 500 mg PO daily
- Cefotaxime: 2 g (peds: 100–150 mg/kg/24 h) i.v. q8h
- Ceftriaxone: 2 g (peds: 100 mg/kg/24 h) i.v. daily
- Doxycycline: 200 mg PO b.i.d. × 3 days, then 100 mg PO b.i.d. for 21–28 days
- Penicillin G: 20–24 mIU i.v. divided q4–6h
- Probenecid: 500 mg PO t.i.d.
- Vaccine (LYMErix) for prevention of disease
  - —A recombinant surface protein
  - —For persons in high/moderate risk areas
  - —For travelers to endemic areas
  - —Three doses (0–1 month to 12 months)

Disposition

ADMISSION CRITERIA

- Meningoencephalitis
- Telemetry/ICU admission for carditis

DISCHARGE CRITERIA

- Patients treated with oral therapy

Miscellaneous

ICD9: 88.81

ICD10: A69.2

SUGGESTED READINGS

Asch ES, Bujak DI, Weiss M, et al. Lyme disease: an infectious and post-infectious syndrome. J Rheumatol 1994;121:157–162.

Preboth M. Infectious Diseases Society of America guidelines on the treatment of Lyme Disease. Am Fam Physician 2001;63:2065, 2067.

Sigal LH. Current recommendations for the treatment of Lyme disease. Drugs 1992;43:683–699.

Steere AC. Lyme disease. N Engl J Med 1989;321:586–596.

Author: Moses Lee

Lymphadenitis, Regional

Clinical Presentation

SIGNS AND SYMPTOMS

- Painful swelling, inflammation/infection of lymph nodes
- Commonly presents simultaneously with acute cellulitis or abscess if pyogenic etiology
- Axillary lymphadenitis
  - —Fever, axillary pain, and acute lymphedema of arms and chest, without features of cellulitis or lymphangitis
- Other forms of infectious lymphadenitis including generalized and chronic are beyond the scope of this chapter

MECHANISM/DESCRIPTION

- Lymph nodes may be swollen and tender as part of the systemic response to infection
  - —Become engorged with lymphocytes and macrophages
  - —May be primarily infected
  - —Infection in a distal extremity may result in painful tender adenopathy proximally
- Acute suppurative lymphadenitis may occur after pharyngeal or skin infection

ETIOLOGY

- Most frequently caused by bacterial infection
- Most common organisms in pyogenic lymphadenitis
  - —Group A β-hemolytic streptococcus
  - —*Staphylococcus aureus*
- Axillary lymphadenitis
  - —*Streptococcus pyogenes*

PEDIATRIC CONSIDERATIONS

- Acute unilateral cervical suppurative lymphadenitis
  - —Most common under age 6 years
  - —Group A streptococci in 75%; also *S. aureus*

Pre-Hospital

N/A

Diagnosis

ESSENTIAL WORKUP

- Lymphadenitis is a *clinical diagnosis,* often part of a larger syndrome (cellulitis)
- History and physical examination to reveal infectious source

LABORATORY

- WBC count is not essential
  - —Possible leukocytosis with left shift or normal

IMAGING/SPECIAL TESTS

- None

DIFFERENTIAL DIAGNOSIS

- Common infections
  - —Scarlet fever
  - —Cat-scratch disease
  - —Fungal
  - —Adenovirus
  - —Herpes zoster
- Unusual infections
  - —Sporotrichosis (rose thorns)
  - —Diphtheria
  - —West Nile fever
  - —Plague
  - —Anthrax
  - —Typhoid
- Venereal infections
  - —Syphilis
  - —Genital herpes
  - —Chancroid
  - —Lymphogranuloma venereum
- Other systematic infections causing generalized lymphadenitis
  - —HIV
  - —Infectious mononucleosis (Epstein-Barr virus [EBV] or cytomegalovirus [CMV])
  - —Toxoplasmosis
- Drug reaction
- Phenytoin
- Allopurinol
- Silicone implants
- Malignancy
- Rheumatologic disorders
- Systemic lupus erythematosus
- Sarcoidosis
- Amyloidosis
- Serum sickness

PEDIATRIC CONSIDERATIONS

- Pediatric differential diagnosis includes
  - —Kawasaki disease
  - —PFAPA syndrome (periodic fever, aphthous stomatitis, pharyngitis, cervical adenitis)

Treatment

INITIAL STABILIZATION

- Ensure ABCs and hemodynamic stability

ED TREATMENT

- Antibiotics based on involved primary organ/suspected pathogen
- Pharyngeal or periodontal origin: oral penicillin or erythromycin
- Skin origin: oral dicloxacillin if mild; more severe use IV nafcillin or IV first-generation cephalosporin
- Other agents based on concurrent or primary infection source
  —Refer to cellulitis and lymphangitis sections
- Drainage of abscesses if present
- Elevation
- Application of moist heat
- Analgesics

MEDICATIONS

- Cefazolin: 1–2 g (peds: 50–100 mg/kg/24 h) IV q6–8h
- Dicloxacillin: 125–500 mg (peds: 12.5–25 mg/kg/24 h) PO q6h
- Erythromycin base: 250–500 mg PO q.i.d. or 333 mg PO t.i.d.
- Erythromycin ethyl succinate: 400 mg (peds: 30–50 mg/kg/24 h) PO q.i.d.
- Nafcillin: (adult only) 1–2 g i.v. q4h
- Penicillin VK: 250–500 mg (peds: 25–50 mg/kg/24 h) PO q6h

Disposition

ADMISSION CRITERIA

- Toxic appearing
- History of immune suppression
- Concurrent chronic medical illnesses
- Unable to take oral medications
- Unreliable patients

DISCHARGE CRITERIA

- Mild infection in a non-toxic-appearing patient
- Able to take oral antibiotics
- No history of immune suppression or concurrent medical problems
- Has adequate follow-up within 24–48 hours

Miscellaneous

OTHER CONSIDERATIONS

- If not found in the context of an acute infection, and not quick to resolve with a course of antibiotics, evaluate for more serious underlying causes (e.g., malignancy)

ICD9: 683

ICD10: I88.9

SEE ALSO: CELLULITIS; LYMPHANGITIS

SUGGESTED READINGS

Boyce JM. Severe streptococcal axillary lymphadenitis. N Engl J Med 1990;323: 655–658.

Henry PH, Longo DL. Enlargement of the lymph nodes and spleen. In: Braunwald E, Fauci AS, Kasper DL, et al., eds. Harrison's principles of internal medicine, 15th ed. New York: McGraw-Hill, 2001:360–365.

Swartz MN. Lymphadenitis and lymphangitis. In: Mandell GE, Bennett JE, Dolin R, eds. Mandell, Douglas and Bennett's principles and practice of infectious diseases, 5th ed. New York: Churchill Livingstone, 2000:1066–1075.

Thomas KT, Feder HM, Lawton AR, et al. Periodic fever syndrome in children. J Pediatr 1999;135(1):15–21.

Authors: John Mahoney; Dolores Gonthier

Lymphangitis

Clinical Presentation

SIGNS AND SYMPTOMS

Acute Lymphangitis

- Warm, tender erythematous streaks develop and extend proximally from a source of infection
- Regional lymph nodes often become enlarged and tender (lymphadenitis)
- Peripheral edema of involved extremity
- Systemic manifestations
  - —Fever
  - —Rigors
  - —Tachycardia
  - —Headache

Chronic (Nodular) Lymphangitis

- Erythematous nodule, chancriform ulcer, or wartlike lesion develops in the subcutaneous tissue at the inoculation site
- Often presents without pain or evidence of systemic infection
- Multiple lesions possible along lymphatic chain

MECHANISM/DESCRIPTION

- Lymphangitis is an *infection of the lymphatics* that drain a focus of inflammation
- Histologically, the lymphatic vessels are dilated and filled with lymphocytes and histiocytes; the inflammation frequently extends into the perilymphatic tissues and may lead to cellulitis or abscess formation

ETIOLOGY

Acute Lymphangitis

- Likely caused by bacterial infection
- Most common organisms
  - —Group A β-hemolytic streptococcus and *Staphylococcus aureus*
- Other organisms
  - —*Pasteurella multocida*
  - —*Spirillum minus* (rat-bite fever)
  - —*Wuchereria bancrofti* (filariasis)

Chronic Lymphangitis

- Usually caused by mycotic, mycobacterial, and filarial infections
- *Sporothrix schenckii* (most common cause of chronic lymphangitis in United States)
  - —Inoculation occurs while gardening or farming (rose thorn)
  - —Organism is present on some plants and in sphagnum moss
  - —Multiple subcutaneous nodules appear along the course of the lymphatic vessels
  - —Typical antibiotics and local treatment fail to cure the lesion
- *Mycobacterium marinum*
  - —Atypical mycobacterium
  - —Grows optimally at 25–32°C in fish tanks and swimming pools
  - —May produce a chronic nodular, single wartlike or ulcerative lesion at the site of an abrasion
  - —Additional lesions may appear in a distribution similar to sporotrichosis
- *Nocardia brasiliensis*
- *Mycobacterium kansasii*
- *Wuchereria bancrofti* (filariasis)

Pre-Hospital

- No specific considerations

Diagnosis

ESSENTIAL WORKUP

- Examination findings
  - —Peripheral infection or traumatic injury, accompanied by fever and erythematous streaks proceeding toward regional lymph nodes, indicates lymphangitis
- Directed at discovering the source of the infection

LABORATORY

- Not necessary to obtain routine labs, except culture
- WBC count is often elevated
- Gram stain and culture obtained from the source lesion may focus antimicrobial selection
- If sporotrichosis or *M. marinum* infection is suspected, the diagnosis should be confirmed by culture of the organism from the wound
- Blood culture may reveal organism

IMAGING/SPECIAL TESTS

- Imaging not commonly performed
- Plain x-ray may reveal abscess formation, subcutaneous gas, or foreign bodies if these are suspected
- Extremity vascular imaging (Doppler ultrasound) can help rule out deep venous thrombosis

DIFFERENTIAL DIAGNOSIS

- Thrombophlebitis
- Differentiation from lymphangitis
  - —Absence of an initial traumatic or infectious focus
  - —No regional lymphadenopathy

PEDIATRIC CONSIDERATIONS

- No unique considerations

Treatment

INITIAL STABILIZATION

- Ensure adequate ABCs and hemodynamic stability

ED TREATMENT

- Antimicrobial therapy should be initiated with first dose in the ED
- To cover both staphylococcus and group A β-hemolytic streptococcus in acute lymphangitis, use a penicillinase-resistant penicillin (oral dicloxacillin or IV nafcillin)
  - —Alternatives: amoxicillin clavulanate or azithromycin
- Penicillin VK may be used when the etiologic agent is known to be group A β-hemolytic streptococcus
  - —Alternative: erythromycin
- Sporotrichosis
  - —Itraconazole or saturated solution of potassium iodide (SSKI)
- *M. marinum*
  - —Localized granulomas are usually excised
  - —Antimicrobial therapy is usually reserved for more severe infections
    - -Limited data on what combination of agents should be employed
    - -Rifampin and ethambutol may be the best choice
- Heat and extremity elevation are also useful adjuncts

MEDICATIONS

- Amoxicillin clavulanate: 500–875 mg (peds: 45 mg/kg/24 h) PO b.i.d. or 250–500 mg (peds: 40 mg/kg/24 h) PO t.i.d.
- Azithromycin (adult and peds): 10 mg/kg up to 500 mg PO on day 1, followed by 5 mg/kg up to 250 mg PO q.d. to complete 5 days
- Dicloxacillin: 125–500 mg (peds: 12.5–25 mg/kg/24 h) PO q6h
- Erythromycin base (adult): 250–500 mg PO q.i.d. or 333 mg PO t.i.d.
- Erythromycin ethyl succinate: 400 mg (peds: 30–50 mg/kg/24 h) PO q.i.d.
- Itraconazole (adult): 100–200 mg PO q.d., continue until lesions resolve (6–12 weeks); peds: not approved for use
- Nafcillin (adult only): 1–2 g i.v. q4h
- Penicillin VK: 250–500 mg (peds: 25–50 mg/kg/24 h) PO q6h
- Saturated solution of potassium iodide (SSKI): 5–10 drops, increase to 40–50 drops (peds: 5–10 drops, increase to 25–40) PO t.i.d. Take in milk, juice, or carbonated beverage to avoid bitter taste

Disposition

ADMISSION CRITERIA

- Toxic appearing
- History of immune suppression
- Concurrent chronic medical illnesses
- Unable to take oral medications
- Unreliable patients

DISCHARGE CRITERIA

- Mild infection in a non-toxic-appearing patient
- Able to take oral antibiotics
- No history of immune suppression or concurrent medical problems
- Adequate follow-up within 24–48 hours

Miscellaneous

ICD9: 457.2, 682.9

ICD10: I89.1

SUGGESTED READINGS

Rex JH, Okhuysen PC. Sporothrix schenckii. In: Mandell GE, Bennett JE, Dolin R, eds. Mandell, Douglas and Bennett's principles and practice of infectious diseases, 5th ed. New York: Churchill Livingstone, 2000: 2695–2698.

Smego RA, Castiglia M, Asperilla MO. Lymphocutaneous syndrome: a review of non-sporothrix causes. Medicine 1999;78(1):38–63.

Swartz MN. Lymphadenitis and lymphangitis. In: Mandell GE, Bennett JE, Dolin R, eds. Mandell, Douglas and Bennett's principles and practice of infectious diseases, 5th ed. New York: Churchill Livingstone, 2000:1066–1075.

Authors: John Mahoney; Owen T. Traynor

Lymphogranuloma Venereum

Clinical Presentation

SIGNS AND SYMPTOMS

Primary Genital Lesions

- Painless genital chancre lasts 2–3 days (rarely, a papule or vesicle)
  - —Initial lesion is rarely noticed
- Incubation: 3–30 days after sexual exposure to *Chlamydia trachomatis*

Inguinal Adenopathy

- Occurs 1–3 weeks after initial inoculation
- Adenopathy is unilateral in two thirds of cases
- Buboes (large inguinal lymph nodes) form in inguinal and femoral chains
- "Groove sign": scarred or coalescent buboes above and below inguinal ligament give a linear depression parallel to the inguinal ligament (seen in 30%)
- Anal-receptive patients may develop hemorrhagic proctocolitis
  - —Perirectal lymphatic inflammation causes fistulae and strictures
- Systemic symptoms (absent with chancroid) may include fever, myalgias, headache, erythema nodosum, nausea, and vomiting
  - —Meningoencephalitis is rare

Chronic Complications

- Genital strictures, perineal and perianal fistulae, and elephantiasis of the ipsilateral leg

ETIOLOGY

- *Chlamydia trachomatis*—serotypes L1, L2, and L3
- AKA struma, tropical bubo, Nicolas-Favre-Durand disease

Pre-Hospital

N/A

Diagnosis

ESSENTIAL WORKUP

- Diagnosis mainly clinical (i.e., thorough history and physical exam)

LABORATORY

- Standard chlamydia DNA probes *do not* test for the lymphogranuloma venereum (LGV) strain
- False-positive VDRL in 20%
- Serologic testing and culture are the standard
  - —Bubo aspiration—specific but expensive and impractical
- Complement fixation titers >1:64 is consistent with LGV infection

DIFFERENTIAL DIAGNOSIS

- Genital herpes (ulcers usually not seen in LGV)
- Syphilis—nodes are nontender, longer incubation
- Chancroid—multiple ulcers, no systemic symptoms
- Granuloma inguinale—lesions are painless and bleed easily

Treatment

INITIAL STABILIZATION

- No field or ED stabilization required

ED TREATMENT

- Antibiotics
  —First line—doxycycline: 100 mg PO b.i.d. until healing occurs
- Contact tracing of partners within the past 30 days
- Aspiration of suppurative nodes is controversial: may prevent chronic sinus drainage due to spontaneous rupture
  —Use 18-gauge needle through lateral intact skin
  —Note that incision and drainage of buboes is contraindicated

MEDICATIONS

- DC recommendations
  —First line—doxycycline: 100 mg PO b.i.d. × 3 weeks
  —Alternative—erythromycin: 500 mg PO q.i.d. × 3 weeks
- Pregnant patients receive erythromycin

Disposition

ADMISSION CRITERIA

- Hospitalization rarely needed (i.e., severe systemic symptoms)

DISCHARGE CRITERIA

- Immunocompetent patient without systemic involvement
- Outpatient follow-up required to confirm diagnosis and cure
  —Rectal infection may require retreatment

Miscellaneous

ICD9: 099.1

ICD10: A55

SUGGESTED READINGS

Borchardt KA, Noble MA. Sexually transmitted diseases. Boca Raton, FL: CRC Press, 1997.

Centers for Disease Control and Prevention: 2002 Guidelines for treatment of sexually transmitted diseases. MMWR 2002;47:RR.

Ernst AA, Marvez-Valls E, Martin DH. Incision and drainage versus aspiration of fluctuant buboes in the emergency department during an epidemic of chancroid. Sex Transm Dis 1995;22(4): 217–220.

Goens JL, Schwartz RA, DeWolf K. Mucocutaneous manifestations of chancroid, lymphogranuloma venereum and granuloma inguinale. Am Fam Physician 1994;49(2):415.

Author: Joel Kravitz

Malaria

Clinical Presentation

SIGNS AND SYMPTOMS

General

- Malaise
- Chills
- Fever
  - —Classic malaria paroxysm
    - -15 minutes to 1 hour of chills
    - -Followed by 2–6 hours of nondiaphoretic fever up to 39°–42°C
    - -Profuse diaphoresis followed by defervescence
    - -Pattern every 48 hours (vivax and ovale) or every 72 hours (falciparum)
  - —Fever pattern may be varied
- Orthostatic hypotension
- Myalgias/arthralgias

Hematology

- Hemolysis
  - —"Blackwater fever"—named from the dark color of the urine partially due to hemolysis in overwhelming falciparum infections
- Jaundice
- Splenomegaly
  - —More common in chronic infections
  - —May cause splenic rupture

CNS

- Headache
- Mental status changes
- Coma
- Seizures

GI

- Emesis
- Diarrhea
- Abdominal pain

Pulmonary

- Shortness of breath
- Rales
- Pulmonary edema

MECHANISM/DESCRIPTION

- Protozoan infection transmitted through the anopheles mosquito
- Incubation period 8–16 days
- Periodicity of disease due to life cycle of protozoan
  - —Exoerythrocytic phase: immature sporozoites migrate to liver where they rapidly multiply into mature parasites (merozoites)
  - —Erythrocytic phase: mature parasites released into circulation and invade RBC
  - —Replication within RBC followed 48–72 hours later by RBC lysis and release of merozoites into circulation, repeating cycle
  - —Fever corresponds to RBC lysis
- *Plasmodium falciparum*
  - —Usually presents as an acute, overwhelming infection
  - —Able to infect red cells of all ages
    - -Results in greater degree of hemolysis and anemia
  - —Causes widespread capillary obstruction
    - -Results in end-organ hypoxia and dysfunction
- More moderate infection in people who are on or who have recently stopped prophylaxis with an agent to which the falciparum is resistant
- Plasmodium vivax and ovale
  - —May present with an acute febrile illness
  - —Dormant liver stages (hypnozoites) that may cause relapse 6–11 months after the initial infection
- *Plasmodium malariae*
  - —May persist in the bloodstream at low levels up to 30 years
- Posttraumatic immunosuppression may cause relapse of malaria in patients who have lived in endemic areas

ETIOLOGY

- Transmission usually occurs from the bite of infected female anopheles mosquito
- North American transmission possible
  - —Anopheles mosquitoes on the east and west coasts of the United States
  - —Transmission may also occur through infected blood products and shared needles
- *P. falciparum* antibiotic resistance
  - —Chloroquine sensitive in the Caribbean, Central America, and the Middle East
  - —Pyrimethamine-sulfadoxine resistance in South America, Africa, southern and southeast Asia, and Indonesia
  - —Mefloquine resistance in southeast Asia

PEDIATRIC CONSIDERATIONS

- Sickle cell trait protective
- Cerebral malaria more common in children

Pre-Hospital

N/A

Diagnosis

ESSENTIAL WORKUP

- Oil emersion light microscopy of a thick-smear Giemsa stain
  - —Demonstrates intraerythrocytic malaria parasites
- Only high degrees of parasitemia will be evident on a standard CBC smear

LABORATORY

- CBC for anemia/thrombocytopenia
- Electrolytes, BUN, creatinine, glucose for
  - —Renal failure
  - —Hypoglycemia
  - —Lactic acidosis
- Urinalysis
- Liver function tests

IMAGING/SPECIAL TESTS

- Chest x-ray
- Immunofluorescence assay (IFA), enzyme-linked immunosorbent assay (ELISA), or DNA probes
  - —Differentiates the type of plasmodium present
  - —5–7% will have mixed infections
- Lumbar puncture/CSF analysis
  - —Performed to distinguish cerebral malaria from meningitis
  - —CSF lactate/protein elevated with malaria
  - —CSF pleocytosis/hypoglycemia absent with malaria

DIFFERENTIAL DIAGNOSIS

- Meningitis
- Encephalitis
- Stroke
- Acute renal failure
- Acute hemolytic anemia
- Sepsis
- Hepatitis
- Viral diarrheal illness
- Hypoglycemic coma
- Heat stroke

Treatment

INITIAL STABILIZATION

- ABCs
- 0.9% NS fluid bolus for hypotension
- Immediate cooling if temperature >40°C
  - —Acetaminophen
  - —Mist/cool-air fans
- Naloxone, D50W (or Accucheck), and thiamine if altered mental status

ED TREATMENT

- Dependent on identifying the type of malaria present
- *Plasmodium vivax, Plasmodium ovale, Plasmodium malariae,* and non-chloroquine-resistant *P. falciparum*
  - —Treated with oral chloroquine in both adults and children
    - -Chloroquine—safe in pregnant women
  - —Chloroquine-sensitive for falciparum, including Central America, Caribbean, and Middle East
  - —Eradicate persistent hypnozoites in vivax and ovale with primaquine beginning after completion of course of chloroquine
- Chloroquine-resistant falciparum infection—PO treatment options
  - —Quinine, *plus*
    - -Tetracycline or doxycycline (avoid in pregnant women and children <8 years old)
    - -Clindamycin (use in pregnant women and children <8 years old)
    - -Pyrimethamine-sulfadoxine
  - —Mefloquine—safety unproved in pregnancy
- IV treatment for severe malaria
  - —Quinidine (rotary isomer of quinine)
  - —Quinine
    - -Not readily available in the United States
    - -Known abortifacient
- Exchange transfusions
  - —Rapidly removes parasitic RBCs, toxins, and red cell debris, replacing them with fresh plasma and RBCs
  - —Efficacy not proved in randomized trials
  - —Consider in seriously ill with *P. falciparum* parasitemias >10%
- Steroids not recommended for cerebral malaria
  - —Dexamethasone worsens both duration of coma and prognosis
- Supportive therapy for complications
- Chemoprophylaxis
  - —Chloroquine
    - -Drug of choice for travel to areas without chloroquine resistance
    - -300 mg PO weekly
    - -Begin 2 weeks prior to departure and continue for 4 weeks after return
  - —Mefloquine
    - -For chloroquine-resistant areas
    - -250 mg PO weekly
    - -Begin 2 weeks before departure and continue for 4 weeks after return
  - —Doxycycline
    - -For chloroquine/mefloquine-resistant areas
    - -100 mg PO daily
    - -Continue for 4 weeks after return
  - —Terminal prophylaxis with 14-day course of primaquine after completing chemoprophylaxis to prevent relapse from hypnozoites of *P. vivax* or *P. ovale*
  - —According to the CDC, since 1992, seven malaria-related deaths have occurred in U.S. citizens who received inadequate prophylaxis when traveling abroad
  - —Vaccine not currently available, but several in field trials

PEDIATRIC CONSIDERATIONS

- In highly endemic areas with minimal lab capability, all children presenting with febrile illness may be treated

MEDICATIONS

- Acetaminophen: 1 g (ped: 15–20 mg/kg) PO
- Chloroquine: 600-mg base initially (1000 mg of chloroquine phosphate) followed by an additional 300-mg (500-mg salt) 6 hours later and again on days 2 and 3 (peds: 10 mg/kg base PO, followed by 5 mg/kg base 6 hours later and on days 2 and 3)
- Clindamycin: 900 mg (peds: 20–40 mg/kg/24 h) PO t.i.d. for 3 days beginning on the third day of quinine therapy
- Dextrose: D50W 1 amp (50 mL or 25 g) (peds: D25W 2–4 mL/kg) i.v.
- Doxycycline: 100 mg PO b.i.d. for 7 days
- Malarone (atovaquone/proguanil)
  - —Prophylaxis: 250 mg/100 mg PO q day
  - —Treatment: 1000 mg/400 mg (4 tablets) PO q day for 3 days
- Mefloquine: 1250-mg single dose (peds: 25-mg/kg single dose)
- Naloxone (Narcan): 2 mg (peds: 0.1 mg/kg) i.v. or i.m. initial dose
- Primaquine phosphate: 15-mg base (peds: 0.3-mg base/kg/24 h) PO for 14 days
- Pyrimethamine-sulfadoxine (Fansidar): 3 tablets PO on last day of quinine treatment
- Quinidine gluconate: 10 mg/kg loading dose (max, 600 mg) in normal saline infused slowly over 1–2 hours, followed by continuous infusion of 0.02 mg/kg/min until patient is able to begin oral therapy
- Quinine: 650 mg PO t.i.d. for 3–7 days
- Quinine dihydrochloride: 20 mg salt/kg loading dose in 5% dextrose over 4 hours, followed by 10 mg salt/kg over 2–4 hours every 8 hours (max, 1800 mg/d) until patient is able to begin oral treatment
- Tetracycline: 250 mg q.i.d. for 7 days
- Thiamine (vitamin B_1): 100 mg (peds: 50 mg) i.v. or i.m.
- Vaccines: a few currently undergoing field trials, release of effective vaccine not expected for several years

Disposition

ADMISSION CRITERIA

- ICU admission for severe *P. falciparum* infection
- Suspected acute *P. falciparum* infection
- Severe dehydration
- Inability to tolerate oral solution/medication
- >3% of RBC containing parasites

DISCHARGE CRITERIA

- Non-*P. falciparum* infection
- Able to tolerate oral medications

Miscellaneous

ICD9: 84.6

ICD10: B54

SUGGESTED READINGS

Hoffman SL. Diagnosis, treatment, and prevention of malaria. Med Clin North Am 1992;76(6):1327–1355.

Stanley J. Malaria. Emerg Med Clin North Am 1997;15:113–155.

Strickland GT. Fever in the returned traveler. Med Clin North Am 1992; 76(6):1375–1391.

White NJ. The treatment of malaria. N Engl J Med 1996;335:800–806.

Author: Kathryn Brinsfield

Malgaigne Fracture

Clinical Presentation

SIGNS AND SYMPTOMS

- Gross pelvic instability, often with anterior iliac crest displaced or mobile
- Shortening of the legs from migration of the hemipelvis
- Ecchymoses, swelling, abrasions, and open wounds involving the hips, groin, buttocks, perineum, pelvis
- Severe pain on pelvic movement, tilt, and compression
- Often presents in the setting of multiple trauma
- Evidence of perineal, urethral, rectal, and vaginal injuries
- See Hemorrhagic Shock
  - —Tachycardia, hypotension, narrowed pulse pressure
  - —Altered mental status, cool and pale extremities

MECHANISM/DESCRIPTION

- Malgaigne fracture indicates that significant forces were applied to the pelvic bones
- Vertical shear forces result in anterior and posterior disruption of the hemipelvis
- Most commonly, these fractures occur as result of vehicular trauma, pedestrian struck by automobile, or falls from great heights
- As many as 20% of all vehicular trauma fatalities have associated Malgaigne fracture
- These fractures are among the most unstable pelvic fractures, with displacement or potential displacement of the entire hemipelvis
- Associated injuries that must be sought include

Pelvic Hemorrhage and Hemorrhagic Shock

- —Intraabdominal
- —Genitourinary and urinary tract
- —Gynecologic, including uterine and vaginal
- —Neurologic
- —Major vessel

ETIOLOGY

- Malgaigne fracture involves at least two breaks in the continuity of the pelvic ring
- Tile type C pelvic fracture resulting in rotational and vertical instability in the pelvic ring (see Pelvic Fracture)
  - —Anterior disruption of symphysis pubis or two to four pubic rami with posterior displacement and instability through sacrum, sacroiliac joint, or ileum
- Both anterior and posterior disruption with real or potential displacement of the intervening fragments or hemipelvis

PEDIATRIC CONSIDERATIONS

- Children can have proportionately greater blood loss with pelvic fractures
- The possibility of nonaccidental trauma should always be considered

Pre-Hospital

CONTROVERSIES

- Use of the pneumatic antishock garment (PASG) is an alternative in victims suspected of having a pelvic fracture, particularly when faced with a prolonged transport time or hemodynamically instability

CAUTIONS

- Aggressive fluid resuscitation must occur before deflation of the PASG abdominal compartment if it has been used

Diagnosis

ESSENTIAL WORKUP

- *Pelvic radiography* is the most valuable initial diagnostic test
- A single AP view of the pelvis should be done early for any major trauma victim
  - —Most Malgaigne fractures will be seen on the AP view of the pelvis
- An *inlet projection* (30-degree caudal angulation) allows visualization of the posterior pelvis and may aid in the assessment of posterior displacement
- Other radiographic signs suggesting the presence of a Malgaigne fracture include
  - —Pubic symphysis disruption with diastasis greater than 15 mm
  - —Symphysis disruption associated with overlapping of the pubis
  - —Symphysis disruption associated with unilateral fracture of both rami
  - —Bilateral breaks of both pelvic rami or markedly displaced unilateral fractures of both rami
  - —A vertical fracture of the sacrum (these fractures rarely occur as isolated pelvic fractures)
  - —Asymmetry of iliac wings
  - —Avulsion of the ischial spine or L-5 transverse process associated with hemipelvis migration

LABORATORY

- Type and cross-match for blood
- Hemoglobin/hematocrit, platelet count, and coagulation studies (prothrombin time [PT] and partial thromboplastin time [PTT])

IMAGING/SPECIAL TESTS

- CT scan further delineates Malgaigne fracture and *retroperitoneal hematoma*
- MRI scan may be indicated with evidence of neurologic injury
- *Abdominal ultrasound* (US) and *diagnostic peritoneal lavage* (DPL) are rapid bedside evaluations for intraperitoneal hemorrhage
  - —Caution must be exercised to avoid false-positive results (higher mortality rate in victims with pelvic fractures who undergo negative laparotomy)
  - —In the setting of Malgaigne fracture, the supraumbilical open approach for DPL should be used

DIFFERENTIAL DIAGNOSIS

- Other pelvic fractures (straddle fracture, open book fracture, severe multiple pelvic fractures; see Pelvic Fracture)
- Intraabdominal injury and hemorrhage

Treatment

INITIAL STABILIZATION

- ABCs of trauma
  - —Aggressive airway management
  - —Avoid using lower extremity IV sites
  - —Aggressive resuscitation with blood or crystalloid, O-negative or type-specific blood if hemodynamically unstable
  - —Immobilize the pelvis to prevent further injury and decrease bleeding
  - —PASG: use in ED is controversial but allows rapid pelvic immobilization and pelvic compression to slow bleeding
  - —External fixator: requires more time to place than PASG but splints pelvis in a similar manner; contraindicated in severely comminuted Malgaigne pelvic fracture
  - —Placement of a stabilization device should not interfere with further workup and care (i.e., DPL)

ED TREATMENT

- Immediate trauma surgery and orthopedics consultation; patient should be NPO
- Pelvic hemorrhage
  - —Angiography and selective vessel embolization; particularly for small vessel arterial bleeding
  - —Direct operative control of pelvic bleeding; most likely necessary for large vessels
- Prioritization of studies: CT, angiography, or surgery
  - —In the hemodynamically *unstable* patient, a rapidly performed US or DPL can determine treatment course with minimal delay; if the US or DPL aspirate is positive, the patient should go for celiotomy with external pelvic fixation followed by selective angiography
  - —If the DPL or US is negative, the patient should undergo external fixation as appropriate, followed by selective angiography
  - —In cases in which the DPL is positive by cell count criteria only, external fixation and angiography may be performed before surgery
  - —In the hemodynamically *stable* patient, the patient can go to CT scan for evaluation of the abdomen, pelvis, and retroperitoneum

MEDICATIONS

- Blood products: cross-matched, type specific, or O negative: 4–6 IU (peds: 10 mL/kg)
- Crystalloid fluids—normal saline or lactated Ringer's: i.v. bolus 2 L (peds: 20 mL/kg)

Disposition

ADMISSION CRITERIA

- All patients with Malgaigne fractures should be admitted given the magnitude of the insult, the instability of the fracture, and the likelihood of pelvic hemorrhage and concomitant injury
- Patients should be admitted to an ICU or monitored setting

DISCHARGE CRITERIA

- No patients with an acute Malgaigne fracture should be discharged from the ED

Miscellaneous

ICD9: 808.43, 808.8

ICD10: S32.7

SEE ALSO: HEMORRHAGIC SHOCK; PELVIC FRACTURE

SUGGESTED READINGS

American College of Surgeons, Committee on Trauma: Advanced Trauma Life Support Program. Chicago: American College of Surgeons, 1997.

Coppola PT, Coppola M: Emergency department evaluation and treatment of pelvic fractures. Emerg Med Clin North Am 2000;18(1):1–27.

Cwinn AA. Pelvis and hip. In: Marx J, ed. Rosen's emergency medicine: concepts and clinical practice, 5th ed. St. Louis: CV Mosby, 2001:625–642.

MacLeod M, Powell JN. Evaluation of pelvic fractures: clinical and radiologic. Orthop Clin North Am 1997;28(3):299–319.

Author: Theodore Chan

Mallory-Weiss Syndrome

Clinical Presentation

SIGNS AND SYMPTOMS

- Multiple bouts of vomiting and retching followed by hematemesis
  —Most bleeding resolves spontaneously
- Also occurs after
  —Seizures
  —Forceful coughing/laughing
  —Lifting
  —Straining
  —Blunt abdominal trauma
  —Childbirth
  —Cardiopulmonary resuscitation
- Most patients have hiatal hernias
- Abdominal pain
  —Found in the presence of gastritis, esophagitis, or gastric ulcer disease

MECHANISM/DESCRIPTION

- Intraluminal mucosal tear of the distal esophagus
- Sudden increase in intraabdominal pressure causes mucosal tear in the distal esophagus or gastric cardia
- Bleeding is arterial and ranges from mild to moderate
- Cause of bleeding may be related to underlying pathology; "mushrooming" of the stomach into the esophagus during retching has been observed endoscopically

ETIOLOGY

- Often found in those who consume alcohol, especially after a recent binge
- Patients with hiatal hernia appear to be at increased risk

PEDIATRIC CONSIDERATIONS

- Rarely found in children

Pre-Hospital

CAUTIONS

- Airway control
  —100% oxygen or intubate if unresponsive or airway patency in jeopardy
- Initiate one or two large-bore IV catheters if hemodynamically unstable or massive hemorrhage
  —Lactated Ringer's (LR) solution or 0.9% NS
  -1 L bolus (20 mL/kg) if hypotensive
- Trendelenburg's position if hypotensive

Diagnosis

ESSENTIAL WORKUP

- Spun hematocrit
- CBC
- Prothrombin time (PT), partial thromboplastin time (PTT)
- Rectal exam for occult blood in stool

LABORATORY

- Electrolytes, BUN, creatinine, glucose
- Amylase/lipase if abdominal pain
- Type and cross-match
  —At least 4 units of packed red blood cells (PRBCs) if bleeding is severe

IMAGING/SPECIAL TESTS

- EKG in elderly or those with cardiac history
- Upright chest x-ray for free air from esophageal or gastric perforation
- Upper endoscopy (esophagogastroscopy)
  —Procedure of choice to locate, identify, and treat the source of bleeding

DIFFERENTIAL DIAGNOSIS

- Nasopharyngeal bleeding
- Hemoptysis
- Esophageal rupture (Boerhaave's syndrome)
- Esophagitis
- Gastritis
- Duodenitis
- Ulcer disease
- Varices
- Carcinoma
- Vascular-enteric fistula

Treatment

INITIAL STABILIZATION

- ABCs
  - —Intravenous access with at least one large-bore catheter; more if unstable
  - —Central catheter placement if unstable for more efficient delivery of fluids and monitoring of central venous pressure
  - —IV fluids of either 0.9% NS (or LR) at 250 mL/h if stable; wide open if hemodynamically unstable
  - —Dopamine for persistent hypotension unresponsive to aggressive fluid resuscitation
- Large-bore Ewald tube placement with evidence of large amount of bleeding
  - —Safe
  - —Will not aggravate Mallory-Weiss tear
  - —Lavage blood from stomach with water while the patient is on side in Trendelenburg's position
- NG tube placement to check for active bleeding
- Transfuse O-negative red blood cells immediately if hypotensive and not responsive to 2 L of crystalloid
- Most bleeding stops spontaneously with conservative therapy

ED TREATMENT

- Transfuse PRBCs if unstable or lowering hematocrit with continued hemorrhage
- Bladder catheter to monitor urine output
- Monitor fluid status closely
- With continuing hemorrhage, arrange for immediate endoscopy
  - —Control bleeding endoscopically via coagulation techniques and application of blood-clotting agents
- Administer intravenous vasopressin in massive bleeding and unavailable endoscopy
- Angiographic infusion of vasopressin can be used in persistent/unresponsive hemorrhage
- Failure of selective perfusion may require gastric embolization in patients of poor surgical risk
- Surgery—last but definitive treatment modality employing techniques to oversew the bleeding site or perform a gastrectomy
- Sengstaken-Blakemore tubes
  - —Avoid because of potential for complications (especially in the presence of hiatal hernia)
  - —May use as last effort when other modalities have failed with mixed results
- Antiemetics, antacids, and H_2 blockers are helpful

MEDICATIONS

- Dopamine: 2–20 μg/kg min i.v. piggyback (IVPB)
- Vasopressin: 0.2–0.4 IU/min IVPB titrating up to 0.9 IU/min as necessary

Disposition

ADMISSION CRITERIA

- ICU admission for
  - —Continued or massive hemorrhage
  - —Hemodynamic instability
  - —Extreme age
  - —Poor underlying medical condition
  - —Complications
- General floor admission if never unstable and minimal bleed that has since cleared

DISCHARGE CRITERIA

- History of minimal bleed that has stopped
- Hemodynamically stable
- Normal/stable hematocrit
- Negative or trace heme-positive stool
- Negative or trace gastric aspirate

Miscellaneous

ICD9: 530.7

ICD10: K22.6

SEE ALSO: GASTROINTESTINAL BLEEDING

SUGGESTED READINGS

Hastings PR, et al. Mallory-Weiss syndrome: review of 69 cases. Am J Surg 1981;142(5); 560–562.

Michel L, et al. Mallory-Weiss syndrome: Evolution of diagnostic and therapeutic patterns over two decades. Ann Surg 1980;192(6):716–721.

Sugawa C, et al. Mallory-Weiss syndrome: a study of 224 patients. Am J Surg 1983; 145(1):30–33.

Younes Z, et al. The spectrum of spontaneous and iatrogenic esophageal injury: perforations, Mallory-Weiss tears, and hematomas. J Clin Gastroenterol 1999;29(4):306–317.

Author: Dino Rumoro

Malrotation

Clinical Presentation

SIGNS AND SYMPTOMS

- Neonates
  —Bilious emesis
  —Abdominal distention
  —Bloody stools
  —Constipation/obstipation
  —Difficulty feeding
  —Poor weight gain
- Older than 1 year
  —Abdominal pain followed by bilious emesis
- Older children and adolescents
  —Chronic vomiting
  —Intermittent colicky abdominal pain
  —Diarrhea
  —Hematemesis
  —Constipation
  —May not exhibit abnormal *physical* findings at the time of presentation (50–75%)
- Adults
  —Symptoms are vague and nonspecific
- Complications
  —Dehydration, acidosis
  —Peritonitis
  —Ischemic bowel
  —Sepsis, shock

MECHANISM/DESCRIPTION

- Usually found in combination with other congenital anomalies (70%)
  —Cardiac, esophageal, urinary, anal
- Associated gastrointestinal anomalies
  —Duodenal stenosis/atresia/web
  —Meckel's diverticulum
  —Intussusception
  —Gastroesophageal reflux
  —Omphalocele or gastroschisis
  —Congenital diaphragmatic hernia
  —Hirschsprung's disease

ETIOLOGY

- Incomplete rotation and fixation of the embryonic intestine as it returns from its extracolonic position during 10th week of gestation
  —Duodenojejunal junction remains right of midline
  —Cecum remains in the upper left abdomen with abnormal mesenteric attachments

Pre-Hospital

CAUTIONS

- Midgut volvulus may result in need for rapid volume and electrolyte replacement/resuscitation to correct severe dehydration and metabolic acidosis

Diagnosis

ESSENTIAL WORKUP

- Diagnosis is suggested by history and physical exam and is delineated by contrast radiography

LABORATORY

- Electrolytes, BUN, creatinine, glucose
  —Assessment of severity of emesis
  —Hypoglycemia in infants with poor feeding and emesis
- CBC
- Urinalysis

IMAGING/SPECIAL TESTS

- Plain abdominal x-rays
  —Diagnostic in fewer than 30%
  —Volvulus likely if accompanied by
    -Duodenal obstruction (requiring no further studies)
    -Gastric distention with paucity of intraluminal gas distally
    -Generalized distention of small bowel loops
  —Upright films in the neonate to demonstrate obstruction of duodenum
  —Triangular gas shadows in the right upper quadrant from the liver edge overlying the air-filled duodenum
- Upper GI contrast studies
  —95% sensitive and 86% accurate
  —Findings
    -Absence of the ligament of Treitz
    -Dilation of the proximal duodenum with termination in conical or beak shape
    -Spiral or corkscrew appearance of the duodenum
    -Proximal jejunum on the right side of the abdomen (although readily displaced in neonates)
    -Thickening of small bowel folds
- Contrast enema
  —If obstruction equivocal
  —Evaluates position of the cecum in midline of upper abdomen or to left of midline
  —More than 20% false-negative results
- Adjuncts (ultrasound, CT, MRI, angiogram ["barber pole sign"]

DIFFERENTIAL DIAGNOSIS

- Early life
  - —Midgut volvulus
  - —Hirschsprung's disease
  - —Necrotizing enterocolitis
- Children—acute abdominal pain with peritoneal signs
  - —Appendicitis
  - —Intussusception
  - —Overwhelming sepsis
- Older children and adults—vague abdominal pain
  - —Irritable bowel syndrome
  - —Peptic ulcer disease
  - —Biliary and pancreatic disease
  - —Psychiatric disorders

Treatment

INITIAL STABILIZATION

- ABCs
- 0.9% NS IV fluid bolus (20 mL/kg) for shock, sepsis, or dehydration
- Initiate antibiotic for signs of sepsis or peritonitis

ED TREATMENT

- Emergent surgical correction when associated with midgut volvulus for
  - —Detorsion of the volvulus
  - —Restoration of intestinal perfusion
  - —Resection of obviously necrotic areas
  - —Replacement of long segments with questionable vascular integrity back into the abdominal cavity for return celiotomy in 36 hours

Disposition

ADMISSION CRITERIA

- Acute abdomen
- Requiring surgery
- Significant dehydration, acidosis
- Sepsis
- Shock

DISCHARGE CRITERIA

- Outpatient evaluation of the stable, minimally symptomatic patient
  - —Surgical evaluation

Miscellaneous

ICD9: 751.4

ICD10: Q43.3

SUGGESTED READINGS

Ford EG, Senac MO, Srikanth MS, et al. Malrotation of the intestine in children. Ann Surg 1992;215(2):172–178.

Kamal I. Defusing the intra-abdominal ticking bomb: intestinal malrotation in children. Can Med Assoc J 2000;162(9): 1315–1317.

Maxson RT, Franklin PA, Wagner CW. Malrotation in the older child: surgical management, treatment, and outcome. Am Surg 1995;61(2):135–138.

Messineo A, MacMillan JH, Palder SB, et al. Clinical factors affecting mortality in children with malrotation of the intestine. J Pediatr Surg 1992;27(10):1343–1345.

Torres AM, Ziegler MM. Malrotation of the intestine. World J Surg 1993;17(3): 326–331.

Author: Andrea Bracikowski

Mandibular Fractures

Clinical Presentation

SIGNS AND SYMPTOMS
- Mandibular pain
- Facial asymmetry, deformity, and dysphagia
- Malocclusion, decreased range of motion of the temporomandibular joint (TMJ), trismus, or a grating sound conducted to the ear

MECHANISM/DESCRIPTION
- Typically due to a direct force
- The most common area fractured is the angle, followed by the condyle, molar, and mental regions
- Because of its thickness, the mandibular symphysis is rarely fractured
- Bilateral mandibular fractures most commonly result from motor vehicle crashes (MVCs)
- Open fractures are common

ETIOLOGY
- The mandible is the third most common facial fracture following nasal and zygomatic fractures
- MVCs, personal violence, contact sports, or industrial accidents
- Patients are often intoxicated and unable to give a clear history of events
- Facial and head lacerations and facial fractures are the most commonly associated injuries

Pre-Hospital

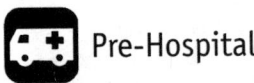

CAUTIONS
- Protect the airway
- Protect the cervical spine
- Preserve any avulsed teeth

Diagnosis

ESSENTIAL WORKUP

Physical Examination
- Inspect the maxillofacial area for obvious deformity, including areas of ecchymosis or swelling
- Malocclusion, trismus, or facial asymmetry
- Loose, fractured, or missing teeth; gross malalignment of teeth; separation of tooth interspaces, bleeding at the base of teeth; gum lacerations between teeth; and ecchymosis or hematoma of the floor of the mouth
- Step-off, bony disruption, or point tenderness with palpation along the entire length of the mandible
- Protrusion or lateral excursion of the jaw
- Interference with normal mandibular function, including decreased range of motion or deviation of the mandible with opening
  - —The examiner should be able to insert three fingers between the mandible and maxilla
  - —Mandible fracture is also suggested by inability of the patient to hold a tongue depressor placed between the teeth when pulled by the examiner, or attempted to be broken by twisting (*positive tongue blade test*)
- Paresthesia of the lower lip or gums strongly indicates a mandibular fracture with secondary damage to the inferior alveolar nerve
- Inability to note motion of the mandibular condyles when palpated through the external ear canals is highly suggestive of a mandibular fracture
- Tenderness of the condyle at the TMJ should increase suspicion of the often-subtle condyle fracture

IMAGING/SPECIAL TESTS
- Plain films or dental panoramic views should be obtained; sensitivity for detecting mandible fractures is equal with either technique
- Plain films including an AP, bilateral obliques, and Towne's view may be obtained
  - —Mandibular views are best for evaluating the condyles and neck of mandible
- Dental panoramic view may be obtained
  - —Panorex best evaluates the symphysis and body
- If condylar fracture is still suspected and not noted on initial radiographs, obtain CT of the condyles in the coronal plane
- Multiple fractures are noted in greater than 50% because of the ringlike structure of the mandible
- Missing teeth that cannot be found mandate a chest radiograph to rule out aspiration
- Obtain cervical spine films if the neck cannot be cleared clinically

DIFFERENTIAL DIAGNOSIS
- Contusions
- Dislocation of the mandible
  - —If a single condyle is dislocated, the jaw will deviate away from the side of the dislocation
  - —If fractured, the jaw will deviate toward the fractured side
- Isolated dental trauma

INITIAL STABILIZATION
- 20–40% of patients with mandibular fractures have associated injuries, and emergency treatment is directed toward immediate, potentially lethal injuries such as airway obstruction, aspiration, major hemorrhage, cervical spine or cord injury, and intracranial injury
- Airway must be protected
- Cervical spine precautions
- If oral intubation cannot be performed secondary to extent of injuries, blind nasotracheal intubation should be performed unless associated facial injuries are present, in which case cricothyrotomy may be indicated

ED TREATMENT
- With the exception of condylar fractures, many mandibular fractures are associated with mucosal, gingival, or tooth socket disruption and should be considered open fractures
  - —Patients should receive antibiotics such as penicillin, clindamycin, or erythromycin to cover intraoral anaerobic pathogens
- Tetanus prophylaxis
- Definitive care usually consists of reduction and fixation by wiring upper and lower teeth in occlusion for 4–6 weeks
  - —Linear, nondisplaced, or greenstick fractures may be treated with soft diet without wiring
- If *mandible dislocation* is present, bilateral downward pressure while the jaw is open is placed on the occlusal surface of the posterior lower teeth while grasping the mandible
  - —The goal is to free the condyle from its anterior position to the eminence
  - —Reduction is facilitated by muscle relaxants (diazepam or midazolam), or anesthetic injection of mastication muscles
  - —A bite block should be used, or the examiner's fingers should be wrapped in gauze to prevent injury

MEDICATIONS

- Acetaminophen: 650 mg (peds: 10–15 mg/kg) PO q4h
- Clindamycin: 150–450 mg PO q.i.d. (peds: 10–20 mg/kg/24 h)
- Diazepam: 10 mg (peds: 0.1–0.2 mg/kg) i.v.
- Erythromycin: 500 mg (peds: 30–50 mg/kg/24 h) PO q.i.d.
- Ibuprofen: 600–800 mg (peds: 20–40 mg/kg/24 h) PO t.i.d. to q.i.d.
- Midazolam: 2–5 mg (peds: safety not established but 0.02–0.05 mg/kg/dose have been used) i.v.
- Penicillin: 500 mg (peds: 25–50 mg/kg/24 h) PO q.i.d.

PEDIATRIC CONSIDERATIONS

- Mandibular fractures are uncommon in children <6 years of age; when they do occur, they are usually greenstick fractures and can be managed with soft diet alone
- The parents should be informed that because any fracture of the mandible has the potential to damage permanent teeth and cause facial asymmetry, long-term follow-up with a specialty consultant is advisable

Disposition

ADMISSION CRITERIA

- Significant displacement or associated dental trauma—open fractures require urgent specialty consultation for possible admission
- The severity of associated trauma may indicate admission
- Any patient with the potential for airway compromise should be admitted
- An unreliable patient with nondisplaced fractures should be admitted for definitive fixation
- In the pediatric population, if the mechanism of injury is not appropriate to the injuries seen, pediatric or child protective services consultation should be obtained

DISCHARGE CRITERIA

- Patients with nondisplaced, closed fractures may be discharged on analgesics and a soft diet
- Patients should be referred to an otorhinolaryngologist or an oral maxillofacial surgeon in a timely fashion

Miscellaneous

ICD9: 802.20

ICD10: S02.6

SUGGESTED READINGS

Alonso LL, Purcell TB. Accuracy of the tongue blade test in patients with suspected mandibular fracture. J Emerg Med 1995;13:297–304.

Luyk NH, Ferguson JW. The diagnosis and initial management of the fractured mandible. Am J Emerg Med 1991;9: 352–359.

Newman J. Medical imaging of facial and mandibular fractures. Radiol Technol 1998;69:417–435.

Schwab RA, Genners K, Robinson WA. Clinical predictors of mandibular fractures. Am J Emerg Med 1998;16:304–305.

Author: David Munter

Marine Envenomation

Clinical Presentation

SIGNS AND SYMPTOMS

Sponges

- Itching and burning a few hours after contact
- Local joint swelling and soft tissue edema
- Fever
- Malaise
- Dizziness
- Nausea
- Muscle cramps
- In severe cases, desquamation in 10 days to 2 months

Coelenterates (Cnidaria—"Jellyfish")

- Mild envenomation
  - —Immediate stinging sensation
  - —Pruritus
  - —Paresthesia, burning sensation
  - —Throbbing
  - —Blistering/local edema/wheal formation
- Moderate/severe
  - —Neurologic
    - -Malaise
    - -Headache
    - -Vertigo/ataxia
    - -Paralysis
    - -Delirium
    - -Seizures
  - —Cardiovascular
    - -Anaphylaxis
    - -Hemolysis
    - -Hypotension
    - -Dysrhythmias
  - —Respiratory
    - -Bronchospasm
    - -Laryngeal edema
    - -Pulmonary edema
    - -Respiratory failure
  - —Musculoskeletal
    - -Muscle cramps or spasm
    - -Arthralgias
  - —Gastrointestinal
    - -Nausea, vomiting, diarrhea
    - -Dysphagia
    - -Hypersalivation/thirst
  - —Ophthalmologic
    - -Conjunctivitis
    - -Corneal ulcers
    - -Elevated intraocular pressure

Echinodermata

Starfish

- Immediate pain
- Bleeding
- Mild edema
- Paresthesias/nausea/vomiting if severe

Sea Urchins

- Intense pain and severe local muscle aches
- Nausea, vomiting
- Paresthesias, hypotension, or respiratory distress with multiple stings

Sea Cucumbers

- Mild contact dermatitis
- Corneal and conjunctival involvement
  - —Severe reactions can lead to blindness

Mollusks

Cone Shells

- Puncture wounds similar to wasp stings
- Sharp burning and stinging
- Paresthesias indicate severe envenomation
- Can evolve into muscular paralysis and respiratory failure, dysphagia, syncope, disseminated intravascular coagulation (DIC)

Stingrays

- Puncture wounds or jagged lacerations
- Local, intense pain, edema, bleeding; necrosis if severe
- Nausea, vomiting, diarrhea
- Diaphoresis
- Headache
- Tachycardia
- Seizures
- Paralysis
- Hypotension
- Arrhythmias

Scorpionfish

- Intense local pain for 6–12 hours
- Erythema may progress to cellulitis
- Headache
- Nausea, vomiting, diarrhea
- Pallor
- Delirium
- Seizures
- Fever
- Hypertension

Catfish

- Local pain, ischemic appearance progressing to erythema
- Swelling, bleeding, and edema
- Local muscle spasms
- Diaphoresis
- Neuropathy/fasciculations/weakness/syncope

Sea Snakes

- Bite initially causes very little pain
- Pinlike pairs of fang marks
- Onset from 5 minutes to 6 hours
- Muscle pain, lower extremity paralysis, arthralgias
- Trismus, blurred vision, dysphagia, drowsiness
- Severe signs include
  - —Ascending paralysis
  - —Aspiration
  - —Coma
  - —Renal and liver failure
- 25% mortality if untreated

MECHANISM/DESCRIPTION

- Sponges
  - —Contain sharp spicules with irritants that cause pruritic dermatitis
- Coelenterates (Cnidaria—"jellyfish")
  - —Contain stinging cells known as nematocysts on their tentacles
  - —Fluid-filled cysts eject a sharp, hollow thread-tube upon contact
  - —Thread-tube penetrates skin and envenomates victim
  - —Box jellyfish can kill within 30 seconds
- Starfish
  - —Very sharp, rigid spines are coated with slimy venom
- Sea urchins
  - —Hollow, sharp spines filled with various toxins
- Sea cucumbers
  - —Hollow tentacles secrete holothurin, a liquid toxin
- Cone shells
  - —Venom injected through a dartlike, detachable tooth
  - —Active peptides interfere with neuromuscular transmission
  - —Presents with puncture wounds similar to wasp stings
- Stingrays
  - —Most common cause of human marine envenomations
  - —Tapered spines attached to tail inject venom into victim
- Scorpionfish
  - —Lionfish usually mild; stonefish can be a life threat
  - —Sharp spines along dorsum and pelvis of fish
    - -Often stepped on inadvertently
    - -Neurotoxic venom
- Catfish
  - —Dorsal and pectoral spines contain venom glands
- Sea snakes
  - —Hollow fangs with associated venom glands
  - —Highly neurotoxic venom blocks neuromuscular transmission

Diagnosis

ESSENTIAL WORKUP

- Careful history/repeat evaluation of wound sites
- Soft tissue radiographs to detect foreign body

LABORATORY

- CBC
- Electrolytes, BUN, creatinine, glucose
- Liver function test
- Urinalysis
- Arterial blood gases if severe symptoms

Treatment

INITIAL STABILIZATION

- ABCs
- Establish IV access with 0.9% NS

ED TREATMENT

General

- Prepared for anaphylactic reactions (EPI/steroids)
- Prepare for intubation if needed
- Benadryl for itch/burn/hives
- Tetanus prophylaxis
- Corticosteroids for severe local reactions
- Narcotic analgesia
  - —Most marine envenomations cause severe pain
- Antibiotic prophylaxis for
  - —Large lacerations or burns
  - —Deep puncture wounds
  - —Grossly contaminated wounds
  - —Elderly or chronically ill
- Antibiotic choices
  - —Trimethoprim-sulfamethoxazole (Bactrim)
  - —Tetracycline
  - —Ciprofloxacin
  - —Third-generation cephalosporin

Sponges

- Gently dry skin and remove spicule
  - —Adhesive tape may aid in removal
- 5% vinegar (or 40–70% isopropyl alcohol) soaks q.i.d. for 10–30 minutes

Coelenterates (Cnidaria—"Jellyfish")

- Rinse wound with saltwater or seawater
  - —Hypotonic solutions trigger more nematocysts
- Do not rub skin—may trigger more nematocysts
- Inactivate toxin with 30-minute soak of 5% vinegar
- Remove remaining nematocysts with razor
- Apply topical anesthetics once nematocysts removed
- Box-jellyfish stings (Australia)—emergent cases
  - —Administer Chironex antivenin
  - —1 ampule (20,000 units) IV diluted 1:5 with crystalloid
- Corticosteroids for severe reactions

Echinodermata

Starfish

- Immerse in nonscalding hot water for pain relief
- Irrigate and explore all puncture wounds
- Prophylactic antibiotics for significant wounds

Sea Urchins

- Immerse in nonscalding hot water for pain relief
- Remove any remaining spines
- Prophylactic antibiotics for significant wounds

Sea Cucumbers

- Immerse in nonscalding hot water for pain relief
- 5% acetic acid soaks
- Ocular involvement
  - —Proparacaine for pain
  - —Copious irrigation with normal saline
  - —Careful slit-lamp exam

Mollusks

Cone Shells

- Hot water immersion for pain relief
- Be prepared for cardiac or respiratory support

Stingrays

- Copious irrigation with removal of any visible spines
- Local suction is controversial
- Hot water soaks for pain relief
- Narcotics for pain control
- High incidence of bacterial infection
  - —Administer prophylactic antibiotics for significant wounds

Scorpionfish

- Hot water soaks for pain relief and venom inactivation
- Copious irrigation, removal of any visible spines
- Local lidocaine or regional block for *severe pain*
- Surgical exploration for deep penetration/ foreign bodies
- Stonefish antivenin for severe envenomations
  - —May cause serum sickness
  - —One 2-mL ampule diluted in 50-mL saline IV slow

Catfish

- Hot water soaks for pain relief and venom inactivation
- Copious irrigation, removal of any visible spines
- Consider local lidocaine, regional block, or narcotics for *severe pain*
- Surgical exploration for deep penetration/ foreign bodies
- Leave puncture wounds open to heal
- Consider prophylactic antibiotics for hand, foot, or deep wounds

Sea Snakes

- Immobilize bitten extremity
- Apply pressure bandage for venous occlusion (pre-hospital)
- Keep victim warm and still
- Polyvalent sea snake antivenin reduces mortality to 3%
  - —May require 3–10 ampules (1000 units each)
  - —Prepare early for assisted ventilation

MEDICATIONS

- Cefixime: 400 mg (peds: 8 mg/kg/24h) PO daily
- Ciprofloxacin: 500 mg PO b.i.d.
- Epinephrine: 0.3–0.5 mL SC of 1:1000 (peds: 0.01 mL/kg)
- Tetracycline: 500 mg PO q.i.d.
- Trimethoprim-sulfamethoxazole (Bactrim DS): 1 tablet (peds: 5 mg liquid (40/200 per 5 mL)/10 kg/dose) PO b.i.d.

Disposition

ADMISSION CRITERIA

- Significant signs of systemic involvement

DISCHARGE CRITERIA

- No signs of systemic illness after 8 hours of observation
- Wound check within 48 hours

Miscellaneous

ICD9: 989.5

ICD10: T63.6

SUGGESTED READINGS

Aldred B, Erickson T, Lioscomb J. Lionfish envenomations in an urban wilderness. Wilderness Environ Med 1996;4:291–296.

Auerbach P. Envenomation by marine life: field guide to wilderness medicine. Stanford, CA: Mosby, 1999:414–432.

Bowman MA, Herman BE. Marine envenomations. In: Strange G, Ahreno W, Lelyveld S, et al., eds. Pediatric emergency medicine. New York: McGraw-Hill, 1996:599–600.

McKinistry DM. Catfish stings in the United States: case report and review. J Wilderness Med 1993;4:293.

Authors: Adam Black; Timothy Erickson

Mastitis

Clinical Presentation

SIGNS AND SYMPTOMS

- Fever usually >39°C
- Chills, rigors, malaise
- Tachycardia
- Breast pain, induration, erythema, warmth; usually unilateral
- Onset typically 2–3 weeks to months postpartum while breast-feeding
- Rare during first postpartum week
- More common in advanced maternal age and patients with diabetes

ETIOLOGY

- *Staphylococcus aureus* most common
- Coagulase-negative *Staphylococcus, Streptococcus* species, *Escherichia coli, Haemophilus influenzae*

Pre-Hospital

N/A

Diagnosis

ESSENTIAL WORKUP

- Physical examination with special attention to detecting abscess; abscess is frequently difficult to detect but is more common in the periaureolar area
  —Purulent nipple discharge with palpation

LABORATORY

- Breast milk culture usually not required

IMAGING/SPECIAL TESTS

- Consider breast ultrasound if abscess is suspected; mammography is not indicated acutely

DIFFERENTIAL DIAGNOSIS

- Breast engorgement: transient fever <39°C of 4–16 hours' duration appearing 48–72 hours postpartum with bilateral nonerythematous bilateral engorgement
- Carcinoma (inflammatory)
- Cyst, tumor
- Abscess formation

Treatment

INITIAL STABILIZATION

- No specific stabilization

ED TREATMENT

- Outpatient oral antibiotics for 10 days
  —β-Lactamase-resistant penicillin, e.g., dicloxacillin (Dynapen)
  —First-generation cephalosporin, e.g., cephalexin (Keflex)
  —Erythromycin if penicillin allergic
- Surgical consultation if evidence of abscess

MEDICATIONS

- Cephalexin: 500 mg q6h PO
- Dicloxacillin: 250 mg q6h PO
- Erythromycin: 500 mg q6h PO
- Clindamycin: 300 mg q6h PO

Disposition

ADMISSION CRITERIA

- Incision and drainage under general anesthesia may be necessary and require admission
- Immunocompromised or evidence of septicemia
- Patients with diabetes may account for one third of mastitis cases; make sure their diabetes is not out of control

DISCHARGE CRITERIA

- Most patients may be managed in the outpatient setting
- Most symptoms resolve within 48 hours of therapy

Miscellaneous

- In simple mastitis, breast-feeding may be continued, including using the affected breast
  —Gently massage to enhance drainage
  —Counsel that this will not harm baby
- Breast support, warm compresses, and analgesia for comfort
- In frank abscess, discontinue breast-feeding until purulent discharge resolves
- Follow-up should be arranged to exclude the diagnosis of inflammatory carcinoma

ICD9: 611.0

ICD10: N61

SUGGESTED READINGS

Calhoun BC, Brost B. Emergency management of sudden puerperal fever. Obstet Gynecol Clin North Am 1995;22(2): 357–367.

Gilbert DN, et al., eds. The Sanford guide to antimicrobial therapy, 22nd ed. Hyde Park, VT: Antimicrobial Therapy, Inc., 2002.

Terregino CA, Greenman RA. Breast disorders. In: Tintinalli J, et al., eds. Emergency medicine: a comprehensive study guide, 5th ed. New York: McGraw-Hill, 2000.

Authors: Marco Coppola; Tim Stallard

Mastoiditis

Clinical Presentation

SIGNS AND SYMPTOMS

- Symptoms
  - —Ear pain
  - —Otorrhea
  - —Mild to severe hearing loss
  - —Fever
  - —Headache
  - —History of irritability in a child
  - —History of recurrent otitis media
- Signs
  - —Tenderness, edema, and erythema over the mastoid
  - —Lateral and inferior displacement of the auricle
  - —Loss of the postauricular crease
  - —Swelling of the posterior and superior ear canal wall
  - —Tympanic membrane abnormalities consistent with severe otitis media
    - -Purulent fluid drainage
    - -Bulging tympanic membrane

MECHANISM/DESCRIPTION

- Mastoiditis is the inflammation and infection of the mastoid air cells caused by acute purulent otitis media
- Middle ear and mastoid air cells are contiguous via the antrum
- Fluid accumulation from closure of channel due to otitis media creates opportunity for infection
- Acute mastoiditis
  - —Occurs to some degree in all cases of otitis media
  - —Manifestation ranges from clinically insignificant inflammation of mastoid air cells to infection and destruction of the bone
  - —Inflammatory changes of the mastoid
  - —Early signs and symptoms are those of acute otitis media
  - —Usually secondary to contamination with infectious material trapped in the mastoid by inflammatory obstruction of the channel between middle ear and mastoid air cells
- Acute mastoiditis with periostitis
  - —As infection progresses, periosteum of the mastoid bone is involved causing periostitis
  - —Subperiosteal abscess may be present
- Acute mastoid ostitis (also called coalescent mastoiditis)
  - —Progression of the infection within the mastoid air cells leads to destruction of the mastoid trabeculae causing coalescence of bony trabeculae
  - —Mastoid empyema or a draining fistula may be present
  - —May progress to severe head and neck complications if untreated
- Masked mastoiditis
  - —Mastoid infection, which lingers after an acute otitis media has been treated
  - —May progress to acute or coalescent mastoiditis
- Chronic mastoiditis
  - —Infection lasting more than 3 months
- Mastoiditis can be a complication of a primary disorder
  - —Leukemia
  - —Mononucleosis
  - —Sarcoma of the temporal bone
  - —Human immunodeficiency virus (HIV)
  - —Kawasaki disease
- Prevalence is equal in males and females

COMPLICATIONS

- Bezold's abscess
  - —Extension of infection to soft tissue below pinna or behind the sternocleidomastoid muscle of neck after erosion through the mastoid tip
- Petrositis
  - —Spread of the infection to the petrous air cells
- Osteomyelitis of the calvarium
- Gradenigo's syndrome
  - —Erosion of the medial temporal bone causing otorrhea, retroorbital pain, and cranial nerve VI paralysis
- Intracranial complications
  - —Subperiosteal abscess
  - —Subdural empyema—extension of infection to CNS with empyema around the tentorium
  - —Sinus thromboses

ETIOLOGY

- Distribution of organisms in acute mastoiditis can differ from that in acute otitis media
  - —*Streptococcus pneumoniae*
  - —Group A streptococcus
  - —*Staphylococcus aureus*
  - —*Haemophilus influenzae*
- Gram-negative enteric bacteria most common with chronic mastoiditis
  - —*Pseudomonas aeruginosa*
  - —*Escherichia coli*
  - —*Proteus mirabilis*
  - —*Bacteroides* species
- Other less common causes
  - —*Mycobacterium tuberculosis*
  - —*Aspergillus* species in immunocompromised states

PEDIATRIC CONSIDERATIONS

- More frequently seen in the pediatric population due to strong association with otitis media
- *S. pneumoniae* most common cause in children

Pre-Hospital

N/A

Diagnosis

ESSENTIAL WORKUP

- Mastoid plain radiographs
  - —Early stage of disease may show hazy or cloudy but intact mastoid
  - —May reveal opacification or coalescence of the mastoid air cells or coalescence as disease progresses
  - —Low sensitivity since may be negative
- CT scan
  - —More useful especially if abscess formation present
  - —Can determine presence and extent of destruction of trabeculae as well as evaluate for the complications of mastoiditis

LABORATORY

- CBC
  - —Leukocytosis
- Cultures of drainage important owing to diversity of organisms
  - —If spontaneous drainage present or after surgical drainage
- Blood culture

IMAGING/SPECIAL TESTS

- MRI
  - —If intracranial involvement suspected but not confirmed by CT
- Lumbar puncture/CSF evaluation for signs of meningitis

DIFFERENTIAL DIAGNOSIS

- Otitis media
- Cellulitis
- External otitis media
- Scalp infection with inflammation of posterior auricular nodes
- Rubella—posterior auricular node enlargement
- Trauma to pinna or postauricular area

Treatment

INITIAL STABILIZATION

- Airway management for signs of airway compromise
- 0.9% NS IV fluid bolus for hypotension/volume depletion

ED TREATMENT

- Otolaryngologist consult for surgical drainage
  - —Drainage is the definitive therapy for acute or coalescent mastoiditis
  - —Emergent drainage if the patient is toxic appearing
  - —Types of surgical procedures
  - —Myringotomy drainage and tympanostomy tube placement
  - —Mastoidectomy and drainage for severe extension (needed in about 50% of cases)
- Initiate IV antibiotics
  - —Semisynthetic penicillins (Unasyn, Timentin) with chloramphenicol
  - —Third-generation cephalosporins (ceftriaxone, cefotaxime)
  - —Imipenem
  - —Given increasing proportion of *S. aureus* as causative organism, should consider including antistaphylococcal agent before culture results
  - —Parenteral antibiotics can be switched to oral after patient afebrile for 36–48 hours
- Administer pain medications
  - —NSAIDs
  - —Oral or parenteral narcotics

MEDICATIONS

- Ampicillin sulbactam (Unasyn): 1.5–3 g i.v. q6h
- Cefotaxime: 1–2 g (peds: 50–180 mg/kg/24 h) i.v. q4–6h
- Ceftriaxone: 1–2 g (peds: 50–75 mg/kg/24 h) i.v. q12–24h
- Chloramphenicol: 50–100 mg/kg/24 h i.v. or PO q6h
- Imipenem: 250 mg–1 g i.v. q6–8h
- Ticarcillin clavulanate (Timentin): 3.1 g i.v. q4–6h

Disposition

ADMISSION CRITERIA

- Clinical suspicion of acute or coalescent mastoiditis
- Subperiosteal abscess
- Toxic appearing

DISCHARGE CRITERIA

- No patient with acute or coalescent mastoiditis should be discharged

Miscellaneous

ICD9: 383.00, 383.9, 383.1

ICD10: H70.9

SUGGESTED READINGS

Biter CN, Kluka EA, Steele RW. Mastoiditis in children. Clin Pediatr 1996;35(8): 391–395.

Bluestone CD, Klein JO, et al., eds. Pediatric otolaryngology. 3rd ed, vol 1. Philadelphia: WB Saunders, 1996:618.

Gliklich RE, Eavey RD, Iannuzzi RA, et al. A contemporary analysis of acute mastoiditis. Arch Otolaryngol Head Neck Surg 1996; 122(2):135–139.

Koranyi K. Mastoiditis. In: Harwood-Nuss A, Wolfson A, Linden C, et al. The clinical practice of emergency medicine, 3rd ed. Philadelphia: Lippincott Williams & Wilkins, 2001:1305–1306.

Luntz M, Brodsky A, Nusem S, et al. Acute mastoiditis—the antibiotic era: a multicenter study. Int J Pediatr Otorhinolaryngol 2001;57:1–9.

Nadol JB, Eavey RD. Acute and chronic mastoiditis: clinical presentation, diagnosis, and management. Curr Clin Top Infect Dis 1995;15:204–229.

Wang N, Ewen, Burg J. Mastoiditis: a case-based review. Pediatr Emerg Care 1998;14:290–293.

Author: Sam Shen

MDMA, Poisoning

Clinical Presentation

SIGNS AND SYMPTOMS

- Overdose
  —Altered mental status
  —Severe sympathomimetic symptoms
- CNS
  —CNS excitation
  —Coma
  —Seizures
  —Cerebral edema
  —Brainstem herniation
- Cardiovascular
  —Hypertension (early)
  —Hypotension (late)
  —Palpitations
  —Ventricular tachycardia and ectopy
- Pulmonary
  —Pulmonary edema
- Metabolic
  —Hyponatremia
  —Hypoglycemia
  —Syndrome of inappropriate antidiuretic hormone (SIADH)
- Musculoskeletal
  —Bruxism
  —Restlessness
  —Rigidity
- Renal
  —Rhabdomyolysis
- Hepatic
  —Jaundice
  —Hepatitis
  —Hepatic necrosis
- Hematologic
  —Disseminated intravascular coagulation (DIC)
- Gastrointestinal
  —Vomiting
  —Diarrhea
  —Abdominal cramping
- Psychiatric
  —Euphoria
  —Flight of ideas
  —Delirium/hallucinations
- Other
  —Hyperthermia
  —Mydriasis
  —Nystagmus

MECHANISM/DESCRIPTION

- MDMA: 3,4-methylenedioxymethamphetamine ("ecstasy")
- Schedule I drug manufactured illegally
- Used recreationally
  —Rave parties
  —Dance clubs
  —College campuses
- Amphetamine-like structure stimulates catecholamine release
- Mescaline-like ring structure enhances serotonergic and dopaminergic activity
- Onset of effects: 15–30 minutes after ingestion
- Duration of effects: 2–6 hours
- Pills commonly contain contaminants
  —Caffeine
  —Ephedrine
  —Dextromethorphan
  —Ketamine
  —Related methylated amphetamines (MDA, MDEA, MDBA, PMA)

Pre-Hospital

CAUTIONS

- A single tablet may cause severe toxicity
- Transport all pills/pill bottles involved in overdose for identification in ED
- Watch for MDMA paraphernalia
  —Pacifiers
  —Glowsticks
  —Surgical masks
- Do not induce emesis owing to risk for CNS depression and aspiration
- Provide respiratory support

Diagnosis

ESSENTIAL WORKUP

- Diagnosis based on clinical presentation and an accurate history
- Obtain a core temperature
- Exclude toxic co-ingestants or contaminants

LABORATORY

- Electrolytes, BUN, creatinine, glucose
- Prothrombin time (PT), partial thromboplastin time (PTT), INR
- Urine dip for blood and myoglobin
- Urine toxicology screen to exclude co-ingestants
  —May cause positive amphetamine and metamphetamine screen
- Quantitative MDMA levels rarely helpful
- Creatine phosphokinase if rhabdomyolysis suspected
- Liver function tests for significant overdose or suspected hepatitis

IMAGING/SPECIAL TESTS

- EKG
  —Sinus tachycardia (most common)
  —Dysrhythmias, conduction disturbances
- Chest x-ray if suspected aspiration pneumonia
- Head CT if suspected intracranial hemorrhage

DIFFERENTIAL DIAGNOSIS

- Cocaine overdose
- Amphetamine overdose
- Antihistamine overdose
- Serotonin syndrome
- Occult head injury
- Sepsis
- Thyroid storm
- Pheochromocytoma

Treatment

INITIAL STABILIZATION

- ABCs
  - —Airway control essential
  - —Administer supplemental oxygen
- Administer naloxone, thiamine, and glucose (or Accu-Chek) if depressed mental status

ED TREATMENT

- Supportive care
- Decontaminate with activated charcoal if recent ingestion
- Monitor core temperature and cardiac rhythm for at least 6 hours
- Hydrate with 0.9% NS IV
- Hypertension
  - —Nitroprusside
  - —Phentolamine
  - —Esmolol
- Hypotension
  - —0.9% NS IV bolus
  - —Trendelenburg's position
  - —Pressors titrated to blood pressure
- Anxiety/restlessness/agitation
  - —Diazepam or lorazepam as needed
- Seizures
  - —Treat initially with benzodiazepines
  - —Phenobarbital for persistent seizures
- Rhabdomyolysis
  - —Hydrate aggressively with 0.9% NS IV
  - —Consider sodium bicarbonate administration
  - —Hemodialysis if renal failure
- Hyperthermia
  - —Standard cooling measures
  - —Treat agitation with benzodiazepines
  - —Consider dantrolene in refractory cases

MEDICATIONS

- Activated charcoal: 1–2 g/kg PO
- Dantrolene: 1–2 mg/kg to max 10 mg/kg i.v.
- Diazepam: 5–10 mg (peds: 0.2–0.5 mg/kg) i.v. every 10–15 minutes
- Esmolol: 500 μg/kg i.v. bolus, then 50 μg/kg/min i.v.
- Lorazepam: 2–6 mg (peds: 0.05–0.1 mg/kg) i.v. every 10–15 minutes
- Naloxone: 0.4–2 mg (peds: 0.1 mg/kg; neonatal: 10–30 μg/kg) i.v. or i.m.
- Nitroprusside: 0.3 μg/kg/min to maximum of 10 μg/kg/min
- Phenobarbital: 10–20 mg/kg i.v. (loading dose)
- Phentolamine 1–5 mg (peds: 0.02–0.1 mg/kg) i.v. bolus every 5–10 minutes

Disposition

ADMISSION CRITERIA

- Seizures
- Persistent cardiovascular instability
- Rhabdomyolysis
- Loss of behavioral control
- DIC

DISCHARGE CRITERIA

- Asymptomatic 6 hours after oral overdose

Miscellaneous

ICD9: 969.7

ICD10: T43.6

SUGGESTED READINGS

Kalant H. The pharmacology and toxicity of "ecstasy" (MDMA) and related drugs. Can Med Assoc J 2001;165(7):917–928.

Schwartz RH, Miller NS. MDMA (ecstasy) and the rave: a review. Pediatrics 1997;100(4):705–708.

Shannon MW. Methylenedioxymethamphetamine (MDMA, "ecstasy"). Pediatr Emerg Care 2000;16(5):377–380.

Authors: Todd Clark; Mark B. Mycyk

Measles

Clinical Presentation

SIGNS AND SYMPTOMS

Incubation (8–12 days)

- Transmission via direct contact or inhalation of infectious droplet

Prodrome (1–2 days)

- Mild respiratory illness
- Koplik's spots
  - —Small white to grayish-blue specks on buccal mucosa
  - —Pathognomonic for rubeola
  - —Transient and disappears within 48 hours after onset of rash

Active Disease

- Cough, coryza, conjunctivitis with fever and rash
- Rash begins on the head and neck and spreads centrifugally downward
  - —Initially pale, then discrete and maculopapular, and ultimately, confluent
  - —Clears in 3–4 days and may desquamate as the rash fades

Complications

- Respiratory
  - —Pneumonia, especially the immunocompromised
  - —Most common cause of fatality
  - —Laryngotracheobronchitis in patients <2 years old
- CNS
  - —Encephalomyelitis
    - -Usually 1–14 days after onset of rash
    - -Fever, headache, vomiting, and stiff neck
    - -Lethargy, stupor, and seizure followed by coma
    - -More than half will have permanent residuals
  - —Subacute sclerosing panencephalitis (SSPE)
    - -Develop weeks to years after infection
    - -Insidiously progressive degeneration of CNS functions
    - -Personality change, intellectual deterioration, motor and visual deficits, coma, and death
- Cardiovascular
  - —Transient myocarditis, pericarditis, and conduction defects
  - —Rarely clinically significant
  - —Congestive heart failure in elderly patients
- Thrombocytopenic purpura
- Otitis media
- Sinusitis

ETIOLOGY

- Negative-strand paramyxovirus
- Humans, only known reservoir
- Highly contagious; outbreaks seen in nonimmunized or underimmunized

Pre-Hospital

CAUTIONS

- Nonimmunized pre-hospital care personnel should be advised of potential risks described above
- Risk for spontaneous abortion and premature birth in nonimmunized pregnant pre-hospital personnel if infected

Diagnosis

ESSENTIAL WORKUP

- Diagnosis is based on clinical findings
- Cough, coryza, and conjunctivitis with fever and subsequent rash

LABORATORY

- CSF analysis for suspected encephalitis
- Viral cultures and antibody testing generally impractical

IMAGING/SPECIAL TESTS

- Chest x-ray for suspected pneumonia

DIFFERENTIAL DIAGNOSIS

- Rubella
  - —Milder course, postauricular nodes, pinker rash, no conjunctivitis
- Scarlet fever
  - —Sand paper textured rash, strawberry tongue, sore throat
- Infectious mononucleosis
  - —Serologic test available
- Roseola
  - —Rash appears after temperature falls
- Erythema infectiosum (Fifth's disease)
  - —No prodrome and without fever
  - —Red flushed cheeks with lacelike rash when fading
- Enterovirus
  - —No respiratory complaints
- Kawasaki disease
  - —Rash on palm and soles
- Secondary syphilis
- Toxic shock syndrome
- Drug reactions
  - —Usually without fever and upper respiratory infection symptoms

Treatment

ED TREATMENT

- Prevention with vaccination is cornerstone of therapy
  - —Two doses of measles vaccine given as MMR
  - —First dose at 12 months and second before school entry
- Oxygenation and airway protection
  - —Pneumonia
  - —Encephalitis
- Antipyretics
- IV rehydration as needed
- Isolate suspected cases
- Postexposure prophylaxis for the nonimmune
  - —Give MMR if <72 hours after exposure
    - -Avoid if pregnant, immunocompromised
  - —Immune globulin 100–400 mg/kg i.v. or 0.25 mL/kg i.m. to 15 mL (max)
    - -If given <6 days after exposure, will prevent or modify measles

Disposition

ADMISSION CRITERIA

- Severe pneumonia
- Dehydration
- Encephalitis
- SSPE
- Immunocompromised patients
  - —AIDS
  - —Immunosuppressive therapy
- Elderly patients with comorbid conditions

DISCHARGE CRITERIA

- Duration of infectivity information:
  - —2 days before symptoms and up to 4 days after onset of rash
  - —Immunocompromised are contagious for the duration of illness

Miscellaneous

ICD9: 55.9

ICD10: B05.9

SUGGESTED READINGS

American Academy of Pediatrics. Measles. In: Pickering LK, ed. 2000 Red book: report of the Committee on Infectious Diseases, 25th ed. Elk Grove Village, IL: American Academy of Pediatrics; 2000:385–396.

Centers for Disease Control and Prevention. Measles, mumps and rubella: vaccine use and strategy for elimination of measles, rubella, and congenital rubella syndrome and control of mumps. Recommendations of the Advisory Committee on Immunization Practices (ACIP). MMWR Morb Mortal Wkly Rep 1998;47(RR-8):1–57.

Gable EK. Pediatric exanthems. Primary Care 2000;27(2):353–369.

Goldman L, ed. Cecil textbook of medicine, 21st ed. Philadelphia: WB Saunders, 2000:1802–1805.

Author: Austen Chai

Meckel's Diverticulum

Clinical Presentation

SIGNS AND SYMPTOMS

Common Presenting Sequelae/ Complications

- Obstruction
- Intussusception
- Diverticulitis
- Hemorrhage
- Volvulus

Gastrointestinal

- Abdominal pain
  - —Location depends on cause
  - —"Appendicitis-like"
- Vomiting
- Changes in bowel movements
- Hematochezia
- Melena
- Peritonitis and septic shock (late complications)

General

- Fever
- Malaise
- Weakness
- Fatigue

Cardiovascular

- Tachycardia (due to pain or blood loss)
- Hypotension and shock (due to bleeding)

MECHANISM/DESCRIPTION

- Most common congenital abnormality of the gastrointestinal tract
- Remnant of the omphalomesenteric duct, which usually regresses by the seventh week of gestation
- Ileal true diverticula
  - —50% contain normal ileal mucosa
  - —50% contain either gastric (most common), pancreatic, duodenal, colonic, endometrial, or hepatobiliary mucosa
- "Rule of two"
  - —2% prevalence in general population
  - —Male-to-female ratio of 2:1
  - —Average length, 2 inches
  - —About 2 feet from the ileocecal valve
- Complications
  - —4% lifetime risk for complications, decreasing with age
  - —Obstruction and diverticulitis in adults
  - —Hemorrhage and obstruction in children
  - —Mean age, 10 years
- Obstruction
  - —Diverticulum attached to the umbilicus, abdominal wall, or other viscera or is free and unattached
  - —Intussusception—diverticulum is the leading edge
  - —Volvulus—persistent fibrous band leads to bowel rotation
- Diverticulitis
  - —Opening obstructed
  - —Bacterial infection follows
  - —Presents like appendicitis (most common preoperative diagnosis with Meckel's diverticulum)

PEDIATRIC CONSIDERATIONS

- Present under the age of 5 years with episodic painless rectal bleeding
- Brisk and bright red bleeding
- Most common ectopic: gastric tissue
  - —Gastric secretions lead to erosions and bleeding

Pre-Hospital

CAUTIONS

- High mortality associated with Meckel's diverticulum is due to a lack of recognition of presenting features, potential for hypotension, and complications
- Transport all patients with rectal bleeding or abdominal pain for evaluation
- IV access with 0.9% NS because patients can become hypotensive and require fluid resuscitation

Diagnosis

ESSENTIAL WORKUP

- Meckel's diverticulum causes a variety of signs and symptoms
  - —Fewer than 10% diagnosed preoperatively
  - —Consider in any patient with recurrent nonspecific abdominal pain, nausea and vomiting, or rectal bleeding
- History/physical exam narrow diagnosis but will not give findings specific to Meckel's diverticulum
- Rectal exam mandatory
- Nasogastric tube placement
  - —Most common cause of lower GI bleeding is upper GI bleeding

LABORATORY

- CBC
  - —Decreased hematocrit due to acute bleeding
  - —Meckel's diverticulum rarely a cause of chronic anemia
  - —Leukocytosis with diverticulitis/ gangrene/perforation
- Electrolytes, BUN, creatinine, glucose
- Type and screen when significant GI bleeding

IMAGING/SPECIAL TESTS

- Abdominal radiographs
  - —No value in diagnosing Meckel's diverticulum
  - —Eliminates other causes of abdominal pain or GI bleeding
- Technetium-99m pertechnetate radioisotope scan
  - —Noninvasive scan that identifies Meckel's diverticulum containing heterotopic gastric mucosa only
  - —90% accurate in children
  - —45% accurate in adults
- Small bowel enteroclysis
  - —75% accuracy
  - —Barium/methyl cellulose introduced through NG tube into distal duodenum or proximal jejunum
  - —Radiologist looks for diverticulum
  - —Increases the ability to detect Meckel's diverticulum in adults
  - —Diverticulum may be short and wide-mouthed, making diagnosis difficult

- Barium enema
  - —Introduces fluid into distal small bowel
  - —Look for diverticulum
- Angiogram for further evaluation of Meckel's diverticulum if radioisotope scan and enteroclysis normal
  - —Blood supply is not always abnormal
- Ultrasound may be useful in nonbleeding presentations
- Laparoscopic evaluation may provide both diagnosis and definitive treatment
- EKG
  - —Eliminate myocardial ischemic causes of abdominal pain
  - —When significant blood loss

DIFFERENTIAL DIAGNOSIS

Abdominal Pain

- Appendicitis
- Volvulus
- Bowel obstruction
- Diverticulitis
- Adhesions
- Internal hernias
- Intussusception

Bleeding

- Intussusception
- Upper GI bleeding
- Diverticulosis
- Hemorrhoids
- Inflammatory bowel disease
- Pseudomembranous colitis
- Polyps

Pediatric Differential Diagnosis

- Abdominal pain
  - —Intussusception
  - —Volvulus
  - —Atresia
  - —Strictures
  - —Malrotation
  - —Adhesions
- Bleeding
  - —Milk allergy
  - —Gastroenteritis
  - —Intussusception
  - —Henoch-Schönlein purpura
  - —Volvulus
  - —Hemolytic-uremic syndrome
  - —Anal fissures
  - —Polyps

Treatment

INITIAL STABILIZATION

- ABCs
- Fluid resuscitation with 0.9% NS in 20 mL/kg bolus amounts
- Cardiac monitoring in older patients

ED TREATMENT

- Stabilization followed by early surgical evaluation
- Hypotension
  - —Aggressive fluid resuscitation
  - —Packed RBC transfusion with brisk rectal bleeding (more common in children)
  - —Pressors for septic shock
- NG tube
- Foley
- Preoperative antibiotics

MEDICATIONS

- Ampicillin sulbactam (Unasyn): 3 g (peds: 100–200 mg ampicillin/kg/24 h) q8h i.v.
- Cefoxitin (Mefoxin): 1–2 g (peds: 100–160 mg/kg/24 h) i.v. q6h
- Dopamine: 2–20 μg/kg/min i.v.

Disposition

ADMISSION CRITERIA

- Presumptive diagnosis of Meckel's diverticulum with diverticulitis, obstruction, intussusception, hemorrhage, or volvulus requires admission and surgical evaluation

DISCHARGE CRITERIA

- None

Miscellaneous

ICD9: 751.0

ICD10: Q43.0

SEE ALSO: APPENDICITIS

SUGGESTED READINGS

Bono MJ. Lower gastrointestinal tract bleeding. Emerg Med Clin North Am 1996;14:547–556.

Martin JP, et al. Meckel's diverticulum. Am Fam Physician 2000;61(4):1037–1042.

Schwartz MW, ed. The 5-minute pediatric consult. Baltimore: Williams & Wilkins, 1997:478–479.

Yahchouchy EY, et al. Meckel's diverticulum. J Am Coll Surg 2001;192(5):658–662.

Author: John Bailitz

Medial Collateral Ligament Strain

Clinical Presentation

SIGNS AND SYMPTOMS

- Tearing sensation and immediate pain medial aspect of knee
  - —Medial pain and tenderness may be more pronounced with partial tears than with complete tears
- Localized swelling
  - —Hemarthrosis signifies tear of capsular portion of medial collateral ligament (MCL) or cruciate injury
- Variable ability to bear weight
  - —May be able to bear weight with complete tear
  - —Patients often describe buckling sensation on weight bearing
- Additional findings with involvement of other ligaments

MECHANISM/DESCRIPTION

- Most commonly injured knee ligament
- Direct trauma to lateral knee
- Most common: valgus stress with external rotary component on flexed knee
  - —From catching a ski tip
  - —Side tackle (football)
- When accompanied by other ligament injury
  - —Hyperextension with external rotation (anterior collateral ligament [ACL] and posterior collateral ligament [PCL] injured first)
  - —Anterior stress (ACL injured first)

PEDIATRIC CONSIDERATIONS

- MCL attaches distal to tibial epiphysis and proximal to femoral epiphysis
- MCL injury *infrequent* before growth plate closure (<14 years old)
- MCL injury may accompany underlying fracture
- Most injuries due to direct trauma producing valgus stress (sports, auto-pedestrian)

Pre-Hospital

CAUTIONS

- Evaluate for knee dislocation
- Document neurovascular status
- MCL injury may be overlooked in the multiple trauma victim
- Immobilize in slight flexion

Diagnosis

ESSENTIAL WORKUP

Complete Knee Examination

- Palpate medial femoral condyle (most common site for MCL tear)
- *Valgus stress testing:*
  - —*In flexion:* grasp lateral aspect of knee and abduct while externally rotating at ankle with knee in 30 degrees of flexion
  - —Joint laxity
  - —Mild: severe partial or complete MCL tear
  - —Moderate: complete MCL tear, possible ACL tear
  - —Marked: complete MCL and ACL tear, possible PCL tear
  - —*In extension:* same as above but with knee extended
  - —Joint laxity: complete MCL rupture with or without ACL and PCL tear
- *Note that*
  - —Underlying fracture should be ruled out before stress test
  - —Reexam in 24 hours may be necessary if severe muscle spasm and ligamentous pain present
  - —Intraarticular instillation of anesthetic and analgesic may be required to perform adequate exam
- Classification of ligament injuries (sprains)
  - —Grade 1: stretched fibers without tear; firm end point on stress testing
  - —Grade 2: extracapsular fibers tear without complete rupture; mild instability but firm end point on stress testing; inability to extend knee fully
  - —Grade 3: complete rupture; no fixed end point on stress testing; hemarthrosis

LABORATORY

- Aspiration of joint effusion may be therapeutic (relieve pain) and diagnostic (hemarthrosis with cruciate tears, fat globules with fractures)

IMAGING/SPECIAL TESTS

- Standard radiographs give no clues to MCL tears but can reveal fractures, effusions, tendon calcifications, osteophytes, and foreign bodies
  - —Views: AP, lateral, oblique, notch view
  - —Fat-fluid level is pathognomonic of fracture
- MRI accurately detects collateral ligament injuries and other intraarticular structures and disorders (menisci, ACL, PCL, osteonecrosis, occult fractures)
- Arthroscopy used by consultant for diagnosis and repair of meniscal and cruciate injuries
- Arteriograms to evaluate vascular integrity for severe associated injuries (e.g., knee dislocation)
- Ultrasound useful to diagnose cysts and popliteal artery aneurysms

DIFFERENTIAL DIAGNOSIS

- Meniscal, other ligament injuries, and fractures may be concomitant
- *Hip injury* may present with knee pain
- Arthritis (rheumatoid, osteoid, septic), cellulitis, bursitis

PEDIATRIC CONSIDERATIONS

- Examine hip and obtain radiograph if any concern for hip pathology (especially slipped capital femoral epiphysis)
- Epiphyseal plate tenderness may signify nondisplaced Salter I fracture

Treatment

INITIAL STABILIZATION

- Maintain joint immobilization in neutral position or position of comfort by pre-hospital personnel

ED TREATMENT

- Grade I or II: intermittent ice, elevation, rest, crutches, compression (splint or knee immobilizer)
- Grade III: as I or II but require definitive orthopedic referral
- Joint aspiration of large hemarthrosis may help relieve pain

MEDICATIONS

- NSAIDs recommended
- Narcotic analgesics as needed
- Joint installation of anesthetic (e.g., bupivacaine 0.25%, 5 mL) with an analgesic (e.g., morphine 1–5 mg diluted to 30 mL) may be required for severe pain

Disposition

ADMISSION CRITERIA

- To manage severe associated injuries

DISCHARGE CRITERIA

- Absence of associated injuries requiring admission
- Ensure compliance with splinting and adequate follow-up

Miscellaneous

ICD9: 844.1

ICD10: S83.7

SUGGESTED READINGS

Casazza BA, Young JL, Rossner KK. Musculoskeletal disorders of the lower limbs. In: Braddom RL, Buschbacher RM, eds. Physical medicine and rehabilitation, 2nd ed. Philadelphia: WB Saunders, 2000:840–841.

Gray SD, Kaplan PA, Dussault RG. Imaging of the knee: current status. Orthop Clin North Am 1997;28(4):643–658.

Sherk HH. Injuries of the knee. In: Fleisher GR, Ludwig, eds. Textbook of pediatric emergency medicine, 4th ed. Philadelphia: Lippincott Williams & Wilkins, 2000.

Simon R, Koenigsknecht SJ. Soft tissue injuries and disorders of the knee. In: Emergency orthopedics: the extremities, 4th ed. New York: McGraw-Hill, 2001:453–461.

Smith BW, Green GA. Acute knee injuries. Part II: diagnosis and treatment. Am Fam Physician 1995;51:799–806.

Stewart C. Knee injuries: diagnosis and repair. Emerg Med Rep 1997;18(1):1–12.

Author: Richard A. Craven

Medial Meniscus Injury

Clinical Presentation

SIGNS AND SYMPTOMS

- Usually present within 24 hours of acute injury
- May report hearing a pop, feeling a tear, catch, lock, or a click
- Usually occurs with rotational force, often when knee is flexed
- Patient may recall the knee "giving way"
- Inability to extend knee fully is common
- Effusion found in 50% and usually occurs over 6–12 hours
- Pain often intermittent/localized to the joint line
- Unlike ligamentous injury, patients often report completion of activities at time of injury

MECHANISM/DESCRIPTION

- Among most common adult knee injuries
- Medial meniscus injury 10 times more common than lateral
- Usually occurs in young active adults or geriatric patient with degenerative meniscus
- Sudden rotary motion of knee without the normal compensatory rotation that is required of the tibia
- Geriatric patients with a degenerative meniscus may recall nothing more than a simple twist or rising from a seated or squatting position.

ETIOLOGY

- Medial meniscus is more firmly attached to the joint capsule and less mobile than the lateral meniscus predisposing it to injury when tensile/compressive forces are applied
- Factors that increase propensity for meniscal injuries include congenital discoid meniscus, atrophy of the surrounding musculature, ligamentous laxity, degenerative meniscus common in elderly people
- Medial meniscal injuries often accompany ligamentous injuries particularly the deep medial collateral ligament to which it is attached
- Tears are the result of tensile or compressive forces between the femoral and tibial condyles
  - —With knee flexion, the femur rotates internally on the flexed tibia, displacing the medial meniscus toward the center of the joint
  - —With rapid forceful extension, the meniscus may be trapped centrally, resulting in peripheral segment stretching or tear
  - —Extension of the tear may result in a free segment that may become displaced into the joint, resulting in a true locked joint

PEDIATRIC CONSIDERATIONS

- Rare in children less than 10 years old, especially with open epiphyses and morphologically normal menisci
- Most pediatric cases are the result of direct trauma

Pre-Hospital

CAUTIONS

- Immediate application of ice packs
- Immobilization in a position of comfort
- Careful neurovascular examination
- Evaluate for dislocations and associated injuries

Diagnosis

ESSENTIAL WORKUP

- Physical examination with special attention to joint line tenderness, which has high predictive value of 75–85%
- Effusion is found in 50% and is typically delayed in onset
- An inability to extend the joint at 20–45 degrees secondary to true or pseudo locking is a common finding
  - —Limitation of extension due to severe pain from muscle spasm/effusion suggests *pseudo* locked joint; *true* locked joint due to torn fragment within the joint occurs in only 30%
- Provocative testing should be deferred until severe pain resolves. Provocative tests include McMurray's, Apley, Steinmann, Childress, and Helfet, among others
- Recent systematic review concludes that physical diagnostic tests have low diagnostic accuracy

IMAGING/SPECIAL TESTS

- Plain x-ray may demonstrate effusion or associated bony abnormalities and is recommended
- MRI has replaced arthrography; diagnostic accuracy is greater than 90–98%, depending on type of injury
- Arthroscopy remains the standard for diagnostic accuracy

Arthrocentesis

- May afford significant symptomatic relief when effusion is present
- Aspiration of bloody fluid suggests cruciate ligament tear or injury to peripheral vascular part of meniscus
- Send fluid for cell count, protein and glucose, Gram stain, culture, and crystals, as indicated

DIFFERENTIAL DIAGNOSIS

- Osteochondral fractures, osteochondritis dissecans, patellofemoral joint syndromes, contusion
- Ligamentous injuries, including anterior and posterior cruciate, medial/lateral collateral ligament
- Iliotibial band syndrome, lumbar radiculopathy, gout and other inflammatory arthropathies

Treatment

INITIAL STABILIZATION

- Application of ice packs decreases pain and inflammation
- Immobilization in position of comfort

ED TREATMENT

- Arthrocentesis may afford relief with large effusions and assist to reduce locked joint
- Arthrocentesis should be followed by application of compressive dressing
- Reduction of locked joint should be performed within first 24 hours after injury
  —With patient seated, hang extremity off edge of examination table at 90 degrees (this alone may reduce locked joint)
  —Applying gentle traction and rotation of tibia usually result in reduction of the locked joint
- NSAIDS, both parenteral and oral, are of utility during acute phase of injury
- Weight bearing and range of motion is permitted as tolerated
- Individuals unable to bear weight or those with severe restriction of range of motion should be placed in a knee immobilizer or crutches as needed
- Definitive treatment by orthopedic consultant; operative versus nonoperative treatment is dependent upon multiple factors such as type of meniscal injury, age of patient, activity level, associated injuries and candidacy for physical therapy

MEDICATIONS

- Ibuprofen: 400–600 mg PO q6h (peds: 5–10 mg/kg/dose q6h
- Ketorolac: 15–30 mg i.v. or i.m. initially followed by 10 mg PO q6h (combined treatment not to exceed 5 days)
- Hydrocodone and acetaminophen combinations (Vicodin, Lortab): 1–2 tablets PO q4–6h PRN

Disposition

ADMISSION CRITERIA

- Intractable pain is suggestive of true locked joint and may require emergent orthopedic referral
- High risk for consequential injuries in unassisted elderly patients who are sent home

DISCHARGE CRITERIA

- Patients capable of following a structured discharge plan

Miscellaneous

ICD9: 959.7

ICD10: S83.6

SUGGESTED READINGS

Koski JA, Meniscal injury and repair: clinical status [Review]. Orthop Clin North Am 2000;31(3):419–436.

Marx J, et al. Rosen's emergency medicine: concepts and clinical practice, 5th ed. St. Louis: CV Mosby, 2002.

Scholten RJ, et al. The accuracy of physical diagnostic tests for assessing meniscal lesions of the knee: a meta-analysis. J Fam Pract 2001;50:938–944.

Simon R, Koeingsknecht SJ. Meniscal injuries. In: Simon R, Koeingsknecht SJ, eds. Emergency orthopedics: the extremities, 4th ed. New York: McGraw-Hill, 2000.

Solomon DH. The rational clinical examination: does this patient have a torn meniscus or ligament of the knee? JAMA 2001;286(13):1610–1620.

Authors: Charles S. Graffeo; Francis L. Counselman

Ménière's Disease

Clinical Presentation

SIGNS AND SYMPTOMS

- Unilateral ear fullness and pressure
- Decreased hearing
- Tinnitus
- Vertigo
  —Intense and whirling in nature
  —Reaching maximum intensity within minutes, slowly subsides over hours
- Horizontal nystagmus, often with a rotational component
- Nausea and vomiting
- Patient typically lies with the affected ear up and avoids looking toward the normal side because doing so exaggerates the nystagmus and dizziness

MECHANISM/DESCRIPTION

- Estimated to affect about 0.1% of U.S. population
- Affects males and females equally
- Family history in greater than 7%
- May develop at any age
  —Peak incidence between the ages of 20 and 50 years
- Classically unilateral, but may be bilateral in up to 40% of cases
- Characterized by recurrent, intermittent attacks or rotatory vertigo, decreased hearing, tinnitus, and sensation of aural pressure
- Attacks occur with little or no warning
- Persists from 5 minutes to several hours
- Close clustering of attacks may occur
- Hearing loss is progressive over time, sensorineural in nature, and initially involves lower frequencies

ETIOLOGY

- Endolymphatic hydrops
  —Progressive dilation of the endolymphatic space
  —Thought to be overproduction or reduced absorption of endolymphatic fluid
  —Long-term therapy directed at decreasing production or enhancing drainage of endolymph
- Immune mechanism
  —Immune complex deposition in endolymphatic sac in patients with Ménière's disease
  —Autoantibodies directed against endolymphatic sac in sera of Ménière's patients

Pre-Hospital

- Vertigo and neurologic symptoms can represent a stroke
  —Rapid transport to ED
- Protect patient from falling
- Maintain in comfortable position
- IV isotonic fluids for patients with vomiting
- Monitor for dysrhythmia

Diagnosis

ESSENTIAL WORKUP

- Complete history and neurologic exam
- Patients with central vertigo or focal neurologic findings require neuroimaging
- Focal findings include new unilateral hearing loss, usually with tinnitus

LABORATORY

- None routinely helpful

IMAGING/SPECIAL STUDIES

- CT or MRI of brain
  —Indicated for any patient with focal neurologic findings or central vertigo
  —The most important diagnosis to exclude is acoustic neuroma
- Patients with Ménière's disease require audiometry and electronystagmography (ENG) testing, but these tests are not necessary to the ED evaluation

DIFFERENTIAL DIAGNOSIS

- Otologic
  —Chronic suppurative otitis media
  —Benign positional vertigo
  —Acoustic neuroma
  —Vestibular neuronitis
  —Otosclerosis
  —Otic capsule dysplasia
- Systemic
  —Vertebrobasilar insufficiency or stroke
  —Basilar migraine
  —Epilepsy
  —Multiple sclerosis
  —Paget's disease
  —Thyroid disease
  —Drugs/medications
  —Autoimmune disorders
  —Syphilis
  —Head injury
  —CNS lesion

Treatment

INITIAL STABILIZATION

- IV hydration with isotonic fluids
- Benzodiazepines
- Antiemetics, benzodiazepines

ED TREATMENT

- Supportive therapy

MEDICATIONS

- Symptomatic
  —Diazepam: 5–10 mg PO, PR, or i.v.
  —Lorazepam: 0.5–2.0 mg PO, i.v., or i.m.
  —Meclizine: 12.5–25 mg PO q8h
  —Metoclopramide: 10 mg i.v. or i.m.
  —Promethazine: 10–25 mg PO, PR, i.v. or i.m.
- Therapeutic (patients with established diagnosis of Ménière's disease)
  —Acetazolamide: 250 mg PO daily
  —Furosemide: 20 mg PO daily
  —Hydrochlorothiazide (HCTZ): 25–50 mg PO daily
  —Triamterene: 100 mg PO daily

Disposition

ADMISSION CRITERIA

- Central cause of vertigo
- Patients refractory to ED therapy

DISCHARGE CRITERIA

- Patient with normal neurologic examination
- Symptoms adequately controlled in ED
- Refer to neurology or ENT clinic for outpatient audiometry and ENG testing
- Recurrent attacks are typical
- Restrict sodium, tobacco, caffeine, and alcohol intake
- Avoid driving, operating dangerous equipment, and working at heights until attacks have resolved and sedating medications have been withdrawn

Miscellaneous

ICD9: 388.31, 386.00, 386.10, 386.20

ICD10: H81.0

SEE ALSO: DIZZINESS

SUGGESTED READINGS

Knox GW, McPherson A. Ménière's disease: differential diagnosis and treatment. Am Fam Physician 1997;55:4:1185–1190.

Saeed SR. Diagnosis and treatment of Ménière's disease. BMJ 1998;316: 368–372.

Thai-Van, et al. Ménière's disease pathophysiology and treatment. Drugs 2001;61:8:1089–1102.

Weber PC, Adkins WY. The differential diagnosis of Ménière's disease. Otolaryngol Clin North Am 1997;30:6:977–986.

Author: Charles Pollack

Meningitis

Clinical Presentation

SIGNS AND SYMPTOMS

General

- Fever
- Meningismus
  - —Kernig's: flexed knee resists extension (bilateral)
  - —Brudzinski's: flexion of neck produces flexion at hips
- Confusion/altered mental state
- Headache
- Photophobia
- Papilledema
- Focal CNS abnormalities
- Seizures
- Petechial rash (meningococcal)
- Associated infections: sinusitis, otitis, pneumonia

Infant/Pediatric

- Fever or hypothermia
- Lethargy
- Weak suck
- Vomiting/dehydration
- Respiratory distress
- Irritability
- Bulging fontanel
- Meningismus: commonly absent when <12 months old

Elderly and Immunocompromised

- Confusion with or without fever
- Less striking symptoms

ETIOLOGY

- Bacterial
  - —Neonates: group B streptococcus, gram-negative bacilli, *Listeria* species infection
  - —Children/adults: *Streptococcus pneumoniae, Neisseria meningitides, Haemophilus influenzae* (now rare due to vaccination)
  - —Elderly/alcoholic: *S. pneumoniae*, gram-negative bacilli, *Listeria* species infection
  - —Neurosurgical patients: staphylococcus- and gram-negative organisms
  - —Transplant recipients and dialysis patients: rising incidence of *Listeria* species infection
  - —AIDS: as above, plus tuberculosis, syphilis
- Viral
- Fungal
- Chemical, drug, or toxin induced

PEDIATRIC CONSIDERATIONS

- Pneumococcus most common cause of bacterial meningitis
- Pneumococcal vaccine now part of childhood immunization schedule
- Dexamethasone reduces sensorineuronal hearing loss due to *H. influenzae*
- Meningitis does not present as uncomplicated febrile seizure

Pre-Hospital

CAUTION

- Administer prophylactic antibiotics to any close personal contacts of patient diagnosed with meningococcal meningitis
  - —Adults
    - -Rifampin: 600 mg PO b.i.d. for 2 days, *or*
    - -Ciprofloxacin: 500 mg PO single dose, *or*
    - -Ceftriaxone: 250 mg i.m. (if pregnant)
  - —Children
    - -Ceftriaxone: 125 mg i.m., *or*
    - -Rifampin: 5 mg/kg if <1 month old and 10 mg/kg if >1 month old

Diagnosis

ESSENTIAL WORKUP

- Initiate treatment immediately based on clinical suspicion
- Give antibiotic therapy before diagnostic procedures
- Routine CT before lumbar puncture (LP) unnecessary, but indicated with
  - —Immunodeficiency/HIV
  - —History of CNS disease (abscess, bleed, mass lesion)
  - —History of seizure <7 days
  - —Focal neurologic deficit
  - —Diminished consciousness/comatose
  - —Elderly
  - —Papilledema
- LP
  - —Do not delay antibiotics for LP
  - —Do not delay LP unless:
    - -Risk for herniation (see above)
    - -Unstable patient
    - -Overlying soft tissue infection
- CSF analysis
  - —Cell count and differential
  - —Gram stain, culture and sensitivity
  - —Protein and glucose
  - —Opening pressure
  - —Latex agglutination
    - -Useful if patient with prior antibiotic treatment
    - -Best if urine and blood also tested
    - -Detects: meningococcus, pneumococcus, group B streptococcus, *H. influenzae, E. coli*, cryptococcus
  - —Polymerase chain reaction
    - -Useful for virus and bacteria
    - -Highly sensitive and specific for herpes simplex virus (HSV)
  - —Repeat cell count as needed for traumatic tap
  - —Interpretation
    - -Culture is diagnostic
    - ->5 WBC/mL is highly sensitive for meningitis
    - -Cell count maybe normal in HIV/AIDS
    - -Neonatal considerations: up to 25 WBC/mL may be normal, normal protein up to 120–170 mg/dL
  - —Typical bacterial meningitis
    - -WBC >100 (usually 1,000–20,000)
    - -Differential >80% PMNs
    - -Protein >200 mg/dL
    - -Glucose <40% of serum
  - —Typical viral meningitis:
    - -WBC <2,000
    - -Differential: initially PMNs, then after 24 hours, predominantly lymphocytes
    - -Protein <200 mg/dL
    - -Glucose—normal
  - —Typical fungal meningitis
    - -WBC <500
    - -Differential—lymphocytes
    - -Protein >200 mg/dL
    - -Glucose—low
  - —Typical tuberculosis meningitis
    - -WBC range, 100–400
    - -Differential—mixed
    - -Protein—variable
    - -Glucose—variable

LABORATORY

- Blood and urine culture
- Serum C-reactive protein
  - —Useful for gram-negative meningitis in pediatric patients
  - —Elevated levels very suggestive of bacterial meningitis
- CBC
- Prothrombin time (PT), partial thromboplastin time (PTT), and platelet
  - —Obtain before LP in severe sepsis or disseminated intravascular coagulation (DIC)
- Electrolytes/glucose
  - —Serum-to-CSF glucose ratio
  - —Assess for metabolic acidosis
- Toxicology studies as needed
- Urinalysis
- Chest x-ray: pneumonia, tuberculosis

DIFFERENTIAL DIAGNOSIS

- Encephalitis
- Brain, spinal, epidural abscess
- Febrile seizure
- CNS/systemic lupus erythematosus (SLE) cerebritis
- Intracranial bleed
- Primary or metastatic CNS malignancy
- Stroke
- Venous sinus thrombophlebitis
- Trauma
- Toxic/metabolic

Treatment

INITIAL STABILIZATION

- Isolate patient
- Airway protection, oxygen as needed
- 0.9% NS bolus to treat dehydration and hypotension
- IV hydrocortisone
  - —For severe hypotension due to Waterhouse-Friderichsen syndrome (meningococcemia)
- Antibiotics
  - —Obtain blood cultures and administer antibiotics promptly
  - —Do not delay to obtain LP or CT

ED TREATMENT

Empiric Antibiotic/Steroid Selection for Bacterial Infection

- Neonate: ampicillin + (cefotaxime or aminoglycoside) + vancomycin
- Age 1 to 3 months : ampicillin + ceftriaxone + vancomycin
- Children >3 months: ceftriaxone + vancomycin + dexamethasone
- Adults: ceftriaxone 2 g q12hr + vancomycin
- Elderly/alcoholism: ceftriaxone 2 g q12h + vancomycin + ampicillin
- Immune impaired: ceftazidime 2 g q8h + vancomycin + ampicillin
- CNS surgery/shunt/trauma: vancomycin 1 g q6-12h + ceftazidime 2 g q8h

Other

- Dexamethasone
  - —Give with or just before first antibiotic dose
  - —Benefit shown for children and against *H. influenzae*
- Vancomycin
  - —Add when concerned about penicillin-resistant pneumococci
- Cefotaxime may be used in place of ceftriaxone
- Meropenem
  - —Alternative choice for children >3 months old and adults
- Vancomycin + (aztreonam or chloramphenicol) + Bactrim
  - —Consider only for severe penicillin allergy (i.e., anaphylaxis)
  - —Do not delay therapy for lesser allergy history
  - —Consult infectious disease specialist

MEDICATIONS

- Amikacin: (peds: 7.5 mg/kg i.v. q8h)
- Ampicillin: 2 g (peds: 50–100 mg/kg q6–8h) i.v. q4h
- Aztreonam: 2 g (peds: 30 mg/kg) i.v. q6–8h
- Bactrim: 4–5 mg/kg TMP i.v. q12h
- Cefotaxime: 75 mg/kg i.v. q8h
- Ceftazidime: 2 g i.v. q8h
- Ceftriaxone: 2 g (peds: 50–100 mg/kg) q12h
- Chloramphenicol: 1 g (peds: 25 mg/kg) i.v. q6h
- Dexamethasone: 0.4 mg/kg i.v. q12h × 2 days
- Gentamicin: (peds: 2.5 mg/kg i.v. q8h)
- Hydrocortisone: 100–300 mg i.v.
- Meropenem: 40 mg/kg q8h
- Tobramycin: (peds: 2.5 mg/kg i.v. q8h)
- Vancomycin: 1 g (peds: 15 mg/kg q6h) q6–12h

Disposition

ADMISSION CRITERIA

- All known or suspected cases of bacterial infections
- Immunocompromised host
- Any toxic appearing patient

DISCHARGE CRITERIA

- Clear viral infection with well-controlled symptoms
- Thorough and specific discharge instructions
- Careful follow-up plan discussed with primary care physician

Miscellaneous

ICD9: 320, 047.9

ICD10: G03.9

SUGGESTED READINGS

Attia J, et al. Does this adult patient have acute meningitis? JAMA 1999;282(2): 175.

Chowdhury MH, Tunkel AR. Antibacterial agents in infections of the central nervous system. Infect Dis Clin North Am 2000;14:2.

Goldman L, ed. Cecil textbook of medicine, 21st ed. Philadelphia: WB Saunders, 2000:1645–1654.

Hasbun R, et al. Computed tomography of the head before lumbar puncture in adults with suspected meningitis. N Engl J Med 2001;345:1727.

Pong A, Bradley JS. Bacterial meningitis and the newborn infant. Infect Dis Clin North Am 1999;13(3):711–733.

Preventing pneumococcal disease among infants and young children. Recommendations of the Advisory Committee on Immunization Practices (ACIP). MMWR Morb Mortal Wkly Rep 2000;49(RR-6):1–35.

Sormunen P, et al. C-reactive protein test is useful in distinguishing Gram stain negative bacterial meningitis from viral meningitis in children. J Pediatr 1999;134:725.

Authors: Patricia Shipley; Austen Chai

Meningococcemia

Clinical Presentation

SIGNS AND SYMPTOMS

"Mild" Meningococcemia (Most Common)

- Preceded by upper respiratory infection (URI)
- Fever, chills, myalgias/arthralgias, malaise
- Often self-limited, resolving in several days
- Can progress to meningitis (mortality rate, 2–10%) or overwhelming sepsis without meningitis

Overwhelming Meningococcal Sepsis (10%)

- High mortality rate (20–60%)
- Sudden onset of illness and rapid progression of clinical course
- Initial presentation may be mild
  - —Mild tachycardia
  - —Mild tachypnea/respiratory symptoms
  - —Mild hypotension
- Fever, chills, vomiting, headache, rash, muscle tenderness
- Toxic appearing
- Infants: lethargy, poor feeding, bulging fontanel
- Rash
  - —Combination of purpura/ecchymosis
    - -May later exhibit coalescence, necrosis/sloughing of the involved skin (purpura fulminans)
  - —Petechiae (over skin, mucous membranes, conjunctivae) seen 50–60%
  - —Macules
  - —Papules (scrapings of papules demonstrate the organism on Gram stain)
- Deteriorate quickly over several hours
  - —Hypotension/shock
  - —Acidosis
  - —Acute respiratory distress syndrome (ARDS)
  - —Disseminated intravascular coagulation (DIC)
- Meningitis may or may not be present
- Waterhouse-Friderichsen syndrome
  - —Bilateral hemorrhagic destruction of adrenal glands
  - —Vasomotor collapse
- Acute renal failure
  - —From prolonged hypotension (low renal perfusion causing acute tubular necrosis)

Chronic Meningococcemia (Uncommon)

- Well appearing
- Recurrent fevers, chills, arthralgias over weeks to months
- Intermittent rash—alone or in combination with
  - —Purpura
  - —Petechiae
  - —Macules
  - —Papules
- Splenomegaly (20%)
- Meningococcal meningitis (25%)
  - —Headache
  - —Fever
  - —Neck stiffness
  - —Confusion
  - —Lethargy
  - —Obtundation

Septic Arthritis

- Occurs during active meningococcemia
- Multiple joints involved
- Joint pain, redness, swelling, effusion, fever, chills
- Extremely limited or no range of motion

Other Meningococcal Infections

- Occur with meningococcal infection elsewhere
- Conjunctivitis—may occur alone
- Sinusitis
- Panophthalmitis
- Urethritis
- Salpingitis
- Prostatitis
- Pneumonia
- Myocarditis/pericarditis

MECHANISM/DESCRIPTION

- Acquired from close contact with an infected individual or an asymptomatic carrier by inhalation of airborne nasopharyngeal droplets carrying the bacteria
- Bacteria attach to and enter nasopharyngeal epithelial cells
- Bacteria spread from the nasopharynx through the bloodstream via entry of vascular endothelium
- Most circulating meningococci eliminated by the spleen—some penetrate endothelial cells at other sites to cause infection (meninges, synovium, conjunctivae)
- Meningococci produce an endotoxin (lipooligosaccharide)
  - —Involved in pathogenesis of the skin, adrenal manifestations, and vascular collapse
- Human oropharynx/nasopharynx—only reservoir
- Carrier usually has developed immunity to serotype-specific antibody (not immune to *all* serotypes)
  - —Age <5 years: 1% carrier rate
  - —Age 20–40 years: 30–40% carrier rate
  - —Lower rate of immunity in children, which is reflected by the higher rates of infection
- Most common in fall and spring
- Increased incidence in military recruits/close living conditions
- Epidemics—ages 5–9 years most/earliest affected

ETIOLOGY

- *Neisseria meningitidis*
  - —Serotypes A, B, C, D, H, I, K, L, X, Y, Z, 29E, and W135
  - —Serotype B most common in United States
  - —>95% of infections caused by A, B, C, Y, and W135
- Available vaccines offer protection against serotypes A, C, Y, W135 (consider in epidemics)

Pre-Hospital

CAUTIONS

- Postexposure prophylactic antibiotics for pre-hospital personnel in close contact with patient

Diagnosis

ESSENTIAL WORKUP

- *Do not allow workup (including delay in lumbar puncture) to postpone administration of antibiotics in suspected cases of meningococcemia*
- Suspect diagnosis in setting of dramatic clinical presentation
- Gram stain and culture of
  - —Peripheral blood, CSF, sputum, urine, joint aspirate, or petechial/papular scrapings
  - —Gram stain: intracellular or extracellular gram-negative diplococci

LABORATORY

- CBC
  - —Elevated WBC initially, later may be suppressed in severe disease
  - —Decreased platelet count when large areas of purpura/petechiae or DIC
- Electrolytes, BUN, creatinine, glucose
- CSF: Gram stain, culture, protein and glucose, cell count with differential
  - —Consistent with bacterial infection in meningococcal meningitis
- Arterial blood gases for acidosis, hypoxia
- Fibrinogen levels, fibrin degradation products, prothrombin time (PT), partial thromboplastin time (PTT) if DIC suspected
- Throat/nasopharyngeal swab
  - —Positive swab does not establish the diagnosis of meningococcemia
- Analysis of buffy-coat layer of peripheral blood for bacteria if sepsis is suspected
- Blood culture
  - —Often negative with chronic meningococcemia
  - —Positive in mild and overwhelming meningococcemia
- Immunoassays (beware false negatives)
- Polymerase chain reaction (PCR), especially useful when antibiotics given before specimen collection

IMAGING/SPECIAL TESTS

- Chest x-ray
  - —If pneumonia suspected
  - —For the source of meningococcal sepsis
  - —To rule out ARDS

DIFFERENTIAL DIAGNOSIS

- Viral exanthem
- Vasculitis
- Mycoplasma
- Rocky Mountain spotted fever
- Toxic shock syndrome
- Henoch-Schönlein purpura
- Idiopathic thrombocytopenic purpura (ITP)

Treatment

INITIAL STABILIZATION

Overwhelming Meningococcal Sepsis

- ABCs—immediate endotracheal intubation for severe acidosis, hypoxia, or decreased mental status
  —Hyperventilate to treat acidosis (target PCO_2 about 25)
- Treat hypotension
  —0.9% NS bolus of 20 mL/kg; cautious rehydration with ARDS, congestive heart failure
  —Begin dopamine or norepinephrine (epinephrine if no response) if hypotensive after 2 L of IV fluids
- Narcan, thiamine, dextrose (Accucheck) for altered mental status
- Initiate IV antibiotics
  —First line: high-dose penicillin (proven meningococcemia) or third-generation cephalosporin (broader coverage pending definitive diagnosis)
  —Second line: ampicillin
  —Third line: chloramphenicol (penicillin-allergic patients)

ED TREATMENT

Overwhelming Meningococcal Sepsis

- Severe acidosis (pH <7.0–7.1 or serum HCO_3 <8–10)
  —Administer IV $NaHCO_3$ along with hyperventilation
- Insert Foley catheter to monitor urine output
- Place in respiratory isolation
- High-dose steroids
  —To protect against cranial nerve injury in the setting of ongoing infection (controversial)
  —Administer with adrenal gland injury
- DIC treatment
  —Administer fresh-frozen plasma and platelet transfusions
  —Heparin not indicated unless significant thrombotic complications evident clinically (e.g., cyanosis or cold digits, low urine output despite adequate volume status, and blood pressure)

Mild Meningococcemia

- Initiate IV antibiotics immediately
- Admission in respiratory isolation

Prophylaxis Options for Close Contacts

- 10-day window of observation
- Rifampin: 600 mg (10 mg/kg) PO q12h × 4 doses
- Single-dose ceftriaxone
  —125 mg i.m. for age <12 yrs
  —250 mg i.m. for age >12 yrs
- Single-dose ciprofloxacin: 500 mg PO adults only
- Serogroup-specific vaccine as adjunct only

MEDICATIONS

- Ampicillin: 2–3 g (peds: 200–400 mg/kg/24 h) i.v. q6h
- Cefotaxime: 2 g (peds: 200 mg/kg/24 h) i.v. q6h
- Ceftriaxone: 2 g (peds: 80–100 mg/kg/24 h) i.v. q12h
- Chloramphenicol: 50–100 mg/kg/24 h i.v. q6h (max, 4 g/d)
- Ciprofloxacin: 500 mg PO
- Dopamine: 5–20 μg/kg/min i.v. titrate to BP
- Epinephrine: 2–10 μg/min i.v. titrate to BP
- Heparin: 3,000–5,000 IU (peds: 80 IU/kg) i.v. bolus followed by 600–1,000 IU/h (peds: 18 IU/kg/h) i.v. drip
- Hydrocortisone (Solu-Cortef): 100 mg (peds: 2 mg/kg) bolus i.v. for adrenal insufficiency
- Dexamethasone: 0.15 mg/kg i.v. for pediatric meningitis
- Norepinephrine: 0.5–30 μg/min i.v. titrate to BP
- Penicillin G: 24 mIU/d (peds: 250,000 IU/kg/24 h) i.v. div. q4h
  —Prophylaxis: 250 mg (peds: 25–37.5 mg/kg) i.m. single dose
- Rifampin: 600 mg (peds: 5–10 mg/kg) PO b.i.d. for 2 days
- Sodium bicarbonate: 2–5 mEq/kg (peds: 0.5–1.0 mEq/kg) i.v. over 30 minutes to 4 hours

Disposition

ADMISSION CRITERIA

- ICU admission for overwhelming sepsis with respiratory isolation
- Respiratory isolation admission for mild meningococcemia

DISCHARGE CRITERIA

- Prophylaxis for close patient contacts

Miscellaneous

ICD9: 36.2

ICD10: A34.0

SEE ALSO: MENINGITIS

SUGGESTED READINGS

Cartwright K. Early management of meningococcal disease. Infect Dis Clin North Am 1999;13(3):661.

Apicella M. Neisseria meningitidis. In: Mandell GL, ed. Principles and practice of infectious disease, 5th ed. New York: Churchill Livingstone, 2000.

Leclerc F, Leteurtre S, Cremer R, et al. Do new strategies in meningococcemia produce better outcomes? Crit Care Med 2000;28(9):S60.

Rosenstein NE. Update on *Haemophilus influenzae* serotype B and meningococcal vaccines. Pediatr Clin North Am 2000; 47(2):337.

Author: Neil Troost

Clinical Presentation

SIGNS AND SYMPTOMS

- Naturally occurring mercury is converted into three primary forms, each with its own toxicologic effects

Elemental Mercury

- Classical triad
  —Tremor
  —Neuropsychiatric disturbance (erethism)
  —Gingivostomatitis
- Acrodynia
  —Idiosyncratic, occurs mainly in children
  —Painful extremities
  —Pink discoloration with desquamation (pink disease)

Inorganic Salts

- Gastrointestinal
  —Abrupt onset of abdominal pain and hemorrhagic gastroenteritis
  —Sore throat
  —Nausea/vomiting
  —Gingivostomatitis
  —Diarrhea
- Acute tubular necrosis in a few days
- Metallic taste
- Acrodynia in chronic exposure

Organic Mercury

- CNS
  —Primarily affected
  —Paresthesias
  —Ataxia
  —Visual field constriction
  —Dysarthria
  —Hearing loss
  —Mental deterioration
  —Paralysis
  —Death
- Symptom onset several weeks after exposure

Inhalation Exposure

- Initial phase (first few days)
  —Fever
  —Chills
  —Muscle aches
  —Dry mouth/throat
  —Headache
- Intermediate phase (2 weeks postexposure)
  —CNS, respiratory, GI, urologic symptoms develop
  —Noncardiogenic pulmonary edema
  —Acute renal failure
  —Seizures
- Late phase
  —Respiratory, GI, urologic symptoms resolve
  —CNS symptoms persist

MECHANISM/DESCRIPTION

- Reacts with sulfhydryl groups, causing enzyme inhibition and alterations in cellular membranes
- Binds to phosphoryl, carboxyl, amide, and amine groups of enzymes

ETIOLOGY

- Manufacturing of chlorine and caustic soda, diuretics, antibacterial agents, antiseptics, thermometers, batteries, fossil fuels, plastics, paints, and pigments
- Contaminated seafood
- Dental exposure

Pre-Hospital

- Remove from toxin exposure
- For altered mental status: dextrose, thiamine, naloxone (Narcan), oxygen

Diagnosis

ESSENTIAL WORKUP

- As per patient complaint and clinical condition
  —Abdominal pain, gastrointestinal bleeding
    -CBC
    -Electrolytes, BUN, creatinine, glucose
    -Prothrombin time (PT), partial thromboplastin time (PTT)
    -Amylase
    -Liver function tests (LFTs)
    -Abdominal x-rays
  —Tremors, neuropsychiatric effects
    -CBC
    -Electrolytes, BUN, creatinine, glucose
    -Toxicology screen
    -Head CT scan
    -Consider lumbar puncture

LABORATORY

Elemental and Inorganic Mercury

- Normal urine levels $<10\ \mu g/L$
- Neurologic effects occur with chronic urine levels >100–$200\ \mu g/L$

Organic Mercury

- Whole blood levels $>200\ \mu g/L$ associated with symptoms
- Organic mercury concentrated in RBCs
  —Compare RBC content to plasma (inorganic) content to help determine which form of mercury is involved

IMAGING/SPECIAL TESTS

- Chest x-ray for noncardiac pulmonary edema
- Abdominal radiograph for presence of mercury with intentional oral ingestion

DIFFERENTIAL DIAGNOSIS

- Multisystem involvement often confused with other heavy-metal intoxications
- Cerebrovascular accident (CVA)
- Senile dementia/Alzheimer's disease
- Parkinson's disease
- Peptic ulcer disease
- Gastrointestinal bleeding
- Pancreatitis
- Shock
- Sepsis
- Late inhalation
  —Emphysema
  —Pneumothorax
  —Acute respiratory distress syndrome (ARDS)

Treatment

INITIAL STABILIZATION

- Secure ABCs and monitoring
- 0.9% NS IV fluid resuscitation if hypotension
  - —Blood transfusion for significant GI hemorrhage
- Naloxone, D50W, thiamine for altered mental status

ED TREATMENT

Elemental Mercury

- For inhalation exposure, observe closely for several hours for the development of noncardiogenic pulmonary edema
- Ingestion of elemental mercury passes through the normal intestinal tract with minimal absorption
- Chelate with oral dimercaptosuccinic acid (DMSA)
  - —Enhances urinary mercury excretion
- Avoid bronchoalveolar lavage (BAL; dimercaprol) because it may cause redistribution of mercury to brain

Inorganic Salt Ingestion

- Administer activated charcoal
- Perform gastric lavage for recent ingestion as indicated
- Do not induce emesis because of risk for serious caustic injury
- Aggressive 0.9% NS IV fluid resuscitation/ blood products for gastrointestinal bleeding and hypovolemic shock
  - —Hydrate and maintain urine output (1 mL/kg/h)
- Chelate with BAL
  - —Early administration may avert severe renal injury
- Oral DMSA efficacy limited secondary to severe gastrointestinal symptoms

Organic Mercury

- Perform gastric lavage and administer activated charcoal
- Provide symptomatic care as needed
- Chelate with oral DMSA
  - —Help decrease tissue levels
- Avoid BAL administration

MEDICATIONS

- Dextrose: D50W 1 amp (50 mL or 25 g) (peds: D25W 2–4 mL/kg) i.v.
- Dimercaprol (BAL): 3 mg/kg i.m. q4–6h for 2 days, then q12h for 7–10 days
- DMSA: 10 mg/kg PO q8h for 5 days, then q12h for 2 weeks
- Naloxone (Narcan): 2 mg (peds: 0.1 mg/kg) i.v. or i.m. initial dose
- Thiamine (vitamin B_1): 100 mg (peds: 50 mg) i.v. or i.m.

Disposition

ADMISSION CRITERIA

- Symptomatic patients

DISCHARGE CRITERIA

- Asymptomatic patients with history of ingestion of elemental mercury and an intact intestinal tract
- Patients with a history of inhalation exposure to elemental mercury who remain asymptomatic after several hours of observation

Miscellaneous

ICD9: 985.0

ICD10: T56.1

SUGGESTED READINGS

Agency for Toxic Substance and Disease Registry. Mercury toxicity. Am Fam Physician 1992;46(6):1731–1741.

Ellenhorn MJ, Schoonwald S, Ordog G, et al. Arsenic. In: Ellenhorn's medical toxicology, 2nd ed. Baltimore: Williams & Wilkins, 1997:1588–1602.

Sue YJ. Mercury. In: Goldfrank LR, Flobaum NA, Lewin RG, eds. Goldfrank's toxicologic emergencies, 6th ed. Norwalk, CT: Appleton & Lange, 1998:1051–1062.

Authors: Meika Neblett; Lisandro Irizarry

Mesenteric Ischemia

Clinical Presentation

SIGNS AND SYMPTOMS

- Variable onset
  - —Acute onset likely with embolic source
  - —Hours to days with thrombotic occlusion (partial or complete)
  - —History of postprandial pain preceding acute onset is associated with thrombotic occlusion (<25%)
- Abdominal pain (85%)
  - —Moderate to severe
  - —Diffuse/poorly localized
  - —Initially may be colicky, becoming constant
  - —Out of proportion to exam
- Nausea/vomiting (75%)
- Diarrhea (may be early bowel ischemia)
  - —Fecal occult blood (75%)
  - —Rapid and forceful bowel evacuation, suggestive of acute arterial occlusion (embolic)
- Abdominal distention (may be only early sign)
- Lower GI bleeding (later stage)
- Altered mental status (30% of elderly patients)
- Abdominal tenderness
  - —Initially not proportionate to pain
  - —Increased with progressive ischemia/perforation
- Signs of systemic toxicity/shock with progressive ischemia

MECHANISM/DESCRIPTION

- Superior mesenteric artery (SMA) supplies entire small intestine (except superior part of the duodenum), right colon, and part of pancreas
- Embolus (50%)
  - —SMA easy target owing to large caliber and narrow angle of take-off from aorta
  - —Left-sided cardiac source in 90% of emboli
- Thrombus (15–25%)
  - —Chronic atherosclerosis
  - —May be precipitated by a low-flow state
- Nonocclusive mesenteric ischemia (NOMI) (20%)
  - —Mesenteric vasospasm in the absence of arterial/venous occlusion
  - —Triggered by systemic hypotension (cardiogenic or hypovolemic shock) to preserve cerebral and cardiac perfusion

ETIOLOGY

- >50 years of age with
  - —Cardiac arrhythmias/valvular disease
  - —Congestive heart failure (chronic, poorly controlled)
  - —Valvular or atherosclerotic heart disease
  - —Recent myocardial infarction
  - —Previous embolic phenomena
  - —Hypotension or hypovolemia
  - —Vasoconstrictive medications (including digitalis)
  - —Cocaine
- High mortality rate (average: 69%)—can be reduced to 25% with aggressive diagnosis and intervention

Pre-Hospital

CAUTIONS

- Cardiac monitor for dysrhythmia

Diagnosis

ESSENTIAL WORKUP

- Plain abdominal films to exclude other disease
- Selective angiography confirms diagnosis

LABORATORY

- *Normal lab values do not rule out the diagnosis*
- CBC
  - —Leukocytosis or left shift (75–98%)
  - —Marked leukocytosis (>20,000) with progression
  - —Hemoconcentration from third spacing
- Arterial blood gases
  - —Metabolic acidosis, suggests intestinal infarction
- Electrolytes, BUN, creatinine, glucose
  - —Anion gap (lactic) acidosis worsening as bowel ischemia and necrosis progresses
- Serum lactate (elevated in 50–90%)
  - —Associated with intestinal necrosis
- Serum amylase (elevated in 25%)
- Cardiac enzymes (evaluate for acute myocardial infarction as trigger)
- Urinalysis

IMAGING/SPECIAL TESTS

- Plain radiographs (positive in 25%)
  - —Cannot be used to exclude mesenteric ischemia
  - —Initially normal
  - —Late in the course: bowel wall thickening, thumbprinting, gas in the portal system or intestinal wall
- Selective angiography (gold standard)
  - —Catheter is placed into the SMA and dye infused
  - —Abrupt cutoff suggests an embolic obstruction
  - —Tapered occlusion suggests a thrombus
  - —"Pruned" arterial tree/"string-of-sausages" sign with vasospasm
- EKG
  - —Dysrhythmias
  - —Myocardial ischemia
- CT
  - —Nonspecific; excludes other causes of abdominal pain
  - —Bowel wall thickening, thumbprinting, gas in the portal system or intestinal wall
  - —Site of occlusion occasionally visualized with IV contrast
- Duplex ultrasonography
  - —Bedside, noninvasive
  - —Useful if celiac axis/SMA adequately visualized and patent
  - —Need highly skilled operator
  - —Difficult to visualize, especially in obese, uncooperative patients, or if extensive bowel gas

DIFFERENTIAL DIAGNOSIS

- Abdominal aortic aneurysm
- Aortic dissection
- Myocardial infarction
- Perforated viscus
- Cholelithiasis
- Urolithiasis
- Bowel obstruction
- Sepsis
- Splenic vein thrombosis
- Pancreatitis

Treatment

INITIAL STABILIZATION

- ABCs
- 100% oxygen; intubate if severe respiratory compromise
- Resuscitate
  - —Cardiac monitor
  - —Insert two large-bore IVs
  - —Use lactated Ringer's if potassium not elevated
  - —Type and cross-match; transfuse if necessary
  - —Foley catheter to follow urine output
  - —Nasogastric tube
- Maximize cardiac status
  - —Treat arrhythmias, congestive heart failure, hypotension, hypovolemia, anemia
  - —Consider blood transfusion to aid in oxygen delivery if ischemia present on EKG
- *Avoid* the use of pressor agents (dopamine/norepinephrine) and digitalis: worsen bowel ischemia
- Swan-Ganz catheter may be necessary to achieve optimal cardiac performance

ED TREATMENT

- Obtain surgical consult as soon as diagnosis is suspected
- NPO
- Bedside ultrasonography of mesenteric vessels, if qualified personnel available during resuscitation (must not delay angiogram or surgery)
- Perform angiogram as soon as possible to confirm the diagnosis and define arterial anatomy
- Papaverine via intraarterial catheter (placed during angiography)
  - —Vasodilator (contraindicated in hypotensive patients)
  - —30–60 mg/h infusion directly into the SMA
  - —Relieves mesenteric vasoconstriction before and after operation
  - —Limits the extent of bowel infarction
- Broad-spectrum antibiotics (cefoxitin or gentamicin plus either clindamycin or metronidazole)
- Heparin sulfate infusion
  - —In all suspected cases, unless contraindicated
  - —Prevents propagation of thrombus
- Definitive management includes arteriotomy with embolectomy or thrombectomy, bypass procedure if there is underlying atherosclerosis, plus resection of necrotic bowel

MEDICATIONS

- Cefoxitin (Mefoxin): 2 g (peds: 120–160 mg/kg/24 h) i.v. q6h
- Clindamycin: 900 mg (peds: 25–40 mg/kg/24 h) i.v. q8h
- Gentamicin: 5–7 mg/kg i.v. load (q24h regimen, check peak/trough levels)
- Heparin sulfate: 80 units/kg IV bolus, followed by 18 units/kg/h infusion
- Metronidazole: 1.0 g (peds: 15 mg/kg) load, followed by 500 mg (7.5 mg/kg) i.v. q6h

Disposition

ADMISSION CRITERIA

- All patients with suspected mesenteric ischemia must go to angiography or the operating room
- Admit suspected mesenteric ischemia to the ICU

DISCHARGE CRITERIA

- Exclude mesenteric ischemia before discharge

Miscellaneous

ICD9: 557.1

ICD10: K55.0

SUGGESTED READINGS

Brandt LJ, Smithline AE. Ischemic lesions of the bowel. In: Feldman M, Scharschmidt BF, Sleisenger MH, eds. Sleisenger and Fordtran's gastrointestinal and liver disease: pathophysiology/diagnosis/management, 6th ed. Philadelphia: WB Saunders, 1998:2009–2020.

Cappell MS. Intestinal (mesenteric) vasculopathy. I. Acute superior mesenteric arteriopathy and venopathy. Gastroenterol Clin North Am 1998;27(4):783–825.

Mansour MA. Management of acute mesenteric ischemia. Arch Surg 1999;134(3):328–330.

McKinsey JF, Gewertz BL. Acute mesenteric ischemia. Surg Clin North Am 1997;77(2):307–318.

Park WM, Gloviczki P, Cherry KJ Jr., et al. Contemporary management of acute mesenteric ischemia: factors associated with survival. J Vasc Surg 2002;35(3):445–452.

Author: Harsh Sulé

Metacarpal Injuries

Clinical Presentation

SIGNS AND SYMPTOMS

- Pain or swelling at the site of injury
- Deformity at the site of injury
- Misalignment of the distal tip of the finger on flexion indicates rotational deformity
- Lines drawn down the longitudinal axis of each digit in flexion normally should converge on the scaphoid volarly
- Limitation of movement secondary to pain and anatomic deformity
- A special category of injury is the direct blow of a closed fist against a human tooth (fight bite); the concern here is violation of the extensor sheath, metacarpophalangeal (MCP) joint, or metacarpal head by a tooth with subsequent infection by oral flora

MECHANISM/DESCRIPTION

- Most of these are caused by crush injuries or by a direct blow with the hand to an object
- The most common fracture is the "boxer's fracture" of the distal fifth metacarpal neck

PEDIATRIC CONSIDERATIONS

- These fractures are rare in children, who do not possess the strength or mass to strike an object hard enough to cause the fracture

Pre-Hospital

CAUTIONS

- Metacarpal injuries should be splinted in a position of comfort; patients with hand injuries seen by pre-hospital personnel should be referred for evaluation by a physician

Diagnosis

ESSENTIAL WORKUP

- Examination should pay specific attention to skin integrity and alignment of the distal phalanges in flexion and extension
- Hand x-rays when fracture suspected

IMAGING/SPECIAL TESTS

- Special radiographic views of the proximal metacarpals and the carpometacarpal joints may be necessary for patients with a suggestive physical exam and no definite fracture on a standard three-view series

DIFFERENTIAL DIAGNOSIS

- Fracture of the metacarpal may be accompanied by dislocation of adjacent phalanges or carpal bones

Treatment

INITIAL STABILIZATION

- Other, more serious injuries should be treated first
- Immobilize hand pending evaluation
- Lacerations should be cleaned as soon as possible and consideration should be given to the possibility of foreign body

ED TREATMENT

- Elevation, rest, and intermittent application of ice for the first 24 hours are appropriate treatment for all hand injuries
- Boxer's fractures usually have some volar flexion of the distal fragment
  —Reduction should be attempted for volar angulation of 40 degrees or more
  —Fractures of the fourth and fifth metacarpals that are stable and with no significant rotational component can be treated with a padded ulnar gutter splint
- Fractures of the index and middle finger metacarpals are more difficult to stabilize
  —Radial gutter splint and early orthopedic referral
- Thumb metacarpal fractures are uniformly complicated and should all be referred very early to a hand surgeon or orthopedist
  —Place in thumb spica splint
- Dislocations should be reduced immediately and splinted; metacarpal dislocations are rare and frequently need open reduction and repair
- Appropriate splinting position for the MCP joint is the intrinsic plus, or "cobra," position
  —MCP joint as close to 90 degrees of flexion as possible
  —Proximal interphalangeal (PIP) and distal interphalangeal (DIP) joints in extension
- Antibiotics for oral flora should be started early for any open injury to the metacarpals suspicious for injury against a tooth

MEDICATIONS

- Mild analgesics may be necessary, and NSAIDS or hydrocodone is usually sufficient
- For human bites or dirty wounds, administer amoxicillin/clavulanate (Augmentin), 875/125 mg PO t.i.d.
  —A cephalosporin or other penicillinase-resistant antibiotic given parenterally is appropriate

PEDIATRIC CONSIDERATIONS

- Epiphyseal injuries mandate orthopedic referral
- Simple torus (buckle) fractures may be splinted and followed by a primary care physician

Disposition

ADMISSION CRITERIA

- Open fractures or dislocations require urgent surgical intervention and should be admitted; all thumb metacarpal fractures or dislocations should be seen by an orthopedist or hand surgeon because of the special importance of the thumb in all activities of the hand
- Infection from a bite wound requires prompt orthopedic consultation, admission for irrigation, débridement, and intravenous antibiotics

DISCHARGE CRITERIA

- Patients with a stable transverse or oblique fracture in a good splint may be discharged for early orthopedic follow-up
- Metacarpal-carpal dislocations are usually unstable enough to require surgery even if reduction is achieved, but this may be semi-urgent rather than emergent
- If a metacarpal fracture produces impaired range of motion or misalignment of the finger, the patient will require surgical repair in the first several days after injury

Miscellaneous

ICD9: 815.00, 834.01, 833.05

ICD10: S69.8

SUGGESTED READINGS

American Society for Surgery of the Hand. The hand: examination and diagnosis, 3rd ed. New York: Churchill Livingstone, 1990.

American Society for Surgery of the Hand. The hand: primary care of common problems, 2nd ed. New York: Churchill Livingstone, 1990.

Antosia RE, Lyn E. The hand. In: Rosen P, et al. Emergency medicine: concepts and clinical practice, 4th ed. St. Louis: Mosby–Year Book 1998:625–668.

Hart RG, Uehara DT, Wagner MJ. Emergency and primary care of the hand. Dallas: American College of Emergency Physicians, 2001.

Author: Matthew Walsh

Methanol, Poisoning

Clinical Presentation

SIGNS AND SYMPTOMS

GI

- Anorexia
- Nausea/vomiting
- Abdominal pain

CNS

- Headache
- Dizziness
- Confusion
- Inebriation
- Coma
- Seizures

Ophthalmologic

- Blurry vision
- Photophobia
- "Snow fields"
- Mydriasis
- Blindness
- Optic disc
  - —Hyperemia or pallor
  - —Papilledema

MECHANISM/DESCRIPTION

- Colorless, volatile liquid
- Absorbed in 30–60 minutes
- Metabolized by the liver
- Half-life 4–8 hours
- Methanol
  - —Inebriating
  - —Nontoxic
  - —Metabolites (formaldehyde and formic acid) produce toxic effects
- Formic acid level determines degree of acidosis, visual symptoms, and mortality
- Formic acid–directly toxic to retinal and optic nerve tissue
- Methanol metabolism
  - —Methanol converted to formaldehyde by the liver enzyme alcohol dehydrogenase
  - —Formaldehyde then rapidly converted to formic acid
  - —Formic acid degraded into carbon dioxide and water by a folate-dependent mechanism
  - —Steps 1 and 3 are rate-limiting steps

ETIOLOGY

Common Sources of Methanol

- Wood alcohol
- Windshield washer fluid
- Antifreeze
- Formalin
- Gasoline ("gasohol")
- Paint solvents
- Household cleaners

Pre-Hospital

CAUTIONS

- Transport all substances that the patient may have ingested

Diagnosis

ESSENTIAL WORKUP

- History of all substances ingested
- Inquire about visual symptoms
- Thorough funduscopic examination
- Drawn *simultaneously*
  - —ABG
  - —Serum methanol, ethylene glycol, isopropyl alcohol, and ethanol levels
  - —Electrolytes, BUN, creatinine, and glucose
  - —Measured serum osmolality (by freezing-point depression)

LABORATORY

- Calculate anion gap = $(Na^+) - (Cl^- + HCO_3^-)$
  - —Normal = 8–12
- Determine osmol gap
  - —Osmol gap = measured osmolality − calculated osmolarity
    - -Calculated osmolarity = $2(Na^+)$ + glucose/18 + BUN/2.8 + ethanol (in mg/dL)/4.6
    - ->10 increased
  - —Osmol gap
    - -Screens for toxic alcohols
    - -Primarily affected by methanol, not methanol metabolites
    - -Increased early in poisoning and normalizes as methanol metabolized
    - -Most sensitive early in poisoning
    - -Normal osmol gap does *not* rule out methanol ingestion
- Toxic alcohol levels *confirm* methanol poisoning
- Ethanol level
  - —Determines the amount of ethanol bolus necessary to attain a therapeutic level
- Urinalysis
  - —Envelope-shaped oxalate crystals
    - -Insensitive but specific finding in ethylene glycol poisoning
  - —Ketones
    - -Due to isopropyl alcohol ingestion, starvation, or diabetic ketoacidosis (DKA)

DIFFERENTIAL DIAGNOSIS

- Increased osmol gap: *ME DIE A*
  - —*M*ethanol
  - —*E*thanol
  - —*D*iuretics (mannitol, glycerin, sorbitol)
  - —*I*sopropyl alcohol
  - —*E*thylene glycol
  - —*A*cetone, ammonia
- Elevated anion gap metabolic acidosis: *ACAT MUDPILES*
  - —*A*lcoholic ketoacidosis
  - —*C*yanide, CO, H_2S, others
  - —*A*SA, other salicylates
  - —*T*oluene
  - —*M*ethanol, metformin
  - —*U*remia
  - —*D*iabetic ketoacidosis
  - —*P*araldehyde, phenformin
  - —*I*ron, INH
  - —*L*actic acidosis from other causes
  - —*E*thylene glycol
  - —*S*tarvation ketosis

Treatment

INITIAL STABILIZATION

- ABCs
- Dextrose (or Accucheck), naloxone, and thiamine for altered mental status

ED TREATMENT

Prevent Further Methanol Absorption

- Gastric lavage if the patient presents within 1 hour of significant ingestion or if comatose
  —Endotracheal intubation may be necessary
- Ipecac-induced emesis not recommended
- Activated charcoal
  —For potential co-ingestants
  —Poorly adsorbs methanol

Prevent Methanol Conversion to Toxic Metabolites

- 4-Methylpyrazole (4-MP, Antizol)
  —Competitive inhibitor of alcohol dehydrogenase
  —FDA approval for use in ethylene glycol poisoning
  —Initiate before methanol level returns if an intentional ingestion or more than a sip
  —Advantages over ethanol infusion
    -No need for continuous infusion
    -No inebriation/CNS depression
    -Ease of dosing
    -No hypoglycemia, no hyponatremia, no hyperosmolality
    -No checking levels
    -Reduced nursing care and monitoring
  —Disadvantages over ethanol infusion
    -More expensive than the cost of the alcohol drip
- Ethanol therapy
  —Initiate before the methanol level returns if a potentially toxic ingestion is highly suspected or confirmed by history
  —Ethanol has greater affinity than methanol for alcohol dehydrogenase
  —Slows metabolism to formaldehyde and formic acid by competitive inhibition
  —Indications for ethanol therapy
    -Intertional methanol ingestion
    -Accidental methanol ingestion of greater than a sip
    -Altered mental status or visual symptoms associated with an unexplained osmol gap or elevated anion gap metabolic acidosis
  —Therapeutic range = 100–150 mg/dL
  —Continue until the methanol level is zero

Enhance Elimination of Methanol and Its Toxic Metabolites

- Hemodialysis
  —Decreases the elimination half-life of methanol to 2.5 hours
  —Removes formaldehyde and formic acid
  —Indications
    -Ingestion of >1 mL/kg of 100% methanol
    -Ophthalmologic manifestations
    -Severe acidosis unresponsive to bicarbonate therapy
    -Persistent electrolyte or fluid imbalance
    -Renal insufficiency
    -Serum methanol level >25 mg/dL
  —Continue hemodialysis until methanol level approaches zero
- Folic acid and folinic acid (leucovorin)
  —Folic acid: cofactor required for the conversion of formic acid to carbon dioxide and water
  —Folinic acid: activated form of folic acid, used only for the initial dose
  —Supplemental folate important in malnourished individuals (alcoholics)

Correct Acid-Base Abnormalities

- Sodium bicarbonate for severe acidosis (pH <7.1)

MEDICATIONS

- 4-Methylpyrazole
  —Loading dose: 15 mg/kg slow infusion over 30 minutes
  —Maintenance dose: 10 mg/kg q12h for 4 doses, then 15 mg/kg q12h until ethylene glycol levels reduced below 20 mg/dL
  —Dosing related to hemodialysis
    -Do not administer a dose at the beginning of dialysis if the last dose was <6 hours previously
    -Administer the next dose if the last dose was >6 hours previously
    -Dose every 4 hours during dialysis
    -If the time between the last dose and the end of dialysis was <1 hour from last dose, do not administer a new dose
    -If the time between the last dose and the end of dialysis was 1–3 hours from last dose, administer one half of next scheduled dose
    -If the time between the last dose and the end of dialysis was >3 hours from last dose, administer next scheduled dose
- Ethanol
  —Oral: 50% ethanol solution (100 proof liquor) via NGT
    -Loading dose 1.5 mL/kg
    -Maintenance dose 0.2–0.4 mL/kg/h
    -Maintenance dose during hemodialysis 0.4–0.7 mL/kg/h
  —IV: 10% ethanol in D5W
    -Loading dose 7.5 mL/kg over 30–60 minutes
    -Maintenance infusion 1–2 mL/kg/h
    -Maintenance infusion during hemodialysis 2–3.5 mL/kg/h
- Folic acid: 50 mg i.v. push (IVP) q4h for 24 hours
- Folinic acid: 1–2 mg/kg i.v.
- Sodium bicarbonate: 1 mEq/kg i.v.
- Thiamine: 100 mg IVP

Disposition

ADMISSION CRITERIA

- Significant methanol ingestion even if initially asymptomatic
- ICU admission for seriously ill patients
- Transfer to another facility if hemodialysis or methylpyrazole is indicated but not readily available

DISCHARGE CRITERIA

- Asymptomatic patient with isolated methanol ingestion if the serum methanol level is undetectable

Miscellaneous

ICD9: 980.1

ICD10: T51.1

SEE ALSO: ETHYLENE GLYCOL, POISONING

SUGGESTED READINGS

Brent J, McMartin K, Phillips S, et al. Fomepizole for the treatment of methanol poisoning. N Engl J Med 2001;344: 424–429.

Ford M, Delaney K, Ling L, et al. Ethylene glycol and methanol. In: Clinical toxicology, 1st ed. Philadelphia: WB Saunders, 2001:757–767.

Jacobsen D, McMartin KE. Antidotes for methanol and ethylene glycol poisonings. J Toxicol Clin Toxicol 1997;35(2):127–143.

Leikin J, Paloucek F. Methanol. Fomepizole. Alcohol. In: Leikin JB, Paloucek F, ed. Leikin and Paloucek's poisoning and toxicology handbook, 3rd ed. Hudson, OH: Lexi-Comp, 2002:810–812, 599–600, 201–202.

Author: Kirk Cumpston

Methemoglobinemia

Clinical Presentation

SIGNS AND SYMPTOMS

- "Chocolate cyanosis" unaffected by supplemental oxygen
  - —Cyanosis evident at methemoglobin (MetHb) of 10–15% of total hemoglobin in nonanemic patient (or 1.5 g methemoglobin/dL blood)
- Tissue hypoxia
  - —Syncope
  - —Altered mental status
  - —Chest pain
  - —Dysrhythmias
  - —Dyspnea
- Brown-red blood color
  - —Unchanged by bubbling oxygen through it

MECHANISM/DESCRIPTION

- Methemoglobin
  - —Oxidation of hemoglobin iron from ferrous (Fe^{2+}) to ferric (Fe^{3+}) state
  - —Decreases total oxygen carrying capacity (functional anemia)
  - —Shifts hemoglobin oxygen-dissociation curve to the left, impairing O_2 release to tissues
  - —Maintained at physiologic level (1–2%) by NADH-methemoglobin (cytochrome b_5) reductase in RBCs
- Congenital methemoglobinemia
  - —NADH-methemoglobin (cytochrome b_5) reductase deficiency (homozygous or heterozygous)
  - —Heterozygous hemoglobin M and other abnormal hemoglobins
- Acquired methemoglobinemia results from oxidant stress on RBCs
  - —Some methemoglobin-inducing agents are direct oxidants (e.g., nitrites)
  - —Many substances produce oxidant injury via *N*-hydroxylamine metabolites
  - —Methemoglobinemia may be delayed relative to initial substance exposure
- Many methemoglobin-inducing agents also cause Heinz body hemolytic anemia (HA)
  - —Due to oxidant injury of RBC proteins
  - —Glucose-6-phosphate dehydrogenase (G6PD) deficient patients have a higher risk
  - —Patients with methemoglobinemia should be worked up for HA
- Methemoglobinemia may serve as a marker for genetic abnormalities
  - —Heterozygous NADH-methemoglobin (cytochrome b_5) reductase deficiency

ETIOLOGY

- Dyes
  - —Aniline dyes
  - —Methylene blue (excessive)
- Antiparasitic drugs (high potential for MetHb formation)
  - —Dapsone
  - —Primaquine
  - —Chloroquine
- Local anesthetics (high potential for MetHb formation)
  - —Benzocaine
  - —Lidocaine
  - —Prilocaine
- Analgesics
  - —Phenazopyridine (Pyridium)
  - —Phenacetin
- Antibiotics
  - —Nitrofurantoin
  - —Sulfones
  - —Sulfonamides
- Nitrates/nitrites
  - —Nitrites (NO_2)
  - —Nitrates (NO_3); e.g., nitroglycerine, via metabolic conversion to nitrites
  - —Nitric oxide (NO)
- Others
  - —Metoclopramide
  - —Naphthalene (mothballs)
  - —Paraquat (a herbicide)
  - —Arsine gas (AsH_3)
  - —Chlorates (ClO_4)
  - —Phenols (e.g., dinitrophenol, hydroquinone)

PEDIATRIC CONSIDERATIONS

- Neonates and younger infants have an increased susceptibility to methemoglobinemia

Pre-Hospital

CAUTIONS

- Bring to the hospital all substances the patient may have ingested
- Question witnesses and observe the scene for household products and other potential co-ingestants
  - —Document and relay findings to emergency medical staff
- Commercial or industrial sites
  - —Obtain relevant Material Safety Data Sheets (MSDS) if available to identify commercial or chemical products
  - —Avoid dermal exposures

Diagnosis

ESSENTIAL WORKUP

- Thorough history
  - —Exposure to a methemoglobin-inducing agent
  - —All substances ingested and the time(s) of ingestion
  - —G6PD deficiency
  - —Medical conditions vulnerable to impaired oxygen delivery (e.g., coronary artery disease)
- Physical exam
  - —Cyanosis
  - —Emphasis on mental status and cardiovascular findings
  - —Icterus or dark-colored urine with accompanying hemolytic anemia
- Pulse oximetry (Pulse Ox) is *inaccurate* in methemoglobinemia
  - —MetHb interferes with Pulse Ox measurement of hemoglobin oxygen saturation
  - —Saturation decreases to approximately 85% with increasingly more severe methemoglobinemia
  - —Pulse ox cannot be used to guide management
- Diagnosis made by *co-oximetry*
  - —MetHb level by co-oximetry is reported as percent of total hemoglobin
  - —Hemoglobin oxygen saturation is accurate only by co-oximetry
- ECG

LABORATORY

- CBC with manual differential count and smear analysis for evidence of hemolytic anemia
- Urinalysis for blood versus intact RBCs to detect presence of free hemoglobin in urine
- Enzyme activity studies or hemoglobin electrophoresis if indicated
- Salicylate and acetaminophen levels for patients with suicidal ingestions
- Pregnancy test

DIFFERENTIAL DIAGNOSIS

- Blue discoloration
  - —Hypoxia
  - —Sulfhemoglobinemia
  - —Cyanide poisoning
  - —Hydrogen sulfide poisoning
  - —Excess methylene blue administration
  - —Tellurium toxicity
  - —Skin contact/staining with blue dye

Treatment

INITIAL STABILIZATION

- ABCs
  - —Administer O_2 by non-rebreather for shortness of breath/chest pain/altered mental status
- Treat based on the patient's condition and not on a specific methemoglobin level

ED TREATMENT

- Decontamination if indicated with activated charcoal for oral ingestions
- Methylene blue
  - —To reverse methemoglobinemia in symptomatic patients
  - —Avoid if possible in patients with G6PD deficiency because it may induce more severe hemolysis
  - —Repeat doses of methylene blue in patients with ongoing absorption or production of methemoglobin-inducing agents
- RBC transfusion
  - —May be necessary to increase blood oxygen carrying capacity
  - —Especially if hemolytic anemia is present
- Exchange transfusion
  - —Especially with neonates/infants
- Hyperbaric oxygen therapy
  - —Increases oxygen delivery to tissues by mass effect, independent of hemoglobin
  - —Use in life-threatening methemoglobinemia if immediately available
- Treatment of other toxin-induced problems

MEDICATIONS

- Activated charcoal: 1 g/kg PO or per NGT
- Methylene blue: 1–2 mg/kg i.v. push over 5 minutes

Disposition

ADMISSION CRITERIA

- Admit all patients with serious symptomatic acquired methemoglobinemia for observation
  - —To evaluate for return of treated methemoglobinemia and development of delayed hemolysis

DISCHARGE CRITERIA

- Known congenital methemoglobinemia if asymptomatic and without significant change in usual methemoglobin level
- Mild, asymptomatic acquired methemoglobinemia if on chronic, stable therapy with a known methemoglobin-inducing agent (e.g., dapsone) with close follow-up
- Mild, asymptomatic acquired methemoglobinemia may be discharged if successfully treated after 4–6 hours observation and no return of methemoglobinemia

Miscellaneous

ICD9: 289.7

ICD10: R82.3

SUGGESTED READINGS

Coleman MD, Coleman NA. Drug-induced methemoglobinemia: treatment issues. Drug Saf 1996;14(6):394–405.

Wright RO, Lewander WJ, Woolf AD. Methemoglobinemia: etiology, pharmacology, and clinical management. Ann Emerg Med 1999;34(5):646–656.

Author: Anne Krantz

Mitral Valve Prolapse

Clinical Presentation

SIGNS AND SYMPTOMS

- Palpitations in 40% of cases
  - —Usually ventricular premature beats or paroxysmal supraventricular tachycardia (PSVT)
- Syncope/presyncope
- Orthostasis
- Chest pain, dyspnea, and fatigue relatively uncommon
- Early to midsystolic click
- Mid or late systolic murmur
  - —Standing or Valsalva moves click closer to S1
- May bring out previously unheard click
  - —Squatting moves click closer to S2
- Scoliosis
- Pectus excavatum
- Narrow anteroposterior diameter of the chest
- Arachnodactyly

MECHANISM/DESCRIPTION

- Prolapse of the mitral valve leaflets into the left atrium during systole
  - —Produces nonejection click heard at the apex
  - —Occurs in two phenotypic patterns
  - —Anatomic form
- Thickened, billowing mitral leaflets
  - —Functional form
- Dynamic systolic expansion of the mitral annulus

ETIOLOGY

- Most are primary, idiopathic
- Female-to-male ratio, 3:1
- Frequently associated with connective tissue disorders
  - —Marfan's syndrome
  - —Ehlers-Danlos syndrome
  - —Osteogenesis imperfecta
  - —Pseudoxanthoma elasticum
  - —Stickler syndrome
  - —Systemic lupus erythematosus (SLE)
  - —Polyarteritis nodosa
  - —Von Willebrand's syndrome
  - —Wolff-Parkinson-White (WPW) syndrome
  - —Duchenne's muscular dystrophy

PEDIATRIC CONSIDERATIONS

- Dysrhythmias, sudden death, and bacterial endocarditis have been reported

Pre-Hospital

- Cardiac monitoring and supplemental oxygen
- IV access

CAUTIONS

- Mitral valve prolapse (MVP) may be associated with preexcitation syndromes
  - —Supraventricular tachydysrhythmias may worsen with treatment that blocks conduction through the atrioventricular (A-V) node
- Bradycardia associated with A-V block may be resistant to atropine and require isoproterenol or cardiac pacing

Diagnosis

ESSENTIAL WORKUP

- Electrocardiogram
  - —Usually normal
  - —Occasionally ST-T wave depression and inversion in leads III and aVF
  - —Premature atrial and ventricular contractions

LABORATORY

- CBC
- Thyroid function tests
- Serum potassium and magnesium

IMAGING/SPECIAL TESTS

- Chest x-ray
  - —Typically normal
  - —May show skeletal abnormalities
  - —If mitral regurgitation is present, may show both left atrial and ventricular enlargement
  - —Calcification of the mitral annulus in patients with Marfan's syndrome
- Holter monitor
- Echocardiogram
  - —Most useful for defining MVP
- Exercise stress test
  - —Indicated for patients with chest pain syndromes
- Myocardial perfusion scintigraphy
- Cardiac catheterization
- Electrophysiologic testing for patients with unexplained syncope or WPW

DIFFERENTIAL DIAGNOSIS

- Anemia
- Thyrotoxicosis
- Pregnancy
- Myocardial infarction/ischemia
- Hypertrophic cardiomyopathy with obstruction
- Papillary muscle dysfunction
- Hypokalemia
- Hypomagnesemia
- Valvular heart disease
- Pheochromocytoma
- Anxiety/panic disorder
- Stress
- Menopause
- Toxicity from cocaine, amphetamines, or other sympathomimetics
- Ventricular tachycardia
- WPW syndrome

PEDIATRIC CONSIDERATIONS

- Toxin/drug ingestion, otherwise same as above

Treatment

INITIAL STABILIZATION

- Intravenous access, oxygen, cardiac monitor, pulse oximetry
- Treat dysrhythmias if present

ED TREATMENT

- Reassurance and explanation of the disease
- Search for underlying causes as listed above
- Patients with tachycardia or severely symptomatic often respond to beta-blockers
- Digoxin is an alternative for SVT and prevention of chest pain and fatigue
- Patients do require endocarditis prophylaxis for even minor procedures

PEDIATRIC CONSIDERATIONS

- Full activity for asymptomatic and uncomplicated MVP

MEDICATIONS

- Propranolol: 1–10 mg i.v. load, then 3 mg/h; 80–640 mg/d PO
- Digoxin: 0.125–0.375 mg PO

Disposition

ADMISSION CRITERIA

- Severe mitral regurgitation
- Severe chest pain with ischemic symptoms
- Syncope or near syncope
- Life-threatening dysrhythmias
- Cerebral ischemic events, including transient ischemic attack (TIA)

DISCHARGE CRITERIA

- Asymptomatic
- No laboratory abnormalities
- No significant mitral regurgitation or dysrhythmias

Miscellaneous

ICD9: 424.0

ICD10: I34.1

SUGGESTED READINGS

Avierinos JF, Gersh BJ, Melton LJ 3rd, et al. Natural history of asymptomatic mitral valve prolapse in the community. Circulation 2002;106(11):1355–1361.

Bonow RO, Carabello B, de Leon AC, et al. ACC/AHA guidelines for the management of patients with valvular heart disease. Executive summary. A report of the American College of Cardiology/American Heart Association Task Force on Practice Guidelines (Committee on Management of Patients With Val. J Heart Valve Dis 1998;7(6):672–707.

Devereux RB, Kramer-Fox R, Kligfield P. Mitral valve prolapse: causes, clinical manifestations, and management. Ann Intern Med 1989;111(4):305–317.

Freed LA, Levy D, Levine RA, et al. Prevalence and clinical outcome of mitral-valve prolapse. N Engl J Med 1999;341(1):1–7.

Hanson EW, Neerhurt RK, Lynch III. Mitral valve prolapse. Anesthesiology 1996;85:178.

Lichodziejewska B, Klos J, Rezler J, et al. Clinical symptoms of mitral valve prolapse are related to hypomagnesemia and attenuated by magnesium supplementation. Am J Cardiol 1997;79(6):768–772.

Savage DD, Devereus RB, Garrison RJ, et al. Mitral valve prolapse in the general population. 2. Clinical features: the Framingham Study. Am Heart J 1983;106:577.

Savage DD, Levy D, Garrison RJ, et al. Mitral valve prolapse in the general population. 3. Dysrhythmias: the Framingham Study. Am Heart J 1983;106:582.

Author: Liudvikas Jagminas

Molluscum Contagiosum

Clinical Presentation

SIGNS AND SYMPTOMS

- Lesions are smooth-surfaced, firm, spherical papules, 3–5 mm in diameter
- May be flesh colored, white, translucent, or light yellow in color
- Distinctive central umbilication in 25%
- Distribution in children: face, trunk, and extremities; healthy adults: genitals and lower abdomen; occasionally perioral; rarely on palms and soles
- Molluscum contagiosum (MC) is commonly seen with HIV infection, causing atypical involvement of face, neck, and trunk, lesions to 1.5 cm, and a progressive course
- Occasional intraocular or periocular involvement presenting as trachoma or chronic follicular conjunctivitis
- Incubation period: 14–50 days
- Patients are usually asymptomatic, with occasional pruritus or tenderness
- 10–25% of patients may have eczematous reaction surrounding the lesions
- Untreated lesions in immunocompetent hosts usually resolve within several months but can last up to 5 years

ETIOLOGY

- MC is caused by a double-stranded DNA poxvirus
- Transmission in children is by direct skin-to-skin contact, fomites, pool or bath water
- Transmission in adults is most often by sexual contact; autoinnoculation common at any age

Pre-Hospital

- Maintain universal precautions

Diagnosis

ESSENTIAL WORKUP

- History and careful skin examination
- Skin biopsy for confirmation

DIFFERENTIAL DIAGNOSIS

- Basal cell carcinoma, histiocytoma, keratoacanthoma, intradermal nevus
- Darier's disease, nevoxanthoendothelioma, syringoma, epithelial nevi, sebaceous adenoma
- Atopic dermatitis, dermatitis herpetiformis, mycosis fungoides, Jessner's lymphocytic infiltration

Treatment

INITIAL STABILIZATION
- Not applicable in routine cases

ED TREATMENT
- Treatment is aimed at destruction or removal of virus-infected epithelial cells and is indicated to prevent autoinoculation and transmission
  - —Avoid being overly aggressive: lesions are self-limited in immunocompetent hosts
- Physical treatment modalities generally most effective
  - —Curettage after local anesthesia with EMLA or ethyl chloride
  - —Cryotherapy with liquid nitrogen
  - —Podophyllin, trichloroacetic acid, cantharidin, and tretinoin applied topically are variably effective
- Griseofulvin and methisazone orally for extensive disease have given mixed results
- No therapy has been effective in halting progression in HIV-infected patients
- Examine sexual partners for MC and other sexually transmitted diseases
  - —Patients should avoid contact sports, swimming pools, shared baths and towels, scratching, and shaving until lesions have resolved
- Reexamine treated patients for recurrence every 2–4 weeks; 2–4 treatments often needed to clear lesions completely

MEDICATIONS
- Cantharidin 0.9% solution with equal parts acetone and flexible collodion: apply topically one to three treatments every 7 days or until resolution
- Podophyllin (podofilox 0.5%): apply topically q 12 hrs for 3 days, withhold for 4 days; repeat 1 week cycle up to four times until resolved
- Trichloroacetic acid (50–80%): apply and cover with bandage 5–6 days
- Tretinoin 0.1%: topically q12h for 10 days or until resolution of lesions

PEDIATRIC CONSIDERATIONS
- For painless therapy in children, use topical EMLA (lidocaine/prilocaine cream) 1 hour before curettage; or use cantharidin, a painless blister-inducing agent

Disposition

ADMISSION CRITERIA
- Widespread disease with extensive superinfection in an immunocompromised host

DISCHARGE CRITERIA
- Patients without extensive superinfection may be safely treated as outpatients

Miscellaneous

ICD9: 078.0

ICD10: B08.1

SUGGESTED READINGS

Allen AL, Siegfried EC. Management of warts and molluscum in adolescents. Adolesc Med 2001;12(2):vi,229–242.

Lewis EJ, Lam M, Crutchfield CE 3rd. An update on molluscum contagiosum. Cutis 1997;60(1):29–34.

Ordoukhanian E, Carrington D. Warts and molluscum contagiosum: beware of treatments worse than the disease. Postgrad Med 1997;101(2):223–226, 229–232, 235.

Smith KJ, Yeager J, Skelton H. Molluscum contagiosum: its clinical, histopathologic, and immunohistochemical spectrum. Int J Dermatol 1999;38(9):664–672.

Author: Guy Tarleton

Monoamine Oxidase Inhibitor, Poisoning

Clinical Presentation

SIGNS AND SYMPTOMS

Monoamine Oxidase Inhibitor (MAOI) Overdose

- Delayed onset (12 hours)
- Initial hypertension with headache
- Hyperadrenergic activity
  - —Tachycardia
  - —Hypertension
  - —Mydriasis
  - —Agitation
- Neuromuscular excitation
  - —Nystagmus
  - —Hyperreflexia
  - —Tremor
  - —Myoclonus
  - —Rigidity
  - —Seizures
- Hyperthermia
- Associated complications
  - —Rhabdomyolysis
  - —Renal failure
  - —Disseminated intravascular coagulation (DIC)
  - —Acute respiratory distress syndrome (ARDS)

MAOI Hypertensive Crisis Syndrome (MAOI Interaction With Drug or Food)

- Hypertension
- Tachycardia or bradycardia
- Hyperthermia
- Headache, usually occipital
- Altered mental status
- Intracranial hemorrhage
- Seizures

Serotonin Syndrome (SS)

- Increased neuromuscular activity
  - —Increased deep tendon reflexes (DTRs; lower extremity may be greater than upper)
  - —Tremor
  - —Myoclonus
  - —Rigidity (when severe)
- Autonomic nervous system hyperactivity
- Hyperthermia
- CNS
  - —Agitation
  - —Hallucinations
  - —Delirium
  - —Coma
- Diarrhea
- SS versus neuroleptic malignant syndrome (NMS)
  - —Both present along a spectrum of severity (mild to severe)
  - —Onset: several hours (SS) versus days (NMS)
  - —GI symptoms: may be present (SS) versus absent (NMS)
  - —Only drug/medication history may differentiate in many cases

ETIOLOGY

MAOI Physiology/Pharmacology

- MAOI pharmacologic actions
  - —Disruption of equilibrium between endogenous monoamine synthesis and degradation resulting in
    - -Increased neural norepinephrine levels
    - -Downregulation of several receptor types
  - —Inhibition of irreversible (noncompetitive) enzyme
  - —Inhibition of other B_6-containing enzymes
- Monoamine oxidase (MAO): principal inactivator of neural bioactive amines
  - —MAO A
    - -Present in the gut and liver
    - -Protects against dietary bioactive amines
  - —MAO B
    - -Present in neuron terminals and platelets
    - -Sympathomimetic amines: type of bioactive amines

MAOI Overdose

- Toxicopharmacology poorly understood
- MAO inhibitors: amphetamine-like in structure
  - —Early: indirect sympathomimetic effect
  - —Late: sympatholytic response (hypotension seen here)

MAOI Hypertensive Crisis Syndrome

- Results from impaired norepinephrine degradation, combined with massive norepinephrine release precipitated by exposure to an indirect- or mixed-acting sympathomimetic agent
- Common precipitants: tyramine, cocaine, amphetamines

Serotonin Syndrome

- Commonly results from exposure to combinations of agents that affect serotonin metabolism or action
- Mechanisms/agents
  - —Increased serotonin synthesis
    - -Tryptophan
  - —Increased serotonin release
    - -Indirect- and mixed-acting sympathomimetic agents
    - -Dopamine receptor agonists
  - —Decreased serotonin reuptake
    - -Selective serotonin reuptake inhibitors (SSRIs)
    - -Tricyclic antidepressants
    - -Newer antidepressants: trazodone, nefazodone, venlafaxine
    - -Meperidine, dextromethorphan, tramadol
  - —Direct serotonin receptor agonist
    - -Buspirone, sumatriptan, lysergic acid diethylamide (LSD)
  - —Decreased serotonin breakdown
    - -MAOIs
  - —Increased nonspecific serotonin activity
    - -Lithium
- SSRIs
  - —Frequently prescribed drugs
  - —Consider SS in patient with vague complaints

PEDIATRIC CONSIDERATIONS

- Serious toxicity after minimal MAOI exposure

Pre-Hospital

CAUTIONS

- Transport all substances the patient may have ingested or used
- Question witnesses and observe the scene for household products and other potential co-ingestants

Diagnosis

ESSENTIAL WORKUP

- History of ingested substances
- Rectal temperature monitoring as indicated
- Blood pressure/cardiac monitoring

LABORATORY

- No laboratory or ancillary tests for
  - —Mild, clinically uncomplicated hypertensive syndromes
  - —Mild, clinically uncomplicated serotonin syndrome
- DIC
  - —CBC
  - —Prothrombin time (PT), partial thromboplastin time (PTT)
  - —Fibrin-split products
- Rhabdomyolysis
  - —Electrolytes, BUN, creatinine, glucose
  - —Urinalysis
  - —Creatine phosphokinase (CPK)
  - —Myoglobin
- Acetaminophen levels on all patients with suicidal ingestion

IMAGING/SPECIAL TESTS

- EKG for abnormal cardiovascular exam
- Chest x-ray for fever and hypoxemia
- Head CT and lumbar puncture (LP) for altered mental status with fever

DIFFERENTIAL DIAGNOSIS

Hyperthermia

- Infection
- Hyperthyroidism
- Heat stroke
- Anatomic thalamic dysfunction
- NMS
- Malignant hyperthermia
- Malignant catatonia
- Ethanol or drug withdrawal
- Anticholinergic toxicity
- Sympathomimetic overdose
- Cocaine-associated delirium/rhabdomyolysis
- Salicylate toxicity
- Theophylline toxicity
- Nicotine toxicity

Hypertension

- Hypoglycemia
- Carcinoid syndrome
- Pheochromocytoma
- Accelerated renovascular hypertension
- Ethanol or drug withdrawal
- Sympathomimetic toxicity

Treatment

INITIAL STABILIZATION

- ABCs
- 0.9% NS IV access
- Dextrose (or Accucheck), naloxone, and thiamine for altered mental status

ED TREATMENT

- GI decontamination
  - —Gastric lavage if within *1 hour* of ingestion or if clinical condition mandates endotracheal intubation
  - —Administer activated charcoal
- Hyperthermia
  - —Aggressive control via mist/fan evaporation cooling
- Severe, malignant hypertension
  - —Nitroprusside (for MAOI overdose)
  - —Calcium channel blocker or phentolamine (for MAOI/food interaction)
    - -Use short-acting IV agent that can be rapidly "turned off"
    - -*Phentolamine contraindicated in MAOI overdose* (results in unopposed beta agonism)
- Hypotension
  - —Initially with 0.9% NS i.v., 1–2 L fluid bolus
  - —If no response, administer norepinephrine
  - —Dopamine theoretically contraindicated
- Arrhythmias (premorbid sign in MAOI overdose)
  - —Treat with lidocaine or procainamide
  - —Bretylium contraindicated
- Seizures
  - —Benzodiazepines (initial)
  - —Barbiturates
  - —Pyridoxine for refractory seizures
- Rigidity
  - —Lorazepam
  - —Paralysis with vecuronium, endotracheal intubation and mechanical ventilation
- ARDS
  - —Oxygen
  - —Intubation and positive end-expiratory pressure (PEEP) as indicated
- DIC
  - —Fresh-frozen plasma
  - —Platelets
  - —Whole-blood transfusions
- Rhabdomyolysis
  - —Urinary alkalinization with sodium bicarbonate bolus and infusion
- Specific treatment for serotonin syndrome
  - —Human data limited to case reports and series
  - —Mainstay: supportive care, discontinuation of offending agents
  - —Nonselective serotonin antagonists
    - -Cyproheptadine

MEDICATIONS

- Activated charcoal: 1–2 g/kg PO
- Cyproheptadine: 4–8 mg PO/per NGT q1–4h until therapeutic response; maximum daily dose: 0.5 mg/kg (peds: 0.25 mg/kg/d; maximum 12 mg/d; safety not established age <2 years)
- Dextrose: D50W 1–2 amp (50–100 mL or 25–50 g) (peds: D25W 2–4 mL/kg) i.v. push (IVP)
- Diazepam: 5–10 mg (peds: 0.1 mg/kg slowly) increments IVP
- Lidocaine: bolus 1–3 mg/kg IVP at 25–50 μg/min, infusion: 1–4 mg/min (peds: 0.5–1 mg/kg IVA 20–50 μg/kg/min) i.v.
- Lorazepam: 1–2 mg increments IVP
- Nitroprusside: 0.3–10 μg/kg/min i.v.
- Norepinephrine: 2–4 μg/min peds: 0.05–0.1 μg/kg/min) i.v.
- Phentolamine: 5 mg (peds: 0.05–0.2 mg/kg/dose) increments IVP
- Sodium bicarbonate: bolus: 1–2 mEq/kg IVP; adult infusion: 3 amp sodium bicarbonate in 1,000 mL D5W at 2–3 mL/kg/h i.v.
- Vecuronium: 0.1 mg/kg IVP

Disposition

ADMISSION CRITERIA

- All MAOI overdose patients require admission to a monitored unit for 24 hours
- ICU admission for seriously ill patients

DISCHARGE CRITERIA

- Resolved mild hypertensive syndrome or resolved mild serotonin syndrome
  - —Discharge after several hours of ED observation

Miscellaneous

ICD9: 969

ICD10: T43.1

SUGGESTED READINGS

Blake AS, Wiley JF. Serotonin syndrome: a new pediatric intoxication. Pediatr Emerg Care 1999;(6):440–443.

Brent J. Monoamine oxidase inhibitors and the serotonin syndrome. In: Haddad LM, Shannon MW, Winchester JF, eds. Clinical management of poisoning and drug overdose, 3rd ed. Philadelphia: WB Saunders, 1998:452–464.

Mills KC. Serotonin syndrome: a clinical update. Crit Care Clin 1997;13(4):763–783.

Author: Anne Krantz (First edition author: Ted Toerne)

Mononucleosis

Clinical Presentation

SIGNS AND SYMPTOMS

Symptoms

- Slow onset over a few days
- Fever
- Headaches
- Nausea/anorexia
- Malaise/arthralgias/myalgias
- Sore throat

Signs

- Exudative discharge on tonsils and pharynx (mimic streptococcal pharyngitis)
- Edematous pharynx
- Lymphadenopathy
- Hepatomegaly, 15–25%
  —Hepatitis is most common complication
- Splenomegaly, 50–60%
  —Splenic rupture occurs rarely when splenic enlargement significant
- Rash (<10%)
  —Nonspecific maculopapular
  —Can be precipitated by treatment with ampicillin

Complications (Rare)

- Meningitis
- Encephalitis
- Transverse myelitis
- Guillain-Barré syndrome
- Cranial and peripheral nerve palsies
- Myocarditis

MECHANISM/DESCRIPTION

- Subclinical infection in childhood (asymptomatic <2 years old)
- More symptomatic in adolescents and adults
- 4–6 week incubation period
- Transmitted by *close* contact between susceptible (Epstein-Barr virus [EBV] antibody-negative) individuals and symptomatic or carrier (asymptomatic) individuals
- Fever and sore throat resolve in 10–21 days
- 10–20% experience persistent malaise and fatigue for several weeks or months

ETIOLOGY

- EBV
  —Herpesvirus
  —Infects only humans
  —By age 35 years, vast majority of people have had EBV infection
- Virus infects and replicates in cells of the oropharynx (causing cytolysis and virus shedding), then B lymphocytes (causing B-cell proliferation)
- Previously infected individuals may shed the virus intermittently from the oropharynx for many months or years
- Virus shedding is more frequent and prolific in immunocompromised patients
- Reactivation of EBV after primary infection is subclinical

Pre-Hospital

N/A

Diagnosis

ESSENTIAL WORKUP

- Monospot test positive in first month
- Bacterial throat culture
  —Excludes concomitant β-hemolytic streptococcal infection (common association)

LABORATORY

- CBC
  —Atypical lymphocytosis
    -Enlarged T lymphocytes, containing eccentrically placed and lobulated nuclei, and vacuolated cytoplasm ($10–20 \times 10^9$)
  —Hematologic complications
    -Anemia (hemolytic or aplastic)
    -Neutropenia
    -Thrombocytopenia
- Liver function tests
  —Elevated transaminases up to three times normal found in 80–85%
- Heterophil antibody test
  —IgM antibodies that bind and agglutinate horse and sheep erythrocytes, and lyse bovine RBCs
  —Increase (positive test) between the second and third week of symptoms
  —Negative test possible in the first week
  —>95% sensitive/specific in adolescents and adults
  —Produced by less than 40–50% of children infected at age <5 years
- EBV titers
  —Use in heterophil antibody-negative/equivocal individuals to make diagnosis
- Anticomplement autofluorescence
- Southern blot
- Polymerase chain reaction (PCR)

IMAGING/SPECIAL TESTS

- CT abdomen for splenic rupture when severe abdominal pain/hypotension

DIFFERENTIAL DIAGNOSIS

- Other viral (especially adenovirus) or bacterial pharyngitis
  —Difficult to distinguish from group A β-hemolytic streptococcal infection
- Superimposed bacterial pharyngitis on primary EBV infection
- Cytomegalovirus
  —Causes syndrome with atypical lymphocytes and hepatosplenomegaly but no heterophil antibodies
- *Toxoplasma gondii*
- HIV
- Hepatitis A, B, and C
- Diphtheria in unimmunized populations

Treatment

INITIAL STABILIZATION

- ABCs if patient unstable
- IV hydration/stabilization if splenic rupture

ED TREATMENT

- Supportive therapy
  - —Hydration (oral/IV)
  - —Analgesics/antipyretics
- Steroids (methylprednisolone)
  - —Not administered routinely
  - —Indicated if pharyngeal/tonsillar edema significant enough to cause airway compromise
- Antiviral therapy no effect on course of illness
- Avoid
  - —Ampicillin, owing to associated rash
  - —Contact sports, owing to possible splenic rupture, for 6–8 weeks
  - —Aspirin, owing to associated Reye's syndrome

MEDICATIONS

- Methylprednisolone (Solu-Medrol): 80–125 mg (peds: 2 mg/kg) i.v.
- Prednisone: 40 mg (peds: 1 mg/kg) PO q.d. for 4 days

Disposition

ADMISSION CRITERIA

- Significant pharyngeal or tonsillar edema to indicate potential airway compromise
- Neurologic or severe hematologic/hepatic complications
- Inability to take orally

DISCHARGE CRITERIA

- No airway compromise
- Mild hematologic complications or mild hepatitis
- Able to tolerate oral fluids

Miscellaneous

ICD9: 075

ICD10: B27.9

SEE ALSO: PHARYNGITIS

SUGGESTED READINGS

American Academy of Pediatrics. Epstein-Barr virus infections. In: American Academy of Pediatrics red book: report of the Committee on Infectious Disease, 25th ed. Elk Grove Village, IL: American Academy of Pediatrics, 2000.

Foerster J. Infectious mononucleosis. In: Lee G, ed. Wintrobe's clinical hematology, 10th ed. Philadelphia: Lippincott Williams & Wilkins, 1999.

Jenson H. Epstein-Barr virus. In: Behrman R, ed. Nelson textbook of pediatrics, 16th ed. Philadelphia: WB Saunders, 2000.

Melio F. Pharyngitis. In: Rosen P, ed. Emergency medicine: concepts and clinical practice, 5th ed. St. Louis: Mosby, 2002.

Author: Neil Troost

Multiple Myeloma

Clinical Presentation

SIGNS AND SYMPTOMS

- Bone pain predominates (with secondary disuse or neurologic sequelae)
  - —Ribs/sternum
  - —Spine
  - —Clavicle
  - —Skull
  - —Shoulder
  - —Hip
- Constitutional symptoms
  - —Anemia
  - —Weakness
  - —Fatigue
  - —Recurrent infection
  - —Weight loss
- Asymptomatic (20%)
  - —Multiple myeloma (MM) found on follow-up of routine blood screening
- Multiple bouts of sepsis secondary to the encapsulated organisms (*Streptococcus pneumoniae, Haemophilus influenzae,* and *Staphylococcus aureus*)

MECHANISM/DESCRIPTION

- Normal cells transform into myeloma cells at the hematopoietic stem cell level
- Pathologic derangements
  - —Tumor cells within marrow lead to bone destruction and cytopenia
  - —Immunodeficiency develops secondary to suppression of normal immune functions
  - —Myeloma proteins lead to hyperviscosity and amyloidosis
  - —Multifactorial renal failure
- Plasma cell secretions activate osteoclasts, leading to
  - —Bone lysis, pathologic fractures, and neurologic impairment
  - —Hypercalcemia (exacerbated by impaired renal function)
- Anemia due to marrow infiltration and renal insufficiency
- Immunocompromised due to
  - —Decrease in the number of normal immunoglobulins
  - —Qualitative and quantitative defects in T- and B-cell subsets
  - —Granulocytopenia
  - —Decreased cell-mediated immunity
- Hyperviscosity secondary to protein accumulation
  - —Leads to high-output congestive heart failure
- Myeloma light chains accumulate in the renal epithelial cells and destroy the entire nephron

ETIOLOGY

- Incidence: 4 cases per 100,000 population
  - —1% of all cancers
  - —15% of all hematopoietic malignancies
  - —10,000 deaths per year
- Mean age at diagnosis is 62 years
- Slightly higher incidence in women and African Americans (reason unknown)

PEDIATRIC CONSIDERATIONS

- MM is rarely seen in children
- Fewer than 2% in patients younger than 40 years of age

Pre-Hospital

CAUTIONS

- Patients with MM who present with back pain or neurologic symptoms
  - —Presume to have a pathologic spinal fracture
  - —Immobilize appropriately

Diagnosis

ESSENTIAL WORKUP

- Official diagnosis requires
  - —Demonstrating pathologic cells in the bone marrow
  - —Monoclonal gammopathy on electrophoresis
  - —Clinical signs such as anemia, renal insufficiency, or lytic bone lesions
- Complications
  - —Pathologic fractures
  - —Hypercalcemia
  - —Renal failure
  - —Recurrent infection
  - —Anemia
  - —Spinal cord compression (10% of all MM patients)

LABORATORY

- CBC
  - —Normochromic, normocytic anemia
  - —Thrombocytopenia
  - —Leukocytosis
- Rouleaux formation on peripheral blood smear
- Electrolytes, BUN, creatinine, glucose
  - —Renal insufficiency
- Serum calcium
  - —Hypercalcemia due to bone resorption
- Urinalysis
  - —Dipstick selects for albumin and not light-chain proteinuria
  - —False-negative screening urinalysis for protein common
- Elevated erythrocyte sedimentation rate (ESR)

IMAGING/SPECIAL TESTS

- Plain radiographs demonstrate
  - —Lytic bone lesions
  - —Pathologic fractures
- Urinary and serum electrophoresis: show a monoclonal protein spike
  - —Quantitative screening for light chain is diagnostic
- Technetium pyrophosphate bone scan
  - —Lights up bone deposition
  - —False-negative scan with MM due to an uncoupling of bone absorption and deposition that results in a negative bone scan even when lytic lesions present
- Bone marrow biopsy: increase in plasma cells
- Cytogenetic screening may offer prognostic significance

DIFFERENTIAL DIAGNOSIS

- Monoclonal gammopathy
- Chronic lymphocytic leukemia
- Non-Hodgkin's lymphoma
- Waldenström's macroglobulinemia
- Bone marrow plasmacytosis includes collagen vascular disease, cirrhosis, immune complex disease, viral illness, papular mucinosis

Treatment

INITIAL STABILIZATION

- Recognition and treatment of
  - —Hypercalcemia
  - —Renal failure
  - —Sepsis
  - —Spinal cord compression
  - —Anemia

ED TREATMENT

- Analgesics mainstay of therapy in ED
- Splint pathologic fracture; immobilize pathologic spine fractures
- Chemotherapy—administer on inpatient/outpatient basis
  - —Early or asymptomatic stages do not need treatment
  - —Chemotherapy in early stage shows no benefit
  - —Melphalan and prednisone combination chemotherapy the most common treatment; symptom relief and decrease in M protein levels in up to 70% of patients
  - —Alternative chemotherapy includes cyclophosphamide with or without prednisone or VAD (vincristine, doxorubicin [Adriamycin], and dexamethasone)
- Prolonged melphalan use may lead to a secondary leukemia
- High-dose chemotherapy with stem cell transplantation has shown promise
- Thalidomide is useful for salvage therapy

Disposition

ADMISSION CRITERIA

- Refractory pain requiring systemic analgesics
- Life-threatening complications of MM, including acute renal failure, hypercalcemia, sepsis, spinal cord compression, hyperviscosity, neutropenia, and cardiac tamponade

DISCHARGE CRITERIA

- Pain controlled with oral analgesics

Miscellaneous

ICD9: 203.0

ICD10: C90.0

SUGGESTED READINGS

Hideshima T, Chauhan D, Podar K, et al. Novel therapies targeting the myeloma cell and its bone marrow microenvironment. Semin Oncol 2001;28:607–612.

Reece DE. New advances in multiple myeloma. Curr Opin Hematol 1998;5: 460–464.

UK Myeloma Forum. Diagnosis and management of multiple myeloma. Br J Hematol 2001;115:522–540.

Zaidi AA, Vesole DH. Multiple myeloma: an old disease with new hope for the future. CA Cancer J Clinicians 2001;51:273–285.

Author: Nicholas Jouriles

Multiple Sclerosis

Clinical Presentation

SIGNS AND SYMPTOMS

- Initial attacks of multiple sclerosis (MS) usually represent a single lesion, are abrupt in onset, and are seen in characteristic patterns (in order of decreasing frequency)
  - —Optic neuritis (pain exacerbated by eye movement progressing to visual loss)
  - —Paresthesias (or a sensory level) in one limb
  - —Limb (usually leg) weakness
  - —Diplopia—internuclear ophthalmoplegia from a lesion of the medial longitudinal fasciculus results in unilateral or bilateral paralysis of adduction of the eye on horizontal gaze
  - —Trigeminal neuralgia
  - —Urinary retention
  - —Vertigo
  - —Transverse myelitis—acute onset of motor and sensory findings at a specific spinal cord level often associated with bladder or bowel incontinence; can be an early manifestation of MS
- Symptoms typically develop abruptly (minute to hours) and last 6–8 weeks
- Most common in young women of northern European descent, increased risk in first-degree relatives
  - —Peak age: 30 years
  - —Female-to-male ratio, 2:1
- Pain is an uncommon symptom in MS (exception: trigeminal neuralgia, early optic neuritis)

MECHANISM/DESCRIPTION

- Recurrent episodes of demyelinization in the CNS cause signs and symptoms that depend upon the location of the lesions; MS occurs in distinct patterns
- *Relapsing recurring multiple sclerosis:* two or more episodes lasting ≥24 hours separated by ≥1 month
- *Primary progressive multiple sclerosis:* slow or stepwise progression over at least 6 months
- *Secondary progressive multiple sclerosis:* initial exacerbations and remissions followed by slow progression over at least 6 months
- *Stable multiple sclerosis:* no progression (without treatment) over at least 18 months

ETIOLOGY

- MS is a chronic demyelinating disease of the CNS; the etiology is not well understood
- Presumed to be a T-cell–mediated autoimmune disease
- There is evidence for a viral "trigger"
- Plaques in the white matter: characterized by an infiltrate of T cells and macrophages
- Persons of northern European origin most often affected (in United States)
- Increased prevalence is seen moving away from equator

Diagnosis

ESSENTIAL WORKUP

- MS is suspected based on history and physical exam; definite diagnosis is not made in ED and requires observation over time and confirmatory testing
- Physical exam: focused on "hard" neurologic signs such as afferent pupillary defect, internuclear ophthalmoplegia, a sensory level, sphincter disturbance (transverse myelitis); the physical exam should reveal *objective* evidence of neurologic dysfunction
- MRI is sensitive but not specific; may see plaques (may also see on CT)
- Lumbar puncture: "oligoclonal bands" on CSF electrophoresis

DIFFERENTIAL DIAGNOSIS

- Signs and symptoms usually *focal;* diffuse symptoms (seizures, syncope, and dementia) seldom due to MS
- Systemic lupus erythematosus: CNS involvement usually in setting of known disease; usually nonfocal
- Sarcoid: CNS manifestations usually with known disease and lung involvement; nonfocal
- Lyme disease: may mimic MS; seek history of rash and tick exposure in geographic areas of high risk; Lyme titers may aid in diagnosis
- Psychiatric illness: diagnosis of exclusion
- Postinfectious or postimmunization demyelination: may mimic MS; usually in children
- MS unlikely in patients with
  - —Normal neurologic exam
  - —Abrupt hemiparesis
  - —Aphasia
  - —Pain predominates
  - —Very brief symptoms (seconds to minutes)
  - —Age <10 or >50 years

Treatment

INITIAL STABILIZATION

- Fever in MS patients should be treated aggressively because it can worsen neurologic manifestations of MS

ED TREATMENT

- Acute optic neuritis or transverse myelitis: high-dose parenteral steroids possibly effective; oral steroids *contraindicated* (oral prednisone has been reported to exacerbate symptoms)
- Exacerbations: high-dose IV methylprednisolone (up to 1 g/d) or other parenteral corticosteroid regimen
- Symptomatic treatment
  —Spasticity: baclofen
  —Tremor: clonazepam
  —Urinary symptoms: treat infection; self-catheterization for increased postvoid residual (PVR); oxybutynin may promote continence between catheterizations
  —Trigeminal neuralgia: carbamazepine
  —Fatigue, general weakness: no specific treatment

MEDICATIONS

- Baclofen: 10 mg PO t.i.d. initially, may increase to 25 mg t.i.d.
- Carbamazepine: 100 mg PO b.i.d. to 200 mg q.i.d.
- Clonazepam: 0.5 mg/day PO, increase in 0.5-mg increments and up to 3 times a day
- Oxybutynin: 5 mg PO b.i.d. or t.i.d.
- Methylprednisolone: 1 g i.v.

Disposition

ADMISSION CRITERIA

- Acute exacerbation that requires IV therapy
- Patients unable to care for themselves due to the severity of their illness or in whom another condition requiring inpatient treatment cannot be effectively ruled out

DISCHARGE CRITERIA

- *Suspected MS:* patients may be referred for outpatient evaluation if their general condition permits and other serious conditions requiring admission have been effectively ruled out
- *Complication of known MS:* discharge if effective outpatient treatment available for the condition

Miscellaneous

ICD9: 340

ICD10: G35

SUGGESTED READINGS

Antel JP, ed. Multiple sclerosis. Neurol Clin 1995;13(1):1–228.

Brod SA, Lindsey JW, Wolinsky JS. Multiple sclerosis: clinical presentation, diagnosis, and treatment. Am Fam Physician 1996;54(4):1301–1311.

Rolak LA. The diagnosis of multiple sclerosis. Neurol Clin 1996;14(2):27–43.

Weinshaker BG. Epidemiology of multiple sclerosis. Neurol Clin 1996;14(2):291–306.

van Oosten BW, Truyen L, Barkhof F, et al. Multiple sclerosis therapy a practical guide. Drugs 1995;49(2):200–212.

Author: Richard S. Krause

Mumps

Clinical Presentation

SIGNS AND SYMPTOMS

Incubation (12–25 days)

- Viral transmission via respiratory droplets and saliva
- Replication in nasopharynx and regional lymph nodes
- Viremia to meninges and glands; salivary, pancreas, testes, and ovaries

Active Illness (1–10 days)

- Nonspecific prodromal symptoms
- May include low-grade fever, headache, malaise, myalgia, anorexia, otalgia, jaw pain
- Up to 20% of infections are asymptomatic but still contagious
- Up to 50% of cases have nonspecific symptoms of upper respiratory tract infection, fever, malaise, anorexia, and headache
- Contagious 3 days before and 4 days after onset of disease
- *Parotitis* (30–40% of patients)
  —Most common manifestation of mumps
  —Painful and tender unilateral or bilateral enlargement of parotid gland
  —May begin as earache or pain at angle of jaw
  —Any salivary gland may be affected
  —Skin overlying swollen gland is nonerythematous
  —Symptoms decrease after 1 week and resolve by 10th day
  —Contagious until swelling resolves
- *Orchitis* (20–50% of postpubertal males)
  —Most common complication in postpubertal males
  —May occur alone, before, during, but most commonly, after parotitis
  —Unilateral or bilateral (up to 30%)
  —Abrupt, painful, tender swelling with nausea, vomiting, and fever
  —Pain and swelling resolve in 1 week
  —Testicular atrophy in up to 50% of patients
  —Sterility rare
- *Oophoritis* (5% of post pubertal females)
  —May mimic appendicitis if right sided
  —Fertility not impaired
- *Pancreatitis* (2–5%)
  —May occur without any other manifestations of mumps
  —Fever, nausea, vomiting, and epigastric pain
  —May see transient hyperglycemia
  —May be complicated by pseudocyst formation and shock
- *CNS involvement*
  —Aseptic meningitis (10–15% of patients)
  —Usually resolves without sequelae in 3–10 days
  —Encephalitis (very rare)
  —Deafness (80% unilateral) with permanent hearing impairment
- *Other*
  —Myocarditis (rarely with symptomatic involvement)
  —Glomerulonephritis
  —Polyarthralgia and arthritis
  —Thrombocytopenic purpura
  —Ocular complaints

ETIOLOGY

- Paramyxovirus, a single-stranded RNA virus
- Human reservoir
- No known carrier state

PEDIATRIC CONSIDERATIONS

- May present as lower respiratory tract infection
- Systemic symptoms less common
- Mumps vaccine with measles and rubella (MMR) should be administered to all children on or after 12 months of age
- Admitted patients should be isolated from unimmunized

Pre-Hospital

CAUTIONS

- Nonimmunized pre-hospital care personnel exposed to mumps should be advised of potential risks

Diagnosis

ESSENTIAL WORKUP
- Diagnosis based on clinical findings

LABORATORY
- Laboratory tests as needed
- CSF for symptomatic CNS involvement
- Hyperamylasemia usually due to parotitis
- Viral cultures
  - —Provides definitive diagnosis
  - —From blood, throat swab, salivary gland secretions, CSF, or urine
  - —Not indicated unless need to confirm diagnosis in absence of parotitis
- Enzyme immunoassay
  - —Rapid detection
  - —Not indicated unless need to confirm diagnosis in absence of parotitis

DIFFERENTIAL DIAGNOSIS
- Bacterial parotitis
  - —Commonly *Staphylococcus aureus*
  - —Erythematous and tender parotid gland
  - —Usually in elderly or immunocompromised
- Calculus parotid
  - —Stone may be palpable or be seen on sialogram
- Cervical adenitis
- Tumors
  - —Older patients
  - —History of indolent course
- Testicular torsion
- Bacterial epididymoorchitis

Treatment

INITIAL STABILIZATION
- IV fluids for vomiting/dehydration

ED TREATMENT
- Prevention with mumps vaccination is cornerstone of therapy
  - —MMR at 1 year of age
- Supportive and symptomatic
  - —Antipyretics
  - —Analgesia
    - -Acetaminophen, NSAIDs, narcotics (for severe pain)
  - —IV fluids for vomiting and dehydration
  - —Ice pack
  - —Scrotal support

Disposition

ADMISSION CRITERIA
- Seriously ill that may require supportive care
- Severe vomiting and dehydration
- Encephalitis
- Severe pancreatitis
- Isolate admitted patients

DISCHARGE CRITERIA
- Virtually all patients
- Contagious until about 9 days after onset of pain

Miscellaneous

ICD9: 72.9

ICD10: B26.9

SUGGESTED READINGS

American Academy of Pediatrics. Mumps. In: Pickering LK, ed. 2000 Red book: report of the Committee on Infectious Diseases, 25th ed. Elk Grove Village, IL: American Academy of Pediatrics, 2000:405–408.

Centers for Disease Control and Prevention. Measles, mumps, and rubella: vaccine use and strategy for elimination of measles, rubella, and congenital rubella syndrome and control of mumps. Recommendations of the Advisory Committee on Immunization Practices (ACIP). MMWR Morb Mortal Wkly Rep 1998;47 (RR-8):1–57.

Goldman L, ed. Cecil textbook of medicine, 21st ed. Philadelphia: WB Saunders, 2000:808–810.

Mandell GL, ed. Principles and practice of infectious disease, 5th ed. Philadelphia: Churchill Livingstone, 2000:1776–1780.

Author: Austen Chai

Munchausen's Syndrome

Clinical Presentation

SIGNS AND SYMPTOMS

- Frequent visits to EDs for what appears to be an acute illness
- Numerous hospital admissions (often prolonged)
- A plausible, but dramatic, case history
- Escalating demands for diagnostic testing and therapeutic interventions
- Gastrointestinal
  - —Vomiting
  - —Diarrhea
  - —Abdominal pain
- Hematologic
  - —Dizziness
  - —Weakness associated with bleeding
  - —Anemia (from self-phlebotomy or abuse of anticoagulants)
- Neurologic
  - —Feigned seizures
  - —Loss of consciousness
- Musculoskeletal
  - —Self-induced wounds
  - —Multiple scars
- Cardiac
  - —Complaints of chest pain
  - —Palpitations
  - —Dysrhythmias
- Renal
  - —Renal colic
  - —Dysuria
  - —Hematuria
- Endocrine
  - —Hypoglycemia (from self-administration of insulin)
  - —Hyperthyroidism (secondary to exogenous administration of thyroxine)
  - —Hyperdynamic states (from use of epinephrine)
- Infectious
  - —From injection of sputum or feces
  - —Factitious fever from manipulation of thermometers
- Pulmonary
  - —Shortness of breath
- Psychiatric
  - —Hostility and evasiveness
  - —Arrival with numerous medical reports, hospital cards, or insurance forms
  - —Pseudologia fantastica (the telling of tall tales)
  - —Masochistic acceptance of painful procedures
  - —Use of medically sophisticated language or jargon
  - —A paucity of verifiable history
  - —An absence of close interpersonal relationships
  - —A history of sadistic and rejecting parents
  - —A history of chronic childhood illness
  - —Employment in a medically related field

MECHANISM/DESCRIPTION

- Intentional production/feigning of physical symptoms motivated by need to assume the sick role

PEDIATRIC CONSIDERATIONS

- Munchausen's syndrome by proxy
  - —A form of child abuse
  - —A parent provides a misleading history or induces illness in child to obtain medical attention

Pre-Hospital

N/A

Diagnosis

ESSENTIAL WORKUP

- The diagnosis is suggested by inconsistencies in the history or the pattern of illness and by the recognition of the above patterns of behavior
- Diligent detective work, including obtaining records from other hospitals and calling on family members who can provide evidence of similar prior presentations
- Direct observation of the patient and a search of the patient's room/belongings that may reveal their method of deception (e.g., insulin vials and syringes)

LABORATORY

- Dependent on the organ system involved
- Testing the stool for phenolphthalein to detect laxative abuse
- Determination of exogenous insulin administration with C3 peptide

IMAGING/SPECIAL TESTS

N/A

DIFFERENTIAL DIAGNOSIS

- True physical illness
- Illness that is the unintentional result of self-destructive acts or surgical interventions
  - —Small bowel obstruction
- Malingering
  - —Where a clear-cut secondary gain (e.g., disability benefits) is present
- Conversion disorder
  - —Typically with neurologic symptoms
    - -Blindness
    - -Hemiparesis
    - -Seizures
  - —Where symptoms are not consciously produced
- Somatization disorder
  - —Multiple somatic complaints
  - —Multiple organ system involvement
  - —Symptoms are not intentionally produced

Treatment

INITIAL STABILIZATION

- Treat obvious threats to life or limb
  - —Hypoglycemia, bleeding, or wounds

ED TREATMENT

- Realize that a satisfactory outcome is rare
- Psychiatric intervention
  - —Identify any true medical emergency or condition
  - —Refer for individual and group therapy
  - —Refer for behavior modification
  - —Blacklist identified patients
- Report cases of Munchausen's syndrome by proxy to child protective services so that the child can have a safe environment
- Pay attention to your own emotional reaction to avoid inappropriate abandonment or treatment

Disposition

ADMISSION CRITERIA

- Admission is often required to stabilize and evaluate serious comorbid physical illness
- Psychiatric admission can be useful but is seldom accepted by the patient

DISCHARGE CRITERIA

- Medical stability
- Not an active threat to harm self
- Appropriate referral for medical and psychiatric follow-up arranged

Miscellaneous

ICD9: 301.51

CORE CONTENT CODE: 14.5.1

ICD10: F68.1

SUGGESTED READINGS

Feldman MD, Ford CV. Factitious disorders. In: Sadock BJ, Sadock VA, eds. Kaplan and Sadock's comprehensive textbook of psychiatry, 7th ed. Philadelphia: Lippincott Williams & Wilkins, 2000:1533–1543.

Robertson MM, Cervilla JA. Munchausen's syndrome. Br J Hosp Med 1997;58(7): 308–312.

Souid AK, Keith DV, Cunningham AS. Munchausen syndrome by proxy. Clin Pediatr (Phila) 1998;37(8):497–503.

Stern TA. Munchausen's syndrome revisited. Psychosomatics 1980;21:329–336.

Authors: Theodore A. Stern; Jeff C. Huffman

Clinical Presentation

SIGNS AND SYMPTOMS (GROUPED BY TOXIN)

Amanitine/Phalloidin

- Nausea
- Vomiting
- Abdominal cramps
- Bloody diarrhea
- Clinical course
  - —Onset of symptoms 6–36 hours
  - —Transient latent phase may last 2 days (no pain)
  - —Can progress to hepatic or renal failure and death in 4–7 days
  - —Most lethal mushroom toxins

Orellanine

- Nausea
- Headache
- Sweating
- Chills
- Low-back pain
- Thirst
- Clinical course
  - —May progress to oliguria and acute renal failure
  - —Markedly delayed onset of symptoms (2–14 days)

Ibotenic Acid/Muscimol

- Anticholinergic symptoms include
  - —Hallucinations
  - —Dysarthria
  - —Ataxia
  - —Muscle cramps
  - —Vomiting
  - —Seizures
  - —Coma
- Clinical course
  - —Relatively rapid onset of 30–60 minutes

Gyromitrin

- First 6 hours
  - —Abdominal cramps
  - —Vomiting
  - —Watery diarrhea
- Later symptoms
  - —Weakness
  - —Cyanosis
  - —Confusion
  - —Seizures
  - —Coma

Muscarine

- Cholinergic symptoms include
  - —Miosis
  - —Salivation
  - —Lacrimation
  - —Sweating
  - —Diarrhea
  - —Flushed skin
  - —Nausea
  - —Bradycardia
  - —Bronchoconstriction
- Onset usually within 1 hour (may be delayed)

Coprine

- Disulfram-like reaction when combined with alcohol
  - —Flushing
  - —Sweating
  - —Nausea
  - —Vomiting
  - —Palpitations
  - —Chest pain
- Begins minutes after combining this toxin with ethanol

Psilocin/Psilocybin

- Visual hallucinations
- Alteration of perception
- Nausea
- Mydriasis
- Tachycardia
- Fever and seizures in children
  - —Rarely fatal (case report of myocardial infarction in 18 years old)

Gastric Irritants

- Group of toxins that cause nausea, vomiting, intestinal cramps, and watery diarrhea
- Onset 30 minutes to 2 hours, usually resolved in 6–12 hours

MECHANISM/DESCRIPTION

Amanitine/Phalloidin

- Species
  - —*Amanita phalloides* ("death cap")
  - —*Amanita virosa/verna* ("destroying angel")
  - —*Gallerina marginata; Gallerina venenata*
- Mechanism
  - —Cyclopeptide toxins inhibit RNA polymerase 2
  - —Which kills GI epithelium, hepatocytes, nephrocytes

Orellanine

- Species
  - —*Cortinarius* (several species)
- Mechanism
  - —Direct renal toxicity

Ibotenic Acid/Muscimol

- Species
  - —*Amanita pantherina* ("the panther")
  - —*Amanita muscaria* ("fly agaric")
- Mechanism
  - —GABA agonists

Gyromitrin

- Species
  - —*Gyromitra esculenta* ("false morels")
  - —Other *Gyromitra* species
- Mechanism
  - —Inhibits pyridoxal phosphate
  - —Damage to RBCs, hepatocytes, neurons

Muscarine

- Species
  - —*Inocybe* (several species)
  - —*Clitocybe* (several species)
- Mechanism
  - —Parasympathomimetic

Coprine

- Species
  - —*Coprinus atramentarius* ("inky caps")
- Mechanism
  - —Blocks acetaldehyde dehydrogenase
    - -Causes disulfram-like reaction if mixed with alcohol

Psilocin/Psilocybin

- Species
  - —*Psilocybe* and *Panaeolus* species as well as others
- Mechanism
  - —Similar structure to lysergic acid diethylamide (LSD)

Gastric Irritants

- Many various mushrooms including those normally considered edible

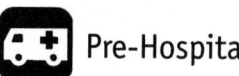

Pre-Hospital

CAUTIONS

- Bring any unconsumed mushrooms or mushroom pieces to the hospital to aid in diagnosis
  - —Refrigerate specimens if possible

Diagnosis

ESSENTIAL WORKUP

- Mushroom description
  - —<3% of cases result in an exact mushroom identification
- Careful history and physical exam
  - —Special detail to the timing of symptom onset

LABORATORY

- CBC
- Prothrombin time (PT), partial thromboplastin time (PTT)
- Electrolytes, BUN, creatinine, glucose
- Urinalysis
- Liver function tests (LFTs)

DIFFERENTIAL DIAGNOSIS

- Symptoms with a late onset (>6 hours) indicate the more lethal toxins
- Always entertain the possibility of multiple species ingestion
- Combination with ETOH may suggest coprine (disulfiram reaction)
- Consider other illicit drugs with visual hallucinations
- Fertilizers, insecticides, fungicides, etc., if mushrooms were found in a public place

Treatment

INITIAL STABILIZATION

- ABCs
- Establish IV 0.9% NS
- Monitor
- Naloxone, D50W (or Accucheck) and thiamine for altered mental status

ED TREATMENT

General

- Decontamination
  - —Activated charcoal (20–50 g) superior to ipecac
    - -Particularly with delayed presentation
  - —Induce vomiting only if
    - -Patients have not yet vomited
    - -Normal mental and respiratory status
    - -Not undergoing hallucinations
- Fluid rehydration and electrolyte replacement as necessary
- Call local poison control center and ask for mycologist
- Obtain specimens (vomitus if needed) for identification

Toxin-Specific Therapy

Amanitine/Phalloidin

- Ewald oral gastric tube aspiration of mushroom fragments
- Administer charcoal every 2–4 hours
- Hypoglycemia and elevated PT
  - —Signs of liver failure
  - —Administer fresh-frozen plasma and vitamin K for coagulation disorders with active bleeding
- Administer calcium in presence of hypocalcemia
- Liver transplant for severe hepatic necrosis
- Consider high-dose penicillin G or silibinin (milk thistle; controversial)

Orellanine

- Closely monitor BUN, creatinine, electrolytes, and urine output
- Lasix contraindicated
  - —Accelerates nephrotoxicity in rats
- Diuresis with alkalinization of urine with $NaHCO_3$
- Hemodialysis/renal transplantation may be needed

Ibotenic Acid/Muscimol

- Usually self-limited toxicity
- Provide supportive care
- Monitor for hypotension
- Treat severe anticholinergic symptoms with physostigmine

Gyromitrin

- Administer pyridoxine in severely symptomatic patients
- Treat seizure with benzodiazepines
- Treat liver dysfunctions as outlined for amanitine/phalloidin group
- Dialysis for renal failure

Muscarinic

- Administer atropine in severe cases

Coprine

- Self-limited toxicity
- Avoid syrup of ipecac (contains alcohol)
- Propranolol for cardiac dysrhythmias

Psylocin/Psilocybin

- Self-limited toxicity
- Monitor if tachycardic
- Dark, quiet room and reassurance
- Do not induce emesis if hallucinating
- External cooling measures if needed in children

GI Irritants

- When poisoning from the above groups not suspected
  - —Administer acetaminophen and antiemetics
  - —Supportive care
- Monitor LFTs in cases in which cyclopeptide-containing mushrooms are suspected

MEDICATIONS

- Activated charcoal slurry: 1–2 g/kg up to 90 g PO
- Atropine: 0.5 mg (peds: 0.02 mg/kg) i.v.; repeat 0.5–1.0 mg i.v. (peds: 0.04 mg/kg) every 10 minutes if secretions recur, to max of 1 mg/kg in children and 2 mg/kg in adults
- Dextrose: D50W 1 amp (50 mL or 25 g) (peds: D25W 2–4 mL/kg) i.v.
- Diazepam (benzodiazepine): 5–10 mg (peds: 0.2–0.5 mg/kg) i.v.
- Ipecac: 30 mL (peds: 15 mL for children <12 years) PO
- Lorazepam (benzodiazepine): 2–6 mg (peds: 0.03–0.05 mg/kg) i.v.
- Naloxone (Narcan): 2 mg (peds: 0.1 mg/kg) i.v. or i.m. initial dose
- Physostigmine: 0.5–2 mg i.m. or i.v. in adults
- Propranolol: 1 mg (peds: 0.01–0.1 mg/kg) i.v.
- Pyridoxine: 25 mg/kg over 30 minutes
- Sorbitol: 1–2 g/kg to a max of 150 g (peds: >1 year: 1–1.5 g/kg as a 35% solution to a max of 50 g) PO mixed in the activated charcoal slurry
- Thiamine (vitamin B_1): 100 mg (peds: 50 mg) i.v. or i.m.

Disposition

ADMISSION CRITERIA

- All symptomatic patients
  - —Protracted vomiting, dehydration, liver or renal toxicity, or seizures
- Transfer to a tertiary medical center for early signs of renal or hepatic failure
- Infants and young children found with mushrooms
  - —Assume ingestion
- ICU admission for known ingestion of an amanitine-containing mushroom
  - —Early liver service consultation

DISCHARGE CRITERIA

- Asymptomatic during 6–8 hours with 24 hours of close home observation available

Miscellaneous

ICD9: 988.1

ICD10: T62.0

SUGGESTED READINGS

Borowiak KS, Ciechanowski K, Waloszczyk P. Psilocybin mushroom (*Psilocybe semilanceata*) intoxication with myocardial infarction. Clin Toxicol 1990;36(1&2): 47–49.

Jacobs J, Von Behren J, Kreutzer, R. Serious mushroom poisonings in California requiring hospital admission, 1990 through 1994. West J Med 1996;165(5):283–288.

McPartland JM, Vilgalys RJ, Cubeta MA. Mushroom poisoning. Am Fam Physician 1997;55(5):1797–1800, 1805–1809, 1811–1812.

O'Donnel M, Fleming S. The renal pathology of mushroom poisoning. Histopathology 1997;30(3):280–282.

Pinson CW, Bradley AL. A primer for clinicians on mushroom poisoning in the West. West J Med 1996;165(5):318–319.

Vetter J. Toxins of *Amanita phalloides*. Toxicon 1998;36:13.

Authors: Adam Black; Timothy Erickson

Myasthenia Gravis

Clinical Presentation

SIGNS AND SYMPTOMS

- Painless, fatigable weakness
- Weakness worse with repeated or sustained muscular activity, improves with rest
- Ocular muscle weakness
  - —Most common initial symptom
  - —Ptosis, diplopia
  - —Inability to keep eyelid shut against resistance
  - —No pupillary changes
- Bulbar and facial muscle weakness
  - —Difficulty with speech, swallowing, chewing
  - —Decreased facial expression
  - —Head droop
- Limb weakness
  - —Proximal limbs or small muscles of the hand
  - —Reflexes and sensory exam normal
- *Myasthenic crisis* defined by respiratory compromise requiring respiratory assistance

MECHANISM/DESCRIPTION

- Bimodal distribution: one peak in second and third decades affecting mostly women, second peak in sixth and seventh decades affecting mostly men
- Evidence of genetic predisposition, possibility of environmental precipitants
- Ocular (15%) or generalized (85%)
- Acute or subacute, with relapses and remissions
- Decreased number of acetylcholine receptors (AChRs) at the neuromuscular junction
- Antibody mediated, although some patients are acetylcholine receptor antibody (AChR Ab) negative
- Associated with thymoma
- *Myasthenic crisis*
  - —Triggers: infection, surgery, trauma, medication changes
  - —More common in untreated and postthymectomy patients
  - —Difficult to distinguish cholinergic crisis from excessive doses of acetylcholinesterase (AChE) inhibitors
    - -Can try *edrophonium test dose,* would improve symptoms in myasthenia gravis but would make symptoms worse in cholinergic crisis
    - -Alternatively, stop all AChE inhibitors, protect the airway, support as needed

ETIOLOGY

- Triggers of myasthenic crisis
  - —Infection
  - —Physical stress/trauma/surgery
  - —Medication changes, e.g., rapid tapering of steroids
- Medications that worsen weakness
  - —Neuromuscular blocking agents
  - —Aminoglycosides
  - —Local anesthetics
  - —Antidysrhythmics (quinine, quinidine, procainamide)
  - —Beta-blockers
- Penicillamine can cause myasthenia gravis as well as other autoimmune conditions

PEDIATRIC CONSIDERATIONS

- Transient neonatal myasthenia
  - —10% of infants of mothers with myasthenia gravis
  - —Transfer of maternal AChR antibodies
  - —Resolves without treatment within a few weeks
- Generalized myasthenia with onset in childhood
  - —50% are seronegative
  - —Often remits spontaneously

Pre-Hospital

- Attention to airway management

Diagnosis

ESSENTIAL WORKUP

- Search for secondary triggers
- Assess for respiratory compromise

LABORATORY

- Workup for infectious source, including chest x-ray
- Electrolytes
- Thyroid function tests
- Assay for anti-AChR Ab
  - —Positive in 85% with generalized disease
  - —Positive in 50% of those with ocular disease

IMAGING/SPECIAL TESTS

- Head CT or MRI to rule out compressive lesions causing cranial nerve findings
- Repetitive nerve stimulation shows characteristic decrement in muscle response
- Chest CT to look for associated thymoma

DIFFERENTIAL DIAGNOSIS

- Drug-induced myasthenia
- Hyperthyroidism
- Electrolyte abnormalities
- Graves' disease
- Lambert-Eaton myasthenic syndrome
- Botulism
- Guillain-Barré syndrome
- Progressive external ophthalmoplegia
- Intracranial mass lesions

Treatment

INITIAL STABILIZATION

- *Myasthenic crisis*
  - —Most important intervention is early intubation and mechanical ventilation
- Focus on airway and respiratory function
- Because respiratory status waxes and wanes, no single parameter can predict the need for respiratory support
- Avoid neuromuscular blocking drugs if possible
  - —Can cause extended period of paralysis
  - —Succinylcholine and other depolarizing agents have a shorter duration of action but should be used with caution
  - —Use versed, etomidate, or thiopental instead

ED TREATMENT

- Treat infections aggressively
- Search for and remove triggers
- Edrophonium (Tensilon) test
  - —Short-acting cholinesterase
  - —Rapid, short-lived (2–5 minutes) improvement in strength
- Myasthenic crisis may require plasmapheresis or intravenous gammaglobulin
- Side effects of AChE inhibitors include bradycardia, GI symptoms (nausea, vomiting, abdominal cramps, diarrhea), and increased bronchial and oral secretions; for adverse reactions to AChE inhibitor, give atropine
- Steroids and immunosuppressive therapy are not used in acute management
- Corticosteroid (high-dose prednisone) produces remission or marked improvement in up to 80%; 30% of patients have initial worsening of symptoms, which last an average of 6 days, and may need inpatient hospitalization for observation while starting high-dose prednisone therapy
- Immunosuppressive drugs (azathioprine, cyclosporine), when used, are usually initiated by neurologist

MEDICATIONS

- Anticholinesterase: dosages variable
- Atropine (to treat AChE inhibitor adverse effects): 0.4–0.5 mg i.v. or i.m.
- Edrophonium (Tensilon): 2 mg i.v. over 15–30 seconds; if no effect after 45 seconds, can give second dose at 8 mg i.v.
- Prednisone: 20–25 mg PO every day or every other day
- Pyridostigmine (Mestinon): 30 mg PO q4–6h (infant: 1–2 mg/kg q4h); for myasthenic crisis, pyridostigmine infusion at 1–2 mg/h

Disposition

ADMISSION CRITERIA

- Myasthenic crisis or questionable respiratory status mandates admission to the intensive care unit (ICU)
- Myasthenic patients with worsening symptoms
- New-onset myasthenic symptoms
- Diagnosis unclear, but myasthenia a possibility

DISCHARGE CRITERIA

- Myasthenic patients who are improving can be discharged in consultation with neurology

Miscellaneous

ICD9: 358.0

ICD10: G60.0

SUGGESTED READINGS

Bedlack RS, Sanders DB. How to handle myasthenic crisis. Postgrad Med 2000;107(4):211–214.

Berrouschot J, Baumann I, Kalischewski P, et al. Therapy of myasthenic crisis. Crit Care Med 1997;25:1228–1235.

Drachman DB. Myasthenia gravis. N Engl J Med 1994;330(25):1797–1810.

Sanders DB, Scoppetta CS. Treatment of patients with myasthenia gravis. Neurol Clin North Am 1994;12(2):343–365.

Thomas CE, et al. Myasthenic crisis: clinical features, mortality, complications, and risk factors for prolonged intubation. Neurology 1997;48(5):1253–1260.

Vincent A, Palace J, Hilton-Jones, D. Myasthenia gravis. Lancet 2001;357 (i9274):2122–2128.

Author: Angela Loh

Myocardial Contusion

Clinical Presentation

SIGNS AND SYMPTOMS

- The clinical picture is varied and nonspecific—from excruciating chest pain and shock to subtle EKG changes without clinical symptoms
- Most common sign is tachycardia out of proportion to the degree of trauma or blood loss
  - —Friction rub may rarely occur
- Retrosternal angina-like chest pain unrelieved by nitroglycerin, often delayed up to 24 hours
  - —May respond to oxygen
- Evidence of significant thoracic trauma such as contusions, abrasions, palpable crepitus, or visible flail segments should heighten suspicion
- Other associated abdominal, skeletal, or CNS injuries may mask the signs and symptoms of myocardial contusion

MECHANISM/DESCRIPTION

- The heart may be compressed between the sternum and vertebrae, swing forward and strike the sternum during deceleration, or be damaged by abdominal viscera upwardly displaced by force on the abdomen
- Pathologically characterized by a discrete and well-demarcated area of hemorrhage
  - —Usually subendocardial
  - —May extend in a pyramidal transmural fashion
  - —Most commonly the anterior wall of the right ventricle or atrium is involved
- Coronary artery occlusion from intimal tearing or adjacent hemorrhage and edema may rarely occur
- Immediate complications include
  - —Life-threatening dysrhythmias
  - —Cardiogenic shock/congestive heart failure (CHF)
  - —Hemopericardium with tamponade
  - —Valvular/myocardial rupture
  - —Intraventricular thrombi
  - —Thromboembolic phenomena
  - —Coronary artery occlusion

ETIOLOGY

- Caused by blunt trauma to the chest, most commonly in high-speed deceleration accidents
  - —May occur in accidents with speeds as low as 20–35 mph
- Also seen in auto-pedestrian injuries, falls, and after prolonged closed chest cardiac massage
- Always consider when multisystem blunt trauma is present; other injuries may be distracting

Pre-Hospital

CAUTIONS

- Pre-hospital personnel must convey accurate information to emergency department personnel concerning the mechanism of injury, motor vehicle status, steering wheel and dashboard damage, use of restraint devices, vehicle speed, and patient position

Diagnosis

ESSENTIAL WORKUP

- No single diagnostic study (other than autopsy findings!) confirms the presence of myocardial contusion
- Only abnormal EKG and CPK-MB correlate directly with complications requiring treatment
- EKG is the best initial screening tool
  - —Most common rhythm is sinus tachycardia (70%)
- A normal EKG does not rule out myocardial damage
- Echocardiography should be performed on all patients with any EKG changes or elevated CPK-MB

LABORATORY

- Sensitivity of CPK-MB isoenzymes varies from 11% to 85%
  - —Specificity decreased in multiple trauma
- CPK-MB levels should be sent on all patients being admitted
- Cardiac troponin and myoglobin assays have not yet been shown to be useful to provide definitive diagnosis

IMAGING/SPECIAL TESTS

- Plain radiography: detects associated injuries such as pulmonary contusion, rib or sternal fractures (particularly important), acute pulmonary edema with normal-sized heart secondary to cardiac decompensation
- Echocardiography: detects wall motion abnormalities and effusions, allows direct visualization of cardiac chambers and valves, but will not visualize small contusions
- Radionuclide angiography: sensitive; detects wall motion abnormalities; allows differentiation between right and left ventricles but is limited in visualizing small areas
- Thallium-201 scintigraphy: sensitive and specific to left ventricular injury but unable to evaluate the right ventricle

DIFFERENTIAL DIAGNOSIS

- Cardiac rupture
- Tamponade
- Valvular damage
- Other traumatic chest wall injury
- Angina or myocardial infarction

Treatment

INITIAL STABILIZATION

- All patients require oxygen, intravenous access, and cardiac monitoring
- The priorities of trauma care take precedence; see the section on Advanced Trauma Life Support (ATLS)

ED TREATMENT

- Dysrhythmias may be treated with the same pharmacologic agents as nontraumatic dysrhythmias
  —SVT: adenosine or verapamil if patient is not hypovolemic
  —Bradycardia: atropine, pacing
  —Ventricular dysrhythmias: electrical conversion, amiodarone, lidocaine, procainamide, bretylium
  —Cardiac arrest: epinephrine, atropine, etc.
  —Rapid atrial fibrillation or flutter: digoxin or diltiazem, if patient not hypotensive
- Prophylactic treatment of dysrhythmias is not indicated
- In cardiogenic shock caused by myocardial contusion, judicious fluid administration, inotropic support (dopamine or dobutamine), and intraaortic balloon counterpulsation may be necessary

MEDICATIONS

- Adenosine: 6 mg (peds: 0.1–0.2 mg/kg) rapid i.v. push (IVP), may repeat 12 mg (peds: 0.2–0.4 mg/kg) every 1–2 minutes × 2 if no response
- Amiodarone: 150 mg (peds: 5 mg/kg load) i.v. over 10 minutes, then 1 mg/min (peds: 5 μg/kg/min) for 6 hours, then 0.5 mg/min (peds: 5 μg/kg/min) for 18 hours
- Atropine: 0.5–1.0 mg (peds: 0.02 mg/kg/dose, minimum 0.1 mg) i.v. or ET
- Bretylium: initial 5 mg/kg i.v., repeat 10 mg/kg if needed; infusion is 1–3 mg/min
- Digoxin: load 0.25 mg (peds: 0.02 mg/kg i.v., then 0.01 mg/kg) i.v. q6h up to 1 mg
- Diltiazem: 0.25 mg/kg (adult and peds) or 20 mg i.v. (adult) over 2 minutes; may rebolus 0.35 mg/kg 15 minutes later
- Dobutamine: 2–15 μg/kg/min (adult and peds)
- Dopamine: 2–20 μg/kg/min (adult and peds)
- Epinephrine: 1 mg (peds: 0.01 mg/kg) i.v. or ET for cardiac arrest (1:10,000 solution)
- Lidocaine: load 1 mg/kg (adult and peds) i.v., then 0.5 mg/kg every 8–10 minutes to max of 3 mg/kg; infusion 1–4 mg/min (peds: 20–50 μg/kg/min) i.v.
- Procainamide: 100 mg (peds: 15 mg/kg/dose) i.v. every 10 minutes or 20 mg/min up to 17 mg/kg
- Verapamil: 0.1–0.3 mg/kg up to 5–10 mg i.v. over 2 minutes; contraindicated in children

Disposition

- Numerous studies show that adverse outcomes, particularly dysrhythmias, are uncommon but generally occur within the first 24 hours
- There is no single test or combination of tests that will accurately predict which patients can be discharged safely from the ED; therefore, all patients in whom there is evidence of myocardial contusion or in whom the diagnosis is seriously being entertained should be admitted

ADMISSION CRITERIA

- Any patient with EKG abnormalities, hemodynamic instability, or other studies suggestive of cardiac contusion must be admitted to a monitored unit for close observation and workup

DISCHARGE CRITERIA

- Patients who are asymptomatic, with no EKG abnormalities or dysrhythmia, may be discharged after a 4- to 6-hour ED observation period

Miscellaneous

ICD9: 861.01

ICD10: S26.8

SUGGESTED READINGS

Kaye P, O'Sullivan I. Myocardial contusion: emergency investigation and diagnosis. Emerg Med J 2002;19(1):8–10.

Maenza RL, Seaberg D, D'Amico F. A meta-analysis of blunt cardiac trauma: ending myocardial confusion. Am J Emerg Med 1996;14(3):237–241.

Markovchick V, Wolfe R. Cardiovascular trauma. In: Rosen P, et al., eds. Emergency medicine: concepts and clinical practice, 4th ed. St. Louis: CV Mosby, 1998: 527–545.

Roxburgh JC. Myocardial contusion. Injury 1996;27(9):603–605.

Author: Robert S. Hamilton

Myocarditis

Clinical Presentation

SIGNS AND SYMPTOMS

- Decreased exercise tolerance
- Fatigue
- Dyspnea
- Palpitations
- Chest discomfort
- Increased jugular venous pulsation
- Decreased pulse pressure
- Fever
- Cyanosis
- Hypotension, tachycardia
- Muffled S1 heart sound
- Diastolic murmurs (unusual)
- Fulminant disease
  - —Rales
  - —Jugular venous distention (JVD)
  - —Peripheral edema
  - —Hepatomegaly

MECHANISM/DESCRIPTION

- Inflammatory disease of the myocardium
- Direct cytotoxic effect of causative agent
- Secondary immune response
- Cytokine expression
- Often results in cardiac dysfunction and heart failure
- 40% of patients report recent viral illness

ETIOLOGY

Infectious

- Viral
  - —Enteroviruses (coxsackie B)
  - —Adenovirus
  - —Herpesvirus (including cytomegalovirus [CMV])
  - —Hepatitis C
  - —Influenza
  - —Mumps
  - —Rubeola
  - —Variola/vaccinia
  - —Yellow fever
  - —Rabies
  - —HIV
- Bacteria
  - —Diphtheria
  - —Tuberculosis
  - —Brucellosis
  - —Psittacosis
  - —Meningococcus
  - —Mycoplasma
  - —Group A streptococcus
- Protozoa
  - —*Treponema cruzi* (Chagas' disease)
    - -Most common cause of heart failure and myocarditis worldwide
    - -20 million persons infected
    - -Central and South America
  - —Toxoplasmosis
  - —Trypanosomiasis
  - —Malaria
  - —Leishmaniasis
- Spirochetes *(Borrelia)* and rickettsial diseases in the United States
  - —Syphilis
- Rickettsial
  - —Scrub typhus
  - —Rocky mountain spotted fever
  - —Q fever
- Bites/stings
  - —Scorpion, snake, black widow venom
- Fungal
  - —Candidiasis
  - —Aspergillosis
  - —Cryptococcosis
  - —Histoplasmosis
  - —Actinomycosis
- Helminthic
  - —Trichinosis
  - —Echinococcosis
  - —Schistosomiasis
  - —Cysticercosis

NONINFECTIOUS

- Drugs
  - —Chemotherapeutic agents (anthracyclines)
  - —Radiation
  - —Hypersensitivity
    - -Sulfamethoxazole, sulfadiazine, and penicillins
  - —Heavy metals
  - —Hydrocarbons
  - —Carbon monoxide
  - —Arsenic
- Autoimmune disorders
  - —Systemic lupus erythematosus (SLE)
  - —Wegener's granulomatosis
  - —Kawasaki disease
- Sarcoidosis
- Peripartum cardiomyopathy
  - —Last month of pregnancy to 5 months postpartum period
- Cardiac rejection

Pre-Hospital

- Standard protocol for management of CHF/pulmonary edema

Diagnosis

ESSENTIAL WORKUP

- EKG
  - —Transient, nonspecific ST- and T-wave changes
  - —Atrial and ventricular dysrhythmias
  - —Heart block and conduction defects common
    - -20% of patients have left bundle branch block
- Chest x-ray
  - —Normal or may demonstrate cardiomegaly, pulmonary edema

LABORATORY

- CBC, erythrocyte sedimentation rate (ESR)
- CPK-MB and lactate dehydrogenase (LDH)
- Cardiac troponin-I or T
- Viral titers; cultures rarely positive
- Mycoplasma, antistreptolysin titers
- Hepatitis panels
- Monospot testing
- CMV serology
- Peripheral blood cultures

IMAGING/SPECIAL TESTS

- Echocardiography
  - —Emergent study for fulminant cases
  - —Ventricular wall motion abnormalities
  - —Left ventricular dilation or increased wall thickness
  - —Left ventricular thrombus (15% of patients)
  - —Abnormal systolic and diastolic filling
  - —Right ventricular enlargement and dysfunction carries a poor prognosis
- Gallium-67- and indium-111-labeled antimyosin antibody scans
- Gadolinium-enhanced MRI
  - —Indicate cardiac inflammation and myocyte necrosis
- Right ventricular endomyocardial biopsy
  - —Appropriate in heart transplant recipients
  - —Polymerase chain reaction amplification of viral genome in endomyocardial tissue

DIFFERENTIAL DIAGNOSIS

- Acute myocardial infarction
- Acute and chronic pulmonary embolus
- Pericarditis
- Adrenal insufficiency
- Severe hypothyroidism and hyperthyroidism
- Sepsis
- Environmental challenges
  - —Hyperpyrexia, hypothermia
  - —Toxin-mediated disease

Treatment

INITIAL STABILIZATION

- Same as for acute CHF/pulmonary edema (see Congestive Heart Failure)
- Treat dysrhythmias if present
- Transvenous pacing for symptomatic heart block

ED TREATMENT

- ACE inhibitors (captopril)
  —Reduce afterload and inflammation
- Digoxin
  —CHF or atrial fibrillation
- Diuretics (furosemide, bumetanide)
- Immunosuppressive therapy (e.g., cyclosporine, prednisone) are of unproved benefit except in patients with immune mediated disease (e.g., SLE)
- Hyperimmunoglobulin therapy improves cardiac function in CMV-associated myopericarditis
- NSAIDs contraindicated in early and acute-phase myocarditis because they increase myocardial damage
- Heparin and warfarin decrease risk for thromboembolic events in patients with depressed LV function or intracardiac thrombus
- Cardiac transplantation
  —5-year mortality or the need for cardiac transplantation rate is 56%
  —About 20–33% of patients recover completely

MEDICATIONS

- Bumetanide: 0.5–1.0 mg i.v./dose
- Captopril (PO)
  —Neonates: 0.025–0.1 mg/dose q.i.d.
  —Infants: 0.15–0.3 mg/kg/dose (max, 6 mg/kg)
  —Children: 0.5–1.0 mg/kg/24 h
  —Adults: initial dose 6.25 mg; can titrate to 50 mg/dose
- Digoxin
  —Infants: 12.5–20.0 μg/kg i.v. or PO
  —2–10 years old: 7.5–15.0 μg/kg i.v.
- Furosemide: 1 mg/kg/dose

PEDIATRIC CONSIDERATIONS

- Intravenous immunoglobulin (IVIG) is an effective treatment option in pediatric viral myocarditis
  —Improved left ventricle function and trend toward better survival

Disposition

ADMISSION CRITERIA

- Symptomatic patients with myocarditis should be admitted
- CHF, dysrhythmia, embolic events, cardiogenic shock
  —Admit to ICU setting

DISCHARGE CRITERIA

- Asymptomatic patient with no evidence of dysrhythmia or cardiac dysfunction

Miscellaneous

ICD9: 429.0

ICD10: I51.4

SUGGESTED READINGS

D'Ambrosio A, Patti G, Manzoli A. The fate of acute myocarditis between spontaneous improvement and evolution to dilated cardiomyopathy: a review. Heart 2001;85:499–504.

Feldman AM, McNamara D. Myocarditis. N Engl J Med 2000;343(19):1388–1398.

Fuse K, Kodama M, Okura Y, et al. Predictors of disease course in patients with acute myocarditis. Circulation 2000;102(23):2829–2835.

Gajarski RJ, Towbin JA. Recent advances in the etiology, diagnosis and treatment of myocarditis and cardiomyopathies in children. Curr Opin Pediatr 1995;7(5): 587–594.

Oakley CM. Myocarditis, pericarditis and other pericardial diseases. Heart 2000;84(4):449–454.

Author: Liudvikas Jagminas

Nasal Fractures

Clinical Presentation

SIGNS AND SYMPTOMS

- Nasal deformity, asymmetry, swelling, or ecchymosis
- Epistaxis: possibly due to septal or turbinate laceration
- Periorbital ecchymosis ("raccoon eyes") from damage to branches of ethmoidal artery, may indicate nasofrontoethmoid complex injury
- Palpable sharp edges, depressions, or other irregularities suggest nasal fracture
- Crepitus or mobility of skeletal parts on palpation indicates a fracture
- *Septal hematoma,* a bluish fluid-filled sac overlying the nasal septum; this is critical to detect because it must be drained expeditiously
- Flattening of the nasal root and widening of the inter canthal distance (telecanthus) is indicative of nasofrontoethmoid complex injury—a serious injury
- Clear rhinorrhea indicates possible CSF leak—rhinorrhea may be delayed in presentation
- Loss of sense of smell suggests significant injury
- Tear duct injuries may be present with abnormal tearing
- Associated eye injuries, including subconjunctival hemorrhage, hyphema, and retinal detachments, may be present

MECHANISM/DESCRIPTION

- Fractures of the nasal skeleton are the most common body fractures
- Most nasal fractures are the result of blunt trauma, frequently from motor vehicle crashes, sports injuries, and altercations
- Lateral forces are more likely to cause displacement than are straight-on blows
- History of trauma with significant force, loss of consciousness, or findings of facial bone injury, frontal bone crepitus, or CSF leak suggest associated injuries

PEDIATRIC CONSIDERATIONS

- Always consider nonaccidental trauma a potential mechanism of injury
- Fractures are rare in children; nasal injuries in children are more likely to be cartilaginous
- Significant injuries in children are not always fully appreciated

Pre-Hospital

CAUTIONS

- Management of the airway takes precedence
- Nasotracheal intubation is contraindicated
- Consider orotracheal intubation or cricothyroidotomy if definitive airway control is needed
- Cervical spine precautions are indicated if there is associated trauma
- Epistaxis can normally be controlled with direct pressure; pinch the nares together

Diagnosis

ESSENTIAL WORKUP

- Physical examination with visual inspection and palpation is most important
- It is critical to identify a *septal hematoma*
- Examine closely for telecanthus: intercanthal width greater than 30-35 mm or wider than the width of one eye may indicate a nasofrontoethmoid fracture and is usually associated with a depressed nasal bridge
- Evaluate the nasolacrimal duct for patency by instilling fluorescein into the eye and looking for fluorescein at the entrance of the lacrimal duct into the nasopharynx under the inferior turbinate (absence implying a duct injury)
- Eyelash "traction test" is simply done by grasping the eyelashes on one eyelid with one's fingers and pulling laterally; if the eyelid margin does not become taut or "bowstring," then the medial portion of the tendon has been disrupted—this test is performed on both the upper and lower eyelids because it is possible for only one portion of the tendon to be selectively injured

IMAGING/SPECIAL TESTS

- Nasal radiographs are rarely indicated because they normally do not alter the initial management
  —Patients with associated facial bone deformity, crepitus, or tenderness may require radiographs
- CT is the test of choice if facial bone fractures or depressed skull fractures are suspected and for diagnosis of nasofrontoethmoid injuries

DIFFERENTIAL DIAGNOSIS

- Nasal fractures may be associated with other facial injuries such as orbital, frontal sinus, maxillary sinus, or cribriform plate fractures, and these more serious injuries must be ruled out
- A nasofrontoethmoid fracture will have frontal crepitus and may have associated telecanthus, nasal bridge depression, or obstruction of the nasolacrimal duct

Treatment

INITIAL STABILIZATION

- Airway: orotracheal intubation or cricothyroidotomy; nasotracheal intubation is contraindicated
- Cervical spine precautions are indicated if there are associated injuries
- Other injuries take precedence; nasal injuries are not normally serious

ED TREATMENT

- Abrasions and lacerations—proper cleansing of facial wounds is essential; lacerations may be sutured
- Bleeding: usually stops spontaneously; packing may occasionally be required, using petroleum jelly gauze, or a nasal pack; posterior packing may be rarely required
- Displaced fractures do not need reduction in the ED unless airway compromise is present
  - —It is preferable to let the swelling go down and reduce the fracture in 3–5 days
- *Septal hematoma* must be drained immediately in the ED
  - —Anesthetize with topical cocaine or lidocaine and vascular constriction with neosynephrine
  - —Attempt to aspirate with an 18- to 20-gauge needle on a 3-mL syringe
  - —Rolling a cotton swab down the septum may facilitate the drainage
  - —Holding the mucosa down against the cartilage must be done to prevent reaccumulation of hematoma
  - —This can be done with petroleum jelly gauze packing
  - —Both nares should be packed to ensure adequate pressure; the packing is left in place for 3–5 days or until follow-up with ENT
  - —Prophylactic antibiotics are prescribed

MEDICATIONS

- Amoxicillin/clavulanate: 500 mg b.i.d. (peds: 40 mg/kg/day b.i.d.) *or*
- Cocaine: topical 4%
- Lidocaine: 1–2% without epinephrine
- Neosynephrine nasal spray
- Trimethoprim-sulfamethoxazole: DS b.i.d. (peds: 40 mg/kg/d sulfamethoxazole)

Disposition

ADMISSION CRITERIA

- Most nasal fractures do not require admission
- Admit patients with nasoethmoid fractures and those with more significant craniofacial injuries

DISCHARGE CRITERIA

- No evidence of significant head, neck, or other injuries
- Follow up with ENT, plastic surgery, or OMF surgeon in 3–5 days for fracture reduction or reevaluation
  - —Patients with septal hematoma should follow up in 24 hours for reevaluation after drainage
- Return for signs of clear rhinorrhea, difficulty breathing, fever, or signs associated with head injury

PEDIATRIC CONSIDERATIONS

- Follow up with specialist sooner because fibrous union begins in only 3–4 days
- Consider contacting Child Protective Services if any suspicion of abuse (i.e., history does not fit injury)

Miscellaneous

ICD9: 802.0

ICD10: S02.2

SUGGESTED READINGS

Cox AJ. Nasal fractures–the details. Facial Plast Surg 2001;16:87–94.

Druelinger L, Guenther M, Marchand EG. Radiographic evaluation of the facial complex. Emerg Med Clin North Am 2000;18:393–410.

Ellis E, Scott K. Assessment of patients with facial fractures. Emerg Med Clin North Am 2000;18:411–447.

Hegtvedt AK, Larsen PE. Isolated nasal fractures. Atlas Oral Maxillofac Surg Clin North Am 1994;2:1–18.

Fedok FG. Comprehensive management of naso-ethmoid—orbital injuries. J Craniomaxillofac Surg 1995;1(4):36–48.

Author: David Munter

Near Drowning

Clinical Presentation

SIGNS AND SYMPTOMS

- Cardiopulmonary arrest
- Cyanosis
- Dyspnea
- Copious pulmonary secretions
- Loss of consciousness
- Cerebral edema/injury
- Evidence of trauma
  —Cervical spine injury
- Hypothermia

Definitions

- Drowning
  —Death by suffocation after submersion in a liquid
  —Death within 24 hours of the accident
- Near drowning
  —Survival beyond 24 hours of submersion accident

Scenario of Drowning

- Unexpected submersion with struggle
- Aspiration of small amount of water
- Laryngospasm
- Hypoxia

Pathophysiology

- Aspiration
  —Small volume of water
  —No significant electrolyte changes
  —Grossly contaminated water: risk for pulmonary infection
- Hypoxemia
  —Metabolic lactic acidosis
  —Multisystem organ dysfunction
  —Myocardial dysfunction
  —Coagulation abnormalities (disseminated intravascular coagulation [DIC])
  —Renal failure
  —CNS dysfunction

Pediatric Considerations

- Hypothermia
  —More common in young children
  —Larger body surface-to-mass ratio
  —Decreases the metabolic rate
  —Survival with full recovery possible (record: 66 minutes)
- Diving reflex
  —Young children more susceptible
  —Potentiated by fear
  —Triggered by submersion of face in cold water
  —Bradycardia ensues: redistribution of blood flow to the heart and brain

Pre-Hospital

CAUTIONS

- Attention to ABCs
- Avoid further aspiration
- Apply cricoid pressure during bag-to-mask ventilation
- Secure airway—intubate
- Strict cervical spine precautions
- 90% survival with appropriate intervention

CONTROVERSIES

- Abdominal thrusts to remove water
  —Increases risk for aspiration
  —Useful if foreign body in airway

Diagnosis

ESSENTIAL WORKUP

- Information from witnesses or EMS personnel at the scene
- Rectal temperature for hypothermia

LABORATORY

- Arterial blood gas
- CBC
- Electrolytes, BUN, creatinine, glucose
  —Usually normal
  —Hyperkalemia
  —Hypernatremia or hyponatremia
- Alcohol and toxicology screen

IMAGING/SPECIAL TESTS

- Chest x-ray
  —Diffuse or focal infiltrates
  —May be normal initially
- Cervical spine series
- EKG
  —Long QT interval

DIFFERENTIAL DIAGNOSIS

- Consider reason for submersion
  —Dysrhythmia (long QT syndrome)
  —Myocardial infarction
  —Seizure
  —Syncope
  —Trauma

PEDIATRIC CONSIDERATIONS

- Consider child abuse/neglect
  —Especially infants in bathtub near drowning

Treatment

INITIAL STABILIZATION

- ABCs
- Remove wet clothing
- Core temperature
  —Initiate rewarming (see Hypothermia)

ED TREATMENT

- Correct hypoxemia
  —Titrate to oxygen saturation
  —Intubate and provide mechanical ventilation with positive end-expiratory pressure
- Evaluate and treat traumatic injuries
- Correct acidosis
  —Administer sodium bicarbonate if pH <7.1
- Cardiopulmonary arrest
  —Initiate advanced cardiac life support (ACLS) measures
  —Continue rewarming efforts
  —Continue resuscitation until core temperature >32°C, or until spontaneous pulse and respirations return
- Importance of admission
  —Delayed pulmonary edema (12 hours later)
  —Delayed neurologic abnormalities

MEDICATIONS (PER ACLS PROTOCOLS)

- Atropine: 1 mg (peds: 0.02 mg/kg) i.v.
- Epinephrine: 1 mg (peds: 0.01 mg/kg) i.v.
- Lidocaine: 1 mg/kg i.v.
- Sodium bicarbonate: 1 mEq/kg i.v.

PEDIATRIC CONSIDERATIONS

- Hypothermia may be protective
  —Aggressive rewarming
  —Aggressive resuscitation
- Evaluate for child abuse/neglect
  —Social service consult
- Prevention is key to treatment
  —Supervision around water
  —Empty pails and buckets
- Family history: sudden death, similar episode
  —Long QT syndrome

Disposition

ADMISSION CRITERIA

- ICU
  —Patients who required CPR or artificial ventilation
  —Abnormal chest radiograph
  —Arterial blood gas abnormalities
  —Glascow coma scale (GSC) <13
- Admit observation status
  —Submersion for >1 minute
  —History of cyanosis or apnea
  —Patients who required brief assisted ventilation
  —GCS ≥13

DISCHARGE CRITERIA

- Questionable history of submersion
  —Observe in ED for 6–8 hours
  —No respiratory distress
  —No neurologic improvement
- Discharge to reliable home
- Home-going instructions
  —Return for shortness of breath or mental status changes

Miscellaneous

ICD9: 994.1

ICD10: W74

SUGGESTED READINGS

Ackerman MJ, Tester DJ, Porter CJ. Swimming, a gene-specific arrhythmogenic trigger for inherited long QT syndrome. Mayo Clin Proc 1999;74:1088–1094.

Causey AL, Tilelli JA, Swanson ME. Predicting discharge in uncomplicated near-drowning. Am J Emerg Med 2000;18:9–11.

Lavelle JM, Shaw KN, Seidl T, et al. Ten-year review of pediatric bathtub near-drowning: evaluation for child abuse and neglect. Ann Emerg Med 1995;25: 344–348.

Sachdeva RC. Near drowning. Crit Care Clin 1999;15(2):281–296.

Zuckerman GB, Gregory PM, Santos-Damiant SM. Predictors of death and neurologic impairment in pediatric submersion injuries. Arch Pediatr Adolesc Med 1998;152:134–140.

Author: Janet Poponick

Neck Injury by Hanging/Strangulation

Clinical Presentation

SIGNS AND SYMPTOMS

Airway Disruption

- Neck ecchymosis or emphysema, dyspnea, dysphonia, stridor, loss of normal cartilaginous landmarks

Neurologic Injury

- Hoarseness, dysphagia, decreased level of consciousness, neurologic deficit

Vascular Injuries

- Expanding hematoma, pulse deficits, bruits, evidence of cerebral infarction, petechiae (on mucosa, skin, eyes)

Cervical Spine Injury

- Respiratory arrest, paralysis

MECHANISM/DESCRIPTION

Strangulation

- Ligature: material used to compress structures of the neck
- Manual: use of physical force to compress structures of neck
- Postural: airway obstruction from body weight (over an object) or position (typically in infants)

Hanging

- Complete: the victim's feet are suspended off the ground
- Incomplete: any position when feet are not freely suspended
  - —Typical: point of suspension placed centrally over the occiput
  - —Atypical: point of suspension not centrally placed over the occiput

Death

- Secondary to direct neurologic injury
- Secondary to mechanical constriction of the neck (arteriovenous compromise or airway compression)
- Secondary to cardiac arrest

ETIOLOGY

Strangulation or Hanging

- Suicide, homicide, accidental
  - —Neck pressure results in venous obstruction causing cerebral hypoxia and then death
  - —Pressure on neck structures may cause airway, soft tissue, and vascular injuries
  - —Rarely may cause upper cervical spine injuries
- Judicial
  - —The victim is dropped a distance equal to his or her height
  - —Forceful distraction of the head from the torso results in a decapitation type of injury (fracture of cervical spine and transection of spinal cord)

Pre-Hospital

CAUTIONS

- Early and aggressive airway management: oxygen, suction, intubation
- Cervical spine stabilization

Diagnosis

ESSENTIAL WORKUP

- Plain radiography
  - —Cervical spine to evaluate for bony injuries as well as soft-tissue swelling and subcutaneous emphysema
  - —Chest to evaluate for subcutaneous emphysema as well as aspiration pneumonitis

LABORATORY

- Pulse oximetry
- ABG: evaluate for evidence of hypoxia or respiratory compromise as indicated
- Hematocrit: check for evidence of significant blood loss
- Type and cross: prepare for transfusion as required if there is vascular disruption

IMAGING/SPECIAL TESTS

- Fiberoptic endoscopy: allows direct visualization for evaluation of endolaryngeal injury; may aid in intubation
- Arteriography: definitive evaluation for potential vascular injuries
- CT scan of the neck: further defines soft-tissue injuries
- Carotid duplex imaging with flow studies
- Surgical exploration

DIFFERENTIAL DIAGNOSIS

Associated Injuries

- Larynx fracture
- Hyoid fracture: most commonly seen in manual strangulation
- Thyroid cartilage disruption
  - —Most commonly an anterior vertical fracture from thyroid cartilage notch to cricothyroid membrane
- Vascular disruption: arterial or venous
- Phrenic nerve injury
- Cervical spine injury
- Hypoxic cerebral injury
- Airway edema
- Aspiration pneumonitis (may be late manifestation)
- Neurogenic pulmonary edema (may be late manifestation)
- Air embolism
  - —Consider when subcutaneous air and vascular injuries are present

PEDIATRIC CONSIDERATIONS

- Structures of the neck are more cartilaginous and mobile than in adults; thus, pediatric patients are more resistant to crush and fracture injuries; however, due to the smaller airway diameter, rapid airway compromise can occur with relatively little edema of the soft tissues

Treatment

INITIAL STABILIZATION

- Early and aggressive airway management with cervical spine precautions is paramount
  - —Early intubation to preclude respiratory compromise
  - —Severe injuries of the larynx may require operative management
- Patient may require emergent tracheostomy
- Cricothyrotomy if severe maxillofacial injuries are present
  - —*Avoid* cricothyrotomy if a hematoma is seen over cricothyroid membrane or evidence of cricotracheal disruption; arrange for emergent tracheostomy (see Larynx Fracture).
- Supplemental humidified oxygen
- Control bleeding with application of direct pressure; do *not* explore in the ED

ED TREATMENT

- IV access
- Consult otolaryngologist in the management of neck soft-tissue injuries
- Elevate head of bed to decrease cerebral edema
- Consider ICP monitoring if evidence of severe hypoxic cerebral injury

MEDICATIONS

Hypoxic Brain Injury

- Mannitol: 0.25–1 g/kg i.v. (for cerebral edema)
- Phenytoin: 15 mg/kg i.v.

Neck Injury with Subcutaneous Emphysema

- Assume that the mucosa of the upper airway communicates with the deep tissues of the neck and administer antibiotics
  - —Ampicillin/sulbactam: 3 g (peds: 100–400 mg/kg/24 h) i.v. q6h
  - —Clindamycin: 600 mg (peds: 25–40 mg/kg/24 h) i.v. q8h

Laryngeal Edema

- Steroids may be useful
  - —Dexamethasone: 4 mg (peds: 0.25–0.5 mg/kg q6h) i.v. q6h

Disposition

ADMISSION CRITERIA

- All patients with strangulation or hanging mechanism injuries must be admitted to a monitored setting to observe for airway compromise (may have delayed onset)
- Prepare for emergent surgical correction of laryngeal injuries
- Initial neurologic status not predictive of outcome

DISCHARGE CRITERIA

- Only patients proven not to have strangulation or hanging injuries may be discharged after appropriate observation in the ED for the development of any airway compromise or mental status changes
- All patients with suspected suicidal or homicidal strangulation injury should have psychiatric or social work consultation

Miscellaneous

ICD9: 959.09

ICD10: W84

SEE ALSO: LARYNX FRACTURE

SUGGESTED READINGS

Iserson KV. Strangulation: a review of ligature, manual and postural neck compression injuries. Ann Emerg Med 1984;13:179–185.

Kaki A, Crosby ET, Lui AC. Airway and respiratory management following non-lethal hanging. Can J Anesth 1997;44:445–450.

McClane GE, Strack GB, Hawley D. A review of 300 attempted strangulation cases, part II: clinical evaluation of the surviving victim. J Emerg Med 2001;21:311–315.

Sabo RA, Hanigan WC, Flessner K, et al. Strangulation injuries in children, part I: clinical analysis. J Trauma 1996;40:68–72.

Authors: Timothy R. Hurtado; David Della-Giustina

Neck Trauma, Blunt, Anterior

Clinical Presentation

SIGNS AND SYMPTOMS

- The presentation of blunt anterior neck trauma varies depending on the mechanism of injury and the structures involved
- Vascular injury
  - —Hemorrhage, ecchymosis, edema
  - —Loss of character of lateral neck profile
  - —Carotid bruit
  - —Neurologic deficits (often delayed)
- Laryngotracheal injury
  - —Voice changes, hoarseness, aphonia
  - —Dyspnea, inspiratory stridor, labored breathing
  - —Subcutaneous emphysema, tenderness to palpation
- Pharyngoesophageal injury
  - —Dysphagia, odynophagia, hematemesis
  - —Tenderness to palpation
  - —Infection, sepsis (delayed presentation)
- Neurologic injury
  - —Central or peripheral nervous system deficits

MECHANISM/DESCRIPTION

- Many injuries may result from blunt anterior neck trauma
  - —Fracture of the thyroid cartilage, vocal cord disruption, or dislocation of airway cartilages
  - —Hematoma of the larynx or trachea, or complete tracheal transection at the junction with the cricoid cartilage
  - —Pharyngoesophageal injury results from hematoma or perforation of the pharynx or esophagus and usually occurs in conjunction with laryngotracheal injury
  - —Presentation is often delayed; injury may be detected only when infection develops
  - —Vascular injuries involving the carotid artery include intramural hematoma, intimal tear, thrombosis, and pseudoaneurysm
  - —Injury may result in ischemic or thromboembolic events
  - —Nervous system injury includes damage to the recurrent laryngeal nerve or injury to the stellate ganglion resulting in *Horner's syndrome*
  - —Cervical spine injury may occur with blunt neck injury

ETIOLOGY

- Motor vehicle accidents
  - —Unrestrained occupants involved in frontal collisions may strike neck on the dashboard or steering wheel
  - —The shoulder harness can also cause shearing injury to the anterior neck
- Assault
  - —Blows from fists, weapons, or other objects to the anterior neck
- "Clothesline injury" is seen when motorcycle, snowmobile, or all-terrain vehicle drivers strike neck on a cord or wire suspended between two objects

PEDIATRIC CONSIDERATIONS

- The head is proportionally larger in children, increasing the risk of acceleration-deceleration injury to the neck

Pre-Hospital

- The airway must be vigilantly monitored, as edema or expanding hematoma can progress to airway compromise
- Early oral intubation is indicated for clinical signs of respiratory distress such as stridor, air hunger, or labored breathing, or if an expanding neck hematoma is present

CAUTIONS

Cervical Spine Stabilization

- Blind nasotracheal intubation should be avoided because of potential rupture of an expanding hematoma and is difficult to perform because of distortion of anatomy

Diagnosis

ESSENTIAL WORKUP
- Inspection of the neck for distortion of anatomy, auscultation for carotid bruits, and palpation to detect tenderness or subcutaneous emphysema
- A neurologic exam should be performed to detect evidence of an ischemic event, spinal cord injury, or peripheral nerve damage
- Cervical spine radiographs
- CXR to rule out associated injury to the thorax

LABORATORY
- Type and cross-match
- Baseline CBC and chemistry panel

IMAGING/SPECIAL TESTS
- Carotid duplex US is a noninvasive, rapid screening test for arterial injury
  - —CT may be used in the stable patient to evaluate laryngotracheal injury and delineate cartilage disruption
- Angiography
  - —Considered the gold standard to evaluate arterial injury
  - —Indicated in the presence of a carotid bruit, large hematoma, CVA with normal head CT scan result or suspected occult vascular injury
- Endoscopy to detect internal soft-tissue defects in the larynx and trachea
- Esophagram or rigid esophagoscopy to rule out pharyngoesophageal injury when odynophagia, hematemesis, or subcutaneous emphysema are present

DIFFERENTIAL DIAGNOSIS
- Vascular injury
- Laryngotracheal injury
- Pharyngoesophageal injury
- PNS or CNS injury
- Cervical spine injury
- Associated head or thoracic trauma

Treatment

INITIAL STABILIZATION

Airway Management with C-spine Control
- Immediate intubation indicated for patients with signs of airway compromise
  - —Orotracheal intubation is the method of choice
- Cricothyroidotomy may be needed if oral intubation fails
- Emergency tracheostomy is preferred in blunt upper airway trauma because cricothyroidotomy may worsen an injury below the level of the cricoid
- Care should be taken to avoid puncturing a neck hematoma during invasive procedures
- Bleeding into the pharynx can be tamponaded by packing the throat with heavy gauze after the airway is secured by intubation
- Unstable patients should go directly to the OR

ED TREATMENT
- Surgical consultation should be obtained for patients with recurrent symptoms, angiographic evidence of vascular injury, or suspected tracheal or esophageal injury
- Once the airway is secured, laryngeal injuries do not require immediate surgical repair
  - —The patient should be placed on voice rest and humidified air and be given prophylactic antibiotics
- Tracheal injury requires prompt surgical repair
- Extensive pharyngeal lacerations and esophageal injuries require immediate surgical repair
- Asymptomatic patients with arterial injury may be observed and do well without intervention
  - —Surgery is indicated for patients with recurrent symptoms or angiographic progression of disease

MEDICATIONS
- *Prophylactic antibiotics* recommended in the presence of laryngotracheal or pharyngoesophageal injury
- Cefoxitin: 2 g i.v. q8h (peds: 80–160 mg/kg/d i.m./i.v. q6h) *or*
- Clindamycin: 600–900 mg i.v. q8h (peds: 25–40 mg/kg/d i.v. q6–8h) *or*
- Penicillin G: 24 million IU/d q4–6h (peds: 150,000–250,000 IU/kg/d q4–6h) *plus*
- Metronidazole: 1 g load then 500 mg i.v. q6h (peds: 30 mg/kg/d i.v. q12h)

Disposition

ADMISSION CRITERIA
- Patients who are symptomatic, have abnormal studies, or significant blunt trauma mechanism must be admitted and observed for at least 24 hours
- Patients with suspicion of airway or vascular injury must be admitted to the ICU

DISCHARGE CRITERIA
- Only patients with the most trivial injuries who have negative studies may be discharged from the ED after thorough evaluation

Miscellaneous

ICD9: 959.09

ICD10: S19.8

SUGGESTED READINGS

Fuhrman GM, Stieg FH, Buerk CA. Blunt laryngeal trauma. J Trauma 1990;30:87.

Jorden RC. Neck trauma. In: Rosen P, et al. eds. Emergency medicine: concepts and clinical practice, 4th ed. St. Louis: CV Mosby, 1998:505–513.

Sweeney TA, Marx JA. Blunt neck injury. Emerg Med Clin North Am 1993;11(1):71–79.

Author: Tamaki Kimbro

Neck Trauma, Penetrating, Anterior

Clinical Presentation

SIGNS AND SYMPTOMS

- Vary depending on the specific structures injured
- Vascular injury
  —Active hemorrhage or hematoma
  —Tracheal deviation, loss of normal anatomic landmarks
  —Pulse deficits in upper extremities
  —Thrills or bruits in neck
- Laryngotracheal injury
  —Respiratory distress
  —Hoarseness, voice changes
  —Hemoptysis
  —Neck pain or tenderness
  —Crepitance
- Pharyngoesophageal injury
  —Dysphagia
  —Odynophagia
  —Hematemesis
- Neurologic injury
  —CNS or PNS deficits

MECHANISM/DESCRIPTION

- Penetrating neck trauma is defined as a wound that penetrates the platysma muscle
- The neck is divided into *three zones* based on superficial landmarks
  —Zone I lies below the cricoid cartilage
    -Penetrating trauma in this zone carries the highest mortality due to injury to thoracic structures
  —Zone II lies between the cricoid cartilage and angle of the mandible
    -Most penetrating neck wounds occur in this zone
    -Zone II wounds have a lower mortality because hemorrhage can be controlled with direct pressure and structures are easily accessible for surgical exploration
  —Zone III lies above the angle of the mandible

ETIOLOGY

- Gunshot wounds
- Stab wounds
- Miscellaneous (glass shards, metal fragments, animal bites)

PEDIATRIC CONSIDERATIONS

- In the pediatric patient, the larynx is located higher in the neck and receives better protection from the mandible and hyoid bone

Pre-Hospital

- Frequent suctioning to clear airway of blood, secretions, or vomitus
- Lateral decubitus or prone positioning may be required to prevent aspiration
- The airway must be vigilantly monitored as edema or expanding hematoma can progress to airway compromise
- Early oral intubation is indicated for clinical signs of respiratory distress, such as stridor, air hunger, or labored breathing, or if an expanding neck hematoma is present

CAUTIONS

- Nasotracheal intubation should be avoided because of potential rupture of an expanding hematoma and is difficult to perform because of distortion of anatomy
- Occlusive dressings should be applied to lacerations over major veins to prevent air embolism

Diagnosis

ESSENTIAL WORKUP

- Careful examination of the wound to determine the extent of injury and if it penetrates the platysma
  —Wounds should never be blindly probed, as this may result in uncontrolled hemorrhage
- Lateral neck radiograph to evaluate soft-tissue injury and detect foreign bodies
- CXR to detect hemopneumothorax, mediastinal air, or bleeding that extends into the upper mediastinum

LABORATORY

- Type and cross-match
- Baseline CBC and chemistry panel

IMAGING/SPECIAL TESTS

- Angiography
  —Considered the gold standard to evaluate arterial injury
  —Indicated for penetrating wounds in zone I or zone III
- Color duplex US is a noninvasive, rapid screening test for arterial injury
- Bronchoscopy can be helpful to evaluate tracheal injury but may increase airway edema and is difficult in patients with respiratory distress
- Esophagram with Gastrografin or dilute barium
  —Low sensitivity
  —Combine with esophagoscopy to exclude injury
  —Indications
    -Wound approaches/crosses midline
    -Subcutaneous air

DIFFERENTIAL DIAGNOSIS

- Vascular injury
- Pharyngoesophageal injury
- Laryngotracheal injury
- PNS or CNS injury
- Cervical spine injury
- Associated head or thoracic trauma

Treatment

INITIAL STABILIZATION

Airway Management with Cervical Spine Control

- Patients who are comatose or in respiratory distress require immediate intubation
- Stable patients without evidence of respiratory distress may be aggressively managed with prophylactic intubation or closely observed with airway equipment at the bedside
- Orotracheal intubation with rapid-sequence induction or sedation is the method of choice for securing the airway in penetrating neck trauma
- Blind nasotracheal intubation is contraindicated with apnea, severe facial injury, or airway distortion because of the risk of puncturing an expanding hematoma
- Endoscopic intubation is contraindicated with active bleeding that may obscure the scope
- Percutaneous transtracheal ventilation may be useful when oral or nasotracheal intubation fails
  —Leaves the airway unprotected and is contraindicated in cases of upper airway obstruction, as it may cause barotrauma
  —Cricothyroidotomy, tracheostomy, or intubation via a penetrating wound may be required in cases of severe facial injury, laryngotracheal injury, or uncontrolled upper airway hemorrhage

Breathing

- Zone I injury can cause pneumothorax or subclavian vein injury and hemothorax, requiring needle decompression and tube thoracostomy

Circulation

- External hemorrhage should be controlled with direct pressure; blind clamping of vessels is contraindicated because of the risk of further neurovascular injury
- Patients with uncontrollable bleeding or hemodynamic instability must go directly to the OR
- After intubation, the throat can be packed with heavy gauze to tamponade the bleeding
- Tube thoracostomy for bleeding into the chest

ED TREATMENT

- NGT should not be placed because of risk of rupturing a pharyngeal hematoma
- Prophylactic antibiotics are recommended (cefoxitin, clindamycin, penicillin G plus metronidazole)
- Surgical consult for all wounds that penetrate the platysma muscle
- Controversy exists in mandatory versus selective surgical exploration in stable patients
  —Mandatory approach
    -Surgical exploration is indicated in all cases of penetrating neck trauma because significant injury may not manifest outward signs or symptoms
  —Selective approach
    -Surgical exploration for specific indications including expanding or pulsatile hematoma, active bleeding, absence of peripheral pulses, hemoptysis, Horner's syndrome, bruit, subcutaneous emphysema, respiratory distress, or air bubbling through a wound
- Tetanus prophylaxis

MEDICATIONS

- Cefoxitin: 2 g i.v. q8h (peds: 80–160 mg/kg/d i.m./i.v. q6h) *or*
- Clindamycin: 600–900 mg i.v. q8h (peds: 25–40 mg/kg/d i.v. q6–8h) *or*
- Penicillin G: 24 million IU/d q4–6h (peds: 150,000–250,000 IU/kg/d q4–6h) *plus*
- Metronidazole: 1 g load then 500 mg i.v. q6h (peds: 30 mg/kg/d i.v. q12h)

Disposition

ADMISSION CRITERIA

- All patients with penetrating neck trauma should be admitted and observed for at least 24 hours
- Observation must take place in a facility capable of providing definitive surgical care
- Patients with injuries suggestive of airway or vascular injury must be admitted to the ICU

DISCHARGE CRITERIA

- Asymptomatic patients who have negative studies may be discharged after at least 24 hours of observation

Miscellaneous

ICD9: 959.09

ICD10: S19.8

SUGGESTED READINGS

Carducci B, Lowe RA, Dalsey W. Penetrating neck trauma: consensus and controversies. Ann Emerg Med 1986;15:208.

Jorden RC. Neck trauma. In: Rosen P, et al. eds. Emergency medicine: concepts and clinical practice, 4th ed. St. Louis: CV Mosby, 1998:505–513.

Kendall JL, Anglin D, Demetriades D. Penetrating neck trauma. Emerg Med Clin North Am 1998;16(1):85–105.

Rathlev NK. Penetrating neck trauma: mandatory versus selective exploration. J Emerg Med 1990;8(1):75–78.

Roon AJ, Christensen N. Evaluation and treatment of penetrating cervical injuries. J Trauma 1979;19:391.

Author: Tamaki Kimbro

Necrotizing Soft Tissue Infections

Clinical Presentation

SIGNS AND SYMPTOMS

- Rapid progression of pain and swelling of involved area
- Pain out of proportion to physical findings
- In first 24 hours, rapid development of local swelling, heat, erythema, and tenderness
- 24–48 hours: purple and blue discoloration, blisters and bullae develop (often hemorrhagic)
- Necrosis of fascia and fat produces a watery, thin, foul-smelling fluid
- Systemic toxicity with fever, tachycardia, and depressed mentation

MECHANISM/DESCRIPTION

- Necrotizing soft-tissue infections are usually caused by toxin-producing, virulent bacteria, characterized by widespread fascial and muscle necrosis with relative sparing of the skin
- Crepitant anaerobic cellulitis: necrotic soft-tissue infection with abundant connective tissue gas
- Progressive bacterial gangrene: slowly progressive erosion affecting the total thickness of skin but not involving deep fascia
- Nonclostridial myonecrosis (synergistic necrotizing cellulitis): aggressive soft-tissue infection of skin, muscle, subcutaneous tissue and fascia
- *Necrotizing fasciitis:* a progressive, rapidly spreading infection with extensive dissection and necrosis of the superficial and deep fascia
- Fournier's gangrene: a mixed aerobic-anaerobic soft-tissue necrotizing fasciitis of the skin of the scrotum and penis in men and the vulvar and perianal skin in women

ETIOLOGY

- Conditions that lead to the development of necrotizing soft-tissue infections
  - —Local tissue trauma with bacterial invasion
  - —Local ischemia and reduced host defenses: more frequently in diabetics, alcoholics, immunosuppressed patients, IV drug users, and patients with peripheral vascular disease
- Polymicrobial etiology including
  - —Group A β-hemolytic streptococcus (GABHS); group B streptococcus, staphylococci, enterococci, bacillus, pseudomonads, *Enterobacter, Bacteroides,* clostridia, and *Vibrio* species
- Possible relationship between the use of NSAIDs and severe invasive GABHS infections has been suggested

PEDIATRIC CONSIDERATIONS

- Neonates: omphalitis and circumcision are predisposing factors
- Children: surgery, trauma, varicella, and congenital and acquired immunodeficiencies are major factors for the development of necrotizing fasciitis; GABHS necrotizing fasciitis as a complication of varicella has been reported

Pre-Hospital

N/A

Diagnosis

ESSENTIAL WORKUP

- Diagnosis can be difficult
- Careful examination for the aforementioned signs and symptoms in high-risk patients
- Necrotizing soft-tissue infections must be suspected in patients who appear very ill and have pain out of proportion to physical findings
- Diagnosis requires incision and probing of tissue

LABORATORY

- CBC with differential, electrolytes, BUN, and creatinine, DIC panel
- Calcium level: hypocalcemia can develop from extensive fat necrosis
- Gram stain and aerobic/anaerobic cultures of wound or tissue biopsy

IMAGING/SPECIAL TESTS

- X-rays to detect soft-tissue gas
- CT scan to delineate extent of spread of the infection

DIFFERENTIAL DIAGNOSIS

- Cellulitis
- Gas gangrene

Treatment

INITIAL STABILIZATION

- ABCs
  - —Control airway as needed
  - —Supplemental oxygen, monitor, evaluate for acid-base disturbances
  - -IV access, CVP line may be needed
  - —Aggressive volume expansion including crystalloid, plasma, packed RBCs, and albumin

ED TREATMENT

- Antibiotics: broad coverage of aerobic gram-positive and gram-negative organisms and anaerobes
  - —Penicillin or cephalosporin, an aminoglycoside, and anaerobic coverage with either clindamycin or metronidazole
  - —Penicillin G if strep or clostridia
  - —Imipenem cilastatin or meropenem if polymicrobial
- Surgical consultation
  - —*Early débridement* of all necrotic tissue with fasciotomy and drainage of fascial planes is paramount
- Hyperbaric oxygen as an adjunct
  - —Early transfer to hyperbaric facility may result in greater tissue salvage
- Observe for major complications including ARDS, renal failure, myocardial irritability, and DIC

MEDICATIONS

- Ceftriaxone: 2 g (peds: 100 mg/kg/24 h; maximum, 4 g) i.v. q24h
- Clindamycin: 900 mg (peds: 40 mg/kg/d q6h) i.v. q8h
- Gentamicin: 2.0 mg/kg (peds: 2.0 mg/kg i.v. q8h) i.v. q8h
- Imipenem-cilastatin: 250–1,000 mg i.v. q6–8h
- Meropenem 1 g (peds: 20–40 mg/kg up to 2 g/dose) i.v. q8h
- Metronidazole: 500 mg (peds: safety not established) i.v. q8h
- Penicillin G: 24 million IU/24 h (peds: 250,000 IU/kg/24 h) i.v. q4–6h

Disposition

ADMISSION CRITERIA

- All patients with a necrotizing soft-tissue infection *must be admitted* for surgical débridement and IV antibiotics; early hyperbaric oxygen therapy is an important adjunct

DISCHARGE CRITERIA

N/A

Miscellaneous

ICD9: 709.8

SUGGESTED READINGS

American Academy of Pediatrics. Committee on Infectious Diseases. Severe invasive group A streptococcal infections: a subject review. Pediatrics 1998;101[Suppl 1; Pt 1):136–140.

Barton LL, Jeck DT, Vaidya VU. Necrotizing fasciitis in children: report of two cases and review of the literature. Arch Pediatr Adolesc Med 1996;150(1):105–108.

Clark LA, Moon RE. Hyperbaric oxygen in the treatment of life-threatening soft-tissue infection. Respir Care Clin North Am 1999;5(2):203–219.

Fontes RA Jr, Oglivie CM, Miclau T. Necrotizing soft-tissue infection. J Am Acad Orthop Surg 2000;8(3):151–158.

Author: Karen Van Hoesen

Needle Stick

Clinical Presentation

SIGNS AND SYMPTOMS

- History of exposure to blood or body fluid
- Mechanisms of exposure
  - —Percutaneous
  - —Mucous membrane
  - —Skin

MECHANISM/DESCRIPTION

- Risk of seroconversion from a single needle-stick exposure without prior immunization
  - —Hepatitis B virus (HBV): 37–62% from HB_sAg-positive and HB_eAg-positive source, 23–37% from HB_sAg-positive and HB_eAg-negative source
  - —Hepatitis C virus (HCV): 2.7–10%
  - —HIV: 0.3%
- Since June 2000, the CDC has received 56 voluntary reports of documented HIV seroconversions in health care workers, with an additional 138 possible occupational infections

ETIOLOGY

- How infectious are various body fluids for HIV?
  - —10–5,000 ppm: plasma/serum
  - —10–1,000 ppm: CSF
  - —10–50 ppm: semen
  - —<1: vaginal secretions, urine, saliva, tears, breast milk
- Factors affecting risk
  - —Viral load, actual injection volume, type and size of needle, portal of entry (depth of inoculation), duration of contact, level of disease in source patient, host susceptibility, barriers (e.g., through gloves)

Pre-Hospital

CAUTIONS

- Pre-hospital personnel should always maintain universal precautions to prevent needle-stick or other body fluid exposure
- Patients with exposure should be evaluated for prophylactic therapy

Diagnosis

ESSENTIAL WORKUP

- Direct and immediate referral from ED triage to occupational health office when available to ensure strictest confidentiality in laboratory testing and treatment
- In the ED after hours, patients with needle-stick exposure must be triaged with high priority, as time is important in the initiation of prophylactic therapy
- Female recipients of body fluid exposure that are considering antiviral therapy must have serum or urine pregnancy testing
- Immunization history

LABORATORY

- To be done with occupational health if possible
  - —Baseline serology for HIV (enzyme immunoassay, Western blot), HBV, HCV
  - —Assess adequacy of HBV vaccination
  - —Obtain consent from source patient for HIV, HBV, HCV testing

IMAGING/SPECIAL TESTS

- Not applicable unless concerned for retained tissue foreign body

DIFFERENTIAL DIAGNOSIS

- Principally concerned with transmission of HBV, HCV, and HIV

Treatment

INITIAL STABILIZATION

- Copious cleaning, wound care
- Direct and immediate referral to occupational health when available to ensure strictest confidentiality in laboratory testing and treatment

ED TREATMENT

- Tetanus prophylaxis if necessary
- If referral to occupational health unavailable, initiate prophylactic therapy in ED
- HIV
  —Antiretroviral prophylaxis with multidrug regimen: zidovudine/lamivudine (Combivir), loprinavir/ritonavir (Kaletra), nevirapine after consideration of risks and benefit
  —Safer sex advice
  —Counseling
- HBV
  —Known HB_sAg-positive source
    -Complete vaccination confirmed by titer: no Rx
    -Incomplete vaccination: HBV vaccine booster
    -Unvaccinated: hepatitis B immune globulin (HBIG) ASAP, begin HBV vaccine series
    -Nonresponder to vaccine: HBIG ASAP, repeat in 30 days; consider revaccination with three-dose series
    -Unknown responder to vaccine with inadequate titer: HBIG ASAP, vaccine booster
  —Known HB_sAg-negative source
    -Vaccinated: no Rx
    -Unvaccinated: HBV vaccine series
  —Unknown source
    -Complete vaccination confirmed by titer: no Rx
    -Incomplete vaccination: HBV vaccine booster
    -Unvaccinated: begin vaccine series
    -Nonresponder to vaccine: HBIG ASAP with revaccination three-dose series, repeat HBIG in 30 days if high-risk exposure
    -Unknown responder to vaccine with inadequate titer: vaccine booster and recheck titer
- HCV
  —Use of immunoglobulins or antivirals (interferon, ribavirin) inconclusive

MEDICATIONS

- Combivir: 1 tab PO b.i.d. × 28 days
- Kaletra: 3 caps PO b.i.d. × 28 days
- Nevirapine: two 200 mg tabs single dose
  —Preferably initiated 1–2 hours postexposure
- Side effects
  —Kaletra: pancreatitis, neutropenia, hepatotoxicity, exfoliative dermatitis
  —Lamivudine: GI sx, headache, fatigue, neuropathy, congestion, cough (caution with trimethoprim-sulfamethoxazole)
  —Nevirapine: Stevens-Johnson syndrome, hepatotoxicity, neutropenia, thrombocytopenia, peripheral neuropathy
  —Protease inhibitors: diabetes
  —Zidovudine: GI symptoms, headache, fatigue, myalgias, marrow suppression, seizure

Hepatitis

- HBIG: 0.06 mL/kg i.m.
- HBV booster: unit-dose vial

Disposition

ADMISSION CRITERIA

- Isolated needle-stick or body fluid exposures need not be admitted

DISCHARGE CRITERIA

- Patients can be managed as outpatients with appropriate follow-up in occupational medicine clinic

Miscellaneous

Prevention

- Universal precautions
- Avoid recapping of needles
- Wear gloves: decreases amount of blood exposure by 50%
- Consider double gloving
- Follow body substance isolation protocols
- HBV vaccination

ICD9: 998.2

ICD10: T75.8

SUGGESTED READINGS

Beltrami EM, Williams IT, Shapiro CN, et al. Risk and management of blood-borne infections in health care workers. Clin Microbiol Rev 2000;13(3):385–407.

Centers for Disease Control and Prevention. Updated U.S. Public Health Service Guidelines for Management of Occupational Exposures to HBV, HCV, and HIV and Recommendations for Postexposure Prophylaxis. MMWR Morb Mortal Wkly Rep 2001;50(RR11):1–42.

Henderson, DK. Risk for exposures to and infection with HIV among health care providers in the emergency department. Emerg Med Clin North Am 1995;13(1):199–211.

Lutwick L. Postexposure prophylaxis. Infect Dis Clin North Am 1996;10(4):899–915.

Author: Gordon Chew

Neonatal Jaundice

Clinical Presentation

SIGNS AND SYMPTOMS

- Yellowish discoloration of skin, tissues such as sclerae, and body fluids in the newborn infant
  - —Indicates an elevated serum bilirubin level
- Increasing levels of bilirubin affect skin color progressing from the face downward
  - —Blanch skin with digital pressure to reveal underlying skin color to correlate level
  - —Face—bilirubin levels >6–8 mg/dL
  - —Feet—bilirubin levels >12–15 mg/dL
- Physical exam clues to some etiologies
  - —Sepsis: lethargy, temperature instability, poor feeding, vomiting, apnea or tachypnea
  - —Hemolytic disease: pallor, hepatoplenomegaly
  - —Extravascular hemolysis: birth trauma associated with cephalohematoma or bruising
  - —Polycythemia: ruddy complexion
  - —Cholestatic jaundice: persistent jaundice for >3 weeks, dark urine or light-colored stools

MECHANISM/DESCRIPTION

- Results from a transient imbalance between rates of bilirubin production and bilirubin elimination
  - —Newborns have higher rates of bilirubin production than adults because of increased RBC mass and shorter RBC life span
  - —Newborns, especially preterm infants, have rate limitations in hepatic conjugation and biliary excretion of bilirubin, increased enterohepatic circulation, and diminished bilirubin binding to albumin- and bilirubin-binding protein
- In the vast majority of newborns, this represents *physiologic jaundice* and is not pathologic
  - —Bilirubin normally increases from 1.5 mg/dL in cord blood to a mean of 6.5 mg/dL on day 3, followed by a gradual decline to normal adult levels of 1.5 mg/dL by day 10 or 12 of life
- However, serum bilirubin levels may rise to dangerous levels requiring therapy; hyperbilirubinemia may be caused by *pathologic conditions*
- Neurotoxic effects of hyperbilirubinemia are seen more commonly with hemolytic disease, less commonly in healthy newborns
  - —*Kernicterus,* or bilirubin encephalopathy, is caused by bilirubin toxicity to the basal ganglia and brainstem nuclei resulting in significant mortality; survivors may have serious neurologic consequences including cerebral palsy and hearing loss
- Risk factors for prolonged or elevated neonatal jaundice
  - —Hemolytic disease
  - —Gestation 35–38 weeks
  - —Low birth weight
  - —Large weight loss after birth
  - —Breast-feeding
  - —Ethnicity: Asian, Native American, Greek Islander
  - —Siblings with hyperbilirubinemia
  - —Family history of G6PD deficiency or hereditary spherocytosis
  - —Maternal diabetes
  - —Perinatal factors: polycythemia, birth trauma, infection

ETIOLOGY

Unconjugated Hyperbilirubinemia

- Physiologic jaundice
- Jaundice in breast-fed infants
  - —*Breast-feeding jaundice*—exaggeration of physiologic jaundice due to inadequate ingestion of breast milk in the first week of life; prolongation up to 8 weeks may be due to factors in breast milk that inhibit hepatic conjugation of bilirubin
- Specific hemolytic conditions
  - —Blood group isoimmunization due to ABO, Rh, and minor blood group incompatibility; ABO is most common: Rh disease is unusual (RhoGAM prevents)
  - —Red cell membrane defects: hereditary spherocytosis
  - —Red cell enzyme deficiencies: G6PD deficiency
- Sepsis: bacterial, viral, or protozoal
- Birth trauma
  - —Increased heme load from resolving cephalohematoma or ecchymosis
- Polycythemia
  - —Due to maternal-fetal transfusion
  - —Fetal-fetal transfusion
  - —Infants of diabetic mothers
- Congenital hypothyroidism
- Defective hepatic conjugation
  - —Gilbert syndrome (familial partial defect in glucuronyl transferase activity) is a common benign condition
  - —Crigler-Najjar syndrome (congenital absence of glucuronyl transferase causes lifelong unconjugated hyperbilirubinemia)
  - —Lucy-Driscoll syndrome (severe unconjugated hyperbilirubinemia thought to be due to inhibition of infant's glucuronyl transferase by unidentified maternal serum factors)

Conjugated Hyperbilirubinemia

- Failure of hepatic excretion of conjugated bilirubin
- Causes include neonatal hepatitis, congenital biliary atresia, extrahepatic biliary obstruction, shock liver from neonatal asphyxia, neonatal hemosiderosis

Pre-Hospital

N/A

Diagnosis

ESSENTIAL WORKUP

- Clinical diagnosis
- Further evaluation is recommended for these newborns with significant jaundice that
  - —Occurs in the first 24 hours of life
  - —Persists beyond the first week of life
  - —Peak bilirubin levels >13–15 mg/dL
  - —Bilirubin is >10% or >2 mg/dL conjugated
- Total serum bilirubin (TSB), direct (conjugated) and indirect (unconjugated) bilirubin levels
- Transcutaneous measurement of bilirubin correlates well with TSB and may be available in some centers

LABORATORY

- Maternal blood type
- Infant blood type
- CBC
- Reticulocyte count
- Microscopic examination of blood smear
- Direct Coombs test on cord blood
  - —Hospital routine vary: some will test newborns from all type O mothers
  - —If not available, direct Coombs test on infant's blood

IMAGING/SPECIAL TESTS

- Further workup is directed at suspected cause
- Red cell enzyme assay
- Liver function tests
- Sepsis evaluation
- Evaluation for obstructive liver disease (direct hyperbilirubinemia): consultation and imaging studies

Treatment

INITIAL STABILIZATION

- 0.9% NS 20 mL/kg, bolus for signs of dehydration

ED TREATMENT

- Treat based on TSB
- Treatment is based on gestational age and cause of jaundice (nonhemolytic vs. hemolytic)
- For *healthy term infants* ≥37 weeks of gestation with no hemolysis
  - —Indications for phototherapy: TSB of ≥15 mg/dL at 24–48 hours, ≥18 mg/dL at 49–72 hours, and 20 mg/dL after 72 hours of life
  - —*Intensive* phototherapy should produce a decline in TSB of 1 to 2 mg/dL within 4–6 hours
  - —Indications for exchange transfusions if *intensive* phototherapy fails: TSB ≥20 mg/dL at 25–48 hours, ≥25 mg/dL after 48 hours
  - —Indications for exchange transfusions: TSB ≥25 mg/dL at 25–48 hours, ≥30 mg/dL after 48 hours
- Term infants who are clinically jaundiced at <24 hours are not considered "healthy" and require evaluation and initiation of intensive phototherapy
- Exchange transfusion may be considered before TSB reaches 20 mg/dL with hemolytic disease or in preterm infants
- Moderate alkalinization (pH 7.45–7.55) by ventilatory strategies or bicarbonate infusion with severe hyperbilirubinemia may help prevent encephalopathy in the inpatient setting
- Treat comorbid illness (sepsis, liver dysfunction, polycythemia, hypothyroidism, and so on)
- Reassurance for physiologic jaundice
- Daily bilirubin levels for infants with borderline bilirubin levels until a decline is documented
- Breast-feeding and *breast milk jaundice*
  - —Most infants can continue to breast-feed
  - —May need supplemental IV hydration if dehydrated
  - —2–3-day cessation of breast-feeding recommended for those infants with *breast milk jaundice* and levels approaching 25 mg/dL with phototherapy
  - —Encourage mother to maintain lactation by use of breast pump or manual expression during period of cessation
- Encourage feeding, whether breast-fed or bottle-fed; supplemental dextrose-water is not useful

Disposition

ADMISSION CRITERIA

- Infants requiring intensive phototherapy
- ICU admission for infants requiring exchange transfusion
- Evidence of significant anemia, sepsis, dehydration, or evidence of obstructive liver disease that may require hospitalization for diagnostic evaluation

DISCHARGE CRITERIA

- Stable infant with hyperbilirubinemia not requiring phototherapy
- Stable infant with uncomplicated nonhemolytic hyperbilirubinemia may have home phototherapy arranged if appropriate follow-up can be ensured

Miscellaneous

ICD9: 774.6

ICD10: P59.9

SUGGESTED READINGS

AAP, Provisional Committee for Quality Improvement and Subcommittee on Hyperbilirubinemia. Practice parameter: management of hyperbilirubinemia in the healthy term newborn. Pediatrics 1994;94:558–562.

AAP, Subcommittee on Neonatal Hyperbilirubinemia. Neonatal jaundice and kernicterus. Pediatrics 2001:763–765.

Dennery PA, Seidman DS, Stevenson DK. Neonatal hyperbilirubinemia. N Engl J Med 2001;344(8):581–590.

Hauth JC, Merenstein GB. Guidelines for perinatal care, 4th ed. Elk Grove Village: AAP, 1997.

Nazarian LF, Robertson WO. Personal reflections on the AAP practice parameter on management of hyperbilirubinemia in the healthy term newborn. Pediatr Rev 1998;19(3):75–77.

Author: Michele Chetham

Neonatal Sepsis

Clinical Presentation

SIGNS AND SYMPTOMS

- Nonspecific history
  - —"Not acting normal"
  - —Feeding poorly
  - —Irritable or lethargic
- General
  - —Toxic appearing
  - —Altered mental status—irritable or lethargic
  - —Apnea or bradycardia
  - —Mottled, ashen, cyanotic, or cool skin
- Vital signs
  - —Hyperthermia/hypothermia
  - —Tachypnea
  - —Tachycardia
  - —Prolonged capillary refill time
- Abdominal distention
- Jaundice
- Bruising or prolonged bleeding

MECHANISM/DESCRIPTION

- Life-threatening infection of the newborn, rarely occurring as late as 3 months of age
- Overwhelmingly bacterial
  - —Rarely viral or fungal infection
  - —Organisms usually present in the maternal perineal flora
- Sepsis syndrome in the neonate
  - —Septic shock
  - —Hypoglycemia
  - —Seizures
  - —DIC
  - —If untreated, cardiovascular collapse and death
- Occurs in 3–5 newborns per 1,000 live births
- Risk factors
  - —Perinatal
    - -History of recent fever (>37.5°C)
    - -Urinary tract infection
    - -Chorioamnionitis
    - -Prolonged rupture of membranes (>18 hours)
    - -Foul lochia
    - -Uterine tenderness
    - -Intrapartum asphyxia
  - —Neonatal
    - -Prematurity
    - -Fetal tachycardia (>180 beats/min)
    - -Male
    - -Twinning (especially second twin)
    - -Developmental or congenital immune defects
    - -Administration of intramuscular iron
    - -Galactosemia
    - -Congenital anomaly (urinary tract, asplenia, myelomeningocele, sinus tract)
    - -Omphalitis

ETIOLOGY

Sepsis

- Bacterial
  - —Group B streptococcus
  - —*Escherichia coli*
  - —*Listeria monocytogenes*
  - —Coagulase-negative *Staphylococcus*
  - —*Treponema pallidum*
- Viral
  - —Herpes simplex is a common viral etiology
  - —Enterovirus
  - —Adenovirus
- Fungi
  - —*Candida* species
- Protozoa
  - —Malaria
  - —Borrelia

Meningitis

- Bacterial
  - —Group B streptococcus
  - —*E. coli* type K1
  - —*L. monocytogenes*
  - —Other streptococci
  - —Nontypeable *Haemophilus influenzae*
  - —Coagulase-positive and coagulase-negative *Staphylococcus*
  - —Less commonly: *Klebsiella, Enterobacter, Pseudomonas, T. pallidum,* and *Mycobacterium tuberculosis*
  - —*Citrobacter diversus* (important cause of brain abscess)
  - —Additional pathogens: *Mycoplasma hominis* and *Ureaplasma urealyticum*
- Viral
  - —Enteroviruses
  - —Herpes simplex virus (type 2 more commonly)
  - —Cytomegaloviruses
  - —*Toxoplasma gondii*
  - —Rubella
  - —HIV
- Fungi
  - —*Candida albicans* and other fungi

Pre-Hospital

CAUTIONS

- Ventilatory support if obtunded, apneic, or respiratory distress
- IV access
- Continuous monitoring

Diagnosis

ESSENTIAL WORKUP

- Sepsis evaluation followed by empiric antibiotics and support
- Determine a source for the infection
- Identify metabolic abnormalities

LABORATORIES

- Bedside glucose determination
- CBC
  - —WBCs elevated or suppressed
  - —Shift to the left
  - —Thrombocytopenia
- Urinalysis
- Cultures as soon as the diagnosis is entertained
  - —Blood, CSF, catheterized or suprapubic urine, stool
- Lumbar puncture
  - —May need to delay if hemodynamically unstable
  - —Cell count, protein, glucose, culture
- Serum glucose needed to exclude hypoglycemia
- ABG and oximetry
  - —Metabolic acidosis is common
- Electrolytes and calcium
  - —Hyponatremia
  - —Hypocalcemia
- DIC panel
  - —Coagulopathy is a late complication
  - —Monitor PT, PTT, and fibrinogen-split products

IMAGING/SPECIAL TESTS

- CXR to rule out pneumonia

DIFFERENTIAL DIAGNOSIS

- Heart disease
  - —Hypoplastic left heart syndrome
  - —Myocarditis
- Metabolic disorders
  - —Hypoglycemia
  - —Adrenal insufficiency (congenital adrenal hyperplasia)
  - —Organic acidoses
  - —Urea cycle disorders
- Intussusception
- Child abuse
- CNS
  - —Intracranial hemorrhage
  - —Perinatal asphyxia
- Neonatal jaundice
- Hematologic emergencies
  - —Neonatal purpura fulminans
  - —Severe anemia
  - —Methemoglobinemia
  - —Malignancy (congenital leukemia)

Treatment

INITIAL STABILIZATION

- Airway management indicated if obtundation, apnea, or respiratory distress
- IV access to administer fluids and pressors as needed
- Continuous monitoring

ED TREATMENT

- Implement empiric treatment for neonatal sepsis if presentation at all consistent, particularly if any risk factors are present
- Administer antibiotics
  - —Ampicillin and gentamicin
  - —Add vancomycin if the patient's condition continues to deteriorate or any suggestion of *Streptococcus pneumoniae*
  - —Cefotaxime may be substituted for gentamicin
- Support for septic shock if present

MEDICATIONS

- Ampicillin: 200 mg/kg/d q6h i.v./i.m. for infants >2 kg birth weight and older than 2 weeks; 150 mg/kg/d q8h if younger than 7 days
- Cefotaxime: 150 mg/kg/d q6h i.v./i.m. for infants >2 kg birth weight and older than 1 week; 150 mg/kg/d q8h i.v./i.m. if 8–28 days of age; 100 mg/kg/d i.v./i.m. q12h if 0–7 days of age
- Gentamicin: 2.5 mg/kg/dose q8h i.v./i.m. if postconceptual age more than 37 weeks and older than 7 days; 2.5 mg/kg/dose q12h if younger than 7 days
- Vancomycin: 15 mg/kg/dose i.v. q8h if postconceptual age more than 37 weeks and older than 7 days; 15 mg/kg i.v. q12h if younger than 7 days

Disposition

ADMISSION CRITERIA

- All patients with suspected sepsis are admitted to the hospital for supportive care, IV antibiotic therapy, and close monitoring

DISCHARGE CRITERIA

N/A

Miscellaneous

ICD9: 771; 790.7

ICD10: P36.9

SUGGESTED READINGS

Anderson MR, Blumer JI. Advances in the therapy for sepsis in children. Pediatr Clin North Am 1997;44:179–205.

Edwards MS. Postnatal bacterial infections. In: Fanaroff AA, Martin RJ, eds. Neonatal-perinatal medicine. Diseases of the fetus and infant, 7th ed. St. Louis: Mosby, 2002:706–722.

Jafari HS, McCracken GH. Sepsis and septic shock: a review for clinicians. Pediatr Infect Dis J 1992;1:739–748.

Shapiro NI, Zimmer GD, Barkin AZ. Sepsis syndrome. In: Marx JA, Hockberger RS, Walls RM, eds. Rosen's emergency medicine: concepts and clinical practice, 5th ed. St. Louis: Mosby, 2002.

Vesikari T, Janas M, Gronroos P, et al. Neonatal septicemia. Arch Dis Child 1985;60:542–546.

Author: Lazaro Lezcano

Nephritic Syndrome

Clinical Presentation

SIGNS AND SYMPTOMS

- Hematuria
  - —Abrupt onset with dysmorphic RBCs and RBC casts
  - —Gross hematuria in 30–40%
- Hypertension
- Edema
  - —Periorbital edema
  - —Generalized edema more common in infants
- Azotemia
- Infection source: upper respiratory tract or skin common—for example, poststreptococcal glomerulonephritis (PSGN)
- CHF
  - —40% occurrence in patients older than 60 years
  - —Rare in children
- Renal failure more common in elderly
- Arthritis, arthralgias, and various skin rashes: PSGN, systemic disease
- Nonspecific manifestations
  - —Malaise
  - —Weakness
  - —Anorexia
  - —Nausea/vomiting

MECHANISM/DESCRIPTION

- Acute glomerulonephritis (AGN) associated with
  - —Abrupt onset of hematuria with RBC casts
  - —Acute renal failure manifested by edema, hypertension, azotemia
  - —Mild proteinuria
- Exact mechanism of AGN unclear
  - —Combination of autoimmune reactivity to specific antigens at renal glomeruli
- Diffuse inflammatory changes occur in the glomeruli

ETIOLOGY

Infectious Causes of Acute Nephritic Syndrome

Poststreptococcal Glomerulonephritis

- Occurs between the ages of 3 and 15 years
- Due to group A β-hemolytic streptococci, nephrigenic strain; risk of developing PSGN approximately 15%
- Preceded by infection: upper respiratory tract (pharynx) > cutaneous infections > all other sources
- *Latent period* between infection and onset of nephritis, thus making diagnosis more difficult
  - —1–2 weeks in pharyngeal infection
  - —2–4 weeks in cutaneous infection
- Renal biopsy usually not necessary for diagnosis
- Antibiotic therapy advised but has not been proven to change course of GN once diagnosis established
- Prognosis
  - —Excellent; >95% recover spontaneously with normalization of renal function within 4 weeks, even with dialysis
  - —Hematuria may persist for up to 6 years
  - —Transient nephrotic phase in 20% of patients during resolution of illness
  - —End-stage renal disease occurs <5%
  - —Rapidly progressive GN (RPGN) is rare, occurring in <1% cases
  - —Most cases resolve spontaneously with no long-term sequelae

Hepatitis Virus–related Glomerular Disease

- Can present with either nephritic or nephrotic symptoms
  - —Nephrotic symptoms more typical

HIV-associated Nephropathy (HIV-AN)

- Can present with either nephritic or nephrotic symptoms
  - —Nephrotic symptoms more typical

Infectious Endocarditis

- Gross or microscopic hematuria, mild proteinuria, and azotemia
- Risk groups: parenteral drug abusers and patients with prosthetic valves
- Antibiotic treatment of infectious endocarditis (IE) results in resolution of GN

Other Infection Sources of GN

- Pulmonary, intraabdominal, cutaneous
- Typically severe infection present for months
- Syphilis, leprosy, schistosomiasis, and quartan malaria

Pre-Hospital

N/A

Diagnosis

ESSENTIAL WORKUP

- Urinalysis to detect
  - —Hematuria, proteinuria, and RBC casts
  - —RBC casts diagnostic of an active glomerular inflammation

LABORATORY

- CBC
  - —Anemia (seen in more chronic cases of GN or other systemic disease)
  - —Acute leukocytosis (indicates infectious process)
- Electrolytes, BUN, creatinine, glucose
  - —Baseline for renal function
  - —Check for hyperkalemia
- Serum albumin
  - —Indicator of severity of proteinuria
- Cultures
  - —Throat, skin, urine, blood
  - —As clinically suspected for infection source

IMAGING/SPECIAL TESTS

- Renal US: kidney-size abnormality
- CXR: enlarged heart, pulmonary edema, hemorrhage, infection
- Renal biopsy
  - —Generally not done for PSGN, as symptoms typically resolve in <2 weeks
  - —Recommended if atypical features of PSGN, persistent abnormal complement levels, persistent hypertension, and proteinuria >3 g/d
  - —Facilitates diagnosis for other causes of nephritis

Special Diagnostic Tests

- Serum complement level (C3, CH_{50}): decreased in IE, shunt nephritis and PSGN
- Streptococcal antibodies
  - —Antistreptolysin (ASO), antistreptokinase (ASK), antideoxyribonuclease B (ADNase B), anti-nicotinyl adenine dinucleotidase (ANADase), and antihyaluronidase (AH)
  - —ASO more reactive in pharyngeal infections
  - —ADNase B, ANADase, and AH more reactive in cutaneous infections
  - —ASK elevated in recent hemolytic streptococcus infections
  - —Titers do not correlate with prognosis of disease
- 24-hour urine protein collection
  - —Proteinuria initially present in 5% of children, 20% adults with PSGN

DIFFERENTIAL DIAGNOSIS

(See Glomerulonephritis, for further information on types of GN)

- Renal
  - —Primary glomerular disease
- Systemic
  - —Goodpasture's syndrome
  - —Vasculitis
  - —Henoch-Schönlein purpura
- Other (rare)
  - —Hemolytic-uremic syndrome
  - —Thrombotic thrombocytopenic purpura
  - —Acute hypersensitivity interstitial nephritis
  - —Guillain-Barré
  - —DPT vaccine
  - —Serum sickness

Treatment

INITIAL STABILIZATION

- ABCs

ED TREATMENT

- Antibiotics for streptococcal infection
  - —Penicillin (erythromycin if penicillin allergic)
  - —Prophylactic antibiotics to siblings of PSGN patients
- Restriction of salt and water intake
- Administer loop diuretics (furosemide)
- Treat pulmonary edema
  - —Oxygen
  - —Morphine
  - —Loop diuretics
- BP stabilization to decrease proteinuria, retard progression of GN
  - —ACE inhibitor
  - —Hypertensive emergency: nitroprusside, diazoxide
- Dialysis for
  - —Severe hyperkalemia
  - —Fluid overload
  - —Uremia

MEDICATIONS

- ACE inhibitor: dependent on drug type chosen
- Diazoxide: 1–3 mg/kg i.v., maximum 150 mg, repeat q15min
- Erythromycin: 250 mg (peds: 30–50 mg/kg/24 h) PO q6h × 7–10 days
- Furosemide: 20–100 mg (peds: 1 mg/kg/dose)
- Morphine sulfate: 2–4 mg (peds: 0.1 mg/kg/dose, maximum 15 mg/dose) i.v. q5min
- Nitroprusside: 0.5–10 μg/kg/min i.v.
- Penicillin
  - —Benzathine penicillin: 1.2 million units (peds: 0.6 million units for <30 kg) i.m.
  - —Penicillin: 2 million units PO q6h × 7–10 days

Disposition

ADMISSION CRITERIA

- Evidence of infectious cause for GN
- Oliguria, anuria
- Uremia
- Elevated creatinine, BUN levels
- Edema
- Hyperkalemia
- Hypertension
- CHF

DISCHARGE CRITERIA

- Mild cases of clinical nephritis in healthy patients with
  - —No comorbid illness
  - —Strict supervision/monitoring of symptoms, diet, urine output, and medication
  - —Close follow-up

Miscellaneous

ICD9: 583.9

ICD10: N05

SEE ALSO: GLOMERULONEPHRITIS; NEPHROTIC SYNDROME; RENAL FAILURE

SUGGESTED READINGS

Campagna DP, Wallace DR. Poststreptococcal glomerulonephritis presenting as impending airway obstruction. Ann Emerg Med 2001;38(4):450–452.

Carithers RL. Hepatitis C and renal failure. Am J Med 1999;107(6B):90S–94S.

Couser WG. Glomerulonephritis. Lancet 1999;353(9163):1509–1515.

Kirpal SC, Sakhuja V. Glomerulonephritis due to other infections. In: Massry SG, Glassock RJ, eds. Textbook of nephrology, 3rd ed. Baltimore: Williams & Wilkins, 1995:703–710.

Korbet SM, Schwartz MM. Human immunodeficiency virus infection and nephrotic syndrome. Am J Kidney Dis 1992;20:97–103.

Author: Shirley Lee

Nephrotic Syndrome

Clinical Presentation

SIGNS AND SYMPTOMS

- Many patients asymptomatic
- Proteinuria
- Peripheral edema
  - —Mild pitting edema to generalized anasarca with ascites
- Hyperlipidemia
- Lipiduria (urine fatty casts and oval fat bodies)
- Postural hypotension/syncope/shock
- Hypertension
- Hematuria
  - —Microscopic or gross hematuria (secondary to renal vein thrombosis)
- Acute renal failure rare
  - —More common in elderly
- Tachypnea, tachycardia, with/without hypotension
  - —Acute onset: suggests pulmonary embolus (PE), secondary to renal or deep veinous thrombosis due to hypercoagulable state
  - —Up to 30% occurrence of PE in membranous glomerulonephritis (GN)
  - —Chronic or exertional tachypnea due to
    - -Pulmonary edema
    - -Pleural effusions
    - -Infection, especially in children on immunosuppressive treatment and frequent exposure to infections such as *Pneumococcus*
  - —Increased respiratory effort due to diaphragm motion restriction secondary to ascites
- Bone fractures (due to underlying osteomalacic bone disease)

MECHANISM/DESCRIPTION

Definition

- Proteinuria >3.5 g/d
- Serum albumin >3 g/dL
- Peripheral edema
- Hyperlipidemia (fasting cholesterol >200 mg/dL)
- Glomerular basement membrane altered by
  - —Immune complexes
  - —Nephrotoxic antibodies
  - —Nonimmune mechanisms
  - —Result
    - -Increased filtration and excretion of albumin and large proteins into Bowman's capsule

Pathophysiology

- Edema due to sodium retention and hypoalbuminemia
- Postural hypotension, syncope, and shock due to severe hypoalbuminemia with plasma volume reduction
- Hypertension, in association with abnormal urinalysis or decrease renal function, indicates
  - —GN
  - —Diabetes mellitus
  - —Connective tissue disease
- Hyperlipidemia due to hepatic lipoprotein synthesis stimulated by decreased plasma oncotic pressure
- Cumulative thromboembolism risk increased to 50% if
  - —Hypovolemia
  - —Low serum albumin (<25 g/L)
  - —High protein excretion (>10 g/24 h)
  - —High fibrinogen levels
  - —Low antithrombin III levels

ETIOLOGY

- Due to primary renal or systemic diseases
- Primary pathologies
  - —Membranous glomerulonephritis (MGN): most common cause in adults; linked to neoplastic disease, therefore need appropriate workup—for example, myeloma
  - —Minimal change disease: primary nephrotic disease in children 75%
  - —Focal segmental glomerulosclerosis (FSGN)
  - —Membranoproliferative glomerulonephritis (MPGN)
  - —Miscellaneous proliferative glomerular nephropathies: 16%
- Secondary pathologies
  - —Account for 20% of causes of nephrotic syndrome
  - —Diabetic nephropathy most common cause of secondary nephrotic syndrome
  - —Diseases can present initially as a nephritic process, with progression to nephrotic syndrome
  - —Rarer causes
    - -Preeclampsia
    - -Drug reaction (NSAIDs, heroin)
    - -HIV
    - -Hepatitis

Hepatitis Virus–related Glomerular Disease

- Hepatitis carrier state associated mainly with membranous GN in children, ages 2–12 years
- In adults, high correlation of hepatitis C with membranoproliferative GN
- Hypertension present in 25% of children, 45% in adults
- Two thirds of children remit 3 years after diagnosis
- In adults, 10–15% require dialysis
- Interferon effective treatment, but many side effects resulting in discontinuation by patients; disease recurs after treatment stopped
- Other therapies: corticosteroids, plasmapheresis, cytotoxic agents

HIV-associated Nephropathy (HIV-AN)

- Main presentation
  - —Proteinuria (nephrotic range) and renal insufficiency
  - —No hematuria present or hypertension present
- >50% of HIV-AN are asymptomatic carriers of HIV
- Focal segmental glomerulosclerosis most common nephropathy
- Collapsing glomerulopathy in seropositive HIV carriers with supernephrotic syndrome (>20-g/d protein loss) result in end-stage renal failure in months
- Despite dialysis, death commonly occurs within a year

Pre-Hospital

N/A

Diagnosis

ESSENTIAL WORKUP

- Urinalysis
  - —Dipstick protein largely positive
    - -Urine specific gravity >1.025 lowers the diagnostic significance of proteinuria
  - —Microscopic analysis for urinary casts and the presence of cellular elements
    - -Oval fat bodies
    - -Free lipid droplets

LABORATORY

- CBC plus differential
  - —Anemia common
  - —Leukocytosis: infection
  - —Leukopenia: neoplastic disease
  - —Thrombocytopenia: liver disease
- PTT, PT, INR
  - —Coagulation profiles abnormal with concurrent liver disease, for example, hepatitis
- D-dimer, fibrinogen, antithrombin III
  - —Suspected thromboembolic event
    - -Often patients asymptomatic with PE or renal vein thrombosis, therefore need high clinical suspicion
- Serum albumin: <3 g/dL
- Serum total protein: <6 g/dL
- Creatinine, BUN: elevated in renal insufficiency
- Lipid profile: elevated total cholesterol, LDL, and VLDL
- Serum glucose: diabetes
- Serum calcium: lowered

IMAGING/SPECIAL TESTS

- Renal US
  - —Not helpful
  - —Used in suspected secondary causes of nephrotic syndrome
- Renal biopsy
  - —Definitive test for patients who do not respond to a short course of corticosteroids
  - —Help discern primary versus secondary pathology and specific therapy

Other Laboratory Tests

- Used to identify systemic disorders
- See also Glomerulonephritis, for review of laboratory tests

DIFFERENTIAL DIAGNOSIS

Proteinuria Resulting from Other Causes

- Renal parenchymal disease
  - —Chronic renal disease
  - —Mechanical nephropathy (obstruction/reflux)
  - —Orthostatic proteinuria
  - —Acute pyelonephritis
  - —Sickle cell disease
- Other causes
  - —CHF
  - —Essential hypertension
  - —Acute febrile illness
  - —Pregnancy (preeclampsia)
  - —Severe obesity

Treatment

INITIAL STABILIZATION

- ABCs
  - —Supplemental oxygen if respiratory distress
  - —IV fluids
    - -Slow rehydration for decreased BP or orthostatic hypotension due to decreased intravascular volume
    - -Active rehydration in the presence of severe hypotension, shock

ED TREATMENT

- Control edema
  - —Restrict sodium intake to 50 mmol (3 g NaCl)/d
  - —Loop diuretic (furosemide): mainstay of therapy, titrate dose until response seen
  - —Thiazides and potassium-sparing diuretics can be used in conjunction to minimize sodium resorption by the nephron tubule—for example, low-dose metolazone
  - —Goal: *slow* diuresis
    - -Aggressive diuresis can precipitate acute renal failure due to hypovolemia and increase the risk of thromboembolic complications
- Thromboembolic prevention/treatment
  - —Heparin: 50–80 IU/kg bolus followed by 18 IU/kg drip i.v.
  - —Consider low-dose ASA 80 mg (may be beneficial, no RCT studies to prove yet)
  - —Support stockings
- Plasmapheresis, for severe cases

Post-ED Treatment

- Glucocorticosteroids: mainstay of treatment for primary nephrotic syndrome
- ACE inhibitor: decreases proteinuria, prevents worsening of renal function, especially diabetic nephropathy
- Cholesterol-lowering agents/dietary manipulation (bile acid resin, lovastatin)
- Cytotoxic agents/cyclosporine: second line in glomerulonephritis treatment, especially in recurrent remissions despite adequate steroid trials
- NSAIDs, reduce proteinuria by decreasing GFR; however, side effects have decreased use of this treatment
- Recombinant erythropoietin for anemia
- Diet manipulation
  - —Protein-restricted diet
    - -*Not* recommended, as does not consistently decrease proteinuria
    - -Associated risk of malnutrition, which worsens prognosis of renal disease
  - —Sodium-restricted diet, recommended to reduce hypertension and edema

MEDICATIONS

- Furosemide: 20–100 mg PO b.i.d. to t.i.d. (peds: 1 mg/kg/dose; maximum 6 mg/kg) i.v.; maximum 2 mg/kg/d
- Heparin: 50–80 IU/kg bolus followed by 18 IU/kg drip i.v.
- Metolazone (Zaroxolyn): 5–20 mg/d PO

Disposition

ADMISSION CRITERIA

- Moderate to severe heart failure, ascites, respiratory compromise
- Signs of comorbid illness, such as undiagnosed malignancy, poorly controlled diabetes, immunocompromised host
- Acute renal failure
- Evidence of thromboembolic event

DISCHARGE CRITERIA

- Patients with no comorbid disease who present with a history and physical compatibility with primary GN, normal vital signs, and normal blood work
- Close follow-up with a nephrologist or general internist for further evaluation and treatment mandatory

Miscellaneous

ICD9: 581.9

ICD10: N04

SEE ALSO: GLOMERULONEPHRITIS; NEPHRITIC SYNDROME; RENAL FAILURE

SUGGESTED READINGS

Glassock RJ, Brenner BM. The major glomerulopathies. In: Wilson et al, eds. Harrison's principles of internal medicine, 13th ed. New York: McGraw-Hill, 1995:1295–1313

Glassock RJ, Cohen AH. The primary glomerulopathies. Dis Mon 1996;42(6):329–383.

Madaio MP, Harrington JT. The diagnosis of glomerular diseases: acute glomerulonephritis and the nephrotic syndrome. Arch Intern Med 2001;161(1):25–34.

Orth SR, Ritz E. The nephrotic syndrome. N Engl J Med 1998;338(17):1202–1211.

Author: Shirley Lee

Neuroleptic Malignant Syndrome

Clinical Presentation

SIGNS AND SYMPTOMS

- Life-threatening condition
- Hallmarks of the disease
  - —Hyperthermia (temperature may be as high as 106–107°F, 41°C)
  - —Altered level of consciousness
  - —Skeletal muscle rigidity, "lead pipe rigidity"
  - —Autonomic instability (tachycardia, labile BP)

MECHANISM/DESCRIPTION

- May develop anytime during therapy with neuroleptics—from a few days to many years after initiating treatment
- Muscular rigidity may result from dopamine antagonism in the nigrostriatal pathway and hyperthermia due to blockage of hypothalamic thermoregulation
  - —May be more likely in the setting of benzodiazepine withdrawal

ETIOLOGY

- Rare complication of treatment with neuroleptic drugs such as phenothiazines, butyrophenones, and thiothixene
- Occurs in approximately 1% of patients treated with neuroleptics (especially haloperidol)
- Has been associated with withdrawal from dopamine agonists in Parkinson's disease

Pre-Hospital

CAUTIONS

- Ventilation may be difficult because of chest wall rigidity
- Cool the patient, and treat seizures if they occur
- Check fingerstick glucose
- Paralysis with a nondepolarizing neuromuscular blocker is preferable to succinylcholine

Diagnosis

ESSENTIAL WORKUP

- An accurate history (especially current medications) and physical exam confirm the diagnosis
- CPK, WBC determination, and liver function tests

LABORATORY

- Electrolytes, glucose, BUN, creatinine, PT/PTT, urine (for myoglobin)
- Lumbar puncture to rule out meningitis

IMAGING/SPECIAL TESTS

- CT scan, EEG if the cause of altered level of consciousness is unclear

DIFFERENTIAL DIAGNOSIS

- Meningitis, encephalitis, sepsis
- Malignant hyperthermia, severe dystonic reaction
- Tetanus
- Heat stroke
- Strychnine poisoning
- Vascular CNS event
- Fatal catatonia
- Thyrotoxicosis
- Rabies
- Central anticholinergic toxicity

Treatment

INITIAL STABILIZATION

- ABCs, IV, O_2, cardiac monitor
- Immediate IV benzodiazepines (diazepam, lorazepam), may require repeated large doses
- If symptoms are not controlled within a few minutes *rapid-sequence intubation* and *neuromuscular blockade* are necessary
  - —Nondepolarizing neuromuscular blockers (vecuronium, rocuronium, pancuronium) are preferable to succinylcholine
- Measures to control hyperthermia
  - —Ice packs, mist and fan, cooling blankets, and so on
- Aggressive IV fluid therapy with lactated Ringer's solution or NS

ED TREATMENT

- Relief of muscle rigidity
  - —Bromocriptine is a dopamine agonist that may play a role in longer term management
  - —Dantrolene is a direct skeletal muscle relaxant that may play a role in longer term management
  - —Neither bromocriptine nor dantrolene has a rapid onset and has not been demonstrated to alter outcome
- Discontinue neuroleptics
- Recognize complications (rhabdomyolysis, respiratory failure, acute renal failure), mortality can be as high as 20%

MEDICATIONS

- Bromocriptine: 20–30 mg/d PO (peds: dose not established)
- Dantrolene (adult/peds): 1–2.5 mg/kg i.v.
- Diazepam: 5–10 mg i.v. (peds: 0.2–0.5 mg/kg/dose, titrate to effect)
- Lorazepam: 2–4 mg i.v. (peds: safety not established, titrate to effect)
- Pancuronium (adult/peds): 0.1–0.15 mg/kg
- Rocuronium (adult/peds): 0.6 mg/kg
- Vecuronium (adult/peds): 0.1–0.3 mg/kg

Disposition

ADMISSION CRITERIA

- All patients should be admitted to ICU

DISCHARGE CRITERIA

- No patients with a diagnosis of neuroleptic malignant syndrome should be discharged

Miscellaneous

ICD9: 333.92

ICD10: G21.0

SUGGESTED READINGS

Bobolakis I. Neuroleptic malignant syndrome after antipsychotic drug administration during benzodiazepine withdrawal. J Clin Psychopharm 2000;20:281–283.

Ebadi M, Srinivasan SK. Pathogenesis, prevention, and treatment of neuroleptic-induced movement disorders. Pharmacol Rev 1995;47(4):575–604.

Sachdev P, Mason C, Hadzi-Pavlovic D. Case control study of neuroleptic malignant syndrome. Am J Psychiatry 1997;154: 1156–1158.

Author: Gary Johnson

Neuroleptic, Poisoning

Clinical Presentation

SIGNS AND SYMPTOMS

- Overdose
  - —Toxic effects are typically mild to moderate
  - —CNS symptoms predominate
- Neurologic
  - —Slurred speech
  - —CNS depression
  - —Agitation
  - —Coma
  - —Seizures
  - —Extrapyramidal symptoms (dystonia, akathisia)
- Cardiovascular
  - —Hypotension
  - —Tachycardia
  - —Prolonged QRS or QTc
  - —Torsades de pointes
- Respiratory
  - —Respiratory depression
- Gastrointestinal
  - —Constipation
  - —Dry mouth
- Genitourinary
  - —Urinary retention
- Hyperthermia
- Ocular: miosis or mydriasis
- Hematologic: anemia, agranulocytosis (clozapine)
- Neuroleptic malignant syndrome (NMS)
  - —Hyperthermia
  - —Skeletal muscle rigidity
  - —Altered mental status
  - —Autonomic dysfunction

MECHANISM/DESCRIPTION

- Neuroleptics used for the management of
  - —Psychotic disorders
  - —Depressive neurosis
  - —Dementia in the elderly
  - —Behavioral problems in children
  - —Antiemetic
- Peak plasma levels within 4 hours
- Dystonia occurs within hours to days of ingestion
- Akathisia occurs within days to weeks of increased dosing

ETIOLOGY

- Typical neuroleptics (phenothiazines, butyrophenones) strongly antagonize dopaminergic receptors
  - —Haloperidol (Haldol)
  - —Chlorpromazine (Thorazine)
  - —Thioridazine (Mellaril)
  - —Fluphenazine (Prolixin)
  - —Promethazine (Phenergan)
  - —Droperidol (Inapsine)
- Atypical neuroleptics have weaker dopaminergic antagonism and moderate serotonergic antagonism
  - —Clozapine (Clozaril)
  - —Risperidone (Risperdal)
  - —Olanzapine (Zyprexa)
  - —Quetiapine (Seroquel)
- Both exhibit strong α-adrenergic antagonism
- Both exhibit anticholinergic activity

Pre-Hospital

CAUTIONS

- Transport all pills/pill bottles involved in overdose for identification in ED
- Do not induce emesis because of risk of CNS depression or seizures

Diagnosis

ESSENTIAL WORKUP

- Monitor vital signs with significant ingestion
- Cardiac monitor/pulse oximetry

LABORATORY

- Electrolytes, BUN, creatinine, glucose
- CBC for clozapine overdose
- Urinalysis
  - —Dip for myoglobin if NMS suspected
- CPK levels if NMS suspected
- Toxicologic screens to exclude common co-ingestants
- Quantitative levels are rarely helpful

IMAGING/SPECIAL TESTS

- EKG
  - —QTc/QRS prolongation
  - —Conduction disturbances
- Abdominal radiograph
  - —Unabsorbed phenothiazine may be radiopaque
  - —Absence of visible tablets does not eliminate possibility of ingestion

DIFFERENTIAL DIAGNOSIS

- Cyclic antidepressant overdose
- Antihistamine overdose
- Cocaine overdose
- Amphetamine overdose
- Opioid overdose
- Occult head injury
- Sepsis

Treatment

INITIAL STABILIZATION

- ABCs
  —Administer supplemental oxygen
  —Administer naloxone, thiamine, D50 (or Accucheck) for altered mental status
  —Intubate if respiratory depression

ED TREATMENT

- Supportive care
- Decontamination
  —Administer a single dose of activated charcoal if recent ingestion
- Hypotension
  —0.9% NS i.v. fluid bolus
  —Trendelenburg
  —Treat resistant hypotension with norepinephrine or phenylephrine
  —Dopamine may be ineffective because of strong β-adrenergic blockade
- Ventricular dysrhythmias
  —Lidocaine sometimes effective
  —Avoid class 1a antidysrhythmics: potential exacerbation of neuroleptic cardiotoxicity
  —Magnesium for prolonged QTc
  —Cardioversion if hemodynamically unstable
- Dystonic reactions
  —Administer diphenhydramine or benztropine mesylate
- Malignant hyperthermia
  —Rapid cooling
  —Administer dantrolene and bromocriptine
- Seizures
  —Treat initially with diazepam
  —Phenobarbital for persistent seizures

MEDICATIONS

- Activated charcoal: 1–2 g/kg
- Benztropine mesylate: 1–2 mg i.v.
- Bromocriptine: 2.5–10 mg q8h PO
- Dantrolene: 1–2 mg/kg q10min i.v. (10 mg/kg max)
- Diazepam: 5–10 mg i.v. q10–15min (0.2–0.5 mg/kg)
- Diphenhydramine: 25–50 mg i.v. (1 mg/kg)
- Lidocaine: loading dose, 1 mg/kg i.v. q5–10min (3 mg/kg max); maintenance dose, 2–4 mg/min i.v.
- Magnesium sulfate: 1–2 g I.V. over 5–15 min
- Norepinephrine: 1–2 μg/kg/min titrate to BP
- Phenobarbital: 10–20 mg/kg i.v. (loading dose)
- Phenylephrine: 40–80 μg/min titrate to BP

Disposition

ADMISSION CRITERIA

- Admit overdose with CNS sedation, agitation, dysrhythmias, or vital sign abnormalities to monitored bed

DISCHARGE CRITERIA

- Asymptomatic after 6 hours of observation
- Patients successfully treated for acute dystonia should be given 3-day course of diphenhydramine to prevent recurrence

Miscellaneous

ICD9: E853.0

ICD10: T43.3

SUGGESTED READINGS

Burns MJ. The pharmacology and toxicology of atypical antipsychotic agents. J Toxicol Clin Toxicol 2001;39(1):1–14.

De Roos FJ. Neuroleptics. In: Ford MD, Delaney KA, Ling LJ, et al, eds. Clinical Toxicology. Philadelphia: WB Saunders, 2001:539–545.

Lewin NA. Neuroleptic agents. In: Goldfrank LR, Flomenbaum NE, Lewin NA, et al, eds. Goldfrank's toxicologic emergencies. Stamford, CT: Appleton & Lange, 1998:943–953.

Author: Mark B. Mycyk

Noncardiogenic Pulmonary Edema

Clinical Presentation

SIGNS AND SYMPTOMS

- Tachycardia
  - —Characteristically seen secondary to decreasing PO_2 levels
- Scattered rhonchi and rales
- Dyspnea
- Tachypnea
- Cyanosis
- Pink, frothy sputum
- The stigmas of left- and right-sided heart failure will *not* be found

MECHANISM/DESCRIPTION

- Functional disruption of the capillary–alveolar membrane from a noncardiac source
- Diffuse injury to either the alveolar epithelium or to the vascular endothelium
- Pulmonary parenchymal changes mimic CHF
  - —Cephalad redistribution of blood flow, pulmonary effusions, and cardiomegaly do *not* develop
- Typically, onset of this edema is within 1–2 hours of noxious insult
- First described by William Osler in 1889 in a patient "poisoned" by morphine
- Approximately 250,000 cases occur each year in the United States

ETIOLOGY

- Cause of capillary leak or alveolar membrane damage is uncertain
- Proposed mechanisms include hypoxia, immunologic effects, or direct toxic effects
- Major causes
  - —Smoke inhalation
  - —Salicylate intoxication
  - —Toxic gas inhalation
  - —Transfusion reaction
  - —Near drowning
  - —DIC
  - —High-altitude pulmonary edema (HAPE)
  - —Radiation pneumonitis
  - —Narcotic abuse
  - —Uremia
  - —Cardiopulmonary bypass
  - —Major trauma
  - —Aspiration
  - —Bacterial pneumonia

Pre-Hospital

- Patent airway
- Adequate oxygenation

CAUTIONS

- Patients will not typically respond to usual measures to treat CHF

Diagnosis

ESSENTIAL WORKUP

- CXR
  - —Classic butterfly pattern of pulmonary edema
  - —Unilateral patchy infiltrates resembling pneumonia
  - —Lack of cardiomegaly
- ABG

LABORATORY

- Electrolytes, BUN, creatinine
- EKG

IMAGING/SPECIAL TESTS

- Echocardiogram may help identify normal cardiac function and ejection fraction

DIFFERENTIAL DIAGNOSIS

- Cardiogenic pulmonary edema
- COPD exacerbation
- Pulmonary embolus
- Restrictive lung disease
- Pneumonia

Treatment

INITIAL STABILIZATION

- Supplemental oxygen (high-flow oxygen)
- IV catheter
- Continuous cardiac monitor
- Continuous pulse oximetry

ED TREATMENT

- The treatment of noncardiogenic pulmonary edema (NCPE) is supportive
- NCPE associated with drug overdose usually responds to high-flow O_2
- Diuretics are *not* used
- Removal of trigger that may have caused NCPE
  —Noxious gas
  —Having patient descend from elevation in cases of HAPE
- Noninvasive ventilatory support (BiPAP, CPAP) may be used if immediately available
  —Measure blood gases frequently
  —If unable to provide adequate oxygenation or ventilation, intubation is required
  —Useful in NCPE caused by drug overdose
- Endotracheal intubation is often necessary
  —Positive end-expiratory pressure (PEEP) of 5–10 cm H_2O
    -NCPE of a neurogenic etiology has a worsened prognosis when PEEP is employed
  —Improved oxygenation
  —Decrease work of breathing
  —To reduce the likelihood of atelectasis, tidal volumes should be on order of 12–15 mL/kg
  —Initially place on 100% O_2
    -Measure PO_2 and decrease FIO_2 accordingly
- Steroids and cyclooxygenase inhibitors have not been proven effective

Disposition

ADMISSION CRITERIA

- All symptomatic patients should be admitted to ICU
  —Symptoms may worsen at any point for up to 3 days after noxious insult

DISCHARGE CRITERIA

- Asymptomatic patients (especially narcotic overdose, HAPE, or aspiration)
  —Observe in ED for 6–12 hours and then discharge with close follow-up scheduled if no evidence of pulmonary edema is present and adequate oxygenation is demonstrated

Miscellaneous

ICD9: 518.4

ICD10: J81

SUGGESTED READINGS

Macias DJ, Brillman JC. Adult respiratory distress syndrome. In: Harwood-Nuss A, Linden C, Luten R, et al, eds. The clinical practice of emergency medicine, 2nd ed. Philadelphia: JB Lippincott Co, 1996:640–643.

McIntyre RC Jr. Thirty years of clinical trials in acute respiratory distress syndrome. Crit Care Med 2000;28(9):3314–3331.

Author: David Jerrard

Nonsteroidal Antiinflammatory Drugs, Poisoning

Clinical Presentation

SIGNS AND SYMPTOMS

Gastrointestinal
- Nausea
- Vomiting
- Epigastric pain

CNS
- Drowsiness
- Dizziness
- Lethargy
- Seizures

Cardiovascular
- Hypotension
- Tachycardia

Pulmonary
- Eosinophilic pneumonia
- Apnea
- Hyperventilation

Renal
- Acute renal failure
- Acute tubular necrosis
- Acute interstitial nephritis

Liver
- Hepatocellular injury
- Cholestatic jaundice

Metabolic
- Mild, short-lived metabolic acidosis

Hypersensitivity
- Aseptic meningitis
- Asthma exacerbation

MECHANISM/DESCRIPTION
- Inhibit cyclooxygenase (COX) that blocks the conversion of arachidonic acid to prostaglandin
- Typically, ingestion of an NSAID is benign
- Fatalities reported with large ingestions
- Greater potential for toxicity with underlying CHF or renal failure
  - —NSAIDs cause sodium and water retention and decrease renal blood flow
  - —Very little overdose experience with the COX-2 inhibitors (celecoxib, rofecoxib, and valdecoxib); treatment should be the same as for the traditional NSAIDs

PEDIATRIC CONSIDERATIONS
- Piroxicam, naproxen, ketoprofen, and mefenamic acid have caused seizures in children

Pre-Hospital

CAUTIONS
- Collect prescription bottles/medications for identification in the ED

Diagnosis

ESSENTIAL WORKUP
- Generally, NSAID ingestion results only in mild toxicity
- Exact identification of drug helpful
  - —Subtle toxicologic differences amongst the NSAIDs

LABORATORY
- Electrolytes, BUN/Cr, glucose
  - —Baseline renal function
  - —Check for metabolic acidosis
- CBC
- ABG for large overdoses
- PT/PTT
  - —False-positive bilirubin/ketone dipstick with etodolac ingestion
- NSAID difficult to detect on toxicology screens
- Plasma ibuprofen levels
  - —Minimal utility
  - —Nomogram for ibuprofen has a poor predictive value

DIFFERENTIAL DIAGNOSIS
- Agents causing metabolic acidosis, altered mental status, and GI irritation
  - —Salicylates
  - —INH
  - —Ethylene glycol
  - —Methanol
  - —Isopropanol

Treatment

INITIAL STABILIZATION

- ABCs
- Naloxone, thiamine, dextrose (or Accucheck) for altered mental status

ED TREATMENT

- Supportive care and GI decontamination
- Gastric lavage
  - If the patient presents within 1 hour of ingestion with an intact gag reflex
  - If no gag reflex is present, protected airway with a cuffed endotracheal tube before lavage
- Avoid syrup of ipecac because NSAIDs may cause CNS depression and seizures in the overdose setting
- Administer activated charcoal and sorbitol early (after lavage completion)
- Extracorporeal methods to enhance elimination are not beneficial due to high degree of plasma protein binding

MEDICATIONS

- Activated charcoal slurry: 1–2 g/kg up to 90 g PO
- Dextrose: D50W 1 amp (50 mL or 25 g) (peds: D25W 2–4 mL/kg) i.v.
- Naloxone (Narcan): 2 mg (peds: 0.1 mg/kg) i.v. or i.m. initial dose
- Sorbitol: 1–2 g/kg to a maximum of 100 g (peds: older than 1 year, 1–1.5 g/kg as a 35% solution to a maximum of 50 g) PO mixed in the activated charcoal slurry; only use for first dose
- Thiamine (vitamin B_1): 100 mg (peds: 50 mg) i.v. or i.m.

Disposition

ADMISSION CRITERIA

- Protracted vomiting, hematemesis
- CNS depression, seizure activity
- Metabolic acidosis
- CHF, hypotension, hypertension
- Renal failure

DISCHARGE CRITERIA

- Nontoxic ingestion in a patient who is asymptomatic 6–8 hours after ingestion

Miscellaneous

ICD9: 965.6

ICD10: T39.3

SUGGESTED READINGS

Paloucek FP, Rynn KO. Nonsteroidal anti-inflammatory drugs (NSAIDs). In: Ford MD, Delaney KA, Ling LJ, et al, ed. Clinical toxicology. Philadelphia: WB Saunders, 2001:281–284.

Seifert SA, Bronstein AC, McGuire TH. Massive ibuprofen ingestion with survival. J Toxicol Clin Toxicol 2000;38:55–57.

Zuckerman GB, Uy CC. Shock, metabolic acidosis, and coma following ibuprofen overdose in a child. Ann Pharmacother 1995;29:869–871.

Author: Michele Kanter

Nursemaid's Elbow

Clinical Presentation

SIGNS AND SYMPTOMS

- Child refuses to use arm
- Elbow slightly flexed with forearm held close to trunk
- Pain with flexion of the elbow
- Pain with forearm supination or pronation
- Absence of point tenderness
- Minimal to no swelling

MECHANISM/DESCRIPTION

- One of the most common injuries of the upper extremity in children younger than 5 years
  —Due to longitudinal traction on an extended, pronated arm
  —Typical history is a sharp pull on the child's outstretched arm such as lifting the child by the wrist
  —Alternatively, caregiver may report history of a fall
- Subluxation of the radial head
  —Annular ligament slips or tears and becomes interposed between the radial head and the capitellum

Pre-Hospital

CAUTIONS

- Place ice on the injured elbow to reduce pain and swelling
- Immobilize in a sling or splint to facilitate transport and prevent further injury
- Assess distal neurovascular status

Diagnosis

ESSENTIAL WORKUP

- Clinical diagnosis
  —Classic history, passive position of arm, and physical exam are sufficient for diagnosis
- Radiographs
  —Not routinely indicated
  —Obtain to exclude or diagnose other injuries if any of the following are present
    -Point tenderness
    -Soft-tissue swelling
    -Deformity
    -Ecchymosis of the elbow
    -Failed reduction

DIFFERENTIAL DIAGNOSIS

- Humerus or radius fracture
- Elbow dislocation
- Joint infection
- Osteomyelitis
- Tumor

Treatment

INITIAL STABILIZATION

- Assess distal motor, sensory, and vascular function

ED TREATMENT

- Two common reduction techniques
- Supination/flexion technique
  —Grasp child's hand in handshake position
  —Stabilize injured elbow with the other hand
  —In a smooth, swift motion, fully supinate the forearm and flex the elbow
- Hyperpronation technique
  —Grasp child's hand in handshake position
  —Stabilize injured elbow with the other hand
  —Hyperpronate and extend the forearm
- Palpable click may accompany successful reduction but is not essential
- Child may cry during the reduction but is frequently pain free and using the arm shortly thereafter
- Second reduction attempt if the child does not use arm 15 minutes after first attempt
- Consider opposing technique for second reduction attempt
- Radiographic studies indicated if the second reduction attempt is unsuccessful
- Perform postreduction neurovascular assessment

MEDICATIONS

- Acetaminophen: 15 mg/kg PO q4h

Disposition

ADMISSION CRITERIA

- None

DISCHARGE CRITERIA

- Discharge to home after child regains full, unrestricted use of the arm
- Patient instructions
  —Inform parents not to pull or lift the child by the hand, wrist, or forearm
  —Warn family of increased incidence of recurrence until the child reaches 5–6 years of age
- Splint with prompt orthopedic referral for any injury of the elbow with a radiographic abnormality; condylar, supracondylar, or displaced fractures need orthopedic evaluation expedited
- Posterior splint with orthopedic follow-up in 24–48 hours, if reduction attempts fail and no radiographic abnormalities can be identified
- Warn family to observe for neurovascular compromise

Miscellaneous

ICD9: 832.0

ICD10: S59.9

SUGGESTED READINGS

Kaufman D. Evaluation of the patient with extremity pain: an evidence based approach. Emerg Med Clin North Am 1999;17(1):77–95.

Macias CG, Bothner J, Wiebe R. A comparison of supination/flexion to hyperpronation in the reduction of radial head subluxations. Pediatrics 1998;102(1):e10.

Macias CG, Wiebe R, Bothner J. History and radiographic findings associated with clinically suspected radial head subluxations. Pediatr Emerg Care 2000;16(1):22–25.

McDonald J, Whitelaw C, Goldsmith LJ. Radial head subluxation: comparing two methods of reduction. Acad Emerg Med 1999;6(7):715–718.

Authors: Daren D. Girard; Daniel L. Savitt

Oculomotor Nerve Palsy

Clinical Presentation

SIGNS AND SYMPTOMS

- Complete
  - —Diplopia, with involved eye deviated laterally and downward
  - —Mydriasis of the involved eye
- Partial
  - —Diplopia with involved eye deviated laterally and downward
  - —Reactive midpoint pupil of the involved eye

MECHANISM/DESCRIPTION

- Complete oculomotor nerve palsy
  - —Compressive lesions such as aneurysms or tumors
  - —Brainstem herniation with compression of the third cranial nerve by the temporal lobe (i.e., increased intracranial pressure)
- Incomplete oculomotor nerve palsy
  - —Vascular infarction of the vasa nervorum of the third cranial nerve

ETIOLOGY

- Intracranial or orbital tumor
- Aneurysm (particularly posterior communicating artery)
- Trauma
- Intracranial hemorrhage
- Diabetes mellitus
- Migraine headache
- Infection, meningitis
- Arteriovenous malformation or fistula
- Cavernous sinus thrombosis
- Neuropathy (e.g., myasthenia gravis and Guillain-Barré)
- Collagen vascular diseases (e.g., sarcoidosis)

PEDIATRIC CONSIDERATIONS

- Trauma is the most common cause of acquired oculomotor nerve palsies
- Congenital oculomotor nerve palsy should be considered in the differential of the pediatric patient; other causes such as diabetes, posterior communicating artery aneurysms, metastatic tumor, and pituitary lesions are less common than in the adult population

Pre-Hospital

- Without associated trauma, there are no specific pre-hospital care issues

Diagnosis

ESSENTIAL WORKUP

- History is of utmost importance in determining etiology; important historical elements include
  - —History of long-standing diabetes mellitus
  - —Head trauma, either recent or distant
  - —Unintentional weight loss
  - —Recent infection involving the upper respiratory tract, eyes, or ears
  - —Severe headache (classical "thunder-clap," or chronic and worsening)
  - —Constitutional symptoms: nausea, vomiting, fever, and so on
- Ophthalmologic examination
  - —Extraocular movements
  - —Exophthalmus
  - —Funduscopic examination to demonstrate papilledema
  - —Direct and consensual pupillary reaction
- Head CT

LABORATORY

- CBC with differential, ESR to rule out infection and malignancy
- ANA, rheumatoid factor, to rule out vasculitis
- Lumbar puncture

IMAGING/SPECIAL TESTS

- CT/MRI of brain, orbit, sinuses
- Doppler imaging for arteriovenous malformations, dural sinus thrombosis
- Cerebral arteriogram rarely useful as most aneurysms are seen on CT or MRI

DIFFERENTIAL DIAGNOSIS

N/A

Treatment

INITIAL STABILIZATION

- Initial stabilization of the posttraumatic patient with oculomotor nerve palsy should concentrate on the underlying traumatic condition
- ABCs
- Any patient with evidence of herniation should have the following measures to control intracranial pressure
  —Intubation using rapid-sequence induction and controlled ventilation to a PCO_2 level of 35–40
  —Elevate the head of the bed 30 degrees
  —Mannitol, furosemide

ED TREATMENT

- Crucial to differentiate between aneurysm and other compressive lesions early in the ED evaluation
  —Differentiation between partial and complete oculomotor nerve palsy guides focus of treatment in the ED
- Depending on the etiology of oculomotor nerve palsy, specific medication regimens should be administered as appropriate
  —Aneurysm: control of severe hypertension with nitroprusside, decrease intracranial pressure with intubation, mannitol, furosemide, and so on
  —Intracranial tumor: control increasing intracranial pressure with intubation, mannitol, and furosemide
  —Decrease inflammation and edema with IV steroids
  —Meningitis: rapid administration of IV antibiotics; IV steroids may be useful to decrease inflammatory response and edema
  —Vasculitis and collagen vascular diseases: decrease inflammatory cell infiltration with intravenous steroids
  —Neuropathy: myasthenia gravis-edrophonium chloride test; Guillain-Barré and others are often a diagnosis of exclusion

MEDICATIONS

- Ceftriaxone: 1–2 g i.v. (peds: 50–100 mg/kg i.v.)
- Dexamethasone: 10 mg i.v. (peds: 0.15–0.5 mg/kg i.v. single dose in ED)
- Edrophonium Cl: 5–8 mg i.v. (peds: 0.15 mg/kg i.v.; one-tenth test dose is given first)
- Furosemide (adults/peds): 1 mg/kg i.v.
- Mannitol (adults/peds): 1 g/kg i.v.
- Methylprednisolone (adults/peds): 1–2 mg/kg i.v. single dose in ED

Disposition

ADMISSION CRITERIA

- Complete oculomotor nerve palsy of any etiology requires admission and emergency neurosurgical evaluation
- Incomplete oculomotor nerve palsy with abnormal CT or MRI, abnormal laboratory studies, or other focal neurologic or constitutional symptoms

DISCHARGE CRITERIA

- Incomplete oculomotor nerve palsy with negative CT or MRI, normal laboratory studies, and otherwise asymptomatic can be referred for urgent outpatient neurologic evaluation

Miscellaneous

ICD9: 378.81

ICD10: G58.8

SUGGESTED READINGS

Henry G, Little N. Neurological emergencies: a symptom oriented approach. New York: McGraw-Hill, 1985.

Ing EB, Sullivan TJ, Clarke MP, et al. Oculomotor nerve palsies in children. J Pediatr Ophthalmol Strabismus 1992;29(6):331–336.

Kodsi SR, Younge BR. Acquired oculomotor, trochlear, and abducent cranial nerve palsies in pediatric patients. Am J Ophthalmol 1992;114(5):568–574.

Richards BW, Jones FR Jr, Younge BR. Causes and prognosis in 4,278 cases of paralysis of the oculomotor, trochlear, and abducens cranial nerves. Am J Ophthalmol 1992;113(5):489–496.

Sammuels MA. Manual of neurologic therapeutics with essentials of diagnosis, 2d ed. Boston: Little, Brown and Company, 1982.

Tiffin PA, MacEwen CJ, Craig EA, et al. Acquired palsy of the oculomotor, trochlear, and abducens nerves. Eye 1996;10[Pt 3]:377–384.

Author: James Leaming

Opiate, Poisoning

Clinical Presentation

SIGNS AND SYMPTOMS

CNS

- CNS depression
- Coma
- Seizures

Gastrointestinal

- Nausea
- Vomiting
- Constipation

Cardiovascular

- Hypotension
- Bradycardia
- Palpitations

Pulmonary

- Respiratory depression
- Bronchospasm
- Pulmonary edema
- Apnea

Other

- Miosis
- Hypothermia

Withdrawal

- Hypertension
- Tachycardia
- Tachypnea
- Abdominal cramps
- Diarrhea
- Piloerection
- Yawning

MECHANISM/DESCRIPTION

- Analgesics for moderate to severe pain
- Bind to μ, κ, and δ opiate receptors in the CNS and PNS
- Physical and psychologic dependence occurs
- Peak plasma levels
  —1–2 hours PO
  —0.5–1 hour IM
  —Seconds-minutes IV or intranasal
- Street preparations of narcotic analogues may contain adulterants
  —Cocaine
  —PCP
  —Strychnine
  —Dextromethorphan
  —Quinine
  —Scopolamine

Pre-Hospital

CAUTIONS

- Transport all pills/pill bottles involved in overdose for identification in ED
- Do not induce emesis because of risk of CNS depression and aspiration
- Provide respiratory support
- Administer naloxone

Diagnosis

ESSENTIAL WORKUP

- Monitor vital signs and pulmonary status with significant exposure
  —Pulse oximetry or ABGs
  —CXR if persistent hypoxia or possible aspiration

LABORATORY

- Plasma opiate levels not clinically useful
  —Treatment based on clinical presentation, not opiate level
- Urine toxicity screen for opioids may not identify some synthetic opioids (methadone)

DIFFERENTIAL DIAGNOSIS

- Clonidine overdose
- Barbiturate overdose
- Benzodiazepine overdose
- γ-Hydroxybutyrate (GHB) overdose
- Neuroleptic overdose
- Occult head injury

PEDIATRIC CONSIDERATIONS

- Neonatal withdrawal
  —Infants born to addicted mothers
  —Onset: 12–72 hours after birth
  —Irritability, tremors, poor feeding, and dehydration
- Diphenoxylate (Lomotil): toxicity—more severe in children than adults and may be fatal

Treatment

INITIAL STABILIZATION

- ABCs
  - —Airway control essential
  - —Administer supplemental oxygen
- Administer naloxone
  - —Reverses respiratory depression and coma in opiate overdoses
  - —Intubate if naloxone does not reverse respiratory depression

ED TREATMENT

Naloxone Administration

- Start with low doses of naloxone for opiate-habituated patients
- High doses of naloxone (10 mg) may be required to reverse the effects of propoxyphene, methadone, and fentanyl
- Administer repeated doses, which reversed symptoms, as needed every 20–60 minutes
- For long-acting opioids, consider an hourly infusion of two-thirds the naloxone dose needed to reverse symptoms

Decontamination

- Administer activated charcoal for oral ingestion
- Administer whole bowel irrigation with polyethylene glycol for asymptomatic body packers

Complications

- Hypotension
  - —0.9% NS i.v. fluid bolus
  - —Trendelenburg
  - —Initiate dopamine for resistant hypotension
- Seizures
  - —Treat initially with diazepam
  - —Administer phenobarbital for persistent seizures
- Treat opiate withdrawal with clonidine or methadone

MEDICATIONS

- Activated charcoal: 1–2 g/kg PO
- Clonidine: 0.1–0.3 mg PO b.i.d. × 10 days; 0.1–0.2 mg/kg/d transdermal patch
- Diazepam: 5–10 mg (peds: 0.2–0.5 mg/kg) i.v. q10–15min
- Dopamine: 2–20 μg/kg/min, titrate to effect
- Methadone: 15–40 mg/d
- Naloxone: 0.4–2 mg (peds: 0.1 mg/kg; neonatal, 10–30 μg/kg) i.v. or i.m.
- Phenobarbital: 10–20 mg/kg i.v. (loading dose)
- Polyethylene glycol: 2 L/h until clear rectal effluent and/or passage of packets

Disposition

ADMISSION CRITERIA

- Symptomatic after oral overdose
- Repeated naloxone dosing or infusion needed to reverse symptoms
- Children younger than 5 years post-diphenoxylate ingestion should be observed for 24 hours

DISCHARGE CRITERIA

- Asymptomatic 6 hours after oral overdose
- Asymptomatic 4 hours after naloxone administration

Miscellaneous

ICD9: 850.0; 850.1; 850.2

ICD10: T460.6

SUGGESTED READINGS

Chamberlain JM, Klein BL. A comprehensive review of naloxone for the emergency physician. Am J Emerg Med 1994;12:650–660.

Kleinschmidt KC, Wainscott M, Ford MD. Opioids. In: Ford MD, Delaney KA, Ling LJ, et al, eds. Clinical toxicology. Philadelphia: WB Saunders, 2001:637–639.

Nelson LS. Opioids. In: Goldfrank LR, Flomenbaum NE, Lewin NA, et al, eds. Goldfrank's toxicologic emergencies. Stamford, CT: Appleton & Lange, 1998:975–995.

Sporer KA. Acute heroin overdose. Ann Intern Med 1999;130:584–590.

Author: Mark B. Mycyk

Opportunistic Infection

Clinical Presentation

SIGNS AND SYMPTOMS

- Signs of systemic inflammatory response syndrome
  - —Temperature >38°C or <36°C
  - —HR >90 beats/min
  - —Respiratory rate >20 breaths/min or PCO_2 <32 mm Hg
  - —WBC >12,000
- Septic shock
- New or worsening fatigue
- Confusion
- Pulmonary symptoms
  - —Tachypnea
  - —Cough
  - —Congestion
  - —Rales
- Genitourinary symptoms
  - —Dysuria
  - —Increased frequency
  - —Urinary retention
- GI symptoms
  - —Vomiting
  - —Diarrhea
  - —Bleeding
- Cardiovascular symptoms
  - —New murmur
  - —Hypotension
  - —Tachycardia

MECHANISM/DESCRIPTION

- Opportunistic infection occurs when the host suffers a decrease in resistance against normally nonpathogenic organisms
- Type of immunocompromise predicts the type of infection that will occur
- Cell-mediated deficiency
  - —Hematologic malignancies
  - —Lymphoma
  - —High-dose glucocorticoid therapy
  - —Autoimmune disorders
  - —Viral infections
  - —Cytotoxic drugs/chemotherapy
  - —Radiation therapy
- Neutrophil impairment/depletion
  - —Cytotoxic drugs
  - —Aplastic anemia
  - —Drug reactions
    - -Dapsone
  - —Neoplastic invasion of bone marrow
  - —Arsenic
  - —Penicillin
  - —Chloramphenicol
  - —Procainamide
  - —Vitamin deficiencies
- Cell-mediated dysfunction associated with intracellular organisms infections
  - —*Legionella*
  - —*Nocardia*
  - —*Salmonella*
  - —Mycobacteria
- Neutrophil disorders associated with
  - —*Staphylococcus* and α-hemolytic *Streptococcus*
  - —Enteric organisms and anaerobes

Pre-Hospital

N/A

Diagnosis

ESSENTIAL WORKUP

- Full workup indicated due to impaired immunity
  - —Signs of infection in the immunocompromised patient may not be present
  - —Can present with subtle signs with rapid deterioration
  - —Signs such as fever must lead to a full evaluation of the patient
  - —Thorough physical exam critical to search for site of infection
- Physical exam
  - —Inspect skin and mucosa carefully for a portal of entry
  - —Examine oral mucosa and perianal area for erythema and palpate for tenderness or crepitus

LABORATORY

- Cultures (aerobic, anaerobic, fungal, viral as indicated)
  - —Urine
  - —Blood
  - —Wound
  - —Fecal
- CBC with differential
  - —Neutropenia or leukocytosis
- Urinalysis for presence of WBC, nitrite, leukocyte esterase
- Electrolytes, BUN/Cr, glucose
  - —Anion gap acidosis suggests severe infection
- ABG for hypoxia/acidosis
- Lactate level
  - —Elevated value suggestive of serious infection
- PT/PTT for evidence of disseminated intravascular coagulation
- CSF analysis if signs of CNS infection

IMAGING/SPECIAL TESTS

- CXR

DIFFERENTIAL DIAGNOSIS

N/A

Treatment

INITIAL STABILIZATION

- ABCs
- Initiate IV 0.9% NS
  —500-mL bolus for hypotension
- Oxygen
- Cardiac monitor for unstable vital signs
- Early initiation of antibiotic therapy

ED TREATMENT

- Strict isolation
- Antibiotics
  —Combination of expanded spectrum penicillin (mezlocillin, ticarcillin, piperacillin) and aminoglycoside (amikacin, tobramycin)
  —Monotherapy with a third-generation cephalosporin (ceftazidime, cefepime), fluoroquinones (levofloxacin, gatifloxacin) or other broad-spectrum antimicrobials (imipenem/cilastatin) may be considered if aminoglycosides contraindicated
  —Vancomycin is not recommended as part of initial therapy unless there is a high incidence of methicillin-resistant organisms in the area
  —Antifungals (amphotericin B, fluconazole) if patient is on adequate antibiotics for 1 week

MEDICATIONS

- Amphotericin B: 0.25 mg/kg i.v. q.d.
- Cefepime: 1–2 g q12h i.v.
- Ceftazidime: 1–2 g (peds: 100–150 mg/kg/24 h) i.v. q8–12h
- Fluconazole: 400 mg first dose then 200–400 mg i.v. q.d. (peds: 3–6 mg/kg/24 h i.v. q12h)
- Gatifloxacin: 400 mg i.v. q.d.
- Imipenem/cilastatin: 500–1,000 mg i.v. q6–8h, maximum 50 mg/kg/d or 4,000 mg/d
- Levofloxacin: 500 mg i.v. q.d.
- Piperacillin: 3 g q4h over 30 minutes
- Ticarcillin: 3 g (peds: 200–300 mg/kg/24 h) i.v. q4h over 30 minutes
- Vancomycin: 1–2 g i.v. q12h (peds: 10–50 mg/kg/24 h i.v. q6h)

Disposition

ADMISSION CRITERIA

- Suspected or confirmed systemic infection

DISCHARGE CRITERIA

- Systemic infection excluded

Miscellaneous

ICD9: N/A

ICD10: N/A

SUGGESTED READINGS

Emmanouilides C, Glaspy J. Opportunistic infections in oncologic patients. Hematol Oncol Clin North Am 1996;10(4):841–860.

Daar ES, Meyer RD. Bacterial and fungal infections. Med Clin North Am 1992;17(1):173–195.

Giamarellou H. Empiric therapy for infections in the febrile, neutropenic, compromised host. Med Clin North Am 1992;79(3):559–578.

Pizzo PA. The compromised host. In: Bennett JC et al, eds. Cecil's textbook of medicine. Philadelphia: WB Saunders, 1996:908–915.

Author: Elicia Sinor Kennedy

Optic Artery Occlusion

Clinical Presentation

SIGNS AND SYMPTOMS

- Sudden painless monocular loss of vision
- "Count fingers" or "light perception" visual acuity (90%)
- Partial field defects
  - —If only a branch of the central retinal artery (CRA) involved
- Normal visual acuity (rare)
  - —If the macula spared by anomalous circulation from the choroid (a cilioretinal vessel)
- Prior episodes of sudden temporary visual loss
  - —Lasts a few seconds to minutes (amaurosis fugax)
  - —Caused by transient embolic phenomena or decreased ocular blood flow

Retinal Appearance

- Emboli visualized within the vascular tree of the retina
  - —Appears as glinting white or yellow flecks (Hollenhorst plaques) within the vessels
- Ischemic edema visible within 15–20 minutes of occlusion
- Affected arteries empty or showing dark red stationary or barely pulsatile segmented rouleaux ("box caring")
- Within 1–2 hours
  - —Opacification of the usually transparent infarcting retinal nerve layer occurs
  - —"Cherry-red spot" remaining over the fovea (only area where there is very thin retina allowing the vascular choroid to show through)

MECHANISM/DESCRIPTION

- CRA
  - —First branch of the ophthalmic artery that arises from the internal carotid artery
  - —Retinal arteries are not innervated but depend on autoregulation (e.g., response to resistance pressure and PCO_2) for dilation and constriction
- Ischemic injury results from obstruction of blood flow by any embolus or thrombus small enough to enter the ophthalmic artery and large enough to block the retinal artery (or one of its branches)
- Unlike cerebral neural tissue that is completely destroyed within 10 minutes of complete ischemia, the nerve layer of the retina may remain viable for up to 2 hours due to the dual circulation of the retina, with the separate choroidal blood flow nourishing the sensitive outer layer of the retina while the inner half is anoxic

ETIOLOGY

- Cause
  - —Embolic phenomena (majority)
  - —Thrombosis
  - —Spasm (postulated but unproven)
- Embolic events related to
  - —Atherosclerotic disease (majority)
  - —Valvular heart disease
  - —Atrial myxoma
  - —Dissection of the ophthalmic artery in the region of the cribriform plate (rare)
- Thrombosis occurs with
  - —Giant cell (temporal) arteritis
  - —Disseminated lupus erythematosus
  - —Other collagen vascular diseases (polyarteritis nodosa)
  - —Risk factors for thrombotic events
    - -Oral contraceptives
    - -Polycythemia vera
    - -Sickle cell disease
    - -Syphilis
    - -Behçet's syndrome
    - -Migraine

Pre-Hospital

N/A

Diagnosis

ESSENTIAL WORKUP

- Accurate funduscopy essential
- Diagnosis made by comparison of the retinas of the two eyes, looking for
  - —Unilateral diffuse pallor
  - —Macular "cherry-red spot"
  - —Focal or diffuse attenuation of the retinal arterioles
  - —"Box caring" the nonmobile or barely pulsatile segmental rouleaux within the retinal vessels
- Do not delay treatment while waiting for laboratory results

LABORATORY

- CBC with differential and platelet count
- PT/PTT
- Electrolytes, BUN/Cr, glucose
- ESR for giant cell arteritis (in patients older than 55 years)
- ANA
- Rheumatoid factor
- RPR
- Hemoglobin electrophoresis
- Serum protein electrophoresis

IMAGING/SPECIAL TESTS

- Carotid artery evaluation by US and Doppler
- Cardiac evaluation
  - —EKG
  - —Echocardiography
  - —Holter monitoring
- Fluorescein angiography or electroretinography to confirm the diagnosis

DIFFERENTIAL DIAGNOSIS

- Acute ophthalmic artery occlusion (treatment is the same as for CRA occlusion)
- Arteritic ischemic optic neuropathy
- Tay-Sachs disease causes "cherry-red spot"
- Central retinal vein occlusion
- Retinal detachment
- Age-related macular degeneration
- Recent inadvertent intraocular injection of gentamicin

PEDIATRIC CONSIDERATIONS

- Cause in young patients: embolism from valvular heart disease

Treatment

INITIAL STABILIZATION

- Initiate treatment *as soon as the diagnosis is made and before the workup proceeds* if the CRA occlusion is <24 hours old
  - —Only immediate treatment may help to salvage or restore sight to the affected eye

ED TREATMENT

- Immediate massage of the globe of the eye
  - —Apply digital pressure to the eye (a few seconds on and off) to dislodge the embolus or thrombus from a larger to a smaller less important vessel
  - —Perform for only 1–2 minutes, as any effect will be noticeable within that time
- Increase CO_2 to dilate the retinal vessels
  - —Initiate rebreathing the patient's own exhalation into a paper bag
  - —Administer Carbogen (95% oxygen, 5% carbon dioxide) q10 min q1–2h
- Urgent ophthalmologic consultation
- Anterior chamber paracentesis with 25-gauge needle
- Administer carbonic anhydrase inhibitor (acetazolamide) or topical β-blockers (timolol) to lower intraocular pressure

MEDICATIONS

- Acetazolamide: 500 mg i.v.
- Timolol 0.25–1.0%: 1 drop to eye
- Consider high-dose systemic corticosteroids if suspected inflammatory arteritis

Disposition

ADMISSION CRITERIA

- Acute CRA occlusion for workup for source of embolic phenomena or thrombosis

DISCHARGE CRITERIA

- Chronic retinal artery occlusion with no evidence of active disease can be worked up as an outpatient

Miscellaneous

ICD9: 362.30

ICD10: H34.2

SUGGESTED READINGS

Haase CG, Buchner T. Microemboli are not a prerequisite in retinal artery occlusive diseases. Eye 1998;12:659–662.

Hayreh SS, Podhajsky PA, Zimmerman B. Ocular manifestations of giant cell arteritis. Am J Ophthalmol 1998;125(4): 509–520.

LaVene D, Halpern J, Jagoda A. Loss of vision. Emerg Med Clin North Am 1995;13(3):539–560.

Morgan A, Hemphill RR. Acute visual change. Emerg Med Clin North Am 1998;16(4):825–843.

Whitmore PV. Sudden painless visual loss, retinal causes. Clin Geriatr Med 1999;15(1):15–24.

Author: G. Carolyn Clayton (First edition author: Evan Liu)

Optic Neuritis

Clinical Presentation

SIGNS AND SYMPTOMS

- Visual loss occurring over days (rarely over hours)
  - —Adults usually unilateral
  - —Bilateral visual loss more common in children
- Retrobulbar pain: increased with movement of the affected eye
- Light, color vision, and depth perception loss more pronounced than visual acuity loss
- Afferent pupillary defect occurring in unilateral cases
- Visual field defects
  - —Central scotoma
- Funduscopic exam usually reveals either
  - —Swollen (papillitis) or normal disk
- Uhthoff's sign
  - —Visual deficit occurring with exercise or increased body temperature
  - —Unusual sign seen occasionally

MECHANISM/DESCRIPTION

- Inflammatory process of the optic nerve, characterized by myelin destruction
- Grouped by site of inflammation
  - —Papillitis: inflammation of the optic disk
  - —Retrobulbar neuritis: inflammation of the optic nerve proximal to the globe

ETIOLOGY

- Between ages 15 and 45 years
- Idiopathic
  - —Most common
  - —Single isolated events
- Multiple sclerosis
  - —20–50% of patients with optic neuritis
- Viral infections
  - —Chicken pox
  - —Measles
  - —Mononucleosis
  - —Herpes zoster
  - —Encephalitis
- Granulomatous inflammation
  - —Tuberculosis
  - —Syphilis
  - —Sarcoidosis
  - —Cryptococcal infection
- Systemic lupus erythematosus
- HIV
  - —Cytomegalovirus
  - —Toxoplasmosis
  - —Histoplasmosis
  - —*Cryptococcus*
- Lyme disease
- Contiguous inflammation of meninges, orbit, sinuses, and intraocular inflammation
- Postviral optic neuritis
  - —Usually occurs 4–6 weeks after a nonspecific viral illness
- Drug induced
  - —Ethambutol
  - —Tamoxifen

Pre-Hospital

N/A

Diagnosis

ESSENTIAL WORKUP

- History
  - —Age
  - —Speed of onset of symptoms
  - —Associated symptoms
  - —Previous episodes
- Check BP
- Complete ophthalmologic and neurologic examination, especially assessment of
  - —Pupillary function
  - —Color vision (Ishihara color plates)
  - —Evaluation of the vitreous body for cells
  - —Dilated retinal exam

LABORATORY

- CBC
- ESR
- RPR, FTA-ABS
- Lyme titer
- ANA
- PPD testing

IMAGING/SPECIAL TESTS

- CXR for tuberculosis
- CT scan or MRI of brain and orbits
  - —Inflammation of the retrobulbar optic nerve during the acute phase may appear as enlargement, thus falsely raising the issue of an optic nerve mass
  - —Visual field testing (preferably automated testing, such as Octopus or Humphrey)

DIFFERENTIAL DIAGNOSIS

- Acute papilledema
- Ischemic optic neuropathy
- Severe systemic hypertension
- Intracranial tumor compressing the afferent visual pathway
- Orbital mass compressing the optic nerve
- Toxic or metabolic neuropathy
  - —Heavy metal poisoning
  - —Anemia
  - —Malnutrition
  - —Alcohols
  - —Chloroquine
  - —INH
- Leber's hereditary optic atrophy

Treatment

INITIAL STABILIZATION

N/A

ED TREATMENT

- Early ophthalmologic and neurologic consultations
- Avoid prednisone, ACTH, and other corticosteroids
  - —Steroid therapy may worsen the course of optic neuritis
  - —Probably not helpful in the treatment of multiple sclerosis

Disposition

ADMISSION CRITERIA

- Bilateral vision loss
- If other sources of acute vision loss cannot be ruled out

DISCHARGE CRITERIA

- Good home support systems
- No other medical or social reason for admission
- Unilateral visual impairment

Miscellaneous

ICD9: 377.3

ICD10: H46

SUGGESTED READINGS

Kosmorsky GS. Sudden painless visual loss, optic nerve and circulatory disturbances. Clin Geriatr Med 1999;15(1):1–13.

Newman NJ. Optic neuropathy. Neurology 1996;46:315–322.

Purvin VA. Optic neuropathies for the neurologist. Semin Neurol 2000;20(1): 97–110.

Van Stavern GP. Management of optic neuritis and multiple sclerosis. Curr Opin Ophthalmol 2001;12(6):400–407.

Author: G. Carolyn Clayton (First edition author: Evan Liu)

Organophosphate, Poisoning

Clinical Presentation

SIGNS AND SYMPTOMS

- Classic presentation: cholinergic toxidrome
  - *DUMBELS*
    - *D*iarrhea/*d*iaphoresis
    - *U*rination
    - *M*iosis/*m*uscle fasciculations
    - *B*radycardia, *b*ronchorrhea, *b*ronchospasm
    - *E*mesis
    - *L*acrimation
    - *S*alivation
- Chronic intermittent exposure, nonspecific symptoms
  - Weakness
  - Fatigue
  - Malaise
  - Anorexia

Mild Exposure

- Visual
  - Miosis
  - Decreased visual acuity
- CNS
  - Headache
  - Dizziness
  - Tremors of tongue and eyelids
  - Anxiety
  - Weakness
- GI
  - Anorexia

Moderate Exposure

- CNS
  - Muscle fasciculation followed by flaccid paralysis
  - Respiratory muscle weakness
  - Incoordination
- GI
  - Nausea
  - Vomiting
  - Abdominal cramps
- Exocrine glands
  - Salivation
  - Lacrimation

Severe Exposure

- Visual
  - Pinpoint nonreactive pupils
- Respiratory
  - Respiratory difficulty
  - Pulmonary edema
- Cardiovascular
  - Bradycardia
  - Heart block
- CNS
  - Convulsion
  - Coma
  - No sphincter tone
- GI
  - Diarrhea

Muscarinic Manifestations

- Respiratory
  - Bronchoconstriction
  - Wheezing
  - Dyspnea
  - Increased bronchial secretion
  - Cough
  - Pulmonary edema
- Cardiovascular
  - Bradycardia
  - Cyanosis
- GI
  - Nausea, vomiting
  - Abdominal pain
  - Diarrhea
  - Tenesmus
  - Fecal incontinence
- Exocrine glands
  - Diaphoresis
  - Salivation
  - Lacrimation
- Pupils
  - Miosis, occasionally unequal
- Ciliary body
  - Blurred vision
- Bladder
  - Frequency
  - Urinary incontinence

Nicotinic Manifestations

- Striated muscle
  - Fasciculation
  - Weakness including respiratory muscles
- Sympathetic ganglia
  - Mydriasis
  - Tachycardia
  - Hypertension
  - Bronchodilation

CNS

- Agitation
- Restlessness
- Tremors
- Confusion
- Depression
- Ataxia
- Weakness
- Coma
- Seizures
- Death

MECHANISM/DESCRIPTION

- Organophosphates (pesticides and nerve agents) irreversibly bind to cholinesterase, causing deactivation of acetylcholinesterase
- Initial accumulation of acetylcholine at neural synapse results in cholinergic overdrive (central and peripheral)
- Predominate effects (muscarinic, nicotinic, CNS) may vary and can overlap
- Death usually secondary to respiratory failure resulting from weakness of respiratory muscles, pulmonary edema, and central depression of respiratory drive

PEDIATRIC CONSIDERATIONS

- *DUMBELS* (symptoms) difficult to differentiate in toddlers
- Common symptoms: miosis, salivation, and muscle weakness
- Seizures found in 25% (3% of adults)

Pre-Hospital

CAUTIONS

- Decontamination is initial priority
  - *DABC*: *d*econtaminate, *a*irway, *b*reathing, *c*irculation
  - Remove all clothes and store as toxic waste (double bagged)
- Protection of health care workers of utmost importance
  - Inpenetrable gloves (neoprene, nitrile), gowns, eye protection
- Decontaminate skin with soap and water
  - Shower or gentle scrubbing ideal if done before entrance into the ED
- Maintain airway and oxygenate
- IV access and place on cardiac monitor

Diagnosis

ESSENTIAL WORKUP

- Inquire about possible exposure, occupation, recent insecticide in home, mislabeled or poorly stored insecticides
  - Obtain original container if suicide attempt
- Look for parasympathetic and CNS signs with muscle weakness or paralysis

LABORATORY

- RBC and plasma cholinesterase levels to confirm diagnosis
  - RBC (true) cholinesterase level is best reflection of synaptic inhibition (a send-out lab)
  - Plasma (pseudo) cholinesterase level not as reliable but more timely
  - Cholinesterase levels
    - Latent exposure: >50% of normal value
    - Mild exposure: 20–50% of normal value
    - Moderate exposure: 10–20% of normal value
    - Severe exposure: <10% of normal value
  - Do not wait for cholinesterase results before administering treatment
- CBC
- Electrolytes, glucose, BUN, creatinine
- ABG when respiratory symptoms

IMAGING/SPECIAL TESTS

- CXR if respiratory difficulty is present or suspect pulmonary edema
- EKG
  - Dysrhythmias (atrial fibrillation, ventricular tachycardia, torsades de pointes, QT prolongation)
  - Bradycardia
  - Heart block
  - ST-T-wave abnormalities
- CT scan of head for altered mental status when diagnosis uncertain

DIFFERENTIAL DIAGNOSIS

Mild to Moderate Exposure

- Gastroenteritis
- Asthma
- Venomous arthropods bite (black widow, scorpion)
- Nonspecific viral syndrome
- Progressive peripheral neuropathy (Guillain-Barré syndrome)
- Carbon monoxide

Severe Exposure

- Narcotic overdose
- Coma and miosis
  - —PCP, meprobamate, phenothiazine, clonidine
  - —Muscarinic-containing mushrooms—cholinergic crisis without nicotinic symptoms
  - —Nicotinic poisoning
- Metabolic and infectious
  - —Ketoacidosis, sepsis, meningitis, encephalitis
  - —Hypoglycemia
  - —Reye's syndrome
- Neurologic
  - —CVA
  - —Subdural or epidural hematoma
  - —Postictal state

Treatment

INITIAL STABILIZATION

- Decontaminate ABCs
  - —Decontamination and protection of staff
  - —Maintain airway and oxygenate
  - —For unstable airway, intubate, and ventilate
  - —IV access with D5W 0.9% NS
- Altered mental status: administer thiamine, glucose, and naloxone (Narcan)

ED TREATMENT

- Atropine
  - —Blocks acetylcholine at muscarinic receptor sites
  - —No effect on nicotinic receptors
  - —Onset of action in 1–4 minutes, peaks at 8 minutes
  - —Goal of therapy/end point
    - -Drying secretions of tracheobronchial tree
  - —Administer test dose 1–2 mg i.v./i.m.
    - -No clinical response: double dose every 5 minutes until muscarinic findings subside
  - —Dose: 1–4 mg i.v. q5min (peds: 0.05–0.2 mg/kg)
  - —Common pitfalls in therapy
    - -Not giving enough atropine
    - -Using pupillary findings (mydriasis) as end point of atropine therapy
    - -Dilated pupils or tachycardia are not contraindications to the administration of atropine
- *Pralidoxime (2-PAM)*
  - —Regenerates cholinesterase by reversing the phosphorylation of the enzyme
  - —Synergistic with atropine and muscarinic signs and symptoms will start to resolve within 10–40 minutes
  - —Side effects include neuromuscular blockade with rapid infusion, respiratory arrest, hypertension, nausea/vomiting, dizziness, and blurred vision
  - —End point is resolution of muscle weakness and fasciculations
  - —Effective only if given before enzyme aging occurs, at which time cholinesterase is permanently inactivated
  - —Onset of aging varies between products
  - —No restriction to its use even if 24–48 hours have passed
- *Supportive care*
  - —Dermal decontamination: remove clothes and flush skin with water
  - —Gastric lavage
    - -Gastric emptying should be done with continuous suction via a NGT
    - -Handle contents with care, and avoid coming in direct contact with it to prevent exposure
  - —Respiratory difficulty
    - -Frequent respiratory secretion suction required
    - -Treat bronchospasm with atropine and not bronchodilators
    - -Tachycardia may result from hypoxia induced by pulmonary secretions and bronchospasm
    - -Atropine will dry secretions and paradoxically lower the heart rate in light of more effective oxygenation
    - -Intubate and ventilate if necessary

MEDICATIONS

- Atropine: 1–4 mg (peds: 0.05–0.2 mg/kg) i.v. q5min (see previous section for details)
- Dextrose: D50W, 1 amp (25 g) of 50% dextrose (peds: 2–4 mL/kg D25W) IVP
- Naloxone (Narcan): 2 mg (peds: 0.1 mg/kg) i.v. or i.m.
- Pralidoxime: 1–2 g (peds: 20–40 mg/kg) dissolved in 0.9% NS over 30-minute i.v.; repeat in 1 hour if necessary, then every 3–8 hours as needed
  - —Some propose a continuous infusion of 500 mg/h to obtain the necessary 4 mg/L effective in treating toxicity

Disposition

ADMISSION CRITERIA

- ICU admission for mild, moderate, or severe exposure confirmed with a response to atropine
- Any symptomatic patient should be admitted for monitoring
- Avoid CNS-depressive effects of opioids, phenothiazines, and antihistamines, as these may potentiate toxicity of organophosphates

DISCHARGE CRITERIA

- Asymptomatic for 6–12 hours after exposure
- Ensure close reliable follow-up and specific instructions when to return for evaluation

Miscellaneous

ICD9: 989.3

ICD10: T60.0

SEE ALSO: HAZMAT, CHEMICAL WEAPONS POISONING

SUGGESTED READINGS

Ford MD, Delaney KA, Ling LJ, et al, eds. Clinical toxicology. Philadelphia: WB Saunders, 2001.

Minton NA, Murray SG. A review of organophosphate poisoning. Med Toxicol 1988;3:350–375.

Tafuri J, Toberts J. Organophosphate poisoning. Ann Emerg Med 1987;16: 193–202.

Williams JL, DeBisschop HC, Verstraete AG, et al. Cholinesterase reactivation in organophosphorus poisoned patients depends on the plasma concentrations of the oxime pralidoxime methylsulphate and of the organophosphate. Arch Toxicol 1993;67:79–84.

Zwiener RJ, Ginsburg CM. Organophosphate and carbamate poisoning in infants and children. Pediatrics 1988;81:121–126.

Author: Sean Bryant

Osgood-Schlatter Disease

Clinical Presentation

SIGNS AND SYMPTOMS

- Pain and swelling over the tibial tuberosity
  - —Often bilateral but unilateral cases more symptomatic
- Pain exacerbated by running, jumping, and kneeling activities
- Increased pain while sitting with knees flexed

MECHANISM/DESCRIPTION

- Inflammation from repetitive stress and secondary partial avulsion injuries at the bone–tendon junction of the patellar tendon into the ossification center of the tibial tuberosity
  - —Fragmentation may lead to heterotopic ossification anterior to the tibial tuberosity
- Fusion of the tubercle to the tibia normally occurs by 18 years of age
  - —Eliminates any further symptoms

ETIOLOGY

- Seen primarily in active adolescent boys between 10 and 15 years of age and girls between 8 and 13 years of age
  - —Two to three times greater incidence in boys
  - —Fivefold greater incidence in very athletic children

Pre-Hospital

N/A

Diagnosis

ESSENTIAL WORKUP

- Clinical diagnosis
  - —Typically pain, swelling, and tenderness localized over the tibial tubercle
  - —Examination of the knee joint unremarkable

IMAGING/SPECIAL TESTS

- Knee radiographs in unilateral cases to exclude potentially serious pathology only if presentation not typical for Osgood-Schlatter disease

DIFFERENTIAL DIAGNOSIS

- Fracture
- Legg-Calve-Perthes disease
  - —Referred hip pain
- Osteochondritis desiccans
- Osteomyelitis
- Patellofemoral syndrome
- Septic joint
- Sinding-Larsen-Johansson syndrome
  - —Apophyseal injury at the inferior pole of the patella
- Slipped-capital femoral epiphysis
  - —Referred hip pain
- Stress fracture
- Tendinitis or bursitis

Treatment

INITIAL STABILIZATION

- Place leg in position of comfort
- Immobilize if necessary to minimize pain

ED TREATMENT

- Mainstay of therapy
  - —NSAIDs
  - —Rest for 2–4 months is recommended
  - —Ice to the affected area after activity
  - —Compress the painful area with an elastic bandage
  - —Elevate the leg
- Mild cases
  - —Avoid overuse until symptomatic improvement
  - —Reassurance of benign, self-limited course
  - —Stretching and strengthening exercises of quadriceps and hamstrings
- Severe cases
  - —Surgical excision of the prominent tibial tubercle or ossicle under the patellar tendon only after complete skeletal maturity

MEDICATIONS

- Ibuprofen: 10 mg/kg PO q6h; maximum 50 mg/kg/d

Disposition

ADMISSION CRITERIA

None

DISCHARGE CRITERIA

- Discharge all patients

Miscellaneous

ICD9: 732.4

ICD10: M92.5

SUGGESTED READINGS

Greene WB, ed. Essentials of musculoskeletal care, 2nd ed. Rosemont, IL: American Academy of Orthopedic Surgeons, 2001:684–685.

Morrissy RT, Weinstein SL, eds. Lovell and Winter's pediatric orthopaedics, 5th ed. Philadelphia: Lippincott Williams & Wilkins, 2001:1280–1281.

Orava S, Malinen L, Karpakka J, et al. Results of surgical treatment of unresolved Osgood-Schlatter lesion. Ann Chir Gynaecol 2000;89(4):298–302.

Peck DM. Apophyseal injuries in the young adult. Am Fam Physician 1995;51(8): 1891–1895.

Author: Raj J. Patel

Osteogenesis Imperfecta

Clinical Presentation

SIGNS AND SYMPTOMS

- Osteogenesis imperfecta refers to multiple heritable defects that lead to brittle bones and are often associated with other connective tissue abnormalities

Bones

- Multiple recurrent fractures (especially in long bones) are the hallmark of this disease
- Fractures may be present at birth or may recur in the elderly
- All bones are affected to some extent (see Imaging/Special Tests)

Eyes

- *Blue sclera* are another hallmark of the disease
- No visual changes are reported

Ears

- Hearing loss usually begins in adolescence; >90% of patients have some deficit by age 30 years
- Hearing loss is generally sensorineural, although some middle ear abnormalities have been demonstrated

Other

- Yellow-brown or blue-gray discoloration and abnormal shape of teeth
- Shares several features with Ehlers-Danlos syndrome: loose joints, valve problems, and vascular abnormalities
- Thyroid abnormalities may be seen
- Extreme cases may result in perinatal death

MECHANISM/DESCRIPTION

- Inherited abnormality of procollagen amino acid sequence
- Bone hypomineralization and incomplete ossification result in brittle bones
- Abnormal collagen affects all connective tissue to varying degrees
- The time course is variable, with most cases involving fractures during childhood followed by quiescence during adolescence and early adulthood

ETIOLOGY

- Procollagen defects result in bone and connective tissue matrix abnormalities
- Defects in different sites on the procollagen protein chain result in more severe forms
- Defects are inherited, either autosomal recessive (generally milder) or autosomal dominant (more severe)
- Lethal cases involve sporadic or new mutations
- Ehlers-Danlos syndrome involves mutations of the same procollagen protein in a different location

PEDIATRIC CONSIDERATIONS

- Most cases involve pathologic fractures during childhood
- Multiple fractures often initiate evaluation for abuse, but the possibility of pathologic fractures also should be considered

Pre-Hospital

- Personnel should obtain information about mechanism or social factors that point toward pathologic fracture versus nonaccidental trauma

Diagnosis

ESSENTIAL WORKUP

- Diagnosis is usually made as a combination of clinical and radiographic findings
- History of repeated fractures or fractures with unimpressive mechanism
- Thorough search for other tender areas and evaluation of eyes, teeth, and joints is important for diagnosis
- Careful examination of neurovascular status distal to fracture

LABORATORY

- Evaluate for metabolic derangements such as hyperparathyroidism, vitamin C or D deficiencies, and calcium/phosphate abnormalities
- DNA studies may be indicated for familial analysis, prenatal testing, and genetic counseling
- Tissue biopsy is controversial but may help differentiate from tumors

IMAGING/SPECIAL TESTS

- Radiographs of fracture sites may reveal osteopenia (usually mild), crumpled long bones ("accordion femora"), or incomplete ossification at physes
- Skeletal survey is mandatory, especially in children
- Skull films may show "wormian" appearance of irregular ossification
- "Popcorn-like" deposits on long-bone ends is a poor prognostic finding
- Formal audiologic testing as an outpatient is required in older patients

DIFFERENTIAL DIAGNOSIS

- Nonaccidental trauma in children
- Ehlers-Danlos syndrome
- Hypophosphatasia
- Achondroplasia
- Scurvy
- Congenital syphilis
- Celiac disease

Treatment

INITIAL STABILIZATION

- ABCs of trauma come first, depending on the mechanism of injury
- Fracture immobilization/splinting

ED TREATMENT

- Specific fracture management dictated by type and location of injury
- Orthopedic consultation regarding the need for traction or operative fixation
- No specific treatment for osteogenesis imperfecta exists at present

MEDICATIONS

- Pain medications as indicated
- Elderly women may benefit from calcium (1–1.5 g/d) and estrogen replacement (0.625 mg/d)

Disposition

ADMISSION CRITERIA

- Admission is determined by multiple trauma or operative needs for fracture repair
- Pediatric patients may need admission to investigate the possibility of nonaccidental trauma

DISCHARGE CRITERIA

- Patients may be considered for outpatient management if isolated fracture is present and appropriate home resources are available
- Most patients should be discharged with orthopedic and primary physician follow-up

Miscellaneous

ICD9: 756.51

ICD10: Q78.0

SUGGESTED READINGS

Chandrasoma P, Taylor CR. Concise pathology. East Norwalk, CT: Appleton & Lange, 1991.

Cole WG. Advances in osteogenesis imperfecta. Clin Orthop 2002;(401): 6–16.

McKusick VA. Heritable disorders of connective tissue, 4th ed. St. Louis: CV Mosby, 1972.

Prockop DJ. Heritable disorders of connective tissue. In: Wilson JD, et al., eds. Harrison's principles of internal medicine, 12th ed. New York: McGraw-Hill, 1991:1860.

Sillence DO. Osteogenesis imperfecta: an expanding panorama of variance. Clin Orthop 1981;(159):11–25.

Author: Daniel Davis

Osteomyelitis

Clinical Presentation

SIGNS AND SYMPTOMS

- Pain: localized, deep, dull, and throbbing
- Chills and fever
- Malaise, nausea, vomiting
- Tenderness to palpation, warmth, erythema, edema, decreased range of motion
- Drainage of sinus tract
- Reluctance to use extremity

MECHANISM/DESCRIPTION

- Osteomyelitis (OM): infection of bone with ongoing inflammatory destruction of bone
- Usually bacterial but fungal OM does exist

ETIOLOGY

Hematogenous OM

- Seeding of bacteria to bone from remote site of infection
- Children have acute OM and adults subacute or chronic
- Hematogenous OM of long bones rarely occurs in adults
- Most children with acute hematogenous OM have no preceding illness
- One third have history of trauma to affected area
- *Staphylococcus aureus* is most common cause of OM in all ages
- Neonates: *S. aureus,* Enterobacteriaceae, group A and B streptococci, and *Escherichia coli*
- Children: *S. aureus,* group A streptococci, *Haemophilus influenzae,* Enterobacteriaceae
  —*Salmonella:* common in sickle cell disease
- Adults: *S. aureus,* Enterobacteriaceae, *Pseudomonas,* gram-negative rods, *Staphylococcus epidermidis*
- Illicit drug users: *Candida, Pseudomonas, Serratia marcescens*
- Prolonged neutropenia: *Candida, Aspergillus, Rhizopus, Blastomyces, Coccidioides*

Hematogenous Vertebral OM

- Uncommon
- Most prevalent in adults older than 45 years
- Involves the disk and vertebra above and below
- Often in setting of long-term urinary catheter placement, IV drug abusers (IVDAs), cancer, hemodialysis, or diabetes
- IVDA: OM of pubic symphysis, sternoclavicular, and sacroiliac joints
- Lumbar vertebrae most common, followed by thoracic, then cervical
- Posterior extension leads to epidural/subdural abscess or meningitis
- Anterior extension may lead to paravertebral, retropharyngeal, mediastinal, subphrenic, retroperitoneal, or psoas abscess

Direct or Contiguous OM

- Organism(s) directly seeded in bone due to trauma; spread from adjacent site of infection or from surgery
- More common in adults and adolescents
- *S. aureus,* Enterobacteriaceae, *Pseudomonas*
- Normal vascularity
  —*S. aureus* and *S. epidermis,* gram-negative bacilli, and anaerobic organisms
- Vascular insufficiency/diabetes
  —Small bones of feet are common sites
  —Infection resulting from minor trauma, infected nail beds, cellulitis, or skin ulceration
  —If ulcer size >2 cm^2 and >3 mm in depth, bone involvement is likely
  —Polymicrobial including anaerobes
  —If bone palpated, high correlation with OM
- Puncture wound through tennis shoe: *S. aureus, Pseudomonas*

Chronic OM

- Osteomyelitis that persists or recurs
- Distinguishing characteristic is necrotic bone
- *S. epidermidis, S. aureus, Pseudomonas aeruginosa, Serratia marcescens, and E. coli*

Pre-Hospital

N/A

Diagnosis

- Standard is culture and bone biopsy
- Polymorphonuclear cells are highly suggestive of OM
- Two of following four need to be present for diagnosis
  —Pus on aspiration
  —Positive bacterial culture from bone or blood
  —Classic signs and symptoms of OM
  —Radiographic changes typical of osteomyelitis

ESSENTIAL WORKUP

- CBC; WBC count (may be elevated but often normal)
- ESR and C-reactive protein (usually elevated)
- Blood cultures (positive in $>50\%$ of children)
- X-rays
- Culture from bone biopsy or aspiration of pus to confirm diagnosis and obtain material for culture
  —Culture of sinus or drainage from wound can be misleading

IMAGING/SPECIAL TESTS

- X-rays
  —Initially normal for 7–10 days after onset of symptoms
  —Earliest finding is periosteal elevation, followed by cortical erosions, then new bone formation
  —40–50% of focal bone loss needed to detect lucency on x-rays, so fewer than a third of cases have diagnostic findings at 10 days
- Bone scan
  —Technetium-99m methylene diphosphonate (^{99m}Tc-MDP)
  —Measures increase in bone metabolic activity
  —95% sensitive but less specific than MRI
  —Bone scan abnormal after 1–2 days of symptoms
  —Negative study 24 hours after onset of symptoms rules out acute OM
- Leukocyte scintigraphy
  —Indium-111-labeled WBCs
  —More specific but less sensitive than bone scan
  —Difficult to distinguish bone inflammation from soft-tissue inflammation (i.e., cellulitis, tumors, inflammatory arthritis)
  —False negative in chronic infection

- CT
  - —Reveals bone edema, cortical destruction, periosteal reaction, small foci of gas or foreign bodies, joint surface damage, and soft-tissue involvement when plain films not helpful
  - —Useful in vertebral OM
- MRI
  - —As sensitive as ^{99m}Tc-MDP scan but more specific
  - —Reveals bone edema, cortical destruction, periosteal reaction, joint surface damage, and soft-tissue involvement before x-rays
  - —Effective in early detection (diagnosis may be evident by MRI before scintigraphy)
  - —Test of choice to identify vertebral OM
  - —Occasional false-positive results in trauma, previous surgical procedures, or neuropathic joint disease

DIFFERENTIAL DIAGNOSIS

- Cellulitis
- Paronychia/felon
- Bursitis, toxic synovitis, septic arthritis
- Extremity fracture
- Acute leukemia, malignant bone tumors
- Mechanical back pain
- Spinal epidural abscess

PEDIATRIC CONSIDERATIONS

- 70–85% of children have fever higher than 38.5°C
- Neonates commonly afebrile
- Only 31% of children will have leukocytosis
- Blood cultures positive in 50%

Treatment

INITIAL STABILIZATION

- Emergent stabilization only if septic

ED TREATMENT

- Empiric antibiotic treatment (nafcillin plus either cefotaxime or ceftriaxone) in ED
  - —Cultures should guide subsequent antibiotic regimen
- Antibiotics: depend on patient's age and organism
- Orthopedic and infectious disease consultation
- Surgical intervention may be needed to optimize treatment (e.g., infected fracture, bone necrosis)
- Parenteral antibiotic treatment for 4–6 weeks

MEDICATIONS

- Neonate to 4 years of age: penicillinase-resistant synthetic penicillin (e.g., nafcillin: 200 mg/kg/d i.v. q4–6h) plus a third-generation cephalosporin (e.g., ceftriaxone: 75 mg/kg/d i.v. q12h); alternative, vancomycin (15 mg/kg i.v. q6h) plus a third-generation cephalosporin
- 4 years of age to adult: penicillinase-resistant synthetic penicillin and third-generation cephalosporin (ceftriaxone: 2 g i.v. q.d.); alternatives: vancomycin, 1 g i.v. q12h, *or* clindamycin, 600–900 mg i.v. q8h (peds: 20–40 mg/kg/d i.v. q6–8h) plus third-generation cephalosporin if gram-negative bacilli are present
- Adult: penicillinase-resistant synthetic penicillin; cefazolin, 2 g i.v. q8h, or vancomycin, 1 g i.v. q12h
- Sickle cell anemia with OM: Cipro, 200–400 mg i.v. q12h, or levo, 500 mg i.v./PO q.d. (*not* in children); alternative: third-generation cephalosporin
- Post-nail puncture through tennis shoe: ceftazidime, 2 g i.v. q.d. (peds: 150 mg/kg/d q8h); alternative: ciprofloxacin
- Posttraumatic OM: nafcillin plus ciprofloxacin; alternatives: vancomycin plus third-generation cephalosporin with antipseudomonal activity

PEDIATRIC CONSIDERATIONS

- Children with hematogenous OM may undergo short-course IV antibiotics and then be changed to oral for additional 1–2 months

Disposition

ADMISSION CRITERIA

- Patients with acute OM should be admitted

DISCHARGE CRITERIA

- Subacute or chronic OM patients may be considered for outpatient management if home IV antibiotics arranged

Miscellaneous

ICD9: 730.20

ICD10: M86.9

SUGGESTED READINGS

Bamberger DM. Diagnosis and treatment of osteomyelitis. Comp Ther 2000;26(2): 89–95.

Carek PJ, Dickerson LM, Sack JL. Diagnosis and management of osteomyelitis. Am Fam Physician 2001;63(12):2413–2420.

Hass DW, McAndrew MP. Bacterial osteomyelitis in adults: evolving considerations in diagnosis and treatment. Am J Med 1996;101(5):550–561.

Jaramillo D, Treves ST, Kasser JR. Osteomyelitis and septic arthritis in children: appropriate use of imaging to guide treatment. AJR Am J Roentgenol 1995;165:399–403.

Lew DP, Waldvogel FA. Osteomyelitis: current concepts. N Engl J Med 1997;336:99–107.

Authors: Boris Lubavin; Federico Vaca

Osteoporosis

Clinical Presentation

SIGNS AND SYMPTOMS

- Usually asymptomatic until pathologic fractures occur
- Fractures with insignificant mechanism or recurrent fractures are hallmark
- Vertebral column most commonly involved
- Multiple compression fractures of vertebral column often lead to kyphosis and scoliosis
- Hip fractures (femoral neck and intertrochanteric fractures) also common

MECHANISM/DESCRIPTION

- Overall decrease in skeletal mass, generally diffuse
- Trabecular bone (especially vertebrae and femur) affected more commonly and earlier
- Disease begins in adolescence, but fractures do not usually manifest until age 50 or older
- Females affected much more commonly than males, especially postmenopause

ETIOLOGY

- Overall increase in resorption over formation of new bone
- Advanced age is most important risk factor
- Inadequate dietary calcium important factor, especially early in life
- Sedentary lifestyle is risk factor (weight bearing on bone favors new bone formation)
- Decreases in estrogen with menopause is a key factor in women
- Other causes include long-term steroid use, alcoholism, methotrexate
- May be a familial or hereditary factor as well

PEDIATRIC CONSIDERATIONS

- Although disease appears to start in adolescence, pediatric patients are asymptomatic

Pre-Hospital

CAUTIONS

- Obtain pre-hospital information on mechanism to help diagnose pathologic nature of fracture
- Avoid aggressive manipulation or movement of patient, as this may exacerbate bony injury

Diagnosis

ESSENTIAL WORKUP

- Fracture without significant mechanism and identification of risk factors is most important
- Careful neurovascular examination distal to femur or other extremity fracture
- Rectal tone and postvoid residual determination should be done in patients with vertebral fractures
- Radiographs of suspected fracture may show osteopenia (late finding in disease)
- Spine films may show old compression fractures
- CT scan should be performed to better evaluate vertebral fractures
  - —Retropulsion, spinal canal compromise is not always apparent on plain films
  - —Make sure CT cuts extend a full level above and below injuries identified on spine radiographs

LABORATORY

- Serum chemistries, such as calcium, parathyroid hormone, and alkaline phosphatase, may help differentiate between illnesses listed later in this chapter

IMAGING/SPECIAL TESTS

- Plain films can identify fractures; however, the age of each fracture may be difficult to determine
- Bone scan or CT help determine the age of fractures, especially in the spine
- Bone densitometry can provide prognostic information and help guide therapy

DIFFERENTIAL DIAGNOSIS

- Multiple myeloma or other metastatic tumor
- Osteogenesis imperfecta (usually apparent in childhood)
- Hyperparathyroidism
- Other demineralizing bone diseases

Treatment

INITIAL STABILIZATION

- Immobilize fractures

ED TREATMENT

- Fractures are treated with the expectation of delayed or incomplete healing
- Prevention is far more effective than treatment
- Long-term therapy is beneficial (see Medications)
- Use of orthotic back braces and vests should be arranged in conjunction with orthopedic spine consultation
- Exercise is also helpful
- Balance must be achieved between osteoporosis risk and steroid or methotrexate therapy

MEDICATIONS

- Alendronate: 10 mg/d
- Calcitonin: 0.5 mg/d s.c. of human, 100 IU/d s.c. of salmon; alternative: nasal spray (100 IU) 1 spray/d in alternate nostrils
- Calcium supplementation (often with vitamin D): 1–1.5 g/d
- Estrogen: 0.625 mg/d (with or without medroxyprogesterone)
- Etidronate: 400 mg/d for 2-week cycles every 15 weeks
- Raloxifene (selective estrogen receptor modulator): 60 mg PO q.d.
- Sodium fluoride: 25 mg b.i.d. with calcium

PEDIATRIC CONSIDERATIONS

- Ensure adequate calcium in diet from early age

Disposition

ADMISSION CRITERIA

- Per normal orthopedic protocols, with special considerations for age and social situation
- Compression fractures are generally stable, but the possibility of a burst fracture with cord compression must be ruled out
- Any cervical fracture or fracture with neurologic symptoms requires admission with emergent consultation with neurosurgery or orthopedics
- Admission may be necessary for pain control and because of decreased ambulation

DISCHARGE CRITERIA

- Per normal orthopedic protocols with special considerations for age and social situation
- Patients with minimal injuries, able to care for themselves at home, or with appropriate assistance, and adequate postoperative pain control may be discharged with orthopedic follow-up

Miscellaneous

ICD9: 733.00

ICD10: M81.9

SUGGESTED READINGS

Chandrasoma P, Taylor CR. Concise pathology. East Norwalk, CT: Appleton & Lange, 1991.

Krane SM, Holick MF. Metabolic bone disease. In: Wilson JD, et al, eds. Harrison's principles of internal medicine, 12th ed. New York: McGraw-Hill, 1991:1921.

North American Menopause Society. Management of postmenopausal osteoporosis: position statement. Menopause 2002;9(2):84–101.

Papaioannou A, et al. Diagnosis and management of vertebral fractures in elderly adults. Am J Med 2002;113(3): 220–228.

Raisz LG. Local and systemic factors in the pathogenesis of osteoporosis. N Engl J Med 1988;318:818–828.

Author: Daniel Davis

Otitis Externa

Clinical Presentation

SIGNS AND SYMPTOMS

- Itching of the external ear canal is usually the first symptom
- Pain in ear or with motion of pinna/tragus
- Swollen, erythematous external ear canal
- Ear drainage
- Decreased auditory acuity
- Clogged sensation in ear
- Pain/swelling in preauricular area

Necrotizing (Malignant) Otitis Externa

- Pain, tenderness, swelling in periauricular area
- Headache
- Otorrhea
- Cranial nerve palsy
  —Facial nerve most affected

MECHANISM/DESCRIPTION

- Inflammation or infection of the auricle, auditory canal, or external surface of the tympanic membrane (TM)
  —Spares the middle ear
- Also called "swimmer's ear" due to the usual history of recent swimming
  —Occasional cases after normal bathing
- Predisposing factors include
  —History of ear surgery or TM perforation
  —Narrow or abnormal canal
  —Humidity
  —Allergy
  —Trauma
  —Abnormal cerumen production
- Necrotizing otitis externa
  —Occurs in elderly, diabetic, or other immunocompromised patients
  —Caused by *Pseudomonas aeruginosa*
  —Infection starts at ear canal and progresses through periauricular tissue toward base of skull

ETIOLOGY

- Often precipitated by an abrasion of the ear canal or maceration of the skin from persisting water or excessive dryness
- *P. aeruginosa, Staphylococcus aureus,* other gram-negative organisms, and fungi play a role in this disease

Pre-Hospital

N/A

Diagnosis

ESSENTIAL WORKUP

- Clinical diagnosis with typical signs/symptoms
  —Pain in ear or with motion of pinna/tragus
  —Otoscopic examination
  —Swollen, erythematous external ear canal
  —Ear drainage
  —Cheesy white or gray green exudate

LABORATORY

- None usually indicated except when possibility of necrotizing otitis externa
  —Signs of systemic toxicity or local spread of infection should be checked
- WBC count
- ESR
- Cultures

DIFFERENTIAL DIAGNOSIS

- Necrotizing otitis externa
- Otitis media
- Folliculitis from obstruction of sebaceous glands
- Otic foreign bodies
- Herpes zoster infection of the geniculate ganglion
- Parotitis
- Periauricular adenitis
- Mastoiditis
- Dental abscess
- Sinusitis
- Tonsillitis
- Pharyngitis
- Temporomandibular joint pain

Treatment

ED TREATMENT

- Clean external ear canal
  —Remove the inflammatory debris by gentle curettage with a cotton-tipped wire applicator
  —Occasional suction with a Fraser suction tip may be necessary
- Insert a cotton or gauze wick 10–12 mm into the canal after cleansing, if the ear canal is very edematous
- Proven or suspected malignant otitis externa
  —Initiate parenteral antibiotics such as a third-generation cephalosporin or an antipseudomonal agent

MEDICATIONS

- Most cases respond well to topical treatment
  —Antiseptic, antiinflammatory, and drying otic drops
  —Eliminates the pathogenic bacteria and allows for rapid healing of the canal
  —Acetic acid solutions such as Domeboro otic (2% acetic acid): 4–6 drops q4–6h
  —Corticosporin otic (hydrocortisone 1%, polymyxin + neomycin) suspension: 4 drops to ear canal q.i.d.; use suspensions and not solutions with suspected tympanic membrane perforation
  —Ofloxacin: 5 drops b.i.d.
- Oral antibiotics
  —Administer to patients with cellulitis of the face or neck, severe edema of the ear canal, concurrent otitis media, or when the tympanic membrane cannot be visualized
  —Treat diabetics and other immunocompromised patients with oral ciprofloxacin and follow closely for symptoms of malignant otitis externa
  —Amoxicillin: 500 mg (peds: 40 mg/kg/d) PO t.i.d.
  —Ciprofloxacin: 500 mg PO b.i.d.
- IV antibiotics for patients with necrotizing otitis externa, severe cellulitis, or septic looking
- Prophylaxis
  —Apply rubbing alcohol or acetic acid (2%) to keep the external ear canal dry and prevent recurrence of infection

Complications

- Chronic use of antibiotics/corticosteroids may lead to overgrowth of fungi such as aspergilli in the ear canal
- Toxicity
- Meningitis
- Facial palsy
- Local spread of infection leading to necrotizing otitis externa
- Osteomyelitis
  - —Requires immediate admission and treatment with IV antibiotics (ciprofloxacin or aminoglycoside/semisynthetic penicillin)
  - —CT/MRI to exclude osteomyelitis

Disposition

ADMISSION CRITERIA

- Necrotizing otitis externa
- Significant involvement of the pinna
- Signs of systemic illness

DISCHARGE CRITERIA

- Most patients
- Close follow-up for patients at risk of otitis externa
- ENT follow-up for worsening of symptoms or failure of initial management
- Patient instructions
  - —Avoid swimming and keep ears completely dry for 3–4 weeks
  - —Apply medications as directed
  - —Return if worse pain, fever, hearing loss develops, or there is any change in mental or neurologic status
  - —Follow-up if symptoms are not improved within 2–3 days

Miscellaneous

- Consider ear canal foreign bodies in children with purulent drainage from edematous, painful ear canals

ICD9: 380.10

ICD10: H60.9

SUGGESTED READINGS

Severance H Jr. Acute otitis externa. In: Harwood-Nuss AL, Linden CH, et al, eds. The clinical practice of emergency medicine, 2nd ed. Philadelphia: Lippincott-Raven Publishers, 1996: 112–115.

Diagnosis and treatment of acute otitis externa: an interdisciplinary update. Ann Otol Rhinol Laryngol Suppl 1999;176: 1–23.

Hughes E, Lee JH. Otitis externa. Pediatr Rev 2001;22(6):191–197.

Sander R. Otitis externa: a practical guide to treatment and prevention. Am Fam Physician 2001;61(5):927–936, 941–942.

Author: Assaad J. Sayah

Otitis Media

Clinical Presentation

SIGNS AND SYMPTOMS

General

- Fever
- Irritability
- Rhinitis
- Vomiting, diarrhea
- Poor feeding

Otolaryngologic

- Ear pain
- Sensation of plugged ear
- Pulling at ear
- Vertigo, tinnitus
- Exclude associated illnesses

Complications

- Recurrent otitis media
  - —Three episodes within 6 months or four or more episodes within 1 year
- Perforated tympanic membrane
- Serous otitis media
- Conductive hearing loss
- Facial nerve injury
- Mastoiditis
- Cholesteatoma
- Meningitis
- Subdural empyema
- Venous sinus thrombosis

MECHANISM/DESCRIPTION

- Infection of the middle ear
- Most commonly occurs in children 6–36 months of age
- Usually associated with (or as a result of) upper respiratory tract infection
- Blockage of eustachian tube
- Predisposing factors
  - —Deficient mucus, cilia, or antibodies
  - —Intubation, especially nasotracheal
  - —American Indians, Eskimos
  - —Down's syndrome
  - —Cleft palate

ETIOLOGY

- Usually infectious
- Viral
  - —Parainfluenza
  - —Respiratory syncytial virus
  - —Influenza
  - —Adenovirus
  - —Rhinovirus
- Bacterial
  - —*Staphylococcus pneumoniae*
  - —*Moraxella catarrhalis*
  - —*Haemophilus influenzae*
  - —*Streptococcus pyogenes*
  - —*Mycoplasma pneumoniae*

Pre-Hospital

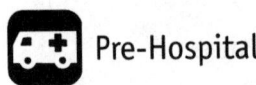

- Assess for associated conditions

Diagnosis

ESSENTIAL WORKUP

- Exclude associated conditions
- Otoscopic examination for appearance and mobility of tympanic membrane
  - —Full visualization essential
  - —Increased vascularity, erythema, purulence
  - —Obscured landmarks—bony, light reflex
  - —Pneumatic otoscopy—mobility, bulging, retracted

LABORATORY

- Cultures unhelpful unless done by tympanocentesis

IMAGING/SPECIAL TESTS

- CT scan of head/sinuses if associated infection is considered
- Tympanocentesis—indications
  - —Severe pain or toxicity
  - —Failure of antimicrobial therapy
  - —Suspicion of suppurative complication
  - —Sick neonate
  - —Immunocompromised patient
- Tympanometry and acoustic otoscopy may be useful with difficult examinations

DIFFERENTIAL DIAGNOSIS

- Infection
  - —Otitis externa
  - —Mastoiditis
  - —Dental abscess
  - —Peritonsillar abscess
  - —Sinusitis
  - —Lymphadenitis
  - —Parotitis
  - —Meningitis
- Trauma
  - —Perforation of the tympanic membrane
  - —Foreign body in ear
  - —Barotrauma
  - —Instrumentation
- Serous otitis media or eustachian tube dysfunction
- Impacted ear cerumen
- Impacted third molar
- Temporomandibular joint dysfunction

Treatment

INITIAL STABILIZATION

- Evaluate and manage associated conditions

ED TREATMENT

- After evaluation antibiotics are usually initiated (most mild cases could resolve without antibiotics)
- Considerations should include recurrent nature of otitis media, lack of clinical response, and resistance patterns in community
- Parenteral antibiotics indicated in febrile toxic children younger than 1 year or with immunocompromise
- Antihistamines and decongestants have no proven efficacy
- Antipyretics and analgesics (avoid local analgesics in perforated tympanic membranes)

MEDICATIONS

- Amoxicillin: 40 mg/kg/d PO t.i.d. × 10 days or 80 mg/kg/d t.i.d. × 7 days
- Amoxicillin-clavulanic acid: 40 mg AMX/kg/d PO t.i.d.
- Azithromycin: 10 mg/kg PO day 1, then 5 mg/kg/d PO days 2–5
- Cefaclor: 50 mg/kg/d PO t.i.d.
- Trimethoprim (TMP)-sulfamethoxazole: 8 mg of TMP/kg/d PO b.i.d.

Disposition

ADMISSION CRITERIA

- Febrile toxic children who are
  - —Younger than 1 year, immunocompromised
  - —Moderately or severely dehydrated
  - —Unable to tolerate oral fluids or medications
  - —Suspected or proven associated significant infection
  - —Suspected abuse
  - —Unreliable caretaker

DISCHARGE CRITERIA

- Children without any of the aforementioned criteria
- Follow-up in 10–14 days to ensure resolution
- Indications for earlier follow-up
  - —Child does not get better in 24–48 hours
  - —Any progression of signs or symptoms
  - —New problems develop including a rash
  - —Any concerns arise

Miscellaneous

ICD9: 382.9

ICD10: H66.9

SUGGESTED READINGS

Barkin RM. Acute otitis media. In: Barkin RM, Rosen P, eds. Emergency pediatrics, 5th ed. St. Louis: CV Mosby, 1999:545–548.

Bauchner H. Ear, ears, and more ears! Arch Dis Child 2001:84(2):185–186.

Hoberman A, Paradise JL. Acute otitis media: diagnosis and management in the year 2000. Pediatr Ann 2000;29(10): 609–620.

Koranyi K. Otitis media and mastoiditis. In: Harwood-Nuss A, et al, eds. The clinical practice of emergency medicine, 2nd ed. Philadelphia: Lippincott-Raven Publishers, 1996:545–548.

Author: Assaad J. Sayah

Otologic Trauma

Clinical Presentation

SIGNS AND SYMPTOMS

- Severe ear pain
- Bleeding
- Auricular deformity
  - —Edema
  - —Hematoma
  - —Laceration
  - —Amputation
- Decreased hearing
  - —Partial loss suggests tympanic membrane (TM) rupture
  - —Complete hearing loss suggests additional injuries to ossicles or inner ear
- Hemotympanum
- Purulent or bloody discharge from ear canal
- Tinnitus
- Vertigo
  - —Inner ear injury
  - —TM perforation in water

MECHANISM/DESCRIPTION

- Ear cartilage has no blood supply and is nutritionally dependent on perichondrium
- Hematomas often disrupt perichondrium and cartilage leading to ischemia, possible perichondritis, necrosis, and cauliflower ear
- Penetrating injuries or animal bites may lead to infection of the cartilage

ETIOLOGY

- Blunt trauma
  - —Often contact sports
- Penetrating trauma
  - —TM perforation from Q-tip swabs
- Blast injury
- Lightning injury
  - —Both TM and ossicular disruption occur in 50% of lightning strikes
- Chemical exposure
- Thermal injury
- Diving injuries
  - —Inner ear barotraumas
  - —TM rupture

Pre-Hospital

- If auricle is amputated, wrap in moist gauze and place in plastic bag

Diagnosis

ESSENTIAL WORKUP

- History—mechanism, associated injuries, allergies, meds, past otologic history
- Physical—search for concomitant injury
  - —Head, cranial nerves, vascular structures, temporal bone
  - —Examine pinna, external ear canal, TM, and hearing

LABORATORY

- Wound culture if signs of infection

DIFFERENTIAL DIAGNOSIS

- Infection
- Hemangioma
- Foreign body ear

Treatment

INITIAL STABILIZATION

- ABCs, full trauma evaluation, and resuscitation as appropriate
- Sterile dressing to injured site

ED TREATMENT

- Anesthesia
  - —Local anesthesia via nerve block to auriculotemporal branch of mandibular nerve, lesser occipital nerve, greater auricular nerve, and auricular branch of vagus nerve; use 1% lidocaine or 0.25% Marcaine
    - -Alternative: inject ring of anesthetic around base of pinna
- Hematoma: drainage imperative to reapproximate perichondrium to cartilage to prevent cartilage necrosis
  - —Aspiration: preferred alterative if clot not yet formed
    - -Use 18–20-gauge needle for aspiration; milk hematoma until totally evacuated
  - —Incision and drainage: more effective with larger and/or clotted hematomas; incise along curvature of pinna with no. 15 scalpel, evacuate and irrigate
    - -Apply pressure dressing to prevent reaccumulation for 3–7 days
  - —Vaseline gauze placed to fill crevices of pinna, gauze placed over and behind pinna, soft gauzed firmly wrapped around head
  - —Alternatively, dental roles sutured into place over incised area
    - -Antistaphylococcal antibiotics
  - —If patient presents again with reaccumulation, reaspiration, consider wick placement

- Laceration
  - —Clean and débride wound, anesthetize as necessary
    - -Superficial abrasions: cleaned, dressed with antibiotic ointment
    - -Simple lacerations: 5.0 or 6.0 monofilament nylon or polypropylene suture, then pressure dressing
    - -May use absorbable suture on medial skin lacerations to avoid having to bend the ear for suture removal
  - —Exposed auricular cartilage
    - -Carefully débride jagged edges, completely cover cartilage to prevent perichondritis
    - -Can remove small amount of cartilage to allow skin coverage
    - -Approximate cartilage first with absorbable sutures at major landmarks; include anterior and posterior perichondrium in stitch
  - —Avulsions: <2 cm total avulsions may be used as graft and survive
    - ->2 cm, consult or urgently refer to otolaryngologist or plastic surgeon; save in subcutaneous pocket
- Management of TM perforation
- Tetanus prophylaxis if necessary
- For hematomas, antistaphylococcal antibiotics for 7–10 days
- For human and animal bites use both penicillin and ceftazidime or Augmentin
- For lacerations prophylactic antibiotics are controversial

MEDICATIONS

- Augmentin (amoxicillin-clavulanate): 875/125 mg PO t.i.d. (peds: 40 mg/kg/d PO t.i.d.)
- Dicloxacillin: 250 mg PO q.i.d.
- Erythromycin: 250 mg PO q.i.d.
- Penicillin VK: 250 mg PO q.i.d.

PEDIATRIC CONSIDERATIONS

- Consider nonaccidental trauma

Disposition

ADMISSION CRITERIA

- Concomitant serious traumatic injuries
- Need for IV antibiotics
- Immunosuppressed persons with serious infections, perichondritis, or chondritis

DISCHARGE CRITERIA

- Able to tolerate oral antibiotics
- Follow up wound suture repair
- Follow up hematomas after 24 hours to determine whether reaccumulation of fluid

Miscellaneous

ICD9: 959.09

ICD10: S09.9

SEE ALSO: TYMPANIC MEMBRANE PERFORATION

SUGGESTED READINGS

Cantrill ST. Facial trauma. In: Rosen P, et al, eds. Emergency medicine: concepts and clinical practice, 4th ed. St. Louis: Mosby–Year Book, 1998.

Lammers RL, Trott AT. Methods of wound closure. In: Roberts, Hedges JR, eds. Clinical procedures in emergency medicine, 3rd ed. Philadelphia: WB Saunders, 1998.

Manthey DE, Harrison BP. Otolaryngologic procedures. In: Roberts, Hedges JR, eds. Clinical procedures in emergency medicine, 3rd ed. Philadelphia: WB Saunders, 1998.

Spring PM, Amedee RG. Ear pain and drainage. In: Calhoun KH, ed. Expert guide to otolaryngology. Philadelphia: American College of Physicians, 2001.

Turbiak TW. Ear trauma. Emerg Med Clin North Am 1987;5(2):243–251.

Author: Shan Liu

Ovarian Cyst/Torsion

Clinical Presentation

SIGNS AND SYMPTOMS

Ovarian Cyst

- Lower quadrant abdominal pain
  - —Sudden, sharp, unilateral
  - —Onset often with exercise, intercourse, trauma, or pelvic exam
- Abdominal tenderness (mild to severe with peritonitis)
- Adnexal tenderness
- Pelvic mass
- Hemorrhagic shock possible
  - —Dizziness, orthostasis, syncope, hypotension, tachycardia
  - —Usually from corpus luteal cyst rupture
- Fever rare

Adnexal Torsion

- *Lower quadrant abdominal pain*
  - —Sudden, sharp, clicky
  - —Unilateral
  - —Radiation to back, flank, or groin
  - —May be chronic or recurrent
- *Nausea, vomiting*
- *Adnexal mass*
- Abdominal tenderness (mild to severe)
- Occasional signs/symptoms
  - —Fever
  - —Leukocytosis
  - —Vaginal bleeding
  - —UTI symptoms

MECHANISM/DESCRIPTION

Ovarian Cyst

- Cysts generally asymptomatic until complicated by hemorrhage, torsion, rupture, or infection
  - —Follicular cysts most common: occur from fetal life to menopause, result from nonrupture of mature follicle or failure of atresia of immature follicle, thin wall predisposes to rupture, unilocular, diameter from 3–8 cm, rupture usually causes minimal or no bleeding
  - —Corpus luteal cysts most significant: result from normal intracystic hemorrhage 2–4 days after ovulation, rapid bleeding causes rupture, gradual bleeding causes enlargement, 3 cm diameter, rupture associated with intraperitoneal bleeding that may be severe

Adnexal Torsion

- Twisting of vascular pedicle of ovary, fallopian tube, or paratubal cyst causes ischemia; occlusion of lymphatics and venous drainage lead to rapid enlargement of adnexa

ETIOLOGY

Ovarian Cyst

- Follicular, corpus luteal, theca lutein, cystic teratoma, endometrioma (chocolate cyst)
- Mittelschmerz: rupture of follicular cyst during ovulation at midcycle
- Rupture of a corpus luteum cyst most commonly occurs just before menses begins, usually days 20–26 of menstrual cycle
- Hemorrhage into cyst or ovary distends capsule and may cause pain without rupture

Adnexal Torsion (Risk Factors)

- Highest frequency in reproductive-age women, especially mid-20s
- Ovarian cysts
- Tumors
  - —Serous cystadenoma most common
  - —Teratomas
- Pelvic surgery
  - —Tubal ligation
  - —Hysterectomy
- Pregnancy
  - —h/o PID

Pre-Hospital

CAUTIONS

- Patients may become hemodynamically unstable so IV essential

Diagnosis

ESSENTIAL WORKUP

- Pregnancy test essential to rule out ectopic pregnancy
- Rapid hemoglobin determination

LABORATORY

- CBC, UA, HCG
- Type and cross PRBCs for patients with significant hemorrhage

IMAGING/SPECIAL TESTS

- US
  - —Demonstrates adnexal cysts and masses
  - —Pelvic free fluid
  - —Enlarged ovary (suggests torsion)
  - —Cystic masses <5 cm in premenopausal women are generally benign and should be reevaluated at end of menstruation
- Doppler
  - —May show decreased flow with torsion
  - —Sensitivity not well established
  - —It is important to document normal blood flow on Doppler in the ED, even though this does not rule out a recent torsion of the ovary
- Culdocentesis
  - —May yield serosanguineous fluid with ruptured cyst
  - —Hematocrit $>15\%$ suggests significant hemoperitoneum
- Laparoscopy is gold standard for torsed adnexa and definitive diagnosis

Special Considerations

- Anticoagulated patients at increased risk of
  - —Hemorrhagic corpus luteal cyst
  - —Significant bleed from ruptured cyst, including with ovulation

DIFFERENTIAL DIAGNOSIS

- DDx for pelvic pain
  - —Ectopic pregnancy
  - —Appendicitis
  - —Renal colic
  - —Diverticulitis
  - —Pelvic inflammatory disease
- DDx for adnexal mass
  - —Benign tumors
  - —Malignant tumors
  - —Polycystic ovaries

Treatment

INITIAL STABILIZATION

- ABCs
  - —Patients in shock should receive supplemental oxygen and intubation as indicated for respiratory failure
  - —IV access and volume replacement with NS or lactated Ringer's solution or blood transfusion when indicated

ED TREATMENT

- Focused on stabilizing the patient and providing analgesia
- Uncomplicated cyst rupture
  - —Analgesia
  - —Observation
- Unstable patients and patients with significant hemorrhage
  - —NPO
  - —Monitor and maintain ABCs
  - —Arrange immediate gynecologic consultation and admission
  - —Unstable patients and patients with torsion require immediate admission to the OR

MEDICATIONS

- Acetaminophen: 325–650 mg q4h (peds: 15 mg/kg, maximum 650 mg PO q4h)
- Ibuprofen: 400–600 mg PO q6h (peds: 5–10 mg/kg/dose PO q6h)
- Morphine sulfate: 2–4 mg i.v. q5min (peds: 0.1 mg/kg/dose q5min, maximum 15 mg)

Disposition

ADMISSION CRITERIA

- Culdocentesis fluid hematocrit >15%
- Significant hemorrhage ascertained by serial hematocrits, orthostasis, culdocentesis, or evidence of shock
- All patients with torsion

DISCHARGE CRITERIA

- Stable patients with a ruptured cyst and without a coagulopathy or evidence of significant hemorrhage can be discharged with close follow-up with a gynecologist

Miscellaneous

ICD9: 620.2; 620.5

ICD10: N83.2

SUGGESTED READINGS

Baker EB, Copas PR. Adnexal torsion: a clinical dilemma. J Reprod Med 1995;40:447–449.

Bernardus RE, et al. Torsion of the fallopian tube: Some considerations on its etiology. Obstet Gynecol 1984;64:675–678.

Copeland LJ, Jarrell JF, eds. Textbook of gynecology, 2nd ed. Philadelphia: WB Saunders, 2000.

Houry D, Abbott JT. Ovarian torsion: a fifteen-year review. Ann Emerg Med 2001;38(2):156–159.

Koonings PP, Grimes DA. Adnexal torsion in postmenopausal women. Obstet Gynecol 1989;73(1):11–12.

Mage G, Canis M, Manhes H, et al. Laparoscopic management of adnexal torsion: a review of 35 cases. J Reprod Med 1989;34(8):520–524.

Tanos, Scheaher JG. Ovarian cysts: a clinical dilemma. Gynecol Endocrinol 1994;8(1):59–67.

Thach AM, Young GP. Pelvic pain. In: Rosen P, Barkin R, eds. Emergency medicine: concepts and clinical practice, 4th ed. Boston: Mosby–Year Book, 1998: 2293–2304.

Author: Kyan J. Berger

Paget's Disease

Clinical Presentation

SIGNS AND SYMPTOMS

Paget's disease involves the resorption of normal bone and its replacement with fibrous and sclerotic tissue. It is also known as osteitis deformans.

- Usually focal, bones most frequently involved include
  - —Pelvis
  - —Femur
  - —Skull
  - —Tibia
  - —Spine
  - —Flat bones
- Many patients are asymptomatic, with the disease discovered by incidental radiographs or elevated alkaline phosphatase levels
- *Acute (resorptive/osteolytic) phase*
  - —*Pathologic fractures*
  - —Pain from acute lysis, pathologic fracture, or resultant arthritis
  - —Hypercalcemia or *renal stones*
  - —*Hypervascularity* may result in significant bleeding complications and hematoma formation if affected bone is fractured
  - —With widespread disease, increased vascularity and blood flow may result in *high-output cardiac failure*
- *Secondary (sclerotic/osteoplastic) phase*
  - —Long-bone involvement may present with swelling or deformity and resultant gait abnormality
  - —Skull involvement may lead to headaches or abnormal skull contours (change in hat size)
  - —Severe skull or spine involvement may result in CNS compression
  - —Hearing loss may result from nerve compression or ossicle involvement
  - —Sarcoma occurs in <1% of patients

MECHANISM/DESCRIPTION

- Occurs in approximately 3% of patients older than 40 years
- Starts with resorptive or osteolytic phase, during which osteoclasts remove otherwise healthy bone
- Hypervascularity begins in the resorptive phase and predisposes to hematoma formation with fracture
- Resorbed bone is eventually replaced by irregular, dense, disorganized trabecular bone in the sclerotic or osteoplastic phase
- Malignant transformation is rare
  - —*Osteosarcoma* is the malignancy of concern
  - —Usually malignant transformation occurs in no more than 1%

ETIOLOGY

- Unknown
- May represent vascular hyperplasia with subsequent inflammation
- Presence of nucleocapsids from measles, canine distemper, or respiratory syncytial virus may implicate a viral etiology
- Familial or genetic component

PEDIATRIC CONSIDERATIONS

- Generally not seen in children

Pre-Hospital

- Pre-hospital personnel should obtain information about mechanism of injury or social factors that suggest pathologic fracture
- Adequate immobilization can limit excessive bleeding around fracture site

Diagnosis

ESSENTIAL WORKUP

- Diagnosis usually suggested by radiographs
- During resorptive phase, lytic lesions are often not seen, except in skull where lesions are well demarcated ("osteoporosis circumscripta")
- Bowing of long bones may occur with resorption and strength loss
- New bone initially appears irregular and spotty and later becomes homogeneous and dense ("ivory pattern")
- Excess bone may be deposited along stress lines leading to cortical irregularities
- A thorough neurologic exam must be documented due to possibility of hematoma formation and mass effect, especially with vertebral or pelvis involvement

IMAGING/SPECIAL TESTS

- CT or MRI defines margins and helps evaluate for neoplasm or hematoma
  - —Spiral CT to detect renal calculi
- Bone scan is most sensitive for diagnosis of Paget's disease
- Radionuclide scans (technetium-99m, gallium-67) may help guide therapy by assessing response to current therapy

LABORATORY

- Alkaline phosphatase is the most dramatic marker of disease activity (especially resorptive phase)
- Calcium and phosphate levels should be checked as well but are usually normal
- EKG if suspect hypercalcemia and a CXR with evidence of high-output cardiac failure
- Increased bone formation may lead to elevations in urine hydroxyproline or serum osteocalcin or procollagen fragments
- Alterations in PTH levels occur as secondary changes during the resorptive/osteolytic phase (low PTH) and the sclerotic/osteoplastic phase (high PTH)

DIFFERENTIAL DIAGNOSIS

- Primary hyperparathyroidism
- Multiple myeloma
- Hodgkin variants
- Acromegaly
- Osteosarcoma

Treatment

INITIAL STABILIZATION

- ABCs are always indicated first, depending on mechanism of injury
- High-output cardiac failure should be treated as indicated in Congestive Heart Failure chapter
- Prompt immobilization of fractures will limit excessive bleeding around fracture site

ED TREATMENT

- Analgesia for the pain of lytic lesions, fractures, or arthritis includes NSAIDs and narcotics
- High-dose prednisone can suppress disease
- Fracture treatment is often more conservative, due to difficulties with bleeding during operative repair
- Orthopedic consultation for severe arthritis and definitive fracture management
- Hypercalcemia may be treated with IV fluids, furosemide (Lasix), calcitonin, inorganic phosphate, etidronate, mitramycin
- Long-term chemotherapy may provide temporary or prolonged remission
- CNS compression requires emergent neurosurgical consultation and possible decompression

MEDICATIONS

- Alendronate: 40 mg/d for 6 months
- Calcitonin: 0.5 mg/d s.c. of human, 100 IU/d s.c. of salmon
- Chemotherapy with plicamycin/mitramycin, dactinomycin, diphosphonate
- Etidronate: 400 mg/d for 6-month cycles
- Furosemide (Lasix): 20–80 mg i.v. for hypercalcemia
- Inorganic phosphate

Disposition

ADMISSION CRITERIA

- Admission as indicated for major trauma or injury, or excessive bleeding
- Orthopedic procedures
- Hypercalcemia
- CNS compressive symptoms

DISCHARGE CRITERIA

- No evidence of significant bleeding, neurologic compromise, or hypercalcemia, and adequate pain control
- Appropriate fracture immobilization and orthopedic follow-up

Miscellaneous

ICD9: 731.0

ICD10: M88.9

SUGGESTED READINGS

Chandrasoma P, Taylor CR. Concise pathology. East Norwalk, CT: Appleton & Lange, 1991.

Favus M. Primer on the metabolic bone diseases and disorders of mineral metabolism. Kelseyville CA: American Society for Bone and Mineral Research, 1990.

Ryan WG. Parathyroid hormone, calcitonin, vitamin D, minerals, and metabolic bone diseases. In: Bone RC, Rosen RL, eds. Quick reference to internal medicine. New York: Igaku-Shoin, 1994:1329.

Schneider D, et al. Diagnosis and treatment of Paget's disease of bone. Am Fam Physician 2002;65(10):2069–2072.

Author: Daniel Davis

Pancreatic Pseudocyst

Clinical Presentation

SIGNS AND SYMPTOMS

Frequency

- Abdominal pain: 86%
- Nausea/vomiting: 72%
- Palpable mass: 49%
- Weight loss: 35%
- Pleural effusion: 15%
- Jaundice: 13%
- Ascites: 11%
- Internal hemorrhage: 7%

Gastrointestinal

- In chronic pancreatitis, pseudocyst heralded by change in typical pain pattern
- Symptoms reflecting structural compression by pseudocyst
  - —Nausea, vomiting, weight loss—duodenal or gastric outlet obstruction
  - —Jaundice—common bile duct compression

Respiratory

- Left lung pleural effusion common

Cardiac

- Commonly occurs with pseudocyst rupture or hemorrhage
- Tachycardia
- Hypotension
- Shock (depending on fluid losses)

Infected Pseudocyst

- Fever
- Chills
- Leukocytosis

Pseudocyst Hemorrhage

- Hypotension
- Expanding abdominal mass
- Usually erodes into splenic or gastroduodenal arteries

Ruptured Pseudocyst

- Abdominal rigidity; severe pain
  - —Occurs when cyst ruptures into peritoneal cavity

MECHANISM/DESCRIPTION

- A cystic collection of fluid with a high content of pancreatic enzymes lacking a true epithelial lining
- Localized in parenchyma of pancreas or adjacent abdominal spaces (lesser peritoneal sac)

ETIOLOGY

- Ethanol abuse and biliary disease account for most cases
- 45 years is average age at diagnosis
- Occurs more frequently in men than in women
- Complication in 2% of acute pancreatitis; up to 10% of chronic pancreatitis

PEDIATRIC CONSIDERATIONS

- Greater than 60% result from blunt trauma
  - —Usually can palpate a mass

Pre-Hospital

N/A

Diagnosis

ESSENTIAL WORKUP

- Laboratory tests not helpful in diagnosis
  - —Useful to anticipate complications

LABORATORY

- Amylase
  - —Normal value in up to 50% of pseudocysts
- CBC
  - —Leukocytosis suggests infected pseudocyst
  - —Low hematocrit with pseudocyst hemorrhage
- Electrolytes, BUN, creatinine, glucose
  - —Hypocalcemia
  - —Hypokalemia with extensive fluid losses
  - —Hypomagnesemia with underlying ethanol abuse
  - —Hyperglycemia

IMAGING/SPECIAL TESTS

- CT scan
  - —Imaging test of choice
  - —Indicated for all cases of newly suspected pseudocyst
- Ultrasound
  - —Useful for follow-up of previously diagnosed pseudocyst to assess pseudocyst dimensions
- Angiography
  - —Helpful in cases of pseudocyst hemorrhage
  - —Usually impractical due to instability of patient

DIFFERENTIAL DIAGNOSIS

- Pancreatic abscess
- Neoplastic pancreatic cysts
- Perforated ulcer
- Ruptured abdominal aortic aneurysm (pseudocyst hemorrhage)
- Myocardial infarction
- Biliary colic
- Intestinal obstruction

Treatment

INITIAL STABILIZATION

- ABCs
  - —Supplemental oxygen
  - —Cardiac monitor
  - —0.9% NS i.v. fluids

ED TREATMENT

- Fluid resuscitation
  - —Fluid losses may necessitate large fluid volumes
  - —Continuously assess vitals, urine output, and electrolytes to ensure rapid and adequate replacement of intravascular volume
  - —Consider CVP monitoring in elderly
- Correct electrolytes abnormalities (hypocalcemia, hypokalemia, hypomagnesemia)
- Blood products
  - —Transfuse immediately in cases of pseudocyst hemorrhage pending definitive surgical treatment
- Analgesia (meperidine)
- Nasogastric suction if intractable nausea/vomiting
- Antiemetics (promethazine)
- Surgical consultation
  - —Emergent surgical consultation mandatory in cases of suspected ruptured pseudocyst or pseudocyst hemorrhage as definitive treatment is emergent laparotomy
  - —Surgical treatment options (pseudocyst >6 cm or persists for >6 weeks)
    - -Observation (no acute intervention)
    - -Surgical excision is possible only in few cases
    - -External drainage in critically ill or when cyst wall is immature (reoccurrence rate 20%)
    - -Internal drainage is preferred method in most patients
    - -Percutaneous drainage
    - -Endoscopic drainage

MEDICATIONS

- Calcium gluconate 10%: 10 mL i.v. over 15–20 minutes
- Magnesium sulfate: 16 mEq (2 g) in 50 mL D5W over 20 minutes
- Meperidine (demerol): 25–50 mg i.v.; 50–75 mg i.m. q3–4h
- Potassium chloride: 10 mEq/h i.v.
- Promethazine: 12.5–25 mg PO/i.m./PR/i.v.

Disposition

ADMISSION CRITERIA

- All newly diagnosed pseudocysts >6 cm
- Pseudocysts <6 cm if symptoms of acute pancreatitis
- Previously known pseudocysts if cyst is increasing in size compared to old studies
- Hemodynamic instability
- Severe abdominal pain
- Fever/infected pseudocyst

DISCHARGE CRITERIA

- Refer stable, asymptomatic patient with pseudocyst <6 cm for urgent surgical clinic follow-up

Miscellaneous

ICD9: 577.2

ICD10: K86.3

SEE ALSO: PANCREATITIS

SUGGESTED READINGS

Aguilar M, Jones RS, Sanfey H. Pseudocysts of the pancreas: a review of 97 cases. Am Surg 1994;60(9):661–668.

Maule W, Reber H. Diagnosis and management of pancreatic pseudocysts, pancreatic ascites, and pancreatic fistulas. In: Go V, et al, eds. The pancreas. New York: Raven Press, 1993:71–78.

Parks RW, Tzovaras G, Diamond T, et al. Management of pancreatic pseudocysts. Ann R Coll Surg Engl 2000;82(6):383–387.

Werner J, Warshaw AL. Pseudocysts, postinflammatory cystic fluid collections, and other non-neoplastic cysts. In: Trede M, et al, eds. Surgery of the pancreas. New York: Churchill Livingstone, 1997: 405–410.

Author: Trevor Lewis

Pancreatic Trauma

Clinical Presentation

SIGNS AND SYMPTOMS

- Abdominal pain, diffuse or epigastric, often out of proportion to physical exam and vital signs
- Soft-tissue contusion in upper abdomen
- Injury to lower ribs or costal cartilage
- Acute abdomen, often associated with other intraabdominal injuries
- Hypotension

MECHANISM/DESCRIPTION

- Most common mechanism is penetrating trauma
- Blunt trauma—deep location of pancreas requires significant force to cause injury
  - —Direct epigastric blow compressing pancreas against the vertebral column
  - —Steering wheel or bicycle handlebars to abdomen

PEDIATRIC CONSIDERATIONS

- Due to smaller body, trauma affects proportionately larger areas leading to multisystem injuries
- Children have less protective muscle and subcutaneous tissue
- Bicycle accidents with trauma from the handlebars can cause significant pancreatic injury
- Children will less often present with hypotension as symptom
- Evaluate for possible child abuse

Pre-Hospital

CAUTIONS

- The extent of pancreatic injury may not be apparent on initial evaluation
- Transport to closest appropriate facility or trauma center

Diagnosis

ESSENTIAL WORKUP

- Concise history, details of incident especially important for blunt trauma
- Physical exam
  - —Inspection for abrasions, contusions, penetrating wounds—must log roll patient for full inspection
  - —Auscultation for presence or absence of bowel sounds
  - —Palpation to determine location and severity of pain, presence of guarding, and rebound tenderness
  - —Rectal exam for occult blood, vaginal, and penile exam as for all trauma patients
  - —Serial physical exams and vital signs for unidentified injuries

LABORATORY

- Blood type, screen, or cross-match
- Hematocrit, WBC count with differential
- Amylase is not a reliable indicator of pancreatic trauma
  - —Serial levels may increase sensitivity but specificity is still poor
  - —Elevated amylase may be an early indicator of potential pancreatic injury
  - —Normal amylase does not rule out pancreatic injury
- Lipase
- Urinalysis
- Pregnancy test
- Alcohol and drug screening if indicated
- PT/PTT, BUN, and creatinine

IMAGING/SPECIAL TESTS

Note that all imaging tests may miss pancreatic injury.

- C-spine, CXR, and pelvis films as for all blunt trauma patients
- Bedside US
- *CT scan* with IV and oral contrast, helical CT if available, which shows better contrast enhancement of pancreatic parenchyma than standard scanning
- DPL to identify intraperitoneal injuries, check fluid for amylase level, still may miss significant pancreatic injury
- ERCP is useful for patients with persistent hyperamylasemia or unexplained abdominal symptoms

DIFFERENTIAL DIAGNOSIS

- 90% of pancreatic injuries are associated with injuries to adjacent structures: liver, stomach, major arteries and veins, spleen, kidney, duodenum, colon, small bowel, common bile duct, and gallbladder

Treatment

INITIAL STABILIZATION

- Follow standard trauma treatment for blunt abdominal trauma (see Abdominal Trauma, Blunt)
  —NGT suction may be especially helpful in setting of pancreatic trauma

ED TREATMENT

- Follow standard trauma treatment for blunt abdominal trauma (see Abdominal Trauma, Blunt)
- Antibiotic treatment for penetrating trauma, and intraabdominal injury that will require operative intervention

MEDICATIONS

- Penetrating trauma: tetanus prophylaxis and broad spectrum antibiotic therapy
- Must cover for colonic bacteria: aerobic *(Escherichia coli, Enterobacter, Klebsiella, Enterococcus)* and anaerobic organisms *(Bacteroides fragilis, Clostridium, Peptostreptococcus)*
- Cefotetan: 2 g i.v. (peds: 20 mg/kg i.v.) + gentamicin: 2 mg/kg i.v. *or*
- Cefoxitin: 2 g i.v. (peds: 40 mg/kg i.v.) + gentamicin: 2 mg/kg i.v. *or*
- Ceftriaxone: 1–2 g i.v. (peds: 50 mg/kg/dose i.v.) + Flagyl: 15 mg/kg i.v. *or*
- Clindamycin: 600 mg i.v. (peds: mg/kg i.v.) + gentamicin: 2 mg/kg i.v.

Disposition

ADMISSION CRITERIA

- All patients with pancreatic injuries must be admitted
- Abdominal pain after blunt trauma requires serial exam and observation for 24 hours
- Intoxicated trauma patient requires admission and serial exams for unidentified injury

DISCHARGE CRITERIA

- Only for very minor trauma and with no evidence of pancreatic or any other intraabdominal injury

Miscellaneous

ICD9: 863.84

ICD10: S36.2

SUGGESTED READINGS

Beckingham IJ. ABC of diseases of liver, pancreas and biliary system: liver and pancreatic trauma. BMJ 2001;322(7289): 783–785.

Bradley EL, Young PR, Chang MC, et al. Diagnosis and initial management of blunt pancreatic trauma. Ann Surg 1998;6: 861–869.

Emmick RH Jr, Peterson SR. Evaluation of pancreatic injury after blunt abdominal trauma. Ann Emerg Med 1996;27(5): 658–661.

Fabian TC. Prevention of infections following penetrating abdominal trauma. Am J Surg 1993;165[Suppl 2A]:14S–19S.

Jurkovich J. Injury to the duodenum and pancreas. In: Feliciano DV, Mattox KL, Moore EE, eds. Trauma, 3rd ed. Norwalk, CT: Appleton & Lange, 1996:473–494.

Novelline RA, Rhea JT, Bell T. Helical CT of abdominal trauma. Radiol Clin North Am 1999;37(3):591–612.

Author: Beth Anne DeGennaro

Pancreatitis

Clinical Presentation

SIGNS AND SYMPTOMS

Frequency

- Abdominal pain: 95–100%
- Epigastric tenderness: 95–100%
- Nausea and vomiting: 70–90%
- Low-grade fever: 70–85%
- Hypotension: 20–40%
- Altered mental status: 20–35%
- Grey Turner/Cullen's sign: <5%
- Subcutaneous fat necrosis: <1%

GI

- Severe, persistent epigastric pain radiating to back
  —Colicky pain or rebound tenderness suggest nonpancreatic source
  —Worse when supine
- Bowel sounds usually decreased or absent
- Cullen's sign
  —Bluish discoloration at umbilicus secondary to hemorrhagic pancreatitis
- Grey Turner's sign
  —Bluish discoloration at flank secondary to hemorrhagic pancreatitis

Respiratory

- Pleuritic chest pain
- Dyspnea
- Lung exam
  —Left pleural effusion (most common)
  —Atelectasis
  —Pulmonary edema
- Hypoxemia (30%)

Cardiac

- Tachycardia
- Hypotension
- Shock

Neurologic

- Irritability
- Confusion
- Coma
- Chvostek and Trousseau signs are rare despite laboratory evidence of hypocalcemia

Ranson's Criteria

- Indicators of morbidity and mortality
  —0–2 criteria: 2% mortality
  —3–4 criteria: 15% mortality
  —5–6 criteria: 40% mortality
  —7–8 criteria: 100% mortality
- Criteria on admission
  —Age older than 55 years
  —WBC count >16,000 IU/L
  —Blood glucose >200 mg/d
  —Serum LDH >350 IU/L
  —SGOT >250 IU/dL
- Criteria during first 48 hours
  —Hematocrit fall >10%
  —BUN increase >5 mg/dL
  —Serum calcium <8 mg/dL
  —Arterial PO_2 <60 mm Hg
  —Base deficit >4 mEq/L
  —Estimated fluid sequestration >6 L

MECHANISM/DESCRIPTION

- Inflammation of the pancreas due to activation, interstitial liberation, and digestion of the gland by its own enzymes
- Acute pancreatitis
  —Exocrine and endocrine function of the gland impaired for weeks to months
  —Glandular function will return to normal
- Chronic pancreatitis
  —Exocrine and endocrine function progressively deteriorate with resultant steatorrhea and malabsorption
  —Dysfunction progressive and irreversible

ETIOLOGY

- Gallstones and alcohol abuse most common etiologies of *acute pancreatitis* (75%)
- Alcohol abuse accounts for 70–80% of *chronic pancreatitis*
- Acute
  —Biliary tract disease
  —Chronic alcoholism
  —Obstruction pancreatic duct
  —Ischemia
  —Drugs
  —Infectious
  —Postoperative
  —Post-ERCP
  —Metabolic diseases
  —After renal transplant
  —Scorpion venom
  —Penetrating peptic ulcer
  —Hereditary
  —Idiopathic
- Chronic
  —Chronic alcoholism
  —Obstruction pancreatic duct
  —Tropical
  —Hereditary
  —Shwachman disease
  —Enterokinase deficiency
  —Enzyme deficiency
  —Idiopathic
  —Hyperlipidemia

PEDIATRIC CONSIDERATIONS

- Etiology mainly viral, trauma, and drugs
- Pancreas well imaged with US

Pre-Hospital

N/A

Diagnosis

ESSENTIAL WORKUP

- Laboratory tests confirm physical diagnosis

LABORATORY

- Amylase
  —Rise within 6 hours of pain onset
  —More than five times upper limit is highly specific for pancreatitis
  —More than 1,000 IU suggests biliary pancreatitis
  —May be normal during acute inflammation due to significant preexisting pancreatic destruction
  —Secreted from various sources
- Lipase
  —Rise within 4–8 hours of pain onset
  —More reliable indicator of pancreatitis than amylase
- Electrolytes, BUN, creatinine, glucose
  —Hypokalemia occurs with extensive fluid losses
  —Hyperglycemia
- CBC
  —Increased hematocrit with fluid losses
  —Decreased hematocrit with retroperitoneal hemorrhage
  —WBC count >12,000 unusual
- Calcium/magnesium
  —Hypocalcemia signifies significant pancreatic injury
  —Hypomagnesemia occurs with underlying alcohol abuse
- Liver function tests
  —Useful for prognostic indicators and if suspected biliary etiology
- Pregnancy test
- ABGs
  —Indicated if hypoxic (assess PO_2) or toxic appearing (assess base deficit)

IMAGING/SPECIAL TESTS

- EKG
  - —Assess electrolyte imbalances, ischemia
- Abdominal series
  - —Excludes free air
  - —May visualize pancreatic calcifications
  - —Most common finding is isolated dilated bowel loop (sentinel loop) near pancreas
- CXR for
  - —Pleural effusion
  - —Atelectasis
  - —Infiltrate
- US if gallstone pancreatitis suspected
- Abdominal CT scan indicated acutely if
  - —High-risk pancreatitis (>3 Ranson's criteria)
  - —Hemorrhagic pancreatitis
  - —Suspicion of pseudocyst
  - —Diagnosis in doubt

DIFFERENTIAL DIAGNOSIS

- Mesenteric ischemia/infarction
- Myocardial infarction
- Biliary colic
- Intestinal obstruction
- Perforated ulcer
- Pneumonia
- Ruptured aortic aneurysm
- Ectopic pregnancy

Treatment

INITIAL STABILIZATION

- ABCs
  - —Supplemental oxygen
  - —Cardiac monitor
  - —IV fluids

ED TREATMENT

- Airway management
  - —Pulmonary complaints necessitate supplemental oxygen
  - —Endotracheal intubation for ARDS or severe encephalopathy
- Fluid resuscitation
  - —Large fluid volumes (up to 5–6 L in first 24 hours) due to fluid losses
  - —Continuously assess vitals, urine output, and electrolytes to ensure rapid and adequate replacement of intravascular volume
  - —Consider CVP monitoring in elderly and when fluid overload is a concern
- Correct electrolyte abnormalities if present
  - —Hypocalcemia (calcium gluconate)
  - —Hypokalemia occurs with extensive fluid losses
  - —Hypomagnesemia occurs with underlying alcohol abuse
- Blood products
  - —In hemorrhagic pancreatitis, transfuse hematocrit to a level of 30%
  - —Fresh-frozen plasma and platelets if coagulopathic and bleeding
- Analgesia
  - —Meperidine is drug of choice
  - —Morphine not recommended due to contraction of sphincter of Oddi
- Nasogastric suction
  - —Not useful in cases of mild pancreatitis
  - —Beneficial in severe pancreatitis or intractable nausea and vomiting
- Antiemetics
- Antibiotics not routinely indicated
  - —Possible benefits in necrotizing pancreatitis
- Surgical consultation
  - —Indicated for severe pancreatitis of biliary origin for possible ERCP

MEDICATIONS

- Calcium gluconate 10%: 10 mL i.v. over 15–20 minutes
- Meperidine (demerol): 25–50 mg i.v., 50–75 mg i.m. q3–4h
- Magnesium sulfate: 16 mEq (2 g) in 50 mL D5W over 20 minutes
- Potassium chloride: 10 mEq/h i.v.
- Promethazine: 12.5–25 mg PO/i.m./PR/i.v.

Disposition

ADMISSION CRITERIA

- Acute pancreatitis with significant pain, nausea, vomiting
- ICU admission for hemorrhagic/necrotizing pancreatitis

DISCHARGE CRITERIA

- Mild acute pancreatitis without evidence of biliary tract disease and able to tolerate oral fluids
- Chronic pancreatitis with minimal abdominal pain and able to tolerate oral fluids

Miscellaneous

ICD9: 577.0; 577.1

ICD10: K85

SEE ALSO: PANCREATIC PSEUDOCYST

SUGGESTED READINGS

Banks PA. Practice guidelines in acute pancreatitis. Am J Gastroenterol 1997;92(3):377–386.

Go V, et al, eds. The pancreas. New York: Raven Press, 1993:575–635.

Heinisch A, Scholmerich J, Leser H. Diagnostic approach to acute pancreatitis: diagnosis, assessment of etiology and prognosis. Hepatogastroenterology 1993;40(6):531–537.

Munoz A, Katerndahl DA. Diagnosis and management of acute pancreatitis. Am Fam Physician 2000;62(1):164–174.

Norton SA, Chevuru CVN, Collins J, et al. An assessment of clinical guidelines for the management of acute pancreatitis. Ann R Coll Surg Engl 2001;83(6):399–405.

Author: Trevor Lewis

Panic Attacks

Clinical Presentation

SIGNS AND SYMPTOMS

- Characteristic, acute episodes of physical symptoms and intense fear that rapidly peak within 10 minutes and resolve in about 20 minutes

Physical Symptoms

- Multiple systems suggest autonomic arousal
- Cardiac
  —Palpitations
  —Tachycardia
  —Chest pain
- Respiratory
  —Shortness of breath
  —Smothering
  —Choking
- Neurologic
  —Tremor
  —Dizziness
  —Light-headedness
  —Feeling faint
  —Numbness
  —Tingling
  —Sweating
  —Chills
  —Flushing
  —Feelings of unreality or detachment
- GI
  —Nausea
  —Cramps
  —Abdominal pain

Intense Fears

- Automatic, stereotypic
- Imminent death
- Humiliation
- Loss of control—"going crazy"

MECHANISM/DESCRIPTION

- Limbic system, norepinephrine release, other neurotransmitters (e.g., serotonin) implicated

Panic Disorder

- Recurrent, unexpected panic attacks with one or more months of persistent
  —Concerns about having another attack
  —Worry about the implications or consequences of the attacks
  —Behavioral change, such as phobic avoidance, related to the attacks
- Episodic, recurrent, or chronic
- Frequently comorbid with depression, substance abuse, disability, suicidal tendency

ETIOLOGY

- Probably genetic
- Risk factors
  —Family history of panic or anxiety
  —Childhood shyness or separation anxiety
  —Major life events in year preceding onset
- May develop in the course of predisposing physical illness or cocaine abuse
  —May persist after the illness or substance use has resolved

Pre-Hospital

N/A

Diagnosis

ESSENTIAL WORKUP

- Known medical conditions
- All medications, including over the counter
- Recreational drugs/alcohol use
- Caffeine consumption
- Age at onset
- Family history of panic, anxiety
- Initiating life events
- Childhood antecedents
- Resultant avoidance
- Response to previous medication trials
- Thorough physical and neurological exam

LABORATORY

- Toxicology screen
- EKG
  —Age older than 40
  —Cardiac symptoms
- CBC
- Electrolytes, BUN/Cr, glucose
- TSH

IMAGING/SPECIAL TESTS

- Echocardiogram for suspected mitral valve prolapse
- Sleep-deprived EEG if seizure suspected

DIFFERENTIAL DIAGNOSIS

- Consider organic causes if
  —Panic presents late in life
  —No childhood antecedents or family history
  —No initiating life events
  —Without avoidance or significant fear
  —With a history of poor response to previous trials of antipanic or antidepressant medication
- Medications
  —Neuroleptics (akathisia)
  —Bronchodilators
  —Digitalis
  —Anticholinergic agents
  —Diet pills
- Respiratory
  —COPD
  —Pulmonary embolus
- Cardiovascular
  —Angina
  —Arrhythmia
  —Anemia
  —Mitral valve prolapse (MVP) may be comorbid with panic
- Substances
  —Stimulant abuse
  —Withdrawal (alcohol, sedative-hypnotics)
  —Excessive caffeine intake
- Endocrine
  —Hyperthyroidism
  —Hypoglycemia
  —Parathyroid disorders
  —Pheochromocytoma

- Neurologic
  - —Complex partial, or limbic seizures (fear, physical symptoms, perceptual distortions)
  - —TIA
- Psychiatric
  - —Other anxiety, stress, or phobic disorders; for example, obsessive-compulsive disorder, posttraumatic stress disorder, or social phobia

Treatment

INITIAL STABILIZATION

- Be calm and reassuring
- Most panic attacks resolve within 20–30 minutes without any treatment
- Fear may trigger another panic attack

ED TREATMENT

- High-potency benzodiazepines
  - —Drugs of choice
  - —Clonazepam
    - -Slow for emergency use
    - -Long acting without rapid onset/offset phenomena
    - -Best choice in this class for maintenance therapy of recurrent panic attacks
  - —Alprazolam
    - -Rapid onset
    - -Rebound anxiety occurs due to short duration and rapid offset
    - -May lead to escalating doses with continued use
  - —Lorazepam
    - -Quick onset
    - -Advantage of sublingual use
    - -Longer effect and less abrupt offset than alprazolam
- Avoid low-potency benzodiazepines
  - —Diazepam
  - —Chlordiazepoxide
- Treat recurrent panic attacks and panic disorder with SSRI, TCA, or MAOI antidepressants, with or without clonazepam
  - —Will not work immediately
  - —Do not need to be started emergently
- Discharge therapy
  - —Several clonazepam tablets in case of repeated attacks
    - -Do not prescribe alprazolam—withdrawal may trigger further attacks
  - —Psychopharmacological and cognitive behavioral therapy evaluation for repeated attacks, or interepisode fear or avoidance, for evaluation

MEDICATIONS

- Alprazolam: 0.5 mg PO
- Clonazepam: 0.5 mg PO in the ED; 0.25–0.5 mg p.o. b.i.d. for initial outpatient therapy
- Lorazepam: 1 mg PO or s.l.

Disposition

ADMISSION CRITERIA

- As medically indicated to rule out organic cause
- Meets criteria for psychiatric admission (suicidal, homicidal)

DISCHARGE CRITERIA

- Most panic attacks do not require inpatient level of care

Miscellaneous

ICD9: 300.01

ICD10: F41.0

SUGGESTED READINGS

APA Work Group on Panic Disorder. Practice guidelines for the treatment of patients with panic disorder. Am J Psychiatry 1998;155[Suppl 5]:1–34.

Glass RM. Panic disorder—it's real and it's treatable. JAMA 2000;19:2573–2574.

Lepola UM, Wade AG, Leinonen EV, et al. A controlled, prospective, 1-year trial of citalopram in the treatment of panic disorder. J Clin Psychiatry 1998;59: 528–534.

Roy-Byrne PP, Katon W, Cowley DS, et al. A randomized effectiveness trial of collaborative care for patients with panic disorder in primary care. Arch Gen Psychiatry 2001;58:869–876.

Roy-Byrne PP, Katon W, Cowley DS, et al. Panic disorder in primary care. Gen Hosp Psychiatry 2000;22:405–411.

Author: B.J. Beck

Paraphimosis

Clinical Presentation

SIGNS AND SYMPTOMS

- Retracted foreskin
- Pain
- Swollen, edematous glans
- Local cellulitis
- Necrosis of glans in untreated cases

MECHANISM/DESCRIPTION

- Paraphimosis is a *urologic emergency*
- It is the entrapment of the retracted foreskin proximal to the glans of the penis
  - —Leads to lymphatic congestion, venous obstruction, which may result in arterial compromise to the glans

ETIOLOGY

- A number of conditions of the foreskin may predispose to paraphimosis, including
  - —Phimosis
  - —Inflammation
  - —Trauma
- Commonly iatrogenic, from failure to replace the foreskin after examination, catheterization, or cleaning

Pre-Hospital

CAUTIONS

- Patients should be transported promptly; do not attempt reduction in the field
- Pre-hospital personnel can be advised to apply an ice pack to the glans with adequate protection of the skin

Diagnosis

ESSENTIAL WORKUP

- Paraphimosis is a clinical diagnosis with the pathognomonic clinical findings described earlier
- Examination should include a search for constricting foreign bodies, constricting bands
- Treatment must not be delayed pending diagnostic laboratory or radiographic studies

IMAGING/SPECIAL TESTS

- If history suggests penile foreign body, x-rays may be obtained once the vascular compromise has been relieved

DIFFERENTIAL DIAGNOSIS

- Foreign bodies constricting the penile shaft may mimic paraphimosis; these include
  - —Hair tourniquets
  - —Wire, string, or other material used for sexual enhancement or punishment
- Balanoposthitis
- Trauma (zipper injuries)
- Acute idiopathic penile edema

Treatment

INITIAL STABILIZATION

- Ice can be applied to the glans while preparing to reduce the prepuce
  —Use the thumb of a glove as an ice-filled condom to aid in direct application
- The incarcerated foreskin must be released as soon as possible to prevent ischemia and necrosis of the glans
- The pain associated with reduction techniques must be managed with conscious sedation, adequate analgesia, and local anesthesia

ED TREATMENT

- Rolled gauze or an elastic wrap may be applied to aid in reducing edema of the glans
- Attempt manual reduction by gentle, steady traction on the foreskin with downward pressure on the glans
- Decrease in glans edema has been obtained with the "puncture" technique, making one or more holes in the swollen foreskin with a small sterile needle, allowing expression of edema fluid; this requires adequate analgesia or anesthesia
- Granulated sugar held on the prepuce may reduce edema through an osmotic effect but may take hours
- Edema may also be reduced by injection of 1-mL aliquots of hyaluronidase using a tuberculin syringe into the edematous prepuce
- Failure of these techniques or the development of ischemia necessitates a dorsal longitudinal slit in the foreskin
- Urologic consultation is required for subsequent circumcision to prevent recurrence

MEDICATIONS

- See Conscious Sedation
- Appropriate analgesics or anesthetics as required

Disposition

ADMISSION CRITERIA

- Necrosis or cellulitis of the penis

DISCHARGE CRITERIA

- Successful reduction with relief of symptoms
- Close urologic follow-up

Miscellaneous

ICD9: 605

ICD10: N47

SUGGESTED READINGS

Barone JG, Fleisher MH. Treatment of paraphimosis using the "puncture" technique. Pediatr Emerg Care 1993;9(5):298–299.

O'Donnell JA II. Phimosis and paraphimosis. In: Barkin RM, et al, eds. Pediatric emergency medicine, 2nd ed. St. Louis: Mosby, 1997:1152–1153.

Pontari MA. Phimosis and paraphimosis. In: Seidman, Hanno PM, eds. Current urologic therapy, 3rd ed. Philadelphia: WB Saunders, 1994:392–397.

Raveenthwan V. Reduction of paraphimosis: a technique based on pathophysiology. Br J Surg 1996;83(9):1247.

Super DM. Phimosis. In: Hoekelman R, et al, eds. Primary pediatric care. St. Louis: CV Mosby, 1987:1232–1234.

Author: Lorne Sherman

Parkinson's Disease

Clinical Presentation

SIGNS AND SYMPTOMS

- "Pill-rolling" resting tremor
- "Cog-wheel" rigidity due to increased muscular tone
- Stooped posture and instability of posture
- Stiffness and slowness of movement
- "Masked face" appearance
- Depression and dementia
- Sudden change in baseline motor function or mental status in a patient with Parkinson's disease may be the only indication of systemic disease such as infection

ETIOLOGY

- Sporadic or idiopathic, degenerative
- Type A encephalitis of von Economo
- CNS viral infections
- Vascular infarction
- Intoxications
  - —Phenothiazine
  - —Butyrophenones
  - —Metoclopramide
  - —Illicit drugs
  - —Carbon monoxide (bilateral infarctions of the globus pallidus)
  - —Manganese

MECHANISM/DESCRIPTION

- Gradually progressive disorder of middle or late life
- Aggregates of melanin-containing nerve cells in the brainstem (substantia nigra locus ceruleus)
- Reactive gliosis with nerve cell loss
- Lewy bodies (eosinophilic intracytoplasmic inclusions)
- *Decreased dopamine* in the caudate nucleus and putamen
- Accelerated *cortical atrophy*
- Can begin unilaterally, but generalizes to symmetric

PEDIATRIC CONSIDERATIONS

- The earliest variants of Parkinson's disease have been found in patients 20 years or older

Pre-Hospital

- None

Diagnosis

ESSENTIAL WORKUP

- *History* is of primary importance, as diagnosis is made based on clinical findings
- Important historical information includes
  - —Onset of symptom, whether gradual or sudden
  - —History of encephalitis, herpes virus infection, or carbon monoxide exposure
- In patients with established Parkinson's disease, sudden change in baseline motor function or mental status should prompt workup for infectious process such as UTI

LABORATORY

- There are no specific or recommended laboratory studies necessary to confirm the diagnosis of Parkinson's disease
- Nonidiopathic Parkinson's disease may require directed laboratory studies relative to the specific disease process
- Urinalysis, CBC, CXR, and other appropriate workup for occult infection in patients with established disease

IMAGING/SPECIAL TESTS

- CT scan/MRI are not required to diagnose Parkinson's disease but are often elements of evaluation for dementia
- CXR may be indicated for any signs of respiratory tract infection

DIFFERENTIAL DIAGNOSIS

- Benign familial tremor
- Major depression
- Wilson's disease
- Huntington's disease
- Alzheimer's disease
- Creutzfeldt-Jacob disease
- Carbon Monoxide poisoning

Treatment

INITIAL STABILIZATION

N/A

ED TREATMENT

- Treatment with antiparkinsonian medications can be initiated in the ED to alleviate symptoms
- Consultation with neurology for recommended medication regimens and ongoing support and monitoring is prudent
- For patients with mild disease, no medication may be required
- For moderate disease involvement including symmetric tremor and postural imbalance, anticholinergic medications and dopaminergic medications should be used
- Treat underlying infection if present

MEDICATIONS

- Amantadine: 100 mg b.i.d.
- Benztropine: 0.5–1 mg t.i.d.
- Bromocriptine: 15 mg q.d.
- Levodopa/dopa carboxylase inhibitor (carbidopa) combination: 25/100 mg q.d.
- Trihexyphenidyl: 1–2 mg q.i.d.

Disposition

ADMISSION CRITERIA

- Patient with intercurrent infections, dehydration, or other medical problems
- Depression with intent to do self-harm
- Medication regimen adjustment

DISCHARGE CRITERIA

- Mild to moderate disease without medications
- Moderate to severe disease with medications and urgent neurologic outpatient follow-up

Miscellaneous

ICD9: 332.0

ICD10: G20

SUGGESTED READINGS

Fahn S, et al. Recent advances in Parkinson's disease. New York: Raven, 1986.

Flint MB, Beal M, Richardson EP, et al. Parkinson's disease. In: Isselbacher KJ, et al, eds. Harrison's principles of internal medicine. New York: McGraw-Hill, 1994.

Lieberman, A. Managing the neuropsychiatric symptoms of Parkinson's disease. Neurology 1998;50[6 Suppl 6]:533–538.

Rajput A, et al. Epidemiology of parkinsonism: Incidence, classification, and mortality. Ann Neurol 1984;16:178.

Author: James M. Leaming

Paronychia

Clinical Presentation

SIGNS AND SYMPTOMS

- Begins as swelling, pain, and erythema in the dorsolateral corner of the nail fold bulging out over the nail plate, which progresses to a subcuticular abscess

MECHANISM/DESCRIPTION

- Disruption of the seal between the nail plate and the nail fold may allow entry of bacteria into the eponychial space
- Inflammation of the nail folds surrounding the nail plate

ETIOLOGY

- Acute paronychia: predominantly *Staphylococcus aureus* but also streptococcal organisms
- Chronic paronychia: predominantly *Candida albicans* but may also be other fungi, atypical mycobacteria; commonly coexisting with *Staphylococcus* species

Risk Factors

- Acute: minor nail trauma such as hangnails, vigorous manicures, nail biting; underlying disease such as diabetes
- Chronic: occupations with persistent moist hands such as dish washers, bartenders; also increased in patients with peripheral vascular disease

PEDIATRIC CONSIDERATIONS

- Frequently anaerobic mouth flora in children from nail biting

Pre-Hospital

N/A

Diagnosis

ESSENTIAL WORKUP

- History and physical exam with special attention to evaluating for concomitant infections such as felon or cellulitis
- Evaluate tetanus status

LABORATORY

- No specific tests are useful

IMAGING/SPECIAL TESTS

- Soft-tissue radiographs if foreign body suspected

DIFFERENTIAL DIAGNOSIS

- Felon
- Herpetic whitlow
- Trauma or foreign body
- Primary squamous cell carcinoma
- Metastatic carcinoma
- Osteomyelitis

Treatment

INITIAL STABILIZATION

- No specific stabilization necessary

ED TREATMENT

Acute Paronychia

- Early paronychia without purulence present may be managed with oral antibiotics
  - —Cephalexin, dicloxacillin
  - —Clindamycin or erythromycin if associated with nail biting or oral contact or allergy
- Early superficial subcuticular abscess
  - —Elevation of the eponychial fold by sliding the flat edge of a no. 11 blade (18-gauge needle or small clamps may be used) gently between the proximal nail fold and the nail plate near the point of maximal tenderness
  - —A digital nerve block or local anesthesia may be necessary
- Partial nail involvement
  - —If the lesion extends beneath the nail, remove a longitudinal section of the nail to allow drainage, followed by Vaseline or iodoform gauze packing for 24 hours
- Runaround abscess
  - —If the lesion extends beneath the base of the nail to the other side, remove one quarter to one third of the proximal nail with two small incisions at the dorsolateral edges of the nail fold, and pack eponychial fold with petroleum or iodoform gauze to prevent adherence
- Extensive subungual abscess
  - —Remove entire nail
- Antibiotics may be used as adjunct
  - —Dicloxacillin or a first-generation cephalosporin such as cephalexin for 5–10 days if any apparent cellulitis, abscess, or systemic signs of infection

Chronic Paronychia

- Eponychial marsupialization involving removal of a crescentic piece of skin just proximal to the nail fold including all thickened tissue down to, but not including, germinal matrix
  - —Topical steroids with a topical antifungal agent have been used with success
  - —Antistaphylococcal treatment should also be considered

MEDICATIONS

- Cephalexin: 500 g PO q.i.d. × 7 days (peds: 40 mg/kg/d PO q6h)
- Clindamycin: 300 mg PO q.i.d. × 7 days (peds: 20–40 mg/kg/d div q6h PO, i.v., i.m.)
- Dicloxacillin: 500 mg PO q.i.d. × 7 days (peds: 12.5–50 mg/kg/d PO q6h)
- Erythromycin: 500 mg PO q.i.d. × 7 days (peds: 40 mg/kg/d q6h PO)

Disposition

ADMISSION CRITERIA

- Patients with uncomplicated paronychia can be managed as outpatients

DISCHARGE CRITERIA

- Patients with uncomplicated paronychia that has been managed in the ED may be discharged with appropriate follow-up instructions
- Patients with packing must return in 24 hours for reevaluation

Miscellaneous

ICD9: 681.9

ICD10: L03.0

SUGGESTED READINGS

Canales FL, Newmeyer WL, Kilgore ES. The treatment of felons and paronychias. Hand Clin 1989;5(4):515–523.

Hochman LG. Paronychia: more than just an abscess. Int J Dermatol 1995;34(6): 385–386.

Moran GJ, Talan DA. Hand infections. Emerg Med Clin 1993;11(3):601–619.

Author: Gene Ma

Patellar Injuries

Clinical Presentation

SIGNS AND SYMPTOMS

Dislocation

- History of feeling knee "go out;" popping, ripping, or tearing sensation
- Pain
- Inability to bear weight
- Obvious lateral deformity of patella
- Mild to moderate swelling
- Often reduced spontaneously before ED evaluation
- Tenderness along patella
- Positive apprehension or Fairbanks sign
  —Attempts to push the patella laterally elicits apprehension

Fracture

- Pain over anterior knee
- Difficulty ambulating
- Increased pain with movement of patella
- Tenderness and swelling over patella
- Difficulty or inability to extend knee
- Palpable defect, crepitus, or joint effusion/hemarthrosis

Patellar Tendon Rupture

- Abrupt onset of severe pain
- Decreased ability to bear weight
- Occasionally hemarthrosis
- Proximally displaced patella
- Incomplete extensor function
- Unable to maintain knee extension against force

Patellar Tendinitis

- "Jumper's knee"
- Pain in area of patellar tendon
- Pain worse from sitting to standing or going up stairs
- Point tenderness at distal aspect of patella or proximal patellar tendon

MECHANISM/DESCRIPTION

Dislocation

- Usually caused by sudden flexion and external rotation of tibia on femur, with simultaneous contraction of quadriceps muscles
- Lateral dislocation of patella most common, with patella displaced laterally over the lateral femoral condyle
- Uncommon dislocations include superior, medial, and rare intraarticular dislocation
- Direct trauma to patella

Fracture

- Direct trauma
  —Most common mechanism of injury
  —Secondary to direct blow or fall on patella
  —Usually results in comminuted or minimally displaced fracture
- Indirect forces
  —Avulsion injury secondary to contraction of the quadriceps tendon
  —Usually results in transverse or displaced fracture (often both)
- Types of patellar fractures
  —Transverse: 50–80% (usually middle or lower third of patella)
  —Comminuted (or stellate): 30–35%
  —Longitudinal: 25%
  —Osteochondral

Patellar Tendon Rupture

- Usually caused by forceful eccentric contraction on a flexed knee (e.g., jump landing and weight lifting)

Patellar Tendinitis

- Overuse syndrome from repeated acceleration, deceleration, jumping, landing

ETIOLOGY

Dislocation

- Risk factors for patellar dislocation
  —Genu valgum ("knock knee")
  —Genu recurvatum (hyperextension of knee)
  —Shallow lateral femoral condyle
  —Deficient vastus medialis
  —Lateral insertion of patellar tendon
  —Shallow patellar groove
  —Patella alta (high-riding patella)
  —Deformed patella
  —Pes planus (flatfoot)
- Common injury in adolescents, especially girls
- The younger the patient at time of initial dislocation, the greater the risk of recurrent dislocation

Fracture

- Direct trauma
- Indirect forces caused by forcible quadriceps tendon contraction
- Male-to-female ratio of 2:1
- Highest incidence in 20–50-year-old age-group

Pre-Hospital

- Patient should be transported in supine position with knee flexed and supported

Patellar Tendon Rupture

- Peak incidence in third and fourth decades
- Risk factors
  —History of patellar tendinitis
  —History of diabetes mellitus, previous steroid injections, rheumatoid arthritis, gout, systemic lupus erythematosus
  —Previous major knee surgery

Patellar Tendinitis

- Microtears of tendon matrix from overuse
- Seen in high jumpers, volleyball and basketball players, and runners

Diagnosis

ESSENTIAL WORKUP

- Radiographs essential
  —Anteroposterior (AP) and lateral views of knee should be obtained
  —Postreduction radiographs should include AP, lateral, and sunrise (or skyline, axial) views to exclude osteochondral fracture (in patellar dislocations)
  —Bipartite patella (patella with accessory bony fragment connected to main body by cartilage) may be mistaken for fracture; comparison view may help differentiate
- For patellar tendon rupture, a high-riding patella (i.e., patella located superior to level of intercondylar notch) observed
- For patellar tendinitis, radiographic findings unlikely with symptoms of <6 months' duration

DIFFERENTIAL DIAGNOSIS

- Patellar subluxation
- Femoral or tibial fracture
- Traumatic bursitis
- Quadriceps tendon rupture

Treatment

INITIAL STABILIZATION

- Patient placed in supine position with knee flexed and supported
- Appropriate history and physical exam to identify any associated injuries (e.g., femoral fracture, hip fracture, posterior hip dislocation)

ED TREATMENT

Dislocation

- For simple lateral patellar dislocation, reduce dislocation by extending the knee gently to 180 degrees
  - —Occasionally may need to apply simultaneous pressure over lateral aspect of patella in medial direction
- For other types of patellar dislocation (superior, medial, intraarticular) do not attempt reduction; obtain orthopedic consultation
- Aspiration of joint with sterile technique necessary if reduction is difficult secondary to hemarthrosis
- If osteochondral fracture present (28–50% of cases), obtain orthopedic consultation
- Although reduction is typically easy to accomplish, procedural sedation or parenteral analgesia may facilitate

Fracture

- Orthopedic consultation when patellar fracture is confirmed
- Initial treatment often consists of long-leg bulky splint and subsequent operative repair

Patellar Tendon Rupture

- Orthopedic consultation, with surgical repair within 2–6 weeks

MEDICATIONS

- Fentanyl citrate: 1–2 μg/kg i.v. (peds: 0.5–1.0 μg/kg i.v.)
- Midazolam HCL: 1–3 mg i.v. (peds: 0.05–0.1 mg/kg, maximum dose 2.5 mg i.v.)
- Morphine sulphate: 2–5 mg/dose i.v. (peds: 0.1–0.2 mg/kg/dose i.v.)
- Meperidine: 50–150 mg i.m. (peds: 0.5–0.8 mg/lb i.m.)
- Toradol: 60 mg i.m.; 30 mg i.v. (peds: 0.5–1 mg/kg/i.v. max 30 mg/dose)

Disposition

ADMISSION CRITERIA

- Patients with superior, medial, or intraarticular dislocation or inability to reduce lateral dislocation require orthopedic consultation in ED and possible admission
- Patellar dislocation associated with a fracture (osteochondral or lateral femoral condyle) requires orthopedic consultation in ED
- Operative intervention indicated if fragments are displaced >4 mm, if patient unable to raise extended leg off bed, or if articular step-off >3 mm
- All open fractures require débridement and irrigation and should be admitted
- For patellar tendon rupture, discuss case with orthopedics

DISCHARGE CRITERIA

- Patients with successful reduction of lateral patellar dislocation and normal postreduction radiographs may be discharged with knee immobilization, crutches, and orthopedic follow-up
- Fracture is displaced <3 mm and patient has full active knee extension
- Knee immobilizer, or bulky long-leg splint, partial to full weight bearing as tolerated with crutches, and orthopedic follow-up within a few days
- For patellar tendinitis, rest, avoid inciting activity, heat, and NSAIDs

Miscellaneous

ICD9: 836.3, 822.0

ICD10: S89.9

SUGGESTED READINGS

Atkin DM, Fithian DC, Marangi KS, et al. Characteristics of patients with primary acute lateral patellar dislocation and their recovery within the first 6 months of injury. Am J Sports Med 2000;28:472–479.

Cash JD, Hughston JC. Treatment of acute patellar dislocation. Am J Sports Med 1988;16:244–249.

Enad JG. Patellar tendon ruptures. South Med J 1999;92:563–566.

Simon RR, Koenigsknecht SJ. The knee, fibular, and patellar dislocations. In: Simon RR, Koenigsknecht SJ, eds. Emergency orthopedics—the extremities, 3rd ed. East Norwalk, CT: Appleton & Lange, 1995:463–470.

Stewart C. Knee injuries: diagnosis and repair. Emerg Med Rep 1997;92:1–12.

Author: Francis L. Counselman

Patent Ductus Arteriosus

Clinical Presentation

SIGNS AND SYMPTOMS

- Asymptomatic when the patent ductus arteriosus (PDA) is small
- CHF
- Wide pulse pressure
- Prominent apical impulse
- Thrill
  - —Maximal in the second left intercostal space
  - —Radiates toward the left clavicle, down the left sternal border, or toward the apex
  - —Systolic or continuous
- Continuous murmur
  - —Humming top or rolling thunder
  - —Begins soon after onset of the first sound, reaches maximal intensity at the end of systole, and wanes in late diastole
  - —Localized to the second left intercostal space or radiates down the left sternal border or to the left clavicle
- Recurrent pulmonary infections
- Retardation of physical growth

MECHANISM/DESCRIPTION

- The ductus arteriosus
  - —Patent vessel in the fetus connects the pulmonary trunk to the descending aorta
  - —Shortly after birth, changes normally provoke contraction, closure, and fibrosis
  - —Sudden increase in the partial pressure of oxygen
  - —Changes in the synthesis and metabolism of vasoactive eicosanoids
- In the preterm infant, patency of the ductus may be life saving
  - —The patent ductus usually has a normal structural anatomy
  - —Results from hypoxia and immaturity
- In the full-term newborn, patency of the ductus is a congenital malformation
  - —Deficiency of both the mucoid endothelial layer and the muscular media of the ductus
  - —As pulmonary vascular resistance falls, aortic blood is shunted into the pulmonary artery
  - —Extent of the shunt reflects the size of the ductus and the ratio of pulmonary to systemic vascular resistances
- Up to 70% of the left ventricular output may be shunted through the ductus to the pulmonary circulation
- Risk factors
  - —Premature birth
  - —Coexisting cardiac anomalies
  - —Conditions resulting in hypoxia
  - —High altitude
  - —Maternal rubella infection
  - —Female-to-male ratio, 2:1

ETIOLOGY

- Prematurity
- Congenital anomaly
- Hypoxia
- Prostaglandins

Pre-Hospital

CAUTIONS

- Supplemental oxygen if evidence of CHF

Diagnosis

ESSENTIAL WORKUP

- Establish the diagnosis with imaging studies
- Rule out complications such as heart failure and endocarditis

LABORATORY

- Unhelpful in making the diagnosis

IMAGING/SPECIAL TESTS

- CXR
  - —Usually normal in infants
  - —In children and adults
    - -Increased intrapulmonary markings
    - -Calcifications
    - -Left ventricle and left atrial enlargement
    - -Dilated ascending aorta
    - -Dilated pulmonary arteries
- EKG
  - —Abnormal if the ductus is large
  - —Left ventricular hypertrophy
  - —Right ventricular hypertrophy is a sign of severity
- Echocardiography
  - —Normal if the ductus is small
  - —Left atrial enlargement
  - —Size of the ductus can be determined by scanning from the suprasternal notch
  - —Doppler studies will determine aortic to pulmonary artery flow during diastole
- Cardiac catheterization
  - —Normal or increased right-sided pressure
  - —Oxygenated blood in the pulmonary artery confirms left-to-right shunting
  - —Injection of contrast into the ascending aorta shows opacification of the pulmonary arteries

DIFFERENTIAL DIAGNOSIS

- Venous hum
  - —Common insignificant bruit
  - —Heard in the neck or anterior portion of the chest
  - —Soft humming sound in systole and diastole
  - —Decreased by light compression of the jugular venous system
- Total anomalous pulmonary venous connection to the innominate vein
  - —Continuous murmur like venous hum
- Aorticopulmonary septal defect
  - —Murmur is often only systolic
  - —Heard at the right upper sternal border
- Ruptured sinus of Valsalva
- Coronary arteriovenous fistulas
- Anomalous origin of left coronary artery from pulmonary artery
- Absence or atresia of pulmonary valve
- Aortic insufficiency with ventricular septal defect
- Peripheral pulmonary stenosis
- Truncus arteriosus

Treatment

INITIAL STABILIZATION

- Small, asymptomatic shunts may not need closure
- Pulmonary support
- Supplemental oxygen

ED TREATMENT

- Sodium and fluid restriction
- Correction of anemia to hematocrit >45%
- Antibiotic prophylaxis for endocarditis
- Preterm infant
  —Usually closes spontaneously
  —Varies with the magnitude of shunting and severity of hyaline membrane disease
  —Pharmacological inhibition of prostaglandin synthesis with indomethacin during the first 2–7 days of life
- Full-term infant and children
  —Surgical closure is required, even in asymptomatic patients, as spontaneous closure is rare
  —Ligation and division
  —Transfemoral catheter technique to occlude PDA with foam plastic plug, or double umbrella

MEDICATIONS

- Indomethacin: 0.2–0.25 mg/kg/dose; repeat every 12–24 hours for three doses

Disposition

ADMISSION CRITERIA

- Presence of a complication
  —Heart failure
  —Endocarditis
  —Pulmonary hypertension

DISCHARGE CRITERIA

- Asymptomatic
- Prophylactic antibiotics
- Close follow-up with plans for early surgical closure

Miscellaneous

ICD9: 747.0

ICD10: Q25.0

SUGGESTED READINGS

Bernstein D. The cardiovascular system. In: Behrnam RE, Kliegman RM, eds. Nelson's textbook of pediatrics, 16th ed. Philadelphia: WB Saunders, 2000: 372–1373.

Burton DA, Cabalka AK. Cardiac evaluation in infants. Pediatr Clin North Am 1994;41: 991–1015.

Friedman WF. Congenital heart disease in infancy and childhood. In: Braunwald E, ed. Heart disease, 5th ed. Philadelphia: WB Saunders, 1997:877–962.

Moore P, Brook MM, Heymann MA. Patent ductus arteriosus. In: Allen HD, et al, eds. Moss and Adams' heart disease in infants, children, and adolescents: including the fetus and young adult, 6th ed. Philadelphia: Lippincott Williams & Wilkins, 2001:652–669.

Author: Steven Lelyveld

Pediatric Trauma

Clinical Presentation

SIGNS AND SYMPTOMS

- Size of child determines potential injuries, nature of signs and symptoms
- Body size
  - —Fat, muscles/connective tissue
    - -Protection from injury
  - —Mass-to-surface area ratio
    - -Insensible water losses; risk of hypothermia, multiple organ injury (kinetic energy of injury dissipated into smaller mass)
- Head
  - —Compliance of bone/soft tissues
  - —Contusions/shearing injuries
  - —Open sutures/fontanelles younger than 2 years
    - -Signs of intracranial hypertension may be delayed or absent
  - —Large head/occiput
    - -Causes cervical spine flexion when supine on adult backboard
- Cervical spine
  - —Weaker cervical muscles, flatter facets, more elastic ligaments, vertebral bodies wedged anteriorly
    - -Risk of dislocation injuries, rotary subluxation, SCIWORA (*s*pinal *c*ord *i*njury *w*ithout *r*adiographic *a*bnormality)
  - —Relatively heavy head
    - -Higher fulcrum of movement; 60–70% of cervical spine injuries in children younger than 8 years occur at C-1 or C-2
- Airway
  - —Large tongue, tonsillar hypertrophy
    - -Airway easily obstructed
  - —Longer, more flexible epiglottis, larynx more anterior/superior
    - -Straight laryngoscope blade for endotracheal intubation
  - —Cricoid cartilage is narrowest portion of airway (younger than 8 years)
    - -Use uncuffed ETTs
  - —Shorter trachea
    - -Right mainstem bronchus intubation common
- Circulation
  - —Cardiac output by heart rate (HR)
    - -Shock/blood loss causes HR compensation
  - —Excellent hemodynamic compensatory mechanisms
    - -Hypotension and bradycardia are signs of severe shock
- Thorax
  - —Chest wall compliance, mobile mediastinum
  - —Implications
    - -Rib fractures/external signs of trauma often absent, internal/pulmonary/cardiac contusions common
    - -Presence of rib fractures suggests high-energy injury
- Abdomen
  - —Rib cage covers less of abdomen, less peritoneal fat
  - —Kidneys more anterior
  - —Bladder is intraabdominal (younger than 2 years)
  - —Implications
    - -Risk of intraabdominal injury, especially spleen, liver, and kidney
- Skeletal
  - —Softer, more porous bones; thicker, stronger periosteum
    - -Bones fracture more easily; fractures tend to be less displaced
  - —Tendons, ligaments, joint capsules stronger than growth plate or bone
    - -Salter-Harris fractures more common than sprains, avulsion fractures more common than ligamentous injuries

MECHANISM/DESCRIPTION

- Pediatric motor vehicle accidents
  - —Air bags deploy at >240 km/h (150 mph); severe injuries and death may occur in front-seat passengers who are younger than 12 years
  - —Seat belts fit adults, may cause intraabdominal or lumbar spine injuries; children may "submarine" (i.e., slide) under the seat belt
- Children struck by motor vehicles; pedestrian/vehicular
  - —Collision often propels child a distance
  - —Secondary injuries, separate from the primary injury, are common
- Pediatric bicycle injuries
  - —Handlebars may impale child, causing severe internal injury
- Falls, crush injuries, direct blow
- Nonaccidental injuries associated with inconsistent history/mechanism (child abuse)
- Smaller blood volume (80 mL/kg)
- Compensation in children excellent with 25–30% loss of blood volume producing few findings; decompensation may occur rapidly
- Psychologic status on patient and family may lead to anxiety and stress
- Leading cause of disability and death in children older than 1 year in the U.S.

Pre-Hospital

- Initial management priorities: stabilization of the airway, breathing, and circulation; when appropriate, immobilization of the cervical spine and extremity fractures, communicate with/transport to receiving facility
- Use pediatric-specific equipment for cervical spine immobilization; adult backboards cause cervical spine malalignment
- Destination policies of regionalized trauma systems may have an impact on destination

Diagnosis

ESSENTIAL WORKUP

- "AMPLE" history
  - —*A*llergies
  - —*M*edications
  - —*P*ast medical history
  - —*L*ast oral intake
  - —*E*vents leading to injury
- Primary survey (modified ATLS protocol)
  - —*A*irway and c-spine immobilization
  - —*B*reathing
  - —*C*irculation and hemorrhage control
  - —*D*isability, check serum dextrose
  - —*E*xposure/environmental control
- Secondary survey
  - —Complete head-to-toe exam, including log-rolling patient, posterior body and rectal exam
  - —"Fingers and tubes in every orifice"
- Standardized pediatric size estimation devices (e.g., Broselow tape) more accurate than physician "guesstimates"

LABORATORY

- No standard set of labs, so individualize to nature and extent of injury and patient's physiologic status; in patients with a major mechanism of injury, a CBC count and type and screen are usually indicated as baseline
- In awake, alert, cooperative patients with mild to moderate abdominal trauma, serial physical exams and a urinalysis are as sensitive as or more sensitive than blood tests
- Consider
  - —CBC, type and screen/cross, PT/PTT, electrolytes, BUN, creatinine, glucose, amylase, lipase, liver transaminases, UA, toxicologic screens, pregnancy test

IMAGING/SPECIAL TESTS

- Standard trauma radiographs
  - —Cervical spine (three views), chest, pelvis
- CT
  - —Study of choice for stable patients with suspected head or abdominal injuries
- US
  - —Utility of bedside US poorly studied in children
  - —Not as sensitive or specific as CT
- Diagnostic peritoneal lavage
  - —Rarely indicated
  - —Consider if abdominal injury suspected, CT unavailable, and vital signs unstable
- Limitations/controversies
  - —Severe injury *cannot* be ruled out by radiographs alone if patient intoxicated or nonverbal or has distracting injuries or altered mental status
  - —Hollow abdominal viscera injuries often missed by CT and US
  - —Utility and timing of oral contrast for abdominal CT is controversial

- Normal anatomic variants mistaken for injuries
  - —Pseudosubluxation (i.e., anterior displacement of C-2 onto C-3) occurs in 20% of children; if spinolaminar line and spinous process tips aligned, true subluxation unlikely
  - —Anterior wedging of vertebral bodies mistaken for compression fractures
  - —Growth plate at base of odontoid process closes between 3 and 6 years old; can be mistaken for fracture
  - —Predental space in children younger than 8 years can be up to 5 mm

DIFFERENTIAL DIAGNOSIS

- Similar to adults, with aforementioned pediatric anatomic/physiologic differences

Treatment

INITIAL STABILIZATION

- Airway, breathing, circulation management as per ATLS protocols and team approach
- May require empiric, aggressive management
- ETT intubation if needed
  - —ETT internal diameter (mm) = 16 + (age [yr]/4); for example, for a 6-year-old, use 5.5 (16 + 6/4) ETT
  - —Depth to insert ETT (cm) = (3) (ETT internal diameter); for example, insert 5.0 ETT to about 15 cm
  - —Ventilator tidal volume: 10–15 mL/kg
- Specialized cervical spine immobilization
  - —Appropriate size collar
  - —Extra shoulder/trunk support *or* board with "cutout" for occiput as needed
- Cardiorespiratory monitoring, pulse oximetry
- Two large-bore IVs; central or intraosseous access as needed
- Keep child warm; hypothermia risk increased

ED TREATMENT

- Close/early collaboration with pediatric/trauma surgeons
  - —90% of pediatric blunt abdominal injuries successfully managed nonoperatively
  - —Intraperitoneal fluid *not* correlated with need for surgery
- Aggressive fluid resuscitation
  - —HR may be only sign of shock
  - —Low risk of fluid overload in healthy children
- Consider
  - —Oropharyngeal or nasopharyngeal airway (tongue control)
  - —ETT intubation if patient to be transferred to another facility and potential for respiratory compromise during transport exists
  - —NGT (if no facial fractures present)
  - —Urinary catheter (if no blood at urethral meatus)
- Fractures: splint, consider immediate reduction if neurovascular compromise present
- Analgesics, sedatives as needed
- CT only if hemodynamically stable
- Careful evaluation for SCIWORA in patients with neck pain, neurologic symptoms
- Parental presence may soothe child, assist in assessment
- Tetanus immunization if indicated

MEDICATIONS

- Blood: 10–20 mL/kg
  - —Indicated if poor response to 60 mL/kg crystalloid or for suspected large blood loss
- Crystalloid: 20-mL/kg bolus, NS or lactated Ringer's, repeat as needed
- Rapid-sequence intubation (RSI)
  - —Atropine: 0.02 mg/kg (minimum, 0.1 mg)
  - —Midazolam: 0.1 mg/kg, *or* etomidate, 0.3 mg/kg
  - —Succinylcholine: 1–2 mg/kg; *or* vecuronium: 0.1–0.2 mg/kg; *or* rocuronium: 0.6–1 mg/kg
- Intracranial hypertension
  - —Lidocaine: 1 mg/kg, for RSI
  - —Mannitol: 0.5–1 g/kg
- Hypoglycemia
  - —D-10: 5–10 mL/kg; or D-25: 2–4 mL/kg

Disposition

ADMISSION CRITERIA

- Multiple trauma or significant mechanism of injury
- Hemodynamic instability
- Airway injury or respiratory distress
- Life- or limb-threatening injury
- Injury requiring surgery
- Neurologic or vascular injury
- Unexplained abdominal pain
- Injuries requiring observation
- Child abuse or poisoning cases requiring admission or observation
  - —Further investigation of social and environmental factors may be required in conjunction with social services before discharge decision
- Unreliable follow-up

DISCHARGE CRITERIA

- Absence of admission criteria
- Reliable adult to observe child at home and timely follow-up available

Miscellaneous

ICD9: 959.9

SEE ALSO: ABUSE, PEDIATRIC

SUGGESTED READINGS

Corbett SW, Andrews HG, Baker EM, et al. ED evaluation of the pediatric trauma patient by ultrasonography. Am J Emerg Med 2000;18:244–249.

Knapp JF. Practical issues in the care of pediatric trauma patients. Curr Prob Pediatr 1998;28:309–320.

Ludwig S, Loiselle J. Anatomy, growth, and development: impact on injury. In: Eichelberger MR, ed. Pediatric trauma: prevention, acute care, rehabilitation. St. Louis: Mosby-Year Book, 1993:39–58.

Rothrock SG, Green SM, Morgan R. Abdominal trauma in infants and children: prompt identification and early management of serious and life-threatening injuries, parts I & II. Pediatr Emerg Care 2000;16:106–115, 189–195.

Sanchez JI, Paidas CN. Childhood trauma, now and in the new millennium. Surg Clin North Am 1999;79:1503–1535.

Author: Thomas H. Chun

Pediculosis

Clinical Presentation

SIGNS AND SYMPTOMS

Head Lice

- Scalp and posterior neck erythema, scaling, and excoriated papules
- Nits (egg casings) attached to hair shafts
- Excoriations may lead to pyoderma, posterior cervical lymphadenopathy, and febrile episodes

Body Lice

- Linear excoriations of neck and trunk
- Pus or serum stains on clothing
- Nits found in seams of clothing

Pubic Lice

- Intense pruritus, particularly at night
- Occasional urticaria with typical flare/wheal formation
- May infest eyelashes and scalp in children
- Characteristic bluish macules (maculae ceruleae) appear infrequently on trunk and thighs

ETIOLOGY

- Infestation by *Pediculus capitis* (head louse), *Pediculus corporis* (body louse), or *Pthirus pubis* (pubic louse)
- Bites are painless
- Signs and symptoms result from host response to saliva and anticoagulant injected during feeding
- Transmitted by direct contact and fomites; pubic lice are transmitted by sexual contact

Pre-Hospital

CAUTIONS

- Maintain universal precautions

Diagnosis

ESSENTIAL WORKUP

- Examine hair for adult lice and nits
- Nits are cemented on hair shafts and are not easily removed
- Head lice and pubic lice infestation is confirmed by differentiating nits from scales, hair casts, and other easily brushed-off artifacts
- Empty nits are not diagnostic of active infection
- Body lice are observed only in very heavy infestation; infestation is confirmed by finding nits in clothing seams

LABORATORY

- Nits may be visualized under low-power microscopy along hair shafts

DIFFERENTIAL DIAGNOSIS

- Scabies
- Contact or allergic dermatitis

Treatment

INITIAL STABILIZATION

- Not applicable for routine cases

ED TREATMENT

Head Lice

- Topical pediculicidal agents: *Permethrin 1% cream rinse* (Nix) is the best first-line agent; it has low toxicity and is ovicidal; *pyrethrin* (Rid) also has low toxicity but is less effective; *lindane shampoo* is effective but may cause CNS toxicity and seizures if applied incorrectly or overused
- All agents require reapplication in 7–10 days if further adult lice or nits noted
- Remove nits with fine-toothed comb
- Examine all members of household; treat infested individuals
- Change clothing and machine wash and dry (using hot cycles) all clothing, towels, linens, and headgear; vacuum floors and furniture; wash combs and brushes in hot water for 10–20 minutes or coat with pediculicide for 15 minutes and wash

Pubic Lice

- Topical pediculicide applied to hairy areas of chest, axilla, and groin
- Remove nits with fine-toothed comb
- Treat sexual contacts simultaneously
- Wash and dry bedding and clothing using hot cycles
- Treat eyelash involvement with topical petrolatum twice daily for 9 days

Body Lice

- Wash and dry bedding and clothing using hot cycles
- Apply topical pediculicide cream or lotions from chin to toes
- Oral antihistamines and topical steroids may help pruritic symptoms of all lice infestations

MEDICATIONS

Antipruritics

- Cetirizine (Zyrtec): age older than 12 years, 5–10 mg PO q.d. (peds: ages 6–11 years, 5–10 mg PO q.d.; ages 2–5 years, 2.5 mg PO q.d.)
- Diphenhydramine (Benadryl): 25–50 mg PO q6h (peds: 5 mg/kg/d q6h)
- Hydroxyzine (Atarax): 25 mg PO q8h (peds: 12.5 mg/dose q6h)

Pediculicides

- Lindane (γ-benzene hexachloride) 1% shampoo: lather for 4 minutes then rinse
  —Lotion: apply chin to toes, wash off after 8 hours; avoid use in children, lactation, pregnancy, or seizure disorder
- Permethrin 1% cream rinse (Nix): apply to scalp and hair, rinse after 10 minutes; reapply in 7–10 days if needed
- Pyrethrin/piperonyl butoxide (Rid): apply to scalp and hair, wash after 10 minutes; repeat in 7–10 days

Disposition

ADMISSION CRITERIA

- Extensive bacterial superinfection; systemic hypersensitivity reaction with cardiorespiratory compromise

DISCHARGE CRITERIA

- Mild to moderate infestation with absence of significant superinfection or hypersensitivity reaction

Miscellaneous

ICD9: 132.9

ICD10: B85.2

SUGGESTED READINGS

Angel TA, Nigro J, Levy ML. Infestations in the pediatric patient. Pediatr Clin North Am 2000;47(4):921–935, viii.

Chosidow O. Scabies and pediculosis. Lancet 2000;355(9206):819–826.

Elston DM. Controversies concerning the treatment of lice and scabies. J Am Acad Dermatol 2002;46(5):794–796.

Potts J. Eradication of ectoparasites in children. How to treat infestations of lice, scabies, and chiggers. Postgrad Med 2001;110(1):57–59, 63–64.

Roberts RJ. Clinical practice. Head lice. N Engl J Med 2002;346(21):1645–1650.

Author: Guy Tarleton

Pelvic Fracture

Clinical Presentation

SIGNS AND SYMPTOMS

- Localized pain, swelling, ecchymoses, tenderness over hips, groin, perineum, and lower back
- Pain on hip movement, ambulation, sitting, standing, defecation
- Tenderness on lateral compression of pelvis, palpation of symphysis pubis or sacroiliac (SI) joints
- Often presents with other traumatic injuries including neurologic, intraabdominal, genitourinary, perineal, rectal, vaginal, and vascular injury
- Gross pelvic instability, deformity, asymmetry in lower extremity
- Evidence of hemorrhagic shock (see Hemorrhagic Shock)
- Inability to actively or passively perform range of motion of involved hip

MECHANISM/DESCRIPTION

Tile Classification System

- Type A: Stable pelvic ring injuries
  - —A1: Avulsion fractures of the innominate bone (ischial tuberosity, iliac crest)
    - -A2-1: Iliac wing fractures (Duverney's fractures) due to direct trauma or lateral compression
    - -A2-2: Isolated rami fractures; commonly seen in falls in the elderly and most common pelvic fracture
    - -A2-3: Four-pillar anterior ring injuries (straddle fracture); fractures of both pubic rami
    - -A3: Transverse fractures of sacrum or coccyx
- Type B: Partially stable pelvic ring injury (rotationally unstable, but vertically stable)
  - —B1: Unilateral open-book fracture; due to anteroposterior compression
    - -Wide separation of symphysis pubis (often >2.5 cm) associated with posterior arch and sacroiliac joint disruption
    - -Increased risk for neurologic and vascular injury
    - -Overall volume of pelvis is increased, allowing expansion of retroperitoneal hematoma
  - —B2: Lateral compression injury
    - -B2-1: Ipsilateral double rami fractures and posterior injury
    - -B2-2: Contralateral double rami fractures and posterior injury (bucket-handle fracture)
    - -B2-3: Bilateral type B injuries
- Type C: Unstable pelvic ring injury—vertical shear (rotationally and vertically unstable), Malgaigne fracture
  - —Anterior disruption of symphysis pubis or two to four pubic rami with posterior displacement and instability thru sacrum, SI joint or ileum
  - —Associated with significant neurologic and vascular injury from involvement of posterior arch of pelvis
  - —C1: Unilateral vertical shear fracture
  - —C2: Unilateral vertical shear combined with contralateral type B injury
  - —C3: Bilateral vertical shear fracture
- Acetabular fractures (posterior lip, central/transverse, anterior column, or posterior column fractures)

ETIOLOGY

- 60% of pelvic fractures due to vehicular trauma, including pedestrians struck by automobiles
- 30% due to falls
- 10% due to crush, athletic, or penetrating injuries
- Mortality rate from pelvic fractures reported is 6–19%
- Increases to nearly 50% with hemorrhagic shock
- Significant pelvic hemorrhage can occur in unstable, high-energy pelvic fractures (Tile type B and C fractures)
  - —Bleeding most commonly arises from posterior injuries involving the venous plexuses
  - —Significant hemorrhage results in retroperitoneal hematoma formation that may tamponade in the enclosed pelvic space

PEDIATRIC CONSIDERATIONS

- Children can have proportionately greater hemorrhage
- Nonaccidental trauma is a concern

Pre-Hospital

CAUTIONS

- Pneumatic antishock garment (PASG) is an option, particularly when faced with a prolonged transport time or hemodynamically unstable
- Aggressive fluid resuscitation must occur before deflation of the PASG

Diagnosis

ESSENTIAL WORKUP

- Pelvic radiology is the most valuable initial diagnostic test
- A single AP view of the pelvis should be obtained as early as possible
  - —Most significant unstable pelvic fractures will be seen on the single AP view
  - —Other views include
    - -Inlet projection: 30-degree caudal view, allows visualization of posterior arch
    - -Outlet projection: 30-degree cephalic angulation, allows visualization of sacrum
    - -Judet oblique views: allows evaluation of acetabulum

LABORATORY

- Type and cross-match
- Hemoglobin/hematocrit, platelet count, and coagulation studies (PT/PTT)

IMAGING/SPECIAL TESTS

- CT scan may further delineate pelvic fracture(s), retroperitoneal hematoma, visceral injuries
- MRI indicated with evidence of neurologic injury
- Diagnostic peritoneal lavage (DPL) is a rapid bedside evaluation for intraperitoneal hemorrhage
  - —In the setting of pelvic fracture, the supraumbilical open approach for DPL should be used
- Abdominal US may be used in place of DPL, but differentiation of intraperitoneal from extraperitoneal hemorrhage from pelvic fracture can be difficult

DIFFERENTIAL DIAGNOSIS

- Normal variants (i.e., os acetabuli epiphyseal line can mimic type I fracture on radiograph)
- Ligamentous injury
- Spinal injury
- Intraabdominal injury and hemorrhage

Treatment

INITIAL STABILIZATION

- ABCs of trauma care
  - —Avoid using lower extremity IV sites
  - —Aggressive resuscitation with blood or crystalloid, O-negative or type-specific blood if hemodynamically unstable
  - —Immobilize the pelvis to prevent further injury and decrease bleeding
  - —PASG: use in ED is controversial but allows rapid pelvic immobilization and pelvic compression to slow bleeding
  - —External fixator requires more time to place than PASG but "splints" pelvis in a similar manner; contraindicated in severely comminuted pelvic fracture
  - —Placement of a stabilization device should not interfere with further workup and care (e.g., DPL)

ED TREATMENT

- Determine which pelvic fractures are stable and unstable
- Type A fractures are generally stable
- Type B and C fractures are unstable

Type A Fractures

- Treated conservatively with bed rest, analgesics, and comfort measures; management decisions may be made in conjunction with orthopedics
- For four-pillar anterior ring injuries, a CT scan should be obtained to evaluate the posterior pelvis
- Ensure there are no other breaks in the pelvic ring

Type B and C Fractures

- Immediate orthopedics consultation; patient should remain NPO
- May require ED pelvic stabilization measures
- Assess for pelvic hemorrhage (see Pelvic Hemorrhage)

Acetabular Fractures

- Immediate orthopedics consultation; patient should remain NPO

Pelvic Hemorrhage

- Angiography and selective vessel embolization
- Direct operative control of pelvic bleeding

Prioritization of Studies: CT, Angiography, or Surgery

- In the hemodynamically *unstable* patient
  - —Open B and C fractures: surgical exploration
  - —Closed fractures: DPL or US can determine management
  - —If the DPL or US result is positive, the patient should go for celiotomy and mechanical stabilization (usually by external pelvic fixation) followed by selective angiography
    - -In cases in which the DPL result is positive by cell count criteria only, external fixation and angiography may be performed before surgery
  - —If the DPL or US result is negative, the patient should undergo external fixation as appropriate, followed by selective angiography
- In the hemodynamically *stable* patient, the patient can go to CT scan for evaluation of the abdomen, pelvis, and retroperitoneum with external fixation as appropriate

MEDICATIONS

- Blood products: 4–6 IU cross-matched, type specific, or O negative (peds: 10 mL/kg)
- Crystalloid fluids: 2-L i.v. bolus of NS *or* lactated Ringer's (peds: 20 mL/kg)

Disposition

ADMISSION CRITERIA

- Hemodynamic instability, and pelvic hemorrhage to the ICU
- Type B or C pelvic fracture
- Acetabular fracture
- Other related injuries (e.g., genitourinary, intraabdominal, neurologic)
- Intractable pain

DISCHARGE CRITERIA

- Type A pelvic fracture; hemodynamically stable with no evidence of other injuries

Miscellaneous

ICD9: 808.8

ICD10: S32.8

SUGGESTED READINGS

American College of Surgeons, Committee on Trauma. Advanced trauma life support program. Chicago: American College of Surgeons, 1997.

Coppola PT, Coppola M. Emergency department evaluation and treatment of pelvic fractures. Emerg Med Clin North Am 2000;18(1):1–27.

Cwinn AA. Pelvis and hip. In: Marx J, et al, eds. Rosen's emergency medicine: concepts and clinical practice, 5th ed. St. Louis: Mosby–Year Book, 2001:625–642.

MacLeod M, Powell JN: Evaluation of pelvic fractures: clinical and radiologic. Orthop Clin North Am 1997;28(3):299–319.

Author: Theodore Chan

Pelvic Inflammatory Disease

Clinical Presentation

SIGNS AND SYMPTOMS

- Lower abdominal pain, usually bilateral
- Vaginal discharge
- Abnormal uterine bleeding
- Dysmenorrhea
- Dysuria
- Dyspareunia
- Nausea and vomiting
- Fever and chills
- Proctitis
- Lower abdominal tenderness
- Decreased bowel sounds
- Bilateral adnexal tenderness
- Cervical motion tenderness
- Purulent endocervical discharge
- Adnexal mass or fullness
- Right upper quadrant tenderness

MECHANISM/DESCRIPTION

- PID is an acute infection of the upper genital tract, including the uterus, fallopian tubes, ovaries, and adjacent structures
- Progressive disease can lead to the formation of a tuboovarian abscess
- *Fitz-Hugh–Curtis syndrome* is a capsular inflammation of the liver that is associated with PID
  —Sharp right upper quadrant abdominal pain that is worse with inspiration, movement, or coughing

ETIOLOGY

- Risk factors
  —Age younger than 35 years
  —Multiple or symptomatic sexual partners
  —Previous episode of PID
  —Intrauterine devices
  —Nonbarrier contraception
  —Oral contraception
  —Instrumentation of the female genital tract
  —African-American ethnicity
- Most common cause of PID is *Neisseria gonorrhoeae* and *Chlamydia trachomatis*
- Other organisms include groups A and B streptococci, staphylococci, gram-negative rods (commonly *Klebsiella* species, *Escherichia coli*, and *Proteus* species), and anaerobes

Pre-Hospital

- No specific pre-hospital considerations
- Appropriate pain management

Diagnosis

ESSENTIAL WORKUP

- History and physical exam including pelvic examination
- Pregnancy test
- Cervical culture for *N. gonorrhoeae* and *C. trachomatis;* swab for Chlamydiazyme

LABORATORY

- CBC, ESR, or C-reactive protein may be elevated but not routinely recommended
- Gram stain of endocervix
- Microscopic exam of vaginal discharge in saline
- Liver enzymes may be elevated in Fitz-Hugh–Curtis syndrome
- Positive UA and/or occult blood in stool decrease the probability of PID

IMAGING/SPECIAL TESTS

- Patients with adnexal fullness or an adnexal mass on exam should have immediate pelvic US to exclude a tuboovarian abscess (TOA)
- Consider obtaining a pelvic US in patients who use an intrauterine device, fail outpatient antibiotic therapy for PID, or who have inadequate pelvic exams due to pain or obesity
- Minimum criteria for clinical diagnosis
  —Lower abdominal tenderness or
  —Uterine/adnexal tenderness or
  —Cervical motion tenderness
- Supportive criteria for diagnosis
  —Fever $>38.3°C$ (101°F)
  —Abnormal cervical/vaginal discharge
  —Intracellular gram-negative diplococci on endocervical Gram stain
  —Leukocytosis $>10,000/mm^3$
  —Elevated ESR or C-reactive protein
  —WBCs or bacteria in peritoneal fluid obtained by culdocentesis or laparoscopy

DIFFERENTIAL DIAGNOSIS

- Ectopic pregnancy
- Acute appendicitis
- Adnexal torsion
- Endometriosis
- Cystitis
- Urolithiasis
- Hemorrhagic corpus luteum cyst
- Adenomyosis uteri
- Pelvic adhesions
- Benign ovarian cyst
- Chronic salpingitis
- Mesenteric vascular disease
- Irritable bowel syndrome

Treatment

INITIAL STABILIZATION

- Manage ABCs and shock as indicated

ED TREATMENT

Outpatient

- Regimen A
  —Ofloxacin or levofloxacin; with or without metronidazole*
- Regimen B
  —Ceftriaxone or cefoxitin/probenecid plus doxycycline; with or without metronidazole*
- Inpatient
  —Doxycycline plus cefoxitin or cefotetan
  —Alternatives include gentamicin plus clindamycin; or metronidazole plus levofloxacin or ofloxacin
  —Continue parenteral antibiotic administration for 24 hours after clinical improvement, followed by oral doxycycline or clindamycin for a total of 14 days
  *Add metronidazole when anaerobes are a particular concern

MEDICATIONS

- Cefotetan: 2 g i.v. q12h
- Cefoxitin: 2 g i.m. single dose (outpatient); 1 g i.v. q6h (inpatient)
- Ceftriaxone: 250 mg i.m. single dose
- Clindamycin: 450 mg PO q.i.d. × 14 days (outpatient); 900 mg i.v. q8h (inpatient)
- Doxycycline: 100 mg PO b.i.d. × 14 days (outpatient); 100 mg i.v. or PO q12h (inpatient)
- Gentamicin: 2 mg/kg loading dose followed by 1.5 mg/kg i.v. q8h
- Levofloxacin: 500 mg PO q.d. × 14 days (outpatient); 500 mg i.v. q24h (inpatient)
- Metronidazole: 500 mg PO b.i.d. × 14 days (outpatient); 500 mg i.v. q8h (inpatient)
- Ofloxacin: 400 mg PO b.i.d. × 14 days (outpatient); 400 mg i.v. q12h (inpatient)
- Probenecid: 1 g PO single dose
- TOAs may require drainage or surgical intervention in addition to antibiotics
- Laparoscopy can be used to lyse adhesions in the acute and chronic stages of Fitz-Hugh–Curtis syndrome

Disposition

ADMISSION CRITERIA

- Uncertain diagnosis and toxic appearance
- Suspected pelvic abscess, including TOA
- Pregnancy
- Adolescence
- Immunodeficiency
- Severe illness (e.g., vomiting or severe pain)
- Failure of outpatient therapy
- Noncompliance
- Consider admission if appropriate clinical follow-up cannot be arranged

DISCHARGE CRITERIA

- Patients who do not meet admission criteria may be treated as outpatients
- Recent studies have shown that in women with mild to moderate PID, there was no difference in reproductive outcomes between women randomized to inpatient versus outpatient treatment

Miscellaneous

ICD9: 614.9

ICD10: N73.9

SUGGESTED READINGS

Centers for Disease Control and Prevention. 2002 guidelines for treatment of sexually transmitted diseases. Centers for Disease Control and Prevention. MMWR Morb Mortal Wkly Rep 2002;51(RR-6).

Lopez-Zeno JA, Keith LG, Berger GS. The Fitz-Hugh-Curtis syndrome revisited. J Reprod Med 1985;30:567–582.

McCormack WM. Pelvic inflammatory disease. N Engl J Med 1994;330:115–119.

Ness RB, et al. Effectiveness of inpatient and outpatient treatment strategies for women with pelvic inflammatory disease: results from the Pelvic inflammatory disease Evaluation And Clinical Health (PEACH) randomized trial. Am J Obstet Gynecol 2002;186(5):929–937.

Pastorek JG. Pelvic inflammatory disease and tubo-ovarian abscess. Obstet Gynecol Clin North Am 1989;16:347–361.

Ross J. Pelvic inflammatory disease. BMJ 2001;322(7287):658–659.

Author: Erich Salvacion

Pemphigus

Clinical Presentation

SIGNS AND SYMPTOMS

- Generalized or focal flaccid bullae (blisters) of the skin and mucosa
- Painful skin erosions with shreds of detached epithelium
- Painful nonhealing oral erosions
- Crusting, partially healing skin erosions from ruptured bullae
- Hypertrophic, hyperplastic erosive plaques with pustules in intertriginous areas (pemphigus vegetans)
- Moist, edematous, exfoliative erosions in seborrheic areas (pemphigus foliaceus)
- Erythematous, scaly, crusting skin lesions in a malar distribution (pemphigus erythematosus)
- Nikolsky's sign (separation of the epidermis with lateral pressure) is characteristic but not diagnostic

MECHANISM/DESCRIPTION

- Pemphigus is an autoantibody-mediated blistering disease of the skin and mucous membranes
  - —If untreated, mortality rates average >73%
- Pemphigus is a rare disease with a worldwide incidence of 0.1–0.5 cases per 100,000
- Two major subtypes exist
  - —Vulgaris, which tends to be more serious with deeper involvement and includes a minor variant, vegetans
  - —Foliaceus, which tends to be milder and more superficial, and which includes two minor variants, erythematosus and herpetiformis
- Pemphigus vulgaris accounts for 80% of all cases
- 70% of patients with vulgaris or vegetans present with oral lesions
- Superficial pemphigus (foliaceus, erythematosus, and herpetiformis) often lack oral lesions and have a better prognosis
- Pemphigus is most common in individuals 40–60 years old but has been reported in people ranging from neonates to 89 years of age

ETIOLOGY

- IgG autoantibodies are directed against pemphigus antigens found in all keratinocytes
- Autoantibodies cause acantholysis (separation of the keratinocytes from each other leading to the loss of cell-cell adhesion), which leads to blistering
- Immunogenetic predisposition secondary to higher frequencies of specific HLA haplotypes contributes to this disease
- Drugs may induce or trigger pemphigus (penicillamine, captopril, rifampin, piroxicam, and phenobarbital)
- Pemphigus may also occur in association with a neoplasm, usually lymphoma (paraneoplastic pemphigus)
- Endemic pemphigus foliaceus (fogo selvagem) may be triggered or transmitted by bites from flying insects

PEDIATRIC CONSIDERATIONS

- Pemphigus is rare in children
- Neonates may develop the disease secondary to transplacental transfer of IgG
- Neonatal pemphigus spontaneously resolves in several weeks as the maternal antibodies are catabolized

Pre-Hospital

CAUTIONS

- Patients with severe pemphigus may require rapid transport and fluid resuscitation similar to severe burn patients secondary to the loss of the skin barrier

Diagnosis

ESSENTIAL WORKUP

- Pemphigus is suspected based on clinical presentation
- Biopsy with histologic and immunofluorescence testing is essential for definitive diagnosis (arrange with a dermatologist)

LABORATORY

- Serum antibody titers, detected by indirect immunofluorescence, are often used as a marker of disease activity; however, the ED physician usually does not order these titers

IMAGING/SPECIAL TESTS

- No diagnostic imaging test exists

DIFFERENTIAL DIAGNOSIS

- Bullous pemphigoid
- Dermatitis herpetiformis
- Erythema multiforme
- Toxic epidermal necrolysis
- Epidermolysis bullosa
- Hand, foot, and mouth disease
- Systemic lupus erythematosus
- Systemic vasculitis
- Oral candidiasis
- Herpes simplex gingivostomatitis
- Erosive lichen planus
- Seborrheic dermatitis

Treatment

INITIAL STABILIZATION

- ABCs
- If severe disease is suspected, a safety net (IV access, pulse oximetry monitor, and cardiac monitor) should be established
- If symptoms of hypotension or sepsis are present, IV fluid resuscitation should be guided by the Parkland burn formula
  - —4 mL of crystalloid per kilogram of body weight per percentage of body surface area involved per 24 hours
  - —Give half of the total calculated fluid over the course of the first 8 hours; the remainder over the next 16 hours
  - —Adjust fluids to keep urine output >0.5 mL/kg/h
- If signs or symptoms of sepsis are present, broad-spectrum antibiotic coverage also should be initiated
- In steroid-dependent patients, stress-dose steroids should be used

ED TREATMENT

- Systemic corticosteroids are the mainstay of therapy
- *Severe disease:* conventional high-dose corticosteroids
  - —If severe symptoms are unresponsive to high-dose PO corticosteroids, consider pulse IV corticosteroids and admission for plasmapheresis
- *Mild to moderate disease* should receive PO prednisone and intralesional triamcinolone acetonide may be used
- *Adjuvant immunosuppressive therapy* may also be added to decrease the symptoms associated with high-dose systemic corticosteroids or in patients with contraindications to steroid therapy
  - —Dapsone, gold, azathioprine, cyclophosphamide, cyclosporine, methotrexate, mycophenolate, and IV immunoglobulins

Steroid Formulations

- Hydrocortisone: 100–300 mg i.v. stress-dose steroids
- Methylprednisolone (pulse IV therapy) (adults): 1 g i.v. over 3 hours q.d.
- Prednisone: 20–400 mg PO q.d. (adults); severe disease, 200–400 mg PO q.d. × 5–10 weeks then taper; mild to moderate disease, 20–80 mg PO q.d.
- Triamcinolone acetonide: 20 mg/mL 0.1-mL injection into each superficial lesion

Disposition

ADMISSION CRITERIA

- Admit to the ICU if any signs and symptoms of shock or sepsis are present, because aggressive fluid resuscitation, wound care, and multiple medications will be required
- Admit to a floor bed if pulse parenteral steroid therapy or plasmapheresis is indicated
- Admit first-time presentations of disease to facilitate treatment and definitive diagnosis

DISCHARGE CRITERIA

- Discharge if mild to moderate disease will not require aggressive steroid management or plasmapheresis
- A follow-up evaluation is essential to monitor the course of the disease and to adjust treatment

Miscellaneous

ICD9: 694.4

ICD10: L10.9

SUGGESTED READINGS

Ahmed AR. Intravenous immunoglobulin therapy in the treatment of patients with pemphigus vulgaris unresponsive to conventional immunosuppressive treatment. J Am Acad Dermatol 2001;45(5):679–690.

Ahmed AR, Sami N. Intravenous immunoglobulin therapy for patients with pemphigus foliaceus unresponsive to conventional therapy. J Am Acad Dermatol 2002;46(1):42–49.

Bystryn JC, Steinman NM. The adjuvant therapy of pemphigus. Arch Dermatol 1996;132:203–212.

Cotell S, Robinson ND, Chan LS. Autoimmune blistering skin diseases. Am J Emerg Med 2000;18(3):288–299.

Korman NJ. New immunomodulating drugs in autoimmune blistering diseases. Dermatol Clin 2001;19(4):637–648.

Odom RB, James WD, Berger TG, et al. Andrews' diseases of the skin: clinical dermatology. Philadelphia: WB Saunders, 2000.

Authors: James T. Vandenberg; Christopher S. Kang

Penile Shaft Fracture

Clinical Presentation

SIGNS AND SYMPTOMS

- Sudden painful sensation in erect penis during sexual intercourse or soon after with loss of erection
  —May hear cracking or crunching sound at the time of trauma
- Swelling and blue-black discoloration at base of penis, usually on one side
- Ecchymosis may also involve scrotum
- Penis flaccid and edematous with angulation away from the side of tear
- Defect in corpus cavernosum may be palpable at the site of tear in tunica albuginea
- Blood at tip of penis or frank hematuria suggests an associated urethral injury
- May have dysuria, inability to void, or an increase in size of the swelling with voiding due to extravasation of urine

MECHANISM/DESCRIPTION

- Traumatic rupture of tunica albuginea, surrounding corpus cavernosum
- Usually unilateral, caused by blunt trauma to erect penis during
  —Sexual intercourse
  —Manipulation
  —Fall on erect penis
- During erection, pressure within corpus cavernosum is maximal, close to arterial pressure, increasing volume in each corpus to maximum, which thins tunica albuginea making it susceptible to rupture
- Penile erection also stretches spongiosum to the limit, which will limit movement vertically, while still allowing lateral movements; this forms a bend at base of penis, making it vulnerable to lateral swing and rupture of corpus cavernosum
- About 25–30% have associated urethral injury, which may be partial or complete

ETIOLOGY

- Peyronie's disease
- Urethritis in past
- Surgical procedure on corpus cavernosum or trauma to corpus cavernosum resulting in weak scar tissue

Pre-Hospital

- Application of ice to penis and elevation to reduce swelling and hematoma

Diagnosis

ESSENTIAL WORKUP

- Urinalysis to evaluate urethral trauma
  —May have frank blood or microscopic hematuria
- Retrograde urethrography—recommended in all cases of suspected urethral trauma
  —Should be done with low pressure during injection, before urethral catheterization
- Cavernosography and MRI of penis may be needed to confirm diagnosis and site of tear

DIFFERENTIAL DIAGNOSIS

- Contusion of penis
- Paraphimosis
- Cellulitis of penis
- Vasculature rupture, especially deep dorsal vein or artery
- Trauma because of constrictive ring or other structure
- Neoplasm of penis

Treatment

INITIAL STABILIZATION

- ABCs if associated trauma present
- Needle suprapubic cystotomy in patients with urethral trauma and full bladder to relieve patient discomfort
- Local treatment: ice packs locally to penis; splinting with tongue blade

ED TREATMENT

- Combined efforts of ED physician and urologist are aimed toward restoration of normal shape of penis and sexual and urinary functions
- ED treatment directed to reduce hemorrhage, prevent further complications
- Prophylactic antibiotic use is unnecessary
- Urethral catheterization in all cases after excluding urethral trauma
- Urologic evaluation and early surgical treatment are essential to prevent complications such as erectile dysfunction, impotence, penile deformity, urethral stenosis
- All patients with suspected or definite diagnosis *must* have early urologic evaluation

MEDICATIONS

- Diazepam: 2–5 mg i.v.
- Lorazepam: 0.5–1.0 mg i.v.
- Meperidine: 1 mg/kg i.v.
- Morphine sulfate: 0.1 mg/kg i.v.

Disposition

ADMISSION CRITERIA

- *All* patients with penile fracture must be hospitalized for prompt surgery

Transfer

- If immediate urologic consultation and treatment unavailable, patient may be transferred to a suitable hospital after initial stabilization, after appropriate criteria for transfer

DISCHARGE CRITERIA

N/A

Miscellaneous

ICD9: 959.1

ICD10: S39.9

SUGGESTED READINGS

Asgari MA, et al. Penile fractures: evaluation therapeutic approaches and long-term results. J Urol 1996;155: 148–149.

Eke N. Fracture of the penis. Br J Surg 2002;89(5):555–565.

Fedel M, et al. The value of MRI in diagnosis of suspected penile fracture with atypical clinical findings. J Urol 1996; 155(6):1924–1927.

Haas CA, et al. Penile fracture and testicular rupture. World J Urol 1999;17(2):101–106.

Author: Stephen R. Hayden

Peptic Ulcer

Clinical Presentation

SIGNS AND SYMPTOMS

- Epigastric pain or tenderness (80–90%)
  - —Burning, gnawing, aching pain
  - —Location: midline, xiphoid, or umbilicus
- Duodenal ulcers
  - —Pain occurs 90 minutes to 3 hours after meals
  - —Usually awakens the patient at night
  - —Food and antacids relieve the pain
- Gastric ulcers
  - —Pain worsens after meals
  - —Nausea and anorexia
- Difficult to differentiate clinically between gastric and duodenal ulcers
- Relief of pain with antacids
- Heme-positive stools
- Complications of PUD
  - —Acute perforation
    - -Rigid "board-like" abdomen
    - -Generalized rebound tenderness
    - -Pain radiation to back or shoulder
  - —Obstruction
    - -Pain with vomiting
    - -"Succussion" splash from retained gastric contents and abdominal distention
  - —Hemorrhage
    - -Hematemesis
    - -Melena
    - -Hypotension
    - -Tachycardia
    - -Skin pallor
    - -Orthostatic changes

MECHANISM/DESCRIPTION

- Produced by a breakdown in the gastric or duodenal mucosal defenses
- Imbalance between production of acid and ability of mucosa to prevent damage

ETIOLOGY

- Major causes
  - —*Helicobacter pylori*
    - -Gram-negative spiral bacteria that live in the mucous layer
    - -Responsible for 90–95% of duodenal ulcers and 80% of gastric ulcers
    - -Increases antral gastrin production and decreases mucosal integrity
  - —NSAIDs
    - -Interfere with prostaglandin synthesis
    - -Lead to a break in the mucosa
  - —Aspirin
  - —Cigarette smoking
  - —Alcohol

Pre-Hospital

CAUTIONS

- Initial stabilization with two large-bore IVs of lactated Ringer's or 0.9% NS to fluid resuscitate for
  - —Perforation with peritonitis
  - —Massive upper GI hemorrhage with hemodynamic compromise
  - —Hypotension

Diagnosis

ESSENTIAL WORKUP

- Careful physical examination including Hemoccult testing and vital signs with orthostatics
- For stable patients oral "GI cocktail" typically relieves pain
  - —Antacid: 30 mL
  - —Viscous lidocaine: 10 mL

LABORATORY

- Normal lab values in uncomplicated ulcer disease
- CBC
  - —Low hematocrit with bleeding
  - —Leukocytosis with perforation/penetration
- Amylase/lipase
  - —Elevated with perforation/penetration
  - —Pancreatitis in differential diagnosis
- Electrolytes, BUN/Cr, glucose for critically ill
- Type and cross-match
  - —For significant blood loss

IMAGING/SPECIAL TESTS

- EKG
  - —For elderly patients
  - —Myocardial ischemia in differential diagnosis
- CXR/abdominal series for
  - —Perforation
  - —Bowel obstruction
- Endoscopy
  - —Procedure of choice
  - —Outpatient unless significant hemorrhage
  - —Allows for biopsies of gastric/duodenal ulcers for the presence of *H. pylori*
  - —Detects malignant gastric ulcers
- Upper GI series
  - —Single contrast barium diagnose 70–80%
  - —Double contrast diagnose 90%
- Gastrin level is elevated in Zollinger-Ellison syndrome

DIFFERENTIAL DIAGNOSIS

- Gastroesophageal reflux
- Biliary colic
- Cholecystitis
- Pancreatitis
- Gastritis
- Abdominal aortic aneurysm
- Aortic dissection
- Myocardial infarction
- Subset with symptoms and no ulcer on endoscopy called "nonulcer dyspepsia"

Treatment

INITIAL STABILIZATION

- For ulcer complications (hemorrhage, perforation, and obstruction)
- ABCs
- Treat hypotension with lactated Ringer's or 0.9% NS i.v. fluid bolus via two large-bore IVs
- NGT for gastric decompression/check for hemorrhage

ED TREATMENT

- Pain control with antacids (GI cocktail) or IV H_2 antagonists
- Avoid narcotics—may mask serious illness
- Promotion of ulcer healing
  - —Antacids
  - —H_2 antagonists (cimetidine, famotidine, ranitidine, nizatidine)
  - —Sucralfate
  - —Prostaglandin congers (misoprostol)
  - —Protease pump inhibitors (omeprazole or lansoprazole)
- Gastric outlet obstruction
  - —Decompress stomach with NGT
  - —IV hydration
- Gastric hemorrhage
  - —IV fluid resuscitation
  - —Blood transfusion depending on loss/hematocrit
  - —Foley catheter to monitor volume status
- Perforation
  - —IV hydration
  - —Foley catheter
  - —Preoperative antibiotics
  - —Emergency surgical consultation
- Treatment of *H. pylori* infection
  - —Invasive or noninvasive testing to confirm infection
  - —Oral eradication antibiotic therapy options
    - -Proton pump inhibitor (omeprazole 20 mg b.i.d.) or lansoprazole 30 mg PO b.i.d. and two antibiotics (clarithromycin 500 mg b.i.d. plus metronidazole 500 mg b.i.d.) for 14 days
    - -H_2 blocker, bismuth subsalicylate (Pepto-Bismol) plus either amoxicillin 1,000 mg b.i.d. or tetracycline 500 mg q.i.d. in combination with either metronidazole 250 mg q.i.d. or clarithromycin 500 mg b.i.d. for 14 days
    - -Most common regimen: omeprazole 20 mg or lansoprazole 30 mg plus clarithromycin 500 mg and amoxicillin 1 g all taken twice a day for 2 weeks

MEDICATIONS

- Bismuth subsalicylate: 525 mg tabs 2 PO q.i.d.
- Cimetidine (H_2 blocker): 800 mg PO q.h.s. for 6–8 weeks
- Famotidine (H_2 blocker): 40 mg PO q.h.s. for 6–8 weeks
- Lansoprazole: 30 mg PO b.i.d. × 2 weeks
- Maalox plus: 2–4 tablets PO q.i.d.
- Misoprostol: 100–200 μg PO q.i.d.
- Mylanta-II: 2–4 tablets PO q.i.d.
- Nizatidine (H_2 blocker): 300 mg PO q.h.s. × 6–8 weeks
- Omeprazole: 20 mg PO b.i.d. × 2 weeks
- Ranitidine (H_2 blocker): 300 mg PO q.h.s. × 6–8 weeks
- Sucralfate: 1 g PO q.i.d. × 6–8 weeks

Disposition

ADMISSION CRITERIA

- Gastric obstruction
- Perforation
- Active upper GI bleed
- Melena
- Uncontrolled pain

DISCHARGE CRITERIA

- Unremarkable physical examination with normal CBC and heme-negative stools
- If heme-positive stools, discharge if stable vital signs, normal hematocrit, and negative NGT aspiration for upper GI hemorrhage

Miscellaneous

ICD9: 533.9

ICD10: K26.9

SEE ALSO: GASTROINTESTINAL BLEEDING

SUGGESTED READINGS

McGuirk TD, et al. Upper gastrointestinal tract bleeding. Emerg Med Clin North Am 1996;14(3):530–533.

Moss SF. Treatment of *H. pylori* infection—who, how and when. Resid Staff Physician 1996;42:11–18.

Smoot DT, et al. Peptic ulcer disease. Prim Care 2001;28(3):487–503.

Author: Marco Cordero

Perforated Viscous

Clinical Presentation

SIGNS AND SYMPTOMS

- Sudden severe abdominal pain
  - —Initially local
  - —Rapidly becoming diffuse
- Rigidity
- Guarding
- Rebound tenderness
- Absent bowel sounds
- Hypovolemic shock
  - —Tachycardia
  - —Hypotension

MECHANISM/DESCRIPTION

- Perforation of any segment of GI tract due to
  - —Inflammation
  - —Ulceration
  - —Shearing/crushing or bursting forces in trauma
  - —Obstruction
- Chemical peritonitis occurs as a result of spillage of gastric or intestinal contents into peritoneal cavity
- Massive outpouring of extracellular fluid into peritoneum follows shortly

ETIOLOGY

- Peptic ulcer disease
- Appendicitis
- Inflammatory bowel disease
- Diverticular disease
- Colon carcinoma
- Foreign body ingestion
- Trauma
- Radiation enteritis

PEDIATRIC CONSIDERATIONS

- Blunt trauma—more common cause of bowel rupture than penetrating trauma in children
  - —Jejunum is the most common site of rupture

Pre-Hospital

CAUTIONS

- Treat hypotension/tachycardia with 500 mL to 1 L bolus (peds: 20 mL/kg) of 0.9% NS

Diagnosis

ESSENTIAL WORKUP

- Upright CXR
  - —Best demonstrates pneumoperitoneum
  - —When in upright position for 5–10 minutes, may detect as little as 1–2 mL of free air under the diaphragm

LABORATORY

- CBC
- Electrolytes, BUN/Cr, glucose
- Amylase/lipase
- Urinalysis

IMAGING/SPECIAL TESTS

- Abdominal radiographs
  - —Left lateral decubitus film
  - —Supine abdomen
    - -Double-wall or "Rigler's" sign: air in intestinal lumen and peritoneal cavity allows for visualization of both serosal (not normally seen) and mucosal surfaces of intestine
- CT abdomen
  - —Small amounts of free air from perforated viscous detected by CT
- EKG

DIFFERENTIAL DIAGNOSIS

- Intraabdominal abscess
- Pneumomediastinum with peritoneal extension
- Pancreatitis
- Peptic ulcer disease
- Inferior wall myocardial infarction
- Cholecystitis

Treatment

INITIAL STABILIZATION

- ABCs
- Correct hypovolemia
  - —Rapid fluid resuscitation with 0.9% NS 1 L in adults (20 mL/kg in children)
  - —Pressure support for persistent hypotension

ED TREATMENT

- NGT
- Foley catheter
- Administer broad-spectrum antibiotics (second-generation cephalosporin)
- Immediate surgical consultation for operative intervention

MEDICATIONS

- Cefoxitin: 1–2 g q6–8h (peds: days 0–7, 40 mg/kg/24 h q12h; day 8 and thereafter, 80–160 mg/kg/24 h q6h) IVPB
- Demerol: 25-mg increments (peds: 1 mg/kg) i.v. p.r.n.
- Morphine sulfate: 2–4-mg increments (peds: 0.1 mg/kg) i.v. p.r.n.

Disposition

ADMISSION CRITERIA

- Suspected or confirmed perforation requires admission and immediate surgical consultation

DISCHARGE CRITERIA

- None

Miscellaneous

ICD9: 799.8

ICD10: K63.1

SEE ALSO: ABDOMINAL PAIN; PEPTIC ULCER

SUGGESTED READINGS

Graff LG, Robinson D. Abdominal pain and emergency department evaluation. Emerg Med Clin North Am 2001;19(1):123–136.

Shaffer H. Perforation and obstruction of the gastrointestinal tract. Radiol Clin North Am 1992;30(2):405.

Sivit C. Gastrointestinal emergencies in older infants and children. Radiol Clin North Am 1997;35(4):865.

Author: Julio Silva

Perianal Abscess

Clinical Presentation

SIGNS AND SYMPTOMS

Local

- Perianal pain
  - —Present constantly
  - —Aggravated by defecation, sitting, and coughing or sneezing
- Perianal swelling in
  - —Perianal abscess
  - —Large ischiorectal abscess
- Intraanal and intrarectal swelling
  - —Intersphincteric abscess
  - —Submucosal abscess
  - —Small, deep ischiorectal abscess
  - —Supralevator abscess

Systemic

- Malaise
- Pyrexia
- Advanced lesions may lead to septic shock

MECHANISM/DESCRIPTION

- Infected anal glands spread to perianal, ischiorectal, supralevator, intersphincteric, or submucosal spaces

ETIOLOGY

- Majority from infected anal glands in the anal crypts
- Foreign body
- Crohn disease
- Abdominal infection (PID or diverticulitis)
- Trauma
- Radiation
- Carcinoma
- Leukemia

PEDIATRIC CONSIDERATIONS

- Rectal duplication may mimic perianal abscess

Pre-Hospital

CAUTIONS

- Sitz baths will reduce pain
- Antibiotics contraindicated, as drainage is the treatment

Diagnosis

ESSENTIAL WORKUP

- Typical signs/symptoms in history
- Abdominal exam for abdominal or pelvic suppurative disease draining to the perineum
- Careful observation of the external anal and perianal region
  - —Any swelling with cellulitis is presumed abscess requiring incision and drainage (I&D)
  - —Identify if drainage has occurred spontaneously
- Gentle rectal exam
  - —To identify deep ischiorectal, supralevator, submucosal, and intersphincteric abscesses
- Vital signs for signs of systemic infection/sepsis
  - —Fever
  - —Tachycardia
  - —Hypotension

LABORATORY

- CBC if suspicion of systemic infection
  - —Leukocytosis
- Glucose for diabetes mellitus

DIFFERENTIAL DIAGNOSIS

- Anal fissure
- Sentinel pile in the posterior midline or anterior midline
- Thrombosed external hemorrhoids
- HIV anal ulcer
- Gonococcal proctitis
- Leukemic infiltrate
- Rectal duplication in children

Treatment

INITIAL STABILIZATION

- None, if no systemic signs
- With systemic signs of sepsis
  - —Treat hypotension with IV fluids/pressors
  - —Broad-spectrum antibiotics
  - —Urgent abscess drainage poststabilization

ED TREATMENT

- Needle aspiration
  - —If it is not clearly an abscess
  - —Use 16-gauge needle
  - —Do not aspirate all of pus
  - —Leave needle in to accurately incise and drain deeper abscesses
- I&D
  - —For visible abscesses
  - —Use local anesthesia with epinephrine
  - —Perform with an elliptical incision, as the pus and necrotic fat is thick and will drain for several days
  - —Large ischiorectal abscesses—caution
    - -Do not I&D if drainage already occurring inside the rectum
    - -I&D of draining abscess may result in high extrasphincteric fistulae
- Operative débridement under anesthesia and IV antibiotics for
  - —Large abscesses (>10 cm)
  - —Large amount of necrotic tissue
  - —Deep internal abscesses
  - —Unable to drain under local anesthetic
  - —Immunosuppressed (HIV, diabetics, transplant recipients, patients on chemotherapy)
- Pain medication/sedation for procedure
- Antibiotics (cefoxitin) for
  - —Systemic toxicity
  - —Large area of cellulitis
  - —Lymphangitis
  - —Immunocompromise

MEDICATIONS

- Cefoxitin: 1–2 g (peds: 100 mg/kg/24 h) i.v. q8h

Disposition

ADMISSION CRITERIA

- Need for operative drainage
- Systemic toxicity/signs of sepsis

DISCHARGE CRITERIA

- Adequate I&D with return of discernible pus
- Ability to ambulate and care for wound

Miscellaneous

ICD9: 566

ICD10: K61.0

SUGGESTED READINGS

Abcarian H, Alexander-Williams J, Christiansen J, et al. Benign anorectal disease: definition, characterization and analysis of treatment. Am J Gastroenterol 1994;89:S182–S193.

Ramanujam P, Prasad ML, Abcarian H. Perianal abscesses and fistulas: a study of 1023 patients. Dis Colon Rectum 1984;27:593–597.

Read DR, Abcarian H. A prospective survey of 474 patients with anorectal abscess. Dis Colon Rectum 1979;22:566–568.

Author: Charles Orsay

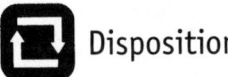

Pericardial Effusion/Tamponade

Clinical Presentation

SIGNS AND SYMPTOMS

- Most are asymptomatic
- Pleuritic chest pain
  —Relieved by sitting forward
- Dyspnea
- Cough
- Fatigue
- Malaise
- Pericardial friction rub
- Signs of shock or right heart failure
- Pulsus paradoxus
  —Fall in systolic BP >10 mm Hg with inspiration
- Dressler's syndrome
  —Fever
  —Chest pain
  —Pericardial friction rub
  —Seen several weeks after a myocardial infarction
- Beck's triad
  —Classic presentation of cardiac tamponade
  —Hypotension
  —Jugular venous distention (JVD)
    -JVD may be absent in hypovolemic patients
  —Muffled heart sounds
  —Beck's triad is present in only one third of patients

MECHANISM/DESCRIPTION

- Pericardial effusion
  —Accumulation of fluid in the pericardial sac
  —Occurs in 10% of cancer patients
- Pericardial tamponade
  —Accumulation of pericardial fluid with elevation of pressure in the pericardial space that results in impairment of ventricular filling and decreased cardiac output
  —Rapid accumulation of 50–200 mL of fluid in the pericardial sac causes hemodynamic compromise and pericardial tamponade
  —Occurs in 2% of patients with penetrating chest trauma

ETIOLOGY

- Medical causes
  —Idiopathic
  —Bacterial, viral, fungal, and parasitic infections
  —Malignancy
  —Uremia
  —Autoimmune/collagen vascular diseases
  —Systemic lupus erythematosus
  —Rheumatoid arthritis
  —Rheumatic fever
  —Scleroderma
  —Radiation therapy
  —Myxedema
  —Drug toxicity (isoniazid, doxorubicin, procainamide, hydralazine, phenytoin)
  —Postmyocardial infarction (Dressler's syndrome)
- Surgical causes
  —Penetrating chest trauma
  —Blunt trauma rarely causes pericardial effusion
  —Thoracic aortic dissection
  —Iatrogenic (cardiac catheterization, post–cardiac surgery, central line placement)

Pre-Hospital

CAUTIONS

- Insert two large-bore IV lines in all cases of suspected cardiac tamponade

Diagnosis

ESSENTIAL WORKUP

- EKG
  —Low voltage
  —Electrical alternans
    -Alternating beat-to-beat variation in QRS amplitude
    -Rare in patients with traumatic pericardial effusions or tamponade
- CXR
  —Enlarged cardiac silhouette only in cases of pericardial effusion/tamponade that develop over time
- Echocardiography
  —Fluid in pericardial sac
  —Transthoracic echo is accurate for penetrating cardiac injury and effusion or tamponade
  —Right ventricular or atrial diastolic collapse—characteristic findings suggestive of tamponade
  —"Sniff" test
    -Inferior vena cava will not collapse in patients with tamponade
    -Suggestive of increased CVP

LABORATORY

- CBC
- Electrolytes, BUN/Cr, glucose for renal failure in suspected uremic pericarditis
- Blood cultures if an infectious source suspected

IMAGING/SPECIAL TESTS

- Chest CT for detecting hemopericardium
- Pericardiocentesis and fluid analysis
  —Further workup for medical causes of pericardial effusion with determination of the etiology of the pericardial fluid
- CVP determination
  —May be used in penetrating chest trauma patients
  —CVP >15 cm H_2O suggests tamponade, but may be normal in the hypovolemic patient
- MRI with gadolinium
- TEE

DIFFERENTIAL DIAGNOSIS

- Other causes of shock
- Myocardial infarction
- CHF
- Pulmonary embolus
- Sepsis
- Tension pneumothorax
- Hemothorax
- Air embolism
- Aortic dissection
- GI tract bleeding
- Ruptured abdominal aortic aneurysm

Treatment

INITIAL STABLIZATION

- IV fluid resuscitation with NS or blood
- Pericardiocentesis for unstable patients to decompress the tamponade
- ED thoracotomy with pericardiotomy for patients in cardiac arrest after penetrating thoracic trauma or those who remain unstable after volume replacement and pericardiocentesis

ED TREATMENT

- Bacterial pericardial effusion
  - —Initiate antibiotic therapy to cover gram-negative and anaerobic organisms and *Staphylococcus aureus*
  - —May require partial surgical resection of the pericardium
- Uremic pericardial effusion
  - —Arrange urgent dialysis
- Dressler's syndrome and postirradiation pericardial effusion
  - —Initiate NSAIDs
- Medical causes of tamponade in patients who are unstable
  - —Perform pericardiocentesis with placement of an indwelling catheter for continued drainage
- Traumatic pericardial tamponade
  - —Consult trauma surgeon immediately
  - —Definitive therapy is thoracotomy in the OR
- Aortic dissection
  - —Immediate surgical consultation for operative repair

MEDICATIONS

- Aspirin: 650 mg PO q4h
- Ibuprofen: 800 mg PO q8h
- Indomethacin: 25–75 mg PO b.i.d.

Disposition

ADMISSION CRITERIA

- ICU admission for acute, symptomatic pericardial effusion/tamponade
- New pericardial effusion

DISCHARGE CRITERIA

- Known effusion in asymptomatic patient

Miscellaneous

ICD9: 429.0

ICD10: I31.3; I31.9

SEE ALSO: CARDIOGENIC SHOCK

SUGGESTED READINGS

Asensio JA, Stewart BM, Murray J, et al. Penetrating cardiac injuries. *Surg Clin North Am* 1996;76:685–724.

Braunwald E. Pericardial diseases. In: Fauci AS, Braunwald E, Isselbacher KJ, et al, eds. *Harrison's principles of internal medicine,* 14th ed. New York: McGraw-Hill, 1998: 1334–1341.

Jouriles NJ. Pericardial and myocardial disease. In: Marx JA, et al, eds. Rosen's emergency medicine: concepts and clinical practice, 5th ed. St. Louis: Mosby, 2002: 1130–1149.

Rosen CL, Wolfe RE. Blunt chest trauma. In: Ferrera PC, et al, eds. Trauma management, an emergency medicine approach. St. Louis: Mosby, 2001:232–258.

Soler-Soler J, Sagrista-Sauleda J, Permanyer-Miralda G. Management of pericardial effusion. Heart 2001;86(2): 235–240.

Tsang TSM, Oh JK, Seward JB. Diagnosis and management of cardiac tamponade in the era of echocardiography. Clin Cardiol 1999;22:442–446.

Authors: Teriggi J. Ciccone; Carlo L. Rosen

Pericarditis

Clinical Presentation

SIGNS AND SYMPTOMS

- Chest pain
  - —Retrosternal or precordial
  - —Usually sharp
  - —Pleuritic
  - —Radiating to the shoulder or the trapezial ridge
  - —Worsened with cough or inspiration
  - —Increased with recumbency
  - —Improved with leaning forward
- Fever
- Mild dyspnea
- Cough
- Hoarseness
- Nausea
- Anorexia
- Tachypnea
- Tachycardia
- Odynophagia
- Friction rub
  - —Heard best at lower left sternal border
  - —Any of three components
    - -Presystolic
    - -Systolic
    - -Early diastolic
  - —Intermittent and exacerbated by leaning forward
- Beck's triad with the accumulation of pericardial fluid
- Muffled heart sounds
- Increased venous pressure (distended neck veins)
- Decreased systemic arterial pressure (hypotension)
- Worsened dyspnea
- Ewart's sign
  - —Dullness and bronchial breathing between the tip of the left scapula and the vertebral column
- Pulsus paradoxus
  - —Exaggerated decrease (>10 mm Hg) in systolic pressure with inspiration
- Constrictive pericarditis
- Signs of both right- and left-sided heart failure
- Pulmonary and peripheral edema
- Ascites
- Hepatic congestion

MECHANISM/DESCRIPTION

- Inflammation, infection, or infiltration of the pericardial sac, which surrounds the heart
  - —Pericardial effusion may or may not be present
- Acute pericarditis
  - —Rapid in onset
  - —Potentially complicated by accumulation of pericardial fluid leading to cardiac tamponade
- Constrictive pericarditis
  - —Results from chronic inflammation causing thickening and adherence of the pericardium to the heart

ETIOLOGY

- Idiopathic (most common)
- Viral
  - —Echovirus
  - —Coxsackie
  - —Adenovirus
  - —Varicella
  - —Epstein-Barr virus
  - —Cytomegalovirus
  - —Hepatitis B
  - —AIDS
- Bacterial
  - —*Staphylococcus*
  - —*Streptococcus*
  - —*Haemophilus*
  - —*Salmonella*
  - —*Legionella*
  - —Tuberculosis
- Fungal
  - —*Candida*
  - —*Aspergillus*
  - —Histoplasmosis
  - —Coccidioidomycosis
  - —Blastomycosis
  - —*Nocardia*
- Parasitic
  - —Amebiasis
  - —Toxoplasmosis
  - —Echinococcosis
- Neoplastic
  - —Lung
  - —Breast
  - —Lymphoma
  - —Leukemia
  - —Melanoma
- Uremia
- Myxedema
- Myocardial infarction, Dressler's syndrome
- Connective tissue disease
  - —Systemic lupus erythematosus
  - —Rheumatoid arthritis
  - —Scleroderma
- Radiation
- Chest trauma
- Postpericardiotomy
- Aortic dissection
- Pancreatitis
- Inflammatory bowel disease
- Drugs
  - —Procainamide
  - —Cromolyn sodium
  - —Hydralazine
  - —Dantrolene
  - —Methysergide
  - —Mesalamine
- Amyloidosis

Pre-Hospital

CAUTIONS

- Differentiation between acute pericarditis and myocardial infarction necessitates rapid transport to the ED for evaluation with a 12-lead EKG
- Treat the hypotensive patient in cardiac tamponade with aggressive pre-hospital fluid resuscitation and rapid transport to point of definitive care

Diagnosis

ESSENTIAL WORKUP

- EKG
  - —Stage 1
    - -ST-segment elevation diffusely except aVR and V_1
    - -ST segments concave up
    - -No reciprocal ST-segment depression in other leads (in contradistinction to the changes seen in acute myocardial infarction)
  - —Stage 2
    - -ST segments return to normal
    - -T waves flatten
    - -PR segments may become depressed
  - —Stage 3
    - -T-wave inversion
  - —Stage 4
    - -Eventual resolution of all changes
    - -Differentiation from myocardial infarction
    - -No Q waves formed
    - -T-wave inversion occurs after the resolution of the ST-segment changes

LABORATORY

- CBC
- Leukocytosis
- ESR may be elevated
- Cardiac enzymes
  - —Helpful in distinguishing pericarditis from myocardial infarction
  - —Reported elevated with the inflammation of pericarditis

IMAGING/SPECIAL TESTS

- CXR
  - —Can be normal
  - —May show enlargement of the cardiac silhouette
  - —No change in heart size until >250 mL of fluid has accumulated in the pericardial sac
- Echocardiography
  - —Diagnostic method of choice for the detection of pericardial fluid
  - —Can detect as little as 15 mL of fluid in the pericardial sac
- Chest CT
  - —Useful for the detection of calcifications or thickening of the pericardium
- Pericardiocentesis
  - —Used to obtain fluid for protein, glucose, culture, cytology, Gram's and acid-fast stains, and fungal smears

DIFFERENTIAL DIAGNOSIS

- Acute myocardial infarction
- Pulmonary embolism
- Pneumothorax
- Aortic dissection
- Pneumonia
- Empyema
- Cholecystitis
- Pancreatitis

Treatment

INITIAL STABILIZATION

- ABCs
- Pericardiocentesis
  - —For hemodynamic compromise secondary to cardiac tamponade
  - —Removal of even a small amount of fluid can lead to a dramatic improvement
  - —Guided by US is the safest technique

ED TREATMENT

- Treatment dependent on the underlying etiology
- Idiopathic, viral, rheumatologic, and posttraumatic
  - —NSAID regimens effective
  - —Corticosteroids reserved for refractory cases
- Bacterial
  - —Aggressive treatment with IV antibiotics along with drainage of the pericardial space
  - —Search for primary focus of infection
  - —Therapy guided by determination of pathogen from pericardial fluid tests
- Neoplastic
  - —Treat underlying malignancy
- Uremia
  - —Intensive 2–6-week course of dialysis
  - —Caution should be used if using nonsteroidal medications
- Expected course/prognosis
  - —Most patients will respond to treatment within 2 weeks
  - —Most have complete resolution of symptoms
  - —Few progress to recurrent bouts with eventual development of constrictive pericarditis or cardiac tamponade

MEDICATIONS

- Aspirin: 350–650 mg PO q3–4h
- Ibuprofen: 400–800 mg PO q6–8h
- Indomethacin: 25–50 mg PO q6h

Disposition

ADMISSION CRITERIA

- ICU
  - —Hemodynamic instability
  - —Cardiac tamponade
  - —Associated malignant dysrhythmia
  - —Any suspicion of myocardial infarction
  - —Severe pain unresponsive to oral medications
  - —Suspicion of bacterial etiology
  - —Patients having undergone pericardiocentesis due to the relatively high incidence of complications

DISCHARGE CRITERIA

- Mild symptoms in patients without any hemodynamic compromise
- Close follow-up
- Able to tolerate a regimen of oral medication

Miscellaneous

ICD9: 423.9

ICD10: I31.9

SEE ALSO: PERICARDIAL EFFUSION/TAMPONADE

SUGGESTED READINGS

Jourilles NJ. Pericardial and myocardial disease. In: Rosen P, et al, eds. Emergency medicine: concepts and clinical practice, 5th ed. St. Louis: Mosby–Year Book, 2002:1130–1138.

Maisch B. The classification of pericardial disease in the age of modern medicine. Curr Cardiol Rep 2002;4(1):13–21.

Maisch B. Myocarditis and pericarditis—old questions and new answers. Herz 1992; 17(2):65–70.

Maisch B. Pericardial diseases, with a focus on etiology, pathogenesis, pathophysiology, new diagnostic imaging methods, and treatment. Curr Opin Cardiol 1994;9:379–388.

Author: Andrew T. McAfee

Perilunate Dislocation

Clinical Presentation

SIGNS AND SYMPTOMS

- Pain in the wrist
- Swelling or mass in the wrist

MECHANISM/DESCRIPTION

- Fall on an outstretched hand usually dorsiflexed
- Dislocation of the carpal bones (usually the capitate) volar or dorsal from the lunate

Pre-Hospital

CAUTIONS

- Consider other more serious injuries
- Dress open wounds
- Immobilize in neutral position
- Elevation, cold to reduce swelling
- Age-appropriate social management

Diagnosis

ESSENTIAL WORKUP

- Physical examination with special attention to skin integrity and neurovascular status, including two-point discrimination
- This diagnosis is often missed by the clinical exam
- Radiographic imaging that includes three views of the wrist

IMAGING/SPECIAL TESTS

- Perilunate dislocation is visualized best on the true lateral view with the distal carpal row dorsal or volar to the lunate and with the lunate in its normal relationship to the radius

DIFFERENTIAL DIAGNOSIS

- Lunate fracture
- Lunate dislocation (dislocation occurs between lunate and distal radius)
- Scapholunate dissociation and other similar ligamentous disruptions
- The scaphoid is frequently fractured with this injury

Treatment

INITIAL STABILIZATION

- Immobilize, ice, elevate pending definitive evaluation
- Identify other, more serious, associated injuries

ED TREATMENT

- Reduction of dislocation
  - —There is frequently a need for operative fixation to reduce and maintain the fracture
  - —It is generally recommended to consult an orthopedist before the first attempt at reduction
  - —The patient is given appropriate conscious sedation
  - —The hand is placed in finger traps and counterweights are used
  - —Finger pressure is placed at the level of the dislocation and the injury is gently exaggerated, then brought to appropriate position, maintaining pressure over the dislocated segment
  - —The wrist is immobilized using a thumb spica or sugar tong splint in neutral position

MEDICATIONS

- Pain control with oral analgesic preparations
- See Conscious Sedation

PEDIATRIC CONSIDERATIONS

- Wrists are rarely sprained in children and the radiograph is difficult to interpret
- Although perilunate dislocation is unusual in pediatric patients, children with wrist pain should be splinted and referred for ongoing evaluation of possible dislocations or fractures; pain in the radial wrist should be splinted with a thumb spica splint
- Consideration of nonaccidental trauma

Disposition

ADMISSION CRITERIA

- Open dislocation, presence of multiple trauma or other, more serious, injuries
- Inability to reduce the dislocation or maintain reduction
- Preference of the consulting orthopedist
- Neurovascular compromise

DISCHARGE CRITERIA

- Closed injuries, adequate reduction, no neurovascular involvement
- Next-day orthopedic follow-up

Miscellaneous

ICD9: 833.00

ICD10: S63.0

SUGGESTED READINGS

American Society for Surgery of the Hand. The hand: primary care of common problems, 2d ed. New York: Churchill Livingstone, 1990:637–649.

Chin HW, Uehara DT. Wrist injuries. In: American College of Emergency Physicians, ed. Emergency medicine: a comprehensive study guide, 5th ed. New York: McGraw-Hill, 2000:1772–1783.

Eisenhauer MA. Forearm and wrist injuries. In: Rosen P, et al, eds. Emergency medicine: concepts and clinical practice, 4th ed. St Louis: Mosby–Year Book, 1998:669–689.

Escarza R, Chin HW. Wrist injuries. In: Hart RG, Uehara DT, Wagner MJ, eds. Emergency and primary care of the hand. Dallas: ACEP, 2001:139–160.

Author: John MacKay

Periodontal Abscess

Clinical Presentation

SIGNS AND SYMPTOMS

- Dental pain
  - —Focal swelling or fluctuance
  - —Tenderness to palpation
  - —Malaise
  - —Fever
  - —Increased mobility
  - —Parulis
    - -Pimple-like lesion on gingiva, representing terminal aspect of a sinus tract
    - -May be seen in chronic abscess
  - —Expression of pus from sinus tract
  - —Trismus generally absent, unless infection has spread to muscles of mastication

MECHANISM/DESCRIPTION

- Periodontal pockets result from progression of periodontal disease and resultant bone loss
- Food and debris accumulate in periodontal pockets
- Coronal epithelial tissues can reattach to the tooth, while bacteria and food debris remain trapped in the pocket, impairing drainage
- Food and debris become secondarily infected in setting of impaired drainage

ETIOLOGY

- Anaerobic and gram-negative pathogens generally are causative agents
- Complications
  - —Osteomyelitis
  - —Dentocutaneous fistula
  - —Cavernous sinus thrombosis
  - —Ludwig's angina
  - —Maxillary sinusitis

Pre-Hospital

N/A

Diagnosis

ESSENTIAL WORKUP

- Physical examination; periodontal abscess is a clinical diagnosis; ancillary testing not essential to make diagnosis

LABORATORY

- Culture of pus recommended for complicated abscess or when the patient is immunocompromised

IMAGING/SPECIAL TESTS

- Panoramic, periapical, or occlusal radiographs may be requested by dental consultant; not essential to make diagnosis, but can confirm and help define extent of abscess
- Electric pulp testing
  - —Performed by dental consultant to verify viability of tooth

DIFFERENTIAL DIAGNOSIS

- Periapical abscess
- Aphthous ulcers
- Oral herpes
- Salivary gland tumors
- Peritonsillar abscess
- Asymptomatic parulis
  - —Fibroma
  - —Pyogenic or peripheral ossifying granuloma
  - —Kaposi's sarcoma

Treatment

INITIAL STABILIZATION

- Assess for airway patency; establish definitive airway via endotracheal intubation or cricothyrotomy/tracheostomy if respiratory distress or inability to handle secretions is present, or if oropharyngeal tissue swelling impairs or threatens airway

ED TREATMENT

- Analgesia with NSAIDs or opiates may be required
- Incision and drainage
  - —Gingiva anesthetized superficially with 2% lidocaine with 1:100,000 epinephrine until blanching occurs
  - —A 1-cm stab incision using a no. 11 scalpel blade is made toward the alveolar bone
  - —Blunt dissection using a mosquito hemostat
  - —Cavity is irrigated with saline
  - —If abscess cavity is sufficiently large, place a ¼-inch iodoform gauze drain or fenestrated Penrose drain for 24–48 hours; to prevent its aspiration, secure the gauze or drain with a silk suture
- Antibiotics
  - —Indicated if abscess is extensive or if systemic signs are present
  - —Penicillin considered first-line empiric therapy
  - —Erythromycin for penicillin-allergic patients
  - —Clindamycin for penicillin-allergic patients or patients not responding to penicillin
- Warm salt-water rinses hourly while awake for 24–48 hours

MEDICATIONS

- Clindamycin: 150–450 mg (peds: 20–30 mg/kg/24 h) PO q6–8h
- Clindamycin: 600–900 mg (peds: 25–40 mg/kg/24 h) i.v. q6–8h
- Erythromycin: 250–500 mg (peds: 30–50 mg/kg/24 h) PO q6–8h
- Penicillin G: 2–24 million U (peds: 100,000–400,000 U/kg/24 h) i.v. q4–6h
- Penicillin VK: 250–500 mg (peds: 15–62.5 mg/kg/24 h) PO q6h

Disposition

ADMISSION CRITERIA

- Severe infection or complication requiring parenteral antibiotics
- Necrosis or cellulitis involving areas with potential airway compromise
- Immunocompromised patients
  - —Neutropenic
  - —Uncontrolled diabetes
  - —Advanced HIV
  - —Cancer patients undergoing chemotherapy
- Ludwig's angina
- Systemic involvement with significant dehydration
- Patients unable to manage infection at home because of physical or mental disability or psychosocial factors

DISCHARGE CRITERIA

- Uncomplicated cases
- Patients are able to obtain dental follow-up in 24–48 hours

Miscellaneous

ICD9: 523

ICD10: K05.2

SEE ALSO: TOOTHACHE

SUGGESTED READINGS

Amsterdam JT. Emergency dental procedures. In: Roberts J, Hedges J, eds. Clinical procedures in emergency medicine, 3rd ed. Philadelphia: WB Saunders, 1998:1149–1163.

Cherehugh V, Tugnait A. Diagnosis and management of periodontal diseases in children and adolescents. Periodontology 2000, 2001;26:146–168.

Nelson LP, Shusterman S. Dental emergencies. In: Fleisher GR, Ludwig S, eds. Synopsis of pediatric emergency medicine. Baltimore: Williams & Wilkins, 1996:760–763.

Van Winkelhoff AJ, Rams TE, Slots J. Systemic antibiotic therapy in periodontics. Periodontology 2000, 1996;10:45–78.

Wayne DB, Trajtenberg CP, Hyman DJ. Periodontal disease: a review for the primary care physician. South Med J 2001;94(9):925–932.

Author: John Sullivan

Periorbital (or Preseptal) Cellulitis and Orbital Cellulitis

Clinical Presentation

SIGNS AND SYMPTOMS

- Both will present with a unilateral, red, swollen eye
- Differences include
  —Anatomic location
  —Extent of deep tissue involvement
  —Etiology and mechanism of infection
  —Associated complications

Periorbital Cellulitis

- Periorbital erythema, warmth, tenderness, and swelling
  —Typically unilateral and involving the upper or the lower lid, rarely involving both
  —Gradual onset
  —Swelling may become predominant symptom leading to obscured vision in affected eye
- Associated with low-grade fever usually <39°C
- Typically nontoxic appearance
- Often preceded by upper respiratory tract infection (URTI)

Orbital Cellulitis

- Painful, red, warm, swollen eye
- Typically involves upper and lower lid
  —About 95% unilateral
- Swelling may obscure vision in the affected eye
- Toxic appearance
- Fever >39°C
- Headache
- Orbital involvement
  —Blurred vision or diplopia
  —Photophobia
  —Restricted, painful extraocular movements
  —Afferent pupillary defect
  —Conjunctival injection
  —Chemosis
  —Proptosis
- Meningismus
- Leukocytosis

MECHANISM/DESCRIPTION

Periorbital Cellulitis

- Periorbital cellulitis is anatomically distinguished by its location isolated to the tissues anterior to the orbital septum
  —Orbital septum is the connective tissue extension of the orbital periosteum that is reflected into the upper and lower eyelids
  —Extension into the tissues deep to the orbital septum is rare, because the septum represents a nearly impenetrable barrier
- Most commonly presents as a complication of URTI and sinusitis
  —Swelling due to inflammatory edema from vascular and lymphatic congestion
  —Not infected tissue
- May occur as a complication of a localized inflammation/infection in the eyelid or adjacent structures
  —Blepharitis
  —Hordeolum
  —Dacryocystitis
  —Surrounding skin disruptions
    -Insect bites
    -Minor trauma
    -Impetigo or other dermatologic disorders

Orbital Cellulitis

- Inflammatory process in the structures posterior to the orbital septum
- Occurs secondary to extension from an adjacent structure
  —Sinusitis
    -Most commonly ethmoid
  —Dental abscess
  —Retained foreign body in the orbit
  —Puncture wounds
  —Orbital fracture
  —Postoperative infection
  —Hematogenous spread from a remote source
  —Rare cause—extension of periorbital cellulitis

ETIOLOGY

Periorbital Cellulitis

- *Streptococcus pneumoniae*
- *Staphylococcus aureus*
- *Streptococcus pyogenes*
- *Moraxella catarrhalis*
- *H. influenzae* (children younger than 5 years)
- Gonococcus
  —May extend from conjunctivitis and/or dacryoadenitis

Orbital Cellulitis

- *S. pneumoniae*
- *S. pyogenes*
  —Currently streptococcal infections are the most common etiology
- *S. aureus*
  —Common in puncture wounds
- *S. pyogenes*
- *Staphylococcus epidermidis*
- Anaerobes
- Bacteroides
- Gram negative
  —Associated with trauma
- Fungal infection—cerebrorhinoorbital phycomycosis (CROP)
  —Life-threatening disease presenting with orbital cellulitis
  —Rapidly fatal in 75% of cases
  —Presentation
    -80% of cases occur in diabetic patients with a recent episode of DKA
    -Toxic appearance
    -Begins in the paranasal sinuses
    -Proliferates in the blood vessels and causes thrombosis and necrosis
    -Bloody nasal discharge
    -Frequently presents with evidence of necrosis of the palate and/or nasal mucosa

PEDIATRIC CONSIDERATIONS

- In children younger than 2 years
  H. influenzae is an important cause of bacteremic periorbital cellulitis
  —Toxic appearance
  —Temperature >39°C
  —Erythematous and violaceous swollen eyelids
  —Dramatic decrease (80%) since Hib vaccine
    -Incidence decreases significantly after two immunizations
  —Preceded by upper respiratory infection

Pre-Hospital

N/A

Diagnosis

ESSENTIAL WORKUP

- Physical exam to rule out orbital involvement
  —Orbital involvement may lead to serious complications
  —High level of suspicion
    -Patients who appear toxic
    -Orbital pain
    -Painful restriction of eye movement
    -Proptosis swelling of upper and lower lids
- Complete neurologic examination to rule out CNS involvement
  —High level of suspicion for CNS penetration
    -Altered mental status
    -Meningismus
    -Visual loss
- Identify complicating medical problems
  —Immunocompromise
  —Diabetes

LABORATORY

- Supportive but not diagnostic
- CBC
  - —WBC <15,000 for periorbital cellulitis
  - —WBC >15,000 may suggest bacteremic periorbital cellulitis
- Blood culture
- Gram stain and culture of tissue aspirate or swab of draining purulent material
  - —Chocolate agar plate should be used when gonorrhea suspected
- Lumbar puncture
  - —Rule out CNS involvement
  - —Consider in patients with
    - -Signs or symptoms of meningismus
    - -Toxic appearance
    - -Patients at risk of *H. influenzae* type B: younger than 4 years and non-Hib vaccinated

IMAGING/SPECIAL TESTS

- CT scan orbits
  - —Indicated if
    - -Suspect orbital cellulitis or traumatic penetration of the orbital septum
    - -Failure to respond to parenteral antimicrobial therapy
  - —Demonstrates extent
    - -Orbital cellulitis
    - -Sinusitis
    - -Orbital emphysema
    - -Subperiosteal abscess
    - -Presence of foreign body

DIFFERENTIAL DIAGNOSIS

Periorbital Cellulitis

- Lack of fever and leukocytosis suggests noninfectious cause
  - —Insect bite
  - —Allergy
- Dacryoadenitis
- Dacryocystitis
- Hordeolum
- Orbital cellulitis

Orbital Cellulitis

- Periorbital cellulitis
- Contusion
- Dacryoadenitis
- Dacryocystitis
- Hordeolum
- Retrobulbar hemorrhage
- Cavernous sinus thrombosis
- Cranial nerve palsy
- Inflammatory orbital pseudotumor
- Grave's disease
- Orbital rhabdosarcoma

Treatment

INITIAL STABILIZATION

- IV fluids for vomiting/dehydration/sepsis
- 0.9% NS 500-mL bolus (20 mL/kg children) for hydration and resuscitation

ED TREATMENT

Periorbital Cellulitis

- Antibiotics
  - —Typically responds to oral antibiotics unless appears bacteremic or toxic
  - —IV antibiotics for severe infections/treatment failures
- Antipyretics and pain medication as needed

Orbital Cellulitis

- Antipyretics
- Pain medication
- Early administration of parenteral antibiotics
- Ophthalmologic consultation
- If sinusitis is the source, consider ENT consultation
- Emergent surgical intervention may be necessary
- If *Bacteroides* is suspected organism
  - —Surgical débridement
  - —Vancomycin
- Tetanus toxoid when appropriate
- If proptosis leaves the cornea exposed
  - —Lubricating drops (Lacri-Lube: 2 drops q2–4h p.r.n.)
- Suspect CROP
  - —Amphotericin B IV at highest tolerated dose
  - —Topical amphotericin B (1 mg/mL) irrigation or nasal packing
  - —Local débridement

MEDICATIONS

Periorbital Cellulitis

- Augmentin: 500 mg (peds: 45 mg/kg/24 h) PO t.i.d.
- Cephalexin: 500 mg (peds: 100 mg/kg/24 h) PO q.i.d.
- Cefazolin: 1 g (peds: 100 mg/k/24 h) i.v. q6–8h
- Cefotaxime: 1–2 g (peds: 150 mg/kg/24 h) i.v. q6–8h
- Clindamycin: 600 mg (peds: 40 mg/kg/24 h) i.v. q6h; 300 mg (peds: 20 mg/kg/24 h) PO q.i.d.
- Dicloxacillin: 500 mg (peds: 100 mg/kg/24 h) PO q.i.d.
- Vancomycin: 500 mg (peds: 40 mg/kg/24 h) i.v. q6h

Orbital Cellulitis

- Ceftriaxone: 1–2 g (peds: 100 mg/kg/24 h) i.v. q12–24 h
- Erythromycin ophthalmologic ointment: applied q4h to lower cul-de-sac
- Gentamicin: 5 mg/kg/24 h i.v.
- Metronidazole: 15 mg/kg i.v. load then 7.5 mg/kg q6h
- Nafcillin: 1–2 g (peds: 100 mg/kg/24 h) i.v. q4h
- Vancomycin: 1 g (peds: 40 mg/kg/24 h) q12h

Disposition

ADMISSION CRITERIA

Periorbital Cellulitis

- Toxicity
- Progression of infection on oral antibiotics
- Unable to arrange follow-up within 24–48 hours
- High risk *H. influenzae* type B

Orbital Cellulitis

- IV antibiotics
- Observation for progression
  - —Without visual findings or restriction
- Surgical incision and drainage

DISCHARGE CRITERIA

Periorbital Cellulitis

- Localized infection and inflammation
- Tolerating oral antibiotics
- Good follow-up

Orbital Cellulitis

- Admit all
  - —High risk of CNS penetration and ophthalmologic complications

Miscellaneous

ICD9: 376.01

ICD10: H05.0

SUGGESTED READINGS

Chang CH, et al. Antibiotic treatment of orbital cellulitis: an analysis of pathogenic bacteria and bacterial susceptibility. J Ocul Pharmacol Ther 2000;16(1):75–79.

Danter EM, Jolly BT. Pediatric ophthalmology. Emerg Med Clin North Am 1995;13(3):669–680.

Ghosh C. Periorbital and orbital cellulitis after *H. influenzae* B vaccination. Ophthalmology 2001;108(9):1514–1515.

Jain A, Rubin PA. Orbital cellulitis in children. Int Ophthalmol Clin 2001;41(4):71–86.

Author: Shari Schabowski

Peripheral Neuropathy

Clinical Presentation

Peripheral neuropathy is a general term for peripheral nerve disorders of any cause.

SIGNS AND SYMPTOMS

- Sensory nerve dysfunction
  - —Numbness, localized tingling, paresthesias, dysthesias
  - —Vibration and position sensations decreased with large-fiber neuropathy
  - —Pain and temperature sensation decreased with small-fiber neuropathy
  - —Deep tendon reflexes decreased secondary to decrease sensation of afferent limb
- Motor nerve dysfunction
  - —Weakness (distal greater than proximal), occasionally fasciculations
  - —Muscle atrophy, diminished tone with long-standing motor nerve involvement
  - —Loss of reflexes secondary to slowing of conduction along motor nerve efferent limb
- Autonomic nerve dysfunction
  - —Orthostasis, constipation, urinary retention, or impotence

Pre-Hospital

CAUTIONS

- Pain control as needed
- Airway protection as indicated

Diagnosis

ESSENTIAL WORKUP

- Studies based on acuteness, severity of neuropathy, and most likely diagnosis
- Neurologic consult early if acute and severe symptoms

LABORATORY

- Basic metabolic panel, CBC count, liver function tests, urinalysis, thyrotropin-stimulating hormone, HIV, or vitamin B_{12} based on individual presentations

IMAGING/SPECIAL TESTS

- CXR, EKG, or lumbar puncture as appropriate
- Electromyographic studies, nerve conduction studies, and nerve biopsy per neurologic consult on admission or outpatient follow-up

DIFFERENTIAL DIAGNOSIS

- Focal
  - —Entrapment
  - —Common sites of compression (carpal tunnel, ulnar, tarsal tunnel, peroneal), myxedema, rheumatoid arthritis, amyloidosis, acromegaly
  - —Compressive neuropathies
  - —Trauma
  - —Ischemic lesions
  - —Diabetes mellitus (DM), vasculitis
  - —Leprosy
  - —Sarcoidosis
  - —Neoplastic infiltration or compression
- Multifocal (mononeuropathy multiplex)
  - —DM
  - —Vasculitis: polyarteritis nodosa, systemic lupus erythematosus, Sjögren syndrome
  - —Sarcoid
  - —Leprosy
  - —Malignancy related
  - —HIV/AIDS
  - —Hereditary predisposition to pressure palsies
- Symmetric
  - —Endocrine (most common is DM, hypothyroidism)
  - —Medications (e.g., isoniazid, lithium, metronidazole, phenytoin, cimetidine, hydralazine, amitriptyline, amiodarone)
  - —Nutritional diseases (e.g., alcoholism, B_{12}/folate deficiency, thiamine)
  - —Critical illness neuropathy
  - —Hypophosphatemia
  - —Guillain-Barré syndrome
  - —Toxic neuropathy (carbon monoxide, acrylamide, carbon disulfide, ethylene oxide, organophosphate esters, lead)
  - —Myelopathy mimicking peripheral neuropathy (e.g., back pain, saddle anesthesia, lower extremity weakness)

Treatment

INITIAL STABILIZATION

- Establish airway protection with severe acute peripheral neuropathy, such as Guillain-Barré syndrome

ED TREATMENT

- Variable depending on acuity of symptoms

MEDICATIONS

- Variable depending underlying diagnosis
- Neurontin is often effective: 300 mg PO TID up to 1800 mg/day

Disposition

ADMISSION CRITERIA

- Respiratory distress or acute gait disturbance
- Intractable pain

DISCHARGE CRITERIA

- Stable respiratory and gait status with outpatient follow-up

Miscellaneous

ICD9: 356.9

ICD10: G62.9

SUGGESTED READINGS

Morgenlander JC. Recognizing peripheral neuropathy. Postgrad Med 1997;102:71–80.

Pascuzzi RM, Fleck JD. Acute peripheral neuropathy in adults. Neurol Clin 1997; 15(3):529–547.

Poncelelet AN. An algorithm for the evaluation of peripheral neuropathy. Am Fam Physician 1998;57:755–764.

Author: Minh V. Le

Peripheral Vascular Disease

Clinical Presentation

SIGNS AND SYMPTOMS

Chronic Arterial Insufficiency

- Claudication
  - —Aching pain in the calves (femoropopliteal occlusion) or buttocks and thighs (aortoiliac region)
  - —Occurs with activity and slowly relieved by rest
  - —Classic claudication present in about half of patients with PVD
- Severe disease presents with limb pain at rest (usually starting in the foot) or rapidly progressive claudication or ulceration
- Physical examination
  - —Absent or decreased peripheral pulses
  - —Delayed capillary refill with cool skin
  - —Increased venous filling time
  - —Bruits
  - —Pallor and dependent rubor of the leg
  - —Muscle and skin atrophy
  - —Thickened nails and loss of dorsal hair
  - —Ulcerations or gangrene with severe disease

Acute Arterial Insufficiency

- Acute limb ischemia (from embolism or arterial thrombosis)
  - —Six *Ps*
    - -Pain (first symptom)
    - -Pallor
    - -Pulselessness
    - -Poikilothermic
    - -Paresthesias (late finding)
    - -Paralysis (late finding)
- Identification of a source of a possible embolic process is crucial

Atheroembolism

- Small atherosclerotic emboli may effect both extremities
  - —Ischemic and painful digits
  - —"Blue toe syndrome"
  - —Livedo reticularis

MECHANISM/DESCRIPTION

- Chronic arterial insufficiency (CAI)
  - —Progressive obstructing atherosclerotic disease
  - —Risks factors include age, smoking, diabetes, hyperlipidemia, and hypertension
  - —15% develop critical leg ischemia
  - —Associated with morbidity and mortality of other forms of atherosclerosis (coronary artery disease, stroke)
  - —Complications: aneurysm, thrombosis, ulceration, limb loss
- Acute arterial insufficiency (AAI)
  - —Caused by either arterial thrombosis (50%) or embolism
  - —Source of arterial thrombosis
    - -Plaques from preexisting CAI thrombose to create AAI
  - —Sources of acute arterial embolus
    - -80% are cardiac emboli from dysrhythmias, valvular heart disease, cardiomyopathy
    - -Aneurysms
    - -Infection
    - -Tumor
    - -Vasculitides or foreign body
- Atheroembolism
  - —Caused by rupture or partial disruption of an atherosclerotic plaque (aorta, femoral, iliac)
  - —Gives rise to cholesterol emboli showers and obstructing arteriolar networks
  - —May be precipitated by invasive arterial procedures such as cardiac catheterization

Pre-Hospital

CAUTIONS

- Maintain hemodynamic stability
- Apply cardiac monitor
- Place the ischemic limb at rest and in a dependent position
- Provide oxygen if low oxygen saturation or pulmonary symptoms

Diagnosis

ESSENTIAL WORKUP

- CAI
  - —Ankle-brachial index (ankle systolic BP divided by arm systolic BP)
  - —Bedside test to determine whether CAI is present
  - —Ratio of <0.9 is abnormal and <0.4 indicates severe disease
- AAI
  - —Physical diagnosis using the six *Ps*
  - —Those with acute-on-chronic arterial insufficiency tolerate limb ischemia better than those without CAI due to well-developed collateral circulation
- Atheroembolism
  - —Clinical diagnosis with affected areas painful, tender, and may be either dusky or necrotic

LABORATORY

- CBC and platelets
- Electrolytes, BUN, creatinine, glucose
- Coagulation studies
- CPK to evaluate for ischemia
- Special tests
  - —Hold blood for special hematologic studies if a hypercoagulable state suspected
  - —Sedimentation rate if vasculitis suspected
  - —Blood cultures if endocarditis possible

IMAGING/SPECIAL TESTS

- Doppler US
  - —Visualizes both venous and arterial systems
  - —Identifies level of arterial occlusion, as well as thrombosis and aneurysm
  - —Sensitivity and specificity $>$80–90% for occlusion of vessels proximal to the popliteal vessels
- Plethysmography
  - —Uses measurements of the volume and character of blood flow to detect areas of CAI
  - —Less widely available than US therefore requires an experienced technician
  - —Approximates US in sensitivity and specificity
- Angiography
  - —Determines details about the anatomy including the level of occlusion, stenosis, and collateral flow
  - —Useful where the diagnosis of AAI is uncertain or before emergent bypass grafting
- CT
  - —CT is useful for diagnosis of occlusive aortic disease or dissection
- MRI
  - —MRI is sensitive for evaluation of CAI and dissection

DIFFERENTIAL DIAGNOSIS

- Acute thrombosis or emboli
- Arterial dissection
- Deep venous thrombosis
- Massive venous insufficiency
- Compartment syndrome
- Buerger's disease
- Spinal stenosis
- Neuropathy
- Bursitis
- Arthritis
- Reflex sympathetic dystrophy

Treatment

INITIAL STABILIZATION

- 0.9% IV fluid bolus for hypotension
- EKG, monitor, pulse oximetry
- Supplemental oxygen

ED TREATMENT

- AAI
  —Limit further clot propagation with heparin
  —Do not anticoagulate patients suspected of having an aortic dissection or symptomatic aneurysm
  —Emergent consultation with a vascular surgeon
    -To determine which diagnostic study will be employed
    -To begin arrangements for operative therapy
  —Options for operative therapy include thrombectomy, embolectomy, regional arterial thrombolysis, or bypass grafting
  —Blood flow to the affected limb must be reestablished within 4–6 hours after onset of ischemic symptoms
  —Complications of AAI include
    -Compartment syndrome
    -Irreversible ischemia requiring amputation
    -Rhabdomyolysis, renal failure
    -Electrolyte disturbances
- Atheroembolism
  —Treat conservatively if a limited amount of tissue is involved and renal function is not significantly compromised
  —No available therapy for the ischemic digits besides supportive wound care and analgesia
  —Amputation for irreversibly necrotic toes
  —Vascular surgeon referral within 12–24 hours of ED visit
  —Prevent further embolic events by a thorough investigation and correction of the source of atheroemboli
- CAI
  —Initiate measures to prevent disease progression
    -Tobacco cessation
    -Aggressive management of hyperlipidemia
    -Exercise therapy
  —Antiplatelet and anticoagulant drugs may help but have not been definitively shown to prevent progression of CAI
  —Invasive therapy
    -Atherectomy
    -Bypass grafting
    -Balloon angioplasty

MEDICATIONS

- Aspirin: 80–325 mg/d
- Heparin: 80 U/kg bolus i.v. followed by 18 U/h i.v.
- Cilostazol: 100 mg b.i.d.
- Clopidogrel: 75 mg/d
- Pentoxifylline: 400 mg t.i.d.

Disposition

ADMISSION CRITERIA

- AAI for evaluation and revascularization
- Rapidly progressive claudication or ischemic pain at rest
  —To undergo heparinization and angiography to rule out an acute thrombosis
- Atheroembolism with large areas involved, significant pain, infection, or renal compromise

DISCHARGE CRITERIA

- Atheroembolism
  —If they have small lesions, adequate pain control, no evidence of renal compromise or superinfection, and follow-up within 24 hours
- CAI
  —No evidence of rapid progression, gangrene, or infection

Miscellaneous

ICD9: 414.0

ICD10: 173.9

SEE ALSO: ARTERIAL OCCLUSION

SUGGESTED READINGS

Dormandy JA, Rutherford RB. Management of peripheral arterial disease. J Vasc Surg 2000;31:S1–S296.

Hiatt WR. Drug therapy: medical treatment of peripheral arterial disease and claudication. N Engl J Med 2001;344: 1608–1621.

Jackson MR, Clagett GP. Antithrombotic therapy in peripheral arterial occlusive disease. Chest 2001;119:283–289.

Mukherjee D, Yadav JS. Update on peripheral vascular diseases: from smoking cessation to stenting. Cleve Clin J Med 2001;68:723–733.

Author: Sally Santen

Peritonsillar Abscess

Clinical Presentation

SIGNS AND SYMPTOMS

Symptoms

- Sore throat
- Unilateral ear pain
- Fever
- Dysphagia
- Trismus
- Muffled voice
- Drooling
- Feeling of oropharyngeal fullness
- Symptoms usually develop 2–4 days after the inciting pharyngitis or upper respiratory tract infection

Signs

- Erythematous
- Bulging tonsil, often displacing the uvula
- Fullness of the superior tonsil and adjacent soft palate
- Tonsillar exudate or fluctuants are not common findings
- Cervical adenopathy
- Torticollis
- Halitosis

MECHANISM/DESCRIPTION

- Most commonly encountered head and neck abscess
- Two theories explain the development of peritonsillar abscess (PTA)
  —Direct bacterial invasion into deeper tissues in the patient with acute pharyngitis
  —Acute obstruction and bacterial infection of small salivary glands present in the superior tonsil
- PTA can occur despite prior antibiotic therapy
- Can happen after tonsillectomy
- Complications
  —Uncommon, but can be life threatening
  —Airway obstruction
  —Sepsis
  —Jugular vein thrombosis ("Lemierre disease")
  —Spontaneous perforation
  —Aspiration
  —Extension to the lateral neck or mediastinum
  —Recurrence in up to 50%

ETIOLOGY

- Affects all age-groups, with highest rates in teens and young adults
- Most common pathogens
  —β-Hemolytic streptococcus
  —Other streptococcal species
  —Anaerobes
  —Staphylococcal species
  —Mixed organisms

PEDIATRIC CONSIDERATIONS

- PTA occurs in children (younger than 18 years) in 24–39% of reported cases
- Presentation and therapy are similar in older children and adults
- Young children may need sedation or general anesthesia if incision and drainage (I&D) or aspiration of the abscess is attempted

Pre-Hospital

CAUTIONS

- Rarely associated with acute airway compromise, but as the diagnosis is likely to be uncertain during transport, patients should be treated as potential airway emergencies
- Apply cardiac and pulse oximetry monitoring
- Place patient in position of comfort
- Administer supplemental oxygen
- Have suction and equipment for bag-valve mask ventilation and intubation readily available
- Initiate IV access in cooperative patients

Diagnosis

ESSENTIAL WORKUP

- PTA is evident by physical examination in most cases, unless trismus obscures full adequate examination

LABORATORY

- Throat culture and Monospot
  —Indicated in persons thought to have streptococcal pharyngitis or Epstein-Barr virus, because this may alter antimicrobial therapy

IMAGING/SPECIAL TESTS

- Soft-tissue lateral neck radiography
  —Useful in excluding other causes of upper airway obstruction, especially in young children at risk for epiglottitis
- CXR in patients with respiratory symptoms or draining abscesses
- CT scanning of the neck
  —Differentiates tonsillar cellulitis from abscess
  —Determines whether deeper tissues of the neck are involved
  —Unnecessary in simple cases of PTA
- Intraoral US
  —Useful in differentiating abscess from cellulitis
  —Useful to localize the fluid collection for aspiration

DIFFERENTIAL DIAGNOSIS

- Peritonsillar cellulitis
- Retropharyngeal abscess
- Croup
- Epiglottitis
- Bacterial tracheitis
- Cervical adenitis
- Lateral neck abscess
- Odontogenic abscess
- Neoplasm (including lymphoma and leukemia)

PEDIATRIC CONSIDERATIONS

- Obtain soft-tissue lateral neck radiograph before oral examination in young children with symptoms of upper airway obstruction

Treatment

INITIAL STABILIZATION

- ABCs
- Administer supplemental oxygen for respiratory distress
- IV hydration with 0.9% NS 500 mL bolus (peds: 20 mL/kg) for dehydration

ED TREATMENT

- Keep NPO in anticipation of drainage procedure
- Administer analgesia
  - —Topical sprays
  - —Parenteral narcotics/NSAIDs
- Perform needle aspiration
  - —Should be performed by person experienced in drainage procedure and adept at advanced airway techniques
    - -More readily accomplished and tolerated than I&D
    - -Cure rates of >85% in children and adults with a single aspiration
    - -Tonsil lies in proximity to the internal carotid artery; sheathing the aspiration needle to prevent introduction of the needle to <0.5 cm is prudent
    - -Aspiration may not always yield abscess fluid; in these patients, medical therapy and timely reexamination is recommended
    - -Repeat aspiration is necessary in 10%
    - -Cooperative patient is essential
    - -Sedation or general anesthesia may be needed for young or uncooperative persons
- Antibiotics
  - —Penicillins or cephalosporins are the initial choice
  - —Clindamycin in patients with penicillin and cephalosporin allergy

MEDICATIONS

- Amoxicillin: 500 mg (peds: 20–40 mg/kg/24 h) PO q.i.d.
- Ampicillin: 2 g (peds: 100–200 mg/kg/24 h) i.v. q6h
- Ceftriaxone: 1 g (peds: 50 mg/kg/24 h) i.v./i.m. q.d.
- Clindamycin
  - —900 mg (peds: 25–40 mg/kg/24 h) i.v. q8h
  - —300 mg (peds: 10–30 mg/kg/24 h) PO t.i.d.
- Penicillin G: 1–2 million U (peds: 50,000 U/kg/24 h) i.v. q4h
- Penicillin VK: 500 mg (peds: 25–50 mg/kg/24 h) PO q.i.d.

PEDIATRIC CONSIDERATIONS

- Children should be exposed to minimal stimulation and accompanied by a parent if feasible
- Do not attempt oropharyngeal examination and IV access in uncooperative children who are maintaining their airway

Disposition

ADMISSION CRITERIA

- Patients unable to maintain oral intake or comply with antibiotic therapy
- Signs of sepsis or complicated PTA

DISCHARGE CRITERIA

- Adequate hydration
- Ability to take antibiotics
- After I&D or aspiration
- Follow-up within 24–48 hours

Miscellaneous

ICD9: 475

ICD10: J36

SEE ALSO: PHARYNGITIS

SUGGESTED READINGS

Friedman NR, Mitchell RB, Pereira KD, et al. Peritonsillar abscess in early childhood. Presentation and management. Arch Otolaryngol Head Neck Surg 1997;123(6):630–632.

Herzon FS. Peritonsillar abscess: incidence, current management practices, and a proposal for treatment guidelines. Laryngoscope 1995;105[Suppl 74, Pt 3]:1–17.

Herzon FS, Nicklaus P. Pediatric peritonsillar abscess: management guidelines. Curr Probl Pediatr 1996;26(8):270–278.

Miziara ID, Koishi HU, Zonato AI, et al. The use of ultrasound evaluation in the diagnosis of peritonsillar abscess. Rev Laryngol Otol Rhinol (Bord) 2001;122(3):201–203.

Scott PM, Loftus WK, Kew J, et al. Diagnosis of peritonsillar infections: a prospective study of ultrasound, computerized tomography and clinical diagnosis. J Laryngol Otol 1999;113(3):229–232.

Author: Lee Shockley

Pertussis

Clinical Presentation

SIGNS AND SYMPTOMS

- Generally three recognized phases with progression
  - —Infants may have indistinct stages
- *Catarrhal stage*
  - —Approximately 1-week duration
  - —Rhinorrhea
  - —Mild cough
  - —Minimal fever
- *Paroxysmal stage*
  - —Classic "whooping" cough, increasing in severity
  - —Coughing spasm that ends with a sudden inflow of air—the "whoop;" unremitting paroxysms
  - —Posttussive emesis
  - —Cyanosis with respiratory distress/failure
  - —Apnea (infants younger than 6 months)
  - —Altered mental status due to hypoxia or encephalitis
- *Convalescent stage*
  - —Waning cough
  - —Improving respiratory status
- Atypical presentations
  - —Often atypical in children younger than 6 months
  - —Partially immunized children have less severe disease
  - —Adult manifestations are often only rhinorrhea, sore throat, persistent cough; often in family members
- Complications
  - —HEENT
    - -Epistaxis
    - -Subconjunctival hemorrhage
  - —Respiratory
    - -Acute respiratory arrest
    - -Pneumonia caused by secondary infection
    - -Pneumothorax
    - -Subcutaneous or mediastinal emphysema with crepitus
    - -Bronchiectasis
  - —GI
    - -Hernia: inguinal or abdominal
    - -Rectal prolapse
  - —Neurologic
    - -Seizures
    - -Encephalitis
    - -Coma
    - -Intracranial hemorrhage
    - -Spinal epidural hemorrhage

MECHANISM/DESCRIPTION

- Acute respiratory tract infection spread by small respiratory droplets
- Bacteria (fimbriae) attach to respiratory epithelial cells and proliferates, producing toxins
  - —Ciliary dysfunction, accumulation of cellular debris, increased mucus production, lymphocytic and granulocytic infiltration
  - —Bronchiolar congestion, obstruction and necrosis
- Incubation period is 6–20 days, usually 7–10 days
- Mostly young children; 24% in children younger than 6 months
- Increasing incidence in adolescents
- Adults are the primary reservoir
- Peak incidence—late summer/fall
- Preventable with diphtheria-tetanus-pertussis (DTP) vaccine
  - —Newly introduced acellular vaccines have fewer side effects and equal efficacy to cellular vaccines
- Uncomplicated cases last 6–10 weeks; half of cases last <6 weeks
- Obstruction of the airway due to mucous plug leading to hypoxia and hypoventilation
- Increased intrathoracic or intracranial pressure
- Secondary bacterial infection may exacerbate respiratory distress/failure
- CNS injury due to encephalitis, increased intracranial pressure, and/or hypoxia
- Mortality
  - —Mortality greatest in those younger than 1 year
  - —1.3% for patients younger than 1 month
  - —0.3% in children between 2 and 11 months
  - —90% is due to secondary bacterial pneumonia

ETIOLOGY

- *Bordetella pertussis*
  - —A fastidious, gram-negative, pleomorphic bacillus

Pre-Hospital

CAUTIONS

- Universal precautions, notably a mask
  - —If exposed, consider chemoprophylaxis of pre-hospital personnel
- Suction in patients with respiratory distress
  - —Complete airway obstruction from a mucous plug is potentially life threatening

Diagnosis

ESSENTIAL WORKUP

- The ED diagnosis should be made on clinical grounds
- Attempt to establish a history of a contact
- Observe the paroxysmal cough with the characteristic whoop
- Use ancillary studies to further support the clinical diagnosis and exclude complications

LABORATORY

- WBC count
  - —Leukocytosis (20,000–50,000 cells/mm^3) with marked lymphocytosis
  - —Elevation of WBC and lymphocytosis parallels severity of cough

IMAGING/SPECIAL TESTS

- CXR
  - —Most often normal
  - —Perihilar infiltrates
  - —Atelectasis
  - —Occasionally characteristic "shaggy" right heart border
  - —Secondary bacterial pneumonia
- Direct immunofluorescence assay (DFA) of nasopharyngeal mucus; false-positive results and negative results
- Immunofluorescent and enzyme immunoassays to exclude respiratory syncytial virus
- Culture of nasopharynx or cough plate on a Bordet-Gengou medium

DIFFERENTIAL DIAGNOSIS

- Infection
  - —Parallel whooping cough syndrome due to *Bordetella parapertussis, Chlamydia trachomatis, Chlamydia pneumoniae, Bordetella bronchiseptica,* or adenovirus
  - —Pneumonia: bacteria, mycoplasma, mycobacterium
  - —Bronchiolitis
- Reactive airway disease
- Foreign body
- Cystic fibrosis

Treatment

INITIAL STABILIZATION

- Oxygen and respiratory support
- Suction mucous plugs

ED TREATMENT

- Universal precautions
  —Specifically requires droplet precautions
- Maintenance of adequate hydration
- Monitor oxygenation during paroxysms; supplement oxygen
- Airway management may be life saving in younger children
- Antibiotics
  —Effective in the catarrhal stage
  —Prevents further transmission in the paroxysmal stage
  —Erythromycin is the first-line agent
  —Alternatively, clarithromycin or trimethoprim-sulfamethoxazole may be used, although the efficacy is unproven; useful if erythromycin is not tolerated
- Corticosteroids and albuterol may reduce paroxysms of coughing, but further studies are required

MEDICATIONS

- Clarithromycin: 7.5 mg/kg PO b.i.d.
- Erythromycin: 10 mg/kg PO q.i.d.
- Trimethoprim-sulfamethoxazole: 4/20 mg/kg PO b.i.d.

Disposition

ADMISSION CRITERIA

- Patients younger than 1 year
- Apnea
- Cyanosis during paroxysms of cough
- Significant associated pneumonia
- Encephalitis

DISCHARGE CRITERIA

- Children without apnea, respiratory compromise, altered mental status, or complications and respiratory
- Warm liquids to reduce coughing spasm
- Remove thick secretions with bulb suction in infants
- Drink lots of fluids
- Avoid cough triggers: cigarette smoke, pollutants, perfumes
- All exposed persons should seek chemoprophylaxis
  —Household and other close contacts should receive 10 days of erythromycin; those younger than 7 years who are unimmunized or received fewer than four doses of DTP vaccine should receive addition immunizations
  —Exposed children, especially incompletely immunized children, should be observed for 20 days and receive chemoprophylaxis and be vaccinated as mentioned
  —Symptomatic children should be excluded from school or work; individuals with pertussis may return after 5 days of erythromycin treatment

Miscellaneous

ICD9: 033.9

ICD10: A37.9

SUGGESTED READINGS

Behrman R, Vaughn V, eds. Nelson's textbook of pediatrics, 13th ed. Philadelphia: WB Saunders, 1987:396–398.

Cattaneo L, Edwards K. *Bordetella pertussis* (whooping cough). Semin Pediatr Infect Dis 1995;6(2):107–118.

Halperin SA, Bartoluss R, Langley JM, et al. Seven days of erythromycin estolate is as effective as fourteen days for the treatment of *Bordetella pertussis* infection. Pediatrics 1997;100:65.

Pickering LK, Peter G, Baker CJ, et al. 2000 red book: report of the Committee on Infectious Diseases, 25th ed. Elk Grove Village, IL: American Academy of Pediatrics, 2000.

Yaari E, et al. Clinical manifestations of *Bordetella pertussis* infection in immunized children and young adults. Chest 1999;115: 1254.

Author: Roger M. Barkin

Phalangeal Injuries, Foot

Clinical Presentation

SIGNS AND SYMPTOMS

- Acute pain, swelling, crepitus, and ecchymosis of affected digit
- Subungual hematomas are often present
- Lacerations or crush-type wounds

MECHANISM/DESCRIPTION

- Usually the result of direct trauma
- Stubbing the toe, kicking a hard surface, or dropping a heavy object onto toes most common mechanisms of injury
- Fifth (or small) toe most commonly affected

Pre-Hospital

N/A

Diagnosis

ESSENTIAL WORKUP

- Radiographs of involved digit
- Lateral view may be most sensitive
- Document neurovascular status of the affected digit

DIFFERENTIAL DIAGNOSIS

- Contusion
- Abrasion/laceration
- Dislocation

Treatment

INITIAL STABILIZATION

- Ice to the affected digit

ED TREATMENT

- Fractures involving the proximal phalanx and interphalangeal (IP) joint of the hallux
  - —Nondisplaced, non-intraarticular fractures may be placed in a short-leg walking cast with toe extension for comfort
  - —Displaced, non-intraarticular fractures should have closed reduction with digital block anesthesia and longitudinal traction, followed by placement in short-leg walking cast with toe extension
  - —Intraarticular fractures of the hallux merit orthopedic consult, as they frequently are treated with ORIF
- Fractures involving the proximal phalanx and IP joint of the lesser toes
  - —Rarely cause long-term disability
  - —Nondisplaced fractures may be treated with splinting or buddy taping, with gauze padding between the taped toes to prevent skin breakdown
  - —Displaced fractures should undergo closed reduction by digital block anesthesia and longitudinal traction, followed by buddy taping or splinting
  - —Hard-sole shoe, weight bearing as tolerated
  - —Oral analgesics for pain
  - —Pain usually resolved by 2–3 weeks
- IP joint dislocations
  - —Closed reduction by digital block anesthesia, longitudinal traction with gentle downward pressure on distal phalanx
  - —Buddy tape to adjacent toe
  - —Unstable or unsuccessful reductions require orthopedic consultation
  - —Oral analgesics for pain
- Distal tuft fractures
  - —Subungual hematomas should be drained
  - —Nail-bed laceration repair may be necessary
  - —Buddy tape digit to adjacent toe
  - —Weight bearing as tolerated
  - —Oral analgesics for pain
  - —Pain usually resolved in 2–3 weeks
- Open fractures
  - —Orthopedic consultation
  - —Prophylactic antibiotics

MEDICATIONS

- Cephalexin: 1 g i.m./i.v. in ED (peds: 50–100 mg/kg i.m./i.v. in ED)
- Ibuprofen: 400–600 mg PO q.i.d. (peds: 5–10 mg/kg PO q.i.d.)

Disposition

ADMISSION CRITERIA

- Intraarticular fractures involving the proximal phalanx of the great toe, unstable or blocked dislocations, and open fractures require orthopedic consultation in the ED

DISCHARGE CRITERIA

- All other fractures may be discharged with orthopedic follow-up in 2–3 weeks to evaluate healing

Miscellaneous

ICD9: 959.7

ICD10: S90.9

SUGGESTED READINGS

Ho K, Abu-Laban RB. Ankle and foot. In: Marx JA, ed. Rosen's emergency medicine: concepts and clinical practice, 5th ed. St. Louis: Mosby–Year Book, 2002: 706–735.

Kensinger DR, Guille JT, Horn BD, et al. The stubbed great toe: importance of early recognition and treatment of open fractures of the distal phalanx. J Pediatr Orthop 2001;21:31–34.

Wedmore IS, Charette J. Emergency department evaluation and treatment of ankle and foot injuries. Emerg Med Clin North Am 2001;18:85–113.

Author: Taylor Y. Cardall

Phalangeal Injuries, Hand

Clinical Presentation

SIGNS AND SYMPTOMS

- Pain in the area of injury, frequently with swelling and ecchymosis
- Deformity, laceration, or amputation of the digit
- Loss of motion in the digit involved

MECHANISM/DESCRIPTION

- The fingers are the body part most frequently injured in athletic or occupational accidents
- Hyperextension injuries most commonly cause ligamentous injury or chip fractures
- Hyperflexion injury to the tip of digits may cause "mallet finger" injury with avulsion fracture at the insertion of the extensor tendon on the distal phalanx
- Crush injuries most commonly cause fractures and diffuse soft-tissue injury
- Amputations at the phalangeal level are rarely re-implanted except on the thumb

PEDIATRIC CONSIDERATIONS

- Injuries may be more difficult to diagnose in children who are unable to cooperate for a full examination; also, open epiphyses make radiographic interpretation less sensitive to bony injury; careful repeated examination and protective splinting are necessary

Pre-Hospital

- Most patients do not require EMS transport solely for phalangeal injury
  —Amputated digits or tissue should be placed in clean moist gauze and keep cool
  —Bleeding should be treated with appropriate direct pressure dressings

CAUTIONS

- Pre-hospital personnel should not attempt to reduce a phalangeal dislocation at the scene unless there will be an unusually long transport time or there is vascular or neurologic compromise
  —Reduction may be successful, but prompt the physician to miss significant ligamentous injuries

Diagnosis

ESSENTIAL WORKUP

- Careful history and complete physical exam
  —Full x-ray series of the affected hand if there is any suggestion of more than a minor superficial injury
- Special attention should be directed at assessing individual tendon status, neurovascular integrity, and identifying rotational deformity
- Examination should be conducted first to assess function, then under anesthesia, and finally with appropriate tourniquet if needed to allow a bloodless field for better examination of lacerated areas
  —For distal digits, an elastic band can be used at the base of the digit

IMAGING/SPECIAL TESTS

- Plain radiography of involved digits including true lateral and oblique views

DIFFERENTIAL DIAGNOSIS

- Tendon laceration/rupture, partial/complete
- Complicated open injuries may include several injuries and the entire hand should be examined carefully
- Beware of lacerations over dorsal metacarpal-phalangeal areas, which may be "fight bites" (human bites)

PEDIATRIC CONSIDERATIONS

- Many fractures in children are torus (buckle) fractures of the phalanges

Treatment

INITIAL STABILIZATION

- Assess for other, more serious injuries
- Immobilize the involved areas by proximal to distal splinting pending definitive evaluation
- Intermittent ice pack application with constant elevation for the first 24 hours
- Dislocations or severely deformed fractures producing vascular compromise should be reduced immediately to a neutral position and immobilized

ED TREATMENT

- Most phalangeal dislocations are dorsal or dorsolateral
  —These may be reduced under digital block, or other appropriate analgesia, by gentle distraction, hyperextension, and guiding the base of the dislocated phalanx into proper position with mild pressure
- Simple impacted transverse or small corner fractures not exceeding 25% of a joint surface and dislocations may be treated with "buddy" splinting in a functional position or with a padded splint in a neutral position
  —Splint for several days, with arrangements for appropriate follow-up within a week
- Unstable fractures (rotational deformity, oblique fractures, fractures involving larger portion of a joint, angulated fractures or significant epiphyseal injuries) should be splinted and referred for urgent orthopedic care
- Any injury with more than a minor subungual hematoma should have the blood released by using a heated paperclip, electric cautery, or a hole drilled in the nail with an 18-gauge needle
  —This injury does not have to be treated as an open injury just because of subungual hematoma
- Nail avulsions need repair of any nailbed lacerations and splinting of the eponychium and germinal matrix to avoid adhesions
  —The avulsed nail can be used or a small piece of gauze or foil can be inserted in the area
- Many other lacerations can be left open with protective cover and allowed to heal secondarily

MEDICATIONS

- Mild analgesics should be offered, with NSAIDs or hydrocodone usually sufficient

Disposition

ADMISSION CRITERIA

- Open joint injuries or fractures are usually admitted for irrigation and débridement and early repair
- Closed injuries requiring surgical management may be admitted for early operative intervention, but it is acceptable to wait for a day or two for semielective repair of clean injuries

DISCHARGE CRITERIA

- Patients with a stable fracture in an appropriate splint may be discharged for orthopedic follow-up

PEDIATRIC CONSIDERATIONS

- If the child does not have significant rotational deformity, simple fractures can be treated with splinting
- Epiphyseal fractures (Salter-Harris injuries) should be referred to an orthopedist

Miscellaneous

ICD9: 959.5

ICD10: S60.9

SUGGESTED READINGS

American Society for Surgery of the Hand. The hand: examination and diagnosis, 3rd ed. New York: Churchill Livingstone, 1990:585–600.

American Society for Surgery of the Hand. The hand: primary care of common problems, 2nd ed. New York: Churchill Livingstone, 1990:437–649.

Antosia RE, Lyn E. The hand. In: Rosen P, et al., eds. Emergency medicine: concepts and clinical practice, 4th ed. St Louis: Mosby-Year Book, 1988:625–668.

Hart RG, Uehara DT, Wagner MJ. Emergency and primary care of the hand. Dallas: American College of Emergency Physicians, 2001:111–122.

Author: Matthew Walsh

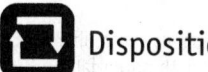

Pharyngitis

Clinical Presentation

SIGNS AND SYMPTOMS

- General
  - —Sore throat
  - —Pharyngeal erythema and exudates
  - —Odynophagia
  - —Dysphagia
  - —Fever
  - —Cervical adenopathy
  - —Diminished oral intake
  - —Fatigue
  - —Soft palate petechiae
  - —Fever
- Viral
  - —Cough
  - —Rhinorrhea
- Group A β-hemolytic streptococcus (GABHS)
  - —Scarlatiniform rash
  - —Headache
  - —Abdominal pain
  - —Nausea
  - —Vomiting
- Diphtheria
  - —Airway-threatening gray pharyngeal membrane
  - —Myocarditis
  - —Cranial and peripheral neuritis
- Mononucleosis
  - —Hepatosplenomegaly
  - —Jaundice
  - —Rash
- Gonococcal pharyngitis
  - —Signs of sexual abuse in children
  - —Recurrent pharyngitis

MECHANISM/DESCRIPTION

- Inflammation/infection of the pharynx
- Third most common complaint for physician visits
- 200 visits per 1,000 population annually in the U.S.
- $300 million annually to diagnose and treat

ETIOLOGY

- Viral
  - —Most common cause of infectious pharyngitis
  - —Rhinovirus (20%)
  - —HIV-1
  - —Acute retroviral syndrome (<1%)
  - —Coronavirus (>5%)
  - —Adenovirus (5%)
  - —Herpes simplex virus (4%)
  - —Influenza (2%)
  - —Parainfluenza (2%)
  - —Epstein-Barr virus (mononucleosis) (<1%)
  - —Cytomegalovirus (<1%)
  - —Coxsackie A (<1%)
- Bacterial
  - —Many bacterial pathogens cause pharyngitis
  - —Focus on organisms with potentially serious sequelae
- *GABHS*
  - —Strep throat
  - —15–30% of childhood pharyngitis
  - —5–10% of adult pharyngitis
  - —Unusual in children younger than 3 years
  - —Peak ages 4–11 years
  - —Peak months January through May, also start of school year
- *Corynebacterium diphtheriae* (diphtheria)
- *Neisseria gonorrhoeae* (gonococcal pharyngitis)
- *Mycoplasma pneumoniae*
- *Chlamydia pneumoniae*
- Syphilis
- Tuberculosis
- Fungal: *Candida* (thrush)
- Noninfectious
  - —Chemical burns
  - —Foreign bodies
  - —Inhalants
  - —Postnasal drip
  - —Lymphoma

Pre-Hospital

CAUTIONS

- Observe/manage airway for respiratory distress
- NS hydration for hypotension/dehydration

Diagnosis

ESSENTIAL WORKUP

- Physical examination
  - —Cannot differentiate GABHS from other organisms
  - —50% false-negative rate for GABHS
  - —75% false-positive rate for GABHS

LABORATORY

- Throat culture
  - —Gold standard
  - —24–48-hour delay for result/treatment
  - —Necessitates recontacting patient/family
  - —False-negative rate for GABHS, 10%
  - —False-positive rate for GABHS, 20%
    - -Due to GABHS carrier state, with superimposed viral pharyngitis
  - —Not recommended routinely for evaluation of adults
- Rapid strep tests (RST)
  - —Convenient
  - —Results within 30 minutes
  - —Sensitivity, 85–95%
  - —Specificity, 96–99%
  - —Treat all positive RST results
  - —Confirm negative RST result by throat culture
  - —Confirmatory culture not routinely recommended for adults
  - —New optical immunoassay *extremely accurate;* negative test results may not require confirmatory culture
  - —Do not reculture to prove eradication after treatment
- Monospot
  - —Detects heterophil antibody for suspected mononucleosis
  - —90% sensitive in patients older than 5 years
  - —75% sensitive in patients aged 2–4 years
  - —Less than 30% sensitive in patients younger than 2 years
- CBC with peripheral smear for suspected mononucleosis
  - —50% lymphocytes, 10% atypical lymphocytes
- Loeffler media culture for *diphtheria*

IMAGING/SPECIAL TESTS

- Lateral neck radiography for suspected epiglottitis, retropharyngeal abscess, or foreign body
- Contrast-enhanced CT scan to identify and define extent of complications such as retropharyngeal abscess

DIFFERENTIAL DIAGNOSIS

- Epiglottitis
- Peritonsillar/retropharyngeal abscess
- Diphtheria
- Ludwig's angina
- HIV acute retroviral syndrome
- Acute leukemia
- Oropharyngeal cancer
- Foreign body
- Postnasal drip

Treatment

INITIAL STABILIZATION

- ABCs
- Volume resuscitation
  —1 L (peds: 20 mL/kg) NS bolus for signs of volume depletion or if patient is unable to tolerate oral solutions

ED TREATMENT

- Antipyretics/analgesics
  —Acetaminophen
  —Ibuprofen
  —Topical analgesics (Chloraseptic spray, lozenges)

GABHS

- Antibiotics for confirmed or highly suspicious
  —Penicillin
  —Erythromycin
  —24–48-hour delay does not increase risk of complications
- Objectives of antibiotic therapy
  —Prevent rheumatic fever (66% risk reduction)
  —Prevent suppurative complications (25–50% reduction)
  —Diminish symptom duration (by mean of 24 hours)
  —Speed return to work or school
  —No clear reduced risk of glomerulonephritis
- Corticosteroids
  —Dexamethasone 10 mg i.m. × 1
  —Symptomatic relief for severe GABHS pharyngitis
- Return to school/work after 24 hours of antibiotics
- Complications
  —*Acute rheumatic fever*
    -Usually occurs $2\frac{1}{2}$ weeks after infection
    -Attack rate 0.5–3.0% in untreated patients
    -Preventable by treatment within 9 days of infection
  —*Poststreptococcal glomerulonephritis*
    -Rarely causes permanent renal failure
  —*Peritonsillar/retropharyngeal abscess*
    -Fewer than 1% of those treated
    -Retropharyngeal abscess primarily before age 3 years
    -Retropharyngeal nodes regress after age 3 years

Diphtheria

- Goals of therapy
  —Prevent airway obstruction by pseudomembrane
  —Treat the infection
  —Counteract exotoxin-mediated myocarditis and neuritis
- Horse antitoxin
  —Dose dictated by illness severity
- Penicillin or erythromycin
- Complications
  —Myocarditis (occurs in two thirds, significant in 10%)
  —Peripheral neuritis usually involves the cranial nerves

Gonococcal Pharyngitis

- Treat per usual sexually transmitted disease protocol
  —Third-generation cephalosporin/azithromycin

MEDICATIONS

- Penicillin
  —Less than 27 kg: pen G benzathine (LA): 0.6 million U i.m. × 1
  —More than 27 kg: pen G benzathine (LA): 1.2 million U i.m. × 1
  —Younger than 12 years: 250 mg PO b.i.d. × 10 days
  —Older than 12 years: 500 mg PO b.i.d. × 10 days
- Erythromycin
  —Erythromycin base: 500 mg PO q.i.d. × 10 days
  —Peds: erythroethylsuccinate: 40 mg/kg/d PO plus t.i.d. × 10 days

Disposition

ADMISSION CRITERIA

- Airway compromise
- Severe dehydration
- Child sexual abuse

DISCHARGE CRITERIA

- Able to tolerate oral intake

Miscellaneous

ICD9: 462

ICD10: J02.9

SUGGESTED READINGS

Bisno AL. Acute pharyngitis. N Engl J Med 2001;344(3):205–211.

Cooper RJ, Hoffman JR, Bartlett JG, et al. Principles of appropriate antibiotic use for acute pharyngitis in adults: background. Ann Emerg Med 2001;37:711–719.

Del Mar CB, Glasziou PP, Spinks AB. Antibiotics for sore throat (Cochrane review). In: The Cochrane library, issue 4. Oxford: Update Software, 2001.

Quayle KS, Fuchs S, Jaffe DM. Otitis and pharyngitis in children. In: Tintinalli J, et al, eds. Emergency medicine: a comprehensive study guide, 5th ed. New York: McGraw-Hill, 2000:786–794.

Stollerman G. Rheumatic fever in the 21st century. Clin Infect Dis 2001;33:806–814.

Authors: Joshua S. Broder; Brian J. Browne

Phencyclidine, Poisoning

Clinical Presentation

SIGNS AND SYMPTOMS

Central Nervous System

- Altered mental status
  - —Agitation
  - —Bizarre/violent behavior
  - —Belligerence
- Coma
- Seizures
- Nystagmus (vertical, horizontal, or rotatory)

Cardiovascular

- Hypertension
- Tachycardia

Musculoskeletal

- Traumatic injury (decreased pain perception)
- Rhabdomyolysis (due to vigorous muscular contraction)

Vital Signs

- Hyperthermia

MECHANISM/DESCRIPTION

- Dissociative anesthetic structurally related to ketamine
  - —Causes decreased perception of pain and agitation
- Half-life of 21–24 hours, but may be longer in overdose
- Enterohepatic recirculation—recirculated into the stomach

ETIOLOGY

- Drug of abuse
  - —Frequently encountered as an adulterant of marijuana
- Street names for PCP include
  - —Angel dust
  - —Wicky stick
  - —Wicky weed
  - —Wacky weed
  - —Embalming fluid
  - —Sherman

PEDIATRIC CONSIDERATIONS

- Exposure in toddlers reported via passive exposure

Pre-Hospital

CAUTIONS

- Use restraints/additional personnel to control combative patient

Diagnosis

ESSENTIAL WORKUP

- Clinical diagnosis based on presentation supported by urine toxicology screen
  - —Dextromethorphan and ketamine may give false positive
- Careful physical exam for occult trauma
- Exclude other causes of altered mental status

LABORATORY

- CBC
- Electrolytes, BUN/Cr, glucose
- Urinalysis
  - —Dip for myoglobin (rhabdomyolysis)
- CPK
  - —If urine dip for blood is positive
- Ethanol level
- Serum osmolality to rule out toxic alcohol ingestion

IMAGING/SPECIAL TESTS

- CXR for aspiration pneumonia
- Extremity/spine radiographs when there is associated trauma
- CT scan of the head when there is head trauma/altered mental status

DIFFERENTIAL DIAGNOSIS

Drugs of Abuse

- Cocaine
- Amphetamines
- Designer drugs
  - —Methcathinone (Cat)
  - —Ecstasy
  - —ICE
- Ketamine
- Other sympathomimetics
- Alcohols

Drugs that Cause Nystagmus

- Lithium
- Carbamazepine
- Sedative-hypnotics
- Alcohols
- Phenothiazines
- Dextromethorphan

Treatment

INITIAL STABILIZATION
- ABCs
- IV
- Cardiac monitor
- Naloxone, thiamine, glucose (or Accu-Chek) if altered mental status
- Protect patient/staff from injury

ED TREATMENT
- Maintain patient in a quiet place; avoid stimulation
- Physical restraints for violent patient
- Sedation
  —Benzodiazepines
  —Butyrophenones (haloperidol) theoretically can lower the seizure threshold
- Activated charcoal/sorbitol if oral co-ingestants
- IV 0.9% NS hydration/mannitol/sodium bicarbonate for rhabdomyolysis

MEDICATIONS
- Activated charcoal slurry: 1–2 g/kg up to 90 g PO
- Ativan (lorazepam): 2 mg i.v. increments
- Dextrose: D50W 1 amp (50 mL or 25 g) (peds: D25W 2–4 mL/kg) i.v.
- Diazepam: 5 mg i.v. increments
- Haloperidol: 5 mg i.m./i.v. increments
- Mannitol: 25–50 g i.v.
- Naloxone (Narcan): 2 mg (peds: 0.1 mg/kg) i.v. or i.m. initial dose
- Sodium bicarbonate: 2 amp diluted in 1 L of D5W, given at 125–250 mL/h (for rhabdomyolysis) to urine pH of 7.0
- Sorbitol: 1–2 g/kg to a max of 100 g (peds: older than 1 year, 1–1.5 g/kg as a 35% solution to a max of 50 g) PO mixed in the activated charcoal slurry—only use for first dose
- Thiamine (vitamin B_1): 100 mg (peds: 50 mg) i.v. or i.m.

Disposition

ADMISSION CRITERIA
- Prolonged altered mental status
- Significant traumatic injuries
- Rhabdomyolysis
- Hyperthermia

DISCHARGE CRITERIA
- Become lucid after a period of observation (6 hours)

Miscellaneous

ICD9: 968.3

ICD10: T41.1

SUGGESTED READINGS

Goldfrank LR, Lewin NA. Phencyclidine. In: Goldfrank LR, Flomenbaum NE, Lewin NA, et al, eds. Goldfrank's toxicologic emergencies, 6th ed. Stamford, CT: Appleton & Lange, 1998.

Moriarty AL. What's "new" in street drugs: "illy." J Pediatr Health Care 1996;10: 41–42.

Patel R, Connor G. A review of thirty cases of rhabdomyolysis-associated acute renal failure among phencyclidine users. Clin Toxicol 1986;23:547–556.

Shannon M. Letter. Pediatr Emerg Care 1998;14:180.

Silber TJ, Iosefsohn M, Hicks JM, et al. Prevalence of PCP use among adolescent marijuana users. J Pediatr 1988;112: 827–829.

Author: Steven Aks

Phenytoin, Poisoning

Clinical Presentation

SIGNS AND SYMPTOMS

- Levels 20–40 μg/mL
  - —Nystagmus
  - —Dizziness
  - —Ataxia
  - —Drowsiness
  - —Nausea/vomiting
  - —Diplopia
  - —Slurred speech
- Levels 40–90 μg/mL
  - —Confusion
  - —Disorientation
- Level >90 μg/mL
  - —Coma
  - —Respiratory depression
  - —Paradoxical seizures
- Hypotension/bradycardia with rapid IV administration
  - —Fosphenytoin injection does not contain propylene glycol
  - —Hypotension/dysrhythmia unlikely with fosphenytoin
- Hypersensitivity reaction following chronic use
  - —Rash
  - —Fever
  - —Neutropenia
  - —Agranulocytosis
  - —Hepatitis
  - —Cholangitis

MECHANISM/DESCRIPTION

- Follows zero-order pharmacokinetics
  - —Small incremental increase in dose can result in a large increase in plasma concentration
- Half-life in overdose—up to 70 hours
- Cardiovascular toxicity from IV administration due to the diluent propylene glycol
- Fosphenytoin, a prodrug for parenteral administration, is metabolized to its active moiety phenytoin

ETIOLOGY

- Phenytoin intoxication results from acute, chronic, or acute on chronic ingestion
- If the etiology of the intoxication is unclear in a patient on phenytoin consider:
  - —Change in the brand of phenytoin
  - —Change in dosage form
  - —Drug interaction

Pre-Hospital

CAUTIONS

- Differentiate phenytoin-induced altered mental status from other potentially serious causes
  - —Head trauma common in seizure population
- Collect/transport prescription bottles and medications to aid in identification and quantification of ingestion

Diagnosis

ESSENTIAL WORKUP

- Determine the time and amount of ingestion
- Phenytoin level
  - —After oral overdose, the peak plasma concentration may not be reached until 24 hours or more post-acute ingestion
  - —Repeat levels every 4 hours until levels have peaked and are declining
  - —Once levels begin declining, check every 24 hours until <30 μg/mL
  - —Fosphenytoin levels are measured as phenytoin
  - —Measure fosphenytoin after conversion to phenytoin is complete (2 hours post-IV infusion/4 hours post-IM injection)
  - —Prior to complete conversion to phenytoin, immunoanalytic techniques may overestimate plasma phenytoin concentrations due to cross-reactivity with fosphenytoin

LABORATORY

- Electrolytes, BUN, Cr, glucose
  - —Check for anion gap metabolic acidosis due to co-ingestant
  - —Determine glucose with altered mental status
  - —Hyperglycemia often present

DIFFERENTIAL DIAGNOSIS

- Intoxication with other CNS depressants
- Guillain-Barré syndrome
- Botulism
- Posterior fossa tumor
- Acute cerebellitis

Treatment

INITIAL STABILIZATION

- ABCs
  —IV access
  —Cardiac monitor (with IV overdose)
- Treat hypotension with IV fluids and Trendelenburg position
  —Dopamine for refractory hypotension
- Treat paradoxical seizures with diazepam

ED TREATMENT

- Gastric lavage if within 1 hour of ingestion
- Activated charcoal
  —Administer single dose
  —Multiple-dose activated charcoal may increase the clearance of phenytoin; does not correlate with clinical improvement in patients with phenytoin toxicity

MEDICATIONS

- Activated charcoal slurry: 1–2 g/kg up to 90 g PO
- Dextrose: D50W 1 amp (50 mL or 25 g) (peds: D25W 2–4 mL/kg) i.v.
- Dopamine: 2–20 μg/kg/min i.v. titrated to desired blood pressure
- Naloxone (Narcan): 2 mg (peds: 0.1 mg/kg) i.v. or i.m. initial dose
- Sorbitol: 1–2 g/kg to a max of 100 g (peds: >1 year old: 1–1.5 g/kg as a 35% solution to a max of 50 g) PO mixed in the activated charcoal slurry—only use for first dose
- Thiamine (vitamin B_1): 100 mg (peds: 50 mg) i.v. or i.m.

Disposition

ADMISSION CRITERIA

- Altered mental status, severe ataxia, increasing phenytoin level
- Level >25 μg/mL
- ICU admission with intoxication from IV phenytoin

DISCHARGE CRITERIA

- Level ≤ 25 μg/mL
- Ambulatory without ataxia

Miscellaneous

ICD9: 966.1

ICD10: T42.0

SUGGESTED READINGS

Browne TR. Fosphenytoin (cerebyx). Clin Neuropharmacol 1997;20:1–12.

Howard CE, Roberts RS, Ely DS, et al. Use of multiple-dose activated charcoal in phenytoin toxicity. Ann Pharmacother 1994;28:201–203.

Kawasaju C, Busgu R, Uekihara S, et al. Charcoal hemoperfusion in the treatment of phenytoin overdose. Am J Kidney Dis 2000;35:323–326.

McKinney PE. Phenytoin. In: Ford MD, Delaney KA, Ling LJ, et al, ed. Clinical toxicology. Philadelphia: WB Saunders, 2001:485–492.

Author: Michele Kanter

Pheochromocytoma

Clinical Presentation

SIGNS AND SYMPTOMS

- 60% have sustained hypertension; 40% hypertensive only during attacks

Hypertensive Crisis

- Classic presentation—paroxysms of:
  - —Hypertension
  - —Headache
  - —Tachycardia
  - —Diaphoresis/anxiety
- Moderate to malignant hypertension
- Chest or abdominal pain
- Cardiac: palpitations
- Tremors
- Diarrhea
- Flushing or pallor

Acute Hemorrhagic Tumor Necrosis

- Acute abdomen
- Marked hypertension followed by declining BP leading to hypotensive shock

Complications

CNS Complications

- Hypertensive encephalopathy
  - —Altered mental status
  - —Focal neurologic signs
  - —Seizures
  - —CVA (infarction, hemorrhagic or embolic)

Cardiac Complications

- Tachydysrhythmias, myocardial infarction
- Orthostatic hypotension due to:
  - —Diminished plasma volume
  - —Blunted sympathetic reflexes

Respiratory Complications

- Cardiogenic or noncardiogenic pulmonary edema

Genitourinary Complications

- Renal artery stenosis (mass effect)
- Renal infarction due to severe vasospasm

Endocrine and Metabolic Complications

- Carbohydrate intolerance (over 50%)
- Hypoglycemia—usually postoperative
- Lactic acidosis in the absence of shock
- Transient thyrotoxicosis
- Hypercalcemia secondary to excess parathyroid hormone (PTH) production
- Diarrhea secondary to excess VIP
- Hypokalemic alkalosis secondary to excess ACTH

MECHANISM/DESCRIPTION

- Hypertensive episode may occur:
  - —Spontaneously
  - —Due to any activity that displaces abdominal contents
  - —Acute hemorrhagic necrosis of the tumor
  - —Precipitation by drugs: TCA, metoclopramide, opiates, histamine, beta-blockers, glucagon

ETIOLOGY

- Catecholamine-producing tumor arising from the chromaffin tissues of the sympathetic nervous system
- Incidence ranges from 0.3% to 1.9%
- 10% extraadrenal in location
- 10% malignant
- Associated with multiple endocrine neoplasia (MEN) IIA and IIB, neurofibromatosis, Von Hippel-Lindau, tuberous sclerosis, Sturge-Weber syndrome
- Alterations occur in levels of circulating catecholamines as well as the cardiovascular response to them

Pre-Hospital

N/A

Diagnosis

ESSENTIAL WORKUP

- EKG abnormalities:
  - —Ischemia
  - —Dysrhythmias—tachydysrhythmia, AFib, VFib

LABORATORY

- CBC
  - —Indicated when abdominal pain/infection
- Electrolytes, BUN, Cr, glucose
  - —Lactic acidosis
  - —Renal failure secondary to hypertension/renal damage
  - —Hyper/hypoglycemia due to impaired response to insulin and effect of catecholamines
- Calcium
  - —Hypercalcemia due to excess PTH
- Urinalysis
  - —Protein in urine due to hypertension

IMAGING/SPECIAL TESTS

- Confirmatory diagnostic studies (usually not in ED)
  - —Plasma catecholamines
  - —24-hour urine for metabolites including metanephrine, normetanephrine, and vanillylmandelic acid
  - —Clonidine suppression test
  - —Glucagon stimulation test
  - —Chromogranin A
  - —Adrenal imaging following biochemical confirmation of diagnosis via CT scan, MRI, MIBG (^{131}I met-iodobenzylguanidine) scan
- CXR for pulmonary edema
- CT scan head if abnormal neurologic exam for CVA, intracranial bleed

DIFFERENTIAL DIAGNOSIS

- Hypertension with associated:
  - —Anxiety
  - —Severe migraines
  - —Hyperthyroidism
  - —MI
  - —Drug abuse (amphetamines, crack, cocaine)
- Alcohol withdrawal
- Monoamine oxidase inhibitor and hypertensive crisis
- Septic shock (pure epinephrine-producing tumor may cause peripheral vasodilation)
- Surgical abdomen (due to tumor necrosis)

Treatment

INITIAL STABILIZATION

- IV access
- Continuous cardiac/blood pressure monitoring

ED TREATMENT

- Hypertensive crisis
  - —Alpha-blockade with phentolamine—first-line agent
  - —Nitroprusside for uncontrolled hypertension
  - —Vigorous fluid resuscitation required as vasoconstriction is relieved
- Beta-blockade (labetalol or esmolol)
  - —For further BP control
  - —If tachycardia develops during induction of alpha-blockade
  - —Caution: institution of beta-blockade without prior α-adrenergic blockade may exacerbate hypertension by antagonizing β-mediated vasodilatation in smooth muscle
- Ventricular tachydysrhythmias
  - —Beta-blockade
  - —Lidocaine
  - —Amiodarone

MEDICATIONS

- Amiodarone: rapid-loading regimen: 5 mg/kg (max: 450 mg) mixed in D5W infused over 10–30 minutes (max rate 30 mg/min)
- Esmolol: load 500 μg/kg over 1 minute, followed by 50 μg/kg/min for 4 minutes; if adequate therapeutic effect not achieved within 5 minutes, repeat loading dose and increase infusion to 100 μg/kg/min; repeat loading dose and titrate infusion rate upward at 50 μg/kg/min q 4–5 minutes as needed; omit further loading doses once nearing therapeutic target
- Labetalol: incremental doses beginning at 20–40 mg i.v.; BP should fall within 5 minutes, with maximum effect at 10 minutes; can double i.v. dose q 30–60 minutes until target reached, with maximum total dose of 300 mg
- Lidocaine: 0.7–1.4 mg/kg IVP, may repeat in 5 minutes; maximum 200–300 mg over 1 hour; follow bolus with infusion of 2–4 mg/min
- Phentolamine: 5–10 mg (peds: 0.05–0.1 mg/kg/dose max 5 mg) i.v., repeat as needed to 20 mg total; can be administered as i.v. drip
- Sodium nitroprusside: 0.5–10.0 μg/kg/min continuous IV infusion, max 800 μg/min; stop infusion if adequate BP control not achieved at 10 μg/kg/min within 10 minutes

Disposition

ADMISSION CRITERIA

- Suspicion of pheochromocytoma in an ill patient mandates alpha-blockade and aggressive volume expansion in a closely monitored setting

DISCHARGE CRITERIA

- Stable patient with mild hypertension, suspicious for pheochromocytoma may be referred for prompt outpatient investigations

Miscellaneous

ICD9: 227.0

ICD10: M8700/0

SUGGESTED READINGS

Dluhy RG. Pheochromocytoma—death of an axiom. N Engl J Med 2002;346(19): 1486–1488.

Gifford R. Management of hypertensive crisis. JAMA 1991;266(6):829–835.

Lenders JW, et al. Biochemical diagnosis of pheochromocytoma: which test is best? JAMA 2002;287(11):1427–1434.

Manger WM, Gifford RW. Pheochromocytoma. J Clin Hypertens (Greenwich) 2002;4(1):62–72.

Salehi A, et al. Pheochromocytoma and bowel ischemia. J Emerg Med 1997;15(1): 35–38.

Werbel S, Ober K. Pheochromocytoma. Med Clin North Am 1995;79(1):131–153.

Author: Steven Friedman

Phimosis

Clinical Presentation

SIGNS AND SYMPTOMS

- Whitish, narrowed preputial opening of the foreskin
- Dysuria, hematuria
- Poor urinary stream
- Edema, erythema, and tenderness of prepuce
- *Balanoposthitis* (inflammation of the glans and foreskin)
- Ballooning of foreskin on urination in severe cases

MECHANISM/DESCRIPTION

- True phimosis is the inability to retract the foreskin over the glans of the penis as a result of scarring
  —The inability to retract a normal, supple foreskin is not true phimosis
- The foreskin is rarely retractable at birth due to normal adhesions between the glans and the inner prepuce.
  —Approximately 90% are retractable by 3 years of age, and 99% are retractable by age 17, as the epithelial cells that comprise smegma are shed
  —Parents should be instructed not to forcibly retract the foreskin

ETIOLOGY

- Possible causes of true phimosis include:
  —Trauma from forcible retraction of the foreskin
  —Repetitive bouts of diaper dermatitis
  —Recurrent balanoposthitis
  —Poorly performed circumcision
  —Congenital anomalies

Pre-Hospital

CAUTIONS

- Pre-hospital personnel and family members should be instructed not to attempt retraction of the foreskin prior to medical evaluation
  —Unwarranted attempts may traumatize a normal, nonretractable prepuce, or convert the situation to a more emergent *paraphimosis*

Diagnosis

ESSENTIAL WORKUP

- In the majority of cases, no workup is necessary
- In patients with severe stenosis, the complication of an *obstructive uropathy* may occur
  —This may result from structural compression, but should be investigated by evaluation of kidney function (BUN and creatinine) and a renal sonogram
- Phimosis secondary to recurrent balanoposthitis should prompt a workup for *diabetes mellitus* (urinalysis, serum glucose, or glucose tolerance test)

DIFFERENTIAL DIAGNOSIS

- Preputial adhesions are normal in young children
- Balanoposthitis without phimosis

Treatment

INITIAL STABILIZATION

- None required in most cases; examination should include an evaluation for potential complications such as *obstruction* and *vascular compromise* to the glans
  —These occur only in the most extreme cases

ED TREATMENT

- Relieve obstructive uropathy, if present, with urethral catheterization or suprapubic aspiration
- If vascular flow to the glans is compromised, a dorsal slit must be made in the foreskin; this is performed with infiltration of local anesthetic without epinephrine at the base of the penile shaft and possibly sedation
  —This is rarely necessary in phimosis
- In uncomplicated cases, provide patients with urologic follow-up for elective dilation of the preputial opening, operative repair, or elective circumcision as necessary
- Potent topical steroids have been reported to successfully reduce phimosis but are inappropriate for emergent cases

MEDICATIONS

- Pain control as required

Disposition

ADMISSION CRITERIA

- Obstructive uropathy
- Severe balanoposthitis with ischemia or necrosis

DISCHARGE CRITERIA

- Ability to urinate
- Adequate urologic follow-up

Miscellaneous

ICD9: 605

ICD10: N47

SUGGESTED READINGS

Dewan PA, Tieu HC. Phimosis: Is circumcision necessary? J Pediatr Child Health 1996;32(4):285–289.

Pontari MA. Phimosis and paraphimosis. In: Seidman EJ, Hanno PM, eds. Current urologic therapy, 3rd ed. Philadelphia: WB Saunders, 1994:392–397.

Super DM. Phimosis. In: Hoekelman R, et al., eds. Primary pediatric care. St. Louis: CV Mosby, 1987:1232–1234.

Author: Lorne Sherman

Pityriasis Rosea

Clinical Presentation

SIGNS AND SYMPTOMS

- *Herald patch:* solitary, erythematous, slightly raised papule 2–10 cm in diameter and seen in 50–90% of cases
- *Secondary eruption:* widespread salmon colored, elliptic, finely scaling 1-cm macular or papular lesions with longest axis along lines of skin tension (a "fir tree" distribution)
  —Generally follows the herald patch by 7–14 days; lesions are concentrated on the trunk and proximal extremities
- Pruritus accompanies the rash in up to 75% of cases
- Prodromal symptoms may be seen in approximately 5% of cases including fever, headache, malaise, arthralgias, and GI symptoms
- Atypical forms of individual lesions occasionally occur including papular, urticarial, pustular, and purpuric

ETIOLOGY

- Unknown; weak evidence exists for an infectious (viral) cause
- Medications including barbiturates, captopril, clonidine, gold, isotretinoin, metronidazole, and penicillamine have been associated with a pityriasis-like eruption

PEDIATRIC CONSIDERATIONS

- Atypical presentations including oral involvement and inverse pityriasis rosea are more common in children
- Oral lesions may include punctate hemorrhages, ulcerations, erythematous macules, and vesicles
- Lesions concentrated on the face and distal extremities with minimal trunk involvement characterize *inverse pityriasis*

Pre-Hospital

N/A

Diagnosis

ESSENTIAL WORKUP

- Syphilis testing: secondary syphilis can mimic pityriasis rosea, so an RPR or VDRL is required if the diagnosis is in question, especially with history of chancre or absence of herald patch
- KOH preparation may be needed to differentiate the herald patch from tinea corporis

DIFFERENTIAL DIAGNOSIS

- Herald patch
  —Nummular eczema
  —Tinea corporis
- Generalized eruption
  —Secondary syphilis
  —Drug eruption
  —Guttate psoriasis
  —Kaposi's sarcoma
  —Lichen planus
  —Occult malignancy
  —Scabies
  —Seborrheic dermatitis
  —Tinea versicolor

Treatment

INITIAL STABILIZATION

- None required

ED TREATMENT

- Pityriasis is treated symptomatically

MEDICATIONS

- Diphenhydramine: adult: 50 mg PO q.i.d.; peds: 5 mg/kg/day divided q.i.d.
- Hydrocortisone: adult: 1% cream t.i.d.; peds: 1% cream t.i.d.
- Prednisone: adult: 15–40 mg qd; peds: 0.25–0.5 mg/kg/qd
- Ultraviolet B (UVB): 5 daily erythemogenic doses

Disposition

ADMISSION CRITERIA

None

DISCHARGE CRITERIA

- Pityriasis rosea is a self-limited disease; admission is not required

Miscellaneous

ICD9: 696.3

ICD10: L42

SUGGESTED READINGS

Allen RA, Janniger CK, Schwartz RA. Pityriasis rosea. Cutis 1995;56(4):198–202.

Bjornborg A. Epidermal-dermal inflammatory conditions of unknown etiology. In: Fitzpatrick TB, et al., eds. Dermatology in general medicine, 4th ed. New York: McGraw-Hill, 1993:1117–1123.

Hartley AH. Pityriasis rosea. Pediatr Rev 1999;20(8):266–269.

Horn T, Kazakis A. Pityriasis rosea and the need for a serologic test for syphilis. Cutis 1987;39(1):81–82.

Parsons J. Pityriasis rosea update: 1986. J Am Acad Dermatol 1986;15(2):159–167.

Author: Nate Rudman

Placenta Previa

Clinical Presentation

SIGNS AND SYMPTOMS

- Vaginal bleeding in second half of pregnancy is placenta previa until proven otherwise
- Painless bright red vaginal bleeding in 70% of patients
- Uterine contraction in 20% of patients
- Occurs at >20 weeks' gestation
- Mean presentation at 30 weeks, one third before 30 weeks
- Frequently no inciting cause
- Initial bleeding is often self-limited and not lethal
- 20% of all antepartum hemorrhage

MECHANISM/DESCRIPTION

- Implantation of the placenta over the internal cervical os
- Uterine enlargement and cervical dilation cause placental vessels near the cervix to tear, resulting in vaginal bleeding
- Placenta previa seen on ultrasound before 28 weeks frequently "migrates" and does not end up as placenta previa at term
- Classifications
  —Total placenta previa: cervical os is completely covered by placenta
  —Partial placenta previa: cervical os is partially covered by placenta
  —Marginal placenta previa: edge of placenta at margin of cervical os
  —Low-lying placenta: placenta edge is close to cervical os

ETIOLOGY

- Unknown
- Incidence: 1/200 births = 0.5% of pregnancies
- Factors affecting location of implantation:
  —Abnormal endometrial vascularization
  —Delayed ovulation
  —Prior trauma to endometrium
- Risk factors:
  —Multiparity
  —Prior C-section (6× increase incident) or other uterine scaring
  —Multiple pregnancies (1/1,500 nulliparas, 1/20 grand multiparas)
  —Increase maternal age
  —Previous placenta previa (4–8% recurrence)
  —Smoking
- Associations:
  —Congenital abnormalities (2× increase incidence)
  —Abnormal fetal presentation (30%)
  —Premature rupture of membranes
  —Vasa previa: fetal vessels course through membranes and cover os
  —Placenta accreta, increta, percreta (growth of placenta into uterine wall)

Pre-Hospital

- Patient with vaginal bleeding at >24 weeks should be transported to a facility that can handle high-risk and premature delivery
- Place patient in left lateral recumbent position if hypotensive in second half of pregnancy
- O_2 and IV as with other patients

Diagnosis

ESSENTIAL WORKUP

- Do not do a digital examination or instrument probing of the cervix in second trimester vaginal bleeding until placenta previa is ruled out
- If OB consult is not readily available, do a partial speculum insertion to identify if blood is from the os or vaginal lesion
- Sonography is diagnostic procedure of choice

LABORATORY

- CBC, platelets
- PT/PTT, FSP, fibrinogen (<300 mg/dL is abnormal)
- Rh status
- Type and cross-match
- Wall clot test—fill red top tube and tape to wall; if no clot in 6 minutes, assume coagulopathy
- Kleihauer-Betke (KB)—detects more than 5 mL of fetal cells in maternal circulation (it takes only 0.1 mL to sensitive mother if Rh negative)

IMAGING/SPECIAL TESTS

- Transabdominal ultrasound—93–97% accurate
  —False negative: obesity, posterior or lateral placenta, fetal head over cervical os
  —False positive: over distended bladder
- Transvaginal ultrasound—100% accurate, generally safe
  —Place probe no more than 3 cm into vagina and do not contact the cervix
- MRI—useful in evaluating placental abnormalities

DIFFERENTIAL DIAGNOSIS

- Placental abruption
- Uterine rupture
- Fetal vessel rupture
- Cervical/vaginal laceration
- Cervical/vaginal lesions
- Congenital bleeding disorder
- Spontaneous abortion
- "Bloody show" of labor

Treatment

INITIAL STABILIZATION

- ABCs
- Two large-bore IVs with NS or LR
- Left lateral recumbent position if hypotensive in second half of pregnancy
- Fluid resuscitation
- Blood transfusion for Hct <30 or hypotension not responding to fluids
- Fetal monitoring (HR <120 or >160 is abnormal)
- Immediate OB consultation

ED TREATMENT

- Volume resuscitation
- Blood transfusion to keep Hct 30–35%
- RhoGAM if indicated
- Fetal monitoring
- Emergent C-section or delivery for continued bleeding or fetal compromise
- Keep NPO and at bed rest until considered stable by OB
- Tocolytics (magnesium sulfate) if preterm labor

MEDICATIONS

- Magnesium sulfate 6 g i.v. over 20 minutes, then 2–4 g/h; adjust to contractions
- RhoGAM 1 vial = 300 μg i.m., for fetal transfusions up to 15 mL of RBS or 30 mL of whole blood (give one vial if mother is Rh negative regardless of KB test, may need more than one vial if KB indicates more than 15 mL of fetal RBC)

Disposition

ADMISSION CRITERIA

- Admit all patients >20 weeks' gestation with vaginal bleeding due to placenta previa

DISCHARGE CRITERIA

- Incidental finding of placenta previa by ultrasound at <28 weeks with no vaginal bleeding or uterine contractions
- Patients at ≥28 weeks with no active bleeding and no uterine contraction may be treated on an outpatient basis after OB consultation to insure follow-up
- Advise: pelvic rest (nothing in vagina) and bleeding precautions

Miscellaneous

ICD9: 641.10

ICD10: 044.1

SUGGESTED READINGS

Cunningham FG, Grant NF, Leveno, KJ, et al. Williams' obstetrics, 21st ed. New York: McGraw-Hill, 2001.

Hacker NF, Moore JG. Essentials of obstetrics and gynecology, 3rd ed. Philadelphia: WB Saunders, 1998.

Marx JA, Hockberger RS, Walls RM, et al. Rosen's emergency medicine concepts and clinical practice. St. Louis: Mosby, 2002.

Neilson JP. Interventions for suspected placenta praevia. Cochrane Library, issue 4. Oxford: Update Software, 2001.

Scott JR, Saia PJ, Hammond CB, et al. Danforth's obstetrics and gynecology, 8th ed. Philadelphia: Lippincott, Williams & Wilkins, 1999.

Author: Roneet Lev

Plague

Clinical Presentation

SIGNS AND SYMPTOMS

- Abrupt onset
- Fever
- Chills
- Cough
- Hemoptysis (usually within 24 hours of symptom onset)
- Dyspnea
- Headache
- Vomiting
- Swollen, tender lymph nodes ("buboes")
- Skin lesion at site of inoculation (e.g., flea bite)
- Confusion
- Abdominal pain
- Oliguria
- Obtundation
- Extensive ecchymoses
- Acral gangrene (digits, nose, penis)

MECHANISM/DESCRIPTION

Three Forms

- Bubonic
  —Spread to humans by flea bite
  —Bacteria multiply in regional lymph nodes
  —Not contagious person-to-person
  —Incubation period 2–8 days
  —Sudden-onset fever, chills, malaise, vomiting
  —Large, painful lymph nodes ("buboes")
  —Skin lesion at site of inoculation
  —Can rapidly progress to septicemia or plague pneumonia if not treated promptly
- Plague pneumonia
  —May be secondary to bubonic form, or primary
  —Inhalation of droplet nuclei into lung
  —Contagious person-to-person
  —Incubation period 1–6 days
  —Fever
  —Cough
  —Chest pain
  —Hemoptysis (usually within 24 hours of symptom onset)
  —Dyspnea
  —Nausea, vomiting, abdominal pain, diarrhea
- Septicemic
  —Not contagious person-to-person
  —Fever
  —Confusion
  —Abdominal pain
  —Oliguria
  —Obtundation
  —Extensive ecchymoses
  —Acral gangrene (digits, nose, penis)
  —Disseminated intravascular coagulation
  —Shock

ETIOLOGY

- Endemic in some populations of small mammals (rats, ground squirrels, prairie dogs)
- Infection with *Yersinia pestis*
- Nonmotile, non-spore-forming, gram-negative bacillus
- Produces a temperature-sensitive coagulase
- Bipolar ("safety pin") staining

Pre-Hospital

CAUTIONS

- Multiple cases of rapidly progressing virulent pneumonia with hemoptysis in young, previously healthy patients should raise suspicion of deliberate dissemination of plague pneumonia
- Plague pneumonia is contagious by droplet route
- Universal and respiratory precautions
- Consider use of Hepa-filter mask

Diagnosis

ESSENTIAL WORKUP

- Notify hospital infection control officer if plague is suspected
- Gram stain of sputum or blood (shows gram-negative bacilli or coccobacilli)
- Wright, Wayson, or Giemsa stain (bipolar uptake)
- Do NOT incise and drain buboes (high risk of aerosolizing infectious material)
- Cultures (sputum, blood, lymph node aspirate) often positive in 24–48 hours
- Specific rapid diagnostic tests may be available through public health departments or the CDC

LABORATORY

- CBC
- Platelet count
- ABG/pulse oximetry
- Coagulation studies (*Y. pestis* can cause disseminated intravascular coagulation)
- Liver function tests (aminotransferases, bilirubin)
- BUN/creatinine

IMAGING/SPECIAL TESTS

- CXR
  —Bronchopneumonia pattern

DIFFERENTIAL DIAGNOSIS

- Anthrax
- Tularemia
- Cat-scratch disease
- Lymphogranuloma venereum
- Chancroid
- Tuberculosis (scrofula)
- Streptococcal adenitis
- Community-acquired pneumonia
- Meningococcal meningitis
- Encephalitis
- Gram-negative sepsis
- Rickettsial infections

Treatment

INITIAL STABILIZATION

- 0.9% NS IV for hypotension/dehydration
- Supplemental oxygen for hypoxia
- Initiate antibiotic treatment

ED TREATMENT

Antibiotic Treatment

- Must be started within 24 hours of symptom onset to minimize mortality
- First-line agents: streptomycin or gentamicin
- Tetracycline
- Doxycycline
- Fluoroquinolones
- Consider adding chloramphenicol if signs and symptoms of meningitis, or patient is unstable

Prophylaxis

- Doxycycline
- Ciprofloxacin

MEDICATIONS

- Chloramphenicol: 25 mg/kg i.v. q6h (peds: 25 mg/kg i.v. q6h)
- Ciprofloxacin: 400 mg i.v. q12h (peds: 15 mg/kg q12h with maximum 1 g daily)
- Doxycycline: 100 mg i.v. q12h (peds <45 kg, 2.2 mg/kg i.v. q12h)
- Gentamicin: 5 mg/kg i.m. or i.v. q24h (peds: 2.5 mg/kg i.m. or i.v. q8h)
- Streptomycin: 1 g i.m. q12h (peds: 15 mg/kg i.m. q12h with maximum 2 g daily)

Prophylaxis (Seven-Day Course)

- Ciprofloxacin: 500 mg PO b.i.d. (peds: 20 mg/kg PO b.i.d.)
- Doxycycline: 100 mg PO b.i.d. (peds <45 kg, 2.2 mg/kg PO b.i.d.)

Notes

- Adjust aminoglycoside doses according to renal function
- Children <2 years should not be treated with chloramphenicol

Disposition

ADMISSION CRITERIA

- Strict respiratory and droplet isolation until patient has been treated with appropriate antibiotics for minimum of 48 hours and is improving clinically

DISCHARGE CRITERIA

None

Miscellaneous

ICD9: 020

ICD10: A20.9

SUGGESTED READINGS

Darling RG, et al. Threats in bioterrorism I: CDC category A agents. Emerg Med Clin North Am 2002;20:273–309.

Inglesby TV, et al. Plague as a biological weapon: medical and public health management. JAMA 2000;283:2281–2290.

McGovern TW, Friedlander AM. Plague. In: Sidell FR, et al., eds. Medical aspects of chemical and biological warfare. Washington, DC: TMM Publications, 1989:479–502.

Author: Leon Gussow

Clinical Presentation

SIGNS AND SYMPTOMS

Herbs

- Shave grass and horsetail
  - —CNS stimulant
  - —Confusion
  - —Ataxia
- Pokeweed, juniper berries, senna
  - —Fulminant gastroenteritis
  - —Abdominal pain/colic
  - —Pokeweed (bradycardia, heart block, tachycardia, VFib)
- Pennyroyal oil
  - —Hepatorenal syndrome
  - —Pulmonary toxicity
  - —Seizures
  - —Coma
  - —Abortifacient
- Sassafras root
  - —Nausea/vomiting
  - —Vertigo
  - —Hallucinations
  - —Shock
  - —Respiratory depression
- Chamomile, chrysanthemums: histamine-releasing/anaphylactic reactions
  - —Angioedema
  - —Bronchospasm
  - —Hypotension
  - —Shock
  - —Death
- Tonka beans, sweet woodruff (natural coumarin)
  - —Hemorrhage
- Nutmeg
  - —Nausea, vomiting
  - —Chest pain
  - —Abdominal pain
  - —Agitation, "feelings of doom"
  - —CNS stimulation, then suppression
  - —Metabolic acidosis
  - —Shock
- Ginseng
  - —Tachycardia
  - —Hypertension
  - —Hypoglycemia
  - —Increased GI motility
- Jimson weed (locoweed, datura)
  - —Anticholinergic toxidrome
    - -Dry mouth, skin, eyes
    - -Dilated pupil
    - -Tachycardia
    - -Altered mental status

Indoor/Outdoor Plants

- Lectins group (castor bean and rosary pea)
  - —CNS depression
  - —Seizures
  - —Severe gastroenteritis
  - —Multisystem organ failure can occur within 24 hours
- Colchicine group (autumn crocus and glory lily)
  - —Three phases:
    - -Gastrointestinal (24 hours): severe abdominal pain, nausea, vomiting, diarrhea
    - -Multisystem failure (2–7 days): ascending paralysis, ARDS, DIC, pancytopenia, cardiac arrhythmias, hepatic insufficiency, delirium
    - -Recovery (>7 days): resolution of organ systems failure, rebound of leukocytosis, alopecia
  - —Requires large amount of plant (>0.8 mg/kg is lethal)
- Solanine group (common nightshade, woody nightshade, potato tubers, Jerusalem cherry)
  - —Symptoms begin 2–4 hours after ingestion
  - —Nausea, vomiting, diarrhea
  - —Headaches
  - —Muscle weakness
  - —Lethargy
  - —Hallucinations
  - —Central nervous system depression

Nicotine-Containing Plants (Tobacco Plants)

- Rapid onset
- Abdominal pain/nausea/vomiting
- Initially tachycardia/hypertension followed by bradycardia/hypotension
- CNS stimulation initially:
  - —Tremor
  - —Seizures
  - —Confusion
  - —Restlessness
- CNS depression later:
  - —Decreased mental state
  - —Coma
- Hypotonia/decreased reflexes/motor paralysis occur sequentially

Grayanotoxin-Containing Plants (Rhododendrons and Azaleas)

- Dose-dependent bradycardia
- Hypotension
- CNS depression
- Most ingestions asymptomatic

Cyanogenic Plants (Seeds of Apples, Pear, and Crab Apple; Lima Beans, Cassava, and Bamboo)

- Headache
- Dyspnea
- Cyanosis
- Convulsions
- Coma, cardiovascular collapse
- Identical to cyanide poisoning due to inhibition of oxidative phosphorylation

Cardiac Glycosides-Containing Plants (Foxglove, Oleander, Yellow Oleander, Lily of the Valley)

- Resembles digoxin toxicity
- Nausea/vomiting
- Alteration in vision
- Cardiac effect
  - —Bradydysrhythmias
  - —Tachydysrhythmias

Aconite (Monkshood, Wolfsbane)

- Sodium channel blockade
- Ventricular dysrhythmias
- Cardiovascular collapse
- Paresthesias, seizures

Hallucinogenics (Marijuana, Morning Glory, Catnip, Peyote, Juniper)

- Mood alteration—euphoria or depression
- Dry mouth/thirst
- Tachycardia
- Toxic psychosis/panic reactions

Gastrointestinal Symptoms

- Irritation of oral mucosa from calcium oxalate crystallization (philodendron)
- Irritation of gastric mucosa (daffodil, narcissus)
- Irritation of intestinal mucosa (pokeweed, horse, chestnut)

PEDIATRIC CONSIDERATIONS

- Often present with lip, tongue, and oropharyngeal irritation and swelling from oxalate crystal-containing plants
  - —Potential for airway compromise
- Usually consume the leaves and seeds
- Nicotine group: 1–2 cigarettes potentially lethal
- Jimson weed:
  - —Seeds highly concentrated
  - —100 seeds = 6 mg of atropine
  - —4–5 g of the leaf lethal
- Yellow oleander:
  - —2 leaves lethal in 12.5-kg child

Pre-Hospital

CAUTIONS

- Nontoxic houseplants
  - —African violet
  - —Aluminum plant
  - —Baby's tears
  - —Bird's nest fern
  - —Corn plant
  - —Creeping Charlie
  - —Creeping Jenny
  - —Gardenia
  - —Grape ivy
  - —Jade plant
  - —Parlor palm
  - —Peacock plant
  - —Piggyback begonia
  - —Prayer plant
  - —Rubber tree
  - —Snake plant
  - —Spider plant
  - —Swedish ivy
  - —Velvet plant
  - —Wandering Jew
  - —Wax plant
  - —Zebra plant
- Collect seeds, leaves, spores in paper bag
- Contact local botanist

CONTROVERSIES
- Syrup of ipecac not recommended in setting of severe GI distress, altered mental status

Diagnosis

ESSENTIAL WORKUP
- Identification of ingested material
- Exact workup depends on plant ingested

LABORATORY
- Electrolytes, BUN, Cr, glucose, LFTs
- ABG
  —Check pH
  —Methemoglobinemia
  —Oxygen saturation
- Digoxin level for cardioglycoside plants
- Cyanide level for cyanogenic plants

IMAGING/SPECIAL TESTS
- EKG: arrhythmias/bradycardia
- CXR

DIFFERENTIAL DIAGNOSIS
- Altered mental status
  —Drug use/alcohol
  —Seizures
  —Trauma
  —CVA
- Digoxin toxicity
- Gastroenteritis
- Agents causing metabolic acidosis (use the mnemonic MUD PILES, as defined in Acidosis)

Treatment

INITIAL STABILIZATION
- ABCs
- 0.9% NS IV
  —Aggressive volume replacement for dehydration/hypotension
  —Initiate pressors (dopamine) for hypotension unresponsive to fluids
- Cardiac monitoring
- Supportive care for most ingestants

ED TREATMENT
- Gastric decontamination
  —Lavage with Ewald tube for recent (<1 hour) ingestion of plant with serious potential toxicity
  —Administer activated charcoal
- Oxalate crystal irritation from Dieffenbacha and philodendron
  —Ice
  —Local wound care
  —Close follow-up
  —Protection of airway
- Gastric decontamination, fluid therapy, and supportive care for
  —Solanine group
  —Lectins group
- Jimson weed poisoning
  —Physostigmine in severe cases or benzodiazepines
  —Consult toxicologist
- Cyanogenic group poisoning
  —Lilly cyanide antidote kit
  —In Europe, hydroxocobalamin and DMAP followed by sodium thiosulfate
- Grayanotoxin group poisoning
  —Atropine for significant bradycardia
- Colchicine group
  —Multidose activated charcoal
- Cardiac glycosides group
  —Digibind may be useful, initial dose 10 vials
  —Correct hyperkalemia
  —Magnesium
- Nicotine group
  —Airway control (due to neuromuscular paralysis)
  —Atropine for symptomatic bradycardia

MEDICATIONS
- Atropine: 0.5 mg (peds: 0.02 mg/kg) i.v., repeat 0.5–1.0 mg i.v. (peds: 0.04 mg/kg)
- DMAP: 3.25 mg/kg i.v.
- Hydroxocobalamin: 50× cyanide dose or 50 mg/kg i.v.
- Magnesium: 2–4 g i.v.
- Physostigmine: 0.5–2 mg i.v.
- Sodium thiosulfate: 150–250 mg/kg

Disposition

ADMISSION CRITERIA
- Cardiac monitoring/dysrhythmias
- Intractable vomiting
- Refractory hypotension
- Evidence of end-organ damage
- Altered mental status

DISCHARGE CRITERIA
- Baseline mental status
- Tolerating fluids
- Normal cardiac activity
- No delayed sequelae

PEDIATRIC CONSIDERATIONS
- Lower threshold to admit children
  —Tend to eat the more concentrated parts
  —Lower doses are lethal
  —Symptoms more nonspecific

Miscellaneous

ICD9: NEC 988.1

ICD10: T62.2

SEE ALSO: DIGOXIN, POISONING; AND ACIDOSIS

SUGGESTED READINGS
Ford M, Delaney K, Ling L, et al. Clinical toxicology, 1st ed. Philadelphia: WB Saunders, 2001:343–351, 909–933.

Graeme K, Braitberg G, Kunkel D, et al. Toxic plants. In: Auerbach PS, ed. Wilderness medicine, 4th ed. St. Louis: Mosby, 2001:1108.

Author: Kirk Cumpston

Pleural Effusion

Clinical Presentation

SIGNS AND SYMPTOMS

- Dyspnea on exertion or at rest
- Decreased breath sounds
- Increased egophony
- Dullness to chest percussion
- Pleural rub
- Primary pathologic process (pneumonia, pulmonary embolus, pancreatitis), not the pleural effusion, is often the source of symptoms

MECHANISM/DESCRIPTION

- Normal conditions
  - —Pleural space contains about 30 mL of clear, protein-free fluid that helps facilitate movement of the pulmonary parenchyma within the thoracic space
  - —Fluid formation and reabsorption is governed by the hydrostatic and colloid forces acting at the parietal and visceral surfaces
  - —Normally, the sum of these forces results in movement of fluid into the pleural space from the parietal surface and reabsorption at the visceral surface
  - —Lymphatics help remove any excess fluid
  - —Alteration of any of the above factors results in excess accumulation and pleural effusion
- Transudative effusion
  - —Results from alteration of systemic hydrostatic and colloid factors
  - —Pleural surface is not involved in the primary pathologic process
- Exudative effusion
  - —Results from pathologic disease of the pleural surface or disruption of lymphatic reabsorption

ETIOLOGY

- Transudative effusions
  - —Hydrostatic factors
    - -Congestive heart failure (right or left ventricular)
    - -Peritoneal dialysis
    - -Cirrhosis
  - —Colloid factors
    - -Acute glomerulonephritis
    - -Myxedema
    - -Hypoproteinemia
    - -Meigs' syndrome
    - -Sarcoidosis
    - -Trauma: hemothorax, chylothorax
    - -Medication: nitrofurantoin, methysergide
- Exudative effusions
  - —Infection
    - -Pneumonia (viral, bacterial, tuberculosis)
    - -Parasitic
    - -Fungal
    - -Neoplasm, metastasis, mesothelioma
  - —Pulmonary embolization or infarction
  - —GI disorders
  - —Pancreatitis
  - —Subdiaphragmatic abscess (hepatic)
  - —Esophageal rupture

Pre-Hospital

CAUTIONS

- Place high-flow oxygen
- Apply cardiac monitor and pulse oximeter
- Initiate IV line access

Diagnosis

ESSENTIAL WORKUP

- CXR
  - —Blunting of the costophrenic angle
  - —Most sensitive radiographic sign
  - —Requires at lease 250 mL of fluid
    - -Lateral decubitus films may reveal a lateral layer of fluid
    - -Presence of subpulmonic effusions may be indicated by loss of supradiaphragmatic vascular markings or an increased space between the gastric bubble and pulmonary parenchyma
    - -Provide hints to the primary source (malignancy, pneumonia)

LABORATORY

- CBC
- Electrolytes, BUN/Cr, glucose
- Pulse oximetry/arterial blood gas
- Coagulation profile
- Pleural fluid analysis
  - —Protein, LDH, and specific gravity
  - —Differentiates between transudative and exudative effusions
  - —Criteria for exudate
    - -Pleural fluid protein/serum protein >0.5
    - -Pleural fluid LDH/serum protein >0.6
- Culture and Gram's stain
- Red cell count
  - —5,000–100,000/mm^3 nonspecific
  - —$>100{,}000/mm^3$ suggestive of malignancy, infarction
- White cell count
  - —1,000–10,000/mm^3 nonspecific
  - —$>10{,}000/mm^3$ suggestive of parapneumonic effusion, pancreatitis, collagen vascular disease, malignancy, or tuberculosis
- Wright stain identifies presence of mesothelial cells, macrophages, plasma cells, lymphocytes, PMNs, eosinophils, and malignant cells
- Cytology identifies malignant cells
- Glucose
  - —Levels $<50\%$ of serum glucose suggestive of rheumatoid/lupus-induced effusion, bacterial
- Empyema, malignancy, or esophageal rupture
- Triglyceride/cholesterol
  - —Triglycerides >110 mg/dL suggestive of chylous effusion from disruption of thoracic duct
- Amylase
  - —Elevated levels suggestive of pancreatitis or esophageal rupture

IMAGING/SPECIAL TESTS

- Ultrasound
  - —Detects smaller fluid volumes than an upright chest x-ray
  - —Indicated as a guide for thoracentesis, particularly if a difficult tap is anticipated
- Diagnostic/therapeutic thoracentesis
  - —Examination of pleural fluid to identify and treat underlying disease
- Method
  - —Position patient upright with arms crossed in front in order to elevate scapula
  - —Identify superior border of effusion via percussion, ultrasound, or egophony
  - —Mark area one interspace below this at the posterior axillary space
  - —Cleanse area with iodophor, dry, and drape for sterile field
  - —Anesthetize with 2% lidocaine
  - —Enter superior border of rib with needle bevel down using 14-gauge syringe/catheter gently aspirating while advancing
  - —Advance catheter through needle once pleural space accessed
    - -Minimum of 100 cc required for basic studies (protein, LDH, cell count, and culture)—more required for cytology and additional studies
  - —After obtaining fluid, withdraw needle, apply pressure, dress, and obtain postprocedural CXR for pneumothorax

Treatment

INITIAL STABILIZATION

- ABCs
- High-flow oxygen for shortness of breath
- Emergency thoracentesis for significant respiratory compromise

ED TREATMENT

- Identify and treat underlying primary pathologic process (CHF, pneumonia, pancreatitis)
- Surgical consult if empyema found for surgical drainage

Disposition

ADMISSION CRITERIA

- Respiratory compromise
- Unknown cause of the effusion
- Primary process requires hospitalization
- Presence of a parapneumonic effusion or empyema
- ICU admission for severe hemodynamic and respiratory compromise

DISCHARGE CRITERIA

- Source of the pleural effusion is known
- No evidence of respiratory compromise exists
- Majority of effusions will resolve if the primary process is treated appropriately

Miscellaneous

ICD9: 511.9

ICD10: J90

SUGGESTED READINGS

Grogan DR, Irwin RS, Corwin RW. Thoracentesis. In: Rippe JM, ed. Intensive care medicine, 2nd ed. Boston: Little, Brown, 1991.

McEwen JI. Pleural disease. In: Rosen P, Barken RM, et al. Emergency medicine: Concepts and clinical practice, 4th ed. St. Louis: CV Mosby, 1998:1511–1528.

Vukich DJ. Diseases of the pleural space. Emerg Med Clin North Am 1989;7(2): 309–24.

Author: Walter G. Belleza

Pneumocystis Carinii Pneumonia

Clinical Presentation

SIGNS AND SYMPTOMS

- Subacute presentation
- Fever
- Cough with none or minimal amount of white sputum
- Dyspnea on exertion or at rest
  —Progressive over days (most common in non-HIV-immunocompromised hosts)
  —Indolent, developing over weeks to months (more common in HIV-positive hosts)
- Chest pain
- Chills
- Fatigue
- Weight loss
- Tachypnea
- Tachycardia
- Crackles and rhonchi on lung examination
- Up to 7% of patients can be asymptomatic
- Patients on inhaled pentamidine prophylaxis may have milder symptoms
  —Increased incidence of pneumothorax
  —Increased incidence of extrapulmonary disease

MECHANISM/DESCRIPTION

- Believed to be transmitted by respiratory-aerosol route
  —Cysts colonize respiratory tract
  —Cysts rupture and multiple trophozoites release and form foamy exudate in alveoli
- Most cases of PCP believed to represent reactivation of latent disease, although person-to-person transmission suggested

ETIOLOGY

- Controversy surrounds the classification of *Pneumocystis* as a parasite or fungus
- *Pneumocystis* occurs in hosts with altered cellular immunity
  —HIV infection (most common, especially when CD4 counts <200 cells/mm^3)
  —Cancer
  —Corticosteroid treatment
  —Organ transplantation
  —Malnutrition

PEDIATRIC CONSIDERATIONS

- PCP in children is typically more severe

Pre-Hospital

CAUTIONS

- Provide supplemental oxygen for symptomatic patients

Diagnosis

ESSENTIAL WORKUP

- Chest x-ray
  —Classically reveals bilateral interstitial or central alveolar infiltrates
  —X-ray normal in up to 25% of patients with PCP
  —Early or mild infection associated with decreased sensitivity
  —Atypical presentations include:
    -Lobar infiltrates
    -Cysts
    -Pneumothoraces
    -Pleural effusions
    -Nodular infiltrates
- High-resolution chest CT
  —Early studies show high sensitivity for PCP in HIV-positive patients
  —Reveals patchy ground-glass attenuation
- Prophylaxis with aerosolized pentamidine is a risk factor for developing predominantly upper lobe infiltrates
- Chest x-ray abnormalities can persist for months after treatment

LABORATORY

- Arterial blood gas
  —Obtain in all cases of PCP
  —Calculate the A-a gradient (usually increased)
  —Adjunctive corticosteroid therapy for A-a gradient >35 or PaO_2 <70
- CBC
- Electrolytes, BUN/Cr, glucose
- LDH
  —Elevated in HIV-positive patients with PCP compared to non-PCP pneumonia
  —Higher levels correlated with poorer prognosis
- Blood cultures

IMAGING/SPECIAL TESTS

- Induced sputum
  - —Definitive diagnosis requires presence of *Pneumocystis* organisms in an appropriately stained respiratory specimen
  - —Specificity approaches 100% but sensitivity depends on quality of induced sputum and lab expertise
  - —Less sensitive in patients on inhaled pentamidine prophylaxis and non–HIV-positive patients
- Bronchoalveolar lavage
  - —Perform if the induced sputum is nondiagnostic and the suspicion for PCP is still high
  - —Sensitivity of 80–100%

DIFFERENTIAL DIAGNOSIS

- Constellation of dyspnea, fever, diffuse radiographic infiltrates, minimal or nonproductive cough, and slow progressive course suggests atypical cause of the pneumonia
  - —Tuberculosis
  - —*Mycoplasma*
  - —*Legionella*
  - —*Chlamydia pneumoniae*
  - —Viral pneumonia (especially CMV)

Treatment

INITIAL STABILIZATION

- ABCs
- Provide adequate oxygenation with nasal cannula up to 100% nonrebreather
- Perform endotracheal intubation in those with refractory hypoxemia despite maximal oxygenation or hypercarbic respiratory failure
- 500–1,000 cc 0.9% NS IV bolus for hypotension, sepsis, dehydration

ED TREATMENT

- Initiate antibiotics
  - —IV Bactrim is the first-line agent
  - —IV pentamidine for those who cannot tolerate Bactrim
  - —Oral therapy is an option for well-appearing patients
  - —Alternative regimens include trimethoprim-dapsone, clindamycin-primaquine, and atovaquone
  - —Continue antibiotics for 21 days
- Adjunctive corticosteroids in patients with A-a gradient >35 or PaO_2 <70
  - —Must start within first 72 hours of treatment
- Isolate suspected PCP patients from others who are immunocompromised

MEDICATIONS

- Atovaquone: 750 mg (peds: dosing not established) PO q12h
- Clindamycin/primaquine: clindamycin 900 mg (peds: dosing not established) i.v. q8h or 300–450 mg PO q6h and primaquine 15–30 mg (peds: dosing not established) PO qd
- Pentamidine: 4 mg/kg/24 hours i.v. over 1 hour (peds: 150 mg/m^2 i.v. qd for 5 days, then 100 mg/m^2 i.v. qd for 16 days)
- Prednisone: 40 mg (peds: dosing not established) PO q12h for 5 days, 40 mg PO qd for 5 days, then 20 mg PO qd for 11 days (i.v. methylprednisolone at 75% of the prednisone dose may be substituted)
- Trimethoprim/dapsone: trimethoprim 15–20 mg/kg/d i.v. divided q8h plus dapsone 100 mg PO qd (peds: dosing not established)
- Trimethoprim/sulfamethoxazole (Bactrim): trimethoprim 15–20 mg/kg/d i.v. divided q6h and sulfamethoxazole 100 mg/kg/d i.v. divided q6 (peds: dosing same)

PEDIATRIC CONSIDERATIONS

- Treatment of choice is IV Bactrim, followed by IV pentamidine
- Dosing for alternative medications not yet established (consult pediatric infectious disease specialist)

Disposition

ADMISSION CRITERIA

- Moderate to severe disease (PaO_2 <70 or A-a gradient >35)
- Inability to digest medications
- Inability to return for careful follow-up

DISCHARGE CRITERIA

- Nontoxic clinical appearance
- Mild disease state (no hypoxemia or A-a gradient)
- Ability to tolerate medications
- Close follow-up arranged
- If results of induced sputum not available, add macrolide to empirical regimen

Miscellaneous

ICD9: 136.3

ICD10: J17.3, B20.6

SUGGESTED READINGS

Moe AA, Hardy WD. Pneumocystis carinii infection in the HIV-seropositive patient. Infect Dis Clin North Am 1994;8(2): 331–364.

Santamauro JT, Stover DE. Pneumocystis carinii pneumonia. Med Clin North Am 1997;81(2):299–318.

Stansell JD, Huang L. Pneumocystis carinii pneumonia. In: Sande MA, Volberding PA, eds. The medical management of AIDS, 5th ed. Philadelphia: WB Saunders, 1997.

Author: Alan M. Kumar

Pneumomediastinum

Clinical Presentation

SIGNS AND SYMPTOMS

- Chest pain
  - —Sharp
  - —Pleuritic
  - —Often positional
- Dyspnea
- Neck pain
  - —Occurs in association with dissection of air into the soft tissues of the neck
  - —Often described as "neck swelling," "neck pain," "throat pain," or "difficulty swallowing"
- Subcutaneous emphysema
- Hamman's crunch
  - —Presence of a crinkling or crepitant sound that varies with the heart beat

MECHANISM/DESCRIPTION

- Presence of air or gas within the mediastinum
- Secondary pneumomediastinum occurs:
  - —Secondary to thoracic barotrauma
  - —As a complication of positive pressure ventilation
  - —In association with esophageal rupture
  - —In association with a mediastinal infection caused by gas-forming organisms
- Primary or spontaneous pneumomediastinum
  - —Occurs secondary to alveolar rupture, followed by dissection of gas toward hilum and mediastinum
  - —Often in the setting of a Valsalva maneuver, in association with bronchospasm or inhalational drug use
- Occasionally unclear triggering etiology

ETIOLOGY

- Relatively rare entity that may occur spontaneously or as a result of trauma or other pathologic processes

Pre-Hospital

N/A

Diagnosis

ESSENTIAL WORKUP

- CXR
  - —Most valuable initial test
  - —Important to include a lateral view because mediastinal air is often missed on the PA view
  - —Excludes pneumothorax
  - —Identification of a pleural effusion or parenchymal infiltrate suggests an esophageal rupture
  - —CXR negative in up to 30% of cases
  - —Chest CT is scan of choice if suspicion is high but CXR is negative

LABORATORY

- CBC if suspicious of mediastinitis

IMAGING/SPECIAL TESTS

- Esophagram with Gastrografin
  - —Study of choice to exclude the diagnosis of esophageal rupture

DIFFERENTIAL DIAGNOSIS

- Pericarditis
- Pulmonary embolus
- Pneumonia
- Coronary ischemia
- Aortic dissection

Treatment

INITIAL STABILIZATION

- Initiate treatment with an IV, oxygen, cardiac monitoring, and pulse oximetry

ED TREATMENT

- Spontaneous pneumomediastinum
  —Does not require specific treatment
  —Efforts should focus on pain relief and reassurance once the diagnosis is confirmed
  —Condition is self-limiting and can be expected to resolve over 2–5 days
- Secondary pneumomediastinum
  —Direct therapy toward underlying cause

Disposition

ADMISSION CRITERIA

- Secondary pneumomediastinum
- Associated pneumothorax
- Possibility of esophageal rupture has not been excluded
- Abnormal vital signs

DISCHARGE CRITERIA

- Patient with spontaneous pneumomediastinum, normal vital signs, and no pneumothorax may be discharged
- Close outpatient follow-up
- Caution against use of inhalational drugs or any activities associated with Valsalva-type or breath-holding maneuvers

Miscellaneous

ICD9: 518.1

ICD10: J98.2

SUGGESTED READINGS

Brody S, Anderson G, Gutman J. Pneumomediastinum as a complication of "crack" smoking. Am J Emerg Med 1988; 6:241–243.

Dekel B, Paret G, Szeinberg A, et al. Spontaneous pneumomediastinum in children: clinical and natural history. Eur J Pediatr 1996;155:695–697.

Panacek E, Singer A, Sherman B, et al. Spontaneous pneumomediastinum: clinical and natural history. Ann Emerg Med 1992;21:1222–1227.

Author: Robert Dart

Pneumonia, Adult

Clinical Presentation

SIGNS AND SYMPTOMS

- Cough
- Sputum production
- Fever
- Chills
- Shortness of breath
- Pleuritic chest pain
- Abnormal vital signs
  - —Tachypnea
  - —Tachycardia
  - —Hypoxia
- Pulmonary examination
  - —Dullness to percussion
  - —Increased tactile fremitus
  - —Egophony
  - —Coarse rales
  - —Rhonchi
  - —However, pneumonia may be present in the absence of signs of consolidation

MECHANISM/DESCRIPTION

- Sixth leading cause of death in the U.S.
  - —#1 infectious cause
  - —4 million cases per year
- Comorbid conditions
  - —Increased age
  - —Cigarette smoking
  - —Chronic obstructive pulmonary disease
  - —Diabetes mellitus
  - —Alcoholism/malnutrition
  - —Immunosuppression
  - —Sickle cell disease
  - —Congestive heart failure
  - —HIV/AIDS
- Complications
  - —Sepsis
  - —Lung abscess
  - —Empyema
  - —Extrapulmonary complications (e.g., meningitis)
  - —Respiratory failure

ETIOLOGY

- *Streptococcus pneumoniae*
- *Haemophilus influenzae*
- *Klebsiella pneumoniae*
- "Atypicals"
  - —*Mycoplasma pneumoniae*
  - —*Chlamydia pneumoniae*
  - —*Legionella* species
- Viruses
  - —Influenza and parainfluenza viruses
  - —Adenovirus
- Nosocomial pneumonia due to above plus:
  - —*Pseudomonas aeruginosa*
  - —*Staphylococcus aureus*
  - —*Enterobacter* species
- Aspiration pneumonias are typically polymicrobial

Pre-Hospital

- Supplemental oxygen
- Intravenous access
- Consider inhaled bronchodilators
- Consider endotracheal intubation in patients with severe respiratory distress

Diagnosis

ESSENTIAL WORKUP

- Patients should first be classified:
  - —Community-acquired versus nosocomial
  - —Age $\geq$60 years old versus age $<$60 years old
  - —The presence of comorbid conditions
  - —Immunocompetent versus immunocompromised
- Pneumonia is both a clinical as well as a radiographic diagnosis

LABORATORY

- Laboratory studies are nonspecific for identifying the etiology of pneumonia
- CBC with differential
  - —WBC count $>$15,000/mm^3 suggests bacterial cause
  - —A very high or very low WBC predicts increased morbidity
- Serum chemistries
- Pulse oximetry
- Arterial blood gas
- Sputum Gram's stain and culture
- Blood cultures

IMAGING/SPECIAL TESTS

- Chest radiography
  - —CXR findings are nonspecific for predicting a particular infectious etiology
  - —May be deferred in young, healthy patients
  - —The absence of CXR findings should not preclude antimicrobial therapy in those with clinical pneumonia
  - —Findings suggestive of pneumonia include:
    - -Segmental or subsegmental infiltrate
    - -Air bronchograms
    - -Abscess formation
    - -Cavitation
    - -Empyema
    - -Pleural effusions
- Diagnostic thoracentesis
  - —Performed for large effusions, enigmatic pneumonias, and patients who fail to respond to standard therapy

DIFFERENTIAL DIAGNOSIS

- Bronchitis
- Spontaneous pneumothorax
- Chronic obstructive pulmonary disease
- Asthma
- Congestive heart failure
- Pulmonary embolism
- Foreign body aspiration
- Occupational or environmental exposure
- Tumor

Treatment

INITIAL STABILIZATION

- Supplemental oxygen
- Intravenous access
- Consider inhaled bronchodilators
- Consider endotracheal intubation in patients in severe respiratory distress
- Fluid resuscitation

ED TREATMENT

- Empiric antimicrobial therapy is necessary before definite etiology is established
  —Symptomatology, radiographic, and laboratory findings are nonspecific for identifying etiologic cause
- Inpatient therapy for healthy adult:
  —Second-generation cephalosporin (cefuroxime) or third-generation cephalosporin (ceftriaxone) or β-lactam and β-lactamase inhibitor combination (ampicillin-sulbactam) plus macrolide (erythromycin or azithromycin)
  —Or extended spectrum fluoroquinolone (levofloxacin)
  —May add clindamycin or metronidazole if aspiration is expected
- Inpatient therapy for critically ill or nosocomial pneumonia may require:
  —Third-generation cephalosporin with antipseudomonal activity (ceftazidime) plus aminoglycoside (gentamicin)
  —May add vancomycin for drug-resistant *S. pneumoniae*
- Outpatient therapy if <60 years old and no comorbidities
  —Macrolide (erythromycin or azithromycin)
  —Or extended spectrum fluoroquinolone (levofloxacin)
- Outpatient therapy if ≥60 years old or with comorbidities
  —Second- or third-generation cephalosporin
  —Or β-lactam and β-lactamase inhibitor combination (amoxicillin-clavulanate)
  —Or extended-spectrum fluoroquinolone (levofloxacin)

MEDICATIONS

- Amoxicillin-clavulanate (Augmentin) 500 mg PO q12h
- Ampicillin-sulbactam (Unasyn) 1.5–3.0 g i.v. q6h
- Azithromycin 500 mg PO on day 1 and 250 mg PO on days 2–5
- Ceftazidime 1 g i.v. q8h
- Ceftriaxone 1–2 g i.v. qd
- Cefuroxime 0.75–1.5 g i.v. q8h
- Clindamycin 150–450 mg PO q.i.d. or 300–900 mg i.v. q.i.d.
- Erythromycin 250–500 mg PO q6h
- Gentamicin 1 mg/kg i.v. q8h
- Levofloxacin 500 mg i.v./PO qd
- Vancomycin 1 g q12h

Disposition

ADMISSION CRITERIA

- Age ≥60 years old
- Significant comorbid illness
  —Chronic obstructive pulmonary disease
  —Diabetes mellitus
  —Chronic renal failure
  —Chronic liver failure
  —Postsplenectomy
  —Immunosuppression
  —Chronic alcohol abuse
  —Malnutrition
  —Pregnancy
- Severe vital sign abnormalities
  —Temperature >38.3°C
  —Heart rate >140
  —Respiratory rate >30
  —PO_2 <60 or PCo_2 >50
- Altered mental status
- Volume depletion
- Previous hospitalization within last year for pneumonia
- Failure to respond to outpatient therapy
- Social conditions that prevent safe outpatient care
- Multiple involvement

DISCHARGE CRITERIA

- Age <60 years
- No comorbid conditions
- Nontoxic appearance
- Normal vital signs
- Primary care follow-up is advised within 72 hours
- Persistent or worsening symptoms should prompt a more aggressive evaluation

Miscellaneous

ICD9: 480, 481, 482

ICD10: J18.9

SUGGESTED READINGS

American Thoracic Society. Guidelines for the initial management of adults with community-acquired pneumonia: diagnosis, assessment of severity, and initial antimicrobial therapy. Am Rev Respir Dis 1993;148:1418–1426.

Bartlett JG, Mundy LM. Community-acquired pneumonia. N Engl J Med 1995;333(24):1618–1624.

Moran GJ, Talan DA. Pneumonia. In: Rosen P, ed. Emergency medicine: concepts and clinical practice, 4th ed. Boston: Mosby-Year Book, 1998:1553–1569.

Pomilla PV, Brown RB. Outpatient treatment of community-acquired pneumonia in adults. Arch Intern Med 1994;154:1793–1802.

Author: Jason Imperato

Pneumonia, Pediatric

Clinical Presentation

SIGNS AND SYMPTOMS

- General (in all ages)
  - —Fever
  - —Hypoxia
  - —Tachycardia
  - —Tachypnea, retractions
  - —Rash (up to 10% of cases); usually maculopapular
  - —Nonspecific symptoms of toxicity
  - —Pulmonary
  - —Cough
  - —Decreased breath sounds, ventilation
  - —Dullness to percussion
  - —Rales
- Infants under 6 months
  - —Altered behavior: listless, irritable
  - —Apnea
  - —Conjunctivitis (*Chlamydia* <1 month old)
  - —Cyanosis
  - —Grunting
  - —Poor feeding
  - —Temperature instability (hypo/hyperthermia)
  - —Vomiting
  - —Pulmonary
    - -Nasal congestion
    - -Nasal flaring
    - -Wheezing
    - -Staccato cough (*Chlamydia*)
- Children over 5 years old
  - —Pleuritic chest pain
  - —Rigors, chills
  - —Productive cough

MECHANISM/DESCRIPTION

- Mechanism is often unknown
- Sources are oropharyngeal aspiration (most common) or hematogenous
- Distribution depends on the organism: interstitial (*Mycoplasma pneumonia*, virus), lobar (*Streptococcus pneumoniae*), abscesses (*Staphylococcus aureus*) or diffuse (*Pneumocystis carinii*)

ETIOLOGY

- *Haemophilus influenza* type b is becoming rare secondary to mass immunization
- Less than 2 weeks
  - —Group B *Streptococcus* species
  - —Enteric gram-negative organisms
  - —Respiratory syncytial virus (RSV)
  - —Herpes simplex virus
  - —*S. aureus*
- Two weeks to 3 months
  - —*Chlamydia trachomatis*
  - —Parainfluenza virus
  - —RSV
  - —*S. pneumoniae*
  - —*S. aureus*
  - —*H. influenza*
  - —*Bordetella pertussis*
- Three months to 8 years
  - —Viral (predominate)
    - -RSV
    - -Parainfluenza virus
    - -Influenza virus
    - -Adenovirus
  - —*S. pneumoniae*
  - —*H. influenza* in unimmunized children
  - —Group A *Streptococcus*
  - —*S. aureus*
  - —*B. pertussis*
- Over 8 years
  - —*M. pneumoniae* most common
  - —Viral
  - —*S. pneumoniae*
- Recent immigrants from developing countries
  - —*Mycoplasma tuberculosis*
  - —*H. influenza*
  - —*B. pertussis*
- Immunocompromised (e.g., HIV, cancer)
  - —*P. carinii*
  - —*Mycoplasma avium complex*
  - —*M. tuberculosis*
  - —*Klebsiella pneumoniae*
  - —*Pseudomonas aeruginosa*
- Less common
  - —Fungal (coccidioidomycosis, histoplasmosis)
  - —Rickettsia (Q fever)

Pre-Hospital

- Oximetry
- Administer high-flow oxygen for respiratory distress
- IV fluids (0.9% NS 20 cc/kg initial bolus) for volume depletion, hypotension
- Support and intubation for respiratory failure

Diagnosis

ESSENTIAL WORKUP

- Oximetry
- Chest radiograph
  - —Gold standard for diagnosis
  - —Should be ordered for patients with signs of lower respiratory tract infection and patients <36 months old with marked leukocytosis or neutrophilia [WBC >20,000 or absolute neutrophil count (ANC) >9,000]
  - —Much overlap between viral and bacterial findings
  - —Viral and *M. pneumoniae* tend to show interstitial infiltrates, often perihilar and peribronchial
  - —Bacterial pneumonias may show focal lobar consolidation, focal alveolar infiltrates, and possibly effusion or pneumatocele
  - —Round pneumonia pathognomonic of *S. pneumonia*
  - —Lateral decubitus films may aid in demonstrating effusion

LABORATORY

- CBC with differential
  - —Patients with bacteremia tend to have leukocytosis with left shift
  - —Sensitivity and specificity are poor
  - —Patients with WBC ≥20,000 or ANC >9,000 are at increased risk of pneumococcal bacteremia
  - —*B. pertussis* usually has elevated WBC with lymphocytosis
- Blood culture
  - —Low yield (<10–20%)
  - —Probably worthwhile in toxic patients requiring hospitalization
- Arterial blood gas (ABG) may be useful in determining degree of respiratory insufficiency in critically ill patients
- Electrolytes to exclude SIADH and in hypotensive children
- Sputum for Gram stain and culture may be obtained in older children with suspected bacterial infection

IMAGING/SPECIAL TESTS

- *Mycoplasma* IgM or cold agglutinin titers
  - —Useful if suspecting this organism
  - —More likely positive with severe illness
- Nasopharyngeal washes for direct fluorescent antibody and culture
  - —Identify RSV, *Chlamydia trachomatis*, and *B. pertussis* infections
- Pleural fluid (if present) for culture, Gram stain, protein, glucose, and cell counts

DIFFERENTIAL DIAGNOSIS

- Reactive airway disease [asthma, bronchiolitis (age <2 years)]
- Aspiration
  - —Gastroesophageal reflux
  - —Vascular ring
  - —H-type tracheoesophageal fistula
  - —Foreign body
  - —Hydrocarbon
- Congestive heart failure
- Congenital
  - —Cystic fibrosis
  - —Sequestered lobe
  - —Congenital lobe absence
  - —Hemangioma
- Neoplasm

Treatment

INITIAL STABILIZATION

- If moderately or severely ill:
  - —Secure airway, as appropriate; intubate for clinical respiratory failure
  - —High-flow oxygen
  - —IV hydration (0.9% NS 20 cc/kg initial bolus) and resuscitation if in shock or hypovolemia
- Monitor
- Apply pulse oximetry; ABG if inadequate ventilation
- Check bedside glucose in severely ill-appearing infants and toddlers
  - —Administer glucose D25 at 2 cc/kg i.v. for toddlers or D10 at 5 cc/kg i.v. for neonates if hypoglycemic

ED TREATMENT

- Perform thoracentesis if pleural effusion compromising respiratory function or for diagnostic tests
- Continue pre-hospital therapy
- Often have concurrent reactive airway disease that needs specific treatment with bronchodilator (albuterol)

Antibiotics

- Initiate IV antibiotic therapy for moderate to severely ill children who require admission
- IV antibiotics
  - —Neonate
    - -Ampicillin and cefotaxime or gentamicin
    - -Erythromycin for suspected *C. trachomatis* or *B. pertussis* pneumonia
  - —Infant 1–2 months of age
    - -Ampicillin and cefotaxime
    - -Erythromycin for suspected *C. trachomatis* or *B. pertussis*
  - —Children 3 months and older
    - -Cefotaxime, cefuroxime, or ceftriaxone
    - -Vancomycin for suspected or confirmed penicillin-resistant *S. pneumoniae*
    - -Erythromycin or clarithromycin for suspected *M. pneumoniae*
- Outpatient empiric antibiotic therapy
  - —Infants <2 months old
    - -Outpatient treatment generally not recommended
  - —Children 3 months–5 years
    - -Amoxicillin
    - -Amoxicillin-clavulanate
    - -Trimethoprim-sulfamethoxazole
    - -Erythromycin-sulfisoxazole
    - -Clarithromycin
  - —Children 5–18 years
    - -Azithromycin
    - -Clarithromycin
- Unusual organisms require specific therapy in coordination with infectious disease consultation

MEDICATIONS

- Albuterol (0.5% solution or 5 mg/mL): nebulizer 0.015 mg (0.03 mL)/kg/dose up to 5 mg/dose q 10–20 min as needed; metered dose inhaler (with spacer) (90 μg/puff) 2 puffs q 10–20 min up to total of 10 puffs
- Amoxicillin: 80 mg/kg/24 hours q12h PO
- Amoxicillin-clavulanate: 30 mg/kg/24 hours q12h PO
- Ampicillin: 100–150 mg/kg/24 hours q6h i.v.
- Azithromycin: 10 mg/kg/24 hours qd × 1 d, then 5 mg/kg/24 hours qd × 4 d
- Cefotaxime: 75 mg/kg/24 hours q8h i.v., max 2 g q8h
- Ceftriaxone: 100 mg/kg/24 hours q12–24h i.v., max 2 g q12h
- Cefuroxime: 100 mg/kg/24 hours q8h i.v., max 2 g q8h
- Clarithromycin: 15 mg/kg/24 hours q12h PO, max 500 g q12h
- Erythromycin: 40 mg/kg/24 hours q6h PO or i.v., max 2 g/d
- Erythromycin-sulfisoxazole: 40 mg/kg/24 hours as erythromycin q8h PO, max 2 g/d
- Gentamicin: 5–7.5 mg/kg/24 hours q8–12h i.v.
- Trimethoprim-sulfamethoxazole: 6–10 mg/kg/24 hours as TMP q12h PO
- Vancomycin: 10 mg/kg/24 hours q6h i.v., max 1,000 mg q6h

Disposition

ADMISSION CRITERIA

- Toxic appearance
- Respiratory distress or failure
- Dehydration/vomiting
- Apnea
- Infants <2 months old
- Infants <6 months old with lobar pneumonia
- Hypoxia [O_2 saturation <92% on room air (sea level)]
- Pleural effusion
- Poor response to outpatient oral therapy
- Immunocompromised children
- Concern about noncompliant parents

DISCHARGE CRITERIA

- Most cases are mild and can be discharged home if no evidence of hypoxia, significant work-of-breathing, dehydration, vomiting, or noncompliance
- Assured follow-up within 1–2 days

Miscellaneous

ICD9: 486, 482.9, 480.9

ICD10: P23.9

SUGGESTED READINGS

Bachur R, Perry H, Harper MB. Occult pneumonias: empiric chest radiographs in febrile children with leukocytosis. Ann Emerg Med 1999;33:166–173.

Baraff LJ. Management of fever without source in infants and children. Ann Emerg Med 2000;36:602–614.

Juvén T, Mertsola J, Waris M, et al. Etiology of community-acquired pneumonia in 254 hospitalized children. Pediatr Infect Dis J 2000;19:293–298.

McCracken GH. Etiology and treatment of pneumonia. Pediatr Infect Dis J 2000;19: 373–377.

Authors: Gary D. Zimmer; Karen P. Zimmer

Pneumothorax

Clinical Presentation

SIGNS AND SYMPTOMS

- Severity of symptoms is generally proportional to size of the pneumothorax
- Chest pain on the ipsilateral side
  - —Sharp, pleuritic pain
  - —Sudden onset
  - —Dull ache in delayed presentations
- Shortness of breath
- Tachypnea
- Heart rate <120 generally seen in simple spontaneous pneumothoraces
- Rarely cough, asymptomatic, or generalized malaise

Tension Pneumothorax

- Hypotension
- Tachycardia, heart rate >120
- Diaphoresis
- Cyanosis
- Cardiovascular collapse
- Tracheal deviation

MECHANISM/DESCRIPTION

- Presence of free air in the intrapleural space
- Spontaneous pneumothorax is due to atraumatic rupture of alveolus, bronchiole, or bleb
- Primary spontaneous pneumothorax (two thirds of incidences)
  - —No underlying pulmonary pathology present
  - —Rupture of small subpleural cyst or bleb
  - —Primarily young and healthy patients (20–40 years old), with tall and thin body habitus
- Secondary spontaneous pneumothorax from underlying pulmonary pathology (see Etiology, below)
- Tension pneumothorax
  - —Air continues to enter pleural space through bronchoalveolar disruption and becomes trapped via "ball-valve" mechanism
  - —Intrapleural pressure increases
  - —Venous return to right heart decreases, resulting in decrease in cardiac output
  - —Mediastinum shifts toward uninvolved side mechanically interfering with right atrial filling
  - —Ventilation compromised and v/q mismatch resulting in hypoxemia

ETIOLOGY

- Idiopathic
- Airway disease
  - —COPD
  - —Asthma
  - —Cystic fibrosis
- Infections
  - —Necrotizing bacterial pneumonia
  - —Tuberculosis
  - —Fungal pneumonia
  - —*Pneumocystis carinii*
- Neoplasm
- Interstitial lung disease
  - —Sarcoidosis
  - —Idiopathic pulmonary fibrosis
  - —Lymphangiomyomatosis
  - —Tuberous sclerosis
  - —Pneumoconioses
- Connective tissue diseases
- Pulmonary infarction
- Endometriosis
- Blunt chest trauma
- Penetrating trauma to neck or trunk
- Iatrogenic
  - —Central line placement
  - —Other vascular access procedure

Pre-Hospital

CAUTIONS

- Suspected tension pneumothorax requires immediate needle thoracostomy

Diagnosis

ESSENTIAL WORKUP

- Tension pneumothorax is a clinical diagnosis
- Initiate intervention for suspected tension pneumothorax immediately; do not wait for CXR confirmation
- Upright chest radiograph (CXR) is the definitive diagnostic test for other than tension pneumothorax
- Patients unable to tolerate upright CXR can be taken in decubitus position with the suspected side up
- Expiratory CXR will improve detection
- A rough estimate of pneumothorax size is sufficient to make clinical decisions

IMAGING/SPECIAL TESTS

- EKG
  - —Often necessary to rule out cardiac etiologies of chest pain
  - —Nonspecific changes include T-wave inversion, left axis deviation, and decreased R-wave amplitude
- Chest CT is very sensitive for small pneumothorax but has little practical advantage over CXR

DIFFERENTIAL DIAGNOSIS

- Exacerbation of COPD
- Asthma
- Pulmonary embolus
- Myocardial infarction
- Pericarditis
- Pneumomediastinum
- Dissection of aortic aneurysm
- Chest wall pain
- Pleuritis
- Acute abdominal processes

Treatment

INITIAL STABILIZATION

- Cardiac monitor
- Pulse oximetry
- Oxygen 100% via nonrebreather face mask
- Intravenous access
- Suspected tension pneumothorax requires either immediate needle thoracostomy or tube thoracostomy
- Needle thoracostomy
  - —Immediate placement indicated in unstable patients with a tension pneumothorax
  - —14- to 18-gauge angiocatheter in the second intercostal space at midclavicular line or 4th or 5th intercostal space at anterior axillary line

ED TREATMENT

- Nontraumatic pneumothorax estimated at <15% collapse and no cardiovascular or respiratory compromise
  - —Observe with 100% oxygen support for 4–6 hours
  - —Repeat CXR and discharge if unchanged
- Simple aspiration
  - —Indications
    - -Simple pneumothorax with only 15–30% collapse
    - -Increase in size of a small pneumothorax during observation
  - —Placement of aspiration catheter (typically 8 Fr) with three-way stopcock
    - -Aspirate air until resistance or 3 L air aspirated
    - -If the pneumothorax is no longer visible on two subsequent chest radiographs at 4-hour intervals, remove catheter
    - -If a final chest radiograph is normal 2 hours after the catheter is removed, the patient may be discharged
    - -A second aspiration may be attempted if the pneumothorax does not resolve
- Heimlich valve
  - —Indicated when <30% collapse after failure of aspiration
  - —Attach Heimlich valve to aspiration catheter or chest tube
- Suction
  - —Indicated when the Heimlich valve fails
  - —Attach aspiration catheter to suction at 20 cm H_2O
  - —Observe in ED for 1 hour
- Tube thoracostomy
  - —Indications
    - -Suspicion of a tension pneumothorax
    - -Gunshot wound to the chest
    - -Clinical evidence of a pneumothorax following blunt chest trauma or penetrating chest trauma
    - -Presence of a pneumothorax of any size in patient receiving positive pressure ventilation
    - -Pneumothorax with >30% collapse
    - -Most cases of secondary pneumothorax
    - -Definitive therapy after needle thoracostomy
  - —Tube size
    - -Small-caliber (7 to 14 Fr) tube for primary spontaneous pneumothoraces
    - -20 to 28 Fr for secondary spontaneous pneumothorax
    - -28 Fr when there is detectable pleural fluid or an anticipated need for mechanical ventilation
  - —Following insertion, the tube should be connected to a water-seal device
  - —A Heimlich valve may be used instead of a water-seal device in stable patients without a pleural effusion
  - —Reexpansion edema is a rare complication requiring supportive care

Disposition

ADMISSION CRITERIA

- Tension pneumothorax
- Chest tube required

DISCHARGE CRITERIA

- <15% collapse, no expansion while in the ED or successful aspiration with catheter removed
  - —Discharge with follow-up in 24 hours and 1 week for CXR to assure reexpansion
- Reliable patients with the thoracic vent and successful aspiration or secured catheter and Heimlich valve
  - —Discharge with 24- and 48-hour follow-up
  - —At 48-hour follow-up
  - —Clamp catheter, observe for 2 hours, and repeat CXR
  - —Remove thoracic vent or catheter if no reexpansion
  - —Observe for 2 hours and repeat CXR
  - —If no reexpansion, discharge with 24-hour and 1-week follow-up
- Discharge instruction include prompt return for new onset of chest pain or dyspnea
- Patients without reexpansion at 1 week require a cardiothoracic surgery consult

Miscellaneous

ICD9: 512.8

ICD10: J93.9

SUGGESTED READINGS

Baumann MH, Strange C, Heffner JE, et al. Management of spontaneous pneumothorax: an American College of Chest Physicians Delphi consensus statement. Chest 2001;119:590.

Light RW. Pleural diseases, 4th ed. Philadelphia: Lippincott Williams & Wilkins, 2001.

Miller AC, Harvey JE. Guidelines for the management of spontaneous pneumothorax. Standards of Care Committee, British Thoracic Society. BMJ 1993;307:114.

Sahn SA, Heffner JE. Spontaneous pneumothorax. N Engl J Med 2000;342:868.

Author: David Feldman

Poisoning

Clinical Presentation

SIGNS AND SYMPTOMS

- Neurologic
  - —Lethargy
  - —Agitation
  - —Coma
  - —Hallucinations
  - —Seizures
- Respiratory
  - —Tachypnea/bradypnea/apnea
  - —Inability to protect airway
- Cardiovascular
  - —Dysrhythmias
  - —Conduction blocks
- Vital signs
  - —Varies depending on toxic substance
  - —Hyperthermia/hypothermia
  - —Tachycardia/bradycardia
  - —Hypertension/hypotension
- Selected toxidromes (see Poisoning, Toxidromes)
  - —Anticholinergic
    - -Altered mental status (confusion, delirium, lethargy)
    - -Dry skin and mucous membranes
    - -Fixed dilated pupils
    - -Tachycardia
    - -Hyperthermia
    - -Flushing
    - -Urinary retention
  - —Cholinergic
    - -Secretory overdrive (salivation, lacrimation, urination, diaphoresis)
    - -Miosis
    - -Bronchospasm/wheezing
  - —Opiate
    - -CNS and respiratory depression
    - -Pinpoint pupils
  - —Sympathomimetic
    - -CNS excitation
    - -Seizures
    - -Tachycardia
    - -Hypertension

MECHANISM/DESCRIPTION

- Pharmacologic mechanism specific to agent

ETIOLOGY

- Intentional
  - —Depression
  - —Suicide
  - —Recreational drug abuse
- Accidental
  - —Common cause in children

PEDIATRIC CONSIDERATIONS

- Accidental ingestions—typically young children (ages 1-5)
- Consider child abuse if inconsistent or suspicious history

Pre-Hospital

CAUTIONS

- Search for clues at scene
  - —Pills/pill bottles
  - —Drug paraphernalia
  - —Witnesses
- Transport all drugs and pill bottles for identification
- Restrain uncooperative patients
- Consider comorbid conditions
  - —Trauma
  - —Medical illness
  - —Environmental exposure

CONTROVERSIES

- Decreased time to activated charcoal (AC) administration when given in the pre-hospital setting
- Home use of ipecac for:
  - —Ingestion of substance known *not* to cause rapid neurologic or respiratory deterioration
  - —Patient whose transit time to health care facility is >1 hour
  - —Consider administration after consultation with the regional poison center

Diagnosis

ESSENTIAL WORKUP

- Accurately identify the ingestant(s)
  - —Send someone to patient's home to obtain the product(s) if necessary
- Accurately identify time of ingestion
- Call poison control center or toxicologist for help

LABORATORY

- Electrolytes, BUN/Cr, glucose
- Calculate anion gap: Na^+-(Cl^+ HCO_3)
  - —Normal anion gap: 8–12
  - —Use mnemonic *A CAT MUD PILES* for elevated anion gap acidosis:
    - -Alcoholic ketoacidosis
    - -Cyanide, carbon monoxide
    - -ASA, other salicylates
    - -Toluene
    - -Methanol, metformin
    - -Diabetic ketoacidosis
    - -Paraldehyde, phenformin
    - -Iron, INH
    - -Lactic acidosis from other causes
    - -Ethylene glycol
    - -Starvation ketosis
- Serum osmolal gap
  - —Calculate osmolal gap if elevated anion gap acidosis from potential toxic alcohol
  - —Most sensitive early in poisoning
  - —Calculated osmolality = 2(Na^+) + glucose/18 + BUN/2.8 + ethanol (in mg/dL)/4.6
  - —Osmolal gap = measured osmolality − calculated osmolality
  - —Use mnemonic *ME DIE A* when osmolal gap >10
    - -Methanol
    - -Ethanol
    - -Diuretics (mannitol, glycerin, sorbitol)
    - -Isopropyl alcohol
    - -Ethylene glycol
    - -Acetone
  - —Normal osmolal gap does not rule out toxic alcohol ingestion
- Pregnancy test
- Acetaminophen level for suicidal ingestions
- Toxicology screen

IMAGING/SPECIAL TESTS

- EKG for dysrhythmias or QRS/QT changes
- CT of head for altered mental status not clearly due to toxin

DIFFERENTIAL DIAGNOSIS

- Causes of altered mental status
  - —Intracranial mass, bleeding
  - —Infection, sepsis
  - —Endocrine abnormalities
  - —Hypothermia
  - —Hypoxia
  - —Metabolic abnormalities
  - —Psychogenic

Treatment

INITIAL STABILIZATION

- ABCs
  - —Endotracheal intubation as needed for airway protection, oxygenation, ventilation, and orogastric lavage
  - —Supplemental oxygen for hypoxia
  - —Pulse oximetry
  - —Cardiac monitor
  - —IV access
- Hypotension
  - —Administer 0.9% NS IV fluid bolus
  - —Trendelenburg
  - —Vasopressors for persistent hypotension
- Bradycardia
  - —Atropine
  - —Cardiac pacing
- If altered mental status, administer coma cocktail: thiamine, D50W (or Accucheck), naloxone

ED TREATMENT

Decontamination

- See Poisoning, Gastric Decontamination
- Prevents systemic absorption of ingested toxin
- Ipecac
  - —Useful pre-hospital, if transit time >1 hour
  - —No advantage over activated charcoal alone
- Orogastric lavage
  - —Consider in potentially lethal ingestions without a known antidote within 1 hour of ingestion
  - —Protected airway essential prior to lavage
- Activated charcoal
  - —Most effective within a few hours of most toxic ingestions
  - —Contraindicated if caustic ingestion, unprotected airway, or bowel obstruction
  - —Drugs not effectively bound to charcoal: metals (borates, bromide, iron, lithium), alcohols, potassium
- Cathartics
  - —Used in combination with first dose (*only*) of activated charcoal to enhance GI transit time
  - —Repeated administration may cause severe electrolyte disturbances
- Whole-bowel irrigation
  - —Polyethylene glycol (Colyte, Go-Lytely) evacuates bowel without causing electrolyte disturbances
  - —Consider in toxins not well adsorbed by charcoal (e.g., iron and lithium), body packers/stuffers, sustained release ingestions
  - —Contraindicated if bowel obstruction, perforation, or hypotension

Enhanced Elimination

- Enhances removal of systemically absorbed toxin
- Multiple-dose activated charcoal
  - —Theophylline
  - —Carbamazepine
  - —Phenobarbital
- Urinary alkalinization
  - —Salicylates
  - —Phenobarbital
- Hemodialysis/hemoperfusion
  - —Lithium
  - —Salicylates
  - —Theophylline
  - —Toxic alcohols

Antidotes

- See Poisoning, Antidotes
- Acetaminophen: *N*-acetylcysteine
- Anticholinergic: physostigmine
- Arsenic: British anti-lewisite (BAL), Ca-EDTA, succimer
- Benzodiazepines: flumazenil
- Beta blockers: glucagon
- Calcium channel blockers: calcium chloride/gluconate, insulin
- Carbon monoxide: oxygen, hyperbaric oxygen
- Coumadin: vitamin K_1
- Cyanide: cyanide antidote kit
- Digoxin: Digibind
- Ethylene glycol: ethanol, 4-methylpyrazole
- Iron: deferoxamine
- Isoniazid (INH): pyridoxine (vitamin B_6)
- Lead: BAL, Ca-EDTA, succimer
- Mercury: Ca-EDTA, succimer
- Methanol: ethanol, 4-methylpyrazole
- Methemoglobinemia: methylene blue
- Opiates: naloxone
- Organophosphates: atropine, pralidoxime
- Tricyclic antidepressants: $NaHCO_3$

Consultation

- Poison control center (national: 1-800-222-1222)
- Local toxicologist
- Psychiatry
- Social services (especially pediatric patients)

MEDICATIONS

- Activated charcoal slurry: 1–2 g/kg PO
- Dextrose: D50W 1 amp (50 mL or 25 g) (peds: D25W 2–4 mL/kg) i.v.
- Naloxone (Narcan): 0.4–2 mg (peds: 0.1 mg/kg) i.v. or i.m. initial dose
- Thiamine (vitamin B_1): 100 mg (peds: 50 mg) i.v. or i.m.

Disposition

ADMISSION CRITERIA

- Altered mental status
- Cardiopulmonary instability
- Suicidal
- Laboratory abnormalities
- Potential for decompensation from delayed acting substance

DISCHARGE CRITERIA

- Psychiatrically clear
- Detoxified

Miscellaneous

ICD9: 977.9

ICD10: T65.9

SEE ALSO: POISONING, ANTIDOTES; POISONING, GASTRIC DECONTAMINATION; AND POISONING, TOXIDROMES

SUGGESTED READINGS

Ford MD, Delaney KA. Initial approach to the poisoned patient. In: Ford MD, Delaney KA, Ling LJ, et al., eds. Clinical toxicology. Philadelphia: WB Saunders, 2001:1–4.

Goldfrank LR, Flomenbaum NE, Weisman RS, et al. Vital signs and toxic syndromes. In: Goldfrank LR, Flomenbaum NE, Lewin NA, et al., eds. Goldfrank's toxicologic emergencies, 6th ed. Norwalk, CT: Appleton & Lange, 1998:277–284.

Hoffman RS, Goldfrank LR. The poisoned patient with altered consciousness. JAMA 1995;274:562–569.

Kulig K. Initial management of toxic substances. N Engl J Med 1992;326: 1678–1682.

Author: Mark B. Mycyk

Poisoning, Antidotes

Clinical Presentation

N/A

Pre-Hospital

N/A

Diagnosis

N/A

Treatment

N-ACETYL CYSTEINE (NAC)

- Indications
  - —Acetaminophen overdose
- Warnings
  - —Unpleasant odor, nausea, vomiting
  - —Most effective if given in first 8 hours postingestion
- Dose
  - —PO: 140 mg/kg, then 70 mg/kg q4h × 17
  - —IV: (consult poison center) 150 mg/kg in 200 mL D5W over 15 minutes, then 50 mg/kg in 500 mL D5W over 4 hours, then 100 mg/kg in 1,000 mL D5W over 16 hours

ATROPINE

- Indications
  - —Bradycardia due to drugs
  - —Organophosphate insecticides
- Warnings
  - —Myasthenia gravis, narrow angle glaucoma, hypertension, coronary ischemia, and urinary obstruction
- Dose
  - —Adult: 0.5–1.0 mg i.v.
  - —Pediatric: 0.02 mg/kg (min 0.1 mg) i.v.
  - —Large repeated doses needed in organophosphate poisoning

BENZTROPINE (COGENTIN)

- Indications
  - —Acute dystonic reactions
- Warnings
  - —Carbamates, myasthenia gravis, narrow angle glaucoma, hypertension, coronary ischemia, and urinary obstruction
- Dose
  - —Adult: 1–2 mg i.v. (for acute reaction) or PO (to prevent reaction)
  - —Pediatric: 0.02 mg/kg i.v. (for acute reaction) or PO (to prevent reaction)

BENZODIAZEPINE

- Indications
  - —Agitation, stimulant drugs, seizures
- Warnings
  - —Respiratory/CNS depression
- Dose
  - —Midazolam
    - -Adult: 1 mg i.v./i.m. q 2–3 min PRN
    - -Pediatric: 0.1 mg/kg i.v./i.m.
  - —Diazepam
    - -Adult: 2–5 mg i.v./i.m., repeat in 10–15 min
    - -Pediatrics: 0.1 mg/kg i.v./i.m.

BICARBONATE, SODIUM

- Indications
  - —Cyclic antidepressant poisoning, metabolic acidosis, urinary alkalinization
- Warnings
  - —May cause CHF, excessive alkalosis, hypokalemia
- Dose
  - —Serum alkalinization:
    - -1 mEq/kg IVP
  - —Urine alkalinization:
    - -100–150 mEq in 1 L DW at 2–3 cc/kg/h i.v., goal urine pH 7–8

BLACK WIDOW SPIDER ANTIVENIN (LACTRODECTUS MACTANS)

- Indications
  - —Severe hypertension, muscle spasms not alleviated by analgesics and muscle relaxants; consider in extremes of age (<5 or >65 years), pregnant women with threatened abortion
- Warnings
  - —Equine serum derived—immediate hypersensitivity, serum sickness 10–14 days
  - —Premedicate for anaphylaxis if know equine serum hypersensitivity
- Dose
  - —1–2 vials i.v. slowly over 15–30 minutes

BOTULIN ANTITOXIN TRIVALENT A,B,E

- Indications
  - —Clinical botulism, prior to onset of paralysis
- Warnings
  - —Only binds free toxins
  - —Not for infant botulism
  - —Equine serum derived—immediate hypersensitivity, serum sickness 10–14 days
  - —Premedicate for anaphylaxis if know equine serum hypersensitivity
- Dose
  - —1–2 vials i.v. q4h for 4–5 doses

CALCIUM

- Indications
  - —Hyperkalemia with cardiac toxicity
  - —Hydrofluoric acid burn
  - —Calcium channel blocker overdose
  - —Citrate, oxalate, phosphate poisoning
- Warnings
  - —Avoid in digoxin toxicity, hypercalcemia
  - —CaCl corrosive to skin, SC tissue
  - —Incompatible with certain IV solutions
- Dose
  - —Adult: 5–10 mL of 10% Ca chloride, or 10–20 mL of 10% Ca gluconate
  - —Pediatric: 0.1–0.2 mL/kg of 10% Ca chloride, or 0.2–0.3 mL/kg of 10% Ca gluconate

CALCIUM EDTA (EDETATE DISODIUM)

- Indications
  - —Lead, chromium, nickel, manganese, zinc toxicity
- Warnings
  - —Nausea, vomiting, chill, nephrotoxicity, hypercalcemia
- Dose
  - —20–30 mg/kg over 24 hours as 6 divided doses or continuous IV infusion, follow Pb level

CORAL SNAKE ANTIVENIN (MICRURUS FULVIUS)

- Indications
  - —Eastern or Texas coral snake
- Warnings
  - —Equine serum derived—immediate hypersensitivity, serum sickness 10–14 days
  - —Premedicate for anaphylaxis if know equine serum hypersensitivity
- Dose
  - —4–10 vials i.v. over 15–30 minutes

CYANIDE ANTIDOTE KIT

- Indications
  - —Cyanide poisoning
- Warnings
  - —Hypotension, methemoglobinemia
- Dose
  - —1. Amyl nitrite: 1–2 amp crushed, inhaled
  - —2. Sodium nitrite:
    - -Adult: 300 mg in 10 mL i.v. over 5 min
    - -Pediatric: 0.3 mL/kg of 3% solution i.v.
  - —3. Sodium thiosulfate:
    - -Adult: 12.5 g i.v., may repeat in 1 hour
    - -Pediatric: 50 mg/kg i.v.

DANTROLENE

- Indications
  - —Malignant hyperthermia
  - —Neuroleptic malignant syndrome
  - —Serotonin syndrome
  - —Muscle rigidity
- Warnings
  - —Muscle weakness, respiratory depression, hepatitis
- Dose
  - —1–2 mg/kg i.v. bolus, repeat q 5–10 min PRN, max 10 mg/kg

DEFEROXAMINE (DESFERAL)

- Indications
  - —Iron toxicity
- Warnings
  - —Do not treat for >24 hours, risk for delayed ARDS
  - —Hypotension if >15 mg/kg/h, flushing, urticaria
- Dose
  - —10–15 mg/kg/h i.v., may increase in severe Fe poisoning

DIGOXIN ANTIBODY (DIGIBIND)

- Indications
  - —Digoxin, digitoxin toxicity
- Warnings
  - —Falsely elevated digoxin levels after use
  - —Development of CHF/atrial fibrillation in patients requiring digoxin
- Dose
  - —1 vial (40 mg) binds 0.6 mg digoxin
  - —# vials = digoxin level (ng/mL) × wt (kg)/100
  - —Dose estimate: acute overdose 10–20 vials, chronic overdose 4–6 vials

DIMERCAPROL (BAL)

- Indications
  - —Arsenic, gold, mercury, lead-induced encephalopathy
- Warnings
  - —Renal toxicity, fever, nausea, vomiting, urticaria, cholinergic symptoms
- Dose
  - —3 mg/kg deep i.m. q4h × 2 days, then q12h × 7 days, follow metal levels
  - —For Pb level >100 μg/dL: 4–5 mg/kg i.m. q4h until Pb <50 μg/dL, in conjunction with EDTA

DIPHENHYDRAMINE (BENADRYL)

- Indications
  - —Antihistamine, acute dystonic reaction
- Warnings
  - —Sedation, excitation in children, anticholinergic symptoms
- Dose:
  - —Adult: 25–50 mg i.v./i.m./PO q4–6h
  - —Pediatrics 0.5–1 mg/kg i.v./i.m./PO q4–6h

DMSA (SUCCIMER, CHEMET)

- Indications
  - —Pediatric lead poisoning
- Warnings
  - —Caution in renal impairment—urinary elimination
  - —Nausea, vomiting diarrhea
- Dose
  - —10 mg/kg PO q8h × 5 days, then q12h × 14 days, then reassess blood lead levels

EPINEPHRINE

- Indications
  - —Angioedema, anaphylaxis, acute asthma, spinal shock, beta-blocker overdose
- Warnings
  - —Dysrhythmias, hypertension, tremor, anxiety
- Dose
  - —Hypotension/shock:
    - -Adult: 1–4 μg/min i.v. infusion
    - -Pediatric: Start i.v. infusion at 0.1 μg/kg/min
  - —Mild-moderate reactions:
    - -Adult: 0.3–0.5 mg s.c.
    - -Pediatric: 0.01 mg/kg s.c.

ETHANOL

- Indications
  - —Methanol or ethylene glycol toxicity
- Warnings
  - —Disulfiram reaction, CNS sedation
  - —Hypoglycemia in pediatric population
  - —Increase dose during dialysis, for chronic alcoholics
- Dose
  - —IV: 10 mL/kg load as 10% solution over 1 hour, then 1 mL/kg/h maintenance
  - —PO: 1.5 mL/kg as 100 proof solution, then 0.3 mL/kg/h maintenance
  - —Goal: ethanol level of 100–150 mg/dL

FLUMAZENIL (ROMAZICON)

- Indications
  - —Benzodiazepine overdose
- Warnings
  - —Contraindicated in TCA overdose
  - —Lowers seizure threshold
  - —Induces benzodiazepine withdrawal
- Dose
  - —Adult: 0.2 mg i.v. slow, repeat q 2–3 min to 1 mg max
  - —Pediatric: 0.01–0.05 mg/kg i.v. over 30 min–1 hour

FOMEPIZOLE (4-MP, ANTIZOL)

- Indications
  - —Methanol or ethylene glycol toxicity
- Warnings
  - —Nausea, dizziness, headache
- Dose
  - —15 mg/kg load, then 10 mg/kg q12h × 4, then 15 mg/kg q12h

GLUCAGON

- Indications
  - —Beta-blocker or calcium channel blocker overdose with bradycardia/hypotension
  - —Hypoglycemia
- Warnings
  - —Nausea, vomiting, hyperglycemia
  - —Hypotension from diluent (phenol-containing)
- Dose
  - —Beta-blocker or calcium channel blocker overdose:
    - -Adult: 5–10 mg i.v. over 1 minute
    - -Pediatric: 0.15 mg/kg i.v. over 1 minute
  - —Hypoglycemia:
    - -Adult: 0.5–1 mg i.m./i.v./s.c.
    - -Pediatric: 0.025–0.1 mg/kg i.m./i.v./s.c. (max 1 mg/dose)

Poisoning, Antidotes

INSULIN/GLUCOSE

- Indications
  - —Calcium channel blocker overdose with severe hypotension/symptomatic bradycardia refractory to other therapies
  - —Hyperkalemia
- Warnings
  - —Experimental therapy: consult a poison control center/medical toxicologist
  - —Follow serum glucose q 15 minutes for 1 hour after the first bolus or after any increase in dose, then q1h
- Dose
  - —Bolus:
    - -0.5–1.0 IU/kg regular insulin, followed by
    - -25 g glucose (1 amp D50)
  - —Maintenance:
    - -Insulin 0.5 IU regular insulin/kg/h, titrate to 1.0 IU regular insulin/kg/h
    - -Glucose D10 start at 100 cc/h (10g/h) and titrate to keep glucose $\geq$100 mg/dL

METHYLENE BLUE

- Indications
  - —Methemoglobinemia with dyspnea or >25%
- Warnings
  - —G6-PD deficiency
- Dose
  - —1–2 mg/kg slow i.v. as 1% solution, repeat in 1 hour

NARCAN

- Indications
  - —Opiate poisoning, empiric treatment of coma
- Warnings
  - —Acute opiate withdrawal, severe agitation
- Dose
  - —Adult: 0.4–2.0 mg i.v. or i.m., repeat to 10 mg
  - —Pediatric: 0.1 mg/kg i.v. or i.m.

OCTREOTIDE

- Indications
  - —Sulfonylurea overdose with hypoglycemia
- Warnings
  - —Use with caution in diabetic patients
- Dose
  - —Adult: 50 μg s.c. q6h
  - —Pediatric: 4-5 μg/kg/d s.c. divided q6h

OXYGEN, HYPERBARIC

- Indications
  - —CO poisoning
- Warnings
  - —TM perforation, seizures due to oxygen toxicity
  - —Difficulty monitoring patient
- Dose
  - —100% oxygen at 2-3 ATM

PENICILLAMINE

- Indications
  - —Arsenic, copper, lead, mercury with/following BAL or EDTA
- Warnings
  - —Contraindicated in penicillin allergy, renal insufficieny
- Dose
  - —Lead
    - -Adult: 250–500 mg/dose PO q8–12h
    - -Pediatric: 25–40 mg/kg/d PO in three divided doses
  - —Arsenic
    - -100 mg/kg/d PO divided in 4 doses for 5 days (maximum: 1 g/day)
  - —Mercury
    - -Adult: 250 mg PO q.i.d.
    - -Pediatric: 20–30 mg/kg/d PO in four divided doses

PHENTOLAMINE

- Indications
  - —Hypertensive crisis: stimulants, sympathomimetics, MAO-tyramine reaction, and extravasated pressors
  - —Reversal of cocaine-mediated vasospasm
- Warnings
  - —Hypertension, tachycardia, dysrhythmias
- Dose
  - —HTN:
    - -Adult: 1–5 mg i.v. bolus
    - -Pediatric: 0.02–0.1 mg/kg bolus
  - —Extravasation:
    - -Adult: 5 mg i.v. bolus diluted in 10–15 mL saline s.c.
    - -Pediatric: 0.1 mg/kg diluted in 10–15 mL saline s.c.

PHYSOSTIGMINE

- Indications
  - —Severe anticholinergic syndrome
- Warnings
  - —Contraindicated in TCA overdose
- Dose
  - —Adult: 0.5–1.0 mg i.v. repeat in 10 min PRN
  - —Pediatric: 0.02 mg/kg i.v. repeat in 10 min PRN

PRALIDOXIME (2-PAM, PROTOPAM)

- Indications
  - —Organophosphate toxicity
  - —Reversal of nicotinic effects
  - —Reactivates enzyme
  - —Use in conjunction with atropine
- Warnings
  - —Myasthenic crisis if myasthenia gravis
  - —Nausea, headache, dizziness, laryngospasm, muscle rigidity
- Dose
  - —Adult: 1–2 g in 100 ml NaCl over 15 min, repeat in 1 hour PRN, repeat in 6 hours if nicotinic symptoms return
  - —Pediatrics: 25–50 mg/kg over 15 min, repeat in 1 hour PRN, repeat in 6 hours if nicotinic symptoms return

PROTAMINE

- Indications
  - —Reversal of heparin anticoagulation
- Warnings
  - —Hypersensitivity in patients with fish allergy
  - —Avoid benzyl alcohol diluent in neonates
- Dose
  - —1 mg for each 100 IU heparin, ½ dose if 30–60 min and ¼ dose if 2 hours after heparin bolus

PYRIDOXINE (VITAMIN B_6)

- Indications
  - —Isoniazid-induced seizures
  - —Gyromitra mushroom
- Warnings
  - —None, nontoxic
- Dose
  - —INH-induced seizures:
    - -Unknown ingested amount: 5 g for adult or 1 g for pediatrics
    - -Dose (mg) = amount INH ingested (mg)
    - -Gyromitra: 25 mg/kg i.v. over 30 min–1 hour

***RATTLESNAKE ANTIVENIN* (CROTALINE)**

- Indications
  - —Significant envenomation by *Crotaline* species: rattlesnake, cottonmouth, water moccasin, pit viper
- Warnings
  - —Equine or ovine derived products—immediate hypersensitivity, serum sickness 10–14 days
  - —Premedicate for anaphylaxis if know equine/ovine serum hypersensitivity
- Dose
  - —Equine-derived (Wyeth-Ayerst polyvalent):
    - -Mild: 5 vials—infuse slowly
    - -Moderate: 10 vials—infuse slowly
    - -Severe: 15 vials—infuse slowly
  - —Ovine-derived (Crofab):
    - -4–6 vials slowly, may repeat dose of 4–6 vials if control of envenomation not achieved, then 2 vials q6h × 3

VITAMIN K (PHYTONADIONE, AQUA MEPHYTON)

- Indications
- Reversal of coumadin anticoagulation
- Warnings
  - —Hypersensitivity from IV administration
- Dose
  - —2–10 mg i.m./s.c./slow i.v., may repeat in 8 hours
  - —2–10 mg PO, may repeat in 12–48 hours

Miscellaneous

ICD9: N/A

ICD10: N/A

Author: Suzan Mazor

Poisoning, Gastric Decontamination

Clinical Presentation

N/A

Pre-Hospital

CAUTIONS

- Ipecac contraindicated in ambulance setting

CONTROVERSIES

- Decreased time to activated charcoal (AC) administration when given in the pre-hospital setting
- Decreased drug absorption in a simulated ingestion while volunteers were lying in the left lateral versus the right lateral decubitus position
- Home use of ipecac in general is not recommended
  —In extremely rare cases (very prolonged transit times, protecting airway, etc.), consider ipecac administration only after consultation with the regional poison control center

Diagnosis

N/A

Treatment

INITIAL STABILIZATION

- ABCs
  —Secure airway for decreased mental status/inability to protect airway
  —IV access/cardiac monitor
- Naloxone, thiamine, dextrose (or Accu-Chek) with altered mental status from overdose

ED TREATMENT

Ipecac

- Derived from the roots of the plant *Cephaelis acuminata*
- Exerts emetic action by direct gastric irritation and centrally mediated chemoreceptive trigger zone stimulation
- Delays administration of activated charcoal
- Offers no advantage over activated charcoal alone when both treatments potentially effective

Dosage

- >12 years old: 30 mL
- Ages 1 through 12 years old: 15 mL
- Ages 6 months through 1 year: 5–10 mL plus 15 mL clear fluid

Indications

- No utility in ED

Adverse Effects

- Vomiting may complicate and worsen the clinical presentation
- Delay to administration of activated charcoal or oral antidotes

Contraindications

- Caustics (acids and alkali)
- Hydrocarbons
- Agents that rapidly depress mental status
- Patients actively vomiting

Orogastric Lavage

- Placement of a large-bore tube (32–36 Fr) in the stomach for removal of ingested toxins
- Effectiveness of orogastric lavage dependent on the time interval since ingestion, timing of the last meal, and toxin ingested
- Protected airway essential prior to any attempts at orogastric lavage

Indications

- Presents within 1 hour of taking a potentially lethal ingestion with no known antidote
- Poisoned intubated patient

Adverse Effects

- Inadvertent intubation of the respiratory tree
- Esophageal or gastric perforation
- Charcoal aspiration
- Patient discomfort

Contraindications

- Large pills (limited by lavage tube port size)
- Caustics (acids and alkali)
- Hydrocarbons
- Agents that rapidly depress mental status
- Unprotected airway

Pediatric Considerations

- Avoid in children
- Unlikely to result in any clinically significant pill extraction secondary to the smaller bore orogastric tube (i.e., 18 Fr)
- Risk of aspiration increased in children

Controversies

- Several randomized controlled trials have documented no benefit when lavage plus activated charcoal is compared to activated charcoal alone

Activated Charcoal

- Prepared by treating heated wood pulp, which creates a large surface area to bind toxins
- Mainstay of gastric decontamination
- Effective when contents have reached the small intestines

Dose

- 1–2 g/kg of body weight or an activated charcoal-to-drug ratio of 10:1; often mixed with sorbitol (see below)
- Oral or nasogastric tube administration

Indications

- Administer in every toxic ingestion (for exceptions see below)
- Optimal for toxic ingestions presenting within 1 hour of ingestion

Adverse Effects

- Vomiting and constipation
- Charcoal aspiration and subsequent charcoal pneumonitis

Contraindications

- Caustic ingestions
- Unprotected airway
- Bowel obstruction or ileus

Drugs Not Effectively Bound to Charcoal

- Metals (borates, bromide, iron, lithium)
- Alcohols
- Potassium
- Potassium cyanide (poorly absorbed)
- Hydrocarbons
- Caustics

Pediatric Considerations

- Mix with a palatable substance (cola or juice) to facilitate intake or administer via gastric tube

Controversies

- Randomized controlled trials have shown a slightly worse outcome and higher complication rate when *asymptomatic* patients received charcoal versus nothing

Multiple-Dose Activated Charcoal (MDAC)

- Used in toxic ingestions that are well absorbed by charcoal and undergo enterohepatic circulation

Dose

- 1 g/kg followed by 0.5 g/kg every 2–6 hours
- *Never* use cathartics in conjunction with multiple-dose activated charcoal

Indications

- Theophylline
- Salicylates
- MDAC may decrease area under the curve for such drugs as phenobarbital, Dilantin, and carbamazepine but has not been proven to improve outcome

Cathartics

- Used in combination with activated charcoal to prevent constipation and to enhance GI transit time
- Limited data available to demonstrate any decreased absorption when a cathartic (sorbitol) is added to activated charcoal
- Cathartics alone are of no proven benefit and should be avoided

Dose

- Magnesium citrate 10% solution: 250 mL (peds: 4 mL/kg)
- Magnesium sulfate: 15–20 g (peds: 250 mg/kg)
- Sorbitol: 0.5–1 g/kg to a max of 100 g of 70% solution (peds: >1 year old: 0.5–1 g/kg as a 35% solution to a max of 50 g) PO mixed in the activated charcoal slurry—only use in first dose

Adverse Effects

- Dehydration
- Hypermagnesemia
- Diarrhea
- Abdominal discomfort

Contraindications

- Preexisting dehydration
- Children
- Renal disease (cathartics containing magnesium)

Whole-Bowel Irrigation

- Cleansing of the bowel

Indications

- Toxins not well absorbed by charcoal—toxic iron and lithium ingestions
- Toxins in sealed containers (body packers) without signs of GI perforation
- Toxic sustained-release product ingestions

Dose

- Polyethylene glycol (Colyte, Go-Lytely)
- Solution at 2 L/h in adults (0.5 L/h in children) until rectal excretions clear
- Administer via a nasogastric tube with activated charcoal as indicated via a continuous or bolus method

Adverse Effects

- Bloating
- Rectal irritation
- Frequent bowel movements

Contraindications

- Mechanical or pharmacologic ileus
- Bowel obstruction
- Intestinal perforation
- Unprotected airway

Disposition

N/A

Miscellaneous

ICD9: 977.9

ICD10: T47.6

SEE ALSO: POISONING; POISONING, TOXIDROMES; AND POISONING, ANTIDOTES

SUGGESTED READINGS

American College of Emergency Physicians. Clinical policy for the initial approach to patients with acute toxic ingestions or dermal or inhalation exposure. Ann Emerg Med 1995;25:570–585.

Ellenhorn MJ, Schoonwald S, Ordog G, et al. Gut decontamination. In: Ellenhorn MJ, ed. Ellenhorn's medical toxicology, 2nd ed. Baltimore: Williams & Wilkins, 1997:66–78.

Perrone J, Hoffman RS, Goldfrank LR. Special considerations in gastric decontamination. Emerg Med Clin 1994;12:285–299.

Pond SM, Lewis-Driver DJ, Williams GM, et al. Gastric emptying in acute overdose: a prospective randomized controlled trial. Med J Aust 1995;163:345–349.

Author: Frank LoVecchio

Poisoning, Toxidromes

Clinical Presentation

SIGNS AND SYMPTOMS

Toxicologic Mnemonics

- Use the following mnemonics to remember the substances and drugs that can present each sign or symptom

Anion Gap Acidosis: A CAT MUD PILES

- AKA
- CO/cyanide
- Acetaminophen
- Toluene
- Methanol
- Uremia
- DKA
- Paraldehyde, phenformin/metformin
- Iron/INH
- Lactic acidosis
- Ethylene glycol
- Salicylates

Increased Osmolar Gap: ME DIE

- Methanol
- Ethylene glycol
- Diuretics (mannitol)
- Isopropyl alcohol
- Ethanol

Seizures: OTIS CAMPBELL

- Organophosphates
- Tricyclic antidepressants
- INH/insulin
- Sympathomimetics, salicylates
- Camphor/cocaine
- Amphetamines, anticholinergic agents
- Methylxanthines (theophylline, caffeine) mushrooms (monomethyl hydrazine group)
- PCP, pethidine (demerol), propoxyphene, plants (nicotine, water hemlock)
- Benzodiazepine withdrawal, GHB
- Ethanol withdrawal
- Lithium, lidocaine
- Lead, lindane

Mydriasis: AAAS

- Antihistamines
- Antidepressants
- Anticholinergics/atropine
- Sympathomimetics

Miosis: COPS

- Cholinergic/clonidine
- Opiates/organophosphates
- Phenothiazines/pilocarpine/pontine bleed
- Sedative hypnotics

Hypertension: CT SCAN

- Cocaine
- Theophylline
- Sympathomimetics
- Caffeine
- Anticholinergics/amphetamines
- Nicotine

Hypotension: CRASH

- Cocaine
- Reserpine
- Antidepressants/aminophylline
- Sedative-hypnotics
- Heroin

Bradycardia: PACED

- Propranolol (beta-blockers)
- Anticholinesterase inhibitors drugs
- Clonidine/calcium channel blockers
- Ethanol/alcohols
- Digoxin/Darvon (opiates)

Tachycardia: FAST

- Free base (cocaine)
- Anticholinergic/antihistamines/ amphetamines
- Sympathomimetics
- Theophylline

Hypothermia: COOLS

- Carbon monoxide
- Opiates
- Oral hypoglycemics
- Liquor
- Sedative hypnotics

Hyperthermia: NASA

- Neuroleptic malignant syndrome, nicotine
- Antihistamines
- Salicylates, sympathomimetics, serotonin syndrome
- Anticholinergics, antidepressants

Rapid respiration: PANT

- PCP, paraquat, pneumonitis
- ASA
- Noncardiogenic pulmonary edema
- Toxin-induced metabolic acidosis

Slow respiration: SLOW

- Sedative-hypnotics (GHB)
- Liquor
- Opiates
- Weed

Diaphoresis: SOAP

- Sympathomimetics
- Organophosphates
- Acetylsalicylic acid
- PCP

Drugs that cause pulmonary edema: MOPS

- Meprobamate, methadone
- Opiates, organophosphates
- Phenobarbital, propoxyphene, phenothiazines
- Salicylates, smoke inhalation, solvents

Toxidromes

Cholinergic: SLUDGE BAM

- Salivation
- Lacrimation
- Urination
- Diarrhea
- Emesis
- Bronchorrhea, bronchospasm, bradycardia (life-threatening)
- Abdominal discomfort
- Miosis

Anticholinergic

- Hyperthermia ("Hot as a hare, red as a beet")
- Dry skin ("Dry as a bone")
- Dilated pupils ("Blind as a bat")
- Delirium ("Mad as a hatter")
- Tachycardia
- Urgency retention

Sympathomimetic
- Diaphoresis
- Mydriasis
- Tachycardia
- Hypertension
- Hyperthermia
- Seizures

Opiate
- Miosis
- Hypovolemia
- Coma
- Bradycardia
- Hypotension

Withdrawal (Alcohol, Benzodiazepine, Barbiturates, Antihypertensives)
- Diarrhea
- Mydriasis
- Piloerection
- Tachycardia
- Lacrimation
- Hypertension
- Yawning
- Cramps
- Hallucinations
- Seizures with alcohol and benzodiazepine withdrawal

Dermatologic

Dry Skin
- Antihistamines
- Anticholinergics

Bullae
- Barbiturates

Acneiform Rash
- Bromides
- Chlorinated
- Aromatic hydrocarbons

Flushed or Red Appearance
- Anticholinergics
- Disulfiram reactions
- Niacin
- Boric acid
- Scombroid poisoning
- Chinese restaurant syndrome
- Carbon monoxide when nearly fatal
- Cyanide (rare)

Cyanosis
- Ergotamines
- Methemoglobinemia forming
  - —Nitrite
  - —Nitrate
  - —Dapsone
  - —Aniline dye
  - —Phenazopyridine

Odors
- Bitter almonds = cyanide
- Carrots = cicutoxins
- Fruity = DKA, isopropanol
- Garlic = organophosphates, arsenic
- Gasoline = petroleum distillates
- Mothballs = naphthalene, camphor
- Pears = chloral hydrate
- Pungent odor = ethchlorvynol
- Oil of wintergreen = methylsalicylate
- Rotten eggs = Hydrogen sulfide
- Peanut butter = Vacor

MECHANISM OF TOXICITY
- Anticholinergic
  - —Adrenergic imbalance results from inhibition of acetylcholine
- Cholinergic
  - —Excess parasympathetic stimulation and *cholinergic crisis* result from inhibition of acetylcholinesterase or increased activity at the acetylcholine receptor
- Opiates
  - —Differ in their agonist and antagonist properties at various opioid receptor sites
  - —μ-Receptor stimulation-full agonist
  - —κ and δ receptors share partial agonist and antagonist properties
- Sympathomimetic
  - —Stimulation of sympathetic effector organs (particularly the CNS)
- Withdrawal
  - —Hyperactivity of sympathetic nervous system predominates

Pre-Hospital

N/A

Diagnosis

N/A

Treatment

N/A

Disposition

N/A

Miscellaneous

ICD9: N/A

ICD10: N/A

SEE ALSO: POISONING; POISONING, ANTIDOTES; AND POISONING, GASTRIC DECONTAMINATION

SUGGESTED READINGS

Bradberry S, Vale A. Multiple-dose activated charcoal: a review of relevant clinical studies. J Toxicol Clin Toxicol 1995;33(5):407–416.

Erickson TB. Toxicology update: a rational approach to managing the poisoned patient. Emerg Med Pract 2001;3(8).

Goldfrank L, Flomenbaum N, Lewin N, et al. Goldfrank's toxicological emergencies, 6th ed. Norwalk, CT: Appleton and Lange, 1998:277–283.

Krenzelok E, Vale A. Summary of American Academy of Clinical Toxicology and European Association of Poison Centres and Clinical Toxicologists position: statements on gut decontamination. J Toxicol Clin Toxicol 1997;35:695–762.

Author: Kirk Cumpston

Polio

Clinical Presentation

SIGNS AND SYMPTOMS

- Fever (37–39°C)
- Malaise
- Anorexia/nausea/vomiting
- Upper respiratory tract symptoms
- Headache, photophobia
- Nuchal rigidity

Neurologic Changes

- Muscle soreness that becomes severe muscle spasm, progressing rapidly to spotty flaccid weakness and paralysis
- Asymmetric paralysis more prominent in the lower than the upper extremities
- Urinary retention (50% of paralytic cases)
- Reflexes
  —Initially hyperactive, then absent
- Apprehensive and irritable, occasionally drowsy
- No sensory loss associated with the motor deficit

MECHANISM/DESCRIPTION

- Caused by poliovirus infection
- Incubation period 9–12 days
- Duration <1 week
- Clinical manifestations are defined as follows:
  —Subclinical (i.e., not apparent) 90–95%
  —*Abortive poliomyelitis* 4–8%
    -Clinically indistinct from many other viral infections (fever, myalgias, malaise)
    -Only suspected to be polio during an epidemic
  —*Nonparalytic poliomyelitis* 1–2%
    -Differs from abortive poliomyelitis by the presence of meningeal irritation
    -Course similar to any aseptic meningitis
  —Paralytic poliomyelitis 0.1%, which is further subdivided:
    -*Spinal paralytic poliomyelitis* (frank polio)
    -*Bulbar paralytic poliomyelitis* (10% of paralytic polio): paralysis of muscle groups innervated by cranial nerves; involves the circulatory and respiratory centers of the medulla with high mortality
    -*Mixed bulbospinal poliomyelitis*
- *Postpoliomyelitis syndrome*
  —New onset of muscle weakness, pain, and atrophy
  —Occurs many years after the active illness, usually in the previously affected limb
  —Gradual progression

ETIOLOGY

- Polioviruses
  —Picornaviruses
  —Small, nonenveloped, RNA viruses of the enterovirus genera
- Fecal-oral route transmission
- Humans are the only natural host and reservoir
- Poliovirus selectively destroys motor and autonomic neurons
- Natural (wild) virus is completely eliminated in North and Latin America
- Oral poliovirus vaccine (OPV)
  —Accounts for only poliomyelitis seen in the U.S. [8–10 cases per year of vaccine-associated paralysis (VAP)]
  —Incidence of VAP: 1 in 700,000
  —Use no longer recommended in U.S.

PEDIATRIC CONSIDERATIONS

- More likely to have a biphasic acute course
  —Viral-type syndrome for 1–2 days
  —Symptom-free period of 2–5 days
  —Then an abrupt onset of the major illness

Pre-Hospital

CAUTIONS

- Rare fatal case comes from respiratory insufficiency, which requires prompt ventilatory support

Diagnosis

ESSENTIAL WORKUP

- Clinical diagnosis
- Differentiate from other causes of acute paralysis
- Notify public health officials when diagnosis suspected

LABORATORY

- CBC
  —WBC normal or mildly elevated
- CSF analysis
  —Abnormalities typical of aseptic meningitis (increased lymphocytes and elevated protein)
  —Poliovirus rarely isolated from the CSF
- Diagnosis confirmed by:
  —Comparing acute to convalescent sera for antigen titers
  —Isolation of virus from blood or CSF

DIFFERENTIAL DIAGNOSIS

- Abortive poliomyelitis is similar to many viral illnesses
- Nonparalytic poliomyelitis is indistinguishable from any viral, aseptic meningitis
- Paralytic poliomyelitis
  —Guillain-Barré (not febrile, symmetrical, not ill appearing)
  —Acute transverse myelitis
  —Diphtheria
  —Botulism
  —Tick paralysis
  —Encephalitis

Treatment

INITIAL STABILIZATION

- Aggressive pulmonary toilet and early intubation mandated for respiratory insufficiency

ED TREATMENT

- Supportive and symptomatic management
- Analgesics for severe muscle pain and spasm
- Bed rest to prevent augmentation or extension of paralysis
- Paralytic poliomyelitis tends to localize to a limb that has been the site of intramuscular injection or injury within 2–4 weeks prior to the onset of infection
  —Avoid any unnecessary tissue damage in suspected cases
- No antiviral agents available

Prevention

- Inactivated polio virus (IPV)
  —Costly
  —Painful
  —No conferred immunity
  —However, no vaccine-associated paralysis (VAP)
- Oral poliovirus vaccine (OPV)
  —Accounted for only poliomyelitis seen in the U.S. [8–10 cases per year of vaccine-associated paralysis (VAP)]
  —Incidence of VAP: 1 in 700,000
  —Confers immunity to unvaccinated contacts by fecal-oral spread
  —Inexpensive
  —No longer recommended

Disposition

ADMISSION CRITERIA

- All acute-phase paralytic poliomyelitis for strict bed rest and observation for respiratory symptoms
  —Isolate from nonvaccinated personnel

DISCHARGE CRITERIA

- No evidence of nervous system involvement and no danger of contact with nonvaccinated population
  —Deterioration of muscle strength usually ends after 3–5 days

Miscellaneous

ICD9: 045.1

ICD10: A80.9

SUGGESTED READINGS

American Academy of Pediatrics. Poliomyelitis prevention: revised recommendations for use of inactivated and live oral poliovirus vaccines. Pediatrics 1999;103:171–172.

Centers for Disease Control. Notice to readers: recommendations of the Advisory Committee on Immunization Practices: revised recommendations for routine poliomyelitis vaccination. MMWR 1999;48:590.

Minor PD. Eradication of polio by vaccination. Virology 2000;268:231–232.

Modlin JF. Poliovirus. In: Mandell GL, Bennett JE, Dolin R, eds. Mandell, Douglas, and Bennett's principles and practice of infectious diseases, 4th ed. New York: Churchill Livingstone, 1995:1613–1620.

Mulder DW. Clinical observations on acute poliomyelitis. Ann NY Acad Sci 1995;753:1–10.

Pascuzzi RM. Poliomyelitis and the postpolio syndrome. Semin Neurol 1992;12(3):193–199.

Racaniello VR, Ren R. Poliovirus biology and pathogenesis. Curr Top Microbiol Immunol 1996;206:305–325.

Author: Philip Shayne

Polycythemia

Clinical Presentation

SIGNS AND SYMPTOMS

General
- Dyspnea
- Weakness
- Sweating
- Weight loss
- Epistaxis
- Pruritus
- Gout
- Erythromelalgia
  —Burning pain in the feet or hands associated with warmth and erythema of the affected areas

Neurologic
- Headache
- Vertigo/dizziness
- Paresthesias
- Scotoma, blurred vision
- Tinnitus
- CVA/TIA

Cardiovascular
- Congestive heart failure/angina
- Hypertension
- Digital artery occlusion
- DVT

Abdominal
- Epigastric discomfort
- Peptic ulcer disease/GI bleed
- Hepatomegaly/splenomegaly

MECHANISM/DESCRIPTION
- Excessive erythropoiesis leading to proliferation of erythroid, myeloid, and megakaryocyte elements in the bone marrow
- Hematocrit >52% = exponential rise in blood viscosity

Classification of Polycythemia
- Relative and stress polycythemia
  —Resulting from decrease in plasma volume
- Primary polycythemia vera
  —Three stages:
    -Proliferative stage: increase in RBCs, megakaryocytes, platelets
    -Stable phase: return of blood counts to normal values due to replacement of marrow by fibrosis
    -Spent phase: extensive marrow fibrosis—peripheral cytopenia
  —Occurs age >60
  —Increase incidence of leukemia later
- Secondary polycythemia
  —Appropriately increased erythropoietin caused by tissue hypoxia
  —Inappropriate autonomous erythropoietin production

Bleeding and Thrombosis
- Increased blood viscosity due to elevated hematocrit
- Platelet abnormalities in 80%
- Decreased factor XII, prekallikrein, and kallikrein inhibitors

Pre-Hospital

N/A

Diagnosis

ESSENTIAL WORKUP
- CBC
  —Elevated RBC mass
  —Low MCV due to decreased iron stores
  —Thrombocytosis with large, hypogranular platelets

LABORATORY
- Bleeding time prolonged in 11% of patients

Diagnostic Criteria
- Category A
  —A1: increased RBC mass
    -Male: >36 mL/kg
    -Female: >32 mL/kg
  —A2: oxygen saturation >92%
  —A3: splenomegaly
- Category B
  —B1: platelets >400,000/mm^3
  —B2: WBC >12,000/mm^3
  —B3: B_{12} >900 pg/mL; unbound vitamin B_{12} binding capacity >2,200 pg/mL
- Diagnosis established by either of these combinations:
  —Presence of all three category A criteria
  —A1 + A2 + any two category B criteria

IMAGING/SPECIAL TESTS
- CT scan if CVA or AMS

DIFFERENTIAL DIAGNOSIS
- Secondary polycythemia
  —Right-to-left shunt congenital heart disease
  —Pulmonary disease
  —Carboxyhemoglobinemia
  —High altitude
  —Decreased tissue oxygen release from high oxygen-affinity hemoglobinopathies
- Inappropriate autonomous erythropoietin production
  —Renal origin: carcinoma, hydronephrosis cyst
  —Other lesions: uterine fibroids, hepatoma of adrenal origin, cerebellar hemangioma
  —Congenital overproduction

Treatment

INITIAL STABILIZATION

- ABCs

ED TREATMENT

- IV rehydration for relative polycythemia (dehydration)
- Pruritus
  - —H_1 blockers: cyproheptadine 4 mg PO t.i.d.
  - —H_2 blockers: cimetidine 300 mg PO t.i.d.
- Hyperuricemia: allopurinol 100–400 mg PO qd

Primary Polycythemia Vera

- Antithrombotic therapy
  - —Low-dose aspirin
- Phlebotomy
  - —For Hct >60%
  - —To bring hematocrit to 45%
  - —500 cc blood withdrawn followed by infusion of 500 cc 0.9% NS
  - —May need to remove 1–1.5 L over 24 hours
- Myelosuppressive therapy
  - —^{32}P (radioactive phosphorus)
  - —Hydroxyurea
  - —Interferon
- Thrombocytosis
  - —Plateletpheresis for platelet count >1,000,000 mm^3 or with thrombosis or hemorrhage
- Splenectomy
  - —If severe thrombocytopenia
  - —Contraindicated if DIC due to uncontrolled hemorrhage
- Surgery with polycythemia
  - —Increased morbidity and mortality
  - —Elective procedures until polycythemia is under control
  - —For emergency surgery, need:
    - -Emergent phlebotomy to lower hematocrit to <45%
    - -Control thrombocytosis with therapeutic plateletpheresis

Cautions

- No studies have shown that lowering the Hct improves survival or reduces rate of thrombotic complications
- Difficult to decrease Hct while maintaining adequate oxygenation (right-to-left shunt or COPD)
- If reduced plasma volume, phlebotomy may worsen hypovolemia and produce shock

Disposition

ADMISSION CRITERIA

- New diagnosis of polycythemia
- Unstable vital signs/underlying medical problems
- Inability to comply with outpatient treatment or follow-up

DISCHARGE CRITERIA

- Previous diagnosis of polycythemia and requiring outpatient phlebotomy
- Stable vital signs

Miscellaneous

ICD9: 238.4

ICD10: D45

SUGGESTED READINGS

Berk PD, Goldberg JD, Fruchtman SM, et al. Therapeutic recommendations in polycythemia vera based on polycythemia vera study group protocols. Semin Hematol 1986;23(2):132–143.

Bilgrami S, Greenberg BR. Polycythemia rubra vera. Semin Oncol 1995;22(4): 307–326.

Braunwald E, Isselbacher K, et al., eds. Harrison's principles of internal medicine, 15th ed. New York: McGraw-Hill, 2001.

Hoffman R, Benz E, Shattil S, et al., eds. Hematology: basic principles and practice, 3rd ed. New York: Churchill Livingstone, 2000.

Landaw S, Williams W. Deciphering polycythemia. Hosp Pract 1996;3:155–166.

Author: Marc Gelman

Postpartum Hemorrhage

Clinical Presentation

SIGNS AND SYMPTOMS

- Ongoing blood loss, usually painless
- Significant hypovolemia, resulting in tachycardia, tachypnea, narrow pulse pressure, decreased urine output, cool clammy skin, poor capillary refill, altered mental status
- Maternal tachycardia and hypotension may not manifest until blood loss exceeds 1,500 mL
- If bleeding is present at other sites, consider coagulopathy

MECHANISM/DESCRIPTION

- *Immediate postpartum hemorrhage (PPH):* hemorrhage occurring within 24 hours of delivery
- *Delayed PPH:* hemorrhage occurring 24 hours or more after delivery, often 1–2 weeks postpartum

ETIOLOGY

- *Immediate PPH:* uterine atony, lower genital lacerations, retained placental tissue, placenta accreta, uterine rupture, uterine inversion, puerperal hematoma, coagulopathies
- *Delayed PPH:* retained products of conception, postpartum endometritis, withdrawal of exogenous estrogen, puerperal hematoma
- Coagulopathies: preexisting ITP, TTP, von Willebrand's disease, DIC

Pre-Hospital

CAUTIONS

- Patients with postpartum hemorrhage may be hemodynamically unstable and require intravenous access and fluid resuscitation

Diagnosis

ESSENTIAL WORKUP

- Abdomen and pelvic examination to access for uterine atony, retained products, or other anatomic abnormality
- Type and cross-match for packed red blood cells (PRBCs)
- Rapid hemoglobin determination

LABORATORY

- CBC
- PT, PTT, platelets, fibrinogen
- Type and cross-match

IMAGING/SPECIAL TESTS

- Ultrasound may be helpful to evaluate for retained products in delayed PPH

DIFFERENTIAL DIAGNOSIS

- Consider puerperal hematomas if perineal, rectal, or lower abdominal pain in conjunction with tachycardia and hypotension

Treatment

INITIAL STABILIZATION

- Attempts to control bleeding and stabilize hemodynamic status proceed simultaneously
- ABC
  - —Supplemental oxygen
  - —Cardiac monitor
- IV fluid resuscitation with normal saline (NS) or lactated Ringer's (LR)
- Foley catheter

ED TREATMENT

- Management of uterine atony
  - —Bimanual massage
  - —Oxytocin (Pitocin) administered IV/IM
  - —Methylergonovine (Methergine) or ergonovine (Ergotrate) IM if oxytocin fails; avoid if known hypertensive; onset in minutes
  - —15-methyl PGF_{2a} (Hemabate) IM if above fails; relatively contraindicated in asthma
  - —Surgery if medical intervention fails
- Inspect closely for genital tract laceration
  - —2 cm or greater require repair
  - —00 or 000 absorbable suture; continuous, locked recommended
- Management of uterine inversion (acute)
  - —Reposition uterus using Johnson maneuver or Harris methods
  - —Use left hand on abdominal wall to stabilize fundus of uterus; place right hand with fingers spread into vagina and push steadily on inverted part to reduce
  - —If unsuccessful, give terbutaline IV or $MgSO_4$ to produce cervical relaxation and reposition
  - —Surgery if unsuccessful or if subacute or chronic inversion
- Management of coagulopathies
  - —FFP, platelets, cryoprecipitate as indicated
  - —Careful attention to volume status
  - —Continuous reassessment

MEDICATIONS

Uterotonics: Stimulate Uterine Contraction to Control Bleeding

- Ergonovine (Ergotrate): 0.2 mg i.m., avoid if known hypertensive
- Methylergonovine (Methergine): 0.2 mg i.m.; 0.2 mg PO q6h; avoid if known hypertensive
- 15-methyl PGF_{2a} (Hemabate): 0.25 mg i.m.; may repeat in 15–60 min
- Oxytocin (Pitocin): 20–40 IU in 1 L NS at 200 mL/h; do not use for resuscitation

Cervical Relaxation: Facilitate Uterine Inversion Reduction

- Magnesium sulfate 20%: 2 g i.v. bolus over 10 min
- Terbutaline: 0.25 mg i.v.; avoid if hypotensive

Disposition

ADMISSION CRITERIA

- All patients with immediate PPH require admission to a closely monitored setting
- Early obstetrics consultation recommended
- Early surgical intervention dependent on etiology
- ICU setting if DIC or evidence of hemodynamic compromise
- Patients with endometritis should be admitted for parenteral antibiotics

DISCHARGE CRITERIA

- Delayed PPH without excessive bleeding that is easily controlled
- Outpatient management with methylergonovine 0.2 mg orally every 6 hours may be considered in consultation and close follow-up with obstetrician

Miscellaneous

ICD9: 666.10

ICD10: 046.8

SUGGESTED READINGS

Druelinger L. Postpartum emergencies. Emerg Med Clin North Am 1994;12(1): 219–237.

Gilstrap LC, Ramin SM. Postpartum hemorrhage. Clin Obstet Gynecol 1994;37(4):824–830.

Kuhn G. Emergencies during pregnancy and the postpartum period. In: Tintinalli JE, Kelen GD, Stapczynski JS, eds. Emergency medicine: a comprehensive study guide, 5th ed. New York: McGraw-Hill, 2000.

Mallon W, Henderson S. Labor and delivery. In: Marx JA, Hockberger RS, Walls RM, eds. Rosen's emergency medicine: concepts and clinical practice, 5th ed. St Louis: Mosby, 2002.

Roberts WE. Emergent obstetric management of postpartum hemorrhage. Obstet Gynecol Clin North Am 1995;22(2): 283–302.

Authors: Marco Coppola; Clyde Turner

Postpartum Infection

Clinical Presentation

SIGNS AND SYMPTOMS

- Persistent fever and chills
- Localized pain and swelling
- Lower abdominal pain
- Foul-smelling lochia, cervical motion tenderness, uterine tenderness
- Absence of other sources of infection; however, in the presence of these signs and symptoms, genital tract infection should be assumed until ruled out

MECHANISM/DESCRIPTION

- *Early postpartum endometritis (PPE):* develops within 48 hours; most often complicating cesarean section
- *Late postpartum endometritis:* develops after 3 days to 6 weeks, usually following vaginal delivery
- *Septic pelvic thrombophlebitis:* diagnosis of exclusion; two distinct clinical presentations, either of which may present with postpartum pulmonary embolus
  - —Acute thrombosis: most common right ovarian vein, usually occurring in first 48 hours as acute, progressive lower abdominal pain
  - —Enigmatic fever: "picket fence" spiking fevers and tachycardia

ETIOLOGY

- Polymicrobial infection result of ascending spread from lower genital tract
- Anaerobic (up to 80%) and aerobic ($\sim$70%)
  - —Gram-positive aerobes: group A, B streptococcus, enterococcus and *Gardnerella vaginalis*
  - —Gram-negative aerobes: *Escherichia coli, Enterobacter*
  - —Anaerobes: bacteroides, *Peptostreptococcus*
  - —Other genital mycoplasmas (urea plasma urealyticum and mycoplasma hominis), *Chlamydia trachomatis*—common in late PPE

Pre-Hospital

N/A

Diagnosis

ESSENTIAL WORKUP

- Abdominal and pelvic examination
- Cervical cultures for chlamydia
- Transcervical endometrial cultures

LABORATORY

- CBC
- Urinalysis and culture
- Blood cultures

IMAGING/SPECIAL TESTS

- CT or MRI for ovarian vein thrombosis—nonurgent
- Ultrasound—sensitive for abscess

DIFFERENTIAL DIAGNOSIS

- Fever from other sources
  - —<6 hours
    - -Early streptococcal infection
    - -Transfusion reaction
    - -Thyroid crisis
  - —<48 hours
    - -Atelectasis
  - —<72 hours
    - -Urinary tract infection
    - -Pneumonia
  - —3–5 days
    - -Mastitis
    - -Breast engorgement
    - -Necrotizing fasciitis
  - —3–7 days
    - -Mastitis
    - -Septic thrombophlebitis
  - —7–14 days
    - -Abscess
  - —>2 weeks
    - -Mastitis
    - -Pulmonary embolism

Treatment

INITIAL STABILIZATION

- ABC
  - —Prompt evaluation of respiratory and hemodynamic status
  - —Supplemental oxygen, cardiac monitor, and pulse oximetry as needed
  - —Venous access; support circulatory status with crystalloid and pressors if needed

ED TREATMENT

- IV antibiotics and close observation
  - —Several choices are appropriate for initial therapy:
    - -Cefoxitin
    - -Ticarcillin/clavulanate (Timentin)
    - -Imipenem cilastatin (Primaxin)
    - -Meropenem
    - -Ampicillin/sulbactam (Unasyn)
    - -Piperacillin/tazobactam *plus* doxycycline
    - -Clindamycin *plus* gentamicin or antipseudomonal third-generation cephalosporin
    - -Trovafloxacin
- Heparin if suspicion or evidence of thrombophlebitis
- Infected wound or abscess should be opened to establish drainage
- Necrotizing fasciitis requires wide surgical débridement, parenteral antibiotics, and adjunctive hyperbaric oxygen therapy
- Peritonitis requires imaging to evaluate cause: AAS, CT

MEDICATIONS

- Ampicillin/sulbactam: 3 g i.v. q6h
- Cefoxitin: 2 g i.v. q6h
- Clindamycin: 900-mg load, then 600 mg i.v. q6–8h
- Gentamicin: 2-mg/kg load, then 1–1.5 mg/kg i.v. q8h
- Heparin: 80-IU/kg loading dose, then 18 IU/kg/h i.v.
- Imipenem cilastatin: 500 mg i.v. q6h
- Meropenem: 1.0 g i.v. q8h
- Mezlocillin: 4 g i.v. q6h
- Piperacillin/tazobactam: 4.5 g i.v. q8h
- Ticarcillin/clavulanate: 3.1 g i.v. q4h
- Trovafloxacin: 300 mg i.v., then 200 mg PO qd

Disposition

ADMISSION CRITERIA

- Patients with endometritis or suspicion for septic pelvic thrombophlebitis should be admitted

DISCHARGE CRITERIA

- Nontoxic, mildly symptomatic patient with late PPE may be considered for outpatient management with erythromycin (500 mg orally q.i.d.) in consultation and close follow-up with obstetrics

Miscellaneous

ICD9: 615.9

ICD10: O23.5

SUGGESTED READINGS

Calhoun BC, Brost B. Emergency management of sudden puerperal fever. Obstet Gynecol Clin North Am 1995;22(2): 357–367.

Druelinger L. Postpartum emergencies. Emerg Med Clin North Am 1994;12(1): 219–237.

Tintinalli J, Kelen G, Stapcynski J, eds. Emergency medicine: a comprehensive study guide, 5th ed. New York: McGraw-Hill, 2000.

Authors: Tim Stallard; Marco Coppola

Preeclampsia/Eclampsia

Clinical Presentation

SIGNS AND SYMPTOMS

Preeclampsia

- Most common in late third trimester

Mild Preeclampsia

- Sudden weight gain may precede other symptoms (>2 lb/wk)
- Hypertension BP 140/90 if unknown baseline; SBP >130 or DBP >80 on two occasions
- Dependent edema progressing to constant edema
- Proteinuria—develops later, wide fluctuation over 24 hours; single urine sample may be negative even in severe cases

Severe Preeclampsia

- Epigastric pain/RUQ pain mimicking cholelithiasis due to hepatocellular necrosis w/edema and stretch of capsule
- Abdominal pain
  - —Nausea and vomiting
- Thrombocytopenia
- Hyperreflexia
- Severe and worsening headache
  - —Visual disturbances including blindness
  - —Hyperreflexia
  - —Oliguria, proteinuria >3+ dipstick, BP >160/110

Eclampsia

- Seizures in patient with pregnancy-induced hypertension (PIH) or preeclampsia
  - —Tonic-clonic activity
- Seizures may occur pre-, peri- or postpartum; majority of postpartum seizures occur within 48 hours but have been documented 10–20 days after delivery
- Unrelenting severe headache +/− visual disturbances typically precede seizures

MECHANISM/DESCRIPTION

PIH-Preeclampsia-Eclampsia Spectrum

- Pregnancy-induced hypertension
  - —Relative or absolute hypertension during pregnancy

Preeclampsia

- Relative or absolute hypertension in pregnancy associated with proteinuria and edema
- Syndrome accompanied by progressive weight gain and diffuse symptoms (see above); number and severity of symptoms correlate with development of eclampsia, subsequent morbidity, and mortality

Eclampsia

- Clinical end point of PIH and preeclampsia
- Up to 2% of preeclamptic women progress to eclampsia

Risk Factors

- Extremes of reproductive age (<20 or >35 years)
- Primigravida
- Multiple gestation
  - —Molar pregnancy, hydrops fetalis
  - —Smoking, hypercholesteremia
- Diabetes, collagen vascular disturbances
- Preexisting renal disease or hypertension (pregnancy-aggravated hypertension; see Differential Diagnosis, below)

ETIOLOGY

- Diffuse arteriolar vasospasm with secondary endothelial activation, microthrombi formation, ischemia
- Heightened vascular permeability
- Exact cause of vasospasm unknown but patients demonstrate increased sensitivity to endogenous vasopressors and decreased prostacyclin production

Pre-Hospital

- Consider eclampsia in any patient >20 weeks pregnant with seizure
  - —Consider in pregnant trauma patient without obvious cause (e.g., single-vehicle MVA)
  - —Transport patient in left lateral recumbent position
- Manage seizures as described below (see below)
- Transport patient to closest facility with high-risk obstetric capability

Diagnosis

ESSENTIAL WORKUP

- History and physical examination with special attention to mental status, neurologic exam, abdominal exam
- Vital signs (blood pressure)
- Stat blood sugar
- Urinalysis for protein

LABORATORY

- Proteinuria on dipstick >1, send urine for 24-hour protein
- Urine sediment for RBC, WBC casts
- PT/PTT, platelets (<150K)
- BUN, creatinine
- Liver function tests
- Urine toxicology—sympathomimetics
- Fetal monitoring/stress test

IMAGING/SPECIAL TESTS

- Emergent ultrasound for EGA, fetal viability
- Head CT after airway stabilization—evaluate for intracranial masses, bleeding
- Lumbar puncture to assess intracranial hemorrhage or infection as cause for seizure

PATHOLOGIC FINDINGS

- Widespread fibrin deposits in small vessels especially kidney and liver
- Microvascular changes in placental flow may effect fetal well-being

DIFFERENTIAL DIAGNOSIS

Preeclampsia

- Chronic hypertension, PIH, pregnancy-aggravated hypertension (chronic hypertension with superimposed PIH or preeclampsia)
- Flare in underlying renal or collagen vascular diseases
- Hydatidiform mole
- Hydrops fetalis
- Concomitant drug abuse

Eclampsia

- Epilepsy
- Encephalitis
- Meningitis
- Encephalopathy
- Brain tumor
- Intracranial hemorrhage
- Hysteria

Treatment

INITIAL STABILIZATION

- ABCs
- Left lateral decubitus position (reduces pressure on IVC, enhancing cardiac return/output)
- 100% O_2, maternal cardiac and tocographic monitoring, fetal monitoring
- Treat seizures—$MgSO_4$ is first choice for seizure prophylaxis and treatment in severe preeclampsia and eclampsia
- Valium and phenytoin are considered second- and third-line treatments for seizures

ED TREATMENT

- Seizure prophylaxis for severe preeclampsia ($MgSO_4$)
  - —Treat hypertension—hydralazine and labetalol are preferred antihypertensive agents
  - —Avoid diuretics—patient is typically intravascularly volume-depleted; diuretics can induce placental hypoperfusion and secondary fetal hypoxia
  - —Obstetrical consult
- Emergent delivery for severe symptoms
- C-section delivery in most severe cases

MEDICATIONS

- Calcium gluconate: 1 g i.v. slowly to reverse hypermagnesemia
- Hydralazine: 5–20 mg i.v.
- Labetalol: 10 mg i.v. initially, then 5–10 mg increments for desired effect
- $MgSO_4$: 2–4 g IVP; followed by 2 g/h i.v. drip *or* 10 mg i.m.; $MgSO_4$ infusion should not exceed 1 g/min; serum Mg goal 4–7 mEq/L; monitor blood pressure, DTRs, and respiratory rate for signs of magnesium toxicity (absent patellar reflex, respiratory depression)
- Phenytoin: 15–18 mg/kg, 25–50 mg/min i.v.
- Valium: 5–10 g i.v. if no analeptic response to $MgSO_4$

Disposition

ADMISSION CRITERIA

- All patients with preeclampsia should be admitted
- Eclamptic patients should be admitted to ICU, labor and delivery, or OR

DISCHARGE CRITERIA

- Patients that are completely asymptomatic with a negative workup (i.e., no proteinuria or other lab abnormalities) may be considered for outpatient management with close Ob-Gyn follow-up

Miscellaneous

PROGNOSIS

- Improved maternal and fetal mortality with aggressive seizure management, early delivery of fetus
  - —Perinatal mortality: 37.9/1,000 births
  - —Neonatal loss largely due to preterm delivery; neonatal mortality and morbidity increased if chronic hypertension or PIH present
  - —In less severe cases, delivery determined by fetal gestational age and lung maturity

ASSOCIATED CONDITIONS

- Renal failure
  - —Pulmonary edema
- Collagen vascular diseases
- Slight increased incidence of abruption

ICD9: 642.40, 780.39

ICD10: 014.9, 015.0

SUGGESTED READINGS

Cunningham FG, MacDonald PC, Grant NF, eds. Williams' obstetrics, 20th ed. Norwalk, CT: Appleton & Lange, 1997.

Evans SD. Preeclampsia/Eclampsia. In: Rosen P, Barkin RM, Hayden SR, et al. eds. Rosen's 5-minute emergency medicine consult, 1st ed. Philadelphia: Lippincott, Williams & Wilkins, 1999.

Houry D, Abbott JT. Acute complications of pregnancy. In: Marx JA, ed. Rosen's emergency medicine, 5th ed. St. Louis: CV Mosby, 2002:2413–2433

Walker JJ. Severe pre-eclampsia and eclampsia. Baillieres Clin Obstet Gynaecol 2000;14(1):57–71.

Author: Elaine M. Sapiro

Preexcitation Syndromes

Clinical Presentation

SIGNS AND SYMPTOMS

- Asymptomatic
- Palpitations
  - —Fast or irregular
- Chest pain
- Dyspnea
- Dizziness
- Nausea
- Diaphoresis
- Tachycardia up to 250 bpm
  - —Rapid and regular (SVT)
  - —Irregular (atrial fibrillation)
- Signs of instability (changes treatment)
  - —Chest pain
  - —Hypotension
  - —Change in mental status
  - —Rales
  - —Cyanosis

MECHANISM/DESCRIPTION

- A group of conditions characterized by an accessory pathway
  - —Connects the atria and the ventricles by bypassing the AV node
  - —Conduction is faster and the refractory period is shorter
  - —Sum of vectors allows for shorter PR intervals
  - —Prototypical pathways are the bundle of Kent and the Mahaim fibers
  - —Allows for early depolarization of the ventricles generating rapid supraventricular tachycardias
- Wolff-Parkinson-White (WPW) syndrome
  - —Type A, or orthodromic, is the most common (70%)
    - -Impulse travels down the AV node and then up the retrograde pathway
    - -A circuit is created that potentiates reentrant tachycardia
  - —Type B or antidromic
    - -Less common than type A
    - -The circuit operates in the opposite direction
- Lown-Ganong-Levine syndrome
  - —Rare preexcitation syndrome with an accessory pathway in the AV node
- The majority of patients with accessory pathways never become symptomatic
- Risk of death is very low (0.1–4%)
  - —Preexcitation with wide complex tachycardia is most at risk for ventricular dysrhythmias
- Prevalence is estimated at 0.1–0.3% of the population
- Men are affected twice as often as women
- Most are young and healthy

PEDIATRIC CONSIDERATIONS

- Most supraventricular tachycardias in children are the result of AV nodal reentry
- 10% are the result of an identified preexcitation syndrome

ETIOLOGY

- Idiopathic
- In association with structural heart disease
  - —Cardiomyopathy
  - —Transposition of the great vessels
  - —Mitral valve prolapse
  - —Ebstein's anomaly

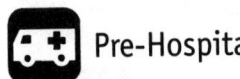

Pre-Hospital

CAUTIONS

- Supplemental oxygen
- Monitor
- Synchronized cardioversion
  - —If signs of instability
  - —Atrial fibrillation with WPW and wide complex tachycardia

CONTROVERSIES

- Pre-hospital use of adenosine
  - —Stable patients do not require emergent conversion
  - —Unstable patients should undergo cardioversion, not adenosine
  - —Recognition of rhythm by paramedics

Diagnosis

ESSENTIAL WORKUP

- The diagnosis is made on the 12-lead EKG
- Preexisting history
- Stable patients must be carefully monitored and reassessed for signs of instability

LABORATORY

- Cardiac enzymes only if signs of ischemia
- Consider electrolytes

IMAGING/SPECIAL TESTS

- EKG
  - —WPW syndrome
  - —Short PR <0.12 seconds
  - —Prolonged QRS >0.10 seconds
  - —*Delta wave*: small slurred upstroke at the beginning of the QRS

DIFFERENTIAL DIAGNOSIS

- AV nodal reentry SVT
- Ventricular tachycardia

Treatment

INITIAL STABILIZATION

- Unstable patients
  - —Synchronized cardioversion starting with 50 Joules
  - —Increase incrementally until sinus rhythm is restored
- Stable patients with wide complex tachycardia
  - —Procainamide

ED TREATMENT

- Stable patients with narrow complex, regular tachycardia
  - —Vagal maneuvers such as a Valsalva
  - —Right carotid artery massage for no more than 10 seconds
    - -Auscultate the artery first for a bruit that would contraindicate this procedure
  - —Fluid replacement and Trendelenburg position if the patient has mild hypotension
  - —Pharmacologic conversion if carotid massage fails
    - -Adenosine
    - -Verapamil
- Irregular wide complex tachycardia
  - —Procainamide or magnesium is effective
  - —Never use calcium channel blockers, beta-blockers, or digoxin
    - -These medications block the AV node
    - -Conduction occurs exclusively down the faster accessory pathway
    - -Precipitation of ventricular dysrhythmias

PEDIATRIC CONSIDERATIONS

- Children may develop ventricular rates up to 320 bpm that are poorly tolerated
- Cardiovert unstable children with 0.5–2 J/kg
- Vagal maneuvers and adenosine are safe in stable children

MEDICATIONS

- Adenosine: 6 mg rapid i.v. push; if ineffective, repeat with 12 mg; peds: 0.1 mg/kg rapid i.v. push; if ineffective, then 0.2 mg/kg i.v. push
- Diltiazem: 0.25 mg/kg i.v. over 2 min followed in 15 min by 0.35 mg/kg i.v. over 2 min
- Esmolol: 0.5 mg/kg over 1 min; maintenance infusion at 0.05 mg/kg/min over 4 min, then 0.1–0.2 mg/kg/min continuously
- Magnesium: 2 g i.v. bolus
- Procainamide: 20 mg/min until arrhythmia controlled, hypotension, or QRS widens by 50% up to a total dose of 17 mg/kg, then 2–6 mg/min
- Verapamil: 2.5–5 mg i.v. bolus over 2 min; may repeat with 5–10 mg every 15–30 min to max of 20 mg

Disposition

ADMISSION CRITERIA

- Patients with signs of instability require admission to a monitored bed
- Failure of outpatient therapy for continuous pharmacologic control or ablation

DISCHARGE CRITERIA

- The majority of patients will be stable and can be discharged once converted to sinus rhythm
- Follow-up should be arranged
- Electrophysiologic studies with possible ablative therapy during the outpatient workup
- Consider low-dose verapamil prophylaxis

Miscellaneous

ICD9: 426.7

ICD10: I45.6

SEE ALSO: WOLFF-PARKINSON-WHITE (WPW) SYNDROME

SUGGESTED READINGS

Rosner MH, Brady WJ Jr, Kefer MP, et al. Electrocardiography in the patient with the Wolff-Parkinson-White syndrome: diagnostic and initial therapeutic issues. Am J Emerg Med 1999;17:705–714.

Tintinalli JE, Ruiz E, Krome RL, eds. Emergency medicine: a comprehensive study guide, 4th ed. New York: McGraw-Hill, 1996.

Wellens HJ, Brugada P, Penn OC. The management of preexcitation syndromes. JAMA 1987;257(17):2325–2333.

Xie B, Thakur RK, Shah CP, et al. Clinical differentiation of narrow QRS complex tachycardia. Emerg Med Clin North Am 1998;16(2):295–330.

Author: Eric Glasser

Pregnancy, Trauma in

Clinical Presentation

SIGNS AND SYMPTOMS

- Abdominal pain
- Uterine contraction
- Vaginal bleeding, leakage of fluid
- Contusion, lap belt marks

MECHANISM/DESCRIPTION

- Fetal and maternal injury specific to pregnancy is evident after the first trimester
  —Increased rate of fetal loss, but not maternal mortality
- Likelihood of fetal injury increases with the severity of maternal insult
- Hypervolemic gestational state frequently leads to an underestimation of blood loss
  —Clinical shock may be apparent only after a 30% maternal blood loss
- Abdominal findings are less evident in the gravid patient
- Minor trauma can also lead to fetal injuries (at least 50% of fetal losses)
- Less frequent bowel injury
- More frequent retroperitoneal hemorrhage due to the engorgement of pelvic organs and veins (also increased severity)
- Increased morbidity and mortality with pelvic fractures due to pelvic and uterine engorgement
- Fetal or uterine trauma includes placental abruption, fetal maternal hemorrhage, premature labor, uterine contusion or rupture (prior C-section), fetal demise, premature membrane rupture, and hypoxemic or anatomic fetal injury (skull fracture)
- Abruption occurs in up to 50% of severe trauma and 1–5% of minor injuries, accounts for up to 50% of fetal loss, and may occur with no external bleeding (20%)
  —Hallmark is uterine contractions
- Fetal/maternal hemorrhage (FMH) occurs in more than 30% of severe trauma
  —Isoimmunization of Rh-negative mothers (with as little as 0.03 cc of FMH)
- Penetrating trauma results in direct injury to fetus, maternal shock, and premature delivery (more devastating to fetus/less maternal mortality: gravid uterus relatively protective)

ETIOLOGY

- Trauma occurs in about 7% of all pregnancies
- Motor vehicle (48–84%)
- Falls
- Direct abdominal trauma
- Penetrating (stab or gunshot)
- Electrical or burn
- Domestic violence (reported at over 14% of all pregnant women)

Pre-Hospital

CAUTIONS

- Patients in late second and third trimester should be transported to a trauma center
- Advise trauma center early of pregnancy and estimated gestational age (EGA) to facilitate early mobilization of fetal monitors, sonography, and of neonatal and obstetric consultants and equipment
- Place patient (while on backboard) in the left lateral recumbent position to avoid supine hypotension (after 24 weeks EGA)
- Mast suit inflation over the abdomen is contraindicated

Diagnosis

ESSENTIAL WORKUP

- Identify maternal condition first
- Follow ATLS guidelines
- Determine the gestational age (EGA) to assess viability
  —Estimate LMP
  —Fundal height (FH); EGA = FH (cm) × 8/7 after week 16
  —Doppler fetal heart tones
  —Sonography (may miss small abruptions)
- Fetal/maternal monitoring for >4–6 hours
  —Abruption does not occur in patients who have no contractions during the first 4 hours of monitoring
  —With >1 contraction/10 min, a 20% abruption incidence is reported
  —The occurrence of bradycardia, poor beat-to-beat variability, or type II "late" deceleration (after the peak of uterine contraction) indicates fetal distress

LABORATORY

- CBC, urinalysis
- Blood gas and electrolyte panel
- Type, Rh, and screening of blood
- The Kleihauer-Betke (KB) stain: identifies FMH in vaginal fluid or blood

IMAGING/SPECIAL TESTS

- Shield the uterus if possible, but *obtain necessary maternal x-rays*
- Fetal radiation injury is less than 1 event/ 1,000/rad exposure
- The rad exposure is estimated at the following:
  —C-spine and chest x-rays: <0.005 rad
  —Femur: <0.012 rad
  —AP pelvis, spine, KUB: 0.14–0.5 rad each
  —IVP: 0.2–0.8 rad
  —CT head: <0.05 rad; thorax: <1 rad; upper abdomen: <3 rad; lower abdomen/pelvis: 3–9 rad
- Ultrasonography
  —Evaluate for solid organ injury or hemoperitoneum, fetal heart activity, gestational age, abruptions, and amount of amniotic fluid
  —Test vaginal fluid with Nitrazine paper (turns blue), and for ferning
- With stable penetrating trauma, triple-contrast CT is advocated, particularly with stab wounds

PEDIATRIC CONSIDERATIONS

- Fetal survival begins at the 24th week (9.9%); it becomes significant after the 26th week (54.7%)

Treatment

INITIAL STABILIZATION

- Direct therapy at the mother with no delays due to pregnancy
- ABCs of trauma care
- Cardiac, pulse-oximetry, and cardiotocographic monitoring
- Tilt patient or board 15–30 degrees to the left (or manually displace uterus to left)

ED TREATMENT

- Use LR for IV fluids; NS may induce a hyperchloremic acidosis
- Replace estimated blood loss in a 3:1 ratio
- Resort to transfusions after 1 L of estimated blood loss or if hypovolemia persists after 2 L of crystalloid
- Nasogastric tube decompression (higher risk of aspiration in pregnancy)
- Foley catheterization to assess urinary output
- If DPL is necessary, use supraumbilical open technique
- Use tocolytic therapy only for hemodynamically stable patients
  - —Contraindicated if cervix dilated >4 cm or if FMH and abruption have not been reasonably ruled out
  - —Use tocolytics only when over 8 contractions/hour have lasted >4 hours
- See Cesarean Section, Emergency
- In minor trauma after the 20th week, fetal and maternal monitoring is best done in the labor and delivery area

MEDICATIONS

- RhoGAM in Rh-negative women (with a positive KB stain, within 72 hours): 50 μg i.m. in women <12 weeks pregnant; 300 μg i.m. in women >12 weeks pregnant
- 24-hour recheck for ongoing FMH: repeat RHIG if needed
- Tocolytics: magnesium sulfate 4 g i.v.
- Avoid aspirin, hypnotics, nonsteroidals, vasopressors
- Contraindicated: chloramphenicol, Dilantin, gentamicin, sulfonamides, tetracyclines

Disposition

ADMISSION CRITERIA

- Vaginal bleeding or amniotic fluid leakage
- Fetomaternal hemorrhage
- Abdominal pain
- Uterine contractions
- Evidence of fetal distress
- Abruption placenta
- Hemoperitoneum or visceral or solid organ injury

DISCHARGE CRITERIA

- All the following criteria must be met
- No uterine contractions for over 4 hours of tocodynamometry
  - —Some authors, however, recommend 24 hours of monitoring
- No evidence of fetal distress
- No vaginal bleeding or amniotic fluid leakage
- No abdominal pain or tenderness
- Timely obstetric follow-up
- Specific instructions to return if any of the above symptoms occur

Miscellaneous

ICD9: 760.5

ICD10: P00.5

SEE ALSO: CESAREAN SECTION, EMERGENCY

SUGGESTED READINGS

ACOG Educational Bulletin. Obstetric aspects of trauma management. Int J Gynecol Obstet 1999;64:87–94.

Curet MJ, et al. Predictors of outcome in trauma during pregnancy: identification of patients who can be monitored for less than 6 hours. J Trauma 2000;49(1):18–24.

Goodwin H, et al. Abdominal ultrasound examination in pregnant blunt trauma patients. J Trauma 2001;50(4):689–694.

Kuhlman RS, Cruikshank DP. Maternal trauma during pregnancy. Clin Obstet Gynecol 1994;37(2):274–293.

Lavery JP, Staten-McCormick M. Management of moderate to severe trauma in pregnancy. Obstet Gynecol Clin North Am 1995;22(1):69–90.

Pearlman MD, Tintinalli JE, Lorenz RP. A prospective controlled study of outcome after trauma during pregnancy. Am J Obstet Gynecol 1990;162:102–110.

Pearlman MD, Tintinalli JE. Evaluation and treatment of the gravida and fetus following trauma in pregnancy. Obstet Gynecol Clin North Am 1991;18:371.

Authors: A. Antoine Kazzi; Christina Matts

Pregnancy, Uncomplicated

- Pregnancy is not a disease process but rather a physiologic state
- All women of reproductive age with abdominal pain are considered pregnant until proven otherwise

Clinical Presentation

SIGNS AND SYMPTOMS

- Amenorrhea
  —The most common cause of secondary amenorrhea in a woman of reproductive age is pregnancy
- Nausea and vomiting (morning sickness)
- Breast tenderness (mastodynia)
- Urinary frequency
- Headache
- Low back pain
- Pica
- Edema of feet and ankles
- Weight gain
- Easy fatigability, generalized malaise
- Increase in abdominal girth

ETIOLOGY

- Preceding signs and symptoms can be explained by elevations in various hormone levels, or changes in anatomy that are a function of the progression of the pregnancy
- Placental human chorionic gonadotropin (HCG)
  —Prevents the normal involution of the corpus luteum at the end of the menstrual cycle
  —Causes the corpus luteum to secrete even larger quantities of estrogen and progesterone
  —Elevated HCG levels are responsible for the nausea and vomiting
- Placental progesterone
  —Causes decidual cells in the endometrium to develop and provide nutrition for the early embryo
  —Decreases contractility of the gravid uterus and risk of spontaneous abortion
  —Helps estrogen prepare the breasts for lactation
- Placental estrogen
  —Responsible for enlargement of uterus, breasts, and mammary ducts
  —Enlargement of female external genitalia, relaxation of pelvic ligaments, symphysis pubis, and sacroiliac joints

MECHANISM/DESCRIPTION

- The changes in pregnancy occur from the production of large amounts of placental hormones; placental progesterone and estrogen
- Feedback mechanisms between maternal and fetal endocrine systems

PEDIATRIC CONSIDERATIONS

- Range for menarche in U.S. is 11–15 years
- Pregnant adolescents who present to the ED may be either unaware of the pregnancy or reluctant to admit it
  —Assume pregnancy in adolescents, regardless of the chief complaint

Pre-Hospital

- Assume that the patient is pregnant
- Administer medications only when necessary to avoid teratogenetic side effects or placental-fetal compromise, i.e., epinephrine
- ACLS or ATLS protocols as indicated
- If greater than 24 weeks' gestation, transport in left lateral decubitus position

Diagnosis

ESSENTIAL WORKUP

- Determine first day of last menstrual period (FDLMP)
  - —40% of women cannot accurately remember their FDLMP
  - —Perform pelvic examination; estimate expected date of delivery by determining uterine fundal height

LABORATORY

- Pregnancy tests: presently, two hormones can be used to assist the clinician in diagnosing and monitoring a pregnancy: the β subunit of human chorionic gonadotropin (HCG) and progesterone (P)
- Measurement of β-HCG
  - —Most urinary pregnancy tests have a sensitivity of 25 mIU/mL
  - —Presently, four main methods are used to determine the serum level of HCG: radioimmunoassay (RIA), immunoradiometric assay (IRMA), fluoroimmunoassay (FIA), and enzyme-linked immunosorbent assay (ELISA)
- Serum progesterone (P) level is an indicator of the viability of the pregnancy and may be utilized to predict the outcome of the pregnancy
  - —A serum P level of <5 ng/mL is indicative of a nonviable pregnancy
  - —P level 25 ng/mL denotes a viable pregnancy

IMAGING/SPECIAL TESTS

- Ultrasonography can estimate gestational age, confirm intrauterine or ectopic pregnancy, evaluate fetal viability, and identify fetal abnormalities
- Vaginal probe ultrasound is contraindicated in premature rupture of membranes and third-trimester vaginal bleeding

DIFFERENTIAL DIAGNOSIS

- Any woman who is of the age to be sexually active who presents to the ED should be assumed to be pregnant until proven otherwise

PEDIATRIC CONSIDERATIONS

- Assume pregnancy in the adolescent regardless of the chief complaint

Treatment

INITIAL STABILIZATION

- ACLS, ATLS measures as needed: oxygen, cardiac monitor, IV access, and fluids
- If greater than 24 weeks' gestation, place in the left lateral decubitus position

ED TREATMENT

- The goal is to optimize maternal condition to improve fetal condition

MEDICATIONS

- First trimester is when organogenesis is occurring
- Fetal malformation continues beyond the first trimester
- Before using any drug, refer to its FDA safety classification in pregnancy
  - —This classification system categorizes drugs as categories A, B, C, D, and X, with category A being the safest and category X being the most toxic
- Analgesics: acetaminophen is the preferred OTC analgesic
- Aspirin and NSAIDs are not teratogenic but are best utilized in consultation with an obstetrician
- Propoxyphene, codeine, hydrocodone, meperidine, and morphine have no known teratogenic affect and can be used for the control of severe pain in pregnancy for short periods of time (3–4 days)
- Antibiotics: selecting the right antibiotic in a gravid female is dependent on three factors:
  - —Maternal drug allergies
  - —Gestational age
  - —Type of infections and associated pathogens

Disposition

ADMISSION CRITERIA

- Pregnant women with the following obstetric complications should be admitted to the hospital:
  - —Hyperemesis gravidarum with inability to tolerate oral fluids
  - —Complicated urinary tract infection
  - —Ectopic or molar pregnancy
  - —Septic abortion
  - —Preterm labor
  - —Premature rupture of membranes
  - —Preeclampsia/eclampsia
  - —Severe pregnancy-induced hypertension
- Pregnant women with medical conditions that would warrant admission in a nongravid female

DISCHARGE CRITERIA

- Women without the above conditions may be discharged from the ED

Miscellaneous

ICD9: V22.2

ICD10: O36.7

SUGGESTED READINGS

Barnhart K, Esposito M, Coutifars C. An update on the medical treatment of ectopic pregnancy. Obstet Gynecol Clin North Am 2000;27:653–667.

Paul M, Schaff E, Nichols M. The roles of clinical assessment, human chorionic gonadotropin assays, and ultrasonography in medical abortion practice. Am J Obstet Gynecol 2000;183(2 suppl):S34–S43.

Romero R, Kadar N, Copel JA. The value of serial human chorionic gonadotropin testing as a diagnostic tool in ectopic pregnancy. Am J Obstet Gynecol 1986;155:392–394.

Authors: James S. Walker; Michael Chamales

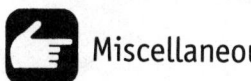

Priapism

Clinical Presentation

SIGNS AND SYMPTOMS

- Penile erection in the absence of sexual arousal that is prolonged and frequently painful
- Urinary retention is possible

MECHANISM/DESCRIPTION

- Engorgement of corpora cavernosa
- *Low-flow priapism* is most common
  - —*Poor venous outflow*
  - —Pain is characteristic
  - —Presence of stagnant, hypoxic blood can lead to ischemia and thrombosis after a few hours
  - —Fibrosis and impotence are late sequelae
- *High-flow priapism* is rare
  - —Penile arterial laceration with *uncontrolled inflow* of arterial blood
  - —Usually painless
  - —Presentation may be later than in low-flow priapism, and ischemia and impotence are uncommon sequelae

ETIOLOGY

- Idiopathic
- Pharmacologic agents
  - —*Intracavernosal injectables* for the treatment of impotence: PGE-1, papaverine, phentolamine
  - —*Psychotropics:* phenothiazines, butyrophenones, trazodone, sedative-hypnotics, selective serotonin uptake inhibitors (SSRIs)
  - —*Antihypertensives:* prazosin, hydralazine, phenoxybenzamine, guanethidine
  - —Rarely implicated agents: sildenafil (Viagra), anticoagulants, cocaine, marijuana, and ethanol
- *Sickle cell anemia, leukemia, polycythemia,* and other hematologic disorders predisposing to sludging of blood may cause low-flow priapism
- *Penile and perineal trauma* can result in arterial laceration and high-flow priapism
- *Spinal trauma* may cause priapism from loss of inhibitory adrenergic tone
- Rare causes: pelvic neoplasms and infections, dialysis, and parenteral nutrition solutions containing a fat emulsion

PEDIATRIC CONSIDERATIONS

- Sickle cell anemia is the cause of the majority of priapism in children

Pre-Hospital

- IV flush
- O_2 administration
- Pain medication

Diagnosis

ESSENTIAL WORKUP

- Cause of priapism can frequently be determined by history
  - —*High-flow priapism*: painless, has a history of trauma
  - —*Low-flow priapism*: painful, has a predisposing condition

LABORATORY

- Complete blood count and coagulation studies
- *Intracavernosal blood gas analysis* can help differentiate high-flow from low-flow priapism
  - —Because of the possibility of penile arterial injury, a urologist best performs this procedure
  - —*High-flow priapism*: near-normal values
  - —*Low-flow priapism*: acidosis and hypoxia (O_2 <30 torr)

IMAGING/SPECIAL TESTS

- *Duplex Doppler ultrasound* can verify and localize the arterial laceration in high-flow priapism
- *Angiography* enables localization and embolectomy of the arterial laceration in high-flow priapism

DIFFERENTIAL DIAGNOSIS

- *Penile erection* from sexual arousal is usually painless and transient
- *Penile implants* are discovered by history and physical examination

PEDIATRIC CONSIDERATIONS

- Sickle cell anemia evaluation may be undertaken in pediatric patients

Treatment

INITIAL STABILIZATION

- Supplemental oxygen
- Analgesia and sedation
- Intravenous hydration
- Urgent urologic consultation

ED TREATMENT

- Management of specific etiologies
  - —*Sickle cell anemia*: RBC transfusion, exchange transfusion, hyperbaric oxygen if other measures fail
  - —*Leukemia*: chemotherapy
  - —*Embolectomy* following angiographic localization of the arterial injury is effective in high-flow priapism
- *Terbutaline* is a β-agonist that may be administered in consultation with a urologist to initiate the treatment of low-flow priapism
- *Intracavernosal injection/aspiration* is an invasive technique that should be performed by an urologist if medical therapy for low-flow priapism fails; if specialty care is unavailable for several hours, the ED physician may perform the procedure as follows:
  - —1. Administer local anesthesia to the glans or perform a pudendal nerve block
  - —2. Prep the penis in a sterile fashion
  - —3. Positioning yourself to the right of the patient, grasp the penile shaft with the left hand
  - —4. Enter the corpus cavernosum with a 19-gauge butterfly needle inserted through the glans laterally to avoid the ventral urethra and the dorsal neurovascular bundle
  - —5. Aspirate blood while "milking" the penile shaft; aspirating both corpora cavernosa is unnecessary as they are connected by shunts; aspirate until arterial blood is obtained; irrigation with saline may be necessary
  - —6. Epinephrine, phenylephrine, or pseudoephedrine may be injected through the butterfly needle if tumescence recurs; monitor heart rate and blood pressure if these agents are utilized, and do not administer them to patients with cardiovascular or cerebrovascular disease or patients taking monoamine-oxidase inhibitors (MAOIs) because of the risk of hypertensive crisis
- *Surgical shunt* (i.e., corpus cavernosum to spongiosum) may be necessary if the above measures fail

MEDICATIONS

- Epinephrine: dilute 1 mg in 100 mL saline; inject 1–3 mL boluses in the corpus cavernosum, up to 10 mL
- Phenylephrine: dilute 1 mg in 100 mL saline; inject 10 mL boluses in the corpus cavernosum
- Pseudoephedrine: 60–100 mg in the corpus cavernosum
- Terbutaline: 0.25–0.5 mg s.c. or 5 mg PO q4–6h

Disposition

ADMISSION CRITERIA

- Persistent priapism despite noninvasive treatments
- Serious underlying disease (sickle cell anemia, leukemia)

DISCHARGE CRITERIA

- Detumescence is complete and has not recurred after several hours of observation
- Urologic consultation has been obtained
- Short-term follow-up has been arranged
- The patient has been advised to return to the ED if tumescence recurs, and the ED physician and the consulting urologist have discussed the possibility of impotence with the patient

Miscellaneous

ICD9: 607.3

ICD10: N48.3

SUGGESTED READINGS

Hakim LS, Kulaksizoglu H, Mulligan R, et al. Evolving concepts in the diagnosis and treatment of arterial high flow priapism. J Urol 1996;155:541–548.

Mulhall JP, Honig SC. Priapism: diagnosis and management. Acad Emerg Med 1996;3: 810–816.

Paulter SE, Brock GB. Priapism. From Priapus to the present time. Urol Clin North Am 2001;28:391–403.

Winter CC, McDowell G. Experience with 105 patients with priapism: update and review of all aspects. J Urol 1988;140: 980–983.

Author: David Barlas

Prostatitis

Clinical Presentation

SIGNS AND SYMPTOMS

- Irritative voiding symptoms (frequency, urgency, dysuria)
- Low back pain
- Perineal, suprapubic, or testicular pain
- Bladder outlet obstruction and urinary retention
- Ejaculatory symptoms such as hematospermia
- *Acute prostatitis*
  - —Fever and chills, malaise, arthralgias, and myalgias
  - —Examination may reveal exquisitely tender, warm, swollen, and firm or boggy prostate; *the acutely inflamed prostate should not be massaged because of the possibility of precipitating hematogenous spread of organisms*
- *Chronic prostatitis* is relapsing dysuria
- Examination is usually normal in chronic prostatitis

MECHANISM/DESCRIPTION

- Five categories:
- Prostatic abscess
  - —Once common after acute prostatitis, now rare except in immunocompromised patients
  - —Fever, rectal symptoms, and leukocytosis despite treatment, along with a fluctuant mass on rectal exam, suggest abscess
- Acute (bacterial) prostatitis
  - —Acute febrile illness in which systemic symptoms may appear days before localizing urinary symptoms appear
  - —Patients may appear toxic and usually have a concurrent cystitis
- Chronic bacterial prostatitis
  - —About 10% of cases of prostatitis
  - —Most common cause of recurrent urinary tract infection in men
  - —White blood cells and bacteria may be present in expressed prostatic secretions (EPSs)
- Chronic nonbacterial prostatitis (also called prostatosis)
  - —Same symptoms as chronic bacterial prostatitis but unable to culture organisms from urine or EPS
- Prostatodynia
  - —Symptoms referable to the prostate but no inflammatory cells are found and no bacteria can be cultured from the urine or prostatic secretions

ETIOLOGY

- Usually a single organism bacterial infection of the prostate
- Acute prostatitis
  - —Age <35 years: *Neisseria gonorrhoeae* and *Chlamydia trachomatis* are usual etiologies
  - —Age ≥35 years: Enterobacteriaceae or *Escherichia coli* (usual), *Klebsiella, Pseudomonas, Enterococcus,* and *Proteus* also seen
  - —Rarely may be caused by *Salmonella, Clostridia,* tuberculosis, or fungi (*Cryptococcus neoformans* in AIDS patients)
- Chronic bacterial prostatitis
  - —Enterobacteriaceae (80%), Enterococcus (15%), and *Pseudomonas aeruginosa*
- Chronic nonbacterial prostatitis:
  - —Possible role for *Chlamydia, Ureaplasma urealyticum, Trichomonas vaginalis,* and *Mycoplasma hominis*

Pre-Hospital

N/A

Diagnosis

ESSENTIAL WORKUP

- Urinalysis (with microscopy) and culture
- Rectal and prostatic examination, do not massage prostate in acute prostatitis

LABORATORY

- *Acute prostatitis:* complete blood count, electrolytes, and blood cultures may be helpful in the acutely ill patient
  - —If <35 years old or suspected sexual transmission, testing for syphilis (VDRL or RPR) is recommended
- *Chronic prostatitis/prostatodynia:* prostatic massage between voiding may be used to capture EPS for Gram stain and culture if organism or white cells not present in the urine

IMAGING/SPECIAL TESTS

- Not indicated in acute prostatitis
- If prostatic abscess suspected, prostatic ultrasound or pelvic computed tomography (CT) scan with intravenous (IV) and rectal contrast will confirm diagnosis
- Pelvic radiographs may reveal prostatic calculi (common in men), which may serve as a nidus for infection in chronic prostatitis

DIFFERENTIAL DIAGNOSIS

- Cystitis
- Pyelonephritis
- Urolithiasis
- Vesicular calculi
- Seminal vesiculitis
- Proctitis
- Perirectal/perianal abscess
- Urethritis
- Epididymitis
- Orchitis
- Prostatic infarction
- Benign prostatic hyperplasia
- Prostatic carcinoma
- Other causes of lower back pain (strain, disc disease, sacroiliac joint disease, etc.)

Treatment

INITIAL STABILIZATION

- Initial resuscitative measures (ABCs) on all patients who are acutely ill, toxic-appearing, or septic

ED TREATMENT

- Prostatic abscess requires urgent urologic consultation and operative management
- Antibiotic therapy should be initiated in ED (see Medications, below)
- Urinary tract instrumentation should be avoided
  —If patient has painful urinary retention in acute prostatitis, suprapubic needle aspiration or suprapubic catheter placement should be performed
- Patients will benefit from adequate IV fluid
- Pain control with NSAIDs and narcotic analgesics as needed
- Stool softeners
- Bed rest
- Irritative voiding symptoms may persist for months after antibiotic therapy and may be treated with NSAIDs

MEDICATIONS

- Analgesia
  —Narcotic/analgesic combinations such as hydroxycodone/acetaminophen 1–2 tabs PO q4h
  —NSAIDs such as ibuprofen 800 mg PO t.i.d.
- Parenteral antibiotic therapy for acute prostatitis
  —Ampicillin/sulbactam: 3 g i.v. q6h
  —Cefotaxime: 2 g i.v. q8h
  —Ceftriaxone: 2 g i.v. qd
  —Ciprofloxacin: 400 mg i.v. b.i.d.
  —Ofloxacin: 200 mg i.v. b.i.d.
  —Piperacillin/tazobactam: 3.375 g i.v. q6h or 4.5 g i.v. q8h
  —Ticarcillin/clavulanate: 3.1 g i.v. q6h
- Antibiotics for outpatient treatment of acute (≤35 years old) prostatitis, suspected etiology *N. gonorrhoeae* or *C. trachomatis*
  —Ceftriaxone 250 mg i.m., then doxycycline 100 mg PO b.i.d. × 10–14 days
  —Levofloxacin 500 mg PO qd for 10–14 days
  —Ofloxacin: 400 mg PO × 1, then 300 mg PO b.i.d. × 10–14 days
- Antibiotics for outpatient treatment of acute (>35 years old), suspected etiology Enterobacteriaceae (coliforms); some authorities recommend treatment for 3–4 weeks
  —Ciprofloxacin 500 mg PO b.i.d. × 14 days
  —Levofloxacin 500 mg PO qd for 14 days
  —Ofloxacin 200 mg PO b.i.d. × 14 days
  —Trimethoprim/sulfamethoxazole: 1 DS tab or 2 regular-strength tablets PO b.i.d. × 14 days
- Outpatient therapy for chronic bacterial prostatitis (Enterobacteriaceae, *Enterococcus*, or *P. aeruginosa*)
  —Ciprofloxacin 500 mg PO b.i.d. × 4 weeks
  —Levofloxacin 500 mg PO qd for 4 weeks
  —Ofloxacin 300 mg PO b.i.d. × 6 weeks
  —Trimethoprim/sulfamethoxazole DS 1 tab PO b.i.d. × 1–3 months
- Prostatodynia/chronic pain syndrome
  —Doxazosin: 1 mg PO qd
  —Peripheral α-adrenergic blocking agents have been used with some success but are controversial; consult a urologist
  —Prazosin: 1 mg PO b.i.d./t.i.d.
  —Terazosin: 1 mg PO qhs

Disposition

ADMISSION CRITERIA

- Acute prostatitis: patients who appear ill or toxic with fever, chills, hypotension, and urinary retention should be admitted for parenteral antibiotics and close observation
- Chronic prostatitis: admission generally not warranted unless patient has signs or symptoms of acute prostatitis

DISCHARGE CRITERIA

- Acute prostatitis: patient must be nontoxic, able to take fluids and oral medications (analgesia and antibiotics), urinate without difficulty, immunocompetent, relatively free of concurrent underlying disease, and have appropriate follow-up care
- Chronic prostatitis: appropriate follow-up care should be available

Miscellaneous

ICD9: 601.9

ICD10: N41.9

SUGGESTED READINGS

Bjerklund Johansen TE. Diagnosis and imaging in urinary tract infection. Curr Opin Urol 2002;12(1):39–43.

Harwood-Nuss AL, Etheredge W, McKenna I. Urologic Emergency. In: Rosen P, et al., eds. Emergency medicine: concepts and clinical practice, 4th ed. St. Louis: CV Mosby, 1998:2227–2260.

Lipsky, Benjamin A. Prostatitis and urinary tract infection in men: what's new; what's true? Am J Med 1999;106(3):327–334.

Lummus WE, Thompson I. Prostatitis. Emerg Med Clin North Am 2001;19(3):691–707.

Robert RO, Lieber MM, Bostwick DG, et al. A review of clinical and pathological prostatitis syndromes. Urology 1997;49:809–821.

Author: Robert S. Hamilton

Pruritus

Clinical Presentation

SIGNS AND SYMPTOMS

- Onset
  - —Shortly after fresh water bathing in swimmer's itch
  - —More intense at night with scabies
  - —Paroxysmal with multiple sclerosis
  - —With sudden changes in temperature in polycythemia vera
- Dermatologic
  - —Absence of rash
  - —Hives
  - —Urticaria
  - —Grouped papules
  - —Interdigital, pubic, axillary, or nipple lesions
  - —Generalized morbilliform eruptions
  - —Discrete weeping patches with vesicles
  - —Dry skin
  - —Jaundice
  - —Excoriations
  - —Prurigo papules
    - -Thickened papular areas of skin from constant rubbing
- Psychogenic
  - —Constant rubbing in areas patient can readily reach

MECHANISM/DESCRIPTION

- Mediated by unmyelinated C fibers in upper portion of dermis
- Peripheral mediators stimulate C fibers and induce itching
  - —Histamine
  - —Serotonin
  - —Trypsin
  - —Proteases
  - —Peptides that release histamine
    - -Bradykinin
    - -Vasoactive intestinal peptide
    - -Substance P
  - —Bile salts
- Prostaglandins (PGE_2, PGH_2) lower threshold to pruritus
- Opiates cause pruritus by acting on central receptors
- No single pharmacologic agent effectively treats all kinds of pruritus
- "Itch-scratch-itch" cycle
  - —Itching triggers scratching, which damages the skin and stimulates nerve endings, thereby producing even greater itching
  - —Pathogenic basis for lichen simplex chronicus and prurigo nodularis

ETIOLOGY

- See Differential Diagnosis

Pre-Hospital

N/A

Diagnosis

ESSENTIAL WORKUP

- Detailed history is key in the ED workup
  - —Onset
  - —Character: paroxysmal, burning, pricking
  - —Time of occurrence, circadian nature
  - —Duration
  - —Severity
  - —Anatomic area
  - —Exacerbating or alleviating factors
    - -Water
    - -Heat
    - -Dryness
    - -Dampness
    - -Coolness
  - —Medications
  - —Use of new topical products
    - -Soap
    - -Hair spray
    - -Lotions
    - -Cosmetics
    - -Perfume
  - —Laundry detergents
  - —Fabric softeners
  - —Family history of atopic dermatitis or skin disease
  - —Personal history of allergies or asthma
  - —Pruritus in other family members
  - —Systemic or associated symptoms
    - -Night sweats, fever, tremors, weight loss, fatigue
  - —Sexual history, history of HIV or AIDS
  - —Social: occupation, hobbies, pets, travel
- Characterization of skin lesions
  - —Diffuse or localized
  - —Location: genitals, interdigital webs, axilla, wrists, etc.
  - —Follicular
    - -Around the hair
    - -Folliculitis
  - —Nonfollicular
    - -Insect bites, scabies
  - —Primary lesions
    - -Papular, pustular, urticarial, or polymorphic
  - —Secondary lesions
    - -Excoriations, lichenification, hyperpigmentation
- Signs of systemic disease on physical examination

LABORATORY

- Laboratory testing should be determined based on specific presentation

IMAGING/SPECIAL TESTS

- Skin biopsy
  - —Performed by dermatologist at follow-up visit

DIFFERENTIAL DIAGNOSIS

Dermatologic

- Xerosis (dry skin)
- Insect infestations
  - —Scabies
    - -Vesicles and burrows on intertriginous areas
  - —Pediculosis
  - —Insect bites
    - -Localized clusters of papules
- Dermatitis
  - —Atopic dermatitis
  - —Contact dermatitis
    - -Includes poison ivy contact
  - —Nummular dermatitis
    - -Round eczematous or vesicular eruption
- Drug-induced
  - —Suspect when pruritus occurs without a rash
  - —Opiates and derivatives
  - —Aspirin
  - —Quinidine
  - —Antimalarials
  - —Phenothiazines
  - —Isoniazid
  - —Vitamin B complex
  - —Estrogens, progestins, testosterone
  - —Tolbutamide
- Lichen planus
  - —Lichenification, hyperpigmentation, skin thickening
- Urticaria
- Eosinophilic folliculitis
- Dermatitis herpetiformis
  - —Burning itch
- Sunburn
- Aquagenic pruritus
- Fiberglass dermatitis
- Seborrheic dermatitis
  - —Scaly plaques on scalp, hairline, eyebrows, central face, and other sebaceous gland-bearing areas like axillae and chest
- Swimmer's itch
  - —Schistosome cercarial dermatitis
  - —Repeated fresh water exposure
  - —Itching starts as water evaporates
  - —Highly pruritic papules develop hours later
- Miliaria rubra

Infectious

- HIV
- Parasites
  - —Hookworm
  - —Onchocerciasis
  - —Ascariasis
  - —Trichinosis

Cholestatic
- Obstructive biliary disease
- Primary biliary cirrhosis
  - —Early sign usually starting on hands and soles
- Hepatic cholestasis secondary to drugs
  - —Chlorpropamide
  - —Estrogens
  - —Phenothiazine
  - —Allopurinol
- Intrahepatic cholestasis of pregnancy
- Extrahepatic biliary obstruction
- Chronic hepatitis, especially hepatitis C

Hematologic
- Polycythemia vera
- Iron-deficiency anemia
- Paraproteinemia
- Waldenström's macroglobulinemia
- Mastocytosis

Neoplastic
- Lymphoma including Hodgkin's disease
- Mycosis fungoides
- Leukemia
- CNS tumors
- Multiple myeloma
- Carcinoid
- Visceral malignancies
  - —Breast, stomach, lung

Metabolic-Endocrine
- Uremia
- Hyperthyroidism
- Hypothyroidism
- Diabetes
- Carcinoid

Neurologic
- Multiple sclerosis
  - —Paroxysmal itching
- Notalgia paraesthetic
  - —Local itch of back, medial shaft scapula
- Brain abscess
- CNS infarct
- Cerebral tumor
- Creutzfeldt-Jakob disease

Renal
- Chronic renal failure
- Chronic hemodialysis

Rheumatologic
- Sjögren syndrome
- Dermatomyositis

Psychiatric
- Stress, anxiety, neurotic excoriation
- Delusions of parasitosis
- Psychogenic pruritus

Treatment

INITIAL STABILIZATION

N/A

ED TREATMENT
- Start with antihistamines for pruritus of undetermined etiology
- Emollients indicated for pruritus secondary to dry skin
- Coolants to alleviate itching: menthol, camphor, eucalyptus oil, calamine lotion
- Substance P evacuators (capsaicin) block C fibers
  - —Burning sensation during first weeks of use
  - —Anesthetic (e.g., EMLA) can be applied prior
- Topical glucocorticoids for contact dermatitis
- Permethrin cream for scabies and lice when rash is suggestive
- Topical antihistamines (doxepin) for eczema, urticaria, bites
- Swimmer's itch
  - —Control with antihistamines, cool compresses, calamine lotion
  - —Topical steroids to suppress intense inflammation
  - —Towel dry immediately after leaving the water as preventative measure
- Discontinue medications that may cause allergic reaction
- Ultraviolet light for uremic pruritus

MEDICATIONS
- Oral antihistamines
  - —Chlorpheniramine: 4 mg (peds: 0.35 mg/kg/24 hours) PO q.i.d.
  - —Diphenhydramine: 25–50 mg (peds: 5 mg/kg/24 hours) PO q.i.d.
  - —Hydroxyzine: 10–25 mg (peds: 2 mg/kg/24 hours) PO q.i.d.
- Topical treatments
  - —Capsaicin 0.025%, 0.075% ointment: apply up to q.i.d.
  - —Doxepin 5% cream: apply q.i.d. for up to 8 days
  - —EMLA (2.5% lidocaine + 2.5% prilocaine): apply prior to capsaicin
  - —Hydrocortisone, 0.5%, 1%, 2.5%: apply up to q.i.d.
  - —Permethrin 5% cream: apply from neck down after bath
    - -Shower thoroughly to remove the medication in 8–12 hours
  - —White petroleum emollients: apply after short bath/shower in warm (not hot) water

Disposition

ADMISSION CRITERIA
- Anaphylaxis
- Generalized exfoliating lesions

DISCHARGE CRITERIA
- Refer patients with skin lesions to primary care physician or dermatologist
- Patients with pruritus without skin lesions should be discharged on antipruritic medication and referred to a physician for an underlying systemic illness
- Practical recommendations for dry skin
  - —Baths with baking soda, bath oils, or colloidal oatmeal
  - —After-bath moisturizers
  - —Avoid dry air (humidity less than 40%)
  - —Avoid irritating textiles (wool)
  - —Avoid alkaline soaps and overwashing
  - —Avoid alcohol and peppery foods (cause vasodilation)
  - —Avoid overexposure to heat, hot water

Miscellaneous

ICD9: 698

ICD10: L29.9

SUGGESTED READINGS

Bueller HA, Bernhard JD. Review of pruritus therapy. Dermatol Nurs 1998;10:101–107.

Greco PJ, Ende J. Pruritus: a practical approach. J Gen Intern Med 1992;7: 340–349.

Leung AK, Wong BE, Chan PY, et al. Pruritus in children. J R Soc Health 1998;118:280–286.

Nowak MA, Tsoukas MM, DeImus FA, et al. Generalized pruritus without primary lesions. Differential diagnosis and approach to treatment. Postgrad Med 2000;107:41–42, 45–46.

Yosipovitch G, David M. The diagnostic and therapeutic approach to idiopathic generalized pruritus. Int J Dermatol 1999;38:881–887.

Author: Christine L. Tsien

Pseudotumor Cerebri

- Also known as idiopathic intracranial hypertension

Clinical Presentation

SIGNS AND SYMPTOMS

Symptoms

- Headache: typically described as constant, bilateral, pressure like, worse in the morning and with Valsalva maneuver
- Nausea and vomiting
- Pulsatile intracranial noise
- Diplopia
- Dizziness
- Scotoma
- Transient visual obscurations lasting seconds
- Blind spots
- Constriction of vision

Signs

- Visual field defects (in up to 90%), most typically inferior nasal visual field loss
- Papilledema
- Lumbar puncture improves symptoms
- Sixth cranial nerve palsy
- Otherwise normal neurologic exam (except for visual changes, abducens palsy, and with very rare exception of seventh cranial nerve palsy)
- Loss of visual acuity

MECHANISM/DESCRIPTION

- Buildup of cerebrospinal fluid (CSF) pressure without mass lesion; no clear cause, two proposed mechanisms:
  —Increased abdominal pressure may decrease CSF drainage through arachnoid granulations by increasing pleural and right heart pressures and thus decreasing venous drainage from the head
  —Vitamin A levels above the saturation of the liver can damage cell membranes in the arachnoid granulations
- Female predominance (7:1)
- Associated with obesity
- Average age of onset 30 years

ETIOLOGY

- Proposed causative agents
  —Obesity
  —Hypervitaminosis A
  —Steroids/steroid withdrawal
  —Tetracycline antibiotics
  —Oral contraceptive pills
  —Hypertension
  —Recent weight gain
  —Chronic carbon dioxide retention with elevated intracranial pressure

PEDIATRIC CONSIDERATIONS

- Usually presents with strabismus as opposed to headache and visual field loss
- Also associated with obesity and medications (tetracycline antibiotics, steroids)

Pre-Hospital

N/A

Diagnosis

ESSENTIAL WORKUP

- Thorough history and physical exam with detailed neurologic assessment and funduscopic exam

LABORATORY

- Lumbar puncture: CSF normal or low protein with a normal cell count
- Opening pressure >25 cm H_2O or >20 cm H_2O in the nonobese, relaxed patient
  —Be sure patient is lying down with measurement of opening pressure
  —Observing respiratory variation ensures good transmission of pressure
- Consider CBC, coagulation studies prior to lumbar puncture

IMAGING/SPECIAL TESTS

- Head CT/MRI to rule out mass lesions (prior to lumbar puncture)
- Improvement of symptoms with lumbar puncture
- Classically the head CT will demonstrate slit-like frontal horns of the lateral ventricles
- MRI recommended in the full workup (can be done as an outpatient), as cerebral venous thrombosis can mimic pseudotumor cerebri in all regards including normal head CT

DIFFERENTIAL DIAGNOSIS

- Migraine headache
- Hypertensive headache
- Anoxic headache
- Tension headache
- Cluster headache
- Subarachnoid hemorrhage
- Aneurysm/arteriovenous malformation
- Meningitis/encephalitis
- Subdural hematoma
- Epidural hematoma
- Tumor
- Abscess
- Trigeminal neuralgia
- Temporal arteritis
- Sinusitis
- Glaucoma
- Central retinal vein/artery occlusion
- Congenital optic nerve head elevation
- Optic nerve drusen
- Labyrinthitis
- Optic neuritis
- Cerebral venous thrombosis
- Chronic carbon dioxide retention

Treatment

INITIAL STABILIZATION

- ABCs
- IV fluid hydration

ED TREATMENT

- Tap off 20–30 cc of CSF, but only if confident of correct diagnosis, and head CT demonstrates open basilar cisterns and 4th ventricle
- Acetazolamide
- Pain control
- Neurology consult
- Ophthalmology consult
- Neurosurgery consult for acute or impending visual loss unresponsive to diuretics (for lumboperitoneal shunt)
- Optic nerve fenestration another surgical option
- Weight loss
- Discontinue any drugs that could be causative
- Typically resolves spontaneously

MEDICATIONS

- Acetaminophen 650 mg–1 g (peds: 15 mg/kg)
- Acetazolamide 500 mg slow release b.i.d. (peds: 25 mg/kg/d divided q.i.d./t.i.d. PO/i.v.)
- Ibuprofen 600–800 mg (peds: 10 mg/kg)
- Lasix 0.5–1 mg/kg i.v./PO
- Morphine 0.1 mg/kg
- Prednisone helpful when severe visual symptoms present, 5-day course recommended (not longer)

Disposition

ADMISSION CRITERIA

- Acute or impending visual loss

DISCHARGE CRITERIA

- In consultation with neurology and ophthalmology
- Appropriate follow-up arranged
- Tolerating oral diuretics
- Pain under control

Miscellaneous

ICD9: 348.2

ICD10: G93.2

SUGGESTED READINGS

Goetz CG, Pappert EJ, eds. Textbook of clinical neurology, 1st ed. Philadelphia: WB Saunders, 1999.

Jones JS, Nevai J Freeman MP, et al. Emergency department presentation of idiopathic intracranial hypertension. Am J Emerg Med 1999;17(6):517–521.

Mouvsas TZ, et al. Current neuro-ophthalmic therapies. Neurol Clin 2001;19(1):145–172.

Rosen P, et al., eds. Emergency medicine: concepts and clinical practice, 5th ed. St. Louis: CV Mosby, 2002.

Author: Ian Reilly

Psoriasis

Clinical Presentation

SIGNS AND SYMPTOMS

- The classic skin lesion is a round red patch with central plaque of silvery white scale that appears on extensor surfaces (psoriasis vulgaris)
  - —The lesions not intensely pruritic, but do itch
- Positive Auspitz sign: new lesions appear in an area of recent skin trauma (Koebner phenomenon); mucous membranes may be affected
  - —The pattern may be gyrate, nummular, annular, arcuate, or circinate
- Scalp lesions may be confused with seborrhea
  - —Lesions that extend beyond the hair borders indicate psoriasis
- Stippling and pitting of nail and oncolysis
  - —Yellow or brown band across the nail will help differentiate psoriasis (+ band) from onychomycosis (− band)
- Classic arthritis (<5% of cases) in the DIP joints of the hands and feet
- Asymmetric oligoarticular arthritis present in 70% with swelling of the juxtaarticular tissue giving a classic "sausage-shape" appearance to the affected digits

MECHANISM/DESCRIPTION

- Autosomal-dominant inheritance pattern
- Caucasians and atopics most affected
- Majority of cases occurring between 10 and 30 years of age
- Equal number of adult male and female cases
- 1,000–2,000 cases per 100,000 population in U.S.
- Defective inhibition of epidermal proliferation and marked increase in cell proliferation and turnover
- Several clinical presentations:
  - —Chronic plaque psoriasis: most common form with classic lesions on the scalp, limbs, and trunk
  - —Guttate psoriasis: occurs more commonly in children, with most lesions found on the trunk
  - —Pustular psoriasis: collections of pustules on one area of the body, usually palms or soles
  - —Erythrodermic psoriasis: the patient may exhibit pustules (von Zumbusch psoriasis) or simple confluent erythroderma
  - —Light-sensitive psoriasis: a Koebner phenomenon response to sunburning
  - —Inverse flexural psoriasis: a variant that causes lesions in flexural areas that don't exhibit scaling due to moisture in these areas
  - —HIV-induced psoriasis: may be a first manifestation of AIDS with an explosive onset of the disease of the erythroderma or pustular variety
  - —Keratoderma blennorrhagicum: psoriasis of the penis seen with Reiter's syndrome with a distinctive winding pattern to the lesion (balanitis circinata)

ETIOLOGY

- Triggers include:
  - —Drugs: lithium, beta-blockers, antimalarials, steroids, NSAIDs, alcohol, tetracycline, penicillin, amiodarone, morphine, procaine, potassium iodide, sulfapyridine, and sulfonamides
  - —Infections: streptococcal pharyngitis, HIV, viral URI
  - —Local trauma: frostbite, sunburn, routine skin breaks
  - —Stress: emotional and physical
  - —Winter (low light exposure)

PEDIATRIC CONSIDERATIONS

- 37% of all cases occur before 20 years of age
- In childhood forms, the female to male cases 2:1
- The younger the patient at onset of disease, the worse the course

Pre-Hospital

N/A

Diagnosis

ESSENTIAL WORKUP

- The diagnosis is clinical and rarely is biopsy necessary; history should address:
  - —Age at first appearance of eruption
  - —Specific location of eruptions
  - —New lesions in sites of recent trauma (Koebner phenomenon)
  - —Drug history
  - —Family history of the disease
  - —Recent illnesses
  - —History of improvement with sun exposure, or if recurrent, success of prior regimens
  - —Systemic symptoms like fevers and chills or joint pain
- Physical examination should concentrate on diagnostic clues the lesions may exhibit:
  - —Scalp lesions that extend beyond the hairline
  - —Nails with pits, staining, and hyperkeratosis
  - —Auspitz sign when plaques are removed
  - —Koebner phenomenon along the lines of recent trauma
  - —"Sausage-shaped" digits from arthritis

LABORATORY

- Elevated sedimentation rate and uric acid
- Decreased serum albumin
- Anemia with vitamin B_{12}, folate, and iron deficiency
- Positive streptococcal cultures and titers
- Hypocalcemia and leukocytosis in pustular disease
- Negative rheumatoid factor
- Key biopsy traits include dilated tortuous capillaries (Auspitz sign), hyperkeratosis, epidermal hyperplasia, and Munro microabscesses

IMAGING/SPECIAL TESTS

- Plain radiographs of the hands or feet may show osteoporosis and bone loss at the distal phalanx, causing the pencil-in-cup deformation at the MTP or MCP joints
  - —Sacroiliitis and ankylosing spondylitis may also be seen on radiographs

DIFFERENTIAL DIAGNOSIS

- Best thought of by region
  - —Scalp: seborrhea
  - —Flexure creases: candidiasis, intertrigo
  - —Nails: onychomycosis
  - —Trunk and extremities: nummular eczema, pityriasis rosea or rubra pilaris, tinea, SLE, syphilis, drug eruption, atopy, mycosis fungoides, squamous cell carcinoma

PEDIATRIC CONSIDERATIONS

- Do not let young age eliminate the diagnosis
- Order streptococcal tests if the history supports the testing

Treatment

INITIAL STABILIZATION

- General resuscitation efforts aimed at correcting fluid and electrolyte abnormalities
- Treating sepsis if present
  - —Cultures of skin, blood, and urine
- Soothing moist compresses are appropriate but occlusive dressings and ointments are contraindicated
- Systemic steroids should not be used as they may predispose to severe complications

ED TREATMENT

- Phototherapy is not an ED treatment modality
- Systemic therapy should be reserved for the acute erythroderma variant with or without pustulosis as noted above
- Dermatology consult should be obtained in all severe cases

MEDICATIONS

- Mild to moderate disease: topical treatment is usually reserved for patients with only 10–20% skin involvement; topical agents include:
  - —Emollients: hydrates and softens plaques; greasier choices work best, but are poorly tolerated by patients for cosmetic reasons
  - —Keratolytics: help to remove plaques; salicylic acid (2–10%) is the mainstay of treatment (caution must be used in applying near the eyes)
  - —Tar preparations: usually used alternatively with topical steroids, with ultraviolet light, or alone; ointments and shampoos are available
  - —Anthralin: may be used in complex treatment regimens with other topical agents and ultraviolet light
  - —Topical corticosteroids: the mainstay of treatment in the U.S.; best results are obtained by rotating drugs and using occlusive dressings; small lesions may be treated with intralesional Kenalog as may psoriatic nails; steroids have been implicated in serious relapses and pustular psoriasis
  - —Vitamin D derivatives: calcipotriene is applied to the lesions twice daily
- Moderate to severe disease: the above-named agents may be employed along with phototherapy and systemic medications
  - —Phototherapy
    - -Ultraviolet B irradiation is combined with coal tar and has reports of 80% remission; ultraviolet B may be used alone in guttate psoriasis
    - -Ultraviolet A irradiation (PUVA) is used with topical agents and systemic agents to gain remission in over 85% of patients using it
  - —Systemic agents: may be used in various combinations with the above modalities
    - -Methotrexate: assess renal, liver, and hematologic function prior to therapy
    - -Etretinate: a retinoid, it causes dryness, scaling, redness, and tenderness of the skin
    - -Systemic corticosteroids: not in favor due to iatrogenic Cushing's syndrome; it may have a role in acute erythrodermic psoriasis where the patient is extremely ill
    - -Cyclosporine: the drug blocks steps in the formation of interleukin-2, thereby preventing clinical expression of the disease; it should not be used with phototherapy

PEDIATRIC CONSIDERATIONS

- The emotional side of this chronic disease may be paramount in children whose body image is being formed
- In general, topical agents are well tolerated, but PUVA and systemic agents are generally avoided in children

Disposition

ADMISSION CRITERIA

- Acute erythroderma and acute pustular psoriasis warrant admission for supportive therapy and systemic treatment as noted above

DISCHARGE CRITERIA

- Patients without the above-mentioned forms may be discharged
- Advise patients the disease is not contagious
- Warn against excessive scrubbing to loosen scale, as it may worsen the disease
- Educate the patient on avoiding medications that trigger relapses
- Refer patients to the National Psoriasis Foundation (telephone 503-244-7404) for further information

PEDIATRIC CONSIDERATIONS

- Except as noted above, no special criteria exist

Miscellaneous

ICD9: 696.1

ICD10: L40.9

SUGGESTED READINGS

Camisa C. Psoriasis: a clinical update on diagnosis and new therapies. Cleve Clin J Med 2000;67(2):105–106, 109–113, 117–119.

Habif T. Psoriasis. In: Habif T, ed. Clinical dermatology, 3rd ed. St. Louis: CV Mosby, 1996:190–212.

Rogers M. Childhood psoriasis. Curr Opin Pediatr 2002;14(4):404–409.

Wood J. Treatment of psoriasis. N Engl J Med 1995;332:581–588.

Author: Stephen R. Hayden

Psychiatric Commitment

Clinical Presentation

SIGNS AND SYMPTOMS

- Civil commitment
  - —Confinement of an individual
- Involuntary commitment
  - —Confinement against the patient's will
- Basis of civil commitment
  - —Danger to self or others
- Psychiatric (civil) commitment:
  - —Refers to an order by a judge for continued hospitalization of an inpatient in a mental health facility for treatment of psychiatric disease against the patient's wishes
  - —Based on danger to self or others by reason of mental illness
- Psychiatric commitment not indicated for other causes of dangerous behavior
  - —Anger
  - —Antisocial behavior
  - —Substance abuse
  - —Medical illness
- Psychiatric commitment usually involves two steps:
  - —Initial involuntary hospitalization in a psychiatric facility, most commonly initiated by a psychiatrist
  - —Petition to the court for psychiatric commitment

MECHANISM/DESCRIPTION

- *Commitment criteria* (check specific laws in your state):
  - —Individual is mentally ill
  - —Failure to hospitalize or discharge from hospital creates likelihood of serious harm
  - —Likelihood of serious harm is defined as:
    - -Substantial risk of physical harm to self: threats or attempts at suicide
    - -Substantial risk of physical harm to other persons: homicidal or violent behaviors, or others are placed in reasonable fear of violent behaviors
    - -Very substantial risk of physical impairment due to inability to protect self due to impaired judgment and reasonable protection not available in community
  - —No less restrictive alternative to hospitalization would attenuate risk

Pre-Hospital

CONTROVERSIES

- Ethical considerations:
  - —Involuntary admission leads to loss of basic rights
  - —*Parens patriae power:* state's authority to care for citizen who cannot care for self
  - —*Police power:* state's authority to detain citizen who is danger to self or someone else

Diagnosis

ESSENTIAL WORKUP

- Psychiatric evaluation through history/mental status exam
  - —History of psychiatric illness
  - —Recent change in behavior or thinking
  - —Dosages of medications
  - —Drugs of abuse: amount and time of last use
  - —Disabling thought patterns: hallucinations, delusions, disorganization
- Assessment of commitment criteria:
  - —Threat of violence toward self
  - —Threat of violence toward others
  - —Inability to care for self or severe deficits in judgment
- Rule out medical causes for mental status change, commonly delirium or substance intoxication/withdrawal
- Complete physical and neurologic exam
- Rule out criminal behavior

LABORATORY

- Appropriate labs and radiology as indicated by history and physical
  - —Electrolytes, BUN, creatinine, glucose
  - —Liver function tests
  - —CBC and differential
  - —Toxicology screens and medication levels
  - —Urinalysis if infection suspected
  - —CT of head if injury or structural CNS pathology suspected

DIFFERENTIAL DIAGNOSIS

- Intoxication or withdrawal
- Delirium
- Dementia
- Traumatic brain injury
- Antisocial behavior

Treatment

INITIAL STABILIZATION

- Initial containment by police
- Transport patient to facility for psychiatric evaluation
- Assure patient and staff safety

ED TREATMENT

- Restrain dangerous patients as needed
  - —Nurse or security guard standing outside the room
  - —Physical restraints
  - —Medications given PO, IM, or IV
  - —Closely observe patients when using physical restraints or involuntary medications
- Determine if patient requires psychiatric hospitalization
- Involuntary psychiatric hospitalization if it is determined that patient is a danger to self or to others, or is gravely disabled, and is refusing hospitalization
- Usually there is a form the physician must sign attesting that the patient meets one of the above-mentioned criteria
- Often leads to 72-hour mandatory hospitalization, which may be followed by petition for psychiatric commitment

MEDICATIONS

- May be necessary for extremely agitated patient

Disposition

ADMISSION CRITERIA

- Involuntary hospitalization: danger to self or to others or gravely disabled

DISCHARGE CRITERIA

- Patients who can care for themselves adequately and have no intention of harm may be discharged after initial psychiatric evaluation
- A patient may be involuntarily hospitalized only if the patient's health or safety, or the health or safety of others, is in danger
- Once the patient is admitted involuntarily, psychiatrist petitions the court for psychiatric commitment
- If court does not grant petition for commitment, patient must be released from the psychiatric facility

Miscellaneous

ICD9: N/A

ICD10: N/A

SUGGESTED READINGS

Behnke SH, Hilliard JT. The essentials of Massachusetts mental health law. New York: WW Norton, 1998.

Folstein MF, Folstein FE, McHugh PR. The "mini-mental state": a practical method for grading the cognitive state of patients for the clinician. J Psychiatr Res 1975;12:189.

Gutheil TG, Appelbaum PS. Clinical handbook of psychiatry and the law, 3rd ed. Philadelphia: Lippincott Williams & Wilkins, 2000.

LaFond JQ. Law and the delivery of involuntary mental health services. Am J Orthopsychiatry 1994;64:209–222.

Nickens HW. Assessment and management of the violent patient. In: Dubin WR, Homke N, Nichory H, eds. Clinics in emergency medicine: psychiatric emergencies, vol 4. Edinburgh: Churchill Livingstone, 1984:101–111.

Schouten R. Psychiatry and the law I: informed consent, competency, treatment refusal, and civil commitment. In: Stern TA, Herman JB, eds. Psychiatry update and board preparation. New York: McGraw-Hill, 2000:415–419.

Authors: Jennifer M. Lafayette; Lawrence Park

Psychosis, Acute

Clinical Presentation

SIGNS AND SYMPTOMS

- Delusions are erroneous beliefs that:
  - —Involve a misinterpretation of perceptions
  - —Are clearly implausible
  - —Are often persecutory, religious, or somatic in nature
- Hallucinations
  - —Sensory experiences that exist only in the mind of the patient
  - —Can involve any sense; auditory and visual are most common
- Disorganized speech
  - —Loose associations
  - —Neologisms
  - —Perseverations
  - —Poverty of content
  - —Word salad
- Disorganized or catatonic behavior
  - —Unable to perform goal-directed behavior
  - —Unaware of the environment
- Negative symptoms
  - —Flattened affect
  - —Poverty of speech
  - —Avolition
    - -Unable to maintain goal-directed activities
- Features suggesting an organic etiology
  - —Sudden onset
  - —>40 years old
  - —Fluctuating course
  - —Confusion
  - —Headaches
  - —Loss of consciousness
  - —Focal neurologic symptoms
  - —Speech difficulties
  - —Abnormal vital signs
  - —Disorientation
  - —Psychomotor retardation
  - —Visual hallucinations
  - —Global impairment of attention and cognitive function
  - —Delusions are disorganized
  - —Labile affect
  - —Incoherent speech
  - —Social immodesty

MECHANISM/DESCRIPTION

- A description of behavior that does not imply a specific cause or diagnosis in general
- The psychosis may be secondary to functional (psychiatric) or organic (medical) causes
- Medical psychoses are generally secondary to systemic or neurologic diseases, or neuroactive medications
- Neurodevelopmental abnormalities in the dopaminergic and serotonergic systems are implicated in functional psychosis

ETIOLOGY

Organic

- Central nervous system
- Encephalopathy
- Seizure
- Head injury
- Neoplasms
- Migraine
- Huntington's chorea
- CVA
- Metabolic
  - —Intoxication or withdrawal
  - —Hypercarbia
  - —Hypoglycemia
  - —Hypoxia
  - —Poisoning
  - —Electrolyte imbalance
- Endocrine
  - —Addison's disease
  - —Thyroid dysfunction
  - —Parathyroid dysfunction
- Other
  - —Autoimmune disorders
  - —Hepatic encephalopathy
  - —Renal failure

Pharmacologic

- Psychoactive agents
- Benzodiazepines
- Chlordiazepoxide
- Antidepressants
- Antiepileptics
- Antibiotics
  - —Isoniazid
  - —Rifampin
- Cardiovascular agents
- Captopril
- Digoxin
- Methyldopa
- Procainamide
- Propranolol
- Reserpine
- Drugs of abuse
  - —Alcohol
  - —Amphetamines
  - —Cocaine
  - —Opioids
  - —Hallucinogens
- Other
  - —Steroids
  - —Heavy metals
  - —Antihistamines
  - —Cimetidine
  - —Disulfiram

Functional

- Brief psychotic disorder
  - —Usually secondary to acute emotional stress
- Schizophreniform disorder
  - —Symptoms present 1–6 months
- Schizophrenia
- Mood disorder with psychotic features or schizoaffective disorder

Pre-Hospital

CAUTIONS

- Prevention of violent behavior must be established before transport
- Consider police backup to reduce risk of violence and to place restraints

CONTROVERSIES

- Chemical restraints are rare in field protocols; may be an adjunct to physical restraints

Diagnosis

ESSENTIAL WORKUP

- The workup is case-specific and is primarily based on the suspected etiology
- Functional and organic etiologies are generally distinguished by features of the history and physical examination described below
- Collateral history is important as the patient history is often unreliable
- Complete physical examination with particular attention to the neurologic examination, vital signs, and mental status examination
- Mental status examination
  —Orientation
  —Memory (short- and long-term)
  —Attention (or calculation)
  —Recall
  —Language
  —Thoughts
  —Perception
  —Mood/affect
  —Judgment

LABORATORY

- Laboratory evaluation is needed in patients at risk for an organic etiology
  —Routine "screening labs" not helpful
  —Specific studies should be guided by the suspected underlying etiologies
  —Serum glucose
  —Toxicologic screen
  —Serum electrolytes
  —Urinalysis

IMAGING/SPECIAL TESTS

- Head CT scan indicated in patients at risk for a neurologic etiology
- Lumbar puncture indicated if signs and symptoms suggest delirium

DIFFERENTIAL DIAGNOSIS

- See Etiology, above

Treatment

INITIAL STABILIZATION

- Prevention of violence
  —See Violence, Management of

ED TREATMENT

- Antipsychotic agents are symptom-specific and therefore useful in both organic or functional psychoses
- High potency, intravenous antipsychotics, such as haloperidol, are most commonly utilized in the ED setting
- Rapid tranquilization may be achieved with the addition of a benzodiazepine
- If a specific organic etiology is identified, therapy should be directed toward the treatment of the medical condition
- Treatment of adverse effects from antipsychotic medications
  —Extrapyramidal symptoms, dystonia, akathisia, pseudoparkinsonism, and tardive dyskinesia
    -Treat with diphenhydramine or benztropine
  —Neuroleptic malignant syndrome is a life-threatening complication
    -Characterized by hyperthermia, muscle rigidity, autonomic instability, and altered consciousness
    -Treat with supportive measures and dantrolene
  —Droperidol has been reported to cause QT prolongation and dysrhythmias

MEDICATIONS

- Antipsychotics
  —Droperidol: 2.5–5.0 mg i.v. or i.m.
  —Haloperidol: 2–5 mg i.v. or i.m. or PO; 0.5–2.0 mg for elderly
  —Risperidone: 1–2 mg PO
- Benzodiazepines
  —Lorazepam 1.0–2.0 mg i.v. or i.m. or PO
- Treatment of medication side effects
  —Benztropine: 2 mg i.m. or i.v.
  —Dantrolene: 1 mg/kg i.v. repeated to symptom resolution or total of 10 mg/kg
  —Diphenhydramine: 50 mg i.v., i.m., or PO

Disposition

ADMISSION CRITERIA

- If the cause is determined to be medical in origin, admission to the appropriate medical service is indicated
- Acute psychosis of psychiatric etiology requires admission to a psychiatric service
- Safety of staff and patient must be maintained in the hospital after disposition from the ED, including possible chemical and physical restraint or a one-on-one sitter
- If the patient is felt to be a danger to either self or others, the patient *cannot* be discharged
- Involuntary commitment is required if patient is uncooperative and a threat to self or others

DISCHARGE CRITERIA

- If the psychotic behavior was caused by a temporary, reversible organic cause (e.g., drug intoxication) and the patient is now deemed to be in control, competent, and not a danger to self or others, the patient may be discharged
- Psychiatric consultation prior to discharge is recommended

Miscellaneous

ICD9: 297, 298, 299

ICD10: F23.9

SEE ALSO: PSYCHOSIS, MEDICAL VS. PSYCHIATRIC

SUGGESTED READINGS

Battaglia J, Moss S, Rush J, et al. Haloperidol, lorazepam, or both for psychotic agitation? A multicenter, prospective, double-blind emergency department study. Am J Emerg 1997;15:335–340.

Hutzler JC, Rund DA. Behavioral disorders: Emergency assessment and stabilization. In: Tintinalli JE, Kelen GD, Stapczynski JS, eds. Emergency medicine: a comprehensive study guide, 5th ed. New York: McGraw-Hill, 2000.

Richards CF, Gurr DE. Psychosis. Emerg Med Clin North Am 2000;18:253–262.

Author: Robert J. Vissers

Psychosis, Medical vs. Psychiatric

Clinical Presentation

SIGNS AND SYMPTOMS

- Psychosis characterized by:
  - —Impaired reality testing
  - —Inappropriate affect
  - —Poor impulse control
  - —Regressive or inappropriate behavior
- Hallucinations
  - —Auditory
  - —Visual
  - —Olfactory
  - —Tactile
- Delusions
  - —False beliefs held strongly by the patient even in the face of reasonable evidence to the contrary
- Affective symptoms include mania and catatonic states
- Focal and diffuse central nervous system (CNS) impairment result in derangements of:
  - —Thinking
  - —Communicating
  - —Perceiving
- Responding inappropriately

MECHANISM/DESCRIPTION

- Wide variety of medical and neurologic illnesses have psychosis as one of their presenting manifestations or that emerge during the course of the illness
- Difficult to determine whether medical or psychiatric illness is the cause of psychotic behavior
- Nature of impairment determines whether a primarily psychiatric disorder or a secondary psychosis based on a medical, neurologic, or toxic etiology
- Evaluation for underlying medical or neurologic condition essential for patients with psychotic presentation without previous history of psychosis

ETIOLOGY

- Age factor
  - —Late adolescence/early adulthood presentation more likely to be schizophrenia
  - —Middle- to late-life presentation more likely to be medical cause
- Etiology of the CNS impairment that results in a psychotic presentation include:
  - —Neurologic disorders
  - —Metabolic conditions
  - —Toxic or drug effects
  - —Nonorganic or psychiatric

Pre-Hospital

N/A

Diagnosis

ESSENTIAL WORKUP

- Careful history and physical examination
- Laboratory investigation for new or previously undiagnosed psychosis
- Use history and physical to guide workup

LABORATORY

- CBC
- Electrolytes, BUN/Cr, glucose
- Toxicology screen
- Ammonium level
- Urinalysis
- Thyroid function tests

IMAGING/SPECIAL TESTS

- CT head
- Lumbar puncture/CSF analysis

DIFFERENTIAL DIAGNOSIS

- Neurologic
  - —Head trauma
  - —Space-occupying lesions
  - —Cerebrovascular disease
  - —Postanoxic encephalopathy
  - —Seizure disorders
- Degenerative diseases
  - —Alzheimer's
  - —Pick's
  - —Huntington's
  - —Parkinsonism
  - —Hydrocephalus
- CNS infections
- Viral
- Herpetic
- Nonherpetic (e.g., rabies, mumps, influenza)
- Cerebral malaria
- Syphilis
- Toxoplasmosis
- Trypanosomiasis
- Schistosomiasis
- Myelin diseases
- Multiple sclerosis
- Leukodystrophies
- Marchiafava-Bignami disease
- Narcolepsy
- Endocrine
- Thyroid disorders
- Parathyroid disorders
- Diabetes mellitus
- Pituitary abnormalities
- Adrenal abnormalities
- Postpartum psychosis
- Metabolic
  - —Electrolyte imbalance
- End-organ failure
  - —Respiratory cardiac
  - —Renal
  - —Hepatic
  - —Pancreatic
- Ketoacidosis
- Porphyria
- Wilson's disease

- Deficiency diseases
  - —Pernicious anemia
  - —Beriberi, Wernicke-Korsakoff syndrome
  - —Pellagra
  - —Pyridoxine deficiency
- Systemic illnesses
  - —Carcinomatosis
  - —Infections, sepsis
- Viral syndromes
  - —Hepatitis
  - —Mononucleosis
- Collagen and autoimmune disorders
- Postoperative states
  - —Delirium
  - —Psychosis
  - —Depression
- Intoxicants
  - —Alcohol
  - —Barbiturates
- Stimulants
- Hallucinogens
- Opiates
- Heavy metals
- Bromide
- Organic phosphates
- Anticholinergic compounds
- Carbon monoxide
- Industrial agents
- Withdrawal states
  - —Alcohol withdrawal (delirium tremens)
  - —Barbiturate withdrawal
- Medication side effects
  - —Antipsychotics
  - —Steroids
  - —Sedative-hypnotics
  - —Antidepressants
  - —Lithium carbonate
  - —Cimetidine
  - —Disulfiram
  - —Belladonna alkaloids
  - —Levodopa
  - —Anticonvulsants
  - —Antituberculous drugs
  - —Antiinflammatory drugs
  - —Antihypertensive agents
  - —Cardiac drugs digitalis lidocaine propranolol procainamide
  - —Idiosyncratic drug reaction of any medication
- Psychiatric
  - —Schizophrenia
  - —Manic-depressive illness
  - —Stress reactions including posttraumatic stress disorder (PTSD)
  - —Intermittent explosive disorder
  - —Impulse control disorder

Treatment

INITIAL STABILIZATION

- ABCs
- If uncooperative and dangerous, control behavior with neuroleptics or benzodiazepines

ED TREATMENT

- Determine if a medical cause for psychosis
- Treat underlying illness
- Psychiatric evaluation for true psychosis
- Control psychotic behavior with psychotropic medications
  - —Treatment approach based on the severity of the psychotic features of the medical or psychiatric illness
  - —Severe behavioral disturbance of medical psychosis requires sedating the patient to adequately attend to the medical workup and treatment
  - —The more behaviorally unstable the patient, the more difficult it is to stabilize medical derangements
- Haloperidol or droperidol in combination with lorazepam
  - —Safest, fastest, and least disruptive of the ongoing mental examination of the patient
  - —Effectively calms and sedates the behaviorally agitated, psychotic, medical patient

MEDICATIONS

- Neuroleptics
  - —Droperidol: 2.5–5 mg i.v.
  - —Haloperidol: 2.5–10 mg i.m./i.v.
  - —Atypical neuroleptics (olanzapine, risperidone, ziprasidone)
- Benzodiazepines
  - —Diazepam: 5–10 mg i.v.
  - —Lorazepam: 0.5–2 mg i.v./i.m.
  - —Midazolam: 1–5 mg i.v.

Disposition

ADMISSION CRITERIA

- Psychosis primarily psychiatric (i.e., schizophrenia/manic depressive)
- Admission same as for involuntary commitment
  - —Suicidal/homicidal behavior
  - —Inability to care for self
  - —Deranged thought pattern that can be threat to self or others
- Psychosis primarily medical etiology
- Admission dictated by specific medical condition and behavior

DISCHARGE CRITERIA

- Stable medical condition
- Not suicidal/homicidal
- Able to care for self
- Decisionally capacitated

Miscellaneous

ICD9: 289.9

ICD10: F29

SEE ALSO: PSYCHOSIS, ACUTE

SUGGESTED READINGS

Cummings JL. Secondary psychoses, delusions, and schizophrenia. In: Cummings JL, ed. Clinical neuropsychiatry. Orlando, FL: Grune & Stratton, 1985:163–182.

Goff D, Henderson DC, Manschreck TC. Psychotic patients. In: Cassem NH, ed. MGH handbook of general hospital psychiatry. St. Louis: Mosby Yearbook, 1997:149–172.

Rundell JR, Wise MG. Concise guide to consultation psychiatry, 3rd ed. Washington, DC: APPI, 2000.

Author: Kathy Sanders

Pulmonary Contusion

Clinical Presentation

SIGNS AND SYMPTOMS

- Dyspnea, tachypnea; onset may be insidious, increasing over time
- Ecchymosis, bony crepitus, and tenderness associated with rib fractures
- Hemoptysis
- Cyanosis, tachycardia, hypotension
- Assume all patients with flail chest have a pulmonary contusion
- Auscultation: initially normal breath sounds progressing to wet rales or absent breath sounds

MECHANISM/DESCRIPTION

- Direct chest wall trauma or sudden deceleration, fall from height, motor vehicle accident, missile wounds
- Direct injury from the transfer of kinetic energy to the lung parenchyma results in disruption of the alveolocapillary membrane
- Microhemorrhage, localized pulmonary edema, and extravasation of blood into the interstitial and alveolar spaces produce arteriovenous shunting, ventilation-perfusion mismatch, decreased lung compliance, hypoxemia, and potential respiratory failure
- The major problem with pulmonary contusion is the ensuing hypoxemia

PEDIATRIC CONSIDERATIONS

- Relatively more elastic chest wall may transmit greater force to the thoracic contents in children

Pre-Hospital

CAUTIONS

- These patients should be routed to the nearest trauma facility
- Patients with significant respiratory distress from pulmonary contusion benefit from early intubation

Diagnosis

ESSENTIAL WORKUP

- Chest radiograph
  —Radiographic findings may not appear until 6–12 hours postinjury
  —Patchy alveolar infiltrates to frank consolidation
  —Associated intrathoracic injury such as rib fractures, pneumothorax, hemothorax, and widened mediastinal silhouette

LABORATORY

- Arterial blood gas may be helpful in assessing the degree of hypoxemia and demonstrate an elevated A-a gradient

IMAGING/SPECIAL TESTS

- Thoracic CT may be a useful adjunct in defining associated thoracic injuries

DIFFERENTIAL DIAGNOSIS

- Adult respiratory distress syndrome (ARDS)
- Pulmonary laceration
- Congestive heart failure
- Pneumonia or other infectious process
- Noncardiogenic causes of pulmonary edema

Treatment

INITIAL STABILIZATION

- ABCs
- Control airway as needed, endotracheal intubation may be indicated for patients with severe hypoxemia (PaO_2 <60 mm Hg on room air, <80 mm Hg on O_2), significant underlying lung disease, or impending respiratory failure
- Early intubation and institution of positive end expiratory pressure (PEEP) is beneficial to correct hypoxemia and acidosis, as well as decrease the work of breathing

ED TREATMENT

- Maintain adequate oxygenation, monitor O_2 saturation and respiratory rate
- In the conscious and alert patient, passive O_2 administration via face mask is first-line therapy; if the patient cannot maintain a PaO_2 >80 mm Hg on high flow oxygen, then continuous positive airway pressure (CPAP) via mask or nasal BiPAP can be attempted
- *Avoid overhydration;* intravenous crystalloid administration needed for resuscitation must be balanced with the risk of increasing interstitial pulmonary edema; frequent reexamination and serial chest radiographs are required to monitor alveolar fluid accumulation

MEDICATIONS

- The benefits of steroids are controversial and remain unproven
- *Prophylactic antibiotics are not indicated*

Disposition

ADMISSION CRITERIA

- Patients with pulmonary contusion must be admitted to the hospital for observation in anticipation of delayed-onset respiratory compromise

DISCHARGE CRITERIA

- Patients with minimal chest trauma, no evidence of respiratory distress or hypoxemia, and clear chest x-ray may be discharged
- Strict instructions should be given to return for shortness of breath, chest pain, or development of any of the above signs and symptoms of pulmonary contusion

Miscellaneous

ICD9: 861.21

ICD10: S27.3

SUGGESTED READINGS

Committee on Trauma, American College of Surgeons. Advanced trauma life support instructor manual, 5th ed. Chicago: American College of Surgeons, 1993.

Vukich D, Markovchick V. Thoracic trauma. In: Rosen P, et al., eds. Emergency medicine: concepts and clinical practice, 4th ed. St. Louis: CV Mosby, 1998:514.

Wilson R. Thoracic trauma. In: Tintinalli J, et al., eds. Emergency medicine: a comprehensive study guide, 4th ed. New York: McGraw-Hill, 1996:1156.

Author: Greg Lampe

Pulmonary Edema

Clinical Presentation

EPIDEMIOLOGY

- 400,000 new cases present yearly
- Prevalence is 1–2% of the general population
- Incidence is greater in males than in females for patients aged 40–75 years
- No sex predilection exists for patients older than 75 years
- Incidence of CHF increases with increasing age and affects 10% of population older than 75
- 30–40% of patients with CHF are hospitalized every year
- 5-year mortality after diagnosis was reported as 60% in men and 45% in women
- Median survival of 3.2 years for males and 5.4 years for females
- Sudden death accounts for up to 45% of all deaths
- In-hospital mortality rate: 19%
- African Americans are 1.5 times more likely to die of CHF than whites
- Mortality approximately 50–60% for noncardiogenic pulmonary edema and up to 80% for cardiogenic shock

SIGNS AND SYMPTOMS

- General
  —Weakness
  —Fatigue
  —Anxiety
  —Diaphoresis
  —Cold, ashen, or cyanotic skin
- Respiratory
  —Dyspnea with exertion is the single most sensitive test
  —Dyspnea at rest is also common
  —Orthopnea, paroxysmal nocturnal dyspnea
  —Cough
    -Pink, frothy sputum
  —Noisy respirations
  —Tachypnea
  —Wheezing, rhonchi, gurgles
  —Moist, crepitant rales noted initially at bases and progressing to apices
  —Dilated alae nasi
  —Inspiratory retraction of the intercostal spaces or supraventricular fossae
  —Cheyne-Stokes respirations
- Cardiovascular
  —Tachycardia
  —Jugular venous distention
  —Abnormal heart sounds
    -Increased P_2, S_3, S_4
  —Nocturnal angina
  —Pulsus alternans—alternating weak and strong pulses
  —Presence of valvular heart disease

MECHANISM/DESCRIPTION

- Imbalance in Starling forces causes an increase in lung fluid secondary to leakage from pulmonary capillaries into the interstitium and alveoli of the lung
- If capacity of lymphatic drainage is exceeded, liquid accumulates in interstitial spaces surrounding bronchioles and lung vasculature, creating CHF
- If increased fluid and pressure tracks into the interstitial space around the alveoli and disrupts the alveolar membrane, the alveoli are flooded causing pulmonary edema
- Systolic dysfunction is characterized by a dilated left ventricle with impaired contractility
- Diastolic dysfunction occurs in a normal or intact left ventricle with impaired ability to relax and receive as well as eject blood
- New York Heart Association classification of CHF
  —Class I: not limited in normal physical activity by symptoms
  —Class II: ordinary physical activity results in fatigue, dyspnea, or other symptoms
  —Class III: marked limitation in normal activity
  —Class IV: symptoms at rest or with any activity

ETIOLOGY

- Six categories:
  —Pulmonary edema secondary to altered capillary permeability
  —Pulmonary edema secondary to increased pulmonary capillary pressure: pulmonary venous thrombosis, stenosis or veno-occlusive disease, and volume overload
  —Pulmonary edema secondary to decreased oncotic pressure found with hypoalbuminemia
  —Pulmonary edema secondary to large negative pleural pressure with increased end expiratory volume
  —Pulmonary edema secondary to lymphatic insufficiency
  —Pulmonary edema secondary to mixed or unknown mechanisms

Specific Etiologies

- *Cardiogenic/altered capillary permeability*
  —Left heart failure
  —Ischemic heart disease
  —Acute myocardial infarction
  —Aortic and mitral valvular disease
  —Hypertensive heart disease
  —Cardiomyopathy
  —Volume overload
  —Arrhythmias
  —Endocarditis
  —Myocarditis
  —Congenital heart disease
  —Acute rheumatic fever and rheumatic heart disease
  —Septal defects
  —High cardiac output states
    -Thyrotoxicosis
    -Beriberi
  —Uremia
- *Respiratory/adult respiratory distress syndrome/altered capillary permeability*
  —Pneumonia
  —Inhaled toxins
  —Circulating foreign substances
    -Snake venom
    -Endotoxins
  —Aspiration
  —Acute radiation pneumonitis
  —Disseminated intravascular coagulation
  —Hypersensitivity pneumonitis
  —Shock lung in association with nonthoracic trauma
  —Acute hemorrhagic pancreatitis
  —Near drowning
- *Hypoalbuminemia/decreased oncotic pressure*
  —Renal failure
  —Hepatic failure
  —Protein-losing enteropathic
  —Severe dermatologic disease with high protein losses
  —Starvation
- *Increased negativity of interstitial pressure*
  —Rapid decompression of a pneumothorax
  —Asthma
- *Lymphatic obstruction*
  —Post-lung transplant
  —Lymphangitic carcinomatosis
  —Fibrosing lymphangitis
- *Mixed or unknown mechanism*
- High-altitude pulmonary edema
- Neurogenic pulmonary edema
- Narcotic overdose
- Pulmonary embolism
- Eclampsia
- Postcardioversion
- Postanesthesia
- Post-cardiopulmonary bypass
- Postextubation

Pre-Hospital

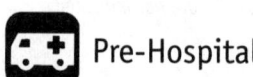

- Intravenous access
- Supplemental oxygen
  —100% non-rebreather mask
- Cardiac monitor
- Pulse oximetry
- Sublingual nitrates
- Furosemide
- Endotracheal intubation may be required in severe cases

CAUTIONS

- Administration of morphine
  —Pulmonary edema may be difficult to distinguish from an acute exacerbation of COPD

Diagnosis

ESSENTIAL WORKUP

- A careful history and physical should determine if the underlying etiology is cardiogenic

LABORATORY

- BNP (B-type natriuretic peptide)
  —A proteohormone secreted by the left ventricle in response to wall tension
  —Promising laboratory parameter for the detection and follow-up of heart failure
  —BNP is available for point of care testing with 10- to 15-minute turnaround time
  —May be helpful in determining whether dyspnea is secondary to COPD or CHF
- Serum electrolytes, BUN, creatinine, urinalysis
  —Hyperkalemia with severe low output states
  —Increased creatinine and dilutional hyponatremia are observed in severe cases
  —Mild azotemia and proteinuria are observed in early and mild-to-moderate disease
- Elevated alanine aminotransferase (ALT), aspartate aminotransferase (AST), or bilirubin suggests congestive hepatopathy
- Cardiac enzymes may be useful if ischemia or infarction is presumed to be the underlying cause
- Serum lipase if pancreatitis is suspected as the underlying cause
- Arterial blood gas may help evaluate hypoxemia, ventilation/perfusion mismatch, hypercapnia, and acidosis

IMAGING/SPECIAL TESTS

Chest Radiograph

- Three phases of pulmonary findings:
  —Pulmonary redistribution
    -Cephalization of vessels
  —Interstitial edema
    -Effusions
    -Kerley B lines
    -Classic butterfly infiltrate
  —Frank alveolar infiltrates
    -May be asymmetric and mistaken for pneumonia

EKG

- Assess for underlying cardiac disorders

Echocardiography

- Excludes acute valvular pathology
- Assessment for focal or global LV dysfunction
- Measurement of cardiac output

DIFFERENTIAL DIAGNOSIS

- Pneumonia
- Asthma
- COPD exacerbation
- Pulmonary embolism
- Hyperventilation syndrome
- Pericardial tamponade
- Pneumothorax
- Pleural effusion

Treatment

INITIAL STABILIZATION

- Intravenous access
- Supplemental oxygen
- Place patient in an upright position
- Cardiac monitor
- Pulse oximetry
- Control airway as needed
- Endotracheal intubation for impending respiratory failure

ED TREATMENT

- Normotensive or hypertensive patients with cardiogenic pulmonary edema
  —Rapid-acting nitrates preferably sublingual or Nitrospray
  —IV nitroglycerin
  —Morphine sulfate
  —Intravenous diuretics
    -Lasix or Bumex
    -IV BNP (Nesiritide) is a balanced vasodilator with no inotropic or chronotropic properties
    -Compared to dobutamine, BNP is not proarrhythmic and has no effect on heart rate and is particularly useful in patients already taking nitrates, as tolerance to Nesritide has not been described
  —Sodium nitroprusside for afterload reduction can be helpful for severe persistent hypertension but is not recommended if cardiac ischemia may be concurrent
  —Noninvasive ventilatory support: continuous or bilevel positive airway pressure (CPAP or Bi-PAP) may decrease the need for intubation, although Bi-PAP may be associated with a higher incidence of AMI
    -Endotracheal intubation for impending respiratory failure
- Hypotensive patients
  —Avoid nitrates, morphine, and diuretics
  —Use agents that increase myocardial contractility
    -Dopamine
    -Dobutamine
    -Amrinone
    -Milrinone
- Renal dialysis patients
  —Emergent renal dialysis is the treatment of choice
  —If rapid dialysis cannot be rapidly achieved
    -IV nitroglycerin
    -IV enalaprilat or oral captopril may be useful

MEDICATIONS

- Bumex: 0.5–1 mg i.v.
- Captopril: 25–50 mg PO t.i.d.
- Dobutamine: begin at 2 μg/kg/min i.v.; titrate to blood pressure, cardiac output, and pulmonary capillary wedge pressure
- Furosemide: 20–80 mg i.v.
- IV enalaprilat: 1.25 mg q6h over 5 minutes
- Morphine sulfate: 2–5 mg i.v.
- Nesiritide: i.v. bolus of 2 μg/kg followed by a continuous infusion of 0.01 μg/kg/min
- Nitroglycerin paste: 1–2 inches; begin drip at 5 μg/min and increase by 5–10 μg/min every few minutes; titrate to blood pressure
- Nitroprusside: begin drip at 10 μg/min and increasing by 5–10 μg/min every few minutes
- Sublingual nitroglycerin or Nitrospray 0.4 mg may give repeatedly as SBP tolerates q 5 min

Disposition

ADMISSION CRITERIA

- Intensive care unit
  —Intubated patients
  —Patients on Bi-PAP
  —Adult respiratory distress syndrome
- Monitored unit
  —New-onset pulmonary edema
  —Electrocardiographic changes
- Observation
  —Known congestive heart failure with mild to moderate disease

DISCHARGE CRITERIA

- Patients with known congestive heart failure presenting with mild pulmonary edema no concomitant complaints suggestive of ischemia
  —Complete resolution of symptoms after ED management
  —Normal oxygenation on room air at the time of discharge
  —No new electrocardiographic changes
- Follow-up arranged within the next 48 hours
- Low-salt diet
- Serial weights to assess fluid accumulation

Miscellaneous

ICD9: 518.4

ICD10: J81

SEE ALSO: CONGESTIVE HEART FAILURE

SUGGESTED READINGS

Braunwald E. Pulmonary edema. In: Braunwald E, ed. Heart disease: a textbook of cardiovascular medicine, 6th ed. Philadelphia: WB Saunders, 2001:503–614.

Evaluation and management of chronic heart failure in the adult: ACC/AHA practice guidelines. J Am Coll Cardiol 2001;38:2101–2113.

Ketai LH, Godwin JD. A new view of pulmonary edema and acute respiratory distress syndrome. J Thorac Imaging 1998;13:147–171.

Pang D, Keenan SP, Cook DJ, et al. The effect of positive pressure airway support on mortality and the need for intubation in cardiogenic pulmonary edema. A systematic review. Chest 1998;114:1186–1192.

Authors: Shamai Grossman; Jonathan Edlow

Pulmonary Embolism

Clinical Presentation

SIGNS AND SYMPTOMS

- Most common
  - —Dyspnea
  - —Pleuritic chest pain
  - —Tachypnea
- General
  - —Fevers (rarely >102.0°F)
  - —Diaphoresis
- Pulmonary
  - —Cough
  - —Hemoptysis (rarely massive)
  - —Rales
- Cardiovascular
  - —Tachycardia
  - —Syncope
  - —Murmur
- Extremities
  - —Cyanosis
  - —Evidence of thrombophlebitis
  - —Lower extremity edema
- Abdominal pain
- Symptoms similar in elderly but typically more subtle if age <40

MECHANISM/DESCRIPTION

- Vast majority arise from thrombi in the deep veins of the lower extremities and pelvis
- Thrombi also originate in renal and upper extremity veins
- After traveling to lungs, size of thrombus determine signs and symptoms

ETIOLOGY

- Most with PE have identifiable risk factor
  - —Recent surgery
  - —Pregnancy
  - —Previous DVT/PE
  - —Stroke or recent paraplegia
  - —Malignancy
  - —Age >50
  - —Obesity
  - —Smoking
  - —Oral contraceptives
  - —Major trauma
  - —Hematologic risk factors
    - -Factor 5 Leiden
    - -Protein C or S deficiency
    - -Antithrombin III deficiency
    - -Antiphospholipid antibody syndrome

PEDIATRIC CONSIDERATIONS

- Thromboembolic disease quite rare in this population
  - —Risk factors in children
  - —Presence of central venous catheter
  - —Immobility
  - —Heart disease
  - —Trauma
  - —Malignancy
  - —Surgery
  - —Infection

Pre-Hospital

CAUTIONS

- Initial supplemental oxygen
- Establish IV access
- Cardiac monitor

Diagnosis

ESSENTIAL WORKUP

- CXR
  - —Used to rule out other causes
  - —Most common findings with PE
    - -Normal
    - -Nonspecific parenchymal abnormality
    - -Atelectasis
  - —Other findings with PE
    - -Pleural effusions
    - -Pleural-based opacities (Hampton hump)
    - -Elevated hemidiaphragm
    - -Local oligemia (Westermark's sign)
- EKG
  - —To rule out cardiac etiology
  - —Usually normal in PE
  - —Other findings include
    - -Nonspecific ST-T wave changes (most common abnormality)
    - -Sinus tachycardia
    - -Left axis deviation
    - -RBBB pattern
    - -S1Q3T3 pattern is uncommon and not specific enough to rule in/out diagnosis

LABORATORY

- ABG
  - —Can show hypoxemia, hypocapnia, respiratory alkalosis, or elevated A-a gradient
  - —PE still possible with normal A-a gradient
  - —Does not aid in diagnosis of PE
- CBC
  - —Anemia may be contributing factor to dyspnea
- D-dimer enzyme-linked immunosorbent assay (ELISA)
  - —High sensitivity (close to 100%) with low specificity for PE
  - —Essential to consider patient population when interpreting results
  - —Negative predictive value 99% in one large study in conjunction with low clinical suspicion

IMAGING/SPECIAL TESTS

- Ventilation-perfusion scan (V/Q)
  - —Results reported in probabilities and correlated to clinical suspicion
  - —Probability of PE with V/Q results:
    - -Normal or near normal V/Q scan: 4% probability for PE
    - -Low probability V/Q scan with low clinical suspicion: 4% probability for PE
    - -Low probability V/Q scan with high clinical suspicion: 16–40% probability for PE
    - -Intermediate V/Q scan: 16–66% probability for PE
    - -High probability V/Q scan with low clinical suspicion: 56% probability for PE
    - -High probability V/Q scan with high clinical suspicion: 96% probability for PE
- Spiral chest CT with IV contrast
  - —Accurate for identifying PE in proximal pulmonary tree
  - —Will not pick up subsegmental PE
  - —Gaining increasing acceptance for diagnosis of PE
- Lower extremity duplex ultrasound
  - —Used in patients who would otherwise require pulmonary angiogram
  - —Presence of DVT requires same anticoagulation as PE
- Pulmonary angiogram
  - —Gold standard for diagnosis
  - —Used when diagnosis not confirmed or excluded
  - —Higher complication rate than other modalities
- Echocardiogram
  - —Used to assess for right heart strain when thrombolysis is an option

DIFFERENTIAL DIAGNOSIS

- Pneumonia
- Cardiac dysrhythmias
- Asthma
- Pneumothorax
- Aortic dissection
- Pericarditis
- Myocardial infarction
- Rib fracture
- Costochondritis
- Anxiety disorder

Treatment

INITIAL STABILIZATION

- ABCs
- Provide supplemental oxygen to maintain adequate oxygen saturation
- Intubate if unable to provide adequate oxygenation
- Administer IV fluids carefully for hypotensive patients
  - —Excessive fluid expansion may worsen right heart failure

ED TREATMENT

- Anticoagulation
  - —Prevents additional thrombus from forming
  - —Stabilizes existent clot to prevent migration
  - —Unfractionated heparin
    - -Mainstay of therapy
    - -Goal to maintain PTT between 1.5 and 2.5 times the control value (60–80 seconds)
  - —Low molecular weight heparin (LMWH)
    - -FDA approved for treatment of DVT with or without PE
    - -Therapeutic goal automatic with weight-based dosing
  - —Warfarin
    - -Oral therapy for long-term anticoagulation
    - -Begin once therapeutic PTT is achieved
    - -Goal is INR of 2–3
- Thrombolysis
  - —Initiate in hemodynamically unstable patients with PE
  - —Consider in stable patients with PE and right heart strain on echo
- Inferior vena cava (IVC) filter
  - —Indicated in patients who have contraindications to anticoagulation or have been therapeutic on anticoagulation but failed prevention of PE
- Surgical or catheter embolectomy
  - —Consider in those with thrombolysis contraindications or failure, or deemed unstable for medical management
  - —Case-by-case basis

MEDICATIONS

- Alteplase: 100 mg (peds: N/A) i.v. over 2 hours
- Enoxaparin: 1 mg/kg (peds: 0.75 mg/kg) s.c. q12h
- Reteplase: 10 U (peds: N/A) i.v. bolus q 30 min × 2
- Streptokinase: 250,000 U (peds: 3,500–4,000 U/kg) i.v. bolus over 30 minutes, then 100,000U (peds: 1,000–1,500 U/kg) i.v. maintenance over 24 hours
- Unfractionated heparin:
  - —Bolus: 80 U/kg (peds: 75 U/kg) i.v. over 10 minutes
  - —Maintenance: 18 U/kg (peds: 20 U/kg) i.v. drip
- Warfarin: 5 mg (peds: 0.05–0.34 mg/kg/d) PO qd; adjust for INR goal 2–3

PEDIATRIC CONSIDERATIONS

- Data on thrombolysis and LMWH limited
- Data suggest longer course of therapy

ADMISSION CRITERIA

- Admit all patients with PE for continued treatment
- Clinically stable patients with a high suspicion for PE, no contraindication to anticoagulation, and a lack of V/Q scanning or angiographic availability may be anticoagulated and studied when resources are available in the morning

DISCHARGE CRITERIA

N/A

Miscellaneous

ICD9: 415.1

ICD10: I26.9

SUGGESTED READINGS

Edlow JA. Emergency department management of pulmonary embolism. Emerg Med Clin North Am 2001;19: 995–1011.

Goldhaber SZ. Pulmonary embolism. N Engl J Med 1999;339:93–104.

PIOPED Investigators. Value of the ventilation/perfusion scan in acute pulmonary embolism. JAMA 1990;263: 2753–2759.

Author: Alan M. Kumar

Purpura

Clinical Presentation

SIGNS AND SYMPTOMS

- Nonblanching lesions from 0.2 to 1 cm in diameter
- Palpable or nonpalpable
- Shape and size
  - —Petechiae (<2 mm)
  - —Macular (2–10 mm)
  - —Ecchymoses (>10 mm)
  - —Annular or erythema multiforme (target lesions)
  - —Irregular (retiform)
- Distribution
  - —Generally more frequent in lower extremities (increased hydrostatic force)
  - —Widespread petechiae and ecchymoses seen with disseminated intravascular coagulation (DIC) and meningococcemia
  - —When oral mucous membranes are involved, consider idiopathic thrombocytopenic purpura (ITP)
- Hypotension
- Altered mental status (AMS)
- Gingival hemorrhage
- Epistaxis
- Hematuria
- Fever
- Malaise
- Arthralgias
- Myalgias
- Purpura fulminans
  - —Large irregular ecchymoses
  - —Fever
  - —Shock
  - —DIC
- Pseudomonas (ecthyma gangrenosum)
  - —Begins as edematous, erythematous papules
  - —Bullae formation in the girdle region
- Disseminated gonococcal infection
  - —Usually <10 lesions, purpuric papules or vesicopustules, extensor surface of hands, dorsal aspect of ankles and toes
  - —Fever
  - —Arthralgias
- Meningococcemia
  - —Small areas of skin infarction cause purpura in irregular pattern
  - —May involve head, palms, soles, mucous membranes including conjunctivae
  - —Fever
  - —Headache
- Rocky Mountain spotted fever (RMSF)
  - —After 4–7 days of generalized symptoms, erythematous macules on distal extremities including palms and soles, then petechial
  - —Fever
  - —Chills
  - —Headache
- Henoch-Schönlein purpura
  - —Extensor aspects of lower extremities and buttocks
  - —Fades in about 5 days
  - —Fever
  - —Arthralgias
  - —Abdominal pain
  - —Hematuria
- Kawasaki's disease
  - —Purpura is rare
  - —Fever, plus four of the following:
    - -Polymorphous exanthema
    - -Peripheral extremity changes
    - -Bilateral conjunctivitis
    - -Changes of lips and mouth
    - -Cervical lymphadenopathy

MECHANISM/DESCRIPTION

- Hemorrhagic lesion that does not blanch completely with pressure, usually red, blue, or purple
- Platelet disorder
  - —Diminished production
  - —Altered distribution
  - —Increased destruction
  - —Abnormal function
- Increased fragility of capillaries or dermal support
- Nonpalpable purpura
  - —Simple hemorrhage or microvascular occlusion with ischemic hemorrhage
  - —Generally platelet disorder
  - —Vasculitic lesions may not be palpable in immunocompromised patients
- Palpable purpura
  - —Generally due to vasculitis
  - —Irregular when due to infectious emboli
  - —Regular lesions with leukocytoclastic emboli
  - —Massive bleeding from a platelet disorder may cause palpable hematomas
- Vasculitis
  - —Autoimmune, small-vessel leukocytoclastic vasculitis
  - —Hypersensitivity to various antigens
  - —Formation of circulating immune complexes deposited in walls of postcapillary venules, activate complement that is chemotactic for polymorphonuclear leukocytes
  - —Enzymes released damage vessel walls and cause leakage of blood

ETIOLOGY

- Nonpalpable purpura
  - —Viral
  - —Echo
  - —Coxsackie
  - —Measles
  - —Parvovirus B19
  - —Drugs
  - —Acetaminophen
  - —Allopurinol
  - —Anticoagulants
  - —Aspirin
  - —Digoxin
  - —Furosemide
  - —Gold salts
  - —Lidocaine
  - —Methyldopa
  - —Penicillin
  - —Phenylbutazone
  - —Quinidine
  - —Quinine
  - —Rifampin
  - —Steroids
  - —Sulfonamides
  - —Thiazides
  - —Nutritional deficiencies
  - —Bone marrow disease
  - —Hypersplenism
  - —ITP
  - —DIC
  - —TTP
  - —Liver or renal insufficiency
  - —Thrombocytosis (>1,000,000)
  - —Spiking elevations of intravascular pressure (childbirth, vomiting paroxysmal coughing)
  - —Hemophilia
  - —Vitamin K deficiency
  - —Solar purpura (limited to sun-exposed areas
  - —Scurvy
- Palpable purpura
  - —Streptococcal pharyngitis
  - —Echovirus type 9
  - —Coxsackie virus
  - —Hepatitis B
  - —Drugs
  - —Allopurinol
  - —ASA
  - —Antiinfluenza vaccines
  - —Cephalosporins
  - —Gold
  - —Hydralazine
  - —Iodides
  - —Metoclopramide
  - —NSAIDs
  - —Penicillin
  - —Phenylbutazone
  - —Phenytoin
  - —Quinidine
  - —Quinine
  - —Streptomycin
  - —Sulfonamides
  - —Thiazides
  - —Ticlopidine
  - —Malignancies
  - —Autoimmune and connective tissue diseases
  - —Gonococcus
  - —Meningococcus
  - —Pseudomonas (ecthyma gangrenosum)
  - —Rocky Mountain spotted fever (RMSF)
  - —In immune-compromised hosts: candida, aspergillus
  - —Occlusion due to microvascular platelet plugs (heparin necrosis)
  - —Cold-related gelling or agglutinations (cryoglobulinemia)
  - —Occlusion due to organisms living in vessels, generally in immunocompromised patients (mucormycosis, aspergillus, disseminated strongyloidiasis)

—Local or systemic coagulation abnormalities: scarlet fever (rarely "strep throat"), *Vibrio vulnificus* bacteremia, "malignant chickenpox," and "black measles" (both rare in U.S.); Coumadin necrosis
—Embolization: cholesterol, crystal, thrombus (atrial myxoma, septic endocarditis, multiple myeloma)

PEDIATRIC CONSIDERATIONS

- Henoch-Schönlein purpura
- Kawasaki's disease

Neonatal

- Extramedullary erythropoiesis (blueberry muffin baby)
- Purpura fulminans (protein C and S deficiency)
- Maternal ITP
- Wiskott-Aldrich syndrome

Pre-Hospital

- Intravenous access and monitor for fever, hypotension, or altered mental status

CAUTIONS

- Respiratory precautions

Diagnosis

ESSENTIAL WORKUP

- Obtain a complete medical history
  —Previous bleeding problems
  —Deep venous thrombosis/pulmonary embolism suggesting factor V Leiden mutation
  —Splenectomy
  —Alcohol abuse
  —Family history of bleeding disorders
  —High-risk medications

LABORATORY

- Platelet count
  —Abnormal counts must be verified by manual examination of a peripheral smear
- DIC screen
  —Indicated when the patient appears toxic
- PT, PTT
- Rapid strep test
- Urinalysis

Studies For Outpatient Management

- Bleeding time
- Hepatitis B and C serologies
- Strep throat culture or ASO titer
- Antinuclear antibodies
- Cryoglobulins
- Platelet function studies
- Serum complements
- Serum protein electrophoresis
- Von Willebrand's disease screen

IMAGING/SPECIAL TESTS

N/A

DIFFERENTIAL DIAGNOSIS

- Secondary purpura (e.g., excoriation of mosquito bite)

Treatment

- Initial stabilization if fever, hypotension, altered mental status, or generalized ecchymoses
  —Airway support
  —Intravenous access
  —Fluid resuscitation
  —Intravenous antibiotics as soon as possible (ceftriaxone)

ED TREATMENT

- Presumptive treatment of bacterial infection
  —Meningococcus: ceftriaxone
  —Pneumococcus: ceftriaxone, consider penicillin
- Prophylaxis for meningococcal infections: rifampin, ciprofloxacin

MEDICATIONS

- Ceftriaxone: 2 g (peds: 100 mg/kg/24 hours) i.v. q12h
- Ciprofloxacin (prophylaxis): 500 mg PO single dose
- Penicillin: 4 million units (peds: 240,000 U/kg/24 hours) i.v. q4h
- Rifampin (prophylaxis): 600 mg PO q12h for 2 days

PEDIATRIC CONSIDERATIONS

- Neonatal sepsis
  —Ampicillin 100 mg/kg/24 hours i.v. q6h *and*
  —Gentamicin 7.5 mg/kg/24 hours i.v. q8h (or cefotaxime 200 mg/kg/24 hours i.v. q6h

Disposition

ADMISSION CRITERIA

- Unstable vital signs
- Altered mental status
- Fever

DISCHARGE CRITERIA

- Exclusion of life-threatening etiologies
  —Serious bacterial infections
  —Critical thrombocytopenia
  —Appropriate close follow-up scheduled
  —Consider follow-up with dermatology (skin biopsy) and hematology

Miscellaneous

ICD9: 287

ICD10: D96.2

SEE ALSO: RASH

SUGGESTED READINGS

Baselga E. Purpura in infants and children. J Am Acad Dermatol 1997;37:673–705.

Cohen YC, Djulbegovic B, Shamai-Lubovitz O, et al. The bleeding risk and natural history of idiopathic thrombocytopenic purpura in patients with persistent low platelet counts. Arch Intern Med 2000;160:1630–1638.

Leung AK, Chan KW. Evaluating the child with purpura. Am Fam Physician 2001;64: 419–428.

Piette WW. Hematologic disorders. In: Freedberg IM, et al., eds. Fitzpatrick's dermatology in general medicine, 5th ed. New York: McGraw-Hill, 1999:1867–1881.

Soter NA. Cutaneous necrotizing venulitis. In: Freedberg IM, et al., eds. Fitzpatrick's dermatology in general medicine, 5th ed. New York: McGraw-Hill, 1999:2044–2053.

Author: Michele B. Wagner

Pyelonephritis

Clinical Presentation

SIGNS AND SYMPTOMS

- Dysuria/urgency/frequency
- Back, flank, or abdominal pain
- Body aches, fever, chills, malaise
- Nausea, vomiting
- Costovertebral angle tenderness or suprapubic tenderness
- Ill/toxic appearing
- Dehydration
- Occult pyelonephritis
  - —Invasion of the upper urinary tract without clinical symptoms
  - —Suspect in lower UTI which doesn't resolve with standard treatment

MECHANISM/DESCRIPTION

- Ascension of bacteria from a lower UTI into the renal parenchyma
- Male/female ratio:
  - —1:5 in first year of life
  - —1:10 in children
  - —1:50 in reproductive years
  - —1:1 in fifth decade and later

ETIOLOGY

- Bacteriology:
  - —*E. coli* 80–95%
  - —*S. saprophyticus* 5–15%
  - —*Proteus mirabilis*
  - —*Klebsiella* species
  - —*Citrobacter freundii*
  - —*Serratia*
  - —*Enterobacter*
  - —*Pseudomonas*
- Predisposing factors:
  - —Recent instrumentation: catheterization, cystoscopy, indwelling urinary catheter
  - —Urinary obstruction: stricture, stone, prostatic enlargement, tumor, other foreign body
  - —Anatomic abnormalities: hypospadias, ureteral ectopia, bifid ureter, renal scarring
  - —Neurologic conditions: neurogenic bladder, spinal cord injury
  - —Abnormal urodynamics
  - —Previous UTIs (in childhood, more than three in past year)
  - —Recent pyelonephritis within 1 year
  - —Diabetes mellitus
  - —Immunosuppression
  - —Pregnancy

PEDIATRIC CONSIDERATIONS

- Fever, irritability, lethargy, poor feeding, or jaundice may be the only symptom in infants
- Enuresis in the previously toilet-trained child
- Hematogenous spread in neonates and immunocompromised children
- Renal scarring
  - —More common sequelae in young children than adults
- Group B streptococci
  - —Etiologic agents in neonates

Pre-Hospital

CAUTIONS

- Treat shock secondary to urosepsis

Diagnosis

ESSENTIAL WORKUP

- Urinalysis
  - —Clean catch or catheterized urine specimen: catheterized specimen if:
    - -Vaginal discharge or bleeding
    - -Contaminated specimen (large number of squamous cells)
  - —Pyuria: 5–10 WBCs, + leukocyte esterase, + nitrates
  - —Hematuria
- Urine culture and sensitivity
  - —Obtain in:
    - -Suspected pyelonephritis
    - -Unclear diagnosis
    - -Treatment failures
    - -Recurrent infections
  - —>100,000 CFU/mL positive
  - —10^2–10^4 CFU considered positive in:
    - -Early infection
    - -Clinical scenario consistent with UTI
    - -Catheter or suprapubic specimen
    - -Males
  - —Identifies bacteria in the event that infection does not respond to empiric therapy
- Assess for dehydration

LABORATORY

- CBC
  - —Optional
  - —Does not rule in or out upper tract infection
- Blood cultures
  - —Not needed; positive cultures do not correlate with more severe disease
  - —Bacteria identified more readily on urine culture

IMAGING/SPECIAL TESTS

- Helical CT
  - —Stranding or inflammation and edema of the parenchyma
  - —Obtain helical CT or renal ultrasound if:
    - -Concomitant stone or obstruction suspected
    - -Diagnosis unclear
    - -Patient very ill or getting worse
    - -At risk for renal emphysema or abscess (diabetes mellitus, elderly)
- Consider elective evaluation of the genitourinary tract in males with pyelonephritis

DIFFERENTIAL DIAGNOSIS

- Lower UTI
- Pelvic inflammatory disease
- Prostatitis
- Epididymitis
- Urethritis
- Nephrolithiasis
- Renal abscess
- Appendicitis
- Diverticulitis
- Cholecystitis
- Lower lobe pneumonia

PEDIATRIC CONSIDERATIONS

- "Bag" urine specimen—don't obtain
  - —Vast majority of positive cultures are contaminants
  - —Helpful only for ruling out disease if culture is negative
- Catheterized or suprapubic specimen with >1,000 CFU is positive
- Blood cultures usually performed for children <1 year of age
- Renal cortical scan using dimercaptosuccinic acid (DMSA)
  - —Sensitive and specific test for diagnosis of pyelonephritis
  - —Decreased cortical uptake without volume loss indicates acute pyelonephritis
- All children with first episode of pyelonephritis should have urinary tract imaging performed later
  - —Renal ultrasound
    - -Within 48 hours if no clinical improvement
    - -Within 3–6 weeks if clinical improvement
  - —Girls 4–10 years old
    - -Radionuclide isocystogram for vesicoureteral reflux
  - —Boys 4–10 years old
    - -Voiding cystourethrogram after urine is sterile and bladder spasm has subsided

Treatment

INITIAL STABILIZATION

- Bolus with 0.9% NS 500 cc–1 L (20 cc/kg ×3 in children) for shock/dehydration

ED TREATMENT

- Parenteral antibiotics for:
  - —Inability to comply with oral therapy
  - —Extremes of age
  - —Failure of oral therapy
  - —Urinary obstruction
  - —Toxicity
  - —Immunosuppression
  - —Pregnancy
  - —Suspected antibiotic resistant organisms
- Empiric intravenous antibiotics
  - —Aminoglycoside (gentamicin) plus ampicillin
  - —Third-generation cephalosporin (ceftriaxone)
  - —Fluoroquinolones—not approved for children
  - —TMP-SMX—not for use in complicated pyelonephritis
  - —In pregnancy
    - -Third-generation cephalosporin
    - -Gentamicin/ampicillin
    - -Cefazolin
    - -Aztreonam
- Outpatient oral antibiotics
  - —For nontoxic and otherwise healthy patient
    - -Fluoroquinolone—7-day course
    - -TMP-SMX—10- to 14-day course
- May administer one dose of parenteral antibiotics prior to oral antibiotics
  - —Assures a prompt cessation of bacterial proliferation
  - —Avoids delays in oral antibiotic administration
  - —No literature addressing efficacy
- Antiemetics for vomiting
- Analgesia for pain

MEDICATIONS

- Oral antibiotics
  - —Cephalexin: 500 mg q.i.d.
  - —Ciprofloxacin: 250 mg b.i.d.
  - —Levofloxacin 250 mg qd
  - —Norfloxacin: 400 mg b.i.d.
  - —Ofloxacin: 200 mg b.i.d.
  - —TMP-SMX: 160 mg/800 mg b.i.d.
- Oral antibiotics for complicated pyelonephritis
  - —Ciprofloxacin 500 mg b.i.d.
  - —Gatifloxacin 400 mg qd
  - —Levofloxacin 500 mg qd
  - —Ofloxacin 200 mg b.i.d.
- IV antibiotics
  - —Ampicillin: 1 g q6h
  - —Cefazolin: 1–1.5 g q8h
  - —Ceftriaxone: 2 g q24h
  - —Ciprofloxacin: 400 mg q12h
  - —Gatifloxacin 400 mg qd
  - —Gentamicin: 2–5 mg/kg load
  - —Imipenem-cilastatin: 0.5–1 g q8h
  - —Levofloxacin 500 mg qd
  - —Ofloxacin 200 mg b.i.d.
  - —Ticarcillin-clavulanate: 3.1 g q6h
  - —TMP-SMX 160 mg/800 mg q12h

PEDIATRIC CONSIDERATIONS

- Oral antibiotic liquid preparations for children
  - —Amoxicillin: 30–50 mg/kg/24 hours t.i.d.
  - —Amoxicillin/clavulanic acid: 45 mg/kg/24 hours t.i.d.
  - —Cefixime: 8 mg/kg/24 hours qd
  - —Cefpodoxime: 10 mg/kg/24 hours b.i.d.
  - —Cephalexin: 50–75 mg/kg/24 hours q.i.d.
  - —Erythromycin/sulfisoxazole: 50 mg EM/kg/24 hours q.i.d.
  - —Loracarbef 15–30 mg/kg/24 hours b.i.d.
  - —TMP-SMZ: 6–12 mg TMP, 30–60 mg SMZ per kg/24 hours b.i.d.
- Parenteral antibiotics for admitted children
  - —Age 0–3 months
    - -Cefotaxime (50–180 mg/kg/d t.i.d.) plus ampicillin (50–100 mg/kg/d q.i.d.)
    - -Gentamicin (1–2.5 mg/kg/d t.i.d.) plus ampicillin
  - —Age >3 months
    - -May substitute ceftriaxone (50–100 mg/kg/d b.i.d. to qd) for cefotaxime

Disposition

ADMISSION CRITERIA

- Unstable vital signs/toxic appearance
- Inability to comply with oral therapy
  - —Nausea/vomiting
  - —Social situation prevents compliance
- Pregnancy
- Indwelling urinary catheter
- Urinary obstruction/anatomic abnormalities
  - —Proximal obstruction (such as a kidney stone) places the patient at high risk for development of a renal abscess or sepsis and so requires emergent urologic consultation
  - —Immunosuppression/diabetes mellitus
  - —Extremes of age (children <2–6 months)
  - —Failure of outpatient therapy/recent antibiotics
- Short-term observation unit
  - —Ideal setting in which to hydrate a patient, control pain and begin IV antibiotics, allowing for early discharge

DISCHARGE CRITERIA

- Ability to maintain oral hydration
- Pain controlled with oral analgesic
- 48–72-hour follow-up

Miscellaneous

ICD9: 590.80

ICD10: N12

SUGGESTED READINGS

Gibly R. Infections of the urinary tract and male genitalia. In: Brillman JC, Quenzer RW, eds. Infectious disease in emergency medicine, 2nd ed. Philadelphia: Lippincott Williams & Wilkins, 1998:602–629.

Hellerstein S. Urinary tract infections: old and new concepts. Pediatr Clin North Am 1993;42(6):1433–1457.

Lipsky BA. Prostatitis and urinary tract infection in men: what's new; what's true? Am J Med 1999;106:327–334.

Stamm WE, Norrby SR. Urinary tract infection: disease panorama and challenges. J Infect Dis 2001;183 (suppl 1):S1–4.

Warren JW, Abrutyn E, Hebel JR, et al. Guidelines for antimicrobial treatment of uncomplicated acute bacterial cystitis and acute pyelonephritis in women. Clin Infect Dis 1999;29:745–758.

Author: Judith Brillman

Pyloric Stenosis

Clinical Presentation

SIGNS AND SYMPTOMS

- Vomiting
  - —Gradual onset, usually beginning at around 3 weeks of age
  - —Progressive, usually becoming projectile
  - —Nonbilious
  - —May be blood tinged (secondary to esophagitis, gastritis, gastric ulceration)
  - —Progressively worsening
  - —Postprandial
- Peristaltic waves moving from left to right in the left upper quadrant, seen best after feeding or just prior to vomiting
- 1.5- to 2-cm olive-shaped mass at the lateral margin of the right rectus abdominis muscle in the right upper quadrant (found in 80% of patients)
  - —Represents the hypertrophied pylorus
  - —Confirms diagnosis
  - —Requires a relaxed abdomen
  - —Best felt immediately after vomiting or after the stomach is emptied via gastric suction as the dilated body of the stomach overlies the pylorus
- Constipation or small amount of stools
- "Lean and hungry" infant early in course; dehydrated and uninterested in feeding late in course; failure to thrive
- Variable dehydration and wasting depending on duration of symptoms
- Jaundice in 8% of children
- Adult presents with vomiting, anorexia, early satiety, and epigastric pain
  - —Physical examination is normal

MECHANISM/DESCRIPTION

- Postnatal hypertrophy and hyperplasia of the circular smooth muscle cell layer causing a thickened pylorus and antrum leads to worsening gastric outlet obstruction
- Neuronal nitric oxide synthase (NOS-1) may be a genetic susceptibility locus
- Administration of erythromycin in infants may increase risk of hypertrophic pyloric stenosis
- Jaundice due to transient glucuronyl transferase deficiency
- Adult: caused by peptic ulcer disease

ETIOLOGY

- Most common cause of gastrointestinal obstruction in infants with an incidence of 1 in 150 males and 1:750 females (average: 3 in 100 live births)
- Males affected five times more commonly than females; firstborn most common
- Familial, 15%
  - —Child of affected parent has 7% incidence
  - —Recurrence risk in subsequent male children is 10%; 2% in females

Pre-Hospital

- IV 0.9% NS 22 cc/kg bolus for volume deficit or hypovolemia

Diagnosis

ESSENTIAL WORKUP

- If "olive" palpable, further diagnostic evaluation is unnecessary and surgical consultation should be sought; otherwise, imaging studies are indicated

LABORATORY

- Electrolytes, BUN/Cr, glucose
  - —Hypokalemic, hypochloremic metabolic alkalosis
  - —Normal electrolytes do not exclude the diagnosis
- Bilirubin
- CBC if blood in emesis
- Urinalysis for hydration

IMAGING/SPECIAL TESTS

- Abdominal ultrasound
  - —Study of choice
  - —Ultrasonic diagnosis hinges on identification and measurement of pyloric muscle mass (3-mm ring thickness with 1.5-cm pylorus channel) and observation of fluid movement through the pylorus
  - —Positive predictive value approaches 100%; 19% false negatives
  - —Serial ultrasounds for equivocal or negative study
- Supine abdominal film
  - —Not diagnostic; rarely helpful
  - —Dilated stomach and no air distal to the pylorus
  - —Most useful with other views to begin evaluation for other abdominal pathology
- Upper GI series
  - —"String sign" representing contrast passing through a narrowed gastric outlet
  - —95% accurate
  - —Remove contrast from the stomach after the study to prevent aspiration

DIFFERENTIAL DIAGNOSIS

- GI anatomic/functional disorder
  - —Gastroesophageal reflux (GER)
  - —Hiatal hernia
  - —Obstruction/atresia
  - —Gastric or duodenal web
- Infection
  - —Gastroenteritis
  - —Urinary tract infection
  - —Sepsis
- Metabolic
  - —Adrenal insufficiency
  - —Inborn error of metabolism
- Feeding problems
  - —Psychosocial: poor maternal interaction or stress
  - —Chalasia
  - —Formula intolerance
  - —Overfeeding
- Drug withdrawal
- Increased intracranial pressure

Treatment

INITIAL STABILIZATION

- IV access
- Rapid bedside glucose test to exclude hypoglycemia
- Correct volume deficit with 20 cc/kg bolus of 0.9% NS IV; may repeat

ED TREATMENT

- Correct electrolyte abnormalities
- Hydrate with dextrose-containing solution after fluid resuscitation at 1–1.5 times maintenance rate
  —Add potassium after ensuring adequate urine output
- Insert nasogastric tube to decompress the stomach
- Restrict oral intake
- Consult pediatric surgeon for pyloromyotomy
- Adult: proton pump antagonist (lansoprazole or omeprazole)

MEDICATIONS (ADULTS)

- Lansoprazole: 30 mg qd PO
- Omeprazole: 20 mg qd PO

Disposition

ADMISSION CRITERIA

- All pediatric patients should be admitted to the hospital for rehydration and surgical correction with either an umbilical pyloromyotomy or laparoscopic pyloromyotomy
- Adult patients: admit as necessary for rehydration; may be scheduled for elective pylorotomy if proton pump inhibitors fail to improve this condition

DISCHARGE CRITERIA

None

Miscellaneous

ICD9: 537.0

ICD10: K31.1

SUGGESTED READINGS

Bishop HC. Diagnosis of pyloric stenosis by palpation. Clin Pediatr 1973;12(4): 226–227.

Garcia VF, Randolph JG. Pyloric stenosis: diagnosis and management. Pediatr Rev 1990;11:292–296.

Heller RM, Hernanz-Schulman M. Application of new imaging modalities to the evaluation of common pediatric conditions. J Pediatr 1999;135:632–639.

Najmaldin A, Tan HL. Early experience with laparoscopic pyloromyotomy for infantile hypertrophic pyloric stenosis. J Pediatr 1995;30:37.

Sleisenger and Fordtran's gastrointestinal and liver disease, 6th ed. Philadelphia: WB Saunders, 1998.

Touloukian RJ, Higgins E. The spectrum of serum electrolytes in hypertrophic pyloric stenosis. J Pediatr Surg 1983;18(4): 394–397.

Author: Kerry B. Broderick

QT Syndrome, Prolonged

Clinical Presentation

SIGNS AND SYMPTOMS

- Syncope
- Near syncope
- Light-headedness
- Dizziness
- Seizure
- Sudden death

MECHANISM/DESCRIPTION

- Alteration in cardiac sodium, potassium, or calcium channel mechanics
- Prolonged ventricular repolarization results in lengthening of QT interval on surface EKG
  - —"Pause-dependent" lengthening due to short-long-short sequence in which a sinus beat is followed by an extrasystole (short), then a post-extrasystolic pause (long), concluding with a ventricular extrasystole (short)
  - —"Adrenergic-dependent" pauses found in congenital cases
- Reentrant rhythm can lead to torsades de pointes, ventricular tachycardia, and ventricular fibrillation
- Hemodynamic compromise following dysrhythmia leads to syncope or death
- Mechanism of magnesium sulfate as treatment unclear
- Congenital form occurs in 1 in 3,000–5,000 with mortality of 6% by age 40 years

ETIOLOGY

- Drugs
  - —Complete list at QTDrugs.org
  - —Class Ia antidysrhythmics—quinidine, procainamide, disopyramide
  - —Class III antidysrhythmics—sotalol, ibutilide, amiodarone
  - —Antibiotics—erythromycin, pentamidine, chloroquine, trimethoprim-sulfamethoxazole
  - —Antifungal agents—ketoconazole, itraconazole
  - —Psychotropic drugs—phenothiazines, haloperidol, risperidone, TCAs
  - —Cisipride
  - —Antihistamines
  - —Organophosphates
- Electrolyte abnormalities
  - —Hypokalemia
  - —Hypomagnesemia
  - —Hypocalcemia
- Cardiac
  - —Bradyarrhythmias
  - —AV block
  - —Mitral valve prolapse
  - —Myocarditis
  - —Myocardial ischemia
- CNS
  - —Subarachnoid hemorrhage
  - —Stroke
- Other
  - —Protein-sparing fasting
  - —Anorexia nervosa
  - —Hypothyroidism
  - —Hypothermia
- Congenital (idiopathic) form
  - —Six genetic loci identified with sporadic cases due to spontaneous mutations
  - —Autosomal-recessive form associated with deafness (Jervell and Lange-Nielsen syndromes)
  - —Autosomal-dominant form not associated with deafness (Romano-Ward syndrome)
  - —Adrenergic stimulation (fright, exertion, delirium tremens, loud auditory stimulus) becomes prodysrhythmic in certain genotypes while sleep-related symptoms found in others
  - —10–15% of carriers have baseline normal QTc
  - —Death occurs in 1% to 2% of untreated patients per year
- Drug-induced QT prolongation may also have a genetic background

PEDIATRIC CONSIDERATIONS

- Diagnosis suspected in the young with syncope, cardiac arrest, or sudden death
- Syncope following emotional stress or exercise suggestive
- Death occurs without preceding symptoms in 10% of pediatric patients

Pre-Hospital

- Supplemental oxygen
- IV access
- Monitor

CAUTIONS

- Stable patients with prolonged QT interval transported without intervention
- Cardioversion for *unstable* patients with *confirmed* torsades de pointes
- Magnesium sulfate for stable patients with evidence of torsades de pointes

Diagnosis

ESSENTIAL WORKUP

- A detailed history
  - —Medications
  - —Congenital deafness
  - —Syncope or sudden death
  - —Family history of syncope or sudden death
- Cardiac monitor
- EKG
  - —QTc (QT corrected for heart rate) >0.44 seconds
  - —Increase in QT variability
  - —T-wave abnormalities (t-wave alternans, biphasic)
  - —Appearance of U waves
  - —Ventricular tachycardia
  - —Ventricular fibrillation
  - —Torsades de pointes

LABORATORY

- Full electrolytes including calcium and magnesium
- Toxicology screen

IMAGING/SPECIAL TESTS

- Echocardiography to exclude other cardiac causes
- EKG stress testing to induce a prolonged QT interval in suspected cases
- Holter monitoring of QTc
- Genetic counseling/testing in suspected congenital forms
- Familial EKG testing

DIFFERENTIAL DIAGNOSIS

- Myocardial infarction
- Hypertrophic cardiomyopathy
- Valvular defect

Treatment

INITIAL STABILIZATION

- IV access
- Monitor
- Determine hemodynamic stability
  - —Unstable patients require immediate cardioversion

ED TREATMENT

- IV magnesium sulfate for torsades de pointes
- IV potassium to serum levels of 4.5–5 mEq/L
- Temporary transvenous cardiac pacing (rates between 90 and 110 beats/min) for recurrences of torsades de pointes refractory to magnesium sulfate therapy (shortens QTc)
- IV isoproterenol for refractory cases of hemodynamically unstable patients with *acquired* long QT (ineffective in congenital cases) and *inability to transvenous pace*
- Must remove any offending medications and correct metabolic derangements
- Consultation with cardiology in those with symptomatic long QT as β-blockers at maximum doses are to be started
- No ED treatment needed (in consultation with cardiology) for those with suspected idiopathic long QT and no history of syncope, family history of sudden cardiac death or ventricular arrhythmias
- Pacemaker or defibrillator placement with or without cervicothoracic stellectomy (to reduce adrenergic stimulation) may be required in high-risk patients
- β-Blockers prevent 70% of cardiac events in congenital cases

MEDICATIONS

- Isoproterenol: 1 μg/min i.v. continuous infusion (peds: 0.1–1.0 μg/kg/min) titrate for effect, up to 10 μg/min
- Magnesium sulfate: 2 g i.v. bolus over 2–3 minutes (peds: 25–50 mg/kg) followed by i.v. infusion at 2–4 mg/min
- Propanolol: 2–3 mg/kg/d PO (peds: 2–3 mg/kg/d) (in consultation with cardiology)

Disposition

ADMISSION CRITERIA

- Symptomatic prolonged QT
  - —Syncope
  - —Cardiac dysrhythmia
- Possible cardiac or ischemic event
- Metabolic abnormality

DISCHARGE CRITERIA

- Asymptomatic prolonged QT in consultation with cardiology

Miscellaneous

ICD9: 427

ICD10: I49.9

SUGGESTED READINGS

Khan IA. Clinical and therapeutic aspects of congenital and acquired long QT syndrome. Am J Med 2002;112:58–66.

Olgin JE, Zipes DP. Specific arrhythmias: diagnosis and treatment. In: Braunwald E, Zipes DP, Libby P, eds. Braunwald: heart disease: a textbook of cardiovascular medicine, 6th ed. Philadelphia: WB Saunders 2001:867–870.

Vincent GM. Ventricular arrhythmias: long QT syndrome. Cardiol Clin 2000;18: 309–325.

Author: Jason Tracy

Rabies

Clinical Presentation

SIGNS AND SYMPTOMS

Prodrome

- Malaise
- Fever
- Headache
- Upper respiratory tract infection (URTI)
- Nonspecific GI complaints
- At site of bite
  - —Pain
  - —Itching
  - —Paresthesia
  - —Spreads to entire limb
  - —Due to virus multiplication in dorsal root ganglion of sensory nerve

Classic (Encephalitic-Furious) Rabies (80%)

- Hydrophobia
  - —Violent reflexive intense contractions of the diaphragm with
    - -Attempts to swallow
    - -Sight of liquid
    - -Blowing air on face (aerophobia)
  - —Possibly exaggerated airway protective reflex
- Fever
- Terror
- Excitement
- Agitation
- Cluster breathing with long periods of apnea
- Respiratory failure
- Cardiac dysrhythmia
- Autonomic instability
- Seizures
- Coma

Paralytic Rabies (20%)

- Ascending paralysis
  - —Symmetric or asymmetric
- Myoedema
- Piloerection
- Fever
- May progress to classic rabies

MECHANISM/DESCRIPTION

- Fatal CNS infection transmitted to humans from animal reservoirs
- Incubation period 4–8 weeks on average (range of days to a year)
  - —Shorter incubation period with bites of the face and neck, with a large inoculum of virus or more virulent strains
- Delay in onset of disease related to multiplication of virus in peripheral tissues (skeletal muscle) before entering nervous system
  - —Virus may be eliminated during this period by host immune mechanisms/prophylactic postexposure immunization
- Virus enters a peripheral nerve and travels centrally by axoplasmic transport
  - —Immune systems unable to suppress once virus enters nervous system

ETIOLOGY

- Small number of human cases in the U.S.
  - —Half of these are acquired outside of the U.S.
- Neurotropic RNA virus of Rhabdovirus family
- Exposure through bite or contact with saliva or neural tissue of natural carrier animal on mucous membrane or nonintact skin
  - —Wildlife (account for 90% of confirmed rabies in the U.S.)—treat as rabid unless negative by laboratory tests
    - -Bats (most common)
    - -Raccoons
    - -Skunks
    - -Foxes
    - -Coyotes
    - -Bobcats
  - —Domestic sources—treat exposure if rabid or suspected rabid (observe animal 10 days)
    - -Cats
    - -Dogs
    - -Ferrets
    - -Livestock
  - —Rodents not natural carriers (but may be infected if bitten by a rabid animal)
    - -Squirrels
    - -Hamsters
    - -Guinea pigs
    - -Gerbils
    - -Chipmunks
    - -Rats
    - -Mice
    - -Rabbits
    - -Hares
- Human–human transmission through corneal transplants

PEDIATRIC CONSIDERATIONS

- Children at greater risk for unrecognized exposure
- Shorter incubation period

Pre-Hospital

CAUTIONS

- Theoretical risk to personnel via human–human transmission
  - —One reported case from human bite

CONTROVERSIES

- Rabies seldom recognized

Diagnosis

ESSENTIAL WORKUP

- Virus isolation from (positive in the first 2 weeks, but confirmation takes 3 weeks)
  - —Saliva
  - —CSF
- Rabies antibody titers
  - —Serum
    - -Any titer confirms diagnosis if patient never vaccinated
    - -Not useful if ever vaccinated
    - -Day 6—earliest positive
    - -Day 13—most positive
  - —CSF is always diagnostic but probably not positive until day 9 or later
- Rabies fluorescent antibody (RFA) for antigen
  - —Hair follicle nerve ending biopsy from nape of neck (50–60% positive)
  - —Brain biopsy
- CSF analysis
  - —Nondiagnostic by usual tests

LABORATORY

- CBC
- Electrolytes, BUN/Cr, glucose
- Blood cultures

IMAGING/SPECIAL TESTS

- CXR for aspiration pneumonia
- Head CT scan for altered mental status

DIFFERENTIAL DIAGNOSIS

- Classic rabies
  - —Tetanus
  - —Delirium tremens
  - —Encephalitis
  - —Psychosis
  - —Hysteria
- Paralytic
  - —Guillain-Barré
  - —Polio
  - —Immune-mediated polyneuritis
  - —Tick-bite paralysis

Treatment

INITIAL STABILIZATION

- ABCs
  - —Intubation for altered mental status/respiratory depression

ED TREATMENT

Prophylaxis

- Local wound cleansing with soap and irrigation with a virucidal agent, such as povidone iodine
- Tetanus prophylaxis if indicated
- Bite of natural rabies carrier (wild) or domestic with aberrant behavior
  - —Consider therapy
    - -Even without known physical contact with bats, when exposure might not have been recognized (sleeping or unattended child, intoxicated or mentally handicapped person in a room with a bat)
    - -With rodents and lagomorphs by individual circumstance because usually not indicated
  - —Rabies immune globulin 20 IU/kg on day 0 (or up to day 7, if initially omitted, do not give after day 7)
    - -Full dose infiltrated locally around wound, if not feasible, then
      - *Remainder of dose IM (deltoid in adults, anterolateral thigh in children)
    - -Do not use RIG if preexposure rabies vaccination
  - —Human diploid cell vaccine (HDCV), rabies vaccine adsorbed (RAV), purified chick embryo cell vaccine (PCEC)
    - -1 mL i.m. on days 0, 3, 7, 14, and 28
    - -Deltoid (do not use gluteal) area in adults
    - -Anterolateral thigh in children
    - -Keep distant from RIG site
  - —Same therapy in pregnancy
  - —Begin, if indicated, regardless of time since exposure
  - —If anaphylaxis before full vaccine series
    - -Consult Centers for Disease Control and Prevention (CDC)
    - -Send titers, if further dose is needed
    - -Pretreat with steroids and diphenhydramine
    - -Before administering dose, establish IV, prepare epinephrine for administration, and set up for possible intubation
    - -Must achieve adequate titers
- Preexposure prophylaxis
  - —Virus laboratory workers, veterinarians, forest rangers, zookeepers
  - —HDCV 0.1 mL i.m. or intradermal

Classic/Paralytic Rabies Therapy

- Supportive care
- Sedation for agitation
- Analgesics
- Almost 100% fatal despite intensive care

Disposition

ADMISSION CRITERIA

- ICU admission for all suspected rabies

DISCHARGE CRITERIA

- Rabies exposure only—discharge after
  - —Appropriate wound management
  - —Prophylaxis

Miscellaneous

ICD9: 71.0

ICD10: A82.9

SUGGESTED READINGS

Centers for Disease Control and Prevention. Human rabies prevention—United States 1999. Recommendations of the Advisory Committee on Immunization Practices (ACIP). MMWR Morb Mortal Wkly Rep 1999;48(RR-1):1–21.

Centers for Disease Control and Prevention. Human rabies-California, Georgia, Minnesota, New York and Wisconsin 2000. MMWR Morb Mortal Wkly Rep 2000;49(49): 1111–1115.

Centers for Disease Control and Prevention. Update: Raccoon rabies epizootic—United States and Canada 1999. MMWR Morb Mortal Wkly Rep 2000;49(2):31–35.

Author: Constance Greene

Radiation Injury

Clinical Presentation

SIGNS AND SYMPTOMS

- Rapidly dividing cells are most radiosensitive
- GI and heme systems most vulnerable

Skin

- With increasing radiation exposure develop
  - —Epilation
  - —Erythema
  - —Dry desquamation
  - —Wet desquamation
- Erythema that develops within 48 hours usually progresses to ulceration or chronic radiodermatitis
- Treat as thermal burn
- Blistering and necrosis occur with severe local exposures and are usually delayed >1 week
- Concomitant radiation exposure greatly increases mortality from thermal burns

Gastrointestinal

- Anorexia/nausea/vomiting/diarrhea
- Dehydration due to transudation of plasma into the GI tract
- Denuded intestinal mucosa a major source of septicemia when combined with bone marrow suppression
- Higher doses result in an earlier onset and more protracted course
  - —<0.5 gray (Gy): onset >6 hours
  - —<2 Gy: onset 2–6 hours
  - —>4 Gy: onset <2 hours
  - —>10 Gy: onset <30 minutes
- High fever with persistent bloody diarrhea is an ominous sign

Hematopoietic

- Pancytopenia due to bone marrow suppression
  - —Anemia is delayed and usually not problematic
  - —Thrombocytopenia with doses exceeding 2–4 Gy after 3–4 weeks
  - —Lymphopenia/neutropenia causing fever and increased risk of infection
- Bone marrow depression develops after a latent phase

CNS

- Headache
- Altered mental status
- Vertigo
- Seizures
- Occurs after massive exposure—associated with near 100% mortality within 48 hours
- Survivable if exposure is limited to the head

MECHANISM/DESCRIPTION

- Acute radiation syndrome results after a major portion of the body is irradiated by deeply penetrating radiation with a dose usually >1 Gy
- Background environmental exposure in US approximately 0.37 rem
- Measuring radiation
  - —Rad (radiation absorbed dose) is a measure of energy imparted to matter
    - -1 rad = 100 ergs/g
    - -1 Gy (international unit of measure) = 100 rad
    - -Various forms of radiation have different biologic effects at the same absorbed dose
    - -Rem (radiation equivalent man) is a measure of the biologic effects of radiation
    - -1 rad = 1 rem for beta and gamma radiation
    - -1 Sievert (Sv) (international unit of measure) = 100 rem

Types of Exposure

- Irradiation
  - —Follows exposure to an external source (e.g., radiation therapy)
  - —No contamination hazard
- Internal contamination (incorporation)
  - —Radioactive material inhaled, ingested, or absorbed through a open wound
  - —Treat as heavy metal ingestion
  - —Blocking, mobilizing, and chelating agents used in treatment
- External contamination
  - —Radioactive material in contact with clothing or skin
  - —Must remove radioactive material
  - —Contain radioactive material to prevent further contamination

ETIOLOGY

- Alpha-, beta-, x-, and gamma-rays emitted during the decay of unstable isotopes
  - —Responsible for acute radiation syndrome
- Alpha particles
  - —Penetration limited to the epidermis
  - —Hazardous only with internal contamination
  - —Difficult to measure with radiation meters
  - —Contamination treated by skin cleaning
- Beta particles
  - —Tissue penetration of a few centimeters possible
  - —Clothing blocks penetration
  - —Measured by radiation meters
  - —Removed by skin cleaning
- Gamma-rays
  - —Primary cause of radiation injury
  - —Deeply penetrating high-energy wave
  - —Measured by radiation meters
  - —Standard lead aprons not protective
- Neutrons
  - —Fourth radioactive particle occurring only around nuclear reactors, weapons, and accelerators
  - —Commonly cause previously stable atoms to become radioactive, creating a source of fallout

Pre-Hospital

CAUTIONS

- Activate disaster plan when predefined criteria met
- Notify receiving hospital early
- If a patient has life-threatening injuries, remove clothing, then transport to ED immediately
- Others should be evacuated from site (preferably upwind) and evaluated for contamination
- Pre-hospital decontamination should be performed if patient stable
  - —Remove/bag clothing (eliminates 90% of contamination) and leave at scene for disposal
  - —Clean skin with soap and water, being careful not to abrade skin
  - —Wound irrigation with 0.9% NS
- Protective clothing including gowns, rubber gloves, masks/face shields, and shoe covers for medical personnel
- Respirators only needed for rescue personnel entering highly contaminated areas
- Exposure of medical personnel <0.01 Gy even for Chernobyl accident workers

Diagnosis

ESSENTIAL WORKUP

- Radiation monitoring to ensure decontamination

LABORATORY

- CBC/platelet count q6h
  - —Baseline important
  - —Consider recent prior radiation exposure if initial counts low
  - —Absolute lymphocyte count at 48 hours correlates with prognosis
    - ->1,200/mm^3, good prognosis
    - -300–1,200/mm^3, fair prognosis
    - -<300/mm^3, poor/critical prognosis
- Save blood for chromosomal analysis in heparinized tube

DIFFERENTIAL DIAGNOSIS

- Burns
  - —Suspect radiation exposure with concomitant GI symptoms or evidence of bone marrow suppression
- Gastroenteritis
- Carbon monoxide poisoning

Treatment

INITIAL STABILIZATION

- ABCs
- Decontamination always secondary to treating life-threatening conditions
- 0.9% NS IV fluid bolus for extensive thermal burns/hypotension

ED TREATMENT

- Ideal treatment area
  - —Separate entrance from rest of ED
  - —Isolated ventilation and wastewater system
  - —Security controlled access to minimize spread of contamination
- Patients can be transported by wrapping them in cloth sheets
- Protect all hospital personnel
  - —Universal precautions with gowns, gloves, shoe covers, masks/face shields
  - —Use radiation survey monitors to prevent contamination
  - —Set up containment and decontamination areas with running water and drainage
  - —Cover floors with disposable paper/plastic
  - —Gather all potentially contaminated items in plastic bags for proper disposal
- Irrigate open wounds with saline followed by 3% hydrogen peroxide if contamination persists
  - —Surgical débridement rarely required for persistent high-count contamination
- Irrigate contaminated eyes and ears
- Gently scrub skin with soap and water 3 minutes (do not abrade)
- Sample collection
  - —Place a moist cotton swab of the nasal mucosa from each side of the nose in separate, sealed plastic bags to evaluate for possible respiratory contamination
  - —Save and refrigerate all urine, feces, and vomit if neutron exposure suspected to help quantitate exposure
- GI tract decontamination for ingestions
  - —Whole-bowel irrigation and activated charcoal within 2 hours of exposure
- Pulmonary decontamination
  - —Consider bronchoalveolar lavage
- Supportive treatment
  - —IV fluids to replace GI losses
  - —Antiemetics (5-HT_3-receptor antagonists) and analgesics
  - —Monitor for need of reverse isolation
  - —Cover severe burns with sterile dressing
  - —Early and broad-spectrum antibiotics for fevers or other signs of infection
  - —Early surgery (within 48 hours) for associated trauma to reduce risk of infection and bleeding
  - —Consider viral prophylaxis (e.g., acyclovir) for serious bone marrow depression
  - —Stimulation of hematopoiesis using growth factors (GCSF, GMCSF) may ultimately be required
  - —Stem cell transfusions and bone marrow transplants useful in selected cases
- Blocking agent potassium iodide prevents thyroid uptake of radioactive ^{131}I ingestion
  - —Indications
    - —>100 rad for adult
    - —>50 rad for child
  - —Blocks 90% ^{131}I if given within 1 hour; 50% if given within 5 hours
- Mobilizing agents increase excretion of radioisotope
  - —Water diuresis for tritium, Na^+, K^+
  - —Methimazole or propylthiouracil for ^{131}I
- Chelating agents reduce availability of radioisotope to tissues
  - —Aluminum reduces absorption of strontium
  - —Barium precipitates radium
  - —EDTA for lead
  - —Penicillamine for lead, copper, cobalt
  - —Prussian blue for thallium, cesium, rubidium
  - —DTPA for plutonium, americium
  - —Deferoxamine for plutonium, iron
  - —Dimercaprol for mercury, arsenic, bismuth, chromium, nickel, lead
- For 24-hour expert assistance contact Radiation Emergency Assistance Center in Tennessee (REAC/TS) 865-576-1005; www.orau.gov/reacts

Illness Categorization for Whole-Body Exposure

- Asymptomatic
  - —<1 Gy exposure
  - —Significant decreases in platelets and WBC counts rare
  - —Discharge after decontamination
- Mild
  - —1–2 Gy exposure
  - —50% with nausea and vomiting within 24–48 hours, absolute lymphocyte count (ALC) at 48 hours >2,000/mm^3
  - —Discharge if asymptomatic, follow daily CBC and platelets
- Degree: Moderate
  - —2–4-Gy exposure
  - —Moderate GI symptoms within 24 hours lasting about 4 days, ALC at 48 hours >1,200/mm^3
  - —Admit for supportive care and observation
- Severe
  - —4–10-Gy exposure
  - —Severe GI symptoms within 24 hours lasting about 7 days, ALC at 48 hours <1,200/mm^3
  - —Median whole-body lethal dose (lethal for 50% of exposed subjects) about 4.5 Gy *with* medical treatment
  - —Lethal for almost all without medical treatment
  - —Admit for reverse isolation, supportive care, infection monitoring/treatment, possible bone marrow transplant
- Fatal
  - —>10–12-Gy exposure
  - —Severe GI symptoms within 30 minutes, CNS symptoms, cardiovascular collapse, ALC at 48 hours <300/mm^3
  - —Death expected within 24 hours to 3 weeks
  - —Admit for palliative care

MEDICATIONS

- Potassium iodide: 130 mg PO (peds: children, 65 mg PO; infants 1–3 months old, 32 mg PO; infants younger than 1 month, 16 mg PO)

Disposition

ADMISSION CRITERIA

- Exposure to a dose of radiation >1 Gy with symptoms
- ALC <1,200/mm^3 at 48 hours

DISCHARGE CRITERIA

- Asymptomatic patients with dose of radiation <2 Gy with close laboratory follow-up

Miscellaneous

ICD9: NEC 990

ICD10: T66

SEE ALSO: CHEMICAL WEAPONS POISONING

SUGGESTED READINGS

Jarrett DG. Medical management of radiological casualties handbook, 1st ed. Bethesda: Armed Forces Radiobiology Research Institute Information Services, 1999. Available online at: *www.afrri.usuhs.mil.*

Markovchick V. Radiation injuries. In: Marx J, et al, eds. Rosen's emergency medicine: concepts and clinical practice, 5th ed. St. Louis: CV Mosby, 2002: 2055–2063.

Mettler FA Jr, Voelz GL. Major radiation exposure—what to expect and how to respond. N Engl J Med 2002;346(20): 1554–1561.

Author: Michael P. Jones

Rapid Sequence Intubation

Clinical Presentation

SIGNS AND SYMPTOMS

N/A

Pre-Hospital

N/A

Diagnosis

ESSENTIAL WORKUP

N/A

DIFFERENTIAL DIAGNOSIS

N/A

Treatment

INITIAL STABILIZATION

Preparation

- Have patient in appropriately monitored area where resuscitation may be instituted
- Assemble appropriate medicines
- Apply cardiorespiratory monitor, pulse oximeter, and BP monitor
- Test laryngoscope blade
  - —Adult: no. 3 to 4 Macintosh (curved) blade
  - —Child younger than 8 years: no. 2 Macintosh blade
  - —Term infant: no. 1 Miller (straight) blade
  - —Premature infant: no. 0 Miller blade
- Obtain ETT
  - —Adult man: 7.5–8.5 French
  - —Adult woman: 7.0–8.0 French
  - —Child: 4+ (age in years/4) or length based (Broselow tape)
    - -Use cuffed ETT for children older than 8 years and adults
    - -Use uncuffed ETT for children younger than 8 years
- Test ETT balloon with 15-mL syringe via inflation
- Use stylet for ETT
  - —Do not extend beyond distal ETT
- At bedside
  - —Bag-valve mask with functioning high-flow oxygen
  - —Functioning suction with Yankhauer tip
- Establish two IV lines

ED TREATMENT

Preoxygenation

- 100% oxygen for 5 minutes as this will allow nitrogen washout and give 3–5 minutes before desaturation below 90% occurs
- Do *not* bag as inflation of the stomach increases aspiration risk

Pretreatment (3 Minutes before Paralytic)

- Vecuronium 1 mg (peds: 0.01 mg/kg to max 1 mg) or rocuronium 0.06 mg/kg i.v.
- Atropine 0.02 mg/kg i.v.
  - —For children younger than 5 years
  - —Before ketamine administration
- Lidocaine 100 mg (peds: 1 mg/kg) i.v.
  - —Increased ICP
  - —Ocular trauma
  - —History of reactive airway disease
- Fentanyl 1-3 μg/kg i.v.
  - —Increased ICP

Induction and Paralysis

- Induction agent immediately before paralytic agent
  - —Etomidate 0.3 mg/kg i.v.
    - -Minimal hemodynamic effects therefore best for hypotensive patients
  - —Thiopental 3–5 mg/kg i.v.
    - -For increased ICP
    - -May cause hypotension, so use in hemodynamically stable patients
  - —Ketamine 1.5–2 mg/kg i.v.
    - -For status asthmaticus
- Paralytic agent
  - —Succinylcholine 1–1.5 mg/kg i.v.
    - -Avoid in ocular trauma, hyperkalemia, 2 days after severe crush injury/burn or congenital neuromuscular disorders and if present use alternative agent
  - —Alternative agents
    - -Rocuronium 0.6–1.2 mg/kg i.v.
    - -Vecuronium 0.15–0.25 mg/kg i.v.
- Immediately apply cricoid pressure and release only after intubation successful

Placement of Endotracheal Tube

- Place tube through vocal cords with direct visualization of the glottis
- Limit attempts to <30 seconds and ventilate briefly with bag-valve mask between attempts
- After placement, the cuff should be inflated and placement confirmed with symmetrical chest expansion, equal breath sounds bilaterally, end-tidal CO_2 monitor and CXR

Special Clinical Situations

- Head injury or penetrating globe injury
  - —Prevent ICP rise
    - -Lidocaine 1.5–2 mg/kg IV
    - -Vecuronium.01 mg/kg IV (defasciculating dose)
    - -Fentanyl 1.0–3.0 μg/kg IVP to prevent sympathetic discharge
  - —Prevent vagally stimulated bradycardia
    - -Atropine 0.01 mg/kg i.v. (minimum dose: 0.1 mg)
  - —Sedation
    - -Etomidate 0.3 mg/kg IVP *or*
    - -Thiopental 4 mg/kg IVP (if hemodynamically stable)
  - —Muscle relaxants/paralytic agents
    - -Succinylcholine 1.5 mg/kg i.v. (2 mg/kg if younger than 10 years) *or*
    - -Vecuronium 0.2 mg/kg i.v.
- Status asthmaticus
  - —Use ketamine as the sedating agent
- Status epilepticus
  - —Use thiopental to sedate (raises seizure threshold) if hemodynamically stable
- Multiple trauma/hemorrhagic shock
  - —Use etomidate for sedation

MEDICATIONS

- Atropine: 0.02 mg/kg
  - —Onset: <1 minute
  - —Indications
    - -For pediatric intubations
    - -When ketamine is used as induction agent
- Etomidate: 0.3 mg/kg
  - —Onset: <1 minute
  - —Duration of action: 5 minutes
  - —Indications
    - -For hemodynamically unstable patients of cardiac and hypovolemic etiology
    - -Asthmatics as it does not release histamine
  - —Cautions
    - -Partial seizures (*not* generalized)
    - -Patients who have *preexisting* adrenal suppression
- Fentanyl: 2–4 μg/kg
  - —Onset: <90 seconds
  - —Duration: 20–30 minutes
  - —Cautions
  - —Respiratory depression (which can be reversed with naloxone 2 mg or peds dose of 0.1 mg/kg)
  - —Hypotension in hypovolemia
  - —Truncal rigidity
  - —Indications
  - —Increased ICP

- Lidocaine: 1.0 mg/kg i.v.
  - —Onset: 1–3 minutes
  - —Indications
    - -Increased ICP
- Rocuronium
  - —Dosage: 0.6 mg/kg i.v.
  - —Onset: 1–3 minutes
  - —Duration: 30–35 minutes
  - —Cautions
    - -Tachycardia
  - —Indications
    - -When succinylcholine is contraindicated as paralytic agent in ocular trauma, hyperkalemia, 2 days after crush or burn injury, or malignant hyperthermia
- Succinylcholine
  - —Dosage: 1.0–1.5 mg/kg i.v.
  - —Onset: <1 minute
  - —Duration: 3–8 minutes
  - —Cautions
    - -Bradyarrhythmias
    - -Increased intraocular or ICP
    - -Hyperkalemia (renal failure, neuromuscular disorders, or rhabdomyolysis)
    - -2 days after burn or crush injury
    - -Malignant hyperthermia
  - —Indication
    - -Paralytic of choice due to rapid onset and short duration of onset
- Thiopental
  - —Dosage: 3.0–5.0 mg/kg i.v.
  - —Onset: 30–60 seconds
  - —Duration: 10–30 minutes
  - —Cautions
    - -Hypotension
    - -Laryngospasm
  - —Indications
    - -For increased ICP in hemodynamically stable patients
- Vecuronium
  - —Dosage
    - -1 mg for defasciculating dose (peds: 0.01 mg/kg)
    - -0.8–0.15 mg/kg for intubating dose
  - —Onset: 2–4 minutes
  - —Duration: 25–40 minutes
  - —Cautions
    - -Prolonged recovery time in obese or elderly or if hepatorenal dysfunction
  - —Indications
    - -When succinylcholine is contraindicated as paralytic agent in ocular trauma, hyperkalemia, 2 days after crush or burn injury, or malignant hyperthermia

Disposition

ADMISSION CRITERIA

- ICU admission for all intubated patients

DISCHARGE CRITERIA

N/A

Miscellaneous

ICD9: N/A

ICD10: N/A

SEE ALSO: AIRWAY MANAGEMENT

SUGGESTED READINGS

Chung D, Lam A. Essentials of anesthesiology, 3rd ed. Philadelphia: WB Saunders, 1997.

Walls RM. Rapid sequence intubation in head trauma. Ann Emerg Med 1993;22:1008.

Walls RM. Airway. In: Marx J, ed. Rosen's emergency medicine: concepts and clinical practice, 5th ed. St. Louis: Mosby, 2002.

Author: Christopher Ross

Rash

Clinical Presentation

Skin lesions are either a primary presenting complaint or an associated finding. Ultimate diagnoses are myriad, and true dermatologic emergencies are limited. Lesion morphology, distribution, chronology, and associated symptoms are of most value.

SIGNS AND SYMPTOMS

- Primary lesion appearance
  - —Macule
    - -Nonraised areas of distinct coloration
    - -Blanching lesions are inflammatory, nonblanching lesions are either altered pigmentation or petechiae/purpura
  - —Papule
    - -Raised, palpable lesions <5 mm in diameter, non-fluid filled
    - -Hemorrhagic, nonblanching lesions palpable purpura
  - —Vesicles
    - -Small, raised, clear fluid-filled lesions (<5 mm)
  - —Bullae
    - -Large, raised, clear fluid-filled lesions (>5 mm)
  - —Pustules
    - -As vesicles and bullae, but containing purulent fluid
  - —Nodule
    - -Solid, raised lesions >5 mm seated in deeper layer of skin and tissue
- Secondary changes
  - —Scaling, lichenification, excoriation, fissuring all result from manipulation/scratching or proliferation/shedding of epidermal cells
  - —Erosions/ulcers from varying degrees of tissue loss (superficial to deep) from loss of vascular supply/tissue integrity
- Distribution
  - —Characterized as central/peripheral, confluent/scattered, mucosal/nonmucosal, presence of palm/sole involvement
- Associated signs/symptoms
  - —Pruritus associated with allergic reactions, systemic and contact
  - —Fever with infection/drug reaction/systemic inflammatory response, viral xanthems common in children
- Vital signs
  - —Abnormal vitals signs, airway compromise, respiratory distress, hemodynamic instability present in severe disease

MECHANISM/DESCRIPTION

- Erythema/red macular lesions from dilatation of superficial vasculature
- Vesicobullous lesions formed by disruption of epidermal/dermal integrity and filling with exudative fluid, commonly allergic/infectious/systemic inflammatory response
- Purpura and petechiae from failure of normal vascular integrity/hemostatic mechanisms
- Nodules from prolonged inflammatory response
- Urticaria from contact/systemic allergic response, histamine release

ETIOLOGY

- Maculopapular
  - —Infections
    - -Viral
    - -Bacterial
    - -Rickettsial
    - -Fungal
    - -Parasites
  - —Allergic reactions
  - —Autoimmune disease
- Purpura/petechiae
  - —Clotting pathway dysfunction
  - —Platelet dysfunction, qualitative or quantitative
  - —Vasculitis
  - —Systemic infection, sepsis
- Vesicobullous
  - —Localized
    - -Allergic reaction
    - -Mechanical/physical trauma: heat, radiation, sunburn
  - —Generalized (systemic)
    - -Infection
    - -Allergic reaction/anaphylaxis
    - -Autoimmune

Pre-Hospital

- Management dictated by presence of hemodynamic instability, airway compromise, and concern for infectious exposure
- IV access and fluid support for hemodynamic instability
- Early identification of life-threatening rashes and highly communicable diseases
  - —Extensive vesicobullous disease
  - —Extensive, diffuse erythematous disease
  - —Petechiae and purpura

CAUTIONS

- Universal precautions, masks if infectious etiology suspected

Diagnosis

ESSENTIAL WORKUP

- History
  - —Age
  - —Immune status (HIV, chemotherapy, diabetes)
  - —Previous episodes/prior history of lesions/reactions
  - —Sick contacts
  - —Chronologic and physical evolution
  - —Associated symptoms, pruritus, fever, abdominal pain, myalgias/arthralgias
  - —Prodrome: fever, headache, cough, odynophagia, rhinorrhea
  - —Environmental exposure: tick bite, unusual flora, diet
  - —Recent change in medication
  - —Family history
- Identify systemic illness
  - —Fever
  - —Abnormal vital signs
  - —Nausea, vomiting, abdominal pain, generalized distribution, altered mental status
  - —Signs/symptoms of local infectious source: pharyngitis, abscess, foreign body, meningismal signs
- Categorize the lesions
  - —Maculopapular
  - —Vesicobullous
  - —Petechial

LABORATORY

- Presence of fever, systemic symptoms, or possible infection warrants blood work
  - —CBC with differential, electrolytes, BUN/creatinine
  - —Blood cultures, viral cultures
  - —Gram's stain and culture of purulent lesions; Tzanck smear or DNA for suspected herpetic lesions
  - —VRDL for suspect syphilis
  - —Lumbar puncture for altered mental status, meningeal signs, suspected meningococcus
- Suspected autoimmune disorders (lupus, RA, JRA, Sjögren syndrome)
  - —CBC, ESR, particular assays in consultation with rheumatologist (ANA, ANCA, etc.)
- Petechiae/purpura warrant complete coagulation evaluation
  - —CBC with platelets
  - —PTT, PT, INR
  - —DIC screen: fibrinogen, fibrin split products, haptoglobin, LDH

IMAGING/SPECIAL TESTS

- CXR indicated for respiratory symptoms, possible infectious/autoimmune etiology
- Biopsy under dermatologic consultation to differentiate allergic/autoimmune/infectious processes
- Nikolsky test: expansion of bullous lesion with lateral stress at margin indicates epidermal/dermal disruptive process
- Scrapings
  - —Indicated to rule out topical fungal infections and parasites
  - —KOH preparation from edge of lesion reveal hyphae
  - —Plain mineral oil to rule out scabies in pruritic linear lesions of hands

DIFFERENTIAL DIAGNOSIS

- Potentially lethal diagnoses
  - —*Diffusely erythematous rashes*
    - -Toxic shock syndrome (TSS): exotoxin, 90% *Staphylococcus aureus,* desquamation 2 weeks after early rash, end organ involvement
    - -Toxic epidermal necrolysis (TEN): constitutional symptoms, adults, drug related, positive Nikolsky test result, full-thickness desquamation, oral lesions prominent
    - -Staphylococcal scalded skin syndrome (SSSS): exotoxin, fever, malaise, flaccid bullae later, superficial desquamation, oral lesions rare, children
    - -Kawasaki syndrome
    - -Generalized exfoliative erythroderma
    - -Lupus
    - -Cutaneous T-cell lymphoma
  - —Vesicobullous lesions
    - -Anaphylaxis
    - -Stevens-Johnson syndrome: continuum with TEN, drug related, constitutional symptoms, mucous membranes involved, symmetric blistering
    - -Toxic epidermal necrolysis
    - -Pemphigus vulgaris: fulminant, usually 40–65 years, painful, flaccid bullae, positive Nikolsky test result, oral lesions, antiepithelial antibody by biopsy
    - -Bullous pemphigoid: more elderly population, oral lesions less common, positive Nikolsky test result, basement membrane antibody by biopsy
    - -Smallpox
    - -Disseminated herpes simplex/zoster/varicella in adults
  - —Maculopapular and local lesions
    - -Gonococcemia: sexually active, polyarthritis, tenosynovitis, hemorrhagic pustules with erythematous base
    - -Secondary syphilis
    - -Erysipelas
    - -Pustular psoriasis
    - -Ecthyma gangrenosum: with gram-negative sepsis, discrete lesions, few in number, peripheral, evolve from macule to pustule to an erythematous base
    - -Envenomations
    - -Malignancy

- —Purpuric and petechial lesions
  - -Meningococcemia
  - -Gonococcemia
  - -Pneumococcemia
  - -DIC
  - -Rocky Mountain spotted fever: pronounced prodrome of fever, headache, myalgia, rash, peripheral, moves to palms/soles, systemic
  - -Babesiosis: similar to RMSF, rash less often, frequent co-infection with Lyme
  - -Henoch-Schönlein purpura
  - -Multiple systemic illness (see Purpura)
- Nonlethal diagnoses
  - —Maculopapular lesions
    - -Psoriasis
    - -Tinea
    - -Pityriasis rosea
    - -Seborrheic dermatitis
    - -Intertrigo
    - -Lichen planus
    - -Lyme disease
    - -Phototoxic and photoallergic reactions
    - -Viral exanthems (mostly in children, see Rash, Pediatric)
    - -Contact dermatitis
    - -Scabies
    - -Eczema
    - -Impetigo
    - -Candidiasis
    - -Urticaria
    - -Nevi
    - -Hypopigmentation
    - -Warts
  - —Vesicobullous lesions
    - -Herpes simplex/zoster (nondisseminated)
    - -Contact allergic dermatitis
    - -Coxsackie
    - -Echovirus
    - -Scabies
    - -Insect bites
  - —Petechial/purpuric lesions
    - -Usually reflect systemic infection/inflammation/vasculitis
    - -Few trivial causes
    - -Actinic purpura in elderly
    - -Traumatic
  - —Pustular lesions
    - -Trivial causes must be localized, have no associated symptoms, and no petechial component
    - -Folliculitis
    - -Candidiasis
    - -Acne

Treatment

INITIAL STABILIZATION

- Aggressive, presumptive management of potentially lethal presentations
  - —Petechial lesions
  - —Fever
  - —Disseminated erythematous or vesicobullous lesions
- Treat for anaphylaxis if acute, urticarial, known exposure, or respiratory distress
- Airway management and respiratory support as indicated
- Early empiric IV antibiotics
- Aggressive fluid resuscitation and pressor support for hemodynamic instability
- Treat disseminated bullous or exfoliative disease as a severe thermal burn
- Identify potential source if sepsis/TNN/TSS suspected (foreign body, abscess, endocarditis)
- Antibiotics
  - —Nafcillin/oxacillin if staphylococcal scalded skin syndrome
  - —Penicillin G and clindamycin if TSS
    - -Removal of the offending agent, supportive care, if any clinical suspicion treat as infectious
  - —Doxycycline or chloramphenicol if Rocky Mountain spotted fever
  - —Ceftriaxone 1 gm i.v. or penicillin G 2 million units i.v. if meningococcemia is suspected as soon as cultures are drawn
- If varicella or disseminated herpes is suspected initiate acyclovir

ED TREATMENT

- Treatment directed for underlying cause
- Symptomatic treatment of pruritus indicated
- Steroid therapy reserved for clear allergic reactions, relapse of known steroid responsive disease, or in consultation with dermatologist
- Allergic reactions treated aggressively
  - —Diphenhydramine
  - —H_2-blocker
  - —Steroids
  - —Epinephrine if respiratory compromise

MEDICATIONS

- Acetaminophen: 625 mg (peds: 60 mg/kg/24 h) PO/p.r. q4–6h
- Acyclovir: 10 mg/kg/dose i.v. q8h
- Cefotaxime: 1–2 g (peds: 100–200 mg/kg/24 h) i.v. q6h
- Ceftriaxone: 1–2 g (peds: 100–200 mg/kg/24 h) i.v. q12h
- Chloramphenicol: 50 mg/kg/24 h) i.v. q12h
- Clindamycin: 900 mg i.v. (peds: 40 mg/kg/24 h) q8h; if staph suspected, treat as SSSS
- Diphenhydramine: 50 mg (peds: 5 mg/kg/24 h) PO/i.m./i.v. q6h
- Doxycycline: 100 mg (peds: older than 8 years, same; younger than 8 years) PO q12h
- Nafcillin/oxacillin: 2 g (peds: 150 mg/kg/24 h) i.v. q4h
- Penicillin G: (peds: 400,000 U/kg/24 h) 2 million units i.v. q2h *or*
- Solu-Medrol: 125 mg (peds: 0.5–2 mg/kg) i.v. q24h

Disposition

ADMISSION CRITERIA

- Potentially lethal diagnoses
- All patients receiving IV antibiotic/fluid support
- Patients with significant bullous/exfoliative disorders
- Associated systemic symptoms
- Metabolic/electrolyte disorders

DISCHARGE CRITERIA

- Limited lesions
- Viral exanthems
- Absence of systemic signs or symptoms may discharge to follow-up with PCP/dermatologist
- Reasons to return
  —Fever
  —Headache
  —Any change or worsening of symptoms

Miscellaneous

ICD9: 709.9

ICD10: R21

SUGGESTED READINGS

Brady WJ, DeBehnke D, Crosby DL. Dermatological emergencies. Am J Emerg Med 1994;12(2):217–237.

Cydulka RK. Dermatologic disorders. In: Marx JA, ed. Marx: Rosen's emergency medicine: concepts and clinical practice. St. Louis, Mosby, 2002.

Fitzpatrick TB, et al. Color atlas and synopsis of clinical dermatology. New York: McGraw-Hill, 1992.

Forstater AT, Neuberger KJ. Life threatening dermatoses. In: Harwood-Nuss A, ed. The clinical practice of emergency medicine. Philadelphia: JB Lippincott Co, 2001.

Habif TP. Clinical dermatology: a color guide to diagnosis and treatment. St. Louis: Mosby, 1996.

Author: Owen Lander

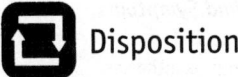

Rash, Pediatric

Clinical Presentation

SIGNS AND SYMPTOMS

Lesion Morphology

- Macule
  - —Localized nonpalpable changes in skin color
  - —Purpura or petechiae if nonblanching when pressure is applied
- Maculopapule
  - —Slightly elevated lesions with localized changes in skin
- Papule
  - —Solid, elevated lesions <5 mm in diameter
  - —Keratotic (rough-surfaced lesion)
  - —Nonkeratotic (smooth lesion)
  - —Palpable purpura if nonblanching when pressure is applied
- Plaque
  - —Solid, elevated lesions >5 mm in diameter
  - —Often results from a confluence of papules
- Nodule
  - —Solid, elevated lesions extending deep into the dermis or subcutaneous tissue >5 mm in diameter
- Wheal
  - —Circular, irregular lesions varying from red to pale
- Vesicle
  - —Clear fluid-filled lesions <5 mm in diameter
- Bullae
  - —Clear fluid-filled lesions >5 mm in diameter
- Pustules
  - —Pus-filled lesions

Secondary Lesions

- Scales
  - —Thin plates of dried cornified epithelium partially separated from the epidermis
- Lichenification
  - —Dried plaques resulting in furrowing of the skin
- Erosion
  - —Moist surface uncovered by rupture of vesicles or bullae
- Excoriation
  - —Linear loss of the skin secondary to trauma
- Ulcer
  - —Deep loss of the skin involving the epidermis and a variable amount of the dermis and subcutaneous tissue

Configuration

- Circles or arcs
- Serpiginous (creeping or wormlike)
- Iris grouping (bull's eye appearance)
- Irregular grouping
- Zosteriform grouping
- Linear grouping
- Retiform grouping

Associated Signs and Symptoms

- Fever
  - —Consider infectious exanthemas
- Pruritus
- Joint pain
- Abdominal pain

MECHANISM/DESCRIPTION

- Most dermatologic emergencies in children are due to an underlying infection
- In children with fever and a rash, viruses account for 72% and bacteria for 20%
- The color of a particular lesion or the entire skin may be due to a number of substances
  - —Red or red-brown lesions result from oxyhemoglobin found in RBCs
  - —The macular erythematous lesions seen in viral exanthema usually represent dilated superficial cutaneous vessels
  - —Purpura and petechiae result from leakage of RBCs out of the vascular space
  - —Hypopigmentation or hyperpigmentation represent postinflammatory change from either increases or decreases in melanin production
  - —Depigmentation refers to the total loss of pigment secondary to an autoimmune effect (vitiligo) or in congenital disorders from a genetic inability to produce melanin (albinism)
- Scales represent a proliferative disorder of epidermal cell turnover

ETIOLOGY

Papulosquamous

- Infections
  - —Viral
  - —Bacterial
  - —Rickettsial
  - —Fungal
- Allergic reactions
- Autoimmune disorders

Purpura and Petechiae

- Clotting disorder
- Platelet disorder
- Vascular fragility disease
- Vasculitis
- Overwhelming infection

Vesicobullous

- Infection
- Drug reaction
- Autoimmune disorder

Ulcer

- Infection
- Vascular insufficiency

Pre-Hospital

- Field management is indicated when there are signs of systemic instability
  - —Airway management using precautions to avoid exposure to respiratory secretions
  - —IV access
  - —Identify rashes with a potentially life-threatening illness or need for special isolation

CAUTIONS

- Mask and gloves should be worn to prevent contagion

Diagnosis

ESSENTIAL WORKUP

- Obtain a detailed history
  - —Age-group
  - —Many conditions occur more commonly at specific ages
  - —Distribution and appearance vary with age
  - —Development, progression, and duration of the rash
  - —Where rash arises first and where it spreads
  - —Lesions synchronous or asynchronous
  - —Associated symptoms
  - —Prodromes—cough, rhinorrhea, pharyngitis, fever, meningismal symptoms
  - —Fever
  - —Pruritus
  - —Family history
  - —Generic dermatoses
  - —Atopic dermatitis
  - —Psoriasis
  - —Immunizations
  - —Exposures
- Classify the rash based on the primary lesions
  - —Papulosquamous
  - —Vesicobullous
  - —Purpuric

LABORATORY

- Indicated if the rash is purpuric
  - —Platelet count
  - —Bleeding time
  - —PTT
  - —PT
  - —DIC screen
- Indicated if fever present
  - —CBC
  - —Electrolytes, BUN, creatinine to evaluate dehydration and scarlatiniforme rash (exclude glomerulonephritis)
  - —Viral culture and titers for suspected exanthems
  - —Bacterial blood cultures for suspected systemic bacterial infection
- Lumbar puncture if meningococcus or other meningitides or encephalitis suspected
  - —Bacterial and viral cultures as appropriate as well as Gram stain

IMAGING/SPECIAL TESTS

- CXR for suspected pulmonary involvement
- Potassium hydroxide preparations
  - —Indicated with scaling lesions to differentiate dermatophytosis from nummular eczema and pityriasis rosea
  - —Superficial scale should be removed from the skin with a scalpel or the edge of a glass slide
  - —The sample should be obtained from the active border of the lesion
  - —Place on a slide and add 1 drop of 10% KOH
  - —Place a coverslip and heat slowly without boiling
  - —Allow the slide to set for a few minutes
  - —Scan for hyphae
- Wood lamp
  - —Useful in dermatophytosis and erythrasma
- Scabies preparations
  - —Most of the mite population resides on the hands and feet in young children
  - —A drop of mineral oil should be placed on the lesion and then scraped with a no. 15 blade
  - —The scraping should be deep enough to produce just a speck of blood
  - —Examine under low power for the mite, ova, larva, or fecal matter

DIFFERENTIAL DIAGNOSIS

Maculopapular Rash

- Solid, skin colored or yellow
  - —Keratotic
  - —Wart
  - —Corn
  - —Callus
  - —Nonkeratotic
  - —Wart
  - —Molluscum contagiosum
  - —Sebaceous cyst
  - —Basal and squamous cell carcinoma
  - —Nevi
  - —Jaundice
- Solid, brown
  - —Café au lait patch
  - —Nevi
  - —Freckle
  - —Melanoma
  - —Photoallergic drug eruption
  - —Phototoxic drug eruption
  - —Tinea nigra palmaris hypopigmentation
- Solid, red, nonscaling
  - —Nonpurpuric
  - —Exanthems
    - -Rubeola
    - -Scarlet fever
    - -Toxin-producing staphylococcal or streptococcal disease
    - -Erythema infectiosum (fifth disease)
    - -Roseola
    - -Rubella
    - -Rubella-like rash (echoviruses, coxsackie A viruses)
    - -Varicella (early manifestations)
    - -Variola (smallpox: early manifestations)
    - -Epstein-Barr virus
    - -Enterovirus
    - -Adenovirus
    - -Mycoplasma
    - -Kawasaki disease
    - -Erythema multiforme
    - -Localized, pruriginous
    - -Insect bites
    - -Scabies
    - -Allergic contact dermatitis
    - -Irritant contact dermatitis

—Purpuric
  -Bacteremia sepsis
  -Meningococcemia
  -*Haemophilus influenzae*
  -Pneumococcemia
  -Gonococcemia
  -Endocarditis
  -Plague
  -DIC
  -Rocky Mountain spotted fever
  -Henoch-Schönlein purpura
  -Idiopathic thrombocytopenic purpura
  -Leukemia
  -Underlying bleeding disorder
  -Ecthyma gangrenosum
  -Rarely, pityriasis rosea
- Solid, red, scaling
  —Without epithelial disruption
    -Tinea corporis, capitis, pedis, or cruris
    -Pityriasis rosea
    -Secondary syphilis
    -Lupus erythematosus
  —With epithelial disruption
    -Papular urticaria
    -Eczema
    -Seborrheic, diaper, contact, or stasis dermatitis
    -Impetigo
    -Candidiasis
    -Tinea corporis, capitis, pedis, or cruris

Vesiculobullous Rash
- Varicella
- Variola (smallpox)
- Herpes simplex
- Herpes zoster
- Hand-foot-and-mouth syndrome
- Scabies
- Drug hypersensitivity, toxic epidermal necrolysis
- Staphylococcal scalded skin syndrome (SSS)
- Bullous impetigo
- Cat-scratch disease
- Dermatitis herpetiformis
- Eczema
- Erythema multiforme
- Impetigo
- Lichen planus

Pustular
- Acne
- Folliculitis
- Candidiasis
- Gonococcemia
- Meningococcemia

With fever, consider
- Infection
- Drug reaction
- Systemic inflammatory disease (JRA, SLE, etc.)

Treatment

INITIAL STABILIZATION
- Aggressive, empiric management of children with a purpuric rash associated with fever or unstable vital signs
  —Airway support, IV access
  —IV antibiotics should be administered as soon as possible
    -Cefotaxime or ceftriaxone
    -Plus doxycycline if Rocky Mountain spotted fever (RMSF) is considered
  —IVF and pressors in the presence of cardiovascular collapse
  —Fluid resuscitation as if burn with SSS or TEN

ED TREATMENT
- Specific ED treatment should be directed to the underlying etiology
- Acetaminophen is indicated in children with fever
- Diphenhydramine should be used when an allergic reaction is suspected

MEDICATIONS

- Acetaminophen: 10–15 mg/kg PO/PR q4–6h
- Cefotaxime: 50 mg/kg i.v. q6h; max dose, 12 g/24 h
- Ceftriaxone: 50 mg/kg i.v. q12h; max dose, 4 g/24 h
- Diphenhydramine: 1.25 mg/kg PO/i.m./i.v. q6h
- RSMF
  —Doxycycline: 100 mg PO/i.v. q12h (older than 8 years) or chloramphenicol 12.5 mg/kg/dose q6h (max, 500 mg/dose)
- Kawasaki disease
  —Immune globulin: 2 g/kg i.v. over 10–12 hours and aspirin 25 mg/kg/dose PO q6h
- Varicella
  —Acyclovir: 800 mg PO q.i.d. (peds: 20 mg/kg/dose) with pulmonary or CNS involvement; give 10–12 mg/kg/dose i.v. q8h in the immunocompromised patient; *no* aspirin should be used
- Toxic shock syndrome or SSS
  —Nafcillin or oxacillin: 2 g i.v. q4h (peds: 200 mg/kg/d i.v. q4h); alternative: cefazolin 2 g i.v. q8h (ped: 100 mg/kg/d i.v. q8h)
- Scarlet fever
  —Penicillin V: 500 mg PO q.i.d. (peds: 250 mg PO q.i.d.) × 10 days; alternative: erythromycin 250–500 mg PO q.i.d. (peds: 12.5 mg/kg/dose PO q.i.d.) × 10 days, or azithromycin 500 mg PO q.d. (peds: 12 mg/kg/d PO q.d.) × 5 days

Disposition

ADMISSION CRITERIA

- Hospital admission is determined by the underlying disorder
- Admit life-threatening conditions: meningococcemia, RMSF, toxic shock syndrome, Kawasaki disease
- Other illnesses associated with systemic illness or potential deterioration; SSS, rubeola, and varicella, as well as others, may require inpatient care

DISCHARGE CRITERIA

- Discharge instructions should be based on the underlying disorder
- Exanthems associated with self-limited entities in stable children
  —Follow-up with PCP or dermatologist should be arranged

Miscellaneous

ICD9: 782.1

ICD10: R21

SEE ALSO: HENOCH-SCHÖNLEIN PURPURA

SUGGESTED READINGS

Barkin RM. Rash. In: Barkin RM, ed. Emergency pediatrics. A guide to ambulatory care. St. Louis: CV Mosby, 1999:285–290.

Mancini AJ. Childhood exanthems: a primer and update for the dermatologist. Adv Dermatol 2000;16:3–37.

Pomeranz AJ. The systematic evaluation of the skin in children. Pediatr Clin North Am 1998;45:49–63.

Author: Bruce Webster

Rectal Prolapse

Clinical Presentation

SIGNS AND SYMPTOMS
- Protruding rectum
- Bleeding
- Mucous discharge
- Sensation of rectal mass
- Tenesmus
- Constipation and incontinence

MECHANISM/DESCRIPTION
- Full-thickness rectum intussuscepts through the rectum to the outside

ETIOLOGY
- Unknown; possibilities include
  —Chronic constipation
  —Outlet obstruction
  —Sphincters with decreased tone
    -Birth trauma
    -Neurologic disease

PEDIATRIC CONSIDERATIONS
- True rectal prolapse unusual in children; more likely intussusception

Pre-Hospital

CAUTIONS
- Reduce pressure on rectum
  —Avoid straining
  —Avoid prolonged sitting

Diagnosis

ESSENTIAL WORKUP
- History with emphasis on bowel obstruction and duration of prolapse
- Rectal examination—must differentiate rectal prolapse, internal hemorrhoids, or intussusception
  —Intussusception identified by placing the examining finger between the protruding rectum and the anus
  —Internal hemorrhoids identified by identifying the folds of mucosa radiating out like spokes in a wheel
  —Folds of mucosa in rectal prolapse are circular

LABORATORY
- No laboratory test necessary for uncomplicated prolapse
- Preoperative tests for acutely incarcerated prolapse with necrosis preoperative
  —CBC
  —Urinalysis
  —Electrolytes, BUN/Cr, glucose

DIFFERENTIAL DIAGNOSIS
- Prolapsed internal hemorrhoids
- Intussusception from above

Treatment

INITIAL STABILIZATION

- No stabilization needed for elective rectal prolapse
- Incarcerated nonreducible prolapse
  - —NPO
  - —IV fluids rehydration
  - —Prepared for surgery

ED TREATMENT

- Reduce prolapse gently
  - —If reduction accomplished without difficulty, correct prolapse electively
  - —If prolapse incarcerated, admission for reduction and surgical correction before the swelling creates a full-thickness necrosis
- If the reduction is easy, recurrence is likely
  - —Elective surgical correction

MEDICATIONS

N/A

Disposition

ADMISSION CRITERIA

- Necrotic or anoxic mucosa on the prolapse
- Inability to easily reduce the prolapse

DISCHARGE CRITERIA

- Chronic, easily reduced rectal prolapse
- Refer to an appropriate surgeon

Miscellaneous

ICD9: 569.1

ICD10: K62.3

SUGGESTED READING

Heine JA, Wong WD. Rectal prolapse. In: Mazier PW, et al, eds. Surgery of the colon, rectum, and anus. Philadelphia: WB Saunders, 1995:515–537.

Author: Charles Orsay

Rectal Trauma

Clinical Presentation

SIGNS AND SYMPTOMS

- Perineal, anal, or lower abdominal pain
- Signs of perforation or peritonitis (guarding, rebound tenderness, fever)
- Pelvic fracture
- Rectal bleeding
- Obstipation
- History of anal manipulation, foreign body insertion, sexual abuse

ETIOLOGY

- Penetrating trauma
  - —Gunshot wounds account for 80%
  - —Knife wounds
  - —Impalement injuries
- Blunt trauma less frequent cause of rectal injury
  - —Motor-vehicle collision
  - —Motorcycle accident
  - —Waterskiing and watercraft accidents (hydrostatic pressure injury)
  - —Falls and crush injuries
  - —Pelvic fractures (bony fragments penetrate rectum)
- Foreign body
  - —Autoeroticism
  - —Assault
  - —Anal intercourse
  - —Ingestion of sharp objects
- Iatrogenic trauma: most common cause of rectal injury
  - —Barium enema: perforation occurs in 0.04% patients, 50% mortality
  - —Colonoscopy: 0.2% perforation rate; increased risk with polypectomy
  - —Urologic and obstetric-gynecologic procedure
  - —Episiotomy

MECHANISM/DESCRIPTION

- Injury to rectal mucosa
- Severity ranges from simple contusion to full-thickness laceration and extension into peritoneum or perineum
- Two thirds of rectum is extraperitoneal

PEDIATRIC CONSIDERATIONS

- Rectal injury can result from thermometer insertion
- Child abuse: follow local reporting laws

Pre-Hospital

CAUTIONS

- ABCs, spinal precautions if blunt trauma
- Fluid resuscitation if blood loss, hypotension
- Do not attempt to remove foreign body from rectum

Diagnosis

ESSENTIAL WORKUP

- History
  - —Time and mechanism of injury
  - —Suspect rectal injury in all patients with gunshot wound, stab wound, or impalement injury to trunk, buttocks, perineum, or upper thigh
  - —Consider in any patient with history of anal manipulation complaining of lower abdominal or pelvic pain
- Physical examination
  - —Inspect and palpate thoroughly the buttocks, anus, and perineum
  - —Identify entrance and exit wounds if penetrating trauma
  - —Perform digital rectal examination to assess for gross blood or guaiac-positive stool; note position of prostate (see Imaging/Special Tests)
  - —Vaginal exam in all female patients: speculum and bimanual mandatory to assess perineal and vaginal integrity
  - —GU exam in male patients
- Anoscopy and sigmoidoscopy
  - —Must be performed if rectal injury is suspected by history or exam
  - —Irrigate and suction feces and blood
  - —Avoid insufflating large amount of air during sigmoidoscopy as it can force stool into peritoneum if proximal bowel perforation exists
- Sexual assault
  - —History of sexual assault requires evidentiary exam to document GU and anal trauma and collect forensic evidence (hairs, sperm sampling)

LABORATORY

- CBC
- Type and screen
- Urinalysis

IMAGING/SPECIAL TESTS

- Supine/upright abdominal films, pelvic x-ray
  - —Evaluate for pneumoperitoneum or extraperitoneal and extrarectal densities suggesting perforation
  - —Identify location, size, and shape of foreign body
  - —Identify pelvic fracture or diastasis of symphysis pubis, which may accompany rectal injury
- Retrograde urethrogram (RUG) if high-riding prostate noted on rectal exam to exclude concurrent urethral injury
- Contrast enema helpful only in situations where perforation is unclear; use water-soluble contrast only, for example, diatrizoate sodium (Gastrografin)

DIFFERENTIAL DIAGNOSIS

- Colon injuries
- GU injuries

Treatment

INITIAL STABILIZATION

- In penetrating or blunt abdominal trauma, follow ATLS protocol: primary survey, resuscitation, secondary survey, and treatment

ED TREATMENT

- Administer tetanus prophylaxis if applicable
- Administer broad-spectrum antibiotics if significant mucosal disruption and/or signs of peritonitis are present (see Medications)
- Place Foley catheter after excluding urethral injury
- Obtain surgical consultation
  - —Peritonitis, all traumatic rectal mucosal lacerations, inability to extract foreign body in ED

Rectal Foreign Body Removal in ED

- Treatment is determined by the location and type of foreign object (<10 cm from anal verge)
- Provide adequate IV sedation and use gentle digital sphincter dilation to increase likelihood of successful ED extraction (60% cases)
- Administer local anesthesia to maximize anal sphincter dilation
- Place patient in lithotomy position
- Use obstetric, ring or biopsy forceps, tenaculum, or suctioning devices to aid extraction while applying suprapubic pressure and having patient bear down during procedure
- Other methods
  - —Foley catheter—pass above foreign body, then inflate balloon and apply gentle traction to release suction and permit extraction
  - —Plaster of Paris—fill hollow object and insert gauze or instrument to serve as "handle"; place above or adjacent to foreign body; when hard, pull on inset handle to permit extraction
- Mandatory sigmoidoscopy to evaluate mucosal injury following extraction

Rectal Foreign Body Removal in OR

- General anesthesia required to remove high-riding or sharp object
- Laparotomy: last resort

MEDICATIONS

- Antibiotics with coverage against gram-negative and anaerobic organisms
  - —Ampicillin/sulbactam: 3 g q6h (peds: 50 mg/kg) i.v.
  - —Cefotetan: 2 g q12h (peds: 40 mg/kg) i.v.
  - —Cefoxitin, 2 g q6h (peds: 80 mg/kg q6h) i.v.
  - —Piperacillin/tazobactam: 3.375 g i.v. (peds: 75 mg/kg)
  - —Ticarcillin/clavulanate: 3.1 g i.v. (peds: 75 mg/kg)
  - —Trovafloxacin: 300 mg i.v. first dose, then 200 mg i.v. q.d. (adults only)
- Additional anaerobic coverage
  - —Clindamycin: 600–900 mg (peds: 10 mg/kg) i.v.
  - —Metronidazole: 1 g (peds: 15 mg/kg) i.v.
- Combination therapy
  - —Ampicillin 500 mg i.v. q6h (peds: 50 mg/kg), gentamicin 3–5 mg/kg/d i.v. t.i.d. (peds and adults), *and* metronidazole 1 g i.v. (peds: 15 mg/kg)
  - —Ciprofloxacin 400 mg i.v. q12h (adults only) *and* metronidazole 1 g i.v.
- Sedation and analgesia
  - —Fentanyl: 2–3 μg/kg i.v. (peds and adults)
  - —Midazolam: 0.01–0.2 mg/kg i.v. (peds and adults)

Disposition

ADMISSION CRITERIA

- Perforation
- Significant bleeding
- Unstable vital signs
- Abdominal pain
- Torn anal sphincter
- Foreign body that requires OR extraction
- Broken glass or other sharp object in rectum requiring surgical removal

DISCHARGE CRITERIA

- Stable vital signs
- No abdominal pain
- Normal sigmoidoscopy/anoscopy exam

Miscellaneous

ICD9: 863.45

ICD10: S36.6

SUGGESTED READINGS

Carrillo EH, Somberg LB, Ceballos CE, et al. Blunt traumatic injuries to the colon and rectum. J Am Coll Surg 1996;183:548–552.

Coates WC. Anorectum. In: Rosen P, et al, eds. Emergency medicine, 5th ed. St. Louis: Mosby, 2002:1343–1359.

Cohen JS, Sackier JM. Management of colorectal foreign bodies. J R Coll Surg Edinb 1996;41:312–315.

Fry RD. Anorectal trauma and foreign bodies. Surg Clin North Am 1994;74(6): 1491–505.

Janicke DM, Pundt MR. Anorectal disorders. Emerg Med Clin North Am 1996;14(4): 757–788.

Ko C. Rectal trauma. In: Rosen P, et al, eds. Five minute emergency consult, 1st ed. Philadelphia: Lippincott Williams & Wilkins, 1999:958–959.

Author: Elaine Sapiro

Red Eye

Clinical Presentation

SIGNS AND SYMPTOMS

- Discharge
- Pruritus
- Pain
- Foreign body sensation
- Ectropion, entropion
- Eyelash against globe (trichiasis)
- Conjunctival injection
- Corneal abrasion, ulcer, or opacity
- Anterior chamber cells or flare
- Photophobia (from movement of an inflamed iris)
- Proptosis
- Preauricular (viral conjunctivitis) lymphadenopathy
- Submandibular lymphadenopathy
- Rosacea (may cause blepharitis)
- Facial or skin lesions (herpes)
- Sinusitis
- Otitis
- Pharyngitis

MECHANISM/DESCRIPTION

- Red eye
  - —May be caused by almost any eye disorder
  - —Often benign
  - —May represent systemic disease
- Pathophysiology
  - —Conjunctival vascular engorgement (common to all nontraumatic red eyes) may be associated with
    - -Inflammatory diseases
      - ∗Uveitis (anterior and posterior)
      - ∗Episcleritis (70% idiopathic)
      - ∗Scleritis (50% associated with systemic disease)
    - -Inflammation/allergy
    - -Histamine release and increased vascular permeability, resulting in swelling of the conjunctiva (chemosis), sometimes with watery discharge and pruritus
    - -Infection
      - ∗Bacterial—purulent mucous discharge
      - ∗Viral—watery or no discharge, pruritus
      - ∗Fungal
    - -Trauma
      - ∗Corneal abrasion
      - ∗Conjunctival hemorrhage
      - ∗Foreign bodies

ETIOLOGY

- Characterize by location of conjunctival injection
  - —Perilimbal
    - -Anterior uveitis (iritis)
  - —Sectorial
    - -Pinguecula
    - -Pterygium
    - -Hemorrhage
    - -Episcleritis
    - -Scleritis
    - -Occult perforation
  - —Diffuse
    - -Bacterial or viral conjunctivitis
    - -Blepharitis
    - -Dry eye syndrome
    - -Acute angle closure glaucoma
    - -Endophthalmitis
- Categorize by the presence of discharge or pain
- With discharge
  - —More common
    - -Conjunctivitis
    - -Allergic reaction
    - -Ophthalmia neonatorum
    - -Blepharitis
  - —Less common
    - -Dacryocystitis
    - -Canaliculitis
- Without discharge
  - —No pain
    - -Subconjunctival hemorrhage
    - -Conjunctival tumor
  - —Mild to moderate pain
    - -Inflamed pinguecula/pterygium
    - -Blepharitis
    - -Dry eye syndrome conjunctivitis
    - -Foreign body
    - -Corneal disorder
    - -Episcleritis
    - -Posterior uveitis
    - -Orbital cellulitis
  - —Moderate to severe pain
    - -Corneal ulcer/abrasion/erosion
    - -Anterior uveitis
    - -Scleritis
    - -Acute angle closure glaucoma
    - -Endophthalmitis

Pre-Hospital

N/A

Diagnosis

ESSENTIAL WORKUP

- Thorough physical examination
- Ophthalmologic
  - —Visual acuity
  - —Pupil examination
  - —Confrontational visual field exam
  - —Extraocular muscle function
  - —Slit-lamp examination with fluorescein
  - —Lid eversion
  - —Funduscopy and tonometry when applicable

IMAGING/SPECIAL TESTS

- Tests should be directed toward the suspected etiology of red eye
- Dacryocystitis: culture discharge
- Corneal ulcers: ophthalmologist may scrape the cornea for cultures
- Bacterial conjunctivitis: obtain conjunctival swab
  - —Moderate discharge: routine culture and sensitivity (usually *Staphylococcus aureus, Streptococcus,* and *Haemophilus influenzae* [children])
  - —Severe discharge: *Neisseria gonorrhoeae* and *Chlamydia*
  - —Treat systemic infection and sexual partners
- Foreign body or orbital disease: plain films or CT scan of the orbits
- Uveitis
  - —If unilateral, nongranulomatous and history and physical are unremarkable: no systemic workup is necessary
  - —If bilateral, recurrent or granulomatous: CBC, ESR, ANA, VDRL, FTA Ab, PPD, ACE level, CXR (sarcoidosis and TB), Lyme titer, and HLA-B27, *Toxoplasma,* and cytomegalovirus titers

DIFFERENTIAL DIAGNOSIS

- Trauma
- Uveitis
- Arthritic disease
- Ankylosing spondylosis
- Ulcerative colitis
- Reiter's syndrome
- TB
- Herpes
- Syphilis
- Sarcoidosis
- *Toxoplasma*
- Cytomegalovirus

Treatment

INITIAL STABILIZATION

N/A

ED TREATMENT

- Direct therapy toward specific etiology
- Differentiate between a corneal abrasion and a corneal ulcer
- Eye patching is no longer routinely recommended for abrasions and is contraindicated for corneal ulcers or abrasions with high infection risk (contact lens wearers, abrasions from tree branches or fingernails)
- Update tetanus immunization for corneal injury
- Do not wear contact lenses
- Do not spread infection from the affected eye to the unaffected eye

Corneal Abrasion

- Non-contact lens wearer
  —Ointment or drops
    -Erythromycin ointment every 4 hours
    -Polytrim drops four times a day
- Contact lens wearers need pseudomonal coverage
  —Ointment or drops
    -Tobramycin ointment every 4 hours
    -Tobramycin, ofloxacin, or ciprofloxacin drops four times a day
- Dilate eyes with cyclopentolate 1–2%, 2–4 drops q.d. to prevent pain from iritis
- Abrasions will heal without patching

Corneal Ulcer

- Non-contact lens wearer
  —Ointment or drops
    -Polytrim ointment four times a day
    -Ofloxacin, ciprofloxacin drops every 2–4 hours
- Contact lens wearers need pseudomonal coverage
  -Tobramycin, ofloxacin, or ciprofloxacin drops every 2–4 hours
  -Tobramycin or ciprofloxacin ointment every hour as needed (optional)
- Severe or vision threatening corneal ulcers
  —Central, larger than 1.5 mm or with significant anterior chamber reaction
  —Treat as aforementioned and add
    -Increased frequency of antibiotic drops (1 drop every 15 minutes for three doses then every 15 minutes for 2–6 hours then every 30 minutes around the clock
  —Ophthalmology consult for further recommendations, which may include
    -Ciprofloxacin 500 mg PO b.i.d.
    -Fortified antibiotic drops (made by ophthalmologist/pharmacy)
- Ulcers from herpes simplex or zoster
  —Add Viroptic 1%, 2 gtt 9 times/d or vidarabine 3% ointment 5 times/d (ointment preferred for children)
- Trauma or uveitis
  —Rule out intraocular foreign body

MEDICATIONS

- Antibiotic drops
  —Ciprofloxacin 0.3%: 1–2 gtt q1–6h
  —Gentamycin 0.3%: 1–2 gtt q4h
  —Ofloxacin 0.3%: 1–2 gtt q1–6h
  —Levofloxacin 0.5%: 1–2 gtt q2h
  —Polytrim: 1 gt q3–6h
  —Sulfacetamide 10%: 0.3% 1–2 gtt q2–6h
  —Tobramycin 0.3%: 1–2 gtt q1–4h
  —Trifluridine 1%: 1 gt q2–4h
- Antibiotic ointments
  —Bacitracin: 500 U/g ½-inch ribbon of ointment q3–6h
  —Ciprofloxacin 0.3%: ½-inch ribbon of ointment q6–8h
  —Erythromycin 0.5%: ½-inch ribbon of ointment q3–6h
  —Gentamycin 0.3%: ½-inch ribbon of ointment q3–4h
  —Neosporin: ½-inch ribbon of ointment q3–4h
  —Polysporin: ½-inch ribbon of ointment q3–4h
  —Sulfacetamide 10%: ½-inch ribbon of ointment q3–8h
  —Tobramycin 0.3%: ½-inch ribbon of ointment q3–4h
  —Vidarabine: ½-inch ribbon of ointment 5 times/d
- Mydriatics and cycloplegics
  —Atropine 1%, 2%: 1–2 gtt q.d. to q.i.d.
  —Cyclopentolate 0.5%, 1%, 2%: 1–2 gtt p.r.n. dilation
  —Homatropine 2%: 1–2 gtt b.i.d. to t.i.d.
  —Phenylephrine 0.12%, 2.5%, 10%: 1–2 gtt t.i.d. to q.i.d.
  —Tropicamide 0.5%, 1%: 1–2 gtt p.r.n. dilation
- Corticosteroid antibiotic combination drops (with ophthalmology consultation)
  —Blephamide: 1–2 gtt q1–8h
  —Cortisporin: 1–2 gtt q3–4h
  —Maxitrol: 1–2 gtt q1–8h
  —Pred G: 1–2 gtt q1–8h
  —TobraDex: 1–2 gtt q2–6h
- Glaucoma agents (always with ophthalmology consultation)
  —Acetazolamide: 250–500 mg PO q.d. to q.i.d.
  —Betaxolol 0.25%, 0.5%: 1–2 gtt b.i.d.
  —Carteolol 1%: 1 gt b.i.d.
  —Levobunolol 0.25%, 0.5%: 1 gt q.d. to b.i.d.
  —Dipivefrin 1%: 1 gt b.i.d.
  —Mannitol: 1–2 g/kg i.v. over 45 minutes
  —Pilocarpine 0.25%, 0.5%, 1%, 2%, 3%, 4%, 6%, 8%, 10%: 1–2 gtt t.i.d. to q.i.d.
    -Only if mechanical closure is ruled out
  —Timolol 0.25%, 0.5%: 1 gt b.i.d.

Disposition

ADMISSION CRITERIA

- Endophthalmitis
- Perforated corneal ulcers
- Orbital cellulitis

DISCHARGE CRITERIA

- Depends on the diagnosis
- If the diagnosis is certain and visual loss will not result, the patient may be discharged without consultation
- Consider telephone or ED consult for
  —Dacryocystitis
  —Corneal ulcer
  —Scleritis
  —Angle closure glaucoma
  —Uveitis
  —Proptosis
  —Orbital cellulitis
  —Vision loss
  —Uncertain diagnosis
  —Gonorrheal conjunctivitis

Miscellaneous

ICD9: N/A

ICD10: N/A

SUGGESTED READINGS

Bertolini J, Pelicio M. The red eye. Emerg Med Clin North Am 1995;13(3):561–579.

Juang P, Rosen P. Ocular examination techniques for the emergency department. J Emerg Med 1997;15:793–810.

Rhee D, Pyfer M. The Wills eye manual: office and emergency room diagnosis and treatment of eye disease, 3rd ed. Philadelphia: Lippincott Williams & Wilkins, 1999.

Author: Pascal Juang

Reiter's Disease

Clinical Presentation

SIGNS AND SYMPTOMS

- History of dysentery, urethritis, or cervicitis 1–6 weeks before disease presentation
- Nonpurulent urethritis
- Conjunctivitis with mild nonpurulent discharge precedes arthritis
- Arthritis
  —Painful
  —Asymmetric and additive
  —Usually beginning in the lower extremities
  —Wrists and distal interphalangeal joints may be involved

Fever

- Weight loss
- Malaise
- Uveitis, iritis
- Low back or buttock pain
- Enthesitis
  —Inflammation of the tendinous insertions into bone
  —"Sausage" digits (dactylitis)
  —Achilles tendinitis
  —Plantar fasciitis
- Oral lesions
  —Painless
  —Transient
  —Often unnoticed
- Balanitis circinata
  —Shallow
  —Painless penile lesions
- Keratoderma blennorrhagica
  —Clear vesicles on an erythematous base that evolve to hyperkeratotic lesions
  —Commonly on soles, palms
- Nail changes
  —Onycholysis
  —Yellowing
  —Hyperkeratosis
- Dysuria, urinary frequency, hematuria
- Rare transient neurologic dysfunction
- Rare dysrhythmia
- Pericarditis or aortic regurgitation in chronic disease

MECHANISM/DESCRIPTION

- A seronegative spondyloarthropathy and reactive arthritis
- The first episode of arthritis usually resolves in 3–6 months
- Recurrence is common
- Rate of chronic disease varies with etiologic organism and presence of HLA-B27
- Classic triad
  —Arthritis
  —Urethritis
  —Conjunctivitis
  —Incomplete forms exist
- Leading cause of inflammatory arthritis in young men
- Mechanism is unclear
  —Antigenic cross-reactivity with HLA-B27
  —Persistent immune response after infection
  —Autoimmune response

ETIOLOGY

- Thought to develop in a genetically susceptible host following bacterial infection such as *Salmonella, Shigella, Yersinia, Campylobacter,* and *Chlamydia*
- Many other agents suggested, including HIV and intravesicular BCG
- Bacterial antigens, chlamydial DNA and RNA have been found in synovial fluid, but no viable organisms (culture negative)
- Men more than women by 5–10:1 in venereal infection
- Men equal women in enteric infection
- Predominantly a disease of the young with peak onset between ages 15 and 35 years
- Strong correlation with HLA-B27, seen in 70–80% of patients
  —Poor prognostic sign for severity, chronicity

PEDIATRIC CONSIDERATIONS

- Rare in the pediatric population
- Diagnosis can be made using adult criteria
- Syndrome is often incomplete, with conjunctivitis as presenting complaint

Pre-Hospital

N/A

Diagnosis

ESSENTIAL WORKUP

- Includes a search for the etiologic infection by history and examination, especially in women where cervicitis is often asymptomatic

LABORATORY

- Arthrocentesis with fluid analysis to rule out an infectious process
  —Synovial fluid shows inflammation with neutrophilic predominance
  —Gram's stain and culture negative
- CBC with differential may show a moderate neutrophilic leukocytosis and anemia
- ESR mildly elevated
- C-reactive protein and C3/C4 levels mildly elevated
- Rheumatoid factor and HLA-B27 may be useful adjuncts
- Urethral or cervical swab for *Chlamydia* infection is mandatory
  —Preferably direct fluorescent antibody or DNA-probes for chlamydial ribosomal RNA
- Stool cultures if ongoing dysentery
- HIV testing should be considered, especially if use of immunosuppressive therapy is contemplated

IMAGING/SPECIAL TESTS

- Plain radiography of affected joints
  —Soft tissue swelling and effusion are common
  —Periosteal spurs with indistinct margins and fluffy periostitis can be seen at the sites of tendinous insertions (enthesitis) especially of lower extremities
  —Joint space narrowing is common in the small joints of the hand
- Plain radiography of lumbar spine, sacroiliac joints
  —Unilateral sacroiliitis in early disease (10%)
  —Bilateral in chronic (70%)
  —Asymmetric spondylitis
  —Syndesmophytes
- Plain radiography of feet
  —Spurs at the insertion of the plantar fascia

DIFFERENTIAL DIAGNOSIS

- Gonococcal arthritis
- Ankylosing spondylitis
- Psoriatic arthritis
- Arthritis related to inflammatory bowel disease
- Undifferentiated spondyloarthropathy
- Lyme disease
- Behçet's syndrome
- Rheumatoid arthritis
- Still's disease
- Sarcoid arthritis
- Gout/pseudogout
- Rheumatic fever
- Viral arthritis

Treatment

INITIAL STABILIZATION

- Supportive care
- IV fluids if hypovolemia due to dysentery
- Ice to inflamed joints

ED TREATMENT

- High-dose NSAIDs are the mainstay of therapy
  —A minimum of 1 month of NSAID treatment at maximum dosage is mandatory before evaluating effectiveness
- Sulfasalazine for NSAID failure or contraindication
- Treat urethritis/cervicitis if present or suspected
  —Partners should also be treated
  —Azithromycin and doxycycline
  —Prolonged (up to 3 months) antibiotic treatment for *Chlamydia*-associated arthritis may improve recovery
- Antibiotics are not indicated for enteric disease
- Local corticosteroids may be helpful for severe arthritis or enthesitis
- In persistent or aggressive disease, immunomodulating therapies may be initiated in consult with a rheumatologist
  —Systemic corticosteroids
  —Azathioprine
  —Methotrexate

MEDICATIONS

- Azathioprine: 1–2.5 mg/kg/d PO q12–24h
- Azithromycin: 1 g (peds: 10 mg/kg) PO × 1 day
- Doxycycline: 100 mg (peds: 5 mg/kg/d, divided) PO q12h × 10 days
- Ibuprofen: 2,400 mg (peds: 20–40 mg/kg/d) PO q6–8h
- Indomethacin: 75–200 mg/d (peds: 1–2 mg/kg/d) PO q6–12h
- Methotrexate: 7.5–25 mg (peds: 0.5–1 mg/kg; maximum, 15–25 mg) PO per week for aggressive unremitting disease
- Sulfasalazine: 1–3 g (peds: 30–60 mg/kg/d; maximum, 2 g) PO q6h, for NSAID failure or contraindication

Disposition

ADMISSION CRITERIA

- Concomitant disease(s) that require admission
- Unremitting pain or inability to ambulate

DISCHARGE CRITERIA

- Most patients can be discharged
- Close follow-up with a rheumatologist or a PCP is required
- Physical therapy and vocational counseling may help

Miscellaneous

ICD9: 099.3

ICD10: M02.3

SUGGESTED READINGS

Amor B. Reiter's syndrome: diagnosis and clinical features. Rheum Dis Clin North Am 1998;24(4):677–695.

Barth WF, Segal K. Reactive arthritis (Reiter's syndrome). Am Fam Phys 1999;60(2):499–503.

Leilisalo-Repo, Marjatta. Prognosis, course of disease, and treatment of the spondyloarthropathies. Rheum Dis Clin North Am 1998;24(4):737–749.

Author: Christine Yang-Kauh

Renal Calculus

Clinical Presentation

SIGNS AND SYMPTOMS

- Sudden onset of severe pain in the costovertebral angle, flank and lateral abdomen
- Colicky or constant pain
  - —Patient cannot find a comfortable position
- Hematuria
- Nausea/vomiting
- Restlessness
- Diaphoresis
- History of prior stone formation
- Abdominal tenderness is not present

MECHANISM/DESCRIPTION

- Urinary tract obstruction
- Intermittent distention of the renal pelvis of proximal ureter produces pain
- Kidney stones
  - —Most common cause of renal colic
- Theories of stone formation
  - —Urinary supersaturation of solute followed by crystal precipitation
  - —Decrease in the normal urinary proteins inhibiting crystal growth
  - —Urinary stasis from a physical anomaly, catheter placement, neurogenic bladder, or the presence of a foreign body
- Stone composition
  - —75%: calcium in conjunction with phosphate and/or oxalate
  - —15%: magnesium phosphate (struvite)
  - —Associated with infections caused by urea-splitting organisms (e.g., *Pseudomonas, Proteus, Klebsiella*) along with an alkalotic urine
  - —5% uric acid
- 90% of urinary calculi radiopaque

ETIOLOGY

- 1% of the population
- Three times more common in men than women

PEDIATRIC CONSIDERATIONS

- Rare in children
  - —When present, indication of an overt metabolic or genetic disorder
- Painless hematuria common presentation (up to 30%)
- Pediatric patients younger than 16 years comprise approximately 7% of all cases of renal stones
- 1:1 sex distribution
- Causes of stone formation
  - —Metabolic abnormalities (50%)
    - -Most common etiologies of stone formation in the pediatric population
  - —Urologic abnormalities (20%)
  - —Infection (15%)
  - —Immobilization syndrome (5%)

Pre-Hospital

CAUTIONS

- Parenteral opiates may be required for pain control with long transport times

Diagnosis

ESSENTIAL WORKUP

Physical Exam

- Obtain vital signs
  - —Fever suggests an occult infection
  - —Hypotension, along with an altered mental status is suggestive of urosepsis
- Abdominal exam
  - —Pain on palpation, rebound tenderness and or guarding suggests a more serious intraabdominal process
  - —Palpate the abdominal aorta for tenderness or pulsatile enlargement suggestive of an aneurysm
- Examine the genitalia for evidence of epididymitis, torsion, or testicular masses

LABORATORY

- Urinalysis
  - —Microscopic hematuria present in >80%
  - —Gross hematuria
  - —Absent urinary blood in 10%
  - —No correlation between the amount of hematuria and the degree of urinary obstruction
  - —WBC/bacteria suggestive of infection
- CBC
  - —WBC >15,000 suggestive of concomitant infection
- Urine culture
- Electrolytes, glucose, BUN, and creatinine
- Pregnancy test when suggestive

IMAGING/SPECIAL TESTS

Computed Tomography

- Helical CT has replaced intravenous pyelogram (IVP) as test of choice
- Detect calculi as small as 1 mm in diameter
- Directly visualizes complications, such as hydroureter, hydronephrosis, and ureteral edema
- Advantages over IVP
  - —Performed rapidly
  - —Does not require IV contrast media
  - —Detects other non-urologic causes of symptoms, such as abdominal aortic aneurysms (AAAs)
- Nonenhanced helical CT in the evaluation of renal colic
  - —Sensitivity of 97%
  - —Specificity of 96%
  - —Accuracy of 97%
- Indications
  - —First-time diagnosis
  - —Persistent pain
  - —Clinical confusion with pyelonephritis

Intravenous Pyelogram

- Establishes diagnosis in 95%
- Demonstrates the severity of obstruction
- Scout film prior may localize stones that would otherwise be obscured by the dye

- Postvoiding film
  - —Useful to identify stones at the ureteral vesicular junction or distal ureter that are obscured by a full bladder

KUB Radiograph

- Indicated when allergy to IVP dye and when renal scanning and US not available
- Assists in locating radiopaque stones and the exclusion of other pathologies in nonpregnant patients
- Difficult to distinguish radiopaque body
  - —Phlebolith
  - —Bowel contents
  - —Obstruction within the urinary tract on the KUB
- Oblique films assist in localizing suspicious calcifications

Ultrasound

- For patients who are not candidates for IV contrast
- Useful in the detection of larger stones and hydronephrosis
- Provides anatomic information only
- Helpful in diagnosing obstruction and localizing stones in the proximal and distal portions of the ureter
- Ability to detect hydronephrosis:
  - —Sensitivity of 85–94%
  - —Specificity of 100%
- Limitations
  - —May miss stones <5 mm in size
  - —May miss an obstruction in the early phase of renal colic
    - -Time delay until the onset of pyelocaliectasis even after total obstruction

Renal Scan

- Useful in patients with a known allergy to contrast media
- Excellent functional test
- Does not provide the anatomic detail of the IVP, US, or CT

DIFFERENTIAL DIAGNOSIS

- Do not miss a catastrophe mimicking renal colic
- Dissecting or rupturing AAA
- Pyelonephritis
- Papillary necrosis (sickle cell disease, NSAID analgesic abuse, diabetes, or infection)
- Renal infarction (vascular dissection or arterial embolus)
- Ectopic pregnancy
- Ovarian cyst/torsion
- Appendicitis (subacute prodrome differentiates)
- Biliary tract disease (RUQ tenderness makes renal calculi unlikely)
- Musculoskeletal strain (worsening of discomfort during physical exam maneuvers)
- Lower lobe pneumonia (auscultate the lungs)

Treatment

INITIAL STABILIZATION

- Rapid dipstick urine test for blood
  - —Positive test in conjunction with clinical findings sufficient to begin analgesic therapy
- Provide adequate analgesia when diagnosis suspected on clinical and laboratory findings

ED TREATMENT

- Hydration
  - —Initiate IV crystalloid infusion with 1 L of NS infused over 30–60 minutes followed by 200–500 mL/h
  - —Bolus volume compromised patients with 500-mL increments until urine output adequate
- Analgesics (demerol, morphine, ketorolac)
- Antiemetics (prochlorperazine, droperidol, Vistaril)

MEDICATIONS

- Hydroxyzine hydrochloride (Vistaril): 25–50 mg i.m. *(not i.v.)* q4–6h
- Ketorolac (Toradol): 30–60 mg i.m. or 30 mg i.v. (alone or with opiates)
- Meperidine (Demerol): 50–100 mg (peds: 1–2 mg/kg/dose) q3–4h i.v./i.m.
- Morphine sulfate: 1–3 mg i.v. may be administered q15min as needed to control pain (peds: 0.1–0.2 mg/kg/dose q2–4h)
- Ondansetron (Zofran): 4 mg IVPB
- Promethazine (Phenergan): 12.5–25 mg i.m./i.v.

Disposition

ADMISSION CRITERIA

- Obstruction in the presence of infection mandates immediate urologic intervention
- Intractable pain with refractory nausea and vomiting
- Severe volume depletion
- Urinary extravasation
- Hypercalcemic crisis
- Solitary kidney and complete obstruction
- Relative admission indications (discuss with urologist)
  - —High-grade obstruction
  - —Renal insufficiency
  - —Intrinsic renal disease
  - —Stone size <5 mm usually pass spontaneously; those >8 mm rarely do

DISCHARGE CRITERIA

- Normal vital signs
- No evidence of concomitant urinary tract infection
- Adequate analgesia
- Able to tolerate po fluids to maintain hydration status
- Reliable patient with an adequate home situation
- Appropriate outpatient follow-up arranged
- Normal renal function
- Provide a urine strainer to collect the stone for possible future stone analysis
- Arrange urologic follow-up

Miscellaneous

ICD9: 592.0

ICD10: N20.0

SUGGESTED READINGS

Javier I, Escobar JL II, Eastman ER, et al. Selected urologic problems. In: Marx, ed. Rosen's emergency medicine: concepts and clinical practice, 5th ed. St. Louis: Mosby, 2002:1414–1421.

Sheley RC, et al. Helical CT in the evaluation of renal colic. Am J Emerg Med 1999;17:279.

Author: Lawrence Heiskell

Renal Failure

Clinical Presentation

SIGNS AND SYMPTOMS

Acute Renal Failure (ARF)

- Typically asymptomatic
  —Diagnosed incidentally from routine BUN/Cr
- Oliguria
  —<400 mL/d
- Fluid overload
  —Dyspnea
  —Hypertension
  —Jugular venous distention
  —Pulmonary edema
  —Peripheral edema
  —Ascites
  —Pericardial effusion
  —Pulmonary effusion
- Nausea/vomiting

Prerenal Failure

- Absolute or relative volume deficit
- Dry mucous membranes
- Hypotension
- Tachycardia
- Low cardiac output
  —CHF
- Systemic vasodilation
  —Sepsis
  —Anaphylaxis

Intrarenal (Intrinsic) Failure

- Renal artery thrombosis
  —Flank or abdominal pain
  —Atrial fibrillation
  —Recent myocardial infarction
- Renal vein thrombosis
  —Nephrotic syndrome (see Nephrotic Syndrome)
  —Pulmonary embolus (see Pulmonary Embolism)
  —Flank pain
- Glomerulonephritis/vasculitis
  —Recent infection
    -Sinusitis
    -Rash (palpable purpura)
    -Pulmonary hemorrhage
- Hemolytic-uremic syndrome (HUS)
  —Preceded by a viral or bacterial infection
  —Upper respiratory infection or diarrhea
- Thrombotic thrombocytopenic purpura (TTP)
  —Headache
  —Confusion
  —Seizures
  —Cranial nerve palsies
  —Coma
- Allergic interstitial nephritis after drug ingestion
  —Fever
  —Rash
  —Arthralgias

Postrenal Failure

- Abdominal or flank pain
- Distended bladder
- Oliguria or anuria

Complications of ARF

Uremic Syndrome

- Pericarditis
- Pericardial effusion
- Cardiac tamponade
- Ileus
- Altered mental status
- Asterixis
- Hyperreflexia
- Restless leg syndrome
- Focal neurologic abnormality
- Seizures

Hematologic Disorders

- Anemia
- Increased bleeding time
- Leukocytosis

MECHANISM/DESCRIPTION

- Decline in glomerular filtration
- Disrupts the extracellular fluid volume, electrolyte, and acid-base status
- Results in accumulation of nitrogenous waste

ETIOLOGY

- Prerenal failure
  —Caused by renal hypoperfusion
  —Renal tissue remains normal unless severe/prolonged hypertension
- Intrarenal failure
  —Caused by diseases of the renal parenchyma
- Postrenal failure
  —Due to acute obstruction of the urinary tract
- Iatrogenic causes include
  —Aminoglycoside antibiotics
  —Radiocontrast material administration

Pre-Hospital

CAUTIONS

- Avoid rapid administration of IV fluid
- Administer calcium/sodium bicarbonate for suspected hyperkalemic cardiac arrest

Diagnosis

ESSENTIAL WORKUP

- Electrolytes
  —Hyperkalemia
  —Hyponatremia
  —Hyperphosphatemia
  —Hypocalcemia
  —Hypermagnesemia
  —Metabolic acidosis
  —Elevated anion gap
- BUN/Cr
  —Elevated
- Urinalysis
  —Centrifuged specimen helps to distinguish between different etiologies of ARF
  —Examined for casts, blood, WBCs, and crystals
- CBC
  —Anemia with chronic renal failure

LABORATORY

Prerenal

- UA
  —Specific gravity >1.018
  —Osmolality >500 mmol/kg
  —Sodium <10 mmol/L
  —Hyaline casts
- BUN/Cr ratio >20
- Rapid recovery renal function when renal perfusion normalized

Intrarenal

- BUN/Cr ratio <10–15
- Glomerulonephritis/vasculitis
  —UA with red cell or granular casts
  —Complement and autoimmune antibodies
- HUS or TTP
  —UA normal
  —Anemia
  —Thrombocytopenia
  —Schistocytes on blood smear
  —Elevated LDH
- Nephrotoxic acute tubular necrosis (ATN)
  —UA
    -Brown granular or epithelial cell casts
    -SG 1.010
    -Urine osmolality <350 mmol/kg
    -Urine Na >20 mmol/L
  —Ethylene glycol ingestion
    -UA: calcium oxalate crystals
    -Anion gap metabolic acidosis
    -Osmolal gap
- Rhabdomyolysis
  —UA: heme positive without red cells
  —Elevated serum K^+, PO_4, myoglobin, CPK-MM, uric acid
  —Decreased serum Ca^{2+}
- Tubulointerstitial disease
- Allergic interstitial nephritis
  —UA with WBC casts, WBCs, RBCs, and proteinuria
  —Systemic eosinophilia

Postrenal

- UA
  - —Usually normal
  - —May have some hematuria but no casts or protein

IMAGING/SPECIAL TESTS

- Intravenous pyelogram
  - —Avoid contrast with renal insufficiency
  - —Predisposes to further renal decompensation
- US
  - —98% sensitive for excluding obstruction
- Helical CT scan without contrast detects for obstruction
- Duplex scan for
  - —Renal artery or vein thrombosis
- Renal arteriogram
  - —Definitive diagnosis or renal artery thrombosis
- Inferior vena cava and renal vessels venogram for
  - —Renal vein thrombosis
- EKG
  - —Severe hypertension
  - —CHF
  - —Hyperkalemia

Treatment

INITIAL STABILIZATION

- ABCs
  - —Supplemental oxygen for hypoxia
- Correct electrolyte disturbances
- Indications for emergent dialysis
  - —Life-threatening hyperkalemia
  - —Intractable hypertension or pulmonary edema
  - —Fluid overload unresponsive to other treatments
  - —BUN >100 mg/dL
  - —Cr >10 mg/dL
  - —Metabolic acidosis (pH <7.2)
  - —Severe uremia—pericarditis
- Avoid nephrotoxins
- Monitor urine output

ED TREATMENT

Prerenal

- Treat hypoperfusion
  - —Consider PRBC for blood loss
- Invasive cardiac monitoring if unable to assess cardiac failure versus hypovolemia
- Administer 0.9% NS fluid challenge cautiously to avoid fluid overload in liver failure with ascites
  - —Response: good indicator of the degree to which hypovolemia is a factor

Intrarenal

- Glomerulonephritis
  - —Immunosuppressive agents (glucocorticoids) or plasma exchange
- ATN—therapeutic options
  - —Low-dose dopamine
  - —Mannitol
  - —Furosemide
  - —Calcium channel blockers
- Acute interstitial nephritis
  - —Withdrawal of causative agent
  - —Treat underlying disease process
- Euvolemic patients with acute oliguric renal failure
  - —Trial of dopamine 0.5–2.5 μg/kg/min

Complications of ATN

- Volume overload
  - —Furosemide (up to 400 mg)
  - —Low dose dopamine
  - —Dialysis
- Hyponatremia
  - —Fluid restriction
- Hyperkalemia
  - —Sodium polystyrene sulfonate for asymptomatic with K^+ >5.5 mEq/L
  - —For K^+ >6.5 mEq/L or EKG abnormalities consistent with hyperkalemia
    - -Calcium gluconate: for cardiac and neuromuscular protection
    - -Glucose and insulin: onset 30–60 minutes, duration several hours
    - -Sodium bicarbonate: onset <15 minutes, duration 1–2 hours
    - -Dialysis for intractable hyperkalemia
- Metabolic acidosis
  - —Consider sodium bicarbonate for pH <7.2 or HCO_3 <15 mEq/L
  - —Dialysis
- Hyperphosphatemia
  - —Calcium carbonate
  - —Aluminum hydroxide
- Myoglobinuria
  - —Mannitol
  - —Sodium bicarbonate to alkalinize the urine
  - —Aggressive fluid resuscitation with 0.9% NS

MEDICATIONS

- Aluminum hydroxide (Amphojel): 500–1,500 mg PO
- Calcium carbonate (Os-Cal): 250–3,000 mg PO
- Calcium gluconate: 10 mL of 10% solution over 5 min i.v.
- Dextrose: D50W 1 amp (50 mL or 25 g) (peds: D25W 2–4 mL/kg) i.v.
- Furosemide: 20–400 mg IVP
- Insulin: 10 IU regular i.v. with dextrose
- Mannitol: 12.5–25 g IVP
- Sodium bicarbonate: 1–2 mEq/kg i.v.
- Sodium polystyrene sulfonate (Kayexalate): 1 g/kg up to 15–60 g PO or 30–50 g retention enema in sorbitol q6h

Disposition

ADMISSION CRITERIA

- New-onset ARF
- Hyperkalemia/significant electrolyte abnormalities
- Fluid overload with hypoxia/CHF

DISCHARGE CRITERIA

- Stable
- Normal electrolytes

Miscellaneous

ICD9: 586

ICD10: N19

SEE ALSO: GLOMERULONEPHRITIS; NEPHRITIC SYNDROME; NEPHROTIC SYNDROME

SUGGESTED READINGS

Albright RC. Acute renal failure: a practical update. Mayo Clin Proc 2001;76(1):67–74.

Brady HR, Brenner BM. Acute renal failure. In: Isselbacher KJ, Braunwald E, Wilson JD, et al, eds. Harrison's principles of internal medicine, 15th ed. New York: McGraw-Hill, 2001:1541–1550.

Brady HR, Singer GG. Acute renal failure. Lancet 1995;346:1533–1540.

Brady HR, Brenner BM, Clarkson MR, et al. Acute renal failure. In: Brenner BM, ed. Brenner and Rector's the kidney, 6th ed. Philadelphia: WB Saunders, 2000: 1201–1262.

Prough DS. Physiologic acid-base and electrolyte changes in acute and chronic renal failure patients. Anesthesiol Clin North Am 2000;18(4):809–833.

Thadhani R, Pascual M, Bonventre JV. Acute renal failure. N Engl J Med 1996;334(22):1448–1460.

Author: Lauren Grossman

Renal Injury

Clinical Presentation

SIGNS AND SYMPTOMS

- Gross hematuria is a common presentation even with minor renal trauma
  —Severity of renal trauma does not correlate with the amount of blood in the urine
- Flank mass or ecchymosis
- Tenderness in the flank, abdomen, or back
- Fracture of the inferior ribs or spinal transverse processes
- Nausea and vomiting

MECHANISM/DESCRIPTION

- Most common of all urologic injuries
- Occurs in approximately 8–10% of all abdominal trauma
  —Majority resulting from blunt trauma including motor-vehicle accidents, falls, domestic violence, and contact sports
- Mechanism of injury and kinematics are important factors in evaluating patients for possible renal injury
- In blunt trauma, note the type and direction (horizontal or vertical) of any deceleration or compressive forces
  —Accounts for 80–85% of all renal injuries and is five times more common than penetrating injury
- In penetrating trauma, note the characteristic of the weapon (type and caliber), distance from the weapon, or the type and length of knife or impaling object
  —Injuries result from a combination of the kinetic energy and shear forces of the penetrating object
- Mechanisms responsible for significant renal injury almost never affect the kidney alone, but most often disrupt and injure other vital organs that can be responsible for patient mortality
- Renal injuries are classified according to type and severity of the injury
  —Grade I: renal contusion; subcapsular hematoma, nonexpanding without parenchymal laceration
  —Grade II: hematoma nonexpanding, perirenal hematoma confined to retroperitoneum; laceration <1 cm parenchymal depth of renal cortex
  —Grade III: laceration >1 cm parenchymal depth of renal cortex without collecting system rupture or urinary extravasation
  —Grade IV: parenchymal laceration extending through renal cortex, medulla, and collecting system; main renal artery or vein with contained hemorrhage
  —Grade V: completely shattered kidney; avulsion of renal hilum that devascularized kidney

PEDIATRIC CONSIDERATIONS

- The kidney is the organ most commonly damaged by blunt trauma in the pediatric population
- Contributing factors include a relatively larger size of kidneys compared with adults and the fact that the tenth and eleventh ribs are not completely ossified until the third decade of life

Pre-Hospital

CAUTIONS

- Obtain details of injury from pre-hospital providers
- IV access
- Penetrating wounds or evisceration should be covered with sterile dressings

Diagnosis

ESSENTIAL WORKUP

- Adults with blunt trauma, microscopic hematuria (>3–5 RBC/HPF) and no evidence of shock (SBP = 90) have an extremely low incidence of major renal injuries and do not require radiographic imaging of the kidneys
  —Unless other major associated intraabdominal injuries coexist
- All adults with blunt renal trauma and gross hematuria, or microhematuria in the presence of shock, require renal imaging for further evaluation of renal injury
- In adults with penetrating renal trauma, the presence or absence of hematuria is of no consequence in predicting upper urinary tract injury
  —Location of penetrating wound in relation to urinary tract is most important factor in deciding need for radiographic imaging
- Important to rule out coexisting injuries

LABORATORY

- Urinalysis: gross hematuria or >50 RBCs/HPF in adults and >20 RBC/HPF in children is suggestive of renal injury
- Baseline laboratory values including hematocrit and Cr/BUN should be obtained

IMAGING/SPECIAL TESTS

- Plain abdominal films may show fractured inferior ribs or transverse processes, a unilateral enlarged kidney shadow secondary to edema or hemorrhage, or absence/obscuring of the psoas margin
- Intravenous pyelogram (IVP)
  —Allows evaluation for renal viability and function
  —Extravasation reflects injury to the collecting system
  —Nonvisualization of a kidney may indicate renal pedicle injury or parenchymal shattering
  —However, often abnormal findings are nonspecific and require more definitive studies, such as CT scan
- US
  —Role in evaluation of renal injury is controversial
  —May show size of perirenal hematoma and whether it is expanding or resolving
  —Otherwise exam is nonspecific and does not provide enough information
- Abdominal CT
  —Contrast-enhanced spiral CT scan (preferred)
  —Superior anatomic detail and diagnostic accuracy of 98% for renal injury
  —Sensitive indicator of minor extravasation, parenchymal laceration, vascular injury, and nonrenal injuries

DIFFERENTIAL DIAGNOSIS

- Renal parenchymal injury
- Renal vascular injury
- Ureteral injury
- Bladder or urethral injury

PEDIATRIC CONSIDERATIONS

- Major blunt renal trauma can occur in the absence of gross hematuria or shock in the pediatric population, thus requiring complete radiographic evaluation for the proper diagnosis and staging of renal injuries after blunt trauma with hematuria
- CT scan is the imaging modality of choice

Treatment

INITIAL STABILIZATION

- ABCs (including C-spine immobilization)
  —Adequate IV access
  —Fluid resuscitation, initially with 2 L of crystalloid (NS or lactated Ringer's solution), followed by blood products as needed
- Rule out potential life-threatening injuries first

ED TREATMENT

- Immediate laparotomy may be appropriate in the acutely injured patient who is hemodynamically unstable with presumed hemoperitoneum and renal injury
- All penetrating renal trauma requires renal exploration unless complete radiographic staging reveals an injury which can be managed nonoperatively in a hemodynamically stable patient
- Management of renal injuries
  —Classes I and II: contusions and minor lacerations with stable vital signs and urographically demonstrated normal renal function can be managed nonoperatively
  —Class III: renal lacerations with urinary extravasation
  —Controversy between operative versus nonoperative management
  —Management should be based on complete radiologic definition of the degree of injury using CT scanning
  —Classes IV and V: shattered kidney or renal pedicle injuries and hemodynamically unstable patients require emergent laparotomy
  —All ureteral injuries require operative repair

Disposition

ADMISSION CRITERIA

- Patients with significant renal injury require hospitalization for definitive laparotomy or observation

DISCHARGE CRITERIA

- Patients with microscopic hematuria only and who are hemodynamically stable with no other traumatic injuries may be discharged with instructions for immediate return if gross hematuria develops
  —Outpatient referral to urologist should be made

Miscellaneous

ICD9: 866.00

ICD10: S37.0

SUGGESTED READINGS

Peterson N. Genitourinary trauma. In: Felicano D, et al, eds. Trauma, 3rd ed. Stamford, CT: Appleton & Lange, 1996:661–694.

Schneider R. Genitourinary system. In: Rosen P, et al, eds. Emergency medicine: concepts and clinical practice, 5th ed. St. Louis: CV Mosby, 2002:437–456.

Stein J, Kaji D, Eastham J, et al. Blunt renal trauma in the pediatric population: Indications for radiographic evaluation. Urology 1994;(44):406–410.

Wessells H, McAninich J. Update on upper urinary tract trauma. AUA Update Series 1996;(15):110–115.

Author: Albert Jin

Reperfusion Therapy, Cardiac

Clinical Presentation

SIGNS AND SYMPTOMS

- See Myocardial Infarction and Unstable Angina
- Therapies
  - —Thrombolytic therapy (see Thrombolytic Therapy for full discussion)
  - —Glycoprotein IIb/IIIa inhibitors
  - —Unfractionated heparin and low-molecular-weight heparin (LMWH)
  - —Percutaneous coronary intervention (PCI); that is, angioplasty and stents

MECHANISM/DESCRIPTION

- Thrombolytics
  - —Reduce morbidity and mortality in ST-segment elevation myocardial infarction (MI)
  - —Maximum benefit is achieved when started within the 6 hours after the infarct
  - —The earlier thrombolytics are started, the greater the myocardium that is salvaged
- PCI
  - —Balloon inflation results in overstretching of the vessel wall and partial disruption of intima, media and adventitia, resulting in enlargement of the lumen and outer diameter of the diseased vessel
  - —Stent placement decreases early and late loss in luminal diameter seen with PTCA
  - —PCI provides greater coronary patency and TIMI III flow then thrombolytics
  - —Lower risk of bleeding then thrombolytics
  - —Immediate knowledge of the extent of disease
  - —Metaanalysis suggests improved survival (4.4% vs. 6.5%) with PCI for ST-segment elevation MI when compared with thrombolytic therapy; however, this may be contingent on operator and institutional expertise
  - —Particularly useful when thrombolytic therapy is contraindicated
  - —PTCA has a 30% restenosis rate in the first 6 months
  - —Stents reduce the restenosis rate to 20%
  - —PCI should be strongly considered within the first 48 hours after a non–ST-segment elevation MI with concomitant use of glycoprotein IIb/IIIa inhibitors
- Glycoprotein IIb/IIIa inhibitors
  - —Antiplatelet agents that bind to the platelet receptor glycoprotein IIb/IIIa and inhibit platelet aggregation
  - —Reduce mortality and reinfarction rate in patients in whom a PCI is planned
  - —Recent data suggest reduced mortality in all patients with unstable angina and non–Q-wave infarction
  - —Not indicated for patients with ST elevation MI, unless also undergoing PCI
- Unfractionated heparin and LMWH are adjuncts in treatment with thrombolytics, glycoprotein IIb/IIIa inhibitors, and PCI
  - —LMWH has been associated with less reocclusion, enhanced late patency, and reduced reinfarction rates when compared with unfractionated heparin

ETIOLOGY

- See Myocardial Infarction and Unstable Angina

Pre-Hospital

- IV access
- Oxygen
- Cardiac monitoring
- Sublingual nitroglycerin for symptom relief

CAUTIONS

- All chest pain should be treated and transported as a possible life-threatening emergency
- Therapy with thrombolytics and glycoprotein IIb/IIIa inhibitors in the field is not currently standard of care

CONTROVERSIES

- Whether to bypass closer EDs in favor of hospitals capable of primary PTCA is controversial
- Local EMS protocols should be followed

Diagnosis

ESSENTIAL WORKUP

- History is critical in assessing the window for use of both thrombolytics and PTCA
- Contraindications to thrombolytic therapy
  - —Active internal bleeding
  - —History of cerebrovascular accident (CVA) in past 6 months
  - —History of a hemorrhagic CVA
  - —Recent (within 2 months) intracranial or intraspinal surgery or trauma
  - —Intracranial neoplasm, arteriovenous malformation, or aneurysm
  - —Known bleeding diathesis
  - —Severe uncontrolled hypertension
  - —Pregnancy
  - —Head trauma within the past month
  - —Trauma or surgery within the last 2 weeks that may result in a closed space bleed
- EKG
  - —Will be normal approximately 50% of the time
  - —Must be compared to prior tracings if available
  - —New ST-segment changes or T-wave inversions are suspicious for unstable angina or non–Q-wave infarct
  - —1-mm depression of the ST segment below the baseline, 80 ms from the J point, is characteristic of unstable angina or non–Q-wave infarct
  - —New left bundle-branch block, or new ST-segment elevation 1 mm in two contiguous limb leads or 2 mm in two contiguous precordial leads suggest Q-wave infarct
- CXR
  - —May be helpful if aortic dissection is being considered
- Heme stool test
  - —Helpful to establish baseline

LABORATORY

- Cardiac enzymes should be elevated and are indicated if the history is suggestive of acute MI
- Baseline creatinine, hematocrit, and coagulation profile are all appropriate in the initial workup

DIFFERENTIAL DIAGNOSIS

- Aortic dissection
- Anxiety
- Biliary colic
- Costochondritis
- Esophageal spasm
- Esophageal reflux
- Herpes zoster
- Hiatal hernia
- Mitral valve prolapse
- MI
- Peptic ulcer disease
- Psychogenic
- Panic disorder
- Pericarditis
- Pneumonia
- Pulmonary embolus

Treatment

INITIAL STABILIZATION

- Place patient on a monitor
- IV access should be obtained
- O_2
- Nitrates

ED TREATMENT

- Aspirin
- β-Adrenergic antagonists, such as metoprolol
- Thrombolytics should be used unless contraindicated and should be used if PCI is not readily available within a 90-minute time frame
- Percutaneous intervention is preferred for both diagnostic and therapeutic options
- PCI and thrombolytic therapy must be used with either unfractionated heparin or an LMWH such as enoxaparin
- LMWH has more predictable kinetics
  —Requires no monitoring
  —Less potential for platelet activation
  —Lower bleeding rate
  —Is at least as effective as unfractionated heparin in the treatment of acute coronary syndromes
- Glycoprotein IIb/IIIa inhibitors

MEDICATIONS

- Aspirin: 160–325 mg PO
- Enoxaparin (Lovenox): 1 mg/kg s.c. q12h
- Glycoprotein IIb/IIIa inhibitors
  —Abciximab (ReoPro) for use before PCI only: 0.25 mg/kg i.v. bolus
  —Eptifibatide (Integrilin): 180 μg/kg i.v. over 1–2 minutes, followed by continuous i.v. infusion of 2 μg/kg/min up to 72 hours
  —Tirofiban (Aggrastat): 0.4 μg/kg/min for 30 minutes, then 0.1 μg/kg/min for 48–108 hours
- Heparin: 80 U/kg i.v. bolus, then 18 U/kg/h
- Metoprolol: 5-mg i.v. bolus and/or 25–50 mg PO
- Thrombolytics
  —APSAC: 30 mg i.v. over 2–5 minutes; patients should also receive methylprednisolone 250 mg i.v.
  —Reteplase (r-tPA): 10 million unit i.v. bolus, and again after 30-minute 10 million unit i.v. bolus; patients should also receive heparin 5,000 IU i.v. bolus then infuse 1,000 IU/h for 48 hours keeping aPTT = 1.5–2.5
  —Streptokinase: 1.5 million unit over 60 minutes; patients should also receive methylprednisolone 250 mg i.v.
  —tPA: 15 mg i.v. bolus, then 0.75 mg/kg (maximum 50 mg) over 30 minutes, then 0.5 mg/kg (maximum 35 mg) over 60 minutes; patients should also receive heparin 5,000 IU i.v. bolus, then infuse 1,000 IU/h for 48 hours keeping aPTT = 1.5–2.5
  —Urokinase: 1.5 IU i.v. over 2 minutes, then 1.5 IU i.v. over next 90 minutes

Disposition

ADMISSION CRITERIA

- All patients being considered for reperfusion therapy should be admitted to a telemetry or ICU setting

DISCHARGE CRITERIA

- No patient being considered for reperfusion therapy should be discharged home from the ED

Miscellaneous

ICD9: N/A

ICD10: N/A

SEE ALSO: ACUTE CORONARY SYNDROME: MYOCARDIAL INFARCTION

SUGGESTED READINGS

Braunwald E, Antman EM, Beasley JW, et al. ACC/AHA guidelines for the management of patients with unstable angina and non-ST-segment elevation myocardial infarction. J Am Coll Cardiol 2000;36:970–1062.

Gibson CM. Primary angioplasty compared with thrombolysis: new issues in the era of glycoprotein IIb/IIIa inhibition and intracoronary stenting. Ann Intern Med 1999;130:841–847.

Lieu TA, Gurley RJ, Lundstrom RJ, et al. Primary angioplasty and thrombolysis for acute myocardial infarction: an evidence based summary. J Am Coll Cadiol 1996;27:737–750.

Ryan TJ, Antman EM, Brooks NH, et al. ACC/AHA practice guidelines for the management of patients with acute myocardial infarction. J Am Coll Cardiol 1996;28:1328–1428. (See also 1999 Web update at *www.acc.org.*)

Schömig H, Kastrati A, Dirschinger J, et al. Coronary stenting plus platelet glycoprotein IIb/IIIa blockade compared with tissue plasminogen activator in acute myocardial infarction. N Engl J Med 2000;343:385–391.

Author: Shamal Grossman

Reperfusion Therapy, Cerebral

Clinical Presentation

SIGNS AND SYMPTOMS

- Dysfunction within a distinct vascular supply territory of the brain warrants consideration for cerebral reperfusion therapy (see Cerebral Vascular Accident)

MECHANISM/DESCRIPTION

- Cerebrovascular accident (CVA) or stroke is a focal interruption of blood supply to the brain
- A transient ischemic attack (TIA) represents symptoms that resolve within 24 hours of onset
- The National Institutes of Health Stroke Scale (NIH-SS) is used to delineate severity of a CVA (by computing the total of subcategory scores, to a maximum of 42) as follows:
  —1a. Level of consciousness (LOC): alert = 0; drowsy = 1; stuporous = 2; coma = 3
  —1b. LOC questions: answers both correctly = 0; one correct = 1; none correct = 2
  —1c. LOC commands: obeys both correctly = 0; one correct = 1; none correct = 2
  —2. Best gaze: normal = 0; partial gaze palsy = 1; forced deviation = 2
  —3. Visual: no visual loss = 0; partial hemianopia = 1; complete hemianopia = 2; bilateral hemianopia = 3
  —4. Facial palsy: normal, symmetric = 0; minor paralysis = 1; partial paralysis = 2; complete paralysis = 3
  —5–8. Best motor (computed for each arm and leg): no drift = 0; drift = 1; some effort against gravity = 2; no effort against gravity = 3; no movement = 4; untestable (e.g., amputation or joint fusion) = 9
  —9. Limb ataxia: absent = 0; present in one limb = 1; present in two limbs = 2
  —10. Sensory (pinprick): normal = 0; partial loss = 1; dense loss = 2
  —11. Best language: no aphasia = 0; mild to moderate aphasia = 1; severe aphasia = 2; mute = 3
  —12. Dysarthria: normal articulation = 0; mild to moderate dysarthria = 1; unintelligible = 2
  —13. Neglect/inattention: no neglect = 0; partial neglect = 1; complete neglect = 2
- Cerebral reperfusion therapy is the use of a thrombolytic agent to effect rapid dissolution of an acute cerebral intravascular occlusion

ETIOLOGY

- Ischemic CVAs are caused by occlusion of a cerebral artery, primarily from thrombotic or embolic events

Pre-Hospital

CAUTIONS

- Assessment in the field for focal neurologic deficits such as facial palsy, motor weakness, or aphasia can quickly ascertain the possibility of a CVA, allowing prearrival mobilization of ED and hospital resources
- Blood glucose testing should be performed
  —Hypoglycemia can cause focal neurologic symptoms that mimic a CVA
  —Hyperglycemia may exacerbate the injury caused by cerebral ischemia
  —Glucose-containing IV fluids should be used with caution

Diagnosis

ESSENTIAL WORKUP

- Stat bedside blood glucose testing
- Immediate noncontrast head CT scan
  —To differentiate between ischemic and hemorrhagic CVA
  —May be normal in the first 24 hours (and especially first 3 hours) of an ischemic CVA
- EKG to assess for dysrhythmia, pericarditis, or myocardial infarction

LABORATORY

- CBC, serum electrolytes and glucose, PT/PTT
- Urine pregnancy test
- Urine toxicology screen

IMAGING/SPECIAL TESTS

- CXR
- Carotid US
- MRI (can detect ischemic CVA <2 hours after onset)
- Cerebral angiography

DIFFERENTIAL DIAGNOSIS

- Intracranial bleed
- Seizure
- Complex migraine
- Bell's palsy, or other focal neuropathies
- Hypoglycemia
- Dural sinus thrombosis
- Intracranial neoplasm
- Intracranial trauma
- Meningitis, encephalitis, or brain abscess
- Vasculitis
- Air embolism or decompression illness
- Spinal cord lesion
- Psychogenic

Treatment

INITIAL STABILIZATION

- Supplemental oxygen to correct hypoxia
- IV access
- Cardiac monitoring and pulse oximetry
- Naloxone, thiamine, and glucose (if hypoglycemic) for altered mental status
- Rapid-sequence intubation if airway protection is warranted

ED TREATMENT

- Exclude other diagnoses in the differential, especially aortic dissection and intracranial hemorrhage (ICH)
- Determine whether the patient meets *inclusion* criteria for IV thrombolytic therapy
  - —Age 18 years or older
  - —Clearly defined onset of symptoms within 3 hours
  - —Noncontrast head CT without evidence of hemorrhage
- Ensure that the patient does not have an *absolute contraindication* to IV thrombolytic therapy
  - —ICH on pretreatment head CT scan
  - —Prior ICH
  - —Clinical presentation consistent with SAH
  - —Known arteriovenous malformation or aneurysm
  - —CVA, serious brain injury, or intracranial surgery within previous 3 months
  - —Active internal bleeding
  - —Major surgery within previous 14 days
  - —Pregnancy
  - —Pericarditis
  - —Known bleeding diathesis: platelet count $<100{,}000/mm^3$; INR >1.7; PT >15 seconds; prolonged PTT; current anticoagulant use; use of heparin within 48 hours
  - —SBP >185 mm Hg
  - —DBP >115 mm Hg
- *Relative contraindications* to IV thrombolytic therapy
  - —Rapid improvement of neurologic symptoms
  - —Mild CVA
  - —GI or GU tract bleeding with 21 days
  - —Recent LP
  - —Recent arterial puncture at a noncompressible site
  - —Seizure at the time stroke was observed
  - —Blood glucose level <50 or >400 mg/dL
- Intraarterial thrombolysis may be considered for patients presenting within 6 hours of symptom onset
- Pretreat BP >185/110 mm Hg with nitroglycerin paste or one to two doses of labetalol; avoid thrombolytic therapy if BP cannot be reduced
- Administer IV tissue plasminogen activator (tPA)
- Avoid antiplatelet agents and anticoagulants for 24 hours after tPA administration
- Monitor arterial BP during the first 24 hours after treatment with tPA
  - —Keep BP <180/105 mm Hg using medication such as labetalol
  - —Nitroprusside for hypertension unresponsive to labetalol or for DBP >140 mm Hg
- Monitor for signs of ICH (a 6% risk with tPA, primarily in patients with a NIH-SS score >20)
- If ICH suspected, obtain emergent head CT to confirm diagnosis; if present, treat as follows:
  - —Discontinue tPA
  - —Obtain blood samples for PT, PTT, platelet count, fibrinogen level
  - —Prepare cryoprecipitate, fibrinogen, and platelets, and infuse as needed
  - —Obtain neurosurgical consultation

MEDICATIONS

- Cryoprecipitate and fibrinogen: 6–8 units
- Labetalol: 10 mg i.v. over 1–2 minutes; repeat or double dose q10min up to a maximum of 150 mg
- Nitroprusside: 0.5–1.0 μg/kg/min, continuous i.v. drip
- Platelets: 6–8 units
- tPA: 0.9 mg/kg i.v., max 90 mg; give 10% of dose as a bolus and infuse remainder over subsequent 60 minutes

Disposition

ADMISSION CRITERIA

- All patients given thrombolytic therapy for a CVA should be admitted to an ICU setting for frequent neurologic checks and vital sign assessments

DISCHARGE CRITERIA

N/A

Miscellaneous

ICD9: N/A

ICD10: N/A

SEE ALSO: CEREBROVASCULAR ACCIDENT

SUGGESTED READINGS

Albers GW. Advances in intravenous thrombolytic therapy for treatment of acute stroke. Neurology 2001;57(S2): S77–S81.

Kothari R, Barsan WG. Stroke. In: Marx JA, et al, eds. Rosen's emergency medicine, clinical concepts & practice, 5th ed. St. Louis: Mosby, 2002:1433–1445.

Lewandowski C, Barsan WG. Treatment of acute ischemic stroke. Ann Emerg Med 2001;37:202–216.

NINDS rt-PA Stroke Study Group. Tissue plasminogen activator for acute ischemic stroke. N Engl J Med 1995;333:1581–1587.

NINDS rt-PA Stroke Study Group. Intracerebral hemorrhage after intravenous t-PA therapy for ischemic stroke. Stroke 1997;28:2109–2118.

Saver JL. Intra-arterial thrombolysis. Neurology 2001;57(S2):S58–S60.

Author: Kama Z. Guluma

Respiratory Distress

Clinical Presentation

SIGNS AND SYMPTOMS

- Tachypnea
- Dyspnea
- Tachycardia
- Anxiety
- Diaphoresis
- Cough ("barking," productive)
- Stridor
- Hoarse voice
- Difficulty swallowing or handling oral secretions
- Upper airway rhonchi (wheezes)
- Lower airway crackles (rales)
- Increased work of breathing
- Accessory and intercostal muscle use
- Hypoxemia
- Hypocapnia or hypercapnia if severe
- Respiratory acidosis
- Cyanosis
- Lethargy, then obtundation

ETIOLOGY

- Upper airway obstruction
  —Epiglottitis
  —Croup syndromes
  —Laryngotracheobronchitis
  —Foreign body
  —Angioedema
  —Retropharyngeal abscess
- Cardiovascular
  —Pulmonary edema/CHF
  —Dysrhythmias
  —Cardiac ischemia
  —Pulmonary embolus
  —Pericarditis
  —Tamponade
- Pulmonary
  —Asthma
  —COPD/emphysema
  —Pneumonia
  —Bronchiolitis
  —Aspiration
  —Adult respiratory distress syndrome (ARDS)
  —Pulmonary edema
  —Pneumothorax
  —Pleural effusion
  —Toxic inhalation injury
- Neuromuscular
  —Guillain-Barré syndrome
  —Myasthenia gravis
- Metabolic/systemic/toxic
- Anaphylaxis
- Anemia
- Acidosis
- Hyperthyroidism
- Sepsis
- Salicylate intoxication
- Drug overdose
- Amphetamines
- Cocaine
- Sympathomimetic
- Obesity
- Psychogenic
  —Anxiety disorder
  —Hyperventilation syndrome

PEDIATRIC CONSIDERATIONS

- Respiratory failure is most common cause of cardiac arrest in infants
- Croup syndromes include
  —Viral
  —Spasmodic
  —Bacterial
  —Congenital defects
  —Noninflammatory causes (foreign body, gastroesophageal reflux, trauma, tumors)
- Most common cause of upper airway obstruction
  —Younger than 6 months: congenital laryngomalacia
  —Older than 6 months: viral croup
- Epiglottitis
  —Highest incidence at ages 2–4 years
  —Abrupt onset
  —Fever
  —Respiratory distress and stridor
  —Difficulty swallowing oral secretions
  —Restlessness and anxiety

Pre-Hospital

CAUTIONS

- Assume a position of comfort for patient
- 100% oxygen
  —Assisted ventilation if obtunded
- Airway adjunct devices (oral or nasal) to maintain patency if tolerated
- Intubation for severe respiratory distress
- Needle aspiration of suspected tension pneumothorax

Diagnosis

ESSENTIAL WORKUP

- Pulse oximetry
- Cardiac and BP monitoring
- Thorough history
  - —Previous history of asthma, COPD, cardiac disease, or dysrhythmia, CHF; foreign body aspiration
  - —Recent fever or upper respiratory tract infection, cough, sputum production, sore throat, systemic disease, anxiety disorder
- Physical examination
  - —Observe: mental status, level of distress, work of breathing, jugular venous pressure, skin color
  - —Feel/palpate: distal pulses, heart PMI, chest wall, peripheral edema
  - —Percuss: lungs for dullness or resonance, abdominal distention or hepatomegaly
  - —Auscultate: heart sounds, lung wheezes or crackles, neck for upper airway stridor, abdomen bowel sounds
- EKG if suspected cardiac etiology

LABORATORY

- ABG for severity and acid-base determination
- CBC
- Electrolytes, BUN/Cr, glucose
- Blood, sputum, urine cultures for fever or sepsis
- Urinary output monitoring for CHF
- Toxicology screen or salicylate level if suspected

IMAGING/SPECIAL TESTS

- CXR for
  - —Pneumonia
  - —Pneumothorax
  - —Hyperinflation
  - —Atelectasis
  - —CHF/pulmonary edema
- Spirometry (peak expiratory flow rates) for asthma, COPD
- Neck radiographs to assess epiglottis and soft tissue spaces, foreign body
- Fiberoptic laryngoscopy to assess epiglottis, vocal cords, and pharyngeal space
- Ventilation/perfusion scan for pulmonary embolus
- Bronchoscopy for foreign body in trachea or bronchus
- Pulmonary artery (Swan-Ganz) catheter for severe CHF, ARDS, pulmonary edema

DIFFERENTIAL DIAGNOSIS

See etiology

PEDIATRIC CONSIDERATIONS

- Evaluate retractions, behavior, respiratory rate, breath sounds, and color
  - —Weak cry, expiratory grunting, nasal flaring, tachypnea, and tachycardia, retractions, and cyanosis in neonates
- CXR/neck radiograph may show "steeple sign" in croup syndromes
- Chest fluoroscopy may be used to assess inspiratory and expiratory excursions if foreign body is suspected

Treatment

INITIAL STABILIZATION

- ABCs
- Ensure patent airway; bag-valve mask assist or intubate for severe distress or arrest
- IV fluids if hypotensive
- 100% oxygen by face mask
  - —Use cautiously in patients with severe COPD or chronic CO_2 retention
- Monitor BP, heart rate, respirations, pulse oximetry
- ACLS for dysrhythmias or arrest

ED TREATMENT

- Treat underlying etiology as appropriate
- CHF or pulmonary edema
  - —Furosemide
  - —Nitroglycerin
  - —Nitroprusside if hypertensive
  - —Pulmonary artery catheter if severe
- Asthma, bronchiolitis, COPD
  - —Bronchodilators
  - —Steroids
  - —Antibiotics for infection
- ARDS, aspiration, toxic lung injury
  - —Mechanical ventilation as needed
  - —Steroids controversial
- Pneumonia
  - —Antibiotics
- Pneumothorax
  - —Needle thoracostomy if suspected tension pneumothorax
  - —Thoracostomy (see Pneumothorax)
- Pleural effusion
  - —Determine etiology
  - —Diagnostic and symptomatic thoracentesis
- Croup
  - —Cool, misted air or oxygen
  - —Steroids
  - —Racemic epinephrine
  - —Antibiotics for bacterial infection
- Epiglottitis
  - —Immediate airway stabilization with intubation or tracheostomy in OR if possible
  - —Antibiotics for *Haemophilus influenzae*
- Anaphylaxis, angioedema
  - —IV steroids
  - —H_1/H_2-blockers
- Retropharyngeal abscess
  - —Drainage
  - —IV antibiotics
  - —ENT consult
- Cardiac
  - —Treat dysrhythmias or ischemia
  - —Pericardiocentesis for tamponade
  - —NSAIDs or aspirin for pericarditis
- Neuromuscular
  - —Support ventilation
  - —Pyridostigmine bromide or neostigmine for myasthenia gravis
- Metabolic/toxic
  - —Treat underlying cause
- Psychogenic
  - —Anxiolytics

PEDIATRIC CONSIDERATIONS

- Transtracheal jet ventilation if unable to intubate (cricothyrotomy not recommended in children younger than 10 years)
- Bronchiolitis
  - —Bronchodilators
  - —Inhaled ribavirin for RSV
  - —Antibiotics for infection
- Spasmodic croup
  - —Very sensitive to misted air
- Bacterial croup (membranous laryngotracheobronchitis)
  - —Treat *Staphylococcus aureus*

Disposition

ADMISSION CRITERIA

- Continued supplemental oxygen requirement
- Cardiac or hemodynamic instability
  - —Requiring IV therapy or hydration
  - —Requiring close airway observation or repeated treatments
- As required by underlying cause or significant comorbid disease

DISCHARGE CRITERIA

- Correction of underlying disease
- Stable airway
- Acute supplemental oxygen not required

Miscellaneous

ICD9: 786.09

ICD10: R06.0

SEE ALSO: DYSPNEA

SUGGESTED READINGS

Williams SA, Hutson HR, Speals HL. Dyspnea. In: *Emergency medicine: concepts and clinical practice,* 4th ed. St. Louis: Mosby, 1998:1460–1469.

Author: Erik D. Barton

Resuscitation, Neonatal

Clinical Presentation

SIGNS AND SYMPTOMS

(requiring resuscitation 2° neonatal distress)

- Apnea or hypoventilation
- Decreased tone or response to stimuli
- Temperature instability
- Shock
  - —Altered mental status
  - —Respiratory distress/failure
    - -Tachypnea/bradypnea
    - -Grunting
  - —Hemodynamic compromise
    - -Tachycardia
    - -Pallor/cyanosis
    - -Cool extremities
    - -Skin mottled, pale, gray, or cyanotic; delayed capillary refill
    - -Weak peripheral pulses
    - -Hypotension
    - -Bradycardia
- Apgar score, low
  - —*A*ppearance (color)
  - —*P*ulse
  - —*G*rimace (reflex irritability)
  - —*A*ctivity (muscle tone)
  - —*R*espirations
  - —Measured at 1 and 5 minutes

MECHANISM/DESCRIPTION

- 6% of all newborns
  - —60% of premature infants weighing <1,500 g
- High-risk pregnancy
  - —Lack of prenatal care
  - —Premature delivery
  - —Maternal history
    - -Perinatal loss
    - -Previous baby with retardation or malformation
  - —Pregnancy-induced hypertension
  - —Gestational diabetes
  - —Prolonged rupture of membranes
  - —Chorioamnionitis
  - —Abruptio placentae
  - —Placentia previa
  - —Breech or face delivery
  - —Trauma induced
  - —Substance abuse
- Meconium aspiration
  - —Sign of intrauterine distress
  - —Occurs in 10–20% of all deliveries
  - —Meconium aspiration syndrome occurs in about 2–5% of these cases
    - -Mortality rate of 40%
- Fetal risk factors for neonatal distress
  - —Multiple births
  - —Meconium stained fluid
  - —Abnormal presentation
  - —Prematurity
  - —Congenital anomalies

ETIOLOGY

- Immediately after delivery
  - —Prematurity
  - —Respiratory
    - -Meconium aspiration
    - -Perinatal aspiration
  - —Inadequate oxygenation/hypoxia
    - -Hypovolemic
  - —Metabolic
    - -Hypoglycemia
    - -Acidosis
  - —Hypothermia
  - —Infection/sepsis
  - —Congenital anomalies
- Delayed
  - —Infection
  - —Dehydration
  - —Anemia
  - —Trauma
  - —Metabolic disease
    - -Inborn error of metabolism
    - -Electrolyte imbalance
  - —Congenital heart disease

Pre-Hospital

- Neonatal kit should be stocked
- Focus on airway, breathing, circulation
- Problems during transport
  - —Hypothermia
  - —Hypoglycemia
  - —Maintaining the airway
    - -Dislodged ETT is a major cause of morbidity during transport
  - —Reassess patient frequently
  - —Maintain IV access

CAUTIONS

- Bradycardia is often an oxygenation problem
- Sudden deterioration; consider pneumothorax from barotrauma

Diagnosis

ESSENTIAL WORKUP

- Assess airway, breathing and circulation
- Detailed physical exam
- Respiratory assessment
  - —Breath sounds
  - —Retractions or stridor
  - —Work of breathing
- Cardiac assessment
  - —Heart sounds
  - —Murmurs
  - —Peripheral pulses
  - —Liver size
  - —Lower extremity BPs
  - —Skin perfusion

LABORATORY

- Bedside serum blood glucose
- If vigorous resuscitation
  - —ABGs
  - —CBC
  - —Electrolytes
  - —Blood cultures, other cultures as indicated

IMAGING/SPECIAL TEST

- CXR
  - —Significant respiratory distress
  - —Congenital heart disease
- Other workup is based on clinical suspicion
  - —Echocardiography
  - —CT/MRI
  - —Lumbar puncture

DIFFERENTIAL DIAGNOSIS

N/A

Treatment

INITIAL STABILIZATION

- Most infants will respond to simple maneuvers
  - —Maintain euthermia
    - -Dry the infant
    - -Remove wet towels
    - -Place the infant in warmer to maintain body temperature
  - —Positioning
    - -Supine with the neck mildly hyperextended (sniffing position)
    - -A 2.5-cm roll under the shoulders
  - —Suctioning
    - -Use a wall suction device or a bulb syringe
    - -Suction the mouth first then the nose
    - -Avoid deep suctioning to prevent vagally mediated bradycardia or apnea
  - —Tactile stimulation
    - -Absence of adequate respirations
    - -Flick soles of feet or rub the back
- Oxygen
  - —100% oxygen is always used
  - —Oxygen toxicity is not a concern during resuscitation
- Positive pressure ventilation (PPV)
  - —Indications
    - -Apnea
    - -Inadequate respirations to maintain oxygenation
    - -Persistent central cyanosis despite delivery of 100% oxygen
    - -Heart rate <100 beats/min
  - —Ventilations are delivered at a rate of 40–60 breaths/min
    - -The initial breath may require up to 70 cm H_2O pressure, and the pop-off valve may need to be bypassed
    - -If available, pressure manometers should be used
  - —After 15–30 seconds, reevaluate
    - -Heart rate >100 beats/min and spontaneous respirations, discontinue PPV
    - -If the heart rate is between 60 and 100 beats/min and increasing, continue PPV
    - -If the heart rate is between 60 and 100 beats/min and not increasing, check the adequacy of the ventilation
    - -If the heart rate remains <60 beats/min, begin chest compressions
  - —Insertion of an orogastric tube is needed with prolonged ventilation
- Tension pneumothorax due to barotrauma
  - —Insertion of a 23–25-gauge catheter or butterfly
  - —Second intercostal space at the midclavicular line
  - —Connect via a three-way stopcock to a 50-mL syringe
- Endotracheal intubation
  - —Indications
    - -Ineffective bag-valve mask ventilation
    - -Need for prolonged ventilation
    - -Meconium aspiration
    - -Known diaphragmatic hernia
    - -Miller 0 (premature infants) or Miller 1 straight blades may be used
    - -Suggested tube size by weight and gestational age
    - -2.5 mm: <1,000 g; <28 weeks
    - -3.0 mm: 1,000–2,000 g; 28–34 weeks
    - -3.5 mm: 2,000–3,000 g; 34–38 weeks
    - -3.5–4.0 mm: >3,000 g; >38 weeks
- Chest compressions
  - —Indications
    - -Heart rate <60 beats/min or heart rate of 60–80 beats/min that is not rapidly increasing
    - -Compressions are delivered at a rate of 120 times/min
- Access
  - —Umbilical venous catheter is the route of choice
  - —Endotracheal route
  - —Instill medications via a feeding tube with saline flush

ED TREATMENT

- Epinephrine
  - —Heart rate <80 beats/min
  - —Adequate ventilation with 100% oxygen
  - —Chest compressions for a minimum of 30 seconds
- Naloxone
  - —Indicated for respiratory depression related to narcotic administration to the mother
  - —May precipitate withdrawal seizures in an infant of a chronically addicted mother
- Sodium bicarbonate
  - —Prolonged resuscitation or documented metabolic acidosis
- Glucose
  - —Serum glucose <35 mg/dL in a term infant or <25 mg/dL in a premature infant
- Hypovolemia
  - —Volume expanders
  - —NS
  - —Ringer's lactate
  - —5% albumin
  - —O-negative blood cross-matched with the mother's blood
- Dopamine
  - —Prolonged resuscitation with continued evidence of shock
  - —Prematurity
  - —Avoid hypothermia, rapid infusion of fluids, and all hypertonic solutions
- Meconium aspiration
  - —Suctioning of the mouth, oropharynx, and then the nose after delivery of the head
  - —Intubate immediately with thick or particulate meconium before any stimulation
  - —Suction the trachea via the ETT until clear
  - —Reintubation followed by repeat suctioning as needed

MEDICATIONS

- Dextrose: 2–4 mL/kg i.v. 10% solution; give slowly over at least 2 minutes
- Dopamine: begin at 5 μg/kg/min, up to 20 μg/kg/min i.v.
- Epinephrine: 0.1–0.3 mL/kg i.v., ET 1:10,000 solution
- Glucagon: 0.1 mg/kg i.m., s.c., i.v. (useful when no vascular access)
- Naloxone: 0.1 mg/kg i.v., ET
- Sodium bicarbonate: 1–2 mEq/kg i.v. 4.2% solution; give slowly over at least 2 minutes
- Volume expanders: 0.9% NS 10 mL/kg bolus

Disposition

ADMISSION CRITERIA

- All neonates requiring resuscitation should be admitted for observation
  - —Neonatal ICU
    - -If more than simple maneuvers
    - -Premature infants for surfactant therapy

DISCHARGE CRITERIA

N/A

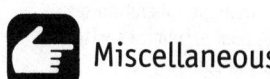

Miscellaneous

ICD9: N/A

ICD10: N/A

SUGGESTED READINGS

Jain L, Vidyasagar D. Controversies in neonatal resuscitation. Pediatr Ann 1995;25:540–545.

Khan NS, Luten RC. Neonatal resuscitation. Emerg Med Clin North Am 1994;12: 239–256.

Kattwinkel J, Niermeyer S, Nadkarni V, et al. ILCOR advisory statement from the pediatric working group of the International Liaison Committee on Resuscitation. Circulation 1999;99: 1927–1938.

Niermeyer S, Van Reempts P, Kattwinkel J, et al. Resuscitation of newborns. Ann Emerg Med 2001;37:S110–S125.

Author: Jeffrey Proudfoot

Clinical Presentation

SIGNS AND SYMPTOMS

- History often nonspecific and obtained from parent/caregiver
- Respiratory failure
  - —Tachypnea
  - —Slow irregular breathing pattern prearrest
  - —Decreased or absent breath sounds; inadequate ventilation
  - —Retractions, accessory muscle use, expiratory grunting, nasal flaring
  - —Mottled skin, cyanosis
  - —Altered level of consciousness (LOC): irritability, agitation, lethargy, weak or absent cry, decreased response to pain
  - —Poor muscle tone
  - —Weak or absent cough or gag reflex
- Early shock (compensated)
  - —Vital signs initially compensated
  - —Orthostatic changes or isolated tachycardia
  - —Slightly delayed capillary refill (>2 seconds)
  - —Warm, dry skin may occur early in septic shock
- Late shock (uncompensated)
  - —Tachycardia, tachypnea, prearrest bradycardia
  - —Hypotension, weak peripheral pulses
  - —Mottled, pale, cool extremities with markedly delayed capillary refill
  - —Decreased urine output progressing to anuria
  - —Decreased LOC, seizures, coma
  - —Fever or hypothermia in septic shock
- Cardiopulmonary arrest
  - —Final common pathway of progressive deterioration of respiratory and circulatory function

MECHANISM/DESCRIPTION

- Respiratory and/or circulatory failure leads to tissue hypoxia, acidosis, and cell death
- Multisystem organ failure subsequently develops

ETIOLOGY

- Respiratory
  - —Upper airway obstruction: croup, epiglottitis, peritonsillar or retropharyngeal abscess, foreign body, tracheitis, congenital anomalies
  - —Lower airway obstruction: asthma, pneumonia, bronchiolitis, foreign body, cystic fibrosis
  - —Thoracic trauma, near drowning
- Hypovolemia: trauma, diarrhea/vomiting, burns
- Cardiovascular: congenital/acquired heart disease, myocarditis, pericarditis, CHF, dysrhythmias
- Infectious: sepsis, meningitis, gastroenteritis, peritonitis
- CNS: status epilepticus, epidural/subdural hematoma
- Metabolic: DKA, hypoglycemia, hypernatremia, hypo/hyperkalemia, acidosis
- Toxicologic: CO poisoning, cardiotoxic agents
- Near sudden infant death syndrome (SIDS)/apparent life-threatening event (ALTE)

Pre-Hospital

- Priority is to stabilize ABCs; monitor
- Avoid prolonged on scene times; rapid transport of critically ill child is crucial
- Recognize respiratory or circulatory failure; intervene early
- Recognize impending arrest and provide life-sustaining procedures during transport
- Timely notification of ED to allow proper preparation
- Gather history from family/bystanders about preceding events, past medical history, medications, allergies

Diagnosis

ESSENTIAL WORKUP

- Airway assessment
  - —Look, listen, feel for air exchange and ventilation; observe for stridor, signs of obstruction
- Breathing assessment
  - —Respiratory rate: tachypnea or slow/irregular pattern (more ominous)
  - —Observe for grunting, nasal flaring, head bobbing, retractions, abdominal distention, chest expansion
  - —Pulse oximetry: reflects hemoglobin oxygen saturation, not necessarily oxygen delivery
  - —Auscultation: assess for wheezing, rales, diminished breath sounds
- Circulation assessment
  - —Pulse: tachycardia or bradycardia (more ominous); orthostatic changes noted early
  - —BP: typical SBP in children = 90 mm Hg + (age in years × 2) mm Hg; hypotension is a late finding, widened pulse pressure in early septic shock
  - —Peripheral pulse presence and strength (brachial/femoral [<1 year] or carotid [>1 year])
  - —Capillary refill: delayed >2 seconds with poor perfusion
  - —Skin: mottled, pale, or cyanotic with poor perfusion
- Mental status assessment
  - —Observe for signs of decreased CNS perfusion: decreased responsiveness, irritability, confusion, agitation, poor muscle tone, sluggish pupillary response, posturing
- Complete set of vital signs including rectal temperature, oximetry, and orthostatics when appropriate
- History from caregivers/parents of onset, progression, inciting, contributing or predisposing trauma/exposure/conditions, associated findings, past medical history, family history, medications, ingestions
- History of preceding events from pre-hospital personnel

LABORATORY

- Workup directed by history, assessment of ABCs, and likely etiologies
- ABG with oximetry to assess oxygenation, ventilation, acid-base status
- Glucose, electrolytes; do bedside glucose
- Other metabolic and toxicology studies as indicated
- Sepsis evaluation including lumbar puncture, urine and blood cultures as indicated

IMAGING/SPECIAL TESTS

- CXR to evaluate pulmonary or cardiac etiologies
- Lateral decubitus or inspiratory/expiratory film or laryngoscopy/bronchoscopy for suspicion of foreign body
- EKG
- Echocardiogram
- Cervical spine films and other trauma studies as indicated
- CT scan of head for neurologic findings

DIFFERENTIAL DIAGNOSIS

- Cardiopulmonary failure in children is usually the result of primary respiratory failure but is the potential end point of all untreated or unresponsive critical illness
- Consider poisoning with acute onset of symptoms, CNS findings, toxidromes, or known exposure
- Consider child abuse when history is inconsistent with the illness or pattern of injury

Treatment

INITIAL STABILIZATION

- Early recognition and stabilization of respiratory failure or shock
- Diagnose and treat immediately life-threatening conditions simultaneously
- Empirical intervention as required
- ABCDE evaluation
  - —Airway: assess patient ability to speak/cry, listen for stridor, observe for trauma
  - —Breathing: observe for tracheal deviation, signs of chest injury or pneumothorax, observe chest excursion, auscultate, apply oxygen
  - —Circulation: evaluate pulses, heart rate, BP, capillary refill
  - —Disability: determine mental status and assess for neurologic deficits; check stat glucose
  - —Exposure/environment: fully expose for rapid skeletal survey while preventing hypothermia
  - —Obtain pertinent history from EMS or family

ED TREATMENT

- Airway
  - —Secure for every resuscitation
  - —Open airway with head tilt, chin lift, or modified jaw thrust (if trauma suspected)
  - —Clear secretions, blood, foreign body with suction
  - —Temporary stabilization with oropharyngeal or nasopharyngeal airway, bag-valve mask assistance; properly performed bag-mask ventilation is effective, particularly when used for short duration
  - —Intubation as necessary using appropriate tube size ([16 + age in years]/4)
  - —Use adjunctive devices, as applicable
  - —Post-intubation: confirm tube placement with colorimetric CO_2 device, continuous $ETCO_2$ monitoring, auscultation, aspiration device
- Rapid-sequence intubation: preoxygenation, pretreatment, paralysis with induction cricoid pressure, intubation, confirmation of placement, post-intubation monitoring
  - —Premedications: atropine to prevent bradycardia, lidocaine following head injury
  - —Induction agents: midazolam, thiopental, etomidate, ketamine
  - —Paralytics: succinylcholine, pancuronium, vecuronium, rocuronium
- Breathing
  - —Oxygenate with supplemental O_2, non-rebreather mask; assist ventilation with bag-valve-mask or control ventilation if intubation performed
  - —Treat conditions that limit ability to oxygenate/ventilate: pneumothorax, hemothorax, cardiac tamponade, circumferential burns
- Circulation
  - —Obtain intravascular access: IV, intraosseous, central access
  - —Fluid resuscitate with crystalloid (NS or lactated Ringer's solution) bolus at 10–20 mL/kg and repeat if necessary; correct hypovolemia
  - —Control obvious sources of bleeding: apply direct pressure, elevate
  - —Consider transfusion of packed RBCs after crystalloid replacement in trauma
  - —Consider vasopressors in decompensated shock: epinephrine, dopamine, norepinephrine
  - —Consider inotropes in compensated shock: dobutamine, milrinone
- Cardiopulmonary resuscitation (CPR)
  - —Provide blood flow to vital organs while restoring spontaneous circulation
  - —Infant younger than 1 year: check for pulse at brachial or femoral artery
  - —Child 1–8 years: check for pulse at carotid artery
- Cardiac dysrhythmias
  - —Usually secondary to respiratory insufficiency or metabolic disturbance
  - —Treat rhythm disturbance as per published algorithms
  - —Unstable tachydysrhythmia may require adenosine, lidocaine, amiodarone, cardioversion or defibrillation
  - —Unstable bradydysrhythmia may require atropine, epinephrine, or pacing
  - —Pulseless rhythms: ventricular fibrillation, pulseless ventricular tachycardia, pulseless electrical activity (PEA), asystole; may require epinephrine, defibrillation, lidocaine
- Continuously monitor patient

MEDICATIONS

First or loading dose

- Adenosine: 0.1 mg/kg
- Amiodarone: 5 mg/kg i.v. rapid
- Atropine: 0.02 mg/kg i.v. minimum 0.1 mg
- Calcium chloride: 20 mg/kg i.v.
- Cardioversion: 0.5 J/kg
- Defibrillation: 2 J/kg initial, then 4 J/kg
- Epinephrine: 0.01 mg/kg i.v. (0.1 mL/kg 1:10,000 i.v.) (first dose); 0.1 mg/kg i.v. (0.1 mL/kg 1:1,000 i.v.) (subsequent or ETT doses) (note: higher dose [0.1–0.2 mg/kg i.v.] may be considered for unresponsive asystolic/pulseless arrest)
- Etomidate: 0.3 mg/kg i.v.
- Ketamine: 1–2 mg/kg i.v.
- Lidocaine: 1–1.5 mg/kg i.v.
- Midazolam: 0.1 mg/kg i.v.
- Naloxone: 0.1 mg/kg i.v.
- Pancuronium: 0.1 mg/kg i.v.
- Rocuronium: 0.6–1.2 mg/kg i.v.
- Sodium bicarbonate: 1 mEq/kg i.v.
- Succinylcholine: 1–1.5 mg/kg i.v.
- Vecuronium: 0.1–0.3 mg/kg i.v.

Disposition

ADMISSION CRITERIA

- All patients with impending or existent respiratory or cardiovascular compromise
- All patients requiring resuscitation
- Survivors of cardiopulmonary arrest require an ICU equipped to manage critically ill children
  - —Continually monitor patients for any signs of decompensation after resuscitation
  - —Consider transferring patient if the child's acuity exceeds hospital capabilities
- Consultation as appropriate depending on specific pathophysiology

DISCHARGE CRITERIA

N/A

Miscellaneous

ICD9: N/A

ICD10: N/A

SUGGESTED READINGS

American Heart Association, Emergency Cardiac Care Committee. guidelines for cardiopulmonary resuscitation and emergency cardiac care, part VI. Pediatric advanced life support. JAMA 1992;268(16):2262–2275.

Bardella IJ. Pediatric advanced life support: a review of the AHA recommendations. American Heart Association. Am Fam Physician 1999;60(6):1743–1750.

Patterson MD. Resuscitation update for the pediatrician. Pediatr Clin North Am 1999;46(6):1285–1303.

Wright JL, Patterson MD. Resuscitating the pediatric patient. Emerg Med Clin North Am 1996;14(1):219–231.

Zaritsky AL, Nadkarn VH, Berg RA, et al. Pediatric advanced life support. Dallas: American Heart Association, 2002.

Authors: Brian Clyne; H. Peter Beauparlant

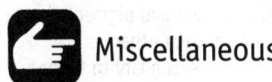

Retinal Detachment

Clinical Presentation

SIGNS AND SYMPTOMS

- Flashes of light
- Floaters
- "Night shade" obscuring visual field
- Peripheral/central vision loss or other visual field defects
- Asymptomatic

MECHANISM/DESCRIPTION

- Three types of retinal detachments
  - —Rhegmatogenous retinal detachments (RRD)
  - —Tractional retinal detachments (TRD)
  - —Exudative retinal detachments (ERD)
- RRD
  - —Most common
  - —Violation of sensory retina allows vitreous to separate the sensory and pigmented parts of retina from each other
  - —Acute event, flashes secondary to tearing of nerve fibers, floaters secondary to bleeding from ruptured retinal vessels
- TRD
  - —Contraction of fibrous vitreous bands pulls the sensory retina off the pigmented retina
  - —Chronic and progressive
  - —Asymptomatic unless hemorrhage or retinal tear occurs
- ERD
  - —Subretinal collections of serous fluid separate retinal layers without violating either layer; affected part of retina changes with head position
  - —Asymptomatic unless macula involved leading to central vision impairment

ETIOLOGY

- RRD
  - —Myopia
  - —Marfan's syndrome
  - —Structural degeneration of underlying anatomy of vitreous body, sensory or pigmented retina
  - —Trauma
- TRD
  - —Proliferative diabetic retinopathy
  - —Vasculopathy
  - —Perforating injury
  - —Chorioretinitis
  - —Retinopathy of prematurity, sickle cell disease or toxocariasis
  - —Trauma
- ERD
  - —Tumors of the choroid or retina (melanoma, retinoblastoma)
  - —Inflammatory disorders (Coates or Harada's disease, posterior scleritis)

Pre-Hospital

N/A

Diagnosis

ESSENTIAL WORKUP

- History
  - —Age
  - —Speed of onset
  - —Associated symptoms
  - —Previous episodes
- Physical
  - —Complete ophthalmologic exam

LABORATORY

- As needed to workup underlying diseases

IMAGING/SPECIAL TESTS

- Visual field testing

DIFFERENTIAL DIAGNOSIS

- Senile retinoschisis
- Juvenile retinoschisis
- Choroidal detachment

Treatment

INITIAL STABILIZATION

N/A

ED TREATMENT

- Bed rest
- Ophthalmologic consultation

Disposition

ADMISSION CRITERIA

- Need for surgical repair

DISCHARGE CRITERIA

- Any retinal detachment seen by an ophthalmologist and deemed safe to go home
- Chronic retinal detachments are repaired over the same time course as it took to create them
- ERD resolves with treatment of the underlying problem

Miscellaneous

ICD9: 361.9

ICD10: H33.2

SUGGESTED READINGS

Albert D, Jakobiec F, Azar D, et al, eds. Principles and practice of ophthalmology, 2nd ed. Philadelphia: WB Saunders, 2000.

Morgan A, Hemphill R. Acute visual change. Emerg Med Clin North Am 1998;16(4):825–843.

Rhee D, Pyfer M, eds. The Wills eye manual office and emergency room diagnosis and treatment of eye disease, 3rd ed. Philadelphia: Lippincott Williams & Wilkins, 1999.

Shingleton B, O'Donoghue M. Blurred vision. N Engl J Med 2000;343(8):556–562.

Whitmore P. Sudden painless visual loss retinal causes. Clin Geriatr Med 1999;15(1):15–23.

Author: David A. Harter

Retropharyngeal Abscess

Clinical Presentation

SIGNS AND SYMPTOMS

- Often preceded by nasopharyngitis or otitis media
- Fever (100%)
- Neck pain
- Torticollis or refusal to move the neck (75%)
  —Aggravated by swallowing
- Muffled voice (if superior to the larynx)
- Dysphagia
- Stridor/drooling (20–40%)
- Cervical adenopathy (100%)
- Pharyngitis (60%)
- Bulging of the posterior pharynx (25%)
- Tenderness moving the trachea and larynx side to side; "tracheal rock"
- Meningismus
- Trismus may or may not be present (usually absent in uncomplicated retropharyngeal abscess)
- Difficult diagnosis in infants
  —Fever
  —Irritability
  —Poor feeding
  —Pain with neck movement
  —Stridor
- Pharynx is erythematous and displaced forward towards the uvula
- Do not palpate the posterior pharynx
  —Spontaneous perforation and aspiration may occur

MECHANISM/DESCRIPTION

- An infection lying between the middle cervical and alar fascia
  —Anterior to the prevertebral fascia, posterior to the pharyngeal mucosa
  —Potential space that extends from the base of the skull to T1-2 in the posterior mediastinum
- Wide spectrum of pathogens
  —Group A *Streptococcus*
  —*Staphylococcus aureus*
  —Anaerobes
  —Acid-fast bacilli
- Primarily a disease of preschool children
  —The posterior pharyngeal nodes regress well before puberty
  —Reported in all age-groups
  —Resurgence of cases in later adulthood
- Complications
  —Septic shock
  —Airway obstruction, asphyxia
  —Mediastinitis
  —Spontaneous perforation
  —Aspiration pneumonia
  —Thrombosis of the internal jugular vein (Lemierre disease)
  —Erosion into the carotid artery
  —Cranial nerve IX, X, or XII palsies
  —Horner's syndrome
- Prognosis with prompt therapy and diagnosis is very good

ETIOLOGY

- Suppurative adenitis of the posterior pharyngeal nodes
- Otitis media
- Sinusitis
- Cervical TB (uncommon)
- Pharyngitis
- Recent upper airway instrumentation
- Upper airway trauma
- Foreign body, especially fish bones
- Pharyngotonsillitis
- Cervical osteomyelitis
- Blunt and penetrating trauma

PEDIATRIC CONSIDERATIONS

- Age 6 months to 4 years
- One half of pediatric cases in children younger than 12 months

Pre-Hospital

CAUTIONS

- The child should be kept calm
- A parent may hold or comfort the child in transport if this is feasible
- Place on pulse oximetry and cardiac monitors
- Provide with supplemental oxygen as needed
- Transport with suction and intubation equipment
- Airway control
  —Before lengthy transports
  —Airway compromise

Diagnosis

ESSENTIAL WORKUP

- Evaluation should occur after the airway is controlled in patients with respiratory compromise
- Determine presence of a fluid collection
- Determine the need for surgical intervention

LABORATORY

- Blood cultures
- CBC
- Throat culture patients with pharyngitis

IMAGING/SPECIAL TESTS

- Soft tissue lateral neck radiographs
  —Taken in inspiration with partial neck extension
  —Crucial in establishing the diagnosis
  —Air fluid level posterior to the pharynx or esophagus
  —Widening of the retropharyngeal space anterior to C2 >7 mm
    -Prevertebral soft tissues that are two times the diameter of vertebral body
  —The retrotracheal space anterior to C6 >14 mm in preschool-aged children or >22 mm in adults
- CXR is used to evaluate for aspiration or mediastinal widening
- Contrasted CT of the neck
  —Delineates the extent of deep space involvement
  —Differentiates abscess formation from cellulitis
  —Detects abnormalities of adjacent vertebra and vasculature

DIFFERENTIAL DIAGNOSIS

- Tonsillopharyngitis
- Epiglottitis
- Tracheitis
- Croup
- Foreign body
- Cervical osteomyelitis
- Epidural abscess
- Retropharyngeal hemorrhage
- Meningitis
- Dystonic reactions
- Other deep space neck infections
- Hematoma
- Osteophyte
- Neoplasm
- Lymphadenopathy

Treatment

INITIAL STABILIZATION

- Standard and surgical airway equipment available
- Patients with significant airway obstruction
- Supplemental oxygen
- Controlled oral intubation or tracheotomy, preferably in an OR
- IV access, but delay to avoid upsetting children when the airway is compromised

ED TREATMENT

- Antibiotics
  —Primarily directed toward gram-positive organisms
  —In selected mild cases, antibiotics alone without surgical drainage may be sufficient
- Patients are made NPO in anticipation of diagnostic or therapeutic intervention
- Surgical consultation
  —Incision and drainage
  —CT-guided aspiration

MEDICATIONS

- Ceftriaxone: 1 g (peds: 50 mg/kg) i.v. *plus*
  —Clindamycin: 600–900 mg (peds: 10 mg/kg) i.v. *or*
  —Ampicillin-sulbactam: 1.5–3.0 g (peds: 50 mg/kg) i.v.
- Penicillin G: 6 million units q6h (50,000 U/kg/d q4–6h) i.v. *plus*
  —Metronidazole: 1 g i.v. load followed by 500 mg i.v. q6h (peds: 7.5 mg/kg/d q6h)

Disposition

ADMISSION CRITERIA

- All patients with retropharyngeal abscess should be admitted with readily available otolaryngologists and anesthesiologists
- Incision and drainage in a controlled setting
- ICU admission
  —Infants and toxic-appearing children
  —Patients with airway compromise
  —Altered mental status
  —Hemodynamic instability
  —Those with evidence of other complications

DISCHARGE CRITERIA

N/A

Miscellaneous

ICD9: 478.24

ICD10: J39.0

SUGGESTED READINGS

Gamage R, Peiris J, Wijegunasinghe D, et al. Retropharyngeal abscess. Arch Neurol 2000;57(10):1521.

Goldenberg D, Golz A, Joachims HZ. Retropharyngeal abscess: a clinical review. J Laryngol Otol 1997;111(6):546–550.

Lalakea M, Messner AH: Retropharyngeal abscess management in children: current practices. Otolaryngol Head Neck Surg 1999;121(4):398–405.

Pontell J, Har-El G, Lucente FE. Retropharyngeal abscess: clinical review. Ear Nose Throat J 1995;74(10):701–704.

Sharma HS, Kurl DN, Hamzah M. Retropharyngeal abscess: recent trends. Auris Nasus Larynx 1998;25(4):403–406.

Author: Lee Shockley

Reye Syndrome

Clinical Presentation

SIGNS AND SYMPTOMS

- Biphasic history marked by an infectious phase (viral illness or prodrome followed by an encephalopathic stage)
- Profuse and repeated vomiting
  - —Typically 4–5 days after the start of the viral illness
- Usually the patient is afebrile
- Tachycardia
- Hyperventilation
- No focal neurologic signs
- Marked behavioral changes, including delirium and combativeness, disorientation and hallucination
- Hepatomegaly in 40% of cases
- Pancreatitis
- Clinical staging of Reye syndrome with Lovejoy's classification
  - —Stage 0
    - -Wakeful
  - —Stage I
    - -Vomiting
    - -Lethargy
    - -Sleepiness
  - —Stage II
    - -Disorientation
    - -Delirium
    - -Combative/stuporous
    - -Hyperventilation
    - -Hyperreflexia
    - -Appropriate response to noxious stimuli
  - —Stage III
    - -Obtunded
    - -Coma
    - -Hyperventilation
    - -Inappropriate response to noxious stimuli
    - -Decorticate posturing
    - -Preservation of pupillary light reflexes
    - -Preservation of oculovestibular light reflexes
  - —Stage IV
    - -Deeper coma
    - -Decerebrate rigidity
    - -Loss of oculovestibular reflexes
    - -Dilated, fixed pupils
    - -Dysconjugate eye movements in response to caloric stimulation
  - —Stage V
    - -Seizures
    - -Absent deep tendon reflexes
    - -Respiratory arrest
    - -Flaccid paralysis
    - -No papillary response
- Infants—atypical presentation
  - —Tachypnea
  - —Apnea
  - —Irritability
  - —Seizures
  - —Hypoglycemia

MECHANISM/DESCRIPTION

- Reversible clinicopathologic syndrome of unknown etiology
- Primary mitochondrial injury
- Decreased enzyme activity
  - —Krebs cycle
  - —Gluconeogenesis
  - —Urea biosynthesis
- Fatty infiltration
  - —Liver
    - -Hyperammonemia due to decreased conversion from ammonia to urea
    - -Hepatorenal syndrome may be the end result
    - -Rapid recovery of liver function in survivors
  - —Brain
    - -Encephalopathy of unclear etiology
    - -Cytotoxic edema
    - -Deteriorating level of consciousness reflects increasing intracranial pressure
    - -Herniation is the most common cause of death
    - -Normal recovery of neurologic function in survivors
  - —Skeletal and myocardial muscle
  - —Fatty infiltration and distorted mitochondria
- Fewer than 10% of cases occurs before the age of 1 year
  - —Average age is 7 years
  - —Peak age is 4–11 years
- Regional differences
  - —Highest incidence in the midwestern states
  - —Lower incidence in the states of the southeast and far west
- More common in whites than in blacks
- Peak incidence is in winter and early spring
- Reye-like syndrome
  - —Describes conditions resulting in defects in urea and fatty acid metabolism, toxicologic injury, and impaired gluconeogenesis

ETIOLOGY

- Not known with certainty
- Multifactorial causes have been epidemiologically implicated
  - —Antecedent viral syndrome
  - —Influenza A or B
  - —Varicella
  - —Diarrhea illness
  - —Genetic predisposition
  - —Exposure to salicylates
  - —Other undefined factors

Pre-Hospital

CAUTIONS

- Decreased mental status
  - —Glucose
  - —Narcan
- Coma
  - —Assist respirations with bag-valve mask

Diagnosis

ESSENTIAL WORKUP

- Establish the presence of encephalopathy and liver abnormalities
- Laboratory testing to assess for characteristic biochemical abnormalities
- Liver biopsy confirms the diagnosis

LABORATORY

- Liver function tests
  - —A threefold or greater rise in AST, ALT
  - —Serum ammonia level greater than 1.5–3 times normal
    - -Transient 24–48 hours after mental status changes
    - -Level >300 μg/dL associated with poor prognosis
  - —Serum bilirubin should be normal or slightly elevated
- Hypoglycemia may be present, especially in infants
- Elevated BUN
- Ketonuria
- The prothrombin time may be prolonged due to decreased liver-dependent clotting factors (II, VII, IX, X)
- Normal platelet count and blood smear
- Negative toxicology screen

IMAGING/SPECIAL TESTS

- Head CT scan
  - —May show diffuse cerebral edema
- Lumbar puncture
  - —Perform after head CT
  - —Edema is diffuse and lumbar puncture is not contraindicated
  - —Measure opening pressure
  - —Less than 8 leukocytes/mm^3
- Percutaneous liver biopsy
  - —Useful in patients with atypical presentation (1 year old, recurrent, familial)
  - —Gastroenterology consult

DIFFERENTIAL DIAGNOSIS

- Inborn errors of metabolism
  - —Disorders of the urea cycle
  - —Disorders of fatty acid oxidation
  - —Systemic carnitine deficiency
  - —Organic acidemias
  - —Disorders of the electron transport chain
- Hypoglycemia
- Toxin exposure
  - —Toxic encephalopathy without liver dysfunction (Gall's syndrome)
  - —Lead
  - —Hydrocarbons
- Drug intoxication
  - —Acetaminophen
  - —Salicylates
  - —Ethanol
- Infection
  - —Sepsis
  - —Meningitis
  - —Encephalitis
  - —Varicella hepatitis
- Trauma, head

Treatment

INITIAL STABILIZATION

- Place on a cardiorespiratory monitor
- Supplemental oxygen
- Rapid-sequence intubation if airway management required
- Glucose if there is altered mental status
  - —10% glucose solution intravenously
  - —Rate of two-thirds maintenance requirement after dehydration corrected
  - —Follow serum glucose hourly; maintain glucose between 125–175 mg/dL
- Avoid early overhydration

ED TREATMENT

- Institute treatment before the liver biopsy
- Vitamin K
  - —Indicated if there is an elevated prothrombin time
- Fresh-frozen plasma
  - —To control bleeding
  - —To correct a severe coagulopathy
- Interventions aimed at lowering intracranial pressure (ICP)
  - —Stage III or greater
  - —Stage II with serum ammonia >300 μg/L
    - -Intubation using rapid-sequence protocol
    - -Hyperventilation
    - -Fluid restriction
    - -Barbiturate coma
    - -Osmotically active agents
      - *Mannitol
    - -Furosemide
    - -Monitor ICP
      - *Subarachnoid bolt
      - *Intraventricular cannula

MEDICATIONS

- D50W: 1–2 mL/kg/dose (0.5–1.0 g/kg) i.v. over the age of 3 years
- D25W: 2–4 mL/kg/dose (0.5–1.0 mg/kg) i.v. under the age of 3 years; maintenance infusion 10% dextrose solution at a rate of 2/3
- Fresh-frozen plasma: 10 mL/kg/dose q12–24h i.v. or p.r.n.
- Lasix: 1 mg/kg i.v.
- Mannitol: 0.25–1.0 g/kg i.v. q4–6h
- Vitamin K: 1–2 mg/dose (infants and children); 2–10 mg/dose (adolescents)
- Pentobarbital: 3–20 mg/kg i.v. slowly while monitoring BP; maintenance infusion 1–2 mg/kg/h; maintain level at 25–40 μg/dL

Disposition

ADMISSION CRITERIA

- All children with suspected Reye syndrome should be admitted to the ICU
- Hospital capable of ICP monitoring

DISCHARGE CRITERIA

N/A

Miscellaneous

ICD9: 331.81

ICD10: G93.7

SUGGESTED READINGS

Belay ED, Bresee JS, Holman RC, et al. Reye's syndrome in the United States from 1981 through 1997. N Engl J Med 1999; 340:1377–1382.

Boenning DA. Reye syndrome. In: Barkin RM, ed. Pediatric emergency medicine, 2nd ed. St. Louis: Mosby-Year Book, 1997: 845–847.

Kaufman RE. Reye's syndrome and salicylate use. By Starko KM, et al, Pediatrics, 1980;66:849–864.

National Institutes of Health Consensus Conference. Diagnosis and treatment of Reye's syndrome. JAMA 1981;246: 2441–2444.

National Patterns of aspirin use and Reye's Syndrome reporting. United States, 1980 to 1985 by Janet B. Arrowsmith, et al, Pediatrics, 1987;79:858–863. Pediatrics, 1998;102:259–262.

Author: Brian Euerle

Rhabdomyolysis

Clinical Presentation

SIGNS AND SYMPTOMS

- Can vary dramatically, reflect underlying disease process
- Obvious crushing injury
- Hypothermia/hyperthermia
- Alert/obtunded
- Muscle pain (only 50%), tenderness, swelling
- Hypovolemic state, dry mucous membrane, poor skin turgor, tachycardia, hypotension
- Decreased urine output
- Change in urine color

MECHANISM/DESCRIPTION

- Syndrome associated with muscle injury and systemic release of its content (CPK)
- Combination of myoglobinuria, hypovolemia, and aciduria lead to acute renal failure
- Direct release of potassium from damaged muscle tissue may lead to dysrhythmias and sudden death

ETIOLOGY

- Muscle injury due to trauma, exercise, seizure, burn, electrical shock
- Hypothermia, hyperthermia
- Prolonged immobile state
- Drugs/toxins (alcohols, cocaine, amphetamines, ecstasy, opiates, antihistamines, barbiturates, PCP, caffeine, carbon monoxide, cholesterol-lowering agents, propofol, succinylcholine, INH, zidovudine, snake venom, bee/hornet venom, etc.)
- Neuroleptic malignant syndrome
- Metabolic disorder (hypokalemia, hypophosphatemia, hyperthyroid state, DKA, hyperosmolar state, hypoxia)
- Infections (viral, bacterial, parasitic, protozoan, rickettsial)
- Genetic disorders (McArdle disease, Tarui disease)
- Immunologic disorders (dermatomyositis, polymyositis)
- Idiopathic

Pre-Hospital

- Need for rapid extrication in case of crush injury
- *Early IV fluids* to prevent complications of restored blood flow to injured limb (hypovolemia, acute renal failure [ARF], hyperkalemia, etc.)

Diagnosis

ESSENTIAL WORKUP

- History and physical are insensitive in making the diagnosis
- Serum CPK level is criterion standard and must be sent if any clinical suspicion exists
- Urine dipstick test positive for heme but absent for RBCs suggests rhabdomyolysis
  - —Because of rapid urinary excretion of myoglobin, up to 26% of patients with rhabdomyolysis have negative urine dipstick test
- Serum electrolytes (potassium, calcium, magnesium, phosphorus, bun, creatinine, uric acid)

LABORATORY

- ABG
- Urine/serum myoglobin is too transient to be useful
- Serum glucose, LDH, SGOT, albumin, toxicology screen in absence of physical injury
- PT/PTT, platelet count, fibrinogen, fibrin-split products if DIC is suspected

IMAGING/SPECIAL TESTS

- MRI is 90–95% sensitive in visualizing muscle injury but does not change initial ED treatment

DIFFERENTIAL DIAGNOSIS

- The following conditions may present with elevated serum CPK but may not lead to complications of rhabdomyolysis
  - —Nontraumatic myopathies
  - —Renal failure
  - —Intramuscular injections
  - —Myocardial injury
  - —Hypothyroidism
  - —Hyperthyroidism
  - —Stroke
  - —Surgery

Treatment

INITIAL STABILIZATION

- ABCs
- Immobilization of trauma/crush injuries
- IV fluids for hypotension and hypovolemia

ED TREATMENT

- Directed toward treating or reversing the cause of rhabdomyolysis
- *Prevent ARF:* IV fluid, mannitol, furosemide (keep urine output >30 cc/hr)
- *Hyperkalemia:* IV fluid, dextrose, insulin, Kayexalate, calcium gluconate, monitor/EKG
- *Acidosis:* bicarbonate IV (keep urine pH >6.5)
- *Overdose:* activated charcoal, lavage, antidote
- *Infection:* broad-spectrum antibiotics
- *Compartment syndrome:* fasciotomy (compartment pressure >35 mm Hg)
- *Neuroleptic malignant syndrome:* dantrolene, bromocriptine
- *Need for hemodialysis:* refractory to treatment, hyperkalemia, hyperphosphatemia, hyperuricemia, volume overload, overdose

MEDICATIONS

- Bicarbonate: 50–100 mL of 8.4% solution i.v. (peds: 1 mEq/kg up to 50–100 mEq)
- Furosemide: 20 mg bolus (peds: 1 mg/kg/dose) i.v.

Disposition

ADMISSION CRITERIA

- *Because it is impossible to predict which patients will develop complications, all patients with significant elevated CPK or with symptoms suggestive of rhabdomyolysis must be admitted*
- Admit to monitored bed for patients with electrolyte abnormalities
- Admit to ICU bed for patients who might require hemodialysis or closer fluid and electrolyte monitoring

DISCHARGE CRITERIA

- No patients suspected of having rhabdomyolysis should be discharged from the ED

Miscellaneous

ICD9: 728.89

SUGGESTED READINGS

Cheney P. Early management and physiologic changes in crush syndrome. Crit Care Nurs Q 1994;17(2):62–73.

Pina EM, Mehlman CT. Rhabdomyolysis—a primer for the orthopaedist. Orthop Rev 1994;23(1):28–32.

Prendergast BD, George CF. Drug-induced rhabdomyolysis—mechanisms and management Postgrad Med J 1993;69(811): 333–336.

Sinert R, Kohl L, Rainone T, et al. Exercise-induced rhabdomyolysis. Ann Emerg Med 1994;23(6):1301–1306.

Vanholder, Sever, Erek, et al. Rhabdomyolysis. J Am Soc Nephrol 2000;11(8):1553–1561.

Viswswaran, Jayarama. Rhabdomyolysis. Crit Care Clin 1999;15(2):415–428.

Zager RA. Rhabdomyolysis and myohemoglobinuric acute renal failure [Editorial Review]. Kidney Int 1996;49(2): 314–326.

Author: Marcelo Sandoval

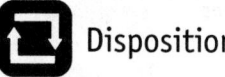

Rheumatic Fever

Clinical Presentation

SIGNS AND SYMPTOMS

- Acute rheumatic fever (ARF) is a clinical diagnosis using the Jones criteria; peak age is 5–15 years
- Two major manifestations *or* one major and two minor manifestations are needed *plus* laboratory evidence of recent group A streptococcal (GAS) pharyngitis
- Other GAS infections do not cause ARF
- Symptoms begin a few weeks after streptococcal pharyngitis
  - —One third of patients are unaware of preceding pharyngitis
- In adults, ARF may present with joint symptoms alone
- In children, the full spectrum of disease—rash, chorea, arthritis, carditis, and fever is more likely
- Spontaneous resolution of ARF within 3 months is the rule, although carditis/valvulitis may persist

Major Manifestations (Jones Criteria)

- *Migratory polyarthritis* in 60–75% of initial attacks
  - —Can involve knees, ankles, elbows, and wrists
  - —Lower extremities joints more commonly involved
  - —Rheumatic arthritis generally responds to salicylates
- *Carditis* occurs in one third of new cases; prednisone used in severe cases
  - —Pericardium, myocardium, and endocardium may be affected (pancarditis)
  - —Myocarditis may lead to heart failure but is frequently asymptomatic
  - —Valvular disease and endocarditis are most serious sequelae of ARF
  - —Carditis heralded by a new murmur, tachycardia, gallop rhythm, pericardial friction rub, or CHF
- *Chorea* occurs in 10% of cases
  - —Sydenham's chorea predominantly affects teenage girls
  - —Purposeless uncoordinated movements of the extremities
  - —Movements more apparent during periods of anxiety and disappear with sleep
  - —Chorea may be the sole manifestation of ARF
- *Erythema marginatum* occurs in <5% of cases
  - —Nonpruritic pink eruptions with central clearing and well-demarcated irregular borders
  - —Usually seen on the trunk and the extremities
- *Subcutaneous nodules* in 10% of patients
  - —Crops of small subcutaneous painless nodules located most commonly on extensor surfaces

Minor Manifestations

- Clinical
  - —Fever (>38°C)
  - —Arthralgia
- Laboratory
  - —Elevated acute-phase reactants
  - —Prolonged PR interval

Supporting Evidence of Recent GAS Throat Infection

- Positive throat culture or rapid antigen test
- Elevated or increasing antibody test—antistreptolysin-O (ASO) titer

ETIOLOGY

- Possible genetic predisposition
- Patients with prior ARF at greater risk for recurrence
- GAS antigens thought to be immunologically cross-reactive with antigens in human tissue
  - —The magnitude of the immune response strongly correlated with the attack rate of rheumatic fever following streptococcal pharyngitis
- Risk factors associated with ARF are the same for streptococcal pharyngitis, including overcrowding, age, dampness, and socioeconomic status
- ARF is rare in the U.S. and remains common in the developing world.

PEDIATRIC CONSIDERATIONS

- In children, cardiac involvement is usually a dominant feature and occurs early
- Chorea is a late finding and is not seen in conjunction with carditis

Pre-Hospital

- Patients with significant CHF may require early airway management

Diagnosis

- The Jones criteria revised in 1992 used for diagnosis of ARF (as described earlier)

ESSENTIAL WORKUP

- CXR
- EKG
- Throat culture
- ASO titer
- Erythrocyte sedimentation rate (ESR) or C-reactive protein
- CBC

LABORATORY

- Rapid antigen test, if positive, but send throat culture if negative
  - —90% of time, throat culture is negative when symptoms develop
- ASO greater than 250 Todd units, though may normally be found up to 300 in healthy school-aged children in crowded urban environments
- Increased PR interval suggests diagnosis
- Approximately 50% of patients will have mild proteinuria or casts in their urine

IMAGING/SPECIAL TESTS

- Echocardiogram may reveal pericardial effusion, valvular disease, or cardiomyopathy

DIFFERENTIAL DIAGNOSIS

- Rheumatoid arthritis
- Infective endocarditis
- Lyme disease
- Reiter's syndrome and other reactive arthritis
- Systemic lupus erythematosus
- Postgonococcal arthritis
- Other infectious causes of arthritis and carditis included are coxsackie B and parvovirus

Treatment

INITIAL STABILIZATION

- In the presence of heart failure, diuretics and digitalis are indicated
- Drainage of malignant pericardial effusion
- In severe carditis, steroids are recommended
- In the case of chorea, haloperidol may be used

ED TREATMENT

- Antibiotic treatment for streptococcal pharyngitis should be given when the diagnosis of ARF is made
  - —IM or PO penicillin, or erythromycin for penicillin allergic
  - —All patients should receive aspirin or NSAIDs for the inflammatory state associated with ARF
  - —ASA/NSAIDs should be continued for 2–3 weeks after ESR approaches near-normal levels
- For *carditis*
  - —Aspirin
  - —Digoxin
  - —Diuretics
  - —Prednisone
- For *chorea*
  - —Haloperidol or sedatives may be used
- Prophylactic regimens for *Streptococcus* include benzathine penicillin G, 1.2 million IU i.m. every month, or penicillin V 250 mg PO b.i.d.
  - —For children without cardiac involvement, 5 years of prophylaxis from the time of the last episode of ARF is generally recommended
  - —Patients with cardiac involvement are placed on life-long prophylactic antibiotics

MEDICATIONS

- Aspirin: 4–8 g/d (peds: 100 mg/kg/d) PO q4–6h
- Digoxin: 0.25–0.5 mg (peds: 0.04 mg/kg) i.v.
- Erythromycin: 250 mg (peds: 30–50 mg/kg/d) q6h PO × 10 days
- Furosemide: 20–80 mg (peds: 1 mg/kg/dose) i.v.
- Haloperidol: 2–10 mg (peds: 0.01–0.03 mg/kg/d) q6h i.m. or PO
- Penicillin (benzathine benzylpenicillin): 1.2 million units (peds: 600,000 units for under 27 kg) i.m. acutely and monthly thereafter (prophylaxis)
- Penicillin VK: 500 mg (peds: 250 mg) PO q8h × 10 days (acute treatment)
- Prednisone: 1–2 mg/kg/d × 14 days; taper steroids for an additional 2 weeks

Disposition

ADMISSION CRITERIA

- Patients with significant carditis or newly diagnosed cases with suspicion of carditis should be admitted to the hospital for stabilization and initiation of treatment

DISCHARGE CRITERIA

- A well-appearing patient who has responded to initial treatment and whose compliance can be ensured
- Chorea is controlled with haloperidol or sedatives; even severe chorea will disappear during sleep

Miscellaneous

ICD9: 390

ICD10: I00

SUGGESTED READINGS

Bisno AL. Rheumatic fever. In: Kelley WN, et al, eds. Textbook of rheumatology, 5th ed. Philadelphia: WB Saunders, 1997: 1225–1239.

Kaplan EL. Rheumatic Fever. In: Braunwald E, et al, eds. Harrison's principles of internal medicine, 15th ed. New York: McGraw Hill, 2001:1340–1342.

Pinals RS. Polyarthritis and fever. N Engl J Med 1994;330(11):769–774.

Stollerman GH. Rheumatic fever. Lancet 1997;349:935–942.

Stollerman GH. Rheumatic fever in the 21st century. Clin Infect Dis 2001: 806–814.

Thatai D, Turi ZG. Current guidelines for the treatment of patients with rheumatic fever. Drugs 1999;57(4):545–555.

Author: Jon D. Mason

Rib Fracture

Clinical Presentation

SIGNS AND SYMPTOMS

- Localized chest pain
- *Point tenderness,* pain referred to fracture site with palpation of the involved rib elsewhere
- Bony crepitus, ecchymosis
- Intercostal muscle spasm
- Localized pain increased with deep inspiration or coughing
- Splinting respirations

MECHANISM/DESCRIPTION

- Direct chest wall trauma, fall from height, motor-vehicle accident, assault
- Ribs usually break at the point of impact or the posterior angle, which is the structurally weakest region
- Pathologic fractures associated with mild trauma and significant underlying disease
- The first three ribs are relatively protected and require significant impact to fracture, indicating possible intrathoracic injury
- Ribs 9 through 12 are relatively mobile and their fracture suggests possible intraabdominal injury

PEDIATRIC CONSIDERATIONS

- A relatively more elastic chest wall makes rib fractures less common in children

Pre-Hospital

CAUTIONS

- Patients with multiple rib fractures (particularly 1–3 or 9–12) should be routed to the nearest trauma center
- Patients with a flail chest should be assumed to have a pulmonary contusion

Diagnosis

ESSENTIAL WORKUP

- Diagnosis is initially made on clinical grounds
- CXR is indicated to rule out associated intrathoracic injury but misses up to 50% of rib fractures
  - —Look for pneumothorax, hemothorax, pneumomediastinum, pulmonary contusion, and widened mediastinal silhouette

IMAGING/SPECIAL TESTS

- Indications for rib x-ray series
  - —Suspected fractures of ribs 1–3 or 9–12
  - —Multiple rib fractures
  - —Elderly patients with preexisting pulmonary disease or suspected pathologic fractures

DIFFERENTIAL DIAGNOSIS

- Rib contusion or intercostal muscle strain
- Costochondral separation
- Sternal fracture and dislocation

Nontraumatic Causes of Chest Pain

- Cardiovascular: myocardial ischemia or infarction, pericarditis, aortic dissection, pulmonary embolus, valvular heart disease
- Pulmonary: infections, inflammation, barotrauma
- Musculoskeletal: costochondritis, cervical or thoracic spine disease
- Gastrointestinal: esophageal reflux or spasm, Mallory-Weiss tear, biliary or renal colic, peptic ulcer disease, gastritis, pancreatitis, hepatitis
- Other: herpes zoster, chest wall tumor

Treatment

INITIAL STABILIZATION

- For simple fractures, generally no significant stabilization is required
- Multiple fractures, elderly patients or significant underlying lung disease
  - —ABCs
  - —Control airway as needed, endotracheal intubation may be indicated for patients with significant underlying lung disease and impending respiratory failure

ED TREATMENT

Simple Fractures

- *Pain control:* adequate pain control is the key to maintaining adequate pulmonary function, avoiding atelectasis and subsequent pneumonia
- *Intercostal nerve blocks* with 0.5% bupivacaine are safe and effective when performed properly, providing 6–12 hours of pain relief
  - —Intercostal nerve block should be performed posteriorly a couple of fingerbreadths from the vertebrae
  - —Inject 0.5–1 mL just under the inferior surface of the rib where the neurovascular bundle runs
  - —Be careful to avoid the intercostal vessels
- Deep breathing or incentive spirometry should be encouraged once adequate pain control is achieved
- *Avoid* binders or banding of the chest wall because these restrict ventilation and promote atelectasis

Multiple Fractures, Elderly Patients, or Significant Underlying Lung Disease

- *Pain control*
- Search for associated injuries, treat exacerbation of underlying lung disease
- *Intercostal nerve blocks* at the involved sites as described earlier with 0.5% bupivacaine for multiple fractures are safe and effective when performed properly, providing 6–12 hours of pain relief

MEDICATIONS

- Combinations of oral NSAIDs and narcotic analgesics are usually effective
- Acetaminophen/codeine (Tylenol 3): 1–2 tabs PO q4–6h
- Acetaminophen/hydrocodone (Vicodin): 1–2 tabs PO q4–6h
- Acetaminophen/oxycodone (Percocet): 1–2 tabs PO q6h
- Bupivacaine 0.5% for intercostal nerve blocks
- Codeine: 30–60 mg PO q4–6h
- Hydromorphone (Dilaudid): 1–2 mg i.v./i.m./s.c. q4–6h
- Ibuprofen (Motrin): 600–800 mg PO q6–8h
- Meperidine (Demerol): 0.75–2.0 mg/kg i.v./i.m. q3–4h
- Morphine sulfate: 0.05–0.1 mg/kg i.v./i.m./s.c. q4–6h
- Naproxen (Naprosyn): 500 mg PO b.i.d.
- For the admitted patient thoracic epidural block or patient-controlled analgesia (PCA) is an effective alternative

Disposition

ADMISSION CRITERIA

- Patients with multiple fractures, fractures of the first three ribs, pneumothoraces, or pneumomediastinum associated with rib fracture, pulmonary contusion, elderly patients, or patients with significant underlying lung disease (COPD, CHF, exacerbated asthma) should be admitted
- Patients whose pain control is inadequate on oral analgesics

DISCHARGE CRITERIA

- Patients with normal pulmonary function, no underlying pulmonary injury and adequate pain control on oral analgesics
- Strict instructions should be given to return for shortness of breath, chest pain, or development of any of the signs and symptoms of pulmonary contusion or pneumothorax

Miscellaneous

ICD9: 807.0

ICD10: S22.3

SUGGESTED READINGS

Committee on Trauma, American College of Surgeons. Advanced trauma life support instructor manual, 5th ed. Chicago: American College of Surgeons, 1993.

Honick, D. Fractures, rib, eMedicine Journal 17 July 2001;2(7). Available at: *www.emedicine.com*.

Vukich D, Markovchick V. Thoracic trauma. In: Rosen P, et al, eds. Emergency medicine: concepts and clinical practice, 4th ed. St. Louis: CV Mosby, 1998:514.

Wilson R. Thoracic trauma. In: Tintinalli J, et al, eds. Emergency medicine: a comprehensive study guide, 4th ed. New York: McGraw-Hill, 1996:1156.

Author: Gregory Lampe

Ring/Constricting Band Removal

Clinical Presentation

SIGNS AND SYMPTOMS

- A constricting band with swollen tissue and skin most commonly on a finger
- Other locations: wrist, ankle, toe, umbilicus, ear lobe, nipple, septum or nares of nose, penis, scrotum, vagina, labia, or tongue
- Pain on manipulation of the appendage or constricting band

MECHANISM/DESCRIPTION

- Untreated, the constricting band may become *embedded* with interruption of skin integrity
- *Primary constricting band:* the band tightened around an appendage causes the swelling and pain, for example, a hair knotted around a toddler's toe
- *Secondary constricting band:* an injury or disease process that causes the swelling and edema that tightens against the band, for example, an impacted ring with an underlying fracture of the finger

ETIOLOGY

- Tourniquet syndrome may result from allergic, dermatologic, iatrogenic, endocrinologic, infectious, malignant, metabolic, physiologic, or traumatic conditions, or it may be pregnancy related

Pre-Hospital

- Remove rings and other potential constricting bands in the pre-hospital setting before the development of the tourniquet syndrome, particularly on regions of extremity trauma
- Elevate involved extremity

Diagnosis

ESSENTIAL WORKUP

- Primary constricting band: diagnosis made by history and physical exam with special attention to neurovascular status
- Secondary constricting band: diagnosis of underlying pathology may be dependent on imaging and laboratory tests

LABORATORY

- Usually not indicated for the acute treatment; however, electrolytes, BUN and creatinine, thyroid function tests, and Tzanck smear of vesicular lesions may be useful in identifying the underlying diagnosis responsible for a secondary constricting band

IMAGING/SPECIAL TESTS

- Plain films for evaluation of underlying fracture or foreign body *after* band removal

DIFFERENTIAL DIAGNOSIS

- *Any* condition causing marked swelling and edema predisposing to the tourniquet syndrome

Treatment

INITIAL STABILIZATION

- Pain management or conscious sedation as needed

ED TREATMENT

- Removal of the constricting band either by advancing the band distally or by division
- The most benign methods should be attempted first
- These adjuvant methods may be used alone or in combination
  - —Elevation of the affected extremity may help decrease vascular congestion
  - —*Cooling* the extremity with ice or cold water to reduce edema and erythema
  - —*Lubrication* with soap or mineral oil to allow slippage over an inflamed or edematous area
  - —*Digital block* with 1–2% lidocaine (without epinephrine) decreases the discomfort of removal and manipulation of an underlying injury
    - -A digital block may increase local swelling
  - —*Gauze* or a *needle holder* may be used to manipulate the band

Distal Edema Reduction by Sequential Compression

- The distal swollen finger, especially the proximal interphalangeal (PIP) joint presents an important obstacle in constricting band removal; distal to proximal edema reduction by sequential compression is achieved by
  - —*Self-adherent tape* wrapped from distal to proximal forms a smooth and decompressed area over which the band is advanced
  - —A *Penrose surgical drain* or a finger cut from a small glove is stretched to fit over the distal swelling before the attempted removal
  - —With lubrication, the proximal end of the drain is pulled under the ring to form a cuff around the ring; the cuff with distal traction applied advances the band over the decompressed area
  - —*Suture material* (no. 0 silk, dental floss, or umbilical tape) is wrapped under tension in a tight layer advancing over the edema in a distal to proximal direction; the proximal tail of the suture material (or floss) is tucked under the ring; with lubrication, the tail under tension is pulled distally and unwound, forcing the ring over the layered suture material and decompressed area

Constricting Band Removal by Division

- A *scissor* may be used to lift then cut the offending fibrous band constricting a toddler's toe or penis
- A *no. 11 scalpel* blade with cutting edge up may be sufficient to cut constricting bands formed by hair, fibers, or plastic ties
- A *handheld wire cutter/stripper* may readily divide small girth metallic rings with minimum discomfort to the underlying injury; this type of removal may impart a crush defect to the ring, making repair difficult
- A *long-handled bolt cutter* available in most ORs or hospital engineering department may be used to divide large girth or broad-sized rings
  - —Long handles provide significant mechanical advantage needed to cut large rings
  - —The reinforced cutting blades may not easily fit through a constricting band with adjacent swollen tissue and skin
- A *standard hand-powered medically approved ring cutter* may be used to divide small girth metallic constricting bands made of soft metals (gold/silver)
  - —This method has the advantage of a cleaner cut for subsequent repair of the ring
  - —The disadvantage is that the handheld ring cutter is labor intensive and may aggravate the pain of an underlying injury with each turn of the handle
- A *motorized high-revolution-per-minute (RPM) cutting device* (a "drill-like" precision cutting tool) may be used to rapidly divide constricting bands irrespective of girth and size of the ring

Cutting Procedure

- The initial cut is made on the band on the volar aspect of the extremity
- A tenacula may be used to further spread the band in softer metals (14–24-karat gold)
- For a second cut, the band should be rotated 180 degrees on the extremity, allowing for the second cut on the band over the volar aspect of the extremity

Motorized Cutting

- *Flammable solvents* removed from the work area
- *Protective eyewear* worn by all persons present including the patient
- A thin *aluminum splint* should be placed between the patient's skin and the ring as a shield to protect underlying tissue
- *Cutting* with the tungsten-carbide cutting disk should be limited to <60-second intervals to avoid excessive heat
  - —*Ice water irrigations* dissipate heat; dry before cutting

Postdivision Care

- Underlying injuries should be irrigated thoroughly to remove metallic dust to avoid foreign body reaction and granuloma formation
- Tetanus prophylaxis

Disposition

ADMISSION CRITERIA

- Neurovascular compromise or injury requiring surgical repair
- Concomitant infection or necrosis

DISCHARGE CRITERIA

- Successful band removal with restoration of circulation

Miscellaneous

ICD9: N/A

ICD10: N/A

SUGGESTED READINGS

Cresap CR. Removal of a hardened steel ring from an extremity swollen finger. Am J Emerg Med 1995;13(3):318–320.

Fasano FJ, et al. Foreign body granuloma and synovitis of the finger: a hazard of ring removal by the sawing technique. J Hand Surg 1987;12A:621–623.

Roberts JR, Hedges JR. Clinical procedures in emergency medicine, 3rd ed. Philadelphia: WB Saunders, 1997.

Rosen P, Chan TC, Vilke GM, et al. Atlas of emergency procedures. St. Louis: Mosby, 2001.

Author: Gary M. Vilke

Rocky Mountain Spotted Fever

Clinical Presentation

SIGNS AND SYMPTOMS

- Fever in nearly all cases
- Triad of fever, headache, and rash in 50%
  - —Often not identified when patient initially presents for care
- Tick bite reported within 14 days of rash in 60–70%
- Rash
  - —Initial rash (3–5 days)
    - -Macular, red, and flat
    - -Blanches under pressure
    - -1–4-mm diameter
  - —In hours to days
    - -Becomes darker, papular, dusky, and palpable
  - —In 2–3 days
    - -Petechial or purpuric
    - -Positive Rumpel-Leede test
    - -May coalesce or ulcerate
  - —In severe disease, necrosis of dependent peripheral parts may occur
  - —Location
    - -Begins in flexor surfaces of wrist and ankles
    - -Spreads centripetal spread
    - -15% with centrifugal spread to palms and soles
- Pulmonary
  - —Nonproductive cough
  - —Chest pain
  - —Dyspnea
  - —Rales
- Gastrointestinal
  - —Associated with fatal Rocky Mountain spotted fever
  - —Secondary to vasculitis
  - —Nausea/vomiting
  - —Abdominal pain/distention
  - —Ileus
  - —Hepatosplenomegaly
- Neurologic
  - —Focal or generalized neurologic manifestation in two thirds
  - —Meningismus
  - —Severe, unremitting headache
  - —Encephalitis
- Other
  - —Generalized edema
  - —Dehydration
  - —Malaise
  - —Myalgia
  - —Retinal hemorrhage and conjunctivitis
- Complications
  - —Disseminated intravascular coagulation (DIC)
  - —Noncardiogenic pulmonary edema
  - —Acute renal failure
  - —Severe or fatal in advance age, male sex, African American, chronic alcohol abuse, G6PD deficiency

MECHANISM/DESCRIPTION

- Rickettsial invasion of small blood vessels
  - —Causes direct vascular damage
  - —Superimposed vascular damage due to immunologic phenomena

ETIOLOGY

- Acute infection by *Rickettsia rickettsii* via tick vector
  - —*Dermacentor andersoni* (wood tick) in the western states
  - —*Dermacentor variabilis* (dog tick) in the eastern states
- Reported in every state with majority in south Atlantic and south-central states
- 90% occur between April and September
- Incubation 2–14 days
- Fatal in 10%
  - —Lower fatality rate in patients reporting a tick bite
- Transmission
  - —Blood meal of an infected female tick (most common)
  - —Tick feces and tick-infected pets (less common)

PEDIATRIC CONSIDERATIONS

- Highest incidence in the 5–9-year-old age-group
- Two thirds of cases occur in children younger than 15 years

Pre-Hospital

N/A

Diagnosis

ESSENTIAL WORKUP

- Clinical diagnosis

LABORATORY

- Serology
  - —Diagnose by single titer >1:64 or fourfold increase
  - —Methods
    - -Immunofluorescent antibody
    - -Complement fixation
    - -Indirect hemagglutination test
    - -Indirect immunofluorescence assay (IFA) is the reference standard
- CBC
  - —Normal WBC count
  - —Thrombocytopenia
  - —Anemia
- Electrolytes, BUN/Cr, glucose
  - —Hyponatremia <130 mEq/L
- Liver profile
  - —Elevated AST
  - —LDH
- ABG for
  - —Hypoxia
  - —Respiratory alkalosis
- Coagulation profile if DIC suspected
- Microbiology
  - —Immunohistologic antibody stain of skin biopsy
  - —Isolation of *R. rickettsii* (time consuming/expensive)
  - —PCR assay
- CSF
  - —Pleocytosis and increased protein

IMAGING/SPECIAL TESTS

- CXR for pulmonary edema
- Echocardiography
  - —Decreased left ventricular contractility

DIFFERENTIAL DIAGNOSIS

- Other tick-borne diseases
  - —Ehrlichiosis: older adults
  - —Relapsing fever
  - —Lyme disease: erythema chronicum migrans (ECM)
  - —Tularemia
  - —Babesiosis
  - —Colorado tick fever
- Infectious diseases
  - —Meningococcemia—late winter, early spring; maculopapular or petechial rash
  - —Measles—late winter, early spring, severe prodrome
  - —Rubella—palms and soles spared
  - —Varicella—does not have rash in the extremities
  - —Infectious mononucleosis—palms and soles spared
  - —Disseminated gonococcal infection—pustular lesions
  - —Typhus—rash starts at the trunk with centrifugal spread
  - —Secondary syphilis
  - —Scarlet fever
  - —Kawasaki disease—red cracked lips
  - —Toxic shock syndrome
  - —Gastroenteritis
  - —Staphylococcal sepsis
- Inflammatory causes
  - —Allergic vasculitis
  - —Thrombotic thrombocytic purpura
  - —Collagen vascular disease
  - —Juvenile rheumatoid arthritis
- Heat illness

Treatment

INITIAL STABILIZATION

- ABCs
- 0.9% NS i.v. fluid bolus for dehydration
- Oxygen for hypoxia

ED TREATMENT

- Correct fluid and electrolyte deficits
- Initiate antibiotic therapy immediately on clinical and epidemiologic findings
  - —Doxycycline—drug of choice
  - —Chloramphenicol in pregnant and allergic patients
  - —Sulfonamides make the infection worse
- Administer acetaminophen for fever
- Administer high-dose steroids for severe cases complicated by extensive vasculitis, encephalitis, or cerebral edema
- Treat complications
  - —DIC
  - —ARDS
  - —CHF

MEDICATIONS

- Acetaminophen: 1 g (peds: 15 mg/kg) PO q4h
- Chloramphenicol: 75 mg/kg/24 h PO or i.v. q6h × 5–7 days and 48 hours after defervescence
- Doxycycline: 100 mg (peds: 2 mg/kg for those younger than 45 kg) PO or i.v. b.i.d. × 5–7 days and 48 hours after defervescence
- Solu-Medrol: 125 mg (peds: 1–2 mg/kg) IVP

PEDIATRIC CONSIDERATIONS

- Doxycycline is used in children due to potential for fatal cases

Disposition

ADMISSION CRITERIA

- Moderate to severe symptoms

DISCHARGE CRITERIA

- Mild, early disease
- Notify family due to clustering

Miscellaneous

ICD9: 82.0

ICD10: A77.0

SUGGESTED READINGS

Bolgiano EB, Sexton J. Tick-borne illness. In: Rosen P, Barkin R, et al, eds. Emergency medicine, 4th ed. St. Louis: CV Mosby, 1998:2598–2629.

Fischer JJ. Rocky mountain spotted fever: when and why to consider the diagnosis. Postgrad Med 1990;87:109–118.

Centers for Disease Control and Prevention on the web: *www.cdc.gov/ncidod/dvrd/rmsf*

Author: Moses Lee

Roseola

Clinical Presentation

SIGNS AND SYMPTOMS

- Sudden, high fever 39.4–41.2°C (103–106°F)
- Febrile seizures in 5–35%
- Absence of physical findings
  —Child looks well
- Temperature normalizes in 3–4 days
- Maculopapular eruption from trunk to arms and neck after temperature normalization
  —Rash fades within 3 days
- Enlarged lymph nodes
- Diarrhea
- Irritability
- Erythematous papules in pharynx (Nakayama's spots)
- Rarely causes severe or fatal disseminating diseases
  —Infectious mononucleosis syndrome of hepatitis
- Reactivation in immunocompromised individuals

MECHANISM/DESCRIPTION

- Incubation period of 5–15 days
- Mode of acquisition unknown
  —Horizontal spread by oral shedding suggested
  —It is spread person to person, but not very contagious
- Pathophysiology
  —Complex immune response (cytokines, antibody responses, T-cell reactivity)

ETIOLOGY

- Exanthem subitum
- Human herpesvirus 6 (HHV-6)
  —Large, double-stranded DNA
  —Closely related to human cytomegalovirus
- Peak incidence at 6–12 months; 90% occurrence within the first year
- Highest incidence in the late spring and early summer

PEDIATRIC CONSIDERATIONS

- Most newborns are seropositive for HHV-6 due to transplacental antibodies
- By age 1–2 years, >90% of infants seropositive

Pre-Hospital

N/A

Diagnosis

ESSENTIAL WORKUP

- Clinical diagnosis
  —High fever in well-appearing child

LABORATORY

- CBC
  —Initial increase in WBC, then normalization with lymphocytosis
- HHV-6 DNA
  —Detected by PCR
  —Available at research level
- IgM appears early, and declines as IgG is produced

DIFFERENTIAL DIAGNOSIS

- Fever of unknown origin
- Scarlet fever
  —"Sandpaper" rash, "Pastia's" lines, and strawberry tongue
- Measles (rubeola)
  —Koplik's spots, cough, coryza, conjunctivitis, and fever
- Rocky Mountain spotted fever
  —Rash begins at ankles and wrists
- Rubella
  —Fever after rash
- Fifth disease (erythema infectiosum)
- Dengue fever
- Pneumococcal bacteremia
- Meningitis

Treatment

INITIAL STABILIZATION

- ABCs

ED TREATMENT

- Supportive
- Antipyretics
  - —Acetaminophen
  - —Ibuprofen

MEDICATIONS

- Acetaminophen: 650 mg (peds: 15 mg/kg) PO q4h
- Ibuprofen: 200–600 mg (peds: 5–10 mg/kg; suspension 100 mg/5 mL; oral drops 40 mg/mL) PO q6h

Disposition

ADMISSION CRITERIA

- Fever in child who is toxic and does not respond to initial supportive care

DISCHARGE CRITERIA

- Usually, all patients may be discharged

Miscellaneous

ICD9: 57.8

ICD10: B09

SUGGESTED READINGS

Asano Y, Yoshikawa T, Suga S, et al. Clinical features of infants with primary human herpesvirus 6 infection (exanthem subitum, roseola infantum). Pediatrics 1994;93:104–108.

Hall CB, Long CE, Schnabel KC, et al. Human herpesvirus-6 infection in children: a prospective study of complications and reactivation. N Engl J Med 1994;331:482–438.

Nelson WE, ed. Textbook of pediatrics. Philadelphia: WB Saunders, 1996:890–892.

Stoeckle MY. The spectrum of human herpesvirus 6 infection: from roseola infantum to adult disease. Annu Rev Med 2000;51:423–430.

Author: Moses Lee

Rubella

Clinical Presentation

SIGNS AND SYMPTOMS

- Acute viral disease
- Low-grade fever
- Malaise
- Headache
- Upper respiratory tract symptoms
- Rash
  - —Rash is fainter than measles rash and does not coalesce
  - —Red macular rash evolving to pink-red maculopapules, with occasional pruritus
  - —Begins in the face with rapid caudal spread
  - —Completed in first day and disappears in 3 days
  - —May have hemorrhagic manifestations
- Lymphadenopathy
  - —Postauricular
  - —Occipital
  - —Posterior cervical
- Complications
  - —Uncommon, tend to occur more in adults
  - —Congenital rubella syndrome (CRS)—infected women in first trimester
  - —Arthritis
    - -More common in women (up to 79%)
    - -Chronic arthritis is rare
    - -Begins after 2–3 days of illness
    - -Knees, wrists, fingers affected
  - —Hemorrhagic manifestations
    - -Secondary to thrombocytopenia
    - -More common in children
  - —Neurologic sequelae
    - -Encephalitis most common in adults

MECHANISM/DESCRIPTION

- Transmission via droplets from respiratory secretions
- Moderately contagious
  - —Especially during rash eruption and infants with CRS
- Up to 50% may be subclinical
- Infants with congenital rubella shed large quantities of virus for several months
- Infectious period 7 days before to 5 days after appearance of rash
- Incubation period: 14–21 days

ETIOLOGY

- Also known as German measles or 3-day measles
- Rubella virus (family: Togaviridae, genus: Rubivirus)
- Live, attenuated virus vaccine indications
  - —All children older than 12 months and entering school
  - —All women of childbearing age

Pre-Hospital

CAUTIONS

- Use Hepa filter mask for potential respiratory transmission

Diagnosis

ESSENTIAL WORKUP

- Clinical diagnosis

LABORATORY

- CBC
  - —Decreased WBC, platelets (more common in children)
- UA
  - —Hematuria
- ELISA to detect rubella IgM
- Rubella antibody titer
  - —Acute and convalescent serum specimens
  - —Hemagglutination-inhibition test most common
  - —Definitive diagnosis in acute infection
  - —Compare infant with maternal sera for CRS
  - —False positives in parvovirus, infectious mononucleosis, rheumatoid factor
- Pharynx
  - —Virus may be isolated from pharynx 1 week before and until 2 weeks after rash onset (valuable epidemiologic tool)
- CSF
  - —Few WBCs (monocytes) in encephalitis

DIFFERENTIAL DIAGNOSIS

- Scarlet fever
  - —"Sandpaper" rash, "Pastia's" lines, and strawberry tongue
- Measles (rubeola)
  - —Koplik's spots, cough, coryza, conjunctivitis, and fever
- Roseola infantum
  - —Spring and fall
- Rocky Mountain spotted fever
  - —Rash begins at ankles and wrists
- Rheumatoid arthritis

Treatment

INITIAL STABILIZATION

- ABCs

ED TREATMENT

- Symptomatic therapy
- Antipyretics and antiinflammatory agents
  —Acetaminophen
  —Ibuprofen
- Isolate rubella patients from susceptible persons (e.g., pregnancy)
- Vaccine
  —Measles-mumps-rubella (MMR) vaccine
  —Rubella vaccine is a live attenuated virus
  —Indications
    -Older than 12 months and entry to school
    -Susceptible postpubertal females
    -High-risk groups (colleges, military, places of employment)
    -Unimmunized contacts
    -Health care workers and women of childbearing age born before 1957
  —Contraindicated in pregnant women
  —Avoid pregnancy for 3 months after vaccination
  —One dose confers, probable lifelong protection
  —Common complaints are fever, lymphadenopathy, and arthralgia
- Immune globulin
  —Will not prevent viremia but may modify symptoms

MEDICATIONS

- Acetaminophen: 650 mg (peds: 15 mg/kg) PO q4h
- Ibuprofen: 200–600 mg (peds: 5–10 mg/kg; suspension 100 mg/5 mL; oral drops 40 mg/mL) PO q6h
- Immune globulin: 0.5 mL reconstituted vial s.c. (0.25–0.50 mL/kg)

Disposition

ADMISSION CRITERIA

- Congenital rubella syndrome
- Encephalitis

DISCHARGE CRITERIA

- Most patients may go home
- Inquire regarding vaccination status of family members

PEDIATRIC CONSIDERATIONS

- Issues of parental education should be considered in nonimmunized child

Miscellaneous

ICD9: 56.9

ICD10: B06.9

SUGGESTED READINGS

Centers for Disease Control. Rubella and congenital rubella—United States, 1984–1986. MMWR Morb Mortal Wkly Rep 1987(b);36:664–675. Available at: *www.cdc.gov/nip/publications/pink/rubella.pdf*.

Maldonado Y. Rubella virus (German or three-day measles). In: Behrman RE, ed. Nelson textbook of pediatrics, 16th ed. Philadelphia: WB Saunders, 2000:951–953.

Reef SE, Frey TK, Theall K, et al. The changing epidemiology of rubella in the 1990s. JAMA 2002;287:464–472.

Author: Moses Lee

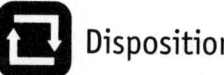

Sacral Fracture

Clinical Presentation

SIGNS AND SYMPTOMS

- Pain in buttocks, perirectal area, and posterior thigh
- Swelling and ecchymosis over the sacral prominence
- Possible sacral nerve dysfunction
  - —Absence or diminished anal sphincter tone is an important finding
  - —Bowel or bladder incontinence

MECHANISM/DESCRIPTION

- Sacral fractures are rarely isolated injuries (<5%)
- They are frequently associated with pelvic fractures
- They are defined by the orientation of the fracture line
- Axial compression
- Direct posterior trauma
- Massive crush injury

Fracture Classification

Transverse

- High sacral
  - —Fall from height
  - —Rare motor weakness
  - —Can see cauda equina syndrome (CES)
- Low sacral
  - —Direct blow
  - —Associated rectal tears
  - —Possible CSF leaks
  - —Rare motor weakness, can see CES

Vertical

- *Alar* (zone 1)
  - —Sciatica
  - —L5 root injury
  - —Neurologic deficit infrequent
- *Foraminal* (zone 2)
  - —Bowel/bladder dysfunction
  - —L5, S1, S2 root injury
  - —Sciatica
  - —Foot drop
  - —Neurologic deficit frequent
- *Canal* (zone 3)
  - —Bowel/bladder dysfunction
  - —Sciatica
  - —L5, S1 root injury
  - —Sexual dysfunction
  - —Neurologic deficit very frequent

Pre-Hospital

- Sacral fractures are frequently associated with other spine and intraabdominal injuries
- Immobilize with backboard and C-spine collar

Diagnosis

ESSENTIAL WORKUP

- History and examination with attention to loss of anal sphincter tone, sensation in the perineum, and bowel and bladder sphincter control
- Sacral fractures rarely occur in isolation, look for associated injuries
- Rectal exam will elicit pain in the sacrum
- Displacement can be assessed with bimanual rectal exam

IMAGING/SPECIAL TESTS

- Only 30% of sacral fractures detected on x-ray
- Rostrally and caudally angulated AP views and cone-down views of the lumbosacral junction may help
- CT scan may better delineate the fracture and associated injuries

DIFFERENTIAL DIAGNOSIS

- Contusion

Treatment

INITIAL STABILIZATION

- ABCs of trauma care
- Early immobilization in unstable pelvis or spine fractures
- Pain control with NSAIDs or narcotic analgesics

ED TREATMENT

- Vertical unstable fractures require a rapid and thorough assessment for life-threatening injuries, and orthopedic consultation (see Pelvic Fracture)
- Nondisplaced isolated sacral fractures are treated symptomatically with bed rest
- Surgery may be required for fractures associated with neurologic injury
- Early orthopedic referral
- Early application of cold compresses

Disposition

ADMISSION CRITERIA

- Critically injured trauma patient with unstable pelvic fracture
- Neurologic impairment

DISCHARGE CRITERIA

- All other types of isolated sacral fractures
- Consider intermediate care for elderly patients

Miscellaneous

ICD9: 805.6

ICD10: S32.1

SEE ALSO: PELVIC FRACTURE

SUGGESTED READINGS

Cwinn AA. Pelvis and hip. In: Rosen P, et al., eds. Emergency medicine: concepts and clinical practice, 4th ed. St. Louis: CV Mosby, 1998:739–762.

Pollack C. Pelvic trauma. In: Harwood-Nuss A, et al., eds. The clinical practice of emergency medicine, 2nd ed. Philadelphia: Lippincott-Raven, 1996.

Simon R, Koenigsknecht S. Traumatic conditions of the hip and fractures of the pelvis. In: Simon R, et al., eds. Emergency orthopedics: the extremities, 4th ed. New York: McGraw-Hill, 2001:356–362, 411–413.

Author: Jaime B. Rivas

Salicylate, Poisoning

Clinical Presentation

SIGNS AND SYMPTOMS

Gastrointestinal

- Nausea
- Vomiting
- Epigastric pain
- Hematemesis

Pulmonary

- Tachypnea
- Noncardiogenic pulmonary edema

CNS

- Tinnitus
- Deafness
- Delirium
- Seizures
- Coma

MECHANISM/DESCRIPTION

- Respiratory alkalosis and metabolic acidosis
  —Secondary to inhibition of Krebs cycle and uncoupling of oxidative phosphorylation
- Dehydration, hyponatremia or hypernatremia, hypokalemia, hypocalcemia
  —Due to increased sweating, vomiting, tachypnea
- Noncardiogenic pulmonary edema
  —Because of a toxic effect of salicylate on the pulmonary endothelium resulting in extravasation of fluids
- Pharmacokinetics of salicylate change from first order to zero order in the overdose setting

PEDIATRIC CONSIDERATIONS

- Children exhibit a faster onset and more severe signs and symptoms than adults
  —Results from the salicylate being distributed more quickly into the target organs such as the brain, kidney, and liver
- Respiratory alkalosis (hallmark of salicylate poisoning in adults) may not occur in children
- Metabolic acidosis occurs quicker in children than adults
- Hypoglycemia more common than hyperglycemia

Pre-Hospital

CAUTIONS

- Morbidity and mortality from chronic salicylate poisoning is much greater than from acute poisoning
  —Manage chronic intoxication more aggressively
- Elderly patients
  —Greater morbidity
  —Respiratory distress/altered mental status indicative of severe toxicity
  —Diagnosis of salicylate intoxication delayed because underlying disease states mask the signs and symptoms

Diagnosis

ESSENTIAL WORKUP

- Guidelines for assessing poisoning severity
  —Acute ingestion of:
    -<150 mg/kg—considered nontoxic
    -150–300 mg/kg—mild to moderately toxic
    ->300 mg/kg—potentially lethal
- Salicylate level
  —At presentation and then every 2 hours until the level begins to decline
  —Make certain units are correct, generally mg/dL
  —In the chronic overdose setting: manage patient on clinical findings and not level alone
    -Clinical findings a better indication of severity than plasma salicylate levels
    -Done nomogram not valid
  —Salicylate levels needed to achieve antiinflammatory effect (20–25 mg/dL) approach toxic levels

LABORATORY

- ABG
  —Respiratory alkalosis
  —Metabolic acidosis
- CBC
- Electrolytes, BUN/Cr, glucose
  —Anion gap metabolic acidosis
  —Hypokalemia
  —Baseline renal function
- Urinalysis
  —Urine pH
- PT/PTT with significant ingestions
- Ferric chloride test
  —Purple color if salicylate present
  —Positive 30 minutes postingestion
- In the presence of salicylate, Phenistix will turn brown-purple and may detect concentrations as low as 20 mg/dL

IMAGING/SPECIAL TESTS

- Abdominal flatplate radiograph for concretions
- CXR for pulmonary edema

DIFFERENTIAL DIAGNOSIS

Acute Salicylate Poisoning

- Considered with change in mental status, unexplained noncardiogenic pulmonary edema, mixed acid-base disorder
  —Methanol
  —Ethylene glycol
  —Conditions causing noncardiogenic pulmonary edema

Chronic Salicylism

- Impending myocardial infarction
- Alcohol withdrawal
- Organic psychoses
- Sepsis
- Dementia

Treatment

INITIAL STABILIZATION

- ABCs
- Naloxone, thiamine, glucose (or Accucheck) for altered mental status
- IV rehydration with 0.9% NS for hypotension

ED TREATMENT

Gastric Decontamination

- Perform gastric lavage for ingestion >150 mg/kg and
  - —Patient comatose (after airway control) or at risk of having seizures
  - —If patient presents within 1-hour postingestion and has an intact gag reflex
    - -If no gag reflex is presented, intubate with a cuffed endotracheal tube prior to performing gastric lavage
- Administer activated charcoal plus sorbitol immediately or postlavage
- Whole-bowel irrigation
  - —For concretions on the KUB
  - —For ingestion of a sustained-release preparation
  - —If the salicylate levels continue to increase despite appropriate management

Enhanced Elimination

- Alkalinization
  - —Enhances elimination of ionized salicylate
  - —Indications
    - -Acidosis
    - -Presence of symptoms
    - -Elevated salicylate levels
  - —1–2 ampules of sodium bicarbonate followed by IV D5W with 3 ampules sodium bicarbonate
    - -Goal: urine pH of 7.5–8 at 3–6 mL/kg/h rate
    - -Add 20–40 mEq KCl per L to avoid hypokalemia
    - -Avoid fluid overload with CHF, coronary artery disease
  - —Closely monitor serum potassium
- Indications for hemodialysis include:
  - —CHF
  - —Noncardiogenic pulmonary edema
  - —CNS depression
  - —Seizures
  - —Unstable vital signs
  - —Severe acid-base disorder
  - —Hepatic compromise
  - —Coagulopathy
  - —Underlying disease state compromising the elimination of salicylate
  - —Absolute salicylate level should not be used as a sole criterion for making a decision to dialyze without considering the patient's clinical status unless the level exceeds 80–100 mg/dL in an acute ingestion
- Lower threshold to dialyze patients with chronic overdose

MEDICATIONS

- Activated charcoal slurry: 1–2 g/kg up to 90 g PO
- Dextrose: D50W 1 amp (50 mL or 25 g) (peds: D25W 2–4 mL/kg) i.v.
- Naloxone (Narcan): 2 mg (peds: 0.1 mg/kg) i.v. or i.m. initial dose
- Sorbitol: 1–2 g/kg to a max of 100 g (peds: >1 year old: 1–1.5 g/kg as a 35% solution to a max of 50 g) PO mixed in the activated charcoal slurry—use only with first dose
- Thiamine (vitamin B_1): 100 mg (peds: 50 mg) i.v. or i.m.

Disposition

ADMISSION CRITERIA

- Monitor patients with salicylate levels >25 mg/dL until level drops below 25 mg/dL and symptoms abate
- ICU admission for altered mental status, metabolic acidosis, pulmonary edema

DISCHARGE CRITERIA

- Salicylate level <25 mg/dL and symptoms have resolved

Miscellaneous

ICD9: 965.1

ICD10: T39.0

SUGGESTED READINGS

Donovan JW, Akhtar J. Salicylates. In: Ford MD, Delaney KA, Ling LJ, et al., ed. Clinical toxicology. Philadelphia: WB Saunders, 2001:275–280.

Juurlink DN, McGuigan MA. Gastrointestinal decontamination for enteric-coated aspirin overdose: what to do depends on who you ask. J Toxicol Clin Toxicol 2000;38: 465–470.

Leatherman JW, Schmitz RG. Fever, hyperdynamic shock and multiple system organ failure: a pseudo-sepsis syndrome associated with chronic salicylate intoxication. Chest 1991;100:1391–1397.

Notarianni L. A reassessment of the treatment of salicylate poisoning. Drug Saf 1992;7:292–303.

Author: Michele Kanter

Sarcoidosis

Clinical Presentation

SIGNS AND SYMPTOMS

- Constitutional
  - —Fatigue
  - —Fever
  - —Anorexia
  - —Weight loss
- Respiratory
  - —Dyspnea
  - —Chest pain
  - —Cough
  - —Hemoptysis (rare)
- Skin
  - —Erythema nodosum
  - —Subcutaneous nodules
  - —Maculopapules
  - —Plaques
  - —Infiltrative scars
  - —Lupus pernio
- Ocular
  - —Acute anterior uveitis
- Neurologic
  - —May affect any aspect but most commonly: cranial nerve palsy (usually CN VII)
- Cardiac
  - —Conduction abnormalities
  - —Congestive heart failure due to infiltrative cardiomyopathy
  - —Papillary muscle dysfunction
  - —Dysrhythmias
  - —Repolarization abnormalities
- Renal
  - —Nephrolithiasis
  - —Nephrocalcinosis
- Lofgren's syndrome
  - —Bilateral hilar adenopathy
  - —Erythema nodosum
  - —Polyarthralgias

PEDIATRIC CONSIDERATIONS

- Children <4 years old classically present with triad of rash, uveitis, and arthritis
- Children ≥ 4 years old present similar to adults

MECHANISM/DESCRIPTION

- Symptoms generally arise due to a local inflammatory reaction associated with noncaseating granulomas

ETIOLOGY

- Unknown

Pre-Hospital

- Oxygen by nasal cannula or non-rebreather

Diagnosis

ESSENTIAL WORKUP

- Physical examination with emphasis on lung, skin, eye, liver, and heart
- Chest x-ray
  - —Stage 0: normal chest radiograph
  - —Stage 1: bilateral hilar lymphadenopathy
  - —Stage 2: lymphadenopathy and pulmonary infiltrates
  - —Stage 3: pulmonary infiltrates only
  - —Stage 4: pulmonary fibrosis
- Pulse oximetry
- Electrocardiogram
- Pulmonary function testing
- Slit-lamp eye examination

LABORATORY

- Serum angiotensin-converting enzyme inhibitor (ACE) level
  - —Caution: may be seen in many disease states
- Basic chemistry panel
- Liver function test: mild, usually asymptomatic, elevation of transaminases
- Serum calcium: hypercalcemia due to oversynthesis of vitamin D
- Urine analysis: hypercalciuria

IMAGING/SPECIAL TESTS

- Biopsy
  - —Demonstrates noncaseating granulomas and exclusion of other diseases producing similar histologic picture

DIFFERENTIAL DIAGNOSIS

- Lymphoma
- Mycobacterial infection
- Parathyroid disease

Treatment

INITIAL STABILIZATION

- Provide adequate oxygenation with nasal cannula or face mask

ED TREATMENT

- Patients should be observed without therapy, if possible, due to the potential of spontaneous improvement
- Initiating steroids in patients demonstrating one of the following:
  —Symptomatic or progressive stage II pulmonary disease
  —Malignant hypercalcemia
  —Severe ocular disease
  —Neurologic or cardiac sarcoid
  —Stage III pulmonary disease
- Consider topical corticosteroids and cycloplegic agents alone for anterior uveitis
- Oxygen if needed for respiratory support

MEDICATIONS

- Prednisone:
  —10–20 mg/d for hypercalcemic nephropathy
  —20–40 mg/d for patients with generally mild to moderate disease
  —40–80 mg/d for neurosarcoid

Disposition

ADMISSION CRITERIA

- Any patient who is hypoxemic
- Patients with moderate to severe symptoms

DISCHARGE CRITERIA

- Life-threatening illness has been ruled out
- Follow-up is established

Miscellaneous

ICD9: 135

ICD10: D86.9

SUGGESTED READINGS

American Thoracic Society. Statement on sarcoidosis. Am J Crit Care Med 1999;160: 736–755.

English J, Patel P, Greer G. Sarcoidosis. J Am Acad Dermatol 2001;44:725–743.

Newman L, Rose C, Maier L. Sarcoidosis. N Engl J Med 1997;336:1224–1234.

Shetty A, Gedalia A. Sarcoidosis: a pediatric perspective. Clin Pediatr 1998;37:707–717.

Author: Tracy Wimbush

Scabies

Clinical Presentation

SIGNS AND SYMPTOMS

- Generalized, intensely pruritic eruption with nocturnal predominance
  —Onset—10–30 days after exposure.
- Reinfestation provokes immediate (1–3 days) pruritus
- Primary lesion: linear papule to 1 cm with a small vesicle containing a black dot at the end
- Found symmetrically in web spaces of fingers, flexor surfaces of elbows and wrist, penis, scrotum, vulva, and areola; head and neck rarely affected in adults but more commonly in infants/children
- Secondary lesions: crusted papules, nodules, excoriations, and secondary impetigo or folliculitis seen on back, shoulders, axilla, waist, buttocks, and flexor aspects of the elbows
- Secondary lesions may be few if patient using topical steroids
- ***Norwegian scabies*** (crusted scabies) is an atypical form of severe scabies seen in handicapped, immunocompromised, and institutionalized patients
  —***Norwegian scabies*** produces gross scaling with hyperkeratotic plaques on hands, feet, scalp, and pressure-bearing areas with heavy infestation but minimal pruritus

ETIOLOGY

- Scabies is produced by the human scabies mite *Sarcoptes scabiei var. hominis* or from animal scabies mites
- Transmitted by direct personal contact or by infected bedding and clothing

MECHANISM/DESCRIPTION

- Mites mate on skin and gravid female burrows into the stratum corneum to lay eggs; animal scabies burrow but cannot reproduce
- Symptoms result from host sensitization to the mite and its products

Pre-Hospital

- No specific considerations in routine cases, maintain universal precautions

Diagnosis

ESSENTIAL WORKUP

- Careful history and skin exam for characteristic lesions
- Obtain skin scraping with mineral oil and a No. 15 blade, observe under low power microscope for mites, eggs, or fecal material

DIFFERENTIAL DIAGNOSIS

- Atopic dermatitis, dermatitis herpetiformis, papular urticaria folliculitis, lichen planus
- Pruritic urticarial papules and plaques of pregnancy (PUPPP)
- Adult linear IgA bullous dermatosis
- Syphilis, pityriasis rosea, impetigo, seborrheic dermatitis, and lymphoma

PEDIATRIC CONSIDERATIONS

- Eruption may be seen from head to toe
- Distribution typically involves the proximal half of the foot and heel
- Neonatal scabies is associated with poor feeding, poor weight gain, and frequent superinfection

Treatment

INITIAL STABILIZATION

- No specific stabilization necessary in routine cases

ED TREATMENT

- Treat patient and all persons in immediate contact with topical scabicide
- Permethrin 5% cream is 89–92% effective and best tolerated
- Crotamiton is 50–60% effective and used when other scabicides are not tolerated
  —Ivermectin (200 μg/kg single oral dose) has shown excellent results though not yet FDA approved for oral use; useful for resistant or crusted scabies
- Lindane 1% is slightly less effective and associated with rare neurotoxicity; legislation will prohibit use in California in 2002, other states pending
- Crusted scabies first requires removal of hyperkeratotic scale with 6% salicylic acid in petroleum jelly to facilitate entry of scabicide
- Machine wash and dry in hot cycles or dry clean all clothes and bedding worn within 2 days of treatment
- Vacuum household floors, carpets, mattresses, and furniture
- Emphasize that itching may continue 1–4 weeks after mites are killed due to skin inflammatory reaction
- Topical steroids and oral antihistamines reduce pruritic symptoms
- Reevaluate after 2 weeks for recurrence; re-treat if live mites found

MEDICATIONS

Scabicides

- Crotamiton 10% lotion or cream: apply topically from neck down in adults and entire skin surface in children qhs for 2 nights, then rinse 48 hours after last application
  —Ivermectin single oral dose of 200 μg/kg gives antiscabetic activity for 6 weeks
- Lindane (γ-benzene hexachloride) 1% lotion or cream: apply topically from neck down and rinse after 8–12 hours, contraindicated in infants, pregnancy, lactation, excessive excoriations, or seizure disorder
- Permethrin 5% cream (Elimite): apply topically from neck down in adults and entire skin in children qhs, rinse off after 8–14 hours

Antipruritics

- Cetirizine (Zyrtec)—low sedating: adult (age >12): 5–10 mg PO qd; peds: not recommended
- Diphenhydramine (Benadryl)—sedating: adult: 25–50 mg PO q6h; peds: 5 mg/kg/ 24 hours divided q6h
- Fexofenadine (Allegra)—nonsedating: adult (age >12): 60 mg PO b.i.d.; peds (age 6–12): 30 mg PO b.i.d.
- Hydroxyzine HCl (Atarax)—sedating: adult: 25 mg PO q8h; peds: 50 mg PO daily divided q6h
- Loratadine (Claritin)—nonsedating: adult and peds >5 years old: 10 mg PO qd; peds 2–5 years old: 5 mg PO qd

Disposition

ADMISSION CRITERIA

- Patients with severe topical or systemic superinfection

DISCHARGE CRITERIA

- Non-toxic-appearing patients with routine symptoms

Miscellaneous

ICD9: 133.0

ICD10: B86

SUGGESTED READINGS

Burkhart CG, Burkhart CN, Burkhart K. An epidemiologic and therapeutic reassessment of scabies. Cutis 2000;65: 233–240.

Chosidow O. Scabies and pediculosis. Lancet 2000;355:819–826.

Potts J. Eradication of ectoparasites in children. How to infestations of lice, scabies and chiggers. Postgrad Med 2001;110:57–59, 63–64.

Author: Guy Tarleton

Scaphoid Fracture

Clinical Presentation

SIGNS AND SYMPTOMS

- Pain and tenderness in the anatomic snuffbox (may be elicited with direct palpation or axial loading of the thumb)
- Alternatively, dorsal wrist pain distal to the radial styloid and decreased range of motion of the wrist and thumb
- Occasionally, incidental damage to the superficial branches of the radial nerve results in sensory changes

MECHANISM/DESCRIPTION

- The scaphoid is the most commonly fractured carpal bone
- Generally results from a *f*all *o*n an *o*utstretched (dorsiflexed) *h*and (FOOSH injury)
- The scaphoid is the stabilizer between the distal and proximal carpal rows; injury may result in arthritis, avascular necrosis, or malunion
- Fractures are missed on initial x-rays 10–15% of the time and delayed diagnosis greatly increases risk of complications
- The blood supply to the scaphoid enters distally; the more proximal the fracture, the higher the risk for avascular necrosis

Pre-Hospital

CAUTIONS

- Evaluate patient for other injuries
- Dress open wounds
- Immobilize in neutral position; ice and elevate

Diagnosis

ESSENTIAL WORKUP

- Appropriate evaluation must include assessment of:
  —Mechanism of injury
  —Point of maximal tenderness
- Examine with special attention to skin integrity and neurovascular status
- Radiographic imaging should include three views of the wrist: PA, lateral, and scaphoid view (wrist prone and in ulnar deviation)

IMAGING/SPECIAL TESTS

- 10–15% of all fractures are not visible on x-ray at the time of injury; follow-up imaging is frequently necessary
- Fracture may be identified by subtle findings such as a displaced fat pad
- Pay special attention to the middle third, or waist, of the bone: 70% of fractures occur here
- A repeat x-ray is required in 7–10 days if the diagnosis is suspected but not confirmed
- A bone scan as early as 3 days postinjury can rule out fracture and allow for earlier rehabilitation; CT or MRI may also be utilized

DIFFERENTIAL DIAGNOSIS

- Bennett's fracture
- Rolando's fracture
- Extraarticular fracture at the base of the thumb metacarpal
- Gamekeeper's thumb
- De Quervain's tenosynovitis
- Perilunate dislocation
- Scapholunate dissociation
- Lunate fracture or dislocation

PEDIATRIC CONSIDERATIONS

- Carpal fractures are rare in children (and in the elderly) as the distal radius usually fails first
- Children with wrist injury should be splinted and referred for appropriate follow-up

Treatment

INITIAL STABILIZATION

- Immobilize thumb in neutral position, ice, and elevate pending definitive evaluation

ED TREATMENT

- Splinting is recommended *any time snuffbox tenderness is present,* whether initial x-rays reveal an obvious fracture or not
  - —Some authorities recommend a long arm splint to prevent rotation at the wrist
  - —Many sources suggest a thumb spica-splint with the thumb in neutral position
- Splint instructions provided to patient
- 72-hour orthopedic referral
- Counsel patient regarding the risk of malunion and avascular necrosis
- If fracture is angulated or is displaced >1 mm, immediate orthopedic referral is required

MEDICATIONS

- Pain control with NSAIDs or oral narcotics

PEDIATRIC CONSIDERATIONS

- Rarely a pediatric injury; carefully evaluate mechanism

Disposition

ADMISSION CRITERIA

- Open fracture, presence of other more serious injuries

DISCHARGE CRITERIA

- Closed injuries, with 72-hour orthopedic follow-up

Miscellaneous

ICD9: 814.01

ICD10: S62.0

SUGGESTED READINGS

American Society for Surgery of the Hand. The hand: primary care of common problems, 2nd ed. New York: Churchill Livingston, 1990:637–649.

Bucholz RW, Heckman JD, eds. Rockwood and Green's fractures in adults, 5th ed. Philadelphia: Lippincott Williams & Wilkins, 2001.

Eisenhauer MA. Wrist and forearm. In: Rosen P, et al., eds. Emergency medicine: concepts and clinical practice, 5th ed. St. Louis: Mosby-Year Book, 2002:535–539.

Perron AD, Brady WJ, Keats TE, et al. Orthopedic pitfalls in the ED: scaphoid fracture. Am J Emerg Med 2001;19(4): 310–316.

Plancher KD. Methods of imaging the scaphoid. Hand Clin 2001;17(4):703–721.

Author: Robyn Heister

Schizophrenia

Clinical Presentation

SIGNS AND SYMPTOMS

Psychotic Symptoms

- The *Diagnostic and Statistical Manual of Mental Disorders* (DSM) criteria require the presence of at least two of the following symptoms for more than 1 month:
- Delusions (fixed, false beliefs)
  - —Bizarre, paranoid, or grandiose
  - —Often involve the conviction that others are tampering with one's mind or body
- Hallucinations
  - —Typically hearing voices
  - —May involve any sensory modality
- Thought disorder
  - —Disorganized speech ranging from odd, idiosyncratic logic to incoherence
- Grossly disorganized or catatonic behavior
- Negative symptoms
  - —Apathy
  - —Flat affect
  - —Social isolation
  - —Anhedonia

MECHANISM/DESCRIPTION

- Genetic component (concordance rate of 50% in monozygotic twins)
- Stressors during second trimester of pregnancy may increase risk
  - —Influenza
  - —Birth complications
- Onset typically early in adulthood
- Substance abuse (alcohol and stimulants) is common
- Approximately 10–15% of patients commit suicide
- Violence may result from impaired judgment, paranoia, and command hallucinations
- Patients with schizophrenia can have abnormally high pain thresholds that can complicate the detection of medical illness
- Premorbid phase
  - —Development of negative symptoms with deterioration of personal, social, and intellectual functioning
- Active phase
  - —Precipitated by a stressful event
  - —Development of active delusions, hallucinations, and bizarre behavior
- Residual phase
  - —Patients are left with impaired social and cognitive ability

Pre-Hospital

CAUTIONS

- Pre-hospital personnel must protect themselves from harm
- Patients can display unpredictable and violent behavior
- Patients may require restraint to protect themselves or EMS crew
  - —Know local laws as they apply to involuntary restraint

Diagnosis

ESSENTIAL WORKUP

- Obtain history from additional sources
  - —Friends or family
  - —Assists in establishing the diagnosis
  - —Evaluate potential dangerousness to self or others
- Medical and neurologic screening
  - —Assessment for drug-induced psychosis (see Psychosis, Medical vs. Psychiatric)
  - —The content of delusions and the nature of auditory hallucinations should be explored to assess safety
  - —Evaluate for acute delirium
    - -Schizophrenia does not affect orientation or memory

LABORATORY

- Toxicology screen
- Electrolytes, BUN, creatinine, glucose, calcium
- Thyroid panel (see Psychosis, Medical vs. Psychiatric)

IMAGING/SPECIAL TESTS

- Head imaging only with suspicion of neurologic etiology

DIFFERENTIAL DIAGNOSIS

- Delirium
- Drug-induced psychosis
- Huntington's chorea
- Temporal lobe epilepsy
- Bipolar (manic depressive) disorder
- Psychotic depression
- Delusional disorder
- Schizotypal personality

Treatment

INITIAL STABILIZATION

- Safety of health care workers and patient is paramount
- Patient may require a quiet room
- Presence of security staff
- Physical or chemical restraints as appropriate
  - —Agitation may be treated with a high-potency antipsychotic and benzodiazepine
    - -Haloperidol or droperidol combined with lorazepam is synergistic
  - —Negative symptoms tend to be less responsive to pharmacotherapy than psychotic symptoms

ED TREATMENT

- Psychiatric consultation after medical evaluation is completed
- High-potency conventional antipsychotic agents (haloperidol, fluphenazine)
  - —Minimal cardiovascular effects (droperidol and thioridazine affect QT interval)
  - —Produce extrapyramidal symptoms
    - -Dystonia
    - -Parkinsonism
    - -Akathisia (restlessness of lower extremities)
- Low-potency conventional agents (chlorpromazine, thioridazine)
  - —Fewer extrapyramidal symptoms
  - —More sedating
  - —Orthostatic hypotension
  - —Anticholinergic side effects
- Atypical antipsychotic agents (risperidone, olanzapine, quetiapine, ziprasidone)
  - —Better tolerated with fewer extrapyramidal symptoms
  - —Risperidone and sertindole can cause orthostatic hypotension
  - —Ziprasidone delays cardiac repolarization (QT interval)
  - —Clozapine is the only agent that is clearly more effective for psychotic symptoms
    - -Requires weekly monitoring of WBC due to agranulocytosis
    - -Highly sedating, anticholinergic, hypotensive
  - —Haloperidol decanoate and fluphenazine decanoate are long-acting depot preparations
- If a conventional antipsychotic agent is administered, patients younger than age 40 should be started on benztropine (Cogentin) 2 mg b.i.d. for 10 days to reduce the risk of dystonic reactions

MEDICATIONS

- Chlorpromazine (Thorazine): 300–800 mg/d
- Clozapine (Clozaril): 200–900 mg/d
- Droperidol: acute agitation; 2.5–10 mg i.v./i.m. repeat q 15–60 min
- Fluphenazine (Prolixin): 5–20 mg/d
- Haloperidol (Haldol): 5–20 mg/d, acute agitation; 5–20 mg i.v./i.m. repeat q 30–60 min
- Lorazepam: acute agitation; 2–4 mg i.v./i.m. repeat q 30–60 min
- Olanzapine (Zyprexa): 10–20 mg/d
- Quetiapine (Seroquel): 250–750 mg/d
- Risperidone (Risperdal): 4–12 mg/d
- Thioridazine (Mellaril): 5–30 mg/d

Disposition

ADMISSION CRITERIA

- Admit if patient is a danger to self or others, or gravely disabled
- Criteria for involuntary hospitalization vary by state
- Patients with new-onset psychosis should also be admitted for evaluation and stabilization

DISCHARGE CRITERIA

- Patients not a danger to self or others and able to perform activities of daily living
- Psychiatric follow-up is arranged
- Psychotic symptoms may persist at time of discharge

Miscellaneous

ICD9: 295.90

ICD10: F20.9

SEE ALSO: PSYCHOSIS, ACUTE

SUGGESTED READINGS

Goff D. A 23 year old man with schizophrenia. JAMA 2002;287:3249–3257.

Goff D, Heckers S, Freudenreich O. Schizophrenia. In: Nemeroff C, ed. Med Clin North Am 2001;85:663–689.

Author: Donald C. Goff

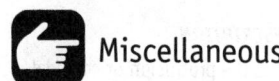

Sciatica/Herniated Disc

Clinical Presentation

SIGNS AND SYMPTOMS

- Pain that radiates from the back into buttocks and lower extremity, with or without nerve dysfunction (sensory or motor deficits)
  - —95% sensitive, 88% specific for herniated disc (HD)
  - —Low back pain (LBP) precedes onset of leg pain; leg pain predominates with time
  - —Sharp, well localized, radiates distal to knee
  - —Exacerbated by activities that increase intradiscal pressure (Valsalva maneuver, cough) or nerve root tension (sitting, straight leg raise)
  - —Relieved by decreasing pressure/tension (lying supine)

MECHANISM/DESCRIPTION

- Herniated Disc is the protrusion of colloidal gel (*nucleus pulposus*) through weakened surrounding fibrous capsule (*annulus fibrosis*)
  - —Peaks 4th–5th decade
  - —2–10% of LBP
  - —95% L5 or S1 nerve root
  - —50–80% improve with conservative management
  - —5–10% require surgery
  - —Risk factors: smoking, repetitive lifting/twisting, vehicular/machinery vibration, obesity, sedentary lifestyle

PEDIATRIC CONSIDERATIONS

- Usually secondary to trauma or serious underlying medical disease; consider complete workup

Pre-Hospital

CAUTIONS

- Full spine precautions for trauma victims

Diagnosis

ESSENTIAL WORKUP

- Complete H&P
  - —Neurologic exam (motor; sensory; DTRs)
    - -*L4 root/L3-4 disc* (knee extension/hip adduction; anteromedial leg/knee/medial malleolus; knee reflex)
    - -*L5 root/L4-5 disc* (great toe and foot dorsiflexion; dorsomedial foot/first web space; no reflex)
    - -*S1 root/L5-S1 disc* (foot plantarflexion; posterior leg/lateral malleolus/ dorsolateral foot; ankle reflex)
  - —Rectal exam (tone, sensation)
  - —*Straight leg raise:* elevate ipsilateral leg by heel 30—60 degrees with or without dorsiflex foot; reproduces radicular pain past knee; 80% sensitive for HD
  - —*Crossed straight leg raise* (pathognomonic): elevate contralateral leg; pain in involved leg; less sensitive but very specific for HD

LABORATORY

- Indicated if clinical suspicion for differential diagnosis (DDx)(esp. tumor/infection), not limited to:
  - —CBC
  - —ESR/CRP
  - —UA

IMAGING/SPECIAL TESTS

- *Postvoid residual (PVR)*
  - —Overflow incontinence: >100 mL, suspect spinal cord compression
- *PA/lateral of LS spine* (help r/o DDx)
  - —Indications:
    - -Extremes of age (<20, >50 years)
    - -Unresolved back pain (>4–6 weeks) despite conservative tx
    - -Red Flags on H&P
  - —Hx: trauma, constitutional symptoms (fever, unexplained weight loss, malaise), h/o cancer, immunocompromise, IVDA, recent bacterial infection, worse at night/awakens patient from sleep
  - —PE: fever, point tenderness, neurologic deficits
- *MRI* (gold standard)
  - —Indications:
    - -Acute severe neurologic deficits (ED)
    - -Suspicion of infectious etiology of back pain (epidural abscess, osteomyelitis, discitis)
    - -Six weeks failed conservative therapy (outpatient basis)
    - -Disc disease (>25%): incidental finding on MRI in asymptomatic patients; no relationship between extent of protrusion and degree of symptoms
- *CT myelogram*
  - —Rarely used alternative for MRI
  - —CT better at bone details

DIFFERENTIAL DIAGNOSIS

- Sciatica
  - —Irritating lesion affecting a lumbosacral nerve anywhere along its route:
  - —*Thalamus/spinothalamic tract:* tumor/hemorrhage
  - —*Spinal cord (myelopathy):* intraspinal tumor/hematoma/infection (epidural abscess, discitis, osteo)
  - —*Root (radiculopathy)*
    - -Intradural: tumor, infection
    - -Extradural: HD, lumbar spine/foraminal stenosis (pseudoclaudication), spondylolisthesis, cyst, tumor, infection
  - —*Plexus (plexopathy):*tumor, aneurysm (AAA), infection (ileopsoas abscess), hematoma (retroperitoneal)
  - —*Peripheral nerve(neuropathy):* toxic/metabolic/nutritional, infection, trauma, ischemia, infiltration, compression, entrapment
- Low back pain/referred pain
  - —Pulmonary: pneumonia, PE
  - —Gastrointestinal: pancreatitis
  - —Genitourinary: pyelo, stone
  - —Gynecologic: ectopic, PID
  - —Vascular: AAA, PVD (claudication)
  - —Orthopaedic: lumbosacral strain, hip/SI joint (infection, fracture, bursitis)
  - —Dermatologic: herpes zoster
  - —Psychologic: functional, secondary gain (drug seeking, disability)

PEDIATRIC CONSIDERATIONS

- $<$10 y/o: infection, tumor, AVM
- $\geq$10 y/o: traumatic HD, spondylolisthesis, Scheuermann's disease, tumor

Treatment

INITIAL STABILIZATION

- Evaluate for neurosurgical emergency

ED TREATMENT

- Pain relief
- Conservative treatment (4–6 weeks)
  - —Minimal to no bed rest or exercise in acute phase
  - —Gradually increase activity, but avoid that which exacerbates pain (heavy lifting, trunk twisting, bodily vibration)
- Unproven therapies: transcutaneous electrical nerve stimulation (TENS), traction, back brace/corset, ultrasound, diathermy, spinal manipulation, acupuncture, massage

MEDICATIONS

- NSAIDs
  - —Celecoxib (Celebrex): 200 mg PO qd
  - —Ibuprofen (Motrin, Advil): 600–800 mg (peds: 5–10 mg/kg/dose) PO t.i.d.–q.i.d.
  - —Ketorolac (Toradol): 15 mg i.v./30 mg i.m. $\times$1
  - —Naproxen (Naprosyn, Aleve): 500 mg PO b.i.d.
  - —Rofecoxib (Vioxx): 25 mg PO qd
- Muscle relaxants (short term)
  - —Cyclobenzaprine (Flexeril): 10–20 mg PO t.i.d.
  - —Diazepam (Valium): 2–10 mg (peds: 0.1 mg/kg/dose) PO t.i.d.–q.i.d.
  - —Methocarbamol (Robaxin): 1,000–1,500 mg PO q.i.d.
- Opioids (short term)
  - —Hydromorphone (Dilaudid): 2–4 mg PO/0.5–2 mg i.m./s.c./slow i.v. q4–6h PRN
  - —Morphine sulfate: 2–10 mg (peds: 0.1 mg/kg/dose) i.m./i.v. $\times$1
  - —Tylenol #3: 1–2 PO q4–6h PRN
  - —Vicodin: 1–2 PO q4–6h PRN

PEDIATRIC CONSIDERATIONS

- Children require surgery more than adults and have a higher success rate

Disposition

ADMISSION CRITERIA

- Severe or progressive neurologic deficit
- Infection/neoplasm
- Unstable fracture
- Inability to manage as outpatient (social situation/pain)

DISCHARGE CRITERIA

- Patient is able to ambulate, follow instructions, has reliable home situation, and planned follow-up

Miscellaneous

ICD9: 722.10

ICD10: M51.1, G55.1

SUGGESTED READINGS

Campana BA. Soft tissue spine injuries and back pain. In: Rosen P, et al., eds. Emergency medicine: concepts and clinical practice, 4th ed. St. Louis: CV Mosby, 1998:878–905.

Della-Giustina DA. Emergency department evaluation and treatment of back pain. Emerg Med Clin North Am 1999;17(4):877–893.

Deyo RA, Weinstein JN. Low back pain. N Engl J Med 2001;344(5):363–370.

Herkowitz HN, Garfin SR, Balderston RA, et al. Rothman-Simone: the spine, 4th ed. Philadelphia: WB Saunders, 1999.

Wheeler AH. Diagnosis and management of low back pain and sciatica. Am Fam Physician 1995;52(5):1333–1341.

Author: Ruth M. Wold

Seborrheic Dermatitis

Clinical Presentation

SIGNS AND SYMPTOMS

- Common, chronic eruptive skin disorder
- Erythematous, greasy, yellow, scaly, and crusting papulosquamous lesions
- Effect areas of high sebaceous gland concentration
- Periods of remission and exacerbation are frequent in adults

Infants

- Onset typically at 1 month of age and usually resolves by 12 months
- Flexural fold involvement may appear as diaper dermatitis, which frequently develops a bacterial or fungal superinfection
- Cradle cap is a thick, greasy, adherent scale on the vertex of the scalp that may be accompanied by inflammation or secondary infection

Young Children

- Blepharitis is a white scale adherent to eyelashes and eyelid margins with characteristic erythema
  - —Resistant to treatment and may persist for years

Adolescents and Adults

- Classic seborrheic dermatitis is characterized by minor itching with greasy, fine, dry, white scaling overlying red inflamed skin
  - —Often exacerbated by avoidance of washing
  - —Usually bilateral and symmetrical, affecting the scalp, forehead, eyebrows, eyelids, external ear canals, posterior auricular folds, posterior neck, and presternal region

ETIOLOGY

- Etiology is most likely multifactorial with genetic, environmental, and hormonal influences
- Cutaneous *Pityrosporum ovale* yeast is increasingly suggested as an important cofactor, which may cause T-cell depression, increased sebum, and activation of the alternate complement pathway
- Disease flares are common with physical and emotional stress or illness
- Medications may induce or aggravate episodes of seborrheic dermatitis including anticonvulsants, buspirone, cimetidine, gold, griseofulvin, haloperidol, interferon-α, lithium, methyldopa, phenothiazines

PEDIATRIC CONSIDERATIONS

- Generalized seborrheic dermatitis may develop in infants immunocompromised due to prematurity or HIV infection

Pre-Hospital

N/A

Diagnosis

ESSENTIAL WORKUP

- Diagnosis is made clinically with thorough history and physical examination

LABORATORY

- Potassium hydroxide preparations of skin scrapings may suggest yeast involvement
- Fungal culture may help exclude tinea capitis as an alternate diagnosis

IMAGING/SPECIAL TESTS

- None required

DIFFERENTIAL DIAGNOSIS

- Atopic dermatitis: characteristically affects antecubital and popliteal fossa in adults
  - —Axillary involvement favors the diagnosis of seborrheic dermatitis
  - —Pruritus, oozing, and weeping support the diagnosis of atopic dermatitis
  - —A strong family history of atopy may suggest the diagnosis; atopic dermatitis is frequently recurrent
- Candidiasis: presence of pseudohypha on cytologic examination with potassium hydroxide is suggestive of candida, but does not exclude the diagnosis of seborrheic dermatitis
- Dermatophytosis: may occur in the groin area; can be difficult to distinguish from seborrheic dermatitis but is generally distributed asymmetrically
- Histiocytosis X: infants affected with acute disseminated histiocytosis X, or Letterer-Siwe disease (Langerhans cell histiocytosis), may display scaling but with associated splenomegaly, reddish-brown papules or vesicles, purpuric lesions, and systemic signs such as fever and adenopathy
- Leiner's disease: complement dysfunction and severe generalized erythematous and exfoliative seborrheic dermatitis with severe diarrhea and failure to thrive
- Lupus: a classic erythematous malar rash of the nose and malar eminences
  - —Chronic, or discoid, lupus erythematosus is characterized by discrete erythematous papules or plaques with a thick adherent scale, which when removed reveals a "carpet tack" appearance
- Psoriasis vulgaris: less likely confined to scalp
- Rosacea: patients usually present with central facial erythema, or forehead involvement
- Tinea capitis: presence of hyphae on cytologic examination with potassium hydroxide is suggestive of tinea
- Tinea versicolor: presence of short hyphae with spores (spaghetti and meatball pattern) on cytologic examination with potassium hydroxide is suggestive of tinea but does not exclude the diagnosis of seborrheic dermatitis

PEDIATRIC CONSIDERATIONS

- Infants with seborrheic dermatitis and cradle cap may present with concurrent atopic dermatitis

Treatment

INITIAL STABILIZATION

- None necessary

ED TREATMENT

- Seborrheic dermatitis is a chronic condition; treatment is not emergent unless secondary infection is present
- Many medications may be utilized
- Patient education, behavior modification, and demonstrating proper cleansing of scaly lesions may be of significant benefit
  —Moderate exposure to sunlight may be beneficial
  —Increase frequency of showering and wash all affected areas

MEDICATIONS

- Scales may be softened with mineral oil, or petrolatum before washing
- For thick scalp scale the patient may apply 10% liquor carbonis detergens (LCD) in Nivea oil (prescription required) at bedtime, then shampoo with Dawn detergent each morning until scale resolves; up to 3 weeks
- Antiseborrheic shampoos containing sulfur, coal tar, or salicylic acid are the most commonly prescribed
  —Sebulex 1–3 times per day
- Zinc pyrithione–based shampoos for more stubborn cases
  —Head and Shoulders, DHS Zinc, Zincon, or X Seb shampoo used daily
- Selenium sulfide shampoos are equally effective
  —Exsel or Selsun
- Low- to midpotency topical glucocorticoids
  —Hydrocortisone 1% lotion: 2–4 times/day—may be applied to scalp as well
- Ketoconazole, where fungal infection is suspected
  —Topical cream applied 1 time each day or 2% shampoo
- In blepharitis, sodium sulfacetamide ophthalmic ointment or solution, and gentle cleansing with baby shampoo may be beneficial

Disposition

ADMISSION CRITERIA

- Seborrheic dermatitis is unlikely to require admission unless severe secondary infection is present
- Immunocompromised patients and those with neurologic disease, such as Parkinson's disease, may have especially severe seborrheic dermatitis
- Severe and sudden attacks of seborrheic dermatitis may be the initial presentation of an immunocompromised patient and warrant admission for further evaluation of the underlying disease process

DISCHARGE CRITERIA

- Patients can be discharged with the recommended medications and appropriate follow-up
- Improvement should be seen within 7–10 days but may take months to resolve completely
- Adolescent and adult forms may persist as a chronic dermatitis
- Provide return precautions for signs of secondary bacterial or fungal infections such as fever, erythema, tenderness, or ulceration
- Consider referral to a dermatologist for severe or refractory cases, or when skin biopsy is required to exclude other causes

PEDIATRIC CONSIDERATIONS

- The prognosis in infants is excellent
- Most infants are free of seborrhea by their first birthday

Miscellaneous

ICD9: 690.10

ICD10: L21.9

SUGGESTED READINGS

Fleisher GR, Ludwig S, eds. Textbook of pediatric emergency medicine, 3rd ed. Baltimore: Williams & Wilkins, 1993.

Habif TP. Clinical dermatology, 3rd ed. St. Louis: CV Mosby, 1996.

Hurwitz S. Clinical pediatric dermatology, 2nd ed. Philadelphia: WB Saunders, 1993.

Janninger CK, Schwartz RA. Seborrheic dermatitis. Am Fam Physician 1995;52:1.

Ruiz-Maldonado R, et al., eds. Pediatric dermatology. Philadelphia: Grune & Stratton, 1989.

Author: Ian Glen Ferguson

Seizures, Adult

Clinical Presentation

SIGNS AND SYMPTOMS

- Altered level of consciousness
- Involuntary, repetitive muscle movements (i.e., tonic posturing or clonic jerking)
- Seizures have abrupt onset; aura may precede a focal seizure
  —Duration is usually 90–120 seconds
  —Impaired memory of the event
  —Postictal state is a brief period of confusion and somnolence following a seizure
- Evidence of recent seizure activity
  —Confusion or somnolence
  —Acute intraoral injury
  —Urinary incontinence
  —Posterior shoulder dislocation
  —Temporary paralysis (Todd's paralysis)
- Other findings may suggest etiology of the seizure
  —Fever and nuchal rigidity (CNS infection)
  —Needle tracks; stigmata of liver disease (drugs and alcohol)
  —Head trauma
  —Papilledema (increased intracranial pressure)
  —Lateralized weakness, sensory loss, or asymmetric reflexes

MECHANISM/DESCRIPTION

Generalized Seizures

- Classically a tonic-clonic (grand mal), which begins as myoclonic jerks followed by loss of consciousness and sustained generalized skeletal muscle contractions
- Nonconvulsive generalized seizures include absence seizures (petit mal), which are brief episodes of sudden immobility and blank stare

Partial Seizures

- Simple: brief sensory or motor manifestations without loss of consciousness (i.e., jacksonian)
- Complex: patients manifest mental and psychological symptoms including affect changes, confusion, automatisms, or hallucinations associated with impairment of consciousness

Status Epilepticus

- Seizure lasting longer than 1 hour or serial seizures that produce an enduring epileptic condition for longer than 1 hour
- Life-threatening emergency with mortality rate of 10–12%

ETIOLOGY

- CNS infections (meningitis, abscess, encephalitis)
- Vascular disease (ischemic or hemorrhagic stroke)
- Neoplasm (primary or metastatic)
- Metabolic abnormalities
- Electrolytes (hypernatremia, hyponatremia, hypocalcemia)
- Hypo/hyperglycemia
- Hypoxia
- Uremia
- Toxins/drugs (lidocaine, TCAs, cocaine, alcohol withdrawal, etc.)
- Eclampsia
- Hypertensive encephalopathy
- Trauma
- Congenital abnormalities
- Idiopathic

PEDIATRIC CONSIDERATIONS

- Febrile seizure is a generalized seizure occurring between 3 months and 5 years of age typically lasting less than 15 minutes in duration
- Associated with a rapid rise in temperature without evidence of CNS infection or other definitive cause

Pre-Hospital

CAUTIONS

- Placing something in the mouth of a seizing patient is contraindicated because it can result in injury to the patient and the bystander
- Anticonvulsant as per local protocol

Diagnosis

ESSENTIAL WORKUP

- A thorough history is the most valuable part of the workup
  —Witness accounts, prior seizures, presence of acute illnesses, past medical problems, and substance abuse
  —Patients with chronic seizure disorder and typical seizure pattern may need to have only serum glucose and anticonvulsant levels checked
  —New-onset seizure mandates workup including electrolytes, head CT, and search for specific underlying cause
  —Patient's condition and resources for follow-up determine whether all these tests need to be done in the ED
- Children with first febrile seizure should receive fever workup as dictated by clinical condition
  —Frequently there is a family history of febrile seizure
  —CBC, blood culture, urinalysis, CXR if any signs of respiratory distress
  —Lumbar puncture for first febrile seizure if age <1 year, any concern about mental status or reliability of exam, or unreliable follow-up

LABORATORY

- Serum anticonvulsant levels
- Other labs as indicated by concomitant disease

IMAGING/SPECIAL TESTS

- Noncontrast head CT for patients with persistent or progressive alteration of mental status, focal deficits, or seizure associated with trauma
- CT scan with contrast should be obtained in HIV-positive patients to rule out toxoplasmosis
- MRI is sensitive for low-grade tumors, small vascular lesions, early inflammation, and early cerebral infarcts, and should be considered as an elective study in new-onset seizures
- EEG may be arranged as an outpatient with neurology

DIFFERENTIAL DIAGNOSIS

- Syncope (may also have incontinence, twitching, and jerking)
- Hyperventilation syndrome
- Psychogenic seizures
- Transient ischemic attacks
- Sleep disorders

PEDIATRIC CONSIDERATIONS

- Children with complicated febrile or new-onset seizures without fever need seizure workup similar to that for adults
- Toxicology screening should be done if there is any suspicion of ingestion or overdose

Treatment

INITIAL STABILIZATION

- ABCs, pulse oximetry, and oxygen; suction available
  - —C-spine precautions
  - —Rapid sequence intubation if patient cannot control airway, hypoxic, or head trauma
  - —IV access, rapid glucose, and if hypoglycemic give IV dextrose 1 amp
  - —Lorazepam or diazepam for actively seizing patients

ED TREATMENT

- Phenytoin or phenobarbital as second-line drugs
- Rectal paraldehyde, or pentobarbital coma for refractory patients
- Treat the underlying cause if identifiable (hypoglycemia, infection, etc.)
- Load with anticonvulsants if levels are low (e.g., phenytoin)
- Fosphenytoin is an option in patients for whom IV Dilantin is considered unsafe
- If no cause is identifiable in new-onset seizure patient, begin single-agent anticonvulsant therapy, e.g., phenytoin
- Notify appropriate department of motor vehicles

PEDIATRIC CONSIDERATIONS

- Fever control with acetaminophen and ibuprofen
- Anticonvulsants are not necessary for febrile seizures
- Anticonvulsants should be prescribed in conjunction with neurologist

MEDICATIONS

- Acetaminophen: 10–15 mg/kg PO or PR
- Diazepam: 0.2 mg/kg i.v. per dose (max 20 mg), 0.5 mg/kg PR
- Fosphenytoin: 15–20 mg/kg at rate of 100–150 mg/min i.v.
- Ibuprofen: 5–10 mg/kg PO
- Lorazepam: 0.1 mg/kg i.v. per dose (max 10 mg)
- Paraldehyde: 0.3–0.5 mL/kg PR 1:1 in mineral oil; peds: 0.3 mL/kg PR 1:2 in mineral oil
- Phenobarbital: 15–20 mg/kg i.v. at rate of 1 mg/kg/min
- Phenytoin: 15–20 mg/kg i.v. at rate of 40–50 mg/min; peds: use rate of 0.5–1.0 mg/kg/min

Disposition

ADMISSION CRITERIA

- Status epilepticus should be admitted to the ICU
- Seizures secondary to underlying disease (e.g., meningitis, intracranial lesion) must be admitted for appropriate treatment and monitoring
- Poorly controlled repetitive seizures should be admitted for monitoring
- Delirium tremens

DISCHARGE CRITERIA

- Patient with normal workup and appropriate neurology follow-up
- Uncomplicated seizure in patient with chronic seizure disorder
- Seizure secondary to reversible cause (e.g., hypoglycemia, alcohol withdrawal)
- Simple febrile seizure

Miscellaneous

ICD9: 780.39

ICD10: R56.8

SUGGESTED READINGS

Bradford JC, Kyriakedes CG. Evaluation of the patient with seizures: an evidence based approach. Emerg Med Clin North Am 1999;17(1):203–220.

Gilad R, Lampl Y, Gabby U, et al. Early treatment of a single generalized tonic-clonic seizure to prevent recurrence. Arch Neurol 1996;53(11):1149–1152.

Roth HL, Drislane FW. Seizures. Neurol Clin 1998;16(2):257–284.

Shepherd SM. Management of status epilepticus. Emerg Med Clin North Am 1994;12(4):941–961.

Stenklyft PH, Carmona M. Febrile seizure. Emerg Med Clin North Am 1994;12(4): 989–999.

Authors: Atul Gupta; Rebecca Smith-Coggins

Seizures, Febrile

Clinical Presentation

SIGNS AND SYMPTOMS

Fever

- Seizure may occur concurrent with recognition of the febrile illness

Seizure

- Generalized tonic-clonic seizure most common
  - —Tonic phase
    - -Muscular rigidity
    - -Apnea and incontinence
    - -Self-limited and last only a few minutes
  - —Other seizure types
    - -Staring with stiffness
    - -Limpness
    - -Jerking movements without prior stiffening

MECHANISM/DESCRIPTION

- Occur between 6 months and 5 years of age associated with fever
  - —No evidence of intracranial infection or other defined cause
  - —Average age of onset is 18–22 months
  - —Children with previous nonfebrile seizures are excluded
- Most common pediatric convulsive disorder
  - —2–4% of young children in U.S.
- Occur in normal children with a systemic viral illness
- High-risk children:
  - —History of febrile seizure in immediate family members
  - —Delayed neurologic development
  - —Males
- Subgroups
  - —Simple febrile seizures
    - -Brief, self-limited lasting <10–15 minutes, resolve spontaneously
    - -Generalized without any focal features
  - —Complex febrile seizures
    - -Duration >15 minutes
    - -Focal features
    - -More than one seizure within a 24-hour period
- Risk of recurrence
  - —One third of cases
  - —Early age of onset, history of febrile or afebrile seizures in first-degree relatives, and temperature <40°C during initial seizure increase the likelihood of recurrence
- Risk of subsequent epilepsy
  - —Greatest for those with abnormal neurologic development, a complex first febrile seizure, or a family history of afebrile seizures
  - —Only slightly greater than the general population if first febrile seizure is simple and neurologic development is normal
  - —Not affected by the use of prophylactic medications

ETIOLOGY

- Common childhood infections
  - —Upper respiratory illnesses
  - —Otitis media
  - —Roseola
  - —Gastrointestinal infections
  - —*Shigella* gastroenteritis

Pre-Hospital

- Protect the airway
- Oxygen
- Support breathing as needed

CAUTIONS

- Keep the child from incurring injury while actively convulsing
- Respiratory insufficiency and apnea occur secondary to overaggressive treatment with benzodiazepines
- Simple febrile seizures are self-limited and generally require no anticonvulsant therapy

Diagnosis

ESSENTIAL WORKUP

- Careful history and physical examination help confirm the diagnosis and rule out other etiologies
  - —Symptoms/evidence of infectious illness
  - —Duration of fever
  - —Medication exposure/toxin
  - —Trauma/occult trauma
  - —Developmental level
  - —Family history of seizures
  - —Complete description of the seizure
  - —Presence of meningismus, tense/bulging fontanelle, preexisting altered mental status
  - —Evidence of focal deficits or increased intracranial pressure

LABORATORY

- Routine laboratory studies are not indicated
- Evaluate for a source of fever if a serious bacterial infections is suspected
  - —White blood cell count
  - —Urinalysis
  - —Blood and urine cultures
- Electrolytes and bedside glucose in infants and children with vomiting or diarrhea

IMAGING/SPECIAL TESTS

- Chest radiograph only in patients with significant respiratory symptoms
- Head CT
  - —Indicated with traumatic injuries, focal neurologic findings, or inability to exclude elevated intracranial pressure
- Lumbar puncture not routinely indicated
  - —Indications:
    - -<12–18 months of age
    - -History or irritability, decreased feeding, lethargy
    - -Physical signs of meningitis
    - -Complex seizure
    - -Prolonged postictal state
    - -Antibiotics altering presentation
    - -Abnormal mentation after postictal state
  - —Indications: >18 month old
    - -Signs/symptoms of central nervous system infection present
- Electroencephalogram
  - -Not helpful in the initial evaluation of febrile seizure
  - -May be indicated if developmental delay, underlying neurologic abnormality, or focal seizure
  - -Does not help predict recurrences or risk for later epilepsy
- Anticonvulsant levels
- Toxicologic studies of blood and urine if history and physical exam suggestive

DIFFERENTIAL DIAGNOSIS

- Febrile delirium
- Febrile shivering with pallor and perioral cyanosis
- Breath-holding spell during febrile event
- Acute life-threatening event
- Other causes of seizure
  —Afebrile seizure occurring during fever event
  —Sudden discontinuance of anticonvulsants
  —Infection
    -Meningitis/encephalitis
    -Acute gastroenteritis, often with dehydration
  —Head trauma
  —Toxicologic
    -Anticholinergics
    -Sympathomimetics
    -Other
  —Hypoxia
  —Metabolic disease
  —Intracranial masses
  —CNS vascular lesions

Treatment

INITIAL STABILIZATION

- Support the airway and breathing
- Benzodiazepines rarely needed
  —Prolonged seizures or compromised patients
  —Lorazepam, diazepam, or midazolam
  —Rectal diazepam or intramuscular midazolam may be easily administered with good efficacy

ED TREATMENT

- Rarely is pharmacologic intervention required; usually self-limited
- Seizures refractory to benzodiazepines
  —Phenytoin or fosphenytoin
  —Phenobarbital
  —Workup to exclude other etiologies
- Administer antipyretics acutely and routinely for at least the next 24 hours
  —Acetaminophen or ibuprofen
- Appropriate antibiotic treatment for specific bacterial disease

MEDICATIONS

- Acetaminophen: 15 mg/kg PO, PR
- Diazepam: 0.2–0.3 mg/kg i.v.; 0.5 mg/kg PR
- Fosphenytoin: 20 mg/kg i.v. over 20 minutes
- Ibuprofen: 10 mg/kg PO
- Lorazepam: 0.1 mg/kg i.v.
- Midazolam: 0.1 mg/kg i.v.; 0.2 mg/kg i.m.
- Phenobarbital: 20 mg/kg i.v. over 20 minutes or i.m.
- Phenytoin: 20 mg/kg i.v. over 30–45 minutes

Disposition

ADMISSION CRITERIA

- Recurrent or prolonged seizures

DISCHARGE CRITERIA

- Simple febrile seizures
  —Normal neurologic examination
  —Source of fever is appropriately treated as outpatient
- Reassurance to parents
- Aggressive treatment of fever with antipyretics is generally recommended despite absence of evidence that this reduces recurrences
- Oral diazepam during febrile illness may reduce risk of recurrence; prophylactic anticonvulsants with other anticonvulsants rarely indicated; controversial

Miscellaneous

ICD9: 780.3

ICD10: R56.0

SEE ALSO: SEIZURES, PEDIATRIC

SUGGESTED READINGS

American Academy of Pediatrics, Provisional Committee on Quality Improvement, Subcommittee on Febrile Seizures. Practice parameter: the neurodiagnostic evaluation of the child with a first simple febrile seizure. Pediatrics 1996;97:769–771.

Depieso AD, Teach SJ. Febrile seizures. Pediatr Emerg Care 2001;17(5):384–387.

Author: John P. Santamaria

Seizures, Pediatric

Clinical Presentation

SIGNS AND SYMPTOMS

Neonates

- Subtle abnormal repetitive motor activity
  - —Facial movements
  - —Eye deviations
  - —Eyelid fluttering
  - —Lip smacking/sucking
- Respiratory alterations
- Apnea
- Seizure activity
  - —Focal or generalized tonic seizures
  - —Focal or multifocal clonic seizure
  - —Myoclonic movements

Older Infants and Children

- Generalized seizures
  - —Tonic-clonic
  - —Tonic
  - —Clonic
  - —Myoclonic
  - —Atonic ("drop")
  - —Absence
- Partial or focal seizures
  - —Simple
    - -Consciousness maintained
    - -Simple partial seizures
      - ∗Motor, sensory, and/or cognitive symptoms
      - ∗Motor activity is focal: one part or side
      - ∗Paresthesias, metallic tastes, and visual or auditory hallucinations
  - —Complex
    - -Consciousness impaired
    - -Complex partial seizure
      - ∗Simple partial seizure progresses with impaired consciousness
      - ∗Aura precedes altered consciousness; auditory, olfactory, or visual hallucination
      - ∗May generalize
- Status epilepticus
  - —Generalized is most common
  - —Sustained partial seizures
  - —Absence seizures
  - —Persistent confusion; postictal period

MECHANISM/DESCRIPTION

- Sudden, abnormal discharges of neurons resulting in a change in behavior or function

ETIOLOGY

- Febrile seizures
- Infection
- Idiopathic
- Trauma
- Toxicologic
  - —Ingestion
  - —Drug action
  - —Drug withdrawal
- Metabolic
  - —Hypoglycemia
  - —Hypocalcemia
  - —Hypo/hypernatremia
  - —Inborn errors of metabolism
- Perinatal hypoxia
- Intracranial hemorrhage
- CNS structural anomaly or malformation
- Degenerative disease

Pre-Hospital

CAUTIONS

- Many conditions may be mistaken for seizures (see Differential Diagnosis, below)
- Immobilize cervical spine if trauma suspected
- Check fingerstick glucose or administer dextrose as appropriate

Diagnosis

ESSENTIAL WORKUP

- Obtain a detailed history
  - —Movements
  - —Duration
  - —State of consciousness
  - —Predisposing conditions/history
- A careful neurologic exam should be performed
- Rapid glucose testing for those in status epilepticus

LABORATORY

- Bedside glucose test
- Performed in young infants and those in status epilepticus
- Select studies in other children reflecting history and physical examination
  - —Electrolytes
  - —BUN
  - —Creatinine
  - —Glucose
  - —Calcium
  - —Magnesium
  - —CBC
  - —Toxicologic screen
- Patients on anticonvulsant therapy
  - —Drug levels
- Febrile seizure
  - —Laboratory studies to evaluate for a serious underlying bacterial infection, if suspected

IMAGING/SPECIAL TESTS

- Head CT
  - —Focal seizure
  - —New focal neurologic abnormality
  - —Suspected intracranial hemorrhage or mass lesion
  - —New-onset status epilepticus without identifiable cause
  - —Not routinely indicated for first afebrile seizure
- Lumbar puncture
  - —Suspicion of meningitis or encephalitis
  - —CT first if suspect increased intracranial pressure
- MRI
  - —Rarely urgently indicated for seizures
- EEG
  - —Generally indicated in children with an afebrile seizure as a predictor of risk of recurrence and classify the seizure type/epilepsy syndrome
  - —Postictal slowing seen within 24–48 hours of a seizure and may be transient; delay EEG if possible

DIFFERENTIAL DIAGNOSIS

Neonates

- Apnea due to other causes
- Jitters or tremors
- Gastroesophageal reflux

Infants and Toddlers

- Breath-holding spells
- Night terrors

Children and Adolescents

- Migraine headache
- Syncope
- Tics
- Pseudoseizures
- Hysteria

Treatment

INITIAL STABILIZATION

- Airway, breathing, and circulation support if actively seizing
- Airway
  - —Oxygen/monitor pulse oximetry
  - —Nasopharyngeal airway preferred over oral airway
  - —Bag-valve-mask support, if hypoventilating or persistently hypoxic
  - —Intubation if seizures are refractory and bag-valve-mask support is unsuccessful
- IV access
- If hypoglycemic, dextrose
- Maintain spine precautions if trauma suspected

ED TREATMENT

Status Epilepticus

- Children
  - —Benzodiazepine
    - -Lorazepam is preferred due to its longer duration of action
    - -Valium is acceptable
    - -If IV access is not available
      - *Diazepam may be given per rectum; use a TB syringe or 14-gauge Angiocath
      - *Midazolam IM is also effective if IV access is not available
  - —Phenytoin
    - -If benzodiazepines fail
    - -For longer-term control
    - -Fosphenytoin easier to administer
  - —Phenobarbital
    - -Use if benzodiazepines and phenytoin fail to break the seizure
    - -Risk of respiratory depression greatly increases if a benzodiazepine has also been given
  - —Alternative therapies in the event of refractory status epilepticus
    - -Paraldehyde (per rectum)
    - -Barbiturate coma
      - *Barbiturate (pentobarbital) coma requires intubation and EEG monitoring to be sure the seizure is suppressed
      - *Associated hypotension
    - -General anesthesia
      - *A final resort
      - *Continuous EEG is needed to be sure the seizure is abolished
- Neonates
  - —Phenobarbital is acceptable first-line therapy
  - —Preferred maintenance drug

MEDICATIONS

- D_{10}: 5 cc/kg i.v. for neonates
- D_{25}: 2 cc/kg i.v. for children
- Diazepam: 0.2–0.3 mg/kg i.v.; 0.5 mg/kg PR
- Fosphenytoin: 20 mg/kg i.v. over 20 minutes
- Lorazepam: 0.1 mg/kg i.v.
- Midazolam: 0.1 mg/kg i.v., 0.2 mg/kg i.m.
- Paraldehyde: 0.3 mL/kg PR mixed 1:1 with cottonseed or olive oil, maximum dose is 5 mL
- Pentobarbital: 10–15 mg/kg i.v. over 1–2 hours; maintenance: 1–3 mg/kg/h i.v.
- Phenobarbital: 20 mg/kg i.v. over 20 minutes
- Phenytoin: 20 mg/kg i.v. over 30–45 minutes

Disposition

ADMISSION CRITERIA

- ICU
  - —Active status epilepticus, intubated, or persistent mental status changes
- Inpatient unit
  - —Status epilepticus resolved in the ED
  - —Underlying cause of seizure not resolved or controlled
  - —Intracranial hemorrhage
  - —Mass lesion
  - —Meningitis/encephalitis
  - —Drug
  - —Toxin ingestions

DISCHARGE CRITERIA

- The child is alert with normal mental status and neurologic exam
- No evidence of an underlying cause requiring hospitalization
- Reliable parent or caregiver
- Home telephone
- Provide seizure precautions and aftercare instructions
- Follow-up with a primary care physician or pediatric neurologist

Miscellaneous

ICD9: 780.3, 780.31

SEE ALSO: SEIZURES, FEBRILE

SUGGESTED READINGS

Cantor RM, Santamaria JP, eds. Pediatric emergency guide. Dallas: American College of Emergency Physicians, 1997.

Hirtz D, et al. Practice parameter: evaluating a first nonfebrile seizure in children—report of the Quality Standards Subcommittee or the American Academy of Neurology, the Child Neurology Society, and the American Epilepsy Society. Neurology 2000;55:616–623.

Roberts MR, Eng-Bourguin J. Status epilepticus in children. Emerg Med Clin North Am 1995;13:489–507.

Vining EPG. Pediatric seizures. Emerg Med Clin North Am 1994;12:973–988.

Author: John P. Santamaria

Sepsis

Clinical Presentation

SIGNS AND SYMPTOMS

- Fever
- Tachycardia
- Tachypnea
- Hypothermia (poor prognosis)
- Hypoxemia
- Diaphoresis

Cardiovascular

- Blood pressure
  —Normal early in sepsis
  —Hypotension when septic shock occurs
- Poor perfusion with septic shock
  —Prolonged capillary refill
  —Cool and clammy extremities

Gastrointestinal/Genitourinary

- Abdominal pain
- Nausea, vomiting
- Diarrhea
- Dysuria/frequency
- Reduced urine output
- Abdominal tenderness
  —Diffuse
  —Localized to right upper quadrant (liver or gallbladder source)
  —Right lower quadrant (appendicitis with or without abscess)
  —Suprapubic area or lower quadrants (urinary tract or pelvic source or diverticulitis)
- Flank pain
  —With pyelonephritis or retroperitoneal abscess

Pulmonary

- Shortness of breath
- Cough (productive or nonproductive)
- Localized wheeze or rales
  —With pneumonia
- Tachypnea
  —Present even when the lungs are not the source of sepsis

Dermatologic

- Any rash is important
- Localized erythema with lymphangitis (streptococcal or staphylococcal cellulitis)
- Rash involving palms of hands and soles of feet (rickettsial infection)
- Petechiae scattered on the torso and extremities (meningococcemia)
- Ecthyma gangrenosum (pseudomonas septicemia)
  —Round, indurated, painless lesion with surrounding erythema and central necrotic black eschar
- Decubitus ulcers
- Indwelling catheter
  —Surrounding skin erythematous with or without purulent drainage

CNS

- Change in mental status
  —Confusion
  —Delirium
  —Coma
- Neck stiffness (meningitis)

MECHANISM/DESCRIPTION

- Systemic inflammatory response syndrome (SIRS)
  —Temperature >38°C or <36°C
  —Heart rate >90 beats/minute
  —Respiratory rate >20/minute or $PaCO_2$ <32 mm Hg
  —WBC >12,000/mm^3, <4,000/mm^3, or >10% band forms
  —Sepsis is the most common cause of SIRS
  —Initially described in ICU patients
  —Neither specific nor sensitive for outpatients
  —Children may have a minor degree of infection but have many of the findings of SIRS (e.g., most children with pneumonia)
- Sepsis with toxicity (septicemia)
  —Two or more of the SIRS
- Septic shock
  —Sepsis-induced hypotension despite fluid resuscitation
    -Systolic BP <90 mm Hg or
    -Reduction of >40 mm Hg from baseline
  —Perfusion abnormalities
    -Acute change in mental status
    -Lactic acidosis
    -Oliguria
    -Poor capillary refill
- Pathophysiology
  —Decreased peripheral vascular resistance due to various mediators of the inflammatory response causing vasodilatation
  —Elevated cardiac output: early appropriate response to vasodilatation
    -Later in septic shock, myocardial depression, and reduced cardiac output (due to injury at the cellular level or mediators acting on the heart)
  —Narrow arteriovenous oxygen difference
  —Multiple organ dysfunction syndrome (MODS) develops if sepsis either untreated or ineffectively treated
    -Pulmonary injury: adult respiratory distress syndrome
    -Renal injury: acute tubular necrosis and kidney failure
    -Hepatic injury and failure
    -Disseminated intravascular coagulation

ETIOLOGY

- Gram-negative bacteria most common
  —*Escherichia coli*
  —*Pseudomonas aeruginosa*
- Gram-positive bacteria
  —Enterococcus species
  —*Staphylococcus aureus*
  —*Streptococcus pneumoniae*
- Fungi (*Candida* species)
- Viruses
- *Legionella* species

PEDIATRIC CONSIDERATIONS

- Major causes of bacterial sepsis
  —*Neisseria meningitis*
  —*Streptococcal pneumoniae*
  —*Haemophilus influenzae*

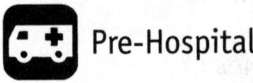

Pre-Hospital

CAUTION

- Aggressive fluid resuscitation for hypotension

Diagnosis

ESSENTIAL WORKUP

- Careful history and physical examination
  - —Guides further evaluation and initiation of appropriate antibiotic therapy

LABORATORY

Septicemia

- Tests should be guided by the clinical presentation
- LP is not needed in all cases
- CBC with differential
- Electrolytes, BUN, Cr, glucose
- Liver function tests
- ABG
  - —Mixed acid-base abnormalities: respiratory alkalosis with metabolic acidosis
- Blood cultures
  - —From two different sites
  - —One may be drawn through an indwelling central line (i.e., Broviac)
- UA and culture

IMAGING/SPECIAL TESTS

- CXR
- CSF analysis
- Cultures
  - —Sputum
  - —Urine
  - —Wound/abscess
  - —CSF
- Lactic acid level
- Lipase
- X-rays of bone and soft tissue underlying any wound for osteomyelitis or gas gangrene
- Abdominal abscess identification
  - —Abdominal ultrasound
  - —CT scan of abdomen

DIFFERENTIAL DIAGNOSIS

- Causes of SIRS
  - —Sepsis (most common)
  - —Pancreatitis
  - —Burns
  - —Multiple trauma
- Adrenal crisis

Treatment

INITIAL STABILIZATION

- ABCs
- Supplemental oxygen to maintain PaO_2 >60 mm Hg
  - —Intubation and mechanical ventilation if shock is present, the pO_2 cannot be maintained, or if the pCO_2 is rising
- Administer 0.9% NS IV fluid to restore circulating blood volume

ED TREATMENT

- Early goal-directed therapy aimed at optimizing preload, afterload, and contractility has been shown to improve outcomes
- Administer antibiotics early based on the most likely organisms or site of infection
- No source identified after initial assessment
  - —Normal immune function
    - -Second- or third-generation cephalosporin and gentamicin
    - -Nafcillin and gentamicin
  - —Immunocompromised host
    - -Piperacillin and gentamicin
    - -Ceftazidime and either nafcillin or vancomycin
- If source identified, or highly suspected, treat the most likely organisms
  - —Pulmonary source
    - -Second- or third-generation cephalosporin and gentamicin, and possibly erythromycin
  - —Intraabdominal source
    - -Ampicillin and metronidazole and gentamicin
    - -Cefoxitin and gentamicin
  - —Urinary tract source
    - -Ampicillin or piperacillin and gentamicin
- Vasopressors
  - —Indicated for persistent hypotension despite fluid administration
    - -Add dopamine if the patient remains hypotensive after 2 L of fluid
  - —Useful to improve renal, mesenteric, cerebral, and coronary flow
    - -Initiate norepinephrine if dopamine not effective

MEDICATIONS

- Ampicillin: 1–2 g (peds: 50–200 mg/kg/24 hours) i.v. q4–6h
- Cefoxitin: 1–2 g (peds: 100–160 mg/kg/24 hours) i.v. q6–8h
- Ceftazidime: 1–2 g (peds: 100–150 mg/kg/24 hours) i.v. q8–12h
- Dopamine: 1–5 μg/kg/min (renal dose); 5–10 μg/kg/min (pressor dose)
- Gentamicin: 1–1.5 mg/kg (peds: 2–2.5 mg/kg q8h) i.v. q8h
- Metronidazole: load with 1 g (peds: 15 mg/kg) i.v., then 500 mg (peds: 7.5 mg/kg) q6h
- Nafcillin: 1–2 g i.v. q4h (peds: 50 mg/kg/24 hours divided q4–6h)
- Norepinephrine: 2–8 μg/min
- Piperacillin: 3–4 g i.v. q4–6h
- Vancomycin: 500 mg (peds: 10 mg/kg) i.v. q6h

PEDIATRIC CONSIDERATIONS

- Antibiotic therapy based on age
  - —<3 months (2 drugs): ampicillin and gentamicin or cefotaxime (50–180 mg/kg/d divided q4–6h)
  - —≥3 months: cefotaxime or ceftriaxone (50–100 mg/kg/d divided q12–24h)
- Initiate vasopressors after no response to 60 mL/kg i.v. fluid
- Avoid hyponatremia and hypoglycemia
- Dexamethasone for children with bacterial meningitis
  - —0.15 mg/kg q6h for 4 days
  - —Potentially may reduce sensorineural hearing loss

Disposition

ADMISSION CRITERIA

- Sepsis with toxicity, septicemia, or septic shock all require admission to ICU

DISCHARGE CRITERIA

- No patient with sepsis should be discharged

Miscellaneous

ICD9: 38.9

ICD10: A41.9

SUGGESTED READINGS

American College of Chest Physicians/Society of Critical Care Medicine Consensus Conference. Definitions for sepsis and organ failure and guidelines for the use of innovative therapies in sepsis. Crit Care Med 1992;20:864.

Bone RC. Diagnosing sepsis: what we need to consider today. J Crit Ill 1996;11:658–665.

Carcillo JA, Cunnion RE. Septic shock. Crit Care Clin 1997;13:553–574.

Cunha BA. Antibiotic treatment of sepsis. Med Clin North Am 1995;79:351–558.

Jacobs RF, Sowell MK, Moss MM, et al. Septic shock in children: bacterial etiologies and temporal relationships. Pediatr Infect Dis J 1990;9:196–200.

Rivers E, Nguyen B, Havstad S, et al. Early goal-directed therapy in the treatment of severe sepsis and septic shock. N Engl J Med 2001;345 (19):1368–1377.

Authors: Kaushal Shah; Richard Wolfe

Serum Sickness

Clinical Presentation

SIGNS AND SYMPTOMS

- Fever
- Rash (urticarial or morbilliform)
- Arthralgias
- Myalgias
- Lymphadenopathy
- Facial and neck edema
- Splenomegaly
- Proteinuria
- Peripheral neuritis
- Myocarditis/pericarditis
- Anaphylaxis

MECHANISM AND DESCRIPTION

- Type III hypersensitivity reaction
- When a foreign protein or drug (the antigen) is injected, the body's immune system responds by forming antibodies to the foreign material and subsequently forms complexes composed of the antigen, antibody, and complement
- These complexes then deposit in tissue, inciting an inflammatory response
  - —C3a and C5a act as anaphylatoxins
  - —C5a is strongly chemotactic for neutrophils
  - —The neutrophils then infiltrate the vessel wall at the site of the immune complex deposition and release enzymes like collagenase and elastase that damage vessel walls
- Occurs 7–10 days after the primary exposure to the antigen
- Usually starts 12–36 hours after ingestion if there is an immunizing exposure
- The time course for this process is 4–14 days

ETIOLOGY

Serum Sickness

- Vaccines containing foreign serum such as rabies
- Antivenom and tetanus inoculations made with horse protein

Serum Sickness–Like Reaction

- Drugs that act as haptens
- Penicillins
- Cephalosporins
- Sulfonamides
- Thiazides
- Gold
- Thiouracils
- Hydantoins
- Phenylbutazone
- Aminosalicylic acid
- Streptomycin

Diagnosis

ESSENTIAL WORKUP

- History of a possible offending agent and time course of 4–14 days before onset of symptoms
- Physical examination revealing rash as well as joint, muscular, cardiac, neurologic, or renal insult

LABORATORY

- Decreased complement levels
- CBC, possible eosinophilia
- Elevated ESR
- Hypergammaglobulinemia
- Proteinuria or hematuria

IMAGING/SPECIAL TESTS

- Biopsy is the only means of definitive diagnosis

DIFFERENTIAL DIAGNOSIS

- Vasculitides (e.g., polyarteritis nodosa, Goodpasture's, Wegener's)
- Rashes (e.g., erythema multiforme, toxic epidermal necrolysis)
- Immunologic (e.g., SLE, polymyositis, anaphylaxis)
- Infectious (e.g., tick-borne disease, Rocky Mountain spotted fever, mononucleosis)

PEDIATRIC CONSIDERATIONS

- Drug-induced hypersensitivity syndrome (DIHS)
  - —Severe systemic involvement may occur
  - —May be a particularly challenging diagnosis given the nonspecific early presentation of fever and rash

Treatment

INITIAL STABILIZATION

- ABCs if a severe systemic reaction is present

ED TREATMENT

- Symptomatic relief until the disease spontaneously resolves in 13 weeks
- Antihistamines
- Antipyretics
- NSAIDs

MEDICATIONS

- Acetaminophen: 325–650 mg PO/PR (peds: 10–15 mg/kg) q4–6h
- Diphenhydramine: 50–100 mg (peds: 5 mg/kg/d, divided) q6–8h
- Ibuprofen: 200–800 mg PO (peds >6 months: 5–10 mg/kg) q6–8h
- Prednisone: 0.052 mg/kg PO (peds: 12 mg/kg) qd, 2 week taper

Disposition

ADMISSION CRITERIA

- Involvement of the airway
- Relapse of symptoms and signs after initial steroids and adrenalin
- Immunosuppression
- Concomitant serious disease
- Sociologic considerations

DISCHARGE CRITERIA

- Stable; most cases are self-limiting in 23 weeks

Miscellaneous

ICD9: 999.5

ICD10: T80.6

SUGGESTED READINGS

LoVecchio F, Curry SC, Welch S, et al. Incidence of immediate and delayed hypersensitivity to *Centruroides* antivenom. Ann Emerg Med 1999;34:615–619.

Piessens WF. Systemic immune complex disease. In: Ruddy S, ed. Kelley's textbook of rheumatology, 6th ed. Philadelphia: WB Saunders, 2001.

Poley GE, Slater JE. Drug and vaccine allergy. Immunol Allergy Clin North Am 1999;19:409–419.

Rosenwasser LJ. The vasculitic syndromes. In: Goldman L, ed. Cecil textbook of medicine, 21st ed. Philadelphia: WB Saunders, 2000:1525–1527.

Winkelstein JA, Fries LF. The complement system and immunopathology. In: Middleton E, ed. Allergy: principles and practice, 5th ed. St. Louis: Mosby Year Book, 1998:63–64.

Author: Kelly J. Corrigan

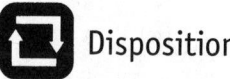

Sexual Assault

Clinical Presentation

SIGNS AND SYMPTOMS

- Victims might not disclose the assault
  - —67% of rape victims do not tell their doctors
  - —Most will reveal history only in response to direct questions
- Tachycardia or pounding heart beat
- Headaches
- Nausea
- Back pain
- Skin problems
- Menstrual symptoms
- Sudden weight change
- Sleeping disorders
- Abdominal pain
- Gagging
- Trouble breathing
- Associated injuries
  - —Of those with injuries, 70% report no injury at presentation
  - —Lacerations of perineum
  - —Vulvar trauma
  - —Laceration of vaginal wall (more common in younger patients near introitus)
  - —Multiple contusions
  - —Abrasions
  - —Human bite
  - —Lacerations or puncture wound to extremity
  - —Burns
  - —Depressed skull fracture

MECHANISM/DESCRIPTION

- Specific legal definition varies from state to state
- Defined as forced sexual contact without consent
  - —Continuum from unwanted touching and fondling to forced penetration of vagina, anus, oral cavity

ETIOLOGY

- 78–82% of female rape victims are raped by someone they know
- 50% of rape victims over 30 years old are assaulted by intimate partner
- Among women suffering physical abuse by a partner, 33–46% report being sexually assaulted
- Age distribution of female rape victims
  - —11–17 years old: 32%
  - —18–24 years old: 22%
  - —>50 years old: 22%

PEDIATRIC CONSIDERATIONS

- Must follow local laws regarding child abuse
- Patient most likely never had a pelvic exam previously
  - —If possible, involve specialist
- Use smallest speculum possible
- Use toys and dolls to have child explain what happened
- Early psychiatric intervention necessary

Pre-Hospital

CAUTIONS

- Assure patient of safety
- Discourage patient from:
  - —Changing clothes
  - —Eating
  - —Drinking
  - —Taking any medication
  - —Gargling
  - —Brushing teeth
  - —Urinating
  - —Defecating
  - —Douching
  - —Showering
- Keep history of assault to a minimum
  - —Repeated histories may retraumatize the patient
- Do not disturb evidence at rape site or on patient
- Do not examine genitalia
- If patient consents, contact local police per local protocol
  - —Including the patient in decision-making will help the patient regain sense of control and start healing

Diagnosis

ESSENTIAL WORKUP

- Obtain written consent prior to any exam, test, or treatment
- Allow patient to pause and proceed at comfortable pace
- Allow advocate to stay with patient during exam with patient's consent

History

- Obtain complete history even if patient does not wish to file charges, including:
  - —Time and place of assault
  - —Race of assailants
  - —Number of assailants
  - —Types of penetration: vaginal, oral, rectal
  - —Assailant ejaculation
  - —Use of force
  - —Victim's activity since assault
    - -Changed clothes
    - -Douched
    - -Bathed
    - -Urinated
    - -Defecated
    - -Ate
    - -Tampon use
  - —Full gynecologic history
  - —Last voluntary intercourse
    - -Sperm may be mobile up to 5 days in cervix and 12 hours in vagina
- Address all physical complaints

Physical Exam

- Use local evidence kit even if victim unsure if reporting to police
- Female chaperone required if male physician
- If clothes soiled, photograph prior to undressing with patient's consent
  - —Note general appearance of clothes
    - -Staining
    - -Tears
    - -Mud
    - -Leaves
    - -Wood's lamp for seminal stains
  - —Have patient disrobe while standing on a sheet and place all clothes in a paper bag
    - -Plastic causes mold and increases bacteria counts
    - -Have only patient handle clothing
    - -Arrange for a change of clothes
- Complete physical should be done with emphasis on:
  - —Abrasions
  - —Lacerations
  - —Bites
  - —Scratches
  - —Foreign bodies
  - —Ecchymoses
  - —Dried semen on skin
- Forensic collection
  - —Fingernail scrapings
  - —Head hair specimens

—If oral penetration, swab between teeth for acid phosphatase and sperm
—Throat culture for gonorrhea/chlamydia if oral sex
- Gynecologic exam
  —Explain all steps and allow patient to pace exam
  —Comb and collect pubic hair per local protocol
  —Lubricate speculum with water
  —Look for genital trauma even in asymptomatic patients
  —May use toluidine blue to identify small pelvic lacerations from traumatic intercourse
    -Best applied to vaginal mucus at introitus
  —Special attention to hymen as one of most common places for trauma
  —Lacerations to vaginal wall near introitus more common in younger patients
  —Aspirate secretions pooled in posterior fornix and place in sterile container to be examined for sperm and acid phosphates
    -If no secretions in posterior fornix, wipe with a cotton tip
    -Swab and microscopically examine for sperm and acid phosphates
  —Swabs for gonorrhea and chlamydia
    -Use of colposcope improves ability to note small lesions and gives ability to photograph findings
- Rectal exam if penetration or attempted penetration
  —Lacerations
  —Fissures
  —Bleeding
  —Gonorrhea and chlamydia cultures

LABORATORY

- Syphilis serology
- Hepatitis band C panel
- Blood type
- Pregnancy test
- Gonorrhea culture
- Chlamydia culture
- Other labs as needed based on injuries

Treatment

INITIAL STABILIZATION

- Treat life-threatening injuries

ED TREATMENT

- Place patient in quiet, private room
- Assure patient of confidentiality regarding name and reason for visit
- Regularly assure patient of safety
- Enforce nonjudgmental behavior by staff
- Designate nursing and medical provider for entire stay who are familiar with evidence collection kit
- Have sexual assault nurse examiner (SANE) perform exam if available
- Contact community or in-hospital advocate to stay with patient while in ED
- Alert hospital security to possibility of assailant presenting to ED
- Contact police if patient consents or local law requires
- Collect evidence as outlined above and according to local law
- Administer pregnancy prophylaxis if not currently pregnant
  —Hormonal therapy if within 72 hours
    -100 μg ethinyl estradiol stat and repeat in 12 hours
    -Decreases risk of pregnancy 60–90%
  —72 hours to 7 days postassault
    -Consult Ob/Gyn consult for possible IUD placement
    -Estimated risk of pregnancy is 2–4% if woman not using contraceptives
- Administer prophylactic therapy for gonorrhea and chlamydia
  —Doxycycline 100 mg PO b.i.d. for 7–10 days
  —Suprax 400 mg PO
- Consider prophylactic therapy for HIV

Disposition

ADMISSION CRITERIA

- Serious traumatic injury

DISCHARGE CRITERIA

- Medical follow-up to check culture results and future HIV testing
- Safe place for patient to go

Miscellaneous

ICD9: V71.5

ICD10: T74.2

SUGGESTED READINGS

Dunn SFM, Gilchrist VJ. Sexual assault. Prim Care 1993;20:359–373.

Dupre AR, Hampton HL, Morrison H, et al. Sexual assault. Obstet Gynecol Surv 1993;45:640–648.

Levine DL, Kaufman LE. Rape and sexual violence: the adult and adolescent female victim. In: Bernstein E, Bernstein J, eds. Case studies in emergency medicine and the health of the public. Boston: Jones & Bartlett, 1996:100–112.

Author: David Levine

Shock

Clinical Presentation

SIGNS AND SYMPTOMS

- Generalized shock
  —Hypotension
  —Decreased peripheral pulses
  —Tachycardia
  —Tachypnea
  —Decreased urine output
  —Diaphoresis
  —Anxiety
  —Obtundation
  —Lethargy
- Hypovolemic shock
  —Cold and clammy extremities
  —Pallor
  —Flattened neck veins
  —Decreased capillary refill
  —Narrowed pulse pressure
- Cardiogenic shock
  —Chest pain/pressure
  —Dyspnea
  —Orthopnea
  —Jugular venous distention
  —Cool, clammy, sweaty extremities
  —Rales
  —Wheezes
  —Dullness at lung bases
  —S3 gallop
- Septic shock
  —Warm flushed extremities
  —Strong pulses
  —Hyperthermia
  —Hypothermia
  —Purpura or petechial rash
- Anaphylactic shock
  —Warm flushed extremities
  —Urticaria
  —Stridor
  —Throat tightness
  —Hoarseness
  —Wheezing
- Neurogenic shock
  —Flaccid paralysis
  —Loss of rectal tone
  —Hypotension with bradycardia

MECHANISM/DESCRIPTION

- Supply of blood flow to tissues inadequate to meet the demands of the tissues
  —Nutrient requirements are not fulfilled
  —Toxic metabolites are not removed
- Main components of blood flow
  —Cardiac output
  —Blood volume
  —Peripheral resistance of arteriolar and venous system (systemic vascular resistance)

Major Categories of Shock

- Hypovolemic shock
  —Blood volume
    -Suspect hemorrhage if acute onset
    -Severe dehydration if progressive onset and elevated HCT, BUN, and creatinine
  —Decrease in central venous pressure (CVP)
  —Resultant decrease in cardiac output leads to compensatory increase of the systemic vascular resistance (SVR) in an attempt to normalize perfusion pressure
- Obstructive (cardiogenic) shock
  —Cardiac output
  —Venous congestion with increase in CVP
  —Increase in SVR
  —Causes of decreased cardiac output:
    -Cardiac dysfunction with reduced contractility
    -Obstruction to inflow of blood to the heart
    -Obstruction to outflow of blood to the heart
- Vasogenic shock
  —Decrease in vascular resistance secondary to excessive immunologic response to infection or antigen
  —Reflexive increase in cardiac output
  —Decreased central venous pressure
- Septic shock
  —An initial infectious insult overwhelms the immune system
  —Biochemical messengers (leukotrienes, histamines, prostaglandins) cause vessel dilatation
  —Capillary endothelium becomes disrupted and the vessels leak
  —Drop in total vascular resistance leads to inadequate tissue perfusion
  —Secondarily, decreased cardiac output resulting in cold septic shock
- Neurogenic shock
  —Spinal chord insults disrupts sympathetic stimulation to vessels
  —Loss of sympathetic tone causes arteriodilation and vasodilatation
  —Lesions proximal to T4 disrupt sympathetic, spares vagal innervation causing bradycardia
- Anaphylactic shock
  —An antigen stimulates the allergic reaction
    -Mast cells degranulate
    -Histamine release along with autocoids stimulate an anaphylaxis cascade
    -Vascular smooth muscle relaxes
    -Capillary endothelium leaks
    -Drop in total vascular resistance leads to inadequate tissue perfusion
- Pharmacologic agents may cause shock through smooth muscle dilation or myocardial depression

ETIOLOGIES

See Differential Diagnosis, below

PEDIATRIC CONSIDERATIONS

- Hypovolemic shock
  —Diarrhea causing volume depletion most common cause of pediatric shock worldwide
- Cardiogenic shock
  —Viral myocarditis
  —Drug ingestions
  —Postoperative cardiac surgery
  —Congenital heart disease
  —Pericardial tamponade
- Septic shock
  —*Haemophilus influenza*
  —*Neisseria meningitidis*
  —Streptococcal pneumonia

Pre-Hospital

- ABCs
- IV access
- Fluid resuscitation for hypotension when cardiogenic shock is *not* suspected

Diagnosis

ESSENTIAL WORKUP

- Identify type or types of shock present
- Identify underlying cause of shock

LABORATORY TESTS

- Hemoglobin/hematocrit
  - —Low hemoglobin and hematocrit—hemorrhage
  - —Very high hematocrit—dehydration
  - —Poor marker with acute hemorrhage
- White blood cell count
  - —High—nonspecific marker of infection
  - —Low—neutropenic infections
- Electrolytes
  - —Low CO_2—acidosis
  - —Increased BUN (GI hemorrhage)
  - —Increased Na, K, Cl, BUN/CR (dehydration)
- Blood glucose
  - —High (DKA or septic shock)
  - —Low (pediatric sepsis)
- PT/PTT
  - —Increased in DIC, septic shock, and liver disease
- Cardiac enzymes
- Urinalysis
  - —High glucose/ketones (DKA or septic shock)
  - —WBCs and bacteria when uroseptic
- Beta-HCG
  - —Women of childbearing age at risk for a ruptured ectopic pregnancy
- Lactic acid level
  - —Anaerobic metabolism of lactic acids when organ demands exceed nutrient supply
  - —Good surrogate marker of shock state

IMAGING/SPECIAL TESTS

- EKG
  - —Assess for ischemia and other disorders of cardiac muscle
  - —Electrical alternans with cardiac tamponade
  - —Right heart strain with pulmonary embolism
- Chest x-ray
  - —Pneumonia
  - —Pulmonary edema
  - —Pneumothorax
  - —Hemothorax
  - —Pulmonary infarction
  - —Traumatic injuries
- Echocardiography
  - —Tamponade
  - —Wall motion abnormalities (myocardial ischemia)
  - —LV collapse (pulmonary embolus)
  - —Aortic dissection
- Abdominal ultrasound
  - —Use to assess for intraperitoneal hemorrhage
  - —Ectopic pregnancy
- CT abdomen
  - —Requires that the patient first be stabilized
  - —In the setting of abdominal trauma and in search for suspicion of abdominal catastrophes and trauma

DIFFERENTIAL DIAGNOSIS

- Hypovolemic shock
  - —Abdominal trauma, blunt or penetrating
  - —Abortion—complete, partial, or inevitable
  - —Anemia—chronic or acute
  - —Aneurysms—abdominal, thoracic, dissecting
  - —Anorexia
  - —Aortogastric fistula
  - —Arteriovenous malformations
  - —Blunt trauma
  - —Bulimia
  - —Burns
  - —Diabetes
  - —Diarrhea
  - —Diuretics
  - —Ectopic pregnancy
  - —Epistaxis
  - —Fractures (especially long bones)
  - —Hemoptysis
  - —Lower GI bleed
  - —Malignancies
  - —Mallory-Weiss tear
  - —Penetrating trauma
  - —Placenta previa
  - —Postpartum hemorrhage
  - —Retroperitoneal bleeds
  - —Severe ascites
  - —Splenic rupture
  - —Toxic epidermal necrolysis
  - —Upper GI bleed
  - —Vascular injuries
  - —Vomiting

- Cardiogenic shock
  - —Cardiomyopathy
  - —Conduction abnormalities and arrhythmias
  - —Myocardial infarction
  - —Myocardial contusion
  - —Myocarditis
  - —Pericardial tamponade
  - —Pulmonary embolus
  - —Tension pneumothorax
  - —Valvular insufficiency
  - —Ventricular septal defect
- Vasogenic shock
  - —Acute respiratory distress syndrome
  - —Abscess
  - —Bacterial infection
  - —Bowel perforation
  - —Cellulitis
  - —Cholangitis
  - —Cholecystitis
  - —Endocarditis
  - —Endometritis
  - —Fungemia
  - —Infected indwelling prosthetic device
  - —Intraabdominal infection or abscess
  - —Mediastinitis
  - —Meningitis
  - —Myometritis
  - —Pelvic inflammatory disease
  - —Peritonitis
  - —Pyelonephritis
  - —Pharyngitis
  - —Pneumonia
  - —Sepsis
  - —Septic arthritis
  - —Thrombophlebitis
  - —Tubo-ovarian
  - —Urinary tract infection
- Anaphylactic
  - —Drug reaction
  - —Food allergy
  - —Insect sting
  - —Radiographic contrast materials
  - —Synthetic products
- Pharmacologic
  - —Antihypertensives
  - —Antidepressants
  - —Benzodiazepines
  - —Cholinergics
  - —Digoxin
  - —Narcotics
  - —Nitrates
- Neurogenic
  - —Spinal chord injury

Treatment

INITIAL STABILIZATION

- Large-bore IV access
- When possible central venous access and monitoring
- Fluid resuscitation in noncardiogenic shock patients
- Control bleeding with temporary measures
  - —Direct pressure
  - —Long bone traction
  - —External fixation of pelvis

ED TREATMENT

Hypovolemic Shock

- Identify source of volume depletion
- Aggressive fluid resuscitation keeping SBP >100 mm Hg until definitive treatment
  - —2–3 L crystalloid initially
  - —Transfuse packed red blood cells (0-negative if type specific unavailable) if 2–3 crystalloids do not correct pressure
- Identify source of bleeding and rapidly move toward definitive treatment
- Dopamine and epinephrine in refractory shock after maximal fluid and blood product resuscitation with delayed hemorrhage control
- Thoracotomy and aortic cross-clamping in refractory shock with penetrating torso trauma

Cardiogenic Shock

- Ease work of breathing with intubation
- Insult specific therapy (e.g., thrombolytics for MI, pericardiocentesis for pericardial tamponade)
- Treat dysrhythmias

Septic Shock

- Aggressive crystalloid fluid resuscitation
- Titrate fluid to urine output >30 cc/h
- Blood product transfusion to maintain Hct 30–35%
- Early antimicrobial therapy
- Inotropic support as needed
  - —Dopamine infusion
  - —Norepinephrine infusion

Anaphylactic Shock

- Intubation for airway compromise
- H-1 blockers (diphenhydramine)
- H-2 blockers (cimetidine)
- Corticosteroids (hydrocortisone or methylprednisolone)
- Nebulized β_2-antagonists for bronchospasm
- Epinephrine
  - —Subcutaneous in noncritical settings
  - —Intravenous drip for immediate life threats or refractory hypotension

Pharmacologic Shock

- Supportive therapy
- Decontamination of overdoses with charcoal
- Inotropic agents as needed
- Drug specific antidotes

Neurogenic Shock

- Supportive therapy
- Traction and fracture stabilization
- Corticosteroids

MEDICATIONS

- Albuterol 2.5 mg/2.5 cc nebulizer PRN
- Calcium gluconate 100–1,000 mg i.v.
- Cimetidine 300 mg i.v.
- Diphenhydramine 50–100 mg i.v. over 3 minutes
- Dobutamine 5–40 μg/kg/min i.v.
  - —Dopaminergic 1–3 μg/kg/min i.v.
  - —Beta effects 3–10 μg/kg/min i.v.
  - —Alpha/beta effects 10–20 μg/kg/min i.v.
  - —Alpha effects 20 μg/kg/min i.v.
- Epinephrine
  - —1–4 μg/min i.v. infusion
  - —SQ/IM 1:1000 0.1–0.3 mg repeat q 5–20 min $\times$ 3 PRN
  - —IV 1:100,000 10 mL over 10 min i.v.
- Glucagon 1–5 mg i.v. bolus initial, then 1–20 mg/h infusion
- Hydrocortisone 5–10 mg/kg i.v.
- Methylprednisolone 1–2 mg/kg i.v.
- Naloxone 0.01 mg/kg initial, titrate to effect
- Norepinephrine start 2–4 μg/min i.v., titrate up to 1–2 μg/kg/min i.v.
- Phenylephrine 40–180 μg/kg/min i.v.

Disposition

ADMISSION CRITERIA

- All patients in shock need to be admitted

ICU Criteria

- All patients with persisting shock need ICU monitoring
- Patients with shock definitively reversed may be admitted to non-ICU setting (e.g., tension pneumothorax that has been decompressed and chest tube placed)

DISCHARGE CRITERIA

- Patients who are in shock should not be discharged home from the ED

Miscellaneous

ICD9 CODE: 785.5, 785.51

ICD10: R57.9

SUGGESTED READINGS

Kline JA. Shock. In: Marx J, et al. eds. Rosen's emergency medicine: concepts and clinical practice. St. Louis: Mosby Year Book, 2000:33–47.

Rivers E, Nguyen B, Havstad S, et al. Early goal directed therapy in the treatment of severe sepsis and septic shock. N Engl J Med 2001;345:1368–1377.

Wheeler AP, Bernard GR. Treating patients with severe sepsis. N Engl J Med 1999;340:207–214.

Author: Nathan Shapiro

Shoulder Dislocation

Clinical Presentation

SIGNS AND SYMPTOMS

- Severe pain in the affected shoulder

Anterior Dislocation

- >90% of shoulder dislocations
- The shoulder is squared off with a prominent acromion process and palpable anterior fullness
- Arm is held in slight abduction and external rotation

Posterior Dislocation

- Often missed
- The coracoid process is prominent with a palpable posterior bulge
- Arm is held in slight adduction and internal rotation

Inferior Dislocation (Luxatio Erecta)

- Rare but easy to identify
- Arm is shortened and fixed above head; the patient's hand looks as if it were raised to ask a question
- Head of humerus may be palpable on the lateral chest wall

MECHANISM/DESCRIPTION

Anterior Dislocation

- Injury is from direct or indirect forces on the abducted and externally rotated arm
- Also may result from direct blow to posterior lateral aspect of shoulder

Posterior Dislocation

- Forces on the adducted and internally rotated arm result in posterior dislocation of humeral head in relation to glenoid fossa
- Most common mechanism is seizure and sudden contraction of all the posterior muscle groups
- Other mechanisms of injury include electrocution and direct blow to anterior shoulder

Inferior Dislocation (Luxatio Erecta)

- Hyperabduction of arm, tear of rotator cuff, and rotation of arm 180 degrees above head
- Commonly seen after a fall from a height where an arm strikes an object on descent and is thrust above the head

PEDIATRIC CONSIDERATIONS

- Dislocation is rare in children; epiphyseal fractures must be ruled out

Pre-Hospital

CAUTIONS

- Neurovascular injury should be identified and the arm splinted in the position of most comfort

Diagnosis

ESSENTIAL WORKUP

- Evaluate neurovascular status of the arm—sensory distribution of the axillary nerve corresponds to the lateral aspect of the shoulder
- Retest neurovascular status after any manipulation
- Dislocation requires prompt treatment, plain films of the shoulder should be obtained immediately
  - —The incidence of posttraumatic arthritis increases with length of time dislocated
- *Even in clinically obvious cases, films should be obtained before manipulation unless there will be a significant delay*
  - —An impacted humeral head fracture may be converted to a displaced humeral head fracture if manipulated
  - —Displaced fracture requires surgical repair and possible prosthesis

IMAGING/SPECIAL TESTS

- At least two views should be obtained
  - —Anteroposterior
  - —Trans-scapular Y or axillary view

Anterior Dislocation

- A posterolateral compression fracture of the humeral head (Hills-Sachs deformity) may be seen; corresponding lesion on glenoid fossa is the Bankart lesion
  - —These do not require treatment
  - —Reduction is not contraindicated
- Fractures of the greater tuberosity of the humeral head are seen in 15–35%; if there is >1 cm displacement after reduction, surgical intervention may be necessary

Posterior Dislocation

- Often missed on anteroposterior film
  - —Degree of overlap on x-ray film is smaller and displaced superiorly producing the "meniscus sign"
  - —Rotated humerus yields "light bulb on a stick" finding on anteroposterior view from lining up lesser and greater tuberosity
- Also, may see a "reverse Hill-Sachs deformity" from compression fracture of the anterior medial humeral head

DIFFERENTIAL DIAGNOSIS

- Fracture of the humeral head
- Fracture of the humeral shaft
- Acromioclavicular injury
- Septic shoulder joint
- Hemarthrosis in shoulder joint

Treatment

INITIAL STABILIZATION

- Exclude more serious injuries
- Ensure no injury to axillary vessels

ED TREATMENT

- Key to successful reduction is adequate analgesia and muscle relaxation
  —Conscious sedation with a short-acting opioid and a benzodiazepine
  —Recent success has also been reported using intraarticular lidocaine (20 mg of 1% lidocaine) injected into shoulder joint

Anterior Dislocation Reduction Techniques

- *Scapular manipulation*
  —Patient seated, traction to arm in horizontal plane, countertraction with other hand with clavicle
  —Second person adducts tip of scapula toward spine, opening shoulder joint
- *Stimson*
  —Patient placed in prone position on stretcher with arm dangling over side, hang 10–15 pounds around wrist; relax muscle over 20–30 minutes
  —Gently manipulate humeral head into place or use scapular manipulation
  —Only one person required
- *Traction/countertraction*
  —Patient in supine position, hold continuous longitudinal traction to arm
  —Gentle countertraction from sheet wrapped through axilla and across chest
  —Arm slightly internally or externally rotated if unsuccessful after several minutes
- *Hennipen*
  —Patient supine, elbow at 90 degrees, gentle, slow external rotation of arm, and finally slow elevation arm above head; must be done slowly with cooperative patient
- Leverage techniques such as the Kocher method are to be avoided because further injury can occur

Posterior Dislocation Reduction Techniques

- May use Stimson or traction/countertraction techniques with manipulation of humeral head anteriorly after muscles are sufficiently relaxed

Inferior Dislocation (Luxatio Erecta) Reduction Techniques

- Patient in supine position, gentle longitudinal traction to distract humeral head, gentle countertraction with sheet draped over trapezius and chest, and arm is slowly rotated from 180 to 0 degrees

Postreduction Care

- Plain films should be repeated after manipulation to confirm successful reduction
- Place in sling and swath or shoulder immobilizer immediately after reduction
- Shoulder should remain immobilized for 2–3 weeks in young patients; immobilization time should be less in older patients because they are at risk of frozen shoulder

MEDICATIONS

- Diazepam: 5–10 mg i.v. (peds: 0.2 mg/kg)
- Fentanyl: 50–100 g i.v. (peds: 2–4 g/kg)
- Meperidine: 50–100 mg i.v. (peds: 1 mg/kg)
- Methohexital: 1–1.5 mg/kg i.v. (peds: not routinely used)
- Midazolam: 2–5 mg i.v. (peds: 0.035–0.1 mg/kg)
- Morphine: 2–8 mg i.v. (peds: 0.1 mg/kg)

Disposition

ADMISSION CRITERIA

- Failure to reduce shoulder may require admission for reduction under general anesthesia or open reduction
- Patients with neurovascular compromise

DISCHARGE CRITERIA

- Successful reductions, confirmed by plain films, may be discharged with shoulder in appropriate immobilizer and with orthopedic follow-up
- Recurrent dislocation may require elective surgery
- Patients with residual neuropraxia from injury or manipulation may be safely discharged with instructions that most symptoms will resolve but should have neurology follow-up

Miscellaneous

ICD9: 831.00

ICD10: S43.0

SUGGESTED READINGS

Beeson MS. Complications of shoulder dislocations Am J Emerg 1999;17:288–295.

Hendley GW. Necessity of radiographs in the emergency department management of shoulder dislocations. Ann Emerg Med 2000;36:108–113.

McNamara RM. Reduction of anterior shoulder dislocations by scapular manipulation. Ann Emerg Med 1993;22:1140–1144.

Riebel GD, McCabe JB. Anterior shoulder dislocation: a review of reduction techniques. Am J Emerg Med 1991;9: 180–188.

Wen D. Current concepts in the treatment of anterior shoulder dislocations. Am J Emerg Med 1999;17:401–407.

Authors: G. Richard Bruno; Wallace Carter

Sick Sinus Syndrome

Clinical Presentation

SIGNS AND SYMPTOMS

- Asymptomatic
- Palpitations/fatigue
- Syncope/presyncope
- Chest pain
- Sudden death
- Bradycardia
- Alternating bradycardia and atrial tachycardia
- Altered mental status
- Transient ischemic attack/stroke
- Shortness of breath

MECHANISM/DESCRIPTION

- Caused by progressive degeneration of the cardiac conduction system
- Characterized by periods of unexplained sinus node dysfunction leading to bradyarrhythmias
- Dysfunction from failure of impulse generation or conduction to atrial tissue
- Syndrome includes
  —Chronic sinoatrial (SA) nodal dysfunction
  —Frequently depressed pacemakers
  —AV nodal conduction disturbances
  —Sluggish return of SA nodal activity after DC cardioversion

ETIOLOGY

Intrinsic Causes

- Coronary artery or SA nodal artery disease
- Cardiomyopathy
- Hypertensive heart disease
- Infiltrative cardiac or collagen vascular disease
- Surgical trauma
- Myocarditis

Extrinsic Causes

- Drugs
- Autonomically mediated syndromes
- Hyperkalemia/hypokalemia
- Ischemia
- Hypothyroidism
- Hypothermia
- Sepsis/infection

Pre-Hospital

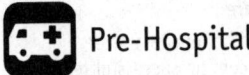

- ALS transport
- Cardiac monitoring
- Transcutaneous pacing for unstable patients

Diagnosis

ESSENTIAL WORKUP

- Ascertaining etiology
- 12-lead EKG

LABORATORY

- Serum electrolytes
- Cardiac markers
- Digoxin level, if appropriate

IMAGING/SPECIAL TESTS

- EKG may show
  —Inappropriate sinus bradycardia
  —Sinus pauses or sinus exit block
  —Atrial fibrillation with slow ventricular response
  —Prolonged pauses after cardioversion or carotid massage
  —Bradyarrhythmias may alternate with supraventricular tachydysrhythmias

DIFFERENTIAL DIAGNOSIS

- Other bradyarrhythmias
- Electrolyte derangements
- Medication toxicity: β-blockers, calcium channel blockers, clonidine, digoxin
- Excessive vagal tone

Treatment

INITIAL STABILIZATION

- Atropine *if* a bradydysrhythmia is causing unstable signs/symptoms: angina, mental confusion, or hypotension
- Transcutaneous pacing if atropine unsuccessful
- If this fails, emergent transvenous pacing

ED TREATMENT

- Supraventricular tachydysrhythmias alternating with bradycardia
  —Unstable
    -Cardiovert
    -Anticipate subsequent profound bradycardia
  —Stable patients
    -Digoxin, diltiazem, verapamil, or magnesium can be used
    -Any medication may cause profound bradycardia
- Bradycardias
  —Discontinuation of medications that alter sinus node function
  —Identifying other remediable causes of SA nodal depression
- Anticoagulation patients with atrial fibrillation and bradycardia/tachycardia syndrome

MEDICATIONS

- Atropine: 0.5 mg i.v. repeat every 5 minutes as necessary, maximum dose of 0.04 mg/kg (peds: 0.02 mg/kg, minimum, 0.1 mg)
- Digoxin: 0.5 mg i.v. initially then 0.25 mg i.v. q4h until desired effect
- Diltiazem: 0.25 mg/kg i.v. over 2 minutes followed in 15 minutes by 0.35 mg/kg i.v. over 2 minutes
- Heparin: load 80 IU/kg i.v.; infusion at 18 IU/kg/h
- Magnesium: 1–2 g i.v.
- Verapamil: 2.5–5 mg i.v. bolus over 2 minutes; may repeat with 5–10 mg every 15–30 minutes to maximum of 20 mg

Disposition

ADMISSION CRITERIA

- New onset
- Symptomatic: CHF, syncope, chest pain
- Persistent bradyarrhythmia or tachydysrhythmia
- Advanced age older than 60 years
- Patients should be admitted to a telemetry floor with cardiology consultation
- Most will require permanent pacing

DISCHARGE CRITERIA

- Asymptomatic otherwise healthy patients can be evaluated as outpatients
- Holter monitoring
- Exercise testing

Miscellaneous

ICD9: 427.81

ICD10: I49.5

SEE ALSO: BRADYDYSRHYTHMIAS

SUGGESTED READINGS

Kaushuk V, Leon A, Forrester J, et al. Bradyarrhythmias, temporary and permanent pacing. Crit Care Med 2000;28:N121–N128.

Mangrum J, DiMarco M. Primary care: the evaluation and management of bradycardia. N Engl J Med 2000;342:703–709.

Rubenstein JJ, Schulman CI, Yurchak PM, et al. Clinical spectrum of the sick sinus syndrome. Circulation 1972;46:5–13.

Authors: Shan Liu; David F.M. Brown

Sickle Cell Disease

Clinical Presentation

SIGNS AND SYMPTOMS

- May present with either
  - —Painful episode
  - —Complications of the disease
  - —Combination of above
- Acute painful episodes
  - —Bone/joint crisis
    - -Pain in extremities, back, sternum, or joints
    - -Variable swelling, warmth
    - -Variable joint effusion
    - -Hand-foot syndrome in infants
  - —Abdominal crisis
    - -Abdominal pain without peritonitis
    - -Variable nausea, vomiting, diarrhea
  - —Priapism—prolonged painful erection
- Complications/progression of disease
  - —Chest crisis (or syndrome)
    - -Pleuritic chest pain
    - -Cough with variable hemoptysis
    - -Dyspnea
    - -Tachypnea
    - -Rales
  - —Splenic sequestration crisis
    - -Abdominal pain
    - -Splenomegaly
    - -Variable nausea, vomiting
    - -Fatigue, lethargy
    - -Pallor
    - -Tachycardia
    - -Hypotension, syncope, shock
  - —Aplastic crisis
    - -Variable fever, headache, nausea, vomiting
    - -Fatigue
    - -Pallor
    - -Tachycardia
  - —Cerebrovascular accident/transient ischemic attack (TIA)
    - -Focal neurologic deficit
    - -Mental status changes
  - —Infections
    - -Fever
    - -Localizing signs

MECHANISM/DESCRIPTION

- Affects multiple organ systems
- Inherited autosomal-recessive disorder caused by a single amino acid substitution in hemoglobin gene
- Abnormal hemoglobin (hemoglobin S) polymerizes under stress, deforms RBC, resulting in hemolysis, vasoocclusion, tissue ischemia, and infarction
- Occurs in people of African, Mediterranean, Middle Eastern, and Indian descent
- Severity is variable, even among the same phenotype
- Vasoocclusion, ischemia, and infarction crises occur in essentially all organ systems
  - —Bone/joint crises
    - -Vasoocclusion of bone microvasculature causes infarction
    - -Dactylitis "hand-foot syndrome" occurs at ages 6–24 months
  - —Chest crisis or syndrome
    - -Vasoocclusion of pulmonary vasculature with infarcts
    - -Fat embolism, viral and bacterial infections may contribute
    - -High mortality (2–14%)
    - -More common in children
    - -Difficult to distinguish from pneumonia
  - —Splenic sequestration
    - -Splenic sinusoids become congested with sickled RBCs and obstruct outflow
    - -High mortality (12–20%)
    - -May be rapidly fatal
    - -More common in children younger than 5 years, rare in adults
  - —Aplastic crisis
    - -Bone marrow suppression usually occurs secondary to viral infection
    - -Increased baseline hemolysis in patients with sickle cell disease requires maximum erythropoiesis
    - -Decrease in hematocrit may be severe
    - -Generally self-limited
    - -More common in children
  - —Cerebrovascular accident/TIA
    - -Secondary to infarction in children; hemorrhage in adults
    - -Peak incidence between ages 9 and 15 years; prevalence 5–20%
    - -Often preceded by TIAs
  - —Bacterial infection
    - -Sepsis is the leading cause of death in patients with sickle cell disease
    - -Ability to fight encapsulated organisms is impaired secondary to decreased splenic function
    - -Children younger than 5 years have 400-fold increase in pneumococcal infections
    - -*Streptococcus pneumoniae, Haemophilus influenzae, Staphylococcus aureus, Escherichia coli,* and *Salmonella* are leading organisms
    - -Sites: lung, central nervous system, bone, kidney
- Genotypes/phenotypes/severity/incidence in African Americans:
  - —SS, sickle cell disease, marked severity, 0.3%
  - —SC, SC disease, mild to moderate severity, 0.1%
  - —Sβthal, β-thalassemia, mild to moderate severity, $<0.1\%$
  - —AS, sickle cell trait, no manifestation of disease, 8%

ETIOLOGY

- Common crisis precipitants
  - —Infection (bacterial and viral)
  - —Dehydration
  - —Hypoxemia
  - —Acidosis
  - —Surgery/trauma
  - —Weather changes
  - —Pregnancy
  - —Toxins

PEDIATRIC CONSIDERATIONS

- Infections commonly precipitate crisis
- Patients immunization history (pneumococcal and *H. influenzae*) must be confirmed
- Acute sickle cell complications in children carry high morbidity and should be screened for aggressively

Pre-Hospital

N/A

Diagnosis

ESSENTIAL WORKUP

- Thorough physical exam

LABORATORY

- CBC
  - —Anemia may be profound
  - —Compare with prior values if available
  - —Leukocytosis is common, does not necessarily indicate infection
- Reticulocyte count
  - —Generally elevated >5.0% in SS individuals
  - —A low count may indicate an aplastic crisis
- Consider the following if indicated
  - —Urinalysis
    - -Asymptomatic hematuria is a common finding
    - -Urinary tract infection may precipitate pain crisis and requires aggressive treatment
  - —Electrolytes, BUN/Cr, glucose
  - —Blood cultures
  - —Type and screen (or cross)

IMAGING/SPECIAL TESTS

- X-rays should be directed to confirm suspected diagnoses
  - —CXR if pneumonia or chest syndrome suspected
  - —Extremities if osteomyelitis suspected
  - —*IV contrast may exacerbate or precipitate a crisis*
- Head CT/MRI to evaluate stroke

DIFFERENTIAL DIAGNOSIS

- Sickle cell crises may mimic or obscure more serious underlying pathology (e.g., acute abdomen, myocardial infarction, nephrolithiasis)
  - —Suspect other diagnoses if pain is more severe or atypical

Treatment

INITIAL STABILIZATION

- Identify and treat high morbidity complications
  - —Sepsis
  - —Splenic sequestration
  - —Chest crisis
  - —CVA
- Assess pain and initiate therapy

ED TREATMENT

- Analgesia
  - —Choice of analgesic agent depends on patient, severity of episode, and prior agents
  - —Evaluate patient frequently and titrate medications accordingly for relief of pain
- Hydration
  - —1.5–2 times maintenance after correction of deficits
  - —Oral hydration if patient can tolerate fluids by mouth
  - —Parenteral IV solution 0.45% NS for adults and children, or 0.2% NS for infants
  - —Monitor fluids closely
- Complication-specific therapy
  - —Oxygen: chest syndrome, pneumonia
  - —Antibiotics: sepsis, pneumonia, osteomyelitis
  - —Acute simple transfusion: sequestration crisis, blood loss, accelerated hemolysis
  - —Exchange transfusion may be required for more severe complications: cerebrovascular accident

MEDICATIONS

- *Severe/moderate pain*
  - —Hydrocodone: 0.15/mg/kg/dose PO q4h
  - —Hydromorphone: 0.01–0.02 mg/kg/dose i.v. q3–4h or 0.04–0.06 mg/kg/dose PO q4h
  - —Ketorolac: 30 mg i.v. initial, then 15–30 mg q6–8h
  - —Meperidine: 0.75–1.5 mg/kg/dose i.v. q2–4h
  - —Morphine: 0.1–0.15 mg/kg/dose i.v. q3–4h or 0.3–0.6 mg/kg/dose PO q4h
- *Mild pain*
  - —Acetaminophen: 1 g (peds: 15 mg/kg/dose) PO q4h
  - —Codeine: 0.5–1 mg/kg/dose PO
  - —Ibuprofen: 800 mg (peds: 5–10 mg/kg/dose) PO q8h

Disposition

ADMISSION CRITERIA

- Refractory pain crisis
- Signs of bacterial infection or fever of undetermined etiology
- Chest syndrome
- Sequestration crisis
- Aplastic crisis
- Cerebrovascular accident or TIA
- Refractory priapism
- Symptomatic anemia

DISCHARGE CRITERIA

- Resolution of pain crisis
- No indications for admission

Miscellaneous

ICD9: 282.60

ICD10: D57.1

SUGGESTED READINGS

Beutler E. Sickle cell anemia. In: Beutler E, et al, eds. Williams hematology, 6th ed. New York: McGraw-Hill, 2001:581–605.

Pollack CV. Emergencies in sickle cell disease. Emerg Med Clin North Am 1993;11:365.

Reed W, Vinchinsky EP. New considerations in the treatment of sickle cell disease. Annu Rev Med 1998;49:461.

Reid C, Carache S, Lubin B, eds. Management and therapy of sickle cell disease. Washington, DC: National Institutes of Health, 1995. Publication no. 95-2117.

Steinberg M. Management of sickle cell disease. N Engl J Med 1999;340(13):1021.

Stephens C. Sickle cell disease: a review of the state-of-the-art emergency management and outcome-effective therapy. Emerg Med Rep 1999;20(18):183.

Wang W, et al. Sickle cell anemia and other sickling syndromes. In: Lee G, et al, eds. Wintrobe's clinical hematology, 10th ed. Baltimore: Lippincott Williams & Wilkins, 1999:1346–1397.

Author: Steven Bowman

Sinusitis

Clinical Presentation

SIGNS AND SYMPTOMS

- Facial pain
- Headache
- Halitosis
- Cough
- Purulent nasal discharge
- Fever
- Edema of the nasal mucous membranes
- Pus in the nares or posterior pharynx
- Warmth, tenderness, and possibly cellulitis over the affected sinus
- Frontal sinusitis
  - —Pain of the lower forehead
  - —Pain worsened when lying on the back and improves when upright
- Maxillary sinusitis
  - —Malar facial pain
  - —Maxillary dental pain
  - —Referred ear pain
  - —Pain worsens with head upright and improves with inclining
- Ethmoid sinusitis
  - —Retroorbital pain
  - —Periorbital edema
- Sphenoid sinusitis (very uncommon)
  - —Pain over the occiput or mastoid
  - —Pain worse when lying on back or bending forward
- Recent history of nasotracheal intubation suggests nosocomial sinusitis
  - —Involves atypical pathogens such as *Pseudomonas* and gram-negative organisms
- Rhinocerebral mucormycosis
  - —Rare but rapidly progressive fungal infection
  - —Occurs in diabetic and other immunocompromised patients
  - —Orbital and facial pain out of proportion to physical signs
  - —Lethargy, headache in a systemically ill appearing patient
  - —Black eschar or pale area on the palate or nasal mucosa

MECHANISM/DESCRIPTION

- Sinusitis is inflammation of the mucous membranes lining the paranasal sinuses
- Acute bacterial sinusitis is diagnosed when signs and symptoms last fewer than 3–4 weeks
- Subacute sinusitis occurs when signs and symptoms last 3 weeks to 3 months
- Chronic sinusitis occurs when signs and symptoms last longer than 3 months in spite of antibiotic treatment
- Nosocomial sinusitis is associated with nasogastric and nasotracheal tubes

ETIOLOGY

- Viral sinusitis is 20 to 200 times more common than bacterial sinusitis
- Complication of simple viral upper respiratory tract infection or allergic rhinitis
- As mucous membranes become inflamed, sinus ostia narrow and block drainage
- Air is absorbed and negative pressure develops, resulting in transudate formation
- Bacteria are trapped and multiply resulting in suppuration and converting the viral infection to a bacterial infection
- Foreign bodies, nasal polyps, tumors, or traumatic fractures can lead to obstruction of ostia
- Immunocompromised patients and patients with impaired mucociliary movement are also predisposed to sinusitis
- Pathogens
  - —Acute sinusitis
    - -*Haemophilus influenzae*
    - -*Streptococcus pneumoniae*
    - -*Moraxella catarrhalis*
    - -*Staphylococcus aureus*
  - —Chronic sinusitis
    - -*Peptostreptococcus*
    - -*Fusobacterium*
    - -*Bacteroides*
    - -*Aspergillus*
  - —Nosocomial sinusitis
    - -*S. aureus*
    - -*Pseudomonas*
    - -*Klebsiella*
  - —Immunocompromised patients with sinusitis
    - -The usual bacterial pathogens
    - -Fungal pathogens (*Aspergillus)*

Complications

- Osteomyelitis
- Extension into the CNS
  - —Seizures
  - —Focal neurologic signs
  - —Cranial nerve palsies
  - —Altered level of consciousness
  - —Meningitis
  - —Subdural empyema
  - —Epidural abscess
  - —Cavernous sinus thrombosis
  - —Brain abscess
- Periorbital cellulitis
- Orbital cellulitis
  - —Periorbital swelling, fever, ptosis, proptosis, papilledema, and painful or decreased extraocular movements
  - —Most frequently a complication of ethmoid sinusitis in children
  - —Cranial nerve III, IV, and VI palsies
- Pott's puffy tumor
  - —A focal, doughy mass localized to the forehead
  - —Indicative of osteomyelitis of the frontal bone

PEDIATRIC CONSIDERATIONS

- Ethmoid and maxillary sinuses are present at birth
- Frontal and sphenoid sinuses do not emerge until age 6–7 years
- Sinusitis is more common in children than adults
- Periorbital/orbital cellulitis is a common complication of ethmoid sinusitis in children
  - —Periorbital swelling, fever, ptosis, proptosis, and painful or decreased extraocular movements

Pre-Hospital

N/A

Diagnosis

ESSENTIAL WORKUP

- Clinical diagnosis based on history and physical exam
- Transillumination is not a reliable indicator of sinus disease
- Imaging is unnecessary in uncomplicated cases (see below)

LABORATORY

- Laboratory studies are not helpful for diagnosis or management

IMAGING/SPECIAL TESTS

- Plain film radiography
  - —Normal plain films do not rule out bacterial involvement
  - —A Water's view may help in the diagnosis of maxillary sinusitis
  - —Opacification or air fluid level in involved sinus
- CT
  - —Preferred to plain films if imaging is necessary
  - —May assist in diagnosing complications of sinusitis

DIFFERENTIAL DIAGNOSIS

- Migraine and cluster headache
- Dental pain
- Trigeminal neuralgia
- TMJ disorders
- Temporal arteritis
- Uncomplicated viral or allergic rhinitis
- Nasal polyp, tumor, or foreign body
- CNS infection

Treatment

INITIAL STABILIZATION

- Toxic-appearing patients may require airway intervention and fluid resuscitation
  —First dose of antibiotics in ED

ED TREATMENT

- Cost-effective approach favors appropriate antibiotic therapy and no testing
- Establishing good drainage with topical or oral decongestants and muco-evacuants
- Reducing edema with topical corticosteroids in chronic sinusitis
- Humidification and saline spray are beneficial adjunct to pharmacologic therapy

Antibiotics

- Reserve antibiotics for patients with
  —Pain and discharge for more than 7 days in spite of decongestant and analgesic treatment
  —Severe symptoms
- Acute sinusitis: antibiotic choices if no antibiotic treatment in the previous month
  —Amoxicillin, amoxicillin-clavulanate, cefpodoxime, or cefuroxime
- Acute sinusitis: antibiotic choices if antibiotic treatment in the previous month (>30% risk of drug resistant *S. pneumoniae*)
  —Amoxicillin-clavulanate, gatifloxacin (adult), levofloxacin (adult), moxifloxacin (adult)
- Acute sinusitis: clinical failure after 3 days of antibiotic treatment
  —Amoxicillin-clavulanate or cefpodoxime (mild to moderate disease)
  —Gatifloxacin, levofloxacin, moxifloxacin (severe disease in adults)
- Acute sinusitis: patient with penicillin or cephalosporin allergy
  —Clarithromycin, azithromycin, trimethoprim-sulfamethoxazole, doxycycline, erythromycin ethyl succinate/sulfamethoxazole, gatifloxacin, levofloxacin, moxifloxacin, or trimethoprim-sulfamethoxazole
- Acute sinusitis: aspergillosis
  —ENT consultation
- Chronic sinusitis
  —Antibiotics are usually not helpful
  —ENT consultation

MEDICATIONS

- Amoxicillin: 250–500 mg PO t.i.d. (peds: 40 mg/kg/d PO t.i.d.)
- Amoxicillin-clavulanate: 250–500 mg PO t.i.d. (peds: 40 mg/kg/d, based on the amoxicillin component, PO t.i.d.)
- Azithromycin: 250–600 mg PO q.d. (peds: 5–10 mg/kg/d, based on the amoxicillin component, PO)
- Cefpodoxime: 100–400 mg PO b.i.d. (peds: 10 mg/kg/d PO b.i.d.)
- Cefuroxime: 250–500 mg PO b.i.d. (peds: 20–30 mg/kg/d PO b.i.d.)
- Clarithromycin: 250–500 mg PO b.i.d. (peds: 7.5 mg/kg/d PO b.i.d.)
- Doxycycline: 100 mg PO b.i.d.
- Erythromycin ethyl succinate-sulfamethoxazole: 50 mg/kg/d (based on the erythromycin component) PO t.i.d. to q.i.d. (peds)
- Gatifloxacin: 400 mg PO q.d. (adult)
- Levofloxacin: 250–500 mg PO q.d. (adult)
- Moxifloxacin: 400 mg PO q.d. (adult)
- Trimethoprim-sulfamethoxazole: 1 double-strength tablet PO b.i.d. (peds: 8–12 mg/kg/d, based on the trimethoprim component, PO b.i.d.)

Decongestants

- Topical: not to be used for 3 days
- Oxymetazoline hydrochloride 0.05%: 2–3 gtt or sprays per nostril b.i.d.
- Phenylephrine hydrochloride 0.5%: 2–3 sprays per nostril q3–4h; oral: if longer than 3 days of treatment
- Pseudoephedrine: 60 mg PO q4–6h

Muco-evacuants

- Guaifenesin: 5–20 mL PO q4h (peds: 5–10 mL/dose if 6–12 years old, 2.5–5 mL if 2–6 years old)

Corticosteroids for Chronic Sinusitis

- Beclomethasone dipropionate: 1 spray/nostril b.i.d./t.i.d.
- Dexamethasone sodium phosphate: 2 sprays/nostril b.i.d./t.i.d.

Disposition

ADMISSION CRITERIA

- Evidence of spread of infection beyond the sinus cavity
- Toxic-appearing patients
- Immunocompromised/diabetic patients with extensive infection
- Multiple sinus involvement
- Frontal sinus involvement
- Extremes of age
- Severe comorbidity
- ENT evaluation and aspiration if patient is severely ill, immunocompromised, or pansinusitis and ill appearing

DISCHARGE CRITERIA

- Most cases of uncomplicated sinusitis may be managed as outpatients
- Follow-up with PCP or ENT if symptoms persist >7 days despite antibiotic therapy

Miscellaneous

ICD9: 473.9

ICD10: J32.9

SUGGESTED READINGS

Combs JT: Antibiotics and sinusitis. Pediatrics 2001;108(6):1387–1388.

Josephson GD, Gross CW. Diagnosis & management of acute & chronic sinusitis. Comp Ther 1997;23(11):708–714.

Poole MD: A focus on acute sinusitis in adults: changes in disease management. Am J Med 1999;106(5A):38S–47S, 48S–52S.

Slavin RG: Sinusitis: current diagnostic and treatment strategies. Am J Ther 1996;3(7):525–528.

Author: Lee Shockley

Skin Cancer

Clinical Presentation

SIGNS AND SYMPTOMS

Basal Cell Carcinoma

- Papule or nodule with waxy or pearly appearance
- Often have central depression or erosion
- May be single or multiple
- Pigmented form may be brownish or stippled
- Usually painless
- Rarely metastasize, may be locally invasive
- Usually appear in sun-exposed areas of skin

Melanoma

- Pigmented skin lesion
- Features suggestive of melanoma: the *ABCDs* of melanoma
  - —*A*symmetry (not regularly round or oval)
  - —*B*order irregularity (notched or poorly defined), *Bleeding* (spontaneous)
  - —*C*olor variegation (shades or combinations of brown, tan, red, white, or blue-black)
  - —*D*iameter >6 mm
- Lesions rarely symptomatic unless ulcerated
- Malignant melanoma
  - —Presentation related to affected organ system
  - —Lymphangitic spread with local to regional lymphadenopathy
  - —Typical visceral sites of hematogenous spread include liver, lung, bone, and brain

MECHANISM/DESCRIPTION

Basal Cell Carcinoma

- Arise from epidermis and cytologically resemble normal basal cells
- >75% of all skin cancers
- Most important risk factor is sun exposure

Melanoma

- Arise from melanin-producing cells
- Most important risk factor is sun exposure, especially sunburns
- Additional risk factors: multiple common melanocytic nevi, atypical nevi, immunosuppression, positive family history, history of nonmelanoma skin cancer (basal cell or squamous cell carcinoma)

Pre-Hospital

N/A

Diagnosis

ESSENTIAL WORKUP

- Suspicious lesions require biopsy, rarely done in ED

LABORATORY

- No specific testing required, liver enzyme/function tests if suspicion of metastatic melanoma

IMAGING/SPECIAL TESTS

- CXR may show pulmonary involvement by metastatic melanoma
- Head or body CT may show visceral involvement by metastatic melanoma

DIFFERENTIAL DIAGNOSIS

- For basal cell carcinoma includes
  - —Squamous cell carcinoma
  - —Bowen's disease
  - —Actinic keratosis
  - —Paget's disease
  - —Benign nevus
  - —Melanoma
- For melanoma includes
  - —Atypical nevus
  - —Common nevus
  - —Actinic keratosis
  - —Pigmented basal cell carcinoma
  - —Squamous cell carcinoma

Treatment

INITIAL STABILIZATION

N/A

ED TREATMENT

- Only specific ED treatment is directed toward possible complications of visceral involvement by metastatic melanoma or locally invasive basal cell carcinoma

Disposition

ADMISSION CRITERIA

- Usually dependent on complications of visceral involvement or invasive spread
- Rarely required due to skin lesions per se

DISCHARGE CRITERIA

- Patients with suspected skin cancer may be discharged with prompt referral to a dermatologist or experienced PCP

Miscellaneous

ICD9: 173.9; 172.9

ICD10: C43.9

SUGGESTED READINGS

Lear JT, Smith AG. Basal cell carcinoma. Postgrad Med J 1997;41:538.

Marks R. An overview of skin cancers: Incidence and causation. Cancer 1995; 75:607–612.

Rivers JK. Melanoma. Lancet 1996;347: 803–807.

Author: Michael K. Doney

Sleep Apnea

Clinical Presentation

SIGNS AND SYMPTOMS

- Snoring in combination with observed apnea
- Daytime drowsiness
- Sleep disturbance
- Irritability
- Predisposing physical features
  —Obesity
  —Craniofacial anomalies
  —Enlarged tonsils
- Signs of chronic disease
  —Hypertension
  —Elevated jugular veins (secondary to pulmonary hypertension)

Associated Emergencies

- Dysrhythmias
- Right and left heart failure
- Hypertension poorly controlled by medical therapies
- Myocardial infarction
- Stroke
- Motor-vehicle accidents

MECHANISM/DESCRIPTION

- Airway closing at the level of nasopharynx or oropharynx during sleep
  —Decreased tone during REM sleep
- Groups at risk
  —Obese
  —Men
  —Age older than 40 years
  —Upper airway anomalies
  —Hypertrophy
  —Myxedema (hypothyroidism)
  —Alcohol/sedative abuse
  —Long-distance truck drivers
- Associated illness
  —Dysrhythmias
  —Right and left heart failure
  —Myocardial infarction
  —Stroke
  —Motor-vehicle accidents

Pre-Hospital

- Supplemental oxygen

Diagnosis

ESSENTIAL WORKUP

- Pulse oximetry
- EKG
- CXR
- A sleep study (polysomnogram)
  —Required for diagnosis
  —Never indicated as part of the emergency evaluation

LABORATORY

- ABG

IMAGING/SPECIAL TESTS

- Lateral neck soft tissue radiograph to rule out other etiologies of upper airway obstruction
- Neck/chest CT rarely indicated in the ED

DIFFERENTIAL DIAGNOSIS

- Central sleep apnea
  —Neurologic, rather than obstructive, cause of apnea during sleep
- COPD
- Asthma
- Left heart failure
- Primary pulmonary hypertension
- Narcolepsy
- Idiopathic hypersomnia

Treatment

INITIAL STABILIZATION

- Chin lift/jaw thrust maneuver, oxygen as needed, oral or nasal airway devices

ED TREATMENT

- Mask ventilation with continuous positive airway pressure (CPAP)
- Endotracheal intubation
  —Often difficult to intubate
  —Early on, plan several possible methods of definitive airway control
  —If intubation required and likely to be difficult, consider blind nasotracheal or fiberoptic-guided nasotracheal intubation in lieu of oral rapid-sequence intubation
  —Be prepared to perform cricothyroidotomy if necessary
  —Use neuromuscular blockade only if successful oral intubation is likely and bag ventilation is easy
- Positive end-expiratory pressure (PEEP) for ventilated patients

MEDICATIONS

- No specific medications useful in ED to treat this chronic disorder
- See Airway Management for details on induction agents and neuromuscular blockade

Disposition

ADMISSION CRITERIA

- Ventilatory failure, especially if intubation was necessary
- Hemodynamic instability

DISCHARGE CRITERIA

- Maintenance of O_2 saturation $>85\%$ for several hours using oxygenation or ventilation equipment available to the patient at home
- Very low likelihood of decompensation overnight
- Patients with sleep apnea who present after motor-vehicle crashes should be managed initially like other blunt trauma patients but at some point require discussion about the increased risk with sleep apnea and require intervention to prevent future accidents

Miscellaneous

ICD9: 780.57

ICD10: G47.3

SUGGESTED READINGS

American Thoracic Society. Sleep apnea, sleepiness, and driving risk. Am J Respir Crit Care Med 1994;150[Suppl 5, Pt 1]: 1463–1473.

Fuchs BD, McMaster J, Smull G, et al. Underappreciation of sleep disorders as a cause of motor vehicle crashes. Am J Emerg Med 2001;19(7):575–578.

Hudgel DW. Treatment of obstructive sleep apnea. Chest 1996;109:1346–1358.

Hung J, Whitford EG, Parsons RW, et al. Association of sleep apnoea with myocardial infarction in men. Lancet 1990;336(8710):261–264.

Man GCW. Obstructive sleep apnea: diagnosis and treatment. Med Clin North Am 1996;80(4):804–820.

Obenza Nishime E, Liu LC, Coulter TD, et al. Heart failure and sleep-related breathing disorders. Cardiol Rev 2000;8(4):191–201.

Pakola SJ, Dinges DF, Pack AI. Review of regulations and guidelines for commercial and noncommercial drivers with sleep apnea and narcolepsy. Sleep 1995;18(9): 787–796.

Ray RM, Senders CW. Airway management in the obese child. Pediatr Clin North Am 2001;48(4):1055–1063.

Strollo PJ, Rogers RM. Obstructive sleep apnea. N Engl J Med 1996;334(2):99–101.

Victor LD. Obstructive sleep apnea. Am Fam Physician 1999;60(8):2279–2286.

Wright J, White J. Continuous positive airways pressure for obstructive sleep apnoea. Cochrane Database Syst Rev 2000;(2):CD001106.

Young T, Peppard PE, Gottlieb DJ. Epidemiology of obstructive sleep apnea: a population health perspective. Am J Respir Crit Care Med 2002;165(9):1217–1239.

Author: Mark Sagarin

Slipped Capital Femoral Epiphysis

Clinical Presentation

SIGNS AND SYMPTOMS

- Older child or adolescent
- Presents with limp or exertional limp
- Pain in the knee, thigh, groin, or hip (referral of pain along the obturator nerve)
  - —Vague and dull for weeks in chronic slipped capital femoral epiphysis (SCFE)
  - —Severe and sudden onset in an acute SCFE
- Commonly presents with the leg externally rotated
- Flexion is restricted (cannot touch thigh to abdomen)
- Often a history of minor trauma

MECHANISM/DESCRIPTION

- Femoral epiphysis translates or "slips" relative to the femoral head/neck
  - —Classified as: Mild (<⅓ translation), moderate (<⅓–½ translation) and severe (>½ translation)
- Peak age at onset 13–15 years for boys and 11–13 years for girls
- Most patients are obese
- Male patients predominate (8:3)
- Approximately one third of cases involve bilateral joints

Pre-Hospital

- Patient should be immobilized for transport, as with suspected hip fracture or dislocation

Diagnosis

ESSENTIAL WORKUP

- Anteroposterior and frog-leg lateral x-ray films of *both* hips should be obtained
  - —Widened or irregular physis
  - —Bird's beak appearance of the actual slipping of the epiphysis off of the femoral head
  - —Klein's line (lateral femoral neck parallel does not transect epiphysis)

LABORATORY

- Without diagnostic radiographic abnormality, the practitioner should consider the following tests to help risk stratify possible alternative diagnoses
- CBC count with differential
- Sedimentation rate
- C-reactive protein

DIFFERENTIAL DIAGNOSIS

- Legg-Calve-Perthes
  - —Typically seen in 4-9-year-old age range
- Septic arthritis of hip
- Osteomyelitis
- Femur or pelvic fractures

Treatment

INITIAL STABILIZATION

- Immobilize hip
- Keep non-weight-bearing
- Do not attempt reduction

ED TREATMENT

- SCFE is an urgent orthopedic condition; delay in diagnosis may lead to chronic irreversible hip joint disability
- Refer immediately to orthopedics for definitive immobilization and operative intervention

Disposition

ADMISSION CRITERIA

- Patients with SCFE require orthopedic admission for urgent operative fixation (usually single central pinning)

DISCHARGE CRITERIA

- None
  —It is too difficult to achieve complete non-weight-bearing status, which is required to prevent further slippage, avascular necrosis, and chondrolysis

Miscellaneous

ICD9: 732.2

ICD10: M93.9

SUGGESTED READINGS

Aronsson DD, Loder RT. Treatment of the unstable (acute) slipped capital femoral epiphysis. Clin Orthop Related Res 1996;322:99–110.

Causey AL, Smith ER, Donaldson JJ, et al. Missed slipped capital femoral epiphysis: illustrative cases and a review. J Emerg Med 1995;13(2):175–189.

Loder RT. Slipped capital femoral epiphysis. Am Fam Physician 1998;57(9):2135–2142.

Author: Judd Glasser

Small Bowel Injury

Clinical Presentation

SIGNS AND SYMPTOMS

- Delays in diagnosis are common secondary to lack of early consistent clinical findings
- Initial presentation may be mild, uniformly patients will progress to manifest serious signs/symptoms
- Awake, alert patients: abdominal tenderness (87–98%), abdominal pain (85%), peritoneal signs (67%)
- Abdominal wall bruising (54%), hypotension (38%), guaiac (+) rectal exam (5%)
- Small bowel injury (SBI) may initially be obscured by abnormal mental status, severe associated injuries
- Progressive abdominal pain, intestinal obstruction, decreased urine output, tachycardia may indicate SBI not initially apparent
- Delays in diagnosis add to morbidity and mortality
  —Mortality with diagnosis within 8 hours is 2%, diagnosis made after 24 hours is 31%

MECHANISM/DESCRIPTION

Penetrating

- Visceral injury (96% gunshot wound, 50% stabbing)
  —Serosal tear, bowel wall hematoma, perforation, bowel transection, mesenteric hematoma/vascular injury

Blunt

- Perforation is twice as common as mesenteric injuries
- Deceleration injury at fixed points like the ligament of Treitz
- Shearing mechanisms near fixed points like the ileocecal junction, adhesions
- Compressive force against anterior spine
- Bursting or "blowout" at antimesenteric margin from sudden closed-loop intraluminal pressure rise
- Mesenteric tears may initially be asymptomatic
- Associated injuries
  —Liver and splenic lacerations, thoracic and pelvic fractures
  —Seat-belt syndrome: abdominal wall ecchymosis, small bowel injury; chance fracture of L-1, L-2

ETIOLOGY

Penetrating

- Small bowel is the second most common injured organ (32%) in anterior abdominal stabbing
- SBI most common in gunshot wounds (49%)
- 80% of SBIs are caused by gunshot wounds, 60% by stab wounds

Blunt

- Third most commonly injured organ (5–10% of all blunt trauma victims)
- Lap belts (incorrect use of restraints is the most important cause)
- Motor-vehicle accidents
- Nonvehicular trauma: abuse/assault, bicycle handlebars, large animal kick

PEDIATRIC CONSIDERATIONS

Penetrating

- Air-gun accidents at close range (<10 feet)

Blunt

- Less common in children (1–8% of all blunt pediatric trauma)
- Wearing both shoulder and lap belts less likely to have intestinal injury

Pre-Hospital

CAUTIONS

- Patients should be transported to the nearest trauma center
- Do not attempt to replace eviscerated abdominal contents, cover with moist gauze, blanket and transport
- Do not remove impaled objects in the abdomen, stabilize the object with gauze and tape and transport

Diagnosis

ESSENTIAL WORKUP

- Initial physical exam noting all wounds and areas of tenderness
- Serial abdominal exams and vital signs
- For stable patients, abdominal CT
- For unstable injury, diagnostic peritoneal lavage (DPL) is superior to US in suggesting hollow viscus injuries

LABORATORY

- No diagnostic test has proven extremely sensitive in predicting SBI
- Baseline CBC, electrolytes, BUN, creatinine, ABG, type and screen, and UA
- Serum amylase, lipase and liver function tests have poor sensitivity for acute injury

IMAGING/SPECIAL TESTS

Plain Radiography (Chest/Abdomen)

- Not useful for SBI
- Poor sensitivity for free air (10–30%); <50% of perforations show free air

Computed Tomography

- CT is the diagnostic standard for solid-organ injury and head trauma but is less sensitive for hollow viscous injuries (up to 30% false-negative CT rate)
- Blunt trauma
  —Used in stable patients
  —Indications in blunt trauma include:
  —Abdominal distention, absent bowel sounds, blood in the NGT
  —Abdominal abrasions or contusions, gross hematuria, lap-belt injury
  —Assault/abuse as mechanism, abdominal tenderness, trauma score <12
  —Specific signs for SBI on CT are pneumoperitoneum and extravasation of luminal or vascular contrast
  —Suggestive signs of SBI include unexplained free intraperitoneal fluid (most sensitive 73%), thickened bowel wall >3 mm (35% sensitive), intramural hematomas (75–88% sensitive), interloop fluid, mesenteric streaking
- Penetrating
  —CT not recommended (sensitivity only 14%, false-negative rate of 18%)

DPL

- Invasive but helpful in unstable patients or clinically suspicious but nondiagnostic abdominal CT
  - —Sensitive for hemoperitoneum but not source specific
  - —Positive if >100,000 RBCs
  - —Lavage amylase (>20 IU/L) and WBC count (>500/mm^3) helpful but late markers of SBI
  - —Lavage microscopy for succus/vegetable matter is specific for SBI but not sensitive
  - —Lavage alkaline phosphatase (>3 IU/L) is reported to be a useful immediate marker of SBI

Ultrasonography

- Little clinical US experience, operator dependent, not sensitive in hollow viscous injury, because air in bowel makes visualization difficult

Laparoscopy

- May play a role in diagnosing SBI in stable patients with progressive signs or symptoms

DIFFERENTIAL DIAGNOSIS

- Hemoperitoneum due to vascular insult
- Solid visceral organ injury or gastric/colon/rectum perforation
- Vertebral injury and associated ileus

PEDIATRIC CONSIDERATIONS

- Delay in diagnosis 1–2 days is common and may increase morbidity

Treatment

INITIAL STABILIZATION

- Standard ATLS protocols including ABCs of multiple trauma care
- Aggressive fluid resuscitation, central line suggested with pressure infusion of warmed IV fluid (lactated Ringer's solution or NS)
- NGT decompression, then administration of CT contrast as indicated
- Eviscerated small bowel should be covered with moist gauze; impaled foreign body should not be removed in ED

ED TREATMENT

- Immediate transfer to OR for patients with an indication for celiotomy
  - —Evisceration, abdominal pain with hypotension, positive DPL or abdominal CT, thoracic abdominal herniation (seen on CXR), impaled foreign body, gunshot wound to the abdomen
  - —Tetanus and antibiotic prophylaxis for penetrating abdominal wounds and blunt injury requiring surgical exploration
- Local wound exploration is safe for abdominal stab wounds
- Serial abdominal examinations and observation
- Judicious analgesia as blood pressure permits once diagnosis established

MEDICATIONS

- Cefotetan (Cefotan): 1–2 g (peds: 20 mg/kg) i.v. *or*
- Cefoxitin (Mefoxin): 1–2 g (peds: 40 mg/kg) i.v. *or*
- Ceftizoxime (Cefizox): 1–2 g (peds: 50 mg/kg) i.v. *plus*
- Flagyl: 500 mg (peds: 7.5 mg/kg) i.v.

Disposition

ADMISSION CRITERIA

- Indication for celiotomy
- Abnormal mental status/intoxication with abdominal injury
- Presence of abdominal pain, tenderness or the "seat-belt sign" requires admission for observation
- Stab and gunshot wounds that violate the abdominal fascia, positive DPL or worsening clinical exams

DISCHARGE CRITERIA

- Minimal mechanism blunt trauma in a nonintoxicated patient with normal exam who has no abdominal pain and adequate follow-up
- Penetrating wounds that do not violate abdominal fascia

Miscellaneous

ICD9: 863.20

ICD10: S36.9

SUGGESTED READINGS

Amoroso TA. Evaluation of the patient with blunt abdominal trauma: an evidenced based approach. Emerg Med Clin North Am 1999;17(1):63–75.

Esinoza R, Rodriguez A. Traumatic and nontraumatic perforation of hollow viscera. Surg Clin North Am 1997;77(6):1291–1304.

Fakhry SM, Brownstein MR, et al. Relatively short delays(less than 8 hours) produced morbidity and mortality in small bowel injuries: an analysis of time to operative intervention in 198 patients from a multicenter experience. J Trauma 2000;48: 408–415.

Malhotra AK, Fabian TC, et al. Blunt bowel and mesenteric injuries: the role of computed tomography. J Trauma 2000;48: 991–1000.

Author: Barry Knapp

Smallpox

Clinical Presentation

SIGNS AND SYMPTOMS

- Caused by *variola,* a DNA orthopox virus
- Declared eradicated by the World Health Organization in 1980
- Last natural case 1977 in Somalia
- Samples of *variola* kept in storage by U.S. and Russia not destroyed
- Threat as a biological weapon
- Virus in environment inactivated within 2 days
- Routine vaccination discontinued in early 1970s
- Incubation period 7–17 days (mean 12 days)
- Sudden-onset febrile illness
  —High fever (often >40°C)
  —Malaise
  —Headache
  —Severe backache
  —Abdominal pain or delirium can occur at onset
- Characteristic exanthema
  —Begins several days after onset of fever
  —Maculopapular rash, progressing to vesicles, pustules, and crusted lesions
  —Distinguishing features (help differentiate from *varicella*)
    -Begins on face and hands, progresses centrally toward trunk
    -Synchronous (all lesions in same stage of development)
    -Commonly involves palms and soles
  —Over 1–2 weeks, scabs separate leaving pitting scars (if patient survives)
  —Lesions involving oropharyngeal mucosa occur approximately 1 day before onset of rash
- Mortality rate 30% in one series
- Death from immune complex toxemia or hypotension

ETIOLOGY

- Large DNA orthopox virus
- No known insect vector
- No known animal reservoir
- Person-to-person transmission
  —Oropharyngeal aerosol as mucosal lesions break down
  —Direct contact with infected material (scabs, clothing, bedding)
- Potential as bioweapon
  —Stable as aerosol
  —Small infectious dose

Pre-Hospital

CAUTIONS

- Strict respiratory and body-surface contact precautions
- In case of outbreak, all medical personnel who may come into contact with infected patients should be vaccinated or revaccinated

Diagnosis

ESSENTIAL WORKUP

- Single case of smallpox would be international health emergency
- Diagnosis probably straightforward after initial (index) case is detected
- Characteristic clinical syndrome and rash

LABORATORY

- Electron microscopy (can detect orthopox virus but cannot specifically diagnose *variola*)
- Polymerase chain reaction technology
- Cell culture
- Serologic tests not useful

DIFFERENTIAL DIAGNOSIS

- *Varicella* (chickenpox)
  —Rash starts centrally on trunk and spreads outward
  —Lesions in different stages of development (papules, vesicles, crusts)
  —Rarely involves palms or soles
- Disseminated molluscum contagiosum (in HIV patients)
- Drug eruptions
- Monkeypox

Treatment

INITIAL STABILIZATION

- ABCs
- IV fluids

ED TREATMENT

- Strict respiratory and contact isolation
- Medical staff caring for smallpox patients should have been recently vaccinated (or revaccinated)
- Hydration
- No antiviral drug has proven efficacy against *variola*
- Treat secondary bacterial infection
- Use public health support and guidelines

Prophylaxis

- Vaccine given within 4 days of initial exposure decreases chances of contracting smallpox or developing severe symptoms or death
- All response teams, health care workers, and other personnel at institutions treating smallpox patients should be vaccinated as soon as possible
- Current smallpox vaccine (as of 2002) associated with significant complications
  —Encephalitis
  —Progressive vaccinia
  —Eczema vaccinatum
  —Generalized vaccinia
  —Accidental eye inoculation
- Certain groups at increased risk of vaccine-related complications
  —Pregnant women
  —Patients with eczema or other similar skin conditions
  —Patients with HIV or hereditary immune deficiency
  —Cancer patients on chemotherapy
- Vaccinia immune globulin (VIG)
  —Treatment for complications related to smallpox vaccine
  —Only very limited supply available from CDC and state health departments
  —Use only for severe complications

MEDICATIONS

- VIG
  —0.6 mL/kg i.m. in divided doses of 24–46 hours
  —May be repeated after 2–3 days

Disposition

ADMISSION CRITERIA

- Will depend on resources and number of potential patients in community
- Need for IV hydration, nutrition, or other hospital-specific therapy
- Admitted patients should be placed in strict respiratory and contact isolation
- Some hospitals may be specifically designated to receive smallpox patients

DISCHARGE CRITERIA

- Many patients may be cared for at home by vaccinated family members or friends

Miscellaneous

ICD9: 050.0

SUGGESTED READINGS

Breman JG, Henderson DA. Diagnosis and management of smallpox. N Engl J Med 2002;346:1300–1308.

Fenner F, Henderson DA, et al. Smallpox and its eradication. Geneva: World Health Organization, 1988.

Henderson DA, et al. Smallpox as a biological weapon: medical and public health management. JAMA 1999;281: 2127–2137.

Author: Leon Gussow

Smoke Inhalation

Clinical Presentation

SIGNS AND SYMPTOMS

- Pulmonary
  - —Cough
  - —Hoarseness
  - —Dyspnea
  - —Wheezing
  - —Rales
- Associated signs (alert to the possibility of significant inhalation injury)
  - —Major burns
  - —Facial burns
  - —Singed nasal hairs
  - —Carbonaceous sputum
- Significant association with significant carbon monoxide exposure and to a lesser extent cyanide (CN) exposure
- May initially be asymptomatic, with symptoms developing over the next 24 hours after injury

CO Toxicity

CO Level/Clinical Manifestations

- 10%: No symptoms
- 20%: Headache, nausea, vomiting, dyspnea on exertion
- 30%: Confusion, lethargy, EKG changes
- 40–60%: Coma
- >60%: Death
- Increased toxicity at lower CO level if exposure prolonged

CN Toxicity

- Seizures
- Coma
- Apnea
- Severe, persistent metabolic acidosis

MECHANISM/DESCRIPTION

- *Upper airway injury:* results in stridor, respiratory arrest
- *Lower airway injury:* results in bronchospasm and noncardiogenic pulmonary edema (ARDS)
- *Cellular asphyxiation:* interference with oxidative phosphorylation by CO and CN results in obtundation, seizures, myocardial ischemia

ETIOLOGY

- Thermal injury
- Chemical insult
- Chemical asphyxiation on a cellular level (e.g., carbon monoxide, CN)

PEDIATRIC CONSIDERATIONS

- Pediatric airway narrower than adult's and more prone to airway compromise from edema
- Fetal hemoglobin especially sensitive to CO toxicity

Pre-Hospital

CAUTIONS

- Intubation for agonal breathing
- 100% oxygen by face mask
  - —Therapeutic maneuver for CO and CN toxicity
- Transport awake, stridorous patients to the nearest ED
  - —Advanced airway management best left to the ED physician unless prolonged transport time
- β-Agonist nebulization for bronchospasm
- IV lactated Ringer's solution or 0.9% NS at high flow rates with major burns
- Cover the patient with major burns with a clean sheet
- Cervical spine and backboard immobilization for traumatized patients
- Pulse oximetry erroneously normal with significant carboxyhemoglobinemia
- Rapid glucose check, consider naloxone, thiamine for patients with altered mental status

Diagnosis

ESSENTIAL WORKUP

- ABG with carboxyhemoglobin level
  - —Hypoxia
  - —Metabolic acidosis
- EKG
  - —Older than 35 years for associated myocardial ischemia
  - —For CO-induced myocardial ischemia
- CXR
  - —Baseline initially normal
  - —Becomes abnormal over 8–24 hours with significant lower airway injury

LABORATORY

- Pulse oximetry erroneously normal with significant carboxyhemoglobinemia
- Pregnancy testing
  - —Management of CO toxicity more aggressive in pregnancy
- Any critically burned patient
  - —Electrolytes, BUN/Cr, glucose
  - —CBC
  - —PT/PTT
  - —CPK, troponin
- CN levels
  - —Not clinically useful
  - —Results come back hours after therapeutic decisions have been made
- Lactate levels as a marker of CN toxicity may be helpful

IMAGING/SPECIAL TESTS

- Bedside peak expiratory flow
- Bronchoscopy
  - —Visualization of upper and lower airway injuries: erythema, edema, ulcerations, desquamation
  - —Used therapeutically to suction out desquamated epithelial debris
- Radionuclide lung scan sometimes used

DIFFERENTIAL DIAGNOSIS

- COPD or asthma exacerbation
- Cardiogenic pulmonary edema
- Toxic gas exposure
- In the setting of trauma: pneumothorax or hemothorax

Treatment

INITIAL STABILIZATION

- 100% oxygen by face mask
- Intubation for
  - —CNS depression
  - —Respiratory distress (stridor/drooling)
  - —Hypoxia
  - —Significant upper airway/facial burns
  - —Unable to protect airway
- IV fluids lactated Ringer's solution or 0.9% NS according to Parkland or similar formula for major burns
- Rapid glucose check, consider naloxone, thiamine for patients with altered mental status

ED TREATMENT

- Intubated patients
  - —Low cuff pressure
  - —Frequent suctioning
  - —Positive end-expiratory pressure
  - —Consider high-frequency ventilation
- Bronchospasm
  - —β-Agonist nebulization
  - —Anticholinergic nebulization
  - —IV steroids only for refractory bronchospasm in patients with asthma or COPD
  - —IV aminophylline: no role
- CO toxicity (see Carbon Monoxide, Poisoning)
  - —100% oxygen decreases the half-life of CO from 4–6 hours to about 90 minutes
  - —Hyperbaric oxygen (HBO) reduces CO half-life to 20 minutes
  - —Fetal hemoglobin has greater affinity for CO
  - —HBO therapy indications: see Carbon Monoxide, Poisoning
- CN toxicity (see Cyanide, Poisoning)
  - —100% oxygen
  - —Sodium thiosulfate portion of the Lilly kit
  - —Amyl nitrite and sodium nitrite portion of Lilly kit
    - -Contraindicated with significant carboxyhemoglobinemia
    - -Inducement of methyl hemoglobinemia further reduces hemoglobin oxygen-carrying capacity
  - —Hydroxocobalamin (probably safe and effective, not yet available in the U.S.)
- No role for prophylactic antibiotics
- No role for steroids unless patient with asthma/COPD with persistent bronchospasm; steroids may worsen outcome in seriously burned patients

MEDICATIONS

- Albuterol nebulization: 2.5–5.0 mg in 2.5 mL NS q20min, or continuous neb 10 mg/h (peds: 0.1–0.3 mg/kg diluted in 2.5 mL NS q20min, maximum 2.5 mg, or continuous neb 0.5 mg/kg/h)
- Dextrose: D50W 1 amp (50 mL or 25 g) (peds: D25W 2–4 mL/kg) i.v.
- Ipratropium bromide: 0.5 mg added to first neb (peds: 0.25 mg/dose for children older than 5 years)
- Methylprednisolone: 125 mg i.v. push (peds: 1–2 mg/kg)
- Naloxone (Narcan): 2 mg (peds: 0.1 mg/kg) i.v. or i.m. initial dose
- Sodium thiosulfate: 50 mL slow IV push:
  - —50-mL ampule, 25% sodium thiosulfate = 12.5 g (peds: 1.65 mL/kg of 25% sodium thiosulfate = 0.41 g/kg)
- Thiamine (vitamin B_1): 100 mg (peds: 50 mg) i.v. or i.m.

Disposition

ADMISSION CRITERIA

- ICU or burn unit
  - —Intubated
  - —Major burn
  - —Continued dyspnea
  - —Hoarseness, odynophagia
  - —Cough with carbonaceous sputum
- General medical admission for 24-hour observation
  - —Persistent cough in otherwise asymptomatic patients
  - —COPD patients or high-risk asthmatics with bronchospasm that has resolved with standard medical therapy in the ED
  - —Otherwise asymptomatic with carbonaceous sputum
  - —Facial burns with significant exposure history
- Consider admission/observation
  - —Underlying illnesses (COPD, CHF, and CAD)
  - —Singed nasal hair
- Transfer severe CO toxicity for HBO therapy

DISCHARGE CRITERIA

- Minimal exposure history, asymptomatic
- Significant exposure history, asymptomatic after 4–6 hours of observation
- Asthmatic, low-risk asthma history, minimal exposure with bronchospasm resolving after one nebulization

Miscellaneous

ICD9: 987.9

ICD10: T59.8

SEE ALSO: CARBON MONOXIDE, POISONING; CYANIDE, POISONING

SUGGESTED READINGS

Ellenhorn MJ, Schoonwald S, Ordog G, et al. Respiratory toxicology. In: Ellenhorn MJ, ed. Ellenhorn's medical toxicology, 2nd ed. Baltimore: Williams & Wilkins, 1997:1448–1531.

Harrigan R. Smoke inhalation injury. In: Bosker G, ed. The emergency medicine reports textbook of adult and pediatric emergency medicine, 1st ed. Atlanta: American Health Consultants, 2000: 1335–1342.

Kirk MA, Holstege CP. Smoke inhalation. In: Goldfrank LR, Flomenbaum NE, et al, eds. Goldfrank's toxicologic emergencies, 6th ed. Stamford, CT: Appleton & Lange, 1988:1539–1549.

Lafferty KA. Smoke inhalation. *www.emedicine.com/emerg/topic538.htm.*

Author: Ross Tannebaum

Snake Envenomation

Clinical Presentation

SIGNS AND SYMPTOMS

Local

- Classic skin changes
  - —One or two puncture wounds
  - —Pain and swelling at the site
- Swelling and edema of the involved extremity
  - —Within an hour in severe envenomations
  - —Tender proximal lymph nodes
- Ecchymosis, petechiae, and hemorrhagic vesicles develop within several hours

Systemic

- Weakness
- Diaphoresis
- Dizziness
- Nausea
- Scalp paresthesias
- Periorbital fasciculations
- Metallic taste
- Severe bites can lead to
  - —Coagulopathies and DIC
  - —Hypotension
  - —Shock
  - —Pulmonary edema
  - —Hematuria
  - —Rhabdomyolysis
  - —Renal failure
  - —Cardiac dysfunction
  - —Thrombocytopenia
- Compartment syndrome in the involved extremity
- Coral snake venom
  - —Primarily neurotoxic
    - -Weakness
    - -Diplopia
    - -Confusion
    - -Respiratory depression
  - —Local effects may be deceivingly minimal

MECHANISM/DESCRIPTION

- Pit viper venom
  - —Mixture of proteolytic enzymes and thrombin-like esterases
    - -Enzymes cause local muscle and subcutaneous tissue necrosis
    - -Esterases have an anticoagulant effect, leading to DIC in severe envenomations
- Bite location
  - —Head or trunk bite—more severe than on the extremities
  - —Lower extremity bites may have a delayed presentation
- Severe envenomation
  - —Direct bite into an artery or vein
  - —All coral snake venom (primarily neurotoxic)
- Bite mark significance
  - —Venomous snake: classically includes one or two puncture marks
  - —Nonvenomous snake: horseshoe-shaped row of multiple teeth marks
- 25% of all pit-viper bites are "dry" and do not result in envenomation

ETIOLOGY

- Venomous snakes indigenous to the U.S.
  - —Pit vipers
    - -Account for 95% of all envenomations
    - -Rattlesnakes, cottonmouths, and copperheads
  - —Coral snakes
    - -More severe envenomations
    - -Western coral snakes are found in Arizona and New Mexico
    - -More venomous eastern coral snakes found in the Carolinas and the Gulf states

PEDIATRIC CONSIDERATIONS

- Small children are most likely target for snake envenomations
- Those who freeze with fear in response to the snake are also more susceptible to multiple envenomations
- Because of their low body weight, smaller children and infants are more vulnerable to severe envenomation

Pre-Hospital

CAUTIONS

- Retreat well beyond striking range of snake
- Immobilize extremity in a functional position at the level of the heart
- Keep physical activity minimal
- Remove rings, watches and all constrictive clothing
- If snake is killed, transport in a closed container
  - —Even a severed head can envenomate

CONTROVERSIES

- Incision and suction of the bite wound is not recommended
  - —Can lead to further wound contamination with human mouth flora
  - —Incision attempts by the inexperienced can lead to severe tendon, nerve, and vascular damage
- Tourniquets, cryotherapy, and electrocautery
  - —Contraindicated due to tissue damage
- Although mechanical suction devices do exist, no clinical human trials support their use

PEDIATRIC CONSIDERATIONS

- Increased urgency in transport to the hospital setting is indicated
  - —Envenomation more likely to be severe
  - —Because of the relatively low body weight of a small child

Diagnosis

ESSENTIAL WORKUP

- History
  - —Description of the snake
  - —Geographic location of the bite
- Physical exam
  - —Careful exam of the wound site and involved extremity
    - -Essential in judging the severity of the envenomation
  - —Careful assessment for anaphylactic reactions

LABORATORY

- CBC
- PT/PTT
- DIC panel
- Electrolytes, BUN/Cr, glucose
- CPK
- Urinalysis
- Type and cross-match with moderate to severe envenomation

DIFFERENTIAL DIAGNOSIS

- Nonpoisonous snakes
  - —Smooth, tapered body
  - —Narrow head
  - —Round pupils
  - —No rattles
- Pit vipers
  - —Triangular or arrow-shaped head
  - —Vertical or elliptical pupils
  - —Rattles
- Coral snakes in United States
  - —"Red on yellow—kill a fellow"
  - —"Red on black—venom lack"

Treatment

INITIAL STABILIZATION

- ABCs (two IVs)
- Vigorous hydration with 0.9% NS to maintain intravascular volume and renal blood flow
- Monitor
- Immobilize the bitten extremity

ED TREATMENT

- Supportive care
- Observe for compartment syndrome
- Repeated measurements of extremity circumference
  —Measure every 15–20 minutes until local progression/swelling subsides
- Analgesia
- Tetanus prophylaxis if needed
- Broad-spectrum antibiotics for moderate to severe envenomations
- Steroids not indicated except for reactions to antivenin (see below)
- Wound severity
  —Minimal
    -Local swelling and tenderness
  —Moderate
    -Extremity swelling
    -Evidence of systemic toxicity
  —Severe
    -Obvious toxicity
    -Unstable vitals
    -Coagulopathy
    -Coral snake
    -Lab abnormalities

Antivenin

Crotalidae Antivenin

- Fundamental treatment for pit viper envenomation
- Effective for rattlesnakes, cottonmouths, and copperheads
- Most effective if given within 4–6 hours of the bite
- Skin test with diluted horse serum (in the antivenin kit) before antivenin administration
- Treatment complications include anaphylaxis and serum sickness
- Dosage (each vial contains 10 mL of antivenin) by wound severity
  —Minimal/moderate: 10 vials
  —Severe: 15–20 vials
- Victims of severe envenomations who develop a positive skin test with horse serum
  —May still receive the antivenin
  —Pretreat with diphenhydramine and corticosteroids
  —Monitor closely for anaphylaxis with epinephrine at the bedside
- CroFab
  —New affinity-purified ovine FAB antibody fragment antivenin
  —May minimize hypersensitivity reactions
  —Undergoing clinical trials

Coral Snake Antivenin

- Effective against the more toxic eastern coral snake, but not against the western coral snakes
- After proper skin testing, three to five vials of antivenin is recommended
- Treatment complications are the same as those with Crotalidae antivenin

Treatment Assistance

- Contact local poison control center, local zoo, or herpetologist
- Call the Antivenom Index at 602-626-6016 in Tucson, Arizona, for assistance in treatment of exotic snakes not indigenous to the U.S.

PEDIATRIC CONSIDERATIONS

- Proportionally more antivenin per body weight
- Children often require standard adult doses

Disposition

ADMISSION CRITERIA

- 24-Hour observation for patients requiring antivenin administration
- ICU admission for
  —Evidence of moderate to severe envenomation, especially in children
  —All victims of coral snake bites

DISCHARGE CRITERIA

- Suspicious bite that shows no signs or symptoms of envenomation for 6–8 hours and has a normal lab panel
  —Discharge with follow-up in 24 hours
  —Observe lower extremity bites for 12 hours because of possible delayed toxicity
  —"Dry" bites occur in up to 25% of pit viper bites

Miscellaneous

ICD9: 989.5

ICD10: T63.0

SUGGESTED READINGS

Erickson T, Herman BE, Bowman MA. Snake envenomations. In: Strange G, Ahrens WR, et al, eds. Pediatric emergency medicine. New York: McGraw-Hill, 2002:676–679.

Gold BS, Dart RC, Barish RA. Current concepts: bites of venomous snakes. N Engl J Med 2002;347:347–357.

Holstege CP, Miller A, Wermuth M, et al. Crotalid envenomation. Crit Care Clin 1997;13:889–921.

Lawrence WT, Giannopoulos A, Hansen A. Pit viper bites: rational management in locales in which copperheads and cottonmouths predominate. Ann Plast Surg 1996;36(3):276–285.

Wuster W, Golay P, Warrell DA. Synopsis of recent developments in venomous snake systematics Toxicon 1997;35(3):319–340.

Authors: Adam Black; Timothy Erickson

Spider Bite, Black Widow

Clinical Presentation

SIGNS AND SYMPTOMS

Local

- Pain
  - —Sharp or burning at the site within minutes of the bite
  - —Usually resolves spontaneously after a few minutes or hours
  - —May become worse and spread proximally from the bite
- Skin findings
  - —Often there is nothing to see or palpate at the wound site but any or all of the following may be observed
    - -Two pinpricks from the spider's fangs
    - -Tender and blanched skin with surrounding erythema ("target lesion")
    - -Urticaria
    - -Piloerection
    - -Swelling
    - -Local sweating

Systemic

- Onset within 20–30 minutes
- Neurologic
  - —Painful muscle cramps and spasms, which can lead to tremors and tonic contractions
  - —Entire body may become progressively involved or symptoms may remain regional
  - —Arm bites may lead to arm and chest muscle tightness and dyspnea
  - —Leg bites tend to cause spasm and rigidity in the thighs and abdomen
    - -Syndrome can be confused with acute abdominal emergencies, particularly in children
- Cutaneous dysesthesia and hyperesthesia
- Autonomic instability with perspiration, nausea, vomiting, tachycardia
- Restlessness, headache, agitation, and a sense of impending death
- Less commonly
  - —Fever
  - —Accelerated or slowed pulse
  - —Hypertension
  - —Dyspnea
  - —Arrhythmias
  - —Pulmonary edema
  - —Seizures
  - —Shock
  - —Acute toxic psychosis

Course

- Rarely fatal
- In most untreated patients, symptoms peak after 2–3 hours and then begin to resolve, occasionally recurring episodically over the following few days
- In otherwise healthy adults, complete resolution of symptoms occurs within 2–3 days
- Persistent neurologic symptoms lasting weeks to months
  - —Fatigue
  - —Generalized weakness or myalgias
  - —Paresthesias
  - —Headache
  - —Insomnia
  - —Impotence
  - —Polyneuritis
- Severity of envenomation depends on
  - —Number of bites
  - —Location of bites
  - —Size and condition of the spider
  - —Age, size, and health condition of the victim

MECHANISM/DESCRIPTION

- Venoms contain potent neurotoxins
  - —Disrupt presynaptic nerve terminal membranes causing neurotransmitter release at the neuromuscular junction (acetylcholine) and in autonomic and cortical tissues (norepinephrine)
  - —Initially, postsynaptic terminals are overstimulated, then blockaded, and neurotransmitters rapidly become depleted
- Morbidity and mortality are dose dependent
- Greatest risk from venom include
  - —Premorbid hypertension or cardiovascular disease
  - —Children (i.e., smaller size for a given dose of venom)

ETIOLOGY

- Black widow found throughout North America, except the far north and Alaska
- Black widow spiders prefer dark, cozy hideaways outdoors and close to the ground
- More bites occur during the warmer months when spiders are defending their webs and egg clutches
- Females are responsible for human envenomations
- Appearance
  - —Black with red markings shaped like an hourglass or a pair of spots on the ventral aspect of the globular abdomen
  - —Females have 25–50-mm leg spans and 15-mm-long bodies

Pre-Hospital

CAUTIONS

- Immobilize the wound site and apply cool compresses or ice for comfort during transport to hospital
- Supportive measures (analgesics, anxiolytics) may be required for patients with systemic symptoms
- Every effort should be made by caregivers at the scene to find and bring in the responsible spider for identification

CONTROVERSIES

- Venom extraction devices (e.g., Sawyer extractor) have been recommended anecdotally but are probably ineffective if >10 minutes has elapsed since the bite

Diagnosis

ESSENTIAL WORKUP

- Diagnosis based on
  - —Clinical presentation
  - —Careful inquiry to elicit the spider bite history
  - —Identification of the spider (if it has been caught)

LABORATORY

- No specific blood tests for black widow spider venom
- WBC can be mildly elevated but is usually normal
- Electrolytes, glucose, calcium, BUN, creatinine, amylase, liver function tests, creatinine kinase, troponin, pregnancy test, and PT/PTT
  - —Appropriate to assess abdominal or chest pain and rule out alternative diagnoses
  - —Usually normal

IMAGING/SPECIAL TESTS

- Abdominal imaging
  - —To rule out other causes of pain
- CXR and ABGs
  - —Indicated in rare cases with pulmonary edema
- EKG and cardiac monitoring
  - —Elderly
  - —Presence of chest pain, unstable vital signs or dysrhythmias
- Calcium gluconate infusion
  - —May provide dramatic but temporary relief
  - —Considered by some to be a good diagnostic test

DIFFERENTIAL DIAGNOSIS

- Acute surgical abdomen (e.g., appendicitis, cholecystitis, pancreatitis)
  - —Black widow spider victims are restless instead of quiet (the posture favored by most patients with peritoneal irritation); the abdominal wall rigidity is also unexpectedly nontender
- Sympathomimetics (e.g., cocaine, amphetamines)
  - —Tetanic muscle contractions uncommon in conscious, nonseizing patients
- Myocardial infarction
- Hypertensive emergency
- Muscular injury or strain
- A high fever and WBC count should prompt consideration of alternatives to spider bites (e.g., infection)

Treatment

INITIAL STABILIZATION

- ABCs
  - —Support airway and respiration if pulmonary edema is present
  - —Stabilize dysrhythmias
- Control seizures

ED TREATMENT

- Cleanse the bite site thoroughly
- Tetanus prophylaxis
- Benzodiazepines for agitation and restlessness
- Antiemetics for nausea and vomiting
- Analgesics
- Muscle cramps/spasm therapy—combinations work synergistically
  - —Benzodiazepines
  - —Narcotics
  - —Calcium gluconate
- Calcium gluconate for muscle cramps
  - —Commonly advocated but consensus is lacking on its utility
  - —Effects may be transient and multiple doses may be required
- Antihypertensive agents for symptomatic hypertension
- Specific antivenin
  - —Indications
    - -Younger than 16 years or older than 65 years or premorbid compromised health status
    - -Symptoms do not respond to symptomatic measures
    - -Significantly increased BP
    - -Respiratory distress
    - -Symptomatic and pregnant
  - —Always perform a skin test for sensitivity to horse serum first (test kit included in the antivenin package)
  - —Watch for hypersensitivity reaction in first 20 minutes
    - -Pretreatment with antihistamines
  - —Due to the small quantity of antivenin used, if serum sickness reactions occur, they are usually mild
  - —Effectiveness is usually apparent within 2 hours of the first treatment and repeated doses are rarely necessary
  - —Antivenin probably helps to prevent persistent neuropathic symptoms and may be worth considering for that indication even if the acute stage illness is mild
  - —Antivenin appears to be beneficial and effective even several days after envenomation and is indicated for persistent symptoms

MEDICATIONS

- Antivenin: 1 ampule (2.5 mL) diluted into 50 mL NS (peds: same dose) i.v. over 1 hour
- Calcium gluconate: 10–20 mL of 10% solution i.v. q2–4h p.r.n.
- Morphine sulfate: 2–10 mg (peds: 0.1 mg/kg) i.v. or i.m. p.r.n. (titrate to patient response)

Disposition

ADMISSION CRITERIA

- Elderly, pregnant or symptomatic young patients
- Significant cardiovascular symptoms and signs, or severe hypertension, particularly in presence of premorbid cardiac disease or chronic hypertension
- Respiratory distress or pulmonary edema
- Persistent symptoms not responding to aggressive management and specific antivenin

DISCHARGE CRITERIA

- Asymptomatic patients with no positive identification of a black widow spider can be released after observation for 1–2 hours
- Asymptomatic patients with no comorbid illness with a positive identification of the black widow spider should be observed for a minimum of 4–6 hours and discharged if their condition does not change
- All discharged patients must be instructed what to watch for in terms of relapsing symptoms and to seek appropriate follow-up if needed
- Discharged patients who received antivenin should be instructed to watch for signs of serum sickness

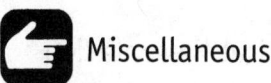

Miscellaneous

ICD9: 989.5

ICD10: T63.3

SUGGESTED READINGS

Allen C. Arachnid envenomations. Emerg Med Clin North Am 1992;10(2):288–291.

Boyer Hassen LV, McNally JT. Spider bites. In: Auerbach PS, ed. Wilderness medicine: management of wilderness and environmental emergencies, 3rd ed. St. Louis: Mosby–Year Book, 1995: 769–786.

Clark MD, et al. Clinical presentation and treatment of black widow spider envenomation: a review of 163 cases. Ann Emerg Med 1992;21(7):782–787.

Miller TA. Latrodectism: bite of the black widow spider. Am Fam Physician 1992;45(1):181–187.

Author: Paul Arnold

Spider Bite, Brown Recluse

Clinical Presentation

SIGNS AND SYMPTOMS

Initial Symptoms

- Usually asymptomatic but may cause minor stinging and burning sensation

Clinical Course

- Local pain with blanching and induration may develop over 1–24 hours
  - —Vast majority of patients recover fully with no sequelae
- Tissue injury may develop at bite site
  - —Blister may form in the center of the blanched area with circumferential erythema
  - —Blister may gradually enlarge and darken with the development of skin and subcutaneous fat necrosis over 3–4 days
  - —Most extensive necrosis develops where increased subcutaneous fat
  - —Lower extremity blisters spread distally under the influence of gravity
  - —Healing by secondary intention may take weeks to months
  - —Rarely evolves into ulcerative necrosis over the following days or weeks
  - —Ulcers can recur even years later
  - —Local response is not dependent on the extent of envenomation and cannot be used to predict the severity of subsequent systemic illness

Systemic Features

- Develop rarely during the first 1–3 days after the bite
- Severity is proportional to the amount of venom injected
- Features include
  - —Fever, chills, malaise
  - —Nausea, vomiting, diarrhea
  - —Myalgias, muscle cramps, arthralgias
  - —Petechial or urticarial rash
- Complications include
  - —Hemolysis leading to hemoglobinuria and acute renal failure
  - —DIC
  - —Shock

MECHANISM/DESCRIPTION

- Venom is a complex cocktail of enzymes and peptides
  - —Causes hemolysis and tissue necrosis
  - —Triggers complement cascades, platelet aggregation, and thrombosis, and release of inflammatory mediators
  - —Result is direct cytotoxic effects, coupled with indirect toxicity due to inflammation and vascular compromise
- Systemic toxicity is due to an inflammatory or allergic response to venom antigenic properties

ETIOLOGY

- Found widely throughout the southern half of North America
- Spider not aggressive
- Humans bitten when they disturb a spider in its habitat, typically any warm and dry location indoors or outdoors such as wood piles, bundles of rags, cellars, or attics
- Spider appearance
  - —Delicate body and legs spanning 10–25 mm
  - —Light- to medium-brown with darker violin-shaped marking visible on the upper aspect of the head
  - —Three pairs of eyes

PEDIATRIC CONSIDERATIONS

- Toxicity proportional to the amount of venom and size of patient
- Children are more vulnerable to a given amount of venom than healthy adults

Pre-Hospital

CAUTIONS

- Immobilize wound site
- Cover with cool compresses
- Transport to hospital when patient experiences immediate onset of symptoms
- Find and bring in the responsible spider for identification
- Supportive measures for patients with systemic symptoms

CONTROVERSIES

- Venom extraction devices (e.g., Sawyer extractor) have been recommended anecdotally but are probably ineffective if >10 minutes has elapsed since bite

Diagnosis

ESSENTIAL WORKUP

- Careful inquiry required to elicit the spider bite history
- Diagnosis based on the clinical presentation and the ruling out of other relevant possibilities

LABORATORY

- No specific tests available
- CBC, electrolytes, BUN, creatinine, PT/PTT for baseline monitoring
- Urinalysis for evidence of systemic hemolysis

IMAGING/SPECIAL TESTS

- Soft-tissue x-ray of bite site
  - —Indicated if the differential includes suspected gas-forming organism, infection of ulcers

DIFFERENTIAL DIAGNOSIS

- Necrotic ulcers
- Other arachnid envenomations
- Soft-tissue infection
- Stevens-Johnson syndrome
- Erythema nodosum
- Diabetic ulcer
- Bed sore
- Lower limb vascular insufficiency with secondary ulcer
- Other etiologies of hemolytic anemia, DIC, anaphylactoid reactions

Treatment

INITIAL STABILIZATION

- IV fluids, oxygen, cardiac monitoring if the patient is experiencing systemic collapse

ED TREATMENT

Local Bite Care

- Supportive and expectant
- Clean/irrigate wound
- Tetanus prophylaxis
- Antibiotics
  - —Appropriate if wound appears infected
  - —Not indicated prophylactically
  - —Antistaphylococcal (first-generation cephalosporin or penicillinase-resistant penicillins)
- Controversial and unproven measures include
  - —Topical or systemic steroids
  - —Dapsone
    - -Screen for G6PD deficiency before initiating
    - -Monitor for methemoglobinemia, hemolysis, and leukopenia during therapy
  - —Hyperbaric therapy
  - —Topical nitroglycerin
  - —Local electric shock
- Specific antivenin
  - —Always perform a skin test for sensitivity to horse serum before using
  - —Watch for hypersensitivity reaction in first 20 minutes
  - —Pretreat with antihistamines
  - —Due to small dose of antivenin, risk of serum sickness is low
  - —Therapeutic value reduced if given >4–6 hours after envenomation
    - -Clinical extent of envenomation exceeds 4–6 hours in all but the most extreme cases
  - —Use controversial due to
    - -Low mortality of brown recluse bites
    - -Risk of side effects from antivenin
- Excision of the necrotic wound
  - —May become necessary at a later date
  - —Not indicated in the first 8 weeks because may cause more severe ulcer formation

Systemic Problem Management

- Analgesics for pain control
- Hemoglobinuria
  - —Treated with IV fluids and alkalinization
  - —Monitor renal, fluid, and electrolyte status carefully
  - —PRBC for significant anemia
- Standard supportive care and interventions should be employed for shock, seizures, DIC, and coma
- Dialysis in the event of acute renal failure

MEDICATIONS

- Antivenin: 1 ampule (2.5 mL) diluted into 50 mL NS (peds: same dose) i.v. over 1 hour
- Dapsone: progressive dosage of 50–500 mg b.i.d. × 2 weeks (peds: 2 mg/kg/24 h PO × 2 weeks)
- Methylprednisolone: 125 mg IVP followed by prednisone 30–50 mg/d × 5 days (peds: methylprednisolone 1–2 mg/kg i.v., prednisone 1–2 mg/kg PO)
- Morphine sulfate: 2–10 mg (peds: 0.1 mg/kg) i.v. or i.m. p.r.n.

PEDIATRIC CONSIDERATIONS

- Use dapsone only in severe cases because of potential for side effects such as
  - —Hepatitis
  - —Methemoglobinemia
  - —Hemolytic anemia
  - —Leukopenia

Disposition

ADMISSION CRITERIA

- Significant local reaction, signs of systemic toxicity, reaction to antivenin
- Lower threshold for children, patients with comorbidities

DISCHARGE CRITERIA

- No evidence of systemic toxicity or severe progression of local wound necrosis after envenomation
- Daily reassessment, including blood work, until 3–4 days after envenomation to guard against the risk of systemic toxicity

PEDIATRIC CONSIDERATIONS

- Longer observation period before disposition of asymptomatic cases because of the higher mortality in this population

Miscellaneous

ICD9: 989.5

ICD10: T14.0

SUGGESTED READINGS

Allen C. Arachnid envenomations. Emerg Med Clin North Am 1992;10:2:288–291.

Forks TP. Brown recluse spider bites. J Am Board Fam Pract 2000;13(6):415–423.

Grendron BP. Loxosceles reclusa envenomation. Am J Emerg Med 1990;8(1):51.

Nishioka S de A. Misdiagnosis of brown recluse spider bite. West J Med 2001;174: 240.

Author: Paul Arnold

Spinal Cord Syndromes

Clinical Presentation

SIGNS AND SYMPTOMS

- Spinal cord syndromes result from localized disruption of neurotransmission and exhibit mixed motor and sensory sparing
- *Anterior cord syndrome*
  - —Bilateral spastic paralysis and loss of pain and temperature sensation below the level of the lesion
  - —Preservation of dorsal column function (proprioception and position sense)
- Brown-Séquard syndrome (lateral cord syndrome)
  - —Ipsilateral spastic paresis and loss of dorsal column function (proprioception and position sense)
  - —Contralateral loss of pain and temperature sensation
  - —Deficits usually begin two levels below the injury
- *Central cord syndrome*
  - —Loss of motor function affects upper extremities more severely than lower extremities
  - —Most profound deficits occur in the distal upper extremities
  - —Sensory loss is more variable
- *Dorsal cord syndrome*
  - —Loss of proprioception, position sensation, and coordination below the level of the lesion
- *Complete cord syndrome*
  - —Flaccid paresis below the level of the injury
  - —Low BP, low heart rate, flushed skin, priapism may be present (loss of sympathetic tone)
- *Sacral sparing is present with incomplete lesions*
- *Sensory deficit levels*
  - —C-2—occiput
  - —C-4—clavicular region
  - —C-6—thumb
  - —C-8—little finger
  - —T-4—nipple line
  - —T-10—umbilicus
  - —L-1—inguinal region
  - —L-5—dorsum of the foot
  - —S-5—perianal area
- *Motor deficit levels*
  - —C-5—elbow flexion
  - —C-7—elbow extension
  - —C-8—finger flexion
  - —T-1—finger abduction
  - —L-2—hip flexion
  - —L-3—knee extension
  - —L-4—ankle dorsiflexion
  - —S-1—ankle plantar flexion

MECHANISM/DESCRIPTION

- Patients with arthritis, osteoporosis, metastatic disease, or other chronic spinal disorders are at risk of developing spinal injuries as the result of even minor trauma
- Anterior cord syndrome
  - —Results from a flexion or axial loading mechanism or direct cord compression from vertebral fractures, dislocations, disc herniation, tumor, or abscess
  - —Rarely caused by a laceration or thrombosis to the anterior spinal artery
- Brown-Séquard syndrome
  - —Hemisection of the spinal cord classically as a result of a penetrating wound
  - —Rarely unilateral cord compression
- Central cord syndrome
  - —Most commonly occurs in elderly patients who have preexisting cervical spondylosis and stenosis
  - —Forced hyperextension causes buckling of the ligamentum flavum, creating a shearing injury to the central portion of the spinal cord
- Dorsal cord syndrome
  - —Associated with hyperextension injuries
- Complete cord syndrome
  - —Blunt or penetrating trauma that results in complete disruption of spinal cord
  - —Symptoms that remain >24 hours generally are permanent

Pre-Hospital

- Full spinal immobilization
- IV access should be established for fluid resuscitation in the setting of neurogenic shock
- Patients should be transported to the nearest trauma center

PEDIATRIC CONSIDERATIONS

- Cervical collars must be the appropriate size for the child, splinting the head and body with towels and tape is a reasonable alternative
- The incidence of spinal cord injury (SCI) without radiographic abnormality is higher in children younger than 8 years

Diagnosis

ESSENTIAL WORKUP

- All areas of clinical suspicion should be imaged with plain radiographs
- CT of the spine when plain films are normal or ambiguous
  - —CT allows assessment of the spinal canal and any impingement by bone fragments
- MRI is the imaging modality of choice for detection of spinal cord damage; in the acute setting, the indications for MRI are
  - —Neurologic deficits not explained by plain films or CT
  - —Clinical progression of a spinal cord lesion
  - —Determination of acute surgical candidacy
  - —Disadvantages of MRI include the inability to adequately monitor the patient while undergoing the study and the incompatibility with certain metal devices

IMAGING/SPECIAL TESTS

- Myelography is used with CT when MRI is not available or cannot be performed

DIFFERENTIAL DIAGNOSIS

- Dorsal root injury
- Peripheral nerve injury
- Guillain-Barré syndrome
- Multiple sclerosis
- Transverse myelitis
- Epidural abscess

Treatment

INITIAL STABILIZATION

- ABCs of trauma care
- Spinal immobilization must be maintained at all times
- Intubation must proceed with in-line spinal immobilization
- IV fluids should be administered at maintenance levels unless shock is present
  - —Spinal trauma may cause hypotension due to loss of sympathetic tone; fluid administration is first-line treatment
  - —Other causes of hypotension (e.g., hemorrhage) should be sought before being attributed to SCI
  - —Generally hypovolemic shock causes tachycardia, whereas neurogenic shock results in bradycardia
  - —If BP does not improve after a fluid challenge and no other cause for hypotension can be found, vasopressor use may be necessary; α-agonist is preferred

ED TREATMENT

- Other injuries must be treated as indicated
- Level of SCI should be determined as a baseline to follow for improvement or deterioration
- A neurosurgeon must be consulted once an SCI is suspected even when plain films are normal; early surgical decompression or immobilization may reduce morbidity
- The patient with an SCI should be managed at an appropriate regional trauma center or spinal center
  - —If necessary, transfer should occur as soon as management of other injuries allow
- High-dose methylprednisolone (MP) is started as soon as possible in the patient with SCI
  - —The greatest benefit is reported when infusion is begun within 8 hours of injury
  - —MP has not been established as having a definitive clinically significant benefit, and high-dose steroids do increase the likelihood of immune system compromise, and GI tract bleeding
  - —To prevent GI tract bleeding with steroid use, concurrently start the patient on IV Pepcid
- IV antibiotics and tetanus prophylaxis are given to patients with a penetrating injury

MEDICATIONS

- MP: 30 mg/kg i.v. loading dose given over 15 minutes in the first hour followed by a 5.4 mg/kg/h continuous infusion for the next 23 hours (adults and peds)
- Pepcid: 20 mg i.v. (peds: 0.6–0.8 mg/kg/24 h q8–12h)
- Phenylephrine: 0.5–2 μg/kg bolus then 50–100 μg/min drip

Disposition

ADMISSION CRITERIA

- All patients with spinal cord syndrome must be admitted to an ICU setting

DISCHARGE CRITERIA

- No patient with symptoms suggestive of SCI should be discharged

Miscellaneous

ICD9: 952.00-952.19

ICD10: T09.3

SUGGESTED READINGS

American College of Surgeons, Committee on Trauma. Advanced trauma life support course for physicians. Chicago: College of Surgeons, 1993:193–203.

Bracken MB, et al. A randomized controlled trial of methylprednisolone or naloxone in the treatment of acute spinal cord injury. N Engl J Med 1990;322(20):1405–1411.

Dumont RJ, Verma S, Okonkwo DO, et al. Acute spinal cord injury, part II: contemporary pharmacotherapy. Clin Neuropharmacol 2000;24(5):265–279.

Gerling MC, Davis DP, Hamilton RS, et al. Effects of cervical spine immobilization technique and laryngoscope blade selection on an unstable cervical spine in a cadaver model of intubation. Ann Emerg Med 2000;36(4):293–300.

Hockberger RS, Kirshenbaum KJ. Spinal trauma. In: Marx JA, et al, eds. Rosen's emergency medicine: concepts and clinical practice, 5th ed. St. Louis: CV Mosby, 2000:329–370.

Author: Judd Glasser

Spine Injury: Cervical, Adult

Clinical Presentation

SIGNS AND SYMPTOMS

- Neck pain, tenderness on palpation
- Numbness, weakness, paresthesias of upper or lower extremities
- Always assume a C-spine injury in any patient with
  - —Altered mental status (unconscious, intoxicated, drugs, or hypoxia) following trauma or if preceding history/events unknown
  - —Inability to communicate (mentally retarded, language barrier, or intubated) following trauma or if preceding history/events unknown
  - —Distracting injury
  - —Blunt trauma involving head or neck

Incomplete Cervical Cord Syndromes (see separate chapter)

- *Brown-Séquard syndrome:* hemisection of cord from penetrating injury (ipsilateral motor paralysis/contralateral sensory hypesthesia)
- *Anterior cord syndrome:* cervical flexion injury causing cord contusion (paralysis/hypesthesia with sparing of position/touch/vibratory sensations)
- *Central cord syndrome:* patients with cervical degenerative arthritis with forced hyperflexion (deficits greater in upper extremities relative to lower extremities)

ETIOLOGY

- Blunt trauma is the major cause of neck injuries
  - —Automobile accidents account for >50%
  - —Falls account for approximately 20%
  - —Sporting accidents account for 15%
  - —Minor trauma in patients with severe arthritis may result in cervical injuries
- Penetrating trauma

MECHANISM/DESCRIPTION

- May have more than one mechanism concurrently

Flexion Injuries

- Simple *wedge fracture:* usually a stable fracture
- *Anterior subluxation:* disruption of the posterior ligament complex without bony injury; potentially unstable injury
- *Clay shoveler fracture:* avulsion fracture of the spinous process of C-7, C-6, or T-1; stable fracture
- Flexion *teardrop fracture:* extremely unstable fracture and may be associated with acute anterior cervical cord syndrome
- *Atlantooccipital dislocation:* unstable injury
- *Bilateral facet dislocation:* can occur from C-2 to C-7; unstable injury

Flexion/Rotation Injuries

- Unilateral facet dislocation "locked" vertebra: stable injury
- Rotary atlantoaxial dislocation: unstable injury

Extension Injuries

- *Extension teardrop fracture:* an avulsion fracture of the anterior inferior corner of the involved vertebral body; unstable in extension and stable in flexion
- *Posterior arch of C-1 fracture:* arch is compressed between the occiput and the spinous process of the axis during hyperextension; unstable fracture
- *Avulsion fracture of the anterior arch of the atlas:* horizontal fracture of C-1 and prevertebral soft-tissue swelling on the lateral C-spine
- *Hangman's fracture:* traumatic spondylolisthesis of the axis involving the pedicles of C-2; unstable fracture
- *Hyperextension dislocation:* described as the syndrome of the paralyzed patient with a radiographically normal appearing C-spine

Extension-Rotation Injury

- Pillar fracture: generally stable fracture

Vertical Compression (Axial Loading) Injuries

- Jefferson fracture: burst fracture of both the anterior and the posterior arch of C-1; extremely unstable fracture
- Burst fracture: a comminuted fracture of the vertebral body with variable retropulsion of the posterior body fragments into the spinal canal

Pre-Hospital

CAUTIONS

- If C-spine injury suspected, immobilize with a hard collar, neck pads, and backboard
- Immobilized patients require constant observation in case of vomiting

CONTROVERSIES

- Immobilize C-spine in patients with penetrating neck wounds only if a neurologic deficit is present
  - —If the weapon is still embedded, immobilize the neck to avoid further injury and *do not* remove the impaling object unless it is directly impeding breathing

Diagnosis

ESSENTIAL WORKUP

- Standard x-rays include three separate views: lateral, anteroposterior, and open-mouth view of the odontoid while still immobilized
- Lateral x-ray must include C1-T1; a swimmer's view may be necessary to view lower levels
- Supine oblique views may help in identifying subtle rotational injuries
- CT should be obtained when C-spine fractures, dislocations, or soft-tissue swelling is seen on plain films or for unexplained neck pain/neurodeficit with normal x-ray
- Flexion-extension views may be needed to evaluate for dynamic ligamentous injuries if static x-rays are negative and patient still complains of significant pain
- MRI has become a valuable tool in evaluation of patients with neurologic deficits

DIFFERENTIAL DIAGNOSIS

- Cervical muscle strain injury (whiplash)
- C-spine dislocation
- Cervical fracture dislocation
- Complex or simple cervical fractures

Treatment

INITIAL STABILIZATION

- Immobilize the spine using a rigid collar and backboard, plus tape/towels or lightweight foam pads along the side of the neck
- ABCs: stabilize the airway, establish IV access, and support circulation
  —Preferred method is careful orotracheal rapid-sequence intubation with in-line spinal immobilization

ED TREATMENT

- Assess patient for other injuries; remember that the abdominal exam in a C-spine–injured patient is unreliable and further objective testing is indicated
- Patients may be clinically cleared and do not require C-spine x-ray if
  —No midline C-spine tenderness present
  —No neurologic deficits present
  —No intoxicating agents
  —No distracting injuries
- If a neurologic deficit is present, consult neurosurgery
- If the x-rays are abnormal, consult neurosurgery or the orthopedic spine service
- If the x-rays are normal but the patient is having severe neck pain, obtain flexion-extension films; if abnormal, consult neurosurgery
- High-dose steroid protocol should be initiated for patients with neurologic deficits due to fractures or dislocations

MEDICATIONS

- High-dose steroid protocol
  —Methylprednisolone: 30 mg/kg i.v. bolus then 5.4 mg/kg/h over the next 23 hours; begin within 8 hours of injury

Disposition

ADMISSION CRITERIA

- C-spine fractures or dislocations associated with a neurologic deficit or any unstable fracture or dislocation should be admitted to the ICU or monitored setting
- Stable C-spine fractures or dislocations should be admitted
- Isolated spinous process fractures that are not associated with any neurologic deficit or instability on plain films
- Simple cervical wedge fractures with no neurologic deficit

DISCHARGE CRITERIA

- Patients with acute cervical strain "whiplash"
- Musculoskeletal injuries that are associated with mild to moderate pain, no neurologic deficit, and normal radiographs
- Patients with radiographically normal C-spine but continuous pain should be discharged with a hard collar and appropriate orthopedic follow-up

Miscellaneous

ICD9: 952.0

ICD10: S14.2

SUGGESTED READINGS

Harris J, Mirvis S. The radiology of acute C-spine trauma, 3rd ed. Baltimore: Williams & Wilkins, 1996.

Hockberger R, Kirshenbaum K. Spine. In: Rosen P, et al, eds: Emergency medicine: concepts and clinical practice, 5th ed. St. Louis: CV Mosby, 2002:329–370.

Hoffman JR, Mower WR, Wolfson AB, et al. Validity of a set of clinical criteria to rule out injury to the cervical spine in patients with blunt trauma. N Engl J Med 2000;343:94–99.

Kathol MH. C-spine trauma. What is new? Radiol Clin North Am 1997;11(3):256–278.

Mower WR, Hoffman JR, Pollack CV Jr, et al. use of plain radiography to screen for cervical spine injuries. Ann Emerg Med 2001;38(1):1–7.

Author: Gary M. Vilke

Spine Injury: Cervical, Pediatric

Clinical Presentation

SIGNS AND SYMPTOMS

- Cervical spine pain
- Limited range of motion
- Neurologic deficit (may be transient)
- May be masked by altered mental status or distracting injury
- Preverbal child may be unable to express symptoms or cooperate with exam

General

- Hypotension
- Bradycardia
- Hypoventilation or apnea

Neck

- Tender to palpation over cervical spine
- Limited range of motion
- Torticollis

Respiratory

- Diaphragmatic breathing

Abdominal

- Ileus
- Fecal incontinence
- Absent rectal tone

Genitourinary

- Priapism
- Urinary retention

Neurologic

- Paresthesias or sensory deficit
- Focal weakness
- Paralysis
  —Partial cord syndromes
  —Quadriplegia
- Absent reflexes

MECHANISM/DESCRIPTION

- 2% of pediatric trauma hospital admissions in the U.S.
- Children younger than 8 years
  —Anatomic differences lead to predominance of C1-3 injuries
  —Relatively larger head
  —Weaker cervical musculature
  —Ligamentous laxity
  —Horizontally oriented facets
- Children age 8–12 years
  —Increased incidence of pancervical injuries
- Children older than 12 years
  —Injury patterns consistent with adults
  —Lower cervical spine injuries more common
  —Evident radiographically
- Spinal cord injury (SCI) without radiographic abnormality (SCIWORA)
  —Occurs in approximately 20% of pediatric cervical spine injuries
  —More common in children younger than 8 years
  —Symptoms may be transient and resolved by time of evaluation
    -Paresthesias
    -Burning sensation down spine
    -Weakness
  —Symptoms often occur immediately after injury but may have delayed onset (minutes to days)

ETIOLOGY

- Motor-vehicle and pedestrian accidents
- Falls
- Sports injuries

Pre-Hospital

CAUTIONS

- Immobilize all infants and children with potential cervical spine injuries
  —Appropriate size cervical collar
  —Tape, towels, padding in combination with car seat or spine board
  —Larger head creates cervical flexion
  —Place padding under neck, shoulders, and back
  —Align external auditory meatus with shoulder

Diagnosis

ESSENTIAL WORKUP

- Obtain cervical spine radiographs if cervical spine tenderness, altered mental status, neurologic deficit (even if transient), distracting injury or mechanism of injury (in preverbal child)
- Remember, the NEXUS C-spine decision rule does not apply to children
- Additional imaging studies (CT, MRI) may be indicated

IMAGING/SPECIAL TESTS

Cervical Spine Radiographs

- Standard initial views: anteroposterior, lateral, and odontoid
- Identifies approximately 80% of fractures, dislocations, and subluxations
- Need to visualize all seven cervical vertebrae
- Normal prevertebral soft-tissue space
  —Space between posterior arch of C-1 and anterior aspect of odontoid process
  —5 mm or smaller in children and 3 mm in adults
- Thickening of prevertebral soft tissue
  —Suggests underlying fracture or ligamentous injury
  —Also occurs with neck flexion, expiration, swallowing
  —Too much variability exists for measurements to be useful
  —Soft tissue below the glottis should be approximately twice as thick as above the glottis
- Pseudosubluxation of C-2
  —Due to ligamentous laxity and often resolves by age of 8 years
  —C-2 anteriorly displaced on C-3
  —Posterior cervical line retains normal relationships
    -Line drawn between anterior aspect of spinous processes of C-1 and C-3 should pass within 2 mm of anterior aspect of spinous process of C-2
    ->2 mm suggests underlying hangman's fracture
    -Can be applied only at C1-3
    -Does not exclude underlying ligamentous injury
- Anterior vertebral wedging of C-3 and C-4
  —May be mistaken for compression fracture
- Epiphyseal growth plates may resemble fractures
  —Posterior arch of C-1 fuses by 4 years of age
  —Anterior arch of C-1 fuses by 10 years of age
  —Base of odontoid fuses with body of C-2 by 7 years of age

Flexion and Extension Views
- Limited utility
- May be useful if suspect occult ligamentous injury
  —Negative cervical spine films
  —No neurologic abnormalities

CT Scan
- Fracture suspected despite negative plain radiographs
- Further definition of fracture identified on plain radiographs
- Differentiating between synchondrosis and fracture

MRI
- Suspected SCI with or without abnormalities found on plain radiographs or CT

DIFFERENTIAL DIAGNOSIS
- Cervical muscle strain
- Torticollis
- Cervical adenitis
- Retropharyngeal abscess
- Meningitis

Treatment

INITIAL STABILIZATION
- Maintain cervical spine immobilization
  —Log roll patient
  —One person devoted to in-line cervical spine immobilization if intubation required

ED TREATMENT
- Methylprednisolone
  —Any trauma patient with neurologic deficit consistent with SCI
- Neurosurgical evaluation
  —True subluxation
  —Fracture
  —Transient or persistent neurologic deficit

MEDICATIONS
- Methylprednisolone: loading dose 30 mg/kg over 15 minutes; maintenance infusion 5.4 mg/kg/h over 23 hours

Disposition

ADMISSION CRITERIA
- Altered mental status
- Signs/symptoms of SCI
- Fracture
- Obtain appropriate consultation
  —Neurosurgery
  —Orthopedics

DISCHARGE CRITERIA
- Completely normal mental status
- No radiographic abnormalities
- No transient or persistent neurologic deficit
- Educate parents
  —SCIWORA can present with delayed onset of symptoms
  —Return if paresthesias, weakness, or paralysis

Miscellaneous

ICD9: 952.0

ICD10: S14.2

SUGGESTED READINGS

Brown RL, Brunn MA, Garcia VF. Cervical spine injuries in children: a review of 103 patients treated consecutively at a level 1 pediatric trauma center. J Pediatr Surg 2001;36(8):1107–1114.

Patel JC, Tepas JJ III, Mollitt DL, et al. Pediatric cervical spine injuries: defining the disease. J Pediatr Surg 2001;36(2): 373–376.

Swischuk LE. Emergency imaging of the acutely ill or injured child, 3rd ed. Baltimore: Williams & Wilkins, 1994: 653–718.

Author: Steven Riley

Spine Injury: Coccyx

Clinical Presentation

SIGNS AND SYMPTOMS

- Tenderness localized over the coccyx
- Ecchymosed over the gluteal fold
- Pain with sitting, especially leaning forward, and with defecation

MECHANISM/DESCRIPTION

- Usually from a fall to a sitting position
- Fall often from standing height
- Can occur during childbirth
- More common in women

Pre-Hospital

CAUTIONS

- Most often isolated injury but if concern for other spinal injury, should have spinal immobilization
- If unstable, need to consider other diagnoses

Diagnosis

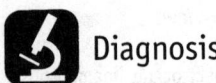

ESSENTIAL WORKUP

- History and exam
- Rectal exam to include evidence of mobility and tenderness to palpation of coccyx
- Check for rectal bleeding, very rare to have rectal perforation
- Should have no evidence of neurologic deficit

IMAGING/SPECIAL TESTS

- Controversial if any radiographic imaging is necessary; concern over unnecessary radiation to gonads when diagnosis can be made clinically
- Radiographs can be hard to interpret because coccyx has normal variant positions that can be confused with a fracture
- Lateral radiograph is best view for fracture and dislocation

DIFFERENTIAL DIAGNOSIS

- Coccygodynia
- Levator ani syndrome
- Pilonidal cyst
- Perirectal abscess

Treatment

INITIAL STABILIZATION

- None usually required; if unstable patient, think of other diagnoses
- Pain medication

ED TREATMENT

- Pain medications
- Reduction of displaced coccyx fracture but rarely successful or necessary
- Patient education: can take years to heal, pain relief with "doughnut" and sitz baths

MEDICATIONS

- Pain medications
- Stool softener

Disposition

ADMISSION CRITERIA

- No medical indications for admission

DISCHARGE CRITERIA

- Coccyx fracture managed as outpatient unless other injury

Miscellaneous

ICD9: 805.6

ICD10: S39.9

SUGGESTED READINGS

Cwinn AA. Pelvis. In: Rosen P, et al, eds. Emergency medicine: concepts and clinical practice, 4th ed. St. Louis: CV Mosby, 2002:625–642.

Gutierrez PR, Mas Martinez JJ, Arenas J. Salter-Harris type I fracture of the sacro-coccygeal joint. Pediatr Radiol 1998;28(9):734.

Author: Gary Schwartz

Spine Injury, Lumbar

Clinical Presentation

SIGNS AND SYMPTOMS

- Pain in lumbar region
- Ecchymosis or deformity overlying lumbar region; localized spinal tenderness; palpable deformity; paraspinal muscle spasm
- Increased interspinous distance by palpation
- "Step-off" (anterior or posterior displacement of spinous process) by palpation
- Neurologic deficits referable to lumbar spinal nerves
  - —Loss of bladder control
  - —Motor: hip flexion (L1-4), leg extension (L-3, L-4), ankle dorsiflexion (L-4, L-5), toe extension (L-5)
  - —Sensory: inguinal crease (L-1), medial thigh (L2-3), knee (L-4), lateral calf (L-5)
  - —Reflexes: knee jerk (L2-4)
- Pain may be masked by associated injuries (e.g., pelvis, calcaneal fractures)
- Multiple injury trauma patients with altered mental status have unreliable exam

MECHANISM/DESCRIPTION

Flexion Compression Fracture

- Wedge compression
  - —<50% anterior compression of the vertebral body, stable injury
  - —No ligamentous injury
  - —No neurologic deficit
- Burst fracture
  - —Vertebral body fracture with retropulsion of bone into the neural canal
  - —Kyphosis on lateral x-ray
  - —Posterior ligamentous injury
  - —Anterior compression, lower extremities, calcaneal fractures
  - —Possible neurologic deficit

Flexion Distraction: "Lap-Belt Injury"

- Abdominal injuries likely
- Chance fracture
  - —Purely bony injury; fracture line through spinous process, pedicles, and vertebral body
  - —No kyphosis on lateral x-ray
  - —No neurologic deficit
- Facet dislocation
  - —Mostly soft-tissue injury; no fracture
  - —Complete disruption of posterior ligaments and intervertebral disc
  - —Neurologic deficit present

Flexion Rotation

- Unstable injury
- Neurologic deficit present

Extension

- Unstable, uncommon
- Disruption of anterior longitudinal ligament and intervertebral disc
- Neurologic sequelae rare but possible

Shear Injuries: "Translational Injuries"

- Anterior, posterior, or lateral translation of superior vertebral segment over the inferior segment
- Complete ligamentous disruption
- Neurologic deficit present

Simple Fractures

- Isolated *spinous process fracture*
  - —Ligamentous disruption
  - —No neurologic deficit
- Isolated *transverse process fracture*
  - —Ligamentous disruption
  - —Neurologic deficit possible; rare isolated root injury

ETIOLOGY

- Blunt trauma with axial distraction, axial compression, or translational forces applied to lumbar region
- Fall from height landing on the feet (associated calcaneal fractures) or on the buttocks
- Motor-vehicle accident

PEDIATRIC CONSIDERATIONS

- Rare reports of child abuse presenting as lower extremity flaccid paralysis due to lumbar spine fracture
- Spinal cord terminates at L-3 in newborn and recedes to T-12 by adulthood; direct cord damage possible in children with high lumbar fractures
- *End-plate avulsion fractures:* adolescent injury usually at L4-5 or L5-S1 level; ligament pulls off vertebral body end plate; associated neurologic findings usually resolve with excision of end-plate fracture

Pre-Hospital

CAUTIONS

- Difficult to determine whether an injury is stable in the field; suspected spinal injuries should be immobilized to prevent further injury

Diagnosis

ESSENTIAL WORKUP

- Lumbar radiographs (described later)
- Careful neurologic examination including assessment of rectal tone, postvoid residual urinary catheterization, bulbocavernosus, and cremasteric reflexes

LABORATORY

- Standard trauma labs as indicated

IMAGING/SPECIAL TESTS

- Lumbar radiography with minimum of anteroposterior and lateral views
  —Characteristics of *unstable* fractures include widening of interspinous, interlaminar or interpedicular distance, kyphosis >20 degrees, translation >2 mm, vertebral body height loss >50%, or articular process fracture
- Radiographs may not help diagnose burst fractures in 25% of cases
- If a fracture is identified, entire spine should be imaged
- Spinous process fracture, transverse process fracture, simple transverse sacral fracture require lumbar *flexion-extension films* if neurologically intact and stable injury
- CT should be performed for further evaluation of suspected fractures or fractures identified on plain films to assess spinal cord integrity

DIFFERENTIAL DIAGNOSIS

- Contusion
- Pathologic fracture (metastatic cancer)
- Osteoporosis
- Pelvic fracture
- Traumatic herniated disc
- Low posterior rib fracture
- Tuberculous spondylitis (Pott's disease)
- Ankylosing spondylitis
- Osteogenesis imperfecta (pediatric)
- Congenital scoliosis with hemivertebra (mistaken for lateral wedge fracture)
- Child abuse

Treatment

INITIAL STABILIZATION

- Immobilization while tending to immediate life-threatening conditions
- ABCs of trauma care

ED TREATMENT

- Maintain spinal immobilization
- High-dose methylprednisolone protocol for any neurologic deficit
- Consultation with orthopedic spine or neurosurgery service
- Appropriate analgesia
- The following "stable" injuries may be treated conservatively if the CT confirms stability of injury and patient is neurologically intact
  —Isolated spinous process, transverse process fracture, chance fractures, anterior wedge compression (<50%) fracture, and "stable" burst fractures
- Total contact orthotic devices may be useful; limited activities; sleep prone; avoid pillows and soft mattresses, which may worsen deformity

MEDICATIONS

- Narcotic pain medication in absence of contraindications
- *High-dose steroid protocol*
  —Methylprednisolone: 30 mg/kg i.v. load over 1 hour, then 5.4 mg/kg/h for the next 23 hours; initiate in ED within 8 hours of injury

Disposition

ADMISSION CRITERIA

- Patients with traumatic lumbar fractures should be admitted for stabilization procedures, parenteral pain control, management of possible ileus, and evaluation for associated injuries

DISCHARGE CRITERIA

- Neurologically intact patients with stable nontraumatic fractures evaluated in conjunction with spine surgeon
- Patients with simple compression (wedge) fractures with no neurologic deficit may be considered for outpatient management if adequate pain control and appropriate follow-up can be arranged
- Simple transverse sacral fracture, isolated spinous process fracture, isolated transverse process fracture may also be considered for outpatient management
- The patient must be neurologically intact with a stable living situation and the CT scan and flexion-extension films must confirm fracture stability

Miscellaneous

ICD9: 805.4

ICD10: S34.2

SUGGESTED READINGS

Campana BA. Soft tissue injuries and back pain. In: Rosen P, Barkin R, eds. Emergency medicine: concepts and clinical practice, 4th ed. St. Louis: CV Mosby, 1998:878–905.

Denis F. Spinal instability as defined by the three-column spine concept in acute spinal trauma. Clin Orthop 1984;189:65–76.

Gabos P, Tuten H, Leet A, et al. Fracture-dislocation of the lumbar spine in an abused child. Pediatrics 1998;101(3): 473–477.

Hockenberger RS, Kirshenbaum KJ, Doris PE. Spinal injuries. In: Rosen P, Barkin R, eds. Emergency medicine: concepts and clinical practice, 4th ed. St. Louis: CV Mosby, 1998:462–505.

Krueger MA, Green DA, Hoyt D, et al. Overlooked spine injuries associated with lumbar process fractures. Clin Orthop 1996;327:191–195.

Petersilge C, Emery S. Thoracolumbar burst fracture: evaluating stability. Semin Ultrasound CT MR 1996;17(2):105–113.

Savitsky E, Votey S. Emergency department approach to acute thoracolumbar spine injury. J Emerg Med 1997;15:49–60.

Author: Bret Ginther

Spine Injury, Thoracic

Clinical Presentation

SIGNS AND SYMPTOMS

- Significant force is required to produce thoracic vertebral fractures
- Pain at the fracture site or impingement of nearby structures by bone fragments
- Because of the stabilizing influence of the rib cage, a tremendous amount of force is required to cause dislocations of the thoracic spine
  - —Concomitant internal injury should be suspected
  - —Thoracic spine fracture-dislocation is less common than thoracolumbar fracture-dislocation but higher incidence of neurologic impairment
- Common signs and symptoms
  - —Localized soft-tissue defect
  - —Pain or tenderness
  - —Localized—pain and tenderness over spinous process
  - —Referred—paraspinal, anterior chest, or abdomen
  - —Paraspinal muscle spasm
  - —Paresthesia or dysesthesia
  - —Weakness (focal or global)
  - —Distal areflexia, flaccid plegia
  - —Bowel or bladder incontinence
  - —Priapism
  - —Loss of temperature control
  - —Spinal shock—hypotension with bradycardia

MECHANISM/DESCRIPTION

- The following forces account for most thoracic fractures and dislocations
  - —Axial compression
  - —Flexion-rotation
  - —Shear
  - —Flexion-distraction
  - —Extension
- Three anatomically distinct columns; if two of the three columns are disrupted, the spinal column is unstable
  - —Posterior column: posterior bony arch and interconnecting ligamentous structures
  - —Middle column: posterior aspects of the vertebral bodies, posterior annulus fibrosis, and the posterior longitudinal ligament
  - —Anterior column: anterior longitudinal ligament, anterior anulus fibrosis, and anterior vertebral body

Major vs. Minor Fractures

- Minor
  - —Isolated articular fracture
  - —Transverse process fracture
  - —Spinous process fracture
  - —Pars interarticularis fracture
- Major
  - —Compression fracture
  - —Burst fracture
  - —Seat-belt injury
  - —Fracture-dislocation
- Compression fracture (anterior or lateral flexion)
  - —Fracture of anterior portion of vertebral body with intact middle column of spine
  - —May be posterior column disruption
  - —Type A: fracture through both end plates
  - —Type B: fracture through superior end plate
  - —Type C: fracture through inferior end plate
  - —Type D: both end plates intact
- Burst fracture (axial loading)
  - —Fracture through middle column of spine
  - —May have spreading of posterior elements and lamina fractures with possible bone fragment retropulsion into the spinal canal and potential neurologic compromise
  - —Type A: fracture through both end plates
  - —Type B: fracture through superior end plate
  - —Type C: fracture through inferior end plate
  - —Type D: burst in middle column with rotational injury leading to subluxation
  - —Type E: burst in middle column with asymmetric compression of anterior column
- Seat-belt injury (flexion-distraction)
  - —Distraction of posterior and middle columns with anterior column intact
  - —Typically caused by lap belts used without shoulder harness
  - —Type A: through bone
  - —Type B: primarily ligamentous
  - —Type C: disruption of bone through middle column
  - —Type D: through ligaments and disc with no middle column fracture
- Fracture-dislocations
  - —Failure of all three columns following compression, tension, rotation, or shear forces
  - —Type A: flexion-rotation; fall from height
  - —Type B: shear—violent force across long axis of trunk
  - —Type C: flexion-distraction; bilateral facet dislocation

ETIOLOGY

- Thoracic spine is rigid due to the rib cage and the costovertebral articulations
  - —The spinal canal is narrowest in the thoracic spine
- Because traumatic thoracic spine fractures require enormous forces, motor-vehicle accidents or falls from height account for most fractures
  - —A small percentage is caused by penetrating injuries (see Spinal Cord Syndromes)
  - —50% of all spinal fractures and 40% of all spinal cord injuries occur at the thoracolumbar junction (T11-L2)

Pre-Hospital

CAUTIONS

- If the patient's positioning initially prevents placement of a long spinal board, then a short board should be placed until the patient is fully extricated
- Patients with neurologic deficit should be transported directly to a trauma center

Diagnosis

ESSENTIAL WORKUP

- Rapid evaluation of airway, breathing, and circulation
- Primary and secondary trauma survey
- Detailed neurologic exam, including rectal tone and perianal sensation
- Thorough spine exam for deformity or tenderness
- Any midline tenderness elicited on examination, distracting injury, or intoxication mandates plain film spine radiography
- If fracture present, determine whether it is stable or unstable
- Assess for bulbocavernous reflex in spinal shock

IMAGING/SPECIAL TESTS

- Midline pain or tenderness, severe motor-vehicle accident, or falls from height are indications for anteroposterior and lateral plain film views of the spine
- Thin-cut CT scanning is indicated in any patient with evidence of spinal fracture or ligamentous injury on plain films to assess spinal canal integrity or in patients with normal plain films and significant pain or tenderness and mechanism for severe injury

DIFFERENTIAL DIAGNOSIS

- Arthritis (degenerative and rheumatoid)
- Ankylosing spondylitis
- Spina bifida
- Congenital malformation
- Neoplasm
- Pathologic fracture

Treatment

INITIAL STABILIZATION

- Follow the ABCs of trauma resuscitation
- Airway intervention should be done with in-line cervical immobilization
- Preserve residual spinal cord function and prevent further injury by stabilizing the spine

ED TREATMENT

- Perform all needed resuscitation and diagnostic tests with the patient in full spinal immobilization
- If spinal cord injury is suspected, administer high-dose steroids and consult a neurosurgeon
- If spinal fracture or ligamentous injury is suspected without neurologic impairment, arrange CT or MRI scanning while consulting neurosurgery or orthopedic surgery
- Pain control should be administered as soon as possible; NSAIDs, opiates, and benzodiazepines are the mainstays of treatment
- Neurogenic hypotension presents with bradycardia or normal heart rate, rather than the tachycardia seen with hypovolemic shock
  —Neurogenic hypotension should be treated with crystalloid bolus but may require vasopressors

MEDICATIONS

- High-dose steroid protocol
  —Solu-Medrol: 30 mg/kg i.v. bolus followed immediately by an infusion of 5.4 mg/kg/h for the next 23 hours if started within 3 hours of injury; continue for 48 hours if started 3–8 hours after injury; not recommended >8 hours after injury
  —H_2-antagonists to prevent gastric irritation

Disposition

ADMISSION CRITERIA

- Patients with significant spinal cord or column injury should be treated in a regional trauma center
- Unstable spinal column injury
- Cord or root injury
- Ileus
- Pain control
- Concomitant traumatic injury

DISCHARGE CRITERIA

- Stable minor fractures after orthopedic or neurosurgical evaluation

Miscellaneous

ICD9: 952.10

ICD10: S24.2

SUGGESTED READINGS

Block BE, et al. Thoracic and lumbar spine injuries in children. Contemp Orthop 1994;29(4):243.

Brandser EA, El-Khoury GY. Thoracic and lumbar spine trauma. Radiol Clin North Am 1997;35(3):533–557.

Chiles BW III, Cooper PR. Acute spinal injury. N Engl J Med 1996;334(8):514–520.

El-Khoury GY, Whitten CG. Trauma to the upper thoracic spine: anatomy, biomechanics, and unique imaging features. AJR Am J Roentgenol 1993;160: 95–102.

Hockberger RS, et al. Spine. In: Rosen P, et al, eds. Emergency medicine: concepts and clinical practice, 5th ed. St. Louis: Mosby, 2002:329–369.

Kinashita H. Pathology of spinal cord injuries due to fracture—dislocations of the thoracic and lumber spine. Paraplegia 1996;34(1):1–7.

Savitsky E, Votey S. Emergency department approach to acute thoracolumbar spine injury. J Emerg Med 1997;15(1):49–60.

Authors: Richard D. Zane; Haritha Challapalli

Splenic Injury

Clinical Presentation

SIGNS AND SYMPTOMS

- Systemic signs from acute blood loss
  - —May present with syncope, dizziness, weakness, confusion
  - —May progress to profound hypotension or shock
- Local signs
  - —LUQ abdominal tenderness
  - —Referred pain to the left shoulder (Kehr's sign)
  - —Abdominal distention, rigidity, rebound tenderness, involuntary guarding
- Contusions, abrasions, or penetrating wounds to the chest, flank, or abdomen may indicate underlying spleen injury
- Fractures of lower left ribs are commonly seen in association with splenic injuries
- Physical exam is neither sensitive nor specific for splenic injury; adjunctive studies are required

MECHANISM/DESCRIPTION

- The spleen is the most commonly injured intraabdominal organ
  - —In nearly two thirds of these cases, it is the only damaged intraperitoneal structure
- Motor-vehicle accidents are the major cause, followed by motorcycle accidents and falls
- Mechanism of injury and kinematics are important factors in evaluating patients for possible splenic injury
- In blunt trauma, note the type and direction (horizontal or vertical) of any deceleration or compressive forces
  - —Injuries are caused by compression of the spleen between the applied force to the anterior abdominal wall and the posterior thoracic cage or vertebral column, producing a crushing effect
- In penetrating trauma, note the characteristic of the weapon (type and caliber), distance from the weapon, or the type and length of knife or impaling object
  - —Injuries result from a combination of the kinetic energy and shear forces of the penetrating object
- Splenic injuries are graded by type and severity of injury
  - —Grade I: superficial laceration
  - —Grade II: more extensive laceration or subcapsular hematoma
  - —Grade III: laceration >3 cm involving trabecular vessels
  - —Grade IV: laceration involving segmental or hilar vessels
  - —Grade V: shattered spleen

PEDIATRIC CONSIDERATIONS

- Poorly developed musculature and relatively smaller anteroposterior diameter increase the vulnerability of abdominal contents to compressive forces
- Rib cage is extremely compliant and less prone to fracture in children but provides only partial protection against splenic injury
- Splenic capsule in children is relatively thicker than that of an adult; parenchyma of spleen seems to contain more smooth muscle than in adults

Pre-Hospital

CAUTIONS

- Obtain details of injury from pre-hospital providers
- Insert two large-bore IVs because hemorrhage is a major threat to life
- Penetrating wounds or evisceration should be covered with moist, sterile dressings

Diagnosis

ESSENTIAL WORKUP

- Physical exam is neither specific nor sensitive for splenic injury
- Adjunctive imaging studies are required

LABORATORY

- No hematologic laboratory studies are specific for diagnosis of injury to the spleen
- Obtain baseline hemoglobin, type, and cross-match

IMAGING/SPECIAL TESTS

- Plain abdominal x-rays are too nonspecific to be of value
- CXR findings suggestive for splenic injury include left lower rib fracture(s), elevation of left hemidiaphragm, or left pleural effusion
- US
  - —Can be done at bedside, especially in patient unstable to go to CT scanner
  - —Primary role is detecting free intraperitoneal blood, which may suggest splenic injury
  - —Does not image solid parenchymal damage well
- Diagnostic peritoneal lavage (DPL)
  - —Extremely sensitive for the presence of hemoperitoneum although nonspecific for source of bleeding and does not evaluate retroperitoneum
- Abdominal CT
  - —Depicts the presence and extent of splenic injury and injuries to adjacent organs, including the retroperitoneum
  - —This modality provides the most specific information in patients stable enough to go to the CT scanner

DIFFERENTIAL DIAGNOSIS

- Intraperitoneal organ injury, especially liver
- Injury to retroperitoneal structures
- Thoracic injury

Treatment

INITIAL STABILIZATION

- ABCs (including C-spine immobilization)
  - —Adequate IV access, including central lines and cutdowns as dictated by the patient's hemodynamic status
  - —Fluid resuscitation, initially with 2 L of crystalloid (NS or lactated Ringer's solution), followed by blood products as needed

ED TREATMENT

- Immediate laparotomy may be appropriate in the acutely injured patient who is hemodynamically unstable with presumed hemoperitoneum and splenic injury
- Most patients with acute splenic injury either are hemodynamically stable or stabilize rapidly with relatively small amounts of fluid resuscitation
- Adjunctive diagnostic procedures supplementing the physical exam should be performed early in the evaluation, followed by laparotomy when indicated by positive diagnostic findings
- Gunshot wounds to the anterior abdomen are routinely explored
- Stab wounds can be managed by local wound exploration, followed by US or DPL when intraperitoneal penetration is demonstrated or equivocal
- Operative versus nonoperative management
  - —Patients with signs and symptoms of intraperitoneal hemorrhage, those with operative indications based on imaging/ diagnostic procedures, and those who fail nonoperative management should undergo laparotomy
  - —Splenectomy versus splenic salvage procedures depends on the grade of splenic injury
  - —Patient selection for nonoperative management includes hemodynamic stability, no evidence of other intraabdominal injury, isolated splenic injury confirmed by imaging study (most commonly CT scan)
  - —Patients older than 55 years should be considered for operative management due to decreased physical tolerance to traumatic insult and reduced physiologic reserve

PEDIATRIC CONSIDERATIONS

- Nonoperative management of splenic injuries is considered safe
- Concerns for overwhelming postsplenectomy infection in patients undergoing splenectomy

Disposition

ADMISSION CRITERIA

- All patients with splenic injury require hospitalization for definitive laparotomy or observation with serial abdominal examinations, serial hematocrit determinations, and bed rest

DISCHARGE CRITERIA

- Only asymptomatic patients objectively demonstrated not to have splenic or other traumatic injury may be discharged

Miscellaneous

ICD9: 865.00

ICD10: S36.0

SUGGESTED READINGS

Dupuy DE, Raptopoulos V, Fink MP. Current concepts in splenic trauma. J Intens Care Med 1995;10:76–90.

Esposito T, Gamelli R. Injury to the spleen. In: Felicano D, et al, eds. Trauma, 3rd ed. Norwalk, CT: Appleton & Lange, 1996: 525–550.

Marx J. Abdominal trauma. In: Rosen P, et al, eds. Emergency medicine: concepts and clinical practice, 5th ed. St. Louis: CV Mosby, 2002:415–436.

Peitzman A, et al. Injury to the spleen. Curr Probl Surg 2001;38(12):932–1008.

Author: Albert Jin

Spondylolysis/Spondylolisthesis

Clinical Presentation

SIGNS AND SYMPTOMS

- Often associated with feeling of stiffness or spasm in paravertebral muscles
- Pain occurs after varying amounts of exercise, with standing, or with coughing
- Relief of pain with rest is variable and slow, and usually requires sitting or stooping
- Pain in the back and proximal legs that is aggravated by standing and walking
- Sitting or forward bending relieves pain
- Hamstring tightness is common
- Neurologic exam usually normal
  - —If abnormal, pain and sensorimotor loss is in a dermatomal distribution
- May have flattening of normal lumbar lordosis

MECHANISM/DESCRIPTION

Spondylolysis

- Bony defect at the pars interarticularis (the isthmus of bone between the superior and inferior facets), which can be unilateral or bilateral
- Type 1: Dysplastic: congenital defect of the neural arch or intraarticular facets
- Type 2: Isthmic: stress fracture from repetitive microtrauma through the neural arch
- Type 3: Degenerative: long-standing segmental instability
- Type 4: Traumatic
- Type 5: Pathologic: generalized or focal bone disease

Spondylolisthesis

- The slipping forward of one vertebra upon another
- Spondylolysis is not a clinical problem but can contribute to spondylolisthesis, which is noted in approximately 5% of the population
- Of those with spondylolysis, 50% will have some degree of spondylolisthesis develop during their lifetime, and 50% of those will be symptomatic
  - —Literature does not associate athletic activity with increased slippage
- Spondylolisthesis predisposes to sciatica
- Spondylolisthesis is divided into four grades based on degree of slippage (Meyerding grading system)
  - —Grade I: up to 25% of the vertebral body width
  - —Grade II: 26–50% of the vertebral body width
  - —Grade III: 51–75% of the vertebral body width
  - —Grade IV: 76–100% of the vertebral body width
- The most common location for spondylolisthesis is L-5 displaced on the sacrum (85–95%), followed by L-4 on L-5

ETIOLOGY

- Unknown; theories include congenital pars anomalies, bone-density alterations, and recurrent subclinical stress injury

PEDIATRIC CONSIDERATIONS

- Spondylolysis is one of the most common causes of serious low back pain in children, although it is most often asymptomatic
- Symptoms most often present during adolescent growth spurt between ages 10 and 15 years
- Seen commonly in athletic teens; particularly in sports involving back hyperextension (e.g., gymnastics, diving, football)
- Acute symptoms are related to trauma
- Spondylolysis in a child younger than 10 years is rare; these patients should be watched for
  - —Constant pain that lasts for several weeks
  - —Pain that occurs spontaneously at night
  - —Pain that interferes repeatedly with school, play, or sports
  - —Pain associated with marked stiffness, limitation of motion, fever, or neurologic signs
  - —Pain at the lumbosacral junction

Pre-Hospital

- Spinal precautions are not needed unless there is a history of recent trauma

Diagnosis

ESSENTIAL WORKUP

- History
  - —Onset of symptoms—often gradual; acute pain generally seen with trauma
  - —Location of pain
  - —Aggravating/alleviating factors: for example, repetitive hyperextending movements
  - —Systemic/neurologic symptoms: minimal, unless significant trauma or "slip"
- Physical exam
  - —Hyperlordotic posture
  - —Tight hamstrings, knees flexed to allow patient to stand upright
  - —Only "typical" finding is one-legged hyperextension; standing on one leg and leaning backward reproduces pain on ipsilateral side
  - —Palpation may reveal step-off with a prominent spinous process of L-5 in significant spondylolisthesis
  - —Neurologic exam is usually normal; if abnormal, consider herniation or spondylolisthesis
  - —Trunk may appear shortened
  - —Rib cage approaches iliac crests

LABORATORY

- Not helpful except for identifying alternative causes

IMAGING/SPECIAL TESTS

- Lumbosacral spine x-rays
  - —Lateral and oblique x-rays of spine most helpful
  - —Spondylolysis will manifest as a radiolucent defect in the pars interarticularis, visible as a "collar" or "broken neck" on the oblique view "Scottie dog"
  - —Majority (85–95%) found at L5-S1 level
  - —Spondylolisthesis will manifest as forward slipping of one vertebral body on another (on lateral)
- SPECT scanning—better specificity for linking back pain to spondylolysis
- CT scan
  - —Pathology more clearly demonstrated than plain films
  - —Can identify other spinal pathology
  - —Can play an important role for orthopedics in management decisions through identification of new stress fractures and healing of old stress fractures
  - —Outpatient evaluation unless history of recent trauma
- MRI
  - —Exact role for MRI in spondylolysis not yet clarified in literature
  - —Useful for defining root impingement and foraminal narrowing

DIFFERENTIAL DIAGNOSIS

- Tuberculosis
- Discitis
- Bone or spinal cord tumor
- Pyelonephritis
- Retroperitoneal infection
- Injury to muscles or joints of back
- Congenital hip dislocation
- Rickets
- Ruptured intervertebral disc
- Vascular claudication

PEDIATRIC CONSIDERATIONS

- Lower threshold for ordering imaging studies
- Progressive slipping more likely to occur than in adults

Treatment

INITIAL STABILIZATION

- Maintain spinal precautions if traumatic spondylolisthesis
- Vigorous attempts at traction should not be pursued

ED TREATMENT

- Pain control and muscle relaxants as clinically needed
- Supportive therapy if symptoms are mild
- Restrict activities if repetitive trauma is likely aggravating cause (e.g., sports) for 3–6 weeks, followed by reintroduction of activity when asymptomatic
- Consider antilordotic braces (controversial) or physical therapy
- Orthopedic consult or referral if symptoms are moderate to severe or unresponsive to supportive care
- Surgical intervention typically consists of spinal fusion in the flexed position
- 50% of symptomatic patients with spondylolisthesis may require surgery
- All symptomatic patients with grade III or IV spondylolisthesis should probably undergo surgery
- Patient education
- Exercises are not of proven benefit

MEDICATIONS

- Muscle relaxants
  —Example: methocarbamol: 1,000–1,500 mg PO q.i.d. (peds: safety and effectiveness for children younger than 12 years not established)
- NSAIDs
  —Example: ibuprofen: 200–800 mg PO q.i.d. (peds: 5–10 mg/kg PO q6h)
- Opioids
  —Example: morphine sulfate: 0.1 mg/kg up to 2–4 mg increments i.v.

PEDIATRIC CONSIDERATIONS

- Activity restriction is not necessary if minimal or no symptoms

Disposition

ADMISSION CRITERIA

- Inability to walk
- Inability to cope at home due to pain or social situation
- Progressive neurologic deficit

DISCHARGE CRITERIA

- Most patients can be treated on outpatient basis
- Orthopedic follow-up arranged
- Social support system in place
- Pain control
- Patient education

PEDIATRIC CONSIDERATIONS

- Close follow-up is mandatory

Miscellaneous

ICD9: 721.90; 756.12

ICD10: M47.9; M43.1

SUGGESTED READINGS

Congeni J, McCulloch J, Swanson K. Lumbar spondylolysis. A study of natural progression in athletes. Am J Sports Med 1997;25(2):248–253.

Nachemson A. Newest knowledge of low back pain. Clin Orthop 1992;279:8.

Satndaert CJ. Spondylolysis. Phys Med Rehab Clin North Am 2000;11(4):785–801.

Skinner H. Disorders, diseases and injuries of the spine. In: Current diagnosis and treatment in orthopedics. Norwalk, CT: Appleton & Lange, 1995:206–211.

Vitek G. Spine conference—spondylolysis and spondylolisthesis. OrthoNews Magazine May 1995. Available at: *www.nmis.com/onm/html/sponconf_spon.htm*.

Authors: Kathleen J. Clem; Joel Kravitz

Spontaneous Bacterial Peritonitis

Clinical Presentation

SIGNS AND SYMPTOMS

- *Often asymptomatic*
- Abdominal pain, usually mild
- Direct or rebound tenderness
- Fever, chills
- Hypothermia
- Onset or worsening of ascites
- Development or worsening hepatic encephalopathy
- Nausea and vomiting
- Hypoactive bowel sounds
- Hypotension
- Worsening liver or renal function

MECHANISM/DESCRIPTION

- Translocation of bacteria through edematous gut mucosa, caused by portal hypertension, into lymph nodes to the peritoneal cavity
- Transient bacteremia, along with low serum complement
- Impaired reticuloendothelial system phagocytic activity and *low ascitic fluid protein* (<1 g/dL), opsonin, and bactericidal activity
- Patients with a total protein concentration <1 g/dL in ascitic fluid have a 20% risk of developing spontaneous bacterial peritonitis (SBP) during the first year after diagnosis of ascites
- 38% survival rate and 69% recurrence rate at 1 year
- SBP in 15–26% of patients hospitalized with ascites

ETIOLOGY

- Usually seen in setting of liver cirrhosis, especially in decompensated jaundiced patients
- Rare in other conditions causing ascites (e.g., nephrotic syndrome and CHF)
- Predominant organisms
  - —*Escherichia coli* (45%)
  - —*Pneumococcus* (20%)
  - —*Klebsiella* (10%)
  - —*Enterobacter*
  - —*Proteus*
  - —*Citrobacter freundii*
  - —*Enterococcus* (5%)
- Polymicrobial is rare (<5%)

Pre-Hospital

CAUTIONS

- IV fluid bolus for unstable vital signs or shock or hypothermia

Diagnosis

ESSENTIAL WORKUP

- Paracentesis
  - —Procedure
    - -10 mL for total protein and cell count
    - -Inject 10 mL of ascitic fluid in each blood culture bottle to maximize the yield (only positive in 50–80% of patients)
  - —Polymorphonuclear (PMN) cell count $>250/\mu L$ diagnostic
  - —Gram stain—infrequently positive
  - —Total protein >10–15 g/L indicates a relatively high concentration of antimicrobial factors and low probability of SBP
  - —Repeat paracentesis after 48 hours of treatment to monitor response

LABORATORY

- CBC
  - —Anemia
  - —Leukocytosis
- Liver profile/liver enzymes
- PT/PTT
  - —Elevated PT
- Blood cultures are infrequently positive
- Spot urine for sodium and creatinine
- Other tests as noted in ascites section
- Serum albumin ascitic gradient (SAAG) remains wide (i.e., >1.1 g/dL)

IMAGING/SPECIAL TESTS

- Abdominal US
  - —Confirms presence of ascites (if volume small)
  - —Helps guide paracentesis
- CXR for pneumonia, CHF, effusion
- Abdominal radiograph for obstruction/perforation

DIFFERENTIAL DIAGNOSIS

- Culture-negative neutrocytic ascites
  - —Ascitic PMN $>250\ \mu L$ but the culture is negative
  - —May progress to SBP—treated similarly
  - —Consider secondary cause TB or malignancy if PMN count does not drop with treatment
- Secondary bacterial peritonitis
  - —Due to perforation or abscess
  - —Multiple organisms, especially anaerobes
  - —Ascitic glucose <50 mg/dL
  - —Ascitic protein >1 g/dL
  - —Ascitic PMN $>10{,}000/\mu L$
- Monomicrobial bacterial ascites
  - —PMN $<250\ \mu L$, but culture is positive
  - —If contamination cannot be ruled out, treat as SBP
- Polymicrobial bacterial ascites
  - —PMN $<250\ \mu L$ but the culture is positive for multiple organisms
  - —Suspicious of accidental gut perforation by the paracentesis needle (rare)
- High ascites WBC ($>500/\mu L$) with lymphocyte prominence favor TB, malignancy or chylous ascites

Treatment

INITIAL STABILIZATION

- ABCs
- Aggressive IV fluid resuscitation and prompt antibiotic treatment for septic shock

ED TREATMENT

- Correct coagulopathy before large-volume paracentesis with large-bore needle
  —Administer 2 units FFP if PT >16
  —Administer 10 IU platelets if platelet count <50,000
- Initiate antibiotic for ascitic fluid PMN >250 μL—*do not* wait for culture result
  —First choice: third-generation cephalosporin (cefotaxime or ceftriaxone)
  —Second-generation cephalosporin, ampicillin and sulbactam combination, or aztreonam provides lesser cure rate
  —*Avoid* aminoglycosides—cirrhotic patients at high risk of nephrotoxicity
- Subsequent antibiotic choice depends on culture and sensitivity result
- Administer antibiotics for 10 days
  —May use 5-day course if the ascitic PMN drops by 50% after 48 hours of treatment
- Higher mortality rate and poor infection resolution seen with
  —Hospital-acquired SBP
  —High BUN
  —High band count in the blood
  —High AST
  —Presence of ileus
- Oral quinolones (ofloxacin or ciprofloxacin) for patients refusing IV antibiotics
  —Not tested in patients who have severe hepatic encephalopathy, GI tract bleed, ileus, septic shock, creatinine level >3 mg/dL
- Predictors of high recurrence rate (up to 69% in 1 year)
  —Ascitic protein <1 g/dL
  —Serum bilirubin >4 mg/dL
  —Prolonged PT
  —Benefit from prophylactic norfloxacin 400 mg/d, or trimethoprim-sulfamethizole 1 D.S. tablet 5 days/wk

MEDICATIONS

- Bactrim DS: 1 tablet 5 days/wk
- Cefotaxime: 2 g (peds: 50–180 mg/kg/24 h) i.v. q8h
- Ceftriaxone: 2 g (peds: 50–75 mg/kg/24 h) i.v. q24h
- Ciprofloxacin: 500 mg PO b.i.d.
- Ofloxacin: 400 mg PO b.i.d.
- Norfloxacin: 400 mg/d

PEDIATRIC CONSIDERATIONS

- Quinolones: not tested in children with SBP

Disposition

ADMISSION CRITERIA

- Admit all patients with SBP with a gastroenterologist consult
- ICU admission if in septic shock or hepatic encephalopathy

DISCHARGE CRITERIA

- Patients refusing inpatient care
  —Administer dose of ceftriaxone followed by oral quinolones for 10 days

Miscellaneous

ICD9: 567.2

ICD10: K65.9

SEE ALSO: HEPATIC ENCEPHALOPATHY; HEPATITIS; HEPATORENAL SYNDROME

SUGGESTED READINGS

Bataller R, Gines P, Arroyo V. Practical recommendations for the treatment of ascites and its complications. Drugs 1997;54(4):571–580.

Garcia-Tsoa G. Treatment of spontaneous bacterial peritonitis with oral ofloxacin: inpatient or outpatient therapy? Gastroenterology 1996;11:1147.

Gilbert JA, Kamath PS. Spontaneous bacterial peritonitis. Mayo Clin Proc 1995;70:365.

Guarner C, Soriano G. Spontaneous bacterial peritonitis. Semin Liver Dis 1997:17;203–217.

McGuire BM, Bloomer JR. Complications of cirrhosis: why they occur and what to do about them. Postgrad Med 1998;103(2): 209–212, 217–218, 223–224.

Author: Craig Houston

Sporotrichosis

Clinical Presentation

SIGNS AND SYMPTOMS

- Several clinical manifestations/syndromes
- Determined by mode of inoculation and host factors

Lymphocutaneous

- Most common manifestation
- Initial lesions appear days to weeks after inoculation
- Begin as papule, become nodular, often ulcerate
  - —Distal extremities more commonly involved
  - —Size: millimeters to 4 cm
  - —Pain is absent or mild
  - —Drainage is nonpurulent
- Systemic symptoms usually absent
- Secondary nodular lesions develop along lymphatics draining original site
- May wax and wane over years if untreated

Fixed Cutaneous

- Plaque-like or verrucous lesion at site of inoculation
- Ulceration uncommon
- Do not manifest lymphangitic progression

Extracutaneous

- Osteoarticular
  - —Most common extracutaneous manifestation
  - —Joint inflammation, effusion, and pain
  - —Single or multiple joint involvement of extremities
  - —Indolent onset, few systemic symptoms
  - —Tenosynovitis, osteomyelitis, and bursitis
- Pulmonary
  - —Syndrome resembles mycobacterial infection
  - —Fever, weight loss, fatigue
  - —Productive cough, hemoptysis
- Less commonly associated sites
  - —Chronic lymphocytic meningitis
  - —Ocular adnexa, endophthalmitis
  - —Genitourinary, sinuses

Multifocal Extracutaneous (Disseminated)

- Low-grade fever, weight loss
- Diffuse cutaneous lesions
- Arthritis/osteolytic lesions/parenchymal involvement
- Can be fatal if untreated
- Often occurs in immunocompromised host

MECHANISM/DESCRIPTION

- Lymphocutaneous/fixed cutaneous
  - —Inoculation of fungus into skin/soft tissue
  - —Secondary to trauma, animal bites/scratches
  - —Increased risk: farmers, gardeners, forestry workers
- Pulmonary
  - —Inhalation of conidia aerosolized from soil/plant decay
  - —Increased risk: alcoholics, diabetics, COPD, steroid use
- Multifocal extracutaneous
  - —Cutaneous inoculation or hematologic spread
  - —Increased risk: HIV/immunosuppressed patients

ETIOLOGY

- Fungal infection caused by *Sporothrix schenckii*
  - —Dimorphic fungus
  - —Occurs as mold on decaying vegetation, moss, and soil in temperate and tropical environments
- Animal vectors, notably cats and armadillos

Pre-Hospital

N/A

Diagnosis

ESSENTIAL WORKUP

- Diagnosis dependent on isolation *S. schenckii* from site of infection

LABORATORY

- Blood tests not indicated with cutaneous disease
- Cultures of sputum, synovial fluid, CSF, blood as indicated by extracutaneous manifestations
- No reliable serologic assays available

IMAGING/SPECIAL TESTS

- Lymphocutaneous/fixed cutaneous
  - —Biopsy reveals pyogranulomatous inflammation, cigar-shaped yeast
- Pulmonary
  - —Chest radiograph reveals cavitary lesions
  - —Gram stain of sputum may yield yeast
  - —Sputum cultures often positive
- Extracutaneous/disseminated
  - —CSF reveals lymphocytic meningitis, increased protein/decreased glucose
  - —Consider bone scan in immunocompromised host

DIFFERENTIAL DIAGNOSIS

- Lymphocutaneous
  - —Leishmaniasis
  - —Nocardiosis
  - —*Mycobacterium marinum*
  - —Tularemia
- Fixed cutaneous
  - —Bacterial pyoderma
  - —Foreign-body granuloma
  - —Inflammatory dermatophyte infections
  - —Blastomycosis
  - —Mycobacteria
  - —Chromoblastomycosis
- Osteoarticular
  - —Rheumatoid arthritis
  - —Gout
  - —TB
  - —Bacterial arthritis
  - —Pigmented villonodular synovitis
- Pulmonary and meningitis
  - —Histoplasmosis
  - —Coccidioidomycosis
  - —Cryptococcal disease
  - —Mycobacterial infections

Treatment

INITIAL STABILIZATION

- Airway/hemodynamic stabilization for severely ill patients with extracutaneous manifestations

ED TREATMENT

Lymphocutaneous/Fixed Cutaneous

- Itraconazole (drug of choice)
  - —Better tolerated
  - —More expensive
  - —Potential for hepatotoxicity
- Saturated solution of potassium iodide (SSKI)
  - —Less expensive
  - —Bitter taste and side effects (anorexia, nausea, diarrhea) lead to limited acceptability
- Local heat therapy (>35°C) inhibits fungal growth
- Therapy may take 3–6 months

Pulmonary

- Itraconazole or amphotericin B in early disease
  - —Effective in about 30% of cases
- More advanced disease often requires resection plus amphotericin B

Osteoarticular

- Itraconazole—first line
- Amphotericin B if refractory

Disseminated

- Itraconazole in stable, immunocompetent patients
- Amphotericin B in following
  - —Acutely ill
  - —Meningitis (may need 5-fluorocystine as adjunct)
  - —Immunosuppressed host

HIV and Sporotrichosis

- Suppressive therapy with itraconazole is recommended after initial infection

MEDICATIONS

- Amphotericin B: start 0.25 mg/kg i.v. q.d., advance to 0.5–1.5 mg/kg i.v. q.d., for 1–2.5-g course
- Itraconazole: 100–200 mg PO q.d. in lymphocutaneous for up to 6 months; 200 mg PO in pulmonary/osteoarticular
- SSKI: 5 gtt in water or juice t.i.d.; increase by 5 gtt/dose each week up to a maximum of 40–50 gtt t.i.d. as tolerated, for 6–12 weeks or until lesions resolve

Disposition

ADMISSION CRITERIA

- Systemic signs/symptoms
- Pulmonary, CNS, multifocal disease
- Immunosuppressed host with disseminated disease

DISCHARGE CRITERIA

- Lymphocutaneous/fixed cutaneous form, nontoxic
- Immunosuppressed host, only if occult disseminated disease ruled out

Miscellaneous

ICD9: 117.1

ICD10: B42.9

SUGGESTED READINGS

Bustamante B, Campos PE. Endemic sporotrichosis. Curr Opin Infect Dis 2001;14(2):145–149.

Kauffman CA. Sporotrichosis. Clin Infect Dis 1999;29:231–237.

Rex JH, Okhuysen PC. *Sporothrix schenckii.* In: Mandel GL, Douglas RG, Bennett JE, eds. Principles and practice of infectious diseases, 5th ed. New York: Churchill Livingstone, 2000:2695–2699.

Winn RE. A contemporary review of sporotrichosis. Curr Top Med Mycol 1995;6:73–94.

Authors: John E. Sather; Robert Powers

Staphylococcal Scalded Skin Syndrome

Clinical Presentation

SIGNS AND SYMPTOMS

- Constitutional symptoms
  - —Malaise
  - —Fever
  - —Irritability
- Diffuse tender scarlatiniform erythema resembling a "sunburn"—erythroderma
- Areas of prominence
  - —Around the flexor areas of the neck
  - —In intertriginous areas, especially axilla and groin
  - —Near the eyes and mouth
- Increased erythema in skin creases
- Facial edema with radial crusting fissures around the eyes, nose, and mouth
- Child may appear well, ill, or overtly toxic
- Flaccid bullae
  - —Within 1–3 days after onset of rash
  - —Initially over flexures
  - —Bullae migrate through epidermis with light lateral pressure; epidermis separates with minor pressure (Nikolsky sign)
  - —Rupture within hours
  - —Epidermis separates with minor trauma
  - —Epidermis is shed in sheets
  - —Denuded areas are moist, sensitive, and painful
  - —Complete healing within 2 weeks
- Purulent conjunctivitis
- Mucous membranes are not affected
- Complications are rare
  - —Hypothermia
  - —Fluid and electrolyte imbalance
  - —Secondary infection
  - —Pneumonia
  - —Septicemia

MECHANISM/DESCRIPTION

- Results from the actions of a soluble epidermolytic exotoxin produced by *Staphylococcus aureus*
  - —Produced at a distant site of infection or colonization
  - —Disseminates hematogenously
  - —Lyses desmosomes of granular cells in the superficial epidermis
  - —Results in generalized intradermal exfoliation
- Disease of infants and children younger than 6 years
  - —Inability to metabolize and excrete toxin efficiently
- Presentation determined by age and extent of the rash
  - —Classic staphylococcal scalded skin syndrome
  - —Pemphigus neonatorum
  - —Bullous impetigo
- Typically, coagulase positive phage group II *Staphylococcus*
  - —Group I and group III also implicated

ETIOLOGY

- Colonization often without overt infection
- Concurrent infection or break of skin barrier
  - —Minor skin abrasions
  - —Circumcision site
  - —Conjunctivitis
  - —Umbilicus/omphalitis
  - —Impetigo
  - —Endocarditis and septicemia
- Often no focus identified

Pre-Hospital

N/A

Diagnosis

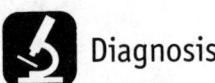

ESSENTIAL WORKUP

- Clinical presentation is diagnostic
- Determine location/source of toxin producing *Staphylococcus*

LABORATORY

- CBC and urinalysis
  - —Assess for sepsis if source is not obvious
- Electrolytes
  - —Indicated if signs of dehydration or extensive rash
- Blood cultures
  - —Rarely positive

IMAGING/SPECIAL TESTS

- Fluid aspirated from bullae
  - —Sterile in staphylococcal scalded skin syndrome
- Skin biopsy or frozen histologic section
  - —Determine level of epidermal/dermal separation
  - —Indicated for children on medications, those older than 6 years, and in cases of mixed rash

DIFFERENTIAL DIAGNOSIS

- Infection
  - —Scarlet fever
    - -Strawberry tongue
    - -Involves the mucous membranes
    - -Painful desquamation does not occur
  - —Bullous impetigo
    - -Turbid or cloudy bullae fluid
  - —Bullous varicella
    - -5 days after the onset of varicella
    - -Tzanck prep or viral base reveals giant cells
  - —Toxic shock syndrome
- Toxic epidermal necrolysis or drug eruption
  - —Much more common in adults
- Dermatologic
  - —Erythema multiforme
  - —Epidermolysis hyperkeratosis
  - —Epidermolysis bullosa
  - —Pemphigus vulgaris
- Scald injury
- Secondary rash of an underlying disorder
  - —Lymphoma
  - —Aspergillosis
  - —Irradiation
  - —Graft-versus-host reaction
  - —Kawasaki disease

Treatment

INITIAL STABILIZATION

- Management is similar to extensive second-degree burn
  - —Large total body-surface area involvement will require IV fluids
- Provide adequate analgesia
- Undress and place child on sterile linen
- Limit handling of child
- Apply moist sterile dressings
- Avoid excess heat loss

ED TREATMENT

- Topical burn creams are of no proven benefit
- Steroids are contraindicated
- IV antibiotics effective against penicillinase-resistant *S. aureus*
  - —Cefazolin
  - —Oxacillin
  - —Nafcillin
- Oral antibiotics for mild involvement
  - —Dicloxacillin
  - —Erythromycin
  - —Cephalexin

MEDICATIONS

- Cefazolin: 50–100 mg/kg/24 h i.v. divided q.i.d.
- Cephalexin: 25–100 mg/kg/24 h PO divided q.i.d.
- Dicloxacillin: 12–25 mg/kg/24 h PO divided q.i.d.
- Erythromycin: 30–50 mg/kg/24 h PO divided q.i.d.
- Nafcillin: 1–2 g i.v. q6h (peds: newborns, 50–100 mg/kg/24 h i.v. divided q6h; children, 100–200 mg/kg/24 h i.v. divided q6h)

Disposition

ADMISSION CRITERIA

- Children younger than 1 year
- All toxic-appearing children
- Widespread skin involvement
- Dehydration and/or electrolyte derangement

DISCHARGE CRITERIA

- Older well-appearing children with mild involvement
- Oral antibiotics for 7 days
- Follow-up within 48 hours

Miscellaneous

ICD9: 695.1

ICD10: L00

SUGGESTED READINGS

Feigin RD, Cherry JD, eds. Textbook of pediatric infectious diseases. Philadelphia: WB Saunders, 1998:1055–1057.

Gemell CG. Staphylococcal scalded skin syndrome. J Med Microbiol 1995;43(5): 318–327.

Ladhani L. Recent developments in staphylococcal scalded skin syndrome. Clin Microbiol Infect 2001;7(6):301–307.

Authors: Timothy J. Mader; J. Brian Liddy

Sternoclavicular Joint Injury

Clinical Presentation

SIGNS AND SYMPTOMS

- Pain localized to the sternoclavicular joint (SCJ) region with the affected arm supported across the chest by the contralateral arm
- Inability to abduct or externally rotate affected arm
- If dislocated, shoulder appears shortened, the head tilts toward injured side due to sternocleidomastoid muscle spasm
- In *anterior dislocation,* medial end of the clavicle is visibly prominent and palpable
- In *posterior dislocation,* there may be a sulcus of the SCJ area through which the lateral border of the manubrium may be palpated
  - —Dislocation may be masked by significant swelling over the sternoclavicular region
  - —Venous congestion in the neck or upper extremities, asymmetric upper extremity pulses, shortness of breath, hoarseness, dysphagia
  - —Signs of shock suggest life-threatening impingement of the posteriorly displaced clavicle upon neurovascular and visceral structures in the mediastinum
- If subluxed or sprained, the SCJ is tender on direct palpation and with shoulder movement but without deformity or significant anteroposterior mobility

MECHANISM/DESCRIPTION

- The SCJ can dislocate in the anterior or posterior direction
- It is among the least frequently injured joints in the body
- Due primarily to trauma from vehicular or athletic injuries through direct or indirect mechanism
- Congenital or atraumatic dislocation rarely seen
- *Anterior dislocation* is more common
  - —Caused by a posteriorly directed force to the anterolateral aspect of the shoulder, resulting in reciprocal anterior displacement of the medial clavicle
- *Posterior dislocation* results from
  - —A direct anterior-to-posterior blow to the medial clavicle, or
  - —An anteriorly directed force to the posterolateral aspect of the shoulder with reciprocal posterior displacement of the medial clavicle
- *Posterior dislocation is a surgical emergency*
  - —Compression of trachea, esophagus, and great vessels in the mediastinum demand immediate reduction

PEDIATRIC CONSIDERATIONS

- The medial epiphyseal growth plates of the clavicles fuse between ages 22 and 25 years
- True dislocations of the SCJ are extremely rare in children because of the strong ligamentous attachments about the medial epiphysis
- Fractures through the medial epiphysis mimic SCJ dislocations
  - —Classified as Salter-Harris type I or II fractures

Pre-Hospital

CAUTIONS

- Attention to airway and vital signs, as well as neurovascular status of the affected extremity
- The affected arm should be splinted in the position of most comfort before transport to the ED

Diagnosis

ESSENTIAL WORKUP

- Complete trauma evaluation for other life-threatening injuries
- Special attention to respiratory, neurologic, and vascular status
- Appropriate analgesia for patient comfort

IMAGING/SPECIAL TESTS

- Routine plain CXRs difficult to evaluate SCJ
  - —May demonstrate asymmetry of the SCJ compared with contralateral side
  - —More useful to assess coexisting bony, pulmonary, and mediastinal injury
- *Rockwood or serendipity view:* x-ray beam aimed at manubrium in a 40-degree cephalic tilt allows view of both SCJs
- US can reliably demonstrate posterior SCJ dislocations
  - —Currently used in OR setting to evaluate the reduction and vascular structures
  - —Advantage of being noninvasive, portable, and simple to use
  - —May be useful in the initial ED evaluation of unstable patients with chest trauma
- *CT scan is best to evaluate the SCJ*
  - —Useful when plain films are inconclusive
  - —Accurately differentiates fractures from dislocations
  - —Demonstrates the position of the medial end of the clavicle in relation to the structures in the mediastinum
  - —Shows detailed anatomy of the structures of the thoracic outlet and mediastinum

DIFFERENTIAL DIAGNOSIS

- Sternoclavicular sprain/subluxation
- Medial clavicle fracture
- Septic joint
- Osteoarthritis

Treatment

INITIAL STABILIZATION

- Endotracheal intubation if acute respiratory distress followed by immediate medial clavicular reduction
- Emergent reduction indicated if hoarseness, dysphagia, sensation of throat tightness, or neurovascular compromise (upper extremity weakness, paresthesia, diminished pulses, signs of shock)
- Orthopedic and thoracic surgical consults mandatory
- Analgesia and sedation as needed

ED TREATMENT

- *Anterior dislocations* may be reduced in the ED
  —Conscious sedation for adequate pain control and muscle relaxation
  —Rolled towel placed between the shoulder blades in the supine position
  -Longitudinal traction applied to the extended ipsilateral arm with the shoulder abducted at 90 degrees
  -Assistant applies gentle inward pressure over the displaced medial end of the clavicle
  -After reduction, immobilize using a well-padded figure-of-eight dressing
  —Many anterior dislocations remain unstable after reduction, but surgery rarely indicated as deformity is mainly cosmetic
- *Posterior dislocations* require prompt reduction best achieved in the operating room under general anesthesia
  —If surgeon not immediately available, emergent reduction in the ED necessary to relieve serious airway, neurologic, or vascular compromise
  -After airway secured, small incision is made directly over the medial head of the clavicle
  -A sterile towel clamp used to grasp the medial clavicular head and gentle anterior traction applied to reduce the dislocation

MEDICATIONS

- Conscious sedation
  —Atropine: (used in pediatric patients in conjunction with ketamine to decrease hypersalivation) (peds: 0.02 mg/kg i.m./i.v., minimum dose of 0.1 mg)
  —Fentanyl: 50–100 μg (peds: 1–2 μg/kg) i.v. q2–3min
  —Ketamine: 3–7 mg/kg i.m. (peds: 0.5–2 mg/kg i.v.)
  —Versed: 1 mg (peds: 0.05–0.1 mg/kg) i.v. q2–3min
- Upon discharge
  —Acetaminophen: 500–1,000 mg q6h p.r.n.
  —Acetaminophen 300 mg with codeine: 30 mg q6h p.r.n.
  —Ibuprofen: 400–800 mg q6h p.r.n. with meals

PEDIATRIC CONSIDERATIONS

- Fractures in the medial clavicle have tremendous capability for healing and remodeling
- Anteriorly displaced epiphyseal fractures of the medial clavicle immobilized with figure-of-eight splint without reduction
- Posteriorly displaced fractures may affect mediastinal structures and uniformly require reduction and surgical intervention

Disposition

ADMISSION CRITERIA

- All posterior dislocations of the SCJ require admission for prompt reduction in the OR and evaluation for potential intrathoracic complications
- Coexisting injury significant enough to warrant hospitalization

DISCHARGE CRITERIA

- SCJ sprains
- Anterior dislocations of the SCJ without neurovascular compromise or other significant injury
- Appropriate outpatient orthopedic follow-up arranged

Miscellaneous

ICD9: 810.01

ICD10: S49.9

SUGGESTED READINGS

Ferrera PC, Wheeling HM. Sternoclavicular joint injuries. Am J Emerg Med 2000;18(1): 58–61.

Medvecky MJ, Zuckerman JD. Sternoclavicular joint injuries and disorders. AAOS Instructional Course Lectures 2000;49:397–406.

Yeh GL, Williams GR. Conservative management of sternoclavicular injuries. Orthop Clin North Am 2000;31(2):189–203.

Authors: Robert S. Chang; Wallace Carter

Stevens-Johnson Syndrome

Clinical Presentation

SIGNS AND SYMPTOMS

- *Prodrome:* fever, headache, malaise, upper respiratory infection (URI) symptoms, arthritis, arthralgias, and myalgias
- *Rash:* target lesions, erythematous or purpuric macules with or without confluence, and small blisters or bullae with skin detachment
- *Mucous membrane:* erosions of the mouth, pharynx, trachea, genitalia, or anus; possibly pseudomembrane formation
- *Eye:* mild to severe conjunctivitis with possible formation of pseudomembranes and corneal ulcers

MECHANISM/DESCRIPTION

- Stevens-Johnson syndrome (SJS) is a severe mucocutaneous disease, which has these features
  - —Blistering of less than 10% of the body surface area
  - —Confluent erosions of at least two mucous membranes
  - —Lesions often involving face, neck, and central trunk regions and entire epidermal layer
- Erythema multiforme, SJS, and toxic epidermal necrolysis (TEN) may be considered variations of the same disease

ETIOLOGY

- The most common causes include medications and infections
  - —Damage to the skin is thought to be mediated by cytotoxic T lymphocytes and mononuclear cells
- *Causative medications:* Sulfonamides, antibiotics, anticonvulsants, oxicams, NSAIDs, and allopurinol have been associated with these severe cutaneous drug reactions
- *Infections:* Mycoplasma pneumonia and herpes simplex are well-recognized causes of erythema multiforme and SJS

Pre-Hospital

CAUTIONS

- Patients with significant cutaneous involvement may sustain fluid loss and require IV crystalloid replacement

Diagnosis

ESSENTIAL WORKUP

- A complete history and physical examination with careful attention to mucous membranes, percentage of blistering, and identification of likely etiology

LABORATORY

- Electrolytes
- Liver enzymes
- Complete blood count
- Urinalysis
- Erythrocyte sedimentation rate (ESR)

IMAGING/SPECIAL TESTS

- Chest radiography if pneumonia is a consideration
- Skin biopsy of lesions and mucous membranes demonstrates necrosis of the entire epidermal layer

DIFFERENTIAL DIAGNOSIS

- Overlapping SJS and TEN (skin detachment between 10% and 30% of the body surface area plus widespread macules or flat atypical target lesions)
- Toxic epidermal necrolysis (skin detachment greater than 30% of the body surface area plus widespread macules or flat atypical targets)
- Pemphigus vulgaris
- Bullous pemphigoid (a chronic bullous eruption most commonly presenting in elderly people)
- Epidermolysis bullosa

PEDIATRIC CONSIDERATIONS

- Staphylococcal scalded skin syndrome is in the pediatric differential diagnosis of severe blistering mucocutaneous diseases
- Bullous impetigo

Treatment

INITIAL STABILIZATION

- ABCs
  - —Endotracheal intubation and ventilatory support may be required for impending respiratory failure (more commonly associated with TEN)
  - —IV fluids

ED TREATMENT

- Recognize and treat underlying infections
  - —Sepsis is the primary cause of death, frequently from Gram-negative pneumonia
- Secondarily infected cutaneous lesions can be treated with débridement of blisters, compresses, and systemic antibiotics
- Corticosteroids are controversial
- Prophylactic antibiotics may be indicated if systemic steroids are given
- Mild systemic symptoms may be treated with acetaminophen or NSAIDs, provided they are not the cause of the mucocutaneous reaction
- Mucous membrane lesions are extremely painful and may require parenteral analgesics
- Large extensive bullae should be débrided, ideally in a burn unit

MEDICATIONS

- Acetaminophen: 650–975 mg PO/PR (peds: 15 mg/kg/dose)
- Acyclovir: 5–10 mg/kg i.v. q8h (for HSV infections)
- Ibuprofen: 300–800 mg PO (peds: 5–10 mg/kg/dose)
- Morphine sulfate: 0.1 mg/kg/dose i.v.

Disposition

ADMISSION CRITERIA

- Patients with SJS should be admitted to the hospital
- Patients with extensive epidermal detachment should be admitted to a burn center or a specialized ICU

DISCHARGE CRITERIA

- Patients with erythema multiforme minor may be discharged with appropriate follow-up

Miscellaneous

ICD9: 695.1

ICD10: L51.1

SUGGESTED READINGS

Fritsch PO, Sidoroff A. Drug-induced Stevens-Johnson syndrome/toxic epidermal necrolysis. Am J Clin Dermat 2000;1(6): 349–60.

Roujeau JC, Kelly JP, Naldi L, et al. Medication use and the risk of Stevens-Johnson syndrome or toxic epidermal necrolysis. N Engl J Med 1995;333: 1600–1607.

Author: James A. Comes

Sting, Bee

Clinical Presentation

SIGNS AND SYMPTOMS

Five Types of Reactions to Stings

- *Local reaction*
  - —Most common type of reaction
  - —Local pain, erythema, and edema at sting site
  - —Symptoms occur immediately and resolve within 1–2 hours
- *Large local reaction*
  - —Similar to local reaction but affects larger area or entire limbs
  - —Peaks at 48 hours and can last several days
  - —Mild to moderate fever
- *Systemic reaction*
  - —Includes anaphylaxis
  - —Can be fatal (usually due to respiratory failure)
  - —Respiratory
    - -Wheezing
    - -Coughing
    - -Stridor
    - -Shortness of breath
    - -Hoarseness
    - -Angioedema
  - —Gastrointestinal
    - -Nausea
    - -Vomiting
    - -Diarrhea
    - -Abdominal pain
  - —Cardiovascular
    - -Hypotension
    - -Chest pain
    - -Tachycardia
    - -Shock
  - —Other
    - -Urticaria
    - -Pruritus
    - -Flushing
  - —Symptoms occur within 15–20 minutes and last up to 72 hours
- *Toxic reaction*
  - —Result of multiple stings and large doses of venom
  - —Symptoms similar to anaphylaxis
- *Unusual reaction*
  - —Due to an unusual immune response
  - —Vasculitis
  - —Nephrosis
  - —Serum sickness
  - —Neuritis
  - —Encephalitis
  - —Reaction delayed (days to weeks after sting)

MECHANISM/DESCRIPTION

- Injection of hymenoptera venom causes
  - —Release of biologic amines
  - —Local or systemic allergic reactions
- Reactions are
  - —Usually IgE-mediated type I hypersensitivity reactions
  - —Rarely type III (Arthrus) hypersensitivity reactions

ETIOLOGY

- Hymenoptera—order of the phylum Arthropoda
- Includes bees, wasps, hornets, and fire ants

Pre-Hospital

CAUTIONS

- Most deaths occur within the first hour due to either respiratory obstruction or anaphylaxis causing cardiovascular and respiratory collapse
- When signs of systemic reactions
  - —Assess for a patent airway
  - —Establish IV access

Diagnosis

ESSENTIAL WORKUP

- History and physical exam—keys to diagnosis
- *No* radiologic or laboratory test will confirm hymenoptera envenomation or anaphylaxis

LABORATORY

- CBC, electrolytes, BUN, creatinine, glucose, arterial blood gases (ABGs)
  - —Not routine
  - —Consider when significant systemic effects present

IMAGING/SPECIAL TESTS

- EKG
  - —When significant systemic effects in patients at risk for cardiovascular disease

DIFFERENTIAL DIAGNOSIS

- Insect bites sometimes cause pain; stings always cause pain
- Cellulitis
  - —Difficult to distinguish between large local reactions and cellulitis
  - —Infections of hymenoptera envenomations are rare and usually caused by wasp envenomations
  - —Local reaction can resemble periorbital cellulitis
- Gout
- Soft tissue trauma
- Systemic/toxic reactions
  - —Pulmonary embolus
  - —Anaphylaxis from a different agent
  - —Hyperventilatory syndrome/anxiety
  - —Acute coronary syndrome

Treatment

INITIAL STABILIZATION

Acute Severe Systemic Reaction/ Anaphylaxis

- ABCs
  - —Intubation/ventilation with rapidly increasing signs of laryngeal compromise
  - —Oxygen
  - —0.9% NS IV access
- Epinephrine SQ/IV
- Antihistamines IV

ED MANAGEMENT

Systemic Reactions

- Epinephrine for respiratory symptoms/ hypotension
- Antihistamines—H_1(diphenhydramine) and H_2(cimetidine) blockers
- Steroids (prednisone, methylprednisolone)
- Inhaled β-agonist for wheezing/shortness of breath
- For persistent hypotension
  - —0.9% NS IV fluid resuscitation
  - —Vasopressor (epinephrine/α-adrenergic) for hypotension resistant to IV fluids
  - —Removal of remnants of stinger at site of envenomation (bees may leave stingers with venom sacs) by scraping, not squeezing

Local Reactions

- Cool compress
- Elevation
- Remove constrictive clothing or jewelry
- Topical antihistamine/topical steroidal cream as needed
- Oral antihistamine or steroids as needed

MEDICATIONS

- Albuterol, β-agonist (inhaled): 3 mg in 5 mL solvent (peds: 0.1 mg/kg of 5 mg/mL concentration) via nebulization
- Cimetidine: 300 mg (peds: 5 mg/kg) i.v., i.m., or PO
- Diphenhydramine:
  - —50–100 mg (peds: 1 mg/kg) i.v. for severe reactions
  - —25–50 mg (peds: 1 mg/kg) PO q.i.d. for severe local reactions
- Epinephrine
  - —0.1 mg (1 mL of 1:10,000 dilution) (peds: 0.01 mg/kg = 0.1 mL/kg of 1:10,000 dilution up to 1 mL) i.v. over 5 minutes for shock
  - —0.3–0.5 mg (0.3 mL to 0.5 mL of 1:1,000 dilution) (peds: 0.01 mg/kg up to 0.5 mg) SQ for severe reactions but not in shock
- Methylprednisolone: 125 mg (peds: 1–2 mg/kg) i.v.
- Norepinephrine: 4–12 μg/min (peds: 0.1 μg/kg/min) titrated continuous infusion
- Prednisone: 60 mg (peds: 1–2 mg/kg) PO

Disposition

ADMISSION CRITERIA

- Worsening symptoms, airway compromise
- Persistent unstable vital signs require ICU admission
- Life-threatening reaction requires 24-hour observation
- Systemic reaction requires a minimum of 6 hours of observation

DISCHARGE CRITERIA

- Minimal isolated local reaction
- Systemic reactions that resolve and do not recur during 6-hour observation period
- Follow-up
  - —Provide patients with life-threatening reactions emergency anaphylaxis kits (EpiPen) (peds: EpiPen Jr. if <15 kg) and medical identification bracelets (Medi-Alert)
  - —Systemic reaction requires follow-up for possible immunotherapy

Miscellaneous

ICD9: 989.5

ICD10: T63.4

SUGGESTED READINGS

Bahna SL. Insect sting allergy: a matter of life and death. Pediatr Ann 2000;29(12): 753–758.

Elgart GW. Ant, bee, and wasp stings. Dermatol Clin 1990;8(2):229–235.Kemp ED. Bites and stings of the arthropod kind. Postgrad Med 1998;103(6):88–104.

McDougle L, Klein G, Hoehler FK. Management of hymenoptera sting anaphylaxis: a preventive medicine survey. J Emerg Med 1995;13:9–13.

Reisman RE. Stinging insect allergy. Clin Allergy 1992;76(4):863–893.

Author: Daniel Wu

Sting, Scorpion

Clinical Presentation

SIGNS AND SYMPTOMS

- Onset within minutes; progresses to maximum severity in about 5 hours
- Scorpion species determines symptomatology

Local Tissue Effects

- Erythema
- Pain
- Hyperesthesia

Autonomic Effects

- Sympathetic symptoms
  - —Tachycardia
  - —Hypertension
  - —Hyperthermia
  - —Pulmonary edema
  - —Agitation
  - —Perspiration
- Parasympathetic effects
  - —Hypotension
  - —Bradycardia
  - —SLUDGE (salivation, lacrimation, urination, defecation, gastric emptying, emesis)

Somatic Effects

- Involuntary muscle contractions
- Restlessness

Cranial Nerve Effects

- Roving eye movements
- Blurred vision
- Nystagmus
- Tongue fasciculations
- Loss of pharyngeal muscle control

MECHANISM/DESCRIPTION

- Scorpion venom is neurotoxic
- Sodium channels altered
- Prolonged firing of neurons
- Automonic, somatic, and cranial nerve excitation occurs
- Symptoms begin within 60 minutes of bite
- Symptoms persist 3–30 hours

ETIOLOGY

- *Centruroides* species found in Southern United States, Mexico, Central America, and Caribbean
- Many other species in Asia, Africa, Israel, South America, and Middle East

PEDIATRIC CONSIDERATIONS

- Can be misdiagnosed with seizures
- Higher mortality and severity of illness

Pre-Hospital

CAUTIONS

- ABCs must be evaluated
- IV access
- Endotracheal intubation, if needed

CONTROVERSIES

- Negative pressure extraction devices have not been evaluated and delay transport

Diagnosis

ESSENTIAL WORKUP

- Identification of scorpion species, if possible
- High clinical suspicion in endemic areas
- Grade severity of envenomation
  - —Grade I: local pain and/or paresthesias at site
  - —Grade II: local pain and pain and/or paresthesias at a remote site
  - —Grade III: Either cranial/autonomic *or* somatic skeletal neuromuscular dysfunction
  - —Grade IV: Both cranial/autonomic *and* somatic skeletal muscle dysfunction

LABORATORY

- Grade I and II envenomations
  - —None
- Grade III and IV envenomations
  - —CBC
  - —BUN, creatinine
  - —Electrolytes
  - —Urinalysis
- Severely agitated patients
  - —Creatine kinase
  - —Urine myoglobin
- Severe respiratory distress
  - —Arterial blood gases (ABGs)

IMAGING/SPECIAL TESTS

- Chest x-ray for respiratory symptoms
- EKG for tachycardia

DIFFERENTIAL DIAGNOSIS

- Snake, spider, insect envenomation
- Tetanus
- Diphtheria
- Botulism
- Overdose/dystonic reaction
- Seizures

Treatment

INITIAL STABILIZATION

- ABCs
- Endotracheal intubation, if necessary
- IV
- O_2
- Monitor

ED TREATMENT

- Mild envenomations: grade I and II
  - —Oral analgesics
  - —Cool compresses
  - —Tetanus prophylaxis
- Severe envenomations: grade III and IV
  - —Antivenom
  - —Tetanus prophylaxis
  - —Hypertensive urgencies/emergencies
    - -Standard therapy such as labetalol
  - —Hypotension
    - -IV fluid resuscitation and pressor therapy with dopamine
  - —Severe agitation
    - -Midazolam
  - —Treatment for rhabdomyolysis, if present

MEDICATIONS

- Antivenom: diluted in saline and given IV
  - —Produced by Arizona State University
  - —For use in Arizona only
  - —Call Arizona Poison Management (602) 253-3334 if considering antivenom therapy
  - —Not FDA approved
  - —Skin test must be performed before administration because of potential for anaphylaxis
- Dopamine: 2–5 μg/kg/min i.v.; increase in 5–10 μg/kg/min as needed
- Labetalol: 20 mg (peds: 0.3–1.0 mg/kg/dose) i.v. every 10 minutes
- Midazolam: 1–2 mg (peds: 0.01–0.05 mg/kg) i.v.
- Tetanus: 0.5 mL i.m. (peds: same dose)

PEDIATRIC CONSIDERATIONS

- Antivenom doses are the same in children because dosage is based on venom burden

Disposition

ADMISSION CRITERIA

- Grade III and IV envenomations require admission to ICU
- If antivenom is given with resolution of symptoms, admit to medical ward or observation unit for minimum 6 hours
- All pediatric patients

DISCHARGE CRITERIA

- Grade I and II envenomations
- Grade III and IV envenomations given antivenom with resolution of symptoms can be discharged after 6 hours of observation
- If patient received antivenom, discuss signs and symptoms of delayed serum sickness
- Discuss possibility of persistence of pain and paresthesias at site
- Encourage patient to return for progression of symptoms

PEDIATRIC CONSIDERATIONS

- Children may not recover as quickly as adults

Miscellaneous

ICD9: 989.5

ICD10: T63.2

SUGGESTED READINGS

Connor DA, Seldon BS. Scorpion envenomation. In: Auerbach PS, ed. Wilderness medicine: management of wilderness and environmental emergencies, 3rd ed. St. Louis: CV Mosby, 1995:831–842.

Curry SC, Vance MV, Ryan PJ, et al: Envenomation by the scorpion Centruroides sculpturatus. J Toxicol Clin Toxicol 1983–84;21(4–5):417–449.

Sofer S. Scorpion envenomation. Intens Care Med 1995;21(8):626–628.

Walter GE, Bilden EF, Gibly RL. Envenomations. Crit Care Clin 1999;15(2): 353–386.

Author: Jessica Freedman

Streptococcal Disease

Clinical Presentation

SIGNS AND SYMPTOMS

- Presents as
  - —*Streptococcal toxic shock syndrome (Strep TSS)*
  - —*Necrotizing fasciitis/myositis*
- *Pain* is the most common initial symptom
  - —Often abrupt in onset and severe
  - —Occurs in 85% of cases
  - —Often requiring IV narcotics
  - —Usually involves an extremity
  - —May mimic peritonitis, pelvic inflammatory disease (PID), pneumonia, acute myocardial infarction (AMI), or pericarditis
- *Fever* is the most common sign
  - —Can present with hypothermia (especially if in shock)
- *Altered mental status* is present in 55%
- *Soft tissue infection* (erythema and swelling) present in 80% of patients
  - —70% progress to necrotizing fasciitis or myositis
    - -Indistinct borders, blisters, bullae
    - -No lymphangitis or lymphadenopathy
    - -Most will require surgical procedure (fasciotomy, surgical débridement, exploratory laparotomy, intraocular aspiration, amputation, or hysterectomy)
- *Influenza-like syndrome* in 20%
  - —Fever
  - —Chills
  - —Myalgias
  - —Nausea, vomiting
  - —Diarrhea
- *Shock*
  - —Present at admission or within 4–8 hours in *all* patients
  - —Persists despite fluids, antibiotics, and pressors in all but 10%
- *Renal failure*
  - —Precedes the onset of shock in many cases
  - —Dialysis often necessary
  - —Kidney function returns to normal within 4–6 weeks in survivors
- *Adult respiratory distress syndrome* (ARDS)
  - —Occurs in 55% of patients and develops after hypotension
  - —Mechanical ventilation required in 90% of patients with ARDS

Strep TSS Case Definition

- Isolation of group A β-hemolytic streptococcus (GABHS) from sterile or nonsterile body site, *and*
  - —Hypotension
  - —Two or more of the following
    - -Renal impairment
    - -Coagulopathy
    - -Liver abnormalities
    - -Acute respiratory distress
    - -Extensive tissue necrosis (necrotizing fasciitis)
    - -Erythematous rash

MECHANISM/DESCRIPTION

- In the late 1980s, an increase in the frequency of an aggressive streptococcal infection that afflicts healthy individuals aged 20–50 years who do not have underlying predisposing diseases
- Dubbed "flesh-eating bacteria" by British press
- Rapid progression of shock and multiorgan dysfunction, with death occurring in many within 1–2 days
- Streptococcal toxic shock syndrome (Strep TSS)
  - —Portal of entry for streptococci
    - -Vagina
    - -Pharynx
    - -Mucosa
    - -Skin
    - -50% of cases the site of entry is unknown
  - —NSAIDs appear to mask or predispose patients to Strep TSS
  - —Most cases occur sporadically
  - —Occasional outbreaks in nursing homes and hospitals
- Necrotizing fasciitis
  - —Mortality rate 30–70%
  - —Infection of the subcutaneous tissue with progressive destruction of the fascia and fat
  - —Often fatal over a course of 24–96 hours
  - —Described by Meleney in 1924, but progression was slower over 7–10 days with lower mortality rate (20%)
- Streptococcal myositis
  - —A rare GABHS infection reported only 21 times from 1900 to 1985
  - —Swelling and erythema develop late
  - —Difficult to differentiate from gas gangrene secondary to *Clostridium* species infection
  - —Mortality rate 80–100%
  - —Aggressive surgical débridement is essential

ETIOLOGY

- Streptococci
  - —Catalase-negative spherical cocci
  - —Divided into two groups: α and β
    - -On ability to lyse red blood cells on an agar plate
  - —β-Hemolytic streptococci fully lyse RBCs
    - -Further divided into Lancefield groups by variations in an antigen in the cell wall (C carbohydrate)
  - —GABHS
    - -Possess another antigen, the M protein, which is associated with the virulence of the bacteria
- Strep TSS
  - —Occurs when a susceptible host is infected with a virulent strain
  - —M protein types 1, 3, and 28 are most common
  - —Possess pyrogenic exotoxins (A, B, and C)
  - —Produce fever and shock via activation of tumor necrosis factor (TNF) and interleukins
  - —Risk factors for development of strep TSS
    - -$<$10 years or $>$60 years of age
    - -Cancer
    - -Renal failure
    - -Leukemia
    - -Severe burns
    - -Corticosteroids
- Necrotizing fasciitis
  - —GABHS is cause in 10%
  - —Mixed anaerobic and aerobic organisms in 70%
  - —*Staphylococcus aureus*, *Clostridium* species, and other enteric organisms

PEDIATRIC CONSIDERATIONS

- Risk factors in children with varicella include:
  - —Home care
  - —Asthma and treatment with albuterol
  - —NSAIDs
  - —Fever after day 2 of varicella
  - —Secondary cases in household

Pre-Hospital

N/A

Diagnosis

ESSENTIAL WORKUP

- Suspect necrotizing fasciitis when pain is out of proportion to examination
- Rapid administration of broad-spectrum antibiotics
- Early surgical consultation

LABORATORY

- CBC with differential
  —Mild leukocytosis with left shift initially
- Electrolytes, BUN, and creatinine
- Calcium level
  —Hypocalcemia in the face of fat necrosis from necrotizing fasciitis
- Urinalysis
  —Hemoglobinuria if renal involvement
- Serum creatine phosphokinase (CPK) that is elevated or rising correlates with necrotizing fasciitis or myositis
- Aerobic and anaerobic blood cultures
- Wound cultures
- Coagulation panel and disseminated intravascular coagulation (DIC) panel

IMAGING/SPECIAL TESTS

- Plain films
  —Gas in soft tissues in 25–75% of cases of necrotizing fasciitis
  —Not commonly associated with GABHS infection
  —More common in mixed anaerobic infections
- CT scan
  —Asymmetric thickening of deep fascia
  —Gas
- MRI
  —High signal intensity of the fascia in T2-weighted images

DIFFERENTIAL DIAGNOSIS

- Sepsis
- Cellulitis
- Erysipelas
- Necrotizing fasciitis/myositis secondary to another pathogen

Treatment

INITIAL STABILIZATION

- ABCs
- Treat shock with fluids and pressors as needed
  —Hypotension is often intractable, and up to 10–20 L/d may be required
- Intubation and mechanical ventilation for
  —ARDS
  —Severe shock
  —Ventilatory failure

ED TREATMENT

- Broad-spectrum antibiotics immediately after cultures
  —Penicillin (or a cephalosporin)
  —Anaerobic coverage (clindamycin or metronidazole)
  —Gram-negative coverage (aminoglycoside, third-generation cephalosporin, or ciprofloxacin)
- Early surgical consultation for débridement
  —Immediate surgery indicated if
  -Extensive necrosis or gas
  -Compartment syndrome
  -Profound systemic toxicity
- Aggressive GABHS infections do not respond well to penicillin
- Clindamycin has been found to be a potent suppressor of bacterial toxin synthesis and inhibits M-protein synthesis
- Reports of successful use of IV immunoglobulin
- Hyperbaric oxygen remains controversial

MEDICATIONS

Invasive Streptococcal Disease

- Clindamycin: 900 mg (peds: 40 mg/kg/d) q6–8h i.v., *and*
- Penicillin G: 4 million units (peds: 250,000 IU/d) i.v. q4–6h, *or*
- Vancomycin: 15 mg/kg q12h (peds: 10 mg/kg q6h) i.v. if penicillin allergy

Polymicrobial Necrotizing Fasciitis and Fournier's Gangrene

- Metronidazole: 15 mg/kg i.v. loading dose, then 7.5 mg/kg i.v. q6h, *and*
- Ticarcillin/clavulanic acid: 3.1 g (peds: 200 mg/kg/d) i.v. q6h, *or*
- Ampicillin/sulbactam: 3 g (peds: 200 mg/kg/d) i.v. q6h, *or*
- Piperacillin/tazobactam: 3.375 g i.v. q6h

Disposition

ADMISSION CRITERIA

- ICU admission for all patients with suspicion of invasive streptococcal infection

DISCHARGE CRITERIA

- None

Miscellaneous

ICD9: 038.0

ICD10: B95.5

SUGGESTED READINGS

Ahmed S, Ayoub E. Severe, invasive group A streptococcal disease and toxic shock. Pediatr Ann 1998;27(5):287–292.

American Academy of Pediatrics, Committee on Infectious Disease. Severe invasive group A streptococcal infections: a subject review. Pediatrics 1998;101(1):136–140.

Stevens DL. The flesh-eating bacterium: what's next? J Infect Dis 1999:179(Suppl 2):S366–374.

Stevens DL. Invasive group A streptococcus infections. Clin Infect Dis 1992;14:2–13.

Author: Scott Sherman

Stridor

Clinical Presentation

SIGNS AND SYMPTOMS

- Anxious
- Audible wheezing or grunting with inspiration
- Increased respiratory rate
- Effort required for inspiration
  - —Nasal flaring
  - —Use of accessory muscles
- Intercostal retractions
- Paradoxical diaphragmatic movement—late
- Dyspnea
- Cough
- Fever
- Drooling
- Sore throat
- "Hot potato" voice—adult
- Trismus
  - —Peritonsillar abscess, retropharyngeal abscess, Ludwig's angina
- Respiratory distress
  - —Agitation
  - —Diaphoresis
  - —Cyanosis
  - —Decreased respiratory rate
  - —Somnolence

MECHANISM/DESCRIPTION

- Impedance of air movement through upper airway causing high-pitched audible wheezing and vibratory harsh sounds on auscultation over larynx during inspiration

ETIOLOGY

- Congenital
  - —Laryngomalacia
- Ectopic thyroid
  - —Laryngeal webs/rings
  - —Vocal cord dysfunction
- Infection
  - —Bacterial tracheitis
  - —Epiglottitis
  - —Viral croup
  - —Peritonsillar abscess
  - —Retropharyngeal abscess
  - —Supraglottitis
  - —Uvulitis—Quincke's disease
  - —Ludwig's angina
  - —Diphtheria
  - —Tetanus
- Extrinsic compression
  - —Trauma
  - —Hematoma
  - —Vascular anomalies (rings)
- Intraluminal obstruction of the trachea
  - —Foreign body
  - —Cyst
  - —Invasive tumors
  - —Squamous cell
  - —Lymphomas
  - —Thyroid carcinomas
  - —Laryngeal or tracheal papilloma
- Subglottic stenosis
  - —Postoperative scarring
  - —After radiation therapy
- Angioedema
- Vocal cord dysfunction
  - —Congenital
  - —Surgical injury
  - —Postintubation trauma
  - —Thyroid malignancy
  - —Mediastinal mass

Pre-Hospital

- Keep child calm, with mother if possible
- Blow-by oxygen
- Maintain adequate airway
- Bag-valve mask if respiratory status deteriorates
- Intubate if bag-valve mask ineffective
- Rapid transport with ED notification

CAUTIONS

- Avoid agitating child
- Rapid deterioration of respiratory status

CONTROVERSIES

- Racemic epinephrine
- Early intubation

Diagnosis

ESSENTIAL WORKUP

- Visualization of the upper airway
  - —Radiographic if symptoms very mild—be careful!
  - —Direct visualization in operating room with a surgeon prepared to perform a cricothyrotomy or tracheostomy is the safest approach

LABORATORY

- Not helpful and may add to agitation in child

IMAGING/SPECIAL TESTS

- Radiograph of lateral neck
  - —Not essential
  - —Only done in extremely mild cases
- Fiberoptic laryngoscopy
  - —Should be performed with an intubating fiberoptic laryngoscope in a setting where a rapid surgical airway can be obtained
- Direct laryngoscopy
  - —Diagnostic study of choice
  - —Should be performed in a setting where a rapid surgical airway can be obtained

DIFFERENTIAL DIAGNOSIS

- Bronchospasm
- Malingering
  - —Patient breathing against a closed glottis

Treatment

INITIAL STABILIZATION

- In children: avoid agitation
- In children: blow-by oxygen
- 100% non-rebreather by face mask

ED TREATMENT

- Airway management
- Stridor defines a difficult airway
  - —Be prepared to perform a surgical airway before intubation
  - —If time permits, perform intubation in operating room with surgeon and pediatric anesthesiologist present
  - —Intubate with tube 1–2 sizes smaller than would be normally used
- Oral awake intubation
  - —Ketamine induction
  - —Patient is sedated but continues to ventilate during procedure
- Avoid blind nasotracheal intubation
- Surgical airway if intubation fails or sudden deterioration in respiratory status occurs
- Postintubation ceftriaxone in cases of infectious etiology
- Sedation/paralysis for duration of intubated status after airway is secured

MEDICATIONS

- Atropine: 0.02 mg/kg i.v.
- Ceftriaxone: 1–2 g i.v.
- Diazepam: 2–10 mg i.v. (peds: 0.2–0.3 mg/kg)
- Etomidate: 0.3 mg/kg i.v.
- Fentanyl: 3 μg/kg i.v.
- Ketamine: 1–2 mg/kg i.v. or 4–7 mg/kg i.m.
- Lidocaine: 1.5 mg/kg i.v.
- Midazolam: 1–5 mg i.v. (0.07–0.30 mg/kg for induction)
- Vecuronium: 0.1 mg/kg i.v.

Disposition

ADMISSION CRITERIA

- All cases of stridor require admission

DISCHARGE CRITERIA

N/A

Miscellaneous

ICD9: 786.1

ICD10: R06.1

SUGGESTED READINGS

Beckman DB. Diagnostic dilemma: vocal cord dysfunction. Am J Med 2001;110(9): 731–741.

Chang AB. A review of cough in children. J Asthma 2001;38(4):299–309.

Konarzewski W. Adult epiglottitis: an under-recognized, life threatening condition. Br J Anaesth 2001;86(3): 456–457.

Levy RJ. Pediatric airway issues. Crit Care Clin 2000;16(3):489–504.

Nakamura H. Acute epiglottitis: a review of 80 patients. J Laryngol Otol 2001;115(1): 31–34.

Verghese ST. Pediatric otolaryngologic emergencies. Anesthesiol Clin North Am 2001;19(2):237–256.

Author: Gregory Ciottone

Subarachnoid Hemorrhage

Clinical Presentation

SIGNS AND SYMPTOMS

- Sudden onset of "worst headache of life," often developing during exertion
- Headache is often occipital in location and different than prior headaches
- "Warning/sentinel" headache
  - —Represents small bleed
  - —20–50% of patients with subarachnoid hemorrhage (SAH)
  - —Occurs days to weeks before current bleed
  - —Onset over seconds, maximum intensity in minutes and lasts hours to days
- Other symptoms include: transient loss of consciousness, buckling of legs, nausea, vomiting (70%), or neck pain instead of headache
- Signs: decreased level of consciousness, seizures (16%) and focal neurologic signs such as retinal hemorrhages (17%), papilledema, cranial nerve III and VI palsies, nuchal rigidity, bilateral leg weakness, nystagmus, ataxia, aphasia, hemiparesis, or left-sided visual neglect

MECHANISM/DESCRIPTION

- Bleeding from cerebral vessels into the CSF
- About 30% of SAHs rebleed within 3 weeks, of which half occur within hours of initial bleed
- Intracerebral hematoma occurs in about 30%
- Hydrocephalus and global cerebral ischemia are other complications of SAH
- Vasospasm occurs in many cases
  - —Those with a localized clot or diffuse hemorrhage to 1 mm at greatest risk

ETIOLOGY

- 85% of nontraumatic SAHs are from rupture of a cerebral aneurysm (most commonly Berry's aneurysm in the circle of Willis)
- Other causes of nontraumatic SAH: arteriovenous malformation (AVM), rupture of a hypertensive intracerebral hemorrhage, or tumor
- Risk factors: increasing age, female gender, African American race, family history, polycystic kidney disease, smoking, hypertension, and heavy drinking
- Most hemorrhages occur before the age of 50 years

PEDIATRIC CONSIDERATIONS

- In children, the etiology is most often an AVM

Pre-Hospital

CAUTIONS

- Rapid progression to unconsciousness can occur, requiring intubation
- The initial neurologic exam is essential, including level of consciousness, Glasgow Coma Scale (GCS) score, and any gross focal deficits
- 12% mortality rate before receiving medical attention

Diagnosis

- Clinical severity on presentation is most important prognosticator
- Hunter-Hess grading system:
  - —Grade I: asymptomatic or mild headache
  - —Grade II: moderate/severe headache, nuchal rigidity, with or without cranial nerve deficit
  - —Grade III: confusion, lethargy, or mild focal symptoms
  - —Grade IV: stupor or hemiparesis
  - —Grade V: comatose or extensor posturing
- World Federation of Neurological Surgeons (WFNS) grading scale for patients with SAH, which places emphasis on level of consciousness as prognosis
  - —Grade I: GCS of 15
  - —Grade II: GCS of 13–14 without focal deficit
  - —Grade III: GCS of 13–14 with focal deficit
  - —Grade IV: GCS of 7–12
  - —Grade V: GCS of 3–6

ESSENTIAL WORKUP

- Neurologic exam including funduscopic exam
- Emergent noncontrast CT scan
- Lumbar puncture is mandatory if CT scan is negative and clinical exam suggests SAH

LABORATORY

- Lumbar puncture
  - —Presence of xanthochromia determined by spectrophotometry is diagnostic of SAH
  - —It takes between 6 and 12 hours for xanthochromia to occur after bleed onset
  - —Presence of erythrocytes in a nontraumatic tap is also diagnostic of SAH
  - —Distinguishing a traumatic tap from a true hemorrhage is suggested by clearing of CSF with subsequent tubes or clear fluid from second lumbar puncture (LP) one interspace higher
  - —CSF pressure should always be measured to distinguish traumatic tap and pseudotumor cerebri or cerebral venous sinus thrombosis from SAH
- Electrocardiogram
  - —~90% of patients with SAH have cardiac dysrhythmias and EKG patterns suggesting ischemia or infarction
  - —Common findings are broad or inverted T waves, QT prolongation, ST elevation/depression, U waves

IMAGING/SPECIAL TESTS

- Noncontrast CT of the head 92–95% sensitive for SAH if performed within 24 hours of symptom onset
  - —Sensitivity decreases with time from onset
- MRI has the advantage of being able to detect aneurysms but is less sensitive for SAH
  - —Other disadvantages include cost, less availability and familiarity with interpretation
- Transcranial Doppler may be useful to detect vasospasm

DIFFERENTIAL DIAGNOSIS

- Subdural/epidural hematoma
- Carotid dissection after neck trauma
- Migraine and tension headaches
- Meningitis
- Dementia
- Brain tumor/abscess

Treatment

INITIAL STABILIZATION

- Airway and breathing: RSI and controlled ventilation with goal PCO_2 of about 35–40 for suspected increased intracranial pressure (ICP)
- Circulation
  - —Obtain central venous access
  - —Maintain mean arterial pressure with crystalloid infusion to optimize cerebral perfusion pressure
  - —If central monitoring acquired, maintain central venous pressure >8 mm Hg or wedge pressure >7 mm Hg
- Urgent neurosurgical consultation
- Type and cross-match

ED TREATMENT

- Rebleeding prevention
  - —Antihypertensives
    - -Generally not recommended because they compromise cerebral perfusion pressure
    - -Severe hypertension >200/110 mm Hg and systemic signs such as heart or renal failure should be controlled
    - -Goal BP, SBP <160 mm Hg and MAP of 110 mm Hg decreases risk for rebleed
  - —Strict bedrest, elevate head of bed 30 degrees
  - —Control pain with mild analgesia
  - —Prevent vomiting and straining with antiemetics and stool softeners
- Vasospasm prevention
  - —Typically occurs 3–12 days after SAH
  - —Begin calcium channel blocker nimodipine for patient in Hunt-Hess grade I, II, and III
  - —Maintain euvolemia and adequate cerebral perfusion pressure
- Hydrocephalus and increased ICP
  - —Intubation and controlled ventilation
  - —Mannitol
- Anticonvulsants—controversial but may decrease risk for rebleeding
  - —Phenytoin
- Antifibrinolytic agents have not been shown to improve outcome by decreasing rebleeds because they also increase brain ischemia
- Neuroprotective drugs—no evidence that they improve outcome

MEDICATIONS

- Anticonvulsants
  - —Diazepam: adult: 5–10 mg i.v. every 10–15 minutes, max 30 mg (peds: 0.2–0.3 mg/kg every 5–10 minutes, max 10 mg)
  - —Lorazepam: 2–4 mg i.v. every 15 minutes PRN (peds: 0.03–0.05 mg/kg/dose, max 4 mg/dose)
  - —Phenytoin load: 1 g i.v., not to exceed 50 mg/min (peds: 15–20 mg/kg i.v., max 1000 mg/24 h)
- Antiemetics
  - —Diphenhydramine (Benadryl): 25–50 mg PO, i.m., or i.v. q6–8h (peds: 5 mg/kg/24 h q6h, max 300 mg/24h)
  - —Prochlorperazine (Compazine): 5–10 mg i.v. or PO q6h (peds: 0.1 mg/kg/dose i.m. or i.v.)
  - —Promethazine (Phenergan): 25–50 mg PO, PR, or i.m. q4h (peds: Phenergan syrup PO—ages 2–6: 1.25 mL q4–6h; ages 6–12: 2.5 mL q4–6h; age >12: 5 mL q4–6h)
- Antihypertensives
  - —Esmolol: adults and peds: 1 mg/kg i.v. load, then 100–150 μg/kg/min
  - —Hydralazine: 10–20 mg i.v. every 30 minutes (peds: safety not established)
  - —Labetalol: 20 mg/min i.v. bolus, then 20–80 mg every 10 minutes, max 300 mg; infusion 0.5–2 mg/min
  - —Mannitol: adults and peds: 0.5–1.0 g/kg i.v. over 30–60 minutes; repeat doses at 0.25 g/kg
  - —Nitroprusside: adults and peds: 0.25–10 μg/kg/min
- Antivasospasm agents
  - —Nimodipine: 60 mg PO q6h for patients with SAH grade I, II, or III

Disposition

ADMISSION CRITERIA

- All patients with positive findings on CT or lumbar puncture should be admitted for vascular imaging and close monitoring
- Patients with onset of symptoms greater than 2 weeks before presentation require special consideration as may have SAH but normal CT and LP

DISCHARGE CRITERIA

- Patients who have a negative CT and lumbar puncture and onset of symptoms less than 2 weeks before presentation to ED may be safely discharged
- All discharged patients should have outpatient follow-up and systematic treatment for headache

Miscellaneous

PROGNOSIS

- Variables associated with outcome: initial presentation, age, and amount of subarachnoid blood on initial CT
- Clinical condition at initial presentation is the most important prognosticator; the Hunter-Hess scale or World Federation of Neurological Surgeons grading scale for SAH
- Fatality rate about 51%
- One third of those who survive SAH remain dependent
- Only 13% of survivors have no significant deficits

ICD9: 430

ICD10: I60.9

SUGGESTED READINGS

Edlow JA, Caplan LR. Avoiding pitfalls in the diagnosis of subarachnoid hemorrhage. N Engl J Med 2000;342(1):29–35.

Schull M. Headache and facial pain. In: Tintinalli JE, et al., eds. Emergency medicine, 5th ed. New York: McGraw-Hill, 2000:1422–1429.

Scott PA, Barsan WG. Stroke, transient ischemic attack, and other central focal conditions. In: Tintinalli JE, et al., eds. Emergency medicine, 5th ed. New York: McGraw-Hill, 2000:1430–1439.

Stieg PE, Kase CS. Intracranial hemorrhage: diagnosis and emergency management. Neurol Clin North Am 1998;16(2):37388.

van Gilin J, Rinkel GJE. Subarachnoid hemorrhage: diagnosis, causes and management. Brain 2001;124:249–278.

Authors: Catherine McLaren; Rebecca Smith-Coggins

Subdural Hematoma

Clinical Presentation

SIGNS AND SYMPTOMS

Acute
- One fifth have diagnosis discovered at autopsy
- Most commonly misdiagnosed as intoxication or cerebrovascular accident (CVA)
- Headache and altered mental status
- Most common clinical signs are hemiparesis or hemiplegia; seen in 40–65%
  - —Subdural hematoma (SDH) opposite motor deficit in 60–85%
- Pupillary abnormality seen in 28–79%
  - —SDH will be on same side of pupillary abnormality in 70–90%
- Seizures may be seen in about 10% initially
- Papilledema in less than one third

Subacute/Chronic
- Less than one half have impaired level of consciousness
- Headaches, nausea, vomiting, and seizures are frequent symptoms
- Presentation is varied and mimics other disease processes

MECHANISM/DESCRIPTION
- Classification
  - —Acute: diagnosis within the first 3 days
  - —Subacute: diagnosis 3 days to 3 weeks
  - —Chronic: diagnosis after 3 weeks
- CT description
  - —Rarely crosses midline but does cross suture lines
  - —Inner margins are often seen to be irregular

Acute
- Most commonly due to acceleration-deceleration forces and less commonly from direct trauma
- Sagittal movement of the head causes stretch of parasagittal bridging veins
- Other bleeding sites include
  - —Laceration of dura
  - —Venous sinus injury
  - —Cortical arteries

Chronic
- Encapsulated hematoma most likely caused by repeated small hemorrhages of bridging veins

ETIOLOGY

Acute
- Most common type of intracranial hematoma (66–70%)
- Represents 26–63% of blunt head injury
- Motor vehicle crash (MVC) is most common cause overall; falls and assault more commonly result in isolated SDH (72%) than does MVC (24%)
- Male-to-female ratio 3:1
- Mean age is 40 years
- Elderly patients and those with seizure disorders are at increased risk
- Mortality is related to presenting signs and symptoms as well as comorbidities:
  - —Less than one half present as *simple extraaxial collection*—22% mortality rate
  - —About 40% of patients will have *complicated SDH* (associated with parenchymal laceration or intracerebral hematoma): mortality rate >50%
  - —Third group *associated with contusion*—mortality rate = 30% with functional recovery of 20%

Chronic
- Most common in babies or old people with atrophy; is associated with infarction in underlying brain
- 75% of patients are >50 years old; mean age of this injury is 63 years
- 20–48% give no history of head injury
- 50% are alcoholic; epilepsy, shunting procedures, and coagulopathy are also associated

PEDIATRIC CONSIDERATIONS
- May occur secondary to trauma at birth
- More commonly occurs from nonaccidental trauma

Pre-Hospital
- Improved outcome related both to transport to regional neurosurgical trauma centers as well as decreased time to treatment
- Hypoxia is found in 30% of patients with severe traumatic brain injury (TBI)
  - —Mechanical airway obstruction is a common finding
  - —Hypoxia is associated with increase in intracranial pressure (ICP)
- Immobilize entire spine: spinal cord injury is found in 10–15% of TBI patients

Diagnosis

ESSENTIAL WORKUP
- Obtain directed history
  - —Mechanism of injury kinetics
  - —Neurologic status: baseline and at-scene
  - —Complicating factors: medical history, medications, allergies, drug use
- Assessment of ABCs
- Rapid neurologic assessment
  - —Glasgow Coma Scale (GCS) (after fluid resuscitation most important)
  - —Brainstem reflexes: anisocoria, papillary light reflex, corneal, gag, oculocephalic/oculovestibular
- Head CT (in coordination of other necessary trauma workup)
- Spinal x-rays

LABORATORY
- ABG, CBC, electrolytes with glucose, prothrombin time (PT), partial thromboplastin time (PTT)
- Blood ethyl alcohol, drug screen

IMAGING/SPECIAL TESTS

Acute
- Characteristic CT finding is crescent-shaped clot overlying hemispheric convexity
- Most (60%) associated with other intracranial lesions

Chronic
- MRI is the test of choice as lesion may be isodense on CT from 2–3 weeks
- CT may show hypodense lesion after 3 weeks

DIFFERENTIAL DIAGNOSIS

Acute
- Diffuse axonal injury
- Cerebral contusion
- Intracerebral bleed
- Subdural hygroma
- Epidural hematoma
- Shaken baby/battered child syndrome

Chronic
- Pseudotumor cerebri
- Brain tumor
- Dementia
- Meningitis
- CVA/transient ischemic attack (TIA)
- Cerebral atherosclerosis
- Toxic, metabolic, respiratory, or circulatory causes

PEDIATRIC CONSIDERATIONS
- Ultrasound can be used to visualize cerebral structures if fontanelles are patent
- Imaging is necessary in infants with persistent vomiting, new seizures, lethargy, irritability, bulging or tense fontanels

Treatment

INITIAL STABILIZATION

- ABCs of trauma care
  - —Hypoxia is a strong predictor of outcome; maintain SAO_2 >95%
  - —Rapid sequence intubation (RSI) is indicated for GCS <9 or for evidence of increased ICP
    - -Routine hyperventilation is no longer recommended due to resultant diminished cerebral perfusion pressure and volume
    - -Maintain PCO_2 35–40 mm Hg
  - —NS to maintain MAP 100–110 is necessary
    - -A single episode of systolic blood pressure <90 is associated to poor outcome
  - —Spine precautions
  - —Elevate head of bed 15–20 degrees (only after adequate fluid resuscitation to avoid resultant decrease in CBF)

ED TREATMENT

Acute

- Early neurosurgical intervention (<4 hours) in comatose patients shows reduced mortality
  - —Burr holes may be used as temporizing measure in deteriorating patients
  - —ICP monitoring is indicated for patients with abnormal CT who are intubated
- Nonoperative treatment may be indicated for small subdurals
  - —<20 mL of blood, <1 cm, midline shift <5 mm, no mass effect, no neurologic deficit
  - —This requires frequent neurologic reassessment
  - —10% go on to require operative intervention
- Maintain euvolemic status with isotonic fluids
  - —Arterial line placement will affect close monitoring of MAP, PO_2, PCO_2
  - —Foley Catheter to monitor I/O status
- Control ICP
  - —Prevent pain, posturing and increased respiratory effort
    - -Sedation with benzodiazepines
    - -Neuromuscular blockade with vecuronium or pancuronium in intubated patients; etomidate is a good induction agent
  - —Mannitol may be used once euvolemic
    - -Shown to increase MAP >CPP and CBF as well as decrease ICP
    - -Keep osmolality between 295 and 310
    - -Use furosemide (Lasix) as an adjunct only if normovolemic
  - —Treat hypertension
    - -Labetalol or hydralazine
- Treat hyperglycemia if present; it is associated with increased mortality in TBI
- Treat and prevent seizures
  - —Diazepam and phenytoin (Dilantin)
- Not considered helpful
  - —Steroids
  - —Antibiotic prophylaxis
  - —Hyperventilation (unless herniation is imminent)
  - —Fluid restriction
  - —Calcium channel blockers
- Factors predictive of worse outcome
  - —Hypotension or delay >4 hours to treatment
  - —Age greater than 50 years
  - —Unconscious at time of OR: mortality rate 40–65%
  - —Pupillary defect
  - —Admission GCS score <8; motor is most predictive
  - —ICP greater than 25 mm Hg postoperatively
  - —Associated parenchymal injuries
  - —SDH >20 mm or increased shift
- Chronic
  - —Operative intervention is indicated for symptomatic patients
    - -Burr holes are placed at maximal hematoma
    - -Shunting may be used in children
    - -Reaccumulation occurs 10–45% of the time
    - -Nonoperative treatment is associated with a >25% risk for necessary operation and prolonged hospitalization

MEDICATIONS

- Diazepam: 5–10 mg i.v. (peds: safety not established)
- Dilantin: adults and peds: load 18 mg/kg at 25-50 mg/min
- Etomidate: 0.3 mg/kg i.v. for induction of RSI
- Hydralazine: 10/mg/h i.v. (peds: safety not established)
- Labetalol: 15-30 mg/h i.v. (peds: safety not established)
- Lasix: adults and peds: 0.5 mg/kg i.v.
- Lidocaine: as preinduction agent, 1.5 mg/kg i.v.
- Mannitol: adults and peds: 0.25–0.5 g/kg i.v. q4h
- Pentobarbital: 1-5 mg i.v. q6h
- Thiopental: As induction agent: 20 mg/kg IV
- Versed: 2-4 mg/h i.v. PRN (peds: safety not established)

Disposition

ADMISSION CRITERIA

- Acute subdural hematomas should be admitted to the OR or ICU by the neurosurgical service
- Subacute subdurals should be admitted to a monitored setting

DISCHARGE CRITERIA

- Patients with chronic subdural hematomas often can be managed as outpatients in conjunction with neurosurgery, adequate home resources, and appropriate follow-up

Miscellaneous

ICD9: 852.20

ICD10: S06.5

SUGGESTED READINGS

Cooper PR, Golfinos JG. Head injury. New York: McGraw-Hill, 2000:1–348.

Marion DW. Head and spinal cord injury: traumatic brain injuries. Neurol Clin 1998;16(2):485–494.

Ono JI, Yamaura A, et al. Outcome prediction in severe head injury: analyses of clinical prognostic factors. J Clin Neurosci 2001;8(2):120–123.

Stieg PE, Kase CS. Neurologic emergencies: intracranial hemorrhage—diagnosis and emergency management. Neurol Clin 1998;16(2):373–390.

Zink BJ. Traumatic brain injury outcome: concepts for emergency care. Ann Emerg Med 2001;37(3):318–332.

Author: Colleen Campbell

Sudden Infant Death Syndrome (SIDS)

Clinical Presentation

SIGNS AND SYMPTOMS

- No significant preexisting signs or symptoms to alert caretakers
- Unpredictable, unpreventable
- Most infants appear normal when put to bed and are subsequently found dead
- Death occurs quickly while the infant is sleeping
- Typically the event is silent; no signs of suffering
- The infant is seemingly healthy and well appearing, well developed, and well nourished
- No clinical or pathologic explanation for death

Apparent Life-Threatening Episode (ALTE)

- Prolonged period of apnea (>20 seconds), lasting long enough to cause changes in skin color—cyanosis, pallor, and occasionally erythema
- Limpness, choking, gagging
- Appears well when evaluated by clinicians after recovery from ALTE; infant should be transported to hospital for evaluation, admission, and monitoring
- Link with sudden infant death syndrome (SIDS) has been suggested but clearly not proved

MECHANISM/DESCRIPTION

- Sudden, unexpected death of an infant less than 1 year old, who was typically well before being placed down to sleep
- Infant death remains unexplained after being thoroughly investigated by autopsy, examination of the death scene, investigation of the circumstances, review of the family and infant medical histories
- The major cause of death in infants from 1 month to 1 year of age; the incidence has declined markedly since the initiation of the "Back to Sleep" program in 1994
  - —1983–1991: 5000–6000 deaths/year in the United States
  - —1999: 2648 deaths in the United States
- Peak occurrence of SIDS between 2 and 4 months of age
  - —88% occur before 5 months of age
  - —2% occur after 12 months of age
- 60:40 male-to-female ratio
- Higher incidence reported in fall and winter
- Practice of infants sleeping on their backs began earlier in Europe, resulting in even greater decline in SIDS deaths in participating countries

ETIOLOGY

- Most likely multifactorial
- Many researchers suggest that SIDS infants have predisposing conditions that make them more vulnerable to normal internal and external stresses that occur in infant life
- Proposed and unproven hypotheses: dysrhythmias, hyperthyroidism, mast cell activation, infection, anemia, mineral and electrolyte abnormalities/imbalances, airway obstruction, suffocation, congenital diseases, neurologic events, occult trauma
- Associations/risk factors for SIDS appear to be environmental and behavioral, including maternal, prenatal, and postnatal

Maternal Influences Prevalent in SIDS Infants

- Prenatal cigarette smoking
- Maternal age <20 years during first pregnancy
- Maternal low weight gain
- Illicit drug use
- Short intervals between pregnancies
- Prenatal illness, sexually transmitted diseases, urinary tract infections

Other Possible Risk Factors and Associations

- Intrauterine growth retardation
- Low birth weight
- Exposure to environmental smoking
- Hyperthermia, including heavy bed linens, blankets
- Bed sharing
- Infant gastrointestinal illnesses and listlessness have been reported in proximity to SIDS deaths

Pre-Hospital

CAUTIONS

- Initiate optimal resuscitation at the scene; transport the infant to ED and continue the protocols en route
- On rare occasion and under medical direction, resuscitations have been aborted and pronounced at the scene; consideration must be given to the emotional, social, and clinical circumstances

ESSENTIAL WORKUP

- SIDS is a diagnosis of exclusion
- A diagnosis of SIDS is preceded by the following workup:

Thorough Investigation of the Death Scene

- Where the infant slept, and conditions in sleeping space (temperature, bedding, bed sharing)
- Position of infant was sleeping; what (if anything) it was doing
- Interview the parents, family members, caregivers
- Collect and examine potentially relevant items from the death scene
- Maintain sensitivity toward family; investigation could be difficult for them

Investigate Infant and Family Case Histories

- History connected to infant: prenatal, perinatal, and postbirth medical history
- Family medical and social history, particularly mother
- Family is very vunerable at the time of the investigation; ultimately, it may help them through grieving process
  - —Could reveal a preventable cause
  - —Could reveal no preventable cause, helping the family to realize that there was nothing that they could have done to prevent the child's death

LABORATORY

- Arterial blood gas (ABG)
- CBC
- Electrolytes, including calcium, magnesium, and phosphorous
- Liver function tests
- Toxicology screen
- Blood culture and other sepsis workup as indicated
- Urinalysis and culture

IMAGING/SPECIAL TESTS

- Chest radiograph, if ongoing resuscitation
- Radiologic skeletal survey to exclude abuse (often done by pathologist)
- Autopsy
  - —Some states require an autopsy in all SIDS cases
  - —Is an important postmortem examination and should be done, especially because SIDS is a diagnosis of exclusion
  - —Involves microscopic examination of vital organs through tissue samples, as well as gross examination
  - —Previous postmortem findings in SIDS cases
    - -Congenital cardiomyopathies
    - -Cardiac rhabdomyomas
    - -Tuberous sclerosis
    - -Rare genetic diseases
    - -Viral myocarditis
    - -Intracranial arteriovenous malformations
- Electrocardiogram of surviving family members may suggest family disorder such as prolonged QT syndrome

DIFFERENTIAL DIAGNOSIS

- Cardiovascular
  - —Dysrhythmia
  - —Myocarditis
  - —Tuberous sclerosis
  - —Cardiomyopathy
  - —Congenital heart disease
- Respiratory
  - —Asphyxiation
  - —Drowning
- Infection
  - —Bronchiolitis/respiratory syncytial virus (RSV)
  - —Bronchopneumonia
  - —Pertussis
  - —Tracheobronchitis
- CNS
  - —Cerebral edema
  - —Subdural hematoma
  - —Meningitis
  - —Encephalitis
  - —Arteriovenous malformation
- Gastrointestinal
  - —Enterocolitis with diarrhea
- Pancreas
  - —Cystic fibrosis
  - —Islet cell hyperplasia
  - —Hypertrophy or neoplasm
- Endocrine
  - —Congenital adrenal hyperplasia/hypoplasia
- Systemic
  - —Dehydration
  - —Sepsis
  - —Intoxication, overdose
  - —Hyperthermia

INITIAL STABILIZATION

- Assess and support airway, breathing, circulation, and blood glucose (bedside)
- Begin and continue resuscitation per established protocols; continue if child viable
- Administer appropriate medications by endotracheal tube if other access unobtainable (lidocaine, epinephrine, atropine, naloxone)
- Monitor vital signs: blood pressure, heart rate, respirations, and oxygen saturation continuously
- Conduct a thorough physical examination; look for accidental as well as intentional trauma

ED TREATMENT

- If the resuscitation is unsuccessful and no obvious diagnosis is found, the parents should not be told that SIDS is the cause of death
  - —When speaking with the parents it is appropriate to include SIDS among the possible causes of death
  - —A diagnosis cannot be made until completion of an autopsy, investigation of circumstances and death scene, and exploration of case medical histories of the infant and family

Family Support

- If resuscitation is unsuccessful, attention should then be focused on the family; if resuscitation is ongoing, communication and support of family is essential
- All family members and caregivers are affected; they experience grief, guilt, failure, and inadequacy
- Some parents want to spend quiet time holding their infants after an unsuccessful resuscitation
- Family is defined variably among different cultures and could be more extensive than nuclear or traditional extended family; ED personnel should attempt to be sensitive to cultural needs and expectations of the family
- Family should be offered support in the ED and supplied with resources of support for beyond the day of their infant's death; the local, state, and national SIDS Foundation resources should be made available

Emergency Personnel Support

- ED debriefing should be conducted for all staff who were involved in the infant's care, including emergency medical service (EMS) personnel; this can be important to allow people to express their feelings and freely process the event in a supportive setting
- The child's primary care physician should be involved in follow-up and supporting family

Disposition

ADMISSION CRITERIA

- Admit all infants who have ALTE for evaluation and monitoring after initial resuscitation and stabilization

DISCHARGE CRITERIA

- None

Miscellaneous

ICD9: 798.0

ICD10: R95

SUGGESTED READINGS

Alteimer WA. A pediatrician's view: crib death and managed care. Pediatr Ann 1995;24:345–346.

American Academy of Pediatrics, Task Force on Infant Sleep Position and Sudden Infant Death Syndrome. Changing concepts of sudden infant death syndrome: implications for infant sleeping environment and sleep position. Pediatrics 2000;24:650–656.

Carroll-Pankhurst C, Mortimer EA Jr. Sudden infant death syndrome, bed baring, parental weight, and age at death. Pediatrics 2001;108:1239–1240.

Dwyer T, Ponsby A. SIDS epidemiology and incidence. Pediatr Ann 1995;24:350–352.

Author: Thea James

Suicide, Risk Evaluation

Clinical Presentation

SIGNS AND SYMPTOMS

- Depressed mood
- Verbalization of suicidal ideation
- Hopelessness
- Helplessness
- Anger/aggression
- Impulsivity
- Psychotic symptoms (command auditory hallucinations)

MECHANISM/DESCRIPTION

- The intentional taking of one's own life
- Suicidal ideation
  - —Passive: no real plan or intent
- Active: with plan and intent to die
- Suicidal gesture: self-injurious behavior not intended to cause death (e.g., superficial cutting, cigarette burns, head banging)
- Reckless behavior: not taking prescribed medications, taking too much of prescribed medications, running into traffic
- *Risk-to-rescue ratio:* lethality of plan compared with likelihood of rescue
  - —High risk-to-rescue ratio indicates increased severity of attempt

ETIOLOGY

- 29,199 suicides in United States (1999)
- 11.4 deaths per 100,000 population
- Two peaks in age group most at risk for suicide:
  - —Age 15–24 years (third leading cause of death in this age group)
  - —Age >60 years (highest rates of any age group, increasing incidence with age)

Risk Factors for Suicidal Behavior

- Alcohol or drug abuse
- History of physical or sexual abuse
- History of head injury or neurologic disorder
- Positive family history of suicide attempt
- Prior psychiatric diagnosis
  - —90% of patients who commit suicide
  - —Depression (bipolar or unipolar)
  - —Substance abuse
  - —Anxiety/panic disorders
  - —Schizophrenia
  - —Personality disorders
- Chronic severe medical illness
  - —Epilepsy
  - —AIDS
  - —Huntington's disease
  - —Stroke
  - —Traumatic brain injury
  - —Cancer
  - —Multiple sclerosis
  - —Spinal cord injuries
  - —Hypertension
  - —Cardiopulmonary disease
  - —Peptic ulcer disease
  - —Chronic renal failure
  - —Cushing's disease
  - —Rheumatoid arthritis
  - —Porphyria
- Gender
  - —Women are 3 times more likely to attempt suicide
  - —Men are 3 times more likely to complete suicide
- Psychological
  - —Impulsivity/aggression
  - —Depression
  - —Anxiety
  - —Hopelessness
  - —Self-consciousness/social disengagement
  - —Poor problem-solving abilities
- Social
  - —Widowed
  - —Divorced
  - —Separated
  - —Lack of social supports
  - —Recent loss of relationship
  - —Anniversary of loss
- Environmental
  - —Rural areas
  - —Access to firearms
  - —Poverty
  - —Unemployment

Risk Factors for Completed Suicide

- Male
- Age >60 years
- White or Native American
- Widowed/divorced
- Living alone
- Unemployment/poverty
- Past suicide attempt

Method of Suicide

- Firearms (most common among men and women, three of five completed suicides)
- Overdose (second most common among women), most common means of suicide attempt (70% of failed attempts are by overdose)
- Hanging (second most common among men)

Populations at Highest Risk for Completing Suicide

- Depression—especially psychotic depression
- Anxiety and panic disorder
- Alcohol or drug intoxication
- Schizophrenia
- Adolescents

Others at Risk for Completing Suicide

- Recent discharge from psychiatric facility
- Past history of suicidal ideation or suicide attempt
- Serious physical illness is present up to 70% of all suicides, particularly in elderly patients
- Prisoners
- Doctors
- Victims of violence/abuse
- Persons expecting secondary gain through attempt

Decreased Risk for Suicide

- Patients with mood disorders (major depression and bipolar disorder) treated with lithium
- Patient with major depression treated with electroconvulsive therapy
- Patients with schizophrenia treated with clozapine
- Patients with major depression treated with selective serotonin reuptake inhibitors (SSRI) *not* shown to decrease suicide rates

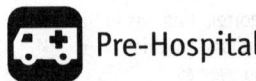

Pre-Hospital

CAUTIONS

- Restraint of potentially dangerous patient who refuses transport to treatment facility: involve police
- Risk to medics on the scene in cases of firearms or other weapons
- Know state and local laws, availability of mobile crisis units, when to involve the police department

Diagnosis

ESSENTIAL WORKUP

- Obtain history to assess risk
  - —Asking about suicide does not increase risk for attempt
- Degree of suicidal ideation
- Plan: immediate risk of self-injury?
  - —Means available to complete plan?
  - —Activity toward initiating plan
  - —Patient's expectations of lethality of plan
- Intent: reasons, goal
- Risk-to-rescue ratio
- Plan or intent to harm others?
- Presence of acute precipitants
  - —Recent losses, lack of social supports
- Risk factors
  - —History of past suicide attempts
  - —Psychiatric review of symptoms: depression, psychosis, panic/anxiety
  - —Chronic medical illness
  - —Alcohol or drug abuse
- Serial assessment of mental status, consistency of responses
- "Why didn't you attempt suicide?"
- Collateral information from outpatient treaters, family, friends

Safety Plan

- Would the patient immediately seek help if suicidal ideation recurred?
- Elimination of means of suicide
- Access to other means of suicide
- Support and supervision in the outpatient setting
- Prompt outpatient follow-up with psychiatric treaters
- Patient investing in not suiciding
- Reasons for living?
- Safety contracts are not useful

LABORATORY

- Blood alcohol level
- Serum toxicology screen: aspirin, acetaminophen, and other medications
- Urine drug screen
  - —Many psychiatric facilities require toxicology screen before placement
- EKG, carbon monoxide (as indicated)

IMAGING/SPECIAL TESTS

- Not routinely indicated

DIFFERENTIAL DIAGNOSIS

- Normal despondency
- Bereavement
- Adjustment disorder with depressed mood
- Major depressive disorder
- Bipolar disorder
- Organic mental disorder (head injury, dementia, delirium)
- Schizophrenia
- Panic and anxiety disorders
- Alcohol or drug abuse
- Borderline personality disorder
- Antisocial personality disorder
- Accidental death
- Attempted homicide

PEDIATRIC/ADOLESCENT SPECIAL CONSIDERATIONS

- Suicide is third leading cause of death among young people 15–24 years of age
- More than 5,000 adolescents commit suicide every year
- Rapidly increasing in young black males, aged 10–14 years
- Less evidence available to link suicide in youth to overt psychiatric illness
- Stresses
  - —Prior attempts
  - —Family disruption
  - —History of psychiatric disorder
  - —Depression
  - —Disciplinary crisis
  - —Broken romance
  - —School difficulties
  - —Bereavement
  - —Rejection
  - —History of physical or sexual abuse
- Early warning signs
  - —Progressive declining schoolwork
  - —Multiple physical complaints
  - —Substance abuse
  - —Disrupted family relations

GERIATRIC CONSIDERATIONS

- Suicide rates highest in age >65 years
- Completed suicide: 83% men
- Risk factors: divorced, widowed, male, social isolation
- Tend to use more lethal methods
- Lower ratio of attempts to completions

Treatment

INITIAL STABILIZATION

- Prevent any ability to elope
- Search the patient
  - —Remove sharp objects, belts, shoelaces, and other articles that could be use for self-injury
- Appropriate supervision

ED TREATMENT

- Voluntary admission to psychiatric facility
- Involuntary admission if patient refuses voluntary
- For involuntary psychiatric admission, patient must have psychiatric disorder and one of the following:
  - —Risk for danger to self
  - —Risk for danger to others
  - —Unable to care for self owing to extremely poor judgment

MEDICATIONS

- Treat underlying psychiatric disorder

Disposition

ADMISSION CRITERIA

- If patient endorses suicidal ideation, with plan and intent, then admission may be needed for safety
- If impulsivity, anger, or aggression hinder ability to control behavior

DISCHARGE CRITERIA

- Patient has no suicidal ideation
- Patient agrees to return to ED immediately or seek psychiatric help if suicidal ideation recurs
- Patient has passive suicidal ideation without plan or intent
- Good support network or placement in appropriate crisis housing
- Appropriate outpatient psychiatric follow-up ensured
- In some cases, patients who express suicidal ideation while intoxicated may be discharged if no longer suicidal once they are sober
- Some patients with borderline personality disorder and chronic suicidal ideation are discharged after careful psychiatric evaluation, in consultation with long-term outpatient caregivers

Miscellaneous

ICD9: 300.9

ICD10: Z91.5

SUGGESTED READINGS

Connor KR, Duberstein PR, Conwell Y, et al. Psychological vulnerability to completed suicide: a review of empirical studies. Suicide and Life-Threatening Behavior 2001;31(4):367–385.

Hoffman D, et al. Depression and suicide assessment. Emerg Med Clin North Am 1991;9(1).

Lagomasino IT, Stern TA. Approach to the suicidal patient. In Stern TA, Herman JB, Slavin PL, eds. The MGH guide to psychiatry in primary care. New York: McGraw-Hill, 1998:15–22.

Mann JJ. A current perspective of suicide and attempted suicide. Ann Intern Med 2002;136(4):302–311.

Authors: Lawrence Park; Jennifer Lafayette

Supraventricular Tachycardia

Clinical Presentation

SIGNS AND SYMPTOMS

- Palpitations (most common)
- Lightheadedness, pressure in the head
- Dyspnea
- Diaphoresis
- Dizziness
- Weakness
- Chest discomfort
- Angina
- Syncope
- Prominent neck veins
- Signs of instability
  - —Mental status changes
  - —Chest pain/ischemia
  - —Acute pulmonary edema
  - —Hypotension

MECHANISM/DESCRIPTION

- Rhythm that originates ectopically above the His bundle
- Rate is greater than 100 beats/min
- Irregular narrow complex supraventricular (SVT)
  - —Atrial fibrillation (AF)
    - -Most common form of SVT seen in the ED
    - -10% of people over 75 years of age have AF
  - —Atrial flutter
  - —Multifocal atrial tachycardia
- Regular narrow complex SVT
  - —Reentrant mechanisms
    - -AV nodal reentry
- 60% of SVT
- Typically present age 30–40 years
- 70% are women
  - -AV reentry involving an accessory pathway
- Wide complex SVT
  - —Aberrant conduction or a bundle branch block is present
  - —Conduction is outside of the normal His-Purkinje system
  - —More common in younger patients without structural disease
  - —Always suspect a ventricular rhythm with a wide complex rhythm

PEDIATRIC CONSIDERATIONS

- SVT is the most common dysrhythmia seen in young adults and children without underlying heart disease
- Aberrant conduction Wolff-Parkinson-White (WPW) syndrome and atrioventricular nodal reentry tachycardia (AVNRT) are the two most common forms of SVT seen in children
- Use verapamil only over 1 year of age

ETIOLOGY

Atrial Tachycardia

- Precipitated by a premature atrial or ventricular contraction
- Electrolyte disturbances
- Drug toxicity
- Hypoxia

Junctional Tachycardia

- AV nodal reentry
- Myocardial ischemia
- Structural heart disease
- Preexcitation syndromes
- Drug and alcohol toxicity

Atrial Fibrillation

- Hypertension
- Coronary artery disease
- Hypothyroidism
- Heavy alcohol intake
- Mitral valve disease
- Chronic pulmonary disease
- Pulmonary embolus
- WPW syndrome
- Hypoxia
- Digoxin toxicity
- Chronic pericarditis
- Idiopathic atrial fibrillation

Atrial Flutter

- Ischemic heart disease
- Valvular heart diseases
- Congestive heart failure
- Myocarditis
- Cardiomyopathies
- Pulmonary embolus
- Other pulmonary disease
  - —Electrolyte abnormalities
  - —Postoperative following cardiac surgery

Multifocal Atrial Tachycardia

- Hypoxic effects of chronic lung disease
- Theophylline toxicity

Pre-Hospital

- Supplemental oxygen
- Intravenous access
- Monitor

CAUTIONS

- Cardioversion must be carried out for severe hemodynamic compromise or cardiovascular collapse

CONTROVERSIES

- Vagal maneuvers (beware of carotid disease)
- Adenosine
  - —Depends on EMS capabilities and field protocols

Diagnosis

ESSENTIAL WORKUP

- Rapid assessment of hemodynamic stability
- A detailed history
  - —Current symptoms
  - —Previous episodes (nature of palpitations, frequency, severity, duration)
  - —Cardiac history
  - —Drug use (illicit, prescription, over-the-counter, and dietary)
- 12-lead EKG with rhythm strip determines management
  - —Rhythm is regular or irregular
  - —QRS complexes are narrow or wide
  - —P waves present or absent
  - —Is there AV dissociation?

LABORATORY

- Studies are indicated when underlying metabolic abnormalities or ischemia is considered
  - —CBC
  - —Electrolytes
  - —Cardiac enzymes
  - —Thyroid function

IMAGING/SPECIAL TESTS

EKG

- Atrial flutter
  - —Regular atrial rate usually greater than 300
  - —Beat-to-beat uniformity of cycle length, polarity, and amplitude
  - —Sawtooth flutter waves directed superiorly and most visible in leads II, III, aVF
  - —AV block, usually 2:1, but occasionally greater or irregular
- Multifocal atrial tachycardia
  - —Three distinctly different P waves with varying PR intervals
- Atrial tachycardia
  - —Rate of 100–200 beats/min
  - —P wave precedes QRS and is morphologically different from the sinus P wave
- Junctional tachycardia
  - —There is usually 1:1 conduction, with ventricular rates equaling the atrial rate
  - —May be either paroxysmal or sustained
  - —Ventricular rates faster than 200 beats/min in an adult suggest an accessory pathway syndrome such as WPW syndrome
  - —Absence of preceding P waves
  - —Often retrograde P waves buried in the QRS
  - —Paroxysmal junctional tachycardia rates range from 120–200 beats/min
  - —Nonparoxysmal junctional tachycardia rates rarely exceed 130 beats/min

Electrophysiologic Testing

- Not indicated during emergency management
- Diagnostic and determines therapy for accessory pathways

DIFFERENTIAL DIAGNOSIS

- Sinus tachycardia
  - —Sepsis
  - —Hypovolemia
  - —Pericardial tamponade
  - —Acute myocardial infarction
  - —Drug intoxication
  - —Infection
- Wide complex tachycardias
  - —Distinguish between supraventricular or ventricular origins

Treatment

INITIAL STABILIZATION

- Intravenous access
- Monitor
- Determination of unstable versus stable patient made by determining whether the patient has organ perfusion (if patient is awake and talking, there is usually time to try other methods before cardioversion even with low BP)

ED TREATMENT

- Atrial fibrillation
  - —Most likely diagnosis when the rhythm is irregular
  - —When unstable, then immediate cardioversion
  - —When stable, rate control is a priority
  - —Beta-blockers or calcium channel blockers, amiodarone, and digoxin
  - —Cardioversion in stable patients should not be attempted unless the dysrhythmia is known to be acute (<24 hours in duration), otherwise anticoagulation is the first step
  - —WPW syndrome
    - -Consider DC cardioversion or amiodarone, flecainide, or procainamide
    - -Avoid adenosine, beta-blockers, calcium channel blockers, and digoxin
- In regular narrow complex SVTs
  - —Vagal maneuvers will occasionally terminate the dysrhythmia
  - —If this is unsuccessful, adenosine is the drug of choice
- Wide complex SVT
  - —Try to determine if ventricular tachycardia or SVT with aberrancy
  - —Verapamil is absolutely contraindicated
  - —Adenosine should be reserved for SVT with aberrancy and is rarely indicated
  - —Electrical cardioversion
  - —Fewer potential complications than antiarrhythmic drugs when mechanism unknown
  - —Antidysrhythmic drugs
  - —IV procainamide and IV amiodarone
  - —Lidocaine is less effective, although sometimes more readily available
  - —Bretylium lacks any evidence of efficacy

MEDICATIONS

- Adenosine: 6 mg rapid IVP; if no response after 1–2 minutes, then 12 mg, 12 mg
- Amiodarone: Load with 15 mg/min over 10 minutes, then 1 mg/min for 6 hours
- Digoxin: 0.5 mg IV initially, then 0.25 mg i.v. q4h
- Diltiazem: 0.25 mg/kg i.v. (usually 10–20 mg) over 2 minutes, followed in 15 minutes by 0.35 mg/kg i.v. over 2 minutes
- Esmolol: 0.5 mg/kg over 1 minute; maintenance infusion: 0.05 mg/kg/min over 4 minutes, then 0.1–0.2 mg/kg/min continuously
- Metoprolol: 5–15 mg slow i.v. push at 5-minute intervals to total of 15 mg
- Procainamide: 20–30 mg/min up to 17 mg/kg, may increase to 50 mg/min for more urgent situations
- Propranolol: 0.1 mg/kg divided into equal doses at 2- to 3-minute intervals
- Sotalol: load 10 mg/min up to 1.0–1.5 mg/kg body weight
- Verapamil: 2.5–5.0 mg i.v. bolus over 2 minutes; may repeat with 5–10 mg every 15–30 minutes to max of 20 mg

Disposition

ADMISSION CRITERIA

- Possible cardiac ischemic event
- Persistent supraventricular tachycardia
- Other underlying metabolic abnormalities

DISCHARGE CRITERIA

- Terminated rhythm without organ hypoperfusion

Miscellaneous

ICD9: 427.0; 427.2; 427.3

ICD10: I47.1

SEE ALSO: PREEXCITATION SYNDROME

SUGGESTED READINGS

Atkins DL, Dorian P, Gonzalez ER, et al. Treatment of tachyarrhythmias. Ann Emerg Med 2001;37:S91–S109.

Chauhan VS, Krahn AD, Klein GJ, et al. Supraventricular tachycardia. Med Clin North Am 2001;85(2):193–223, x.

Connors S, Dorian P. Management of supraventricular tachycardia in the emergency department. Can J Cardiol 1997;13(Suppl A):19A–24A.

Gupta AK, Thakur RK. Wide QRS complex tachycardias. Med Clin North Am 2001;85(2):245–266, ix–x.

Obel OA, Camm AJ. Supraventricular tachycardia: ECG diagnosis and anatomy. Eur Heart J 1997;18(Suppl C):C2–C11.

Authors: Jamie Collings; James Adams

Sympathomimetic, Poisoning

Clinical Presentation

SIGNS AND SYMPTOMS

Vital Signs

- Tachycardia
  - —Bradycardia possible for cocaine and some other decongestants
- Increased blood pressure
  - —Severely intoxicated individuals may be hypotensive
- Tachypnea
- Hyperthermia
  - —Often present, may be severe, and is often overlooked

CNS

- Anxiety
- Headache
- Agitation
- Altered mentation
- Diaphoresis
- Seizures
- Stroke

Cardiovascular

- Palpitations
- Chest pain
- Myocardial ischemia or infarction
- Tachydysrhythmias
- Cardiovascular collapse
- Murmur (endocarditis)

Other

- Dilated pupils
- Dry mucous membranes
- Urinary retention may cause enlarged bladder
- Needle track marks or abscesses on extremities should be sought
- Increased or decreased bowel sounds
- The presence of diaphoresis and bowel sounds may help to differentiate sympathomimetic toxicity from anticholinergic poisoning

MECHANISM/DESCRIPTION

- Direct or indirect stimulation of adrenergic receptors in the sympathetic and central nervous systems
- Often no correlation between dose used and degree of toxicity
- Cocaine may in addition block sodium channels of cardiac myocytes, leading to "tricyclic" or class 1a-type dysrhythmias

ETIOLOGY

- Sympathomimetic toxicity can result from the use of any sympathetically active drug, including
  - —All amphetamines, methamphetamines, and derivatives (e.g., "ecstasy" or MDMA)
  - —Cocaine
  - —Phencyclidine (PCP)
  - —Lysergic acid diethylamide (LSD)
  - —Decongestants (rare)
- Drug delivery routes: inhalation, injection, snorting, or ingestion

PEDIATRIC CONSIDERATIONS

- Sympathomimetic poisoning in children may present similarly to meningitis or other systemic illness

Pre-Hospital

CONTROVERSIES

- Extreme agitation and violent behavior may require restraints
  - —Overzealous use of restraints in significantly intoxicated sympathomimetic patients has led to airway compromise and difficulty with oxygenation
- Treat cocaine-related cardiac ventricular dysrhythmias similarly to tricyclic antidepressant poisoning using sodium bicarbonate
  - —Lidocaine use may help but should be avoided if possible due to its potential for lowering seizure thresholds and its sodium channel interactions
- Benzodiazepines to control agitation or seizures, and possibly even tachycardia and dysrhythmias in some cases

Diagnosis

ESSENTIAL WORKUP

- Continuously monitor vital signs/cardiac rhythm
- EKG and chest x-ray for chest pain or shortness of breath

LABORATORY

- Electrolytes, BUN, creatinine, glucose
- Arterial blood gas (ABG)
  - —For severe signs or symptoms
  - —Acidosis may precipitate dysrhythmias or renal dysfunction in rhabdomyolysis
- Urine dip for myoglobin
- Creatine phosphokinase (CPK) when rhabdomyolysis suspected
- Urine toxicology
  - —Of limited utility in adults because tests can be positive for 3 or more days after use
  - —Some sympathomimetic compounds used for weight reduction, for narcolepsy, or as decongestants can cross-react with assays for amphetamines
  - —LSD will not show up on most urine toxicology screens
- Blood toxicology testing is of no value
- Cardiac enzymes
  - —For EKG abnormalities and in those admitted for chest pain

IMAGING/SPECIAL TESTS

- Cranial CT scanning for abnormal neurologic examinations or seizures

DIFFERENTIAL DIAGNOSIS

- Meningitis
- Hypertensive encephalopathy
- Anticholinergic poisoning
- Alcohol or sedative-hypnotic withdrawal
- Organic psychosis
- Heatstroke
- Sepsis
- Thyroid storm
- Hypoglycemia

PEDIATRIC CONSIDERATIONS

- Urine toxicology screening may be the only way to discover sympathomimetic poisoning in children presenting with altered mental status
- Ritalin and other sympathomimetics used for attention-deficit hyperactivity disorder (ADHD) may cross-react with the assay for amphetamines

Treatment

INITIAL STABILIZATION

- ABCs
- IV 0.9% NS
  - —Administer at least 2 L of crystalloid to hypotensive individuals
- Monitor cardiovascular function
- Treat seizures, acute agitation, or severe hypertension with *liberal* IV benzodiazepines
- Treat EKG changes or histories consistent with myocardial ischemia with aspirin, nitrates, anticoagulant, or thrombolytics as indicated

ED TREATMENT

Elimination

- Activated charcoal orally if exposure was through ingestion or "body packing"
- Whole-bowel irrigation with polyethylene glycol solution for "body packers"

Cardiovascular

- Treat severe hypertension with nitroprusside, phentolamine, labetalol, or other related antihypertensive therapies
  - —The use of β-receptor antagonists alone may result in worsening hypertension from unopposed α stimulation (labetalol has some α-receptor antagonistic activity and can be used)
- Benzodiazepines may aid in controlling dysrhythmias and hypertension
- Sodium bicarbonate is the treatment of choice for ventricular dysrhythmias and heart blocks indicative of sodium channel blocking effects with cocaine poisoning (such as widened QRS complex on EKG)
- Lidocaine for ventricular dysrhythmias refractory to alkalinization, benzodiazepines, and supportive care
- β-Receptor antagonists (especially esmolol) for ventricular tachydysrhythmias

Other

- Butyrophenones (e.g., haloperidol) *with caution* to manage agitation
  - —May lower seizure thresholds and may prolong QT duration
- Treat hyperthermia aggressively
- Alkalinize urine or use diuretics for rhabdomyolysis

MEDICATIONS

- Activated charcoal: 1 g/kg
- Diazepam: 5–10 mg i.v. (peds: 0.2–0.3 mg/kg i.v. or 0.5 mg/kg PR) as needed
- Esmolol: 50–200 μg/kg/min i.v. infusion
- Haloperidol: 2.5–10 mg i.v. or i.m.
- Labetalol: 20 mg i.v. every 10 minutes up to 300 mg
- Lidocaine: 1–2 mg/kg i.v. followed by infusion of 1–3 mg/min as needed
- Lorazepam: 1–2 mg (peds: 0.05–0.15 mg/kg) i.v. or i.m. as needed
- Nitroprusside: 0.5–10 μg/kg/min i.v. infusion
- Phentolamine: 0.05–0.1 mg/kg/dose to max 5 mg i.v.
- Sodium bicarbonate: 1–2 amps (peds: 1 mEq/kg) i.v. bolus; infusion may be indicated for rhabdomyolysis

Disposition

ADMISSION CRITERIA

- Body packers or stuffers
- Severe manifestations of toxicity (seizures, dysrhythmias, hyperthermia, rhabdomyolysis, severe hypertension, or severely altered mental status) to a monitored bed
- Ischemic chest pain

DISCHARGE CRITERIA

- Mildly intoxicated patients can be observed and treated in the ED until resolution of altered mentation and other clinical manifestations

Miscellaneous

ICD9: 971.2

ICD10: T44.9

SUGGESTED READINGS

Callaway CW, Clark RF. Hyperthermia in psychostimulant overdose. Ann Emerg Med 1994;24:68–76.

Chiang WK. Amphetamines. In: Goldfrank LR, et al., eds. Goldfrank's toxicologic emergencies, 6th ed. Stamford, CT: Appleton & Lange, 1998:1091–1103.

Derlet RW, Albertson TE. Emergency department presentation of cocaine intoxication. Ann Emerg Med 1989;18:182–186.

McCarron M, Schulze BW, Thompson GA, et al. Acute phencyclidine intoxication: incidence of clinical findings in 1000 cases. Ann Emerg Med 1981;10:237–242.

Richards CF, Clark RF, Holbrook T, et al. The effects of cocaine and amphetamines on vital signs in trauma patients. J Emerg Med 1995;13:59–63.

Authors: Richard Clark; Sean Patrick Nordt

Syncope

Clinical Presentation

SIGNS AND SYMPTOMS

- Transient loss of consciousness associated with loss of postural tone
- Prodromal symptoms
  - —Lightheadedness
  - —Diaphoresis
  - —Dimming vision
  - —Nausea
- The following findings suggest an underlying life threat
  - —Sudden event without warning
  - —Chest pain

MECHANISM/DESCRIPTION

- Ultimately, it is the lack of oxygen to the brainstem reticular activating system, which results in a loss of consciousness and postural tone
- Most commonly an inciting event causes a drop in cardiac output
- Cerebral perfusion is reestablished by autonomic regulation as well as the reclined posture, which results from the event
- Accounts for 3% of ED visits
- Elderly with highest incidence as well as increased morbidity

ETIOLOGY

- Cardiac dysfunction
  - —Typically sudden and without prodromal symptoms
  - —Tachydysrhythmias or bradydysrhythmias
  - —Aortic stenosis
  - —Hypertrophic cardiomyopathy
  - —Pulmonary embolus
  - —Typically sudden and without prodromal symptoms
- Hypovolemia
  - —Acute hemorrhage (see Hemorrhagic Shock)
  - —Severe dehydration
- Vasovagal reflex
  - —Commonly incited by pain or fear
  - —Prodromal findings are usually present
  - —Typically involves an inappropriately withdrawn sympathetic response, which is replaced with vagal stimulation
  - —Tilt-table testing is the gold standard in the diagnosis of vasovagal syncope
- Orthostatic syncope
  - —Iatrogenic
    - -Beta-blockers
    - -Diuretics
    - -Hypovolemia
- Neurologic
  - —Transient spike in intracranial pressure (ICP) that exceeds cerebral perfusion pressure
  - —Postsyncopal headache is almost universal
  - —May be presentation of a subarachnoid hemorrhage

Pre-Hospital

CAUTIONS

- Oxygen
- Cardiac monitoring
- IV access

Diagnosis

ESSENTIAL WORKUP

- EKG immediately upon arrival to check for
  - —Ischemia
  - —Dysrhythmias
  - —Block
  - —Long QT interval
  - —Wolff-Parkinson-White syndrome
- Detailed history and physical examination will determine diagnosis in 85% of those who eventually obtain a diagnosis
- 6 Ps of a syncope history:
  - —1. Pre-Prodrome activities
  - —2. Prodrome symptoms—visual symptom, nausea
  - —3. Predisposing factors—age, chronic disease
  - —4. Precipitating factors—stress, postural symptoms
  - —5. Passerby witness—what did they see?
  - —6. Postictal phase, if any—suggests seizure
- Physical examination
  - —Evaluate for trauma
  - —Orthostatic vital signs
  - —Check for difference in blood pressure in both arms suggesting aortic dissection or subclavian steal syndrome
  - —Careful cardiovascular examination, including murmurs, bruits, and dysrhythmias
  - —Rectal examination to check for GI bleeding
  - —Urine pregnancy test in reproductive age female
  - —Careful neurologic examination

LABORATORY

- Driven by history and physical examination
- CBC in suspected occult hemorrhage
- Cardiac enzymes in suspected ischemia
- Pregnancy test in reproductive age female
- Electrolytes in patients with profound dehydration or diuretic use

IMAGING/SPECIAL TESTS

- EKG and monitoring until cardiac etiology ruled out
- Chest x-ray if congestive heart failure, dissection, or massive pulmonary embolism suspected
- Head CT if abnormal neurologic examination or transient ischemic attack (TIA) suspected
- Echocardiogram if concern for structural defects

DIFFERENTIAL DIAGNOSIS

- Seizure is most commonly mistaken for syncope
  - —Key differentiating factor is postictal confusion
  - —Brief tonic movements and urinary incontinence may be seen with syncope
- Hypoxemia
- Hypoglycemia
- Toxicologic
- Stroke

Treatment

INITIAL STABILIZATION

- Advanced cardiac life support (ACLS) interventions for unstable patients
- Oxygen
- Cardiac monitoring
- IV access with normal saline fluid bolus in suspected hypovolemia
- Consider coma cocktail—dextrose, thiamine, and naloxone for persistent altered mental status

ED TREATMENT

- ACLS interventions for dysrhythmias
- Standard regimens for acute MI
- Control blood pressure for subarachnoid hemorrhage and aortic dissection

MEDICATIONS

- Dextrose: D50W 1 amp (50 mL or 25 g) (peds: D25W 2–4 mL/kg i.v.)
- Naloxone: 2 mg i.v. or i.m. (peds: 0.1 mg/kg)
- Thiamine: 100 mg i.v. or i.m. (peds: 50 mg)

Disposition

ADMISSION CRITERIA

- Suspected cardiac syncope must be admitted to monitored bed
- GI bleeds consider ICU bed
- Admit elderly patients with syncope

DISCHARGE CRITERIA

- Vasovagal or orthostatic syncope may be evaluated on outpatient basis with close follow-up, if patient is reliable and has a good social structure
- Driving restrictions until cleared

Miscellaneous

ICD9: 780.2

ICD10: R55

SUGGESTED READINGS

Hayes OW. Evaluation of syncope in the emergency department. Emerg Med Clin North Am 1998;16(3):601–615.

Meyer MD. Evaluation of the patient with syncope: an evidence based approach. Emerg Med Clin North Am 1999;17(1): 189–201.

Oh JH. Psychiatric illness and syncope. Cardiol Clin 1997;15(2):269–275.

Panther R, et al. Echo in the diagnostic evaluation of syncope. J Am Soc Echo 1998;11(3):294–298.

Authors: Sam Keim; Stephen Hocheder

Syndrome of Inappropriate Antidiuretic Hormone Secretion (SIADH)

Clinical Presentation

SIGNS AND SYMPTOMS

- Serum sodium <130 mEq/L
  - —Weakness
  - —Lethargy
  - —Weight gain
  - —Headache
  - —Anorexia
- Sodium serum <120 mEq/L
  - —Mental status change
  - —Seizure
  - —Coma
- Chronic hyponatremia: 50% asymptomatic
- High mortality when hyponatremia develops acutely

MECHANISM/DESCRIPTION

Normal Regulation of Water Balance

- Antidiuretic hormone (ADH)
  - —Integral part of the homeostatic mechanism that controls water balance
  - —Increases water permeability of the kidney collecting tubules resulting in water reabsorption
  - —Released when hypothalamic osmoreceptors, left atrial stretch receptors, and carotid baroreceptors detect water deprivation

Hyponatremia

- Serum sodium <135 mEq/L
- Excess extracellular water *relative* to sodium
- Depletional hyponatremia
  - —Sodium depletion can be caused by diet, GI losses, diuretic use, renal or adrenal disease
  - —Often accompanied by extracellular fluid volume depletion
  - —Hyponatremia associated with clinical signs of dehydration
  - —Increased hematocrit, BUN, creatinine
  - —Urinary sodium excretion <20 mEq/L
- Dilutional hyponatremia
  - —Increased extracellular water in presence of normal or increased total body sodium
  - —Can be caused by increased fluid intake (oral, IV), drugs that cause water retention, and medical conditions causing water retention
  - —Euvolemia or edema
  - —Normal or decreased hematocrit, BUN, creatinine
  - —Urinary sodium excretion >20 mEq/L
  - —Inappropriate ADH secretion is a form of dilutional hyponatremia

Definition of SIADH

- ADH secretion in absence of hyperosmolality or hypovolemia
- Criteria for definition
  - —Hyponatremia
  - —Hyposmolality of the plasma
  - —Continued renal excretion of sodium in absence of diuretics
  - —No clinical evidence of volume depletion
  - —Urine osmolality greater than appropriate with respect to plasma osmolality
  - —Normal renal, adrenal, and thyroid function
- Inappropriate ADH secretion can originate from the hypothalamus or extrahypothalamic tissue

Common Causes of SIADH

- Diuretic hormone–producing tumors
  - —Neoplastic
  - —Bronchogenic
  - —Pancreatic
  - —Prostatic
  - —Pituitary
  - —Thymoma
  - —Lymphoma
- Pulmonary disease
  - —Asthma
  - —Pneumonia
  - —Tuberculosis
- CNS disorders
  - —Infection
  - —Cerebrovascular accident (CVA)
  - —Trauma
- Common drugs
  - —Fluoxetine
  - —Tricyclic antidepressants
  - —Antipsychotics
  - —Antiemetics
  - —Anticonvulsants
- Other
  - —Positive pressure ventilation
  - —AIDS
  - —Idiopathic

Pre-Hospital

N/A

Diagnosis

ESSENTIAL WORKUP

- Exclude depletional hyponatremia
- Exclude other causes of dilutional hyponatremia
- Electrolytes, BUN, creatinine, glucose
  - —Hyponatremia (serum sodium <135 mmol/L)
  - —Serum hyposmolality (serum osmolality <280 mOsm/kg)
- Urine osmolality
  - —Inability to excrete a dilute urine
  - —Urine osmolality >100 mOsm/kg
- Urine sodium
  - —Continued urinary excretion of sodium
  - —Urinary sodium >20 mEq/L
- Exclude other causes of hyponatremia

LABORATORY

- Serum protein
- Lipid levels
- Serum osmolality
- Liver and thyroid function test
- Morning cortisol level

IMAGING/SPECIAL TESTS

- Chest x-ray and CT head to screen for pathology causing SIADH

DIFFERENTIAL DIAGNOSIS

Causes of Hyponatremia

- Increased extracellular fluid (dilutional hyponatremia)
  - —Renal failure
  - —Cardiac failure
  - —Liver cirrhosis
- Normal extracellular fluid (dilutional hyponatremia)
  - —SIADH
  - —Physical and emotional stress
  - —Myxedema
  - —Sheehan's syndrome
  - —Reset osmostat syndromes
- Decreased extracellular fluid (depletional hyponatremia)
  - —Excessive sweating
  - —Vomiting
  - —Diarrhea
  - —Third-space sequestration
  - —Diuretics
  - —Aldosterone deficiency (Addison's disease)
  - —Salt-losing nephropathies (renal tubular acidosis)
- Pseudohyponatremia
  - —Hyperproteinemia
  - —Hyperlipidemia
  - —Hyperglycemia

Syndrome of Inappropriate Antidiuretic Hormone Secretion (SIADH)

Treatment

INITIAL STABILIZATION

- Severe symptomatic hyponatremia with CNS manifestations
- Endotracheal intubation for patients in need of airway protection
  —Intravenous access
  —Naloxone, thiamine, dextrose (or Accucheck)
  —Treat seizures with benzodiazepines
- Proceed to hyponatremia treatment

ED TREATMENT

- Initial treatment of hyponatremia caused by SIADH is the same for all causes of euvolemic/hypervolemic hyponatremia
- Mildly symptomatic hyponatremia, chronic hyponatremia with minimal symptoms, asymptotic hyponatremia
  —Serum sodium usually >125 mEq/L
  —Fluid restriction 800–1000 mL/d alone or in conjunction with
    -0.9% NS infusion
    -IV furosemide
  —Correct serum sodium by no more than 0.5 mEq/L/h
  —Too rapid correction of serum sodium levels can induce central pontine myelinolysis, associated with development of bulbar palsy, quadriplegia coma, and death
- Severe hyponatremia
  —Symptomatic patient, serum sodium <125 mEq/L
  —Increase serum sodium by no more than 12 mEq/L in first 24 hours at rate of 0.5–1 mEq/L/h
  —Target level 125 mEq/L
  —Treat patients with significant neurologic symptoms with 3% saline solution
  —Serum sodium laboratory testing every 1–2 hours
- Acute life-threatening hyponatremia
  —Serum sodium usually <120 mEq/L
  —Associated with seizures or coma
  —Clinical goal: stop seizure, improve neurologic status
  —Therapeutic goal: same as for severe hyponatremia
  —Administer 3% saline solution
  —IV furosemide to promote a prompt diuresis and induce a negative fluid balance
  —Once serum sodium 125 mEq/L, further IV fluid should be in form of 0.9% saline solution
  —Restoration of serum sodium to normal levels should take place over >48 hours
- Most effective treatment of SIADH is successful eradication of the underlying cause
- Drugs that inhibit the secretion or the renal effect of ADH
- Indicated when SIADH not self-limited and cause cannot be removed
- Demeclocycline (blocks renal effect of ADH)

MEDICATIONS

- Demeclocycline: 300 mg PO b.i.d.
- Hypertonic saline solution (3% NaCl): 250–500 mL
  —25–100 mL/h
  —Limit rate in rise of serum sodium to 0.5–1.0 mEq/L/h
  —Discontinue when a resolution in hyponatremic seizure is obtained, or serum sodium 125 mEq/L reached
  —Rise in serum sodium by 4–6 mEq/L usually sufficient to stop seizures
- Isotonic saline solution (0.9% NS): standard maintenance rates
- Lasix: 1 mg/kg up to 20–40 i.v. push

Disposition

ADMISSION CRITERIA

- Severe life-threatening hyponatremia
- Symptomatic hyponatremia
- Serum sodium <125 mEq/L regardless of symptoms
- New-onset SIADH in which underlying cause must be diagnosed and treated
- Complications secondary to the underlying cause of SIADH
- Patient's compliance an issue

DISCHARGE CRITERIA

- Asymptomatic chronic hyponatremia
  —Serum sodium >125 mEq/L
  —No unstable comorbid factors
  —Known diagnosis of SIADH

Miscellaneous

ICD9: 253.6

ICD10: E22.2

SEE ALSO: HYPONATREMIA

SUGGESTED READINGS

Fried LF, Palevsky PM. Hyponatremia and hypernatremia. Med Clin North Am 1997; 81(3):585–609.

Miller M. Syndrome of excess antidiuretic hormone release. Crit Care Clin 2001;17(1): 11–23.

Sorensen JB, Anderson MK, Hansen HH. Syndrome of inappropriate secretion of antidiuretic hormone (SIADH) in malignant disease. J Intern Med 1995;238(2):97–110.

Spigset O, Hedenmalm K. Hyponatremia and the syndrome of inappropriate antidiuretic hormone secretion (SIADH) induced by psychotropic drugs. Drug Saf 1995;12(3):209–225.

Author: John McCourt

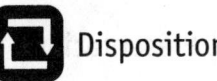

Synovitis, Toxic

Clinical Presentation

SIGNS AND SYMPTOMS

- Unilateral hip pain, acute onset
- Painful limp
- Limitation of hip medial rotation and abduction
- Pain in anteromedial thigh and knee
- Refusal or inability to bear weight
- Preferred external rotation, abduction, and flexion
- Pain over anterior portion of hip with palpation
- Low-grade fever
- Possible upper respiratory infection recent or current
- Nontoxic appearing

MECHANISM/DESCRIPTION

- Acute inflammation of the hip joint in children associated with joint effusion
- Disease process is self-limiting
- Number one cause of hip pain in children younger than 10 years of age
- Also referred to as *transient synovitis* and *irritable hip syndrome*
- Age group most affected is 3–6 years
- 2:1 male predominance
- Right hip is affected more than the left

ETIOLOGY

- Cause of toxic synovitis is unknown
- Infectious etiology is suspected because there is a preceding upper respiratory illness in a large number of cases

Pre-Hospital

N/A

Diagnosis

ESSENTIAL WORKUP

- CBC, erythrocyte sedimentation rate (ESR), C-reactive protein (CRP)
  —Normal or elevated
- If two out of following four criteria are present, there is a 95% sensitivity and 91% specificity for septic arthritis
  —Severe pain and spasm
  —Temperature >38°C
  —ESR >20 or CRP >1
  —Tenderness on palpation
- An elevated CBC or ESR does not differentiate toxic synovitis from septic arthritis or osteomyelitis
  —If both CBC and ESR/CRP are normal, more serious causes of hip pain are less likely
- Plain hip films (AP and frog-leg view)
  —Usually normal
  —May detect an effusion or other causes of hip pain
- Ultrasound to rule out joint effusion if high suspicion for septic arthritis
  —If a joint effusion is present, an ultrasound-guided joint aspiration should be performed to rule out septic arthritis

IMAGING/SPECIAL TESTS

- Joint aspiration
  —Not necessary if the patient is afebrile with a normal CBC and ESR/CRP
  —Abnormal joint fluid analysis indicates septic arthritis (see Arthritis, Septic)
  —Patients with septic arthritis rarely present without one of these elevated values
- MRI (rarely indicated)
  —Very useful in diagnosing Legg-Calvé-Perthes disease
  —Can detect abnormalities in toxic synovitis
  —Recent study suggested that signal intensity alteration in the bone marrow of the affected hip might differentiate toxic synovitis from septic arthritis
- Bone scan
  —Used to differentiate Legg-Calvé-Perthes disease from toxic synovitis
  —Can detect osteomyelitis
  —The increased radiation is usually reserved for recurrent cases or cases in which the diagnosis is still in question
  —Negative bone scan decreases the likelihood of infection, fracture, or tumor

DIFFERENTIAL DIAGNOSIS

- Septic arthritis
- Osteomyelitis
- Soft tissue infection
- Legg-Calvé-Perthes disease
- Slipped capitol femoral epiphysis
- Juvenile rheumatoid arthritis
- Rheumatic fever
- Chondrolysis
- Gaucher's disease
- Osteosarcoma
- Ewing's sarcoma
- Osteoid osteoma
- Leukemia
- Tuberculosis of the hip
- Fracture
- Lyme disease
- Psoas abscess
- Sickle cell crisis

PEDIATRIC CONSIDERATIONS

- Second event may occur in 4–17% within 6 months of initial event
- Association of toxic synovitis with Legg-Calvé-Perthes disease
  - —2–10% of patients with toxic synovitis later develop Legg-Calvé-Perthes disease
  - —Suggested that toxic synovitis may represent an early stage of Legg-Calvé-Perthes disease

Treatment

ED TREATMENT

- Conservative treatment
- Bed rest in position of comfort—flexion and external rotation
- Initiate NSAIDs
- Antibiotics and steroids are not indicated
- Some authors recommend no weight-bearing for 7–10 days following improvement and return of normal hip function citing increased risk for recurrence
- Close follow-up essential with repeat radiographs due to association with Legg-Calvé-Perthes

MEDICATIONS

- Ibuprofen: 200–600 mg (peds >6 months old: 5–10 mg/kg) PO q6h

Disposition

ADMISSION CRITERIA

- Patients with severe joint pain or a large effusion may require hospitalization for bed rest and analgesics

DISCHARGE CRITERIA

- All patients who have been excluded for more serious diagnosis of hip pain and diagnosed with toxic synovitis can be discharged from the hospital with good follow-up

Miscellaneous

ICD9: 727.00

ICD10: M67.3

SUGGESTED READINGS

Della-Giustina K, Della-Giustina D. Emergency department evaluation and treatment of pediatric orthopedic injuries. Emerg Med Clin North Am 1999;17(4):895–922.

Do T. Transient synovitis as a cause of painful limps in children. Curr Opin Pediatr 2000;12:48–51.

Eich G, et al. The painful hip: evaluation of criteria for clinical decision-making. Eur J Pediatr 1999;158:923–928.

Hoffer FA, Zawin JK, Rand FF, et al. Joint effusion in children with an irritable hip: US diagnosis and aspiration. Radiology 1993;187:459–463.

Koop S, Quanbeck D. Three common causes of childhood hip pain. Pediatr Clin North Am 1996;43:1053–1066.

Lee S, et al. Septic arthritis versus transient synovitis at MR imaging: preliminary assessment with signal intensity alterations in bone marrow. Radiology 1999;211:459–465.

Spock A. Transient synovitis of the hip joint in children. Pediatrics 1959;24:1042.

Tachidjian MS. Acute transient synovitis of the hip. In: Tachidjian MS, ed. Pediatric orthopedics. Philadelphia: WB Saunders, 1990:1461–1465

Authors: Dick Kuo; James Colletti

Syphilis

Clinical Presentation

SIGNS AND SYMPTOMS

Primary

- Chancre
  - —At site of inoculation
  - —10–60 days postexposure
  - —Classic is a *painless* chancre—clean based, circular, with sharply defined borders
  - —Commonly found on penis, vulva, and rectum, but may see extravaginally
  - —May become painful if secondary infection
  - —Usually solitary
  - —Usually heals spontaneously without therapy in 4–5 days but might last up to 6 weeks
- Rubbery, nontender regional adenopathy
  - —May occur 4 weeks postexposure
- Rectal chancre
  - —Painful or painless
  - —Rectal irritation/discharge
  - —Painless enlargement of lymph nodes

Secondary

- Rash
  - —Dull, diffuse, maculopapular, symmetric rash
  - —Classically involving the palms and soles
  - —Starts on the trunk and on flexor surfaces
  - —Appears 6 weeks after primary chancre heals
  - —May mimic virtually any dermatologic condition
- Flu-like symptoms
  - —Fever
  - —Chills
  - —Lethargy
- Lymphadenopathy
- Condylomata lata
  - —Papular lesions seen in intertriginous areas
  - —Flat rectal warts found at this stage
- Less common
  - —Patchy alopecia
  - —Syphilitic meningitis
- Loss of the lateral third of the eyebrows
- Painless mucosal lesions (mucous patches)
- Resolves spontaneous within 1–2 months

Latent

- No clinical signs of syphilis, and CSF is normal
- Positive serologic test
- "Late latent" not infectious except for fetal transmission in pregnant women
- May persist for lifetime of patient or develop into tertiary

Tertiary

- Occurs years after the initial infection, sometimes up to 20 years
  - —Destructive stage of the disease
- Neurosyphilis
  - —Asymptomatic
    - -CSF abnormalities in absence of clinical symptoms
    - -CSF pleocytosis, protein elevation, reactive VDRL
  - —Meningitis
    - -Aseptic
    - -Involves the base of brain
    - -Unilateral/bilateral cranial nerve palsies
  - —General paresis
    - -Progressive dementia
    - -Loss of cortical function
  - —Tabes dorsalis (neuropathy)
    - -Degeneration of posterior columns/posterior roots of spinal cord
    - -Progressive loss of reflexes, vibratory/position sensation
    - -Progressive ataxia
    - -Argyll Robertson pupils
    - -Urinary incontinence
- Cardiovascular
  - —Thoracic aneurysm (ascending most common)
  - —Aortic insufficiency
- Destructive lesions of skeletal structure or skin

Congenital Syphilis

- Rash
- Rhinitis
- Hepatosplenomegaly
- Lymphadenopathy
- Many asymptomatic initially

MECHANISM/DESCRIPTION

- Sexually transmitted disease, 70,000 new cases per year
- Enters the body through mucous membranes and nonintact skin
- Spirochetes multiply at site of inoculation and enter local lymphatics, regional lymph nodes, and bloodstream
- Focal endarteritis
  - —Primary pathologic lesion
- Replication and hematogenous spread produces secondary syphilis
- Granulomatous reaction occurs in secondary and tertiary syphilis
- Cofactor in transmission of HIV
- Infectious during primary and secondary stages

ETIOLOGY

- *Treponema pallidum*
  - —Causative agent
  - —Spirochete bacteria
- Increased prevalence in the past 10 years secondary to sexual behavior associated with drug use

Pre-Hospital

N/A

Diagnosis

ESSENTIAL WORKUP

- Serologic tests
  - —Nontreponemal tests: RPR (rapid plasma regain); VDRL (Venereal Disease Research Laboratories)
    - -Correlate with disease activity
    - -Usually positive 2–4 weeks after the chancre appears
    - -Many early false-negatives results, especially $\leq$7 days after primary chancre
    - -Repeat negative tests in 2 weeks
    - -2% false-positive rate
    - -Four-fold change in titer is clinically significant
    - -100% sensitive in secondary
    - -Will become nonreactive after successful treatment
  - —Treponemal antibody test: FTA-ABS (fluorescent treponemal antibody absorbed) and MHA-TP (hemagglutination assay for antibody to *T. pallidum*)
    - -More sensitive and specific than nontreponemal tests
    - -False positive as high as 1% when screening normal population
    - -Used as confirmatory test
    - -Stays positive for life even with treatment
    - -More costly and harder to perform

LABORATORY

- Darkfield microscopy
  - —Used to identify treponemes from samples of primary and secondary lesions
  - —Recommended with suspicious early lesions because of false-negative serology in early primary
  - —Ointments and creams applied to lesions may lead to a false-negative microscopy
  - —Oral specimens are unsuitable
- CSF analysis
  - —For tertiary syphilis
  - —Positive VDRL
  - —>5 lymphocytes/mL
  - —Protein >45

DIFFERENTIAL DIAGNOSIS

Genital Ulcer

- Chancroid
- Genital herpes
  —Vesicles
  —Multiple
- Lymphogranuloma venereum
- Granuloma inguinale
- Superficial fungal infection
- Carcinoma

Secondary Syphilis

- Pityriasis rosea
- Drug rash
- Acute febrile exanthems
- Psoriasis
- Lichen planus
- Scabies
- Infectious mononucleosis

Treatment

INITIAL STABILIZATION

- Lower blood pressure/IV access for aortic dissection

ED TREATMENT

- Treatment other than penicillin-associated with increased relapse rate
- Desensitize those allergic to penicillin
- Pregnancy
  —Treat with penicillin as above for stage/latency
  —Admit women allergic to penicillin to desensitize before penicillin administration
- Jarish-Herxheimer reaction
  —Transient febrile reaction to therapy
  —May be due to liberation of antigens from spirochetes or activation of complement cascade
  —Occurs in the first few hours with a peak at 8 hours and resolution in 24 hours
  —Symptoms include
    -Fever
    -Myalgia
    -Headache
    -Malaise
    -Worsening of syphilitic rash
  —Treat with antipyretics
  —No serious sequelae
- Recommend testing
  —Of sexual partners
  —For concomitant sexually transmitted diseases including HIV
  —Repeat serologic testing in 6 and 12 months

MEDICATIONS

- Early primary, secondary, latent <1 year antibiotic options
  —Benzathine penicillin G: 2.4 million units i.m. (best)
  —Doxycycline: 100 mg PO b.i.d. × 14 days
  —Tetracycline: 500 mg PO q.i.d. × 14 days
- Latent: >1 year duration (except neurosyphilis) antibiotic options
  —Benzathine penicillin G: 2.4 million units i.m. weekly for 3 weeks (best)
  —Doxycycline: 100 mg PO b.i.d. × 4 weeks
  —Tetracycline: 500 mg PO q.i.d. × 4 weeks
- Neurosyphilis
  —Penicillin G: 3–4 million units i.v. q4h × 10–14 days
  —Procaine penicillin: 2.4 million units i.m. daily, *plus* probenecid, 500 mg PO q.i.d. for 10–14 days
- Congenital
  —Penicillin G: 50,0000 μ/kg i.v. q8–12h for 10–14 days, *or*
  —Procaine penicillin: 50,000 μ/kg i.m. daily for 10–14 days

Disposition

ADMISSION CRITERIA

- Neurosyphilis requiring IV antibiotic therapy
- Pregnant women allergic to penicillin requiring desensitization before initiation of penicillin

DISCHARGE CRITERIA

- Follow-up care
  —Measure for falling titers, 6 months, and 1 year after therapy
  —Tertiary/latent (>1 year) needs serology 3, 6, 12, and 24 months after treatment to measure for falling titers

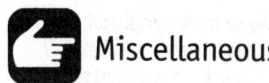

Miscellaneous

ICD9: 97.9

ICD10: A53.9

SUGGESTED READINGS

Berger RE. Sexually transmitted disease. Adv Urol 1997;2:97.

Drugs for sexually transmitted infections. Med Lett Drugs Therapeutics 1999;41: 85–90.

Kreipe RE. Sexually transmitted disease in adolescents. Pediatr Infect Dis J 1998;17: 921–922.

McKinzie J. Sexually transmitted disease. Emerg Med Clin North Am 2001;19(3): 723–743.

Author: David Levine

Systemic Lupus Erythematosus

Clinical Presentation

SIGNS AND SYMPTOMS

Systemic

- Fatigue
- Fever
- Weight loss
- Dyspnea

Skin

- Malar rash (butterfly facial)
- Discoid rash (raised red patches)
- Photosensitivity rash (subacute cutaneous lupus)

Joints

- Joint pain
- Arthritis
  - —Defined as two or more peripheral joints with warmth, tenderness, or effusion
  - —Polyarthritis, symmetric, or migratory

Heart

- Chest pain
- Pericardial rub
- Murmur

Vascular

- Vasculitis
- Thrombosis
- Atherosclerosis
- Peripheral vascular disease

Lungs

- Dyspnea
- Tachypnea
- Pleural rub
- Rales

Nervous System

- Psychosis
- Depression
- Headache
- Seizures
- Peripheral neuropathies
- Stroke
- Cranial nerve deficits

Gastrointestinal

- Painless oral ulcers
- Abdominal pain
- Guarding or rebound tenderness
- Positive stool guaiac suggests mesenteric ischemia

MECHANISM/DESCRIPTION

- Multisystem autoimmune disease with systemic complications
  - —Arthritis
  - —Cardiac
    - -Endocarditis
    - -Myocarditis
    - -Congestive heart failure
    - -Conduction abnormalities
    - -Atherosclerosis
    - -Myocardial infarction
  - —Renal
    - -Glomerulonephritis
    - -Renal failure
  - —Pulmonary
    - -Pleural effusion (usually exudative)
    - -Pneumonitis
    - -Pulmonary hemorrhage
    - -Pulmonary embolism
    - -Pneumonia
    - -Pleuritis
    - -Pulmonary edema
    - -Pulmonary hypertension
  - —Neurologic
    - -Lupus cerebritis
  - —Vascular
    - -Vasculitis
    - -Thrombosis
    - -Atherosclerosis
  - —Gastrointestinal
    - -Peritonitis
    - -Mesenteric vasculitis and ischemia
    - -Pancreatitis
- More common in females than males (ratio, 5:1)
- More common in African Americans
- Peak onset is between ages 15 and 40 years
- Higher frequency among first-degree relatives

ETIOLOGY

- Autoantibody production against cell nucleus and cytoplasmic structures leading to inflammatory changes, vasculitis, and immune complex deposition in multiple organ systems
- A significant percentage of patients have an associated antiphospholipid syndrome
  - —Characterized by antibodies against cellular phospholipid components
  - —Tendency toward recurrent vascular thrombosis
- Lupus is a chronic disease with exacerbating factors
  - —Infection
  - —Sun exposure
  - —Trauma
  - —Medications
  - —Stress
  - —Diet
  - —Pregnancy
- Drug-induced lupus
  - —Chlorpromazine
  - —Methyldopa
  - —Procainamide
  - —Hydralazine
  - —Isoniazid

Pre-Hospital

CAUTIONS

- Do not mistakenly categorize these patients as purely psychiatric or nonemergent

Diagnosis

ESSENTIAL WORKUP

- History and physical examination
- Four of the eleven criteria from the following list are needed to make the diagnosis
  - —Malar rash
  - —Discoid rash
  - —Photosensitivity rash
  - —Oral ulcers
  - —Arthritis
  - —Serositis
  - —Neurologic disorders
  - —Hematologic disorders
  - —Immunologic disorders
  - —Renal disorders
  - —Antinuclear antibodies

Major Flare-Ups

- CBC
- Electrolytes, BUN, creatinine, glucose
- Urinalysis
- Erythrocyte sedimentation rate (ESR)
- Chest x-ray, EKG, and pulse oximetry for cardiorespiratory symptoms

LABORATORY

- CBC
  - —Leukopenia, thrombocytopenia, and hemolytic anemia
  - —Degree of hematologic disorders suggests degree of disease activity
- ESR
  - —May be elevated during acute exacerbations, but this test tends to remain high months after a flare-up has ceased
- Partial thromboplastin time (PTT)
  - —May be elevated owing to lupus anticoagulant
- Urinalysis
  - —Protein
  - —Casts
  - —Hematuria
  - —WBCs
- Amylase is elevated in mesenteric ischemia and pancreatitis
- Send antinuclear antibody (ANA) or fluorescent antinuclear antibody (FANA), RF, ASO titer if diagnosis unclear
- Anti-Sm and Anti-dsDNA are diagnostic,
- A false-positive VDRL is supportive of the diagnosis
- Joint aspirate typically shows fluid with fewer than 3,000 WBCs

IMAGING/SPECIAL TESTS

- Chest x-ray
  - —Pneumonitis
  - —Pneumonias
  - —Pleural effusion
  - —Cardiomegaly
- EKG
- Echocardiogram

DIFFERENTIAL DIAGNOSIS

- Hypotension may be due to shock secondary to a major flare-up or secondary to acute steroid withdrawal in the known lupus patient
- Other autoimmune diseases
  - —Rheumatic fever
  - —Rheumatoid arthritis
  - —Dermatomyositis
  - —Overlap syndromes
- Skin changes
  - —Urticaria
  - —Erythema multiforme
- Idiopathic thrombocytopenic purpura (ITP)
- Multiple sclerosis
- Epilepsy

Treatment

INITIAL STABILIZATION

- ABCs

ED TREATMENT

- Mainstays include NSAIDs, antimalarials, corticosteroids, and immunosuppressive drugs
- Special attention must be given to CNS and renal involvement as well as infections; these are the main determinants of morbidity and mortality
  - —Atherosclerosis is a leading cause of death in the older lupus patients
- *Mild flare-ups:* arthralgias, myalgias, and fatigue, rash
  - —NSAIDs, ASA, topical steroids for rash, sunscreen
  - —If not sufficient, begin low-dose prednisone
- *Major flare-ups:* life- or organ-threatening
  - —Methylprednisolone
  - —Anticoagulation for thrombosis; give blood products early if needed
  - —Psychotropics for neuropsychiatric symptoms
  - —Anticonvulsants for seizures
  - —If poor response, consult rheumatology before starting cytotoxic medications such as azathioprine or cyclophosphamide
- *Chronically*
  - —Prednisone taper
  - —NSAIDs
  - —Antimalarials: a rheumatologist should initiate quinacrine, chloroquine
  - —Methotrexate, hormonal therapy, thalidomide, and monoclonal antibodies are under investigation

MEDICATIONS

- Adult dosages (for pediatric medications consult rheumatologist)
  - —Methylprednisolone: 15 mg/kg/d i.v. up to 1 g
  - —Prednisone: <0.5 mg/kg/d PO for minor flare
- Pediatric dosages
  - —Ibuprofen: 5–10 mg/kg/dose divided q6h
  - —Prednisone: 0.5 mg/kg/d divided q.d. or b.i.d.

Disposition

ADMISSION CRITERIA

- Patients who have end-organ disease such as renal or CNS involvement, pericarditis, pancreatitis, or gastrointestinal symptoms
- Those with severe end-organ or life-threatening manifestations should be admitted to the ICU
- Patients with lupus should be treated as immunocompromised and suspected or diagnosed infections should be treated aggressively

DISCHARGE CRITERIA

- Patients may be discharged home with mild flare-ups if afebrile, well hydrated, and not ill-appearing
- ESR should not be used as a disposition criteria as it may be elevated long after a flare-up has subsided
- Lupus is a chronic disease and patients must be followed adequately by a rheumatologist or a capable primary care physician

Miscellaneous

ICD9: 710.0

ICD10: M32.9

SUGGESTED READINGS

Boumpas DT, Austin HA 3rd. Systemic lupus erythematosus: emerging concepts. Part 1: Renal, neuropsychiatric, cardiovascular, pulmonary, and hematologic disease. Ann Intern Med 1995;122(12):940–950.

Boumpas DT, Fessler BJ. Systemic lupus erythematosus: emerging concepts. Part 2. Dermatologic and joint disease, the antiphospholipid antibody syndrome, pregnancy and hormonal therapy, morbidity and mortality, and pathogenesis. Ann Intern Med 1995;123(1):42–53.

Gladman DD, Urowitz MB. Systemic lupus erythematosus. B. Clinical and laboratory features. In: Klippel JH, ed. Primer on the rheumatic diseases, 11th ed. Atlanta: Arthritis Foundation, 1997:251–257.

Hahn BH. Management of systemic lupus erythematosus. In: Kelley WN, et al., eds. Textbook of rheumatology, 5th ed. Philadelphia: WB Saunders, 1997: 1040–1056.

Lahita RG. Clinical presentation of systemic lupus erythematosus. In: Kelley WN, et al., eds. Textbook of rheumatology, 5th ed. Philadelphia: WB Saunders, 1997: 1028–1039.

Ruiz-Irastorza G, Khamashta MA. Systemic lupus erythematosus. Lancet 2001;357: 1027–1032.

Author: Steven Furer

Tachydysrhythmias

Clinical Presentation

SIGNS AND SYMPTOMS

- Asymptomatic
  - —Frequent with supraventricular tachycardia (SVT)
  - —Rare with sustained ventricular tachycardia (VT)
- Palpitations
- Lightheadedness
- Dyspnea
- Diaphoresis
- Dizziness
- Weakness
- Chest discomfort
- Angina
- Syncope
- Prominent neck veins
- VT
  - —Splitting of heart sounds
  - —Gallop rhythm
- Ventricular fibrillation (VF)
  - —Sudden loss of consciousness
  - —Absent pulse, heart rate, and blood pressure
- Signs of instability
  - —Hypotension
  - —Pulmonary edema
  - —Chest pain
  - —Mental status changes

MECHANISM/DESCRIPTION

- Any disturbance of the heart's rhythm resulting in a rate greater than 100 beats/min
- Caused by disorders of impulse formation or conduction
- Reentry is the most common underlying mechanism for tachydysrhythmias
  - —Ventricular dysrhythmias result from a reentrant circuit established as a result of drugs, ischemia, metabolic abnormalities, or scarred or infiltrated myocardial tissue
  - —Supraventricular dysrhythmias usually result from reentrant pathways or AV nodal reentry

Tachycardia

- Narrow complex regular rhythm at a rate of 100–150 beats/min
- Infants and young children can obtain rates of 170–225 beats/min
- Functional response to physiologic stress
- Caused by increased catecholamine tone or decreased vagal stimulation

SUPRAVENTRICULAR TACHYARRHYTHMIA

- Supraventricular tachycardia (SVT)
  - —A narrow complex tachycardia that originates above the His bundle
  - —One of the most frequent cardiac disturbances evaluated in the ED
  - —Most common dysrhythmia seen in young adults and children without underlying heart disease
  - —Wide complex tachycardias can be supraventricular in origin
- Irregular
  - —Atrial fibrillation
  - —Atrial flutter
  - —Multifocal atrial tachycardia
- Regular
  - —Atrial tachycardia
    - -Any rapid dysrhythmia from a nonsinus focus above the AV node
  - —Junctional tachycardia
    - -Regular tachycardia without preceding depolarization waves

Ventricular Tachycardia

- Three or more consecutive ventricular ectopic beats at a rate of 100 beats/min
- Most common initiating rhythm in sudden death in patients with previous myocardial infarction
- Always suspect a ventricular rhythm with a wide complex rhythm, especially in the older patient
- Sustained VT that persists for 30 seconds or more and polymorphic VT require termination because they are usually unstable and degenerate into VF
- Need to distinguish between monomorphic VT and SVT with aberrant conduction

Torsades De Pointes

- Paroxysmal form of VT with undulating axis and prolonged baseline QT interval
- Secondary to either congenital or acquired abnormalities of ventricular repolarization
- Often the result of drug therapy or electrolyte disturbances

Ventricular Fibrillation

- EKG shows oscillations without evidence of discrete QRST morphology
- Accounts for 80–85% of sudden cardiac deaths
- Frequently results from degeneration of sustained VT

ETIOLOGY

- Sinus tachycardia
  - —Acute myocardial infarction
  - —Anemia
  - —Anxiety
  - —Congestive heart failure
  - —Drug intoxication
  - —Hyperthyroidism
  - —Hypovolemia
  - —Hypoxia
  - —Infection
  - —Pain
  - —Pericardial tamponade
  - —Pulmonary embolism
- Atrial tachycardia
  - —Precipitated by a premature atrial or ventricular contraction
  - —Electrolyte disturbances
  - —Drug toxicity
  - —Hypoxia
- Junctional tachycardia
  - —AV nodal reentry
  - —Myocardial ischemia
  - —Structural heart disease
  - —Preexcitation syndromes
  - —Drug and alcohol toxicity
- Irregular narrow complex SVTs
  - —Atrial fibrillation
    - -Hypertension
    - -Coronary artery disease
    - -Hypothyroidism
    - -Heavy alcohol intake
    - -Mitral valve disease
    - -Chronic pulmonary disease
    - -Pulmonary embolus
    - -Wolf-Parkinson-White syndrome
    - -Hypoxia
    - -Digoxin toxicity
    - -Chronic pericarditis
    - -Idiopathic atrial fibrillation
  - —Atrial flutter
    - -Ischemic heart disease
    - -Valvular heart disease
    - -Congestive heart failure
    - -Myocarditis
    - -Cardiomyopathies
    - -Pulmonary embolus
    - -Other pulmonary disease
    - -Electrolyte abnormalities
    - -After cardiac surgery
  - —Multifocal atrial tachycardia
    - -Hypoxic effects of chronic lung disease
    - -Theophylline toxicity
- VT
  - —Dilated cardiomyopathy
  - —Cardiac ischemia
  - —Hypoxia
  - —Cardiac scarring/fibrosis
  - —After cardiac surgery or congenital anomaly repair
  - —Digoxin toxicity
  - —Long QT syndrome
  - —Electrolyte abnormalities
- Torsades de pointes
  - —Drug toxicity (class IA and IC agents)
  - —Hypokalemia
  - —Hypomagnesemia
  - —Congenital QT prolongation
- VF
  - —Acute myocardial infarction (most common)
  - —Chronic ischemic heart disease
  - —Hypoxia
  - —Acidosis
  - —Anaphylaxis
  - —Electrocution
  - —Shock
  - —Hypokalemia
  - —Initiation of quinidine therapy
  - —Massive hemorrhage

Pre-Hospital

- Supplemental oxygen
- Intravenous access
- Monitor

CAUTIONS

- Cardioversion must be carried out in severe hemodynamic instability or evidence of end-organ hypoperfusion with supraventricular or ventricular tachydysrhythmias

CONTROVERSIES

- Vagal maneuvers (beware of carotid disease)
- Adenosine
  —Depends on EMS capabilities and field protocols

Diagnosis

ESSENTIAL WORKUP

- Determination of unstable versus stable patient
- A detailed history
  —Current symptoms
  —Previous episodes
  —Cardiac history
  —Drug use
- 12-lead EKG and rhythm strip to categorize the tachycardia
  —Determine whether the rhythm is regular or irregular
  —Determine whether the complexes are narrow or wide
  —P waves present or absent
  —AV dissociation, sinus capture beats, fusion beats

LABORATORY

- Studies are indicated when underlying metabolic abnormalities or ischemia is considered
  —CBC
  —Electrolytes
  —Cardiac enzymes
  —Thyroid function tests

IMAGING/SPECIAL TESTS

EKG

- Atrial flutter
  —Regular atrial rate usually greater than 300
  —Beat-to-beat uniformity of cycle length, polarity, and amplitude
  —Sawtooth flutter waves directed superiorly and most visible in leads II, III, aVF
  —AV block, usually 2:1, but occasionally greater or irregular
- Multifocal atrial tachycardia
  —Three distinctly different P waves with varying PR intervals
- Atrial tachycardia
  —Rate of 100–200 beats/min
  —P wave precedes QRS and is morphologically different from the sinus P wave
- VT
  —QRS is usually 0.12 seconds and often 0.14 seconds
- Torsades de pointes
  —Ventricular rate greater than 200 beats/min
  —QRS structure displays an undulating axis, with the polarity of the complexes appearing to shift around the baseline
  —Occurrence is often in short episodes of less than 90 seconds
- VF
  —EKG shows oscillations without evidence of discrete QRST morphology
  —Oscillations are usually irregular and occur at a rate of 150–300 beats/min
  -When the amplitude of most oscillations is 1 mm, the term "coarse" is used
  -"Fine" VF is used for oscillations <1 mm

Electrophysiologic Testing

- Diagnostic but not required emergently
- Determines therapy for accessory pathways

DIFFERENTIAL DIAGNOSIS

- See Etiology

Tachydysrhythmias

Treatment

INITIAL STABILIZATION

- Intravenous access (after cardioversion if needed)
- Open airway, oxygen, positive-pressure ventilation (if indicated)
- Monitor/rhythm assessment
- Basic life support in patients with loss of consciousness or sudden death
- Cardioversion/defibrillation as indicated by specific rhythm

ED TREATMENT

- Irregular narrow complex
  —Rate control
  —Beta-blockers or calcium channel blockers
  —Anticoagulation if onset is greater than 24 hours
    -Cardioversion for severe hemodynamic compromise
    -Once rate control has been achieved, the patient must be anticoagulated if onset of dysrhythmia is greater than 24 hours
- Regular narrow complex tachydysrhythmia
  —Vagal maneuvers are often employed initially and occasionally terminate the dysrhythmia
  —Adenosine
    -Rapid onset and short half-life
    -90% effective in terminating SVTs
    -May be diagnostic by slowing the rate and revealing an underlying atrial fibrillation
- Stable wide complex tachycardia
  —Try to determine whether VT or SVT with aberrancy
  —Administration of AV nodal-blocking agents may result in VF
    -Verapamil contraindicated
    -Adenosine may be okay because of ultrashort duration but should be reserved for SVT with aberrancy
  —Electrical cardioversion should be utilized owing to fewer potential complications than antidysrhythmic drugs when mechanism unknown
  —Antidysrhythmic drugs include IV procainamide and IV amiodarone
  —Lidocaine is less effective although sometimes more readily available
  —Bretylium lacks evidence of efficacy
  —In patients with Wolff-Parkinson-White (WPW) syndrome
    -Administration of AV nodal-blocking agents may result in VF
    -DC cardioversion or amiodarone, flecainide, or procainamide
- Polymorphic VT with prolonged QT (torsades de pointes)
  —Correct abnormal electrolytes
  —Magnesium, overdrive pacing, isoproterenol, phenytoin, or lidocaine
- Polymorphic VT with normal baseline QT interval
  —Treat ischemia and correct electrolytes
  —Beta-blockers, lidocaine, amiodarone, or procainamide
  —If cardiac function impaired, amiodarone or lidocaine; then synchronized cardioversion
- Monomorphic VT
  —With preserved cardiac function, procainamide or sotalol; then amiodarone or lidocaine
  —With poor ejection fraction, amiodarone or lidocaine; then synchronized cardioversion
- VT or pulseless VT
  —Defibrillation up to 3 times (200 J, 200–300 J, 360 J)
  —If persistent or recurrent VF/VT then intubate, establish IV, and look for underlying causes
  —Epinephrine: 1 mg i.v. push; repeat every 3–5 minutes, or vasopressin
  —Attempt to defibrillate at 360 J
  —Consider antidysrhythmics: amiodarone, lidocaine, magnesium, or procainamide
  —Continue attempts to defibrillate

MEDICATIONS

- Adenosine: 6 mg rapid i.v. push; if no response after 1–2 min, then 12 mg
- Amiodarone: 15 mg/min over 10 minutes, followed by 1 mg/min over the next 6 hours and then 0.5 mg/min over 18 hours
- Digoxin: load 0.25 mg i.v. q6h to 1 mg
- Epinephrine: 1 mg bolus administration every 3–5 minutes
- Lidocaine: 1–1.5 mg/kg bolus i.v. push, 0.5–0.75 mg/kg every 5–10 minutes, max 3 mg/kg
- Magnesium sulfate: 1–2 g i.v. push
- Procainamide: VF/VT, 100 mg i.v. every 5 minutes; if successful, then 1–4 mg/min infusion; tachycardia, 20–30 mg/min up to 17 mg/kg
- Vasopressin: 40 units i.v. push once
- Verapamil: 2.5–5 mg over 2 minutes, then 5–10 mg every 15–30 minutes

Disposition

ADMISSION CRITERIA

- VT or VF
- Possible cardiac ischemic event
- Persistent SVT
- Other underlying metabolic abnormalities

DISCHARGE CRITERIA

- Terminated supraventricular rhythm without organ hypoperfusion

Miscellaneous

ICD9: 427.0; 427.1; 427.2

ICD10: I41.9, R00.0

SEE ALSO: SUPRAVENTRICULAR TACHYCARDIA; VENTRICULAR TACHYCARDIA

SUGGESTED READINGS

Atkins DL, Dorian P, Gonzalez ER. Treatment of tachyarrhythmias. Ann Emerg Med 2001;37:S91–S109.

Connors S, Dorian P. Management of supraventricular tachycardia in the emergency department. Can J Cardiol 1997;13(Suppl A):19A–24A.

Obel OA, Camm AJ. Supraventricular tachycardia: ECG diagnosis and anatomy. Eur Heart J 1997;18(Suppl C):C2–C11.

Authors: Jamie Collings; Lynn Schrader; James Adams

Temporal Arteritis

Clinical Presentation

SIGNS AND SYMPTOMS

- May present with acute, subacute, or chronic symptoms
- Headache is the single most frequent symptom
  —Often boring or lancinating in quality
  —Often described as unilateral over a temple
- Tongue or jaw claudication upon mastication are common symptoms
- Constitutional symptoms
  —Fatigue
  —Malaise
  —Anorexia
  —Weight loss
  —Weakness
  —Arthralgias
  —Low-grade fever
- Visual findings
  —Develop weeks to months after the onset of other symptoms
  —May fluctuate, but visual impairment does not usually improve over time, even with treatment
  —Diplopia
  —Ptosis
  —Extraocular muscle weakness
  —Scotomata
  —Blurred vision
  —Amaurosis fugax
  —Blindness
- Sore throat, dysphagia, and cough
- Scalp tenderness, especially over the temporal artery
- Pulsations over temporal artery
  —Increased pulsations early in disease
  —Decreased pulsations late in the disease
- Erythema, warmth, swelling, or nodules over scalp arteries
- Bruits or decreased pulses over large arteries
- Rare findings
  —Respiratory symptoms
  —Ischemic chest pain
  —Congestive heart failure
- Neurologic problems
  —Occurs in up to one third of patients
  —Neuropathies
  —Transient ischemic attacks
  —Cerebral vascular accidents
- Occult manifestations include
  —Glossitis
  —Lingual infarction
  —Tongue infarction
  —Raynaud's phenomenon
  —Tumor-like lesions
    -Breast
    -Ovarian
    -Uterine mass
- 40% do not present with the classic features of headache, scalp tenderness, visual changes, or jaw claudication
- Frequently associated with polymyalgia rheumatica (up to 50%)
  —Stiffness
  —Aching pain in the proximal muscles
  —Worse in the morning and decreasing with exercise
- Associated synovitis, especially in the knees, is common

MECHANISM/DESCRIPTION

- Temporal arteritis most commonly causes inflammation of arteries originating from the arch of the aorta
- Other vessels, including veins, are sometimes involved
- Although usually clinically silent, involvement of the thoracic aorta occurs in a significant minority of patients, and aortic aneurysm may result
- Thoracic aortic aneurysm is a late manifestation with an incidence 17 times those without temporal arteritis
- Abdominal aortic aneurysm is about twice as common in those with temporal arteritis
- Pathologic specimens feature patchy mononuclear granulomatous inflammation resulting in a markedly thickened intima and occlusion of the vessel lumen
- Occlusive arteritis may involve thrombosis of the ophthalmic artery resulting in ischemic optic neuritis and visual loss
- Inflammation of arteries supplying the muscles of mastication results in jaw claudication
- Hepatic involvement is seen in about 25% of cases

ETIOLOGY

- Age is the greatest risk factor
  —Rare in patients <50 years old
  —>90% are >60 years old
- Increased prevalence in Northern latitude
- Two to four times more common in women
- Rare in African American patients, common in whites
- Genetic predisposition is linked to HLA-DR4—60% prevalence
- Annual incidence has risen 10% from 1981 to 1998
- There is a strong association with polymyalgia rheumatica

Pre-Hospital

CAUTIONS

- Symptoms may be confused with stroke
- Initiate appropriate monitoring and oxygen
- Patients may be hypotensive from one of the rare sequelae (aortic dissection, abdominal aortic aneurysm, or myocardial infarction)

Diagnosis

- Presence of any three or more of the following in patients with vasculitis
  —Erythrocyte sedimentation rate greater than 50
  —Age greater than 50 years
  —New onset of headache, or change in quality of headache
  —Tenderness or decreased pulsation of temporal artery
  —Abnormal artery biopsy

ESSENTIAL WORKUP

- Focused physical examination with emphasis on
  —Temporal artery and scalp abnormalities
  —Complete neurologic examination
  —Ophthalmic examination including visual acuity and visual field testing
- Funduscopy
  —Often normal initially
  —Iritis and fine vitreous opacities may be early findings
  —Optic nerve edema
  —Hyperemia of the disk
  —Pallor
  —Hemorrhage
  —Scattered cotton-wool spots
  —Vessel engorgement and exudates are seen later
- Any pulse differences in the extremities or bruits over large arteries should be noted

LABORATORY

- Elevated erythrocyte sedimentation rate
- C-reactive protein above 2.45 mg/dL
- A mild normochromic anemia is typical; platelets tend to be elevated, white cell count can be normal or slightly elevated, and differential is usually normal
- Liver function tests and prothrombin time (PT) may be elevated; creatine phosphokinase (CPK), tests of renal function, and urinalysis are generally normal
- Elevation in interleukin-6 (IL-6) is seen during flares

IMAGING/SPECIAL TESTS

- Temporal artery biopsy
  - —Multiple sections should be done in 24–48 hours and no longer than 96 hours after initiation of steroids
  - —Gold standard for diagnosis
- Doppler ultrasound
  - —Decreased blood flow in temporal, facial, and ophthalmic arteries
- Angiogram
  - —Smooth, tapered occlusions or stenosis
- MRI
  - —Indicated for examination of large arteries

DIFFERENTIAL DIAGNOSIS

- Vasculitides
  - —Polyarteritis nodosa
  - —Hypersensitivity vasculitis
  - —Systemic lupus erythematosus (SLE)
  - —Takayasu's arteritis
  - —Wegener's granulomatosis
- Thrombosis of retinal, ophthalmic, or temporal arteries
- Lyme disease

Treatment

INITIAL STABILIZATION

- Although rare, patients may present with vascular catastrophe such as aortic dissection or myocardial infarction and need appropriate aggressive early management

ED TREATMENT

- Steroids
  - —Strong clinical indications if started before temporal artery biopsy
  - —Early treatment significantly reduces the incidence of blindness
  - —Steroids effectively control systemic and local symptoms within days to weeks
  - —Treatment with prednisone may continue for years—usual disease length, 3–4 years
  - —Sustained steroid therapy may accelerate osteopenia, cause cataracts, and potentiate hyperglycemia and hypertension
- Symptomatic pain management with NSAIDs or salicylates
- Referral to rheumatology
- Referral to ophthalmology if associated with visual symptoms

MEDICATIONS

- Ibuprofen: 400 mg PO every 4 hours
- Methylprednisolone (Solu-Medrol): 125 mg i.v.
- Prednisone: 60–100 mg PO per day that is not tapered for several weeks

Disposition

ADMISSION CRITERIA

- Patients with impending vascular complications
- Patients with associated acute visual loss

DISCHARGE CRITERIA

- Less symptomatic patients without evidence of end-organ involvement
- Able to be seen in follow-up within 1–2 days

Miscellaneous

CONTROVERSIES

- Viral and bacterial association has been postulated with parvovirus, human parainfluenza virus, and *Chlamydia pneumoniae*
- It is believed that the infectious agent causes an immunologic response in genetically predisposed individuals
- Methotrexate, in combination with reduced doses of steroids, has had varying results; investigation is ongoing to determine whether methotrexate reduces the total steroid requirement and reduces relapses

ICD9: 446.5

ICD10: M31.6

SUGGESTED READINGS

Hunter GG. Clinical features of GCA/PMR. Clin Exp Rheumatol 2000;18:s6–s8.

Hunter GG. Giant cell arteritis and polymyalgia rheumatica. Med Clin North Am 1997;81(1):195–219.

Levine SM, Hellmann DB. Giant cell arteritis. Curr Opin Rheumatol 2002; 14:3–10.

Meskimen S, Cook TD, Blake RI. Management of giant cell arteritis and polymyalgia rheumatica. Am Fam Physician 2000;61:2061–2067.

Nesher G. Neurologic manifestations of giant cell arteritis. Clin Exp Rheumatol 2000;18:s24–s26.

Author: Andrew Aronson

Temporomandibular Joint Injury/Syndrome

Clinical Presentation

SIGNS AND SYMPTOMS

- Preauricular pain
  - —Constant
  - —Dull and aching
  - —May be referred to the ipsilateral ear, head, or neck
  - —Exacerbated by mandible movement (pathognomonic)
  - —More conspicuous at night and may cause insomnia
  - —Tenderness over the muscles of mastication and temporomandibular joint (TMJ)
- Joint sounds
  - —Popping or clicking sensation with TMJ articulation
  - —A palpable or audible click with opening and closing
- Malalignment and limited range of motion
  - —Dentoskeletal malocclusion or lateral deviation
  - —Open or closed locking of the jaw

MECHANISM/DESCRIPTION

- TMJ dysfunction is poorly understood
  - —Multifactorial: bruxism, trauma, malocclusion
- TMJ pain
  - —Originates from the joint (capsulitis, traumatic arthritis, acute disk displacement) or muscles of mastication (spasm)
- TMJ clicking
  - —Highly correlated with disk displacement
  - —May be normal finding; present as a transient finding in 30–40% of the population
- TMJ motion
  - —Typical range is 42–55 mm (maxillary to mandible incisors)
  - —Limited by adhesions within the joint or disk displacement or trismus from muscle spasm
- TMJ locking
  - —Open locking (dislocation): typically from yawning consequent to joint laxity and easily reduced
  - —Closed locking: results from disk displacement and is difficult to correct

Pre-Hospital

- Provide comfort and reassurance

Diagnosis

ESSENTIAL WORKUP

- Diagnosis based on clinical presentation
- Exclude other causes of headache and facial pain

LABORATORY

- No specific laboratory tests are indicated

IMAGING/SPECIAL TESTS

- Panorex is the screening radiograph of choice
  - —May demonstrate fracture or intraarticular pathology (i.e. tumor, or degenerative joint disease), but usually unremarkable

DIFFERENTIAL DIAGNOSIS

- Acute coronary syndrome
- Carotid artery dissection
- Intracranial hemorrhage (subarachnoid hemorrhage)
- Temporal arteritis
- Trigeminal or glossopharyngeal neuralgia
- Vascular headache
- Intraoral and dental pathology
- Herpes zoster
- Salivary gland disorder, otitis, and sinusitis
- Elongated styloid process pain

Treatment

INITIAL STABILIZATION
N/A

ED TREATMENT
- Acute therapeutic options
  - —Patient reassurance and education—"usually mild and self-limited"
  - —Analgesics and anxiolytics
  - —Urgent reduction of open or closed locking (Montgomery 2000)—may require procedural sedation
  - —Physical therapy—moist heat or ice packs
- Outpatient management
  - —Combination pharmacotherapy
  - —Home physical therapy—moist heat or ice packs and mechanically soft diet
  - —Referral to dentist or oral-maxillofacial surgeon

MEDICATIONS
- Narcotic analgesics
- NSAIDs
- Anxiolytics
- Muscle relaxants
- Sedative-hypnotics

Disposition

ADMISSION CRITERIA
N/A

DISCHARGE CRITERIA
- Treat as outpatients with pain medication, muscle relaxants, and warm compresses

Miscellaneous

ICD9: 524.60

ICD10: K07.6

SUGGESTED READINGS
Gray RJM, Davies SJ. Emergency treatment of acute temporomandibular disorders: part I. Dent Update 1997;24:170–173.

Gray RJM, Davies SJ. Emergency treatment of acute temporomandibular disorders: part II. Dent Update 1997;24:186–189.

Montgomery MT. Extraoral facial pain. Emerg Med Clin North Am 2000;18(3):577–600.

Author: Timothy J. Mader

Tendinitis

Clinical Presentation

SIGNS AND SYMPTOMS

- The classic inflammatory signs include pain, warmth, erythema and swelling
- Pain will resolve quickly after initial movement only to become a throbbing pain after exercise
- Findings may include decreased range of motion, deformity, instability, pain on motion, and tenderness to palpation
- There is a poor distinction between tendinitis and tenosynovitis

MECHANISM/DESCRIPTION

- Defined as inflammation of the tendon only
- *Overuse syndrome:* mechanical overload or repetitive microtrauma to the musculotendinous unit is secondary to intrinsic and extrinsic factors
  —Intrinsic factors: inflexibility, muscle weakness, or imbalance
  —Extrinsic factors: excessive deviation, frequency, or activity
- Chemotactic and vasoactive chemical mediators are released, causing vasodilation and cellular edema and increasing the number and activity of polymorphonuclear (PMN) cells
- If no further injury occurs, the process may last from 48 hours to 2 weeks
- Continuous irritation causes fibrosis, resulting in tendon thickening and stenosing tenosynovitis

Supraspinatus Tendinitis

- Supraspinatus and other rotator cuff tendons anatomically sit between the humerus and acromion, which cause compression
- Overuse of the extremity may lead to microtrauma of the tendon fibers
- Neer's classification:
  —*Stage 1*
    -Age <25 years, involved in sports requiring repetitive overhead motion (e.g., swimmers, pitchers)
    -Edema and hemorrhage within and around the tendon
    -Flexion-abduction motion will elicit pain ("dull aches")
  —*Stage 2*
    -Age 25–40 years
    -Pain is constant and worsens at night
    -Active motion is limited by pain
    -Passive range of motion is preserved
    -Exam shows diffuse pain, fibrosis, and thickening of the tendon
  —*Stage 3*
    -Partial or complete tendon tears
    -Raising the humerus in a forced forward flexion while preserving scapular rotation causes impingement

Calcific Tendinitis

- Age over 40 with unknown etiology
- Any tendon of the rotator cuff can be affected, but there is a predisposition for the supraspinatus
- Most cases are asymptomatic and are found on routine radiographs
- Calcium is deposited within the tendon over time; the calcium undergoes spontaneous resorption, causing pain
- Acute attacks of calcified tendinitis may develop secondary to crystal release from the tendon, often after trauma

Bicipital Tendinitis

- Patients complain of pain to the anterior shoulder, which radiates down the radius
- Patients complain of discomfort when rolling on the shoulder while sleeping or trying to reach a hip pocket or back zipper
- Focal tenderness is between the greater and lesser tuberosities of the humerus
- *Yergason's test:* pain increases when the patient is asked to resist supination of the wrist with the elbow at 90 degrees to the arm against the body
- *Speeds test:* Pain along the bicipital groove, resulting from resisted forward flexion and forearm supination of an extended elbow

Lateral Epicondylitis (Tennis Elbow)

- A rotational repetitive motion causes pain
- Dull ache on the outside of the elbow that increases with grasping and twisting
- Results from inflammation at the insertion of the common extensor tendon onto the lateral epicondyle of the humorous
- Resisted active dorsiflexion of the wrist on extension of the middle finger against resistance can reproduce pain with the elbow extended
- Soft tissue calcification may be seen
- Inflammation and microtrauma at the site of insertion of the flexor carpi-radialis on the medial epicondyle (bowlers, golfers, pitchers)
- Active flexing of the wrist against resistance causes pain

de Quervain's Tendinitis

- Inflammation of the abductor pollicis longus and extensor pollicis brevis
- *Finkelstein's test:* the thumb is held in the palm by the fingers and the wrist is deviated in the direction of the ulna; pain occurs on radial styloid
- Osteoarthritis of the carpal metacarpal joints or gonococcal (GC) tenosynovitis causes the same pain

Trigger Finger

- Proximal portion of the flexor tendon sheath on the palmer surface over the base of the metacarpal head becomes stenosed and catches as the finger is moved
- Symptoms vary from pain to locking in flexion

Achilles Tendinitis

- Overuse injury commonly seen in males
- Trauma or systemic disease causing inflammation
- Tendon sheath becomes inflamed and tendon inflammation follows
- With repeated stress, scar tissue formation and degeneration of the tendon will occur
- Patient will have pain, reduced range of motion, or morning stiffness

Achilles Tendon Rupture

- Seen more commonly in 30- to 40-year-old recreational athletes
- Complaining of a "popping sensation," acute weakness, and inability to continue the activity; usually complain of having the sensation of being kicked
- May initially have a gap by palpation, followed by ecchymosis and a "boggy" sensation
- Inability to plantar-flex the foot reveals complete rupture
- *Thompson's test:* patient lies prone with the feet hanging over the edge of the bed; the physician squeezes the calf muscles and looks for plantar flexion

PEDIATRIC CONSIDERATIONS

- It is rare to have tendinitis when a growth plate is open; concern for epiphyseal fracture
- Apophysitis occurs in children at an ossification center subject to traction
  —Little League elbow: at the medial epicondyle
  —Osgood-Schlatter syndrome: at the tibial tubercle
- *Avascular necrosis* presents with pain and swelling around a joint and can occur in pediatric patients at various locations
  —Well-recognized sites of avascular necrosis are the capitellum of the humerus, the head of the femur, the tarsal navicular, and the metatarsal head
  —The diagnosis is made by plain radiograph

Pre-Hospital

- Immobilize affected part if acute injury
- Ice, elevation

Diagnosis

ESSENTIAL WORKUP

- Accurate physical examination
- Radiographs to evaluate for fracture in acute injury

IMAGING/SPECIAL TESTS

Radiographs

- Extraarticular from articular etiologies
- SECONDS: **s**oft tissue swelling, **e**rosions, **c**alcifications, **o**steoporosis, **n**arrowing, **d**eformity, and **s**eparation

Ultrasound

- Evaluate joint effusions
- More sensitive than MRI
- Limited use in the emergency setting
- Loss of fibular echotexture, focal tendon thickening, diffuse thickening, focal hypoechoic areas, extended hypoechogenecity, irregular and ill-defined borders, microruptures, and peritendinous inflammatory edema

Scintigraphy

- Technetium-99m pertechnetate phosphate (binds with plasma protein) and concentrates in joint space (bursitis)
- Not often performed through ED

MRI

- Can demonstrate change in attenuation of involved structure
- Not often performed through ED

DIFFERENTIAL DIAGNOSIS

- Septic arthritis
- Fracture
- Osteoarthritis

Treatment

INITIAL STABILIZATION

- Immobilize involved structure
- Ice (20-minute intervals), elevation
- Pain relief

ED TREATMENT

- Recommend limited activity initially
- A one-time local steroid injection may be indicated
- NSAIDS are mainstay
- Range-of-motion exercises
- Referral for physical therapy may be beneficial

MEDICATIONS

- Ibuprofen: 400–800 mg PO q68h (peds: 10 mg/kg PO q6h)

Disposition

ADMISSION CRITERIA

- Inpatient care only necessary for acute operative intervention

DISCHARGE CRITERIA

- Most patients can be managed effectively in the outpatient setting
- Referral for orthopedic consultation, physical therapy

Miscellaneous

ICD9: 726.90

ICD10: M77.9

SUGGESTED READINGS

Anderson SJ, et al. Intensive training and sports specialization in young athletes. Pediatrics 2000;106(1):154–157.

Gibbon WW, Wakefield RJ. Ultrasound in inflammatory disease. Radiol Clin North Am 1999;37(4):633–639.

Hoffman J, Blake R. Emergency department evaluation and treatment of the shoulder and humerus. Emerg Med Clin North Am 1999;17(4):859–877.

Micheli LJ, Glassman R, Klein M. The prevention of sports injuries in children. Clin Sports Med 2000;19(4):821–834, ix.

O'Donnell JA, Gelone SP. Fluoroquinolones. Infect Dis Clin North Am 2000;14(2): 489–513, xi.

Rosen P, ed. Emergency medicine concepts and clinical practices, 5th ed. St Louis: Mosby, 2002:1599–1607.

Steele M. Tendonitis. eMedicine Journal 10/23/2001, Vol. 2, Number 10. (Electronic medical journal at: *http://www.imedicine.com*).

Teefey SA, Middleton WD, Yamaguchi K. Shoulder sonography, state of the art. Radiol Clin North Am 1999;37(4):767–785.

Winter TC III, Teefey SA, Middleton WD. Musculoskeletal ultrasound, an update. Radiol Clin North Am 2001;39(3):465–483.

Author: James Killeen

Tendon Laceration

Clinical Presentation

SIGNS AND SYMPTOMS

- Soft tissue damage: swelling, ecchymosis, or hemorrhage
- Pain is the cardinal symptom
  - —Combined with a functional deficit, an abnormal resting position of the extremity, or large joint instability augments the suspicion for tendon injury

MECHANISM/DESCRIPTION

Divided Into External Versus Internal Trauma

- External trauma further subdivided into
  - —Penetrating trauma (gunshot wounds, glass, knives, or foreign bodies)
  - —Blunt trauma (crushing force or avulsion from hyperextension of a joint)
- Internal trauma entrapment/laceration from underlying bony fracture (rare)

ETIOLOGY

- Open tendon injuries grossly categorized into upper versus lower extremity
- Upper extremity injuries frequently related to the workplace, home, an assault, or attempted suicide
- Lower extremity injuries most often allied with work or motor vehicle crash (MVC)

PEDIATRIC CONSIDERATIONS

- Same characteristics as adults
- The healing process is usually quicker and often associated with complete return to preinjury function as compared with adults

Pre-Hospital

- Do not remove foreign bodies in the field
- Immobilize and transport
- Contact medical control before any attempted reduction
  - —Assess distal neurovascular status for compromise

Diagnosis

ESSENTIAL WORKUP

- A careful history, thorough clinical examination
- History should include mechanism, time of injury, hand position during injury, hand dominance, drug allergies, medication, past medical history, and tetanus status
- Physical exam should follow the orthopedic scheme of "look, feel, move"
- Perform neurovascular exam before anaesthetizing
- Further explore tendons and wounds after anesthesia (1% lidocaine or 0.5% bupivacaine) in a bloodless, well-lit field
- Tendons near lacerations must be explored through complete range of motion to best elucidate tendon injuries distal or proximal to a skin wound
- Examine each digit separately
- Knowledge of the zones of flexor and extensor tendon injuries (Verdan's classification) is helpful in relaying information to the hand specialist
- Flexor digitorum profundus (FDP) injuries present with inability to flex the distal interphalangeal (DIP) joint; exam involves holding proximal interphalangeal (PIP) joint of effected digit in full extension, while the patient attempts to flex DIP
- Flexor digitorum superficialis (FDS) injuries present with inability to flex the PIP joint of a digit
  - —Usually established via the "standard superficialis tendon test," that is, holding the uninjured digits in full extension while the patient attempts to flex the affected finger at the PIP joint
  - —If the profundus is functioning properly, injury of the FDS can be masked
  - —The *DIP extension test* may make this diagnosis more apparent; the patient is asked to make a precision pinch between the thumb and the injured finger and then asked to flex the PIP joint so that the DIP is hyperextended (confirms the integrity of the FDS)
  - —Forearm and wrist flexors: inability to flex ulnar or radial side of wrist or to flex the wrist while opposing the thumb to the little finger
- Extensor tendon injury found by weakness or lack of extension of the distal phalanx against resistant indicates partial or complete disruption of tendon
  - —Best determined with patient placing palm on flat surface and asking the patient to attempt to extend the fingers individually
  - —Palpate each tendon
  - —Loss of normal tension is indicative of injury

LABORATORY

- Wounds more than 12 hours after injury or with signs of infection should be cultured

IMAGING/SPECIAL TESTS

- X-rays needed when radiopaque foreign bodies or fractures are suspected
- High-frequency ultrasound is a valuable tool in the identification of intact versus complete tendon lacerations while partial tendon lacerations may prove difficult to image
- Ultrasound guidance in foreign body location may be helpful

DIFFERENTIAL DIAGNOSIS

- Partial lacerations are common but more difficult to diagnosis than complete disruptions since they may demonstrate intact function
- Alterations of the normal resting hand position may indicate partial laceration
- Lacerations over the metacarpophalangeal (MP) joint should be considered the result of a human bite until proved otherwise
  - —Look for associated extensor tendon injury while MP joint flexed
- Lacerations over the PIP joint may involve the lateral bands or the central slip of the extensor mechanism (boutonniere deformity results from improper repair)
- Avulsion of the FDP distally may be present with or without an associated avulsion fracture
  - —Suspect when a grasping finger is hit by a speeding object ("jammed" finger)
- Disruption of the extensor tendon distal to the central slip results in a mallet finger deformity

Treatment

INITIAL STABILIZATION

- Evaluate extremity and control hemorrhage with direct pressure
- Remove all jewelry or constricting bands

ED TREATMENT

- Tetanus toxoid as needed
- Broad-spectrum antibiotic, such as a first-generation cephalosporin, e.g., cefazolin
- Copious irrigation with 1 L NS or an NS/povidone-iodine (Betadine) solution mixed 50:1
- Remove all foreign bodies and debride avascular tissue
- Partial tendon lacerations that involve more than 20% of the cross-sectional area of the tendon must be repaired
- *All* suspected flexor tendon lacerations require consultation and repair by a hand surgeon, ideally within 12 hours
- If a surgeon is not promptly available, after irrigation the skin can be closed without repair of tendon, injured hand immobilized with a bulky volar dressing and splint with the wrist in 20–30 degrees of flexion, the metacarpal (MC) joint in 60–70 degrees of flexion, and the interphalangeal (IP) joints in 10–15 degrees of flexion
- Simple extensor tendon lacerations may be repaired in the ED
  - —Use a 4-0 or 5-0 nonabsorbable suture in a figure-of-eight or a modified Kessler stitch
- Tendon lacerations over the PIP joint may result in a boutonniere deformity and should be referred to a hand surgeon
- Tendon lacerations of the wrist and distal forearm require repair by a hand surgeon owing to retraction of the proximal end
- The superficial nature of multiple tendons, nerves, and vessels on the volar aspect of the wrist renders them easily vulnerable to penetrating trauma
  - —The "spaghetti wrist" or "full house" describes a volar wrist laceration with at least 10 structures involved (requires prompt hand surgeon consultation)
- Tendon lacerations associated with fractures require referral for operative repair
- Tendon lacerations associated with human bites must be copiously irrigated, with patient placed on broad-spectrum antibiotics and hand immobilized and elevated

MEDICATIONS

- Cefazolin: 1 g i.v. piggyback (peds: 100 mg/kg/d i.m. or i.v. divided q6h, followed by 40 mg/kg/d PO q.i.d. for 5–7 days)
- Tetanus toxoid: 0.5 mL i.m. (peds: <7 years old: DPT preferred; ≥ 7 years old: TD if immunization series not completed), TIG, as required, 250 IU i.m.

Disposition

ADMISSION CRITERIA

- Infected tendon lacerations must be admitted for operative débridement
- Any extensor tendon injury secondary to human bite must be admitted for operative débridement and IV antibiotics
- Any significant flexor tendon laceration must be admitted for timely operative repair or transferred to the nearest hand surgeon

DISCHARGE CRITERIA

- Any patient with an extensor tendon laceration that is not infected, nor associated with other significant injury or underlying fracture, that was repaired by the ED physician and that is properly splinted, may be discharged with timely surgical follow-up
- Any patient with an extensor tendon laceration requiring surgeon referral for repair (wrist, forearm, PIP joint) and that has been properly treated, and splinted, with the patient placed on antibiotics, may be discharged for timely surgical follow-up

Miscellaneous

ICD9: 848.9

ICD10: T14.6

SUGGESTED READINGS

Dogan T, Celebiler O, Gurunluoglu R, et al. A new test for superficialis flexor tendon function. Ann Plast Surg 2000;45(1):93–96.

Hudson DA, de Jager LT. The spaghetti wrist: simultaneous laceration of the median and ulnar nerves with flexor tendons at the wrist. J Hand Surg (Brit) 1993;18B:171–173.

Jozsa LG, Kannus P. Human tendons: anatomy, physiology and pathology. Champaign: Human Kinetics, 1997.

Lee DH, Robbin ML, Galliott R, et al. Ultrasound evaluation of flexor tendon lacerations. J Hand Surg (Am) 2000;25A:236–241.

Perron AD, Brady WJ, Keats TE, et al. Orthopedic pitfalls in the emergency department: closed tendon injuries of the hand. Am J Emerg Med 2001;19(1):76–80.

Stahl S, Kaufman T, Bialik V. Partial lacerations of flexor tendons in children: primary repair versus conservative treatment. J Hand Surg (Brit) 1997;22B:377–380.

Authors: Elisa Aumont; Verena Valley

Tenosynovitis

Clinical Presentation

SIGNS AND SYMPTOMS

- Cardinal signs of Kanavel include:
  - —Tenderness and symmetric swelling along flexor tendon sheath (sausage digit)
  - —Flexed posture of the digit
  - —Severe pain with passive extension of the finger

Hand

- *de Quervain's tenosynovitis*
  - —Repetitive motion (i.e., assembly line workers, carpentry, or weeding)
  - —Pain in the radial aspect of the wrist becomes worse with activity and better with rest
  - —Pain on palpation along the radial aspect of the wrist
  - —Pain with passive range of motion of the thumb
  - —*Finkelstein's test* is where pain occurs with ulnar deviation of the wrist with the thumb cupped in a closed fist
- *Volar flexor tenosynovitis* (trigger finger)
  - —Most commonly affects the thumb or ring finger
  - —Most common in middle-aged women
  - —Locking of the involved finger in flexion is followed by sudden release
  - —Tenderness at proximal end of the tendon sheath in the distal palm
  - —Crepitation and catching of the tendon when the finger is flexed
- *Gonococcal tenosynovitis*
  - —Vaginal or penile discharge often absent, but fever, chills, malaise, or polyarthralgia are common
  - —Erythema, tenderness to palpation, and painful range of motion of the involved tendon
  - —Fever is common
  - —Dermatitis with hemorrhagic macules or papules on the distal extremities or trunk

Ankle

- *Stenosing tenosynovitis*
  - —Inferior retinaculum of the peroneus tendon with thickening of the sheath on exam
  - —Motion increases the pain
- *Rheumatoid tenosynovitis*
  - —Posterior tibial and flexor hallucis longus and peronei tendons commonly involved
  - —Anteriorly the anterior tibial tendon is involved
  - —Motion increases the pain
  - —Spontaneous rupture may occur
- *Achilles tenosynovitis* (excessive use of the calf muscle)
  - —Commonly seen in ballet dancers and long-distance runners
  - —Swelling, tenderness, and fine crepitus on motion of the foot
  - —Patients will usually hold the foot in equinus for comfort
  - —Passive dorsiflexion will elicit pain

MECHANISM/DESCRIPTION

Definition

- Inflammation of the tendon and tendon sheath, which is caused by inflammation, overuse or infection

ETIOLOGY

- *de Quervain's tenosynovitis* is caused by overuse
- *Volar flexor tenosynovitis* has an unknown etiology
- *GC tenosynovitis: Neisseria gonorrhoeae*
- *Nongonococcal infectious tenosynovitis*
  - —*Staphylococcus aureus* and *Streptococcus* species are the most common agents in penetrating injuries
  - —*Pasteurella multocida* in cat bites
  - —*Eikenella corrodens* in human bites
  - —*Pseudomonas* species are seen in patients with diabetes or marine-associated injuries
  - —*Mycobacterium* species in immunocompromised patients
- Infection can be introduced directly into the tendon sheaths through a skin wound or via hematogenous spread
- Flexor tenosynovitis (FTS) is caused by inflammation and distention of the synovial sheaths
- Penetrating injury especially at the proximal and distal flexion creases of the finger (most superficial site) is the most common mechanism
- High-pressure "injection" injury to the hands or fingers from air tools, paint sprayers, or hydraulic equipment may appear minor on the surface but are associated with a high incidence of FTS

Pre-Hospital

- Elevation and immobilization of the affected extremity should be performed in the pre-hospital setting

Diagnosis

ESSENTIAL WORKUP

- Careful history and physical should include mechanism (puncture wound, high pressure, or environmental exposure) and onset and progression of symptoms
- High-pressure injection injuries mandate emergent evaluation by a hand surgeon
- Assess tetanus status and comorbid factors

LABORATORY

- CBC, erythrocyte sedimentation rate (ESR) for infectious etiology
- GC cultures (urethra, cervix, rectum, or pharynx) may be useful, and liver function tests (LFTs) may be elevated with disseminated *Neisseria gonorrhoeae* infection

IMAGING/SPECIAL TESTS

- Radiographs are low yield, except if soft tissue foreign body is suspected
- MRI has proved accurate in the diagnosis of tenosynovitis, but it is expensive and generally unnecessary

DIFFERENTIAL DIAGNOSIS

- Ankle, soft tissue injuries
- Bursitis
- Carpal tunnel syndrome
- Cellulitis
- Compartment syndrome
- Endocarditis
- Felon
- Gonorrhea
- Gout and pseudogout
- Hand infections
- High-pressure hand injuries
- Soft tissue hand injuries
- Soft tissue knee injuries
- Reiter's syndrome
- Rheumatic fever
- Rheumatoid arthritis

Treatment

INITIAL STABILIZATION

- ABCs (septic patient)
- Elevation and immobilization of the affected extremity
- IV access
- Tetanus status

PROCEDURE

- Arthrocentesis is indicated if joint effusion is present
  - —Cultures are negative in 50% of patients
  - —Most GC arthritis is monoarticular; 25% of cases are polyarticular
  - —Joint fluid glucose is normal
  - —White blood cell (WBC) counts usually are less than 50,000, and a Gram stain is positive in 25% of patients

ED TREATMENT

Hand

- *de Quervain's tenosynovitis*
  - —Rest, NSAIDs, and thumb spica splint
  - —Lidocaine/corticosteroid injection if condition is unresponsive to conservative therapy
- *Volar flexor tenosynovitis*
  - —Peritendon lidocaine/corticosteroid injection is the treatment of choice
  - —May need surgical tendon release
- *GC tenosynovitis*
  - —Admit for IV antibiotic therapy
  - —Penicillin or first-generation cephalosporin for initial therapy
  - —Second-generation cephalosporin as alternative
  - —Surgical drainage may be indicated
  - —Pain management
- *Nongonococcal infectious tenosynovitis*
  - —If diagnosis is equivocal, the patient should be admitted for IV antibiotic therapy and consultation with a surgical specialist
  - —Cover for *Staphylococcus, Streptococcus* species as well as anaerobic bacterial infection
  - —Coverage for *Pseudomonas* species for the diabetic or immunocompromised patient
  - —Pain management

Forearm

- *Traumatic tenosynovitis*
  - —Rest, ice, elevation, immobilization
  - —NSAIDs

Ankle

- *Stenosing tenosynovitis*
  - —Rest, ice, elevation, immobilization
  - —NSAIDs
- *Rheumatoid tenosynovitis*
  - —Rest, ice, elevation, immobilization
  - —NSAIDs
- *Achilles tenosynovitis*
  - —Decrease activity
  - —Heel pad
  - —Stretching exercises of the Achilles complex
  - —Ice after exercise and NSAIDs
  - —For persistent pain, a short leg walking cast may be used for 10 days
  - —Surgical intervention may be required to release the thickened tenosynovium for comfort

MEDICATION

- Cefazolin: 1–2 g i.v. q8h (peds: 50–100 mg/kg/d i.v. divided q8h)
- Cefotetan: 1–2 g i.v. q12h (peds: 50–100 mg/kg/d i.v. divided q12h)
- Cefoxitin: 1–2 g i.v. q8h (peds: 80–160 mg/kg/d i.v. divided q6–8h)
- Ceftriaxone: 1–2 g i.v. q12h (peds: 50–100 mg/kg/d i.v. divided q12h)
- Clindamycin: 600–900 mg i.v. q8h (peds: 20–40 mg/kg/d divided q8h)
- Penicillin G: 12–24 million IU i.v. divided q4–6h (peds: 100,000–400,000 IU/kg/d IV divided q4–6h)
- Piperacillin (Zosyn): 3.375 g i.v. q6h (peds: safety not established)
- Ticarcillin (Timentin): 3.1 g i.v. q6h (peds: safety not established)
- Tobramycin: 1 mg/kg i.v. q8h *or* 5 mg/kg i.v. q24h (peds: 2–2.5 mg/kg i.v. q8h)

Disposition

ADMISSION CRITERIA

- Patients with flexor tenosynovitis require immediate consultation with a hand specialist and admission
- Surgical débridement is indicated if the patient is not markedly improved within the first 24 hours, or physical findings are not resolved within 48 hours
- The hand surgeon may attempt continuous catheter irrigation of the tendon sheath instead of surgical drainage

DISCHARGE CRITERIA

- Patients may be discharged only after an evaluation from a surgical specialist
- Inflammatory forms of tenosynovitis

Miscellaneous

ICD9: 727.00

ICD10: M65.9

SUGGESTED READINGS

Hausman MR, Lisser SP. Hand infections. Orthop Clin North Am 1992;23(1):171–185.

Rosen P, ed. Emergency medicine concepts and clinical practices, 5th ed. St. Louis: Mosby, 2002:1599–1607.

Siegel DB, Gelberman RH. Infections of the hand. Orthop Clin North Am 1988;19(4): 779–789.

Simon RR, Koenigsknecht SJ, eds. Emergency orthopedics: the extremities, 3rd ed. Upper Saddle River, NJ: McGraw-Hill/Appleton & Lange, 1995.

Steele M. Tenosynovitis. eMedicine Journal 9/17/2001, Vol. 2, Number 9. (electronic medical journal at: *http://www.imedicine.com*).

Author: James Killeen

Testicular Torsion

Clinical Presentation

SIGNS AND SYMPTOMS

- Sudden onset of unilateral testicular pain and tenderness followed by scrotal swelling and erythema
- Less commonly, torsion may present with pain in the inguinal or lower abdominal area
- Up to 40% of patients may describe previous (more than 2 weeks prior) similar episodes of testicular pain that remitted spontaneously, representing spontaneous torsion and detorsion
- The affected testicle may lie transversely as opposed to the normal vertical lie
- Nausea and vomiting occur in 50% of cases, and low-grade fever occurs in 25%
- There is a bimodal distribution with peak incidences in infancy and adolescence
  - —85% of cases of testicular torsion occur between the ages of 12 and 18 years, with a mean of 13 years
  - —Torsion is rare after age 30 years but still possible
- Symptoms of urinary infection (dysuria, frequency, and urgency) are absent
- In distinguishing torsion from epididymitis, localization of tenderness is helpful early in the course; however, once significant scrotal swelling occurs, the anatomy becomes indistinct, and some form of testicular flow study or surgical exploration is required
- The cremasteric reflex is frequently absent with testicular torsion
- The classic Prehn's sign, which consists of relief of pain on elevation of the testicle in epididymitis and worsening or no change in the pain with torsion, is considered unreliable

ETIOLOGY

- Most patients have a congenital abnormality of the genitalia, with a high insertion of the tunica vaginalis on the spermatic cord and a redundant mesorchium that permit increased mobility and twisting of the testicle on its vascular pedicle
- The anatomic abnormality is generally bilateral, so that both testicles are susceptible to torsion

MECHANISM/DESCRIPTION

- Rotation generally occurs medially and ranges from incomplete (90–180 degrees) to complete (540–720 degrees) torsion
- Depending on the degree of torsion, vascular occlusion occurs, and the result is infarction of the testicle after more than 6 hours of warm ischemia
  - —Testicular salvage is 100% with less than 6 hours ischemia, 70% at 6 to 12 hours, and less than 20% after 12 hours; nevertheless it is still worthwhile to attempt to salvage the torsed testicle up to 24 hours after the onset of torsion
- Testicular infarction leads to atrophy and may ultimately decrease fertility

PEDIATRIC CONSIDERATIONS

- Testicular torsion has been described in utero and in virtually every pediatric age group
- The peak incidence occurs in late childhood and adolescence, with a smaller peak in infancy

Pre-Hospital

CAUTIONS

- There is no definitive treatment that can be rendered in the field; however, pre-hospital personnel need to recognize the urgency of acute testicular pain in young patients
- These patients should be transported to the ED immediately because the outcome is time dependent

Diagnosis

ESSENTIAL WORKUP

- The presentation of an "acute scrotum" in a child or adolescent requires rapid assessment and immediate consultation with a urologist
- These patients require noninvasive flow studies or surgical exploration to confirm torsion
- 25–30% of these patients ultimately prove to have testicular torsion

LABORATORY

- Urinalysis is usually normal, but up to 20% of cases of torsion have pyuria
- Elevated WBC count with a left shift is present in 50% of cases
- There are no laboratory tests specific for testicular torsion

IMAGING/SPECIAL TESTS

- The criterion standard imaging modality has traditionally been technetium-99m pertechnetate radionuclide scans, which show decreased flow in the torsed testicle compared with the unaffected side
  - —Epididymitis will reveal increased flow due to inflammation
  - —This technique has overall sensitivity and specificity rates of 98% and 100%, respectively
- Because of the frequent time delays in obtaining nuclear scans, use of Doppler ultrasound to assess testicular blood flow has increasingly replaced nuclear scanning as a less invasive, more readily available test with comparable accuracy
  - —Several modalities are available, including color-flow Doppler, power Doppler, and pulsed Doppler with mechanical sector scanning, although none of these modalities has demonstrated superiority
  - —Color-flow Doppler is the most commonly available
  - —Use of Doppler contrast material may soon become available and should enhance the accuracy of this modality
  - —Overall sensitivity and specificity rates for color-flow Doppler are 86–100% and 97–100%, respectively, although the accuracy tends to be lower in infants
- There are limitations of all flow studies in that they reflect only the current state of perfusion; consequently, a spontaneously detorsed testicle may show normal or even increased flow and yet still be at high risk for recurrent torsion

DIFFERENTIAL DIAGNOSIS

- Epididymitis/orchitis
- Torsion of the appendix testis
- Testicular trauma or rupture of the testicle
- Incarcerated inguinal hernia
- Testicular tumor
- Acute hydrocele
- Henoch-Schönlein purpura
- Other intraabdominal conditions (appendicitis, pancreatitis, renal colic may rarely present with testicular pain)

PEDIATRIC CONSIDERATIONS

- All imaging techniques designed to evaluate testicular blood flow have technical limitations when applied to infants because the testicular vessels are very small and the amount of blood flow to the testicle under normal conditions is minimal
- Scrotal exploration may be required

Treatment

INITIAL STABILIZATION

- Intravenous fluid, analgesics as appropriate

ED TREATMENT

- Establish the diagnosis and mobilize appropriate urologic care
  —Applying an ice pack to the scrotum relieves pain and can prolong the viability of the ischemic testicle
- In situations in which definitive care is likely to be delayed beyond 4-5 hours from the onset of torsion, manual detorsion may be attempted
  —This is accomplished by externally rotating the affected testicle (opposite the usual medial direction of torsion) until pain is relieved or normal anatomy is restored; all patients who undergo manual detorsion must be surgically explored

Disposition

ADMISSION CRITERIA

- Any patient with confirmed testicular torsion (based on unequivocal clinical findings or positive flow studies) must be admitted for scrotal exploration and bilateral orchiopexy
- Flow studies that are inconclusive and technical failures mandate further investigation by surgical exploration of the scrotum
- Admission for urgent surgical exploration of an acute scrotum is mandatory if there is any potential delay in obtaining a flow study
  —Patients in whom apparent spontaneous detorsion has occurred should undergo semiurgent exploration for bilateral orchiopexy

DISCHARGE CRITERIA

- Patients with negative scrotal exploration and those with normal flow studies can be discharged with appropriate urologic follow-up
- Appropriate parameters for return to ED must be discussed because of the possibility of intermittent torsion
- Patients with an obvious diagnosis other than testicular torsion (e.g., a nonincarcerated inguinal hernia) can be referred for elective care

Miscellaneous

ICD9: 608.2

CORE CONTENT CODE: 19.2.2.4, 13.13.3.1

ICD10: N44

SUGGESTED READINGS

Al Mufti RA, Ogedegbe AK, Laferty K. The use of Doppler ultrasound in the clinical management of acute testicular pain. Br J Urol 1995;76:625–627.

Burgher SW. Acute scrotal pain. Emerg Med Clin North Am 1998;16:781–809.

Coley BD, Frush DP, Babcock DS, et al. Acute testicular torsion: comparison of unenhanced and contrast enhanced power Doppler US, color Doppler US, and radionuclide imaging. Radiology 1996;199:441–446.

Rabinowitz R, Hulbert WC Jr. Acute scrotal swelling. Urol Clin North Am 1995;22: 101–105.

Sidhu PS. Clinical and imaging features of testicular torsion: role of ultrasound. Clin Radiol 1999;54:343–352.

Author: Edward Newton

Tetanus

Clinical Presentation

SIGNS AND SYMPTOMS

Local

- Persistent rigidity of the muscles in proximity to a wound
  - —May be mild
  - —May persist for months and resolve
  - —May evolve to generalized form (13%)

Generalized

Initial Presentation

- Trismus (initial)
- Irritability
- Restlessness
- Diaphoresis
- Dysphagia

Later Manifestations

- Muscle group rigidity
  - —Sudden burst of tonic contractions of muscle groups causing
    - -Opisthotonos
    - -Flexion and adduction of the arms
    - -Clenching of fists
    - -Extension of the lower extremities
  - —Diaphragmatic spasm or paralysis
    - -May compromise respiration
- Hypersympathetic state
  - —Begins in the second week
  - —Prominent cause of mortality
  - —Dysrhythmias
  - —Blood pressure changes
  - —Diaphoresis
  - —Hyperthermia
  - —Rhabdomyolysis
  - —Laryngeal spasm

Cephalic

- Uncommon variant (6%)
- Follows head injury or otitis media
- Spasm of lower cranial and facial muscles
  - —Cranial nerve palsies, CN VII most common
- May progress to generalized tetanus

Neonatal

- Irritability
- Poor suck
- Facial grimacing
- Muscle spasms with touch
- A form of generalized tetanus resulting from traditional practices of putting dirt or dirty rags on umbilical stump
- Very high mortality rate (50–100%)
- Incubation period 1–2 weeks

MECHANISM/DESCRIPTION

- Rare disease in the United States
- Incubation period
  - —Inoculation to the appearance of the first symptoms
    - -48 hours to 3 or more weeks
    - -<7 days—poor prognosis
  - —Period of onset
    - -Poor prognosis if <48 hours from first symptom to first reflex spasm
- Neonatal tetanus
  - —Due to infected umbilical stump
  - —Symptom onset in second week of life when maternal antibodies decrease
- Admission signs associated with poor prognosis
  - —Fever
  - —Tachycardia
- Mortality in the United States: 7.5% if <60 years, 18% if >60 years, 0% if completely immunized

ETIOLOGY

- *Clostridium tetani*
  - —Slender, motile, anaerobic gram-positive rod with a terminal spherical spore
- Spore characteristics
  - —Resistant to oxygen, moisture, temperature extremes
  - —Can survive indefinitely
  - —Ubiquitous in soil and feces
- When inoculated into a wound or devitalized tissue or injected IV as a contaminant of street drugs, the spores germinate, and if the oxygen tension is low, they proliferate and produce toxins
- Toxins
  - —Tetanolysin
    - -Damages tissue
    - -Reduces oxidation-reduction potential
    - -Allows greater logarithmic growth of organisms
  - —Tetanospasmin
    - -Responsible for the clinical manifestations
    - -Released by manipulation of wound

Pre-Hospital

CAUTIONS

- Careful airway management required
  - —Endotracheal intubation complicated by
    - -Trismus
    - -Vocal cord paralysis
    - -Facial/neck muscle rigidity
- Excessive stimulation may provoke tetany of musculature

Diagnosis

ESSENTIAL WORKUP

- Clinical diagnosis
  - —Suspected in all cases of trismus
  - —No wound recalled in one fifth of cases
  - —Full tetanus immunization almost eliminates diagnosis

LABORATORY

- CBC
- Electrolytes, BUN, creatinine, glucose
  - —For hypocalcemia
- Strychnine level
- Arterial blood gas (ABG), pulse oximetry
  - —For oxygenation status
- Wound culture for *C. tetani*
  - —Positive in one third
- *C. tetani* titers
  - —Will only be useful after the fact

IMAGING/SPECIAL TESTS

- CSF analysis
  - —Normal with tetanus
  - —For meningitis
- CT brain for altered mental status
  - —Normal

DIFFERENTIAL DIAGNOSIS

- Strychnine poisoning
- Dystonic reaction to dopamine blockade
- Meningitis
- Rabies
- Encephalitis
- Peritonitis
- Alveolar abscess
- Tetany/hyperventilation syndrome
- Hysteria
- Dislocated mandible/temporomandibular joint (TMJ) syndrome
- Bell's palsy (cephalic form, before trismus)

Treatment

INITIAL STABILIZATION

- ABCs
  - —Prophylactic intubation
  - —Require neuromuscular blockade due to trismus
  - —Establish IV 0.9% NS
  - —Monitor BP and cardiac rhythm (autonomic instability)

ED TREATMENT

- Administer benztropine or diphenhydramine to rule out dystonic reaction
- Human tetanus immune globulin (HTIG)
  - —500 IU i.m., adult and pediatric
  - —Administer *before* débridement of wound
  - —Neutralizes toxins that have not yet entered neurons
  - —No effect on toxin already bound in CNS
- Surgical débridement of the wound
  - —Delay until several hours after the administration of HTIG
- Antibiotics to eliminate remaining bacteria
  - —Metronidazole
  - —Second line, penicillin G, erythromycin, tetracycline, or chloramphenicol
- Supportive care
  - —Treat muscle spasms with benzodiazepines; if large doses fail, can administer dantrolene
  - —Nondepolarizing neuromuscular blockage may be required (vecuronium preferred) in severe cases
  - —Meticulous airway support to prevent aspiration/pneumonia
- Autonomic instability therapy
  - —Occurs during the second or third week
  - —Tachydysrhythmia and hypertension
    - -No treatment universally effective
    - -Alpha- and beta-blockers can be tried, but may cause worsening
    - -Clonidine, magnesium, morphine, fentanyl, and epidural anesthesia may be tried
  - —Hypotension
    - -Rule out septicemia and hypovolemia
    - -Initiate dopamine or dobutamine when low cardiac output
  - —Bradycardia
    - -Temporary pacemaker more effective than atropine
  - —Treat rhabdomyolysis if it occurs

Prophylaxis

- HTIG (tetanus immune globulin)
  - —250 IU i.m.
  - —Separate site from tetanus-diphtheria toxoid (Td)
  - —Unimmunized or incompletely immunized in presence of wound
- Td, 0.5 mL i.m.
  - —Unimmunized or incompletely immunized
  - —Diphtheria, pertussis, and tetanus vaccine (DPT) or Td for children under 7
  - —>5 years since booster

PEDIATRIC CONSIDERATIONS

- For prophylaxis, use DPT or TD instead of Td in children under 7 years

MEDICATIONS

- Benztropine: 1–2 mg i.v.
- Chloramphenicol: 1.0 g (peds: 50–100 mg/kg/24 h) i.v. q6h
- Chlorpromazine: 10–50 mg i.m.
- Diazepam (benzodiazepine): 5–10 mg (peds: 0.2–0.4 mg/kg) i.v.
- Diphenhydramine: 50 mg i.v.
- Dobutamine: 2.5–15 μg/kg/min i.v.
- Dopamine: 2–20 μg/kg/min i.v.
- Doxycycline: 100 mg i.v. q12h
- Erythromycin: 500 mg i.v. q6h
- Labetalol: 20 mg (peds: 0.3–1 mg/kg/dose) i.v. every 10 minutes up to 300 mg PRN—start infusion 2 mg/min (peds: 0.4–1 mg/kg/hr max 3 mg/kg/hr as needed)
- Metronidazole: 1.0 g (peds: 15 mg/kg) load, followed by 500 mg (7.5 mg/kg) i.v. q6h
- Penicillin G potassium: 1.2 million IU (peds: 100,000 IU/kg/24 h) i.v. q6h for 10 days
- Propranolol: 0.5–1 mg (peds: 0.01–0.1 mg/kg) i.v.

Disposition

ADMISSION CRITERIA

- All patients should be admitted, usually to intensive care settings

DISCHARGE CRITERIA

- None for suspected generalized tetanus

Miscellaneous

ICD9: 37.0

ICD10: A35

SUGGESTED READINGS

Bleck TP, Brauner JS. Tetanus. In: Scheld WM, Whitely RJ, Durack DT, eds. Infections of the central nervous system, 2nd ed. Philadelphia: Lippincott-Raven, 1997:629–653.

Centers for Disease Control. Tetanus surveillance—United States, 1995–1997. MMWR Morb Mortal Wkly Rep 1998;47:1–13.

Hsu SS, Groleau G. Tetanus in the emergency department: a current review. J Emerg Med 2001;20,4:359–365.

Author: Constance Greene

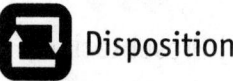

Theophylline, Poisoning

Clinical Presentation

SIGNS AND SYMPTOMS

Cardiovascular

- Sinus or supraventricular tachycardias
  - —Multifocal atrial tachycardia
  - —Caused by β_1-receptor stimulation
- Hypotension
  - —In acute or acute-on-chronic ingestions only
  - —Associated with theophylline >35 mg/L
  - —Caused by β_2-receptor stimulation
  - —May be refractory to fluids, positioning, and conventional vasopressors

Central Nervous System

- Tremor
- Mental status changes
- Seizures with theophylline level
  - —>100 mg/L in acute overdose
  - —>30 mg/L in acute-on-chronic intoxication
  - —As low as 20 mg/L in chronic intoxication
  - —Usually refractory to and may be enhanced by phenytoin

Gastrointestinal

- Nausea, vomiting
  - —Protracted and refractory to usual antiemetics at usual doses
- Abdominal pain
- Pharmacobezoar
  - —From sustained-release dosage forms in acute ingestions
  - —Delays peak concentrations

Miscellaneous

- Hypokalemia
  - —As low as 1.5 mEq/L
- Hyperglycemia
- Leukocytosis
- Hypercalcemia, hypophosphatemia, hypomagnesemia

MECHANISM/DESCRIPTION

- Acute overdose
  - —Ingestion within an 8-hour interval in a patient in whom no prior detectable theophylline would be found
- Acute-on-chronic overdose
  - —Single excessive dose in a patient previously receiving usual therapeutic doses for ≥24 hours
- Chronic intoxication
  - —Accumulation of theophylline >20 mg/L associated with prior therapeutic use for ≥24 hours secondary to
    - -Drug-drug, drug-diet, or drug-disease interactions
    - -Due to use of serial excessive doses
- Electrolyte shifts and hypotensive effects only occur in acute overdoses
  - —Tachyphylaxis to these effects occurs with maintenance therapy
  - —Due to cellular shifts between extracellular and intracellular fluids

ETIOLOGY

- Acute ingestions require larger concentrations to achieve specific toxic effects than acute-on-chronic or chronic overdoses
- Drug-drug interactions
  - —Inhibiting theophylline metabolism
    - -H_2-receptor antagonists
    - -Macrolide antibiotics
    - -Fluoroquinolones
    - -Allopurinol
    - -Influenza vaccine
    - -Interferons
  - —Enhances theophylline metabolism (leads to toxicity when discontinued)
    - -Carbamazepine
    - -Barbiturates
    - -Smoking
    - -Rifampin
- Chronic theophylline accumulation
  - —Uncontrolled congestive heart failure
  - —Liver disease (cirrhosis or severe hepatitis)
  - —Acute viral infections

Pre-Hospital

CAUTIONS

- Bring pill bottles/pill samples in suspected overdose

Diagnosis

ESSENTIAL WORKUP

- Serum theophylline concentration
  - —≥20 mg/L confirms diagnosis
- Detailed history to differentiate acute from acute-on-chronic from chronic intoxication

LABORATORY

- Theophylline level
  - —Repeat every 2 hours until declining to confirm immediate absorption is complete and "peak" value has occurred
  - —Serious morbidity in acute overdose if ≥100 mg/L
  - —Massive caffeine concentrations can yield detectable and/or "toxic" theophylline determinations with conventional laboratory testing
- CBC
- Electrolytes
  - —Transient hypokalemia
- Serum acetaminophen level

IMAGING/SPECIAL TESTS

- KUB
  - —Undissolved sustained-release tablets or pharmacobezoars may appear as radiopacities
  - —Bead-filled capsules may appear as radiolucencies
- Ultrasound of the stomach may detect intact sustained-release dosage forms

DIFFERENTIAL DIAGNOSIS

- Caffeine/β-agonist bronchodilator overdose
- Amphetamines
- Sympathomimetic
- Anticholinergic
- Drug withdrawal syndromes
- Pheochromocytoma
- Thyrotoxicosis

Treatment

INITIAL STABILIZATION

- ABCs
  —Cardiac monitor
  —0.9% NS IV fluid rehydration
- Naloxone, thiamine, and D-50-W (or Accu-Chek) for altered mental status

Cardiovascular

- Initiate beta-blockers or calcium channel blockers for rate control with supraventricular tachyarrhythmias
  —Theophylline toxicity is refractory to adenosine
- 0.9% NS IV fluid resuscitation for hypotension
  —With treatment failure, consider beta-blocker to reverse theophylline-induced β_2-receptor–stimulated vasodilation
- Treat ventricular dysrhythmias conventionally

Seizures

- Administer benzodiazepines
- Phenytoin contraindicated

ED TREATMENT

- Decontamination
- Perform gastric lavage for severe (≥50 mg/kg) acute overdoses presenting within 1 hour of ingestion
- Administer activated charcoal
- Administer cathartics with the first dose of activated charcoal
- Multidose charcoal
  —Especially with sustained-release products
  —Binds theophylline, which back-diffuses to the small intestine
  —For mild to moderate toxicity
  —10–25 g q1–2h until theophylline level ≤20 mg/L
- Initiate whole bowel irrigation with sustained-release products
  —Administer until a clear, colorless rectal effluent or serum theophylline <20 mg/L
- Treat protracted vomiting with metoclopramide or $5HT^3$-receptor antagonists
- Avoid ipecac

Electrolyte Disturbances

- Treat hypokalemia in acute ingestions cautiously
  —Not pathophysiologic owing to β-receptor–mediated intracellular shift of extracellular potassium
  —Aggressive correction leads to symptomatic hyperkalemia as theophylline concentrations decrease
- Most electrolyte imbalances respond to beta-blocker therapy
  —Generally not indicated owing to the absence of associated morbidity and the potential for beta-blocker–induced bronchospasm in pulmonary patients

Extracorporeal Elimination

- Hemoperfusion—more efficacious
- Hemodialysis—faster availability
- Initiate hemodialysis or hemoperfusion if theophylline level
  —≥100 mg/L in acute ingestions
  —≥60 mg/L in acute-on-chronic or chronic intoxications

MEDICATIONS

- Activated charcoal: 1 g/kg PO, if dose ingested is known, 10 g/1gm theophylline ingested, no one dose more than 100 g
- Diazepam: 0.1 mg/kg i.v. every 5–10 minutes until seizures abate up to 30 mg
- Diltiazem: 0.25 mg/kg i.v. bolus, can repeat after 15 minutes, then 5–15 mg/h infusion
- Esmolol: 500 μg/kg i.v. bolus, followed by 50 μg/kg/min infusion, increase by 50 μg/kg/min increments to max of 200 μg/kg/min
- Metoclopramide: 10 mg i.v. bolus can repeat to maximum of 1 mg/kg
- Ondansetron: 0.15 mg/kg i.v. bolus up to max of 32 mg total
- Polyethylene glycol (high molecular weight): 1–2 L/h via NGT

Disposition

ADMISSION CRITERIA

- Acute overdoses with serum theophylline concentrations >100 mg/L
- Acute-on-chronic or chronic theophylline with either a serum concentration >60 mg/L or >60 years old
- Seizures, or fluid and vasopressor refractory hypotension in a patient with serum theophylline concentration >30 mg/L
- Serial unchanged or rising serum theophylline concentrations (two or more) >30 mg/L an acute or acute-on-chronic ingestion of sustained-release theophylline

DISCHARGE CRITERIA

- Two consecutive (2 or more hours apart) declining serum theophylline concentrations with the most recent concentration <30 mg/L
- Mildly symptomatic patient without comorbid illness or evidence of intention to do self-harm with theophylline level <30 mg/L

Miscellaneous

ICD9: 974.1

ICD10: T48.6

SUGGESTED READINGS

Henderson A, Wright DM, Pond SM. Management of theophylline overdose patients in the intensive care unit. Anaesth Intensive Care 1992;20:56–62.

Shannon MW. Comparative efficacy of hemodialysis and hemoperfusion in severe theophylline intoxication. Acad Emerg Med 1997;4:674–678.

Shannon MW. Life-threatening events after theophylline overdose. Arch Intern Med 1999;159:989–994.

Stork CM, Howland MA, Goldfrank LR. Concepts and controversies of bronchodilator overdose. Emerg Med Clin North Am 1994;12:415–436.

Author: Frank Paloucek

Thoracic Outlet Syndrome

Clinical Presentation

SIGNS AND SYMPTOMS

Vascular Compression

- Ischemic symptoms
  - —Cool
  - —Claudication
  - —Color changes
- Diminished pulse
- Venous engorgement
- Edema

Neurogenic

- True neurogenic
  - —Pain
  - —Paresthesias
  - —Numbness
  - —Weakness of the arm and hand
    - -Usually in C8–T1 nerve distribution
  - —Vasomotor symptoms
- Disputed neurogenic
  - —Includes above symptoms but not in a neuroanatomic distribution
  - —Protean of other complaints of the shoulder, neck, head, and chest

General

- Symptoms
  - —May be exacerbated by repetitive use or positional (i.e., working overhead)
  - —Usually insidious in onset and progressive
  - —Can occur or worsen suddenly after trauma
- Supraclavicular tenderness
- May have a bruit in supraclavicular area

MECHANISM/DESCRIPTION

- Encompassing diagnosis for a variety of chronic complaints of the upper extremity, shoulder, and neck unified by the underlying pathophysiology of neurovascular compression
- Prevalence is higher in females
- Right extremity is more commonly affected
- Bilateral involvement is common
- Neurologic symptoms, ischemia or edema of the upper extremity
- Vascular compression thoracic outlet syndrome (TOS) occurs in about 5% of patients
- Neurogenic TOS
  - —About 95% of patients
  - —True (1–3%)—those with objective findings
  - —Disputed (90%)—those with no or limited objective findings

ETIOLOGY

- Compression of the neurovascular components (brachial plexus, subclavian artery, and vein) of the upper extremity as they pass through the thoracic outlet
- Compression results from cervical ribs and other congenital anomalies, trauma, or abnormal tone of the shoulder suspensory musculature

Pre-Hospital

N/A

Diagnosis

ESSENTIAL WORKUP

- Rule out cardiac ischemia
  - —EKG
- Tests for diminished strength or sensation
  - —Elevated arm stress test (EAST)
    - -Arms abducted 90° from the thorax and elbows flexed at 90°
    - -Shoulders braced slightly back of the frontal plane
    - -Fists are open and closed for 3 minutes
    - -Early heaviness and fatigue of the arm
    - -Gradual onset of hand numbness
    - -Progressive aching through the arm and top of shoulder
    - -Evaluates arterial, venous, and neurologic TOS
    - -If radial pulse is normal during the test, a neurologic cause should be suspected
  - —Adson's test
    - -Arm down, patient rotates head toward extremity, looks up, and inhales
    - -Not as reliable as EAST
- During testing
  - —Check for pulse diminution
  - —Reproduction/exacerbation of symptoms
- None of these tests is very sensitive or specific

LABORATORY

N/A

IMAGING/SPECIAL TESTS

- Perform as outpatient except in case of limb-threatening ischemia
- Chest radiograph
  - —Assess for anatomic abnormalities
    - -First rib
    - -Cervical rib
    - -Clavicle deformity
  - —Pulmonary disease
- Cervical spine series
  - —Fracture
  - —Scoliosis
- Arteriogram
  - —Indications
    - -Obliteration of the radial pulse on EAST
    - -BP is 20 mm Hg less than the opposite limb
    - -Suspected subclavian stenosis
    - -Bruit or abnormal supraclavicular pulsations
    - -Peripheral emboli in the upper extremity
- Venography
  - —Indicated if edema, peripheral unilateral cyanosis, or distended thoracic and extremity veins
- Neurogenic thoracic outlet syndrome (TOS)
  - —No gold standard test—diagnosis remains mostly clinical
  - —Nerve conduction studies helpful in confirming the clinical diagnosis and in identifying other disorders in the differential diagnosis
  - —MRI required to assess for spinal cord disease or a herniated cervical disk

DIFFERENTIAL DIAGNOSIS

- Cardiac ischemia
- Cervical spondylosis or disk disease
- Carpal tunnel syndrome or nerve entrapments
- Pancoast's tumor; other neck/mediastinum malignancies
- Neuritis
- Myositis
- Raynaud's disease
- Multiple sclerosis or degenerative spinal cord disease
- Shoulder inflammatory diseases—arthritis, rotator cuff injury, bicipital tendonitis
- Atherosclerotic or thromboembolic disease

Treatment

INITIAL STABILIZATION

N/A

ED TREATMENT

- Symptomatic relief
  - —NSAIDs
  - —Steroids
  - —Muscle relaxants
    - -Cyclobenzaprine
    - -Methocarbamol
    - -Diazepam
  - —Soothing liniments or ointments
- Initial management
  - —Usually conservative involving physical therapy and medications
- Surgery for failure of medical therapy
  - —70–90% of patients experience some to complete relief postoperatively

MEDICATIONS

- Cyclobenzaprine (Flexeril): 10 mg PO t.i.d.
- Diazepam: 5 mg PO t.i.d.
- Ibuprofen: 800 mg PO t.i.d.
- Methocarbamol (Robaxin): 1,000–1,500 mg PO t.i.d.

Disposition

ADMISSION CRITERIA

- Limb-threatening ischemia

DISCHARGE CRITERIA

- Follow-up arranged with a neurologist, thoracic surgeon, or orthopedist

Miscellaneous

ICD9: 353.0

ICD10: G54.0

SUGGESTED READING

Atasoy E. Thoracic outlet compression syndrome. Orthop Clin North Am 1996;27:265–303.

Author: Chris Moore

Thrombotic Thrombocytopenic Purpura

Clinical Presentation

SIGNS AND SYMPTOMS

Five Major Clinical Features: The Classic Pentad

- Thrombocytopenia
  - —Platelet count <20,000/mm^3
- Microangiopathic and hemolytic anemia
  - —Hb <10 g/dL (<6 g/dL in 40%)
- Neurologic symptoms
  - —Presenting complaint in 60%, occur in 90%
  - —Typically fluctuating
  - —Headache
  - —Altered mentation (confusion, stupor, coma)
  - —Behavioral or personality changes
  - —Focal sensory or motor deficits or aphasia
  - —Seizures
  - —Spontaneous intracranial hemorrhage
- Renal insufficiency
  - —Usually mild
  - —Creatinine <3.0 mg/dL
- Fever
  - —Occurs in acute episodes and prodromal syndromes

Symptoms

- General
  - —Weakness
  - —Fatigue
  - —Fever
  - —Malaise
- Hemorrhage
  - —Easy bruising
  - —Epistaxis
  - —Menorrhagia
  - —GI bleeding
  - —Loss or change in vision
- GI complaints
  - —Nausea
  - —Anorexia
  - —Diarrhea
  - —Abdominal pain
- Neurologic
  - —Headache
  - —Confusion
  - —Seizure
  - —Behavioral or personality changes
  - —Focal sensory or motor deficits or aphasia
- Changes in vision or blindness

Signs

- Purpura
- GI hemorrhage: hematemesis, hematochezia, melena
- Epistaxis
- Jaundice
- Shock
- Altered mental status (confusion, stupor, coma)
- Focal sensory or motor deficits
- Pulmonary infiltrates and edema
- Alteration of vision, retinal hemorrhage or detachment, occlusive retinopathy (Purtscher's retinopathy)
- Abnormalities of cardiac conduction

Classic Course

- Acute onset
- Fulminant course lasting days to a few months
- Nearly always fatal outcome without treatment
  - —>90% mortality without treatment
  - —Reverses to >90% survival with modern treatment

MECHANISM/DESCRIPTION

- Systemic endothelial cell damage of uncertain stimulation with apoptosis of the microvascular endothelial cells
- Release of von Willebrand's factor (vWF) multimers, with deficiency of vWF multimer cleaving protease and formation of ultralarge vWF multimers
- Platelet aggregation and fibrin deposition occurring in the arterioles and capillaries leading to microthrombi and obstruction to blood flow
- Platelet aggregation leads to
  - —Consumption of platelets in excess of the bone marrow's ability to respond producing thrombocytopenia
  - —Widespread microvascular hyaline thrombotic lesions
- Microvasculature obstruction with platelet aggregates leads to
  - —Red cell hemolysis
  - —Accumulation of heme breakdown products
  - —Anemia
- End-organ ischemia results from the diffuse thrombosis in small vessels
  - —Most common in heart, brain, kidney, pancreas, and adrenal glands
  - —Lungs and liver relatively spared

ETIOLOGY

- Unknown primary stimulant but results in abnormal activation and failure of control of coagulation pathway
- Deficiency of vWF-cleaving protease identified but not specific to thrombotic thrombocytopenic purpura (TTP) or hemolytic-uremic syndrome (HUS)
- Clinical presentations include
  - —Idiopathic
  - —Familial, chronic or relapsing
  - —Drug-induced
    - -Allergic or immune mediated (quinine, ticlopidine, clopidogrel)
    - -Dose-related toxicity (mitomycin C, cyclosporine)
  - —Pregnancy, postpartum associated
  - —Bone marrow transplantation associated
  - —Infection
- More common in the third to sixth decades of life
- Uncommon in the pediatric or geriatric populations
- Women affected about twice as frequently as men

Pre-Hospital

N/A

Diagnosis

ESSENTIAL WORKUP

- Clinical diagnosis
  - —Due to success of treatment base on identification of the two major findings:
    - -Thrombocytopenia
    - -Microangiopathic hemolytic anemia
    - -Exclude other major differential diagnoses
- Comprehensive history and physical exam with directed laboratory testing targeted at identification of the major symptoms and signs, complications, and exclusion of major differential diagnoses
- Identify possible drug-associated disease and avoid reexposure

LABORATORY

- CBC/platelet count/reticulocyte count
  - —Anemia: hemoglobin <10 g/dl
  - —Thrombocytopenia <20,000/mm^3
  - —Increased reticulocyte count
- Coagulation studies
  - —Normal
- Peripheral blood smear
  - —Macroangiopathic changes
  - —Schistocytes
  - —Helmet cells
  - —Nucleated RBCs
- Coombs' test
  - —Negative direct Coombs' test
- Electrolytes, BUN, creatinine, glucose
  - —Mild elevation of BUN, creatinine
  - —Hyperkalemia due to RBC lysis
- Lactate dehydrogenase (LDH)
  - —Elevated 5–10 times
  - —Elevated owing to both hemolysis and diffuse tissue ischemia
- Bilirubin
  - —Increased unconjugated bilirubin
- Urinalysis
  - —Hematuria (microscopic to gross)

IMAGING/SPECIAL TESTS

- Biopsy
  - —Confirms diagnosis
  - —Reveals hyaline lesions in small vessels
  - —Contraindicated during fulminant presentation (hemorrhage risk)
- CT head
  - —For altered mental status to rule out intracranial hemorrhage
- Electroencephalography (EEG)
  - —To predict need for anticonvulsant therapy

DIFFERENTIAL DIAGNOSIS

- HUS
  - —Triad of thrombocytopenia, schistocytosis, and renal dysfunction
  - —Neurologic symptoms unusual
  - —Often preceded by infectious prodrome and diarrhea
  - —Pediatric variant usually related to toxin producing *Escherichia coli* infection
  - —Adult variant responds to treatment similarly to TTP
- Disseminated intravascular coagulation
  - —Causes the deposition of fibrin in microvasculature and not hyaline
  - —Coagulation studies abnormal
- Idiopathic thrombocytopenic purpura (ITP)
  - —No evidence of hemolysis
  - —LDH and bilirubin normal
- Pregnancy-related thrombocytopenia
  - —Preeclampsia, eclampsia
  - —Pregnancy-associated hemolysis
  - —HELLP (hemolysis, elevated liver enzymes, and low platelets)
- Evans' syndrome
  - —Autoimmune hemolytic anemia
  - —Prominence of microspherocytes rather than schistocytes
  - —Positive direct Coombs' test
- Malignant hypertension
- Bacterial sepsis
- Subacute bacterial endocarditis
- Autoimmune disorders (e.g., systemic lupus erythematosus [SLE])
- Disseminated malignancy
- Heparin-associated thrombocytopenia
- Prosthetic valves or severely calcified aortic stenosis

Treatment

INITIAL STABILIZATION

- ABCs
- 0.9% NS IV fluid resuscitation for shock or GI hemorrhage
- RBC transfusions
  - —For significant anemia or bleeding complications
- Platelet transfusions
  - —Reserve for life-threatening hemorrhage (e.g., CNS bleeds) or required invasive procedures
  - —May aggravate the thrombotic, microvascular obstructive process and worsen the end-organ ischemia and shock

ED TREATMENT

- *Fresh-frozen plasma* (FFP) or fresh-unfrozen plasma
  - —Initiated as bridge to exchange transfusions upon diagnosis of TTP
  - —Success rate approaching 64%
  - —Provides a platelet-antiaggregating factor absent or diminished in the patient's own serum
  - —Used prophylactically to prevent recurrence in the chronic relapsing variant
- *Plasma exchange transfusions*
  - —Most important component of treatment
  - —Combination of plasmapheresis and infusion of FFP
  - —Plasmapheresis removes
    - -Immune complexes responsible for endothelial damage and initiation of TTP
    - -Circulating proaggregation factors promoting platelet aggregation
  - —Perform daily until
    - -Platelet count normalizes
    - -Neurologic symptoms improve
    - -LDH normalizes
    - -Improvement of renal function may lag behind other findings
    - -Taper frequency based on empiric judgment of response, may need to resume if relapse occurs
  - —Complications include
    - -Allergy or serum sickness
    - -Secondary infection
    - -Hypotension
- *Corticosteroids*
  - —Unproven therapeutic benefit
  - —May limit immunologically mediated endothelial damage and decrease splenic sequestration of platelets and damaged RBCs
  - —Supportive benefit if adrenal glands damaged through hemorrhage or ischemia
- *Antiplatelet or immunosuppressive drugs*
  - —Aspirin and dipyridamole most commonly used
  - —Sulfapyrazine, dextran, and vincristine use has been reported
  - —Utilized with variable effectiveness
  - —Can worsen bleeding complications
  - —Heparin is ineffective
- *Splenectomy*
  - —Historically recommended
  - —Of uncertain efficacy
- Dialysis
  - —For renal failure
- *Alternatives in refractory cases*
  - —Increase frequency or volume of exchange transfusion
  - —Add or increase corticosteroid dose or antiplatelet dose
  - —Consider other immunosuppressive treatment
  - —Consider splenectomy

MEDICATIONS

- Aspirin: 325–650 mg PO q4–6h
- Dipyridamole: 75–100 mg PO q.i.d.
- FFP
  - —Plasma infusion: 30 mL/kg/d (75–100 mL/h)
  - —Plasma exchange transfusion: 3–4 L/d
    - -Exchange one plasma volume per day
    - -If resistant case may increase to b.i.d. exchange and/or to 1.5 plasma volume per exchange
    - -Consider using cryosupernant plasma (devoid of additional vWF)
- Methylprednisolone: 0.75 mg/kg q12h
- Prednisone: 1–2 mg/kg/d (high dose up to 200 mg/d)
- Vincristine: 2 mg i.v. q4–7d for four doses

Disposition

ADMISSION CRITERIA

- Newly diagnosed serious platelet disorder, especially with bleeding complications or altered mental status or renal dysfunction
- ICU admission for TTP with active bleeding or neurologic findings
  - —Transport to a tertiary care center with appropriate specialty care facilities

DISCHARGE CRITERIA

- None

Miscellaneous

ICD9: 446.6

ICD10: M31.1

SUGGESTED READING

Elliot MA, Nichols WL. Thrombotic thrombocytopenic purpura and hemolytic uremic syndrome. Mayo Clin Proc 2001;76(11):1154–1162.

George JN. How I treat patients with thrombotic thrombocytopenic purpura: hemolytic uremic syndrome. Blood 2000;96(4):1223–1229.

Liu J, Hutzler, Li C, Pechet L. Thrombotic thrombocytopenic purpura (TTP) and hemolytic uremic syndrome (HUS) the new thinking. J Thromb Thrombolysis 2001;11(3):261–272.

Medina PJ, Sipols JM, George JN. Drug-associated thrombotic thrombocytopenic purpura: hemolytic uremic syndrome Curr Opin Hematol 2001;8(5):286–293.

Author: Timothy Pavek

Thumb Fractures

Clinical Presentation

SIGNS AND SYMPTOMS

- Pain, swelling, and deformity of the thumb
- Exam should include the thenar eminence for pain or deformity
- The thumb may be rotated at the fracture site
- The base of the thumb may appear radially deviated relative to the rest of the hand in the resting position
- Occasionally, there may be damage to the thumb digital nerves

MECHANISM/DESCRIPTION

Distal Phalangeal Fractures

- Blunt trauma, hyperextension of the thumb, axial loading of the thumb
- *Tuft fracture* is a fracture similar to that in other digits in which the distal phalanx is crushed and fragmented; it may open or closed and associated with nailbed injury; it is treated as a soft tissue injury

Proximal Phalangeal Fractures and Thumb Metacarpal Fractures

- Blunt trauma to the thumb, axial loading of the thumb with the metacarpal phalangeal joint flexed, hand closed, or the thumb metacarpal-phalangeal joint otherwise stabilized
- *Bennett's fracture* is an oblique intraarticular fracture of the ulnar aspect of the base of the thumb metacarpal with the larger distal fragment displaced
  —The oblique fracture involves the ulnar surface and the metacarpal-carpal joint. The ulnar fragment is maintained in its anatomic position, and the larger distal fragment is pulled radially and proximally by its tendon insertions
- *Rolando's fracture* is a comminuted Y- or V-shaped intraarticular fracture of the ulnar base of the thumb metacarpal with the large distal fragment displaced

Pre-Hospital

CAUTIONS

- Dress open wounds
- Immobilization in neutral position
- Elevation, cold to reduce swelling
- Age-appropriate social management

Diagnosis

ESSENTIAL WORKUP

- Radiography as noted below

IMAGING/SPECIAL TESTS

- Avoid stress testing of thumb metacarpal-phalangeal joint (i.e., to test for gamekeeper's thumb) until plain radiography is completed

DIFFERENTIAL DIAGNOSIS

- Extraarticular fracture of the base of the thumb metacarpal
- Scaphoid fracture
- Gamekeeper's thumb

PEDIATRIC CONSIDERATIONS

- Fractures to the thumb occur in children, but as in all childhood fractures, one should consider nonaccidental trauma

Treatment

INITIAL STABILIZATION

- Immobilize thumb pending definitive evaluation

ED TREATMENT

- Thumb spica splint with the thumb in neutral position (as if holding a soda can)
- Splint instructions provided to patient
- 72-hour orthopedic referral
- Counsel patient that there is a high likelihood of the need for operative repair

MEDICATIONS

- Pain control with oral analgesic preparations (some theoretical consideration of decreased bone healing with NSAIDs)

Disposition

ADMISSION CRITERIA

- Open fracture, presence of multiple trauma, or other more serious injuries

DISCHARGE CRITERIA

- Closed injuries, 72-hour orthopedic follow-up with frequent need for operative fixation

Miscellaneous

ICD9: 816.00

ICD10: S62.5

SUGGESTED READINGS

American Society for Surgery of the Hand. The hand: examination and diagnosis, 2nd ed. New York: Churchill Livingstone, 1983.

American Society for Surgery of the Hand. The hand: primary care of common problems, 2nd ed. New York: Churchill Livingstone, 1990.

Antosia RE, Lyn E. The Hand. In: Rosen P, et al., eds. Emergency medicine: concepts and clinical practice, 4th ed. St. Louis: Mosby–Year Book, 1998:625–668.

Chaffin TH. Phalangeal fractures. In: Hart RG, Uehara DT, Wagner MJ, eds. Emergency and primary care of the hand. Dallas: ACEP 2001:111–122.

Sullivan JH, Tsonis GD. Metacarpal fractures. In: Hart RG, Uehara DT, Wagner MJ, eds. Emergency and primary care of the hand. Dallas: ACEP 2001:99–110.

Author: John MacKay

Tibial/Fibular Shaft Fracture

Clinical Presentation

SIGNS AND SYMPTOMS

- Pain: usually immediate, severe, and well localized to the fracture site
- Deformity: visible or palpable at the fracture site
- Inability to bear weight if tibia involved; may be able to walk if isolated fibula fracture
- Significant soft tissue damage with high-energy trauma
- Compartment syndrome
- Possible foot drop on affected leg from peroneal nerve injury as it wraps around fibular head

MECHANISM/DESCRIPTION

- High-energy versus low-energy injury
  —Amount of soft tissue injury is prognostic and is determined by the degree of energy involved
- Indirect force: frequently low-energy trauma
  —Rotary and compressive forces often result in oblique and spiral fractures (e.g., skiing, fall, child abuse)
- Direct force: high-energy trauma
  —Direct blow to leg often results in transverse and comminuted fractures (e.g., pedestrian versus auto, motor vehicle crash [MVC])
  —Bending force over a fulcrum often produces comminution with a wedge-shaped butterfly fragment (e.g., skier's boot top, football tackle, MVC)

Fracture Description

Tibia

- Extent of soft tissue damage
  —Open versus closed
  —Gustilo-Anderson classification of open fractures
  —Type I: wound <1 cm; little soft tissue damage; no crush injury
  —Type II: wound >1 cm; moderate soft tissue damage; little or no devitalized soft tissue
  —Type III: severe soft tissue injury; A—adequate soft tissue coverage of bone; B—tissue loss/periosteal stripping; C—neurovascular injury requiring surgical repair
- Anatomic location
  —Proximal, middle, or distal third
  —Articular extension
- Displacement
- Degree of shortening
- Angulation
- Configuration
  —Spiral, transverse, or oblique
  —Comminuted, with butterfly fragment or multiple fragments

Fibula

- Proximal: may be associated with peroneal nerve injury, or disruption of ankle syndesmosis (Maisonneuve's fracture)
- Middle
- Distal

PEDIATRIC CONSIDERATIONS

- Rely on parents for historical information
- Child may present limping with no obvious deformity
- Nonphyseal fracture patterns
  —Compression (torus)
  —Incomplete tension-compression (greenstick)
  —Plastic/bowing deformity of fibula may occur with complete tibia fracture
  —Complete fractures
- Tibial shaft fractures may extend to physis in Salter-Harris II pattern
- *Bicycle spoke injury:* Usually occurs in child riding on handlebars or rear fender
  —Foot and lower leg get caught between frame and wheel spoke
  —Crush injury is the primary problem
  —Initial benign appearance of the soft tissues is often deceiving, and full-thickness skin loss can occur within days
  —Orthopedic surgery consultation should be obtained on all spoke injury patients with associated fractures
- *Toddler's fracture:*
  —Spiral fracture involving the distal third of the tibia with intact fibula secondary to rotational force (turning on planted foot)
  —Age range is 9 months to 6 years, most often when learning to walk
  —Fractures in midshaft or more transverse are suspicious of non accidental trauma

Pre-Hospital

CAUTIONS

- Look for associated injuries in high-energy mechanisms
- Assess for neurologic or vascular compromise
  —Reduction may be necessary of grossly deformed leg with vascular compromise in attempt to reestablish circulation
- Adequate immobilization is essential to prevent further injury

Diagnosis

ESSENTIAL WORKUP

- Careful assessment of soft tissues
- Careful neurovascular examination (compare with contralateral side)
- Assessment for compartment syndrome
- Examine for associated injuries
  —Completely expose patient and put into gown
- Radiography
  —Anteroposterior and lateral views of the leg, including knee and ankle

Compartment Syndrome

- Relatively common complication of tibia fractures and may not appear until 24 hours after injury
- Signs and symptoms
  —Pain disproportionate from that expected
  —Swollen, tight compartment, with pain on palpation of compartment
  —Pain on passive stretch of toes
  —Sensory deficit
  —Motor weakness is a late finding
  —*Pulselessness is not a sign of compartment syndrome,* i.e., palpable pulses are almost always present in compartment syndrome unless there is underlying arterial injury
- Four leg compartments: anterior, lateral, deep posterior, and superficial posterior
  —Anterior compartment: deep peroneal nerve (sensation of first web space, ankle and toe dorsiflexion), anterior tibial artery (feeds dorsalis pedis artery)
  —Lateral compartment: superficial peroneal nerve (sensation of dorsum of foot, foot eversion)
  —Deep posterior compartment: tibial nerve (sensation to sole of foot, ankle, and toe plantarflexion), posterior tibial and peroneal arteries
  —Superficial posterior compartment: branch of sural cutaneous nerve (sensation to lateral foot)

IMAGING/SPECIAL TESTS

- Compartment pressures if compartment syndrome suspected (consult orthopedic surgery)
  —Pressures >30 mm Hg are an indication for fasciotomy

DIFFERENTIAL DIAGNOSIS

- Adults
  —Stress fracture
  —Pathologic fracture
  —Osteomyelitis
- Children
  —Sarcoma
  —Pathologic fracture
  —Osteomyelitis
  —Child abuse

PEDIATRIC CONSIDERATIONS

- May need to obtain oblique radiographs to detect nondisplaced fracture

Treatment

INITIAL STABILIZATION

- ABCs, advanced trauma life support (ATLS) protocol for multiple trauma victim
- Elevate and immobilize extremity
- Apply ice
- Strict NPO
- IV sedation/analgesia if necessary after initial evaluation

ED TREATMENT

- Closed fractures
  - —Gentle attempt at reduction if fracture displaced (do not attempt multiple reductions)
  - —Immobilization with well-padded long-leg posterior splint with knee in 10–20 degrees of flexion (avoid circumferential cast)
  - —If pain persists after immobilization, suspect complication (e.g., compartment syndrome or nerve compression)
  - —Crutches
- Open fractures
  - —Remove contaminants and cover wound with moist sterile dressing
  - —Antibiotics
  - —Tetanus prophylaxis
  - —Immobilization with well-padded long-leg posterior splint
  - —Immediate orthopedic surgery consultation for débridement and fracture fixation
- Isolated fibula fracture
  - —Usually treated symptomatically with padded splint, elevation, ice, and non-weight-bearing status until swelling is resolved
  - —Crutches if non-weight-bearing

MEDICATIONS

- Cefazolin for open fractures: 2 g i.v. loading dose (peds: 50 mg/kg, gram-positive cocci coverage)
- Gentamicin plus cefazolin if Gustilo-Anderson type III: 2–5 mg/kg i.v. loading dose (peds: 2.5 mg/kg, adds gram negative rod coverage)
- Penicillin G if farming accident: 10 million IU i.v. loading dose (peds: 75,000 IU/kg, *Clostridium* species coverage)
- Tetanus toxoid: 0.5 mL and tetanus immune globulin: 250 units i.m. as indicated by the type of wound and the number of primary immunizations
- Vancomycin if penicillin allergy: 1 g i.v. loading dose (peds: 10 mg/kg)

Disposition

ADMISSION CRITERIA

- Multiple trauma
- High-energy mechanism
- Soft tissue involvement
  - —Low threshold for admission and observation for compartment syndrome
- All open fractures
- Displaced, angulated, transverse, shortened, comminuted, and otherwise unstable fractures
- Intraarticular involvement
- Neurovascular compromise
- Inadequate pain control
- Pathologic fracture
- Nonaccidental trauma in children

DISCHARGE CRITERIA

- Minimally displaced fracture with low-energy injury mechanism
- Close orthopedic follow-up
- Return parameters for compartment syndrome in a reliable patient
- Additional consideration: if fracture is more than 24 hours old, compartment syndrome is unlikely if it has not occurred, and discharge criteria may be more liberal

Miscellaneous

ICD9: 823.80, 823.81

ICD10: S82.2

SUGGESTED READINGS

Mubarak SJ, Owen CA, Hargens AR, et al. Acute compartment syndromes: diagnosis and management with aid of the wick catheter. J Bone Joint Surg 1978;60A(8): 1091–1095.

Russel TA. Fractures of the tibia and fibula. In: Rockwood CA, Green DP, Bucholz RW, et al., eds. Rockwood and Green's fractures in adults, 4th ed. Philadelphia: Lippincott-Raven, 1996:1593–1652.

Trafton PG. Tibial shaft fractures. In: Browner BD, Jupiter JB, Levine AM, et al., eds. Skeletal trauma: fractures, dislocations, ligamentous injuries, 2nd ed. Philadelphia: WB Saunders, 1998: 2187–2293.

Watson JT. Treatment of unstable fractures of the shaft of the tibia. J Bone Joint Surg 1994;76A(10):1575–1584.

Authors: Tyler Vadeboncoeur; Seth K. Williams

Tibial Plateau Fracture

Clinical Presentation

SIGNS AND SYMPTOMS

- Painful, swollen knee
- Inability to bear weight
- Knee effusion (hemarthrosis)
- Limited active and passive range of motion of the knee
- Tenderness along the proximal tibia and joint line
- Possible varus or valgus deformity of the knee
- Possible joint instability due to associated ligamentous injury

MECHANISM/DESCRIPTION

- Synonym: tibial condylar fracture
- Fracture or depression of the proximal tibial articulating surface
- Valgus or varus force applied in combination with axial loading
  —*Lateral* plateau fractures occur classically after a pedestrian is struck by a vehicle bumper on the lateral aspect of the knee with a medially directed force
  —*Medial* plateau fractures are much less common and require significant force to occur
- Younger patients are more resistant to depressed plateau fractures
- Elderly patients are more prone to depression type fractures
- Fall from a height causing femoral condyles to impact on tibial surface
- Violent twisting force (e.g., skiing)
- Associated injuries include
  —Ligamentous (collaterals, cruciates)
  —Meniscal
  —Neurovascular (peroneal nerve and popliteal vessels)

PEDIATRIC CONSIDERATIONS

- Tibial plateau fractures are rare in children because of the dense cancellous bone of the tibial plateau

Schatzker's Classification of Plateau Fractures

- *Type 1:* split fracture of the *lateral* tibial plateau *without* depression of the plateau
  —Occurs in younger patients in whom the cancellous bone of the plateau resists depression
  —Usually occurs from a valgus force to the knee in combination with axial load
- *Type 2:* combination of a split fracture *and* depression of all or a portion of the remaining *lateral* plateau
  —The mechanism is similar to the above, but these patients tend to be in their fourth decade of life or older and have weaker subcondral bone
- *Type 3:* local depression of the articulating surface of the *lateral* plateau
  —Dependent on location, size, and degree of depression these injuries may be unstable
- *Type 4:* fracture/depression of the *medial* plateau
  —Requires much more force (varus and axial loading) for this injury to occur
  —Be suspicious for associated injuries
  —Damage to the popliteal artery, peroneal nerve, lateral collateral ligament, medial meniscus, and cruciate ligaments must be considered
- *Type 5: bicondylar* fracture
  —High-energy injury associated with popliteal vessel injury, peroneal nerve injury, and development of compartment syndrome
- *Type 6: bicondylar,* grossly comminuted fracture of the plateau with diaphyseal-metaphyseal dissociation
  —Occurs from a violent force, usually a fall from a height, with associated neurovascular injuries and compartment syndrome

Pre-Hospital

CAUTIONS

- In high-energy mechanisms, associated major life-threatening injuries take precedence
- Immobilize to prevent further neurologic or vascular injury

Diagnosis

ESSENTIAL WORKUP

Physical Examination

Decision Aids for the Use of Radiography

- *Ottawa Knee Rule* (knee radiographs are indicated if any of the following are present):
  —1. Age >55 years (Ottawa Knee Rule has not been validated in patients <18 years old)
  —2. Tenderness of the fibular head
  —3. Isolated patellar tenderness
  —4. Inability to flex to 90 degrees
  —5. Inability to *transfer* weight for four steps both immediately after the injury and in the ED
  —Limping is allowed
- *Pittsburgh Knee Rule* (knee radiographs are indicated in fall or blunt trauma mechanism and the following are present)
  —1. Age <12 or >55 years (Pittsburgh Knee Rule should be applied with caution to patients <18 years old)
  —2. Inability to bear weight fully for four steps on both toe pads and heel pad of each foot
  —Limping is *not* allowed
- Neurovascular examination
  —High-energy mechanism (medial plateau or bicondylar fractures) carry risk for neurovascular injury and compartment syndrome
  —Check popliteal, posterior tibial, and dorsalis pedis pulses
  —Check integrity of peroneal nerve—ankle and toe dorsiflexion and sensation in webspace between great and second toes
- Plain radiography
  —Anteroposterior (AP) and cross-table lateral views of the knee and proximal tibia
  —Cross-table lateral view may demonstrate lipohemarthrosis (fat-fluid level)
  —Oblique views may identify fractures not apparent on other films
  —Pay attention to areas of ligamentous attachment where avulsion fractures may take place, i.e., medial and lateral femoral condyles, tibial spine (intercondylar eminence), and fibular head

IMAGING/SPECIAL TESTS

- Tibial plateau view: AP view with the knee in 10–15 degrees of flexion helps visualize depressions
- Sunrise view of the patella may be useful in identifying fractures of the patella not visualized on AP or lateral views
- CT scan may reveal occult fractures not seen on plain radiographs and further delineate the extent of fractures
- MRI can be used to better elucidate soft tissue injuries
- Arthrocentesis to look for fat globules if mechanism strongly suggests fracture and effusion present without x-ray findings
- Arteriography is indicated if
  —High-energy mechanism
  —Schatzker's type 4, 5, or 6 fracture
  —Alteration in distal pulses
  —Expanding hematoma
  —Bruit
  —Injury to anatomically related nerves
- Compartment pressure measurements are indicated if
  —Pain not over fracture site
  —Pain on passive stretch
  —Paresthesias
  —Abnormality of pulses
  —Pressures greater than 30 mm Hg are an indication for emergent orthopedic consultation for fasciotomy

DIFFERENTIAL DIAGNOSIS

- Knee dislocation
- Proximal fibula fracture
- Femoral condyle fracture
- Patella fracture
- Tibial subcondylar fracture
- Tibial tuberosity fracture
- Tibial spine fracture
- Cruciate ligament tears
- Collateral ligament tears
- Meniscal tears

PEDIATRIC CONSIDERATIONS

- Include oblique views as part of routine radiography

Treatment

INITIAL STABILIZATION

- Stabilization of the multiple-injury trauma patient
- Long-leg splint
- Ice
- Elevation

ED TREATMENT

- Non-weight-bearing
- Pain control
- Nondisplaced fractures or minimally displaced (<8 mm) *lateral* plateau fractures without ligamentous injury
  —Aspiration of hemarthrosis and injection of local anesthetic
  —Examination for ligamentous instability
  —If knee is *stable:*
  —Compressive dressing
  —Ice and elevation for 48 hours
  —Non-weight-bearing/crutches
  —If knee is *unstable,* then urgent orthopedic consultation is warranted
- Open fractures
  —Remove contaminants
  —Apply moist sterile dressing
  —Assess tetanus immunity
  —Antibiotics
  —Emergent orthopedic consultation

MEDICATIONS

- Open fractures
  —Cefazolin: 2 g i.v. (peds: 50 mg/kg)
  —Gentamicin: 2–5 mg/kg i.v. (peds: 2.5 mg/kg)
  —Tetanus toxoid if indicated
  —Vancomycin: 1 g i.v. loading dose (peds: 10 mg/kg) if penicillin allergy

Disposition

ADMISSION CRITERIA

- Open fractures for débridement, irrigation, and i.v. antibiotics
- Comminuted, bicondylar fractures for traction
- High-energy mechanisms for observation of neurovascular status and development of compartment syndrome
- Pain control

DISCHARGE CRITERIA

- Nondisplaced or minimally displaced, stable fractures of the lateral plateau

Miscellaneous

ICD9: 823.00

ICD10: S82.1

SUGGESTED READINGS

Seaberg DC, Yealy DM, Lukens T, et al. Multicenter comparison of two clinical decision rules for the use of radiography in acute, high-risk knee injuries. Ann Emerg Med 1998;32:8–13.

Simon RR, Koenigsknecht SJ. Emergency orthopedics: the extremities, 4th ed. New York: McGraw-Hill, 2001.

Stiell IG, Greenberg GH, Wells GA, et al. Prospective validation of a decision rule for the use of radiography in acute knee injuries. JAMA 1996;275(8):611–615.

Watson JT, Wiss DA. Fractures of the proximal tibia and fibula. In: Bucholz RW, Heckman JD, eds. Rockwood and Green's fractures in adults, 5th ed. Philadelphia: Lippincott Williams & Wilkins, 2001: 1801–1838.

Author: Binh T. Ly

Tinea Infections, Cutaneous

Clinical Presentation

SIGNS AND SYMPTOMS

- Tinea capitis
  - —Disease of children spread through hand-to-scalp contact
  - —Alopecia
  - —May manifest as a kerion—a boggy inflammatory mass that exudes pus
  - —"Black dots" from infected hairs broken off at the scalp
- Tinea corporis ("ringworm")
  - —Arms, legs, and trunk
  - —Sharply marginated, annular lesion with raised margins and central clearing
  - —Hair follicle involvement may produce indurated papules and pustules
  - —Lesions may be single, multiple, or concentric
  - —Pets are often a vector
- Tinea cruris ("jock itch")
  - —Erythematous, scaly, marginated patches involving the perineum, thighs, and buttocks
  - —Associated with heat, humidity, perspiration, and tight-fitting undergarments
  - —The scrotum and penis spared
- Tinea pedis ("athlete's foot")
  - —Scaling, maceration, or fissuring between the toes
  - —Initially third, fourth, or fifth web space, may involve plantar surfaces
  - —Risk factors include elderly patients, immunocompromised patients, hot and humid climates, and infrequent changes of socks
  - —Foul odor may indicate secondary bacterial infection
  - —More common in adults than children
  - —"Trichophytid" reaction: vesicular eruption remote from the infection involving hands, mimics dyshidrotic eczema
- Tinea unguium (onychomycosis)
  - —Yellow or brown discoloration with thickening and debris under the nails
  - —Onycholysis: loosening of the nail from its bed
  - —May involve the plantar surface of the foot
- Tinea versicolor
  - —Most common in warm months
  - —Round or oval superficial brown, yellow, or hypopigmented macules that may coalesce
  - —Upper trunk, arms, and neck
  - —Facial involvement is common in children

MECHANISM/DESCRIPTION

- Superficial fungal infections of the hair, skin, or nails, which rarely invade below the stratum corneum

ETIOLOGY

- Most common organisms are dermatophytes (microsporum, trichophyton, and epidermophyton)
  - —*Malassezia furfur*, a yeast, is the etiologic agent of tinea versicolor
- Trauma or maceration of the skin may allow fungal entry into skin

PEDIATRIC CONSIDERATIONS

- Fungi can be spread from toys and hair-care items
- Tinea unguium is rare in children and is associated with Down's syndrome, immunosuppression, and tinea pedis or capitis

Pre-Hospital

N/A

Diagnosis

ESSENTIAL WORKUP

- Diagnose by clinical exam
- Wood's lamp is insensitive because not all fungi fluoresce
  - —Trichophyton does not fluoresce
  - —Microsporum fluoresces bright yellow-green
  - —*Malassezia* (tinea versicolor) fluoresces yellow-orange
  - —Erythrasma (nontinea corynebacterial infection) will fluoresce coral red
- Microscopy
  - —Cleanse area with 70% ethanol and scrape active margin of lesion with #10 or #15 scalpel blade
  - —Place scrapings on a glass slide, add a drop of 10–20% potassium hydroxide solution, and cover with a coverslip
  - —The presence of budding yeast or hyphae confirms the diagnosis
- Fungal cultures are of limited value in that they may take up to 6 weeks to grow

DIFFERENTIAL DIAGNOSIS

- Tinea capitis: impetigo, pediculosis, alopecia areata, seborrheic dermatitis, and psoriasis
- Tinea corporis: impetigo, herpes simplex, Lyme disease, verruca vulgaris, psoriasis, discoid eczema, herald patch of pityriasis rosea, erythema multiforme, urticaria, seborrheic dermatitis, and secondary syphilis
- Tinea cruris: impetigo, seborrheic dermatitis, psoriasis, candidal infection, irritant and allergic contact dermatitis, and erythrasma
- Tinea pedis: scabies, erythrasma, candida, allergic and contact dermatitis, psoriasis, and bacterial interdigital infection
- Tinea unguium: psoriasis, dermatitis, lichen planus, and congenital nail dystrophy
- Tinea versicolor: vitiligo, secondary syphilis

PEDIATRIC CONSIDERATIONS

- Brushing the hair with a toothbrush or rolling a moistened cotton swab may be easier, less traumatic ways to obtain fungal elements for culture or microscopy

Treatment

INITIAL STABILIZATION

- None required except in immunocompromised patients

ED TREATMENT

- Tinea capitis
  - —Oral terbinafine is first-line treatment
  - —Oral ketoconazole, itraconazole, and griseofulvin are alternatives
  - —Selenium sulfide shampoo, once per day, may enhance the elimination of spores
  - —Kerion may respond more rapidly with addition of prednisone
- Tinea corporis
  - —Topical antifungal therapy with clotrimazole, miconazole, or other topical antifungal for 4–6 weeks
  - —Alternative therapy is ketoconazole
- Tinea cruris
  - —Topical antifungal therapy (see tinea corporis)
  - —Area should be kept dry with loose undergarments and fragrance-free talcum powder
  - —Pruritus can additionally be treated with a low-potency corticosteroid such as topical hydrocortisone
  - —Resistant disease may be treated with oral ketoconazole
- Tinea pedis
  - —Topical antifungals for mild cases
  - —Oral fluconazole is alternative
  - —Acute vesicular tinea pedis may respond to drying agents (Burow's), or topical corticosteroids
  - —Prevention includes drying between toes and using talcum or antifungal powders
- Tinea unguium
  - —Itraconazole or fluconazole are first line treatments
  - —Nail removal may be necessary
  - —Ciclopirox 8% nail lacquer in combination with oral therapy shown to provide improved outcomes
- Tinea versicolor
  - —2.5% selenium sulfide solution is first-line therapy
  - —Topical antifungals or oral ketoconazole
  - —Alternatives are fluconazole and itraconazole
- Immunocompromised patients may require systemic antifungals for any cutaneous fungal infection

MEDICATIONS

- Ciclopirox 8% nail lacquer: apply cream to affected nails daily for 1–2 weeks (peds: same)
- Clotrimazole: apply cream to affected area 2–3 applications/day for 1–3 weeks (peds: same)
- Fluconazole: tinea unguium: 150 mg/wk pulse therapy for 3 months for fingernails, 6 months for toenails; tinea corporis, cruris, and pedis: 150 mg PO weekly for 1–4 weeks; tinea versicolor: 400 mg PO single dose; peds: none (may cause hepatotoxicity)
- Griseofulvin: tinea capitis: 500 mg PO q.d. for 4–6 weeks (peds: 11 mg/kg up to 500 mg PO q.d. until hair regrows, usually 6–8 weeks); most specialists now using 20–25 mg/kg/d for 6–8 weeks for improved efficacy
- Itraconazole: tinea capitis: adults and peds: 3–5 mg/kg PO q.d.; tinea unguium: 200 mg PO q.d. for 3 months; tinea versicolor: 400 mg PO q.d. for 3 days (peds: 3–5 mg/kg/d for 4–6 weeks) (tinea capitis); contraindicated with terfenadine
- Ketoconazole: tinea capitis, corporis: 200 mg PO q.d. for 4 weeks (peds: 3.3–6.6 mg/kg PO q.d. for 4 weeks) (contraindicated with terfenadine and astemizole); soda increases absorption 65%
- Miconazole: apply cream to affected area 2–3 applications per day for 1–3 weeks (peds: same)
- Prednisone: adults: none (peds: 1 mg/kg PO q.d. for 2 weeks)
- Selenium sulfide: 2.5% shampoo to affected area for 10–15 minutes for 1–2 weeks (peds: same)
- Terbinafine: tinea unguium: 250 mg PO daily for 6 weeks for fingernails, 12 weeks for toenails (peds: <20 kg—67.5 mg/d, 20–40 kg—125 mg/d, >40 kg—250 mg/d at same interval as adult; tinea pedis: 250 mg PO daily for 2 weeks (peds: 3–4 mg/kg/day for 2 weeks); tinea capitis: 250 mg/d for 4 weeks
- Tolnaftate: apply cream to affected area 2–3 applications per day for 1–3 weeks (peds: same)

PEDIATRIC CONSIDERATIONS

- Topical preparations are preferred

Disposition

ADMISSION CRITERIA

- Invasive disease in the immunocompromised host
- Kerion with secondary bacterial infection

DISCHARGE CRITERIA

- Most patients may be managed as outpatients
- Children may returned to school once appropriate treatment has been initiated

Miscellaneous

ICD9: 110.9

ICD10: B35.9

SUGGESTED READINGS

Bergus GR, Johnson JS. Superficial tinea infections. Am Fam Physician 1993;48:259–268.

Elewski BE. Cutaneous mycoses in children. Br J Dermatol 1996;134(Suppl 46):7–11.

Elewski BE. Tinea capitis: a current perspective. J Am Acad Dermatol 2000;42(1):1–20.

Gupta AK, Baran R. Ciclopirox nail lacquer: the first prescription topical therapy for onychomycosis. J Am Acad Dermatol 2000;43:S96–102.

Lesher J. Oral therapy of common superficial fungal infections of the skin. J Am Acad Dermatol 1999;40:S31–34.

Moossavi M, Bagheri B. Systemic dermatologic therapy: systemic antifungal therapy. Dermatol Clin 2001;19:35–52.

Rezabek GH, Friedman AD. Superficial fungal infections of the skin. Drugs 1992;43(5):674–682.

Wargon O. Tinea of the skin, hair and nails. Med J Aust 1996;164:552–556.

Authors: Steve C. Patterson; Mark G. Richmond

Toluene, Poisoning

Clinical Presentation

SIGNS AND SYMPTOMS

Acute

- Neurologic
  —Depression
  —Euphoria
  —Ataxia
  —Seizures
- Cardiac
  —Fatal arrhythmias
- Pulmonary
  —Chemical pneumonitis
- Gastrointestinal
  —Abdominal pain
  —Nausea, vomiting
  —Hematemesis
- Renal
  —Distal renal tubular acidosis
  —Hematuria
  —Proteinuria
- Musculoskeletal
  —Diffuse weakness

Chronic

- Neurologic
  —Peripheral neuropathies
  —Encephalopathy
  —Optic atrophy
  —Clonus
- Cardiac
  —Congestive heart failure
  —Cardiomyopathy
- Renal
  —Distal renal tubular acidosis
  —Renal failure
- Musculoskeletal
  —Rhabdomyolysis

MECHANISM/DESCRIPTION

- Rapidly absorbed by inhalation
- Readily crossing the blood-brain barrier, reaching high concentrations in the brain
- Alveolar excretion and liver metabolism
- Methods of intoxication
  —"Sniffing"—simple inhalation of substance directly from container
  —"Huffing"—vapors inhaled through cloth saturated with substance
  —"Bagging"—inhaling vapors from bag containing substance
- Toxic range
  —100 ppm—impairment of psychomotor and perceptual performance
  —500–800 ppm—headache, drowsiness, nausea, weakness, and confusion
  —>800 ppm—convulsions, ataxia, staggering gait for several days
  —10,000–30,000 ppm—anesthesia within 1 minute

ETIOLOGY

- Volatile hydrocarbon
- Abused for its euphoric effect
- Used as an organic solvent—found in
  —Glue
  —Coolants
  —Paints and paint thinners
  —Petroleum products
  —Aerosolized household products
  —Correction fluid

PEDIATRIC CONSIDERATIONS

- Prevalent in the adolescent age group
  —Inexpensive "high" with readily available sources
  —Many psychosocial problems
  —Develop chronic neurologic dysfunction

Pre-Hospital

CONTROVERSIES

- Forced emesis is not indicated
  —Aspiration due to decreased level of consciousness

CAUTIONS

- Rapid onset of toxicity
- Death possible with sudden cardiac dysrhythmias

Diagnosis

ESSENTIAL WORKUP

- Physical clues to diagnosis
  - —Presence of agent on lips, nose, or clothes (gold paint has the highest concentration)
  - —Perioral eczematous dermatitis from chronic huffing or bagging can be covered by a beard
  - —Odor of agents

LABORATORY

- Arterial blood gas (ABG)
  - —Acidosis
  - —Hypoxia if chemical pneumonitis
- Electrolytes, BUN, creatinine, glucose
  - —Hypokalemia
  - —Normal or high anion gap metabolic acidosis
  - —Hyperchloremia
  - —Impaired renal function
- Calcium and phosphorus
  - —Severe hypocalcemia/hypophosphatemia common
- Urinalysis
  - —Check for myoglobin (rhabdomyolysis)
  - —Hematuria and protein often present
- Creatinine kinase if suspect rhabdomyolysis
- Alcohol level—often a co-ingestant
- Liver enzymes, prothrombin time (PT) and partial thromboplastin time (PTT) if hepatic dysfunction suspected

IMAGING/SPECIAL TESTS

- EKG—atrial and ventricular dysrhythmias
- Chest x-ray
  - —Indicated if dyspnea or low oxygen saturation
  - —Chemical pneumonitis
- Urine for hippuric acid (metabolite of toluene)
- CT
  - —For altered mental status/chronic exposure
  - —Cerebral/cerebellar atrophy

DIFFERENTIAL DIAGNOSIS

- Alcohol intoxication
- Methanol
- Ethylene glycol
- Salicylate
- Heavy-metal exposure (especially lead)
- Guillain-Barré syndrome
- Metabolic abnormalities

Treatment

INITIAL STABILIZATION

- ABCs
- Cardiac monitor
- 0.9% NS IV access
- Naloxone, thiamine, and check glucose if altered mental status

ED TREATMENT

- Treat cardiac dysrhythmias in a standard fashion
- Correct metabolic abnormalities
  - —Potassium
  - —Calcium
  - —Phosphate
- Acidosis resolves with IV fluids
- If rhabdomyolysis
  - —Maintain high urine output
  - —Alkalinize urine
- Gastric decontamination for oral ingestion
  - —Charcoal does not bind hydrocarbons well

MEDICATIONS

- Dextrose: D50W, 1 amp (50 mL or 25 g) (peds: D25W, 2–4 mL/kg) i.v.
- Naloxone (Narcan): 2 mg (peds: 0.1 mg/kg) i.v. or i.m. initial dose
- Thiamine (vitamin B_1): 100 mg (peds: 50 mg) i.v. or i.m.

Disposition

ADMISSION CRITERIA

- Altered mental status
- Dysrhythmias
- Hepatic dysfunction
- Renal failure
- Rhabdomyolysis
- Severe metabolic derangements

DISCHARGE CRITERIA

- After 4–6 hours observation
  - —Mental status at baseline
  - —No evidence of cardiac, metabolic, or neurologic derangement

Miscellaneous

ICD9: 982.0

ICD10: T52.2

SUGGESTED READINGS

Filley C, Kleinschmidt-demasters B. Toxic leukoencephalopathy. N Engl J Med 2001;345(6):425–432.

Ford M, Delaney K, Ling L, et al. Clinical toxicology, 1st ed. Philadelphia: WB Saunders, 2001:806–809.

Leikin J, Paloucek F. Leikin and Paloucek's poisoning and toxicology handbook, 3rd ed. Lexi-Comp, 2002:1195–1196.

Author: Kirk Cumpston

Toothache

Clinical Presentation

SIGNS AND SYMPTOMS

- Tooth pain
  - —May be referred to jaw, ear, face, eye, and neck
  - —Pain often associated with chewing, changes in temperature and recumbency
- Malodorous breath
- Fever and chills
- Foul taste in mouth
- Dental caries
- Pain on percussion/palpation of tooth and gums
- Abscess
- Facial swelling or erythema
- Cervical adenopathy
- Trismus
  - —Decreased maximal interincisal opening
  - —Normal, 35–50 mm

MECHANISM/DESCRIPTION

- Pain caused by irritation to the root nerves located in the pulpal tissues

ETIOLOGY

- Dental
  - —Dental caries (hard structures demineralized by bacteria)
  - —Pulpitis (inflamed pulp secondary to infection)
  - —Periapical abscess (necrotic pulp and subsequent abscess)
  - —Postextraction pain (dry socket, infection)
  - —Root canal pain
  - —Cracked-tooth syndrome (pain, cold sensitivity, crack difficult to visualize)
- Periodontal disease
  - —Gingivitis and periodontitis (gingivitis with loss of periodontal ligament attachment)
  - —Periodontal abscess (gum boil)
  - —Pericoronitis (gingival inflammation from malerupted tooth)
  - —Acute necrotizing ulcerative gingivitis (gingival pain, ulcers with/without pseudomembranes)
  - —Denture stomatitis
  - —Herpetic gingivostomatitis
  - —Aphthous ulcers (canker sores)
  - —Traumatic ulcers

Pre-Hospital

- Maintain patent airway in patients with severe facial swelling or trismus
- The patient should sit up if possible

Diagnosis

ESSENTIAL WORKUP

- Medical and dental history
- Drug allergies, especially antibiotics
- Assess need for predental procedure antibiotic prophylaxis
  - —Rheumatic fever
  - —Cardiac valve replacements
  - —Orthopedic joint replacements
  - —Mitral valve prolapse or valvular heart disease
- Physical examination should include
  - —Inspection and palpation of lips, salivary glands, floor of the mouth, lymph nodes of the neck
  - —Identify periodontal abscess
  - —Evaluate for deep-space infection
  - —Teeth should be percussed for tenderness and mobility
  - —Dental numeric system used in adults
    - -Maxillary: right to left 1–16; mandibular: left to right 17–32

LABORATORY

- None needed except for signs of systemic toxicity or deep fascial space infections

IMAGING/SPECIAL TESTS

- Periapical x-rays and Panorex if deeper abscess suspected
- CT scan of the orofacial area and neck if deep fascial space infection suspected

DIFFERENTIAL DIAGNOSIS

Nonodontogenic

- Sinusitis
- Otitis media
- Pharyngitis
- Peritonsillar abscess
- Temporomandibular joint (TMJ) syndrome (usually present with pain around the ear)
- Trigeminal neuralgia
- Vascular headache
- Herpes zoster
- Myocardial infarction

PEDIATRIC CONSIDERATIONS

- Tooth eruption in an infant or child may cause oral pain, irritability, low-grade fevers, diarrhea, and decreased food intake

Treatment

INITIAL STABILIZATION

- Airway management for deep-space infection and airway compromise
- Early pain management as indicated

ED TREATMENT

- Appropriate analgesia
- Dental anesthetic field block
  —Injected along the buccal surface of the affected tooth
  —Specific nerve block for multiple teeth
  —Long-acting anesthetic (e.g., bupivacaine)
- Antibiotics if dental infection is present
  —Penicillin is the antibiotic of choice
  —Clindamycin for penicillin allergy or for predominance of anaerobes
  —Erythromycin and other macrolides are third-line agents
- Localized periapical and periodontal abscesses should be incised, drained, and irrigated
  —Drain may be placed for 24 hours
- Saline rinses at home four times a day and dental referral in 24 hours

MEDICATIONS

- Antibiotics
  —Clindamycin: 150–450 mg PO q6h (peds: 25–30 mg/kg/24 h [max, 2 g] q6h)
  —Erythromycin: 500 mg PO q6h (peds: 30–50 mg/kg/24 h [max, 2 g] q6h)
  —Penicillin VK: 500 mg PO q6h (peds: 25–50 mg/kg/24 h [max, 3 g] q6h
- Analgesics
  —Acetaminophen: 650–1,000 mg PO q4h (peds: 15 mg/kg/dose q4h)
  —Acetaminophen and codeine #3: 1–2 tabs PO q4–6h (peds: elixir: codeine 12 mg/5 mL)
  —Acetaminophen and oxycodone: 1–2 tab PO q6h (peds: 0.05–0.15 mg/kg/dose [max, 10 mg])
  —Ibuprofen: 400–800 mg PO q8h (peds: 10 mg/kg PO q6h)
  —Ketorolac: adults: 30 mg i.v., 60 mg i.m. q6h (peds: 1 mg/kg/dose i.m.)
  —Morphine sulfate: 2–8 mg SQ or i.v. q2h (peds: 0.1 mg/kg/dose SQ or i.v. q2h)

PEDIATRIC CONSIDERATION

- Teething infants may be helped by over-the-counter topical anesthetics

Disposition

ADMISSION CRITERIA

- Severe facial swelling
- Suspicion of deep fascial space infections (e.g., Ludwig's angina, retropharyngeal abscess)
- Facial cellulitis proximal to the eye
- Extensive trismus
- Dehydration
- Evidence of systemic toxicity

DISCHARGE CRITERIA

- Toothaches and localized dental infections can be discharged from the ED

Miscellaneous

ICD9: 525.9

ICD10: K08.8

SUGGESTED READINGS

Amsterdam JT. Dental disorders. In: Rosen P, et al., eds. Emergency medicine: concepts and clinical practice. St. Louis: Mosby–Year Book, 2002:2680–2697.

Heir GM. Facial pain of dental origin: a review for physicians. Headache 1987; 27(10):540–547.

Hodgdon A. Toothache and common periodontal problems. In: Harwood-Nuss A, ed. The clinical practice of emergency medicine. Philadelphia: Lippincott Williams & Wilkins, 2001:75–78.

Klokkevold P. Common dental emergencies: evaluation and management for emergency physicians. Emerg Med Clin North Am 1989;7(1):29–63.

Author: Colin B. Devonshire

Torticollis

Clinical Presentation

SIGNS AND SYMPTOMS

- Intermittent painful spasms of sternocleidomastoid (SCM), trapezius, and other neck muscles
- Head is rotated and twisted to one direction
- Pure flexion (anterocollis) or extension (retrocollis) is *rare*
  - —Represents symmetric involvement of muscles
- Neck movements vary from jerky to smooth
- Symptoms usually aggravated by standing, walking, or stressful situations
- Usually does not occur with sleep
- Congenital form
  - —First sign may be a firm, nontender, enlargement of the SCM muscle visible at birth
- Psychological factors (e.g., depression, anxiety) may play a role

MECHANISM/DESCRIPTION

- "Twisted neck"
- A fixed or dynamic posturing of the head and neck in tilt, rotation, and flexion
- Synonym: cervical dystonia

ETIOLOGY

Local

- Acute wry neck
  - —Develops overnight without provocation
  - —Most prevalent
  - —Self-limited, symptoms resolve in 1–2 weeks
- Cervical spine
  - —Fracture
  - —Dislocation, subluxation
  - —Infections
  - —Spondylosis
  - —Tumor
  - —Scar tissue–producing injuries
  - —Ligamentous laxity in atlantoaxial region
- Inflammatory disease causing muscular damage
  - —Myositis
  - —Lymphadenitis
  - —Tuberculosis
- Infections of surrounding soft tissues
  - —Nasopharyngeal abscess
  - —Retropharyngeal abscess
  - —Cervical adenitis
  - —Tonsillitis
  - —Mastoiditis
  - —Sinusitis
  - —Posttrauma

Compensatory

- Tilt with essential head tremor (patient tilts head to suppress tremor)
- Ocular muscle palsy

Central

- Idiopathic spasmodic torticollis
  - —Female >male
  - —Onset 31–60 years old
- Dystonias
  - —Torsion dystonia
  - —Generalized tardive dystonia
  - —Wilson's disease
  - —L-Dopa therapy
  - —Acute (neuroleptic drugs)

PEDIATRIC CONSIDERATIONS

Local

- Congenital
  - —Odontoid hypoplasia
  - —Hemivertebrae
  - —Spina bifida
  - —Arnold-Chiari syndrome
  - —Pseudotumor of infancy
  - —Hypertrophy or absence of cervical musculature
- Otolaryngologic
  - —Vestibular dysfunction
  - —Otitis media
  - —Cervical adenitis
  - —Pharyngitis
  - —Retropharyngeal abscess
  - —Pharyngitis
  - —Mastoiditis
- Esophageal reflux
- Syrinx with spinal cord tumor
- Trauma
  - —Cervical fracture/dislocation
  - —Clavicular fractures
- Juvenile rheumatoid arthritis

Compensatory

- Strabismus (fourth cranial nerve paresis)
- Congenital nystagmus
- Posterior fossa tumor

Central

- Dystonias
  - —Torsion dystonia
  - —Drug induced
  - —Cerebral palsy

Pre-Hospital

- Ensure patent airway
- Cervical spine precautions for any history of trauma
- Support head

Diagnosis

ESSENTIAL WORKUP

- Geared toward diagnosing life-threatening etiologies above
- Distinguish torticollis from other causes of neck stiffness (meningismus)
- Good medication/ingestion history
- *Cervical spine films* to evaluate for fracture except patients with chronic paroxysmal episodes

LABORATORY

- No specific tests helpful

IMAGING/SPECIAL TESTS

- CT or MRI of cervical spine diagnostic of retropharyngeal abscess, tumor

DIFFERENTIAL DIAGNOSIS

- CNS infections
- Tumors of soft tissue or bone
- Basal ganglia disease
- Abscess of cervical glands
- Myositis of cervical muscles
- Cervical disk lesions

Treatment

INITIAL STABILIZATION

- Cervical spine immobilization if fracture is suspected
- If airway management is necessary, RSI/paralytics is procedure of choice

ED TREATMENT

- Drug (e.g., phenothiazine) induced
  - —Diphenhydramine or benztropine
- Acquired
  - —If less than 1 week in duration, recommend soft collar and rest
  - —If less than 1 month in duration, consult orthopedics for possible traction
- Miscellaneous
  - —Physical therapy
  - —Massage
  - —Local heat
  - —Analgesics
  - —Sensory biofeedback
  - —Transepidermal neurostimulation (TENS)
  - —Surgery

MEDICATIONS

- Benztropine (for drug-related dystonia): 1–2 mg i.m. or slow i.v., followed by 3–5 days PO
- Botulinum toxin A (used for failed drug therapy): 50–200 IU i.m.
- Clonazepam (second-line drug): 0.5 mg PO t.i.d.
- Diphenhydramine (for drug-related dystonia): 25–50 mg i.v. or i.m., followed by 3–5 days PO (peds: 5 mg/kg/24 h div q6h i.v., i.m., or PO)
- Trihexyphenidyl (a first-line drug): 2–5 mg/d PO, advance to 30 mg/d
- Valium: 2–5 mg i.v., 2–10 mg PO t.i.d. (peds: 0.1–0.2 mg/kg/dose i.v. or PO q6h)

PEDIATRIC CONSIDERATIONS

- Congenital
  - —Operative division of involved muscle if physical therapy (e.g., passive stretching) is unsuccessful by 1 year of age

Disposition

ADMISSION CRITERIA

- Cervical spine fracture
- Diagnosis is in doubt
- Infectious causes
- Toxic appearance
- Unable to maintain adequate fluid intake
- No support system

DISCHARGE CRITERIA

- None of the above and symptoms adequately controlled with oral meds

Miscellaneous

ICD9: 723.5

ICD10: M43.6

SUGGESTED READINGS

Dauer WT, Burke RE, Greene P, et al. Current concepts on the clinical features, aetiology and management of idiopathic cervical dystonia. Brain 1998;121:547–560.

Duane DD. Spasmodic torticollis. Adv Neurol 1988;49:135–150.

Kahn ML, Davidson R, Drummond DS. Acquired torticollis in children. Orthop Rev 1991;20:667–674.

Smith DL, DeMario MC. Spasmodic torticollis: a case report and review of therapies. J Am Board Fam Pract 1996;9: 435–441.

Author: Andrew Chang

Toxic Epidermal Necrolysis

Clinical Presentation

SIGNS AND SYMPTOMS

- Prodrome: 2 to 3 days of low-grade fever, erythema, cutaneous tenderness, anorexia, malaise, myalgias, arthralgias, conjunctivitis, pruritus, pharyngitis, dysuria, vomiting, and diarrhea
- Mucous membranes: commonly affected 1–3 days before skin lesions (oropharynx >eyes >genitalia >anus)
- Skin: rash usually begins on face (scalp usually spared) and trunk as erythematous macules, irregular target-like bullae, or diffuse ill-defined erythema; widespread epidermolysis, denuding of skin surfaces, flaccid bullae, and sheetlike sloughing of epidermis generally progress over 3–4 days, but can progress rapidly over hours
  - —Nikolsky's sign—the separation of epidermis from dermis (the skin denudes and sloughs) with lateral pressure on the skin
- Ocular lesions (pseudomembranes, synechiae or adhesions, keratitis, corneal erosions)

MECHANISM/DESCRIPTION

- One of the most fulminant and potentially fatal of all dermatologic disorders
- Skin sloughing at the dermal-epidermal interface results in the equivalent of a second-degree burn; can affect up to 100% of total body surface area (TBSA)
- May extend to involve GI mucosa (esophagitis, GI bleeding), respiratory mucosa (dyspnea, bronchial hypersecretion, respiratory failure), and renal epithelium (glomerulonephritis)
- Thought to be a combination of type III and IV hypersensitivity reactions
- Classification system is controversial; one view is that toxic epidermal necrolysis (TEN) is the extreme presentation in continuum of erythema multiforme (EM)/Stevens-Johnson syndrome (SJS)/TEN
  - —<10% TBSA coverage constitutes SJS, 10–30% overlap zone, >30% TEN
- More common in elderly patients (more medications), HIV patients (more medications, immunocompromised), and bone marrow transplant recipients
- Mortality rate is about 25%, usually from secondary infection
- Prognostic factors include neutropenia, age, TBSA, BUN, need for mechanical ventilation

ETIOLOGY

- Dose-independent drug reactions are the usual cause of TEN
  - —Drugs introduced within 1–3 weeks are most likely candidates
  - —Frequently implicated drugs include sulfonamides, anticonvulsants, NSAIDs, penicillins, allopurinol, hydantoins
- Others: infections (systemic herpes, mycoplasmal infections), graft-versus-host disease, malignancies, immunizations, idiopathic cases (4%)

Pre-Hospital

CAUTIONS

- Transport to facility with burn center
- Gentle care during transport to avoid skin trauma
- IV catheter avoided for short transport if hemodynamically stable (more sterile conditions in ED)
- Avoid adhesive material

Diagnosis

ESSENTIAL WORKUP

- Diagnosis is made clinically
  - —Based on history and characteristic skin and mucous membrane lesions
- Ophthalmology consultation for evaluation and removal of pseudomembranes and adhesions

LABORATORY

- No confirmatory laboratory tests
- CBC: normocytic anemia, leukocytosis, lymphopenia/neutropenia, thrombocytopenia may be present
- Electrolyte derangements if extensive fluid losses
- Prerenal azotemia
- Urinalysis may show hematuria (urethral mucosal erosion, glomerulonephritis) or casts (acute tubular necrosis [ATN])
- Erythrocyte sedimentation rate (ESR) may be elevated secondary to systemic inflammation

IMAGING/SPECIAL TESTS

- Biopsy by consulting dermatologist to rule out autoimmune bullous diseases, staphylococcal scalded skin syndrome (SSSS), and other diagnoses
  - —Results not immediately available to ED physician
- Patch test being developed but usefulness is limited
- Chest x-ray if pneumonitis is suspected

DIFFERENTIAL DIAGNOSIS

- Staphylococcal scalded skin syndrome (SSSS)
- Stevens-Johnson syndrome (SJS): affects <10% of TBSA
- Autoimmune bullous diseases (pemphigus vulgaris, bullous pemphigoid)
- Scarlet fever
- Toxic shock syndrome
- Chemical or thermal scalds
- Kawasaki syndrome
- Differentiation of TEN from SSSS
  - —*Mucous membranes:* involved with TEN and usually absent with SSSS
  - —*Skin cleavage:* Dermal-epidermal junction in TEN; intraepidermally in SSSS (both can exhibit a positive Nikolsky's sign)
  - —*Pain:* painful in TEN; painless in SSSS
  - —*Age:* TEN is generally a disease of adults (but may occur in children); SSSS primarily affects children
  - —*Etiology:* TEN most often represents an idiosyncratic, drug-induced, dose-independent reaction and hence does not require treatment with antibiotics; SSSS is the result of an infection and requires antibiotics

Treatment

INITIAL STABILIZATION

- ABCs
- If intubation is required, gentle technique to minimize mucosal damage
- Peripheral IV preferred over central line
- Cardiac monitor, pulse oximeter, nasogastric tube, Foley catheter
- Meticulous sterile technique

ED TREATMENT

- Identify and stop any causative medication
- Aggressive fluid resuscitation with lactated Ringer's solution as in burn care (Parkland formula)
  —Keep urine output >0.5 mL/kg/h
- Pain control with IV opiates
- Warming measures and frequent core temperature evaluation
- Antibiotics are usually withheld because TEN is usually drug induced
- If available, cover with biologic dressings (e.g., Biobrane)
  —Reduce pain, decrease caloric and evaporative losses, facilitate healing
- Antibiotic drops to eyes
- Timely admission to burn unit/ICU
- Timely dermatology and ophthalmology consultation
- Prophylactic antibiotics are not recommended because the cause of TEN is usually drug related
- Systemic corticosteroids are no longer recommended
  —Retrospective studies show no benefit and suggest greater risk for death from infection

MEDICATIONS

- Cyclosporine: 3 mg/kg/day may result in more rapid reepithelialization and less probability of multiorgan failure
- Cyclophosphamide: 100–300 mg/d
- Intravenous immunoglobulin: 0.2–0.4 g/kg/d; disease progression was rapidly reversed in 10 patients

Disposition

ADMISSION CRITERIA

- All patients with suspected TEN should be admitted
- Transfer to facility with burn unit has been shown to improve outcome
- If transfer is not possible or burn unit is unavailable, then admit to ICU

DISCHARGE CRITERIA

N/A

Miscellaneous

ASSOCIATED CONDITIONS

- Sepsis
- Disseminated intravascular coagulation (DIC)
- Pneumonia
- ATN
- Shock
- Impaired thermoregulation

SYNONYMS

- Lyell's syndrome
- Fixed drug necrolysis
- Epidermolysis necroticans combustiformis
- Epidermolysis bullosa

ICD9: 695.1

ICD10: L51.2

SUGGESTED READINGS

Becker DS. Toxic epidermal necrolysis. Lancet 1998;351(9113):1417–1420.

Craven NM. Management of toxic epidermal necrolysis. Hosp Med 2000;61:778–781.

Ringheanu M, Laude TA. Toxic epidermal necrolysis in children—an update. Clin Pediatr 2000;39:687–694.

Smoot EC 3rd. Treatment issues in the care of patients with toxic epidermal necrolysis. Burns 1999;25:439–442.

Stella M, Cassano P, Bollero D, et al. Toxic epidermal necrolysis treated with intravenous high-dose immunoglobulins: our experience. Dermatology 2001;203(1): 45–49.

Viard I, Wehrli P, Bullani R, et al. Inhibition of toxic epidermal necrolysis by blockade of CD95 with human intravenous immunoglobulin. Science 1998;16(282): 490–493.

Wolkenstein P, Revuz J. Toxic epidermal necrolysis. Dermatol Clin 2000;18:485–495.

Authors: Stephen Anderson; Andrew Chang

Toxic Shock Syndrome

Clinical Presentation

SIGNS AND SYMPTOMS

Criteria for Diagnosis

- Fever >38.9°C
- Hypotension (systolic BP <90 mm Hg) or shock
- Diffuse, blanching nonpruritic macular erythroderma rash with subsequent desquamation 5–12 days after the resolution of rash (painless "sunburn")
- Clinical involvement of *at least three* of the following
  —Renal
    -Increase in BUN and creatinine 2 times normal or
    -Sterile pyuria without evidence of infection
  —Hepatic
    -Total BR, alanine transaminase (ALT), aspartate transaminase (AST) elevated to more than 2 times normal values
  —Hematologic
    -Thrombocytopenia <100,000/mm^3
  —Gastrointestinal
    -Profuse diarrhea or
    -Vomiting
  —Musculoskeletal
    -Severe myalgias or
    -Twofold increase in creatine phosphokinase (CPK)
  —Mucosal inflammation
    -Conjunctival, vaginal, or pharyngeal hyperemia
  —CNS
    -Disorientation, confusion, or hallucinations

Other

- Tachycardia
- Hyperemic mucous membranes
- Pharyngitis/conjunctivitis
- Can rapidly progress to multisystem dysfunction
- Associated with tampon use in menstruating females usually between the third and fifth day of menses
- Fatality rate: 2.7%

MECHANISM/DESCRIPTION

- Severe acute life-threatening illness caused by toxin-producing strains of *Staphylococcus aureus*
- Exotoxin, toxic shock syndrome toxin (TSST-1)
  —Produced by 20% of *S. aureus* isolates
  —Significant factor in the production of symptoms associated with toxic shock syndrome (TSS)
- Biologic properties of TSST-1 include the ability to
  —Induce fever directly on the hypothalamus or indirectly via interleukin-1 (IL-1) and tumor necrosis factor (TNF) production
  —Promote T-lymphocyte superantigenization and overstimulation
  —Induce interferon production
  —Enhance delayed hypersensitivity
  —Suppress neutrophil migration and immunoglobulin
  —Enhance host susceptibility to endotoxins
- Massive vasodilation occurs
  —Causes rapid movement of serum proteins and fluids from the intravascular to the extravascular space

ETIOLOGY

- Initially a disease of young, healthy menstruating females
- 25% of nonmenstruating TSS associated with postpartum *S. aureus* vaginal infections
- Males constitute one third of patients with TSS
- *S. aureus* enters the body in TSS in a variety of clinical settings
  —Nasal packing (nasal tampons)
  —Surgical wounds and infected abrasions
  —20–40% of the adult population carries *S. aureus* in the nasal vestibule

Pre-Hospital

CAUTIONS

- Fluid resuscitation as for hypovolemia or septic shock

Diagnosis

ESSENTIAL WORKUP

- Clinical diagnosis using diagnostic criteria with the absence of other causes of illness

LABORATORY

- CBC
- Electrolytes, BUN, creatinine, glucose
  —Elevated BUN and creatinine
- Calcium, magnesium
  —Hypocalcemia/hypomagnesemia often present
- Urinalysis
  —Normal or sterile pyuria without evidence of infection
- Arterial blood gas (ABG)
- CPK
  —Two-fold increase
- Hepatic function
  —Elevated total bilirubin, AST, ALT
- Prothrombin time (PT), partial thromboplastin time (PTT), platelets
  —Thrombocytopenia <100,000 platelets/mm^3
- Blood, urine, throat, and CSF cultures as indicated

IMAGING/SPECIAL TESTS

- Chest x-ray
- Investigation of other etiologies
  —Serology for Rocky Mountain spotted fever (RMSF), rubeola, and leptospirosis
  —VDRL
  —Monospot
  —Antinuclear antibody
  —Hepatitis B surface antigen

DIFFERENTIAL DIAGNOSIS

- Staphylococcal scalded skin syndrome
  - —In children <5 years old
  - —Initial macular rash followed by the formation of ill-defined bullae that can be rubbed off revealing a shiny, moist, glistening epidermis (Nikolsky's sign)
- Scarlet fever
  - —Preceding streptococcal pharyngitis
  - —Rash begins on the upper chest, neck, and back spreading to the remainder of the trunk, sparing the palms and soles
  - —Hypotension absent
- Kawasaki disease
  - —Fever, conjunctival hyperemia, and erythema of the mucous membranes
  - —Not associated with renal failure, hypotension, or thrombocytopenia
- Stevens-Johnson syndrome
  - —Severe, multisystem involvement
  - —Mucosal involvement prominent with involvement of the mouth, conjunctivae, vagina, anus, and urethral meatus
- Leptospirosis
  - —Transmitted through contact with infected animals
  - —Fever, headache, severe myalgias, and conjunctivitis
  - —Truncal rash that only desquamates in children
- RMSF
  - —Rash is pink and macular, beginning on the wrists, palms, ankles, and soles of the feet spreading to the trunk and face
  - —Petechiae appear after 4 days

Treatment

INITIAL STABILIZATION

- ABCs
  - —Adult respiratory distress syndrome (ARDS) may complicate TSS and require mechanical ventilation with positive end-expiratory pressure
- Aggressive management of circulatory shock with IV fluids and pressors

ED TREATMENT

- Management depends on severity

Hypotension

- Aggressive fluid replacement
  - —During the first 24 hours may require 4–20 L of crystalloid and fresh-frozen plasma (colloid)
  - —*Caution:* large amounts of IV fluids and pressor agents used to treat refractory hypotension can result in the rapid onset of pulmonary edema
  - —Pressors (dopamine) if fluid correction fails to restore normal arterial pressure

Infection Management

- Search for and treat the focus of infection
- Remove the source of infection (e.g., tampon, nasal, or wound packing)
- Some authorities recommend women with tampon-related TSS to have vaginal irrigation with saline or povidone-iodine solution
- Early surgical/gynecologic consultation if drainage or débridement of infectious sites necessary
- Antibiotics
  - —Recommended but have not been shown to not alter the course
  - —Antibiotic choices
    - -Clindamycin (preferred)
    - -β-Lactamase-resistant penicillins (nafcillin or excelling)
    - -Cefazolin
    - -Vancomycin
- Intravenous immunoglobulin (IVIG) treatment
  - —Initiate if no response to fluids, pressors, and antibiotics in patients with pulmonary edema and hypotension

MEDICATIONS

- Cefazolin (Ancef): 1 g (peds: 50–100 mg/kg/24 h) i.v. q6h
- Clindamycin: 600–900 mg (peds: 20–40 mg/kg/24 h) i.v. q6–8h
- Dopamine: 2–20 μg/kg/min i.v., titrate to BP
- Nafcillin: 1.5 g (peds: 100 mg/kg/24 h) i.v. q4h
- Oxacillin: 1–2 g (peds: 50–100 mg/kg/24 h) i.v. q4h
- Vancomycin: 500 mg (peds: 10 mg/kg) i.v. q6h

Disposition

ADMISSION CRITERIA

- ICU admission for critically ill/shock

DISCHARGE CRITERIA

- None

Miscellaneous

ICD9: 785.5, 785.59

ICD10: A48.3

SUGGESTED READINGS

Centers for Disease Control and Prevention. Toxic-shock syndrome—United States. MMWR Morb Mortal Wkly Rep 1999;48 (LMRK):60–70.

Hauser AR. Another toxic shock syndrome: streptococcal infection is even more dangerous than the staphylococcal form. Postgrad Med 1998;104:31–43.

Marx JA, et al., eds. Rosen's emergency medicine clinical practice, 5th ed. St. Louis: Mosby, 2002:1806–1810.

Author: Lawrence Heiskell

Toxoplasmosis

Clinical Presentation

SIGNS AND SYMPTOMS

- Four types of infection

Immunocompromised Host

CNS

- Subacute presentation (90%)
- Encephalitis
- Headache
- Altered mental status
- Fever
- Seizures
- Cranial nerve palsies
- Spinal cord lesions
- Cerebellar signs
- Meningitis-like symptoms
- Movement disorders
- Neuropsychological symptoms
  - —Psychosis
  - —Paranoia
  - —Dementia
  - —Anxiety
  - —Agitation

Pulmonary

- Pneumonitis
- Prolonged febrile illness
- Nonproductive cough
- Dyspnea

Immunocompetent Host

- 10% with symptoms
- Lymphadenopathy
- Fever
- Malaise
- Headache
- Sore throat
- Night sweats
- Maculopapular rash
- Urticaria
- Self-limited process; resolves in 2–12 months
- Rarely presents with pneumonitis or encephalitis

Ocular Toxoplasmosis

- Blurred vision
- Scotoma
- Pain
- Photophobia
- Retina
  - —Small clusters of yellow-white, cotton-like patches

Congenital Toxoplasmosis

- Results from an asymptomatic acute infection during pregnancy
- First trimester
  - —Spontaneous abortion
  - —Stillbirth
  - —Severe disease up to 25% of the time
- Second or third trimester
  - —50–60% chance of acquiring congenital toxoplasmosis
  - —2% fatal
- Most asymptomatic at birth
- Delayed onset
  - —CNS disease
  - —Ocular disease (blindness months–years later)
  - —Lymphadenopathy
  - —Hepatosplenomegaly

MECHANISM/DESCRIPTION

- *Toxoplasma gondii*—intracellular protozoan parasite
  - —Three forms
    - -Tachyzoite: asexual invasive form
    - -Tissue cyst: persists in tissues of infected hosts during chronic phase
    - -Oocyst: contains sporozoites and produced during sexual cycle in cat intestine
- Transmission
  - —Ingesting tissue cysts or oocysts
    - -Ingesting undercooked meat
    - -Vegetables contaminated with oocysts
    - -Contact with cat feces, through cat or soil
  - —Transplacental
  - —Blood product
  - —Organ transplantation

ETIOLOGY

- 70% of adults seropositive
- Asymptomatic in most immunocompetent patients
- Chorioretinitis
  - —Usually secondary to congenital transmission
  - —Does not become symptomatic until 20–30 years of age

Pre-Hospital

N/A

Diagnosis

ESSENTIAL WORKUP

- Diagnose via
  - —Isolation of organism
    - -Blood
    - -CSF for encephalitis
    - -Bronchoalveolar lavage for pneumonitis
    - -Amniotic fluid
    - -Aqueous humor
  - —Detection of tachyzoites in tissues or body fluids
  - —Demonstrating characteristic lymph node pathology
- Thorough ocular examination
  - —Retinal examination
  - —Visual acuity

LABORATORY

- CBC
  - —Atypical lymphocytes
- Arterial blood gas (ABG)/pulse oximetry for pulmonary symptoms

IMAGING/SPECIAL TESTS

- Chest x-ray for pulmonary symptoms
- CT head with contrast
  - —Multiple bilateral hypodense ring enhancing lesions
- MRI brain
  - —High signal abnormalities on T2-weighted images
- Immunoglobulin M (IgM) antibodies
  - —Absence excludes diagnosis in immunocompetent host
  - —Diagnoses acute infection
  - —Appear in 5 days
  - —Disappear in weeks–months
  - —Neonatal testing differentiates from maternal infection
- IgG antibodies
  - —High number of false-positive and false-negative results
  - —Common tests
    - -Sabin-Feldman dye test
    - -Indirect fluorescent antibody
    - -Agglutination
    - -Enzyme-linked immunosorbent assay (ELISA) test
- Brain biopsy for encephalitis—definitive diagnosis

DIFFERENTIAL DIAGNOSIS

- Cryptococcal meningitis
- CNS lymphoma
- *Pneumocystis carinii* pneumonia
- Cytomegalovirus retinitis

Treatment

Initial Stabilization

- Treat seizures in standard fashion with diazepam and phenytoin
- Initiate oxygen if hypoxia due to pneumonitis

ED TREATMENT

Immunocompetent

- Toxoplasmic lymphadenitis
  —No antibiotics unless symptoms severe and persistent
- Treat symptomatic patients with
  —Pyrimethamine and folinic acid plus sulfadiazine or clindamycin for 2–4 weeks
  —Reassess to determine if longer therapy needed

Immunocompromised

- Confirmed acute infection by serology/symptoms
  —Treat with pyrimethamine and folinic acid plus sulfadiazine or clindamycin for 4–6 weeks after resolution of symptoms
  —Alternative medications
    -Trimethoprim-sulfamethoxazole
    -Pyrimethamine and folinic acid plus dapsone
- CNS symptoms plus a lesion on CT or MRI
  —Treat empirically with pyrimethamine and folinic acid plus sulfadiazine or clindamycin
  —Brain biopsy or CSF to confirm diagnosis
  —Administer anticonvulsants only if confirmed prior seizures
    -Poorer outcome for patients on anticonvulsants
- Chronic asymptomatic infection
  —No therapy required
  —Prophylaxis options for toxoplasmosis in AIDS patients
    -Trimethoprim-sulfamethoxazole: 1 tablet daily or 2 tablets twice a week
    -Pyrimethamine (75 mg/week) and dapsone (200 mg/week)
    -Fansidar (pyrimethamine-sulfadoxine) 3 tablets every 2 weeks

Ocular

- Treat with pyrimethamine and sulfadiazine for 1 month
  —May add clindamycin
- Administer systemic steroids with macula or optic nerve involvement

Acute Acquired Infection in Pregnancy

- Initially treat with spiramycin pending confirmatory tests
- After the infection is documented, initiate treatment with
  —Sulfadiazine in the first 16 weeks
  —Pyrimethamine and sulfadiazine after 16 weeks
- Studies suggest maternal-fetal transmission is rapid and treatment may have little effect
- Treat congenital infection with sulfadiazine, pyrimethamine, and folinic acid for 12 months

MEDICATIONS

- Clindamycin
  —600 mg (peds: 20–40 mg/kg/24 h) i.v. q6h
  —300 mg (peds: 8–20 mg/kg/24 h) PO q6h
- Dapsone: 100 mg PO daily
- Folinic acid: 5–10 mg PO daily in conjunction with pyrimethamine
- Pyrimethamine: 100 mg b.i.d. on first day loading dose, then 25–50 mg PO daily (peds: 1 mg/kg/24 h PO b.i.d. for 1–2 days, then 0.5 mg/kg/24 h)
- Sulfadiazine: 500 mg–2 g (peds: 100–200 mg/kg/24 h) PO q6h
- Trimethoprim-sulfamethoxazole: 5 mg/kg of trimethoprim component IV or PO q6h

Disposition

ADMISSION CRITERIA

- Acute infection with severe systemic symptoms
- Immunocompromised patients with
  —Toxoplasmosis encephalitis
  —Pneumonitis
  —Sepsis

DISCHARGE CRITERIA

- Immunocompetent patients with
  —Mild symptoms
  —Ocular
- Maternal/congenital infection with mild symptoms

Miscellaneous

ICD9: 130.9

ICD10: B58.9

SUGGESTED READINGS

Chang HR. The potential role of azithromycin in the treatment of prophylaxis of toxoplasmosis. Int J STD AIDS 1996;(Suppl 1):18–22.

Fung HB, Kirschenbaum HL. Treatment regimens for patients with toxoplasmic encephalitis. Clin Ther 1996;18: 1037–1056.

Ramsey RG, Bean AD. Neuroimaging of AIDS. I. Central nervous system toxoplasmosis. Neuroimaging Clin North Am 1997;7:171–186.

Rodriguez JC, Martinez MM, et al. Evaluation of different techniques in the diagnosis of toxoplasma encephalitis. J Med Microbiol 1997;46:597–601.

Subauste CS, Remington JS. In: Bennet JC, Plum F, eds. Cecil's textbook of medicine. Philadelphia: WB Saunders, 1996:1907.

Author: Kathryn Brinsfield

Transfusion Complications

Clinical Presentation

SIGNS AND SYMPTOMS

General

- Fever
- Chills
- Burning at infusion site
- Urticaria/pruritus/skin erythema
- Anaphylaxis—occurs in 1 of 20,000 transfusions

Pulmonary

- Dyspnea
- Bronchospasm
- Respiratory distress/failure

Cardiovascular

- Tachycardia
- Hypotension
- Substernal chest pain/tightness

GI

- Nausea
- Vomiting
- Diarrhea

Hematologic

- Bleeding
- Hemoglobinuria
- Oozing from surgical wounds
- Jaundice
- Disseminated intravascular coagulation (DIC)

Miscellaneous

- Low back pain
- Renal failure (oliguria/anuria)

MECHANISM/DESCRIPTION

Acute Intravascular Hemolytic Transfusion Reaction

- Mortality and morbidity correlate with the amount of incompatible blood transfused
- Occurs immediately from
  —ABO incompatibility
  —Blood type identification error
  —Incompatible transfused cells immediately destroyed by antibodies
- Intravascular hemolysis causing activation of the coagulation system leading to inflammation, shock, and DIC
- Mediators (cytokines) released during inflammatory response
- Renal failure
  —Cytokines cause local release of endothelin in kidney causing vasoconstriction
  —Leads to parenchymal ischemia and acute renal failure
- Respiratory failure due to pulmonary edema/adult respiratory distress syndrome (ARDS)
  —Free hemoglobin (Hb) causes vasoconstriction in pulmonary vasculature

Other Transfusion-Related Complications

- Hemolysis due to Rh incompatibility
  —Mild, self-limiting
  —1/200 units transfused
- Febrile nonhemolytic transfusion reaction
  —Temperature increases at least 1°C, with chills
  —Antigen-antibody reaction to transfused blood components (WBCs, platelets, plasma)
  —Usually mild
  —Occurs with multiple transfusions or multiparous women
- Allergic transfusion reaction
  —Occur in 1% of transfusions
  —Usually seen with immunoglobulin A (IgA)-deficient patients

Delayed Reactions

- Infection
  —Blood screened for HIV, hepatitis B, hepatitis C
  —Blood treated to inactivate viruses
  —Risk for transmission
    -HIV: 1/150,000 units
    -Hepatitis B: 1/50,000 units
    -Hepatitis C: 1/10,000 units
- Delayed extravascular hemolytic reaction
  —Occurs 7–10 days after transfusion
  —Antigen-antibody reaction that develops after transfusion
  —Coombs' test is positive
  —Usually asymptomatic
  —Blood bank analysis detects antibody
- Noncardiogenic pulmonary edema
  —1/5,000 transfusions
  —Incompatibility of transfused WBC antibodies
  —Reaction develops within 4 hours of transfusion
- Electrolyte imbalance
  —Hypocalcemia: calcium binds to citrate
  —Hypokalemia: citrate metabolized to bicarbonate, which drives potassium intracellular
- Graft-versus-host disease
  —Usually fatal (>90%)
  —Immunologically competent lymphocytes transfused into immunoincompetent host
  —Host unable to destroy new WBCs
  —Donor WBCs recognize host as foreign and attack host's tissues

Pre-Hospital

N/A

Diagnosis

ESSENTIAL WORKUP

- Recognize clinical findings of transfusion reaction
- Recheck identifying information of blood and patient for compatibility

LABORATORY

- CBC
- Electrolytes, BUN, creatinine, glucose
  —For electrolyte abnormalities
- Prothrombin time (PT), partial thromboplastin time (PTT)
- Serum calcium
- Fibrinogen, fibrin degradation products
- Bilirubin (direct/indirect)
- Coombs' test
- Hemoglobinemia
  —Pink or red supernatant of plasma or serum indicates hemolysis
- Urinalysis
  —Hemoglobinuria: dipstick-positive blood without RBC on micro

Lab Findings Indicating Hemolysis

- Thrombocytopenia (<100,000)
- Fibrinogenopenia (<150 mg/L)
- Fibrin degradation products
- Prolonged activated PTT (aPTT)
- Spherocytosis

Lab Findings Indicating Hemolysis Due to Rh Incompatibility

- Coombs' test is positive
- Elevated indirect bilirubin
- Posttransfusion hemoglobin/hematocrit does not show expected rise

IMAGING/SPECIAL TESTS

- Chest x-ray: diffuse patchy infiltrates without cardiomegaly
- EKG for arrhythmia, signs of electrolyte abnormality

DIFFERENTIAL DIAGNOSIS

- Sepsis
- Anaphylaxis/allergic reaction due to medication

Treatment

INITIAL STABILIZATION

- Immediately stop the infusion
  - —Severity of reaction proportional to amount of blood infused
  - —ABCs
  - —Supplemental oxygen—intubation and ventilation if needed
- Recheck blood-identifying information—patient's bracelet, blood labels, call blood bank

ED TREATMENT

- Hypotension
  - —0.9% NS hydration with two large-bore IVs
  - —Trendelenburg's position
  - —Dopamine
- Prevention of renal failure
  - —Maintain urine output of 100 mL/h
  - —Adequate hydration
  - —Furosemide or mannitol if oliguric
  - —Dopamine infusion: 2 μg/kg/min
- Febrile reactions
  - —Antipyretics (acetaminophen/NSAID)
  - —Antihistamine (diphenhydramine) IV
  - —Steroids (Solu-Medrol)
- Allergic reactions
  - —Antihistamine (diphenhydramine) IV
  - —Epinephrine for respiratory symptoms
  - —Steroids (Solu-Medrol)
- Redraw blood sample for repeat ABO/Rh typing, direct antiglobulin testing
- Foley catheter to monitor urine output
- Replete calcium if hypocalcemia develops
- Treat DIC

MEDICATIONS

- Calcium gluconate: 10 mL of 10% (peds: 100 mg/kg/dose) solution slow i.v. push
- Dopamine: 2–20 μg/kg/min i.v.
- Diphenhydramine: 25–50 mg (peds: 1.25 mg/kg) i.m., i.v., or PO
- Epinephrine (1:1000): 0.3–0.5 mL (peds: 0.01 mL/kg) SC
- Mannitol: 1–2 g/kg i.v.
- Solu-Medrol: 125 mg (peds: 2 mg/kg) i.v.

Disposition

ADMISSION CRITERIA

- Acute hemolytic transfusion reaction, pulmonary complications, anaphylaxis, sepsis require ICU monitoring
- Delayed hemolytic transfusion reactions for evaluation/treatment

DISCHARGE CRITERIA

- Uncomplicated febrile or allergic reaction

Miscellaneous

ICD9: 999.8

ICD10: T80.9

SUGGESTED READINGS

Braunwald E, Isselbacher K, et al., eds. Harrison's principles of internal medicine, 15th ed. New York: McGraw-Hill, 2001.

Capon SM, Goldfinger D. Acute hemolytic transfusion reaction, a paradigm of the systemic inflammatory response: new insights into pathophysiology and treatment. Transfusion 1995;35(6):513–520.

Hoffman R, Benz E, Shattil S, et al., eds. Hematology: basic principles and practice, 3rd ed. New York: Churchill Livingstone, 2000.

Isersion KV. Transfusion reactions and complications. In: Harwood, Nuss A, eds. *Clinical practice of emergency medicine.* Philadelphia: Lippincott-Raven, 1996: 917–920.

Kruskall MS, Mintz PD, Bergin JJ, et al. Transfusion therapy in emergency medicine. Ann Emerg Med 1988;17:327–335.

Storer DI. Blood and blood component therapy. In: Rosen P, Barkin R, eds. Emergency medicine: concepts and clinical practice, 5th ed. St. Louis: CV Mosby, 2002.

Author: Marc Gelman

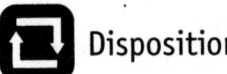

Transient Ischemic Attack

Clinical Presentation

SIGNS AND SYMPTOMS

- The vessel involved dictates neurologic deficits
- Motor and sensory symptoms—paralysis, weakness, clumsiness, numbness, and paresthesias
- Carotid artery (anterior circulation)
  - —Manifests signs and symptoms of both anterior cerebral artery (ACA) and middle cerebral artery (MCA)
- ACA
  - —Motor and sensory—contralateral leg greater than arm, can also involve face
  - —Speech—anarthria (speechlessness), dysarthria, perseveration
  - —Vision—amaurosis fugax, or blurred vision on one side of field of vision of both eyes opposite to side of diseased artery
  - —Contralateral neglect
- MCA
  - —Motor and sensory—contralateral arm and face greater than leg
  - —Speech—if dominant hemisphere involved—receptive or expressive aphasia, or both
  - —Mentation—inattention, neglect, apraxia
  - —Vision—homonymous hemianopsia, gaze preference to side of infarct
- Vertebrobasilar artery (posterior circulation)
  - —Hallmark—crossed neurologic deficits—ipsilateral cranial nerves deficits and contralateral motor weakness or crossed sensory deficits
  - —Vision—diplopia
  - —Other features: dizziness, vertigo, and dysphagia
  - —Wallenberg's syndrome—ipsilateral cranial nerve deficits, contralateral motor weakness, gait and limb ataxia, and incomplete Horner's syndrome (anhydrosis usually absent)
  - —"Drop attack"—sudden onset of inability to walk, often with vertigo, headache, neck pain, and nausea and vomiting

MECHANISM/DESCRIPTION

- Transient ischemic attack (TIA)—a temporary neurologic deficit that resolves within 24 hours (80% resolve in less than 30 minutes)
- Contrast with other ischemic neurologic conditions:
  - —Reversible ischemic neurologic deficit (RIND)—transient deficits lasting longer 24 hours but eventually resolves entirely
  - —Stroke in evolution—neurologic deficits that continue to worsen over minutes to hours
  - —Completed stroke—persistent deficit after 3 weeks despite improvement

ETIOLOGY

- Transient hypoperfusion of portion of brain from
  - —Embolus from heart or proximal atherosclerotic plaque
  - —Thrombus formation in involved vessel
  - —Vasculopathies—carotid or vertebral dissection
  - —Hypercoaguable states—antiphospholipid antibody syndrome and protein C and S deficiency

PEDIATRIC CONSIDERATIONS

- Etiology in children most commonly involves congenital heart disease, sickle cell anemia, meningitis, and acute and congenital hemiplegia of childhood
- Moyamoya disease—rare primary vascular disease defined by diffuse cerebral arterial narrowing that manifests as reoccurring TIAs

Pre-Hospital

CAUTIONS

- Initial assessment of neurologic deficits is crucial because they may completely resolve before arrival at ED
- Avoid glucose-containing fluids unless a low glucose level is confirmed

Diagnosis

ESSENTIAL WORKUP

- Neurologic evaluation that assesses level of consciousness, vision, cranial nerves, motor and sensory, coordination, speech, and signs of neglect
- Non contrast head CT to rule out hemorrhage
- Cardiac monitoring and EKG to diagnose atrial fibrillation, other cardiac abnormalities
- Glucose level

LABORATORY

- Hypoglycemia can manifest with neurologic deficits similar to that of stroke/TIA and therefore should be assessed early
- CBC: assess for anemia or signs of hyperviscosity (elevated hematocrit)
- Electrolytes: some abnormalities can mimic stroke or are common comorbid states of TIA
- Coagulation studies: as baseline for possible anticoagulation therapy
- Tox screen: particularly in younger symptomatic patients for cocaine or amphetamine induced ischemia
- EKG: check for atrial fibrillation and acute myocardial infarction (AMI)

IMAGING/SPECIAL TESTS

- Noncontrast head CT
  - —Has a sensitivity of greater than 90% for subarachnoid bleed
  - —Ischemic evidence on CT often does not appear unless imaged >6 hours after symptom onset
- Carotid duplex scan—indicated when a high-grade carotid obstruction is suspected or crescendo TIAs; it can detect stenosis of >60% but cannot distinguish 95% from 100% occlusion; positive findings would suggest candidacy for emergent carotid endarterectomy or anticoagulation
- EKG—may demonstrate cardioembolic phenomenon (mural thrombus, tumor, or valvular vegetation)
- MRI—Picks up ischemic changes earlier than CT but is less sensitive for hemorrhage; also is a better study for posterior bleeds
- Angiography—gold standard for detection of both stenosis and aneurysm of cerebral blood vessels; however, cost, availability, and invasiveness preclude its use; MRA in future may replace angiography as better study for posterior fossa and less invasive

DIFFERENTIAL DIAGNOSIS

- Subarachnoid/intracerebral hemorrhage
- Subdural/epidural hematoma
- Giant arteritis
- Air embolism
- Migraine headache
- Todd's paralysis
- Ménière's disease
- Brain tumor/mass
- Dementia
- Wernicke's encephalopathy
- Carotid dissection after neck trauma
- Hypoglycemia
- Diabetic ketoacidosis/hyperosmolar coma

PEDIATRIC CONSIDERATIONS

- Differential diagnosis in children includes
  —Severe dehydration with associated hypernatremia
  —Todd's paralysis
  —Moyamoya disease
  —Acute infantile hemiplegia

Treatment

INITIAL STABILIZATION

- Airway: support as needed
- Breathing: oxygen
- Circulation: careful hydration avoiding cerebral edema and decreased cerebral blood flow (CBF)

ED TREATMENT

- Hypertension—only severe (>220/120 mm Hg) should be treated with nitroprusside because it allows for careful titration but may increase intracranial pressure; labetalol and angiotensin-converting enzyme (ACE) inhibitors can be used for gradual pressure reduction
  —Be careful not to precipitously drop BP
- Early evaluation to prevent transient ischemia becoming infarct
- Neurology consult
- Anticoagulation—aspirin, heparin (may be used with neurology consultation if patient is having recurrent symptoms)
- Thrombolytic therapy—may be appropriate for those with progressive symptoms (see Cerebrovascular Accident)

MEDICATIONS

- Aspirin: 30 mg–1 g PO
- Heparin: 5000 IU SC q8–12h, or 5,000–7,500 IU i.v. bolus; 1,000 IU/h infusion
- Labetalol: 20 mg/min i.v. bolus, then 20–80 mg every 10 minutes, max, 300 mg; infusion 0.5–2 mg/min
- Mannitol: 1 g/kg over 20 minutes if impending herniation is suspected
- Nitroprusside: adults and peds: 0.25–10 μg/kg/min
- Thrombolytics: controversial in TIA; refer to institutional protocol

Disposition

ADMISSION CRITERIA

- New onset of TIA warrants admission for evaluation and workup
- Workup should include evaluation for a surgically reversible cause and medical treatment with anticoagulants

DISCHARGE CRITERIA

- Completely asymptomatic patients with extensively investigated condition may be discharged as long as appropriate follow-up is ensured

PEDIATRIC CONSIDERATIONS

- All children with TIA require admission for close monitoring of blood pressure, fluid status, and neurologic status in pediatric intensive care

Miscellaneous

PROGNOSIS

- 5–20% of those who experience a TIA will have a stroke in 1 month and 50% within 1 year
- High risk for recurrence: known high-grade lesion, cardioembolic source, crescendo TIA (3 TIAs in 72 hours), and TIAs despite antiplatelet therapy
- 30 mg–1 g of aspirin daily reduces risk of stroke by 20% after prior stroke or TIA

ICD9: 425.9

ICD10: G45.9

SUGGESTED READINGS

Albers GW, et al. Supplement to the guidelines for the management of transient ischemic attacks: a statement from the Ad Hoc Committee on Guidelines for the Management of Transient Ischemic Attacks, Stroke Council, American Heart Association. 1999.

Barsan WG, Kothari R. Stroke. In: Rosen P, et al., eds. Emergency medicine: concepts and clinical practice, 4th ed. St. Louis: Mosby–Year Book, 1998:2184–2195.

Scott PA, Barsan WG. Stroke, transient ischemic attack, and other central focal conditions. In: Tintinalli JE, et al., eds. Emergency medicine, 5th ed. New York: McGraw-Hill, 2000:1430–1439.

Authors: Catherine McLaren; Rebecca Smith-Coggins

Transplant Rejection

Clinical Presentation

SIGNS AND SYMPTOMS

Bone Marrow Transplant Rejection

- Systemic
  - —Fever
  - —Generalized wasting
- Respiratory
  - —Dyspnea
  - —Cough
  - —Chest pain
- Skin
  - —Rash
  - —Mucositis
  - —Keratoconjunctivitis,
- Gastrointestinal
  - —Dysphagia
  - —Abdominal pain
  - —Diarrhea
  - —Jaundice

REJECTION OF SOLID ORGAN TRANSPLANTS

- Kidney
  - —Progressive systemic hypertension
  - —Fever
  - —Swelling
  - —Tenderness over the allograft
  - —Decreased urine output
- Heart
  - —Fever: temperature >38°C
  - —Shortness of breath
  - —Rales
  - —Nausea, vomiting
  - —Chest pain
  - —Hypotension or poorly controlled hypertension
  - —New arrhythmia
- Lung
  - —Cough
  - —Dyspnea
  - —Fever
  - —Rales
  - —Rhonchi
- Liver
  - —Fever
  - —Right upper quadrant pain

MECHANISM/DESCRIPTION

Bone Marrow Transplant Rejection

- Respiratory insufficiency with pulmonary infiltrates and hypoxia
  - —Acute graft-versus-host disease (immune attack of donor marrow on lung tissue)
  - —Interstitial pneumonitis from cytomegalovirus (CMV) and *Pneumocystis, Aspergillus, Mycobacteria,* and *Nocardia* species infections
  - —Chronic graft-versus-host disease (incidence, 25–50% of patients)

Rejection of Solid Organ Transplants

- Kidney
  - —Early rejection caused by T and B lymphocytes, which attack microvasculature and impair graft perfusion
  - —Chronic rejection from progressive nephrosclerosis of renal vessels
- Heart
  - —Acute rejection occurs in 75–85% of patients within the first 3 months
  - —Chest pain is not related to ischemia because the heart is denervated
  - —Accelerated atherosclerosis, however, is the hallmark of chronic rejection and presents as congestive heart failure (CHF), ventricular dysrhythmias, hypotension, syncope, or sudden death
- Lung
  - —Rejection develops early
  - —Only 25–40% develop chronic rejection
  - —Diffuse infiltrates are seen in early acute rejection, but when rejection occurs >1 month after transplantation, radiographs may be normal or unchanged
  - —Chronic rejection mimics upper respiratory infection or bronchitis
  - —Transplanted lungs have impaired mucociliary clearance, depressed cough reflex (because transplanted lungs are denervated), and defective alveolar macrophages and are susceptible to infection
  - —CMV pneumonia is the most common pathogen in transplanted lungs
  - —The most common fungal infection is from aspergillus
- Liver
  - —Commonly follows reduction in immunosuppression regimen
  - —Ascending cholangitis can occur because the biliary stent is left in place for months after surgery and can be colonized

Pre-Hospital

CAUTIONS

- Avoid aggressive fluid resuscitation
  - —Administer what is necessary to maintain baseline state of hydration

Diagnosis

ESSENTIAL WORKUP

- CBC
- Blood cultures
- Urinalysis
- Chest x-ray

Kidney

- Electrolytes, BUN, creatinine
- Renal ultrasound

Heart

- EKG
  - —Commonly demonstrates two P waves because the native sinus node is left in place
  - —Decreased QRS voltage, new S3, or new CHF or atrial arrhythmias suggests rejection
- Arterial blood gas (ABG)
- Echocardiogram

Lung

- ABG
- Pulmonary function tests
- Bronchoscopy/biopsy

Liver

- Liver function tests
  - —Late acute rejection presents with elevated bilirubin and transaminases
- Ultrasound, CT
- Immunosuppressive medication levels (i.e., cyclosporine)

IMAGING/SPECIAL TESTS

- In consultation with appropriate specialist

DIFFERENTIAL DIAGNOSIS

- Infection
  - —Exposure before transplantation
    - -Tuberculosis
    - -Histoplasmosis
    - -Coccidioidomycosis
    - -Blastomycosis
    - -Strongyloides stercoralis
    - -Hepatitis B and C
    - -HIV
    - -CMV
    - -Epstein-Barr virus (EBV)
    - -Varicella zoster
    - -Herpes simplex
  - —Community-acquired exposure after transplantation
    - -Influenza
    - -Primary varicella
    - -Salmonellosis
    - -Tuberculosis
    - -Fungal infections
    - -Legionellosis
    - -Nocardiosis
    - -Cryptococcosis
    - -CMV
    - -EBV
  - —Nosocomial exposure
    - -Aspergillosis
    - -Legionellosis

Treatment

INITIAL STABILIZATION

- ABCs
- Shock state treated with IV fluids and pressor agents
- Treat hypertensive crisis like other hypertensive emergencies

ED TREATMENT

- For kidney, heart, lung and liver rejection, administer 500–1000 mg methylprednisolone i.v.
- Treatment decisions should be made in consultation with the patient's oncologist, transplant surgeon, or organ specialist
- Avoid blood transfusions because these need special screening to prevent transmission of disease
- Pressors and inotropics work as usual in the transplanted heart
- Atropine will have no effect on bradycardia because there is no vagal innervation
- Use dopamine, epinephrine drips, or external pacing to increase heart rate if bradycardia is symptomatic

Disposition

MEDICATION

- Common regimens are cyclosporine, prednisone, and azathioprine or tacrolimus (formerly known as FK506), and prednisone
  —Azathioprine (3–5 mg/kg/d PO)
    -Bone marrow suppression
    -Nausea, vomiting, stomatitis, pancreatitis, and cholestatic hepatitis
  —Cyclosporine (5–10 mg/kg/d PO)
    -Dose-related nephrotoxicity
    -Monitor drug levels and renal function
    -Severe hypertension from renal arterial spasm
    -Levels increased by drugs that inhibit cytochrome P-450 (macrolides, fluconazole, cimetidine), NSAIDs, angiotensin-converting enzyme (ACE) inhibitors, and calcium channel blockers
  —Methotrexate (15 mg/d PO)
    -Nausea, vomiting, stomatitis, diarrhea, hepatotoxicity, pneumonitis
  —Steroids
    -GI bleeding, glucose intolerance, skeletal myopathy, and adrenal suppression
  —Tacrolimus (FK506): levels increased by macrolides, quinolones, NSAIDs, fluconazole, cimetidine, omeprazole.
    -Neurotoxicity: headache, tremors, insomnia, dysarthria, seizures, and coma
    -Also causes glucose intolerance and may require insulin therapy
  —Mycophenolate mofetil: may reduce incidence of chronic allograft nephropathy, with less hypertension and hyperuricemia than earlier regimens

Disposition

ADMISSION CRITERIA

- Admit all transplant recipients with fever, shortness of breath, signs or symptoms of rejection, abdominal pain, or other signs of organ infection
- Admit to the ICU patients who are septic or have cardiopulmonary compromise

DISCHARGE CRITERIA

- Nontoxic patients in whom rejection or serious infection has been excluded may be discharged with close follow-up

Miscellaneous

ICD9: 996.52

ICD10: T86.9

SEE ALSO: CARDIAC TRANSPLANTATION COMPLICATIONS

SUGGESTED READINGS

Andrews PA. Renal transplantation. Br Med J 2002;324:530–534.

Deng MC. Cardiac transplantation. Heart 2002;87:177–184.

Jain A, Khanna A, Molmenti EP, et al. Immunosuppressive therapy. Surg Clin North Am 1999;79:59–76.

Noble-Jamieson G, Barnes N. Diagnosis and management of late complications after liver transplantation. Arch Dis Child 1999;81:446–451.

Petri WA Jr. Infections in heart transplant recipients. Clin Infect Dis 1994;18:141.

Sternbach GL, et al. Emergency department presentation and care of heart and heart/lung transplant recipients. Ann Emerg Med 1992;21:1140.

Suthanthiran M, Strom TB. Mechanisms and management of acute renal allograft rejection. Surg Clin North Am 1998; 78:77–94.

Sweny P, Burroughs AK. Infections in solid organ transplantation. Curr Opin Infect Dis 1994;7:436.

Author: Mark Langdorf

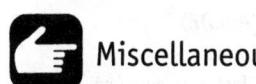

- Standardized approach for rapid assessment of the trauma patient
- While presented here as a sequential method for gathering information, it is important to understand that many of the steps can be performed simultaneously, and life-threatening injuries must be immediately addressed and treated before going on to the next level
- With any change in the patient's status, the primary survey should be repeated

Clinical Presentation

SIGNS AND SYMPTOMS

Primary Survey (ABCDE)

Airway, Cervical Spine

- Look, listen, and feel from nose/mouth to trachea/bronchial tree to assess patency
- Evaluate gag reflex
- Cervical spine must be immobilized
- Ability to speak or the effective movement of air with respiration indicates patency
- Gurgling, stridor, wheezing, snoring, choking, or absence of air movement requires immediate intervention
- Manage airway compromise before next step in primary survey

Breathing

- An awake, alert patient with normal speech and good air movement suggests effective breathing
- Symmetric chest wall rise/fall, equal breath sounds, normal respiratory rate, and oxygen saturation >95% suggest effective breathing
- Asymmetric chest movement, unequal breath sounds, abnormal respiratory rate, decreased oxygen saturation, inadequate air movement, or an obtunded patient suggests ineffective breathing
- Decreased unilateral breath sounds, tracheal shift, hyperexpansion, hyperresonance to percussion, subcutaneous air, hypoxia, or hemodynamic compromise raises concerns for tension pneumothorax
  - —Manage immediately with needle thoracostomy followed by tube thoracostomy
- Decreased breath sounds with dullness to percussion suggest hemothorax

Circulation

- Adequate circulating blood volume must be maintained
- Primary assessment includes blood pressure, heart rate, pulse quality, and end-organ function (mentation, urine output, capillary refill)
- Tachycardia and oliguria indicate early shock; hypotension is a late finding
- Classes of hemorrhagic shock (see Hemorrhagic Shock)

Disability

- Assess level of consciousness, gross motor function, pupil size/reactivity
- Glasgow Coma Scale (GCS) is most commonly used; score of 8 or less indicates severe head injury/coma
- Spinal cord injuries are grossly assessed by observing movement of all extremities
- Pupil size and reactivity to light is a measure of brainstem function

Exposure

- Patient should be undressed completely

Secondary Survey

- Once the primary survey has been completed with the patient stabilized at each level, a complete physical exam from head to toe is performed
- "Tubes and fingers in every orifice"

PEDIATRIC CONSIDERATIONS

- See Pediatric Trauma

Pre-Hospital

- Triage to a major trauma center is dictated by local protocols
  - —Injuries with the potential need for acute surgical, neurosurgical, or orthopedic intervention should be transported to a major trauma center
- Primary survey should be performed on scene and en route

Diagnosis

- Initial stabilization should begin simultaneously with essential workup

ESSENTIAL WORKUP

- Primary and secondary survey
- Cervical spine and chest x-rays are mandatory for major trauma patients; pelvis x-rays should be performed with clinical suspicion of pelvic trauma or with hemodynamic instability
- Hemoglobin/hematocrit, arterial blood gas, tube for blood typing
- Urine dip for blood (and subsequent urinalysis if positive)
- Urine pregnancy test for any female patient of childbearing age

LABORATORY

- Baseline coagulation and chemistry studies with massive injury or hemorrhage

IMAGING/SPECIAL TESTS

- Loss of consciousness, posttraumatic amnesia (anterograde or retrograde), or persistent altered level of consciousness is indication for head CT
- Significant blunt and penetrating chest trauma requires objective evaluation of the heart and great vessels with echocardiography, CT scan, angiography, or direct visualization
- Blunt abdominal trauma requires objective evaluation: diagnostic peritoneal lavage, ultrasound, or CT depending on patient's condition
- Extremity injury
  - —X-rays
  - —Suspected vascular damage requires angiography or duplex ultrasound

Treatment

INITIAL STABILIZATION

- The initial treatment should parallel the primary survey with injuries treated before addressing the next assessment level

Airway With Cervical Spine Control

- Jaw thrust, suctioning, and oropharyngeal or nasopharyngeal airways provide initial airway support
- Rapid sequence intubation is the airway management option of initial choice for multiple trauma patients (see Rapid Sequence Intubation)
  - —Nasotracheal intubation or cricothyroidotomy may be necessary

Breathing

- 100% oxygen and respiratory monitoring
- Tension pneumothorax should be diagnosed clinically and decompressed emergently with a needle thoracostomy below the axilla or above the second rib
  - —Tube thoracostomy should follow
- Open chest wounds should be covered with an adherent dressing and a tube thoracostomy performed
- Respiratory distress from flail segment or pulmonary contusion should prompt early intubation with mechanical ventilation and positive end-expiratory pressure

Circulation

- Two large-bore IVs with constant hemodynamic and cardiac monitoring
  - —Alternatives include central lines, venous cutdowns (saphenous or femoral), or pediatric intraosseous lines
- Aggressive fluid replacement with 3 parts fluid for every 1 part circulatory volume loss; adjust fluids based on ongoing assessment
  - —2 L initial bolus in adults, 20 mL/kg in children
- Whole blood, or autotransfused blood for class III and class IV hemorrhagic shock or uncontrolled bleeding
- Pericardial tamponade requires emergent pericardiocentesis/pericardial window
- External bleeding should be managed with direct pressure

Disability

- Head injury with GCS of 8 or less should initiate treatment for elevated intracranial pressure (ICP) with mannitol; rapid sequence induction and intubation or surgical airway, oxygenation, and controlled ventilation (to a PCO_2 of 35 mm Hg)
- Elevate head 20–30 degrees, maintaining spine immobilization

ED TREATMENT

- Definitive treatment is often surgical: prompt stabilization, early recognition of the need for operative intervention, and appropriate trauma surgical consultation are paramount

MEDICATIONS

- See Rapid Sequence Intubation

PEDIATRIC CONSIDERATIONS

- Intraosseous lines are an alternative to IV lines for fluids and medications

Disposition

ADMISSION CRITERIA

- Most major trauma patients should be admitted for observation, monitoring, and further evaluation
- Patients with significant injuries or hemodynamic instability should be admitted to an ICU
- Patients requiring frequent assessments should be admitted to a monitored setting

DISCHARGE CRITERIA

- Minor trauma patients with negative objective workup may be observed in the emergency department for several hours and then discharged

Miscellaneous

ICD9: 959.80

ICD10: T07

SUGGESTED READINGS

Committee on Trauma, American College of Surgeons. Advanced trauma life support. St. Louis: Mosby, 1997.

Gin Shaw SL, Jordan RC. Multiple trauma. In: Marx J, et al., eds. Rosen's emergency medicine: concepts and clinical practice, 5th ed. St. Louis: Mosby, 2002.

Krantz BE. Initial assessment. In: Feliciano DV, et al., eds. Trauma. Stamford, CT: Appleton & Lange, 1996:123.

Author: Daniel Davis

Trichomonas

Clinical Presentation

SIGNS AND SYMPTOMS

Female

- Vaginitis
  - —Malodorous, profuse; in most, itchy discharge
    - -Usually yellow-green
    - -May be gray, white, or frothy
  - —Inflammation of vaginal walls
- Cervix
  - —Stippled
  - —Punctate hemorrhages with strawberry coloring
- Dysuria (20%)
- Abdominal pain
- Elevated vaginal pH (>5.5)
- Dyspareunia

Male

- Usually asymptomatic
- Urethritis in minority
  - —Scant discharge
  - —Dysuria
  - —20% of nonspecific urethritis in males caused by trichomonas
- Prostatitis
- Epididymitis
- Reversible sterility

MECHANISM/DESCRIPTION

- Sexually transmitted disease
- Causes urogenital infections in males and females
  - —May contribute to adverse pregnancy outcome such as premature rupture of membrane or preterm labor
- Prevalence
  - —5 million cases/year in United States
  - —15% in women seen in STD clinics

ETIOLOGY

- *Trichomonas vaginalis*
  - —Causative agent
  - —Flagellated protozoan
  - —Most commonly isolated from the urethra, bladder, and Skene's gland

Pre-Hospital

N/A

Diagnosis

ESSENTIAL WORKUP

- Saline wet mount of cervical smears or spun urine
  - —Motile, pear-shaped flagellated trichomonas
    - -Slightly larger than leukocytes
    - -Seen in 60% of females with active infection
  - —Many polymorphonuclear neutrophils (PMNs)

LABORATORY

- Culture
  - —Prostate message before collecting culture in males most sensitive
- Immunofluorescence and immunoassay available but expensive

DIFFERENTIAL DIAGNOSIS

- Urinary tract infection
- Gonorrhea
- Chlamydia
- Candidal vaginitis
- Nonspecific vaginitis

Treatment

INITIAL STABILIZATION

N/A

ED TREATMENT

- Nonpregnant patients
  - —Metronidazole: 2-g single dose (90–95% cure rate)
  - —Resistant infections:
    - -Metronidazole: 500 mg PO b.i.d. for 7 days
    - -Metronidazole: 375 mg PO b.i.d. for 7 days is FDA approved but no clinical data comparing to 500 mg
  - —Metronidazole gel less efficacious
  - —No alternate if allergic—use desensitization
- Pregnant patients
  - —In the first-trimester: clotrimazole, 100-mg vaginal suppository for 7 days
    - -70% effective
  - —After first trimester: use metronidazole as above
  - —Some sources state metronidazole safe in all stages of pregnancy
- Avoid concomitant alcohol use with metronidazole
  - —May precipitate Antabuse reaction
- Recommend testing
  - —Of sexual partners
  - —For concomitant sexually transmitted diseases including HIV

Disposition

ADMISSION CRITERIA

- None

DISCHARGE CRITERIA

- All patients

Miscellaneous

ICD9: 131.9

ICD10: A59.9

SEE ALSO: URETHRITIS

SUGGESTED READINGS

Berger RE. Sexually transmitted diseases. Adv Urol 1997;2:97.

Center for Disease Control and Prevention. 1998 Guidelines for treatment of sexually transmitted disease. MMWR Morb Mortal Wkly Rep 1998;47:RR1–116.

Drugs for sexually transmitted infections. Med Lett Drugs Therapeutics 1999;41: 85–90.

Kreipe RE. Sexually transmitted diseases in adolescents. Pediatr Infect Dis J 1998;17: 921–922.

McKinzie J. Sexually transmitted disease. Emerg Med Clin North Am 2001;19(3): 723–743.

Author: David Levine

Tricyclic Antidepressant, Poisoning

Clinical Presentation

SIGNS AND SYMPTOMS

- Rapid deterioration may occur
- Classic tricyclic antidepressant (TCA) compounds (imipramine, amitriptyline, nortriptyline)—greatest cardiovascular toxicity
- Newer agents (serotonergic agents)—less overall toxicity in overdose

Central Nervous System (CNS)

- Stimulation or depression
- Stimulation
  - —Tremulousness
  - —Agitation
  - —Fasciculation
  - —Seizures (resulting acidemia may lead to worsening cardiovascular toxicity)
- Depression
  - —Drowsiness
  - —Lethargy
  - —Coma

Cardiovascular System

- Hypotension
- Tachycardia (early; due to blockade of norepinephrine reuptake and anticholinergic effects)
- Bradycardia (late; due to catecholamine depletion state)
- EKG changes
  - —QRS widening (>100 milliseconds)
  - —Rightward shift in terminal 40 milliseconds in frontal plane axis
- Dysrhythmias
  - —Supraventricular tachycardia (SVT)
  - —Ventricular arrhythmias

Anticholinergic Effects (Less Common)

- Dilated pupils
- Decreased bowel sounds
- Urinary retention

MECHANISM/DESCRIPTION

- Primary mechanism of TCA toxicity
  - —Sodium channel blocking effect (quinidine-like effect)
  - —Inhibition of norepinephrine reuptake
  - —Alpha-blockade
  - —Anticholinergic effect
- Selective serotonin reuptake inhibitors (SSRIs)
  - —Wider margin of safety than TCA
  - —Less CNS/cardiovascular toxicity
- Nonselective serotonin reuptake inhibitors
  - —Serotonin and norepinephrine reuptake inhibitors (SNRIs)
  - —Can cause cardiac dysrhythmias or seizures
  - —Venlafaxine (Effexor)

ETIOLOGY

- Tricyclic antidepressants
  - —Amitriptyline
  - —Nortriptyline
  - —Imipramine
  - —Doxepin
- Newer-generation antidepressants (nontricyclic)
  - —Have different toxic profile than the TCAs
  - —Dibenzoxazepines
    - -High CNS toxicity
    - -Lower cardiovascular toxicity than TCA
    - -Amoxapine (Asendin)
- Triazolopyridines: trazodone
- Tetracyclics: maprotiline (Ludiomil)
- SSRIs
  - —Lack anticholinergic effects
  - —Fluoxetine (Prozac)
  - —Sertraline (Zoloft)
  - —Paroxetine (Paxil)

Pre-Hospital

CAUTIONS

- Do not be lulled into false sense of security with a well-appearing patient
  - —Rapid onset of altered mental status, seizures, and dysrhythmias occur
- Perform endotracheal intubation if any evidence of compromise
- Secure IV access
- Administer sodium bicarbonate if any evidence of QRS widening (>100 milliseconds)
  - —1 ampule in adults
  - —1-2 mEq/kg in children
- Ipecac contraindicated (risk for aspiration with development of depressed mental status, or seizure)

Diagnosis

ESSENTIAL WORKUP

- EKG: factors associated with TCA poisoning
  - —Sinus tachycardia (almost always present at sometime after poisoning)
  - —QRS widening
    - ->100 milliseconds associated with seizure
    - ->160 milliseconds associated with ventricular dysrhythmia
  - —QT prolongation
  - —PR prolongation
  - —Rightward shifting of the terminal 40 milliseconds QRS axis
  - —R-wave amplitude in aVR <3 mm
- Continuous cardiac monitor

LABORATORY

- CBC
- Electrolytes, BUN, creatinine, glucose
- Arterial blood gas (ABG)
- Urine toxicology screen
  - —Rule out other toxins

IMAGING/SPECIAL TESTS

- Chest x-ray for aspiration pneumonia/pulmonary edema
- TCA levels
  - —Not useful
  - —Do not correlate well with the degree of toxicity
  - —Qualitative screen appropriate to confirm ingestion if necessary

DIFFERENTIAL DIAGNOSIS

Drugs That Cause Coma

- Alcohols
- Alcohol withdrawal
- Anticholinergics
- Lithium
- PCP
- Opioids
- Phenothiazines
- Sedative hypnotics
- Salicylates

Cardiotoxic Drugs

- Antidysrhythmics (category IA)
- Digoxin toxicity
- Sympathomimetics
- Anticholinergics

Drugs That Cause Seizures

- Alcohol withdrawal
- Anticholinergics
- Camphor
- Isoniazid
- Lindane
- Lithium
- Phenothiazines
- Sympathomimetics
- Toxic alcohols

Treatment

INITIAL STABILIZATION

- ABCs
  - —Low threshold to intubate patients with altered mental status
- IV 0.9% NS
- Oxygen
- Cardiac monitor
  - —For wide complex rhythm (QRS >100 msec) bolus sodium bicarbonate
- Naloxone, thiamine, glucose (Accu-Chek) for altered mental status
- Flumazenil contraindicated in combined TCA/benzodiazepine overdose

ED TREATMENT

Cardiac Toxicity

- QRS widening (>100 msec)
  - —Bolus with 1 amp (peds: 1–2 mEq/kg) of sodium bicarbonate; repeat if sudden increase in QRS width
  - —Maintain arterial pH of 7.45–7.5 with hyperventilation
  - —Initiate sodium bicarbonate infusion if hyperventilation alone does not reach target pH
- Dysrhythmia
  - —Sinus tachycardia requires no treatment
  - —Bolus 1–2 amps of sodium bicarbonate (1–2 mEq/kg in children) for sudden change in rhythm
  - —Follow advanced cardiac life support (ACLS) protocol with addition of sodium bicarbonate boluses
    - -Lidocaine is the second-line agent after sodium bicarbonate
  - —Use of class IA (procainamide) and IC agents and physostigmine contraindicated

Hypotension

- 0.9% NS fluid bolus
- Norepinephrine
  - —Preferred pressor (over dopamine)
  - —Counters the alpha-blockade better
  - —Dopamine requires higher doses

Decontamination

- Gastric lavage
  - —For recent ingestion (<1–2 hours)
  - —Performed when airway has been secured in the lethargic patient
- Administer activated charcoal with sorbitol
- Ipecac contraindicated

Seizure

- Diazepam first-line followed by phenobarbital/phenytoin
- Neuromuscular paralysis with short-acting agent (rocuronium/vecuronium) for refractory seizures (monitor electroencephalogram [EEG])
- Sodium bicarbonate bolus to prevent acidosis

MEDICATIONS

- Activated charcoal slurry: 1–2 g/kg up to 90 g PO
- Dextrose: D50W, 1 amp (50 mL or 25 g) (peds: D25W, 2–4 mL/kg) i.v.
- Diazepam (benzodiazepine): 5–10 mg (peds: 0.2–0.5 mg/kg) i.v.
- Dopamine: 2–20 μg/kg/min i.v. infusion titrated to desired effect
- Lorazepam (benzodiazepine): 2–6 mg (peds: 0.03–0.05 mg/kg) i.v.
- Naloxone (Narcan): 2 mg (peds: 0.1 mg/kg) i.v. or i.m. initial dose
- Norepinephrine: 4–12 μg/min (peds: 0.05–0.1 μg/kg/min) i.v. infusion titrated to desired effect
- Sodium bicarbonate: 1–2 amps i.v. push (peds: 1–2 mEq/kg); drip—add 3 amps to 1 L of D5W (efficacy of a drip is unknown)
- Sorbitol: 1–2 g/kg to a max of 150 g (peds: >1 year old: 1–1.5 g/kg as a 35% solution to a max of 50 g) PO mixed in the activated charcoal slurry
- Thiamine (vitamin B_1): 100 mg (peds: 50 mg) i.v. or i.m.

Disposition

ADMISSION CRITERIA

- Symptomatic patients observed more than 6 hours
- Altered mental status
- Dysrhythmia or conduction delay
- Seizure
- Heart rate >100 beats/min 6 hours after ingestion
- Co-ingestion requiring prolonged observation

DISCHARGE CRITERIA

- Asymptomatic after 6 hours observation
- No alteration in mental status
- Normal EKG with heart rate <100 beats/min
- Active bowel sounds; tolerated activated charcoal
- Psychiatry clearance if there has been a suicide attempt or gesture

Miscellaneous

ICD9: 969.0

ICD10: T43.0

SUGGESTED READINGS

Brent J. Serotonin reuptake inhibitors, newer antidepressants, and the serotonin syndrome. In: Ford M, Delaney C, Ling L, et al., eds. Clinical toxicology, 1st ed. Philadelphia: WB Saunders, 2001.

Ellison DW, Pentel PR. Clinical features and consequences of seizures due to cyclic antidepressant overdose. Am J Emerg Med 1989;7:5.

Gueye P, Hoffman JR, Taboulet P. Empiric use of flumazenil in comatose patients: limited applicability of criteria to define low risk. Ann Emerg Med 1996;27:730.

Lavoie FW, Gansert GG. Value of Initial ECG findings and plasma drug levels in cyclic antidepressant overdose. Ann Emerg Med 1990;19:696.

Liebelt EL, Francis PD, Woolf AD. ECGT lead aVR versus QRS interval in predicting seizures and arrhythmias in acute tricyclic antidepressant toxicity. Ann Emerg Med 1995;26:195–201.

McCabe JL, Cobaugh DJ, Menegazzi JJ, et al. Experimental tricyclic antidepressant toxicity: a randomized, controlled comparison of hypertonic saline solution, sodium bicarbonate and hyperventilation. Ann Emerg Med 1998;32:329–333.

Weisman R. Cyclic antidepressants. In: Goldfrank LR, Flomenbaum NE, Lewin NA, et al., eds. Goldfrank's toxicologic emergencies, 6th ed. Stamford, CT: Appleton & Lange, 1998.

Author: Steven Aks

Trigeminal Neuralgia

Clinical Presentation

SIGNS AND SYMPTOMS

- *Brief, intense, lancinating* pain (tic douloureux)
- *Unilateral* in the distribution of a branch of the trigeminal nerve in the face is most common; however, bilateral trigeminal neuralgias do occur
- May occur without provocation or may be initiated by tactile stimulation of a particular area on the face, lips, tongue, or scalp
- Pain seldom lasts more than a few seconds to several minutes
- Occurs almost exclusively in the middle-aged or elderly patient and is more common in females than males
- Associated sensory loss in the effected region may be found
- *Paroxysmal pattern* of pain lasting weeks in duration

MECHANISM/DESCRIPTION

- Idiopathic
- Redundant or tortuous blood vessel in the posterior fossa resulting in irritation of the nerve root
- Space-occupying lesion causing direct compression of the nerve
- Bilateral tic douloureux in younger adult can be seen in multiple sclerosis
- Irritation of the nerve during exacerbation of herpes zoster associated with rash in same distribution

ETIOLOGY

- Primary *idiopathic* is most common
- Multiple sclerosis
- Rarely with herpes zoster
- Space-occupying lesions (aneurysm, neurofibroma, meningioma)

PEDIATRIC CONSIDERATIONS

- Not commonly seen in pediatric population

Pre-Hospital

N/A

Diagnosis

ESSENTIAL WORKUP

- Diagnosis is made clinically; history is of primary importance, including
  —Onset, duration of pain
  —Associated constitutional symptoms
  —Visual disturbances
  —Associated paraesthesias
  —History of trauma
- Cranial nerve examination for both sensory and motor function is crucial, including visual acuity
- Neurologic examination for focal deficits
- Skin examination for presence of rash or other abnormalities
- Dental and oral examination

LABORATORY

- No specific tests for trigeminal neuralgia

IMAGING/SPECIAL TESTS

- Idiopathic trigeminal neuralgia (tic douloureux) does not require any special imaging
- The presence of focal cranial nerve or neurologic findings suggests possible intracranial etiologies for the patient's pain; CT or MRI should be obtained

Treatment

INITIAL STABILIZATION

- Pain management with narcotic medication is often necessary as other treatments require several days before demonstrating efficacy

ED TREATMENT

- Should focus on pain control and patient comfort
- Recurrent or refractory tic douloureux may require surgical intervention
- Carbamazepine is the mainstay of treatment of trigeminal neuralgia
  —Gastrointestinal intolerance may be seen in up to one-third of patients
- Narcotic analgesia
- Phenytoin is a second-line medical therapy that has been used with varying efficacy

MEDICATIONS

- Carbamazepine: begin with 100 mg b.i.d.; can be increased to 600 mg b.i.d. for symptom control
- Phenytoin: starting doses should be 300 mg daily and increased to control pain

PEDIATRIC CONSIDERATIONS

- No specific pediatric considerations are relevant

Disposition

ADMISSION CRITERIA

- Trigeminal neuralgia with presence of other focal neurologic findings or positive CT or MRI studies requires emergent neurologic or neurosurgical consultation
- Refractory or recurrent trigeminal neuralgia not responding to outpatient pain management or anticonvulsant therapy may require admission for surgical intervention and ablation of the trigeminal nerve

DISCHARGE CRITERIA

- Patients without any focal neurological findings and improved pain control in the ED may be managed as outpatients

Miscellaneous

ICD9: 350.1

ICD10: G50.0

SUGGESTED READINGS

Dalessio DJ. Trigeminal and glossopharyngeal neuralgia. In: Johnson RT, ed. Current therapy in neurologic disease, 2nd ed. Philadelphia: Decker, 1987:62–65.

Henry G, Little N. Neurological emergencies: a symptom oriented approach. New York: McGraw-Hill, 1985.

Selby G. Diseases of the fifth cranial nerve. In: Dyck PJ, et al., eds. Peripheral neuropathy, 2nd ed. Philadelphia: WB Saunders, 1984:1244–1265.

Sweet WH. The treatment of trigeminal neuralgia (tic douloureux). N Engl J Med 1986;315:174.

Author: James M. Leaming

Tuberculosis

Clinical Presentation

SIGNS AND SYMPTOMS

Pulmonary Tuberculosis

- Fever
- Malaise
- Weight loss
- Night sweats
- Chronic cough
- Hemoptysis
- Shortness of breath

Extrapulmonary Tuberculosis

- Central nervous system infections
  —Meningeal irritation and cranial nerve defects
  —Malaise
  —Intermittent headache
  —Low-grade fever
  —Confusion
  —Meningismus
  —Diplopia
  —Hyponatremia (due to SIADH)
  —Acute ischemic stroke
- Pericardial infection
  —Pleuritic chest pain increased with recumbency
- Renal infection
  —Fever
  —Flank pain
  —Sterile pyuria
- Spinal tuberculosis (Pott's disease)
  —Back pain/stiffness
  —Fever
  —Point tenderness
  —Decreased range of motion
- Miliary tuberculosis
  —Multiorgan system involvement
  —Diffuse adenopathy
  —Hepatomegaly
  —Splenomegaly
  —Weight loss
  —Fever

MECHANISM/DESCRIPTION

- Infection with *Mycobacterium tuberculosis,* an acid-fast bacillus, resulting in disease
- Most common route of infection is by droplet nuclei inhaled through the respiratory tract
- Primary infection
  —Initial infection with bacilli occurs when organisms enter the alveoli, then spread via regional lymph nodes to the bloodstream
  —Patients are usually asymptomatic
  —Positive reaction to purified protein derivative (PPD) indicates past exposure or infection
- Reactivation tuberculosis
  —Characterized by a chronic wasting disease
  —Malaise
  —Low-grade fever
  —Weight loss
  —Night sweats
  —Cough

ETIOLOGY

- Tuberculosis affects about one third of the world's population (90 million new cases in past decade worldwide, with about 30 million deaths)
- Three tuberculosis epidemics
  —Global resurgence
  —HIV-infected patients
  —Multidrug-resistant tuberculosis
- Conditions that predispose the individual to developing tuberculosis include
  —HIV infection and other immunocompromised states
  —Drug and alcohol abuse
  —Poverty
  —Homelessness
  —Institutionalization
  —Immigration from a high-prevalence area

Pre-Hospital

CAUTIONS

- Place patient in respiratory isolation (negative flow)
- Place a mask on the patient to prevent respiratory spread of the disease
- Initiate treatment with an IV, oxygen, and pulse oximetry
- Endotracheal intubation may be required in patients with severe hemoptysis or respiratory compromise
- Providers should wear submicron-particulate filter masks
- Inform close contacts

Diagnosis

ESSENTIAL WORKUP

- Diagnosis difficult due to the variety of clinical presentations

Chest Radiography

- Most valuable test for diagnosing active pulmonary tuberculosis
- In primary disease, parenchymal infiltrates with unilateral hilar adenopathy are the classic findings
- Reactivation tuberculosis typically appears as cavitary lesions with or without calcification usually in upper lung segments
- Chest x-ray may be nondefinitive in AIDS patients
- Unilateral pleural effusion in both primary and reactivation tuberculosis
- Tracheal deviation with scarring or atelectasis
- Ghon's focus—calcified scar/healed primary focus of infection

Skin Testing

- Inject 0.1 mL of PPD subcutaneous in the forearm
- Positive test indicates prior or current infection with mycobacterium
- Test results read between 48 and 72 hours after administration
- Interpretation of positive
  —>5 mm induration
    -Close contacts with tuberculosis
    -Positive chest x-ray
    -HIV
  —>10 mm induration
  —High-risk groups
    -Immigrants from high-prevalence countries
    -Immunosuppressed
    -Health care workers
    -Prison inmates
    -Institutionalized
  —>15 mm induration
    -Low-risk individuals

LABORATORY

- CBC
- Electrolytes, BUN, creatinine, glucose
- Pulse oximetry/arterial blood gas for respiratory symptoms

IMAGING/SPECIAL TESTS

- Sputum staining for acid-fast bacilli (Ziehl-Neelsen stain)
  —Provides a quick presumptive diagnosis
- Sputum, CSF, blood, urine, or peritoneal fluid culture
  —Gold standard for diagnosis of tuberculosis
  —Average time for positive culture is 3–6 weeks
- Spinal tap with CSF analysis
  —For suspected tuberculous meningitis
  —WBC range 0–1,500/mm^3 with lymphocyte predominance
  —Elevated protein
  —Low to normal glucose
- Spine radiographs for Pott's disease
  —May be normal
  —Anterior wedging of two involved vertebral bodies and destruction of disk
- CT
  —Better define extent of disease

DIFFERENTIAL DIAGNOSIS

- Bacterial or viral pneumonia
- Lung abscess
- Primary lung cancer
- Lymphoma
- Granulomatous disease (sarcoidosis)

Treatment

INITIAL STABILIZATION

- ABCs
  —Control airway as needed
  —With severe hemoptysis, endotracheal intubation with a double-lumen tube can be used to confine bleeding to one lung while rapid surgical consult is obtained
  —While preparing for intubation, roll patient to the bleeding side to protect the nonbleeding lung
  —Inflate the balloon on the bleeding side and ventilate the nonbleeding side
  —Oxygenate the patient with 100% oxygen
- Isolate patients in negative pressure rooms with at least six air exchanges per hour

ED TREATMENT

- *Isolation* and strict respiratory precautions
- Initiate therapy directed toward area of tubercular involvement

Antituberculosis Medications

- Treatment is dependent on the suspicion of multidrug resistance
- Any regimen must contain multiple drugs to which the tuberculous bacteria is susceptible
- Directly observed therapy may be necessary to ensure compliance in certain populations
- Standard therapy (no suspected resistance)
  —2 months of
    -Isoniazid
    -Rifampin
    -Pyrazinamide
  —Then 4 months of
    -Isoniazid
    -Rifampin
- Suspected/known drug resistance
  —Individualize with infectious disease consult
  —Need at least three susceptible medications to tuberculosis
  —Options
    -Isoniazid
    -Rifampin
    -Pyrazinamide
    -Ethambutol or streptomycin
    -Plus at least two additional drugs (paraaminosalicylic acid, ethionamide, cycloserine, capreomycin, kanamycin, thiacetazone)
- Preventative therapy for positive skin test converters
  —Healthy adults: 6 months isoniazid
  —Children: 9 months of isoniazid
  —HIV: 12 months of isoniazid
  —Isoniazid resistance suspected: 9 months of rifampin
  —Multidrug-resistance suspected: 6 months of ethambutol/quinolone and pyrazinamide

Disposition

ADMISSION CRITERIA

- Respiratory compromise
- Suspicion of diagnosis
- Inability to comply with outpatient therapy
- Involuntary admission for noncompliant outpatients occurs
  —Be aware of respective state laws concerning involuntary admission (consult infectious disease specialist)

DISCHARGE CRITERIA

- Without respiratory compromise
- Home isolation procedure compliance
- Ability and willingness to comply with long-term therapy
- Notification of the public health authorities is mandatory

Miscellaneous

ICD9: 011.9

ICD10: A16.9

SUGGESTED READINGS

American Thoracic Society. Diagnostic standards and classification of tuberculosis. Am Rev Respir Dis 1990;142:725.

American Thoracic Society. Treatment of tuberculosis and tuberculosis infection in adults and children. Am J Respir Crit Care Med 1994;149:1359.

Iseman MD. Treatment of multidrug-resistant tuberculosis. N Engl J Med 1993; 329:784.

Iseman MD. Tuberculosis. In: Bennett JC, et al., eds. Cecil's textbook of medicine, 20th ed. Philadelphia: WB Saunders, 1996:1683–1689.

Neville K, Bromberg A, Bromberg R, et al. Escalating threat from tuberculosis: the third epidemic. Thorax 1995;50(Suppl 1): 537–542.

Author: Christopher A. Lipinski

Tularemia

Clinical Presentation

SIGNS AND SYMPTOMS

- Abrupt onset
- Fever: temperature >101°F
- Chills
- Headache
- Anorexia
- Myalgias
- Vomiting
- Diarrhea
- Abdominal pains
- Sore throat
- Ulcer at site of tick
- Regional lymphadenopathy
- Secondary skin rash
- Primary tularemia pneumonia
  —Substernal burning
  —Nonproductive cough

MECHANISM/DESCRIPTION

- Inoculated cutaneously from as few as 50 organisms through inapparent skin lesions
- 3–5 day incubation period

Six Forms

- Ulceroglandular
  —From tick bites or animal contact
  —Large tender regional lymph nodes
  —Red painful papule, reactive ulcer
  —Fever
- Glandular
  —Tender regional lymphadenopathy with no local lesions
- Ocular glandular
  —Entry through conjunctiva
  —Unilateral
  —Edema, conjunctivitis, injection, chemosis with periauricular, submandibular, or cervical lymphadenopathy
- Pharyngeal
  —From contaminated food/water
  —Severe throat pain
  —Exudative pharyngitis with ulceration
  —Regional lymph node involvement
- Typhoidal
  —Unapparent point of entry
  —Fever
  —Severe diarrhea
  —Bowel necrosis
  —Pulmonary infiltrates
- Pulmonic
  —Secondary to inhalation especially in sheep shearers, farmers, or lab workers
  —Fever
  —Dry cough
  —Pleuritic chest pain
  —Chest x-ray: lobar infiltrate, hilar adenopathy, pleural effusion, or a miliary pattern

ETIOLOGY

- Transmission
  —Tick
  —Mosquito bite
  —Skinning, dressing, and eating infected rabbits, muskrat, beaver, squirrels, and birds
  —Airborne transmission (laboratory workers, bioterrorism)
  —Lawn mowing and brush cutting

Pre-Hospital

CAUTIONS

- Clusters or disease in unusual areas should raise suspicion of biologic agents
- Universal and respiratory precautions are recommended

Diagnosis

ESSENTIAL WORKUP

- Diagnosis based on clinical manifestations/serologic studies
- Agglutinin titers
  —Antibody titer >1:160 with skin ulcer for 2 weeks—diagnostic
  —Four-fold rise in second titer obtained 2 weeks later confirms diagnosis

LABORATORY

- Routine lab tests nonspecific
- CBC
  —Normal WBC in uncomplicated disease
- Sedimentation rate is elevated
- Gram stain or tissue biopsies often negative
  —Tissue may show caseation necrosis similar to tuberculosis
- Culture
  —Source
    -Blood
    -Pleural fluid
    -Lymph node
    -Wound
    -Sputum
    -Gastric aspirate
  —If special media used, inform lab personnel
- ABG/pulse oximetry for suspected pneumonia

IMAGING/SPECIAL TESTS

- Enzyme-linked immunosorbent assay (ELISA)
  —Antigen prep useful although not positive until the second week of illness
- Polymerase chain reaction of purulent specimens may provide rapid diagnosis
- Tularemia skin test
  —Delayed hypersensitivity reaction
  —Positive skin test similar to tuberculin test response
- Chest x-ray for pulmonary symptoms
  —Lobar infiltrate
  —Hilar adenopathy
  —Pleural effusion
  —Miliary pattern

DIFFERENTIAL DIAGNOSIS

- Tuberculosis
- Cat-scratch disease
- Syphilis
- Chancroid
- Lymphogranuloma venereum
- Toxoplasmosis
- Sporotrichosis
- Rat-bite fever
- Anthrax
- Plague
- Herpes simplex infection
- Ocular symptoms
  —Adenoviral infection
- Pharyngeal symptoms
  —Diphtheria, bacterial pharyngitis
  —Infectious mononucleosis
  —Adenoviral infection
- Typhoidal tularemia mistaken for
  —Salmonella
  —Brucellosis
  —Legionella
  —Q fever
  —Malaria
  —Disseminated fungal or mycobacterial infections
- Pneumonic form mistaken for
  —Mycoplasma
  —Legionella
  —Chlamydia
  —Tuberculosis

Treatment

INITIAL STABILIZATION

- 0.9% NS IV fluid for hypotension/dehydration
- Supplemental oxygen for hypoxia
- Administer acetaminophen for fever
- Initiate antibiotic therapy

ED TREATMENT

Antibiotic

- First-line agent: streptomycin or gentamicin
- For tularemic meningitis
  —Add chloramphenicol or third-generation cephalosporin (ceftriaxone)
- Tetracycline
  —Oral agent
  —Only bacteriostatic
  —High level or relapse
- Third-generation cephalosporins and fluoroquinolones as primary treatment
  —Frequent failures
- Treat documented exposures, particularly in lab workers: one dose streptomycin i.m.
- Do not treat tick bites prophylactically

MEDICATIONS

- Ceftriaxone: 1–2 g (peds: 50–100 mg/kg/24 h) q24h
- Ciprofloxacin: 500 mg PO b.i.d.
- Chloramphenicol: 50–100 mg/kg/24 h i.v. divided q6h
- Gentamicin: 3–5 mg/kg/24 h i.v. q8h for 7–14 days
- Streptomycin: 7.5–10 mg/kg (peds: 20–40 mg/kg/24 h q12h i.m.) q12h i.m. or i.v. for 7–14 days

Disposition

ADMISSION CRITERIA

- ICU admission for advanced age, neutropenic, or presenting with typhoidal tularemia
- Isolation not necessary

DISCHARGE CRITERIA

- Mild cases
  —Treat with IM/PO therapy

Miscellaneous

ICD9: 21.9

ICD10: A21.9

SUGGESTED READINGS

Cross JT, Jacobs RF. Tularemia: treatment failures with outpatient use of ceftriaxone. Clin Infect Dis 1993;17:976–980.

Enderlin G, et al. Streptomycin and alternative agents for the treatment of tularemia. Clin Infect Dis 1994;19:42–47.

Fredricks DN, Remington JS. Tularemia presenting as community acquired pneumonia. Arch Intern Med 1996;156: 2137–2140.

Spach DH, et al. Tick-borne diseases in the United States. N Engl J Med 1993;329: 936–947.

Author: Kathryn Brinsfield

Tumor Compression Syndromes

Clinical Presentation

SIGNS AND SYMPTOMS

Spinal Cord Compression

- May have symptoms for many months before acute presentation
- Back pain
  - —Axial
  - —Referred
  - —Radicular
  - —May occur at any level
  - —Aggravated by
    - -Straining
    - -Movement
    - -Straight-leg raising
    - -Neck flexion
    - -Rest may make pain worse (contrary to degenerative joint disease, where rest improves pain)
- Rarely, weakness or ataxia are the presenting complaints
- Progression of symptoms leads to
  - —Paralysis
  - —Sensory disturbances
  - —Incontinence
- Once symptoms do develop, progression is rapid
  - —30% of patients with advanced symptoms are paraplegic in 1 week

Superior Vena Cava (SVC) Obstruction

- Facial plethora and edema
- Periorbital edema
- Conjunctival suffusion
- Facial swelling
- Shortness of breath
- Thoracic and neck vein distention
- Increased intracranial pressure with severe disease
- Headache
- Blurred vision
- Altered mental status
- Coma
- Papilledema

Inferior Vena Cava (IVC) Obstruction

- Edema of the lower limbs
- Evidence of extensive collateral flow

MECHANISM/DESCRIPTION

Spinal Cord Compression

- 5% of all patients dying of cancer will have some degree of spinal cord compression at autopsy, but only 1% of all patients will have this complication diagnosed during life
- The level of compression
  - —Cervical: 10%
  - —Thoracic: 70%
  - —Lumbar: 20%
- Between 10% and 38% of patients may have multiple, noncontiguous levels, especially if associated with breast or prostate cancer
- Anterior or anterolateral aspect of the cord most often affected
- Site of the metastases
  - —Vertebral column (85%)
    - -Body usually, but also pedicle and posterior arch
  - —Paravertebral spaces (10–15%)
  - —Epidural space (rare)

ETIOLOGY

Spinal Cord Compression

- More than 50% of cases are metastases from lung, breast, or prostate cancer
- Other common causes include multiple myeloma, kidney, melanoma, thyroid, lymphoma, and sarcoma
- In children, common causes are sarcoma, neuroblastoma, germ cell tumors, lymphoma
- Median survival for patients with epidural compression is 7 months, with a 36% probability of a 1-year survival

SVC Obstruction

- Most often secondary to bronchogenic carcinoma or postirradiation fibrosis
- Small cell lung cancer most common cause

Pre-Hospital

N/A

Diagnosis

ESSENTIAL WORKUP

History

- Previous history of malignant disease
- Prolonged history of back pain, worse with rest
- Development of neurologic symptoms

Physical Examination

- Careful neurologic examination, including sensory testing
- Assessment of rectal tone
- Assessment of maximal area or areas of bony tenderness

LABORATORY

- Required on a case-by-case basis to assess comorbid conditions (anemia)

IMAGING/SPECIAL TESTS

- Chest x-ray
  - —For SVC compression
  - —Mass present in 10%
  - —Pleural effusion in 25%
- Plain spinal radiography
  - —Will show 85% of metastases causing compression
  - —A normal spine (or one showing just degenerative changes) on plain radiology does not exclude the diagnosis of possible cord compression
- CT
  - —More sensitive and specific than plain radiography and radionucleotide imaging in distinguishing benign from malignant disease in spinal compression syndrome
  - —To identify mass and impingement in vena cava obstruction
- MRI
  - —Investigation of choice to assess extension into the epidural space
  - —Indicated in patients with cancer and unexplained back pain, even in the absence of neurologic signs and normal (or degenerative changes only) plain radiographs
  - —25% of adult patients and as many as 65% of pediatric patients with a radiculopathy in this setting will be found to have evidence of spinal cord compression
  - —Early diagnosis using MRI may be a cost-effective option in the investigation of patients with possible spinal cord compression
- Myelography for patients unable to undergo MRI (pacemaker, severe claustrophobia)

DIFFERENTIAL DIAGNOSIS

- Intervertebral disk disease
- Osteoporotic vertebral fractures
- Spondylosis
- Spondylitis
- Epidural abscess
- Primary bone tumors
- Arteriovenous malformations
- Neurologic diseases
- Multiple sclerosis
- Amyotrophic lateral sclerosis
- Transverse myelitis
- Spinal infarction

Treatment

INITIAL STABILIZATION

- Early diagnosis and treatment are the key to an improved outcome
  - —Level of neurologic dysfunction on presentation is a key factor in the prognosis for spinal cord compression
- Avoid IV line placement in upper extremities if severe SVC compression present

ED TREATMENT

Spinal Cord Compression

- Corticosteroids (dexamethasone)
  - —Administer in ED
  - —Higher doses alleviate the pain more rapidly, but studies indicate no significant difference in outcome with regard to sphincter function or ambulation between the dose schedules
- Radiotherapy
  - —Definitive treatment modality
- Pain medication with narcotics
- Oncology, radiotherapy, and neurosurgical consultation for further management of tumor/malignancy

SVC Compression

- Manage the underlying malignancy with either radiotherapy or chemotherapy
- Elevate head
- Diuretics associated with transient symptomatic improvement
- Administer steroids if respiratory compromise
- Use of stents to hold the vein open has been reported to be successful in relieving symptoms
- Urgent oncology referral

MEDICATIONS

- Dexamethasone: 1 mg/kg loading dose, followed by 4–24 mg q6h

Disposition

ADMISSION CRITERIA

- All patients with spinal cord or acute vena caval compression

DISCHARGE CRITERIA

- None

Miscellaneous

ICD9: 336.9

ICD10: T79.5

SUGGESTED READINGS

Boogerd W, van der Sande JJ. Diagnosis and treatment of spinal cord compression in malignant disease. Cancer Treat Rev 1993;19:129–150.

Byrne TN. Spinal cord compression from epidural metastases. N Engl J Med 1992;327:614–619.

Johnston RA. The management of acute spinal cord compression. J Neurol Neurosurg Psychiatry 1993;56:1046–1054.

Jordan JE, Donaldson SS, Enzmann DR. Cost effectiveness and outcome assessment of magnetic resonance imaging in diagnosing cord compression. Cancer 1995;75:2579–2586.

Stock KW, Jacob AL, Proske M, et al. Treatment of malignant obstruction of the superior vena cava with the self-expanding Wallstent. Thorax 1995;50:1151–1156.

Author: Martin J. Carey

TymPanic Membrane Perforation

Clinical Presentation

SIGNS AND SYMPTOMS

- Ear pain (mild)
- Decreased hearing (partial)
- Severe pain or complete hearing loss in the affected ear suggests additional injuries
- Purulent or bloody discharge from ear canal
- Tinnitus
- Vertigo (especially if perforation occurs in water)

MECHANISM/DESCRIPTION

- Infection (acute otitis media)
- Blunt trauma (slap to the ear)
- Penetrating trauma (Q-tip)
- Rapid pressure change (diving, flying)
  - —Rupture usually occurs between 100 and 400 mm Hg (at a depth of 2.6 feet, there is a pressure differential of 60 mm Hg)
- Extreme noise (blast)
- Lightning
- Acute necrotic myringitis (β-hemolytic streptococcus)
- Acid burns
- Slag burns (welding or metalworking)

Pre-Hospital

N/A

Diagnosis

ESSENTIAL WORKUP

- Clinical examination
  - —Direct visualization of tympanic membrane with otoscope
  - —Test hearing in both ears
  - —Note any nystagmus with changes of position or pressure on the tragus occluding the canal (fistula sign)

IMAGING/SPECIAL TESTS

- Insufflation via pneumatic otoscope
  - —Small perforations may be evident only as an immobile tympanic membrane
  - —Holding pressure for 15 seconds (the fistula test) may cause nystagmus or vertigo if the pressure is transmitted through the middle ear and into a labyrinthine fistula
- Weber test (tuning fork on midline bone)
  - —Sound should be equal or louder in the injured ear, consistent with decreased conduction
  - —Sound localizing to the opposite side of injury indicates possible otic nerve injury
- Rinne's test
  - —Usually normal (air conduction detected after bone conduction fades) or shows a small conductive loss
- Cranial CT
  - —Obtain if clinically indicated to rule out temporal bone fracture

DIFFERENTIAL DIAGNOSIS

- Temporal bone fracture
- Serous otitis media
- Infectious otitis media
- Otitis externa
- Cerumen impaction
- Barotrauma
- Acoustic trauma
- Foreign body
- Child abuse

Treatment

INITIAL STABILIZATION

- ABCs of trauma care
  - —Immobilize cervical spine and investigate for intracranial injury when indicated

ED TREATMENT

- Remove debris from the ear canal
  - —Do not irrigate because this may force more debris into the middle ear
  - —If the tympanic membrane is not visible because of impacted cerumen and suspicion for perforation is high, then remove cerumen by manual disimpaction or suctioning
- If clinically indicated, obtain CT scan to rule out temporal bone fracture
- Prescribe antibiotics if there is evidence of infection (use broad-spectrum antibiotic if patient has been scuba diving)
  - —Antibiotic choices (7–10 days administration)
    - -Amoxicillin
    - -Trimethoprim-sulfamethoxazole
    - -Cefixime
    - -Augmentin
  - —Prophylactic antibiotics not indicated
- Analgesics if needed for pain
- Do not prescribe topical steroids
- Urgent ENT consultation (indications)
  - —Vertigo
  - —Sensorineural hearing loss
  - —Severe tinnitus
  - —Active and significant bleeding
  - —Facial paralysis
- Arrange outpatient ENT follow-up
  - —After detailed examination and formal audiometric tests, most otolaryngologists follow the perforation with monthly examinations
  - —Operative repair (patch or tympanoplasty) reserved for the 10–20% that do not heal spontaneously
- Provide detailed discharge instructions
  - —Occlude the ear canal with cotton coated in petroleum jelly or antibiotic ointment when showering to prevent entry of water into the middle ear, which can be painful
  - —Swim only with fitted earplugs
  - —Avoid forceful blowing of the nose
- Expected outcome
  - —Most perforations heal spontaneously in a few days to several months; in one study of children, 70% closed within 1 week, and 94% closed within 1 month
  - —Perforations caused by molten metal or electrical burns are less likely to heal spontaneously
  - —Forceful entry of water, as in a water-skiing accident, is more likely to lead to infection
  - —Complications include infection, dislocation of ossicles, perilymph leak, and cholesteatoma

MEDICATIONS

- Amoxicillin: 250–500 mg (peds: 20–40 mg/kg/24 h) PO t.i.d.
- Augmentin: 250–500 mg (peds: 20–40 mg/kg/24 h) PO t.i.d.
- Cefixime: 400 mg (peds: 8 mg/kg/24 h) q.d.
- Trimethoprim-sulfamethoxazole (Bactrim DS): 1 tablet (peds: 6–12 mg/kg/24 h TMP) PO b.i.d.

Disposition

ADMISSION CRITERIA

- Associated injuries requiring admission
- Severe vertigo impairing ambulation

DISCHARGE CRITERIA

- Almost all patients will be discharged

Miscellaneous

ICD9: 384.20

ICD10: H72.9

SUGGESTED READINGS

Berger G. Nature of spontaneous tympanic membrane perforation in acute otitis media in children. J Laryngol Otol 1989;103: 1150–1153.

Gladstone HB, Jackler RK, Varav K. Tympanic membrane wound healing: an overview. Otolaryngol Clin North Am 1995; 28:913–933.

Kristensen S. Spontaneous healing of traumatic tympanic membrane perforations in man: a century of experience. J Laryngol Otol 1992;106:1037–1050.

Kristensen S, Juul A, Gamelgaard NP, et al. Traumatic tympanic membrane perforations: complications and management. Ear Nose Throat J 1989;68: 503–516.

Ott MC, Lundy LB. Tympanic membrane perforation in adults: how to manage and when to refer. Postgrad Med 2001;110: 81–84.

Turbiak T. Ear trauma. Emerg Med Clin North Am 1987;5:243–251.

Author: Andrew Chang

Ultraviolet Keratitis

Clinical Presentation

SIGNS AND SYMPTOMS

- Foreign body sensation
- Increased lacrimation
- Photophobia
- Severe pain
- Blepharospasm
- Decreased visual acuity
- 6- to 10-hour latent period between exposure and the onset of symptoms
- Worse symptoms associated with increased exposure time and more intense exposure

Ocular Findings

- Conjunctival injection
- Corneal edema
- Iritis (cell and flare in the anterior chamber or spasm of the pupillary sphincter)
- Diffuse bilateral punctate uptake or confluence of fluorescein in an interpalpebral pattern—pathognomonic
  —Sloughing of large portions of the cornea may obliterate this finding later in severe cases

MECHANISM/DESCRIPTION

- Prolonged exposure to ultraviolet radiation leads to corneal edema and sloughing, followed by secondary inflammation of the iris
- Sources of ultraviolet radiation
  —Sun lamps
  —Welder's arcs
  —Reflected sunlight (water or snow—worse at high altitude)

Pre-Hospital

N/A

Diagnosis

ESSENTIAL WORKUP

- Accurate history including
  —Type of exposure
  —Timing and duration of exposure
- Visual acuity
- Complete ocular exam including
  —Extraocular movements
  —Conjunctiva/sclera/corneas with fluorescein
  —Anterior chambers (checking for cell and flare)
  —Lenses
  —Eversion of the lids to check for foreign bodies

LABORATORY

N/A

IMAGING/SPECIAL TESTS

- Orbit radiographs/ultrasound/CT/MRI for suspected intraocular foreign body

DIFFERENTIAL DIAGNOSIS

- Foreign body of the cornea or eyelids
- Intraocular foreign body
- Corneal abrasion
- Chemical exposures
- Thermal burns

Treatment

INITIAL STABILIZATION

- Topical anesthesia helps to obtain
  - —More accurate documentation of visual acuity
  - —More thorough eye exam and fluorescein staining
  - —Do not prescribe on outpatient basis—interferes with healing and worsens keratitis

ED TREATMENT

- Initiate short-acting cycloplegic for iritis, which usually develops
- Apply topical broad-spectrum antibiotic ointment (preferred) or drops
- Apply eye patch in severe cases
  - —Soft double patching with mild pressure for patient comfort
  - —If both eyes involved, either patch both eyes or patch the eye that is more severely affected
- Analgesics (acetaminophen/NSAIDs/codeine/oxycodone)
- Tetanus prophylaxis if needed

MEDICATIONS

- Topical anesthetics
  - —Proparacaine (Ophthaine) 0.5% (onset, 20–30 seconds; duration, 15 minutes)
  - —Tetracaine (Pontocaine) 0.5% (onset, 30–60 seconds; duration, up to 20 minutes)
- Topical antibiotics
  - —Fluoroquinolones
  - —Gentamicin, tobramycin
  - —Sulfacetamide
- Topical cycloplegics
  - —Cyclopentolate 0.5% (onset, 30–60 minutes; duration, up to 24 hours)
  - —Homatropine 2% (onset, 40 minutes to 3–4 hours; duration, 24–48 hours)

Disposition

ADMISSION CRITERIA

- Patients requiring bilateral patching with severely decreased visual acuity and whose social circumstances make it impossible for the patient to take care of his or her own needs

DISCHARGE CRITERIA

- Nearly all patients may be discharged from the ED following treatment with cycloplegics, topical antibiotics, and patching
  - —Lesions usually heal completely within 24 hours
- Ophthalmologist referral for patients who have other eye disorders, or for those who fail to improve significantly after 24 hours

Miscellaneous

ICD9: 370.20

ICD10: H16.8

SEE ALSO: CORNEAL ABRASION

SUGGESTED READINGS

Daxecker F, Blumthaler M, Ambach W. Keratitis solaris and sunbeds. Ophthalmologica 1995;209(6):329–330.

Tenkate TD. Occupational exposure to ultraviolet radiation: a health risk assessment. Rev Environ Health 1999;14(4):187–209.

Torok PG, Mader TH. Corneal abrasions: diagnosis and management. Am Fam Physician 1996;53(8):2521–2529.

Author: G. Carolyn Clayton

Urethral Trauma

Clinical Presentation

SIGNS AND SYMPTOMS

- Prior history of trauma
- Pelvic pain, inability to void
- Blood at the meatus, high-riding prostate, perineal or genital swelling

MECHANISM/DESCRIPTION

- Females: injuries to the urethra are rare owing to the short, unexposed, and mobile urethra
  - —Usually occur at the bladder neck
- Males: urethra is divided into sections
  - —Posterior urethra
    - -Prostatic
    - -Membranous
    - -Injuries more common
  - —Anterior urethra
    - -Bulbar
    - -Penile
    - -Rarely injured owing to its mobility
- Posterior injuries are much more common and have the classification system detailed below
- *Classification of posterior urethral injuries*
  - —Type I: urethra stretched but not ruptured
  - —Type II: prostatic/membranous portions ruptured (either partially or completely); urogenital diaphragm intact
  - —Type III: both the prostatic/membranous urethra and urogenital diaphragm are ruptured, frequently with damage to the proximal bulbar urethra

ETIOLOGY

- Females
  - —Childbirth or vaginal surgery
  - —Straddle injuries
  - —Rare with pelvic fracture
- Males
  - —Trauma, especially straddle injuries
  - —Mutilation injuries
  - —Sexual activity
  - —Instrumentation
  - —About 95% of posterior urethral injuries are caused by pelvic fractures
  - —As many as 25% of pelvic fractures have concomitant urethral injuries

POTENTIAL COMPLICATIONS

- Impotence
- Incontinence
- Strictures
- Infection

PEDIATRIC CONSIDERATIONS

- Urethral damage, frequently caused by traumatic mechanisms similar to adults
- Nonaccidental trauma or sexual abuse, especially females, may be contributory
- Most posterior urethral injuries are type I

Pre-Hospital

- Similar considerations as for major trauma victims

Diagnosis

ESSENTIAL WORKUP

- Female
  - —A meticulous vaginal examination to exclude vaginal laceration as the bleeding source
  - —Radiographic evaluation of the integrity of the urethra should be performed before urinary catheter placement if urethral injury is suspected
  - —If this is not possible, suprapubic aspiration or cystostomy should be done
- Male
  - —Determine whether the prostate is normally positioned (not high-riding) and examine for blood at the external meatus
  - —Radiographic evaluation of the integrity of the urethra should be performed before urinary catheter placement if urethral injury is suspected
  - —If this is not possible, suprapubic aspiration or cystostomy should be done

LABORATORY

- Urinalysis
- Hematocrit
- BUN and creatinine

IMAGING/SPECIAL TESTS

- Retrograde urethrography (RUG)
  - —Water-soluble contrast is injected via a catheter-tipped syringe at the urethral meatus
  - —Extravasation of contrast and its relation to the prevesical space and urogenital diaphragm should be noted
  - —Proximity of the extravasation to the meatus and the bladder should be appreciated
  - —If the urethral tear is complete, there will be no contrast within the bladder, and marked extravasation will occur
  - —A partial tear will demonstrate contrast material within the bladder
  - —Excretory urethrography to define proximal urethral tears
- Cystography
  - —40% of urethral injuries have concomitant bladder injuries

DIFFERENTIAL DIAGNOSIS

- Perineal and vaginal trauma
- Bladder trauma
- Ureter or kidney trauma

PEDIATRIC CONSIDERATIONS

- If an examination of the introitus and perineum cannot easily be performed, examination under anesthesia should occur
- An examination in the OR, in addition to being better tolerated by the patient, allows the physician to rule out sexual abuse and to confirm that the injury is consistent with the history
- The workup of male pediatric patients should also include an examination in the operating room if an adequate ED examination does not occur or if suspicion of abuse exists

Treatment

INITIAL STABILIZATION

- ABCs of trauma care take precedence

ED TREATMENT

- After RUG, the urologist should be contacted
- Urethral contusions, lacerations, and avulsions are best managed by an experienced urologist
- Catheter placement, if appropriate, or suprapubic aspiration/cystostomy followed by laboratory evaluation comprise the ED treatment

MEDICATIONS

- No specific medications for this injury

Disposition

ADMISSION CRITERIA

- Concurrent closed head injury, blunt abdominal trauma, or pelvic fracture
- Need for operative management of urethral, penile, or bladder injuries

DISCHARGE CRITERIA

- Isolated urethral injuries frequently may be managed in the outpatient setting after appropriate urinary catheterization or suprapubic cystostomy with urologic follow-up

Miscellaneous

ICD9: 867.0

ICD10: S37.3

SUGGESTED READINGS

Avanoglu A, Ulman I, Herek O, et al. Posterior urethral injuries in children. Br J Urol 1996;77:598–600.

Carter CT, Schafer N. Incidence of urethral disruption in females with traumatic pelvic fractures. Am J Emerg Med 1993;11(3):218–220.

Goldman SM, Sandler CM, Corriere JN Jr, et al. Blunt urethral trauma: a unified, anatomical mechanical classification. J Urol 1997;157:85–89.

Lynch JM, Gardner MJ, Albanese CT. Blunt urogenital trauma in prepubescent female patients: More than meets the eye. Pediatr Emerg Care 1995;11(6):372–375.

Watnik NF, Coburn M, Goldberger M. Urologic injuries in pelvic ring disruptions. Clin Orthop 1996;329:37–45.

Author: Kenneth Bramwell

Urethritis

Clinical Presentation

SIGNS AND SYMPTOMS

- Urethral discharge, dysuria, cloudy first portion of urine
- Pyuria
- Inguinal adenopathy may be present

MECHANISM/DESCRIPTION

- Symptoms usually develop 1–2 weeks after exposure but can take up to 4–6 weeks
  —Initially minimal or absent in many patients
- Urethritis may develop after exposure to a partner with a sexually transmitted disease, bacterial vaginosis, or a urinary tract infection
- Urethritis may also develop after orogenital contact

ETIOLOGY

- Sexually transmitted diseases
- The most common causes are
  —*Neisseria gonorrhoeae* (20%)
  —*Chlamydia trachomatis* (30–50%)
  —*Ureaplasma urealyticum* (10–40%)
- Rarer causes include *Trichomonas vaginalis*, candidal species, herpes simplex virus, genital warts, and foreign bodies
- Sometimes no cause is identified

POTENTIAL COMPLICATIONS

- Recurrent infections
- Ascending urinary tract infections including pelvic inflammatory disease and epididymoorchitis
- Fallopian tube damage and infertility
- Arthritis
- Conjunctivitis, uveitis, and blindness

PEDIATRIC CONSIDERATIONS

- Urethritis in children should arouse suspicion of child abuse

Pre-Hospital

N/A

Diagnosis

ESSENTIAL WORKUP

- Urethral swabs for *N. gonorrhea,* and *Chlamydia* species will confirm the diagnosis
- An RPR or VRDL should be drawn because sexually transmitted diseases frequently occur together

LABORATORY

- Gram stain and cultures from urethral swabs should be reviewed when the patient is reevaluated by their physician after treatment
- Urinalysis should be performed after urethral swabs to identify urinary tract infections

IMAGING/SPECIAL TESTS

- No specific tests

DIFFERENTIAL DIAGNOSIS

- Urinary tract infection
- Prostatitis
- Epididymitis
- Orchitis
- Pelvic inflammatory disease
- Reiter's syndrome

PEDIATRIC CONSIDERATIONS

- Because *N. gonorrhoeae* infects the entire vaginal vault in prepubescents, a speculum examination is not required; external examination and cultures are sufficient

Treatment

INITIAL STABILIZATION

- Most patients will not require significant stabilization

ED TREATMENT

- Treatment may be given empirically based on probable etiologic causes
- Patients should be treated for both gonorrhea and chlamydia

MEDICATIONS

- Gonorrhea
  —Cefixime: 400 mg PO
  —Ceftriaxone: 125 mg i.m. or i.v. (peds: ceftriaxone 25–50 mg/kg i.m.)
- Chlamydia
  —Azithromycin: 1 g PO (peds: 10 mg/kg PO day 1, 5 mg/kg PO days 2–5
  —Doxycycline: 100 mg PO b.i.d. for 7 days
  —Erythromycin base: 500 mg PO q.i.d. for 10 days (peds: 40 mg/kg/day div. q6h for 10 days)
- Single-dose oral therapy is preferred
- The quinolones have been reported as equivalents but do not have adequate activity against *Ureaplasma* species to treat these infections

Disposition

ADMISSION CRITERIA

- Patients should not require admission for urethritis unless other complaints or infections so mandate

DISCHARGE CRITERIA

- All patients should be discharged with follow-up arranged at an outside clinic or with their physician

PEDIATRIC CONSIDERATIONS

- If child abuse is suspected, child protective services must be involved, and the child should be admitted if a safe home situation cannot be ensured

Miscellaneous

ICD9: 597.80

ICD10: N34.2

SUGGESTED READINGS

Ingram DL. Neisseria gonorrhoeae in children. Pediatr Ann 1994;23(7):341–345.

Ness RB, Markovic N, Carlson CL, et al. Do men become infertile after having sexually transmitted urethritis? An epidemiologic examination. Fertil Steril 1997;68(2): 205–213.

Nickel P, Naher H. Nongonococcal urethritis. Curr Probl Dermatol 1996; 24:97–104.

Authors: Kenneth Bramwell; Roscoe Nelson

Urinary Retention

Clinical Presentation

SIGNS AND SYMPTOMS

- History of chronic voiding hesitancy
  - —Decreased size and force of urine stream
  - —Difficulty holding or initiating urinary stream
  - —Feeling of incomplete bladder emptying or postvoid residual
  - —Interruption of urinary stream
- Lower abdominal pain
- Distended and tender bladder

MECHANISM/DESCRIPTION

- Normal micturition *sequence*
  - —As the bladder fills, sensory stretch signals are conducted to the sacral cord through the pelvic nerves and then back through the parasympathetics, supplying the body and neck of the bladder
  - —Once the micturition reflex becomes powerful enough, an inhibitory reflex through the somatic pudendal nerves from S-2 to S-3 causes relaxation of the external urethral sphincter
  - —Urination occurs if inhibition is more powerful than the voluntary constriction signals
- Acute urinary retention (AUR)
  - —Sudden inability to void urine, resulting in bladder distention
- More common in men with advancing age than women, less common in children
- Atonic bladder
  - —More common in women
  - —Decompensated bladder that has resulted from years of infrequent voiding
  - —Destruction of sensory nerve fibers from the bladder to spinal cord that prevents transmission of stretch signals and prevents micturition reflex contractions
  - —Loss of bladder control occurs despite intact neurogenic connections to the brain
  - —Bladder fills to capacity and overflows a few drops at a time (overflow incontinence)
- Automatic bladder
  - —From damage of the spinal cord above the level of S-2 to S-3
  - —Micturition inhibited due to "spinal shock" from the sudden loss of facilitory impulse from the brainstem and cerebrum
  - —Intermittent straight catheterization facilitates the return of the excitability of the micturition reflex by preventing physical bladder injury
- Neurogenic bladder
  - —From partial damage in the spinal cord or brainstem that interrupts inhibition
  - —Sacral centers are in a constant state of excitation that even a small quantity of urine results in frequent and relatively uncontrollable micturition

ETIOLOGY

- Benign prostatic hypertrophy: most common in men
- Multiple sclerosis and diabetes: most common in women and may be an early manifestation of neurologic disease in children
- Bladder outlet obstruction
  - —Benign prostatic hypertrophy
  - —Prostate
  - —Cancer
  - —Acute prostatitis
  - —Stones
  - —Blood clots
  - —Prostatic congestion
- Detrusor muscle failure
  - —Acute spinal cord injury
  - —Elderly patients
  - —Sympathomimetics
- Neurologic causes
  - —Detrusor hyperactivity with impaired contractility
  - —Multiple sclerosis
  - —Parkinson's
  - —Stroke
  - —Herniated disk
  - —Diabetes melitis
  - —Dementia
  - —Myasthenia gravis
  - —Brain tumor
  - —Landry-Guillain-Barré syndrome
  - —Bladder neck dysfunction
- Urethral stricture
  - —Meatal stenosis
  - —Phimosis
  - —Paraphimosis
  - —Foreign body constriction
- Gynecologic
  - —Posturethropexy
  - —Postvaginal delivery
  - —Infectious
  - —Periurethral abscess
  - —Urinary tract infection
  - —Constipation
- Medications that cause AUR
  - —β-Agonists
  - —α-Adrenergic stimulator
  - —Narcotics
  - —Anticholinergics
  - —Musculotropic relaxants

PEDIATRIC CONSIDERATIONS

- AUR uncommon in children
- Cystitis most common cause
- Less common cause include phimosis, paraphimosis, and meatal stenosis
- Exclude testicular torsion

Pre-Hospital

N/A

Diagnosis

ESSENTIAL WORKUP

- Thorough history and physical examination
- Urinalysis

LABORATORY

- Electrolytes, BUN, creatinine, and glucose
- For renal failure
  - —Prostate-specific antigen
  - —Urine culture

IMAGING/SPECIAL TESTS

- Ultrasound
- CT scan
- Intravenous pyelography (IVP)

Treatment

INITIAL STABILIZATION

- Urinary drainage by catheterization
- Caution with history of urethral stricture or traumatic catheter insertion
- Defer catheterization in patient with pelvic fracture, prostate displacement on rectal examination, or blood at the urethral meatus until retrograde urethrogram
- Suprapubic catheter if urethral catheterization contraindicated or impossible
- Palpable bladder essential

ED TREATMENT

- Drain out and monitor urine output
- Place leg Foley bag before discharge if Foley is to remain indwelling
- Initiate therapy for underlying cause of AUR
  - —Rapid decompression following catheter placement may result in transient gross hematuria in the chronically distended edematous bladder
- Postobstructive diuresis
  - —Complication of AUR in the catheterized patient
  - —Occurs from a combination of factors, including osmotic diuresis, involvement of natriuretic and diuretic factors, disorder nephron function, altered tubular permeability, and disturbance of sodium-regulating hormones
  - —Hypovolemic or hypotensive may result in severe cases
- Observe for 4–6 hours all patients with chronic or insidious obstructive voiding symptoms and urinary retention with particular attention to hourly intake, urinary output, and vital signs

PEDIATRIC CONSIDERATIONS

- Bladder decompression via Foley catheter or suprapubic bladder aspiration (SPA)
- Estimate the expected bladder capacity in ounces by age in years plus 2

MEDICATIONS

- Baclofen (Lioresal) for external sphincter emptying: 5 mg PO t.i.d., max 80 mg/d (peds: 2–7 years old: 10–15 mg/24 h div. q8h; titrate to max dose 40 mg/24 h; >8 years old: max dose 60 mg/d div. q8h)
- Belladonna and opium (B and O) suppositories to alleviate the constant urge to urinate secondary to bladder spasm, frequently accompanying an indwelling catheter: 1 PO q4–6h
- Bethanechol (Urecholine) acts on the detrusor to empty the bladder: 10–50 mg PO b.i.d./q.i.d.; SC: 5 mg (peds: PO 0.6 mg/kg/24 h div. q6–8h; SC: 0.15–0.2 mg/kg/24 h div. q6–8h)
- Dantrolene (Dantrium) for external sphincter emptying: initial: 25 mg PO q.d., increase frequency to t.i.d. to q.i.d., then increase dose by 25 mg/dose at 4–7 day intervals (peds [not indicated <5 years old]: >5 years old: initial: 0.5 mg/kg/dose PO b.i.d.; increment: increase frequency to t.i.d. to q.i.d. at 4- to 7-day intervals, then increase doses by 0.5 mg/kg)
- Diazepam (Valium) for external sphincter emptying: i.m. or i.v. 2–10 mg/dose q3–4h PRN, PO: 2–10 mg/dose q6–8h PRN (peds: i.m. or i.v.: 0.04–0.2 mg/kg/dose q2–4h (max dose: 0.6 mg/kg within an 8-hour period; PO: 0.12–0.8 mg/kg/24 h div. q6–8h)
- Doxazosin mesylate (Cardura) for vesical outlet emptying: initial 1 mg PO q.d., after 24 hours, increase to 2 mg PO q.d. then to 4, 8, 16 mg q.d.
- Meperidine HCl (Demerol) for external sphincter relaxation: PO, i.m., i.v.: 50–150 mg/dose q3–4h PRN (peds: PO, i.m., i.v.: 1.0–1.5 mg/kg/dose q3–4h PRN, max dose: 100 mg)
- Oxybutynin (Ditropan) for storage: 5 mg PO b.i.d. to t.i.d.
- Phenoxybenzamine HCl (Dibenzyline) for vesical outlet emptying: 10 mg PO, increase dosage every other day, usually to 20–40 mg, b.i.d. to t.i.d.
- Prazosin HCl (Minipress) for vesical outlet emptying: initially 1 mg PO b.i.d. to t.i.d., slow increase to 20 mg/d in divided doses
- Pseudoephedrine (Sudafed) for vesical outlet storage: 30–60 mg/dose PO q6–8h, max dose 240 mg/24 h (peds: <12 years old: 4 mg/kg/24 h PO div. q6h)
- Terazosin (Hytrin) for vesical outlet emptying: start 1 mg PO q.h.s., max 20 mg/d
- Trimethoprim without sulfa (Trimpex or Proloprim) for the duration of catheter insertion, if it is to remain indwelling for more than 5 days: 100 mg tablets q.d. or b.i.d.

Disposition

ADMISSION CRITERIA

- Significant postobstructive diuresis requiring IV fluids, electrolyte, and urine output monitoring

DISCHARGE CRITERIA

- Good health with support system
- No clinical or laboratory evidence of infection
- Urology follow-up

Miscellaneous

ICD9: 788.20

ICD10: R33

SUGGESTED READINGS

Escobar JI II, Eastman ER, Hardwood-Nuss AL. Acute urinary retention. In: Marx J, Hockberger R, Walls R, et al. eds. Rosen's emergency medicine, 5th ed. St. Louis: Mosby, 2002.

Gausehe M. Genitourinary surgical emergencies. Pediatr Ann 1996;25(8): 458–464.

Nyman MA, et al. Management of acute urinary retention: rapid vs gradual decompression and risk of complications. Mayo Clin Proc 1997;72:951.

Peter JR, Steinhardt GF. Acute urinary retention in children. Pediatr Emerg Care 1993;9:205–207.

Samm BJ, Dmochowski RR. Urologic emergencies. Postgrad Med 1996;100(4): 177–184.

Author: Anthony Huynh

Urinary Tract Fistula

Clinical Presentation

SIGNS AND SYMPTOMS

- Vesicointestinal fistulas
  - —Chronic or recurrent urinary tract infections
  - —Most infections are caused by *Escherichia coli*
  - —Mixed organisms account for one third of infections
  - —Pneumaturia—60% occurrence rate
  - —Fecaluria—40% occurrence rate
  - —Abdominal pain
  - —Change in bowel habits
- Vesicovaginal, urethrovaginal, and ureterovaginal fistulas
  - —Constant leakage of urine from the vagina; described as watery vaginal discharge
  - —Malodorous urine
  - —Perineal dermatitis and maceration
  - —Severe perineal pain if fistula is a complication of radiation therapy
  - —Ureterovaginal fistula
  - —Abdominal pain
  - —Flank tenderness
  - —Fever
  - —Drainage of urine through the operative site
- Vesicocutaneous fistula
  - —Constant leakage of urine from bladder through fistula to skin
  - —Usually located in perineal region
  - —Perineal dermatitis and maceration at site of leakage

MECHANISM/DESCRIPTION

- Fistula formation can occur between any part of the urinary tract and contiguous structures
- Communications between the urinary tract and gastrointestinal tract, external perineum, and female reproductive organs are most common
- Urinary fistulas
  - —Not the result of primary urologic disease
  - —Due to rather a complication of gynecologic surgery, childbirth, and gastrointestinal disorders

ETIOLOGY

- Vesicointestinal fistulas
  - —Complication of a primary gastrointestinal disease
  - —Diverticulitis: 50–60% of cases
  - —Colon cancer: 20–25% of cases
  - —Crohn's disease: 10% of cases
  - —Radiation enteritis: 7% of cases
  - —Pelvic trauma: 5% of cases
  - —Bladder cancer: 4% of cases
  - —Other causes
    - -Appendicitis
    - -Gynecologic cancers
    - -Tuberculosis
- Vesicovaginal, urethrovaginal, and ureterovaginal fistulas
  - —Gynecologic surgery: 80% of cases
  - —Occurs 10–14 days after surgery
  - —Obstetric complication: 8–10% of cases
  - —Pelvic irradiation: 6% of cases
  - —Pelvic trauma: 4% of cases
- Vesicocutaneous fistula
  - —Cervical or uterine cancer
  - —Bladder cancer
  - —Advanced prostatic cancer

Pre-Hospital

N/A

Diagnosis

ESSENTIAL WORKUP

- Vesicointestinal fistulas
  - —Thorough history points to diagnosis
- Vesicovaginal, urethrovaginal, and ureterovaginal fistulas
  - —Clinical diagnosis
  - —Speculum exam may reveal a small, reddened area of granulomatous tissue at site of fistula opening
  - —If uncertain whether vaginal discharge contains urine, give phenazopyridine (Pyridium), 200 mg orally, and perform speculum exam 1 hour later
  - —Orange discoloration of discharge confirms fistula
- Vesicocutaneous fistula
  - —Clinical diagnosis with thorough physical examination

LABORATORY

- Urinalysis
  - —Undigested food residue with vesicointestinal fistulas
  - —Bacteria with vesicovaginal, urethrovaginal, and ureterovaginal fistulas
  - —Bacteria and white blood cells with vesicocutaneous fistula
- Urine culture
  - —*E. coli* major pathogen with vesicointestinal fistulas
  - —One third infected with multiple organisms
  - —Mixed organisms with vesicovaginal, urethrovaginal, and ureterovaginal fistulas
  - —To exclude infection with vesicocutaneous fistula

IMAGING/SPECIAL TESTS

- Cystoscopy with or without fistulography is a very reliable means of diagnosis
- CT scan has sensitivity close to 100% in diagnosing vesicointestinal fistulas

DIFFERENTIAL DIAGNOSIS

- Vesicointestinal fistulas
  - —Recurrent urinary tract infection
  - —Other causes of pneumaturia
  - —Urinary tract infection with gas-forming organism such as clostridia
  - —Fermentation of glucose in urine
  - —Recent urinary tract instrumentation
- Vesicovaginal, urethrovaginal, and ureterovaginal fistulas
  - —Urinary incontinence
  - —Copious vaginal discharge
- Vesicocutaneous fistula
  - —Urinary incontinence

Treatment

INITIAL STABILIZATION

- Treat urosepsis with IV fluid bolus and IV antibiotics

ED TREATMENT

- Vesicointestinal fistulas
  - —Rule out complications from patient's primary disease
  - —Obtain cultures if signs of urinary tract infection
  - —Initiate broad-spectrum antibiotic if infection found
  - —Antibiotic resistance is common
  - —Most patients have received multiple antibiotics for recurrent or chronic urinary tract infections
  - —Urologic referral for definitive surgical therapy
- Vesicovaginal, urethrovaginal, and ureterovaginal fistulas
  - —Place Foley catheter for any patient suspected of having a genitourinary fistula
  - —Treat perineal dermatitis and skin maceration with
  - —Antifungal creams such as nystatin, clotrimazole, or miconazole
  - —Protective ointment applied to protect skin from moisture
  - —Initiate broad-spectrum antibiotics if a urinary tract infection is present
  - —Third-generation cephalosporin, fluoroquinolone, or amoxicillin/clavulanate acid
  - —Prompt urology and gynecology referral
- Vesicocutaneous fistula
  - —Place Foley catheter
  - —Treat dermatitis and skin maceration with
  - —Antifungal creams such as nystatin, clotrimazole, or miconazole
  - —Protective ointment applied to protect skin from moisture
  - —Initiate broad-spectrum antibiotics if a urinary tract infection is present
  - —Third-generation cephalosporin, fluoroquinolone, or amoxicillin/clavulanate acid
  - —Prompt urology referral

MEDICATIONS

- Amoxicillin/clavulanate: 875 mg PO b.i.d. or 500 mg PO t.i.d.
- Ampicillin/sulbactam: 3 g i.v. q6h
- Cefaclor: 500 mg PO t.i.d.
- Cefixime: 400 mg PO q.d.
- Ceftriaxone: 2 g i.v. q.d.
- Ciprofloxacin: 400 mg i.v. or 500 mg PO b.i.d.
- Levofloxacin (Levaquin): 500 mg PO q.d.

Disposition

ADMISSION CRITERIA

- Presence of urosepsis or septic shock
- Unable to take oral antibiotics
- Dehydration
- Complications from primary gastrointestinal disease or pelvic malignancies
- Bowel obstruction
- Malnutrition

DISCHARGE CRITERIA

- No evidence of urosepsis or shock
- Able to administer oral antibiotics if urinary tract infections present
- Able to care for Foley catheter

Miscellaneous

ICD9: 599.1

ICD10: N36.0

SUGGESTED READINGS

Diver CP, Anderson DN, Findlay K, et al. Vesico-colic fistulae in Grampian Region: presentation, assessment, management, and outcome. J R Coll Surg Edinb 1997;42:182–185.

Lee RA, Symonds RE, Williams TJ. Current status of genitourinary fistula. Obstet Gynecol 1988;72(3):313–19.

McVay KT, Marshall FF. Urinary fistulas. In: Gillenwater J, et al., eds. Adult and pediatric urology, 3rd ed. St. Louis: CV Mosby, 1996.

Moos RL, Ryan JA. Management of enterovesical fistulas. Am J Surg 1990;159:514–517.

Shobeiri SA, Chesson RR, Echols KT. Cystoscopic fistulography: a new technique for the diagnosis of vesicocervical fistula. Obstet Gynecol 2001;98(6):1124–1126.

Author: Anthony Huynh

Urinary Tract Infections, Adult

Clinical Presentation

SIGNS AND SYMPTOMS

- *Lower urinary tract infection (UTI):* cystitis
  - —Dysuria, frequency, urgency
  - —Hesitancy
  - —Suprapubic pain
  - —Hematuria
- *Upper UTI:* pyelonephritis
  - —Symptoms of cystitis
  - —Fever, chills
  - —Flank pain
  - —Costovertebral angle tenderness (CVAT)
  - —Nausea, vomiting, anorexia
  - —Leukocytosis
- Pyelonephritis: up to 50% may be without clinical symptoms (silent upper tract disease)
  - —Symptom duration greater than 5 days and being homeless are risk factors for upper UTI
- *Elderly people:*
  - —Altered mental status
  - —Anorexia
  - —Decreased social interaction
  - —Abdominal pain
  - —Nocturia
  - —Incontinence

MECHANISM/DESCRIPTION

- Colonization of urine with uropathogens and invasion of genitourinary tract (GU)
- Defined as urinary symptoms with $\geq 10^2$ to 10^5 CFU/mL of uropathogen and $\geq$10 WBC/mm^3
- *Uncomplicated cystitis* (criteria)
  - —Females aged 13 to 50 years
  - —Symptoms <2–3 days
  - —Not pregnant
  - —Afebrile (temperature <38°C)
  - —No flank pain
  - —No CVAT
  - —Fewer than four UTIs in past year
  - —No recent instrumentation or previous GU surgery
  - —No functional/structural GU abnormality
  - —No immunocompromising comorbidity
  - —Neurologically intact
- *Complicated cystitis*
  - —Male gender
  - —Patients with anatomic, functional, or metabolic abnormalities of GU tract
  - —Postvoid residual urine
  - —Catheters
  - —Resistant pathogens
  - —Recent antimicrobial use
- *Uncomplicated pyelonephritis*
  - —Renal parenchymal infection
  - —Dysuria, frequency, urgency
  - —Fever, chills, myalgias
  - —Flank, back or abdominal pain
  - —CVAT
  - —Nausea, vomiting
  - —Leukocytosis (common)
- *Complicated pyelonephritis*
  - —Renal parenchymal infection
  - —Temperature >40°C
  - —Urosepsis with septic shock
  - —Intractable nausea, vomiting
  - —Diabetes
  - —Pregnancy
  - —Immunosuppression
  - —Asymptomatic (occult)

ETIOLOGY

- Organisms colonize periurethral area and subsequently infect the GU tract
- Risk factors
  - —Behavior: sexual intercourse, spermicides, diaphragms
  - —Elderly females/postmenopausal state due to less efficient bladder emptying, instrumentation
  - —Elderly males due to prostatic hypertrophy and instrumentation
- *Organisms*
  - —*Escherichia coli* (80–85%)
  - —*Staphylococcus saprophyticus* (10%)
  - —Other (10%): *Klebsiella* species, *Proteus mirabilis, Enterobacter* species, *Pseudomonas aeruginosa,* group D streptococci

PEDIATRIC CONSIDERATIONS

- See Urinary Tract Infection, Pediatric

Pre-Hospital

N/A

ESSENTIAL WORKUP

- Urinalysis (dipstick test, microscopy)
- Females: pregnancy test
- Females: rule out urethritis, vaginitis, pelvic inflammatory disease (PID)
- Males: rule out urethritis, epididymitis, prostatitis
- Males: inquire about anal intercourse and HIV status
- Urologic evaluation in young healthy males with first UTI is *not* necessary

LABORATORY

- *Rapid urine screen:* urine dipstick (leukocyte esterase + nitrite)
  - —Laboratory urinalysis/microscopy unnecessary if pyuria and bacteriuria confirmed by dipstick
  - —Leukocyte esterase: sensitivity, 75–96%; specificity, 94–98%
  - —Nitrite: sensitivity, 35–85%; specificity, 92–100%
  - —Both tests have excellent negative predictive values
- *Urinalysis/microscopy:* obtain if rapid urine screen unavailable or negative in patients with presumed UTI
  - —10 WBC/mm^3 in clean-catch midstream urine indicates infection
  - —Bacteria detected in unspun urine indicates >10^5 CFU/mL
- *Indications for urine culture*
  - —Complicated UTIs
  - —Persistent signs/symptoms after 2 to 3 days of treatment
  - —Recurrence (relapse versus reinfection)
  - —Recently hospitalized patients
  - —Nosocomial infections
  - —Pyelonephritis
- Additional labs dictated by clinical setting

IMAGING/SPECIAL TESTS

- Indicated for complicated upper tract disease, see Pyelonephritis
- Helical CT, intravenous pyelogram (IVP), or renal ultrasound if concomitant stone or obstruction suspected

DIFFERENTIAL DIAGNOSIS

- Pyelonephritis
- Urethritis
- Vulvovaginitis
- PID, cervicitis
- Prostatitis
- Epididymitis
- Nephrolithiasis
- Appendicitis
- Diverticulitis

Treatment

INITIAL STABILIZATION

Urosepsis, Septic Shock

- ABCs, crystalloid resuscitation, cultures, vasopressors as needed
- Antibiotics (fluoroquinolone or antipseudomonal penicillin with aminoglycoside or carbapenems, or third-generation cephalosporin with antipseudomonal activity)

Stable Patients

- *Prevalence of uropathogens resistant to trimethoprim-sulfamethoxazole (TMP-SMX), amoxicillin, first-generation cephalosporins is increasing (up to 30%)*
- Antibiotics of choice:
  —Fluoroquinolones (95% susceptibility rates)
  —TMP-SMX (10% to 20% resistance)
  —Nitrofurantoin (15% to 20% resistance)
- Fluoroquinolones indicated first-line treatment in women:
  —Sulfonamide intolerance
  —Failed recent treatment
  —Live in areas with significant resistance to TMP-SMX (>10–20%)
  —Live in areas with unknown TMP-SMX resistance rates
- Second- or third-generation oral cephalosporins may be reasonable alternates (cefuroxime, cefixime) in specific circumstances
  —Require 7-day treatment regimens
- Asymptomatic bacteriuria in pregnancy requires treatment with 3- to 7-day course of antibiotics using nitrofurantoin, TMP-SMX, amoxicillin, or cephalexin
- Fosfomycin also safe and effective in pregnancy
- Treat symptom of *dysuria* with phenazopyridine
- Treatment of upper tract disease: *rule of 2s*
  —Administer 2 L of IV fluid, 2 tablets of Tylenol #3, 2 g of ceftriaxone or 2 mg/kg of gentamicin
  —If fever drops by 2°C and patient can retain 2 glasses of water, discharge with prescription for fluoroquinolone for 2 weeks, with follow-up in 2 days

MEDICATIONS

- Uncomplicated cystitis, 3–5 day regimen; outpatient treatment of upper tract disease, 10–14 day regimen
- Amoxicillin: 500 mg PO q12h or 875 mg PO q12h
- Cefixime: 400 mg PO q.d. or 200 mg PO q12h
  -Can be used to treat gonorrhea (400 mg PO single dose) or chlamydia infection (300 mg PO q12h for 7 days) when diagnosis of UTI versus sexually transmitted disease is unclear
- Ceftazidime: 1–2 g i.v. q8–12h
- Ceftriaxone: 1–2 g i.v. or i.m. q24h
- Cefuroxime: 250–500 mg PO q12h
- Cephalexin: 250–500 mg PO q6h
- Ciprofloxacin: 100–500 mg PO q12h
  —Uncomplicated pyelonephritis, PO = i.v. efficacy; 500 mg PO q12h for 7 days is more effective than TMP-SMX
- Fosfomycin: 3 g single dose
- Gentamicin: 2 mg/kg i.v. q8h
- Levofloxacin: 250 mg PO q24h
- Nitrofurantoin: 100 mg PO q12h (sustained release)
- Norfloxacin: 400 mg PO q12h or 800 mg PO q24h
- Ofloxacin: 200 mg PO q12h or 400 mg i.v. q12h
- Phenazopyridine: 200 mg PO t.i.d. for 2 days
- TMP-SMX: 160 mg/800 mg PO q12h or 8–10 mg/kg i.v. q12h
  -For symptomatic treatment of dysuria; may turn urine and contact lenses orange

Disposition

ADMISSION CRITERIA

- Inability to comply with oral therapy
- Unstable vital signs
- Toxic appearance
- Pyelonephritis with intractable symptoms, extremes of age, immunosuppression, urinary obstruction, significant comorbid disease, outpatient treatment failure
- Pyelonephritis in early pregnancy with good follow-up may be treated as outpatients

DISCHARGE CRITERIA

- Well appearing
- Stable vital signs
- Can maintain oral hydration
- Can comply with oral therapy
- No significant comorbid disease
- Adequate follow-up (48–72 hours) as needed
- Healthy patients with uncomplicated pyelonephritis who respond to treatment in ED according to rule of 2s

PEDIATRIC CONSIDERATIONS

- See Urinary Tract Infection, Pediatric

Miscellaneous

ICD9: 599.0

ICD10: N39.0

SUGGESTED READINGS

Gupta K, Scholes D, Stamm WE. Increasing prevalence of antimicrobial resistance among uropathogens causing acute uncomplicated cystitis in women. JAMA 1999;281(8):736–738.

Hooton TM. Practice guidelines for urinary tract infection in the era of managed care. Int J Antimicrob Agents 1999;11:241–245.

Hooton TM, Stamm WE. Diagnosis and treatment of uncomplicated urinary tract infection. Infect Dis Clin North Am 1997;11(3):551–581.

Stamm WE, Hooton TM. Management of urinary tract infections in adults. N Engl J Med 1993;329(18):1328–1334.

Warren JW, Abrutyn E, Hebel JR, et al. Guidelines for antimicrobial treatment of uncomplicated acute bacterial cystitis and acute pyelonephritis in women. Clin Infect Dis 1999;103(4):843–852.

Authors: Paul Szucs; Barnet Eskin

Urinary Tract Infection, Pediatric

Clinical Presentation

SIGNS AND SYMPTOMS

- Often nonspecific
- Neonates
  - —Manifestations of sepsis
  - —Feeding difficulties
  - —Irritability, listlessness
  - —Fever, hypothermia
- 1 month–3 years of age
  - —Fever
  - —Irritability
  - —Vomiting, diarrhea
  - —Abdominal pain
  - —Poor feeding, failure to thrive
  - —Hematuria
- >3 years of age
  - —Dysuria
  - —Frequency
  - —Enuresis
  - —Pain: abdominal, suprapubic, back, costovertebral (CVA)
  - —Fever
  - —Hematuria
  - —Malodorous cloudy urine
  - —Systemic toxicity: high fever and chills with CVA tenderness
- *Complications*
  - —Recurrent urinary tract infection (UTI)
  - —Pyelonephritis
  - —Chronic renal failure
    - -Incidence of scarring greatest in children <1 year old
    - -Scarring prevented by early detection and intervention
  - —Perinephric abscess
  - —Bacteremia/sepsis
  - —Urolithiasis

MECHANISM/DESCRIPTION

- Bacteria colonize via retrograde contamination of rectal or perineal flora
  - —Infants—often hematogenous spread
  - —Older children—vesicoureteral reflux major risk
- UTI is defined by culture with >10,000 organisms/mL on a catheterized or suprapubic specimen
- In infants 0–3 months old, UTI is associated with a 30% incidence of sepsis
- Predisposing factors
  - —Poor perineal hygiene
  - —Short urethra of female
  - —Female > male
  - —Infrequent voiding
  - —Constipation
  - —Sexual activity
  - —Circumcision probably reduces risk

ETIOLOGY

- UTI found in 4–7% of febrile infants
- Bacterial agents
  - —*Escherichia coli* accounts for 90%
  - —*Klebsiella pneumoniae*
  - —*Staphylococcus aureus*
  - —*Enterobacter* species
  - —*Proteus* species
  - —*Pseudomonas aeruginosa*
  - —*Enterococcus* species

Pre-Hospital

N/A

Diagnosis

ESSENTIAL WORKUP

- Urinalysis with microscopic RBC and WBC counts, and smear for bacteria
  - —Urinalysis alone has low diagnostic sensitivity in infants
  - —Causes of pyuria besides UTI include chemical (bubble bath) or physical (masturbation) irritation, dehydration, renal tuberculosis, trauma, acute glomerulonephritis, respiration infections, appendicitis, pelvic infection, and gastroenteritis
  - —Leukocyte esterase correlates with presence of pyuria
  - —Positive nitrite test indicates presence of bacteria capable of fixing nitrate
  - —Gram stain of urinary sediment may be useful
- Urine culture
  - —Catheterized or suprapubic tap specimens required; clean-catch midstream sample only useful in cooperative child
  - —Specimen should be cultured within 30 minutes or refrigerated
  - —Bagged urine samples should be used for urinalysis only (70% contamination rate)
  - —False-negative results may be caused by dilution, improper culture medium, recent antimicrobial therapy, fastidious organisms, bacteriostatic agent in urine, complete obstruction of ureter
- Urine collection method
  - —Clean-catch in cooperative male children
  - —Plastic bag collection adequate for urinalysis
  - —Clean the perineum (females) and glans (males) before application
  - —Can be used to rule out an infection if patient is not placed on antibiotics empirically
- Positive culture usually needs to be confirmed by suprapubic or catheterized specimen since contamination is common
  - —Bladder catheterization
    - -Acceptable in all infants
    - -Higher success rate than suprapubic aspiration
    - -Aseptic technique essential
  - —Suprapubic aspiration
    - -Most useful in infants
    - -Full bladder optimal
    - -Less commonly used than catheter

LABORATORY

- CBC and blood culture for young children with fever or nonspecific symptoms and no source on exam
- Electrolytes, BUN, creatinine
  - —Check if dehydration, pyelonephritis, or recurrent infection

IMAGING/SPECIAL TESTS

- Children requiring radiologic evaluation
  - —Infants <3 months of age
  - —Males (increased association with anomaly)
  - —Clinical signs and symptoms consistent with pyelonephritis
  - —Clinical evidence of renal disease
  - —After second documented lower tract UTI in females
- Voiding cystoureterogram (VCUG) and ultrasound
  - —UTI is associated with vesicoureteral reflux and other genitourinary abnormalities
  - —Nuclear cystogram is often substituted for VCUG in females
  - —Further evaluation with nuclear medicine studies depends upon the grade of vesicoureteral reflex and response to treatment

DIFFERENTIAL DIAGNOSIS

- Infection
  - —Volvovaginitis
  - —Viral cystitis
  - —Urethritis (*Neisseria gonorrhea or Chlamydia trachomatis*)
  - —Glomerulonephritis
  - —Appendicitis
- Trauma
  - —Chemical irritation
  - —Perineal
  - —Sexual abuse
  - —Genitourinary
  - —Masturbation
  - —Foreign body
- Nephrolithiasis
- Diabetes

Treatment

INITIAL STABILIZATION

- Treat infants <3 months old presumptively for sepsis until blood and other appropriate cultures are final
- Airway intervention for septic/acidotic infants with depressed respiratory drive
- 20 mL/kg bolus 0.9% NS for dehydration, hypovolemia, or sepsis; may repeat

ED TREATMENT

- Initiate IV antibiotics in all infants <3 months old
  - —Ampicillin and gentamicin in neonates
  - —Cephalosporins after 4–8 weeks of age
- Outpatient oral antibiotic for 7–10 days for children discharged
  - —Amoxicillin
  - —Amoxicillin/clavulanate
  - —Ampicillin
  - —Cephalexin
  - —Nitrofurantoin
  - —Trimethoprim-sulfamethoxazole (TMP-SMX)

MEDICATIONS

- Amoxicillin: 40 mg/kg/24 h PO q8h
- Amoxicillin/clavulanate: 40 mg/kg/24 h PO q8h
- Ampicillin: 100 mg/kg/24 h i.v. q6h
- Cefotaxime: 100 mg/kg/24 h i.v. or i.m. q6–8h
- Ceftriaxone: 50 mg/kg/24 h q12–24 h i.v. or i.m.
- Cephalexin: 50 mg/kg/24 h PO q6–12h
- Gentamicin: 2.5 mg/kg/dose i.v. q8h if full-term and age >7 days; 2.5 mg/kg/dose i.v. q12h if full-term and age 0–7 days (special dosing regimens in infants <36 weeks postconceptual age)
- Nitrofurantoin: 5–7 mg/kg/24 h PO q6h
- TMP-SMX (Bactrim, Septra suspension): 5 mL liquid (of 40/200 per 5 mL) per 10 kg per dose PO b.i.d.

Disposition

ADMISSION CRITERIA

- Infants <3 months of age
- Dehydration
- Ill appearance/toxicity/sepsis
- Suspected pyelonephritis
- Urinary obstruction
- Male with febrile UTI
- Vomiting, inability to retain medications
- Immunocompromised patient
- Renal insufficiency
- Foreign body (indwelling catheter)
- Pregnant

DISCHARGE CRITERIA

- Sufficiently hydrated
- Low risk for sepsis or meningitis
- Able to take oral antibiotics; compliant

Miscellaneous

ICD9: 599.0

ICD10: P39.3

SUGGESTED READINGS

American Academy of Pediatrics, Subcommittee on Urinary Tract Infection. Practice parameter: the diagnosis, treatment and evaluation of the initial urinary tract infection in febrile infants and young children. Pediatrics 1999;103:843.

Dick PT, Feldman W. Routine diagnostic imaging for childhood urinary tract infection: a systematic overview. J Pediatr 1996;15128.

Hoberman A, Han-Pu C, Keller DM, et al. Prevalence of urinary tract infection in febrile infants. J Pediatr 1993;123(1): 17–23.

Nelson DS, Gurr MB, Schunk JE: Management of febrile children with urinary tract infections. Am J Emerg Med 1998;16:643–647.

Schlager T, Lohr J. Urinary tract infection in outpatient febrile infants and children younger than five years of age. Pediatr Ann 1993;22:505–509.

Author: Suzanne Z. Barkin

Urticaria

Clinical Presentation

SIGNS AND SYMPTOMS

- Transient, pruritic, well-circumscribed skin eruptions consisting of erythematous or white, nonpitting, edematous plaques (wheals), which may be surrounded by an erythematous ring (flare); may see bullae or purpuric lesions with intense swelling
- Lesions are various sizes and shapes, haphazard distribution, may become confluent
- Wheals usually resolve in 3–4 hours
- New lesions evolve as old ones resolve
- *Acute:* <6 weeks
- *Chronic:* >6 weeks
- May be associated with systemic features—hypotension, flushing, headache, dizziness, respiratory distress
- May be part of *anaphylactic* reaction (respiratory distress and hypotension) or *angioedema* (edema of lower dermis—swelling of face and tongue)

MECHANISM/DESCRIPTION

- Skin mast cell release of inflammatory mediators, primarily histamine, resulting in increased vascular permeability and pruritus
- Edema of the epidermis, upper dermis, and mid dermis

ETIOLOGY

Acute

- Drugs: especially penicillin, sulfa, aspirin, NSAID, angiotensin-converting enzyme (ACE) inhibitors
- Foods or additives
- Insect bites, stings
- Connective tissue, endocrine, or neoplastic disorders
- Pregnancy, menstrual cycle
- Infections, particularly virus (including hepatitis), bacteria, fungus, parasite
- Inhalant or contact allergen
- Emotional stress
- Physical urticaria: more than 20 identified types, including
  - —Dermographism: most common form; reaction to skin pressure, linear wheals under tight clothing or on areas scratched with a firm object
  - —Cholinergic: monomorphic wheals 2–3 mm with bright red flare and intense pruritus
  - —A response to elevated core temperature (hot bath, fever, exercise, occlusive dress, or emotional stress)
  - —Other rare forms include cold-induced (may be fatal in cold immersions), delayed pressure, solar, aquagenic, vibratory, and idiopathic

Chronic

- 75% idiopathic
- Often an unrecognized recurring physical urticaria

PEDIATRIC CONSIDERATIONS

- Urticaria is frequently the result of reactions to foods in infants
- Swelling of distal extremities and acrocyanosis may be prominent in infants
- Bullae may form in the center of the wheal, especially on legs and buttocks

Pre-Hospital

CAUTIONS

- Patients with severe allergic reactions can progress rapidly to respiratory failure

Diagnosis

ESSENTIAL WORKUP

- *Complete history and physical exam:* lesion appearance, location, timing, duration, acute versus chronic, associated symptoms, triggers, coexisting diseases, allergies, medications, environment, exposures, and new foods; characteristics and location of hives, evaluate for sources of infection and signs of systemic diseases

LABORATORY

- Acute cases: not needed
- Chronic cases: evaluate for subclinical infection or systemic disease (CBC with differential, erythrocyte sedimentation rate, thyroid-stimulating hormone [TSH] and thyroid functions, urinalysis, liver function tests, hepatitis panel)
- Skin biopsy if urticarial vasculitis suspected (not done in ED)

IMAGING/SPECIAL TESTS

- Acute cases: not needed
- Chronic cases: chest, sinus, or dental radiographs may help identify subclinical infection
- Dermographism: scratch skin with a tongue blade, observe for linear wheal
- Cholinergic: exercise challenge to raise core temp
- Solar: expose to sunlight
- Cold: place an ice cube on skin for 5 minutes
- Aquagenic: apply tap water at differing temperatures

DIFFERENTIAL DIAGNOSIS

- Anaphylaxis
- Angioedema
- Insect bites, stings
- Infection
- Contact or allergic dermatitis
- Rash (varicella and other viral exanthems)
- Erythema multiforme
- Vasculitis
- Urticaria pigmentosa
- Systemic lupus erythematosus

Treatment

INITIAL STABILIZATION

- Severe reaction: ABCs, oxygen, parenteral or inhaled β-agonist, IV crystalloid, and vasopressors as needed
- See Anaphylaxis and Angioedema

ED TREATMENT

- Treatment largely symptomatic except in severe reactions
- Significant mucosal edema: suspect angioedema (see Angioedema)
- Prolonged, painful, or nonblanching lesions: suspect vasculitis (see Vasculitis)
- Avoid offending agent
- *β-Agonist* (parenteral or inhaled): severe hives, angioedema, or systemic features
- *H_1-receptor antagonist* (first or second generation): *mainstay of treatment*
- *H_2-receptor antagonist:* may be beneficial as adjunct to H_1-blocker when no response to H_1-blocker alone
- *Corticosteroid* (oral): severe or refractory cases
- *Tricyclic antidepressants:* potent histamine blockers
- Avoid aspirin, NSAIDs, and opiates—may exacerbate condition
- Concurrent use of ketoconazole or macrolides alters hepatic metabolism of antihistamine; use with caution
- Chronic urticaria unresponsive to antihistamines may respond to colchicine or dapsone; topical steroids are not effective

MEDICATIONS

β-Agonist

- Albuterol (0.5% solution): 0.5 mL nebulized every 20 minutes PRN (peds: 0.01–0.05 mL/kg/dose [max 0.5 mL/dose] nebulized every 20 minutes PRN)
- Epinephrine (1:1000 solution): 0.1–0.5 mg SC or i.m. every 10–15 minutes PRN (peds: 0.01 mg/kg, SC [max single dose not to exceed 0.3 mg] every 15 minutes PRN)
- Terbutaline: 0.25 mg SC every 15–30 minutes PRN (max 0.5 mg q 4 hrs); (peds, <12 years old: 0.005–0.01 mg/kg [max 0.4 mg/dose] SC every 15–20 minutes × 3 PRN)

H_1-Receptor Antagonist (First Generation—Sedating)

- Diphenhydramine hydrochloride (Benadryl): 25–50 mg PO, i.v., or i.m., up to q6h (peds: 5 mg/kg/24 h divided q.i.d. [max 300 mg/24 h])
- Hydroxyzine hydrochloride (Atarax): 25–50 mg PO or i.m. up to q.i.d. (peds: 2 mg/kg/24 h PO divided q.i.d. or 0.5–1 mg/kg i.m. q4–6h PRN)

H_1-Receptor Antagonist (Second Generation—Less Sedating, Not as Effective)

- Cetirizine (Zyrtec): adult and peds ≥6 years old: 5–10 mg PO q.d. (peds: 2–6 years old: 2.5 mg q.d. to b.i.d.)
- Loratadine (Claritin): 10 mg PO b.i.d.
- Fexofenadine (Allegra): 60 mg PO b.i.d.

H_2-Receptor Antagonist (Suggested Dosage)

- Cimetidine (Tagamet): 300 mg PO, i.v., or i.m. b.i.d. (peds: infants <1 year: 10–20 mg/kg/24 h PO, i.v., or i.m. divided q.i.d.; >1 year old: 20–40 mg/kg/24 h PO, i.v., or i.m. divided q.i.d.)
- Famotidine (Pepcid): 20 mg i.v. q12h or 20–40 mg PO q.h.s. (peds: 0.6–0.8 mg/kg/24 h i.v. [max 40 mg/24h] divided q8–12h or 1–1.2 mg/kg/24 h [max 40 mg/24 h] PO divided q8–12h)
- Ranitidine (Zantac): 150 mg PO b.i.d. (peds: neonate: 2–4 mg/kg/24 h PO divided q8–12h or 2 mg/kg/24 h i.v. divided q6–8h; infants and children 4–5 mg/kg/24 h PO divided q8–12h or 2–4 mg/kg/24 h i.v. or i.m. divided q6–8h)

Corticosteroid

- Prednisolone: 50 mg PO q.d. for 3 days (peds: 0.5–2 mg/kg/24 h [max 80 mg/24 h] divided q.d. to b.i.d. for 3–5 days)
- Prednisone: 40 mg PO q.d. or 20 mg PO b.i.d. for 3–5 days (peds: 1–2 mg/kg/24 h [max 80 mg/24 h] divided q.d. to b.i.d. for 3–5 days)

Tricyclic Antidepressant

- Doxepin (Sinequan): 10–25 mg PO t.i.d. (peds: not approved for under 12 years of age)

Disposition

ADMISSION CRITERIA

- Respiratory distress or failure
- Refractory hypotension or shock
- Severe refractory cases requiring IV medications
- Other systemic disease or infection

DISCHARGE CRITERIA

- Normal ventilation and oxygenation
- Normal blood pressure
- Absence of other condition requiring admission
- Symptoms controlled
- Adequate ability of caregivers at home to monitor for further exacerbations

Miscellaneous

ICD9: 708.9

ICD10: L50.9

SUGGESTED READINGS

Habif TP. Skin disease diagnosis and treatment. St. Louis: Mosby, 2001.

Hurwitz S. Clinical pediatric dermatology. Philadelphia: WB Saunders, 1993:516–519.

Mahmood T. Urticaria. Am Fam Physician 1995;51(4):811–816.

Mahmood T. Physical urticarias. Am Fam Physician 1994;49(6):1411–1414.

Sveum RJ. Urticaria. Post Grad Med 1996;100(2):77–84.

Author: Jeffrey Horton

Vaginal Bleeding

Clinical Presentation

SIGNS AND SYMPTOMS

- Vaginal bleeding
  - —Variable amounts
  - —May be associated with fetal tissue/clots
- Lightheadedness
- Weakness
- Thirst
- Acute hypotension or tachycardia
  - —May have altered mentation with significant pelvic bleeding due to ectopic pregnancy or ruptured ovarian cyst
  - —Abdominal distention or tenderness

MECHANISM/DESCRIPTION

- Common presenting complaint in the ED
- Most cases are due to benign causes
- Some patients will have potentially life-threatening conditions
- Most important principles in evaluating women with vaginal bleeding
  - —*All women capable of childbearing might be pregnant*
  - —Menstrual and sexual history *do not* rule out pregnancy

ETIOLOGY

- Pregnancy related
  - —Early pregnancy
  - —Ectopic pregnancy (occurs in 2% of pregnancies)
  - —Abortion (threatened, incomplete, complete, missed, inevitable, septic)
  - —Molar pregnancy
  - —Trauma
  - —Later pregnancy
  - —Placenta previa
  - —Placental abruption
  - —Molar pregnancy
  - —Labor
  - —Trauma
  - —Immediate postpartum
  - —Postpartum hemorrhage
  - —Uterine inversion
  - —Early postpartum
  - —Retained placenta
  - —Endometritis
- Nonpregnant patients
  - —Dysfunctional uterine bleeding
  - —Structural abnormalities
  - —Uterine fibroids
  - —Cervical/endometrial polyps
  - —Pelvic tumors
  - —Atrophic endometrium (most common cause of postmenopausal bleeding)
  - —Rare for systemic disorders to present solely with vaginal bleeding (von Willebrand's disease, idiopathic thrombocytopenic purpura [ITP])
  - —Trauma

Pre-Hospital

CAUTIONS

- Establish IV 0.9% NS with 1-L fluid bolus for significant bleeding or hypotension
- Administer high-flow oxygen in pregnant or unstable patients
- In later pregnancy
  - —Uterine contractions may be transiently terminated with terbutaline 0.25 mg SQ
  - —Place woman in left-lateral decubitus position to prevent occlusion of inferior vena cava by uterus

Diagnosis

ESSENTIAL WORKUP

- Qualitative pregnancy test; point-of-care testing, i.e., urine pregnancy test preferred
- Pelvic examination
  - —Essential for all women with vaginal bleeding
  - —If necessary, delay examination pending an ultrasound to rule out placenta previa for vaginal bleeding present in later pregnancy
  - —Speculum/bimanual exam; assess if cervical os open or closed
  - —Deferred if patient is near-term with possible rupture of fetal membranes and without other indications for emergent bimanual examination
- Pregnancy test for all patients with childbearing potential
- Early pregnancy
  - —Type and Rh
  - —Ultrasound (US) to confirm intrauterine pregnancy
  - —Quantitative β-human chorionic gonadotropin (β-hCG) if ultrasound is nondiagnostic
  - —Hematocrit (Hct) if significant bleeding
  - —Type and cross-match if ectopic pregnancy or low Hct
  - —Urinalysis
- Later pregnancy
  - —Type and Rh
  - —Ultrasound if no fetal heart tones, no documented intrauterine pregnancy, or unknown lie of placenta
  - —Hct if significant bleeding
  - —Type and cross-match if placenta previa/abruption or low Hct
  - —Disseminated intravascular coagulation (DIC) panel if placental abruption—platelets, prothrombin time (PT), partial thromboplastin time (PTT), fibrinogen, fibrin-split products
- Early postpartum
  - —Ultrasound for retained products
  - —Hct
  - —β-hCG if concerned about retained tissue

LABORATORY

- Hct for nonpregnant women with significant bleeding
- Platelet count for suspected thrombocytopenia
- PT/PTT for suspected coagulopathy

IMAGING/SPECIAL TESTS

- Send any passed tissue to pathology
- Endometrial sampling if older than 35–40 years or there are other risk factors for endometrial cancer

Treatment

INITIAL STABILIZATION

- ABCs
- Oxygen for significant bleeding or unstable patient
- Establish two large-bore IVs and initiate fluid bolus (1–2 L) for hypotensive patients
  —Transfuse blood if continued hypotension from blood losses despite intravenous fluid resuscitation
- Cardiac/pulse oximeter monitors

ED TREATMENT

- If unstable with surgical condition, transfer patient to operating room as soon as possible
- RhoGAM for vaginal bleeding, pregnancy, and Rh-negative mother
  —RhoGAM: 1 vial i.m. if >13 weeks pregnant
  —MICRhoGAM (50 μg) i.m. if <13 weeks pregnant

EARLY PREGNANCY

- US positive for ectopic
  —Definitive treatment with surgery or methotrexate as per the standard at the treating institution
- US positive for intrauterine pregnancy (IUP) without concerns of heterotopic pregnancy (1/2600–1/30,000)
  —Discharge patient for obstetric follow-up
- US indeterminate for IUP or ectopic with β-hCG greater than institutional discriminatory zone (likely 1000–2000 IU)
  —Cannot exclude an ectopic pregnancy
  —If hemodynamically stable with little bleeding, close outpatient obstetric-gynecologic follow-up within 48 hours for repeat β-hCG
  —Strict return parameters
- US indeterminate for IUP or ectopic with β-hCG less than institutional discriminatory zone (likely 1000–2000 IU)
  —Patient stable with low risk for ectopic, then discharge with repeat β-hCG and obstetric follow-up in 2 days
  —Patient may still have an ectopic pregnancy
- Complete abortion
  —Discharge if stable without significant ongoing bleeding
- Incomplete abortion
  —Obstetric consult
  —Dilation and curettage (D&C) versus expectant management
- Missed abortion
  —Expectant management initially
  —D&C for infection, bleeding, or retained products of conception
- Septic abortion
  —IV antibiotics and admission
- Molar pregnancy
  —Chemotherapy, very responsive in early stages of disease

Later Pregnancy

- Placenta previa
  —Usually expectant management
  —Obstetric consult for possible admission
- Placental abruption
  —Induction of labor if large
  —Can lead to fetal/maternal death
  —May require cesarean section

Immediate Postpartum

- Uterine inversion
  —Prevent by avoiding strong traction on umbilical cord after delivery
  —Replace uterus immediately
  —Occasionally requires operative management
- Postpartum hemorrhage
  —Extraction of placenta if retained
  —Hysterectomy if uncontrolled life-threatening bleeding

Early Postpartum

- Retained tissue
  —D&C
- Endometritis
  —IV antibiotics

Nonpregnant

Menses

- NSAIDs and supportive care

Dysfunctional Uterine Bleeding (DUB)

- <35–40 years of age
  —If known anovulatory DUB, Provera, 10 mg PO q.d. for first 10 days of menstrual cycle—warn patient of a withdrawal bleed
  —Oral contraceptive pill q.i.d. for 7 days
  —Discharge if stable
- >35–40 years of age
  —Uterine sampling necessary before initiation of hormonal treatment to rule out endometrial cancer
  —US for any masses felt on exam
- Structural abnormalities
  —Fibroids or uterine tumors conservative management or lumpectomy/hysterectomy
  —Ultrasound for workup of other pelvic masses
  —Pap smear/biopsy for cervical lesions

MEDICATIONS

- DUB: Provera 10 mg PO q.d. for first 10 days of menstrual cycle—warn patient of a withdrawal bleed
- MICRhoGAM (50 μg) i.m. if <13 weeks pregnant
- RhoGAM: 1 vial i.m. if >13 weeks pregnant

Disposition

ADMISSION CRITERIA

- Ectopic pregnancy not meeting methotrexate discharge criteria or if patient is unstable
- Uterine inversion
- Septic abortion
- Placental abruption
- Postpartum hemorrhage
- Endometritis
- Dysfunctional uterine bleeding
  —Unstable
  —Significant symptomatic or life-threatening anemia
- Newly diagnosed molar pregnancy

DISCHARGE CRITERIA

- Stable vital signs
- Confirmed intrauterine pregnancy if pregnant
- Ectopic pregnancy meeting institutional methotrexate discharge criteria
- Low-risk patient for ectopic pregnancy with pregnancy without findings of IUP on ultrasound with β-hCG below discriminatory zone

Miscellaneous

ICD9: 623.8

ICD10: N93.9

SUGGESTED READINGS

Alexander JD, Schneider FD. Vaginal bleeding associated with pregnancy. Primary Care: Clinics in Office Practice 2000;27(1):137–151.

American College of Emergency Physicians. Clinical policy for the initial approach to patients presenting with a chief complaint of vaginal bleed. Ann Emerg Med 1997;29:435–458.

Bravender T, Emans SJ. Menstrual disorders. Dysfunctional uterine bleeding. Pediatr Clin North Am 1999;46(3):545–553.

Kaplan BC, Dart RG, Moskos M, et al. Ectopic pregnancy: prospective study with improved diagnostic accuracy. Ann Emerg Med 1996;28:10–17.

Shwayder JM. Pathophysiology of abnormal uterine bleeding. Obstet Gynecol Clin North Am 2000;27(2):219–234.

Author: Carla Valentine

Vaginal Bleeding in Pregnancy

Clinical Presentation

SIGNS AND SYMPTOMS

- Minimal spotting to frank hemorrhage
  - —Dark or bright red in color
  - —Watery, blood tinged mucus, clots or tissue
  - —Pain or painless
  - —Placenta previa
    - -Classically painless, bright red hemorrhage
  - —Abruptio placenta
    - -Classically painful, dark red hemorrhage
  - —Spontaneous abortion
    - -Classically crampy, diffuse pelvic pain
  - —Ectopic pregnancy
    - -Classically sharp pelvic pain with lateralization
- Origin of bleeding from vagina, cervix, uterus, or placenta
- Life-threatening conditions may present as only mild vaginal bleeding
- Patency of os
  - —Threatened abortion—os closed
  - —Inevitable abortion—os open
  - —Incomplete abortion—os open or closed
  - —Complete abortion—os closed
  - —Missed abortion—os closed
- Frank hemorrhage
  - —Pallor
  - —Tachycardia
  - —Hypotension
  - —Orthostatic changes in pulse or BP
  - —Change in mentation
- Signs of hemodynamic instability may be absent due to pregnancy related physiologic increase in blood volume
- 5–10% of spontaneous abortions require blood transfusions

MECHANISM/DESCRIPTION

- Obstetric hemorrhage
  - —Leading cause of maternal/fetal morbidity and mortality
  - —Vaginal bleeding due to pregnancy mandates investigation for potential complications
- Early pregnancy hemorrhage (<20 weeks)
  - —Common reason for ED visit
  - —Occurs in 30% of all pregnancies
  - —50% lead to spontaneous abortion
- Antepartum hemorrhage (>20 weeks)
  - —Requires evaluation in 5–10% of these pregnancies
- Postpartum hemorrhage
  - —Defined as blood loss that causes 10% drop from baseline hematocrit or one that requires blood transfusion
- Risk factors
  - —Advanced maternal age
  - —Substance abuse (cocaine, tobacco)
  - —Pelvic inflammatory disease (PID)
  - —Intrauterine diethylstilbestrol (DES) exposure
  - —Intrauterine device (IUD) use
  - —Previous cesarean section
  - —Previous termination of pregnancy, dilation and curettage (D&C)
  - —Previous ectopic pregnancy
  - —Increased parity
  - —Multiple gestation
  - —Diabetes
  - —Minority race
  - —Trauma

ETIOLOGY

- Early pregnancy (<20 weeks)
  - —Physiologic bleed (common)
  - —Spontaneous abortion (50%)
  - —Threatened, inevitable, incomplete, missed, and septic abortion
  - —Ectopic pregnancy (2–5%)
  - —Hydatiform mole (<0.1%)
  - —Blighted ovum or anembryonic pregnancy
  - —Subchorionic bleed
  - —Incompetent cervix
  - —Cervical/vaginal trauma or pathology
  - —Ruptured hemorrhagic corpus luteal cyst
- Antepartum hemorrhage (>20 weeks)
  - —Bloody show (most common)
  - —Abruptio placenta (30%)
  - —Placenta previa (20%)
  - —Vasa previa
  - —Preterm premature rupture of membrane (PROM)
  - —Postcoital bleed
  - —Cervical/vaginal trauma or pathology
  - —Uterine rupture (uncommon)
- Postpartum hemorrhage
  - —Uterine atony (most common)
  - —Retained products of conception
  - —Uterine rupture
  - —Vaginal/cervical laceration/hematoma

Pre-Hospital

CAUTIONS

- Unstable vital signs warrant aggressive resuscitation and continuous cardiac monitoring in females of childbearing age with vaginal bleeding
- In late pregnancy position patient on left side to decrease uterine compression of vena cava

Diagnosis

ESSENTIAL WORKUP

- History
  - —Last menstrual period
  - —Parity
  - —Intensity and duration of bleeding
  - —Previous obstetric-gynecologic complications
  - —Last intercourse
- Physical exam
  - —Vital signs
  - —Fetal heart tone (FHT)—auscultated with Doppler past 10 weeks' gestation and with fetoscope past 18 weeks' gestation
  - —Pelvic exam
    - -Evaluate source and intensity of bleeding
    - -Determine patency of cervical os
    - -Assess uterine size or tenderness
    - -Check for uterine fibroids or adnexal masses
  - —Late pregnancy
    - -Do not perform pelvic exam unless in controlled OR setting
    - -Placenta previa or vasa previa has to be ruled out by sonography before speculum or digital exam
    - -Fatal hemorrhage may ensue
  - —Bedside ultrasound (if available) to evaluate for intrauterine pregnancy

LABORATORY

- CBC
  - —Dilutional "anemia" is a normal physiologic change in pregnancy, blood volume expands by 45%
- Quantitative β-human chorionic gonadotropin (β-hCG) (correlate with ultrasound findings)
  - —β-hCG doubles every 48 hours in normal early pregnancy until 10 weeks of gestation
- Typing and Rh
- Type and screen; type and cross-match if significant bleed
- Liver function test
  - —If suspect DIC or before initiation of methotrexate therapy
- BUN, creatinine in abruption
- Prothrombin time (PT), partial thromboplastin time (PTT), and DIC panel in missed abortion
- Blood culture in septic abortion
- Urine/blood toxicology

IMAGING/SPECIAL TESTS

- Transvaginal ultrasound
  - —Standard of care in evaluation of early pregnancy bleed
  - —Confirms intrauterine pregnancy (IUP)
  - —Can rule out ectopic pregnancy by showing IUP
  - —Proves ectopic pregnancy by showing fetal pole outside uterus
  - —Suggests ectopic pregnancy by detecting free fluid in cul de sac or adnexal mass
  - —Detects retained products of conception
  - —Detects gestational sac at 5 weeks or β-hCG = 1,800 IU, yolk sac at 6 weeks and cardiac activity at 6.5 weeks of gestation
- Culdocentesis
  - —Identifies free fluid in cul de sac
  - —Limited use with ultrasound available
- Suction D&C
  - —Indicated if incomplete, missed, or septic abortion; mole pregnancy; and to evacuate retained products
- Laparoscopy/laparotomy
  - —Definitive diagnosis and treatment of ectopic pregnancy

Treatment

INITIAL STABILIZATION

- *ABCs*
- Oxygen
- Pulse oximetry
- Cardiac monitor
- Two large-bore IV lines with 0.9% NS or lactated Ringer's solution infusion
- Blood transfusion as indicated

ED TREATMENT

- Administer RhoGAM if patient is Rh-negative
- Ectopic pregnancy
  - —Unstable: consider bedside US with emergent OB consultation for laparoscopy/laparotomy
  - —Stable: perform US; if confirms or suggestive of ectopic pregnancy, obtain OB consultation for surgery or methotrexate therapy
- Threatened abortion
  - —Patient evaluation
  - —No strenuous activity, no douching or intercourse while bleeding
  - —Seek medical advice if increased bleeding, pain, passed tissue or fever
  - —Save passed tissue for later analysis
  - —Arrange follow-up with OB within 24–72 hours
- Complete abortion
  - —Consider PO doxycycline or flagyl therapy for 10 days
  - —Arrange follow-up with OB within 24–72 hours if bleeding minimal
  - —If bleeding is heavy, consider oxytocin IV or methylergovonine maleate (Methergine) PO/IM and obtain emergent OB consultation
- Inevitable/incomplete/missed abortion
  - —Obtain emergent OB consult for D&C
- Septic abortion
  - —Initiate broad-spectrum antibiotic therapy
  - —Obtain blood culture
  - —Emergent OB consultation for D&C
- Grief counseling for fetal loss

MEDICATION

- Doxycycline: 100 mg PO b.i.d.
- Flagyl: 500 mg PO b.i.d.
- Methylergovonine maleate (Methergine): 0.2 mg PO or i.m. q.i.d. PRN
- Methotrexate: 50 mg/m^2 i.m. single dose—initiated by OB consultant
- Oxytocin: 10 units in 500 mL NS i.v. at 120–240 mL/h
- RhoGam: $<$12 weeks—50 μg i.m.; $>$12 weeks—300 μg i.m.

Disposition

ADMISSION CRITERIA

- Early pregnancy
  - —Unstable vital signs or significant hemorrhage
  - —Ruptured ectopic pregnancy
  - —Suspected ectopic pregnancy with symptoms
  - —Incomplete abortion (open os)
  - —Septic abortion
- Late pregnancy
  - —These patients require monitoring in OB unit

DISCHARGE CRITERIA

- Threatened abortion (closed os) with stable symptoms
- Asymptomatic, hemodynamically stable patient with small unruptured ectopic pregnancy after OB consultation
- Controlled bleeding from local vaginal/cervical source

Miscellaneous

ICD9: 623.8

ICD10: 046.0

SUGGESTED READINGS

Alexander JD. Vaginal bleeding associated with pregnancy. Primary Care 2000;27(1): 137–151.

Eisinger SH. Early pregnancy bleeding: a rational approach. Clin Fam Practice 2001;3 (2).

Nadukhovskaya L, Dart R. Emergency management of the nonviable intrauterine pregnancy. Am J Emerg Med 2001;19: 495–500.

Turner LM. Vaginal bleeding during pregnancy. Emerg Med Clin North Am 1994;12:45–54.

Willis D. Bleeding in pregnancy. In: Benrubi GI, ed. Obstetric and gynecologic emergencies. Philadelphia: JB Lippincott, 1994:127–138.

Author: Shirin H. Trachiotis

Vaginal Discharge/Vaginitis

Clinical Presentation

SIGNS AND SYMPTOMS

- Abnormal discharge
- Vulvovaginitis
  —Localized pain
  —Erythema
  —Edema
- Dysuria
- Pruritus
- Asymptomatic
- Excoriations
- Abnormal odor

MECHANISM/DESCRIPTION

- Overgrowth of normal vaginal bacteria
- Infecting bacteria or viruses
- Chemical irritation
- Atrophic/hypoestrogenism

ETIOLOGY

- Candidal infection
- Chemical irritant
- *Chlamydia trachomatis* infection
- Foreign body
- *Gardnerella* species infection, bacterial vaginosis
- Herpes simplex virus (HSV)
- Lichens sclerosis (atrophic)
- *Neisseria gonorrhoeae* infection
- Trichomonal vaginitis

PEDIATRIC CONSIDERATIONS

- Chemical irritant, foreign body most likely
- Strongly suspect child abuse if sexually transmitted cause

Pre-Hospital

N/A

Diagnosis

ESSENTIAL WORKUP

- History
  —Description and duration of symptoms
  —Description of discharge if any
  —Timing with regard to menses
  —Sexual history of patient and partners if possible
  —Use of oral contraceptives and/or antibiotics
  —Likelihood of pregnancy
- Physical
  —Abdominal exam to assess for tenderness
  —Inspection of vulva
  —Speculum and bimanual exam of pelvis

LABORATORY

- Urinalysis
- β-Human chorionic gonadotropin (β-hCG)
- pH of discharge with Nitrazine paper (normal in premenopausal adults is between 3.5 and 4.1)
- Saline wet prep exam of discharge at 400×: clue cells (*Gardnerella* species), trichomonads (*Trichomonas* species)
- KOH wet prep exam of discharge for pseudohyphae (*Candida* species)
- Endocervical swab for gonorrhea (chocolate agar) or chlamydia, urine test for chlamydia
- Tzanck smear for multinucleated giant cells of HSV, but unroofing of lesions highly painful for patient
  —Diagnosis by visualization of lesions alone adequate

IMAGING/SPECIAL TESTS

N/A

DIFFERENTIAL DIAGNOSIS

- Urinary tract infection
- Pelvic inflammatory disease (PID)
- Anal disease

PEDIATRIC CONSIDERATIONS

- Ask about new irritants: bubble bath, soap, and laundry detergent
- Consider sexual assault

Treatment

INITIAL STABILIZATION

N/A

ED TREATMENT

- Candidiasis: single oral dose fluconazole vs. 3–7 days of intravaginal imidazole drug
  - —Routine treatment of male sex partner: no
- Chemical irritant
  - —Avoid irritant
  - —Use sitz baths, cotton underwear
- Chlamydial
  - —One dose azithromycin (for vaginitis/cervicitis, not adequate for PID) vs. 10–14 days of doxycycline, tetracycline, ofloxacin or erythromycin
  - —Treat for presumed concurrent gonococcal infections
  - —Routine treatment of male sex partners: yes
- Foreign body: removal of foreign body; may necessitate sedation for removal and appropriate antibiotics if infection present
- *Gardnerella* species infection, bacterial vaginosis
  - —Single high dose vs. 1 week of lower dose metronidazole vs. vaginal metronidazole gel for 5 days
  - —Clindamycin cream for first-trimester pregnant patients because some experts believe flagyl PO is contraindicated
  - —Advise no alcohol intake if taking metronidazole up to 24 hours after treatment
  - —No routine treatment of male sex partners
- Gonococcal
  - —One dose treatment with ceftriaxone, cefixime, ciprofloxacin, ofloxacin, norfloxacin, or spectinomycin
  - —Treat for presumed concurrent chlamydial infection
  - —Routine treatment of male sex partners
- HSV
  - —Acyclovir for 10 days for initial attack
  - —5 days for recurrences (5 times per day lose dose, 3 times per day higher dose)
  - —Lidocaine jelly for topical relief
  - —Routine treatment of male sex partners: only if symptomatic; however, patient and partner may be shedding viral particles *without symptoms*
- Lichen sclerosis
  - —Referral to gynecologist for estrogen cream and further treatment
- *Trichomonas* species infection
  - —Same metronidazole recommendations as bacterial vaginosis
  - —Clotrimazole cream for pregnancy
  - —Routine treatment of male sex partners: yes
- Advise patient to use condoms until partner is evaluated and treated for sexually transmitted diseases

MEDICATIONS

- Acyclovir: first occurrence—200 mg PO 5 times per day for 10 days or 400 PO 3 times per day for 10 days
  - —Recurrent—200 mg PO 5 times per day for 5 days or 400 PO 3 times per day for 5 days
  - —Suppressive—400 mg PO b.i.d. up to 1 year
- Azithromycin: 1 g PO × 1
- Cefixime: 400 mg PO × 1
- Ceftriaxone: 125 mg i.m. or 250 mg i.m. × 1
- Ciprofloxacin: 500 mg PO × 1
- Clindamycin 2% cream: 1 applicator PV q.h.s. for 7 days
- Clotrimazole 1% cream: 2–100 mg tabs PV q.h.s. × 3 days or 1–150 mg tabs PV × 1 or 1 app PV q.h.s. for 7–14 days
- Doxycycline: 100 mg PO b.i.d. for 7 days (class D)
- Fluconazole: 150 mg PO × 1
- Erythromycin ethyl succinate: 800 mg PO q.i.d. for 7 days
- Erythromycin base: 500 mg PO q.i.d. for 7 days
- Itraconazole: 200 mg PO b.i.d. for 1 day
- Metronidazole: 2 g PO × 1 or 500 mg PO b.i.d. for 7 days (class D)
- Metronidazole 0.75% gel: 0.75% gel PV b.i.d. for 5 days
- Miconazole: 200 mg PV q.h.s. for 3 days
- Miconazole: 5 g 2% cream PV q.h.s. for 7 days or 100 mg supp PV q.h.s. for 7 days
- Norfloxacin: 800 mg PO × 1
- Ofloxacin: 400 mg PO × 1 or 300 mg PO b.i.d.
- Spectinomycin: 2 g i.m. × 1
- Tetracycline: 500 mg PO q.i.d. for 7–10 days (class D)
- Terconazole: 80 mg supp q.h.s. for 3 days or 5 g of 0.8% cream PV q.h.s. for 3 days or 5 g of 0.4% cream PV for 7 days
- Tioconazole: 5 g of 6.5% cream PV for 7 days

PEDIATRIC CONSIDERATIONS

- If sexual abuse is suspected, report

Disposition

ADMISSION CRITERIA

- Disseminated gonococcal infection
- Sepsis secondary to foreign body
- PID toxicity
- Pain control, consequent inability to urinate or stool (HSV)

DISCHARGE CRITERIA

- Most can be discharged; follow-up in about 1 week is suggested

Miscellaneous

ICD9: 616.10

ICD10: N76.0

SUGGESTED READINGS

Botash AS. Vaginitis. Emedicine July 27 2001;2(7).

Egan ME, Lipsky MS. Diagnosis of vaginitis. Am Fam Physician 2000;62(5):1095–1104.

Quan M. Vaginitis: meeting the clinical challenge. Clin Cornerstone 2000;3(2): 36–37.

Author: Michelle A. Finkel

Valvular Heart Disease

Clinical Presentation

SIGNS AND SYMPTOMS

- Mitral stenosis
  - —Exertional dyspnea
  - —Fatigue
  - —Palpitations
  - —Paroxysmal nocturnal dyspnea
  - —Orthopnea
  - —Hemoptysis
  - —Systemic emboli
  - —Pulmonary edema
  - —Malar flush ("mitral facies")
  - —Prominent jugular a waves
  - —Right ventricular lift
  - —Loud S1
  - —Opening snap
  - —Low-pitched diastolic rumble
- Mitral regurgitation
  - —Acute
    - -Acute pulmonary edema
    - -Jugular venous pressure (JVP) exhibits cannon a waves and giant v waves
    - -Harsh apical crescendo-decrescendo murmur radiating to the axilla
    - -Palpable thrill at apex
    - -S3 and S4
  - —Chronic
    - -Palpitations
    - -Atrial fibrillation
    - -Dyspnea
    - -Orthopnea
    - -Nocturnal paroxysmal dyspnea
    - -Edema
    - -Systemic emboli
    - -Normal JVP
    - -Left ventricular hypertrophy
    - -Apical high-pitched pansystolic murmur
    - -Decreased or obscured S1
    - -Widely split S2
    - -S3
- Aortic stenosis
  - —Exertional angina
  - —Syncope (during exercise)
  - —Congestive heart failure (initially diastolic failure, then systolic)
  - —Arrhythmias
  - —Harsh crescendo-decrescendo systolic murmur at aortic focus radiating to carotids
  - —Absent aortic component of S2
  - —Delayed upstroke in peripheral pulse (pulsus parvus et tardus)
  - —S4 gallop
  - —Ejection click
- Aortic regurgitation
  - —Fatigue
  - —Dyspnea
  - —Paroxysmal nocturnal dyspnea
  - —Orthopnea
  - —Chest pain
  - —Edema
  - —Acute pulmonary edema
  - —High-pitched decrescendo diastolic murmur at aortic area
  - —Wide pulse pressure
  - —De Musset's sign (head bobbing with systole)
  - —Quincke's pulse (nail bed pulsations)
  - —Austin Flint murmur (soft diastolic rumble)

MECHANISM/DESCRIPTION

- Mitral stenosis
  - —Obstruction of diastolic blood flow into the left ventricle (LV)
- Mitral regurgitation
  - —Inadequate closure of the leaflets allows retrograde blood flow into the left atrium (LA)
  - —Acute
    - -Pressure overload in LA and pulmonary veins causing acute pulmonary edema
  - —Chronic
    - -LV volume overload with dilatation and hypertrophy with LA enlargement
- Aortic stenosis
  - —Resistance to ejection and systolic gradients increase
  - —Progressive increase in LV systolic pressure
- Aortic regurgitation
  - —Acute
    - -Acute LV pressure and volume overload leading to left heart failure and pulmonary edema
  - —Chronic
    - -Chronic volume overload with LV dilation and hypertrophy

ETIOLOGY

- Mitral stenosis
  - —Rheumatic fever
  - —Cardiac tumors
  - —Rheumatologic disorders (lupus, rheumatoid arthritis)
  - —Myxoma
  - —Congenital defects
  - —Calcification
- Mitral regurgitation (acute)
  - —Ruptured papillary muscle (infarction, trauma)
  - —Papillary muscle dysfunction (ischemia)
  - —Ruptured chordae tendineae (trauma, endocarditis, myxomatous)
  - —Valve perforation (endocarditis)
- Aortic stenosis
  - —Congenital aortic stenosis (major cause in persons <30 years old)
  - —Congenital bicuspid valve
  - —Rheumatic aortic stenosis
  - —Calcific aortic stenosis
- Aortic regurgitation (acute)
  - —Acute
    - -Rheumatic fever
    - -Infective endocarditis
    - -Rupture of sinus of Valsalva
  - —Acute aortic dissection
    - -Following valve surgery
    - -Trauma

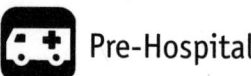

Pre-Hospital

CAUTIONS

- Avoid vasodilators in aortic stenosis
- May result in profound and irreversible hypotension

Diagnosis

ESSENTIAL WORKUP

- Thorough cardiopulmonary examination
- EKG
  - —Mitral stenosis
    - -Left atrium enlargement
    - -Right ventricular (RV) hypertrophy
  - —Acute mitral regurgitation
    - -Q-wave inferior, posterior, or lateral
  - —Aortic stenosis
    - -LVH most common
    - -Left atrium enlargement
    - -Interventricular conduction delay
  - —Aortic regurgitation
    - -Acute = LV strain
    - -Chronic = LV hypertrophy and strain
- CXR
  - —Mitral stenosis
    - -Enlarged LA
    - -Prominent pulmonary veins
  - —Mitral regurgitation
    - - LV and LA enlargement in chronic cases
    - -Pulmonary edema and normal LV and LA dimensions in acute cases
  - —Aortic stenosis
    - -LVH
    - -Aortic calcification
    - -Pulmonary congestion
  - —Aortic regurgitation
    - -Acute = normal heart, pulmonary edema
    - -Chronic = enlarged LV and dilated aorta

IMAGING/SPECIAL TESTS

- Echocardiogram
  - —Valvular anatomy
  - —Aortic root size
  - —Enlarged LV
  - —LV function
  - —Estimate of regurgitation
- Cardiac catheterization for acute mitral regurgitation/aortic regurgitation
- Spiral CT scan to exclude aortic dissection with acute aortic regurgitation

Treatment

INITIAL STABILIZATION

- IV access, oxygen, monitor, pulse oximetry
- Mitral stenosis
  —Treat symptoms of congestive heart failure
  —Rate control if in atrial fibrillation
- Mitral regurgitation
  —Differentiate between acute and chronic MR
- Aortic stenosis
  —Gentle diuresis if CHF
  —Mild hydration if hypotensive and not in CHF
  —Avoid nitrates
- Aortic regurgitation
  —Distinguish cause of pulmonary edema (acute mitral regurgitation vs. acute aortic regurgitation)

ED TREATMENT

- Mitral stenosis
  —Digoxin
  —β-Blockers
  —Heparin (if new onset atrial fibrillation)
  —Diuretics
  —Endocarditis prophylaxis/education
- Mitral regurgitation
  —Acute
    -Afterload reduction (nitroglycerin, morphine, or sodium nitroprusside)
    -Diuresis
    -Intra-aortic balloon pump (temporizing for urgent surgery)
  —Chronic
    -Diuresis
    -Nitrates
    -Hydralazine
    -Angiotensin-converting enzyme inhibitor
    -Digoxin
    -β-Adrenergic blocker (ventricular rate control)
    -Calcium antagonist (ventricular rate control)
    -Heparin (if atrial fibrillation)
    -Endocarditis prophylaxis
- Aortic stenosis
  —Limited once symptomatic
  —Digoxin
  —Consideration for valve replacement or valvuloplasty
  —Intra-aortic balloon pump (temporize for surgery)
  —Endocarditis prophylaxis education
- Aortic regurgitation
  —Chronic
    -Preload and afterload reduction
    -Digoxin
    -Diuretics
    -Endocarditis prophylaxis education
  —Acute
    -Preload and afterload reduction
    -Intra-aortic balloon pump
    -Urgent surgery

MEDICATIONS

- Bumetanide: 0.5–1.0 mg q2–3h PRN; infusion 0.08–0.3 mg/h; PO 0.5–2 mg t.i.d. q.d.
- Digoxin: 0.5 mg i.v. bolus, then 0.25 mg i.v. q2h up to 1 mg
- Diltiazem: 0.25 mg/kg IV over 2 min (repeat in 15 min PRN with 0.35 mg/kg) then 5–15 mg/hr
- Enalapril IV: 1.25 mg q 6 hrs; po 2.5–10 mg bid
- Esmolol: 500 μg bolus IV, then 50–400 μg/kg/min
- Furosemide: 20–80 mg IV q 1–2 hrs
- Heparin: 80 IU/kg IV bolus, then 18 IU/kg/hr drip, adjust to maintain PTT 1.5–2X control (INR 2–3)
- Hydralazine: 10–25 mg q 2–4 hrs IV
- Metoprolol: 5 mg IV
- Nitroglycerin: IV start at 20 μg/min and titrate to effect (up to 300 μg/min); SL 0.3–0.6 mg PRN; Topical 1–2 inches of 2% q 6 hrs
- Phentolamine: 5 mg IV bolus, then 1–2 mg/min IV infusion
- Propranolol: 1 mg IV
- Sodium nitroprusside: 0.5 μg/kg/min; increase in increments of 0.5–1.0 μg/kg/min q 5–10 min up to 10 μg/kg/min

Disposition

ADMISSION CRITERIA

- New onset atrial fibrillation
- Congestive heart failure/pulmonary edema
- Hemodynamically unstable
- Acute mitral or aortic regurgitation
- Cardiac ischemia
- Angina
- Syncope
- Arrhythmias

DISCHARGE CRITERIA

- Hemodynamic stability
- Unchanged ECG
- Resolution of CHF symptoms with diuresis
- Chronic mitral regurgitation

Miscellaneous

ICD9: 746.9

ICD10: I38

SEE ALSO: HEART MURMUR

SUGGESTED READINGS

Carabello BA, Crawford FA. Valvular heart disease. N Engl J Med 1997;337:32–41.

Cheitlin MD, Douglas PS, Parmley WW. Task Force 2: acquired valvular heart disease. J Am Coll Cardiol 1994;24:874–880.

Roldan CA, Shively BK, Crawford MH. Value of the cardiovascular examination for detecting valvular heart disease in asymptomatic subjects. Am J Cardiol 1996;77:1327–1331.

Author: Liudvikas Jagminas

Varicella

Clinical Presentation

SIGNS AND SYMPTOMS

- Varicella, commonly known as chicken pox, causes a spectrum of five basic disease patterns depending on specific group infected

Neonates

- Congenital varicella syndrome—occasionally follows maternal zoster infection
  - —Cicatricial skin lesions
  - —Limb hypoplasia or paresis
  - —Microcephaly
  - —Ophthalmic lesions

Children (2–12 Years of Age)

- Prodrome of low-grade fever (100–103°F) and malaise precedes rash by 1–2 days
- Classic exanthem
  - —Lesions begin on the trunk and face, spreading to entire body
  - —Vesicles, pustules, and small scabs on erythematous bases in varying stages of evolution
  - —Round or oval, 0.5–1.0 cm in diameter
  - —Duration of vesicle formation 3–5 days
  - —Pruritus, anorexia, and listlessness
  - —10- to 21-day incubation period
  - —Infectious from 48 hours before vesicle formation until all vesicles are crusted (typically 4–5 days)

Adolescents and Adults

- Extracutaneous manifestations in 5–50%
- Presents similarly to disease in children but generally of greater severity

Immunocompromised Patients

- More numerous lesions that may have hemorrhagic base
- Absolute neutrophil counts (ANCs) and absolute lymphocyte counts (ALCs) <500 are the best predictors of complicated disease
- Healing may take 3 times longer
- Lesions last 3 times as long
- Extracutaneous manifestations, especially pneumonia, common

Pregnant Patients

- Prevalent in young expectant women (14–19 years of age)
- Produces a more severe disease presentation
  - —Risk to the fetus of congenital varicella syndrome greatest if infection in first half of pregnancy
  - —Maternal disease severity greatest if infection in second half of pregnancy

Extracutaneous Manifestations

- Pneumonitis
  - —25 times more common in adults
  - —Most common in adult smokers and immunocompromised children
  - —Occurs 3–5 days after onset of rash
  - —Early signs—continued eruption of new lesions, fever, and new-onset cough
  - —Tachypnea, dyspnea, cyanosis, pleuritic chest pain, and hemoptysis
- Cerebellar ataxia
  - —Cerebellar ataxia may develop 5 days after rash
  - —Ataxia, vomiting, slurred speech, fever, vertigo, nystagmus, and tremor
- Cerebritis
  - —Develops 3–8 days after appearance of rash; duration about 2 weeks
  - —Progressive malaise, headache, meningismus, vomiting, fever, delirium, and seizures
- Reye's syndrome
  - —Vomiting, restlessness, irritability, and progressive deterioration in mental status from cerebral edema
  - —Aspirin use may be associated
  - —Myocarditis, nephritis, bleeding diatheses, and hepatitis

MECHANISM/DESCRIPTION

- 90% of children are infected by 15 years of age
- Adults have a 15 times greater risk for death owing to chicken pox than children
- Most common in late winter and early spring

ETIOLOGY

- DNA virus characterized by latency in dorsal root ganglia and periodic reactivation
- Virus is transmitted by respiratory route
- Humans are only known reservoir

PEDIATRIC CONSIDERATIONS

- Classic disease of childhood
- Do not use aspirin for treatment of fever
- Perinatal disease occurs in the mother from 5 days predelivery to 48 hours postdelivery
  - —Has a high neonatal mortality

PRE-HOSPITAL PRECAUTIONS

- Nonimmune transport personnel must avoid respiratory or physical contact with patients
- Transport personnel with varicella or herpes zoster should not come in contact with immunocompromised or pregnant patients

Diagnosis

ESSENTIAL WORKUP

- History and physical are sufficient in uncomplicated cases
- If confirmation necessary, obtain a tissue culture
- Pneumonitis
  - —Chest x-ray classically demonstrates 2- to 5-mm peripheral densities, may coalesce and persist for weeks
- Reye's syndrome
  - —Ammonia level peaks early, may normalize in 48–72 hours
  - —Liver function tests, transaminases will be elevated
  - —Prothrombin time (PT), partial thromboplastin time (PTT)
- Cerebritis
  - —Lumbar puncture demonstrates lymphocytic pleocytosis and elevated levels of protein

LABORATORY

- Serologic tests for varicella antibodies
  - —Latex agglutination most sensitive (sensitivity ≥95%)
  - —Enzyme-linked immunosorbent assay (ELISA) (sensitivity ranges from 86–97%, specificity from 82–99%)

IMAGING/SPECIAL TESTS

- Liver biopsy—definitive test for Reye's syndrome

DIFFERENTIAL DIAGNOSIS

- Impetigo
- Disseminated herpes
- Disseminated coxsackievirus
- Measles
- Rickettsial disease

Treatment

INITIAL STABILIZATION
- ABCs
- Protect airway if obtunded

ED TREATMENT
- Neonatal/Infant
  —Varicella-zoster immunoglobulin (VZIG) for infants if maternal varicella develops <7 days before delivery or up to 28 days after delivery
  —Maternal zoster not an indication for VZIG to infant
- Children (2–12 years old)
  —Treat with antipyretics and antipruritics
  —Closely cropped nails and good hygiene help prevent secondary bacterial infections
- Acyclovir
  —Controversial, not generally needed for uncomplicated cases
  —Must be initiated within 24 hours of disease onset to be efficacious
  —Reduces total lesions by 25%
  —Adequate immunity still develops
  —Currently regarded as safe during pregnancy
- Prophylaxis with VZIG
  —All pregnant women with significant exposure to varicella-zoster virus (VZV)
    -Living in same household as a person with active chickenpox or herpes zoster
    -Face-to-face contact >5 minutes with person infected with chickenpox or zoster
  —72 hours postexposure for maximal effect, although may provide benefit up to 96 hours postexposure for immunocompromised patients
  —Ineffective once clinical illness is established
- Adolescents/adults
  —Symptomatic with antipyretics and antipruritics
  —Acyclovir when initiated within 24 hours of rash decreases progression to disseminated disease
- Pregnant women
  —VZIG as noted above
  —Acyclovir, when initiated during incubation period or within 24 hours of onset of rash
    -Prophylaxis after exposure is 84% protective against infection
  —IV acyclovir for pneumonitis or other complications
    -Respiratory, neurologic, hemorrhagic rash, or continued fever after 6 days
- Immunocompromised patients
  —Acyclovir recommended
  —Must be initiated within 72 hours of disease onset
  —Decreases progression to disseminated disease
  —Foscarnet for acyclovir-resistant disease
  —Interferon
  —Prophylaxis with VZIG for the nonimmune immunocompromised patient (see above for recommendations)
- Extracutaneous
  —IV acyclovir, or foscarnet if viral resistance

MEDICATIONS
- Acyclovir
  —Uncomplicated: 800 mg PO 5 times a day for 7 days; adolescents (13–18 years old): 20 mg/kg per dose q.i.d. for 7 days (peds: 20 mg/kg suspension PO q.i.d. for 5 days [max 800 mg PO q.i.d.])
  —Immunocompromised: 10 mg/kg i.v. q8h infused over 1 h *or* 800 mg PO 5 times a day for 7 days (peds: 10–12 mg/kg i.v. q8h infused over 1 h *or* 500 mg/m^2 i.v. q8h)
- Diphenhydramine: 25–50 mg i.v., i.m., or PO q4h (peds: 5 mg/kg/d elixir 12.5 mg/5 mL)
- Foscarnet: 40 mg/kg q8h over 1 hour for 10 or more days (peds: same)
- Hydroxyzine: 25–50 mg i.m. or PO q4–6h (peds: 0.5 mg/kg q4–6h suspension 10 and 25 mg/5 mL)
- Varicella-zoster immune globulin (VZIG): 625 IU i.m. (peds: 1 vial per 10 kg i.m. to a max dose of 5 vials [each vial contains 125 IU])

PEDIATRIC CONSIDERATIONS
- Avoid treating with salicylates, which may produce Reye's syndrome

Disposition

ADMISSION CRITERIA
- Patients with pneumonia any evidence of respiratory failure should be admitted to an ICU
- Immunocompromised patients: ICU versus ward, depending on severity of illness
- All admitted patients must be kept in isolation
- Newborns need to be admitted for IV acyclovir; neonatal ICU vs. ward depending on disease severity

DISCHARGE CRITERIA
- Immunocompetent children without evidence of Reye's syndrome or secondary bacterial infection
- Adults with no evidence of extracutaneous disease

PEDIATRIC CONSIDERATIONS
- Parents need to be cautioned regarding risk for secondary bacterial infection and possible progression to sepsis

Miscellaneous

ICD9: 052.9

ICD10: B01.9

SUGGESTED READINGS

Advisory Committee on Immunization Practices. Prevention of varicella. Updated Recommendations of the Advisory Committee on Immunization Practices (ACIP). MMWR Morb Mortal Wkly Rep 1999;48:RR-6.

Dunkle LM, Balfour HH. A controlled trial of acyclovir for chickenpox in normal children. N Engl J Med 1991;325:1539–1544.

Feldman S. Varicella-zoster virus pneumonitis. Chest 1994;106(Suppl): 22S–27S.

Heuchan A, et al. The management of varicella-zoster virus exposure and infection in pregnancy and the newborn period. MJA 2001;174:288–292.

Tucker JR, Linakis JG. Complications of varicella: varicella-associated cerebritis in a child. Case report and review. J Emerg Med 1993;11:535–538.

Whitley RJ. Therapeutic approaches to varicella-zoster virus infections. J Infect Dis 1992;166(Suppl 1):S51–S57.

Authors: Steve C. Patterson; Mark G. Richmond

Varices

Clinical Presentation

SIGNS AND SYMPTOMS

General

- Weakness and fatigue
- Tachycardia
- Tachypnea
- Hypotension
- Cool, clammy skin; prolonged capillary refill

Abdominal

- Significant active upper GI bleeding
  - —Hematemesis
  - —Hematochezia
  - —Melena
  - —20–40% of total blood volume loss possible
- Abdominal pain
- Stigmata of severe hepatic dysfunction
  - —Jaundice
  - —Spider angiomata
  - —Palmar erythema
  - —Pedal edema
  - —Hepatosplenomegaly
  - —Ascites
- History of portal hypertension
  - —Most commonly alcoholic cirrhosis
  - —Others, including sarcoidosis, primary biliary cirrhosis, schistosomiasis, Budd-Chiari syndrome, severe congestive heart failure (CHF)

Cardiovascular

- Chest pain/shortness of breath

CNS

- Syncope—common presentation
- Confusion and agitation at initial presentation
- Lethargy and obtundation—later finding

MECHANISM/DESCRIPTION

- Portal-systemic shunts that develop with elevated portal venous pressures caused by cirrhosis of the liver (in adults)
- Bleeding typically occurs when portal pressure exceeds 12–18 mm Hg
- Finding of large varices at endoscopy—important risk factor for bleeding

ETIOLOGY

- 10–30% of all causes of upper gastrointestinal (UGI) bleeding
- Up to 90% of UGI bleeding in patients with cirrhosis
- Variceal hemorrhage occurs in 30% of patients with cirrhosis
  - —30% of initial episodes are fatal
  - —70% have recurrent bleeding

PEDIATRIC CONSIDERATIONS

- Massive hematemesis—typical initial presentation
  - —Hypotension may be a late finding
- Etiology
  - —Intrahepatic obstruction from biliary cirrhosis (most common)
  - —α_1-Antitrypsin deficiency
  - —Hepatitis
  - —Cystic fibrosis

Pre-Hospital

CAUTIONS

- Aggressive airway management
  - —AMS or massive hemoptysis
  - —Consider intubation early in transport
  - —Facilitates emergent endoscopy
- Treat hypotension with two large-bore IVs (18-gauge or larger) and 0.9% NS infusion
- Cardiac and pulse oximetry monitoring

CONTROVERSIES

- Normal saline replacement is of concern because adults with cirrhosis also often have significantly impaired renal excretion
- Overhydration can increase venous and portal hypertension, leading to increased rebleeding and fluid overload

PEDIATRIC CONSIDERATIONS

- In children <6 years old, use intraosseous access after three peripheral attempts or 90 seconds if patient is unstable
- Vital signs changes may be a very late finding in children
  - —Subtle changes in mental status, capillary refill, mild tachycardia, or orthostatic changes may indicate significant blood loss
  - —Overaggressive correction in infants can very quickly lead to significant electrolyte abnormalities

Diagnosis

ESSENTIAL WORKUP

- Gastric tube placement
  - —Determines whether patient is actively bleeding
  - —Facilitates a better endoscopic exam
  - —Will not increase or cause esophageal variceal bleeding
- Emergent endoscopy

LABORATORY

- Arterial blood gas for
  - —Acidosis
  - —Hypoxemia
- CBC
  - —Hematocrit (Hct) may be inaccurate with rapid bleeding
- Electrolytes, BUN, creatinine, glucose
  - —Evaluate renal function
  - —Increased BUN may be due to blood in GI tract
  - —Monitor electrolyte imbalances (sodium and potassium)
- Prothrombin time (PT), partial thromboplastin time (PTT), and platelets
  - —Coagulopathy
  - —Prolonged bleeding times
  - —Thrombocytopenia
  - —Type and cross-match—6–8 units
  - —Significant transfusion requirements

IMAGING/SPECIAL TESTS

- Chest x-ray (portable) for aspiration/perforation
- Abdominal radiographs if obstruction suspected
- EKG for myocardial ischemia

DIFFERENTIAL DIAGNOSIS

- Bleeding/perforated peptic ulcer
- Erosive gastritis
- Mallory-Weiss syndrome
- Boerhaave's syndrome
- Aortoenteric fistula
- Gastric varices

Treatment

INITIAL STABILIZATION

- ABCs with aggressive airway control/ intubation
  - —Avoid succinylcholine if hyperkalemia
- Insert two large-bore IVs and initiate 1–2 L (20 mL/kg) 0.9% NS bolus for hypotension
- Establish central IV access with invasive intravascular monitoring for hypotension not responsive to initial fluid bolus
- Replace blood loss as soon as possible
  - —Initiate with O-negative blood until type-specific blood available
  - —10 mL/kg bolus in children
  - —Fresh-frozen plasma and platelets may be required
- Place gastric tube (nasally or orally)

ED TREATMENT

- Emergent endoscopic evaluation required—use pharmacologic and tamponade devices as temporizing measures

Pharmacologic Measures

- Octreotide: first line
  - —Complications: hyperglycemia and abdominal cramping
- Vasopressin: replaced by octreotide secondary to high incidence of vascular ischemia

Balloon Tamponade

- Sengstaken-Blakemore and Minnesota tubes
- Applies direct pressure to the suspected bleed
- Temporary benefit in experienced hands with risk for esophageal ulceration with extended use

Endoscopy

- Procedure of choice in acute esophageal bleeding
- Esophageal band ligation equivalent to sclerotherapy with fewer complications
  - —May be difficult to visualize in cases of massive bleeding
- Sclerotherapy with massive bleeding
- Administer antibiotics at time of procedure to decrease risk for spontaneous bacterial peritonitis
  - —Cefotaxime or ceftriaxone

Refractory Bleeding

- Interventional radiology: transjugular intrahepatic portosystemic shunt (TIPS) procedure
- Surgical options: portacaval shunt, variceal transection and stomach devascularization, liver transplantation

PEDIATRIC CONSIDERATIONS

- Most pediatric bleeding stops spontaneously
- Direct medical intervention at patient support and emergent endoscopic evaluation

MEDICATIONS

- Cefotaxime: 2 g (peds: 50–180 mg/kg/24 h) i.v. q8h
- Ceftriaxone: 2 g (peds: 50–75 mg/kg/24 h) i.v. q24h
- Octreotide: 50-μg bolus then 50-μg/h infusion for 5 days

Disposition

ADMISSION CRITERIA

- ICU admission for actively bleeding varices
- Recent history of variceal bleeding
- High risk for early rebleeding
  - —Age >60 years, renal failure, initial hemoglobin <8

DISCHARGE CRITERIA

- Nonbleeding varices

Miscellaneous

ICD9: 454.9

ICD10: I83.9

SEE ALSO: GASTROINTESTINAL BLEEDING

SUGGESTED READINGS

Hegab AM, Luketic VA. Bleeding esophageal varices. Postgrad Med 2001;109(2):75–89.

McGuirk TD, Coyle WJ. Upper gastrointestinal tract bleeding. Emerg Med Clin North Am 1996;14:523–545.

Sharara AI, Rockey DC. Gastroesophageal varices. N Engl J Med 2001;345(9): 689–681.

Author: John Bailitz

Vasculitis

Clinical Presentation

SIGNS AND SYMPTOMS

Prepulseless Early Phase

- Fever
- Fatigue
- Weight loss
- Diffuse aches and pains
- Nondestructive oligoarthritis and neuropathy

Large Arteries—Takayasu's Arteritis

- Diminished pulses and bruits over several large arteries
- Pulse discrepancy >30 mm Hg between the left and right arms
- Cool upper extremities with claudication and ulceration
- Posturally dependent visual blurring, diplopia
- Severe or resistant hypertension (secondary to renal artery stenosis)
- Abdominal angina (from mesenteric artery stenosis)
- Myocardial ischemia
- Aortic valve dilation
- Congestive heart failure
- Facial or scalp ulcerations
- Hair loss
- Stroke
- Syncope
- Visual loss
- Postural dizziness

Medium and Small Arteries

- Palpable purpura (nodules, ulcers, livedo papules)
- Three of the following 10 criteria are needed to diagnosis polyarteritis nodosa (PAN)
  - —Weight loss >4 kg
  - —Livedo reticularis
  - —Testicular pain or tenderness
  - —Myalgias or weakness
  - —Mononeuropathy or polyneuropathy
  - —Diastolic BP >90 mm Hg
- Churg-Strauss syndrome
  - —Variant of PAN in patients with asthma
  - —Allergic rhinitis and eosinophilia

Small Arteries (Hypersensitivity Vasculitis)—Henoch-Schönlein Purpura (HSP)

- Palpable purpura
- Abdominal pain or cramping
- Nausea and vomiting
- Diarrhea or constipation (frequently accompanied by the passage of blood or mucus per rectum)
- Rarely intussusception
- Hematuria

MECHANISM/DESCRIPTION

- Acute or chronic inflammation and necrosis of blood vessels
- Immune complexes are deposited in vessel walls
- The complement system is activated and stimulates accumulation of polymorphonuclear cells at the site and release of lysosomal enzymes
- Vessel wall damage and necrosis occurs
- Many factors influence the clinical picture
  - —Size of immune complexes
  - —Size of blood vessels affected
  - —Site of deposition
  - —Degree of permeability of the affected vessels
  - —Usually there is multiorgan dysfunction
  - —Single-organ system involvement may occur

ETIOLOGY

Large Arteries

- Takayasu's arteritis
  - —Seen in young (10–30 years of age) Asian females
  - —Affects aorta, proximal portions of its major branches and pulmonary arteries
  - —Streptococcal or tuberculous infections
- Temporal arteritis
- Arteritis associated with Reiter's syndrome and ankylosing spondylitis

Medium Arteries

- Polyarteritis nodosa
  - —May involve any organ system
  - —Predilection for the renal and visceral arteries
- Wegener's granulomatosis
- Behçet's disease
- Kawasaki disease

Small Arteries

- HSP
- Hypersensitivity vasculitis
- Mixed cryoglobulinemia
- Goodpasture's syndrome
- Erythema nodosum

Secondary Causes

- Connective tissue disorders
- Malignancy
- Infectious Epstein-Barr virus
- Lyme disease
- Serum sickness

Pre-Hospital

N/A

Diagnosis

ESSENTIAL WORKUP

- History and physical examination
- CBC, erythrocyte sedimentation rate (ESR), urinalysis, BUN, creatinine

LABORATORY

- Mild leukocytosis
- ESR >20 mm/h
- Anemia of chronic disease with hemoglobin <12
- ANA and ANCA titers
  - —Both are generally elevated
  - —Elevated ANCA especially sensitive for Wegener's disease
- Positive tissue biopsy
- Hepatitis B antigen
  - —30% of patients with PAN will be positive
  - —Usually the ANCA is negative except with Churg-Strauss
- Urinalysis
  - —Proteinuria and hematuria can occur with HSP

IMAGING/SPECIAL TESTS

- Arteriography
  - —Takayasu's arteritis
    - -Irregular vessel walls
    - -Stenosis
    - -Poststenotic dilation
    - -Aneurysms
    - -Occlusion
    - -Increased collateral circulation
  - —PAN
    - -Mesenteric arteriography shows multiple berrylike aneurysms
- Serial CT scans
  - —Used in the early phases
- MRI
- Digital subtraction angiography

DIFFERENTIAL DIAGNOSIS

- Thrombosis
- Antiphospholipid antibody syndrome
- Extensive according to specific to presenting symptom
  - —Renal failure
  - —Arthritis
  - —Purpura
  - —Congestive heart failure

Treatment

INITIAL STABILIZATION

- Initial stabilization is directed toward congestive heart failure, myocardial infarction, and pulmonary edema

ED TREATMENT

- Corticosteroids
- Cytotoxic agents such as cyclophosphamide in patients who fail to respond to steroid treatment with Takayasu's arteritis or PAN
- Treat CHF or hypertension with diuretics or an angiotensin-converting enzyme (ACE) inhibitor such as captopril in patients with Takayasu's arteritis

MEDICATIONS

- Captopril (Capoten): 12.5–25 mg PO t.i.d. initially (peds: 0.5–1 mg/kg/d in 3 doses, max 6 mg/kg/d)
- Cyclophosphamide: 2 mg/kg/d (up to 4 mg/kg) (peds: dose as per consultant)
- Furosemide: 40–100 mg i.v. (peds: 1 mg/kg i.v.)
- Prednisone: 40–60 mg/d (peds: 1–2 mg/kg/d)

Disposition

ADMISSION CRITERIA

- Patients with evidence of severe disease and end-organ dysfunction should be admitted
- Consult for procedures to revascularize ischemic organs

DISCHARGE CRITERIA

- Less symptomatic patients without evidence of end-organ involvement

Miscellaneous

ICD9: 447.6

ICD10: I77.6

SUGGESTED READINGS

Allen NB, Bressler PB. Diagnosis and treatment of the systemic and cutaneous necrotizing vasculitis syndromes. Med Clin North Am 1997;81(1):243–259.

Hunder GG. Giant cell arteritis and polymyalgia rheumatica. Med Clin North Am 1997;81(1):195–215.

Numano F, Okawara M, Inomata H, et al. Takayasu's arteritis. Lancet 2000;356: 1023–1025.

Roberti I, Reisman L. Vasculitis in childhood. Pediatr Nephrol 1993;7: 479–487.

Sercombe CT. Systemic lupus erythematosus and the vasculitides. In: Marx J, ed. Rosen's emergency medicine: concepts and clinical practice, 5th ed. St. Louis: Mosby, 2002.

Sneller MC, Fauci AS. Pathogenesis of vasculitis syndromes. Med Clin North Am 1997;81(1):221–237.

Author: Andrew Milsten

Venous Insufficiency

Clinical Presentation

SIGNS AND SYMPTOMS

- Subcutaneous venous varicosity
- Profuse bleeding from a varicosity
- Dependent lower extremity edema
- Dull, aching pain
- Hyperpigmentation
- Lipodermatosclerosis (thickened, indurated skin)
- Venous ulceration

MECHANISM/DESCRIPTION

- Highly prevalent disease with a chronic, progressive course
- Risk factors include
  - —Obesity
  - —Age
  - —Immobility
  - —Deep venous thrombosis (DVT) or phlebitis
  - —Vascular trauma
  - —Homelessness

ETIOLOGY

- Long and short saphenous veins, their perforating branches, and direct vessels drain into the deep venous system of the leg
- Normal venous flow is from superficial to deep veins
- Bicuspid venous valves moderate intravascular pressures during muscle contraction (25 mm Hg) and maintain unidirectional blood flow from the superficial to deep venous systems
- Development of venous hypertension is the common final pathway
- Major anatomic abnormality is valvular incompetence
- May be a primary (intrinsic), secondary (obstruction from DVT), or congenital defect
- Regurgitant blood flow and elevated venous pressures (60–90 mm Hg) during muscle contractions distend superficial veins
- A vicious cycle develops as distended vessels distort, causing further valvular dysfunction
- Perivascular fibrin cuff formation inhibits oxygen diffusion while endothelial dysfunction allows water, red blood cells, and proteins to leak into the extracellular matrix
- Eventually fibrosis, protein leakage, and diminished oxygen diffusion leads to sclerosis, hypoxia, and ulceration of overlying tissue

Pre-Hospital

CAUTIONS

- Control bleeding with direct pressure
- Note the estimated blood loss at the scene

Diagnosis

ESSENTIAL WORKUP

- History and clinical manifestations (edema, skin changes, ulceration) will confirm the diagnosis
- Determine the time course of the disease
- Worsening erythema, swelling, and pain suggest cellulitis
- Asymmetric swelling, cyanosis, and pain suggest DVT
- Poor peripheral pulses and low ankle-brachial index (ABI) suggest concurrent peripheral arterial disease

LABORATORY

- Hematocrit for substantial or prolonged blood loss

IMAGING/SPECIAL TESTS

- Duplex Doppler ultrasonography if DVT or popliteal cysts are suspected
- ABIs to assess for peripheral arterial disease
  - —Ankle systolic pressure divided by brachial systolic pressure
  - —ABI <0.9 indicates peripheral arterial disease
  - —Will affect management because compression/elevation is relatively contraindicated

DIFFERENTIAL DIAGNOSIS

- Edematous states
  - —Congestive heart failure
  - —Hypoalbuminemia, liver disease
  - —Nephrotic syndrome
  - —Hypothyroidism (myxedema)
- Lower extremity swelling
  - —DVT, postphlebitis syndrome
  - —Lymphatic obstruction
  - —Popliteal cyst
- Lower extremity ulceration
  - —Peripheral arterial disease
  - —Diabetic foot ulcer

Treatment

INITIAL STABILIZATION

- Control bleeding with direct pressure
- Refractory bleeding may require figure-of-eight stitch

ED TREATMENT

- Mechanical therapy
  - —Leg elevation above the level of the heart
  - —Compression stockings (contraindicated with peripheral arterial disease)
  - —Pneumatic compression devices
- Wound care
  - —Dressings speed wound healing by providing a moist environment for epithelialization
  - —Reduces pain, odor, and exudative deposits
  - —Should be applied before initiating compressive treatment
  - —Topical solutions include povidone-iodine (Betadine), sodium hypochlorite (Dakin's solution), and acetic acid (Burow's solution)
  - —Compression bandages embedded with zinc oxide paste (Unna boot) are effective
  - —Topical antibiotics do not improve wound healing
  - —Systemic antibiotics are indicated if clinical evidence of cellulitis is present
- Surgery
  - —Consider surgical referral for cases refractory to medical management

MEDICATIONS

- Amoxicillin/clavulanate: 875/125 mg PO b.i.d.
- Aspirin: 325 mg PO q.d. (may accelerate wound healing)
- Cephalexin: 500 mg PO q.i.d.
- Dicloxacillin: 500 mg PO q.i.d.

Disposition

ADMISSION CRITERIA

- Failed outpatient cellulitis therapy
- Bleeding not controlled by direct pressure
- Noncompliant patients who are unable or unwilling to change dressing material

DISCHARGE CRITERIA

- Most patients can safely be discharged home and treated as an outpatient
- Must ensure close follow-up with primary care provider
- May need home services to help with dressing material

Miscellaneous

ICD9: 459.8

ICD10: I87.2

SUGGESTED READINGS

Beauchamps DR, Townsend CM. Sabiston textbook of surgery, 16th ed. Philadelphia: WB Saunders, 2001:1435–1443.

Guyton AC, Hall JE. Textbook of medical physiology, 10th ed. Philadelphia: WB Saunders, 2000:158–159.

Scott TE, LaMorte WW, Gorin DR, et al. Risk factors for chronic venous insufficiency: a dual case-control study. J Vasc Surg 1995; 22:622.

Author: Calvin Brown

Ventricular Fibrillation

Clinical Presentation

SIGNS AND SYMPTOMS

- Loss of consciousness
- Seizure
- Pulseless
- Apnea
- Cyanosis

MECHANISM/DESCRIPTION

- Heart stops effective pumping, brain perfusion ceases, and the patient loses consciousness
- Ventricular fibrillation (VF)
  —Totally disorganized depolarization and contraction of small areas of the ventricle, without effective ventricular pumping
- EKG or cardiac monitor
  —Absence of QRS complexes and T waves
  —Presence of low-amplitude baseline undulations that are variable in both amplitude and periodicity

ETIOLOGY

- Initial rhythm in about 50–70% of patients sustaining sudden cardiac death in the pre-hospital setting
  —Most often a result of severe myocardial ischemia or infarction
  —Complication of a cardiomyopathy
    -Up to 50% of patients with dilated cardiomyopathy suffer an episode of VF
  —In hypertrophic cardiomyopathy, unexpected sudden death occurs with reported frequency of up to 3% per year
- Other less common causes of VF
  —Blunt chest trauma
  —Hypothermia
  —Iatrogenic myocardial irritation from pacemaker placement or a pulmonary artery catheter
- VF often preceded by ventricular tachycardia (VT)
- Predisposition to VT
- Drug toxicities (cyclic antidepressants, digitalis)
- Hereditary QT prolongation,
- Metabolic abnormalities that prolong the QT interval (hyperkalemia, hypocalcemia)
- Idiopathic ventricular fibrillation (10–15%) including the subgroup of patients with Brugada's syndrome

PEDIATRIC CONSIDERATIONS

- Primary ventricular dysrhythmias extremely rare in children
- VF usually results from a respiratory arrest, hypothermia, or near drowning

Pre-Hospital

CAUTIONS

- Patients in VT or supraventricular tachycardia may deteriorate rapidly if defibrillated without EKG synchronization
- In hypothermic cardiac arrest (core temperature $<30°C$), if the patient remains in VF after the delivery of the first three shocks, rewarm the patient before further attempts of defibrillation
- Precordial thump is an acceptable intervention for witnessed arrest when the victim has no pulse and a defibrillator is not *immediately available* to the healthcare provider
- Do not defibrillate awake patients

CONTROVERSIES

- Biphasic automatic external defibrillation (AED)
  —Multicenter study showed that low-energy (150 J) biphasic AED resulted in superior defibrillation rate compared with the monophasic AED, resulting in return of spontaneous circulation in a greater percentage of patients
  —The rates of survival to hospital admission and discharge did not differ between the two groups
- CPR before defibrillation for prolonged VF
  —Data from animal studies and review of previous pre-hospital studies showed that CPR first (90 seconds of CPR before defibrillation attempt) improved survival

ESSENTIAL WORKUP

- Cardiac monitor

LABORATORY

- Laboratory tests are not useful during the resuscitation
- After successful resuscitation
  —Electrolytes including magnesium and calcium
  —Cardiac enzymes
  —Toxicologic screen

DIFFERENTIAL DIAGNOSIS

- Asystole
  —Fine VF may appear to be asystole on a single EKG lead
  —Check one other lead to make sure there are no fine fibrillations present

Treatment

INITIAL STABILIZATION

- Immediate defibrillation
  - —200 J first attempt (or the equivalent biphasic joules)
  - —200–300 J second attempt (or the equivalent biphasic joules)
  - —360 J third attempt (or the equivalent biphasic joules)
- Initiate CPR and airway management with intubation
- Establish IV access
  - —Administer epinephrine, 1.0 mg i.v. or 2–2.5 mg via endotracheal tube (ETT)
  - —Vasopressin, 40 U i.v. single dose, can be given one time only as first drug before epinephrine
- After the epinephrine or vasopressin, repeat defibrillation with 360 J (or equivalent biphasic joules) within 30–60 seconds
  - —If VF persists, consider antiarrhythmics, amiodarone, lidocaine, magnesium, or procainamide
- Further rounds of defibrillation can be given 30–60 seconds after each round of medications
- Epinephrine is initiated 10–20 minutes after vasopressin

ED TREATMENT

- If the patient is successfully resuscitated, start continuous infusion of the last antiarrhythmic agent administered to the patient
- Begin an evaluation for the cause of the VF, recognizing that the most likely is myocardial ischemia

MEDICATIONS

- Amiodarone: 300 mg i.v. bolus, repeat 150 mg i.v. every 3–5 minutes
- Epinephrine
  - —1:10,000 concentration: 1mg i.v., repeat every 3–5 minutes
  - —1:1,000 concentration: 2–2.5 mg in 10 mL NS via ETT
- Lidocaine: l mg/kg i.v. bolus, repeat 0.5 mg/kg
  - —Lidocaine infusion: 2–4 mg/min (30–50 μg/kg/min)
  - —Lidocaine via ETT: 2.0–2.5 mg in 10 mL NS
- Magnesium sulfate: 1–2 g in 10 mL D5W i.v. bolus
- Procainamide: 20–50 mg/min until arrhythmia suppressed, hypotension, QRS widens by 50%, or a total dose of 17 mg/kg is reached
  - —Procainamide infusion: 1–4 mg/min
- Vasopressin: 40 U i.v. one time only

Disposition

ADMISSION CRITERIA

- All patients who survive to the coronary care unit

DISCHARGE CRITERIA

- None

Miscellaneous

ICD9: 427.41

ICD10: I49.0

SEE ALSO: CARDIAC ARREST

SUGGESTED READINGS

American Heart Association. Guidelines 2000 for cardiopulmonary resuscitation and emergency cardiovascular care. Circulation 2000;102:195.

ArKern KB, Halperin HR, Field J. New guidelines for cardiopulmonary resuscitation and emergency cardiac care. JAMA 2001;285:1267.

Blum FC. Adult medical resuscitation. In: Howell J, et al., eds. Emergency medicine. Philadelphia: WB Saunders, 1997.

Cummins RO, ed. ACLS provider manual. Dallas: American Heart Association, 2001.

Author: Ra'ed Hijazi

Ventricular Peritoneal Shunts

Clinical Presentation

SIGNS AND SYMPTOMS

Shunt Obstruction

- *Headache,* nausea, malaise, general weakness, irritability
- Decreased level of consciousness (LOC) or coma
- Increased head size or bulging fontanel
- New-onset seizures, increased seizure frequency
- Autonomic instability, decreased upward gaze
- Apnea/respiratory arrest
- Papilledema: rare

Overdrainage Syndrome

- Severe headache, focal neurologic signs, malaise, seizures, coma
  - —Signs and symptoms may be postural
- Rapid overdrainage may cause upward shift of the brainstem, causing apnea, bradycardia, hypotension, syncope, laryngospasm
- Subdural hygroma or hematoma, chronic overdrainage, pneumocranium

Shunt Infections

- Signs and symptoms of shunt obstruction
- Fever (may be absent), meningeal signs, local signs of infection (erythema, swelling, tenderness), peritonitis
- Infections usually occur soon after shunt placement (about 80% within 6 months)

Slit Ventricle Syndrome

- Episodic headache, alternating periods of normal behavior and lethargy, headache, nausea and vomiting

MECHANISM/DESCRIPTION

- *Obstruction:* shunt malfunction produces impaired drainage of CSF and results in increased intracranial pressure (ICP)
  - —Rate of ICP increase determines severity
- *Overdrainage syndrome:* assuming upright posture increases CSF outflow and causes decreased ICP and post-lumbar puncture (LP)-like headache
- *Infection:* a shunt is a foreign body and a conduit between CSF and the peritoneal cavity
  - —Staphylococcal epidermidis and other staphylococcal species: about 75% of infections
- *Slit ventricle syndrome:* prolonged overdrainage causes decreased ventricular size and intermittent increases in ICP owing to proximal obstruction

PEDIATRIC CONSIDERATIONS

- If cranial sutures are open, CSF may accumulate without much ICP increase, producing relatively nonspecific signs and symptoms

Pre-Hospital

CAUTIONS

- Patients with shunt malfunction are at risk for apnea and respiratory arrest
- Oxygen should be applied with close monitoring of respiratory status
- If increased ICP is suspected, transport with head elevated to 30 degrees

Diagnosis

ESSENTIAL WORKUP

Suspected Shunt Malfunction

- Manipulation of the pumping chamber:
  - —Chamber should compress easily and refill within 3 seconds
  - —Failure to compress easily implies distal obstruction; failure to fill implies proximal obstruction (up to 40% of malfunctioning shunts compress/fill normally)
- *Shunt series:* radiographs of skull, chest, and abdomen aid diagnosis of disconnection, malposition, or kinking of shunt components
- Head CT

Suspected Infection

- Aspiration of CSF from shunt reservoir (in consult with neurosurgeon)
  - —May be performed using sterile technique and 23-gauge butterfly needle
  - —Aspirate slowly 5–10 mL CSF for the studies noted below

LABORATORY

- Electrolytes, anticonvulsant levels, renal function, blood count, and glucose aid in the differential diagnosis of seizures and altered mental status

SUSPECTED INFECTION

- Analysis of CSF from the shunt reservoir for culture, cell count, Gram stain, glucose and protein levels
  - —CSF analysis may be normal early, especially with prior antibiotic treatment
- Blood cultures

IMAGING/SPECIAL TESTS

- Cranial CT: catheter position, ventricular size, subdural hematoma or hygroma, other causes of elevated ICP
  - —Enlarged ventricles: shunt malfunction
  - —Smaller ventricles: overdrainage
- Ultrasound: may be used to assess ventricular size and position of catheter tip
- Shunt manometry: high pressure (>20 cm H_2O) implies distal shunt obstruction

DIFFERENTIAL DIAGNOSIS

- Seizure disorder (idiopathic, toxic, metabolic)
- Infections: non–shunt-related CNS infection, systemic infections
- Metabolic abnormalities: hypoglycemia, hyponatremia, hypoxia
- Intoxication/poisoning
- Head trauma

Treatment

INITIAL STABILIZATION

Signs of Impending Herniation

- Rapid sequence intubation (see Conscious Sedation and Rapid Sequence Intubation) and mild hyperventilation to PCO_2 about 35
  - —Pretreat with lidocaine (pediatric: plus atropine)
  - —Thiopental/etomidate for induction
  - —Paralytic choice is controversial
  - —Depolarizing agents (succinylcholine) may increase ICP a few mm Hg, though this may not be clinically significant
  - —Use pretreatment dose of nondepolarizing agent if depolarizing agent chosen
  - —Nondepolarizing agents (vecuronium, rocuronium) may be preferable
- Forced pumping of shunt chamber
- Flush the device with 1 mL saline to remove distal obstruction
- Slow drainage of CSF from the reservoir to achieve pressure <20 cm H_2O
- IV mannitol to lower ICP
- *Ventricular puncture* is procedure of last resort if above unsuccessful and neurosurgeon unavailable
- *Status epilepticus* is treated with benzodiazepines (lorazepam)

ED TREATMENT

- Early neurosurgeon consultation
- Shunt malfunction
  - —Elevate head of bed to 30 degrees
  - —Medical management with diuretics (mannitol, furosemide) may be appropriate in certain mild cases
- Overdrainage syndrome
  - —Supine position
  - —Correct volume depletion
- Shunt infection
  - —Systemic antibiotics (vancomycin *plus* cefotaxime *or* gentamicin if gram-negative suspected)

MEDICATIONS

- Atropine: 0.02 mg/kg i.v. (min 0.1 mg)
- Cefotaxime: 30 mg/kg i.v. (newborn: 50 mg/kg i.v.)
- Furosemide: 1 mg/kg i.v.
- Gentamicin: 2–5 mg/kg i.v.
- Lidocaine: 1 mg/kg i.v.
- Mannitol: 1.0 mg/kg i.v.
- Rocuronium: 0.6–1 mg/kg i.v.
- Succinylcholine: 1.5 mg/kg i.v.
- Vancomycin: 15 mg/kg i.v.
- Vecuronium: 0.1–0.3 mg/kg i.v.

Disposition

ADMISSION CRITERIA

- Patients with shunt complications require neurosurgical consultation and admission to an ICU or other closely monitored setting

DISCHARGE CRITERIA

- If shunt malfunction is ruled out, disposition depends on diagnosis and patient condition

Miscellaneous

ICD9: 996.2

SUGGESTED READINGS

Guertin SR. Cerebrospinal fluid shunts: evaluation, complication, and crisis management. Pediatr Clin North Am 1987;34(1):203–217.

Key CB, Rothrock SG, Falk JL. Cerebrospinal fluid shunt complications: an emergency medicine perspective. Pediatr Emerg Care 1995;11(5):265–273.

Madsen MA. Emergency department management of ventriculoperitoneal cerebrospinal fluid shunts. Ann Emerg Med 1986;15(11):1330–1343.

McLaurin RL, Frame PT. Treatment of cerebrospinal fluid shunts. Rev Infect Dis 1987;9(3):595–603.

Author: Richard S. Krause

Ventricular Tachycardia

Clinical Presentation

SIGNS AND SYMPTOMS

- Asymptomatic
- Syncope/near syncope
- Lightheadedness/dizziness
- Shortness of breath
- Palpitations
- Chest discomfort/pain
- Diaphoresis
- Cannon A waves
- Hypotension
- Congestive heart failure
- Beat-to-beat variability of systolic blood pressure
- Variability in heart tones, especially S1

MECHANISM/DESCRIPTION

- Rapid and regular depolarization of the ventricles independent of the atria and the normal conduction system
- Reentry
  —Structural heart disease most common
  —Seen in dilated cardiomyopathy, ischemia, and infiltrative heart disease, previous myocardial infarction, scarring
  —May be pharmacologically induced
  —Usually produces a regular and monomorphic rhythm
- Triggered automaticity
  —Minority of ventricular tachycardia (VT)
  —Caused by repetitive firing of a ventricular focus
- Torsades de pointes
  —Polymorphic form of VT
  —Alternating electrical polarity and amplitude
  —Prolongation in repolarization necessary
  —Usually pharmacologically induced
- Regardless of the mechanism, all VT may degenerate to ventricular fibrillation (VF)

ETIOLOGY

- Wide complex tachycardia
  —80% likelihood of being VT
  —20% supraventricular tachycardia (SVT) with a baseline left bundle branch block (LBBB) or aberrancy
- Wide complex tachycardia and a history of myocardial infarction
  —>95% likelihood of being VT
- Incidence of nonsustained VT
  —0–4% in the general population
  —Up to 60% of patients with dilated cardiomyopathy
- Associated with increased risk for sudden cardiac death (SCD)

PEDIATRIC CONSIDERATIONS

- Primary cardiac arrest and VT are rare in children
- Usually secondary to hypoxia and acidosis
- VT is tolerated for longer periods in children than adults and is less likely to degenerate to VF
- Infants in VT most commonly present with congestive heart failure
- VT in children results from
  —Cardiomyopathy
  —Congenital structural heart disease
  —Congenital prolonged QT syndromes
  —Coronary artery disease secondary to vasculitis
  —Toxins, poisons, drugs
  —Severe electrolyte imbalances, especially of potassium

Pre-Hospital

CAUTIONS

- Transport stable patients suspected of being in VT without attempting to convert them
- *Synchronized* cardioversion for unstable patients with a pulse
- Defibrillation for pulseless VT

CONTROVERSIES

- Lidocaine
  —No benefit in the prevention of VT in patients with isolated premature ventricular contractions (PVCs), regardless of the frequency
  —Infusions are no longer advanced cardiac life support (ACLS) protocol

Diagnosis

ESSENTIAL WORKUP

EKG

- Most important initial test to differentiate VT from SVT with aberrancy or LBBB
- VT
  —Three or more consecutive QRS complexes with a ventricular rate over 100 beats/min and a QRS duration >120 milliseconds
- Torsades de pointes
  —Polymorphic VT that rotates its axis every 10–20 beats
- Criterion to determine VT
  —AV dissociation (present in 60–75%)
  —Fusion beats (P wave partially activates ventricle in advance of next VT cycle, capture beats (P wave totally activates ventricle)
  —Uniform morphology (except in the case of torsades)
  —Extreme axis deviation (−90 to +180 degrees)
  —QRS >140 milliseconds, with right bundle branch block (RBBB) morphology; or QRS >160 milliseconds, with LBBB morphology, but >160 suggests VT regardless of bunch branch morphology
  —QRS concordance in the precordial leads
  —Brugada's criteria: (99% sensitivity, 97% specificity)
    -R-S interval absent in all precordial leads
    -R-S interval >100 milliseconds in any precordial lead
    -AV dissociation
  —V-1 R wave >30 milliseconds; R-S interval >70 milliseconds, slurred, notched S
  —Wide QRS with LBBB in precordium
- Indicators of SVT with aberrancy include
  —Normal-axis QRS <140 milliseconds
  —Absence of Q waves
  —RBBB in V1 with rsR' triphasic pattern
  —NB: slowing of impulse conduction velocity seen with antiarrhythmic drugs is more pronounced at faster rates so may result in wide-complex SVT (SVT with aberrancy)

LABORATORY

- Cardiac enzymes
- Electrolytes, BUN, creatinine, glucose
- Magnesium level
- Calcium level
- Digoxin level if toxicity suspected

IMAGING/SPECIAL TESTS

- Esophageal pacing catheters
  —May be able to detect atrial activity to establish AV dissociation and therefore diagnose VT
  —Catheters can then be used to overdrive pace if needed

DIFFERENTIAL DIAGNOSIS

- SVT with aberrancy or baseline LBBB
- Proarrhythmia secondary to antidysrhythmia medications; suspect if
  - —VT morphology is different than previous episodes of VT
  - —Medications have recently been started or changed
  - —QT interval is prolonged
  - —Torsades de pointes
  - —If VT continues to recur after cardioversion

Treatment

INITIAL STABILIZATION

- Pulseless VT: defibrillate immediately and follow the ventricular fibrillation treatment plan

ED TREATMENT

- Unstable patient
  - —Definition
    - -Chest pain
    - -Hypotension
    - -Evidence of worsening heart failure
  - —Initiate immediate synchronized cardioversion with 100 J, quickly progressing to 200 J, 300 J, and 360 J if no response
    - -If the VT is polymorphic, begin cardioversion at 200 J
  - —Sedate the patient before cardioversion if at all possible
  - —If unable to terminate the VT, administer lidocaine and repeat the cardioversion
  - —Antitachycardia overdrive pacing if torsades
  - —After successful return of sinus rhythm, begin amiodarone
- Stable patient, monomorphic VT
  - —Normal cardiac function at baseline
    - -Procainamide *or* sotalol; may also consider amiodarone or lidocaine
  - —Impaired cardiac function at baseline
    - -Amiodarone bolus, then infusion *or* lidocaine, then synchronized cardioversion
- Stable patient, polymorphic VT
  - —Normal QT interval at baseline
    - -Correct electrolyte abnormalities
    - -Treat ischemia if present
    - -Then begin *one* of the following: beta-blockers, lidocaine, amiodarone, procainamide, or sotalol
  - —Prolonged QT/torsades de pointes
    - -Correct electrolytes
    - -Magnesium sulfate *or* overdrive pacing *or* one of the following: isoproterenol, phenytoin, lidocaine
    - -Isoproterenol is used to overdrive the tachycardia if the patient has no history of coronary artery disease
    - -Temporizing measure until external pacing available
  - —Impaired cardiac function at baseline
    - -Amiodarone bolus *or* lidocaine bolus then synchronized cardioversion

MEDICATIONS

- Adenosine: 6 mg i.v. push followed by 12 mg i.v. push if needed in 1–2 minutes (peds: 1 mg/kg, max 6 mg; note: does not convert VT, no longer ACLS protocol)
- Amiodarone: 150mg IV bolus over 10 minutes, may repeat; max cumulative dose 2.2 g i.v/24 h; infusion 540 mg i.v. over 18 hours (0.5 mg/min) (peds: 5 mg/kg i.v. or i.o. over 20–60 minutes, max 15 mg/kg/d
- Isoproterenol: 2–10 μg/min, titrate to heart rate (peds: 0.1 μg/kg/min); note: do not give with epinephrine, may precipitate VT/VF
- Lidocaine: 1–1.5 mg/kg bolus i.v. push first dose, 0.5–0.75 mg/kg second dose, and every 5–10 minutes for a max of 3 mg/kg; tracheal administration 2–4 mg/kg; maintenance infusion 1–4 mg/min if converted (peds: 1 mg/kg bolus with infusion 20–50 μg/kg/min)
- $MgSO_4$: 2 g in D5W over 5–10 min followed by infusion of 0.5 to 1.0g/hour IV, titrate to control torsades
- Procainamide: 20–30 mg/min until converted or for a total maximum total dose of 17 mg/kg; maintenance infusion 1–4 mg/min

PEDIATRIC CONSIDERATIONS

- Begin cardioversion at 1 J/kg, 2 J/kg, and 4 J/kg as needed

Disposition

ADMISSION CRITERIA

- Admit sustained VT to a critical care setting
- Admit nonsustained VT and a history of myocardial infarction or dilated cardiomyopathy for electrophysiologic studies

DISCHARGE CRITERIA

- Rare patients with nonsustained VT and a previous evaluation that revealed no structural heart disease can be discharged
  - —At low risk for SCD
- Patients with automatic internal cardiac defibrillators that are well functioning can also be discharged

Miscellaneous

ICD9: 427.1

ICD10: I47.2

SUGGESTED READINGS

Alpert MA, Mukeiji V, Bikkina M, et al. Pathogenesis, recognition, and management of common cardiac arrhythmias. South Med J 1995;88(1):1–21.

Brady WJ, Skiles J. Wide QRS complex tachycardias; ECG differential diagnosis. Am J Emerg Med 1999;17(4):376–381.

Brugada P, Brugada J, et al. A new approach to the differential diagnosis of a regular tachycardia with a wide QRS complex. Circulation 1991;83:1649–1659.

Fogel RI, Prystowsky EN. Management of malignant ventricular arrhythmias and cardiac arrest. Crit Care Med 2000;28(10):165–169.

Gupta AK, Thakur RK. Wide complex tachycardias. Med Clin North Am 2001;85(2).

Hazanski MF, Cummins RO, Field JM. American Heart Association handbook of emergency cardiovascular care. 2000.

Passman R, Kadish A. Polymorphic VT, long QT syndrome and torsades de pointes. Med Clin North Am 2001;85(2).

Walid SI, Natale A. Ventricular tachycardia syndromes. Med Clin North Am 2001;85(2).

Author: Jennifer Audi

Vertigo

Clinical Presentation

SIGNS AND SYMPTOMS

- "Dizzy" describes a variety of experiences, including
  - —Sensations of motion
  - —Weakness, fainting
  - —Lightheadedness
  - —Unsteadiness
  - —Depression
- True vertigo
  - —Sensation of disorientation in space combined with a sensation of motion
  - —Hallucination of movement either of the self or the external environment
  - —Most patients have an organic basis for these symptoms
- Peripheral vertigo
  - —Sudden onset
  - —Severe symptoms
  - —Intermittent episodes lasting seconds to minutes, occasionally hours
  - —Horizontal or horizontorotary nystagmus (also positional, fatigues, and suppressed by fixation)
  - —Normal neurologic exam
  - —Sometimes associated hearing loss or tinnitus
- Central vertigo
  - —Gradual onset
  - —Mild continuous symptoms
  - —All varieties of nystagmus (horizontal, vertical, rotatory)
  - —Absence of hearing loss
  - —No positional association
  - —Presence of neurologic findings
- Nausea and vomiting often associated with vertigo
- Ataxia

ETIOLOGY

Peripheral

- Benign paroxysmal positional
  - —Uncertain etiology
  - —Dependent on head position
  - —Fatigues
- Acute labyrinthitis
  - —Associated with hearing deficit
  - —Sudden onset
  - —May be serous, acute suppurative, toxic, or chronic
  - —Ototoxic drugs
    - -Aminoglycosides
    - -Antimalarials
    - -Erythromycin
    - -Furosemide
- Ménière's disease
  - —Episodic vertigo, hearing loss, and tinnitus
- Vestibular neuronitis
  - —Severe vertigo and symptoms resolving over days to weeks
  - —No hearing deficits
  - —Highest incidence in third to fifth decade
- Acoustic neuroma
  - —Tumor of Schwann's cells enveloping the eighth cranial nerve (CN VIII)
  - —Develops into central cause
  - —Progressive unilateral hearing deficits and tinnitus
  - —May also involve CN V, VII, or X
- Trauma
  - —Rupture of tympanic membrane, round window, labyrinthine concussion, or development of perilymphatic fistula can all have severe symptoms
- Otitis media and serous otitis with effusion
- Foreign body in ear canal

Central

- Cerebellar hemorrhage
  - —Sudden onset of headache, vertigo, vomiting, and ataxia
  - —Visual paralysis to affected side
  - —Ipsilateral CN VI paralysis
- Vertebrobasilar artery insufficiency
  - —Dysarthria
  - —Ataxia
  - —Numbness of the face
  - —Hemiparesis, headache
  - —Diplopia/visual disturbances
  - —Disturbances may be transient or exacerbated by movement of the neck
  - —Consider in elderly patients with isolated new-onset vertigo without an obvious cause
- Cerebellar infarction
  - —Nausea
  - —Vomiting
  - —Ipsilateral nystagmus
  - —Ataxia
- Trauma
  - —Vertiginous symptoms common after whiplash injury
  - —Postconcussive syndrome or damage to labyrinth or CN VIII secondary to basilar skull fracture
- Temporal lobe epilepsy
  - —Associated with hallucinations, aphasia, trancelike states, or convulsions
  - —More common in younger patients
- Vertebrobasilar migraines
  - —Prodrome of vertigo, dysarthria, ataxia, visual disturbances, or paresthesias followed by headache
  - —Often a family history of migraines or similar attacks
- Tumor
- Multiple sclerosis
  - —Onset between 20 and 40 years of age
  - —All forms of nystagmus
  - —May have abrupt onset of severe vertigo and vomiting
  - —History of other vague and varying neurologic signs or symptoms
- Subclavian steal syndrome
  - —Exercise of an arm causing shunting of blood from vertebral and basilar arteries into the subclavian artery, resulting in vertigo or syncope
  - —Secondary to a stenotic subclavian artery
  - —Diminished unilateral radial pulse or differential systolic blood pressure between arms
- Hypoglycemia
  - —Suspect in diabetic patient or any other patient with unexplained symptoms or mental status change

Pre-Hospital

N/A

Diagnosis

ESSENTIAL WORKUP

- Ask patient describe the sensation without using the word "dizzy"
- Determine whether the cause is a peripheral or a central process using patient's clinical presentation (see above)
- Detailed physical exam
  - —Auscultation of the carotid and vertebral arteries for bruits
  - —Pulses and pressures in both arms
  - —Inspection of the ears
  - —Evaluation of hearing (Weber's and Rinne's tests)
  - —Ocular assessment (pupils, fundi, visual acuity, nystagmus)
  - —Cardiac auscultation
  - —Full neurologic examination

LABORATORY

- Electrolytes, BUN, creatinine, glucose

IMAGING/SPECIAL TESTS

- EKG
- Head CT/MRI for evaluation of suspected tumor, central cause, or posttraumatic cause
- Angiography for suspected vertebrobasilar insufficiency

DIFFERENTIAL DIAGNOSIS

- Diabetes mellitus
- Hypothyroidism
- Drugs (e.g., alcohol, barbiturates, salicylates)
- Hyperventilation
- Cardiac (i.e. arrhythmia, myocardial infarction, or other etiologies of syncope)
- Peripheral vascular disease (i.e., hypertension, orthostatic hypotension, vasovagal)
- Motion sickness

Treatment

INITIAL STABILIZATION

- ABCs
- IV access for dehydration/vomiting
- Monitor
- Finger-stick blood glucose

ED TREATMENT

- Based on accurate diagnosis
  - —Central etiologies require more aggressive workup than peripheral
  - —Symptomatic treatment for peripheral vertigo with appropriate follow-up
- Administer medication to control vertiginous symptoms—options
  - —Diphenhydramine
  - —Meclizine
  - —Promethazine
  - —Diazepam
- Initiate IV antibiotics for acute bacterial labyrinthitis

MEDICATIONS

- Diazepam (Valium): 2.5–5 mg i.v. q8h or 2–10 mg PO q8h
- Diphenhydramine (Benadryl): 25–50 mg i.v., i.m., or PO q6h
- Meclizine (Antivert): 25 mg PO q6h PRN
- Promethazine (Phenergan): 12.5 mg i.v. q6h or 25–50 mg i.m, PO, or PR q6h

Disposition

ADMISSION CRITERIA

- Cerebellar infarct/hemorrhage
- Vertebrobasilar insufficiency
- Acute suppurative labyrinthitis
- Intractable nausea/vomiting
- Inability to ambulate

DISCHARGE CRITERIA

- Patient with peripheral etiology and stable

Miscellaneous

ICD9: 780.4

ICD10: R42

SEE ALSO: DIZZINESS; LABYRINTHITIS

SUGGESTED READINGS

Derebery MD. The diagnosis and treatment of dizziness. Med Clin North Am 1999; 83:10.

Gizzi M, Riley E, Molinari S. The diagnostic value of imaging the patient with dizziness. Arch Neurol 1996;53:1299–1304.

Gomez CR, et al. Isolated vertigo as a manifestation of vertebrobasilar ischemia. Neurology 1996;47:94–97.

Herr R, et al. A directed approach to the dizzy patient. Ann Emerg Med 1989;18:6: 664–672.

Olshaker S. Vertigo. In: Marx J, et al., eds. Rosen's emergency medicine: concepts and clinical practice. St. Louis: CV Mosby, 2001:123–131.

Wolf JS, et al. Success of the modified Epley maneuver in treating benign paroxysmal/vertigo. Laryngoscope 1999;109:900.

Authors: Jonathan S. Olshaker; Aryeh J. Pessah

Violence, Management of

Clinical Presentation

SIGNS AND SYMPTOMS

- Behaviors suggesting impending violence
  - —Provocative behavior
  - —Anger
  - —Pacing
  - —Loud speech
  - —Tense posture
  - —Pounding, clenching of fists

MECHANISM/DESCRIPTION

- ED is clinical area likely to experience violent episodes owing to 24-hour access
- First contact of victims and perpetrators of violence
- High prevalence of intoxicated patients and psychiatric patients
- Only reliable predictors
  - —Male gender
  - —Alcohol or drug abuse
- No difference exists in
  - —Ethnicity
  - —Language
  - —Age
  - —Education
  - —Employment status
  - —Medical diagnosis

ETIOLOGY

- Functional
  - —Psychiatric
    - -Schizophrenia
    - -Affective
    - -Antisocial
    - -Borderline
    - -Paranoid
    - -Adjustment disorders
  - —Antisocial behavior
- Organic
  - —CNS
    - -Delirium
    - -Dementia
    - -Infection
    - -Seizures
    - -Cerebrovascular accident
    - -Head injury
  - —Metabolic
    - -Hypoglycemia
    - -Hypoxia
    - -Hypothermia or hyperthermia
    - -Endocrine disorders
  - —Drugs
    - -Alcohol and sedatives (withdrawal, intoxication)
    - -Cocaine
    - -LSD
    - -PCP
    - -Anticholinergics
    - -Steroids

Pre-Hospital

CAUTIONS

- Restrain potentially violent patients
- Seek police aid in control of violent/dangerous patients

Diagnosis

ESSENTIAL WORKUP

Predict Violence

- Identify prodromes of violence
    - -Begins with anxiety
    - -Then defensiveness
    - -Then physical aggression
  - —History
    - -Previous threats and violence
    - -Psychiatric history
    - -Substance abuse
    - -Self-mutilation
    - -Verbalized threats
    - -Plans of violence
- Physical
  - —Focus on identifying and distinguishing between associated functional and medical conditions
  - —Attention to the neurological exam, vital signs, and mental status exam
  - —Often cannot be performed until the patient is safely restrained

LABORATORY

- CBC if infectious etiology for behavior
- Electrolytes, BUN, creatinine, glucose if metabolic or toxic etiology suspected
- Drug screen if ingestion likely

IMAGING/SPECIAL TESTS

- CT head for altered mental status or head trauma

Treatment

INITIAL STABILIZATION

- Prevention of violence
  - —Deterrence
    - -Signs stating weapons not permitted
    - -Visible security personnel
    - -Metal detectors
    - -Secure single public entrance
  - —Triage to an appropriate assessment room
    - -Sparse, solid walls
    - -Lockable
    - -Visible
    - -Exits clear of obstruction
    - -Equipment free
    - -Panic button
  - —Never underestimate the potential for violence
  - —ED protocols for violent situations
  - —Educate staff on preventing, recognizing, and dealing with potentially violent situations
- Approaching the potentially violent patient
  - —Immediately assess safety
  - —Call security and employ physical or chemical restraint if the patient is violent or threatening, or if there is an immediate perceived danger
  - —Remove any weapons before interview
  - —Maintain open exit for patient and physician
  - —Maintain distance of 6–8 feet
  - —Allow patient to ventilate
  - —Develop therapeutic alliance
    - -Be nonjudgmental, peace offering
  - —Use submissive posture
    - -Avoid eye contact
  - —Leave immediately and initiate seclusion or restraint if there is any destabilization

ED TREATMENT

Verbal Deescalation

- Situation can be verbally controlled, particularly if there is an identifiable situational precipitant

Isolation

- Temporarily isolate patient in an appropriate room before more definitive restraint, or to prevent elopement

Physical Restraints

- Required for patient's safety, the safety of others, and to allow physical examination
- Performed by several trained personnel, by protocol, with clear documentation of indications and rechecks

Chemical Restraint

- Least restrictive and potentially therapeutic
- If uncooperative, patients often require physical restraint first
- Neuroleptic agents (haloperidol) or benzodiazepines (lorazepam)
  - —May use combination if single agent ineffective
  - —Administer every 15 to 30 minutes until desired effect reached
  - —Side effects of neuroleptics include
    - -Dystonic reactions (treat with diphenhydramine or benztropine)
    - -Neuroleptic malignant syndrome (rare)
    - -QT prolongation and torsades de pointes (rare)

Duty to Warn

- Doctor can owe a duty to warn a third party when that third party is in danger because of the medical or psychological condition of the patient

MEDICATIONS

- Benztropine: 2 mg i.m. or i.v.
- Diphenhydramine: 50 mg i.v., i.m., or PO
- Droperidol: 2.5–5 mg i.v. or i.m.
- Haloperidol: 5–10 mg i.v. or i.m.; 0.5–2 mg for elderly
- Lorazepam: 1–2 mg i.v., i.m., or PO

Disposition

ADMISSION CRITERIA

- Violence secondary to an associated organic cause that is not temporary or reversible in the ED
- Psychiatric admission
  - —Violent psychiatric patient requires psychiatric consultation
  - —Patient is felt to be a danger to either self or others
  - —Involuntary commitment if uncooperative

DISCHARGE CRITERIA

- Violent behavior was caused by a temporary, reversible organic cause (e.g., drug or alcohol intoxication), and the patient is now deemed to be in control, competent, and not a danger to self or others
  - —Psychiatric consultation before discharge recommended
  - —If violent act is due to antisocial behavior, not an organic or psychiatric condition, patient may be discharged into police custody, with the warning that the patient may be a danger to self or others

Miscellaneous

ICD9: N/A

ICD10: N/A

SUGGESTED READINGS

American Council of Emergency Physicians. Protection from physical violence in the emergency department. ACEP policy statement, reapproved October 2001.

Blanchard JC, Curtis KM. Violence in the emergency department. Emerg Med Clin North Am 1999;17:717–31.

Hill S. Petit J. The violent patient. Emerg Med Clin North Am 2000;18:301–315.

McCoy MC. Violence in the emergency department. In: Tintinalli JE, Kelen GD, Stapczynski JS, eds. Emergency medicine: a comprehensive study guide, 5th ed. New York: McGraw-Hill, 2000.

Author: Robert J. Vissers

Visual Loss

Clinical Presentation

SIGNS AND SYMPTOMS

- Flashing lights
- New floaters
- Decreased vision
- Afferent pupillary defect
- Visual field defects
- Eye pain
- Limitation or pain with eye movements
- Conjunctival injection or discharge
- Corneal opacity
- Cataract
- Optic nerve head swelling
- Pale retina with a cherry-red spot
- Palpable temporal artery with or without tenderness
- Carotid bruits
- Neurologic symptoms consistent with intracranial or vascular processes
- Heart murmur

MECHANISM/DESCRIPTION

- Categorize visual loss by the properties associated with the decrease in visual function
- Transient (<24 hours)
  - —Seconds
    - -Papilledema usually (bilateral)
  - —Minutes
    - -Transient ischemic attack (amaurosis fugax) (unilateral)
    - -Vertebrobasilar artery insufficiency (bilateral)
  - —Minutes to an hour
    - -Migraine
    - -Sudden blood pressure changes
- Persistent (>24 hours)
  - —Sudden and painless
    - -Artery or vein occlusion
    - -Vitreous hemorrhage
    - -Retinal detachment
    - -Optic neuritis and temporal arteritis
  - —Gradual and painless (weeks to years)
    - -Cataract
    - -Presbyopia
    - -Refraction error
    - -Open-angle glaucoma
    - -Chronic retinal disease
    - -Macular degeneration
    - -Diabetic or cytomegalovirus (CMV) retinopathy
    - -CNS tumor
  - —Painful
    - -Corneal abrasion or ulcer
    - -Angle closure glaucoma
    - -Optic neuritis
    - -Iritis/uveitis
    - -Keratoconus with hydrops
- Monocular
  - —Pathology anterior to optic chiasm
- Binocular
  - —Pathology posterior to optic chiasm
- Associated with systemic neurologic symptoms or visual field defects
  - —CVA (especially posterior and occipital circulation)
  - —Mass lesions (pituitary adenomas, aneurysm, meningioma, other tumors)
- Malingering

ETIOLOGY

- Decrease in visual function, i.e., visual acuity, visual fields, blurry vision
  - —Vision loss has many etiologies and can be caused by multiple body systems
- Visual system causes
  - —Eyelid or tear film abnormality
  - —Anterior segment (cornea, anterior chamber, iris, lens)
  - —Posterior segment (vitreous, retina, optic nerve)
  - —Posterior to the eye (optic nerve, chiasm, radiations)
- Neurologic causes
  - —Cerebral (CVA) or intracranial pathology (mass lesion)
  - —Multiple sclerosis
  - —Optic neuritis
- Cardiovascular system
  - —Embolic
  - —Thrombotic
  - —Ischemic
  - —Hypertensive events
- Immunologic system
  - —Infectious
    - -HIV optic neuropathy, CMV retinitis
  - —Autoimmune causes (uveitis, temporal arteritis)
- Endocrine
  - —Diabetic retinopathy leading to vitreous hemorrhage or acute glaucoma
  - —Thyroid disease may cause diplopia (muscle hypertrophy) or corneal erosions
- Toxic
  - —Methanol (acute severe loss, subacute optic atrophy)
  - —Licorice (transient loss, self limited)
  - —Digitalis (flashing lights, color changes)
  - —Amiodarone (rare cause of optic neuropathy)

Pre-Hospital

N/A

Diagnosis

ESSENTIAL WORKUP

- Thorough physical examination
- Ophthalmologic
  - —Visual acuity
  - —Pupil exam
  - —Confrontational visual field exam
  - —Extraocular muscle function
  - —Slit-lamp examination
  - —Funduscopy
  - —Tonometry
- Cardiovascular
  - —Murmurs
  - —Carotid bruits
- Neurologic exam
  - —Optic chiasm and intracerebral lesions
  - —Occipital and posterior circulation lesions
- General
  - —Manifestations of immune, endocrine, or toxic disorders

IMAGING/SPECIAL TESTS

- Tests should be directed toward the suspected etiology of visual loss
- Dilated fundus exam may be performed to assess for posterior segment disease
- Erythrocyte sedimentation rate and temporal artery biopsy may be obtained if temporal arteritis is suspected
- Brain CT, MRI, MR angiography and transcranial Doppler may be used to evaluate neurologic symptoms and vertebrobasilar artery flow
- Cardiac and carotid ultrasound should be obtained urgently if a retinal artery occlusion is diagnosed

DIFFERENTIAL DIAGNOSIS

- Trauma
- Conjunctivitis with discharge
- Neurologic lesion

Treatment

INITIAL STABILIZATION

- Two conditions for which treatment must begin in minutes
  - —Central retinal artery occlusion (CRAO)
  - —Chemical burn

ED TREATMENT

- Direct therapy toward cause of visual loss
- Ophthalmology consultation for visual loss with an uncertain diagnosis

CRAO

- Clinical criteria
  - —Unilateral, painless, acute loss of vision
  - —Afferent pupillary defect
  - —Pale fundus with a cherry-red spot
  - —Counting fingers to light perception in 94% of patients
- Therapy
  - —Maneuvers lower intraocular pressure, allowing the embolus to move to the periphery
  - —Ocular massage
  - —Acetazolamide: 500 mg i.v. or PO
  - —Topical beta-blocker (timolol or levobunolol 0.5%) b.i.d.
  - —Anterior chamber paracentesis by an ophthalmologist
  - —Referral for cardiac and carotid artery workup
  - —Rule out temporal arteritis

Chemical Burn

- Clinical criteria
  - —Alkali worse than acids
  - —White eye (vessels already sloughed) worse than red eye (vessels intact)
  - —Treat mace, cements, plasters, solvents
- Therapy
  - —Copious irrigation of the eyes with lactated Ringer's solution or NS (nonsterile water is acceptable if others not available) for at least 30 minutes
    - -Do not try to neutralize acids with alkalis, and vice versa
    - -Moist cotton-tipped applicator to sweep furnaces of residual chemical precipitants
    - -Dilate with cycloplegic (atropine, cyclopentolate, tropicamide)
    - -Do not use phenylephrine; it will vasoconstrict already ischemic conjunctival blood vessels
    - -Erythromycin ointment every 1-2 hours while awake
    - -Artificial tears every 1 hour
    - -Check intraocular pressure

MEDICATIONS

- Antibiotic drops
  - —Ciprofloxacin 0.3%: 1-2 gtt q1-6h
  - —Gentamicin 0.3%: 1-2 gtt q4h
  - —Ofloxacin 0.3%: 1-2 gtt q1-6h
  - —Levofloxacin 0.5%: 1-2 gtt q2h
  - —Polymyxin (Polytrim): 1 gtt q3-6h
  - —Sulfacetamide 10%, 0.3%: 1-2 gtt q2-6h
  - —Tobramycin 0.3%: 1-2 gtt q1-4h
  - —Trifluridine 1%: 1 gtt q2-4h
- Antibiotic ointments
  - —Bacitracin: 500 units/g ½-inch ribbon of ointment q3-6h
  - —Ciprofloxacin 0.3%: ½-inch ribbon of ointment q6-8h
  - —Erythromycin 0.5%: ½-inch ribbon of ointment q3-6h
  - —Gentamicin 0.3%: ½-inch ribbon of ointment q3-4h
  - —Neosporin: ½-inch ribbon of ointment q3-4h
  - —Polymyxin (Polysporin): ½-inch ribbon of ointment q3-4h
  - —Sulfacetamide 10%: ½-inch ribbon of ointment q3-8h
  - —Tobramycin 0.3%: ½-inch ribbon of ointment q3-4h
  - —Vidarabine: ½-inch ribbon of ointment 5 times/day
- Mydriatics and cycloplegics
  - —Atropine 1%, 2%: 1-2 gtt q.d. to q.i.d.
  - —Cyclopentolate 0.5%, 1%, 2%: 1-2 gtt PRN dilation
  - —Homatropine 2%: 1-2 gtt b.i.d. to t.i.d.
  - —Phenylephrine 0.12%, 2.5%, 10%: 1-2 gtt t.i.d. to q.i.d.
  - —Tropicamide 0.5%, 1%: 1-2 gtt PRN dilation
- Corticosteroid–antibiotic combination drops (with ophthalmology consultation)
  - —Blephamide (prednisolone): 1-2 gtt q1-8h
  - —Cortisporin (hydrocortisone; neomycin sulfate; bacitracin zinc; polymysin B sulfate): 1-2 gtt q3-4h
  - —Maxitrol (dexamethasone; neomycin sulfate; polymyxin B sulfate): 1-2 gtt q1-8h
  - —Pred-G (prednisolone acetate; gentamicin sulfate): 1-2 gtt q1-8h
  - —TobraDex (dexamethasone; tobramycin; chlorobutanol): 1-2 gtt q2—26h
- Glaucoma agents (always with ophthalmology consultation):
  - —Acetazolamide: 250-500 mg PO q.d. to q.i.d.
  - —Betaxolol 0.25%, 0.5%: 1-2 gtt b.i.d.
  - —Carteolol 1%: 1 gtt b.i.d.
  - —Dipivefrin 1%: 1 gtt b.i.d.
  - —Levobunolol 0.25%, 0.5%: 1 gtt q.d. to b.i.d.
  - —Mannitol: 1-2 g/kg i.v. over 45 minutes
  - —Pilocarpine 0.25%, 0.5%, 1%, 2%, 3%, 4%, 6%, 8%, 10%: 1-2 gtt t.i.d. to q.i.d.
    - -Only if mechanical closure is ruled out
  - —Timolol 0.25%, 0.5%: 1 gtt b.i.d.

Disposition

ADMISSION CRITERIA

- Ruptured globe
- Hyphema (depending on severity)
- Significant cardiac, carotid, or neurologic disease

DISCHARGE CRITERIA

- If the diagnosis is certain and visual loss will not progress

Miscellaneous

ICD9: 369.9

ICD10: H54.7

SUGGESTED READINGS

Juang P, Rosen P. Ocular examination techniques for the emergency department. J Emerg Med 1997;15:793–810.

La Vene D, Halpern J, Jagoda A. Loss of vision. Emerg Med Clin North Am 1995;13(3):539–560.

Rhee D, Pyfer M. The Wills eye manual: office and emergency room diagnosis and treatment of eye disease, 3rd ed. Philadelphia: Lippincott Williams & Wilkins, 1999.

Author: Pascal S. C. Juang

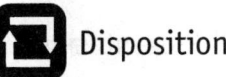

Vitreous Hemorrhage

Clinical Presentation

SIGNS AND SYMPTOMS

- Sudden painless unilateral loss or decrease in vision
- Appearance of dark spots ("floaters") in visual axis
  —Above sometimes accompanied by flashing lights, and the floaters move with head movements
- Blurred vision, decreased visual acuity
- Loss of "red reflex"
- Inability to visualize fundus
- Mild afferent papillary defect

MECHANISM/DESCRIPTION

- Vitreous hemorrhage is a secondary diagnosis and identification of a specific cause is necessary for successful treatment to occur
  —Retinal vessel tear secondary to vitreous separation
  —Sudden tearing of vessels due to trauma
  —Spontaneous bleeding due to neovascularization

ETIOLOGY

- Blunt or penetrating trauma
- Retinal break/tear/detachment
- Any proliferative retinopathy
- Diabetes mellitus
- Sickle cell disease
- Retinal vein occlusion
- Eales' disease
- Senile macular degeneration
- Retinal angiomatosis
- Retinal telangiectasia
- Peripheral uveitis
- Subarachnoid or subdural hemorrhage
- Intraocular tumor

Pre-Hospital

N/A

Diagnosis

ESSENTIAL WORKUP

- History with special attention to preexisting systemic disease and trauma
- Complete ocular exam including
  —Slit lamp
  —Tonometry
  —Dilated funduscopic exam

LABORATORY

- CBC
- Prothrombin time (PT), partial thromboplastin time (PTT), coagulation studies if indicated
- Electrolytes, BUN, creatinine, glucose

IMAGING/SPECIAL TESTS

- B-scan ultrasound when no direct retinal view is possible to rule out retinal detachment or intraocular tumor
- Fluorescein angiography to define the cause
- CT scan/AP/lateral orbital films to rule out intraocular foreign body

DIFFERENTIAL DIAGNOSIS

- Vitreitis (WBC in the vitreous)
- Retinal detachment without hemorrhage

Treatment

INITIAL STABILIZATION

- Bed rest with head of bed elevated
- No Valsalva maneuvers (lifting, stooping, or heavy exertion)

ED TREATMENT

- Urgent ophthalmologic consultation with treatment based on the etiology of the hemorrhage and carried out by the consultant
  —Laser photocoagulation or cryotherapy for proliferative retinal vascular diseases
  —Repair retinal detachments
- Avoid NSAIDs, aspirin, and other anticlotting agents
- Delayed vitrectomy for blood that does not clear with time

Disposition

ADMISSION CRITERIA

- Retinal break or detachment

DISCHARGE CRITERIA

- Retinal break/retinal detachment excluded as etiology of hemorrhage

Miscellaneous

ICD9: 379.23

ICD10: H43.1

SUGGESTED READINGS

Duguid G. Managing ocular flashes and floaters. Practitioner 1998;242:302–304.

Ferrone PJ, de Juan E. Vitreous hemorrhage in infants. Arch Ophthalmol 1994;112: 1185–1189.

Mohamad-Reza D, Werner MS, et al. Spontaneous and traumatic vitreous hemorrhage. Ophthalmology 1993;100: 1377–1383.

Rhee DJ, Pyfer MF, eds. The Wills eye manual: office and emergency room diagnosis and treatment of eye disease, 3rd ed. Philadelphia: Lippincott Williams & Wilkins, 1999.

Shingleton BJ, O'Donoghue MW. Blurred vision. N Engl J Med 2000;343(8):556–562.

Author: David Harter

Volvulus

Clinical Presentation

SIGNS AND SYMPTOMS

- Bowel obstruction
  - —Colicky, cramping abdominal pain (90%)
  - —Abdominal distention (80%)
  - —Obstipation (60%)
  - —Nausea and vomiting (28%)
- Presence of gangrenous bowel
  - —Increased pain
  - —Peritoneal signs: guarding, rebound and rigidity
  - —Fever
  - —Blood on digital rectal exam
- Cecal volvulus
  - —Sudden onset of pain and distention
  - —Asymmetric abdominal distention
  - —Often a palpable mass in the left upper quadrant/mid-abdomen
- Sigmoid volvulus
  - —More insidious onset

MECHANISM/DESCRIPTION

- Axial twist of a portion of the gastrointestinal tract around its mesentery causing partial or complete obstruction of the bowel
- Anatomic predisposition: redundant/freely mobile segment, with close approximation of points of fixation of bowel
- Precipitated by pathologic distention of the colon
- Blood supply compromised by venous congestion leading to gangrene of the bowel, and potential infarction due to arterial obstruction

ETIOLOGY

- Third most common cause of colonic obstruction (10–15%) following tumor and diverticular disease
- Sigmoid (75%)
  - —Due to redundant sigmoid colon with narrow mesocolon base
  - —Most common in elderly/institutionalized/chronic bowel motility disorders
  - —Associated with chronic constipation and concomitant laxative use
- Cecal volvulus (22%)
  - —More common in young adults
  - —Due to improper congenital fusion of the mesentery with the posterior parietal peritoneum, causing the cecum to be freely mobile in varying degrees
  - —Associated with increased gas production (malabsorption and pseudoobstruction)
- Transverse colon and splenic flexure (3%)
- Gastric volvulus (rare) associated with diaphragmatic defects

PEDIATRIC CONSIDERATIONS

- Midgut volvulus
  - —Due to congenital *malrotation* in which the midgut fails to rotate properly in utero as it enters the abdomen
  - —Entire midgut from the descending duodenum to the transverse colon rotates around its mesenteric stalk, including the superior mesenteric artery
  - —Common in neonates (75% <1 month old; 6–20% >1 year old)
  - —Sudden onset of bilious emesis (97%) with abdominal pain
  - —May have previous episodes of feeding problems/bilious emesis
  - —In children >1 year old, associated with failure to thrive and alleged intolerance to feedings
  - —Constipation
  - —Mild distention since obstruction higher in GI tract
  - —May not appear toxic based on degree of ischemia

Pre-Hospital

N/A

Diagnosis

ESSENTIAL WORKUP

- Plain abdominal radiograph
  - —Suggestive, but often inconclusive
  - —Diagnostic finding present in <70% of cases
  - —Sigmoid volvulus: inverted U-shaped loop of dilated colon arising from the pelvis
  - —Cecal volvulus: dilated and displaced cecum in the left abdomen (kidney shaped), often with dilated loops of small bowel

LABORATORY

- May give clues as to the presence of gangrenous bowel, but normal laboratory values do not exclude the diagnosis
- CBC
  - —Leukocytosis (WBC >20,000) suggests strangulation with infection/peritonitis
- Electrolytes, BUN, creatinine, glucose
  - —Anion gap acidosis due to lactic acidosis
  - —Prerenal azotemia due to dehydration
- Urinalysis
  - —Elevated specific gravity and ketones

IMAGING/SPECIAL TESTS

- Barium enema
  - —"Bird's beak" deformity at the site of torsion
  - —Perform cautiously owing to perforation risk
  - —May be therapeutic
- CT scan
  - —"Whirl" sign in cecal volvulus
  - —May be useful in sigmoid volvulus to determine extent of obstruction

DIFFERENTIAL DIAGNOSIS

- Obstruction due to colonic tumor or diverticulitis
- Small bowel obstruction
- Ileus
- Intussusception
- Appendicitis, pelvic inflammatory disease (PID) and salpingitis, especially for cecal volvuli

PEDIATRIC CONSIDERATIONS

- Evaluate any child with signs/symptoms of obstruction (including bilious vomiting and abdominal pain) for malrotation, even if they appear nontoxic
- Delay in diagnosis >1–2 hours results in gangrenous bowel necessitating large resection and leading to permanent parenteral nutrition with its associated complications
- Diagnosis of midgut volvulus
  - —Duodenum lies entirely to the right of the spine on plain films
  - —"Double-bubble" sign on an upright film due to distended stomach and proximal duodenal loop
  - —Established by upper gastrointestinal swallow: coiled spring/corkscrew appearance of jejunum in the right upper quadrant

Treatment

INITIAL STABILIZATION

- ABCs
- Aggressive fluid resuscitation with 0.9% NS bolus of 20 mL/kg
- Nasogastric tube
- Foley catheter

ED TREATMENT

- Prepare patient for the operating room
- Correct hypovolemia and electrolyte abnormalities
- Preoperative antibiotics

Definitive Therapy

Sigmoid Volvulus

- Nontoxic patient
  —Reduce volvulus nonoperatively with sigmoidoscopy (60% successful, 40–50% recurrence)
  —Follow with elective sigmoid resection and primary anastomosis (<3% recurrence)
- Toxic patient
  —Emergent resection of sigmoid and any gangrenous bowel, with placement of end-colostomy

Cecal Volvulus

- Emergent operative reduction followed by cecectomy and primary anastomosis (preferred), or cecopexy if the cecum is still viable (higher recurrence)

MEDICATIONS

- Ampicillin sulbactam (Unasyn): 3 g (peds: 100–200 mg ampicillin/kg/24 h) i.v. q6h
- Cefoxitin (Mefoxin): 2 g (peds: 80–160 mg/kg/24 h) i.v. q6h

PEDIATRIC CONSIDERATIONS

- Laparotomy within 1–2 hours to reduce risk for ischemia
- Surgical detorsion of bowel with resection of gangrenous bowel and a Ladd procedure is performed to prevent recurrent volvulus

Disposition

ADMISSION CRITERIA

- Admit all suspected of having a volvulus with a surgical consult

DISCHARGE CRITERIA

- None

Miscellaneous

ICD9: 560.2

ICD10: K56.2

SUGGESTED READINGS

Frizelle EA, Wolff BG. Colonic volvulus. Adv Surg 1996;29:131–139.

Madiba TE, Thomson SR. The management of sigmoid volvulus. Diseases of the Colon and Rectum. 2000;45(2):74–80.

Madiba TE, Thomson SR. The management of cecal volvulus. Diseases of the Colon and Rectum. 2002;45(2):264–267.

Rolandelli RH, Roslyn JJ. Colon and rectum. In: Townsend CM Jr. Sabiston textbook of surgery, 16th ed. Philadelphia: WB Saunders, 2001;947–950.

Turnage RH, Bergen PC. Intestinal obstruction and ileus. In: Feldman M, Scharschmidt BF, Sleisenger MH. Sleisenger and Fordtran's gastrointestinal and liver disease: pathophysiology/diagnosis/management, 6th ed. Philadelphia: WB Saunders, 1998;1799–1808.

Author: Harsh Sulé

Vomiting, Adult

Clinical Presentation

SIGNS AND SYMPTOMS

- Presaged by nausea
- Diaphoresis
- Pallor
- Tachycardia or bradycardia
- Symptoms/signs of an underlying cause
  - —Fever
  - —Papilledema
  - —Nuchal rigidity
  - —Chest pain
  - —Respiratory distress
  - —Abdominal pain
  - —Diarrhea
  - —Headache
  - —Nystagmus
  - —Focal neurologic deficits

MECHANISM/DESCRIPTION

- Forceful retrograde expulsion of gastric contents up the esophagus and out of the mouth
- Coordinated action of many muscles
  - —Breathing is held
  - —The diaphragm descends
  - —The anterior abdominal wall contracts
  - —The pelvic diaphragm is raised
  - —The pylorus is closed
  - —The esophageal sphincter is opened
- Regulated by a specialized area in the medulla
  - —Requires an intact brainstem and functioning somatic musculature
  - —Aspiration will not occur immediately in the neurologically normal patient

ETIOLOGY

- Gastrointestinal
  - —Nearly any GI pathology
- Metabolic/endocrine
  - —Ketoacidosis (i.e., diabetic, alcoholic patient)
  - —Thyrotoxicosis
  - —Uremia
  - —Metabolic alkalosis
  - —Adrenal insufficiency
  - —Hyperparathyroidism
- Drugs/toxicologic
  - —Antibiotics
  - —Opioids
  - —NSAIDs
  - —Chemotherapeutic agents
  - —Digoxin
  - —Alcohols (i.e., ethanol, methanol, isopropyl)
  - —Anticholinergics
- Neurologic
  - —CNS mass
  - —CNS bleeding
  - —Cerebral edema
  - —Hydrocephalus
  - —CNS infections (i.e., meningitis, encephalitis)
  - —Concussion
  - —Vascular headaches
  - —Posterior fossa cerebrovascular accident (CVA)
- Vascular
  - —Myocardial infarction or ischemia
  - —Mesenteric ischemia
  - —Ovarian torsion
  - —Testicular torsion
- Ophthalmologic
  - —Glaucoma
  - —Postsurgical
- ENT
  - —Labyrinthitis
  - —Ménière's disease
- Psychiatric
  - —Bulimia
  - —Anorexia nervosa
  - —Anxiety disorder
- Other
  - —Urolithiasis
  - —Pregnancy, hyperemesis gravidarum
  - —Motion sickness

Complications

- Hypovolemia
- Metabolic alkalosis
- Hypokalemia
- Mallory-Weiss tears
- Boerhaave's syndrome

Pre-Hospital

CAUTIONS

- Identify hemodynamic or airway compromise
- Intravenous access and fluid resuscitation in volume depleted patients
- Position patient to avoid aspiration

Diagnosis

ESSENTIAL WORKUP

- The history and physical examination should suggest possible underlying causes
- Many patients will require ancillary studies

LABORATORY

- β-Human chorionic gonadotropin (β-hCG) in women of childbearing age

IMAGING/SPECIAL TESTS

- Directed by history and physical examination findings
  - —EKG in elderly diabetic or other patients at high risk for coronary artery disease (CAD)
  - —Cranial CT scan in patients with neurologic findings

DIFFERENTIAL DIAGNOSIS

- Regurgitation
- Hemoptysis

Treatment

INITIAL STABILIZATION

- Large-bore intravenous access
- Supplemental oxygen
- Place patient upright or in lateral decubitus position
- Airway control indicated to prevent aspiration in patients with altered mental status

ED TREATMENT

- Fluid resuscitation with isotonic crystalloid in hypovolemic patients
  - —Avoid overhydration
  - —Caution in patients with potentially increased intracranial pressure
- Decompress stomach with nasogastric tube if intractable vomiting
- Antiemetics

MEDICATIONS

- Droperidol: 0.625–2.5 mg i.v. or i.m.
- Metoclopramide: 10 mg i.v. or i.m.
- Ondansetron: 4–32 mg i.v.
- Prochlorperazine: 5–10 mg i.v. or i.m. or 25 mg PR
- Promethazine: 25–50 mg i.v., i.m., or PR
- Trimethobenzamide: 200 mg i.m. or PR

Disposition

ADMISSION CRITERIA

- Serious underlying etiologies
- Intractable vomiting
- Inability to take PO

DISCHARGE CRITERIA

- Response to treatment
- Able to keep oral fluids down
- Close follow-up arranged, especially in elderly patients

Miscellaneous

ICD9: 787.0

ICD10: R11

SUGGESTED READINGS

Brown HG. Anatomy of vomiting. Br J Anaesth 1963;35:163.

Heilenbach T. "Nausea and vomiting." In: Marx J, et al., eds. Rosen's emergency medicine: concepts and clinical practice. St. Louis: CV Mosby, 2001:178–185.

Author: Myles Greenberg

Vomiting, Pediatric

Clinical Presentation

SIGNS AND SYMPTOMS

General

- Appearance variable depending on the underlying cause
- Signs of dehydration, including tachycardia, tachypnea, pallor, decreased perfusion, and shock
- Altered mental status may occur secondary to shock, hypoglycemia, or extraabdominal conditions (sepsis, inborn error of metabolism, increased intracranial pressure, toxicologic poisoning)

Vomiting Characteristics

- Assess color, composition, onset, progression, and relationship to intake and position
- Nonbilious emesis is caused by a lesion proximal to the pylorus
- Bilious (green) emesis indicates obstruction below the ampulla of Vater; in infants, bilious emesis is associated with a more serious underlying condition (malrotation, volvulus, intussusception, bowel obstruction); may also be due to adynamic ileus or sepsis.
- Bloody emesis involves a lesion proximal to the ligament of Treitz; bright red bloody emesis has little or no contact with gastric juices due to an active bleeding site at or above cardia
- "Coffee-ground" emesis results from reduction of heme by gastric juices
- Feculent odor suggests lower obstruction or peritonitis
- Undigested food in emesis suggests an esophageal lesion or one at or above the cardia
- Gastroesophageal reflux (GER): begins shortly after birth, remains relatively constant, usually with normal weight gain
- Hypertrophic pyloric stenosis: begins insidiously at 3–4 weeks and progresses, becoming increasingly forceful (projectile) after feedings
- Obstruction and/or ischemic bowel (malrotation with midgut volvulus, intussusception, necrotizing enterocolitis): sudden onset associated with rapid progression to appearing ill out of proportion to the duration of illness; abdomen distended and tender

Abdominal

- Distention suggests obstruction
- Peritoneal signs suggest perforation

Complications

- Aspiration
- Mallory-Weiss tear
- Boerhaave's syndrome

MECHANISM/DESCRIPTION

- Forceful retrograde expulsion of gastric contents through the mouth; characterized by nausea, retching, and emesis; no gastric contents are expelled during retching
- Emesis results from sustained contraction of abdominal muscles and diaphragm; at the same time, the pylorus and antrum contract

ETIOLOGY

Neonate/Infant

- Gastrointestinal/mechanical: gastroesophageal reflux (GER), meconium ileus, necrotizing enterocolitis, hypertrophic pyloric stenosis, intussusception, malrotation with midgut volvulus, Hirschsprung's disease, congenital obstructions (atresias, stenoses, and webs), hernia, foreign body/bezoar, paralytic ileus
- Metabolic/endocrine: inborn errors of metabolism (amino acidurias, fatty acid oxidation disorders, urea cycle defects), uremia, congenital adrenal hyperplasia, kernicterus
- Neurologic: CNS bleeding (often due to trauma), tumor, hydrocephalus
- Infectious: otitis media, urinary tract infection (UTI), pneumonia, sepsis, meningitis/encephalitis
- Feeding problems: chalasia, improper technique (overfeeding, improper position), milk allergy
- Other: toxicologic, nonaccidental trauma

Child/Adolescent

- Gastrointestinal: gastroenteritis, obstruction (hernia, adhesions, intussusception, foreign body, bezoar), pancreatitis, appendicitis, peritonitis, paralytic ileus, trauma (duodenal hematoma)
- Metabolic/endocrine: diabetic ketoacidosis, uremia, adrenal insufficiency
- Infectious: gastroenteritis, UTI, sinusitis, upper respiratory infection (URI), sepsis, meningitis, encephalitis, pneumonia, hepatitis
- Neurologic: CNS mass/tumor, CNS bleeding (often due to trauma), cerebral edema, concussion, migraine, kernicterus
- Other: toxicologic, (nonaccidental) trauma, pregnancy, bulimia

Pre-Hospital

- Evaluation/treatment of hypovolemia and hypoglycemia

Diagnosis

ESSENTIAL WORKUP

N/A

LABORATORY

- As indicated by differential considerations
  - —Metabolic assessment (glucose, electrolytes)
  - —Infection assessment (CBC, culture—urine)
  - —Pregnancy tests for females of childbearing age

IMAGING/SPECIAL TESTS

- As indicated by differential considerations
- Abdominal radiographs (flat plate, upright and decubitus) helpful for evaluation of obstruction or perforation
- Pelvic and abdominal ultrasound for evaluation of hypertrophic pyloric stenosis, intussusception, appendicitis as well as pelvic pathology
- Abdominal CT scan helpful for evaluation of appendicitis, mass/tumor often requiring contrast

Treatment

INITIAL STABILIZATION

- Fluid resuscitation with 0.9% NS IV; caution if concern about increased intracranial pressure
- Determine bedside finger-stick glucose

ED TREATMENT

- Continue fluid resuscitation and correction of electrolyte imbalance if present
- Decompress stomach with nasogastric or orogastric tube if abdomen distended or vomiting persistent
- Continue evaluation for underlying cause
- Consider antiemetic medications
- Surgical consultation if acute abdomen; antibiotics if peritonitis or other systemic infection present

MEDICATIONS

- Antiemetics helpful once the underlying cause of vomiting has been determined; less frequently used in young children
- Antiemetic options in children:
  —Metoclopramide: 10 mg (0.1 mg/kg/dose) PO q6h
  —Ondansetron: 4–8 mg (0.1 mg/kg/dose) i.v. q6h
  —Prochlorperazine: 2.5–5 mg (0.1 mg/kg/dose) i.v., i.m., or PR q6h
  —Promethazine: 12.5–25 mg (0.25 mg/kg/dose) PO, PR, or i.m. q6h

Disposition

ADMISSION CRITERIA

- Unstable vital signs, including persistent tachycardia or other evidence of hypovolemia
- Serious etiologic condition
- Inability to exclude serious etiologic conditions
- Intractable vomiting or inability to take oral fluids
- Inadequate social situation or follow-up

DISCHARGE CRITERIA

- Stable; able to tolerate oral fluids
- Benign etiology considered most likely
- Serious or potentially important etiologies excluded
- Parental understanding of instructions to advance clear liquids slowly and return for continued vomiting, abdominal distention, decreased urination, fever, lethargy, or unusual behavior

Miscellaneous

ICD9: 787.03

ICD10: P92.0

SEE ALSO: DIARRHEA, PEDIATRIC

SUGGESTED READINGS

Hostetler MA, Bracikowski A. Gastrointestinal disorders. In: Marx JA, Hockerberger RS, Walls RM, et al., eds. Emergency medicine: concepts and clinical practice, 5th ed. St. Louis: Mosby, 2000: 2296–2315.

Hostetler MA, Schulman M. Necrotizing enterocolitis presenting in the emergency department: case report and review of differential considerations for vomiting in the neonate. J Emerg Med 2001;21(2): 165–170.

Irish MS, Pearl RH, Caty MG, et al. The approach to common abdominal diagnoses in infants and children. Pediatr Clin North Am 1998;45(4):729–772.

Kimura K, Loening-Baucke V. Bilious vomiting in the newborn: rapid diagnosis of intestinal obstruction. Am Fam Physician 2000;61(9):2791–2798.

Pearl RH, Irish MS, Caty MG, et al. The approach to common abdominal diagnoses in infants and children. Part II. Pediatr Clin North Am 1998;45(6):1287–1326.

Author: Mark A. Hostetler

von Willebrand's Disease

Clinical Presentation

SIGNS AND SYMPTOMS

- Most common presenting symptom—mucosal bleeding
  - —Recurrent epistaxis
  - —Bruising at multiple sites
  - —Gingival bleeding
  - —Menorrhagia
  - —GI bleeding
  - —Most often in children and adolescents
- Milder forms—mucosal bleeding
- Severe forms—deep-tissue bleeding (similar to hemophilia)
  - —Hemarthrosis
- Great variation in the frequency and severity of symptoms, even within the same family

MECHANISM/DESCRIPTION

- Caused by an abnormality of von Willebrand's factor (vWF)
- vWF
  - —Cofactor for platelet adhesion
  - —Facilitates platelet adhesion by interaction of platelet receptor and the subendothelial matrix
  - —Protects factor VIII procoagulant from proteolytic degradation in the plasma
- von Willebrand's disease (vWD) subtype categories
  - —Type I: quantitative defect
    - -Mild to moderate decrease in vWF plasma levels, but normal structure
    - -Proportionate decrease in activity
    - -Most common type (70%)
    - -Genetic transmission: autosomal dominant
  - —Type II: qualitative defect
    - -Lacks high-molecular-weight multimers
    - -Impaired ability to mediate platelet adhesion
    - -Caused by decreased vWF synthesis or increased destruction
    - -Genetic transmission: autosomal dominant or recessive
  - —Type III: total (or near) absence of vWF
    - -Markedly defective hemostasis
    - -Greatly reduced levels of factor VIII procoagulant
    - -Absent levels of vWF
    - -1 case per 1,000,000 population
    - -Genetic transmission: autosomal recessive

ETIOLOGY

- Most common congenital bleeding disorder (1% of the population)
- vWD may occur secondary to
  - —Hypothyroidism
  - —Wilms' tumor
  - —Congenital heart disease
  - —Systemic lupus erythematosus (SLE)
  - —Thalassemia
  - —Myeloproliferative disorders
  - —Drugs (ciprofloxacin, tetracycline, valproic acid, griseofulvin)
- vWD is associated with sickle cell anemia, hereditary hemorrhagic telangiectasia, hemophilia A, thrombocytopenia, platelet dysfunction, factor XII deficiency

Pre-Hospital

N/A

Diagnosis

ESSENTIAL WORKUP

- Screen for vWD if
  - —Large bruises
  - —Bruises at multiple sites
  - —Positive family history
- Prothrombin time (PT), partial thromboplastin time (PTT), platelet count, bleeding time, and ristocetin test

LABORATORY

- Bleeding time prolongation
  - —50% of type I
  - —All of type II and type III
- PT: normal
- PTT: normal or prolonged if vWD occurs concurrently with factor II, factor XII, or factor VIII procoagulant deficiency
- CBC: platelet count normal

IMAGING/SPECIAL TESTS

- Ristocetin test
  - —Used to measure vWF activity
  - —Causes vWF to bind platelets; degree of agglutination proportional to the concentration of vWF
- vWF plasma concentration
  - —Can be measured directly
  - —Decreased in types I and III; normal or decreased in type II

DIFFERENTIAL DIAGNOSIS

- Platelet defects
- Collagen vascular disease
- Medications (aspirin, NSAIDs, and antiplatelet agents)
- Normal platelet count rules out thrombocytopenia
- Normal PT and PTT excludes clotting deficiencies

Treatment

INITIAL STABILIZATION

- Use local measures to control bleeding

ED TREATMENT

- Avoid antiplatelet medications
- Use desmopressin (DDAVP) to treat bleeding or in preparation for surgery
- Patient education and coordination between the primary care provider and a potential surgeon is essential
- Desmopressin (DDAVP)
  - —Causes a two- to five-fold increase in plasma vWF or factor VIII procoagulant levels by release of vWF from endothelial storage sites
  - —IV or intranasally administration
  - —Works within 30 minutes and lasts 6–8 hours
  - —First-line agent for type I vWD—excellent response to DDAVP
  - —Types II and III—little or no response to DDAVP
- Virus-inactivated factor VIII, vWF concentrate
  - —Used for types II and III and patients unresponsive to DDAVP
- Tranexamic acid (Cyklokapron), ϵ-aminocaproic acid (Amicar), or topical thrombin
  - —For dental procedures, epistaxis, and mucous membrane bleeding
  - —Use as adjunct to DDAVP or concentrate
- Cryoprecipitate
  - —Contains factor VIII and vWF
  - —Best for types II and III vWD bleeding
  - —Best if made from known donors to minimize risk for virus transmission
  - —Rarely used given advent of concentrate
- Recombinant factor VIII contains no vWF

Intervention Strategy

- Type I—DDAVP
- Types II and III
  - —Factor VIII, vWF concentrate
  - —DDAVP contraindicated in type IIB secondary to transient thrombocytopenia
- Type III with alloantibodies
  - —Recombinant factor VIII continuous infusion
  - —Limited treatment experience
- Adjuncts—Amicar, Cyklokapron to any mucosal or cutaneous bleed

MEDICATIONS

- Amicar: 50–60 mg/kg q6h
- Cryoprecipitate: 2–3 bags/10 kg q12h
- Desmopressin (DDAVP): 0.3 μg/kg (up to 20 μg total) i.v, i.n., or SC
- Factor VIII, vWF concentrate: 20–60 IU/kg
- Fresh-frozen plasma: 10–20 mL/kg
- Tranexamic acid: 25 mg/kg i.v. q6h

Disposition

ADMISSION CRITERIA

- Refractory or potential life-threatening bleeding
- Observe type III vWD after major trauma, especially trauma to the head or spinal cord, to rule out occult bleeding

DISCHARGE CRITERIA

- No bleeding

Miscellaneous

ICD9: 286.4

ICD10: D68.0

SUGGESTED READINGS

Association of Hemophilia Clinic Directors of Canada. Hemophilia and von Willebrand disease. 1. Diagnosis, comprehensive care and assessment. Can Med Assoc J 1995; 153:19–25. 2. Management. Can Med Assoc J 1995;153:147–157.

Federici AB, Mannucci PM. Advances in the genetics and treatment of von Willebrand's disease. Curr Opin Pediatr 2002;14:22–33.

Mannucci PM. Treatment of von Willebrand disease. Thromb Haemost 2001;86: 149–153.

Michaels JJ, Budde U, van der Planken M, et al. Acquired von Willebrand disease: clinical features, aetiology, pathophysiology, classification and management. Best Practice and Research Clinical Haematology 2001;14:401–436.

Werner EJ. von Willebrand disease in children and adolescents. Pediatr Clin North Am 1996;43:683–707.

Authors: Jno Disch; Nicholas Jouriles

Warts

Clinical Presentation

SIGNS AND SYMPTOMS

- Pedunculated growths, often with cauliflower-like appearance
- Flesh-colored to slightly pigmented or red
- In men, usually on glans penis, shaft, scrotum, or anus
- In women, found on labia, vagina, cervix, or anus
- May extend into urethra, bladder, or rectum
- Can develop in mouth or throat if oral sexual contact

ETIOLOGY

- Human papillomavirus (HPV), usually subtypes 6 and 11

PATHOLOGY

- Self-limiting benign epithelial tumors lasting months to years
- Virus not eradicated by treatment and often causes warts to reappear later

TRANSMISSION

- Direct sexual contact
- Contact with contaminated objects
- Autoinnoculation

Pre-Hospital

CAUTIONS

- Maintain universal precautions

Diagnosis

ESSENTIAL WORKUP

- Diagnosis made by characteristic appearance of lesions
  - —If difficult to see, may add acetic acid to suspected area, which will cause infected areas to whiten and become more visible
- Screen for other sexually transmitted diseases

LABORATORY

- Pregnancy test for females

DIFFERENTIAL DIAGNOSIS

- Condyloma latum (secondary syphilis)
- Herpes simplex
- Prominent glands around head of penis

Treatment

INITIAL STABILIZATION

- None required

ED TREATMENT

- If available may use podophyllin, trichloroacetic acid, 5-fluorouracil cream, or alternative therapies listed below
- Alternative treatments
  —Cryotherapy with liquid nitrogen or dry ice
  —Electrocautery
  —Laser therapy
  —Surgical excision
- Provide appropriate referral

MEDICATIONS

- 5-Fluorouracil 5% topical cream: apply b.i.d.
  —Do not use in pregnancy
- Imiquimod cream: apply 3 times/week for up to 16 weeks
- Podophyllin 20–25% in benzoin: weekly topical application
  —Protect surrounding normal tissue with petroleum jelly
  —Wash off 1–4 hours later
  —Do not use in pregnancy—highly toxic and teratogenic
- Trichloroacetic acid, topical 85%
  —Wash off several hours later

Disposition

ADMISSION CRITERIA

- Disseminated cases in immunocompromised patients may require admission

DISCHARGE CRITERIA

- Most patients may be treated as outpatients

Miscellaneous

ASSOCIATED CONDITIONS

- Linked to carcinoma of the penis, vulva, anus, and cervix
- May produce laryngeal papillomatosis in infants from viral exposure at birth

SYNONYMS

- Genital warts
- Condyloma acuminata
- Venereal warts

ICD9: 078.19

ICD10: B07

SUGGESTED READINGS

Centers for Disease Control and Prevention. Sexually transmitted diseases treatment guidelines. MMWR Morb Mortal Wkly Rep 2002;51:1–78.

Miller KE, Graves JC. Update on the prevention and treatment of sexually transmitted diseases. Am Fam Physician 2000;61:379–386.

Pearson GW, Langely RG. Topical imiquimod. J Dermatol Treat 2001;12: 37–40.

Author: Gary M. Vilke

Weakness

Clinical Presentation

SIGNS AND SYMPTOMS

Altered Physical Strength

- Assessment of strength
  - —1: No contraction
  - —2: Active movement, with gravity eliminated
  - —3: Active movement against gravity
  - —4: Active movement against gravity and resistance
  - —5: Normal power
  - —Fatigability
- Change in muscle tone
  - —Flaccidity (the absence of normal muscle tone)
  - —Spasticity
  - —Rigidity
- Abnormal deep tendon reflexes (DTRs)
- Abnormal plantar reflexes
  - —Muscle atrophy
    - -Generalized
    - -Focal
- Difference of >1 cm in the leg and thigh and >0.5 cm in the forearm and arm
- Visual changes
  - —Diplopia
  - —Drooping eyelids

Systemic Findings

- Fatigue
- Dizziness
- Paresis
- Paresthesias
- Hoarse voice
- Dysphagia
- Confusion
- Fever
- Chest pain
- Dyspnea
- Cough
- Weight loss
- Rash
- Dysuria
- Upper respiratory infection (URI) symptoms

MECHANISM/DESCRIPTION

- Lack of physical strength or energy
- An inability to carry out a desired movement with normal force because of a reduction in strength of the muscles
  - —Differentiate from dyspraxia, which is due to a failure in the motor centers in the cortex
- Subjective sensation caused by neuromuscular disorders, systemic disorders, and psychiatric illness
- Most common neuromuscular causes
  - —Myasthenia gravis (5 to 14.2 cases per 100,000)
  - —Guillain-Barré syndrome (0.75 to 2 cases per 100,000)
- 1,500 new cases of acute flaccid paralysis in United States. per year not due to trauma, stroke, or malignancy

Categories of Neuromuscular Disorders

- Upper motor neuron (UMN) lesions
  - —DTRs increased
  - —Plantar reflexes upgoing
  - —Increased muscle tone
  - —Muscle atrophy absent
- Lower motor neuron (LMN) lesions
  - —DTRs decreased to absent
  - —Plantar reflexes absent or normal
  - —Decreased muscle tone
  - —Muscle atrophy present
  - —Fasciculations
- Neuromuscular junction (NMJ) or muscle fiber lesions
  - —DTRs normal
  - —Plantar reflexes normal or absent

ETIOLOGY

Neuromuscular Disorders

- UMN lesions
  - —Multiple sclerosis
  - —Amyotrophic lateral sclerosis
  - —Transverse myelitis
  - —Poliomyelitis
- LMN lesions
  - —Guillain-Barré syndrome
  - —Toxic neuropathies
  - —Diphtheria
  - —Porphyria
  - —Seafood toxins
- NMJ lesions
  - —Myasthenia gravis
  - —Lambert-Eaton syndrome
  - —Botulism
  - —Periodic paralysis
  - —Tick paralysis
  - —Electrolyte imbalance

Nonneuromuscular Disorders

- Dehydration
- Simple fatigue
- Chronic fatigue syndrome
- Fibromyalgia
- Anxiety/psychogenic
- Malignancy
- Cerebrovascular accident
- Head or neck trauma
- Infection/sepsis
- Myocardial ischemia
- Endocrine abnormalities
  - —Hypothyroidism
  - —Adrenal insufficiency
- Toxins
  - —Medications
  - —Environmental
  - —CO poisoning
- Systemic lupus erythematosus
- Polymyalgia rheumatica

Pre-Hospital

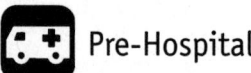

- Supplemental oxygen
- Intravenous access
- Consider endotracheal intubation in patients with severe respiratory distress

Diagnosis

ESSENTIAL WORKUP

- Clinical suspicion gathered through history and physical exam guides further testing
  - —Generalized versus focal
  - —Acute versus chronic
  - —Proximal versus distal
  - —Ascending versus descending
  - —Symmetric versus asymmetric
  - —Improved versus worsened with activity

LABORATORY

- Serum glucose
- CBC
- Electrolytes
- BUN and creatinine
- Toxin screen
- Urinalysis
- Thyroid function tests (rule out hypothyroidism)
- Erythrocyte sedimentation rate (ESR) (rule out rheumatologic cause)

IMAGING/SPECIAL TESTS

- EKG (rule out acute coronary syndrome)
- Chest x-ray (rule out infectious etiology)
- CT or MRI head (rule out intracranial pathology)
- Bedside spirometry
  - —Forced vital capacity, negative inspiratory force, peak expiratory force
  - —May identify those with impending ventilatory failure
- Lumbar puncture
  - —In suspected Guillain-Barré syndrome
    - -Albumin-cytologic dissociation in CSF (protein >400, WBC <10) is virtually diagnostic
- Tensilon test
  - —Distinguishes myasthenic crisis from cholinergic crisis in myasthenia gravis

Treatment

INITIAL STABALIZATION

- Supplemental oxygen
- Intravenous access
- Endotracheal intubation for impending ventilatory failure

ED TREATMENT

- Neurology consult if needed
- When the diagnosis is determined, specific therapies can be applied
  - —Plasma exchange and/or intravenous immunoglobulin (IVIG) for Guillain-Barré syndrome
  - —Hydrocortisone for adrenal insufficiency
  - —Potassium supplementation for hypokalemia
  - —Dextrose for hypoglycemia
  - —Specific antitoxins for botulism and diphtheria

MEDICATIONS

N/A

Disposition

ADMISSION CRITERIA

- All patients with new-onset neuromuscular problems should be admitted for definitive diagnosis
- Any evidence of impending ventilatory or circulatory compromise warrants ICU admission

DISCHARGE CRITERIA

- Resolution of symptoms
- Stable vital signs
- Definitive diagnosis and correction of abnormality

Miscellaneous

ICD9: N/A

ICD10: N/A

SUGGESTED READINGS

Chew WM, Birnbaumer DM. Evaluation of the elderly patient with weakness: an evidence based approach. Emerg Med Clin North Am 1999;17(1):265–278.

LoVecchio F, Jacobson S. Approach to generalized weakness and peripheral neuromuscular disease. Emerg Med Clin North Am 1997;15(3):605–623.

Reiser RC, Weakness. In Marx J, et al. eds: Rosen's emergency medicine: concepts and clinical practice, 5th ed. St. Louis: Mosby, 2002:119–123.

Author: Jason Imperato

West Nile Virus

Clinical Presentation

SIGNS AND SYMPTOMS

- Severity of illness
  - —Asymptomatic—80%
  - —Flu-like illness—20%
  - —Encephalitis <1%
- Clues to presence of disease in area:
  - —Aseptic meningitis/encephalitis in late summer/early fall where West Nile Virus found
- Most infections asymptomatic or mild, flu-like illness
  - —Incubation 3–14 days
  - —Symptoms last 3–6 days
- Age ≥50 years: significant risk for severe disease
  - —Encephalitis/meningitis
- General
  - —Fever
  - —Malaise
  - —Anorexia
  - —Headache
- Neurologic
  - —Altered mental status
  - —Profound motor weakness
    - -Can present as flaccid paralysis
    - -May resemble Guillain-Barré syndrome
  - —Ataxia
  - —Extrapyramidal signs
  - —Cranial nerve palsies
  - —Seizures
- Gastrointestinal
  - —Nausea, vomiting
  - —Pancreatitis (rare)
  - —Fulminant hepatitis (rare)
- Musculoskeletal
  - —Myalgia
- Hematologic
  - —Lymphadenopathy
- Dermatologic
  - —Rash (maculopapular or morbilliform on neck, trunk, extremities)
- Cardiovascular
  - —Myocarditis (rare)
- Ophthalmologic
  - —Optic neuritis

ETIOLOGY

- Vector-borne virus
- Transmitted by infected mosquitoes late summer/early fall
- Wild birds natural host
- Found throughout much of United States, Europe, and Israel

Pre-Hospital

CAUTIONS

- Universal precautions
  - —Transmission through blood exposure unclear
  - —Infection after transplant/transfusion reported, currently under investigation

Diagnosis

ESSENTIAL WORKUP

- CSF and serum for serology (IgM antibody-capture enzyme-linked immunosorbent assay [ELISA]) and culture
  - —Procedures for submitting samples vary by state
  - —Refer to local public health department for guidelines

LABORATORY

- CSF
  - —Pleocytosis with lymphocyte predominance
  - —Elevated protein
  - —Normal glucose
- CBC
  - —WBC often normal or mildly elevated
  - —Anemia can occur
- Chemistry
  - —Hyponatremia sometimes seen; etiology uncertain, possibly syndrome of inappropriate antidiuretic hormone (SIADH)

IMAGING/SPECIAL TESTS

- CT head usually negative
- MRI
  - —One third of patients show enhancement of leptomeninges and/or periventricular white matter

DIFFERENTIAL DIAGNOSIS

- Other causes of meningitis
  - —Bacterial
  - —Viral
  - —Tuberculous
  - —Fungal
- Other causes of encephalitis
  - —Other arboviruses, especially St. Louis encephalitis virus
  - —Enterovirus
  - —Herpes simple virus (HSV)
  - —Cytomegalovirus (CMV)
  - —Epstein-Barr virus (EBV)
  - —Mumps virus
- Intracranial abscess
- Nonspecific viral syndrome
- Gastroenteritis

Treatment

INITIAL STABILIZATION

- ABCs
- Seizure precautions

ED TREATMENT

- Supportive care
- IV fluids for signs of dehydration
- For signs of meningitis, administer antibiotics pending results of CSF
- Administer antipyretics and pain medications
- Interferon-α2b and ribavirin
  —Effective in vitro
  —No controlled studies

Disposition

ADMISSION CRITERIA

- Neurologic symptoms
- Dehydration

DISCHARGE CRITERIA

- No signs of encephalitis or meningitis
- Able to tolerate oral solutions

Miscellaneous

ICD9: 066.3

ICD10: B34.9

SEE ALSO: MENINGITIS; ENCEPHALITIS

SUGGESTED READINGS

Asnis DS, Connetta R, Waldman G, et al. The West Nile virus encephalitis outbreak in the United States (1999–2000): from Flushing, New York, to beyond its borders. Ann N Y Acad Sci 2001;951:161–171.

Hayes CG. West Nile virus: Uganda, 1937, to New York City, 1999. Ann N Y Acad Sci 2001;951:25–37.

Hubálek Z, Halouzka J. West Nile fever—a reemerging mosquito-borne viral disease in Europe. Emerg Infect Dis 1999;5:643–650.

Nash D, Mostashari F, Fine A, et al. The outbreak of West Nile virus infection in the New York City area in 1999. N Engl J Med 2001;344:1807–1814.

Petersen LR, Marfin AA. West Nile Virus: a primer for the clinician. Ann Intern Med 2002;137:173–179.

Petersen LR, Roehrig JT. West Nile virus: a reemerging global pathogen. Emerg Infect Dis 2001;7:611–614.

Weiss D, Carr D, Kellachan J, et al. Clinical findings of West Nile virus infection in hospitalized patients, New York and New Jersey, 2000. Emerg Infect Dis 2001;7:654–658.

Author: Roy Hanaki

Wheezing

Clinical Presentation

SIGNS AND SYMPTOMS

- A whistling sound made while breathing
  - —Diffuse
    - -As with reactive airway disease or pulmonary edema
  - —Focal
    - -As with pneumonia or pulmonary embolism
- Dyspnea
- Respiratory distress
- Chest pain
- Cough
- Sputum production
  - —Frothy (pulmonary edema)
- Stridor
- Fever
- Cyanosis
- Tachypnea
- Tachycardia

MECHANISM/DESCRIPTION

- Result of turbulent airflow
  - —High-pitched sound with dominant frequency at 400 Hz
    - -Gas flowing through constricted airways analogous to a vibrating reed
  - —Resonant vibration of the bronchial walls when airflow velocity reaches critical values
- Caused by airway narrowing between 2 and 5 mm
  - —Wheezing is very low pitched, with airway diameters of 5 mm
  - —Airways of <2 mm are unable to transmit sound because the energy is lost as friction heat
- Airway narrowing is caused by a combination of one or more of the following
  - —Constriction (as with reactive airway disease)
  - —Peribronchial interstitial edema
  - —Inflammation
  - —Obstruction

ETIOLOGY

Pulmonary—Small Airway

- Asthma
- Acute respiratory distress syndrome
- Anaphylaxis
- Aspiration pneumonia
  - —Wheezing occurs early in the disease due to intense bronchospasm following the event
- Byssinosis
  - —Occupational lung disease of textile workers exposed to cotton dust
- Hyperventilation
- Pneumonia
- Chronic obstructive pulmonary disease (COPD)
- Chronic cor pulmonale
- Chemical pneumonitis
- Carcinoid tumors
- Pulmonary edema
- Pulmonary embolism
  - —Rarely associated with wheezing
  - —Focal
- Forced exhalation in normal patients
- Sleep apnea

Pulmonary—Large Airway

- Vocal cord dysfunction (paralysis, paradoxical movement)
- Foreign body
- Epiglottitis
  - —Wheezing associated with stridor in 10% of cases
- Diphtheria
- Smoke inhalation
- Bronchial tumor

Pediatric

- Viral bronchiolitis in patients younger than 3 years of age
- Asthma
- Croup
- Foreign body aspiration
- Congenital abnormalities
- Cystic fibrosis
- Congestive heart failure

Pre-Hospital

- Supplemental oxygen
- Initiate pulse oximetry and cardiac monitoring
- Initiate therapy for underlying condition when indicated
  - —Asthma
  - —Pulmonary edema
- Intubate for respiratory failure or anticipated respiratory failure

Diagnosis

ESSENTIAL WORKUP

- Pulse oximetry
- Peak flow
- Chest x-ray

LABORATORY

- Arterial blood gas
  - —Sometimes used to determine whether patient is fatiguing by noting falling oxygenation, rising CO_2, and acidosis
  - —Clinical assessment is a more reliable indicator of the need for airway management
- WBC
  - —Elevated WBC does not distinguish infection from other disorders as stress causes demargination
  - —WBC is also elevated in noninfected patients taking steroids
  - —A normal WBC does not rule out an underlying pneumonia

IMAGING/SPECIAL TESTS

- Peak expiratory flow
  - —To assess function of small airways
  - —Use to determine severity and track the progress of therapy in patients with reactive airway disease
- Chest x-ray
  - —Assess for diagnosis of pulmonary conditions
    - -Pneumonia
    - -Foreign body aspiration
  - —Assess for pulmonary edema
- EKG
  - —Useful when patient at risk for cardiac ischemia
  - —Indicated in all cases in which wheezing is caused by pulmonary edema
- Soft tissue neck
  - —Used to assess for foreign body or obstructing mass
- Bronchoscopy
  - —Indicated when obstruction is thought to be causal
  - —Used to retrieve an inhaled foreign body or diagnose an underlying tumor

DIFFERENTIAL DIAGNOSIS

N/A

Treatment

INITIAL STABILIZATION

- ABCs
- Intubation for impending airway failure
  - —Prepare for possible foreign body in airway
  - —Anticipate difficult airway

ED TREATMENT

- Supplemental oxygen
- Treat the underlying condition
- Bronchodilators
  - —Reversibility following the use of β-agonists such as albuterol or terbutaline suggests reactive airway disease
- Trial of steroids indicated if wheezing is caused by bronchospasm or noninfectious inflammation
- Heliox
  - —Less dense than air or oxygen alone
  - —Decreases work of breathing
  - —More efficacious in large airway disease
  - —Not as effective for small airway disease
- Magnesium sulfate
  - —Evidence for benefit only in moderate to severe asthmatics
- Ketamine
  - —For intubation of the asthmatic patient

MEDICATIONS

- Albuterol: 2.5 mg in 2.5 mL NS every 20 minutes inhaled (peds: 0.1–0.15 mg/kg/dose every 20 minutes; minimum dose 1.25 mg)
- Methylprednisolone: 60–125 mg i.v. (peds: 1–2 mg/kg/dose i.v. or PO q6h for 24 hours)
- Prednisone: 40–60 mg PO (peds: 1 mg/kg/d in single or divided doses)
- Racemic epinephrine: (peds 0.25–0.5 mL nebulized for croup)
- Terbutaline: 0.25 mg SC q0.5h for 2 doses (peds: 0.01 mg/kg up to 0.3 mg SC)

Disposition

ADMISSION CRITERIA

- Hypoxia
- Persistent or worsening wheezing
- Underlying condition requires hospital admission

DISCHARGE CRITERIA

- Improvement or resolution of wheezing
- Adequate oxygenation

Miscellaneous

ICD9: 786.09

ICD10: R06.2

SEE ALSO: ASTHMA, ADULT

SUGGESTED READINGS

Boushey HA, Corry DB, Fahy JV. Asthma. In: Murray JF, Nadel JA, eds. Textbook of respiratory medicine, 3rd ed. Philadelphia: WB Saunders, 2000:1247–1288.

Dorland's illustrated medical dictionary, 28th ed. Philadelphia, WB Saunders, 1994.

Fiz JA, et al. Detection of wheezing during maximal forced exhalation in patients with obstructed airways. Chest 2000;122(1): 186–191.

White MV. Differential diagnosis in the difficult asthmatic. Immunol Allergy Clin North Am 2001;21(3).

Author: Stephen Epstein

Wilms' Tumor

Clinical Presentation

SIGNS AND SYMPTOMS

History

- Abdominal pain
- Gross hematuria

Abdomen

- Abdominal mass that is usually smooth and 5–10 cm in size
  - —Usually does not cross midline

Vital Signs

- Hypertension (60%) due to renal ischemia from tumor pressure on the renal artery

Cardiac/Pulmonary

- Congestive heart failure may be present

Complications

- Before surgery: massive bleeding from ruptured tumor, "acute abdomen," bowel obstruction
- After nephrectomy: bowel obstruction (5.1%), urinary tract infection, pneumonia, hemorrhage (1.9%), vascular injury (1.5%)
- During and after chemotherapy: neutropenia with fever, renal insufficiency, anemia, thrombocytopenia, hepatotoxicity, venoocclusive disease of liver (VOD)
- Acquired von Willebrand's syndrome is rarely associated with Wilms' tumor

MECHANISM/DESCRIPTION

- Solid tumor (nephroblastoma) of the kidney, accounting for 5–6% of childhood tumors in the United States
- Incidence: 7 cases per million children per year
- Mean age at diagnosis: 3.2 years (median: 2.6 years; range: 3 months–16 years)
- Male predominance: 1.3:1
- Overall 5-year survival: 83% (95% CI: 80–85%)
- Relapse rate: 22%
- Stages (10-year survival)
  - —I: Limited to kidney (94%)
  - —II: Spread by direct extension (86%)
  - —III: Spread via lymphatic drainage (71%)
  - —IV: Spread via hematogenous metastasis (36%)
  - —V: Involves both kidneys
- Favorable versus unfavorable histology
  - —10-year survival with unfavorable histology is 36%

ETIOLOGY

- Abnormal proliferation of metanephric blastema without normal differentiation into tubules and glomeruli

Pre-Hospital

N/A

Diagnosis

ESSENTIAL WORKUP

- Urinalysis: hematuria in 25% of patients
- Ultrasound can identify mass and distinguish cystic from solid tumor

LABORATORY

- Renal function tests
- CBC
- INR/partial thromboplastin time (PTT)

IMAGING/SPECIAL TESTS

- CT or MRI scan of abdomen to diagnose and stage the disease
- Chest x-ray and chest CT scan evaluating for metastases

DIFFERENTIAL DIAGNOSIS

- Infection: urinary tract infection
- Anatomic: urinary tract anomaly, hydronephrosis, renal cyst
- Neoplasm: neuroblastoma, renal cell carcinoma, sarcoma, lymphoma

Treatment

INITIAL STABILIZATION

- Resuscitation as appropriate, including management of hypertension, CHF, anemia, renal failure

ED TREATMENT

- Pediatric oncologic/genitourinary referrals after initiating diagnostic evaluation
- Definitive treatment
  —Surgical removal of affected kidney
  —Chemotherapy reflecting type and stage
    -Stage I with favorable histology: vincristine *or* vincristine plus actinomycin D
    -Stage II with favorable histology: same agents with longer course than stage I
    -Stages III and IV with favorable histology and any stage with unfavorable histology: radiation and vincristine and actinomycin D plus doxorubicin

Disposition

ADMISSION CRITERIA

- Hypertension, congestive heart failure
- Renal insufficiency
- Significant anemia
- Pulmonary findings
- Poor compliance
- Lack of timely follow-up

DISCHARGE CRITERIA

- Normal blood pressure
- Normal renal function
- Near-normal hematocrit
- Normal cardiac and pulmonary examination
- Reliable parents
- Rapid follow-up available

Miscellaneous

ICD9: 189.0

ICD10: C64

SUGGESTED READINGS

Blakely ML, Ritchey ML. Controversies in the management of Wilms' tumor. Semin Pediatr Surg 2001;10:127–131.

Czauderna P, Katski K, Kowalczyk J, et al. Venoocclusive liver disease (VOD) as a complication of Wilms' tumour management in the series of consecutive 206 patients. Eur J Pediatr Surg 2000;10:300–303.

Grodzinski J, Weirich A, Tournade MF, et al. Primary nephrectomy for emergency: a rare event in the International Society of Pediatric Oncology Nephroblastoma Trial and Study no. 9. Eur J Pediatr Surg 2001;11:36–39.

Plesko I, Kramarova E, Stiller CA, et al. Survival of children with Wilms' tumour in Europe. Eur J Cancer 2001;37:736–743.

Ritchey ML, Shamberger RC, Haase G, et al. Surgical complications after primary nephrectomy for Wilms' tumor: report from the National Wilms' Tumor Study Group. J Am Coll Surg 2001;192:63–68.

Yip WC, Ho TF, Yip YY, et al. Value of abdominal sonography in the assessment of children with abdominal pain. J Clin Ultrasound 1998;26:397–400.

Author: Joseph Kahn

Withdrawal, Alcohol

Clinical Presentation

SIGNS AND SYMPTOMS

- Onset of symptoms 6–8 hours after cessation of drinking
- Agitation/tremor (most common)
- Anxiety
- Depression
- Anorexia
- Nausea, vomiting
- Confusion
- Hallucinations (up to 25% incidence)
  —Visual (most common)
  —Auditory
  —Olfactory
  —Tactile
- Seizures (5–25% of withdrawing alcohol-dependent patients)
  —Peak time between 13 and 24 hours after cessation of drinking
  —Occurs up to 96 hours after cessation
  —Typically occur singularly (40%)
  —Generalized tonic-clonic activity
  —Usually self-limited (only 3% develop status seizures)
- Sleep disturbances (insomnia and nightmares)
- Delirium tremens
  —Onset in 48 to 72 hours after cessation of drinking
  —Severe sympathetic hyperactivity
  —Temperature
  —Tachycardia
  —Tremor
  —Altered sensorium
  —Occurs in up to 5% of withdrawing alcoholics
- Diaphoresis
- Flushing
- Tachycardia
- Hypertension
- Tachypnea
- Fever
- Hyperreflexia
- Stigmata of chronic alcohol abuse
  —Spider angiomata
  —Rhinophyma
  —Hepatomegaly
  —Cirrhosis
  —Ascites
  —Muscle wasting

MECHANISM/DESCRIPTION

- Withdrawal syndrome primarily affects persons who are habituated (tolerant) to chronic ethanol ingestion who either cease their drinking or markedly reduce their consumption
- Characterized by a hyperadrenergic state that develops 6–8 hours after the cessation of drinking and may last up to 5 days
- Enhanced excitatory neurotransmission
  —Increased levels of plasma and urine catecholamines
  —Decreased inhibitory activity of presynaptic α_2 receptors
- Symptom severity determined by the amount of endogenous norepinephrine released during withdrawal

ETIOLOGY

- The most common withdrawal syndrome seen in the ED
- Predisposing factors: acute, prolonged, and chronic ethanol ingestion; malnutrition
- Dose dependence
- Amount and chronicity of alcohol intake related to the severity of the syndrome
  —"Kindling" hypothesis: withdrawal episodes become progressively more severe

Pre-Hospital

CAUTIONS

- Cardiac monitoring
- Blood glucose if abnormal mental status
- Physical or chemical restraints for agitation
- Seizure precautions

CONTROVERSIES

- Physical or chemical restraints for agitation

Diagnosis

ESSENTIAL WORKUP

- Rapid blood glucose

LABORATORY

- Electrolytes, BUN, creatinine, glucose
- Alcohol level (Breathalyzer or serum sample)
- Drug screen if co-ingestion suspected

IMAGING/SPECIAL TESTS

- CT scan of the brain
  —Abnormal mental status
  —Head trauma
  —First-time seizure
  —Focal or status seizures
- Lumbar puncture and CSF analysis if meningitis suspected

DIFFERENTIAL DIAGNOSIS

- Withdrawal from sedative-hypnotic drugs
- Head trauma
- Epilepsy
- Encephalopathy
- Hypoglycemia
- Hyperthyroidism
- Sepsis
- Meningitis
- Encephalitis
- Sympathomimetic overdose
- Pheochromocytoma
- Anticholinergic poisoning
- Psychosis
- Electrolyte disorders
- Mercury poisoning
- Lithium overdose
- Cyclic antidepressant overdose
- Phenytoin overdose

Treatment

INITIAL STABILIZATION

- ABCs
- Correct hypoglycemia
- IV fluids
- Initiate tranquilization to prevent the progression of the syndrome to more severe levels and to relieve the symptoms
- Administer thiamine

ED TREATMENT

Restore Inhibitory Tone to the CNS

- Benzodiazepines
  - —Standard therapy
  - —High doses required owing to cross-tolerance with chronic ethanol ingestion
  - —Administer aliquots and follow the patient's response
- Barbiturates
  - —Alternatives to benzodiazepines
  - —May also have a synergistic effect in patients with apparent "benzodiazepine resistance"
- Butyrophenone antipsychotics
  - —Haloperidol (low doses)
  - —Indicated as adjuncts in the hallucinating patient but do not replace treatment with adequate quantities of benzodiazepines or barbiturates
  - —Best avoided in the nonhallucinating patient
- Beta-blockers
  - —Propranolol and atenolol
  - —Used to relieve some of the signs and symptoms
  - —Considered adjunctive therapy but do not replace treatment with adequate quantities of benzodiazepines or barbiturates
  - —Avoid in patients with contraindications (asthma, bradycardia, or CHF)
- Clonidine
  - —Adjunct to treat the hyperadrenergic signs and symptoms of alcohol withdrawal but do not replace treatment with adequate quantities of benzodiazepines or barbiturates
- Anticonvulsive prophylaxis
  - —Phenytoin is not useful in alcohol-withdrawal patients who do not also have an underlying seizure disorder that is not alcohol related

Identify and Correct Fluid, Electrolyte, and Nutritional Deficiencies

- Administer glucose for hypoglycemia or alcoholic ketoacidosis
- Treat hypovitaminosis syndromes due to malnutrition with thiamine and folate
- Correct electrolyte abnormalities
- Replete magnesium
  - —25% of chronic alcoholic patients are total-body magnesium depleted owing to malnutrition and increased renal losses
  - —Hypomagnesemic state makes replenishment of potassium difficult and may lower patient's seizure threshold
- Bed rest, minimal physical stimulation
- Minimal use of physical restraints after adequate sedation to decrease the risk for rhabdomyolysis associated with agitation and struggling

MEDICATIONS

- Chlordiazepoxide: 25–100 mg PO for mild reactions; 25 mg i.v. in repeated doses as necessary for more severe reactions
- Clonidine: 0.1–0.2 mg PO q4–6h
- Clorazepate: 15–30 mg PO q8–12h
- Diazepam: 5–20 mg PO for mild reactions; 5–10 mg i.v.
- Folate: 1 mg i.v. or PO
- Glucose: 5% solution in i.v. fluids; 25 g i.v. bolus in hypoglycemic patients
- Haloperidol: 2–10 mg PO, i.v., or i.m.
- Lorazepam: 7 mg/d PO for mild reactions; 2 mg i.v. in repeated doses as necessary for more severe reactions
- Magnesium sulfate: 2–6 g in i.v. solutions, except in renal failure
- Pentobarbital: 260 mg i.v. loading dose followed by 130 mg in repeated doses every 30 minutes titrated to light sedation
- Propranolol: 0.5–1 mg i.v.; 10–40 mg PO
- Thiamine: 100 mg i.v.

Disposition

ADMISSION CRITERIA

- Moderate to severe symptoms or persistent symptoms should be admitted to a medical facility
- Severe symptoms (impending delirium tremens [DTs]), DTs, or patients who fail to resolve their symptoms with moderate amounts of medication should be admitted to an intensive care unit

DISCHARGE CRITERIA

- Mild to moderate symptoms that can be controlled with oral medications
  - —Having patients self-administer their medications is fraught with failure and is strongly discouraged

Miscellaneous

ICD9: 291.81

ICD10: F10.3

SUGGESTED READINGS

Chang PH, Steinberg MB. Alcohol withdrawal. Med Clin North Am 2001;85(5): 1191–1212.

Holbrook AM, Crowther R, Lotter A, et al. Diagnosis and management of acute alcohol withdrawal. CMAJ 1999;160(5): 675–680.

Jaeger TM, Lohr RH, Pankratz VS. Symptom-triggered therapy for alcohol withdrawal syndrome in medical inpatients. Mayo Clin Proc 2001;76(7):695–701.

Myrick H, Brady KT, Malcolm R. New developments in the pharmacotherapy of alcohol dependence. Am J Addict 2001;10(1):3–15.

Williams D, McBride AJ. The drug treatment of alcohol withdrawal symptoms: a systematic review. Alcohol Alcohol 1998;33(2):103–115.

Author: Lee Shockley

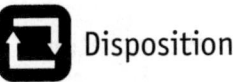

Withdrawal, Drug

Clinical Presentation

SIGNS AND SYMPTOMS

GABA-minergic (Benzodiazepines, Barbiturates, Alcohol)

- Anxiety
- Depression
- Agitation
- Tremulous
- Anorexia
- Nausea, vomiting
- Confusion
- Hallucinations
- Seizures
- Sleep disturbances (insomnia and nightmares)
- Physical signs
  —Diaphoresis
  —Flushing
  —Tachycardia
  —Hypertension
  —Orthostatic hypotension
  —Tachypnea
  —Fever
  —Hyperreflexia, myoclonus
  —Seizures, delirium, and autonomic instability
    -Markers of severe withdrawal

Opiates

- Mild withdrawal
  —Drug craving
  —Lacrimation
  —Rhinorrhea
  —Yawning
  —Diaphoresis
  —Anxiety
  —Restlessness
  —Myalgias, arthralgias
  —Dysphoria
  —Mydriasis
  —Piloerection
- More severe withdrawal
  —Nausea, vomiting
  —Diarrhea
  —Abdominal pain
  —Mild increase in blood pressure, pulse, and respiratory rate

Sympathomimetics

- Postexcitation syndrome, not true withdrawal because continuous use of the drug does not prevent the syndrome
  —Crash (extreme exhaustion that follows binge usage)
    -Lethargy
    -Psychomotor retardation
    -Increased appetite or anorexia
    -Sleep disturbances
    -Muscle twitching
    -Depression
    -Fatigue and dysphoria may last 6–18 weeks in the abstinent patient
  —Extinction (episodically evoked cravings that can last for months to years after abstinence)

MECHANISM/DESCRIPTION

- GABA-minergic withdrawal
  —Requires physical dependence
  —Characterized by a hyperadrenergic state that develops in 3–7 days after the cessation of the drug
  —Enhanced excitatory neurotransmission
  —Increased levels of plasma and urine catecholamines
  —Decreased inhibitory activity of presynaptic α_2 receptors
  —Symptom severity determined by the amount of endogenous norepinephrine released during withdrawal
  —Severe withdrawal can be life-threatening
- Opiate withdrawal
  —Requires physical dependence
  —Decrease in the exogenous opioid binding causes a catecholamine release in the locus ceruleus
  —Syndrome may be temporarily disabling and very uncomfortable
  —Not life-threatening
  —Onset within 4–8 hours for heroin, 36–72 hours for methadone
  —Opiate antagonists administration (e.g., naloxone) can precipitate withdrawal (usually only lasting 20 to 60 minutes)
- Sympathomimetic postexcitation syndrome
  —Causes tiredness, depression, and dysphoria
  —Neurotransmitter depletion
  —No serious metabolic or neurologic complications
  —May be associated with an increased suicide risk and cravings for the drug, which often result in cycles of binges and transient abstinence

PEDIATRIC CONSIDERATIONS

- Opiate withdrawal
  —Neonatal seizures

Pre-Hospital

CAUTIONS

- Initiate cardiac monitoring
- Determine blood glucose if abnormal mental status
- Physical or chemical restraints for agitated patients

Diagnosis

ESSENTIAL WORKUP
- Thorough physical examination to determine nature of withdrawal
- Blood glucose

LABORATORY
- Electrolytes, BUN, creatinine, glucose
- Drug screens may be useful if polysubstance abuse is suspected

IMAGING/SPECIAL TESTS
- Lumbar puncture and CSF analysis for withdrawal patients in whom meningitis suspected
- CT scan of the brain for
  - —Abnormal mental status
  - —Head trauma
  - —Focal seizures
  - —Status seizures

DIFFERENTIAL DIAGNOSIS
- GABA-minergic
  - —Head trauma
  - —Epilepsy
  - —Encephalopathy
  - —Hypoglycemia
  - —Hyperthyroidism
  - —Sepsis, meningitis
  - —Encephalitis
  - —Sympathomimetic overdose
  - —Pheochromocytoma
  - —Anticholinergic poisoning
  - —Psychosis
  - —Electrolyte disorders
- Opiates
  - —Sedative-hypnotic and ethanol withdrawal
  - —Gastrointestinal diseases
- Sympathomimetics
  - —Alcohol or sedative-hypnotic intoxication
  - —Acute psychiatric disease (depression or psychosis)
  - —Head trauma
  - —CNS infection

Treatment

INITIAL STABILIZATION
- ABCs
- Correct hypoglycemia with glucose
- Initiate IV fluid for dehydration

ED TREATMENT
- Sedative-hypnotic withdrawal
  - —Reinstitution of therapy or the substitution of a sedative-hypnotic drug with a long half-life to facilitate detoxification
  - —Beta-blocking agents
  - —Adjuncts to lessen the adrenergically mediated symptoms
- Opiate withdrawal
  - —Phenothiazines and butyrophenones for nausea and vomiting
  - —Clonidine reduces the signs and symptoms of opiate withdrawal
  - —Combination therapy with clonidine and the long half-life antagonist naltrexone may shorten the withdrawal duration by as much as 50% without increasing the severity of symptoms
  - —Benzodiazepines
    - -May help ease some of the symptoms
  - —Rapid opiate detoxification (ROD) or ultra-rapid opiate detoxification (UROD) protocols (high-dose naloxone treatment while under general anesthesia) followed by antiemetics, sedatives, clonidine, and naltrexone; the safety and efficacy of these protocols have not been proved
- Sympathomimetics withdrawal
  - —Supportive therapy

MEDICATIONS
- Chlordiazepoxide: 25–100 mg PO for mild reactions; 25 mg i.v. in repeated doses as necessary for more severe reactions
- Clonidine: 0.1–0.2 mg PO q4–6h
- Clorazepate: 15–30 mg PO q8–12h
- Diazepam: 5–20 mg PO for mild reactions; 5–10 mg i.v. in repeated doses as necessary for more severe reactions
- Droperidol: 1.25–5.0 mg i.v.
- Glucose: 5% solution in i.v. fluids; 25-g i.v. bolus in hypoglycemic patients
- Haloperidol: 2–10 mg PO or i.v.
- Lorazepam: 7 mg/d PO for mild reactions; 2 mg i.v. in repeated doses as necessary for more severe reactions
- Methadone: 5–20 mg/d PO
- Naltrexone: 50 mg/d PO
- Pentobarbital: 100 mg i.v. in repeated doses as necessary for more severe reactions
- Promazine: 25 mg i.m. every 30 minutes as needed, up to 125 mg
- Propranolol: 0.5–1.0 mg i.v.; 10–40 mg PO

Disposition

ADMISSION CRITERIA
- Sedative-hypnotic
  - —Moderate severe or persistent symptoms
  - —Seizures
  - —Psychosis during withdrawal
  - —Severe autonomic instability or delirium should be admitted to an intensive care unit
- Opiates
  - —Medical conditions that may complicate withdrawal
  - —Intractable vomiting
- Sympathomimetics
  - —Extremely lethargic or minimally responsive must be admitted
  - —Suicidal patients require psychiatric evaluation and possible admission

DISCHARGE CRITERIA
- Able to tolerate oral solutions
- Not suicidal

Miscellaneous

ICD9: 292.0

ICD10: F10.19

SEE ALSO: WITHDRAWAL, ALCOHOL

SUGGESTED READINGS

Hamilton RJ, Olmedo RE, Shah S, et al. Complications of ultrarapid opioid detoxification with subcutaneous naltrexone pellets. Acad Emerg Med 2002;9(1):63–68.

O'Connor PG. Rapid and ultrarapid opioid detoxification techniques. JAMA 1998;279(3):229–234.

Olmedo R, Hoffman RS. Withdrawal syndromes. Emerg Med Clin North Am 2000;18(2):273–288.

Upthegrove RA, Naik PC. Pharmacological management of opiate withdrawal. Hosp Med 2001;62(5):277–281.

Williams H, Salter M, Ghodse AH. Management of substance misusers on the general hospital ward. Br J Clin Pract 1996;50(2):948.

Woods JH, Winger G. Current benzodiazepine issues. Psychopharmacology (Berl) 1995;118(2): 107–115; discussion, 118, 1201.

Author: Lee Shockley

Wolff-Parkinson-White Syndrome

Clinical Presentation

SIGNS AND SYMPTOMS

- Asymptomatic
- Palpitations
- Dyspnea
- Dizziness
- Nausea
- Abnormal heart rate
  - —Rapid and regular (supraventricular tachycardia [SVT])
  - —Irregular (atrial fibrillation)
- Signs of instability
  - —Chest pain
  - —Hypotension
  - —Change in mental status
  - —Rales

MECHANISM/DESCRIPTION

- Syndrome caused by ventricular preexcitation via the accessory atrioventricular (AV) pathway, the bundle of Kent
- Conduction may be anterograde, retrograde, or both
- Type A or orthodromic is the most common (70%)
  - —Impulse travels down the AV node and then up the retrograde pathway
  - —A circuit is created that potentiates reentrant tachycardia
- Type B or antidromic
  - —Less common than type A
  - —The circuit operates in the opposite direction

ETIOLOGY

N/A

Pre-Hospital

CAUTIONS

- Supplemental oxygen
- Monitor
- Synchronized cardioversion if signs of instability

CONTROVERSIES

- Pre-hospital use of adenosine
  - —Stable patients do not require emergent conversion
  - —Unstable patients should undergo cardioversion and *should not* receive adenosine

Diagnosis

ESSENTIAL WORKUP

- Wolff-Parkinson-White (WPW) syndrome should be considered the underlying etiology in all cases of tachydysrhythmia
- The diagnosis should be based on the characteristic EKG findings once the patient has converted to a sinus rhythm
- Electrophysiology studies to assess for radioablation or surgery should be performed on outpatient basis

LABORATORY

N/A

IMAGING/SPECIAL TESTS

- EKG in sinus rhythm
  - —Short PR, <0.12 seconds
  - —Prolonged QRS, >0.10 seconds
  - —Delta wave
    - -Small slurred upstroke at the beginning of the QRS
  - —EKG morphology will depend on the degree of preexcitation

DIFFERENTIAL DIAGNOSIS

- AV nodal reentry SVT
- Ventricular tachycardia

Treatment

INITIAL STABILIZATION

- Unstable patients
  - —Synchronized cardioversion starting with 50 J/min
  - —Increase incrementally until sinus rhythm is restored

ED TREATMENT

- Stable patients with *narrow* complex, regular tachycardia
  - —Vagal maneuvers such as Valsalva
  - —Right carotid artery massage for no more than 10 seconds
    - -Auscultate the artery first for a bruit, which would contraindicate this procedure
  - —Fluid replacement and Trendelenburg position if the patient has mild hypotension
  - —Pharmacologic conversion if carotid massage fails
    - -Adenosine
- Stable patients with irregular *wide* complex tachycardia
  - —Procainamide is the drug of choice
  - —Never use calcium channel blockers, beta-blockers, or digoxin
    - -These medications prolong the refractory period of the AV node, increasing the rate of transmission through the accessory pathway and resulting in fatal ventricular dysrhythmias

MEDICATIONS

- Adenosine: 6 mg rapid i.v. bolus over 1–2 seconds; if ineffective, repeat with 12 mg (peds: 0.1 mg/kg rapid i.v. push, repeat with 0.2 mg/kg)
- Procainamide: 6–13 mg/kg i.v. at 0.2–0.5 mg/kg/min until either arrhythmia controlled, QRS widens 50%, or hypotension, then 2–6 mg/min, maximum dose of 1,000 mg

Disposition

ADMISSION CRITERIA

- Patients with signs of instability require admission to a monitored bed
- Failure of outpatient therapy for continuous pharmacologic control or ablation

DISCHARGE CRITERIA

- Most patients will be stable and can be discharged once converted to sinus rhythm
- Follow-up should be arranged with a cardiologist

Miscellaneous

ICD9: 426.7

ICD10: I45.6

SEE ALSO: PREEXCITATION SYNDROME

SUGGESTED READINGS

Al-Khatib SM, Pritchett EL. Clinical features of Wolff-Parkinson-White syndrome. Am Heart J 1999;(3 Pt 1):403–413.

Shah CP. Clinical approach to wide QRS complex tachycardias. Emerg Med Clin North Am 1998;16:331–360.

Xie B, Thakur RK, Shah C, et al. Emergency management of cardiac arrhythmias: clinical differentiation of narrow QRS complex tachycardias. Emerg Clin North Am 1998;16:295–330.

Zipes DP. Specific arrhythmias: diagnosis and treatment. In: Braunwald E, ed. Heart disease: a textbook of cardiovascular medicine, 5th ed. Philadelphia: WB Saunders, 1997:667–675.

Author: Mitch Adelstein

Wound Ballistics

Clinical Presentation

SIGNS AND SYMPTOMS

- Severe underlying tissue damage and life-threatening injury may occur with even small-entrance wounds

MECHANISM/DESCRIPTION

- Wounding potential of a bullet is determined by its mass and velocity
- The type and severity of a wound is determined not only by the wounding potential but also by the construction and shape of the bullet, its orientation upon striking the body, any deformity or fragmentation it undergoes, and what tissues the bullet traverses
- The traditional distinction between low and high muzzle *velocity* bullets does not necessarily differentiate the kind and severity of wounding
  —A civilian hunting rifle or a large-caliber handgun with a hollow-point bullet may produce a more severe wound than a round with a full metal jacket from a "high-velocity" military rifle
- Bullets wound by two main mechanisms: *crush and stretch*
- The sonic pressure wave that precedes the bullet has no role in wounding
- The bullet crushes the tissue it directly passes through, forming the *permanent cavity*
- *Stretch* is produced by the radial energy transferred from the bullet as it slows down in tissue, forming the *temporary cavity*
- A bullet is stabilized in flight from *spin* transmitted by the rifling in the barrel
  —This spin minimizes *yaw,* which is the angle between the long axis of the bullet and its flight vector
  —Without spin, a bullet would yaw to its most stable flight configuration, which is base and center of mass forward
  —This configuration is not aerodynamically efficient
  —As a bullet enters tissue, the spin of the bullet is reduced and the bullet will yaw
  —When yaw is 90 degrees, a bullet crushes the maximal amount of tissue, slows down the most, and maximal stretch injury occurs
- Bullets designed to deform in tissue (soft point, hollow point) will expand on impact into a mushroom shape, increasing the amount of crush injury and moving the center of mass of the bullet forward
- Jacketed bullets prevent lead stripping in the barrel that occurs at high muzzle velocities
  —Jacketed bullets do not deform but may fragment
  —Fragmentation increases surface area and crush injury
  —Bullets striking bone often fragment and may cause bone fragments to become secondary projectiles
- Wound severity is also dependent on *tissue composition and thickness*
  —Organs consisting of minimally elastic, near water-density tissue (brain, liver) may be greatly injured by the temporary cavity formation, as may fluid-filled (heart, bowel) and dense organs (bone)
  —More elastic tissue such as lung and skeletal muscle may absorb the energy from temporary cavity formation and sustain minimal damage
  —Extremities are often not thick enough for the bullet to yaw fully
  —Temporary cavity formation is minimal and rarely is responsible for significant tissue injury
  —Most damage is caused by direct crush injury of the bullet, its fragments, or secondary projectiles
  —Short-range shotgun blasts produce severe wounds with compromise of the blood supply
  —In short-range shotgun injuries, although the entrance wounds may be close together, the pellets may be greatly scattered in tissue secondary to the pellets striking each other
- Stab wounds with knives and other sharp instruments are low-energy wounds with tissue injury from direct weapon contact

Pre-Hospital

- Field personnel can provide information about weapon type and size, distance and angle between the weapon and victim
- Gunshot and stab wounds to the chest with unstable vital signs warrant a needle thoracostomy in the side of the chest with the entrance wound in order to relieve a potential tension pneumothorax, and if no improvement, a needle thoracostomy should be placed in the contralateral hemithorax
- Impaled objects or projectiles should not be removed; immobilize with tape and gauze and transport
- Clothing should be preserved, if possible; clothing should be cut around holes made by the projectiles to preserve evidence
- The patient should be transported to the closest trauma center for definitive care
- In some systems, the hypotensive patient may be taken directly to the operating room

Diagnosis

ESSENTIAL WORKUP

- Radiographs taken in the AP and lateral projections help localize the bullet, and with placement of a marker at the entrance wound, the trajectory can be estimated
  - —Additionally, any fragments, fractures, pneumothoraces, or hemothoraces will be identified
- Evaluate for entrance and exit wounds
  - —May estimate trajectory and potential for tissue damage
  - —Exit wounds are often stellate and larger than entrance wounds unless energy is dissipated at skin surface by special bullet type (e.g., hollow point)
  - —With high-velocity projectiles, exit wound may be much more extensive than entrance wound
  - —Because of the elasticity of the skin, the bullet can often be palpated subcutaneously if it did not exit
  - —It is not always possible to differentiate entrance from exit wounds; clinicians do this poorly, so that wounds should be only described fully in the medical record; classification as entrance or exit wounds should be avoided

IMAGING/SPECIAL TESTS

- The extent of tissue injury is often only apparent on surgical exploration
- See chapters on penetrating chest and abdominal trauma for further diagnostic considerations

Treatment

INITIAL STABILIZATION

- ABCs of trauma care

ED TREATMENT

- Impaled objects or projectiles should be removed only in the operating room
- The care of such patients in the ED includes initial stabilization, estimation of tissue injury based on the above principles, and initiation of appropriate diagnostic workup
- Wound care includes appropriate exploration, irrigation, and débridement of devitalized tissue
- All bullets are contaminated with bacteria and are *not* sterilized by being fired; therefore, all nongrazing bullet wounds warrant empiric antibiotics
- Early trauma, orthopedic, and vascular surgery consultation is necessary
- For further treatment considerations, see penetrating chest and abdominal trauma chapters

Disposition

ADMISSION CRITERIA

- Patients with neurovascular compromise and extensive tissue damage must be admitted for appropriate surgical intervention
- Patients with injury to the head, neck, torso, or abdomen should be admitted
- Patients with injury from high-velocity projectiles or gunshot wounds should be admitted to a monitored setting for observation of neurovascular status

DISCHARGE CRITERIA

- Patients with minor penetrating extremity trauma, or stabbing victims found not to have significant injury may be discharged with appropriate follow-up

Miscellaneous

ICD9: E922.9

ICD10: W43

SEE ALSO: ABDOMINAL TRAUMA, PENETRATING; CHEST TRAUMA, PENETRATING

SUGGESTED READINGS

Fackler, ML. Gunshot wound review. Ann Emerg Med 1996;28:194–203.

Hollerman JJ, Fackler ML. Wound ballistics. In: Tintinalli JE ed. Emergency medicine: a comprehensive study guide, 5th ed. New York: McGraw Hill, 1999:1722–1729.

Swan KG, Swan RC. Principles of ballistics applicable to the treatment of gunshot wounds. Surg Clin North Am 1991;71: 221–239.

Author: Brian Snyder

Appendix A: Incompetence, Determination of

Clinical Presentation

SIGNS AND SYMPTOMS

- Inability to make rational decisions about medical treatment

MECHANISM/DESCRIPTION

- Competence
  - —Legal term to be defined by a judge
  - —In a medical context, refers to a patient's ability to make rational decisions about medical treatment
- A patient who lacks such ability is said to be *incompetent* or *decisionally incapacitated*
- Someone other than the patient declared incompetent must assume responsibility for making medical decisions for that patient
  - —Depending on circumstances, this role will be assumed by a family member, the physician, or the court

Pre-Hospital

CAUTIONS

- Patients ordinarily have the right to accept or reject treatment as they see fit
  - —This right is not absolute
  - —Right may be denied if the patient is thought to be incompetent, especially in case of a true emergency
- Rules vary widely from state to state
  - —Familiarity with local statutes essential

Diagnosis

ESSENTIAL WORKUP

- Diagnosis is a legal, not a medical, condition
  - —Law presumes individuals to be competent until proved otherwise
  - —Patient may be declared incompetent only through judicial procedures
- *When the patient's condition necessitates immediate treatment,* physician may be forced to make a presumptive determination of competence without the benefit of judicial decision of legal counsel
- In most states, individuals <18 years old are considered incompetent as a matter of law
  - —A parent, guardian, or judge must consent to medical treatment on behalf of the patient
  - —Exceptions: when the patient is emancipated or when a true emergency exists
- Incompetence rules vary widely from state to state
  - —Familiarity with local statutes essential

Incompetence Evaluation

"Method of Decision" Test

- Most widely accepted by the courts
- Presence of decision test
  - —Patient deemed competent so long as the patient makes a decision when one is called for
  - —Quality of decision is irrelevant
- Method of decision test
  - —Patient deemed competent so long as a reasonable basis exists for reaching the decision
  - —Patients who base their decisions on irrelevant issues are considered incompetent
- Nature of decision test
  - —Patient is deemed competent so long as the decision seems rational to the examiner
- General incompetence test
  - —Patient is deemed competent so long as the patient is fit to function in the world generally, rather than as a patient
  - —These conditions render the patient incompetent
    - -Intoxication
    - -Mental retardation
    - -Psychosis

"Sliding Scale" Test

- Uses a variable standard
- As the potential consequences of the patient's decisions become more serious, a more stringent standard of competence is required
  - —A patient demonstrating questionable competence might be allowed to refuse care so long as the associated risk to his/her health is small
  - —A patient with a life-threatening illness would be allowed to refuse treatment only if clearly competent

LABORATORY

- As appropriate for medical condition
- CBC
  - —For infection
  - —Anemia
- Electrolytes, BUN, creatinine, glucose
  - —For ingestion
- Metabolic abnormalities
- Toxicology screen

Treatment

INITIAL STABILIZATION

- Physical restraint
  - —For potentially uncooperative patients and when, if the patient's competence is in question, refusal of care would seriously jeopardize the patient's health
- Independent second opinion, psychiatric consult, or consultation with hospital counsel
  - —Useful as a safeguard against liability
  - —Whenever a patient's autonomy is abridged owing to incompetence, the reasons must be clearly documented

ED TREATMENT

- No test of competence is valid in all parts of the United States
- Practitioners should familiarize themselves with locally accepted standards
- Most competence tests require at a minimum demonstration of the following
  - —Ability to communicate a choice and to maintain that choice long enough for the chosen course of action to be implemented
  - —Ability to understand relevant information
    - -Best evaluated by asking the patient to paraphrase the information provided
  - —Appreciation of the situation and its consequences, including comprehension of the following
    - -Nature of the medical condition
    - -Recommended treatment
    - -Treatment alternatives
    - -Risks and benefits of accepting or refusing the proposed treatment
  - —Ability to manipulate information rationally
- Patient's conclusion must be logically consistent with the starting premise

Disposition

ADMISSION CRITERIA

- As medically justified

DISCHARGE CRITERIA

- Because forced treatment and the deprivation of decision-making rights represent a serious infringement of the patient's liberty, every effort must be made to assist the patient to demonstrate competence

Miscellaneous

ICD9: N/A

SUGGESTED READINGS

Appelbaum P, Grisso T. Assessing patient's capacities to consent to treatment. N Engl J Med 1988;319(25):1635–1638.

Borak J, Veilleux S. Informed consent in emergency settings. Ann Emerg Med 1984;13(9):731–735.

Drane J. Competency to give informed consent. JAMA 1984;252(7):925–927.

Lavoie F. Consent, involuntary treatment, and the use of force in an urban emergency department. Ann Emerg Med 1992;21(1): 25–32.

Authors: Jay Weaver; Kathryn Brinsfield

Appendix B: COBRA/Patient Transfer Issues

Clinical Presentation

SIGNS AND SYMPTOMS

Enforcement Procedures

- Following a violation
  - —Medicare participation of the physician or hospital is terminated in 23 days
  - —Notice of termination is published in newspapers at 19 days
  - —To prevent this a plan of correction must be submitted, implemented, and approved
    - -If corrective plan is accepted, reevaluation is made within 90 days
  - —Appeals take up to 3 years, and funding is not reinstated during the process
  - —Hospitals that fail to report violations by other hospitals have been cited
  - —Application of standards vary in different regions of the United States

Office of Inspector General (OIG) Enforcement

- Operates separately from the Health Care Financing Administration (HCFA)
- Receives and uses HCFA and Professional Review Organization (PRO) findings
- If violation is found, it issues a civil monetary penalty (CMP)
  - —$50,000 per violation for both hospitals and physicians
  - —$25,000 for hospitals with less than 100 beds
  - —CMP not covered by malpractice insurance

MECHANISM/DESCRIPTION

- Consolidated Omnibus Budget Reconciliation Act (COBRA)
  - —Also known as the Emergency Medical Treatment and Labor Act (EMTALA)
  - —Federally mandated standards of practice for hospitals and physicians
  - —Passed in 1986; amended in 1988, 1989, and 1994
  - —Initially motivated by the issue of patient dumping
    - -Denial of care or transfer of patients based on inability to pay for care
- COBRA preempts state law
- 700 hospitals (or 1 in 6 hospitals) have received COBRA enforcement actions from HCFA
- Few have received termination of funding; 1 did in 1996 for following an HMO procedure
- Costs for plans and actions to make corrections, for consultants, lawyers, equipment, and personnel
  - —Generally about $150,000 for small hospitals
  - —$1.8 million for one 400–500 bed hospital
  - —Several hundred civil suits have been filed with some verdicts and settlements of more than $3 million

ETIOLOGY

- COBRA duties of a hospital
  - —Provide a Medical Screen Examination (MSE) to all patients who present to its premises regardless of ability to pay
  - —Provide stabilizing care
  - —Not to transfer unstable patients
  - —Transfer only for medical necessity
  - —Maintain an on-call system for specialists
  - —Accept requests for in-coming transfers
- Medical screening exam
  - —Provide all necessary testing and on-call services
  - —Determine presence of an Emergency Medical Condition (EMC)
  - —Address affected and potentially affected areas and known chronic conditions
  - —Florida law requires all necessary treatment and surgery
  - —All necessary definitive treatment should be rendered
  - —Only true follow-up care may be referred to physicians offices or clinics
  - —Triage without an MSE is not acceptable
  - —Screening of psychiatric patients must rule out trauma, disease, or organic condition
  - —Screening of intoxicated patients must rule out trauma, toxic, psychological, and medical causes
  - —Use of nonphysician medical screening personnel is discouraged but not prohibited
- Emergency medical condition
  - —Broader under COBRA than typical medical usage
  - —Any condition that is a danger to the health and safety of the patient or unborn fetus
  - —Includes conditions that may result in risk for impairment or dysfunction of any body part
  - —Undiagnosed acute pain that is sufficient to impair normal function
  - —Pregnancy with contractions
  - —Symptoms of substance abuse
  - —Psychiatric disturbances, i.e., severe depression, inability to comprehend danger or care for one's self
- Managed care conflicts with COBRA
  - —Third-party payers do not have the authority to authorize treatment, only payment
  - —Hospitals that follow HMO and insurance company procedures do so at their own risk and will be held to COBRA compliance
  - —It is acceptable to obtain information during the routine registration process, but the information must not be acted on
  - —No advance approval may be obtained from a third-party payer or employer
  - —Calls to insurance companies and employers have resulted in citations
  - —Handing a phone to the patient to speak to his/her insurance company has resulted in citations
  - —Transfers may not be based on medical care organization (MCO) direction or policy

Pre-Hospital

N/A

Diagnosis

ESSENTIAL WORKUP

- HCFA—responsible for investigation and partially responsible for enforcement
- OIG of the Department of Health and Human Services (DHHS) is responsible for other enforcement aspects
- Violations also may be reported to Office of Civil Rights, Internal Revenue Service (IRS), Joint Commission on Accreditation of Healthcare Organizations (JCAHO)
- Civil suits are heard in state and federal courts
- Possible violations must be reported by receiving hospitals within 72 hours
- Other sources of information regarding violations
  —Physician complaints
  —Patient complaints
  —EMS system complaints
  —Routine site visits
  —Newspaper articles
  —PRO screens
  —State reporting

LABORATORY

N/A

IMAGING/SPECIAL TESTS

N/A

DIFFERENTIAL DIAGNOSIS

N/A

Treatment

N/A

Disposition

ADMISSION CRITERIA

- HCFA conducts investigation

DISCHARGE CRITERIA

- PRO
  —Acts as a nonbinding advisor to OIG
  —Does not generally affect HCFA findings
  —Goes by standard medical practice rather than HCFA
  —Tension exists between PRO and HCFA offices
- State enforcement
  —Agencies have varying familiarity with HCFA
  —COBRA enforcement is increasing
  —State agencies are often required to comply with federal inspections, including COBRA
  —Actions under COBRA

Summary

- Evaluation of patients must not be based on insurance status
- MCOs cannot refuse care, only payment
- MSE must be performed regardless of approval from patients' insurance company
- Transfers and acceptances of transfers must be based on medical needs
- Patients may refuse or request transfers

Miscellaneous

ICD9: N/A

ICD10: N/A

SUGGESTED READINGS

Bitterman RA. What is an "appropriate" medical screen examination under COBRA? ED Leg Lett 1997;8(3):35–44.

Bitterman RA. Dealing with managed care under COBRA. Emerg Phys Leg Bull 1997;7(4):1–8.

COBRA statute: 42 USC §1395.

COBRA regulations 48924: special responsibilities of Medicare hospitals in emergency cases. Frew Consulting Group. COBRA Online at: *www.medlaw.com/novnl.htm*.

Author: Steven Crespo

Commonly Used Drugs in the Emergency Department

- *Acyclovir* (Zovirax): 5–10 mg/kg i.v. q8h
  —Genital herpes: first episode: 400 mg PO q8h; prophylaxis: 400 mg PO q12h
  —Zoster: 800 mg PO 5 times/d for 10 days
  —Varicella: 20 mg/kg up to 800 mg PO q6h for 5 days
- *Adenosine* (Adenocard): 6 mg i.v. followed by flush through central line if possible; if no response after 1–2 minutes, then repeat with 12 mg (peds: initial dose 50 μg/kg followed by 100–200 μg/kg if needed)
- *Aminophylline:* load 6 mg/kg i.v. over 20–30 minutes; infusion 1 g in 250 mL D5W (4 mg/mL) at 0.5–0.7 mg/kg/h
- *Amoxicillin* (Amoxil): 250–500 mg PO q8h (peds: 40 mg/kg/d divided in 3 doses)
- *Atropine:* 0.5–1.0 mg i.v./ET (peds: 0.02 mg/kg)
- *Azithromycin* (Zithromax): 500 mg i.v. per day; oral (adult/peds): 10 mg/kg up to 500 mg the first day, then 5 mg/kg up to 250 mg q.d. for 4 days
  —Chlamydia: 1,000 mg PO single dose
- *Benzathine penicillin* (Bicillin LA): 1.2 million IU i.m. (dose lasts 2–4 weeks) (peds: 300,000–600,000 IU if less than 27 kg; 900,000–1.2 million IU if greater than 27 kg)
- *Bretylium* (Bretylol): initial 5 mg/kg i.v., repeat 10 mg/kg if needed; infusion 500 mg in 50 mL D5W (10 mg/mL) at 1–3 mg/min (7–21 mL/h)
- *Bumetanide* (Bumex): 0.5–1.0 mg i.v./i.m.
- *Carbamazepine* (Tegretol): 200–600 mg PO q12h
- *Cefazolin* (Ancef, others): 0.5–1.5 g i.v./i.m. q6–8h (peds: 25–50 mg/kg/d divided q6–8h; may go up to 100 mg/kg/d for severe infections)
- *Cephalexin* (Keflex, others): 250–500 mg PO q6h (peds: 25–50 mg/kg/d)
- *Ceftriaxone* (Rocephin): 1–2 g i.v./i.m. q24h (peds: 50–75 mg/kg/d [max 2 g], 100 mg/kg/d for meningitis)
  —For gonorrhea: 125 mg/i.m. single dose (250 mg for pelvic inflammatory disease)
- *Charcoal* (activated): 0.5–1.0 g/kg PO as load; can repeat if needed
- *Chloral hydrate* (Noctec): 25–50 mg/kg PO up to 1000 mg
- *Chlordiazepoxide* (Librium): 5–25 mg PO, larger doses may be required for ethanol withdrawal
- *Cimetidine* (Tagamet): 300 mg i.v./i.m./PO q6h, 400 mg PO q12h, or 400–800 mg every night
- *Ciprofloxacin* (Cipro): 200–400 mg i.v. q12h; oral: 250–750 mg q12h
  —Gonorrhea: 250 mg PO single dose
- *Clarithromycin* (Biaxin): 250–500 mg PO q12h (peds: 7.5 mg/kg PO q12h)
- *Clindamycin* (Cleocin): 600–900 mg i.v. q8h; i.m. dosing should be 600 mg or less; oral: 150–450 mg PO q6h (peds: 20–40 mg/kg/d i.v. divided in 3–4 doses, or 8–20 mg/kg/d PO divided in 3–4 doses)
- *Clonidine* (Catapres): hypertension: 0.1 mg PO q12h up to 2.4 mg/d (rebound hypertension can follow abrupt withdrawal)
  —Addiction therapy: 0.1 mg PO q8h
- *Codeine:* 0.5 mg/kg up to 15–60 mg PO i.m. q4–6h
- *Cyclobenzaprine* (Flexeril): 10 mg PO q8h
- *Deferoxamine* (Desferal): iron poisoning: infusion up to 15 mg/kg/h; higher doses may be used in serious poisonings; use for greater than 36 hours may lead to pulmonary toxicity
- *Dexamethasone* (Decadron): croup: 0.6 mg/kg i.m.
  —Acute pharyngitis: 10 mg i.m.
- *Diazepam* (Valium): 0.2–0.4 mg/kg up to 5–10 mg i.v.; alcohol withdrawal treatment may require higher doses
- *Digoxin* (Lanoxin): 0.25 mg i.v. q6h up to 1 mg for treatment of atrial fibrillation
- *Digoxin immune Fab* (Digibind): 2–10 vials i.v.; may repeat 10 vials if no response (40 mg/vial)
- *Diltiazem* (Cardizem, others): bolus 0.25 mg/kg or 20 mg i.v. over 2 minutes; rebolus 15 minutes later (if needed) 0.35 mg/kg or 25 mg; infusion 5–15 mg/h
- *Diphenhydramine* (Benadryl): 25–50 mg i.v./i.m./PO q6h (peds: 5mg/kg/d div q6h)
- *Dobutamine* (Dobutrex): 250 mg in 250 mL D5W (1 mg/mL) at 2.5–15 μg/kg/min
- *Dopamine* (Intropin): 400 mg in 250 mL D5W (1600 μg/cc) at 2–20 μg/kg/min
- *Doxycycline* (Vibramycin, Doryx): 200 mg PO/i.v. initially, then 50–100 mg q12h
- *Droperidol* (Inapsine): 1.25–2.5 mg i.v./i.m. q3–6h
- *Epinephrine:* 1 mg i.v./ET for cardiac arrest (1:10,000 solution)
  —Anaphylaxis or allergy dose 0.3–0.5 mg SC (1:1,000 solution), may repeat in 15–20 minutes
- *Erythromycins*
  —Erythromycin base (E-Mycin): 250–500 mg PO q6h, 333 mg PO q8h, or 500 mg PO q12h
  —Erythromycin ethylsuccinate (EES): 400 mg PO q6h (peds: 30–50 mg/kg/d PO divided in 4 doses)
  —Erythromycin lactobionate: 15–20 mg/kg/d (max 4 g) i.v. divided q6h
- *Esmolol* (Brevibloc): 5 mg in 50 mL (10 mg/mL), load with 500 μg/kg over 1 minute, then infuse 50–200 μg/kg/min (for 70-kg patient, load with 35 mg, infuse at 100 μg/kg/min)
- *Etomidate* (Amidate): induction dose 0.3 mg/kg i.v. over 30–60 seconds
- *Famciclovir* (Famvir): genital herpes: 125 mg PO q12h for 5 days
  —Zoster: 500 mg PO q8h for 7 days
- *Famotidine* (Pepcid): 20 mg i.v. q12h; oral 20–40 mg every night
- *Fentanyl* (Sublimaze): 2–3 μg/kg up to 50–75 μg i.v.
- *Fluconazole* (Diflucan): vaginal candidiasis: 150 mg PO single dose
  —Candidiasis: 200 mg i.v./PO, then 100–200 mg q.d.
- *Flumazenil* (Romazicon): 0.2 mg i.v. every 1–3 minutes up to 1 mg until benzodiazepine sedation reversed
- *Fosphenytoin* (Cerebyx): load 15–20 mg/kg (phenytoin equivalents) i.v./i.m. no faster than 100–150 mg/min
- *Furosemide* (Lasix): 1 mg/kg up to 20–40 mg i.v.
- *Gentamicin* (Garamycin): 1–2 mg/kg i.v./i.m. as load and 1 mg i.m./i.v. q8h
  —Alternative dosing is 5–7 mg/kg once daily
- *Glucagon:* for hypoglycemia, 1 mg i.v./i.m./SC
- *Glycopyrrolate* (Robinul): 0.1–0.2 mg i.v./i.m., 1–2 mg PO q6–8h
- *Haloperidol* (Haldol): 2–5 mg i.v./i.m.
- *Heparin:* load 80 IU/kg i.v., then mix infusion 25,000 IU in 250 mL D5W (100 IU/mL) and start at 18–20 IU/kg/h (peds: load 50 IU/kg i.v.)
- *HIV prophylaxis (triple therapy):* initiate as soon as possible (ideally <1 hour) after exposure to HIV
  —Zidovudine (AZT, Retrovir): 300 mg PO q12h
  —Lamivudine (3TC, Epivir): 150 mg PO q12h
  —*And either* indinavir (Crixivan): 800 PO q8h *or* saquinavir (Invirase): 600 mg PO q8h
- *Hydralazine* (Apresoline): 10–40 mg i.v./i.m. q4–6h
- *Hydroxyzine* (Vistaril, others): 0.5 mg/kg up to 50–100 mg i.m. q4–6h
- *Ibuprofen* (Motrin, others): 200–800 mg PO q6h (peds: for children older than 6 mo: 5–10 mg/kg PO q6h)
- *Indomethacin* (Indocin): 25–50 mg PO q8h
- *Insulin* (Humulin, others): maintenance: 0.5–1 unit/kg/d, extremely variable

—DKA: begin with 0.1 IU regular/kg i.v. bolus followed by infusion of 0.1 IU regular/kg/h
—Extreme hyperkalemia: 5–10 IU regular i.v. concurrently with glucose

- *Itraconazole* (Sporanox): start 200 mg PO q.d., max 400 mg/d
- *Ketamine* (Ketalar): 1–2 mg/kg i.v. over 1–2 minutes or 4 mg/kg i.m.
  —Concurrent atropine (0.02 mg/kg) suggested to reduce hypersalivation
- *Ketorolac* (Toradol): 30 mg i.v./i.m. q6h as needed; first i.m. dose may be 60 mg
- *Labetalol* (Trandate, Normodyne): 20 mg i.v. every 10 minutes to 300 mg
- *Lidocaine* (Xylocaine): load 1–1.5 mg/kg i.v., then 0.5 mg/kg every 8–10 min as needed to max of 3 mg/kg; maintenance infusion 2 g in 250 mL D5W (8 mg/mL) at 1–4 mg/min (7–30 mL/h) (peds: 20–50 μg/kg/min)
- *Lorazepam* (Ativan): 0.5–2 mg i.v./i.m./PO q8h; higher doses may be required for ethanol withdrawal
- *Magnesium sulfate:* for eclampsia 1–4 g i.v. over 2–4 minutes; infusion 5 g in 250 mL D5W (20 mg/mL)
- *Mannitol* (Osmitrol): 1.5–2 g/kg over 30–60 minutes
- *Meperidine* (Demerol, others): 1–2 mg/kg i.v. or i.m. up to 150 mg q3–4h
- *Methocarbamol* (Robaxin): 1000–1500 mg PO q6h
- *Methylprednisolone* (Solu-Medrol): 10–125 mg i.v./i.m. (peds: 1–2 mg/kg/d div q.d. or b.i.d.)
- *Metronidazole* (Flagyl): trichomonal infection: 2 g PO single dose
  —Giardia infection: 250 mg PO q8h for 5 days
- *Midazolam*(Versed): sedation: 1–5 mg i.v./i.m., usually administered 1 mg q2–3 min as needed (peds: sedation 6 months–5 years of age: 0.05–0.1 mg/kg up to 0.6 mg/kg i.v.; 6–12 years of age: 0.025–0.05 mg/kg up to 0.4 mg/kg i.v.; may also be administered i.m.
- *Morphine sulfate:* 0.1 mg/kg i.v. or i.m. up to 15 mg for analgesia q3–4h; 2–4 mg i.v. for adjunct treatment of congestive heart failure
- N-*acetylcysteine* or NAC (Mucomyst): acetaminophen poisoning: load with 140 mg/kg PO followed by 70 mg/kg q4h for 17 doses
- *Nalmefene* (Revex): 0.5 mg/70 kg i.v. or i.m. for reversal of opioid toxicity
- *Naloxone* (Narcan): 0.01 mg/kg up to 2 mg i.m., i.v., ET for treatment of opioid toxicity; may require up to 10 mg to reverse some opioids
- *Naproxen* (Naprosyn, others): 250–500 mg PO q12h
- *Nitroglycerin* (intravenous, Tridil): 50 mg in 250 mL D5W (200 μg/mL), begin at 5 μg/min (2 mL/h), titrate up as needed
- *Nitroprusside sodium* (Nipride): 50 mg in 250 mL D5W (200 μg/mL), start at 0.3 μg/kg/min (for 70-kg adult 6 mL/h)
- *Norepinephrine* (Levophed): 4 mg in 500 mL D5W (8 μg/mL) at 2–4 μg/min; 20 mL/h = 3 μg/min
- *Pancuronium* (Pavulon): 0.1 mg/kg i.v.
- *Pediazole* (erythromycin ethylsuccinate 200 mg and sulfisoxazole 600 mg/5 mL): 50 mg/kg/d (based on EES dose) PO q6h
- *Phenobarbital:* load 15–20 mg/kg i.v. at 25–50 mg/min
- *Phentolamine* (Regitine): 5 mg bolus for hypertension related to pheochromocytoma; repeat as needed
  —For extravasation: 5–10 mg in 10 mL saline local injection
- *Phenylephrine* (Neo-Synephrine): 50 μg boluses i.v., followed by infusion of 20 mg in 250 mL D5W (80 μg/mL) at 40–180 μg/min (35–160 mL/h)
- *Phenytoin* (Dilantin): load 15–20 mg/kg i.v. up to 1,000 mg, no faster than 50 mg/min (mix in NS)
- *Physostigmine* (Antilirium): reversal of antimuscarinic poisoning: 0.5 mg i.v. q5–10 minutes up to 2.0 mg max; may cause severe bradycardia or seizures
- *Prednisone:* 1–2 mg/kg PO q.d.
- *Procainamide* (Pronestyl): 100 mg i.v. every 10 minutes, or infuse at 20 mg/min until either dysrhythmia resolves, QRS widens more than 50% baseline, 1,000 mg infused, or patient becomes hypotensive; mix 2 g in 250 mL D5W (8 mg/mL), maintenance infusion 2–6 mg/min (15–45 mL/h)
- *Prochlorperazine* (Compazine): 5–10 mg i.v./i.m. (i.v. should be over 2–5 min)
- *Propofol* (Diprivan): 40 mg i.v. every 10 seconds until sedation (2–2.5 mg/kg)
- *Ranitidine* (Zantac): 50 mg i.v. q6–8h; oral: 150 mg q12h or 300 mg every night
- *RhoGAM* (RHO immune globulin): 1 vial i.m. within 72 hours if mother Rh-negative
  —Microdose (MICRhoGAM) if spontaneous abortion at less than 12 weeks' gestation
- *Rocuronium* (Zemuron): 0.6 mg/kg i.v.
- *Sodium bicarbonate:* 1 mEq/kg up to 50–100 mEq i.v.
- *Sodium polystyrene sulfonate* (Kayexalate): 1 g/kg up to 15–60 g PO or 30–50 g retention enema (in sorbitol) q6h as needed
- *Succinylcholine* (Anectine): 1–1.5 mg/kg up to 150 mg i.v. (peds: 2 mg/kg i.v. preceded by atropine 0.02 mg/kg)
- *Sumatriptan* (Imitrex): 6 mg SC; may repeat after 1 hour to max of 12 mg/d; oral: 25 mg; if no response, may repeat 25–100 mg q2h to max 300 mg/d
- *Thiopental* (Pentothal): induction dose 3–5 mg/kg i.v.
- *Thrombolytics*
  —Alteplase (t-PA, Activase): 15 mg i.v. bolus, then 0.75 mg/kg (max 50 mg) over 30 minutes, then 0.5 mg/kg (max 35 mg) over next 60 minutes
  —Anistreplase (APSAC, Eminase): 30 IU i.v. over 2–5 minutes
  —Reteplase (Retevase): 10.8 IU i.v. over 2 minutes; repeat in 30 minutes
  —Streptokinase (Streptase, Kabikinase): 1.5 million IU i.v. over 60 minutes
- *Trimethoprim-sulfamethoxazole* (Bactrim, Septra, Cotrim, others): 1 double-strength tab PO q12h (peds: 5 mL liquid per 10 kg per dose q12h)
- *Vecuronium* (Norcuron): 0.1 mg/kg i.v.
- *Verapamil* (Isoptin, Calan): 0.1–0.3 mg/kg up to 5–10 mg i.v. over 2 minute for supraventricular tachycardia (SVT)

Coordinated by Richard F. Clark

Index

Page numbers followed by "f" denote figures; those followed by "t" denote tables.

V

W

Rapid-Sequence Intubation

1. Preoxygenate with 100% oxygen
2. Lidocaine: 1 mg/kg i.v. push (optional for severe HTN/↑ICP/bronchospasm)
3. Defasciculating dose (optional—see table below)
4. Atropine: 0.02 mg/kg i.v. push (for children $<$ 5 years old)
5. WAIT 3 MINUTES
6. Succinylcholine: 1.5 mg/kg i.v. push
7. Sedative agent (optional): etomidate 0.2–0.4 mg/kg or thiopental* 3–5 mg/kg (for ↑ICP) i.v. push
8. Apply cricoid pressure
9. WAIT 30 SECONDS
10. Intubate when optimal conditions achieved

*Avoid in trauma and hypovolemia.

Neuromuscular Blocking Agents

Agent	*Dosage (paralytic)*	*Dosage (fas pro*)*	*Onset*	*Duration*
Succinylcholine	RSI: 1–2 mg/kg		30–60s	4–6 min
Rocuronium	RSI: 0.6–1.2 mg/kg M: 0.6 mg/kg	0.06 mg/kg	2 min	30 min
Vecuronium	RSI: 0.015–0.25 mg/kg M: 0.1 mg/kg	0.01 mg/kg	2.5–5 min	25–40 min
Atracurium	M: 0.4 mg/kg	0.04 mg/kg	3–5 min	20–35 min
Pancuronium	M: 0.1 mg/kg	0.01 mg/kg	3–5 min	45–60 min

*fas pro, fasciculation prophylaxis/defasciculating dose; RSI, rapid-sequence intubation; M, maintenance dose.

Sedative and Induction Agents

Sedative	*Dosage IVP*	*Onset*	*Duration*
Etomidate	0.2–0.6 mg/kg	60 s	3–5 min
Fentanyl	*induction:* 2–10 μg/kg *sedation (titrate):* 2–4 μg/kg	60 s	30–60 min
Ketamine	2.0 mg/kg	30–60 s	15 min
Midazolam	*induction:* 0.07–0.3 mg/kg *sedation (titrate):* 0.02–0.04 mg/kg	2 min	1–2 h
Thiopental	3–5 mg/kg	20–40 s	5–10 min

Pediatric Vital Signs and Resuscitation Equipment Sizes

	Term	6 months	1 year	2 years	5 years	10 years
Approximate Weight	2–4 kg	8 kg	10 kg	13 kg	20 kg	35 kg
Vital Signs						
BP (systolic) mm Hg	60 ± 10	89 ± 29	96 ± 30	99 ± 25	99 ± 20	112 ± 19
HR	125	130	125	115	100	75
RR	40 ± 10	38 ± 10	39 ± 11	28 ± 4	27 ± 6	21 ± 4
Resuscitation						
Defibrillation	8 J	16 J	20 J	26 J	40 J	70 J
Cardioversion	2–4 J	4–8 J	5–10 J	7–13 J	20–40 J	25–70 J
Suction catheter	8F	8–10F	8–10F	10F	10F	12F
Airway						
Laryngoscope blade	1 (st)	1–2 (st)	1–2 (st)	2 (st/c)	2 (st/c)	2-3 (st/c)
Endotracheal tube (mm)	3.0–3.5	3.5–4.0	4.0–4.5	4.5	5.0–5.5	6.5
Lip–tip length (mm)	10.5	12	12	13.5	16.5	19.5
Tubes						
Nasogastric tube	5/6	8	10	10	10–12	12
Urinary catheter	5 feeding tube	5–8 feeding tube	8 feeding tube	10 Foley	10 Foley	10 Foley
Chest tube (French)	10–12	14–20	16–20	14–24	20–28	28–32

Temperature Conversion: Celsius ↔ Fahrenheit

Celsius	Fahrenheit	Celsius	Fahrenheit
34.2	93.6	38.6	101.4
34.6	94.3	39.0	102.2
35.0	95.0	39.4	102.9
35.4	95.7	39.8	103.6
35.8	96.4	40.2	104.3
36.2	97.1	40.6	105.1
36.6	97.8	41.0	105.8
37.0	98.6	41.4	106.5
37.4	99.3	41.8	107.2
37.8	100.0	42.2	108.0
38.2	100.7	42.6	108.7

$°F = 9/5 \times °C + 32$

Weight Conversion: Pounds ↔ Kilogram

10 lb	4.53 kg	110 lb	49.89 kg
20 lb	9.07 kg	120 lb	54.43 kg
30 lb	13.60 kg	130 lb	58.96 kg
40 lb	18.14 kg	140 lb	63.50 kg
50 lb	22.68 kg	150 lb	68.04 kg
60 lb	27.21 kg	160 lb	72.57 kg
70 lb	31.75 kg	170 lb	77.11 kg
80 lb	36.28 kg	180 lb	81.64 kg
90 lb	40.82 kg	190 lb	86.18 kg
100 lb	45.36 kg	200 lb	90.72 kg

$kg = lb \times 2.2$